Medical Physiology

Medical Physiology
A Cellular and Molecular Approach

UPDATED SECOND EDITION

Walter F. Boron, MD, PhD
Professor
David N. and Inez Myers/Antonio Scarpa Chairman
Department of Physiology and Biophysics
Case Western Reserve University
Cleveland, Ohio

Emile L. Boulpaep, MD
Professor
Department of Cellular and Molecular Physiology
Yale University School of Medicine
New Haven, Connecticut

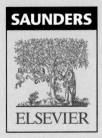

SAUNDERS

ELSEVIER

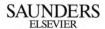

1600 John F. Kennedy Blvd.
Ste 1800
Philadelphia, PA 19103-2899

MEDICAL PHYSIOLOGY: A CELLULAR AND MOLECULAR APPROACH
ISBN: 978-1-4377-1753-2

International Edition
ISBN: 978-0-8089-2449-4

Previous editions copyrighted 2003, 2005, 2009

Library of Congress Cataloging-in-Publication Data
Medical physiology : a cellular and molecular approach / [edited by] Walter F. Boron, Emile L. Boulpaep. – 2nd ed.
    p. ; cm.
  Includes bibliographical references and index.
  ISBN 978-1-4377-1753-2
  1. Human physiology—Textbooks.   I. Boron, Walter F.   II. Boulpaep, Emile L.
  [DNLM: 1. Physiology.   2. Cell Physiology.   3. Genomics. QT 104 M4894 2009]
QP34.5.B65 2009
612–dc22

2008000942

Acquisitions Editor: Elyse O'Grady
Developmental Editor: Andrew Hall
Publishing Services Manager: Patricia Tannian
Senior Project Manager: John Casey
Design Manager: Steven Stave

Printed in United States

Last digit is the print number: 9   8   7   6   5   4   3   2

CONTRIBUTORS

Michael Apkon, MD, PhD
Associate Clinical Professor
Department of Pediatrics
Yale University School of Medicine
New Haven, Connecticut

Peter S. Aronson, MD
Professor
Section of Nephrology
Department of Internal Medicine
Yale University School of Medicine
New Haven, Connecticut

Eugene J. Barrett, MD, PhD
Professor
Department of Internal Medicine
University of Virginia School of Medicine
Charlottesville, Virginia

Paula Barrett, PhD
Professor
Department of Pharmacology
University of Virginia School of Medicine
Charlottesville, Virginia

Henry J. Binder, MD
Professor of Medicine
Professor of Cellular and Molecular Physiology
Department of Internal Medicine
Yale University School of Medicine
New Haven, Connecticut

Walter F. Boron, MD, PhD
Professor
David N. and Inez Myers/Antonio Scarpa Chairman
Department of Physiology and Biophysics
Case Western Reserve University
Cleveland, Ohio

Emile L. Boulpaep, MD
Professor
Department of Cellular and Molecular Physiology
Yale University School of Medicine
New Haven, Connecticut

Lloyd Cantley, MD, FASN
Professor
Department of Internal Medicine
Yale University School of Medicine
New Haven, Connecticut

Michael J. Caplan, MD, PhD
Professor
Department of Cellular and Molecular Physiology
Yale University School of Medicine
New Haven, Connecticut

Barry W. Connors, PhD
Professor and Chair
Department of Neuroscience
Brown University
Providence, Rhode Island

Arthur DuBois, MD
Professor Emeritus of Epidemiology and Public Health
    and Cellular and Molecular Physiology
John B. Pierce Laboratory
New Haven, Connecticut

Gerhard Giebisch, MD
Professor Emeritus of Cellular and Molecular
    Physiology
Department of Cellular and Molecular Physiology
Yale University School of Medicine
New Haven, Connecticut

Fred S. Gorelick, MD
Professor
Section of Digestive Diseases
Department of Internal Medicine
Yale University School of Medicine
New Haven, Connecticut

Peter Igarashi, MD
Professor
University of Texas Southwestern Medical Center
    at Dallas
Dallas, Texas

Ervin E. Jones, MD, PhD
Department of Obstetrics and Gynecology
Yale University School of Medicine
New Haven, Connecticut

W. Jonathan Lederer, MD, PhD
Director, Medical Biotechnology Center and Department
    of Physiology
University of Maryland Biotechnology Institute
University of Maryland School of Medicine
Baltimore, Maryland

Christopher R. Marino, MD
Professor of Medicine and Physiology
University of Tennessee Health Science Center
Chief, Medical Service
VA Medical Center
Memphis, Tennessee

Edward J. Masoro, PhD
Professor Emeritus of Physiology
University of Texas Health Science Center at San Antonio
San Antonio, Texas

Edward G. Moczydlowski, PhD
Professor and Chair
Department of Biology
Clarkson University
Potsdam, New York

Kitt Falk Petersen, MD
Associate Professor
Section of Endocrinology
Department of Internal Medicine
Yale University School of Medicine
New Haven, Connecticut

Bruce R. Ransom, MD, PhD
Professor and Chair
Department of Neurology
University of Washington Health Sciences Center
Seattle, Washington

Adrian Reuben, MBBS, FRCP, FACG
Director of Liver Studies
Department of Gastroenterology and Hepatology
Medical University of South Carolina
Charleston, South Carolina

George B. Richerson, MD, PhD
Professor
Department of Neurology
Yale University School of Medicine
New Haven, Connecticut

Steven S. Segal, PhD
Professor
Department of Medical Pharmacology and Physiology
University of Missouri School of Medicine
Columbia, Missouri

Gerald I. Shulman, MD, PhD
Professor
Section of Endocrinology
Department of Internal Medicine
Yale University School of Medicine
New Haven, Connecticut

John T. Stitt, PhD
Professor Emeritus of Epidemiology and Public Health
John B. Pierce Laboratory
New Haven, Connecticut

Frederick J. Suchy, MD
Professor and Chair
Pediatrics, Hepatology
Mount Sinai Medical Center
New York, New York

Erich E. Windhager, MD
Professor
Department of Physiology and Biophysics
Weill Medical College
Cornell University
New York, New York

PREFACE TO THE SECOND EDITION

We are very grateful for the enthusiastic reception with which the academic community received the first edition of our book. In producing this second edition, three guiding principles have remained the same as before. First, create a modern textbook of physiology that provides the expertise of several authors but the consistency of a single pen. Second, weave an integrative story that extends from the level of DNA and proteins to the level of cells, tissues, and organs, and finally to the interaction among organ systems. Third, illustrate important physiological principles with examples from pathophysiology, thereby putting physiology in a clinical context. In addition, we have strived to improve the book along the lines suggested by our readers. Moreover, we have updated the material—reflecting new molecular insights— as well as the presentation of this material. The result is two new chapters, new authors for seven chapters, the reordering or reorganization of several chapters, and—throughout the book—countless improvements to the text. In addition, the second edition includes 65 new or redrawn figures as well as enhancements to 488 others.

In Section II (The Physiology of Cells and Molecules), fresh insights into genetics led to substantial revisions in Chapter 4 (Regulation of Gene Expression). Moreover, advances in genomics and the understanding of genetic diseases led to the creation of new tables to organize families of transporter proteins in Chapters 5 (Transport of Solutes and Water) and ion channels in Chapter 6 (Electrophysiology of the Cell Membrane).

In Section III (The Nervous System), new molecular developments led to major changes in Chapter 15 (Sensory Transduction). In Section IV (The Cardiovascular System), we have added new Chapter 18 on Blood. In Section V (The Respiratory System), we have shifted some pulmonary function tests into Chapter 26 (Organization of the Respiratory System). In Section VI (The Urinary System), genomic progress led to a new table on amino-acid transporters. In Section VII (The Gastrointestinal System), Chapter 45 (Nutrient Digestion and Absorption) now contains a section on nutritional requirements. In Section VIII (The Endocrine System), we have renamed Chapter 48 to Endocrine Regulation of Growth and Body Mass to reflect updated coverage of the regulation of appetite. In Section IX (The Reproductive System), we have modified figures to clarify mitosis versus meiosis in males versus meiosis in females, as well as to clarify the development of the follicle. Finally, in Section X (The Physiology of Cells and Molecules), we have largely rewritten Chapter 58 (Metabolism), with special emphasis on energy interconversion (e.g., gluconeogenesis); energy capture after ingestion of carbohydrate, protein, or fats; and the integrative response to fasting. Moreover, we have added new Chapter 62 (The Physiology of Aging).

To create the second edition, we recruited as new authors several outstanding scientist-educators: Lloyd Cantley (Chapter 3), Gerald Shulman and Kitt Petersen (Chapter 58), John Stitt (Chapter 59), Arthur DuBois (Chapter 61), and Edward Masoro (Chapter 62). In addition, two previous authors picked up additional chapters: Edward Moczydlowski (Chapter 9) and Steven Segal (Chapter 60).

Online Access. The Web site **www.StudentConsult.com** offers the reader access to the online edition of the textbook, with the ability to search, bookmark, post notes, download highlighted text to a handheld device, access all of the images in the book, and more. The hundreds of "mouse" icons in the text direct the reader to "webnotes" that likewise are available on the **Student Consult** website. These webnotes provide derivations of mathematical equations, amplification of concepts, supplementary details, additional clinical illustrations, and links that may be of interest (e.g., biographies of famous physiologists).

Acknowledgments. A textbook is the culmination of successful collaborations among many individuals. First, we thank our authors. Second, we thank Philine Wangemann, who made invaluable suggestions for the Vestibular and Auditory Transduction subchapter in Chapter 15. Third, we thank our colleagues who provided advice on parts of the book: Samuel Cukierman, Sarah Garber, and Mark Shapiro (Chapters 6-8); R. John Solaro and John Walsh (Chapter 9); T. Richard Nichols (Chapter 16); Don McCrimmon and Frank Powell (Chapter 32); Franz Beck, Gerhard Burkhardt, Bruce Koeppen, Patricia Preisig, Luis Reuss, James Schafer, Jurgen Schnermann, James Wade, and Carsten Wagner (Chapters 33-40); Mark Donowitz (Chapter 44); Charles Mansbach (Chapter 45); as well as Harold Behrman and Richard Ehrenkranz (Chapters 53-57).

We thank all of our readers who sent us their suggestions.

At the art studio Dartmouth Publishing Inc, we thank Stephanie Davidson for developing new figures and updating others, while maintaining the textbook's aesthetic appeal originally established by JB Woolsey and Associates.

At Elsevier, we are very grateful to William R. Schmitt, Acquisitions Editor, for his trust and endurance. Andrew Hall, Developmental Editor, was the project's communications hub, responsible for coordinating all parties working on the textbook, and for assembling the many elements that comprised the final product. His meticulous care was indispensable. We thank Sharon Lee, Project Manager, for overseeing production of the textbook.

Finally, at Yale University and Case Western Reserve University we thank Charleen Bertolini, who used every ounce of her friendly, good-humored, and tenacious personality to keep our authors—and us—on track.

As we did in the First Edition, we again invite the reader to enjoy learning physiology. If you are pleased with our effort, tell others. If not, tell us.

PREFACE TO THE FIRST EDITION

We were intrigued by an idea suggested to us by W.B. Saunders: write a modern textbook of physiology that combines the expertise of a multi-author book with the consistency of a single pen. Our approach has been, first, to recruit as writers mainly professors who teach medical physiology at the Yale University School of Medicine, and then to recast the professors' manuscripts in a uniform style. After much effort, we now present our book, which we hope will bring physiology to life and at the same time be a reliable resource for students.

Target Audience. We wrote *Medical Physiology* primarily as an introductory text for medical students, although it should also be valuable for students in the allied health professions and for graduate students in the physiological sciences. The book should continue to be useful for the advanced medical student who is learning pathophysiology and clinical medicine. Finally, we hope that physicians in training, clinical fellows, and clinical faculty will find the book worthwhile for reviewing principles and becoming updated on new information pertinent for understanding the physiological basis of human disease.

Content of the Textbook. Aside from Part I, which is a brief introduction to the discipline of physiology, the book consists of nine major Parts. Part II (Physiology of Cells and Molecules) reflects that, increasingly, the underpinnings of modern physiology have become cellular and molecular. Chapters 2, 4, and 5 would not be present in a traditional physiology text. Chapter 2 (Functional Organization of the Cell), Chapter 4 (Signal Transduction), and Chapter 5 (Regulation of Gene Expression) provide the essentials of cell biology and molecular biology necessary for understanding cell and organ function. The other chapters in Part II cover the *cellular* physiology of transport, excitability, and muscle—all of which are classic topics for traditional physiology texts. In this book we have extended each of these subjects to the *molecular* level. The remainder of the book will frequently send the reader back to the principles introduced in Part II.

Parts III to IX address individual organ systems. In each case, the first chapter provides a general introduction to the system. Part III (Cellular Physiology of the Nervous System) is untraditional in that it deliberately omits those aspects of the physiology of the central nervous system that neuroscience courses generally treat and that require extensive knowledge of neuroanatomical pathways. Rather, Part III focuses on cellular neurophysiology, including synaptic transmission in the nervous system, sensory transduction, and neural circuits. In addition, Part III also treats two subjects—the autonomic nervous system and the neuronal microenvironment—that are important for understanding other physiological systems. Finally, Part X (The Physiology of Everyday Life) is an integrated, multisystem approach to metabolism, temperature regulation, exercise, and adaptations to special environments.

Emphasis of the Textbook. Some important aspects of physiology remain as fundamentally important today as when the pioneers of physiology discovered them a century or more ago. These early observations were generally phenomenological descriptions that physiologists have since been trying to understand at a mechanistic level. Where possible, a goal of this textbook is to extend this understanding all the way to the cell and molecule. Moreover, although some areas are evolving rapidly, we have tried to be as up to date as practical. To make room for the cellular and molecular bricks, we have omitted some classic experimental observations, especially when they were of a "black-box" nature.

Just as each major Part of the textbook begins with an introductory chapter, each chapter generally first describes—at the level of the whole body or organ system (e.g., the kidney)—how the body performs a certain task and/or controls a certain parameter (e.g., plasma K^+ concentration). As appropriate, our discussion then progresses in a reductionistic fashion from organ to tissue to cell and organelles, and ultimately to the molecules that underlie the physiology. Finally, most chapters include a discussion of how the body regulates the parameter of interest at all levels of integration, from molecules to the whole body.

Creating the Textbook. The first draft of each chapter was written by authors with extensive research and/or teaching experience in that field. The editors, sitting shoulder to shoulder at a computer, then largely rewrote all chapters line by line. The goal of this exercise was for the reader to recognize, throughout the entire book, a single voice—a unity provided by consistency in style, in organization, in the sequence for presenting concepts, and in terminology and notation, as well as in consistency in the expression of standard values (e.g., a cardiac output of 5 liters/min). The editors also attempted to minimize overlap among chapters by making extensive use of cross references (by page, figure, or table number) to principles introduced elsewhere in the book.

After the first round of editing, Dr. Malcolm Thaler—a practicing physician and accomplished author in his own right—improved the readability of the text and sometimes added clinical examples. Afterwards, the editors again went through the entire text line by line to decide on the material to be included in specific illustrations, and to match the main text of the book with the content of each figure. The editors then traveled to Philadelphia to visit the art studio of JB Woolsey and Associates. Over many visits, John Woolsey and the editors together developed the content and format for each of the approximately 760 full-color illustrations used in the textbook. These meetings were unique intellectual and pedagogical dialogues concerning the design of the figures. To a large extent, the figures owe their pedagogical style to the creativity of John Woolsey.

The illustrations evolved through several iterations of figure editing, based on suggestions from both the editors and authors. This evolution, as well as text changes requested by authors, led to yet a third round of editing of the entire book, often line by line. Throughout this seemingly endless process, our goal has been to achieve the proper balance among reader friendliness, depth, and accuracy.

Special Features. Compared with other major textbooks of physiology, a much larger fraction of the space in this book is devoted to illustrations. Thus, although our textbook may appear thick, it actually has fewer text words than most other leading medical physiology books. Virtually all illustrations in our book are in full color, conceived de novo, with consistent style and pedagogy. Many of the figures feature "dialogue balloons" that tell a story. The illustrations are also available in digital format on the Evolve Web site (http://evolve.elsevier.com/productPages/s_417.html) for use in the classroom.

The textbook makes considerable use of clinical boxes—highlighted on a color background—that present examples of diseases illustrating important physiological principles. The text includes over 2000 cross references that send the reader from the current page to specific pages, figures, or tables elsewhere in the book for relevant concepts or data. The text also includes hundreds of web icons, which direct the reader to our website at **http://www.wbsaunders.com/ MERLIN/BandB/**. These web links provide derivations of mathematical equations, amplification of concepts, material that was deleted for the sake of brevity from earlier drafts of the textbook, and clinical illustrations not included in the clinical boxes.

The website will also contain several other features, including summaries for each subchapter, an expanded list of references (sometimes with direct links to the primary literature), other links that may be of interest to the physiology student (e.g., biographies of famous physiologists), late-breaking scientific developments that occur after publication of the book, and—alas—the correction of errors. Finally, we invite the reader to visit our website to comment on our book, to point out errors, and to make other helpful suggestions.

Acknowledgments. A textbook is the culmination of successful collaborations among many individuals. First, we would like to thank our authors. Second, we acknowledge the expert input of Dr. Malcolm Thaler, both in terms of style and clinical insight. We also thank Dr. Thaler for emphasizing the importance of telling a "good story." The textbook's aesthetic appeal is largely attributable to JB Woolsey and Associates, particularly John Woolsey and Joel Dubin.

At W.B. Saunders, we are especially thankful to William R. Schmitt—Acquisitions Editor—for his trust and patience over the years that this book has been in gestation. At the times when the seas were rough, he steered a safe course. Melissa Dudlick—Developmental Editor at W.B. Saunders—was the project's nerve center, responsible for day-to-day communication among all parties working on the textbook, and for assembling all of the many components that went into making the final product. Her good humor and careful attention to detail greatly facilitated the creation of the textbook. We thank Frank Polizzano—Publishing Services Manager at W.B. Saunders—for overseeing production of the textbook.

Before this textbook was completed, the author of Part X (The Physiology of Everyday Life), Ethan Nadel, passed away. We are indebted to those who generously stepped up to carefully check the nearly finished manuscripts for the final four chapters: Dr. Gerald Shulman for Chapter 57, Dr. John Stitt for Chapter 58, the late Dr. Carl Gisolfi for Chapter 59, and Dr. Arthur DuBois for Chapter 60. In addition, Dr. George Lister provided expert advice for Chapter 56. We are also grateful to Dr. Bruce Davis for researching the sequences of the polypeptide hormones, to Mr. Duncan Wong for expert information-technology services, and to Mrs. Leisa Strohmaier for administrative assistance.

We now invite the reader to enjoy the experience of learning physiology. If you are pleased with our effort, tell others. If not, tell us.

CONTENTS

xi

INTRODUCTION

CHAPTER 1

FOUNDATIONS OF PHYSIOLOGY

Emile L. Boulpaep and Walter F. Boron

WHAT IS PHYSIOLOGY?

Physiology is the dynamic study of life. Physiology describes the "vital" functions of living organisms and their organs, cells, and molecules. For centuries, the discipline of physiology has been closely intertwined with medicine. Although physiology is not primarily concerned with structure—as is the case of anatomy, histology, and structural biology—structure and function are inextricably linked because the living structures perform the functions.

For some, physiology is the function of the whole person (e.g., exercise physiology). For many practicing clinicians, physiology may be the function of an individual organ system, such as the cardiovascular, respiratory, or gastrointestinal system. For still others, physiology may focus on the cellular principles that are common to the function of all organs and tissues. This last field has traditionally been called general physiology, a term that is now supplanted by "cellular and molecular physiology." Although one can divide physiology according to varying degrees of reductionism, it is also possible to define a branch of physiology—for example, comparative physiology—that focuses on differences and similarities among different species. Indeed, comparative physiology may deal with all degrees of reductionism, from molecule to whole organism. In a similar way, medical physiology deals with how the human body functions, which depends on how the individual organ systems function, which depends on how the component cells function, which in turn depends on the interactions among subcellular organelles and countless molecules. Thus, medical physiology takes a global view of the human body; but in doing so, it requires an integrated understanding of events at the level of molecules, cells, and organs.

Physiology is the mother of several biological sciences, having given birth to the disciplines of biochemistry, biophysics, and neuroscience as well as their corresponding scientific societies and journals. Thus, it should come as no surprise that the boundaries of physiology are not sharply delineated. Conversely, physiology has its unique attributes. For example, physiology has evolved over the centuries from a more qualitative to a more quantitative science. Indeed, many of the leading physiologists were—and still are—trained as chemists, physicists, mathematicians, or engineers.

Physiological genomics is the link between the organ and the gene

The life of the human body requires not only that individual organ systems do their jobs but also that these organ systems work "hand in hand" with each other. They must share information. Their actions must be interdependent. The cells within an organ or a tissue often share information, and certainly the individual cells must act in concert to perform the proper function of the organ or tissue. In fact, cells in one organ must often share information with cells in another organ and make decisions that are appropriate for the health of the individual cell as well as for the health of the whole person.

In most cases, the sharing of information between organs and between cells takes place at the level of atoms or molecules. Cell-to-cell messengers or intracellular messengers may be atoms such as H^+ or K^+ or Ca^{2+}. The messengers may also be more complex chemicals. A cell may release a molecule that acts on a neighboring cell or that enters the bloodstream and acts on other cells a great distance away. In other cases, a neuron may send an axon a centimeter or even a meter away and rapidly modulate, through a neurotransmitter molecule, the activity of another cell or another organ. Cells and organs must interact with one another, and the method of communication is almost always molecular.

The grand organizer—the master that controls the molecules, the cells, and the organs and the way they interact—is the genome. Traditionally, the discipline of physiology has, in its reductionistic journey, always stopped at about the level of cells and certain subcellular organelles as well as their component and controlling molecules. The discipline of physiology left to molecular biology and molecular genetics the business of how the cell controls itself through its DNA. The modern discipline of physiology has become closely intertwined with molecular biology, however, because DNA encodes the proteins in which physiologists are most interested. Very often, physiologists painstakingly develop elegant strategies for cloning of the genes relevant to physiology. Sometimes, brute force approaches, such as the Human Genome Project in the United States, hand the physiologist a candidate gene, homologous to one of known function, on a silver platter. In still other cases, molecular biologists may clone a gene with no known function. In this case, it may be up to the physiologist to determine the *function* of the gene product, that is, to determine its *physiology*.

Physiological genomics (or functional genomics) is a new branch of physiology devoted to understanding of the roles that genes play in physiology. Traditionally, physiologists have moved in a reductionistic direction from organ to cell to molecule to gene. One of the most fascinating aspects of physiological genomics is that it has closed the circle and linked organ physiology directly with molecular biology. Perhaps one of the most striking examples is the knockout mouse. Knocking out the gene encoding a protein that, according to conventional wisdom, is very important will sometimes have no obvious effect or sometimes unexpected effects. It is up to the physiologist, at least in part, to figure out why. It is perhaps rather sobering to consider that to truly understand the impact of a transgene or a knockout on the physiology of a mouse, one would have to carefully re-evaluate the totality of mouse physiology. To grasp the function of a gene product, the physiologist must retrace the steps up the reductionistic road and achieve an integrated understanding of that gene's function at the level of the cells, organs, and whole body. Physiology is unique among the basic medical sciences in that it is both broad in its scope (i.e., it deals with multiple systems) and integrative in its outlook.

In some cases, important physiological parameters, such as blood pressure, may be under the control of many genes. Certain polymorphisms in several of these many genes could have a cumulative effect that produces high blood pressure. How would one identify which polymorphisms of which genes may underlie high blood pressure? This sort of complex problem does not easily lend itself to a physiologist's controlled studies. One approach would be to study a population of people, or strains of experimental animals, and use statistical tools to determine which polymorphisms correlate with high blood pressure in a population. Indeed, epidemiologists use statistical tools to study group effects in populations. However, even after the identification of variants in various genes, each of which may make a small contribution to high blood pressure, the physiologist has an important role. First, the physiologist, performing controlled experiments, must determine whether a particular genetic variant does indeed have at least the potential to modulate blood pressure. Second, the physiologist must determine the mechanism of the effect.

Cells live in a highly protected milieu intérieur

In his lectures on the phenomena of life, Claude Bernard wrote in 1878 on the conditions of the constancy of life, which he considered a property of higher forms of life. According to Bernard, animals have two environments: the milieu extérieur that physically surrounds the whole organism; and the milieu intérieur, in which the tissues and cells of the organism live. This internal environment is neither the air nor the water in which an organism lives but rather—in the case of the human body—the well-controlled liquid environment that Bernard called "the organic liquid that circulates and bathes all the anatomic elements of the tissues, the lymph or the plasma." In short, this internal environment is what we today call the extracellular fluid. He argued that physiological functions continue in a manner indifferent to the changing environment because the milieu intérieur isolates the organs and tissues of the body from the vagaries of the physical conditions of the environment. Indeed, Bernard described the milieu intérieur as if an organism had placed itself in a greenhouse.

According to Bernard's concept of milieu intérieur, some fluids contained within the body are not really inside the body at all. For example, the *contents* of the gastrointestinal tract, sweat ducts, and renal tubules are all outside the body. They are all continuous with the milieu extérieur.

Bernard compares a complex organism to an ensemble of anatomical elements that live together inside the milieu intérieur. Therefore, in Part II of this textbook, we examine the physiology of these cells and molecules. In Chapter 2 ("Functional Organization of the Cell"), we begin our journey through physiology with a discussion of the biology of the cells that are the individual elements of the body. Chapter 3 ("Signal Transduction") discusses how cells communicate directly through gap junctions or indirectly by molecules released into the extracellular fluid. These released molecules can bind to receptors on the cell membrane and initiate signal transduction cascades that can modify gene transcription (a genomic response) and a wide range of other cell functions (nongenomic responses). Alternatively, these released molecules can bind to receptors in the cytoplasm or nucleus and alter the transcription of genes. In Chapter 4 ("Regulation of Gene Expression"), we examine the response of the nucleus. Chapter 5 ("Transport of Solutes and Water") addresses how the plasma membrane separates the cell interior from Bernard's milieu intérieur and establishes the composition of the cell interior. In the process of establishing the composition of the intracellular fluid, the plasma membrane also sets up ion and voltage gradients across itself. Excitable cells—mainly nerve and muscle cells—can exploit these gradients for the long-distance "electrical" transmission of information. The property of "excitability," which requires both the perception of a change (a signal) and the reaction to it, is the topic of Chapters 6 to 9. In Part III, we examine how the nervous system exploits excitability to process information.

Another theme developed by Bernard was that the "fixité du milieu intérieur" (the constancy of the extracellular fluid) is the condition of "free, independent life." He explains that organ differentiation is the exclusive property of higher organisms and that each organ contributes to "compensate and equilibrate" against changes in the external environment. In that sense, each of the systems discussed in Parts IV to VIII permits the body to live within an adverse external environment because the cardiovascular system, the respiratory system, the urinary system, the gastrointestinal system, and the endocrine system create and maintain a constant internal environment. Individual cell types in various organ systems act in concert to support the constancy of the internal milieu, and the internal milieu in turn provides these cells with a culture medium in which they can thrive.

The discipline of physiology also deals with those characteristics that are the property of a living organism as opposed to a nonliving organism. Four fundamental properties distinguish the living body. First, only living organisms exchange matter and energy with the environment to continue their existence. Several organ systems of the body participate in these exchanges. Second, only living organisms can receive signals from their environment and react accordingly. The principles of sensory perception, processing by the nervous system, and reaction are discussed in the chapters on excitability and the nervous system. Third, what distinguishes a living organism is the life cycle of growth and reproduction, as discussed in the chapters on reproduction (Part IX). Finally, the living organism is able to adapt to changing circumstances. This is a theme that is developed throughout this textbook but especially in the chapters on everyday life (Part X).

Homeostatic mechanisms—operating through sophisticated feedback control mechanisms—are responsible for maintaining the constancy of the milieu intérieur

Homeostasis is the control of a vital parameter. The body carefully controls a seemingly endless list of vital parameters. Examples of tightly controlled parameters that affect nearly the whole body are arterial pressure and blood volume. At the level of the milieu intérieur, tightly regulated parameters include body core temperature and plasma levels of oxygen, glucose, potassium ions (K^+), calcium ions (Ca^{2+}), and hydrogen ions (H^+). Homeostasis also occurs at the level of the single cell. Thus, cells regulate many of the same parameters that the body as a whole regulates: volume, the concentrations of many small inorganic ions (e.g., Na^+, Ca^{2+}, H^+), and energy levels (e.g., ATP).

One of the most common themes in physiology is the **negative feedback mechanism** responsible for homeostasis. Negative feedback requires at least four elements. First, the system must be able to sense the vital parameter (e.g., glucose) or something related to it. Second, the system must be able to compare the input signal with some internal reference value called a set-point, thereby forming a difference signal. Third, the system must multiply the error signal by some proportionality factor (i.e., the gain) to produce some sort of output signal (e.g., release of insulin). Fourth, the output signal must be able to activate an effector mechanism (e.g., glucose uptake and metabolism) that opposes the source of the input signal and thereby brings the vital parameter closer to the set-point (e.g., decrease of blood glucose levels to normal). Sometimes the body controls a parameter, in part, by cleverly employing positive feedback loops.

A single feedback loop often does not operate in isolation but rather as part of a larger network of controls. Thus, a complex interplay may exist among feedback loops within single cells, within a tissue, within an organ or organ system, or at the level of the whole body. After studying these individual feedback loops in isolation, the physiologist may find that two feedback loops act either synergistically or antagonistically. For example, insulin lowers blood glucose levels, whereas epinephrine and cortisol have the opposite effect. Thus, the physiologist must determine the relative weights of feedback loops in **competition** with one another. Finally, the physiologist must also establish **hierarchy** among various feedback loops. For example, the hypothalamus controls the anterior pituitary, which controls the adrenal cortex, which releases cortisol, which helps control blood glucose levels.

Another theme of homeostasis is **redundancy**. The more vital a parameter is, the more systems that the body mobilizes to regulate it. If one system should fail, others are there to help maintain homeostasis. It is probably for this reason that genetic knockouts sometimes fail to have their expected deleterious effects. The result of many homeostatic systems controlling many vital parameters is a milieu intérieur with a stable composition.

Whether at the level of the milieu intérieur or the cytoplasm of a single cell, homeostasis occurs at a price: energy. When a vital parameter (e.g., the blood glucose level) is well regulated, that parameter is not in equilibrium. **Equilibrium** is a state that does not involve energy consumption. Instead, a well-regulated parameter is generally in a **steady state**. That is, its value is constant because the body or the cell carefully matches actions that lower the parameter value with other actions that raise it. The net effect is that the vital parameter is held at a constant value.

An important principle in physiology, to which we have already alluded, is that each cell plays a specialized role in the overall function of the body. In return, the body—which is the sum of all these cells—provides the milieu intérieur appropriate for the life of each cell. As part of the bargain, each cell or organ must respect the needs of the body as a whole and not run amok for its own greedy interests. For example, during exercise, the system that controls body core temperature sheds heat by elaborating sweat for evaporation. However, the production of sweat ultimately reduces blood volume. Because the body as a whole places a higher **priority** on the control of blood volume than on the control of body core temperature, at some point the system that controls blood volume will instruct the system that controls body core temperature to reduce the production of sweat. Unfortunately, this juggling of priorities works only if the individual stops exercising; if not, the result may be heat stroke.

The **adaptability** of an organism depends on its ability to alter its response. Indeed, flexible feedback loops are at the root of many forms of physiological adaptation. For instance, at sea level, experimentally lowering the level of oxygen (the sensory stimulus) in the inspired air causes an increase in breathing (the response). However, after **acclimatization** at high altitude to low oxygen levels, the same low level of oxygen (the same sensory stimulus) causes one to breathe much faster (a greater response). Thus, the response may depend on the previous history and therefore the "state" of the system. In addition to acclimatization, genetic factors can also contribute to the ability to respond to an environmental stress. For example, certain populations of humans who have lived for generations at high altitude withstand hypoxia better than lowlanders do, even after the lowlanders have fully acclimatized.

Medicine is the study of "physiology gone awry"

Medicine borrows its physicochemical principles from physiology. Medicine also uses physiology as a reference state: it is essential to know how organs and systems function in the healthy person to grasp which components may be malfunctioning in a patient. A large part of clinical medicine is simply dealing with the abnormal physiology brought about by a disease process. One malfunction (e.g., heart failure) can lead to a *primary* pathological effect (e.g., a decrease in cardiac output) that—in chain reaction style—leads to a series of *secondary* effects (e.g., fluid overload) that are the appropriate responses of physiological feedback loops. Indeed, as clinician-physiologists have explored the basis of disease, they have discovered a great deal about physiology. For this reason, we have tried to illustrate physiological principles with clinical examples, some of which are displayed in clinical boxes in this text.

Physiologists have developed many tools and tests to examine normal function. A large number of functional tests—used in diagnosis of a disease, monitoring of the evolution of an illness, and evaluation of the progress of therapy—are direct transfers of technology developed in the physiology laboratory. Typical examples are cardiac monitoring, pulmonary function tests, and renal clearance tests as well as the assays used to measure plasma levels of various ions, gases, and hormones. Refinements of such technology in the hospital environment, in turn, benefit the study of physiology. Thus, the exchange of information between medicine and physiology is a two-way street. The understanding of physiology summarized in this book comes from some experiments on humans but mostly from research on other mammals and even on squids and slime molds. However, our ultimate focus is on the human body.

REFERENCES

Bernard C: Leçons sur les phénomènes de la vie communs aux animaux et aux végétaux. Cours de physiologie générale du Museum d'Histoire Naturelle. Paris: Baillière et Fils, 1878.

Cannon WB: The Wisdom of the Body. New York: Norton, 1932.

Smith HW: From Fish to Philosopher. New York: Doubleday, 1961.

PHYSIOLOGY OF CELLS AND MOLECULES

CHAPTER 2

FUNCTIONAL ORGANIZATION
OF THE CELL

Michael J. Caplan

In the minds of many students, the discipline of physiology is linked inextricably to images from its past. This prejudice is not surprising because many experiments from physiology's proud history, such as those of Pavlov and his dogs, have transcended mere scientific renown and entered the realm of popular culture. Some might believe that the science of physiology devotes itself exclusively to the study of whole animals and is therefore an antique relic in this era of molecular reductionism. Nothing could be further from the truth. Physiology is and always has been the study of the homeostatic mechanisms that allow an organism to persist despite the ever-changing pressures imposed by a hostile environment. These mechanisms can be appreciated at many different levels of resolution.

Certainly it would be difficult to understand how the body operates unless one appreciates the functions of its organs and the communication between these organs that allows them to influence one another's behaviors. It would also be difficult to understand how an organ performs its particular tasks unless one is familiar with the properties of its constituent cells and molecules.

The modern treatment of physiology that is presented in this textbook is as much about the interactions of molecules in cells as it is about the interactions of organs in organisms. It is necessary, therefore, at the outset to discuss the structure and characteristics of the cell. Our discussion focuses first on the architectural and dynamic features of a generic cell. We then examine how this generic cell can be adapted to serve in diverse physiological capacities. Through adaptations at the cellular level, organs acquire the machinery necessary to perform their individual metabolic tasks.

STRUCTURE OF BIOLOGICAL MEMBRANES

The surface of the cell is defined by a membrane

The chemical composition of the cell interior is very different from that of its surroundings. This observation applies equally to unicellular paramecia that swim freely in a fresh-water pond and to neurons that are densely packed in the cerebral cortex of the human brain. The biochemical processes involved in cell function require the maintenance of a precisely regulated intracellular environment. The cytoplasm is an extraordinarily complex solution, the constituents of which include myriad proteins, nucleic acids, nucleotides, and sugars that the cell synthesizes or accumulates at great metabolic cost. The cell also expends tremendous energy to regulate the intracellular concentrations of numerous ions. If there were no barrier surrounding the cell to prevent exchange between the intracellular and extracellular spaces, all of the cytoplasm's hard-won compositional uniqueness would be lost by diffusion in a few seconds.

The requisite barrier is provided by the **plasma membrane**, which forms the cell's outer skin. The plasma membrane is *impermeable* to large molecules such as proteins and nucleic acids, thus ensuring their retention within the cytosol. It is *selectively permeable* to small molecules such as ions and metabolites. However, the metabolic requirements of the cell demand a plasma membrane that is much more sophisticated than a simple passive barrier that allows various substances to leak through at different rates. Frequently, the concentration of a nutrient in the extracellular fluid is several orders of magnitude lower than that required inside the cell. If the cell wishes to use such a substance, therefore, it must be able to *accumulate* it against a concentration gradient. A simple pore in the membrane cannot concentrate anything; it can only modulate the rate at which a gradient dissipates. To accomplish the more sophisticated feat of creating a concentration gradient, the membrane must be endowed with special machinery that uses metabolic energy to drive the *uphill* movements of substances—**active transport**—into or out of the cell. In addition, it would be useful to rapidly modulate the permeability properties of the plasma membrane in response to various metabolic stimuli. Active transport and the ability to control passive permeabilities underlie a wide range of physiological processes, from the electrical excitability of neurons to the resorptive and secretory functions of the kidney. In Chapter 5, we will explore how cells actively transport solutes across the plasma membrane. The mechanisms through which the plasma membrane's dynamic selectivity is achieved, modified, and regulated are discussed briefly later in this chapter and in greater detail in Chapter 7.

The cell membrane is composed primarily of phospholipids

Our understanding of biological membrane structure is based on studies of red blood cells, or erythrocytes, that were conducted in the early part of the 20th century. The erythrocyte lacks the nucleus and other complicated intracellular structures that are characteristic of most animal cells. It consists of a plasma membrane surrounding a cytoplasm that is rich in hemoglobin. It is possible to break open erythrocytes and release their cytoplasmic contents. The plasma membranes can then be recovered by centrifugation, providing a remarkably pure preparation of cell surface membrane. Biochemical analysis reveals that this membrane is composed of two principal constituents: lipid and protein.

Most of the lipid associated with erythrocyte plasma membranes belongs to the molecular family of **phospholipids**. In general, phospholipids share a **glycerol** backbone, two hydroxyl groups of which are esterified to various **fatty acid** or **acyl groups** (Fig. 2-1A). These acyl groups may have different numbers of carbon atoms and also may have double bonds between carbons. For glycerol-based phospholipids, the third glycerolic hydroxyl group is esterified to a **phosphate** group, which is in turn esterified to a small molecule referred to as a **head group**. The identity of the head group determines the name as well as many of the properties of the individual phospholipids. For instance, glycerol-based phospholipids that bear an ethanolamine molecule in the head group position are categorized as **phosphatidylethanolamines** (Fig. 2-1A).

Phospholipids form complex structures in aqueous solution

The unique structure and physical chemistry of each phospholipid (Fig. 2-1B) underlie the formation of biological membranes and explain many of their most important properties. Fatty acids are nonpolar molecules. Their long carbon chains lack the charged groups that would facilitate interactions with water, which is polar. Consequently, fatty acids dissolve poorly in water but readily in organic solvents; thus, fatty acids are **hydrophobic**. On the other hand, the head groups of most phospholipids are charged or polar. These head groups interact well with water and consequently are very water soluble. Thus, the head groups are **hydrophilic**. Because phospholipids combine hydrophilic heads with hydrophobic tails, their interaction with water is referred to as **amphipathic**.

When mixed with water, phospholipids organize themselves into structures that prevent their hydrophobic tails from making contact with water while simultaneously permitting their hydrophilic head groups to be fully dissolved. When added to water at fairly low concentrations, phospholipids form a **monolayer** (Fig. 2-1C) on the water's surface at the air-water interface. It is energetically less costly to the

A PHOSPHATIDYLETHANOLAMINE

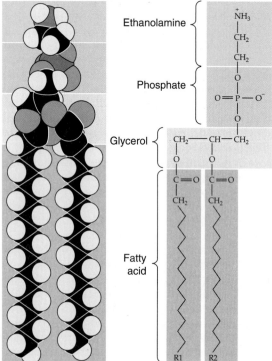

B PHOSPHOLIPID ICON

This icon is used in this text to represent this and other phospholipid molecules.

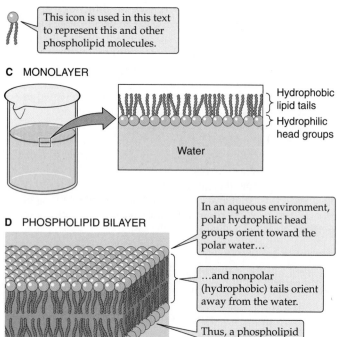

Figure 2-1 Phospholipids.

system for the hydrophobic tails to stick up in the air than to interact with the solvent.

At higher concentrations, phospholipids assemble into **micelles**. The hydrophilic head groups form the surfaces of these small spheres, whereas the hydrophobic tails point toward their centers. In this geometry, the tails are protected from any contact with water and instead are able to participate in energetically favorable interactions among themselves. At still higher concentrations, phospholipids spontaneously form **bilayers** (Fig. 2-1D). In these structures, the phospholipid molecules arrange themselves into two parallel sheets or **leaflets** that face each other tail to tail. The surfaces of the bilayer are composed of hydrophilic head groups; the hydrophobic tails form the center of the sandwich. The hydrophilic surfaces insulate the hydrophobic tails from contact with the solvent, leaving the tails free to associate exclusively with one another.

The physical characteristics of a lipid bilayer largely depend on the chemical composition of its constituent phospholipid molecules. For example, the width of the bilayer is determined by the length of the fatty acid side chains. Dihexadecanoic phospholipids (whose two fatty acid chains are each 16 carbons long) produce bilayers that are 2.47 nm wide; ditetradecanoic phospholipids (bearing 14-carbon fatty acids) generate 2.3-nm bilayers. Similarly, the nature of the head groups determines how densely packed adjacent phospholipid molecules are in each leaflet of the membrane.

Detergents can dissolve phospholipid membranes because like the phospholipids themselves, they are amphipathic. They possess very hydrophilic head groups and hydrophobic tails and are water soluble at much higher concentrations than are the phospholipids. When mixed together in aqueous solutions, detergent and phospholipid molecules interact through their hydrophobic tails, and the resulting complexes are water soluble, either as individual dimers or in mixed micelles. Therefore, adding sufficient concentrations of detergent to phospholipid bilayer membranes disrupts the membranes and dissolves the lipids. Detergents are extremely useful tools in research into the structure and composition of lipid membranes.

The diffusion of individual lipids within a leaflet of a bilayer is determined by the chemical makeup of its constituents

Despite its highly organized appearance, a phospholipid bilayer is a fluid structure. An individual phospholipid molecule is free to diffuse within the entire leaflet in which it resides. The rate at which this two-dimensional diffusion occurs is extremely temperature dependent. At high temperatures, the thermal energy of any given lipid molecule is greater than the interaction energy that would tend to hold adjacent lipid molecules together. Under these conditions, lateral diffusion can proceed rapidly, and the lipid is said to be in the **sol state**. At lower temperatures, interaction energies exceed the thermal energies of most individual molecules. Thus, phospholipids diffuse slowly because they lack the energy to free themselves from the embraces of their neighbors. This behavior is characteristic of the **gel state**.

The temperature at which the bilayer membrane converts from the gel to the sol phase (and vice versa) is referred to as the **transition temperature**. The transition temperature is another characteristic that depends on the chemical makeup of the phospholipids in the bilayer. Phospholipids with long, saturated fatty acid chains can extensively interact with one another. Consequently, a fair amount of thermal energy is required to overcome these interactions and permit diffusion. Not surprisingly, such bilayers have relatively high transition temperatures. For example, the transition temperature for dioctadecanoic phosphatidylcholine (which has two 18-carbon fatty acid chains, fully saturated) is 55.5°C. In contrast, phospholipids that have shorter fatty acid chains or double bonds (which introduce kinks) cannot line up next to each other as well and hence do not interact as well. Considerably less energy is required to induce them to participate in diffusion. For example, if we reduce the length of the carbon chain from 18 to 14, the transition temperature falls to 23°C. If we retain 18 carbons but introduce a single, double bond (making the fatty acid chains monounsaturated), the transition temperature also falls dramatically.

By mixing other types of lipid molecules into phospholipid bilayers, we can markedly alter the membrane's fluidity properties. The *glycerol-based* phospholipids, the most common membrane lipids, include the phosphatidylethanolamines described earlier (Fig. 2-1A) as well as the **phosphatidylinositols** (Fig. 2-2A), **phosphatidylserines** (Fig. 2-2B), and **phosphatidylcholines** (Fig. 2-2C). The second major class of membrane lipids, the **sphingolipids** (derivatives of *sphingosine*), are made up of three subgroups: **sphingomyelins** (Fig. 2-2D), **glycosphingolipids** such as the galactocerebrosides (Fig. 2-2E), and **gangliosides** (not shown). Cholesterol (Fig. 2-2F) is another important membrane lipid. Because these other molecules are not shaped exactly like the glycerol-based phospholipids, they participate to different degrees in intermolecular interactions with phospholipid side chains. The presence of these alternative lipids changes the strength of the interactions that prevent lipid molecules from diffusing. Consequently, the membrane has a different fluidity and a different transition temperature. This behavior is especially characteristic of the cholesterol molecule, whose rigid steroid ring binds to and partially immobilizes fatty acid side chains. Therefore, at modest concentrations, cholesterol decreases fluidity. However, when it is present in high concentrations, cholesterol can substantially disrupt the ability of the phospholipids to interact among themselves, which increases fluidity and lowers the gel-sol transition temperature. This issue is significant because animal cell plasma membranes can contain substantial quantities of cholesterol.

Bilayers composed of several different lipids do not undergo the transition from gel to sol at a single, well-defined temperature. Instead, they interconvert more gradually over a temperature range that is defined by the composition of the mixture. Within this transition range in such multicomponent bilayers, the membrane can become divided into compositionally distinct zones. The phospholipids with long-chain, saturated fatty acids will adhere to one another relatively tightly, which results in the formation of regions with "gel-like" properties. Phospholipids bearing

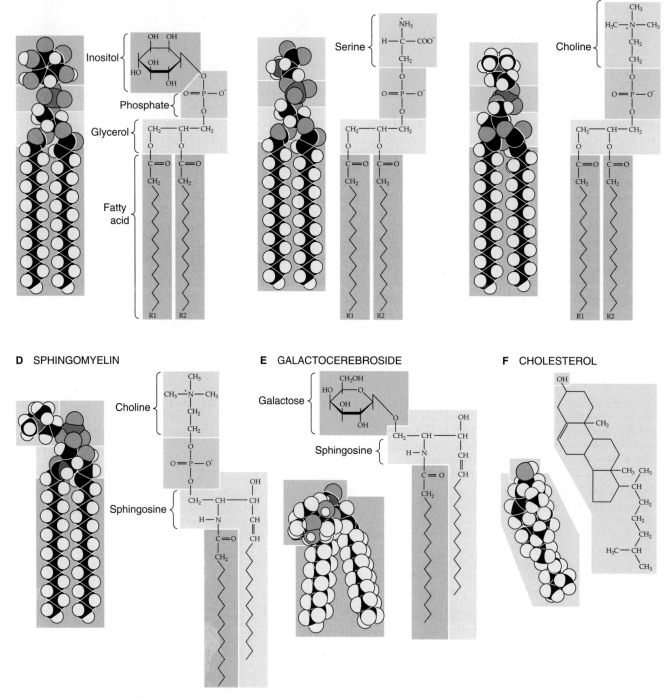

Figure 2-2 Structures of some common membrane lipids.

short-chain, unsaturated fatty acids will be excluded from these regions and migrate to sol-like regions. Hence, "lakes" of lipids with markedly different physical properties can exist side-by-side in the plane of a phospholipid membrane. Thus, the same thermodynamic forces that form the elegant bilayer structure can partition distinct lipid domains within the bilayer. As discussed later, the segregation of lipid lakes in the plane of the membrane may be important for sorting membrane proteins to different parts of the cell.

Although phospholipids can diffuse in the plane of a lipid bilayer membrane, they do not diffuse between adjacent leaflets (Fig. 2-3). The rate at which phospholipids spontaneously "flip-flop" from one leaflet of a bilayer to the other is extremely low. As mentioned earlier, the center of a bilayer membrane consists of the fatty acid tails of the phospholipid molecules and is an extremely hydrophobic environment. For a phospholipid molecule to jump from one leaflet to the other, its highly hydrophilic head group would have to transit

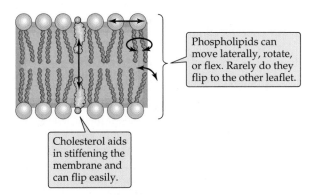

Phospholipids can move laterally, rotate, or flex. Rarely do they flip to the other leaflet.

Cholesterol aids in stiffening the membrane and can flip easily.

Figure 2-3 Mobility of lipids within a bilayer.

this central hydrophobic core, which would have an extremely high energy cost. This caveat does not apply to cholesterol (Fig. 2-3), whose polar head is a single hydroxyl group. The energy cost of dragging this small polar hydroxyl group through the bilayer is relatively low, thus permitting relatively rapid cholesterol flip-flop.

Phospholipid bilayer membranes are impermeable to charged molecules

The lipid bilayer is ideally suited to separate two aqueous compartments. Its hydrophilic head groups interact well with water at both membrane surfaces, whereas the hydrophobic center ensures that the energetic cost of crossing the membrane is prohibitive for charged atoms or molecules. Pure phospholipid bilayer membranes are extremely impermeable to almost any charged water-soluble substance. Ions such as Na^+, K^+, Cl^-, and Ca^{2+} are insoluble in the hydrophobic membrane core and consequently cannot travel from the aqueous environment on one side of the membrane to the aqueous environment on the opposite side. The same is true of large water-soluble molecules, such as proteins, nucleic acids, sugars, and nucleotides.

Whereas phospholipid membranes are impermeable to water-soluble molecules, small *uncharged* polar molecules can cross fairly freely. This is often true for O_2, CO_2, NH_3, and, remarkably, water itself. Water molecules may, at least in part, traverse the membrane through transient cracks between the hydrophobic tails of the phospholipids, without having to surmount an enormous energetic barrier. The degree of water permeability (and perhaps that of CO_2 and NH_3 as well) varies extensively with lipid composition; some phospholipids (especially those with short or kinked fatty acid chains) permit a much greater rate of transbilayer water diffusion than others do.

The plasma membrane is a bilayer

As may be inferred from the preceding discussion, the membrane at the cell surface is, in fact, a phospholipid bilayer. The truth of this statement was established by a remarkably straightforward experiment. In 1925, Gorter and Grendel measured the surface area of the lipids they extracted from erythrocyte plasma membranes. They used a device called a Langmuir trough in which the lipids are allowed to line up

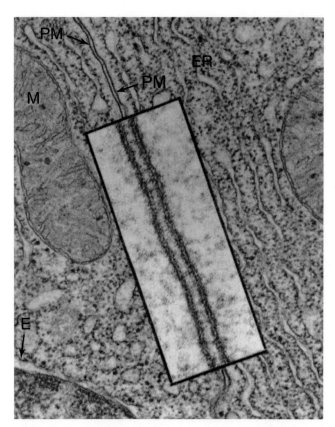

Figure 2-4 Transmission electron micrograph of a cell membrane. The photograph shows two adjacent cells of the pancreas of a frog (magnification ×43,000). The *inset* is a high-magnification view (×216,000) of the plasma membranes (PM) of the cells. Note that each membrane includes two dense layers with an intermediate layer of lower density. The dense layers represent the interaction of the polar head groups of the phospholipids with the OsO_4 used to stain the preparation. ER, endoplasmic reticulum; M, mitochondrion. *(From Porter KR, Bonneville MR: Fine Structure of Cells and Tissues, 4th ed. Philadelphia: Lea & Febiger, 1973.)*

at an air-water interface (Fig. 2-1C) and are then packed together into a continuous monolayer by a sliding bar that decreases the surface available to them. The area of the monolayer that was created by the erythrocyte lipids was exactly twice the surface area of the erythrocytes from which they were derived. Therefore, the plasma membrane must be a bilayer.

Confirmation of the bilayer structure of biological membranes has come from x-ray diffraction studies performed on the repetitive whorls of membrane that form the myelin sheaths surrounding neuronal axons (see Chapter 11). The membrane's bilayer structure can be visualized directly in the high-magnification electron micrograph depicted in Figure 2-4. The osmium tetraoxide molecule (OsO_4), with which the membrane is stained, binds to the head groups of phospholipids. Thus, both surfaces of a phospholipid bilayer appear black in electron micrographs, whereas the membrane's unstained central core appears white.

The phospholipid compositions of the two leaflets of the plasma membrane are not identical. Labeling studies performed on erythrocyte plasma membranes reveal that the surface that faces the cytoplasm contains phosphatidyletha- nolamine and phosphatidylserine, whereas the outward- facing leaflet is composed almost exclusively of phosphatidylcholine. As is discussed later in this chapter, this asymmetry is created during the biosynthesis of the phos- pholipid molecules. It is not entirely clear what advantage this distribution provides to the cell. It appears likely that the interactions between certain proteins and the plasma mem- brane may require this segregation. The lipid asymmetry may be especially important for those phospholipids that are involved in second-messenger cascades (see Chapter 3). Finally, the phospholipids that are characteristic of animal cell plasma membranes generally have one saturated and one unsaturated fatty acid residue. Consequently, they are less likely to partition into sol-like or gel-like lipid domains than are phospholipids that bear identical fatty acid chains.

Membrane proteins can be integrally or peripherally associated with the plasma membrane

The demonstration that the plasma membrane's lipid com- ponents form a bilayer leaves open the question of how the membrane's protein constituents are organized. Membrane proteins can belong to either of two broad classes, peripheral or integral. **Peripherally associated membrane proteins** are neither embedded within the membrane nor attached to it by covalent bonds; instead, they adhere tightly to the cyto- plasmic or extracellular surfaces of the plasma membrane (Fig. 2-5A). They can be removed from the membrane,

however, by mild treatments that disrupt ionic bonds (very high salt concentrations) or hydrogen bonds (very low salt concentrations).

In contrast, **integral membrane proteins** are intimately associated with the lipid bilayer. They cannot be eluted from the membrane by these high- or low-salt washes. To dislodge integral membrane proteins, the membrane itself must be dissolved by adding detergents. Integral membrane proteins can be associated with the lipid bilayer in any of three ways. First, some proteins actually span the lipid bilayer once or several times (Fig. 2-5B, C) and hence are referred to as **transmembrane proteins**. Experiments performed on eryth- rocyte membranes reveal that these proteins can be labeled with protein-tagging reagents applied to either side of the bilayer.

The second group of integral membrane proteins is embedded in the bilayer without actually crossing it (Fig. 2- 5D). A third group of membrane-associated proteins is not actually embedded in the bilayer at all. Instead, these lipid- anchored proteins are attached to the membrane by a cova- lent bond that links them either to a lipid component of the membrane or to a fatty acid derivative that intercalates into the membrane. For example, proteins can be linked to a special type of glycosylated phospholipid molecule (Fig. 2- 5E), which is most often glycosylphosphatidylinositol (**GPI**), on the outer leaflet of the membrane. This family is referred to collectively as the **glycophospholipid-linked proteins**. Another example is a direct linkage to a fatty acid (e.g., a myristyl group) or a prenyl (e.g., farnesyl) group that inter- calates into the inner leaflet of the membrane (Fig. 2-5F).

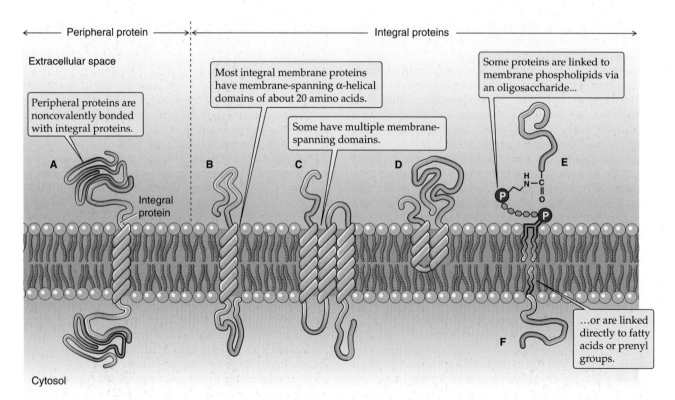

Figure 2-5 Classes of membrane proteins. In **E,** protein is coupled by a GPI linkage.

The membrane-spanning portions of transmembrane proteins are usually hydrophobic α helices

How can membrane-spanning proteins remain stably associated with the bilayer in a conformation that requires at least some portion of their amino acid sequence to be in continuous contact with the membrane's hydrophobic central core? The answer to this question can be found in the special structures of those protein domains that actually span the membrane.

The side chains of the eight amino acids listed in the upper portion of Table 2-1 are hydrophobic. These aromatic or uncharged aliphatic groups are almost as difficult to solvate in water as are the fatty acid side chains of the membrane phospholipids themselves. Not surprisingly, therefore, these hydrophobic side chains are quite comfortable in the hydrophobic environment of the bilayer core. Most **membrane-spanning segments**—that is, the short stretch of amino acids that passes through the membrane once—are composed mainly of these nonpolar amino acids, in concert with polar, uncharged amino acids.

The hydrophobic, membrane-spanning segments of transmembrane proteins are specially adapted to the hydrophobic milieu in which they reside. The phospholipid molecules of the membrane bilayer actually protect these portions of transmembrane proteins from energetically unfavorable interactions with the aqueous environment. Transmembrane proteins tend to be extremely insoluble in water. If we separate the membrane-spanning segments of these proteins from the amphipathic phospholipids that surround them, these hydrophobic sequences tend to interact tightly with one another rather than with water. The resulting large protein aggregates are generally insoluble and precipitate out of solution. If, however, we disrupt the phospholipid membrane by adding detergent, the amphipathic detergent molecules can substitute for the phospholipids. The hydrophobic membrane-spanning sequences remain insulated from interactions with the aqueous solvent, and the proteins remain soluble as components of **detergent micelles**. This ability of detergents to remove transmembrane proteins from the lipid bilayer—while maintaining the solubility and native architectures of these proteins—has proved important for purifying individual membrane proteins.

Transmembrane proteins can have a single membrane-spanning segment (Fig. 2-5B) or several (Fig. 2-5C). Those with a single transmembrane segment can be oriented with either their amino (N) or their carboxyl (C) termini facing the extracellular space. Multispanning membrane proteins weave through the membrane like a thread through cloth. Again, the N or C termini can be exposed to either the cytoplasmic or extracellular compartments. The pattern with which the transmembrane protein weaves across the lipid bilayer defines its membrane **topology**.

The amino acid sequences of membrane-spanning segments tend to form α helices, with ~3.6 amino acids per turn of the helix (Fig. 2-5B). In this conformation, the polar atoms of the peptide backbone are maximally hydrogen bonded to one another—from one turn of the helix to the next—so they do not require the solvent to contribute

hydrogen bond partners. Hence, this structure ensures the solubility of the membrane-spanning sequence in the hydrophobic environment of the membrane. Whereas most transmembrane proteins appear to traverse the membrane with α-helical spans, it is clear that an intriguing subset of membrane polypeptides makes use of a very different structure. The best studied member of this class is the porin protein, which serves as a channel in bacterial membranes. As discussed in Chapter 5, the membrane-spanning portions of porin are arranged as a β barrel.

In the case of multispanning membrane proteins, their transmembrane helices probably pack together tightly (Fig. 2-5C). Molecular analysis of a number of known membrane-spanning sequences has helped in the development of algorithms predicting the likelihood that a given amino acid sequence can span the membrane. These algorithms are widely used to assess the likelihood that newly identified genes encode transmembrane proteins and to predict the number and location of membrane-spanning segments.

Many membrane proteins form tight, noncovalent associations with other membrane proteins in the plane of the bilayer. These **multimeric proteins** can be composed of a single type of polypeptide or of mixtures of two or more different proteins. The side-to-side interactions that hold these complexes together can involve the membrane-spanning segments or regions of the proteins that protrude at either surface of the bilayer. By assembling into multimeric complexes, membrane proteins can increase their stability. They can also increase the variety and complexity of the functions that they are capable of performing.

Some membrane proteins are mobile in the plane of the bilayer

As is true for phospholipid molecules (Fig. 2-3), some transmembrane proteins can also diffuse within the surface of the membrane. In the absence of any protein-protein attachments, transmembrane proteins are free to diffuse over the entire surface of a membrane. This fact was demonstrated by Frye and Edidin in 1970 (Fig. 2-6). They labeled the surface proteins of a population of *mouse* lymphocytes with a lectin (a plant protein that binds strongly to certain sugar groups attached to proteins) that was linked to the fluorescent dye fluorescein. They also tagged the surface proteins of a second population of *human* lymphocytes with a lectin that was conjugated to a different fluorescent dye, rhodamine. Because fluorescein glows green and rhodamine glows red when excited by the light of the appropriate wavelengths, these labeling molecules can be easily distinguished from one another in a fluorescence microscope. Frye and Edidin mixed the two lymphocyte populations and treated them with a reagent that caused the cells to fuse to each other. Immediately after fusion, the labeled surface proteins of the newly joined cells remained separate; half of the fused cell surface appeared red, whereas the other half appeared green. During a period of ~30 minutes, however, the green and red protein labels intermixed until the entire surface of the fused cell was covered with both labeling molecules. The rate at which this intermingling occurred increased with temperature, which is not surprising, given the temperature dependence of membrane fluidity.

Table 2-1 Classification of the Amino Acids Based on the Chemistry of Their Side Chains

	Name	3-Letter Code	Single-Letter Code	Structure of the Side Chain	Hydropathy Index*
Nonpolar	Alanine	Ala	A	$-CH_3$	+1.8
	Valine	Val	V	$-CH(CH_3)_2$	+4.2
	Leucine	Leu	L	$-CH_2CH(CH_3)_2$	+3.8
	Isoleucine	Ile	I	$-CH-CH_2-CH_3$ with CH_3	+4.5
	Proline	Pro	P		−1.6
	Phenylalanine	Phe	F	$-CH_2-$ (benzene ring)	+2.8
	Tryptophan	Trp	W	$-CH_2-$ (indole ring)	−0.9
	Methionine	Met	M	$-CH_2-CH_2-S-CH_3$	+1.9
Polar uncharged	Glycine	Gly	G	$-H$	−0.4
	Serine	Ser	S	$-CH_2-OH$	−0.8
	Threonine	Thr	T	$-CH-CH_3$ with OH	−0.7
	Cysteine	Cys	C	$-CH_2-SH$	+2.5
	Tyrosine	Tyr	Y	$-CH_2-$ (benzene ring) $-OH$	−1.3
	Asparagine	Asn	N	$-CH_2-C=O$ with NH_2	−3.5
	Glutamine	Gln	Q	$-CH_2-CH_2-C=O$ with NH_2	−3.5
Polar, charged, acidic	Aspartate	Asp	D	$-CH_2-C=O$ with O^-	−3.5
	Glutamate	Glu	E	$-CH_2-CH_2-C=O$ with O^-	−3.5
Polar, charged, basic	Lysine	Lys	K	$-CH_2-CH_2-CH_2-CH_2-NH_3^+$	−3.9
	Arginine	Arg	R	$-CH_2-CH_2-CH_2-NH-C-NH_2$ with NH_2^+	−4.5
	Histidine	His	H	$-CH_2-$ (imidazole ring)	−3.2

*Kyte and Doolittle generated these values (arbitrary scale from -4.5 to +4.5) by averaging two kinds of data. The first is an index of the energy that is required to transfer the side chain from the vapor phase into water. The second indicates how likely it is to find the side chain buried in (as opposed to being on the surface of) 12 globular proteins, whose structures were solved by x-ray crystallography. A positive value indicates that the side chain is hydrophobic.

Note: The portion shown in red is part of the peptide backbone.

From Kyte J, Doolittle RF: A simple method for displaying the hydropathic character of a protein. J Mol Biol 1982; 157:105-132.

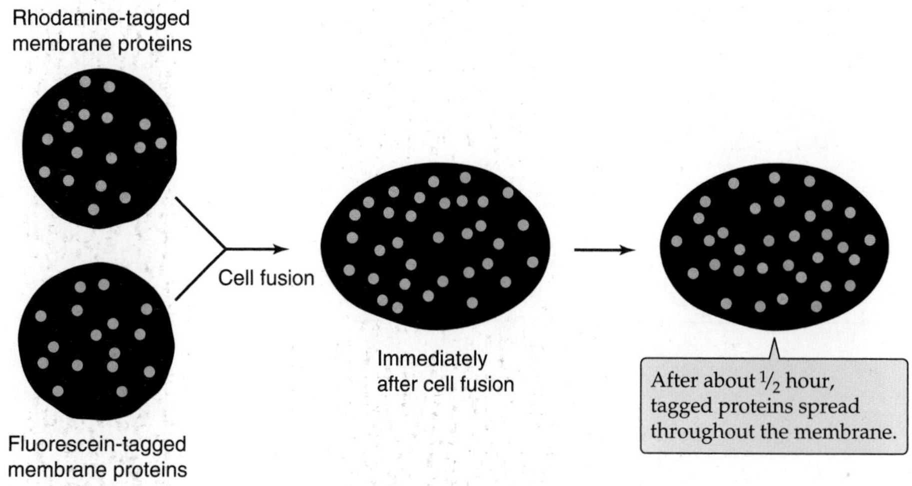

Rhodamine-tagged
membrane proteins

Figure 2-6 Diffusion of membrane proteins within the plane of the cell membrane. The surface proteins of a *human* lymphocyte are tagged with a lectin conjugated to rhodamine, a fluorescent dye; the surface proteins of a *mouse* lymphocyte are tagged with a lectin linked to fluorescein, another fluorescent dye. Immediately after fusion of the two cells, the labeled surface proteins remained segregated. However, the membrane proteins intermingled during a period of ~30 minutes.

Cell fusion

Immediately
after cell fusion

After about $1/2$ hour, tagged proteins spread throughout the membrane.

Fluorescein-tagged
membrane proteins

Because transmembrane proteins are large molecules, their diffusion in the plane of the membrane is much slower than that of lipids. Even the fastest proteins diffuse ~1000 times more slowly than the average phospholipid. The diffusion of many transmembrane proteins appears to be further impeded by their attachments to the cytoskeleton, just below the surface of the membrane. Tight binding to this meshwork can render proteins essentially immobile. Other transmembrane proteins appear to travel in the plane of the membrane by directed processes that are much faster and less directionally random than diffusion is. Motor proteins that are associated with the cytoplasmic cytoskeleton (discussed later) appear to grab onto certain transmembrane proteins, dragging them in the plane of the membrane like toy boats on strings. Finally, like phospholipids, proteins can diffuse only in the plane of the bilayer. They cannot flip-flop across it. The energetic barrier to dragging a transmembrane protein's hydrophilic cytoplasmic and extracellular domains across the bilayer's hydrophobic core is very difficult to surmount. Thus, a membrane protein's topology does not change over its life span.

FUNCTION OF MEMBRANE PROTEINS

Integral membrane proteins can serve as receptors

All communication between a cell and its environment must involve or at least pass through the plasma membrane. For the purposes of this discussion, we define communication rather broadly as the exchange of any signal between the cell and its surroundings. Except for lipid-soluble signaling molecules such as steroid hormones, essentially all communication functions served by the plasma membrane occur through membrane proteins. From an engineering perspective, membrane proteins are perfectly situated to transmit signals because they form a single, continuous link between the two compartments that are separated by the membrane.

Ligand-binding receptors comprise the group of transmembrane proteins that perhaps most clearly illustrate the concept of transmembrane signaling (Fig. 2-7A). For water-

soluble hormones such as epinephrine to influence cellular behavior, their presence in the extracellular fluid compartment must be made known to the various intracellular mechanisms whose behaviors they modulate. The interaction of a hormone with the extracellular portion of the hormone receptor, which forms a high-affinity binding site, produces conformational changes within the receptor protein that extend through the membrane-spanning domain to the intracellular domain of the receptor. As a consequence, the intracellular domain either becomes enzymatically active or can interact with cytoplasmic proteins that are involved in the generation of so-called second messengers. Either mechanism completes the transmission of the hormone signal across the membrane. The transmembrane disposition of a hormone receptor thus creates a single, continuous communication medium that is capable of conveying, through its own structural modifications, information from the environment to the cellular interior. The process of transmembrane signal transduction is discussed in Chapter 3.

Integral membrane proteins can serve as adhesion molecules

Cells can also exploit integral membrane proteins as **adhesion molecules** that form physical contacts with the surrounding extracellular matrix (i.e., cell-matrix adhesion molecules) or with their cellular neighbors (i.e., cell-cell adhesion molecules). These attachments can be extremely important in regulating the shape, growth, and differentiation of cells. The nature and extent of these attachments must be communicated to the cell interior so that the cell can adapt appropriately to the physical constraints and cues that are provided by its immediate surroundings. Numerous classes of transmembrane proteins are involved in these communication processes. The **integrins** are examples of matrix receptors or **cell matrix adhesion molecules**. They comprise a large family of transmembrane proteins that link cells to components of the extracellular matrix (e.g., fibronectin, laminin) at adhesion plaques (Fig. 2-7B). These linkages produce conformational changes in the integrin molecules that are transmitted to their cytoplasmic tails. These tails, in turn, communicate the linkage events to

A   LIGAND-BINDING RECEPTOR

B   CELL-MATRIX ADHESION MOLECULE (INTEGRIN)

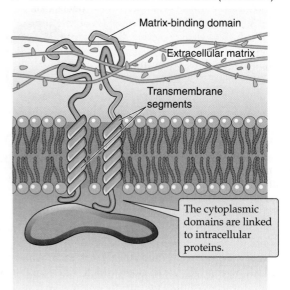

N

Ligand-binding domain

7 transmembrane segments

The cytoplasmic domain interacts with the intracellular proteins.

C

The helical domains form a compact unit in the membrane.

Matrix-binding domain

Extracellular matrix

Transmembrane segments

The cytoplasmic domains are linked to intracellular proteins.

Figure 2-7   Integral membrane proteins that transmit signals from the outside to the inside of a cell. **A,** The ligand may be a hormone, a growth factor, a neurotransmitter, an odorant, or another local mediator. **B,** An integrin is an adhesion molecule that attaches the cell to the extracellular matrix.

various structural and signaling molecules that participate in formulating a cell's response to its physical environment.

In contrast to matrix receptors, which attach cells to the extracellular matrix, several enormous superfamilies of **cell-cell adhesion molecules** attach cells to each other. These cell-cell adhesion molecules include the Ca^{2+}-dependent cell adhesion molecules (cadherins) and Ca^{2+}-independent neural cell adhesion molecules (N-CAMs). The **cadherins** are glycoproteins (i.e., proteins with sugars attached) with one membrane-spanning segment and a large extracellular domain that binds Ca^{2+}. The **N-CAMs**, on the other hand, generally are members of the immunoglobulin superfamily. The two classes of cell-cell adhesion molecules mediate similar sorts of transmembrane signals that help organize the cytoplasm and control gene expression in response to intercellular contacts. Some cell-cell adhesion molecules belong to the **GPI-linked class** of membrane proteins. These polypeptides lack a transmembrane and cytoplasmic tail. It is not clear, therefore, how (or if) interactions mediated by this unique class of adhesion molecules are communicated to the cell interior.

Adhesion molecules orchestrate processes that are as diverse as the directed migration of immune cells and the guidance of axons in the developing nervous system. Loss of cell-cell and cell-matrix adhesion is a hallmark of metastatic tumor cells.

Integral membrane proteins can carry out the transmembrane movement of water-soluble substances

Earlier in this discussion, we noted that a pure phospholipid bilayer does not have the permeability properties that are normally associated with animal cell plasma membranes. Pure phospholipid bilayers also lack the ability to transport substances uphill. Transmembrane proteins endow biological membranes with these capabilities. Ions and other membrane-impermeable substances can cross the bilayer with the assistance of transmembrane proteins that serve as pores, channels, carriers, and pumps. **Pores** and **channels** serve as conduits that allow water, specific ions, or even very large proteins to flow passively through the bilayer. **Carriers** can either facilitate the transport of a specific molecule across the membrane or couple the transport of a molecule to that of other solutes. **Pumps** use the energy that is released through the hydrolysis of adenosine triphosphate (ATP) to drive the transport of substances into or out of cells against energy gradients. Each of these important classes of proteins is discussed in Chapter 5.

Channels, carriers, and pumps succeed in allowing hydrophilic substances to cross the membrane by creating a hydrophilic pathway in the bilayer. Previously, we asserted that membrane-spanning segments are as hydrophobic as the fatty acids that surround them. How is it possible for these *hydrophobic* membrane-spanning domains to produce the *hydrophilic* pathways that permit the passage of ions through the membrane? The solution to this puzzle appears to be that the α helices that make up these membrane-spanning segments are amphipathic. That is, they possesses both hydrophobic and hydrophilic domains.

For each α helix, the helical turns produce alignments of amino acids that are spaced at regular intervals in the sequence. Thus, it is possible to align all the hydrophilic or hydrophobic amino acids along a single edge of the helix. In **amphipathic helices**, hydrophobic amino acids alternate with hydrophilic residues at regular intervals of approximately three or four amino acids (recall that there are ~3.6 amino acids per turn of the helix). Thus, as the helices pack together, side-by-side, the resultant membrane protein has distinct hydrophilic and hydrophobic surfaces. The hydrophobic surfaces of each helix will face either the membrane lipid or the hydrophobic surfaces of neighboring helices. Similarly, the hydrophilic surfaces of each helix will face a common central pore through which water-soluble particles can move. Depending on how the protein regulates access to this pore, the protein could be a channel, a carrier, or a pump. The mix of hydrophilic amino acids that line the pore presumably determines, at least in part, the nature of the substances that the pore can accommodate. In some instances, the amphipathic helices that line the pore are contributed by several distinct proteins—or subunits—that assemble into a single multimeric complex. Figure 2-8 shows an example of a type of K⁺ channel that is discussed in Chapter 7. This channel is formed by the apposition of four identical subunits, each of which has six membrane-spanning segments. The pore of this channel is created by the amphipathic helices

as well as by short, hydrophilic loops (P loops) contributed by each of the four subunits.

Integral membrane proteins can also be enzymes

Ion pumps are actually enzymes. They catalyze the hydrolysis of ATP and use the energy released by that reaction to drive ion transport. Many other classes of proteins that are embedded in cell membranes function as enzymes as well. Membrane-bound enzymes are especially prevalent in the cells of the intestine, which participate in the final stages of nutrient digestion and absorption (see Chapter 45). These enzymes—located on the side of the intestinal cells that faces the lumen of the intestine—break down small polysaccharides into single sugars, or break down polypeptides into shorter polypeptides or amino acids, so that they can be imported into the cells. By embedding these enzymes in the plasma membrane, the cell can generate the final products of digestion close to the transport proteins that mediate the uptake of these nutrient molecules. This theme is repeated in numerous other cell types. Thus, the membrane can serve as an extremely efficient two-dimensional reaction center for multistep processes that involve enzymatic reactions or transport.

Many of the GPI-linked proteins are enzymes. Several of the enzymatic activities that are classically thought of as extracellular markers of the plasma membrane, such as **alkaline phosphatase** and **5′-nucleotidase**, are anchored to the external leaflet of the bilayer by covalent attachment to a GPI. The biological utility of this arrangement has yet to be determined. However, the GPI linkage is itself a substrate for

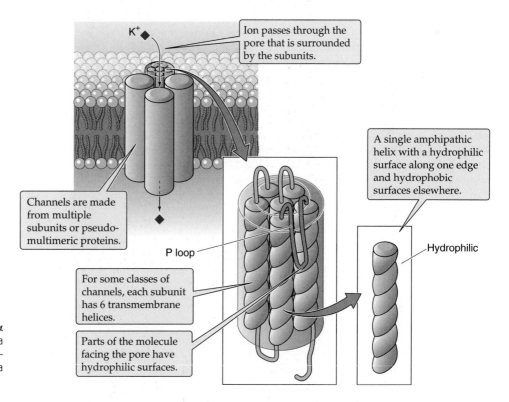

Figure 2-8 Amphipathic α helices interacting to form a channel through the cell membrane. This is an example of a potassium channel.

K⁺

Ion passes through the pore that is surrounded by the subunits.

A single amphipathic helix with a hydrophilic surface along one edge and hydrophobic surfaces elsewhere.

Channels are made from multiple subunits or pseudo-multimeric proteins.

P loop

Hydrophilic

For some classes of channels, each subunit has 6 transmembrane helices.

Parts of the molecule facing the pore have hydrophilic surfaces.

enzymatic cleavage. Phospholipase C, which is present at appreciable levels in the serum, can cleave the covalent bond between the protein and its lipid anchor, thereby releasing the protein from the membrane. The released protein subsequently behaves like a soluble polypeptide.

Integral membrane proteins can participate in intracellular signaling

Some integral proteins associate with the cytoplasmic surface of the plasma membrane by covalently attaching to fatty acids or prenyl groups that in turn intercalate into the lipid bilayer (Fig. 2-5F). The fatty acids or prenyl groups act as hydrophobic tails that anchor an otherwise soluble protein to the bilayer. These proteins are all located at the *intra*cellular leaflet of the membrane bilayer and often participate in intracellular signaling and growth regulation pathways. The family of lipid-linked proteins includes the small and heterotrimeric guanosine triphosphate (GTP)–binding proteins, kinases, and oncogene products (see Chapter 3). Many of these proteins are involved in relaying the signals that are received at the cell surface to the effector machinery within the cell interior. Their association with the membrane, therefore, brings these proteins close to the cytoplasmic sides of receptors that transmit signals from the cell exterior across the bilayer. The medical relevance of this type of membrane association is beginning to be appreciated. For example,

denying certain oncogene products their lipid modifications—and hence their membrane attachment—eliminates their ability to induce tumorigenic transformation.

Peripheral membrane proteins participate in intracellular signaling and can form a submembranous cytoskeleton

Peripheral membrane proteins attach loosely to the lipid bilayer but are not embedded within it. Their association with the membrane can take one of two forms. First, some proteins interact through **ionic interactions** with phospholipid head groups. Many of these head groups are positively or negatively charged and thus can participate in salt bridges with adherent proteins.

For a second group of peripheral membrane proteins, attachment is based on the direct binding of peripheral membrane proteins to the extracellular or cytoplasmic surfaces of integral membrane proteins (Fig. 2-5A). This form of attachment is epitomized by the cytoskeleton. For instance, the cytoplasmic surface of the erythrocyte plasma membrane is in close apposition to a dense meshwork of interlocking protein strands known as the **subcortical cytoskeleton**. It consists of a long, fibrillar molecule called spectrin, short polymers of the cytoskeletal protein actin, and other proteins including ankyrin and band 4.1 (Fig. 2-9).

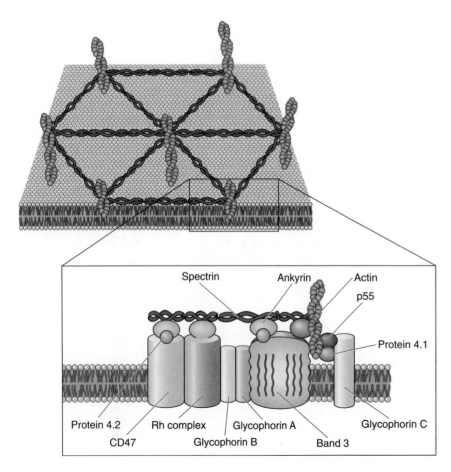

Figure 2-9 Attachments of the cell membrane to the submembranous cytoskeleton in red blood cells. Integral membrane proteins form the bridges that link the cell membrane to the interlocking system of proteins that form the subcortical cytoskeleton.

Two closely related isoforms of **spectrin** (α and β) form dimers, and two of these dimers assemble head-to-head with one another to form spectrin heterotetramers. The tail regions of spectrin bind the globular protein **band 4.1**, which in turn can bind to actin fibrils. Each **actin** fibril can associate with more than one molecule of band 4.1 so that, together, spectrin, actin, and band 4.1 assemble into an extensive interlocking matrix. The protein known as **ankyrin** binds to spectrin as well as to the cytoplasmic domain of **band 3**, the integral membrane protein responsible for transporting Cl⁻ and HCO_3^- ions across the erythrocyte membrane. Thus, ankyrin is a *peripheral* membrane protein that anchors the spectrin-actin meshwork directly to an *integral* membrane protein of the erythrocyte.

The subcortical cytoskeleton provides the erythrocyte plasma membrane with strength and resilience. People who carry mutations in genes encoding their components have erythrocytes that do not have the characteristic biconcave disk shape. These erythrocytes are extremely fragile and are easily torn apart by the shear stresses (see Chapter 17) associated with circulation through capillaries. It would appear, therefore, that the subcortical cytoskeleton forms a scaffolding of peripheral membrane proteins whose direct attachment to transmembrane proteins enhances the bilayer's structural integrity.

The subcortical cytoskeleton is not unique to erythrocytes. Numerous cell types, including neurons and epithelial cells, have submembranous meshworks that consist of proteins very similar to those first described in the erythrocyte. In addition to band 3, transmembrane proteins found in a wide variety of cells (including ion pumps, ion channels, and cell adhesion molecules) bind ankyrin and can thus serve as focal points of cytoskeletal attachment. In polarized cells (e.g., neurons and epithelial cells), the subcortical cytoskeleton appears to play a critically important role in organizing the plasma membrane into morphologically and functionally distinct domains.

CELLULAR ORGANELLES AND THE CYTOSKELETON

The cell is composed of discrete organelles that subserve distinct functions

When a eukaryotic cell is viewed through a light microscope, a handful of recognizable intracellular structures can be discerned. The intracellular matrix, or cytoplasm, appears grainy, suggesting the presence of components that are too small to be discriminated by this technique. With the much higher magnifications available with an electron microscope, the graininess gives way to clarity that reveals the cell interior to be remarkably complex. Even the simplest nucleated animal cell possesses a wide variety of intricate structures with specific shapes and sizes. These structures are the **membrane-enclosed organelles**, the functional building blocks of cells.

Figure 2-10 illustrates the interior of a typical cell. The largest organelle in this picture is the **nucleus**, which houses the cell's complement of genetic information. This structure, which is visible in the light microscope, is usually round or

oblong, although in some cells it displays a complex, lobulated shape. Depending on the cell type, the nucleus can range in diameter from 2 to 20 μm. With some exceptions, including skeletal muscle and certain specialized cells of the immune system, each animal cell has a single nucleus.

Surrounding the nucleus is a web of tubules or saccules known as the **endoplasmic reticulum (ER)**. This organelle can exist in either of two forms, rough or smooth. The surfaces of the rough ER tubules are studded with **ribosomes**, the major sites of protein synthesis. Ribosomes can also exist free in the cytosol. The surfaces of the smooth ER, which participates in lipid synthesis, are not similarly endowed. The ER also serves as a major reservoir for calcium ions. The ER membrane is endowed with a Ca^{2+} pump that uses the energy released through ATP hydrolysis to drive the transport of Ca^{2+} from the cytoplasm into the ER lumen (see Chapter 5). This Ca^{2+} can be rapidly released in response to messenger molecules and plays a major role in intracellular signaling (see Chapter 3).

The **Golgi complex** resembles a stack of pancakes. Each pancake in the stack represents a discrete, flat saccule. The number and size of the saccules in the Golgi stack vary among cell types. The Golgi complex is a processing station that participates in protein maturation and targets newly synthesized proteins to their appropriate subcellular destinations.

Perhaps the most intriguing morphological appearance belongs to the **mitochondrion**, which is essentially a balloon within a balloon. The outer membrane and inner membrane define two distinct internal compartments: the intermembrane space and the matrix space. The surface of the inner membrane is thrown into dramatic folds called *cristae*. This organelle is ~0.2 μm in diameter, placing it at the limit of resolution of the light microscope. The mitochondrion is the power plant of the cell, a critical manufacturer of ATP. Many cellular reactions are also catalyzed within the mitochondrion.

The cell's digestive organelle is the **lysosome**. This large structure frequently contains several smaller round vesicles called **exosomes** within its internal space.

The cytoplasm contains numerous other organelles whose shapes are not quite as distinguishing, including **endosomes**, **peroxisomes**, and **transport vesicles**.

Despite their diversity, all cellular organelles are constructed from the same building blocks. Each is composed of a membrane that forms the entire extent of its surface. The membranes of the subcellular organelles are what can be visualized in electron micrographs. The biochemical and physical properties of an organelle's limiting membrane dictate many of its functional properties.

The nucleus stores, replicates, and reads the cell's genetic information

The nucleus serves as a cell's repository for its complement of chromosomal DNA. To conceive of the nucleus as simply a hermetically sealed vault for genetic information, however, is a gross oversimplification. All of the machinery necessary to maintain, to copy, and to transcribe DNA is in the nucleus, which is the focus of all of the cellular pathways that regulate gene expression and cell division. Transcriptional control is

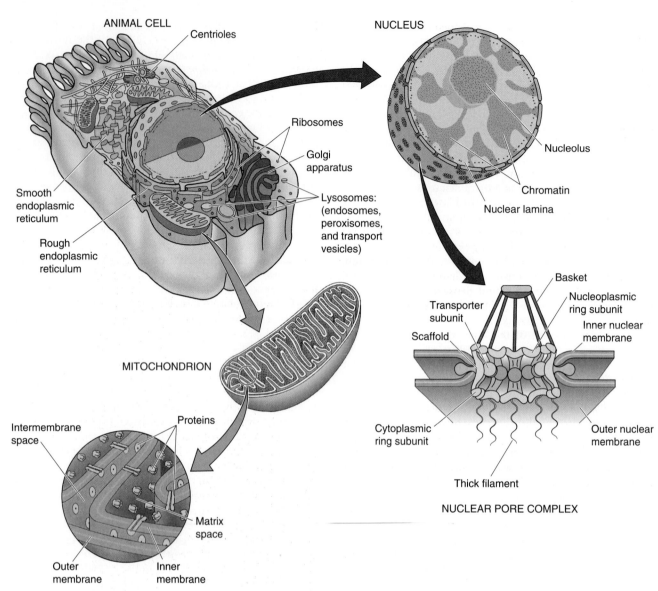

Figure 2-10 Ultrastructure of a typical animal cell.

discussed in Chapter 4. The focus of this section is nuclear structure.

The nucleus is surrounded by a double membrane (Fig. 2-10). The **outer membrane** is studded with ribosomes and is continuous with the membranes of the rough ER. The **inner membrane** is smooth and faces the intranuclear space, or nucleoplasm. The space between these concentric membranes is continuous with the lumen of the rough ER. The inner and outer nuclear membranes meet at specialized structures known as **nuclear pores**, which penetrate the nuclear envelope and provide a transport pathway between the cytoplasm and the nuclear interior (see Chapter 5). All RNA transcripts that are produced in the nucleus must pass through nuclear pores to be translated in the cytoplasm. Similarly, all the signaling molecules that influence nuclear function as well as all proteins of the nuclear interior (which are synthesized in the cytoplasm) enter the nucleus through nuclear pores.

Nuclear pores are selective in choosing the molecules that they allow to pass. Cytoplasmic proteins destined for the nuclear interior must be endowed with a **nuclear localization sequence** to gain entry. Several nuclear localization sequences have been characterized, and all seem to share common structural elements. For example, they all have short stretches of four to eight basic amino acids that can be located anywhere in the protein's sequence. Evidence implies that the ability of these signals to mediate nuclear localization can be modulated by phosphorylation, which suggests that the entry of proteins into the nucleus may be under the control of the cell's second-messenger systems.

The selectivity of the nuclear pore is surprising, considering its size. The outer diameter of the entire nuclear pore is ~100 nm, considerably larger than the proteins whose passage it controls. The nuclear pore's specificity is provided by the **nuclear pore complex** (**NPC**), an intricate matrix of protein that is distributed in a highly organized octagonal array. In its resting state, the NPC forms an aqueous channel that is ~9 nm in diameter, restricting the movement of any protein larger than 60 kDa. However, when it is confronted with a protein bearing a nuclear localization signal or a messenger RNA (mRNA) transcript, the pore complex can dilate to many times this size. The mechanisms by which the pore's permeability is regulated remain unknown. The NPC has a barrier that prevents the diffusion of intrinsic membrane proteins between the outer and inner membranes of the nuclear envelope. Thus, although the inner and outer nuclear membranes are continuous with one another at nuclear pores, their protein contents remain distinct.

Between mitoses, the chromosomal DNA is present in the nucleus as densely packed heterochromatin and more loosely arrayed euchromatin. **Chromatin** is a complex between DNA and numerous DNA-binding proteins, which organize the chromosome into a chain of tightly folded DNA-protein assemblies called **nucleosomes** (see Chapter 4). Interspersed within the nucleoplasm are round, dense **nucleoli**, where the transcription of ribosomal RNA and the assembly of ribosomal subunits appear to occur.

The interior surface of the inner nuclear membrane is apposed to a fibrillar protein skeleton referred to as the **nuclear lamina**. This meshwork, composed of proteins known as *lamins*, is presumably involved in providing structural support to the nuclear envelope. The nuclear lamina may also play a role in orchestrating **nuclear reassembly**. During mitosis, the nuclear envelope breaks down into small vesicles, and the contents of the nucleoplasm mix with the cytoplasm. After mitosis, these vesicles fuse with one another to regenerate the double-walled nuclear membrane. The means by which these vesicles find one another and assemble correctly is the subject of intense study. Similarly, the mechanisms involved in maintaining the compositional discreteness of the inner and outer membranes during vesiculation and reassembly have yet to be determined. After reconstitution of the nuclear envelope, the proteins of the nucleoplasm are re-imported from the cytoplasm through the nuclear pores by virtue of their nuclear localization sequences.

Lysosomes digest material that is derived from the interior and exterior of the cell

In the course of normal daily living, cells accumulate waste. Organelles become damaged and dysfunctional. Proteins denature and aggregate. New materials are constantly being brought into the cells from the extracellular environment through the process of endocytosis (discussed later). In specialized cells of the immune system, such as macrophages, the collection of foreign materials (in the form of pathogens) from the extracellular milieu is the cellular raison d'être. If this material were allowed to accumulate indefinitely, it would ultimately fill the cell and essentially choke it to death. Clearly, cells must have mechanisms for disposing of this waste material.

The lysosome is the cell's trash incinerator. It is filled with a broad assortment of degradative enzymes that can break down most forms of cellular debris. **Proton pumps** embedded within the lysosome's limiting membrane ensure that this space is an extremely acidic environment, which aids in protein hydrolysis. A rare group of inherited disorders, called

lysosomal storage diseases (see the box on page 43 about this topic), result from the deficiency of lysosomal enzymes that are involved in the degradation of a variety of substances.

The lysosomal membrane is specially adapted to resist digestion by the enzymes and the acid that it encapsulates, thus ensuring that the harsh conditions necessary for efficient degradation are effectively contained. Loss of lysosomal membrane integrity may underlie some clinically important inflammatory conditions, such as gout.

Material that has been internalized from the cell exterior by endocytosis is surrounded by the membrane of an **endocytic vesicle**. To deliver this material to the lysosome, the membranes of the endocytic vesicles fuse with the lysosomal membrane and discharge their cargo into the lysosomal milieu.

Intracellular structures that are destined for degradation, such as fragments of organelles, are engulfed by the lysosome in a process called **autophagy**. Autophagy results in the formation of membrane-enclosed structures within the lysosomal lumen; hence, the lysosome is often referred to as a multivesicular body.

The mitochondrion is the site of oxidative energy production

Oxygen-dependent ATP production—or oxidative phosphorylation—occurs in the mitochondrion. Like the nucleus, the mitochondrion (Fig. 2-10) is a double-membrane structure. The inner mitochondrial membrane contains the proteins that constitute the electron transport chain, which generates pH and voltage gradients across this membrane. According to the "chemiosmotic" model (see Chapter 5), the inner membrane uses the energy in these gradients to generate ATP from adenosine diphosphate (ADP) and inorganic phosphate.

The mitochondrion maintains and replicates its own genome. This circular DNA strand encodes **mitochondrial transfer RNAs (tRNAs)** and (in humans) 13 **mitochondrial proteins**. Several copies of the mitochondrial genome are located in the inner mitochondrial matrix, which also has all of the machinery necessary to transcribe and to translate this DNA, including ribosomes. Whereas the proteins encoded in mitochondrial DNA contribute to the structure and function of the mitochondrion, they account for a relatively small fraction of total mitochondrial protein. Most *mitochondrial* proteins are specified by nuclear DNA and are synthesized on *cytoplasmic* ribosomes.

The two mitochondrial membranes enclose two distinct compartments: the intermembrane space and the inner mitochondrial matrix space. The **intermembrane space** lies between the two membranes; the **inner mitochondrial matrix space** is completely enclosed by the inner mitochondrial membrane. These compartments have completely different complements of soluble proteins, and the two membranes themselves have extremely different proteins.

In addition to its role in energy metabolism, the mitochondrion also serves as a reservoir for intracellular Ca^{2+}. It is not clear whether—under physiological conditions—the mitochondrion releases Ca^{2+} from this reservoir. The mitochondrial Ca^{2+} stores are released as a consequence of energy starvation, which leads to cell injury and death. Finally, the mitochondrion plays a central role in the process called **apoptosis**, or programmed cell death (see Chapter 62). Certain external or internal signals can induce the cell to initiate a signaling cascade that leads ultimately to the activation of enzymes that bring about the cell's demise. One of the pathways that initiates this highly ordered form of cellular suicide depends on the participation of the mitochondrion. Apoptosis plays an extremely important role during tissue development and is also involved in the body's mechanisms for identifying and destroying cancer cells.

The cytoplasm is not amorphous but is organized by the cytoskeleton

Our discussion thus far has focused almost exclusively on the cell's membranous elements. We have treated the cytoplasm as if it were a homogeneous solution in which the organelles and vesicles carry out their functions while floating about unimpeded and at random. Rather, the cytoplasm is enormously complex with an intricate local structure and the capacity for locomotion.

The cytoplasmic **cytoskeleton** is composed of protein filaments that radiate throughout the cell, serving as the beams, struts, and stays that determine cell shape and resilience. On the basis of their appearance in the electron microscope, these filaments were initially divided into several classes (Table 2-2): thick, thin, and intermediate filaments as well as microtubules. Subsequent biochemical analysis has revealed that each of these varieties is composed of distinct polypeptides and differs with respect to its formation, stability, and biological function.

Intermediate filaments provide cells with structural support

Intermediate filaments are so named because their 8- to 10-nm diameters, as measured in the electron microscope, are intermediate between those of the actin *thin* filaments and

Table 2-2   Components of the Cytoskeleton

	Subunits	Diameter (nm)
Intermediate filaments	Tetramer of two coiled dimers	8-10
Microtubules	Heterodimers of α and β tubulin form long protofilaments, 5 nm in diameter	25
Thin filaments	Globular or G-actin, 5 nm in diameter, arranged in a double helix to form fibrous or F-actin	5-8
Thick filaments	Assembly of myosin molecules	10

the myosin *thick* filaments. As with all of the cytoskeletal filaments that we will discuss, intermediate filaments are polymers that are assembled from individual protein subunits. There is a very large variety of biochemically distinct subunit proteins that are all structurally related to one another and that derive from a single gene family. The expression of these subunit polypeptides can be cell type specific or restricted to specific regions within a cell. Thus, **vimentin** is found in cells that are derived from mesenchyme, and the closely related **glial fibrillary acidic protein** is expressed exclusively in glial cells (see Chapter 11). **Neurofilament proteins** are present in neuronal processes. The **keratins** are present in epithelial cells as well as in certain epithelially derived structures. The **nuclear lamins** that form the structural scaffolding of the nuclear envelope are also members of the intermediate filament family.

Intermediate filament monomers are themselves fibrillar in structure. They assemble to form long, intercoiled dimers that in turn assemble side-to-side to form the tetrameric subunits. Finally, these tetrameric subunits pack together, end-to-end and side-to-side, to form intermediate filaments. Filament assembly can be regulated by the cell and in some cases appears to be governed by phosphorylation of the subunit polypeptides. Intermediate filaments appear to radiate from and to reinforce areas of a cell that are subject to tensile stress. They emanate from the **adhesion plaques** that attach cells to their substrata. In epithelial cells, they insert at the **desmosomal junctions** that attach neighboring cells to one another. The toughness and resilience of the meshworks formed by these filaments is perhaps best illustrated by the **keratins**, the primary constituents of nails, hair, and the outer layers of skin.

Microtubules provide structural support and provide the basis for several types of subcellular motility

Microtubules are polymers formed from heterodimers of the proteins α and β **tubulin** (Fig. 2-11A). These heterodimers assemble head to tail, creating a circumferential wall of a microtubule, which surrounds an empty lumen. Because the tubulin heterodimers assemble with a specific orientation, microtubules are polar structures, and their ends manifest distinct biochemical properties. At one tip of the tubule, designated the **plus end**, tubulin heterodimers can be added to the growing polymer at three times the rate that this process occurs at the opposite **minus end**. The relative rates of microtubule growth and depolymerization are controlled in part by an enzymatic activity that is inherent in the tubulin dimer. Tubulin dimers bind to **GTP**, and in this GTP-bound state they associate more tightly with the growing ends of microtubules. Once a tubulin dimer becomes part of the microtubule, it hydrolyzes the GTP to guanosine diphosphate (GDP), which lowers the binding affinity of the dimer for the tubule and helps hasten disassembly. Consequently, the microtubules can undergo rapid rounds of growth and shrinkage, a behavior termed *dynamic instability*. Various cytosolic proteins can bind to the ends of microtubules and serve as caps that prevent assembly and disassembly and thus stabilize the structures of the microtubules. A large and diverse family of **microtubule-associated proteins** appears

A MICROTUBULE AND ITS MOLECULAR MOTORS

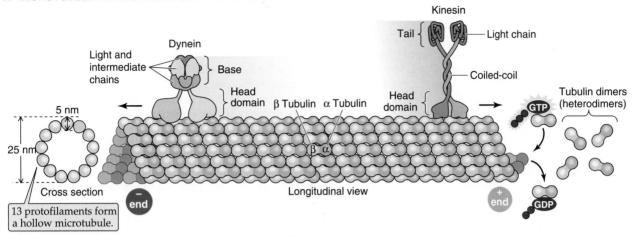

B MICROTUBULE-ORGANIZING CENTER   **C** MOTILE CILIUM

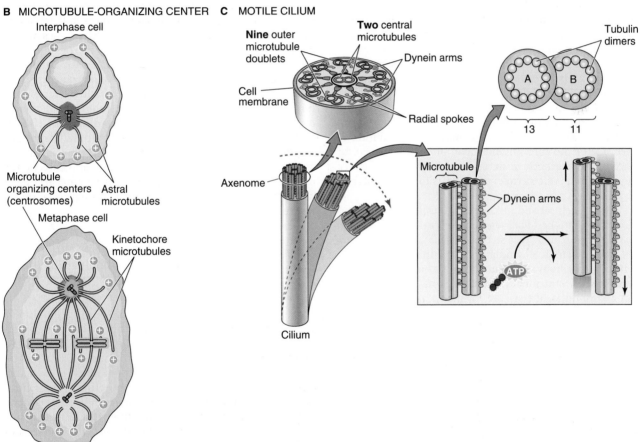

Figure 2-11 Microtubules. **A,** Heterodimers of α and β tubulin form long protofilaments, 13 of which surround the hollow core of a microtubule. The microtubule grows more rapidly at its plus end. The molecular motor dynein moves along the microtubule in the plus-to-minus direction, whereas the molecular motor kinesin moves in the opposite direction. ATP is the fuel for each of these motors. **B,** The microtubules originate from a microtubule-organizing center or centrosome, which generally consists of two centrioles *(green cylinders)*. **C,** A motile cilium can actively bend as its microtubules slide past each other. The molecular motor dynein produces this motion, fueled by ATP.

to modulate not only the stability of the tubules but also their capacity to interact with other intracellular components.

In most cells, all of the microtubules originate from the microtubule-organizing center or **centrosome**. This structure generally consists of two **centrioles**, each of which is a small (~0.5 μm) assembly of nine triplet microtubules that are arranged obliquely along the wall of a cylinder (see upper portion of Fig. 2-11B). The two centrioles in a centrosome are oriented at right angles to one another. The minus ends of all of a cell's microtubules are associated with proteins that surround the centrosome, whereas the rapidly growing plus ends radiate throughout the cytoplasm in a star-like arrangement ("astral" microtubules).

Microtubules participate in a multitude of cellular functions and structures. For example, microtubules project down the axon of neurons. Microtubules also provide the framework for the lacy membranes of the ER and Golgi complex. Disruption of microtubules causes these organelles to undergo dramatic morphological rearrangements and vesicularization. Microtubules also play a central role in cell division. Early in mitosis, the centrioles that make up the centrosomes replicate, forming two centrosomes at opposite poles of the dividing nucleus. Emanating from these centrosomes are the microtubules that form the **spindle fibers**, which in turn align the chromosomes (see lower portion of Fig. 2-11B). Their coordinated growth and dissolution at either side of the chromosomes may provide the force for separating the genetic material during the anaphase of mitosis. A pair of centrioles remains with each daughter cell.

The architectural and mechanical capacities of microtubules are perhaps best illustrated by their role in motility. An electron microscopic cross section of a cilium demonstrates the elegance, symmetry, and intricacy of this structure (Fig. 2-11C). Every cilium arises out of its own **basal body**, which is essentially a centriole that is situated at the ciliary root. **Cilia** are found on the surfaces of many types of epithelial cells, including those that line the larger pulmonary airways (see Chapter 26). Their oar-like beating motions help propel foreign bodies and pathogens toward their ultimate expulsion at the pharynx. At the center of a cilium is a structure called the **axoneme**, which is composed of a precisely defined 9 + 2 array of microtubules. Each of the 9 (which are also called outer tubules) consists of a complete microtubule with 13 tubulin monomers in cross section (the A tubule) to which is fused an incomplete microtubule with 11 tubulin monomers in cross section (the B tubule). Each of the 2, which lie at the core of the cilium, is a complete microtubule. This entire 9 + 2 structure runs the entire length of the cilium. The same array forms the core of a flagellum, the serpentine motions of which propel sperm cells (see Chapter 56).

Radial spokes connect the outer tubules to the central pair, and outer tubules attach to their neighbors by two types of linkages. One is composed of the protein dynein, which acts as a **molecular motor** to power ciliary and flagellar motions. **Dynein** is an ATPase that converts the energy released through ATP hydrolysis into a conformational change that produces a bending motion. Because dynein attached to one outer tubule interacts with a neighboring

outer tubule, this bending of the dynein molecule causes the adjacent outer tubules to slide past one another. It is this sliding-filament motion that gives rise to the coordinated movements of the entire structure. To some extent, this coordination is accomplished through the action of the second linkage protein, called nexin. The **nexin** arms restrict the extent to which neighboring outer tubules can move with respect to each other and thus prevent the dynein motor from driving the dissolution of the entire complex.

The utility of the dynein motor protein is not restricted to its function in cilia and flagella. Cytoplasmic dynein, which is a close relative of the motor molecule found in cilia, and a second motor protein called kinesin provide the force necessary to move membrane-bound organelles through the cytoplasm along microtubular tracks (Fig. 2-11A). The ability of vesicular organelles to move rapidly along microtubules was first noted in neurons, in which vesicles carrying newly synthesized proteins must be transported over extremely long distances from the cell body to the axon tip. Rather than trust this critical process to the vagaries of slow, nondirected diffusion, the neuron makes use of the kinesin motor, which links a vesicle to a microtubule. **Kinesin** hydrolyzes ATP and, like dynein, converts this energy into mechanical transitions that cause it to "walk" along the microtubule. Kinesin will move only along microtubules and thereby transport vesicles in the **minus-to-plus direction**. Thus, in neurons, kinesin-bound vesicles move from the microtubular minus ends, originating at the centrosome in the cell body, toward the plus ends in the axons. This direction of motion is referred to as anterograde fast axonal transport. **Cytoplasmic dynein** moves in the opposite **plus-to-minus** (or retrograde) direction.

The motor-driven movement of cellular organelles along microtubular tracks is not unique to neurons. This process, involving both kinesin and cytoplasmic dynein, appears to occur in almost every cell and may control the majority of subcellular vesicular traffic.

Thin filaments (actin) and thick filaments (myosin) are present in almost every cell type

Thin filaments, also called microfilaments, are 5 to 8 nm in diameter. They are helical polymers composed of a single polypeptide called globular actin or **G-actin**. Thin filaments are functionally similar to microtubules in two respects: (1) the actin polymers are polar and grow at different rates at their two ends, and (2) actin binds and then hydrolyzes a nucleotide. However, whereas tubulin binds GTP and then hydrolyzes it to GDP, actin binds ATP and then hydrolyzes it to ADP. After G-actin binds ATP, it may interact with another ATP-bound monomer to form an unstable dimer (Fig. 2-12A). Adding a third ATP-bound monomer, however, yields a stable trimer that serves as a nucleus for assembly of the polymer of fibrous actin or **F-actin**. Once it is part of F-actin, the actin monomer hydrolyzes its bound ATP, retaining the ADP and releasing the inorganic phosphate. The ADP-bound actin monomer is more likely to disengage itself from its neighbors, just as GDP-bound tubulin dimers are more likely to disassemble from tubulin. Even though the length of the F-actin filament may remain more or less constant, the polymer may continually grow at its plus end but

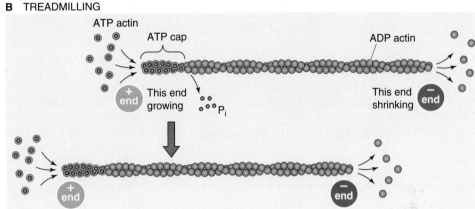

A FORMATION OF F-ACTIN

ATP-bound   Unstable
G-actin   actin dimer

ATP

G-actin   Stable actin
molecule   oligomer

Activation   Nucleus   Assembly
                 formation

F-actin
filament

P_i

B TREADMILLING

ATP actin   ATP cap   ADP actin

+ end   This end   This end   − end
         growing P_i shrinking

+ end   − end

Figure 2-12 Thin filaments. **A,** Single molecules of G-actin form F-actin filaments. **B,** F-actin can grow at the plus end while shrinking at the minus end, with no change in length.

disassemble at its minus end (Fig. 2-12B). This "treadmilling" requires the continuous input of energy (i.e., hydrolysis of ATP) and illustrates the unique dynamic properties of actin filament elongation and disassembly.

Thick filaments are composed of dimers of a remarkable force-generating protein called myosin. All **myosin** molecules have helical tails and globular head groups that hydrolyze ATP and act as motors to move along an actin filament. The energy liberated by ATP hydrolysis is invested in bending the myosin molecule around a pivot point called the hinge region, which marks the junction between the globular and tail regions. By means of this bending, myosin, like the dynein and kinesin that interact with microtubules, acts as a molecular motor that converts chemical into mechanical energy.

In muscle, the myosin molecules are in the **myosin II** subfamily and exist as dimers with their long tails intertwined (Fig. 2-13A). In muscle, each of the two myosin II heads binds two additional protein subunits that are referred to as myosin **light chains**. Non-muscle cells, in addition to myosin II, may have a variety of other, smaller myosin molecules. These other myosins, the most widely studied of which is **myosin I**, have shorter tails and, at least in some cases, act as molecular motors that move vesicles along actin filaments.

In muscle, the myosin II dimers stack as antiparallel arrays to form a bipolar structure with a bare central region that contains only tails (Fig. 2-13A). The ends of the thick filament contain the heads that bend toward the filament's central region. The pivoting action of the myosin head groups drags the neighboring thin filament (Fig. 2-13B), which includes other molecules besides actin. This sliding-

filament phenomenon underlies muscle contraction and force generation (Fig. 2-13C).

Actin as well as an ever-growing list of myosin isoforms is present in essentially every cell type. The functions of these proteins are easy to imagine in some cases and are less obvious in many others. Many cells, including all of the fibroblast-like cells, possess actin filaments that are arranged in **stress fibers**. These linear arrays of fibers interconnect adhesion plaques to one another and to interior structures in the cell. They orient themselves along lines of tension and can, in turn, exert contractile force on the substratum that underlies the cell. Stress fiber contractions may be involved in the macroscopic contractions that are associated with wound healing. Frequently, actin filaments in non-muscle cells are held together in bundles by cross-linking proteins. Numerous classes of cross-linking proteins have been identified, several of which can respond to physiological changes by either stabilizing or severing filaments and filament bundles.

In motile cells, such as fibroblasts and macrophages, arrays of actin-myosin filaments are responsible for **cell locomotion**. A Ca^{2+}-stimulated myosin light chain kinase regulates the assembly of myosin and actin filaments and thus governs the generation of contractile force. The precise mechanism by which these fibers cooperate in causing the cell to crawl along a substrate remains poorly understood.

In contrast to fibroblasts and circulating cells of the immune system, cells such as neurons and epithelial cells generally do not move much after their differentiation is complete. Despite this lack of movement, however, these cells are equipped with remarkably intricate actin and myosin filament networks. In some cases, these cytoskeletal elements

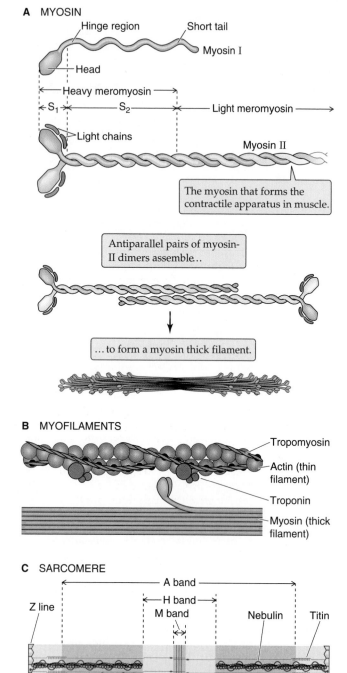

Figure 2-13 Thick filaments. **A,** Myosin I is one of a large number of widely distributed myosins that have short tails. Myosin II is the myosin that participates in muscle contraction. **B,** The pivoting action of the myosin head, fueled by ATP, moves the thick filament past the thin filament. **C,** In skeletal and cardiac muscle, the sarcomere is the fundamental contractile unit.

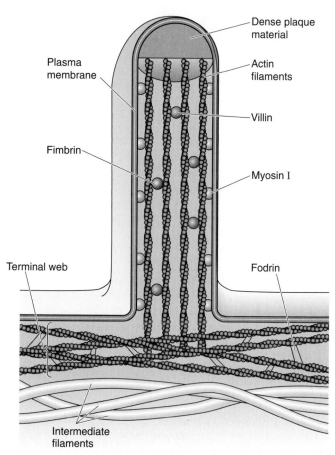

Figure 2-14 Actin filaments at the brush border of an epithelial cell.

permit the cell to extend processes to distant locations. This is the case in neurons, in which the growth and migration of axons during development or regeneration of the nervous system bear a striking morphological resemblance to the crawling of free-living amoebae. The tip of a growing axon, known as a **growth cone**, is richly endowed with contractile fibers and is capable of the same types of crawling motions that characterize motile cells.

In **epithelial cells**, the role of the actin-myosin cytoskeleton is somewhat less obvious but still important to normal physiological function. The **microvilli** at the apical surfaces of many epithelial cell types (e.g., those that line the renal proximal tubule and the small intestine) are supported by an intricate scaffolding of actin filaments that form their cores (Fig. 2-14). This bundle of actin fibers is held together and anchored to the overlying plasma membrane by a variety of cross-linking proteins, including various myosin isoforms. The roots of the microvillar actin filament bundles emerge from the bases of the microvilli into a dense meshwork of cytoskeletal filaments known as the **terminal web**. Included among the components of the terminal web network are **fodrin** (the nonerythroid homologue of spectrin) and myosin. It remains unclear whether the myosin in the terminal web is present simply to interconnect the actin filaments of neighboring microvilli or if this actin-myosin complex is capable of generating contractile movements.

Actin and myosin filaments also form an **adhesion belt** that encircles the cytoplasmic surface of the epithelial plasma membrane at the level of the **tight junctions** that interconnect neighboring cells. These adhesion belts are apparently capable of contraction and thus cause epithelial cells that normally form a continuous sheet to pull away from one another, temporarily loosening tight junctions and creating direct passages that connect the luminal space to the extracellular fluid compartment.

Actin and myosin also participate in processes common to most if not all cell types. The process of cytokinesis, in which the cytoplasm of a dividing cell physically separates into two daughter cells, is driven by actin and myosin filaments. Beneath the cleavage furrow that forms in the membrane of the dividing cell is a contractile ring of actin and myosin filaments. Contraction of this ring deepens the cleavage furrow; this invagination ultimately severs the cell and produces the two progeny.

SYNTHESIS AND RECYCLING OF MEMBRANE PROTEINS

Secretory and membrane proteins are synthesized in association with the rough endoplasmic reticulum

Transmembrane proteins are composed of hydrophobic domains that are embedded within the phospholipid bilayer and hydrophilic domains that are exposed at the intracellular and extracellular surfaces. These proteins do not "flip" through the membrane. How, then, do intrinsic membrane proteins overcome the enormous energetic barriers that should logically prevent them from getting inserted into the membrane in the first place?

The cell has developed several schemes to address this problem. Mammalian cells have at least three different membrane insertion pathways, each associated with specific organelles. The first two are mechanisms for inserting membrane proteins into peroxisomes and mitochondria. The third mechanism inserts membrane proteins destined for delivery to the plasma membrane and to the membranes of organelles (the endomembranous system) other than the peroxisome and mitochondrion. This same mechanism is involved in the biogenesis of essentially all proteins that mammalian cells secrete and is the focus of the following discussion.

The critical work in this field centered on studies of the rough ER. The membrane of the **rough ER** is notable for the presence of numerous ribosomes that are bound to its cytosol-facing surface. Whereas all nucleated mammalian cells have at least some rough ER, cells that produce large quantities of secretory proteins—such as the exocrine cells of the pancreas, which function as factories for digestive enzymes (see Chapter 43)—are endowed with an abundance of rough ER. Roughly half of the cytoplasmic space in an exocrine pancreatic acinar cell is occupied by rough ER.

In early experiments exploring cell fractionation techniques, membranes that were derived from the rough ER were separated from the other membranous and cytoplasmic components of pancreatic acinar cells. The mRNAs associated with rough ER membranes were isolated and the proteins they encoded were synthesized by in vitro translation. Analysis of the resultant polypeptides revealed that they included the cell's entire repertoire of *secretory* proteins. It is now appreciated that the mRNA associated with the ER also encodes the cell's entire repertoire of *membrane* proteins, with the exception of those destined for either the peroxisome or the mitochondrion. When the same experiment was performed with mRNAs isolated from ribosomes that are freely distributed throughout the cytoplasm, the products were not *secretory* proteins but rather the soluble *cytosolic* proteins. Later work showed that the ribosomes bound to the ER are biochemically identical to and in equilibrium with those that are free in the cytosol. Therefore, a ribosome's subcellular localization—that is, whether it is free in the cytosol or bound to the rough ER—is somehow dictated by the mRNA that the ribosome is currently translating. A ribosome that is involved in assembling a secretory or membrane protein will associate with the membrane of the rough ER, whereas the same ribosome will be free in the cytosol when it is producing cytosolic proteins. Clearly, some **localization signal** that resides in the mRNA or in the protein that is being synthesized must tell the ribosome what kind of protein is being produced and where in the cell that production should occur.

The nature of this signal was discovered in 1972 during studies of the biosynthesis of immunoglobulin light chains. Light chains synthesized in vitro, in the absence of rough ER membranes, have a 15–amino acid extension at their amino terminus that is absent from the same light chains synthesized and secreted in vivo by B lymphocytes. Similar **amino-terminal extensions** are present on most secretory or membrane proteins but never with the soluble proteins of the cytosol. Although they vary in length and composition, these extensions are present on most acids that are interspersed with occasional basic residues. These **signal sequences**, as they have come to be known, serve as the localization devices discussed earlier. As it emerges from a ribosome and is freely floating in the cytosol, the signal sequence of a nascent protein (Fig. 2-15, stage 1) targets the ribosome-mRNA complex to the surface of the rough ER where the protein's biogenesis will be completed. Ribosome-mRNA complexes that lack a signal sequence complete the translation of the mRNA—which encodes neither secretory nor membrane proteins—without attaching to the rough ER. For his work on signal sequences, Günter Blobel received the 1999 Nobel Prize for Physiology or Medicine.

Why does the cell bother to segregate the synthesis of different protein populations to different cellular locales? Proteins that are destined either to reside in a membrane or to be secreted are inserted into or across the membrane of the rough ER at the same time that they are translated; this is called **cotranslational translocation**. As the nascent polypeptide chain emerges from the ribosome, it traverses the rough ER membrane and ultimately appears at the ER's luminal face. There, an enzyme cleaves the amino-terminal signal sequence while the protein is still being translocated. This is why proteins that are synthesized in vitro in the absence of membranes are longer than the same proteins that are produced by intact cells.

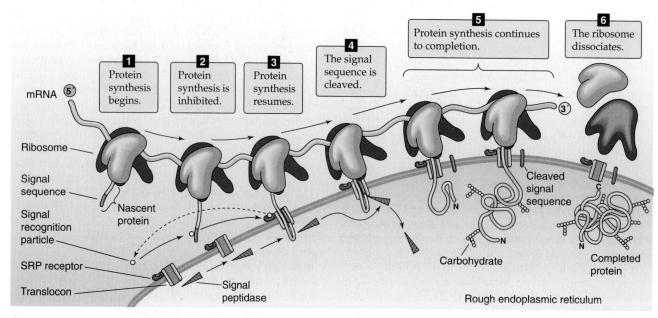

Figure 2-15 Synthesis and translocation of a secretory protein.

Simultaneous protein synthesis and translocation through the rough endoplasmic reticulum membrane requires signal recognition and protein translocation machinery

The information embodied within a signal sequence explains how a nascent protein can direct a cell to complete that protein's translation at the time of translocation in the rough ER. However, the signal sequence by itself is not sufficient. Two critical pieces of targeting machinery are also necessary to direct the ribosome and its attached nascent peptide to the ER. The first is a ribonucleoprotein complex called the **signal recognition particle (SRP)**, which binds to the signal sequence on the nascent peptide (Fig. 2-15, stage 2). The SRP is composed of seven distinct polypeptides and a short strand of RNA. When the SRP binds to a nascent chain, it also binds a GTP molecule. The second vital piece of targeting machinery is a transmembrane component of the rough ER, the **SRP receptor**, also called the **docking protein**. Interaction between a signal sequence and the SRP, and subsequently between the SRP–nascent peptide–ribosome complex and the docking protein, directs the nascent chain to the rough ER's translocation apparatus.

Because the membrane of the rough ER has a finite number of docking sites, the cell must coordinate the synthesis of secretory and membrane proteins with the availability of docking sites. If all docking sites were occupied, and if the synthesis of nascent secretory and membrane proteins were allowed to continue unabated, these nascent peptides would be synthesized entirely in the cytoplasm on free ribosomes. As a consequence, these newly synthesized proteins would never arrive at their proper destination. The SRP serves as a regulatory system that matches the rate of secretory and membrane protein syntheses to the number of unoccupied translocation sites. By associating with a nascent

signal sequence, the SRP causes the ribosome to halt further protein synthesis (Fig. 2-15, stage 2). This state of **translation arrest** persists until the SRP–nascent peptide–ribosome complex finds an unoccupied docking protein with which to interact. Thus, SRP prevents secretory and membrane proteins from being translated until their cotranslational translocation can be ensured. Because SRP interacts only with nascent chains that bear signal sequences, ribosomes that synthesize proteins destined for release into the cytosol never associate with SRP, and their translation is never arrested. Thus, SRP serves as a highly specific spatial and temporal sorting machine, guaranteeing the accurate and efficient targeting of secretory and membrane proteins.

How does the cell terminate the translation arrest of the SRP–nascent peptide–ribosome complex? When this complex interacts with a docking protein (Fig. 2-15, stage 3), one of the SRP's subunits hydrolyzes the previously bound GTP, thereby releasing the SRP from a successfully targeted nascent peptide–ribosome complex. In this way, the docking protein informs the SRP that its mission has been accomplished and it can return to the cytosol to find another ribosome with a signal peptide. A second GTP hydrolysis step transfers the nascent peptide from the docking protein to the actual translocation tunnel complex. GTP hydrolysis is a common event and is involved in the transmission of numerous cellular messages (see Chapter 3). In this case, the two separate instances of GTP hydrolysis serve a quality-control function because the activation of the GTPase activity depends on the delivery of the nascent peptide to the appropriate component in the translocation apparatus.

Adjacent to the docking protein in the membrane of the rough ER is a protein translocator termed a **translocon** (Fig. 2-15, stage 3), which contains a tunnel through which the nascent protein will pass across the rough ER membrane. It appears that delivery of a nascent chain to the translocon causes the entrance of the translocator's tunnel, which is normally closed, to open. This opening of the translocon also allows the flow of small ions. The electrical current carried by these ions can be measured by the patch-clamp technique (see Chapter 6). By "gating" the translocon so that it opens only when it is occupied by a nascent protein, the cell keeps the tunnel's entrance closed when it is not in use. This gating prevents the Ca^{2+} stored in the ER from leaking into the cytoplasm.

Because the tunnel of the translocon is an aqueous pore, the nascent secretory or membrane protein does not come into contact with the hydrophobic core of the ER membrane's lipid bilayer during cotranslational translocation. Thus, this tunnel allows hydrophilic proteins to cross the membrane. As translation and translocation continue and the nascent protein enters the lumen of the rough ER, an enzyme called **signal peptidase** cleaves the signal peptide, which remains in the membrane of the rough ER (Fig. 2-15, stage 4). Meanwhile, translation and translocation of the protein continue (Fig. 2-15, stage 5). In the case of **secretory proteins** (i.e., *not* membrane proteins), the peptide translocates completely through the membrane. The ribosome releases the complete protein into the lumen of the rough ER and then dissociates from the rough ER (Fig. 2-15, stage 6).

Proper insertion of membrane proteins requires start-transfer and stop-transfer sequences

Unlike soluble proteins, nascent *membrane proteins* do not translocate completely through the membrane of the rough ER (Fig. 2-16A, stage 1). The current concept is that the hydrophobic amino acid residues that will ultimately become the transmembrane segment of a membrane protein also function as a **stop-transfer sequence** (Fig. 2-16A, stage 2). When a stop-transfer sequence emerges from a ribosome, it causes the translocon to disassemble, releasing the hydrophobic membrane-spanning segment into the hospitable environment of the rough ER membrane's hydrophobic core (Fig. 2-16A, stage 3). In the meantime, the ribosomal machinery continues to translate the rest of the nascent protein. If the signal peptidase cleaves the amino terminus at this time, the end result is a protein with a *single transmembrane segment*, with the amino terminus in the lumen of the rough ER and the carboxyl terminus in the cytoplasm (Fig. 2-16A, stage 4).

There is another way of generating a protein with a single transmembrane segment. In this case, the protein lacks a signal sequence at the N terminus but instead has—somewhere in the middle of the nascent peptide—a bifunctional sequence that serves both as a signal sequence that binds SRP and as a hydrophobic membrane-spanning segment. This special sequence is called an **internal start-transfer sequence**. The SRP binds to the internal start-transfer sequence and brings the nascent protein to the rough ER, where the internal start-transfer sequence binds to the translocon in such a way that the more positively charged residues that flank the start-transfer sequence face the cytosol. Because these positively charged flanking residues can either precede or follow the hydrophobic residues of the internal start-transfer sequence, either the carboxyl (C) terminus or the N termi-

nus can end up in the cytosol. If the more positively charged flanking residues are at the *carboxyl*-terminal end of the internal start-transfer sequence (Fig. 2-16B), the protein will be oriented with its *carboxyl* terminus in the cytosol. If the more positively charged flanking residues are at the *amino*-terminal end of the internal start-transfer sequence (Fig. 2-16C), the protein will be oriented with its *amino* terminus in the cytosol.

By alternating both *stop-transfer* sequences (Fig. 2-16A) and *internal start-transfer* sequences (Fig. 2-16B, C), the cell can fabricate membrane proteins that span the membrane more than once. Figure 2-16 shows how the cell could synthesize a multispanning protein with its N terminus in the cytosol. The process starts just as in Figure 2-16C, as the translation machinery binds to the rough ER (Fig. 2-16D, stage 1) and the protein's first internal start-transfer sequence inserts into the translocon (Fig. 2-16D, stage 2). However, when the first stop-transfer sequence reaches the translocon (Fig. 2-16D, stage 3), the translocon disassembles, releasing the protein's first two membrane-spanning segments into the membrane of the rough ER. Note that the first membrane-spanning segment is the internal start-transfer sequence and the second is the stop-transfer sequence. In the meantime, an SRP binds to the second internal start-transfer sequence (Fig. 2-16D, stage 4) and directs it to the rough ER (Fig. 2-16D, stage 5) so that cotranslational translocation can once again continue (Fig. 2-16D, stage 6). If there are no further stop-transfer sequences, we will end up with a protein with three membrane-spanning segments.

Several points from the preceding discussion deserve special emphasis. First, translocation through the ER membrane can occur only cotranslationally. If a secretory or membrane protein were synthesized completely on a cytoplasmic ribosome, it would be unable to interact with the translocation machinery and consequently would not be inserted across or into the bilayer. As discussed later, this is not true for the insertion of either peroxisomal or mitochondrial proteins. Second, once a signal sequence emerges from a ribosome, there is only a brief period during which it is competent to mediate the ribosome's association with the ER and to initiate translocation. This time constraint is presumably due to the tendency of nascent polypeptide chains to begin to fold and acquire tertiary structure very soon after exiting the ribosome. This folding quickly buries hydrophobic residues of a signal sequence so that they cannot be recognized by the translocation machinery. Third, because the translocation channel appears to be fairly narrow, the nascent protein cannot begin to acquire tertiary structure until after it has exited at the ER's luminal face. Thus, the peptide must enter the translocation tunnel as a thin thread immediately after emerging from the ribosome. These facts explain why translocation is cotranslational. In systems in which posttranslational translocation occurs (e.g., peroxisomes and mitochondria), special adaptations keep the newly synthesized protein in an unfolded state until its translocation can be consummated.

Finally, because the protein cannot flip once it is in the membrane, the scheme just outlined results in proteins that are inserted into the rough ER membrane in their final or "mature" topology. The number and location of a membrane protein's transmembrane segments, as well as its cytoplasmic

A SINGLE MEMBRANE-SPANNING SEGMENT, CYTOPLASMIC C TERMINUS

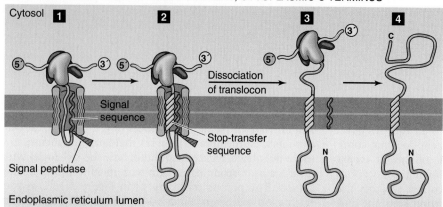

B SINGLE MEMBRANE-SPANNING SEGMENT, CYTOPLASMIC C TERMINUS (ALTERNATE MECHANISM)

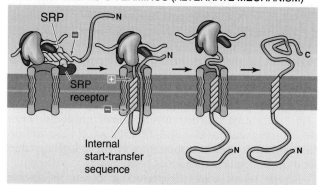

C SINGLE MEMBRANE-SPANNING SEGMENT, CYTOPLASMIC N TERMINUS

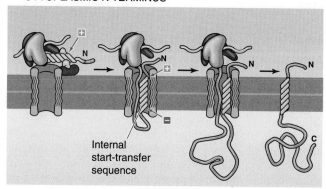

D MULTIPLE MEMBRANE-SPANNING SEGMENTS

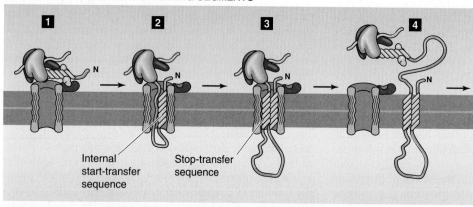

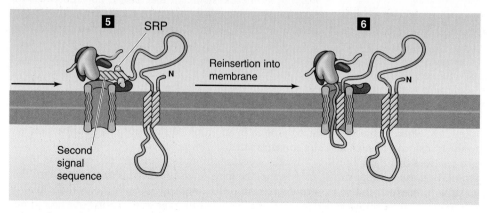

Figure 2-16 Synthesis of integral membrane proteins. **A,** Like a secreted protein, the membrane protein can have a cleavable signal sequence. In addition, it has a stop-transfer sequence that remains in the membrane as a membrane-spanning segment. **B,** The emerging protein lacks a signal sequence but instead has an *internal start-transfer sequence,* which is a bifunctional sequence that serves both as a signal sequence that binds signal recognition particles and as a hydrophobic membrane-spanning segment. In this example, the positively charged region flanking the internal start-transfer sequence is on the *carboxyl*-terminal end of the internal start-transfer sequence. Therefore, the C-terminal end is in the cytoplasm. **C,** The example is similar to that in **B** except that the positively charged region flanking the internal start-transfer sequence is on the *amino*-terminal end of the internal start-transfer sequence. **D,** The emerging peptide has alternating internal start-transfer and stop-transfer sequences.

and extracytoplasmic loops, are entirely determined during the course of its cotranslational insertion into the ER membrane. The order in which signal, internal start-transfer, and stop-transfer sequences appear in a membrane protein's primary structure completely determines how that protein will be arrayed across whatever membrane it ultimately comes to occupy.

Newly synthesized secretory and membrane proteins undergo post-translational modification and folding in the lumen of the rough endoplasmic reticulum

As a newly synthesized secretory or membrane protein exits the tunnel of the translocon and enters the lumen of the rough ER, it may undergo a series of **post-translational modifications** that will help it to acquire its mature conformation. The first alteration, as discussed earlier, is cleavage of the signal sequence (if present) and is accomplished very soon after the signal sequence has completed its translocation. Other covalent modifications that occur as translocation continues include glycosylation and formation of intramolecular disulfide bonds. **Glycosylation** refers here to the enzymatic, en bloc coupling of preassembled, branched oligosaccharide chains that contain 14 sugar molecules (Fig. 2-17A) to asparagine (Asn) residues that appear in the sequence Asn-X-Ser or Asn-X-Thr (X can be any amino acid

except proline). These **N-linked sugars** (N is the single-letter amino acid code for asparagine) will go on to be extensively modified as the protein passes through other organellar compartments. The addition of sugar groups to proteins can serve numerous functions, which include increasing the protein's stability and endowing it with specific antigenic, adhesive, or receptor properties.

Disulfide bond formation is catalyzed by **protein disulfide isomerase**, an enzyme that is retained in the ER lumen through noncovalent interactions with ER membrane proteins. Because the cytoplasm is a reducing environment, disulfide bonds can form only between proteins or protein domains that have been removed from the cytosolic compartment through translocation to the ER's interior. Other, more specialized modifications also take place in the lumen of the rough ER. For example, the ER contains the enzymes responsible for the **hydroxylation** of the proline residues that are present in newly synthesized collagen chains.

The ER also catalyzes the formation of **GPI linkages** to membrane proteins (Fig. 2-17B). GPI-linked proteins are synthesized as transmembrane polypeptides, with a typical membrane-spanning region. Shortly after their translation, however, their lumen-facing domains are cleaved from the membrane-spanning segments and covalently transferred to the GPI phospholipid. They retain this structure and orientation throughout the remainder of their journey to the cell surface. A defect in the synthesis of GPI-linked proteins

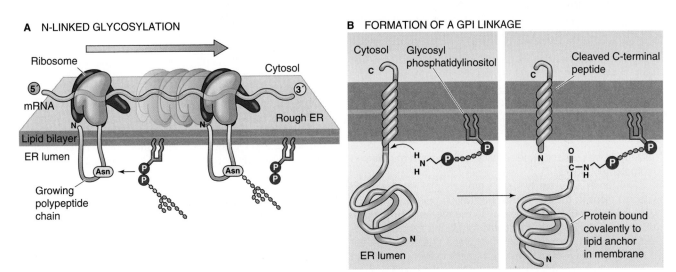

Figure 2-17 Post-translational modifications of integral membrane proteins. **A,** An enzyme in the ER lumen attaches a preassembled, branched, oligosaccharide chain to an asparagine (Asn or N) residue on the nascent protein. **B,** An enzyme in the ER lumen cleaves the protein and couples the protein's new terminal carboxyl group to the terminal amino group on the GPI molecule.

underlies the human disease paroxysmal nocturnal hematuria (see the box on this topic).

Perhaps the most important maturational process for a nascent chain emerging into the ER lumen is the acquisition of **tertiary structure**. The folding of a secretory or membrane protein is determined during and immediately after its cotranslational translocation. The progress of protein folding influences—and is influenced by—the addition of sugar residues and the formation of disulfide bridges. Proteins fold into conformations that minimize their overall free energies. Their extramembranous surfaces are composed of hydrophilic residues that interact easily with the aqueous solvent. Hydrophobic residues are hidden in internal globular domains where they can be effectively isolated from contact with water or charged molecules. Left to its own devices, a linear strand of denatured protein will spontaneously fold to form a structure that reflects these thermodynamic considerations. Thus, protein folding requires no catalysis and can occur without help from any cellular machinery. However, the cell is not content to allow protein folding to follow a random course and instead orchestrates the process through the actions of molecular chaperones.

The **chaperones** constitute a large class of ATP-hydrolyzing proteins that appear to participate in a wide variety of polypeptide-folding phenomena, including the initial folding of newly synthesized proteins as well as the refolding of proteins whose tertiary structures have been damaged by exposure to high temperature (i.e., heat shock) or other denaturing conditions. Chaperones bind to unfolded protein chains and stabilize them in an unfolded conformation, thus preventing them from spontaneously folding into what might be an energetically favorable but biologically useless arrangement. Using energy that is provided through ATP hydrolysis, the chaperones sequentially release domains of unfolded proteins and thus allow them to fold in an ordered fashion. Distinct subclasses of chaperones are present in several cell compartments, including the cytoplasm, the mitochondrion, and the lumen of the rough ER. Newly synthesized secretory and membrane proteins appear to interact with ER chaperones as they exit from the tunnel of the translocon and subsequently disengage from the chaperones to assume their mature tertiary structure.

The acquisition of tertiary structure is followed quickly by the acquisition of **quaternary structure**. As noted earlier

Paroxysmal Nocturnal Hematuria

The list of proteins embedded in the plasma membrane through a GPI linkage is remarkably long and ever-growing. In red blood cells, the inventory of GPI-linked proteins includes a pair of polypeptides, decay-accelerating factor (DAF) and CD59, which help protect the erythrocytes from being accidentally injured by constituents of the immune system. One of the mechanisms that the immune system uses to rid the body of invading bacteria involves the activation of the **complement cascade**. Complement is a complex collection of proteins that circulate in the blood plasma. The complement system recognizes antibodies that are bound to the surface of a bacterium or polysaccharides in the bacterial membrane. This recognition initiates a cascade of enzymatic cleavages that results in the assembly of a subset of complement proteins to form the membrane attack complex, which inserts itself into the membrane of the target organism and forms a large pore that allows water to rush in (see Chapter 5). The target bacterium swells and undergoes osmotic lysis. Unfortunately, the complement system's lethal efficiency is not matched by its capacity to discriminate between genuine targets and normal host cells. Consequently, almost every cell type in the body is equipped with surface proteins that guard against a misdirected complement attack.

DAF and CD59 are two such proteins that interfere with distinct steps in the complement activation pathway. Because GPI linkages couple both proteins to the membrane, any dysfunction of the enzymes that participate in the transfer of GPI-linked proteins from their transmembrane precursors to their GPI tails in the ER would interfere with the delivery of DAF and CD59 to their sites of functional residence at the cell surface. One of the proteins that participates in the synthesis of the GPI anchor is a sugar transferase encoded by the phosphatidylinositol glycan class A (PIG-A) gene. This gene is located on the X chromosome. Because every cell has only one working copy of the X chromosome (although female cells are genetically XX, one of the two X chromosomes is inactivated in every cell), if a spontaneous mutation occurs in the PIG-A gene in a particular cell, that cell and all of its progeny will lose the ability to synthesize GPI-linked proteins.

In **paroxysmal nocturnal hemoglobinuria** (i.e., hemoglobin appearing in the urine at night, with a sharp onset), a spontaneous mutation occurs in the PIG-A gene in just one of the many precursor cells that give rise to erythrocytes. All of the erythrocytes that arise from this particular precursor, therefore, are deficient in GPI-linked protein synthesis. Consequently, these cells lack DAF and CD59 expression and are susceptible to complement attack and lysis. For reasons that are largely unknown, the complement system is somewhat more active during sleep, so the hemolysis (lysis of erythrocytes) occurs more frequently at night in these patients. Some of the hemoglobin released by this lysis is excreted in the urine.

Because the PIG-A gene product is required for the synthesis of *all* GPI-linked proteins, the plasma membranes of affected red blood cells in patients with paroxysmal nocturnal hemoglobinuria are missing a number of different proteins that are found in the surface membranes of their normal counterparts. It is the lack of DAF and CD59, however, that renders the cells vulnerable to complement-mediated killing and that creates the symptoms of the disease. Paroxysmal nocturnal hemoglobinuria is an uncommon disease. Because it is the result of an acquired mutation, it is much more likely to occur in people of middle age rather than in children. Patients with paroxysmal nocturnal hemoglobinuria are likely to become anemic and can suffer life-threatening disorders of clotting and bone marrow function. It is a chronic condition, however, and more than half of patients survive at least 15 years after diagnosis.

in this chapter, many membrane proteins assemble into oligomeric complexes in which several identical or distinct polypeptides interact with one another to form a macromolecular structure. Assembly of these multimers occurs in the ER. It is unknown whether the oligomeric assembly process occurs entirely spontaneously or if, like folding, it is orchestrated by specialized cellular mechanisms. Cells clearly go to great trouble to ensure that proteins inserted into or across their ER membranes are appropriately folded and oligomerized before allowing them to continue with their postsynthetic processing. As discussed later, proteins destined for secretion from the cell or for residence in the cell membrane or other organellar membranes depart the ER for further processing in the membranous stacks of the **Golgi complex.** This departure is entirely contingent on successful completion of the protein folding and assembly operations.

Misfolded or unassembled proteins are retained in the ER and ultimately degraded. The ER chaperone proteins play a critical role both in identifying proteins with incorrect tertiary or quaternary structures and in actively preventing their egress to the Golgi complex. Proteins that have not folded or assembled correctly are destroyed through a process known as **ERAD** (endoplasmic reticulum–associated degradation). The sequential, covalent addition of **ubiquitin** monomers results in the formation of a branched-chain ubiquitin polymer that marks these proteins for destruction. Ubiquitin is a small protein of 76 amino acid residues. The process known as **retrotranslocation** removes ubiquitin-tagged proteins from the ER membrane, and a large cytoplasmic complex of proteolytic enzymes—the **proteosome**—degrades the ubiquitinated proteins.

Secretory and membrane proteins follow the secretory pathway through the cell

The rough ER is the common point of origin for the cell's secretory and membrane proteins. Most of these proteins are not retained in the rough ER but depart for distribution to their sites of ultimate functional residence throughout the cell. As is true for their arrival in the rough ER, the departure of these proteins is a highly organized and regimented affair. In fact, the rough ER is the first station along the **secretory pathway,** which is the route followed (at least in part) by all secretory and membrane proteins as they undergo their post-translational modifications (Fig. 2-18).

The elucidation of the secretory pathway occurred in the 1960s, mainly in the laboratory of George Palade. For his contribution, Palade was awarded the 1975 Nobel Prize in Physiology or Medicine. This work also exploited the unique properties of pancreatic acinar cells to illuminate the central themes of secretory protein biogenesis. Because ~95% of the protein that is synthesized by pancreatic acinar cells are digestive enzymes destined for secretion (see Chapter 43), when these cells are fed radioactively labeled amino acids, the majority of these tracer molecules are incorporated into secretory polypeptides. Within a few minutes after the tracer is added, most of the label is associated with a specialized subregion of the rough ER. Known as **transitional zones,** these membranous saccules are ribosome studded on one surface and smooth at the opposite face (Fig. 2-18). The smooth side is directly apposed to one pole of the pancake-like membrane stacks (or cisternae) of the **Golgi complex.** Smooth-surfaced carrier vesicles crowd the narrow moat of cytoplasm that separates the transitional zone from the Golgi. These vesicles "pinch off" from the transitional zone and fuse with a Golgi stack. From this first or *cis*-Golgi stack, **carrier vesicles** ferry the newly synthesized proteins sequentially and vectorially through each Golgi stack, ultimately delivering them to the *trans*-most saccule of the Golgi. Finally, the newly synthesized secretory proteins appear in **secretory vesicles** (also called secretory granules in many tissues).

The journey from the rough ER to the secretory vesicle takes ~45 minutes in pancreatic acinar cells and requires the

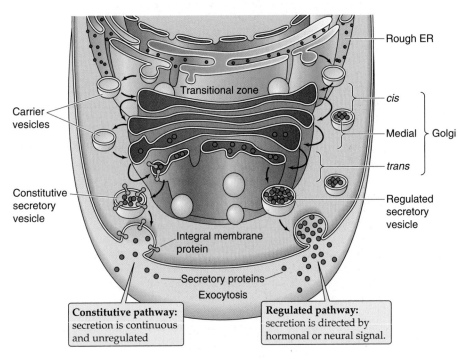

Figure 2-18 The secretory pathway. After their synthesis in the rough ER, secretory and membrane proteins destined for the plasma membrane move through the Golgi stacks and secretory vesicles. In the constitutive pathway, vesicles fuse spontaneously with the plasma membrane. In the regulated pathway, the vesicles fuse only when triggered by a signal such as a hormone.

Rough ER

Transitional zone

Carrier vesicles

cis

Medial } Golgi

trans

Constitutive secretory vesicle

Regulated secretory vesicle

Integral membrane protein

Secretory proteins

Exocytosis

Constitutive pathway: secretion is continuous and unregulated

Regulated pathway: secretion is directed by hormonal or neural signal.

expenditure of metabolic energy. Each nucleated eukaryotic cell possesses a secretory pathway that shares this same general outline, although the specific features reflect the cell's particular function. The secretory pathway of the pancreatic acinar cell, for example, is specially adapted to accommodate the controlled secretion of protein by the so-called **regulated pathway**. Instead of being released from the cell continuously as they are produced, newly synthesized secretory proteins are held in *specialized secretory vesicles* that serve as an intracellular storage depot. This type of storage occurs in several cells, including those of endocrine and exocrine secretory tissues, and neurons. When the cells receive the requisite message, the storage vesicles fuse with the plasma membrane, sometimes at a specialized structure called a porosome, in a process known as **exocytosis**. The vesicles then dump their contents into the extracellular space. In the case of the pancreatic acinar cells, the enzymes are secreted into the pancreatic ductules and then make their way to the site of digestion in the duodenum (see Chapter 43).

Most cell types, however, deliver newly synthesized secretory and membrane proteins to the cell surface in a *continuous* and *unregulated* fashion, which is referred to as the **constitutive pathway**. Specialized cells that have the capacity for regulated delivery also send an important subset of their secretory and membrane protein synthetic products to the cell surface constitutively. The regulated and constitutive secretory pathways are identical except for the final station of the Golgi complex. At this point, the "regulated" proteins divert to the specialized secretory vesicles described in the previous paragraph. The "constitutive" proteins, at the *trans*-most cisterna of the Golgi complex, sort into other secretory vesicles, which move directly to the cell surface. There, the constitutive *membrane proteins* are delivered to the plasma membrane, and the constitutive *secretory proteins* are immediately exocytosed.

This section has provided a broad overview of the secretory pathway. In the following sections, we examine the details of how newly synthesized proteins move between organellar compartments of the secretory pathway, how the proteins are processed during this transit, and how they are sorted to their final destination.

Carrier vesicles control the traffic between the organelles of the secretory pathway

As the preceding discussion suggests, the secretory pathway is not a single, smooth, continuous highway but rather a series of saltatory translocations from one discrete organellar compartment to the next. Each of these steps requires some orchestration to ensure that the newly synthesized proteins arrive at their next terminus.

The cell solves the problem of moving newly synthesized proteins between membranous organelles by using membrane-enclosed carrier vesicles (or vesicular carriers). Each time proteins are to be moved from one compartment to the next, they are gathered together within or beneath specialized regions of membrane that subsequently evaginate or pinch off to produce a carrier vesicle (Fig. 2-18). Secretory proteins reside within the lumen of the carrier vesicle, whereas membrane proteins span the vesicle's own encapsulating bilayer. On arrival at the appropriate destination, the

carrier vesicle fuses with the membrane of the acceptor organelle, thus delivering its contents of *soluble* proteins to the organelle's lumen and its cargo of *membrane* proteins to the organelle's own membrane. Carrier vesicles mediate the transport of secretory and membrane proteins across the space between the ER's transition zone and the *cis*-Golgi stack and also between the rims of the Golgi stacks themselves. The movement between one vesicular compartment and the next is mediated by the cytoskeleton and molecular motors that were discussed earlier.

A few critical facts deserve emphasis. First, throughout the formation, transit, and fusion of a carrier vesicle, no mixing occurs between the vesicle lumen and cytosol. The same principle applies to the carrier vesicle's membrane protein passengers, which were inserted into the membrane of the rough ER with a particular topology. Those domains of a membrane protein that are exposed to the cytosol in the rough ER remain exposed to the cytosol as the protein completes its journey through the secretory pathway.

Second, the flow of vesicular membranes is not unidirectional. The rate of synthesis of new membrane lipid and protein in the ER is less than the rate at which carrier vesicles bud off of the ER that is bound for the Golgi. Because the sizes of the ER and Golgi are relatively constant, the membrane that moves to the Golgi by carrier vesicles must return to the ER. This return is again accomplished by vesicular carriers. Each discrete step of the secretory pathway must maintain vesicle-mediated backflow of membrane from the acceptor to the donor compartment so that each compartment can retain a constant size.

Finally, we have already noted that each organelle along the secretory pathway is endowed with a specific set of "resident" membrane proteins that determines the properties of the organelle. Despite the rapid forward and backward flow of carrier vesicles between successive stations of the secretory pathway, the resident membrane proteins do not get swept along in the flow. They are either actively retained in their home organelles' membranes or actively retrieved by the returning "retrograde" carrier vesicles. Thus, not only the size but also the composition of each organelle of the secretory pathway remains essentially constant despite the rapid flux of newly synthesized proteins that it constantly handles.

Specialized protein complexes, such as clathrin and coatamers, mediate the formation and fusion of vesicles in the secretory pathway

The formation of a vesicle through evagination appears to be geometrically indistinguishable from its fusion with a target membrane. In both cases, a cross-sectional view in the electron microscope reveals an "omega" profile, which is so named because the vesicle maintains a narrow opening to the organellar lumen that resembles the shape of the Greek letter omega (Ω). However, different problems are confronted during the formation and fusion of membrane vesicles.

Vesicle Formation in the Secretory Pathway To form a spherical vesicle from a planar membrane, the mechanism that pulls the vesicle off from the larger membrane must grab onto the membrane over the entire surface of the nascent vesicle. The mechanism that achieves this makes use of a scaffolding that is composed of coat proteins. The cell has at least two and probably more varieties of coat proteins. The best characterized of these is clathrin, which mediates the formation of secretory vesicles from the *trans* Golgi. Clathrin also mediates the internalization of membrane from the cell surface during the process of endocytosis, which is the reverse of exocytosis. Another major protein coat, which is involved in nonselective trafficking of vesicles between the ER and Golgi and between the stacks of the Golgi, is a protein complex known as *coatamer*. Both clathrin and coatamer proteins form the borders of a cage-like lattice.

In the case of **clathrin**, the coat proteins preassemble in the cytoplasm to form three-armed "triskelions" (Fig. 2-19A). A triskelion is not planar but resembles the three adjoining edges of a tetrahedron. As triskelions attach to one another, they produce a three-dimensional structure resembling a geodesic dome with a roughly spherical shape. A triskelion constitutes each vertex in the lattice of hexagons and pentagons that form the cage.

The triskelions of clathrin attach indirectly to the surface of the membrane that is to be excised by binding to the cytosolic tails of membrane proteins. Mediating this binding are adapter proteins, called adaptins, that link the membrane protein tails to the triskelion scaffold. The specificity for particular membrane proteins is apparently conferred by specialized adaptins. Triskelions assemble spontaneously to form a complete cage that attaches to the underlying membrane and pulls it up into a spherical configuration. Completion of the cage occurs simultaneously with the pinching off of the evaginated membrane from the planar surface, forming a closed sphere.

The pinching off, or fission, process appears to involve the action of a GTP-binding protein called dynamin, which forms a collar around the neck of the forming vesicle and may sever it. The fission process must include an intermediate that resembles the structure depicted in Figure 2-19A. According to the prevalent view, each of the lumen-facing leaflets of membrane lipids fuse, leaving only the cytoplasmic leaflets to form a continuous bridge from the vesicle to the donor membrane. This bridge then breaks, and fission is complete.

Once formed, the clathrin-coated vesicle cannot fuse with its target membrane until it loses its cage, which prevents the two membranes from achieving the close contact required

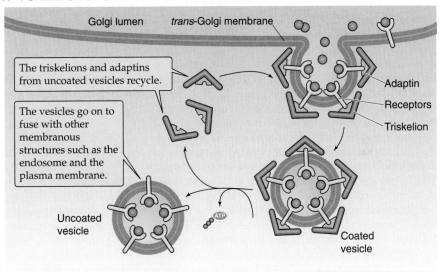

Figure 2-19 Vesicle formation and fusion. **A,** Clathrin mediates the formation of secretory vesicles that bud off from the *trans* Golgi as well as the internalization of membrane from the cell surface during the process of endocytosis. **B,** A complex of proteins forms a bridge between the vesicle and the target membranes. ATP provides the fuel for fusion. The Rab appears to be a molecular switch. NSF, *N*-ethylmaleimide–sensitive factor; SNAP, soluble NSF attachment protein; SNARE, SNAP receptor.

to permit fusion. Because formation of the clathrin cage is spontaneous and energetically favorable, dissolution of the cage requires energy. Uncoating is accomplished by a special class of cytoplasmic enzymes that hydrolyze ATP and use the energy thus liberated to disassemble the scaffold (Fig. 2-19A).

The function of **coatamers** is similar to that of clathrin in that coatamer forms a cage around the budding membrane. However, coatamer coats differ from clathrin in several respects. First, coatamer coats are composed of several coatamer proteins, one of which is related to the adaptins. Second, unlike the spontaneous assembly of the clathrin triskelions, assembly of the coatamer coat around the budding vesicle requires ATP. Third, a coatamer-coated vesicle retains its coat until it docks with its target membrane.

Vesicle Fusion in the Secretory Pathway   Membrane fusion occurs when the hydrophobic cores of two bilayers come into contact with one another, a process that requires the two membranes to be closely apposed. Because the cytoplasmic leaflets of most cellular membranes are predominantly composed of negatively charged phospholipids, electrostatic repulsion prevents this close apposition from occurring spontaneously. To overcome this charge barrier and perhaps to assist in targeting as well, a multicomponent protein complex forms and acts as a bridge, linking vesicular membrane proteins to membrane proteins in the target bilayer (Fig. 2-19B). Investigators have established the components of this complex by use of three approaches: studies of the membrane fusion steps involved in vesicular transport between successive Golgi stacks, genetic analysis of protein secretion in yeast, and molecular dissection of the protein constituents of the synaptic vesicles of nerve terminals. In each case, the same proteins are instrumental in attaching the donor and target membranes to one another.

The central components of the bridge are proteins known as **SNAREs** (so named because they act as receptors for the SNAPs discussed in the next paragraph). There are SNAREs in both the vesicular membrane (v-SNAREs) and the membrane of the target organelle (t-SNAREs). The best studied SNARE family members are those that participate in the fusion of neurotransmitter-containing synaptic vesicles with the plasma membrane of the axons in neurons (see Chapter 8). In that setting, the v-SNARE is known as synaptobrevin, and proteins known as syntaxin and SNAP-25 together act as t-SNAREs. The t-SNAREs and v-SNAREs bind to each other extremely tightly, pulling the vesicular and target membranes close together. This proximity alone may be sufficient to initiate fusion, although this point remains controversial. In cells that employ rapid and tightly regulated membrane fusion, such as neurons, increases in the cytoplasmic concentration of Ca^{2+}, sensed by the SNARE fusion complex, trigger fusion (see Chapter 8). Although the nature of the fusion event itself remains unclear, clues have emerged about its regulation. Fusion requires the participation of a class of small GTP-binding proteins called **Rabs** that are important for signaling. Rabs appear to act as molecular switches that assemble with the SNARE fusion complex when they are binding GTP but dissociate from the complex after they hydrolyze the GTP to GDP. Rab-GTP must associate with the fusion complex for fusion to occur. Numerous Rab isoforms exist, each isoform associated with a different vesicular compartment and a distinct membrane-to-membrane translocation step.

Once fusion occurs, the former vesicle generally loses its spherical shape rapidly as it becomes incorporated into the target membrane. This "flattening out" is the result of surface tension, inasmuch as the narrow radius of curvature demanded by a small spherical vesicle is energetically unfavorable. After fusion, it is also necessary to disassemble the v-SNARE/t-SNARE complex so that its components can be reused in subsequent fusion events. The dissociation step involves the activity of two additional components that participate in the SNARE complex. The first is an ATP-hydrolyzing enzyme; because it is inhibited by the alkylating agent N-ethylmaleimide (NEM), it was named NEM-sensitive factor (NSF). Soluble NSF attachment proteins (the SNAPs mentioned before), which target NSF to the SNARE complex, are the second. Hydrolysis of ATP by NSF causes dissociation of the SNARE complex, thus regenerating the fusion machinery. Homologues of the neuronal t-SNARE and v-SNARE proteins are found in almost every cell type in the body and are thought to participate in most if not all membrane fusion events.

Newly synthesized secretory and membrane proteins are processed during their passage through the secretory pathway

While in the rough ER, newly synthesized secretory and membrane proteins undergo the first in a series of posttranslational modifications. As discussed earlier, this first group includes glycosylation, disulfide bond formation, and the acquisition of tertiary structure. On delivery to the *cis* stack of the Golgi complex, these proteins begin a new phase in their postsynthetic maturation. For many proteins, the most visible byproduct of this second phase is the complete remodeling of their N-linked sugar chains, originally attached in the rough ER.

Of the 14 sugar residues transferred en bloc to newly synthesized proteins during N-linked glycosylation, nine are mannose and three are glucose (Fig. 2-20A). Enzymes called glucosidases and one called a mannosidase are associated with the luminal face of the ER; these enzymes remove the three glucose residues and one mannose. As proteins arrive from the ER, mannosidases in the *cis* Golgi attack the N-linked sugar trees, thereby shearing off all except two N-acetylglucosamine and five mannose residues. As the proteins pass from the *cis*-Golgi cisterna to the medial cisterna and ultimately to the *trans*-Golgi cisterna, another mannosidase removes two additional mannose residues, and other enzymes add sugars to the stump of the original sugar tree in a process referred to as **complex glycosylation**.

The addition of new sugars occurs one residue at a time and is accomplished by enzymes called **sugar transferases** that face the lumens of the Golgi stacks. Each sugar is transported from the cytoplasm to the Golgi lumen by a carrier protein that spans the Golgi membrane. Throughout the maturation process, the N-linked sugar chains are always exposed only to the luminal face of the Golgi.

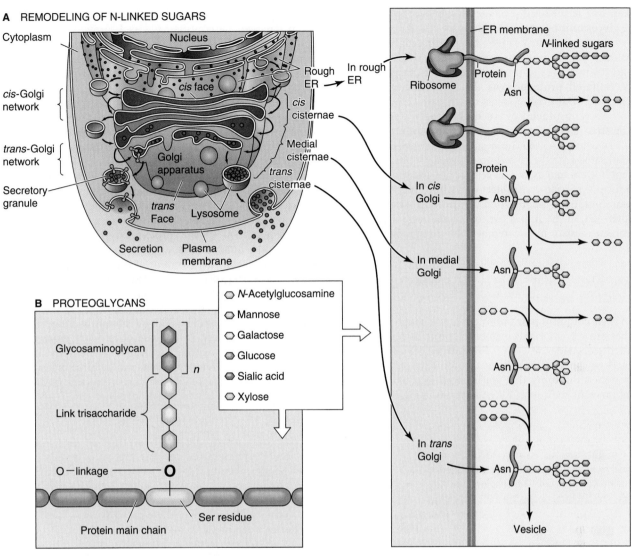

A   REMODELING OF N-LINKED SUGARS

Cytoplasm
Nucleus
cis-Golgi network
cis face
Rough ER
cis cisternae
Medial cisternae
trans-Golgi network
Golgi apparatus
trans cisternae
Secretory granule
trans Face
Lysosome
Secretion
Plasma membrane

In rough ER
ER membrane
N-linked sugars
Ribosome
Protein
Asn

In *cis* Golgi
Protein
Asn

In medial Golgi
Asn

Asn

In *trans* Golgi
Asn

Vesicle

B   PROTEOGLYCANS

Glycosaminoglycan

Link trisaccharide

O—linkage

Protein main chain

Ser residue

n

- N-Acetylglucosamine
- Mannose
- Galactose
- Glucose
- Sialic acid
- Xylose

Figure 2-20   Modification and assembly of the sugar chains on proteins in the Golgi. **A,** Remodeling of N-linked sugars. **B,** Proteoglycans. A trisaccharide links glycosaminoglycan chains to the protein by the -OH group of a serine residue. The glycosaminoglycan is made up of *n* repeating disaccharide units, one of which is always an *amino* sugar.

Each cisterna of the Golgi is characterized by a different set of sugar transferases and sugar transporters. Thus, each Golgi compartment catalyzes a distinct step in the maturation of the N-linked chains. Complex glycosylation, therefore, proceeds like an assembly line from one modification station to the next. Because proteins have different shapes and sizes, however, the degree to which a sugar chain of any given polypeptide has access to each transferase can vary quite extensively. Thus, each protein emerges from the assembly line with its own particular pattern of complex glycosylation. The Golgi's *trans*-most cisterna houses the enzymes responsible for adding the terminal sugars, which cap the N-linked chain. The final residue of these terminal sugars is frequently *N*-acetylneuraminic acid, also known as sialic acid. At neutral pH, sialic acid is negatively charged. This acidic sugar residue therefore is responsible for the net negative electrostatic charge that is frequently carried by **glycoproteins**.

The Golgi's function is not limited to creating N-linked sugar tree topiaries. It oversees a number of other post-translational modifications, including the assembly of O-linked sugars. Many proteins possess **O-linked sugar chains**, which attach not to asparagine residues but to the hydroxyl groups (hence, O) of serine and threonine residues. The O-linked sugars are not preassembled for en bloc transfer the way that the original 14-sugar tree is added in the rough ER in the case of their N-linked counterparts. Instead, the O-linked sugars are added one residue at a time by sugar transferases such as those that participate in the remodeling of complex N-linked glycosylation. O-linked chains frequently carry a great deal of negatively charged sialic acid.

Proteoglycans contain a very large number of a special class of O-linked sugar chains that are extremely long (Fig. 2-20B). Unlike other O-linked sugars that attach to the protein core by an *N*-acetylglucosamine, the sugar chain in a proteoglycan attaches by a xylose-containing three-sugar "linker" to a serine residue on the protein backbone. One or more **glycosaminoglycan** side chains are added to this linker, one sugar at a time, to form the mature proteoglycan.

As the sugar chains grow, enzymes can add sulfate groups and greatly increase the quantity of negative charge that they carry. **Sulfated proteoglycans** that are secreted proteins become important components of the extracellular matrix and are also constituents of mucus. Proteoglycan chains can also be attached to membrane proteins that eventually reach the plasma membrane. The negatively charged sugars that are associated with the glycosaminoglycan groups, which are present both in mucus and on cell surface glycoproteins, can help form a barrier that protects cells from harsh environmental conditions such as those inside the stomach (see Chapter 42). In the upper portion of the respiratory tract, the mucus assists in the removal of foreign bodies (see Chapter 26).

Newly synthesized proteins are sorted in the *trans*-Golgi network

From their common point of origin at the rough ER, newly synthesized secretory and membrane proteins must be distributed to a wide variety of different subcellular destinations. How can a cell recognize an individual protein from among the multitudes that are inserted into or across the membranes of the rough ER and ensure its delivery to the

site of its ultimate functional residence? Such a sorting operation has two prerequisites: (1) each protein to be sorted must carry some manner of address or "sorting signal" that communicates its destination, and (2) the cell must possess machinery capable of reading this sorting signal and acting on the information it embodies.

Little is known about the molecular correlates of sorting signals, and even less is established about the sorting machinery. However, for many proteins, it is clear that sorting occurs in the *trans*-Golgi network (TGN). The *trans*-most cisterna of the Golgi complex is morphologically and biochemically distinct from the other Golgi stacks. Viewed in cross section, it appears as a complex web of membranous tubules and vesicles (Fig. 2-21). This structure befits the TGN's apparent function as a staging area from which carrier vesicles depart to transport their specific protein cargoes to one of many distinct subcellular locales.

Sorting machinery within or at the TGN appears to segregate classes of proteins—each bound for a common destination—into small discrete clusters. Each cluster is subsequently incorporated into a separate carrier vesicle, which evaginates from the TGN membrane and mediates the final stage of delivery. In the case of *secretory proteins*, this clustering happens within the lumen of the TGN. In fact, such clusters of secretory proteins can be directly visualized in the electron microscope. *Membrane proteins* gather into two-dimensional clusters in the plane of the TGN mem-

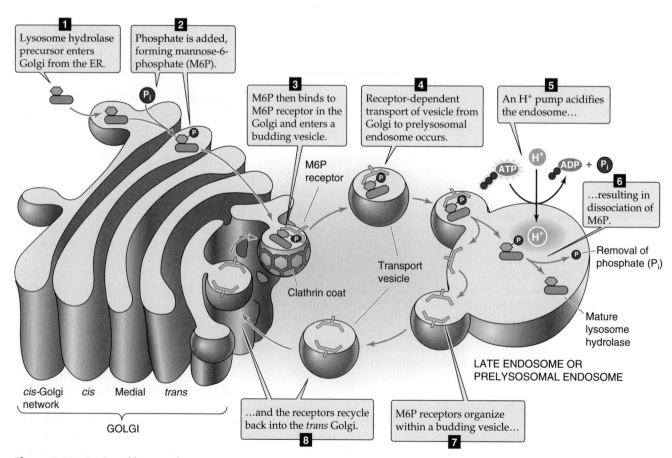

Figure 2-21 Sorting of lysosomal enzymes.

brane. Carrier vesicles incorporate these clusters into their own bilayers. Proteins bound for different destinations co-cluster in different subdomains of the TGN. Secretory and membrane proteins that are earmarked for the same destination can cluster in the same subdomain of the TGN and can be incorporated into the same carrier vesicle. Therefore, the TGN appears to function as a cellular transportation terminal that is able to direct groups of passengers who are carrying the same tickets to a common waiting area and ultimately to load them onto a common shuttle. Ticket agents herd passengers bearing different tickets into different waiting lounges.

A mannose 6-phosphate recognition marker is required to target newly synthesized hydrolytic enzymes to lysosomes

The most thoroughly established sorting paradigm is the pathway for newly synthesized lysosomal enzymes. Like secretory proteins, lysosomal enzymes carry amino-terminal signal sequences that direct their cotranslational translocation across the membrane of the rough ER. Their N-linked glycosylation and folding proceed in the usual fashion, after which they join all of the other simultaneously synthesized proteins in the Golgi complex (Fig. 2-21, stage 1).

A special sugar transferase in the *cis*-Golgi cisterna recognizes newly synthesized lysosomal enzymes and adds a unique sugar. This enzyme adds *N*-acetylglucosamine phosphate to the mannose residues at the termini of the lysosomal enzymes' N-linked sugar trees. This enzyme differs from the usual sugar transferases in that it adds a *phospho*-sugar group to the mannose residue, rather than just a sugar. This enzyme is also unique in recognizing specific amino acid sequences that are exclusively in these lysosomal enzymes. A second *cis*-Golgi enzyme removes the additional *N*-acetylglucosamine sugar, leaving its phosphate group behind. As a result, the sugar trees of the lysosomal enzymes terminate in mannose 6-phosphate residues (Fig. 2-21, stage 2).

A special class of mannose 6-phosphate receptors, localized predominantly in the elements of the *trans* Golgi, recognize proteins that carry mannose 6-phosphate groups (Fig. 2-21, stage 3). This recognition step constitutes the first stage of the cosegregation and clustering process discussed earlier. The mannose 6-phosphate receptors are transmembrane proteins. Their luminal portions bind to the newly synthesized lysosomal enzymes, whereas their cytoplasmically facing tails possess a particular signal that allows them to interact with adaptins and hence to be incorporated into clathrin-coated vesicles. The assembly of the clathrin lattice causes the mannose 6-phosphate receptors to cluster, along with their associated lysosomal enzymes, in the plane of the TGN membrane. Completion of the clathrin cage results in the formation of a vesicle whose membrane contains the mannose 6-phosphate receptors that bind their cargo of lysosomal enzymes.

After departing the TGN, these transport vesicles lose their clathrin coats (Fig. 2-21, stage 4) and fuse with structures referred to as late endosomes or **prelysosomal endosomes**. Proton pumps in the membranes of these organelles ensure that their luminal pH is acidic (Fig. 2-21, stage 5).

When exposed to this acidic environment, the mannose 6-phosphate receptors undergo a conformational change that releases the mannose 6-phosphate–bearing lysosomal enzymes (Fig. 2-21, stage 6). Consequently, the newly synthesized enzymes are dumped into the lumen of the prelysosomal endosome, which will go on to fuse with or mature into a lysosome. The empty mannose 6-phosphate receptors join vesicles that bud off from the lysosome (Fig. 2-21, stage 7) and return to the TGN (Fig. 2-21, stage 8). The luminal environment of the TGN allows the receptors to recover their affinity for mannose 6-phosphate, thus allowing them to participate in subsequent rounds of sorting.

Disruption of lysosomal sorting can be produced in several ways. For example, a drug called **tunicamycin** blocks the addition of N-linked sugars to newly synthesized proteins and thereby prevents attachment of the mannose 6-phosphate recognition marker. Compounds that elevate the luminal pH of the prelysosomal endosomes prevent newly synthesized enzymes from dissociating from the mannose 6-phosphate receptors and consequently block recycling of the receptor pool back to the TGN. The resulting shortage of unoccupied receptors allows mannose 6-phosphate–bearing proteins to pass through the TGN unrecognized (see the box titled Lysosomal Storage Diseases). Thus, instead of diverting to the lysosomes, these lysosomal enzymes continue along the secretory pathway and are ultimately released from the cell by constitutive secretion.

Cells internalize extracellular material through the process of endocytosis

The same fundamental mechanisms in the secretory pathway that produce vesicles by evaginating regions of Golgi membrane can also move material in the opposite direction by inducing vesicle formation through the invagination of regions of the plasma membrane. Vesicles created in this fashion are delimited by membrane that had formerly been part of the cell surface, and their luminal contents derive from the extracellular compartment.

This internalization process, referred to as **endocytosis**, serves the cell in at least four ways. First, certain nutrients are too large to be imported from the extracellular fluid into the cytoplasm by transmembrane carrier proteins; they are instead carried into the cell by endocytosis. Second, endocytosis of hormone-receptor complexes can terminate the signaling processes that are initiated by numerous hormones. Third, endocytosis is the first step in remodeling or degrading of portions of the plasma membrane. Membrane that is delivered to the surface during exocytosis must be retrieved and ultimately returned to the TGN. Fourth, proteins or pathogens that need to be cleared from the extracellular compartment are brought into the cell by endocytosis and subsequently condemned to degradation in the lysosomes. Because endocytosed material can pursue a number of different destinies, there must be sorting mechanisms in the endocytic pathway, just as in the secretory pathway, that allow the cell to direct the endocytosed material to its appropriate destination.

Fluid-phase endocytosis is the uptake of the materials that are dissolved in the extracellular fluid (Fig. 2-22, stage 1) and not specifically bound to receptors on the cell surface.

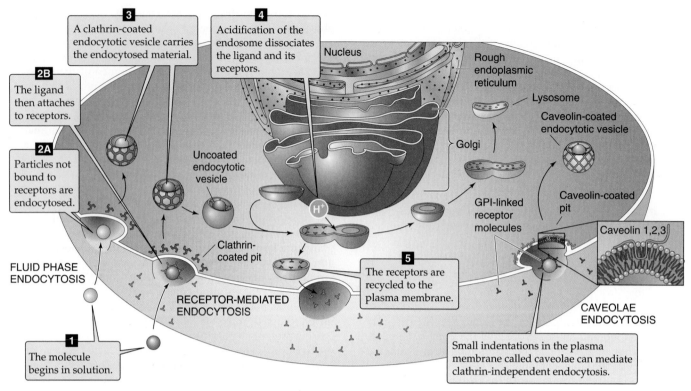

3 A clathrin-coated endocytotic vesicle carries the endocytosed material.

4 Acidification of the endosome dissociates the ligand and its receptors.

2B The ligand then attaches to receptors.

2A Particles not bound to receptors are endocytosed.

Nucleus

Rough endoplasmic reticulum

Lysosome

Caveolin-coated endocytotic vesicle

Uncoated endocytotic vesicle

Golgi

Caveolin-coated pit

Clathrin-coated pit

GPI-linked receptor molecules

Caveolin 1,2,3

FLUID PHASE ENDOCYTOSIS

5 The receptors are recycled to the plasma membrane.

RECEPTOR-MEDIATED ENDOCYTOSIS

CAVEOLAE ENDOCYTOSIS

1 The molecule begins in solution.

Small indentations in the plasma membrane called caveolae can mediate clathrin-independent endocytosis.

Figure 2-22 Endocytosis.

This process begins when a clathrin cage starts to assemble on the cytoplasmic surface of the plasma membrane. Earlier we discussed the physiology of clathrin-coated vesicles in the *secretory* pathway (Fig. 2-19). The clathrin attaches to the membrane through interactions with adaptin proteins, which in turn adhere to the cytoplasmic tail domains of certain transmembrane polypeptides. Construction of the cage causes its adherent underlying membrane to invaginate and to form a coated pit (Fig. 2-22, stage 2A). Completion of the cage creates a closed vesicle, which detaches from the cell surface through the process of membrane fission (Fig. 2-22, stage 3). The resultant vesicle quickly loses its clathrin coat through the action of the uncoating ATPase and fuses with an organelle called an **endosome.**

Receptor-mediated endocytosis is responsible for internalizing specific proteins

Most of the proteins that a cell seeks to import by endocytosis are present in the extracellular fluid in extremely low concentrations. Furthermore, the volume of extracellular fluid that is internalized by an individual coated vesicle is very small. Consequently, the probability that any particular target molecule will enter the cell during a given round of fluid-phase endocytosis is low. To improve the efficiency of endocytosis and to ensure that the desired extracellular components are gathered in every endocytic cycle, the cell has devised a method for concentrating specific proteins at the site of endocytosis before initiating their uptake.

This concentration is achieved in a process known as **receptor-mediated endocytosis**, in which molecules to be internalized (Fig. 2-22, stage 1) bind to cell surface receptors with high affinity (Fig. 2-22, stage 2B). Through this interaction, the substrates for endocytosis become physically associated with the plasma membrane, thus greatly enhancing the probability that they will be successfully internalized. Cells increase this probability even further by ensuring that the receptors themselves cluster in regions of the membrane destined to be endocytosed. The cytoplasmic tails of these receptors are endowed with recognition sequences that allow them to serve as binding sites for adaptins. Consequently, these receptors congregate in regions of the cell membrane where clathrin cages are assembling and are incorporated into coated pits as they are forming. The affinity of these receptors for the endocytic machinery ensures that their ligands are internalized with maximum efficiency.

Most endocytic receptors are constitutively associated with coated pits and are endocytosed whether or not they have bound their specific ligands. The cytoplasmic tails of certain receptors, however, interact with adaptins only when the receptor is in the bound state. For example, in the absence of epidermal growth factor (EGF), the EGF receptor is excluded from regions of the membrane in which coated pits are assembling. Modifications induced by ligand binding alter these receptors' tails, which allows them to participate in coated vesicle formation and hence in endocytosis.

After the clathrin-coated vesicle forms (Fig. 2-22, stage 3), it quickly loses its clathrin coat, as described earlier for fluid-phase endocytosis, and fuses with an endosome. Although endosomes can be wildly pleomorphic, they frequently have a frying pan–like appearance in which a round vesicular body is attached to a long tubular "handle" (Fig. 2-22, stage

Lysosomal Storage Diseases

The experimental elucidation of lysosomal enzyme sorting was achieved only because of the existence of a remarkable, naturally occurring human disease that was traced to a genetic defect in the sorting machinery. In lysosomal storage diseases, the absence of a particular hydrolase—or group of hydrolases—from the lysosome prevents the lysosomes from degrading certain substances, resulting in the formation of overstuffed lysosomes that crowd the cytoplasm and impede cell function.

In I-cell disease, most hydrolases are missing from the lysosomes of many cell types. As a result, lysosomes become engorged with massive quantities of undigested substrates. The enormously swollen lysosomes that characterize this disease were named inclusion bodies, and the cells that possess them were designated inclusion cells, or I cells for short. Whereas I cells lack most lysosomal enzymes, the genes that encode all of the hydrolases are completely normal. The mutation responsible for I-cell disease resides in the gene for the phosphosugar transferase that creates the mannose 6-phosphate recognition marker (Fig. 2-21). Without this enzyme, the cell cannot sort any of the hydrolases to the lysosomes. Instead, the hydrolases pass through the *trans*-Golgi network unnoticed by the mannose 6-phosphate receptors and are secreted constitutively from the affected cells. Certain cell types from I-cell individuals can sort newly synthesized hydrolases normally, suggesting that alternative, as yet unelucidated pathways for the targeting of lysosomal enzymes must also exist.

In some other lysosomal storage diseases, *specific* hydrolases are not missorted but rather are genetically defective. For example, children who suffer from **Tay-Sachs disease** carry a homozygous mutation in the gene that encodes the lysosomal enzyme **hexosaminidase A** (HEX A). Consequently, their lysosomes are unable to degrade substances that contain certain specific sugar linkages. Because they cannot be broken down, these substances accumulate in lysosomes. Over time, these substances fill the lysosomes, which swell and crowd the cytoplasm. The resulting derangements of cellular function are toxic to a number of cell types and ultimately underlie this disease's uniform fatality within the first few years of life. Carriers of the Tay-Sachs trait can be detected either by HEX A enzyme testing or by DNA analysis of the HEX A gene. Among the Ashkenazi Jewish population, in which 1 in 27 individuals is a carrier, three distinct HEX A mutations account for 98% of all carrier mutations.

most of the endocytosed membrane components and return them to the plasmalemma. However, substances that a cell wishes to degrade must be routed to lysosomes and prevented from escaping back to the surface. The sophisticated sorting operation required to satisfy both of these conditions takes place in the endosome.

Proton pumps embedded in its membrane ensure that like the lysosome, the endosome maintains an acidic luminal pH (Fig. 2-22, stage 4). This acidic environment initiates the separation of material that is destined for lysosomal destruction from those proteins that are to be recycled. Most endocytic receptors bind their ligands tightly at neutral pH but release them rapidly at pH values below 6.0. Therefore, as soon as a surface-derived vesicle fuses with an endosome, proteins that are bound to receptors fall off and enter the endosomal lumen. The receptor proteins segregate in the membranes of the handles of the frying pan–shaped endosomes and are ultimately removed from the endosome in vesicles that shuttle them back to the cell surface (Fig. 2-22, stage 5). The soluble proteins of the endosome lumen, which include the receptors' former ligands, are ultimately delivered to the lysosome. This sorting scheme allows the receptors to avoid the fate of their cargo and ensures that the receptors are used in many rounds of endocytosis.

The **low-density lipoprotein (LDL) receptor** follows this regimen precisely. On arrival of the LDL-laden receptor at the endosome, the acidic environment of the endosome induces the LDL to dissociate from its receptor, which then promptly recycles to the cell surface. The LDL travels on to the lysosome, where enzymes destroy the LDL and liberate its bound cholesterol.

A variation on this paradigm is responsible for the cellular uptake of iron. Iron circulates in the plasma bound to a protein called **transferrin**. At the mildly alkaline pH of extracellular fluid, the iron-transferrin complex binds with high affinity to a transferrin receptor in the plasma membranes of almost every cell type. Bound transferrin is internalized by endocytosis and delivered to endosomes. Instead of inducing *transferrin* to fall off its receptor, the acid environment of the endosome lumen causes *iron* to fall off transferrin. **Apotransferrin** (i.e., transferrin without bound iron) remains tightly bound to the transferrin receptor at an acidic pH. The released iron is transported across the endosomal membrane for use in the cytosol. The complex of apotransferrin and the transferrin receptor recycles to the cell surface, where it is again exposed to the extracellular fluid. The mildly alkaline extracellular pH causes the transferrin receptor to lose its affinity for apotransferrin and promptly releases it. Thus, the cell uses the pH-dependent sorting trick twice to ensure that both the transferrin receptor and apotransferrin recycle for subsequent rounds of iron uptake.

Certain molecules are internalized through an alternative process that involves caveolae

Clathrin-coated pits are not the only cellular structures involved in receptor-mediated internalization. Electron microscopic examination of vascular endothelial cells that line blood vessels long ago revealed the presence of clusters of small vesicles that display a characteristic appearance, in close association with the plasma membrane. These **caveolae**

4). The cytoplasmic surfaces of the handles are often decorated with forming clathrin lattices and are the sites of vesicular budding.

Endocytosed proteins can be targeted to lysosomes or recycled to the cell surface

In many cell types, endocytosis is so rapid that each hour, the cell internalizes a quantity of membrane that is equivalent in area to the entire cell surface. To persist in the face of this tremendous flux of membrane, the cell must retrieve

were thought to be involved in the transfer of large molecules across the endothelial cells, from the blood space to the tissue compartment. Actually, caveolae are present in most cell types. The caveolae are rich in cholesterol and sphingomyelin. Rather than having a clathrin lattice, they contain intrinsic membrane proteins called **caveolins**, which face the cytosol (Fig. 2-22). In addition, caveolae appear to be rich in membrane-associated polypeptides that participate in intracellular signaling, such as the Ras-like proteins as well as heterotrimeric GTP-binding proteins (see Chapter 5). They are also enriched in the receptor for folate, a vitamin required by several metabolic pathways (see Chapter 45). Unlike the receptors in the plasma membrane discussed earlier, the **folate receptor** has no cytoplasmic tail that might allow it to associate with coated pits. Instead, it belongs to the GPI-linked class of proteins that are anchored to the membrane through covalent attachment to phospholipid molecules. It appears that caveolae mediate the internalization of folate. In fact, a large number and variety of GPI-linked proteins are embedded in the outer leaflet of the caveolar membrane that faces its lumen.

The role of caveolae in the uptake of other substances, the significance of the large inventory of GPI-linked proteins in caveolae, and the functions served by their cache of signaling molecules remain to be determined. It is clear, however, that the caveolae represent a novel endocytic structure that participates in pathways distinct from those involving coated vesicles and endosomes.

SPECIALIZED CELL TYPES

All cells are constructed of the same basic elements and share the same basic metabolic and biosynthetic machinery. What distinguishes one cell type from another? Certainly, cells have different shapes and molecular structures. In addition, out of an extensive repertory of molecules that cells are capable of making, each cell type chooses which molecules to express, how to organize these molecules, and how to regulate them. It is this combination of choices that endows them with specific physiological functions. These specializations are the product of cell differentiation. Each of these cell types arises from a **stem cell**. Stem cells are mitotically active and can give rise to multiple, distinct cellular lineages; thus, they are referred to as *pluri*potent. Clearly, the zygote is the ultimate stem cell because through its divisions, it gives rise to every cell lineage present in the complete organism. Specific cell types arise from stem cells by activating a differentiation-specific program of gene expression. The interplay of environmental signals, temporal cues, and transcription factors that control the processes of cellular differentiation constitutes one of the great unraveling mysteries of modern biology.

Epithelial cells form a barrier between the internal and external milieu

How can an organism tightly regulate its internal fluid environment (i.e., internal milieu) without allowing this environment to come into direct and disastrous contact with the external world (i.e., external milieu)? The body has solved these problems by arranging a sheet of cells—an **epithelium**—between two disparate solutions. Because of their unique subcellular designs and intercellular relationships, epithelial cells form a dynamic barrier that can import or expel substances, sometimes against steep concentration gradients.

Two structural features of epithelia permit them to function as useful barriers between two very different solutions (Fig. 2-23). First, epithelial cells connect to one another by tight junctions, which constrain the free diffusion of solutes and fluids around the epithelial cells, between the internal and external compartments. Second, the tight junctions define a boundary between an apical and a basolateral domain of the plasma membrane. Each of these two domains is endowed with distinct protein and lipid components, and each subserves a distinct function. Thus, the surface membranes of epithelial cells are polarized. In Chapter 5, we discuss the mechanisms by which polarized epithelial cells exploit their unique geometry to transport salts and water from one solution to the other. However, it is worth touching on a few of the cellular specializations that characterize polarized epithelia and permit them to perform their critical roles.

The **apical membranes** of the epithelial cells (Fig. 2-23) face the lumen of a compartment that is often topologically continuous with the outside world. For example, in the stomach and intestine, apical membranes form the inner surface of the organs that come into contact with ingested matter. The apical membranes of many epithelial cells, including those lining kidney tubules, are endowed with a single nonmotile cilium. Known as the **central cilium**, this structure may sense the mechanical deformation associated with fluid flow. Mutations that disrupt individual components of the central cilium are associated with cystic disease of the kidney, in which the normal architecture of the kidney is replaced by a collection of large fluid-filled cysts.

The **basolateral membranes** of epithelial cells face the extracellular fluid compartment—which indirectly makes contact with the blood—and rest on a basement membrane. The **basement membrane** is composed of extracellular matrix proteins that the epithelial cells themselves secrete and include collagens, laminin, and proteoglycans. The basement membrane provides the epithelium with structural support and, most important, serves as an organizing foundation that helps the epithelial cells to establish their remarkable architecture.

Each epithelial cell is interconnected to its neighbors by a variety of **junctional complexes** (Fig. 2-23). The lateral surfaces of epithelial cells participate in numerous types of cell-cell contacts, including tight junctions, adhering junctions, gap junctions, and desmosomes.

Tight Junctions   A **tight junction** (or *zonula occludens*) is a complex structure that impedes the passage of molecules and ions *between* the cells of the epithelial monolayer. This pathway between the cells is termed the **paracellular pathway**. Although the complete molecular structure of the tight junction has yet to be elucidated, it is clear that its functional properties are related to its intriguing architecture (Fig. 2-23). Viewed by transmission electron microscopy, tight junctions include regions of apparent fusion between

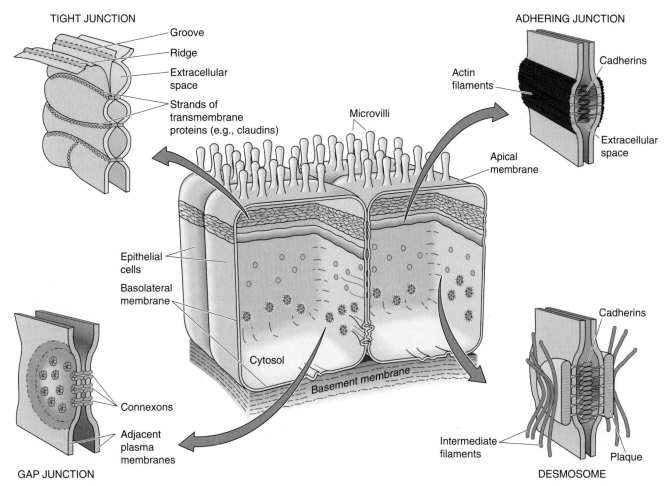

Figure 2-23 Epithelial cells. In an epithelial cell, the tight junction separates the cell membrane into apical and basolateral domains that have very different functional properties.

the outer leaflets of the lipid bilayer membranes of neighboring epithelial cells. Freeze-fracture electron microscopy reveals that the tight junction comprises parallel strands of closely packed particles, which presumably represent the transmembrane proteins participating in the junction's formation. The degree of an epithelium's impermeability—or "tightness"—is roughly proportional to the number of these parallel strands. The **claudins**, a large family of proteins, are the principal structural elements of the tight junction. Interactions between the claudins present in the apposing membranes of neighboring cells form the permeability barrier (see Chapter 5).

Tight junctions play several roles. First, they are **barriers** in that they separate one compartment from another. In some epithelial cells, such as those of the renal thick ascending limb, the tight junctions form an essentially impenetrable boundary that completely blocks the flow of ions and water between cells. In contrast, the tight junctions of the renal proximal tubule are leaky, permitting significant transepithelial movement of fluid and solutes.

Second, tight junctions can act as selective **gates** in that they permit certain solutes to flow more easily than others. Examples are the leaky tight junctions of tissues such as the proximal tubule. As discussed in Chapter 5, the permeability and selectivity of an epithelium's tight junctions are critical variables for determining that epithelium's transport characteristics. Moreover, the permeability properties of the gate function of tight junctions can be modulated in response to various physiological stimuli. The inventory of claudins expressed by an epithelium appears to determine in large measure the permeability properties of the tight junctions.

Third, tight junctions act as **fences** that separate the polarized surfaces of the epithelial plasma membrane into apical and basolateral domains. The presence of distinct populations of proteins and lipids in each plasma membrane domain is absolutely essential for an epithelium to mediate transepithelial fluid and solute transport (see Chapter 5).

Adhering Junction An adhering junction (or *zonula adherens*) is a belt that encircles an entire epithelial cell just below the level of the tight junction. Epithelial cells need two pieces of information to build themselves into a coherent epithelium. First, the cells must know which end is up. The extracellular matrix (see earlier) provides this information by defining which side will be basolateral. Second, the cells must know that there are like neighbors with which to establish cell-cell contacts. Adhering junctions provide epithelial cells with clues about the nature and proximity of their neighbors. These cell-cell contacts are mediated by the extracellular domains of members of the **cadherin** family, transmembrane proteins discussed earlier. Epithelial cells will organize themselves into a properly polarized epithelium—with differentiated apical and basolateral plasma membranes—only if the cadherins of neighboring cells have come into close enough apposition to form an adhering junction. Formation of these junctions initiates the assembly of a subcortical cytoskeleton, in which **anchor proteins** (e.g., vinculin, catenins, α-actinin) link the cytosolic domains of cadherins to a network of **actin filaments** that is associated with the cytosolic surfaces of the lateral membranes. Conversely, the disruption of adhering junctions can lead to a loss of epithelial organization. In epithelial tumors, for example, loss of expression of the adhering junction cadherins tends to correlate with the tumor cell's loss of controlled growth and its ability to **metastasize**, that is, to leave the epithelial monolayer and form a new tumor at a distant site in the body.

Gap Junctions   Gap junctions, which are discussed in Chapter 6, are channels that interconnect the cytosols of neighboring cells. They allow small molecules (less than ~1000 in molecular weight) to diffuse freely between cells. In some organs, epithelial cells are interconnected by an enormous number of gap junctions, which organize into paracrystalline hexagonal arrays. Because ions can flow through gap junctions, cells that communicate through gap junctions are electrically coupled. The permeability of gap junctions, and hence the extent to which the cytoplasmic compartments of neighboring cells are coupled, can be regulated in response to a variety of physiological stimuli.

Desmosome   A desmosome (or *macula adherens*) holds adjacent cells together tightly at a single, round spot. Desmosomes are easily recognized in thin-section electron micrographs by the characteristic dense plaques of intermediate filaments. The extracellular domains of transmembrane proteins in the **cadherin** family mediate the interaction of adjacent cells. **Anchor proteins** link the cytosolic domains of the cadherins to **intermediate filaments** that radiate into the cytoplasm from the point of intercellular contact (Fig. 2-23). These filaments interact with and organize the cytoplasmic intermediate filaments, thus coupling the structurally stabilizing elements of neighboring cells to one another. Epithelial cells are often coupled to adjacent cells by numerous desmosomes, especially in regions where the epithelium is subject to physical stress.

Epithelial cells are polarized

In many epithelia, the apical surface area is amplified by the presence of a **brush border** that is composed of hundreds of finger-like, microvillar projections (Fig. 2-23). In the case of the small intestine and the renal proximal tubule, the membrane covering each microvillus is richly endowed with enzymes that digest sugars and proteins as well as with transporters that carry the products of these digestions into the cells. The presence of a microvillar brush border can amplify the apical surface area of a polarized epithelial cell by as much as 20-fold, thus greatly enhancing its capacity to inter-

act with, to modify, and to transport substances present in the luminal fluid.

The basolateral surface area of certain epithelial cells is amplified by the presence of **lateral interdigitations** and **basal infoldings** (Fig. 2-23). Although they are not as elegantly constructed as microvilli, these structures can greatly increase the basolateral surface area. In epithelial cells that are involved in large volumes of transport—or in transport against steep gradients—amplifying the basolateral membrane can greatly increase the number of basolateral Na-K pumps that a single cell can place at its basolateral membrane.

Although the morphological differences between apical and basolateral membranes can be dramatic, the most important distinction between these surfaces is their protein composition. As noted earlier, the "fence" function of the tight junction separates completely different rosters of membrane proteins between the apical and basolateral membranes. For example, the Na-K pump is restricted to the basolateral membrane in almost all epithelial cells, and the membrane-bound enzymes that hydrolyze complex sugars and peptides are restricted to apical membranes in intestinal epithelial cells. The polarized distribution of transport proteins is absolutely necessary for the directed movement of solutes and water across epithelia. Furthermore, the restriction of certain enzymes to the apical domain limits their actions to the lumen of the epithelium and therefore offers the advantage of not wasting energy putting enzymes where they are not needed. The polarity of epithelial membrane proteins also plays a critical role in detecting antigens present in the external milieu and in transmitting signals between the external and internal compartments.

The maintenance of epithelial polarity involves complex intermolecular interactions that are only beginning to be understood. When tight junctions are disrupted, diffusion in the plane of the membrane leads to intermingling of apical and basolateral membrane components and thus a loss of polarity. The subcortical cytoskeleton beneath the basolateral surface may play a similar role by physically restraining a subset of membrane proteins at the basolateral surface.

However, such mechanisms for stabilizing the polarized distributions of membrane proteins do not explain how newly synthesized proteins come to be distributed at the appropriate plasma membrane domain. We give two examples of mechanisms that cells can use to direct membrane proteins to either the basolateral or apical membrane. The first example focuses on protein-protein interactions. As noted during our discussion of the secretory protein pathway, the sorting operation that separates apically from basolaterally directed proteins apparently occurs in the TGN. Some proteins destined for the basolateral membrane have special amino acid motifs that act as sorting signals. Some of these motifs are similar to those that allow membrane proteins to participate in endocytosis. Members of the adaptin family may recognize these motifs during the formation of clathrin-coated vesicles at the TGN and segregate the basolateral proteins into a vesicle destined for the basolateral membrane.

Another example of mechanisms that cells use to generate a polarized distribution of membrane proteins focuses on lipid-lipid interactions. In many epithelia, GPI-linked proteins are concentrated exclusively at the apical surface. It appears that the phospholipid components of GPI-linked proteins are unusual in that they cluster into complexes of fairly immobile gel-phase lipids during their passage through the Golgi apparatus. We saw earlier how lakes of phospholipids with different physical properties may segregate within a membrane. The "glycolipid rafts" of GPI-linked proteins incorporate into apically directed vesicles so that sorting can occur through lipid-lipid interactions in the plane of the membrane rather than through protein-protein interactions at the cytoplasmic surface of the Golgi membrane. From these two examples, it should be clear that a number of different mechanisms may contribute to protein sorting and the maintenance of epithelial polarity.

REFERENCES

Books and Reviews

Goldstein JL, Brown MS, Anderson RGW, et al: Receptor-mediated endocytosis: Concepts emerging from the LDL receptor system. Annu Rev Cell Dev Biol 1985; 1:1-39.

Mellman I: Endocytosis and molecular sorting. Annu Rev Cell Dev Biol 1996; 12:575-625.

Palade GE: Intracellular aspects of the process of protein synthesis. Science 1985; 189:347-358.

Rodriguez-Boulan E, Powell SK: Polarity of epithelial and neuronal cells. Annu Rev Cell Dev Biol 1992; 8:395-427.

Rothman JE: The protein machinery of vesicle budding and fusion. Protein Sci 1995; 5:185-194.

Sheetz MP: Microtubule motor complexes moving membranous organelles. Cell Struct Funct 1996; 21:369-373.

Journal Articles

Frye LD, Edidin M: The rapid intermixing of cell surface antigens after formation of mouse-human heterokaryons. J Cell Sci 1970; 7:319-335.

Griffiths G, Hoflack B, Simons K, et al: The mannose 6-phosphate receptor and the biogenesis of lysosomes. Cell 1988; 52:329-341.

Kyte J, Doolittle RF: A simple method for displaying the hydropathic character of a protein. J Mol Biol 1982; 157:105-132.

Walter P, Ibrahimi I, Blobel G: Translocation of proteins across the endoplasmic reticulum. I. Signal recognition protein (SRP) binds to in vitro assembled polysomes synthesizing secretory protein. J Cell Biol 1981; 91:545-550.

CHAPTER **3**

SIGNAL TRANSDUCTION

Lloyd Cantley

The evolution of multicellular organisms necessitated the development of mechanisms to tightly coordinate the activities among cells. Such **communication** is fundamental to all biological processes, ranging from the induction of embryonic development to the integration of physiological responses in the face of environmental challenges.

As our understanding of cellular and molecular physiology has increased, it has become evident that all cells can receive and process information. External **signals** such as odorants, chemicals that reflect metabolic status, ions, hormones, growth factors, and neurotransmitters can all serve as **chemical messengers** linking neighboring or distant cells. Even external signals that are not considered chemical in nature (e.g., light and mechanical or thermal stimuli) may ultimately be transduced into a chemical messenger. Most chemical messengers interact with specific **cell surface receptors** and trigger a cascade of secondary events, including the mobilization of diffusible intracellular **second-messenger systems** that mediate the cell's response to that stimulus. However, hydrophobic messengers, such as steroid hormones and some vitamins, can diffuse across the plasma membrane and interact with **cytosolic or nuclear receptors**. It is now clear that cells use a number of different, often intersecting intracellular signaling pathways to ensure that the cell's response to a stimulus is tightly controlled.

MECHANISMS OF CELLULAR COMMUNICATION

Cells can communicate with one another by chemical signals

Early insight into signal transduction pathways was obtained from studies of the endocrine system. The classic definition of a **hormone** is *a substance that is produced in one tissue or organ and released into the blood and carried to other organs (targets), where it acts to produce a specific response.* The idea of endocrine or ductless glands developed from the recognition that certain organs—such as the pituitary, adrenal, and thyroid gland—can synthesize and release specific chemical messengers in response to particular physiological states.

However, many other cells and tissues not classically thought of as endocrine in nature also produce hormones. For example, the kidney produces 1,25-dihydroxyvitamin D_3, and the salivary gland synthesizes nerve growth factor.

It is now recognized that intercellular communication can involve the production of a "hormone" or chemical signal by one cell type that acts in any (or all) of three ways, as illustrated in Figure 3-1: on distant tissues (**endocrine**), on a neighboring cell in the same tissue (**paracrine**), or on the same cell that released the signaling molecule (**autocrine**). For paracrine and autocrine signals to be delivered to their proper targets, their diffusion must be limited. This restriction can be accomplished by rapid endocytosis of the chemical signal by neighboring cells, its destruction by extracellular enzymes, or its immobilization by the extracellular matrix. The events that take place at the neuromuscular junction are excellent examples of paracrine signaling. When an electrical impulse travels down an axon and reaches the nerve terminal (Fig. 3-2), it stimulates release of the neurotransmitter acetylcholine (ACh). In turn, ACh transiently activates a ligand-gated cation channel on the muscle cell membrane. The resultant transient influx of Na^+ causes a localized positive shift of V_m (i.e., depolarization), initiating events that result in propagation of an action potential along the muscle cell. The ACh signal is rapidly terminated by the action of acetylcholinesterase, which is present in the synaptic cleft. This enzyme degrades the ACh that is released by the neuron.

Soluble chemical signals interact with target cells by binding to surface or intracellular receptors

Four types of chemicals can serve as extracellular signaling molecules: **amines**, such as epinephrine; **peptides and proteins**, such as angiotensin II and insulin; **steroids**, including aldosterone, estrogens, and retinoic acid; and other **small molecules**, such as amino acids, nucleotides, ions (e.g., Ca^{2+}), and gases (e.g., nitric oxide).

For a molecule to act as a signal, it must bind to a **receptor**. A receptor is a protein (or in some cases a lipoprotein) on the cell surface or within the cell that specifically binds a

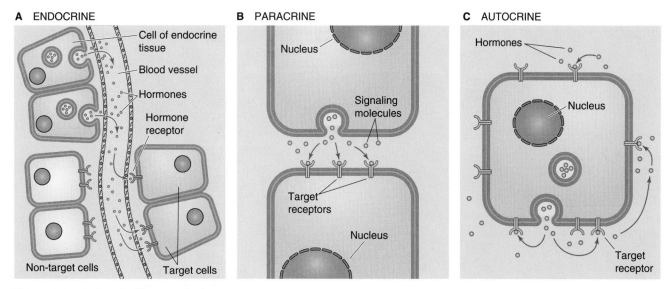

Figure 3-1 Modes of cell communication.

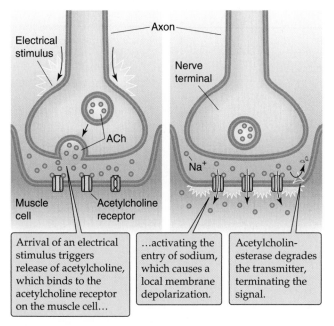

| Arrival of an electrical stimulus triggers release of acetylcholine, which binds to the acetylcholine receptor on the muscle cell… | …activating the entry of sodium, which causes a local membrane depolarization. | Acetylcholine-esterase degrades the transmitter, terminating the signal. |

Figure 3-2 Example of paracrine signaling. The release of ACh at the neuromuscular junction is a form of paracrine signaling because the nerve terminal releases a chemical (i.e., ACh) that acts on a neighboring cell (i.e., the muscle).

signaling molecule (the ligand). In some cases, the receptor is itself an ion channel, and ligand binding produces a change in V_{m}. Thus, the cell can transduce a signal with no machinery other than the receptor. In most cases, however, interaction of the ligand with one or more specific receptors results in an association of the receptor with an effector molecule that initiates a cellular response. Effectors include enzymes, channels, transport proteins, contractile elements, and transcription factors. The ability of a cell or tissue to respond to a specific signal is dictated by the complement of receptors it possesses and by the chain of intracellular reactions that

are initiated by the binding of any one ligand to its receptor. Receptors can be divided into four categories on the basis of their associated mechanisms of signal transduction (Table 3-1).

1. **Ligand-gated ion channels.** Integral membrane proteins, these hybrid receptor/channels are involved in signaling between electrically excitable cells. The binding of a neurotransmitter such as ACh to its receptor—which in fact is merely part of the channel—results in transient opening of the channel, thus altering the ion permeability of the cell.

2. **G protein–coupled receptors.** These integral plasma membrane proteins work indirectly—through an intermediary—to activate or to inactivate a separate membrane-associated enzyme or channel. The intermediary is a heterotrimeric guanosine triphosphate (GTP)–binding complex called a G protein.

3. **Catalytic receptors.** When activated by a ligand, these integral plasma membrane proteins are either enzymes themselves or part of an enzymatic complex.

4. **Nuclear receptors.** These proteins, located in the cytosol or nucleus, are ligand-activated transcription factors. These receptors link extracellular signals to gene transcription.

In addition to these four classes of membrane signaling molecules, some other transmembrane proteins act as messengers even though they do not fit the classic definition of a receptor. In response to certain physiological changes, they undergo regulated intramembrane proteolysis within the plane of the membrane, liberating cytosolic fragments that enter the nucleus to modulate gene expression. We discuss this process later in the chapter.

Signaling events initiated by plasma membrane receptors can generally be divided into six steps:

Step 1: **Recognition** of the signal by its receptor. The same signaling molecule can sometimes bind to more than one

Table 3-1 Classification of Receptors and Associated Signal Transduction Pathways

Class of Receptor	Subunit Composition of Receptor	Ligand	Signal Transduction Pathway Downstream from Receptor

Ligand-gated ion channels (ionotropic receptors)	Heteromeric or homomeric oligomers	*Extracellular*
		  GABA
		  Glycine
		  ACh: muscle
		  ACh: nerve
		  5-HT
		  Glutamate: non-NMDA
		  Glutamate: NMDA
		  ATP (opening)
		Intracellular
		  cGMP (vision)
		  cAMP (olfaction)
		  ATP (closes channel)
		  IP_3
		  Ca^{2+} or ryanodine
			Ion Current
			$Cl^- > HCO_3^-$
			$Cl^- > HCO_3^-$
			Na^+, K^+, Ca^{2+}
			Na^+, K^+, Ca^{2+}
			Na^+, K^+
			Na^+, K^+, Ca^{2+}
			Na^+, K^+, Ca^{2+}
			Ca^{2+}, Na^+, Mg^{2+}
			Na^+, K^+
			Na^+, K^+
			K^+
			Ca^{2+}
			Ca^{2+}

Receptors coupled to heterotrimeric ($\alpha\beta\gamma$) G proteins	Single polypeptide that crosses the membrane seven times	*Small transmitter molecules*
		  ACh
		  Norepinephrine
		Peptides
		  Oxytocin
		  Parathyroid hormone
		  Neuropeptide Y
		  Gastrin
		  Cholecystokinin
		Odorants
		Certain cytokines, lipids, and related molecules
			$\beta\gamma$ *Directly activates downstream effector:*
			  Muscarinic ACh receptor activates atrial K^+ channel
			α *Activates an enzyme:*
			  Cyclases that make cyclic nucleotides (cAMP, cGMP)
			  Phospholipases that generate IP_3 and diacylglycerols
			  Phospholipases that generate arachidonic acid and its metabolites

Catalytic receptors	Single polypeptide that crosses the membrane once May be dimeric or may dimerize after activation	ANP TGF-β NGF, EGF, PDGF, FGF, insulin, IGF-1 IL-3, IL-5, IL-6, EPO, LIF, CNTF, GH, IFN-α, IFN-β, IFN-γ, GM-CSF CD45	Receptor guanylyl cyclase Receptor serine/threonine kinases Receptor tyrosine kinase Tyrosine kinase–associated receptor Receptor tyrosine phosphatase

Intracellular (or nuclear) receptors	Homodimers of polypeptides, each with multiple functional domains
	
	Heterodimers of polypeptides, each with multiple functional domains
		Steroid hormones
		  Mineralocorticoids
		  Glucocorticoids
		  Androgens
		  Estrogens
		  Progestins
		Others
		  Thyroid hormones
		  Retinoic acid
		  Vitamin D
		  Prostaglandin
			Bind to regulatory DNA sequences and directly or indirectly increase or decrease the transcription of specific genes

kind of receptor. For example, ACh can bind to both ligand-gated channels and G protein–coupled receptors. Binding of a ligand to its receptor involves the same three types of weak, noncovalent interactions that characterize substrate-enzyme interactions. *Ionic bonds* are formed between groups of opposite charge. In *van der Waals* interactions, a transient dipole in one atom generates the opposite dipole in an adjacent atom, thereby creating an electrostatic interaction. *Hydrophobic interactions* occur between nonpolar groups.

Step 2: **Transduction** of the extracellular message into an intracellular signal or second messenger. Ligand binding causes a conformational change in the receptor that triggers the catalytic activities intrinsic to the receptor or causes the receptor to interact with membrane or cytoplasmic enzymes. The final consequence is the generation of a **second messenger** or the activation of a catalytic cascade.

Step 3: **Transmission** of the second messenger's signal to the appropriate effector. These effectors represent a diverse array of molecules, such as enzymes, ion channels, and transcription factors.

Step 4: **Modulation of the effector.** These events often result in the activation of protein **kinases** (which put phosphate groups on proteins) and **phosphatases** (which take them off), thereby altering the activity of other enzymes and proteins.

Step 5: **Response** of the cell to the initial stimulus. This collection of actions represents the summation and integration of input from multiple signaling pathways.

Step 6: **Termination** of the response by feedback mechanisms at any or all levels of the signaling pathway.

Cells can also communicate by direct interactions

Gap Junctions   Neighboring cells can be electrically and metabolically coupled by means of gap junctions formed between apposing cell membranes. These water-filled channels facilitate the passage of inorganic ions and small molecules, such as Ca^{2+} and $3',5'$-cyclic adenosine monophosphate (cAMP), from the cytoplasm of one cell into the cytoplasm of an adjacent cell. Mammalian gap junctions permit the passage of molecules that are less than ~1200 Da but restrict the movement of molecules that are greater than ~2000 Da. Gap junctions are also excellent pathways for the flow of electrical current between adjacent cells, playing a critical role in cardiac and smooth muscle.

The permeability of gap junctions can be rapidly regulated by changes in cytosolic concentrations of Ca^{2+}, cAMP, and H^+ as well as by the voltage across the cell membrane or membrane potential (V_m) (see Chapter 5). This type of modulation is physiologically important for cell-to-cell communication. For example, if a cell's plasma membrane is damaged, Ca^{2+} passively moves into the cell and raises $[Ca^{2+}]_i$ to toxic levels. Elevated *intracellular* $[Ca^{2+}]$ in the damaged cell triggers closure of the gap junctions, thus preventing the flow of excessive amounts of Ca^{2+} into the adjacent cell.

Adhering and Tight Junctions   **Adhering junctions** form as the result of the Ca^{2+}-dependent interactions of the extracellular domains of transmembrane proteins called **cadherins** (see Chapter 2). The clustering of cadherins at the site of interaction with an adjacent cell causes secondary clustering of intracellular proteins known as **catenins**, which in turn serve as sites of attachment for the intracellular **actin cytoskeleton**. Thus, adhering junctions provide important clues for the maintenance of normal cell architecture as well as the organization of groups of cells into tissues.

In addition to a homeostatic role, adhering junctions can serve a signaling role during organ development and remodeling. In a cell that is stably associated with its neighbors, a catenin known as β-catenin is mainly sequestered at the adhering junctions, minimizing concentration of free β-catenin. However, disruption of adhering junctions by certain growth factors, for example, causes β-catenin to disassociate from cadherin. The resulting rise in free β-catenin

levels promotes the translocation of β-catenin to the nucleus. There, β-catenin regulates the transcription of multiple genes, including ones that promote cell proliferation and migration.

Similar to adhering junctions, **tight junctions** (see Chapter 2) comprise transmembrane proteins that link with their counterparts on adjacent cells as well as intracellular proteins that stabilize the complex and also have a signaling role. The transmembrane proteins—including claudins, occludin, and junctional adhesion molecule—and their extracellular domains create the diffusion barrier of the tight junction. One of the integral cytoplasmic proteins in tight junctions, zonula occludin 1 (ZO-1), colocalizes with a serine/threonine kinase known as WNK1, which is found in certain renal tubule epithelial cells that reabsorb Na^+ and Cl^- from the tubule lumen. Because WNK1 is important for determining the permeability of the tight junctions to Cl^-, mutations in WNK1 can increase the movement of Cl^- through the tight junctions (see Chapter 35) and thereby lead to hypertension.

Membrane-Associated Ligands   Another mechanism by which cells can directly communicate is by the interaction of a receptor in the plasma membrane with a ligand that is itself a membrane protein on an adjacent cell. Such membrane-associated ligands can provide spatial clues in migrating cells. For example, an **ephrin** ligand expressed on the surface of one cell can interact with an Eph receptor on a nearby cell. The resulting activation of the Eph receptor can in turn provide signals for regulating such developmental events as axonal guidance in the nervous system and endothelial cell guidance in the vasculature.

Second-messenger systems amplify signals and integrate responses among cell types

Once a signal has been received at the cell surface, it is typically amplified and transmitted to specific sites within the cells through second messengers. For a molecule to function as a second messenger, its concentration, or window of activity, must be finely regulated. The cell achieves this control by rapidly producing or activating the second messenger and then inactivating or degrading it. To ensure that the system returns to a resting state when the stimulus is removed, counterbalancing activities function at each step of the cascade.

The involvement of second messengers in catalytic cascades provides numerous opportunities to **amplify** a signal. For example, the binding of a ligand to its receptor can generate hundreds of second-messenger molecules, which can in turn alter the activity of thousands of downstream effectors. This modulation usually involves the conversion of an inactive species into an active molecule or vice versa. An example of such a cascade is the increased intracellular concentration of the second messenger **cAMP**. Receptor occupancy activates a G protein, which in turn stimulates a membrane-bound enzyme, **adenylyl cyclase**. This enzyme catalyzes the synthesis of cAMP from adenosine triphosphate (ATP), and a 5-fold increase in the intracellular concentration of cAMP is achieved in ~5 seconds. This sudden rise in cAMP levels is rapidly counteracted by its breakdown to adenosine 5′-monophosphate by **cAMP phosphodiesterase**.

Second-messenger systems also allow **specificity** and **diversity**. Ligands that activate the same signaling pathways in cells usually produce the same effect. For example, epinephrine, adrenocorticotropic hormone (ACTH), glucagon, and thyroid-stimulating hormone induce triglyceride breakdown through the cAMP messenger system. However, the same signaling molecule can produce distinct responses in different cells, depending on the complement of receptors and signal transduction pathways that are available in the cell as well as the specialized function that the cell carries out in the organism. For example, ACh induces contraction of skeletal muscle cells but inhibits contraction of heart muscle. It also facilitates the exocytosis of secretory granules in pancreatic acinar cells. This signaling molecule achieves these different endpoints by interacting with distinct receptors.

The diversity and specialization of second-messenger systems are important to a multicellular organism, as can be seen in the coordinated response of an organism to a stressful situation. Under these conditions, the adrenal gland releases epinephrine. Different organ systems respond to epinephrine in a distinct manner, such as activation of glycogen breakdown in the liver, constriction of the blood vessels of the skin, dilation of the blood vessels in skeletal muscle, and increased rate and force of heart contraction. The overall effect is an **integrated response** that readies the organism for attack, defense, or escape. In contrast, complex cell behaviors, such as proliferation and differentiation, are generally stimulated by combinations of signals rather than by a single signal. Integration of these stimuli requires **crosstalk** among the various signaling cascades.

As discussed later, most signal transduction pathways use elaborate cascades of signaling proteins to relay information from the cell surface to effectors in the cell membrane, the cytoplasm, or the nucleus. In Chapter 4, we discuss how signal transduction pathways that lead to the nucleus can affect the cell by modulating gene transcription. These are **genomic** effects. Signal transduction systems that project to the cell membrane or to the cytoplasm produce **nongenomic** effects, the focus of this chapter.

RECEPTORS THAT ARE ION CHANNELS

Ligand-gated ion channels transduce a chemical signal into an electrical signal

The property that defines this class of multisubunit membrane-spanning receptors is that the signaling molecule itself controls the opening and closing of an ion channel by binding to a site on the receptor. Thus, these receptors are also called **ionotropic receptors** to distinguish them from the metabotropic receptors, which act through "metabolic" pathways. One superfamily of ligand-gated channels includes the ionotropic receptors for ACh, serotonin, γ-aminobutyric acid (GABA), and glycine. Most structural and functional information for ionotropic receptors comes from the *nicotinic* ACh receptor (AChR) present in skeletal muscle (Fig. 3-2). The *nicotinic* AChR is a cation channel that consists of four membrane-spanning subunits, α, β, γ, and δ, in a

stoichiometry of 2:1:1:1. This receptor is called nicotinic because the nicotine contained in tobacco can activate or open the channel and thereby alter V_m. Note that the nicotinic AChR is very different from the *muscarinic* AChR discussed later, which is not a ligand-gated channel. Additional examples of ligand-gated channels are the IP3 receptor and the Ca^{2+} release channel (also known as the ryanodine receptor). Both receptors are tetrameric Ca^{2+} channels located in the membranes of intracellular organelles.

RECEPTORS COUPLED TO G PROTEINS

G protein–coupled receptors (GPCRs) constitute the largest family of receptors on the cell surface, with more than 1000 members. GPCRs mediate cellular responses to a diverse array of signaling molecules, such as hormones, neurotransmitters, vasoactive peptides, odorants, tastants, and other local mediators. Despite the chemical diversity of their ligands, most receptors of this class have a similar structure (Fig. 3-3). They consist of a single polypeptide chain with seven membrane-spanning α-helical segments, an extracellular N terminus that is glycosylated, a large cytoplasmic loop that is composed mainly of hydrophilic amino acids between helices 5 and 6, and a hydrophilic domain at the cytoplasmic C terminus. Most small ligands (e.g., epinephrine) bind in the plane of the membrane at a site that involves several membrane-spanning segments. In the case of larger protein ligands, a portion of the extracellular N terminus also participates in ligand binding. The 5,6-cytoplasmic loop appears to be the major site of interaction with the intracellular G protein, although the 3,4-cytoplasmic loop and the cytoplasmic C terminus also contribute to binding in some cases. Binding of the GPCR to its extracellular ligand regulates this interaction between the receptor and the G proteins, thus transmitting a signal to downstream effectors. In the next four sections of this subchapter, we discuss the general principles of how G proteins function; three major

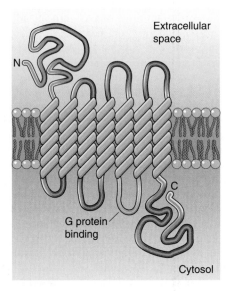

Figure 3-3   Receptor coupled to a G protein.

second-messenger systems that are triggered by G proteins are then considered.

GENERAL PROPERTIES OF G PROTEINS

G proteins are heterotrimers that exist in many combinations of different α, β, and γ subunits

G proteins are members of a superfamily of **GTP-binding proteins**. This superfamily includes the classic heterotrimeric G proteins that bind to GPCRs as well as the so-called small GTP-binding proteins, such as Ras. Both the heterotrimeric and small G proteins can hydrolyze GTP and switch between an active GTP-bound state and an inactive guanosine diphosphate (GDP)–bound state.

Heterotrimeric G proteins are composed of three subunits, α, β, and γ. At least 16 different α subunits (~42 to 50 kDa), 5 β subunits (~33 to 35 kDa), and 11 γ subunits (~8 to 10 kDa) are present in mammalian tissue. The α subunit binds and hydrolyzes GTP and also interacts with "downstream" effector proteins such as adenylyl cyclase. Historically, the α subunits were thought to provide the principal specificity to each type of G protein, with the βγ complex functioning to anchor the trimeric complex to the membrane. However, it is now clear that the βγ complex also functions in signal transduction by interacting with certain effector molecules. Moreover, both the α and γ subunits are involved in anchoring the complex to the membrane. The α subunit is held to the membrane by either a myristyl or a palmitoyl group; the γ subunit is held by a prenyl group.

The multiple α, β, and γ subunits demonstrate distinct tissue distributions and interact with different receptors and effectors (Table 3-2). Because of the potential for several hundred combinations of the known α, β, and γ subunits, G proteins are ideally suited to link a diversity of receptors to a diversity of effectors. The many classes of G proteins, in

Table 3-2 Families of G Proteins

Family/Subunit	% Identity	Toxin	Distribution	Receptor	Effector/Role
α_s $\alpha_{s(s)}$ $\alpha_{s(l)}$	100	CTX	Ubiquitous	β-adrenergic, TSH, glucagon	↑ Adenylyl cyclase ↑ Ca^{2+} channel ↑ Na^+ channel
α_{olf}	88	CTX	Olfactory epithelium	Odorant	↑ Adenylyl cyclase Open K^+ channel
G_i α_{i1} α_{i2} α_{i3}	100 88	PTX PTX PTX	~Ubiquitous Ubiquitous ~Ubiquitous	M_2, α_2-adrenergic, others	↑ IP_3, DAG, Ca^{2+}, and AA release ↓ Adenylyl cyclase
α_{O1A} α_{O1B}	73 73	PTX PTX	Brain, others Brain, others	Met-enkephalin, α_2-adrenergic, others	
α_{t1} α_{t2}	68 68	PTX, CTX PTX, CTX	Retinal rods Retinal cones	Rhodopsin Cone opsin	↑ cGMP-phosphodiesterase
α_g α_z	67 60	PTX, CTX (?)	Taste buds Brain, adrenal, platelet	Taste (?) M_2 (?), others (?)	? ↓ Adenylyl cyclase
G_q α_q α_{11} α_{14} α_{15} α_{16}	100 88 79 57 58		~Ubiquitous ~Ubiquitous Lung, kidney, liver B cell, myeloid T cell, myeloid	M_1, α_1-adrenergic, others Several receptors	↑ PLCβ1, β2, β3 ↑ PLCβ1, β2, β3
G_{12} α_{12} α_{13}	100 67		Ubiquitous Ubiquitous		

CTX, cholera toxin; M_1 and M_2, muscarinic cholinergic receptors; PTX, pertussis toxin; TSH, thyrotropin (thyroid-stimulating hormone).

conjunction with the presence of several receptor types for a single ligand, provide a mechanism whereby a common signal can elicit the appropriate physiological changes in different tissues. For example, when epinephrine binds β_1-adrenergic receptors in the heart, it *stimulates* adenylyl cyclase, which increases heart rate and the force of contraction. However, in the periphery, epinephrine acts on α_2-adrenergic receptors coupled to a G protein that *inhibits* adenylyl cyclase, thereby increasing peripheral vascular resistance and consequently increasing venous return and blood pressure.

Among the first effectors found to be sensitive to G proteins was the enzyme adenylyl cyclase. The heterotrimeric G protein known as **G_s** was so named because it stimulates adenylyl cyclase. A separate class of G proteins was given the name **G_i** because it is responsible for the hormone-dependent inhibition of adenylyl cyclase. Identification of these classes of G proteins was greatly facilitated by the observation that the α subunits of individual G proteins are substrates for adenosine diphosphate (ADP) ribosylation catalyzed by bacterial toxins. The toxin from *Vibrio cholerae* activates G_s, whereas the toxin from *Bordetella pertussis* inactivates the cyclase-inhibiting G_i (see the box titled Action of Toxins on Heterotrimeric G Proteins).

For their work in identifying G proteins and elucidating the physiological role of these proteins, Alfred Gilman and Martin Rodbell received the 1994 Nobel Prize in Physiology or Medicine.

G protein activation follows a cycle

In their inactive state, heterotrimeric G proteins are a complex of α, β, and γ subunits in which GDP occupies the guanine nucleotide–binding site of the α subunit. After ligand binding to the GPCR (Fig. 3-4, step 1), the activated receptor interacts with the $\alpha\beta\gamma$ heterotrimer to promote a conformational change that facilitates the release of bound GDP and simultaneous binding of GTP (step 2). This GDP-GTP exchange stimulates dissociation of the complex from the receptor (step 3) and causes disassembly of the trimer into a free α subunit and $\beta\gamma$ complex (step 4). The free, active GTP-bound α subunit can now interact in the plane of the membrane with downstream effectors such as adenylyl cyclase and phospholipases (step 5). Similarly, the $\beta\gamma$ subunit can now activate ion channels or other effectors.

The α subunit terminates the signaling events that are mediated by the α and $\beta\gamma$ subunits by hydrolyzing GTP to GDP and inorganic phosphate (P_i). The result is an *inactive* α-GDP complex that dissociates from its downstream effector and reassociates with a $\beta\gamma$ subunit (Fig. 3-4, step 6), thus completing the cycle (step 1). The $\beta\gamma$ subunit stabilizes α-GDP and thereby substantially slows the rate of GDP-GTP exchange (step 2) and dampens signal transmission in the resting state.

The RGS (for "regulation of G protein signaling") family of proteins appears to enhance the intrinsic guanosine triphosphatase (GTPase) activity of some but not all α subunits. Investigators have identified at least 15 mammalian RGS proteins and shown that they interact with specific α subunits. RGS proteins bind the complex $G\alpha/GDP/AlF_4^-$, which is the structural analogue of the GTPase transition state. By stabilizing the transition state, RGS proteins may promote GTP hydrolysis and thus the termination of signaling.

As noted earlier, α subunits can be anchored to the cell membrane by myristyl or palmitoyl groups. Activation can result in the removal of these groups and the release of the α subunit into the cytosol. Loss of the α subunit from the membrane may decrease the interaction of G proteins with receptors and downstream effectors (e.g., adenylyl cyclase).

Activated α subunits couple to a variety of downstream effectors, including enzymes, ion channels, and membrane trafficking machinery

Activated α subunits can couple to a variety of enzymes. A major enzyme that acts as an effector downstream of activated α subunits is **adenylyl cyclase** (Fig. 3-5A). This enzyme can be either activated or inhibited by G protein signaling, depending on whether it associates with the GTP-bound form of $G\alpha_s$ (stimulatory) or $G\alpha_i$ (inhibitory). Thus, different hormones—acting through different G protein complexes—can have opposing effects on the same intracellular messenger.

G proteins can also activate enzymes that break down cyclic nucleotides. For example, the G protein called **transducin**, which plays a key role in phototransduction (see Chapter 15), activates the cyclic guanosine monophosphate (cGMP) **phosphodiesterase**, which catalyzes the breakdown of cGMP to GMP (Fig. 3-5B). Thus, in retinal cells expressing transducin, light leads to a decrease in $[cGMP]_i$.

G proteins can also couple to **phospholipases**. These enzymes catabolize phospholipids, as discussed in detail later in the section on G protein second messengers. This superfamily of phospholipases can be grouped into phospholipases A_2, C, or D on the basis of the site at which the enzyme cleaves the phospholipid. The G protein α_q subunit activates phospholipase C, which breaks phosphatidylinositol bisphosphate (PIP_2) into two intracellular messengers, membrane-associated diacylglycerol and cytosolic IP_3 (Fig. 3-5C). Diacylglycerol stimulates protein kinase C, whereas IP_3 binds to a receptor on the endoplasmic reticulum membrane and triggers the release of Ca^{2+} from intracellular stores.

Some G proteins interact with **ion channels**. Agonists that bind to the β-adrenergic receptor activate the L-type Ca^{2+} channel in the heart and skeletal muscle (see Chapter 7). The G protein G_s directly stimulates this channel as the α subunit of G_s binds to the channel, and G_s also indirectly stimulates this channel through a signal transduction cascade that involves cAMP-dependent protein kinase.

A clue that G proteins serve additional functions in **membrane trafficking** (see Chapter 2) in the cell comes from the observation that many cells contain intracellular pools of heterotrimeric G proteins, some bound to internal membranes and some free in the cytosol. Experiments involving toxins, inhibitors, and cell lines harboring mutations in G protein subunits have demonstrated that these intracellular G proteins are involved in vesicular transport. G proteins have been implicated in the budding of secretory vesicles from the *trans*-Golgi network, fusion of endosomes, recruitment of non–clathrin coat proteins, and transcytosis and apical secretion in polarized epithelial cells. The receptors

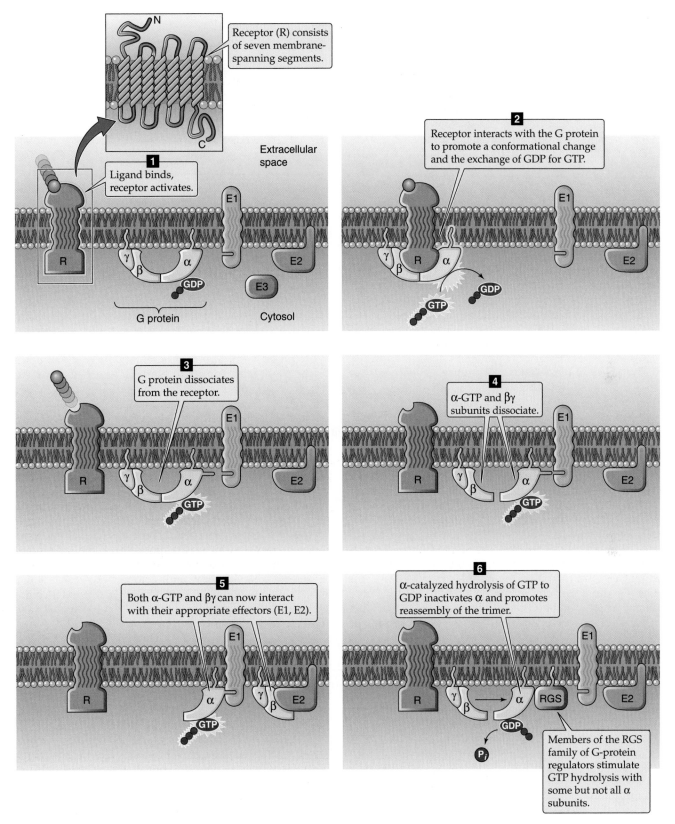

Figure 3-4 Enzymatic cycle of heterotrimeric G proteins.

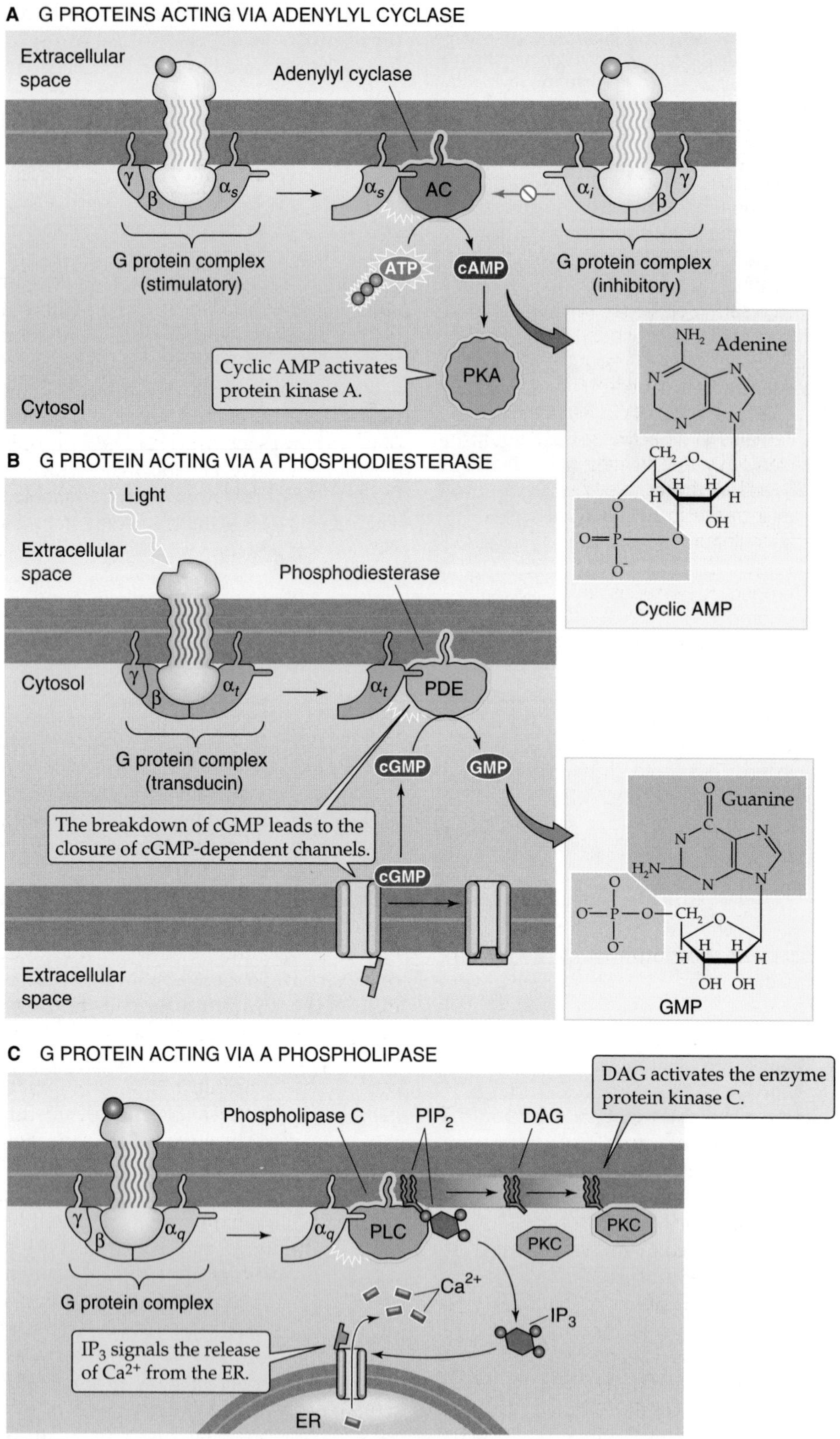

A   G PROTEINS ACTING VIA ADENYLYL CYCLASE

B   G PROTEIN ACTING VIA A PHOSPHODIESTERASE

C   G PROTEIN ACTING VIA A PHOSPHOLIPASE

Figure 3-5   Downstream effects of activated G protein α subunits. **A,** When a ligand binds to a receptor coupled to α_s, adenylyl cyclase (AC) is activated, whereas when a ligand binds to a receptor coupled to α_i, the enzyme is inhibited. The activated enzyme converts ATP to cAMP, which then can activate protein kinase A (PKA). **B,** In phototransduction, a photon interacts with the receptor and activates the G protein transducin. The α_t activates phosphodiesterase (PDE), which in turn hydrolyzes cGMP and lowers the intracellular concentrations of cGMP and therefore closes the cGMP-activated channels. **C,** In this example, the ligand binds to a receptor that is coupled to α_q, which activates phospholipase C (PLC). This enzyme converts PIP_2 to IP_3 and diacylglycerol (DAG). The IP_3 leads to the release of Ca^{2+} from intracellular stores, whereas the diacylglycerol activates protein kinase C (PKC). ER, endoplasmic reticulum.

Action of Toxins on Heterotrimeric G Proteins

Infectious diarrheal disease has a multitude of causes. **Cholera toxin,** a secretory product of the bacterium *Vibrio cholerae,* is responsible in part for the devastating characteristics of cholera. The toxin is an oligomeric protein composed of one A subunit and five B subunits (AB_5). After cholera toxin enters intestinal epithelial cells, the A subunit separates from the B subunits and becomes activated by proteolytic cleavage. The resulting active A1 fragment catalyzes the ADP ribosylation of $G\alpha_s$. This ribosylation, which involves transfer of the ADP-ribose moiety from the oxidized form of nicotinamide adenine dinucleotide (NAD^+) to the α subunit, inhibits the GTPase activity of $G\alpha_s$. As a result of this modification, $G\alpha_s$ remains in its activated, GTP-bound form and can activate adenylyl cyclase. In intestinal epithelial cells, the constitutively activated $G\alpha_s$ elevates levels of cAMP, which causes an increase in Cl^- conductance and water flow and thereby contributes to the large fluid loss characteristic of this disease.

A related bacterial product is **pertussis toxin,** which is also an AB_5 protein. It is produced by *Bordetella pertussis,* the causative agent of whooping cough. Pertussis toxin ADP-ribosylates $G\alpha_i$. This ADP-ribosylated $G\alpha_i$ cannot exchange its bound GDP (inactive state) for GTP. Thus, α_i remains in its GDP-bound inactive state. As a result, receptor occupancy can no longer release the active α_i-GTP, so adenylyl cyclase cannot be inhibited. Thus, both cholera toxin and pertussis toxin increase the generation of cAMP.

and effectors that interact with these intracellular G proteins have not been determined.

The βγ subunits of G proteins can also activate downstream effectors

Considerable evidence now indicates that the βγ subunits can also interact with downstream effectors. The neurotransmitter ACh released from the vagus nerve reduces the rate and strength of heart contraction. This action in the atria of the heart is mediated by *muscarinic* M_2 AChRs (see Chapter 14). These receptors can be activated by muscarine, an alkaloid found in certain poisonous mushrooms. *Muscarinic* AChRs are very different from the *nicotinic* AChRs discussed earlier, which are ligand-gated channels. Binding of ACh to the muscarinic M_2 receptor in the atria activates a heterotrimeric G protein, resulting in the generation of both activated $G\alpha_i$ as well as a free βγ subunit complex. The βγ complex then interacts with a particular class of K^+ channels, increasing their permeability. This increase in K^+ permeability keeps the membrane potential relatively negative and thus renders the cell more resistant to excitation. The βγ subunit complex also modulates the activity of adenylyl cyclase and phospholipase C and stimulates phospholipase A_2. Such effects of βγ can be independent of, synergize with, or antagonize the action of the α subunit. For example, studies using

various isoforms of adenylyl cyclase have demonstrated that purified βγ stimulates some isoforms, inhibits others, and has no effect on still others. Different combinations of βγ isoforms may have different activities. For example, $\beta_1\gamma_1$ is one tenth as efficient at stimulating type II adenylyl cyclase as is $\beta_1\gamma_2$.

An interesting action of some βγ complexes is that they bind to a special protein kinase called the **β-adrenergic receptor kinase (βARK).** As a result of this interaction, βARK translocates to the plasma membrane, where it phosphorylates the ligand-receptor complex (but not the unbound receptor). This phosphorylation results in the recruitment of **β-arrestin** to the GPCR, which in turn mediates disassociation of the receptor-ligand complex and thus attenuates the activity of the same β-adrenergic receptors that gave rise to the βγ complex in the first place. This action is an example of **receptor desensitization.** These phosphorylated receptors eventually undergo endocytosis, which transiently reduces the number of receptors that are available on the cell surface. This endocytosis is an important step in **resensitization** of the receptor system.

Small GTP-binding proteins are involved in a vast number of cellular processes

A distinct group of proteins that are structurally related to the α subunit of the heterotrimeric G proteins are the **small GTP-binding proteins.** More than 100 of these have been identified to date, and they have been divided into five groups including the Ras, Rho, Rab, Arf, and Ran families. These 21-kDa proteins can be membrane associated (e.g., Ras) or may translocate between the membrane and the cytosol (e.g., Rho).

The three isoforms of Ras (N, Ha, and Ki) relay signals from the plasma membrane to the nucleus through an elaborate kinase cascade (see Chapter 4), thereby regulating gene transcription. In some tumors, mutation of the genes encoding Ras proteins results in constitutively active Ras. These mutated genes are called **oncogenes** because the altered Ras gene product promotes the malignant transformation of a cell and can contribute to the development of cancer (oncogenesis). In contrast, Rho family members are primarily involved in rearrangement of the actin cytoskeleton; Rab and Arf proteins regulate vesicle trafficking.

Similar to the α subunit of heterotrimeric G proteins, the small GTP-binding proteins switch between an inactive GDP-bound form and an active GTP-bound form. Two classes of regulatory proteins modulate the activity of these small GTP-binding proteins. The first of these includes the **GTPase-activating proteins (GAPs)** and neurofibromin (a product of the neurofibromatosis type 1 gene). GAPs increase the rate at which small GTP-binding proteins hydrolyze bound GTP and thus result in more rapid inactivation. Counteracting the activity of GAPs are **guanine nucleotide exchange proteins (GEFs)** such as "son of sevenless" or SOS, which promote the conversion of inactive Ras-GDP to active Ras-GTP. Interestingly, cAMP directly activates several GEFs, such as Epac (exchange protein activated by cAMP), demonstrating crosstalk between a classical heterotrimeric G protein signaling pathway and the small Ras-like G proteins.

G PROTEIN SECOND MESSENGERS: CYCLIC NUCLEOTIDES

cAMP usually exerts its effect by increasing the activity of protein kinase A

Activation of G_s-coupled receptors results in the stimulation of adenylyl cyclase and a rise in intracellular concentrations of cAMP (Fig. 3-5A). The downstream effects of this increase in $[cAMP]_i$ depend on the specialized functions that the responding cell carries out in the organism. For example, in the adrenal cortex, ACTH stimulation of cAMP production results in the secretion of aldosterone and cortisol; in the kidney, vasopressin-induced changes in cAMP levels facilitate water reabsorption (see Chapters 38 and 50). Excess cAMP is also responsible for certain pathologic conditions. One is **cholera** (see the box on page 57, titled Action of Toxins on Heterotrimeric G Proteins). Another pathologic process associated with excess cAMP is **McCune-Albright syndrome**, characterized by a triad of (1) variable hyperfunction of multiple endocrine glands, including precocious puberty in girls, (2) bone lesions, and (3) pigmented skin lesions (café au lait spots). This disorder is caused by a somatic mutation that constitutively activates the G protein α_s subunit in a mosaic pattern.

cAMP exerts many of its effects through **cAMP-dependent protein kinase A (PKA)**. This enzyme catalyzes transfer of the terminal phosphate of ATP to certain **serine or threonine residues** within selected proteins. PKA phosphorylation sites are present in a multitude of intracellular proteins, including ion channels, receptors, and signaling pathway proteins. Phosphorylation of these sites can influence either the localization or the activity of the substrate. For example, phosphorylation of the β_2-adrenergic receptor causes receptor desensitization in neurons, whereas phosphorylation of the cystic fibrosis transmembrane conductance regulator (CFTR) increases its Cl^- channel activity.

To enhance regulation of phosphorylation events, the cell tightly controls the activity of PKA so that the enzyme can respond to subtle—and local—variations in cAMP levels. One important control mechanism is the use of **regulatory subunits** that constitutively inhibit PKA. In the absence of cAMP, two catalytic subunits of PKA associate with two of these regulatory subunits, resulting in a heterotetrameric protein complex that has a low level of catalytic activity (Fig. 3-6). Binding of cAMP to the regulatory subunits induces a conformational change that diminishes their affinity for the catalytic subunits, and the subsequent dissociation of the complex results in activation of kinase activity. In addition to the short-term effects of PKA activation noted before, the free catalytic subunit of PKA can also enter the nucleus, where substrate phosphorylation can activate the transcription of specific PKA-dependent genes (see Chapter 4). Although most cells use the same catalytic subunit, different regulatory subunits are found in different cell types.

Another mechanism that contributes to regulation of PKA is the targeting of the enzyme to specific subcellular locations. Such targeting promotes the preferential phosphorylation of substrates that are confined to precise locations within the cell. PKA targeting is achieved by the

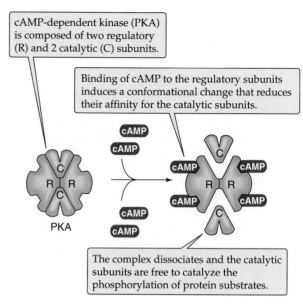

Figure 3-6 Activation of protein kinase A by cAMP.

association of a PKA regulatory subunit with an **A kinase anchoring protein** (AKAP), which in turn binds to cytoskeletal elements or to components of cellular subcompartments. More than 35 AKAPs are known. The specificity of PKA targeting is highlighted by the observation that in neurons, PKA is localized to postsynaptic densities through its association with AKAP79. This anchoring protein also targets calcineurin—a protein phosphatase—to the same site. This targeting of both PKA and calcineurin to the same postsynaptic site makes it possible for the cell to tightly regulate the phosphorylation state of important neuronal substrates.

The cAMP generated by adenylyl cyclase does not interact only with PKA. For example, olfactory receptors (see Chapter 15) interact with a member of the G_s family called G_{olf}. The rise in $[cAMP]_i$ that results from activation of the olfactory receptor activates a cation channel, a member of the family of **cyclic nucleotide–gated (CNG) ion channels**. Na^+ influx through this channel leads to membrane depolarization and the initiation of a nerve impulse.

For his work in elucidating the role played by cAMP as a second messenger in regulating glycogen metabolism, Earl Sutherland received the 1971 Nobel Prize in Physiology or Medicine. In 1992, Edmond Fischer and Edwin Krebs shared the prize for their part in demonstrating the role of protein phosphorylation in the signal transduction process.

This coordinated set of phosphorylation and dephosphorylation reactions has several physiological advantages. First, it allows a single molecule (e.g., cAMP) to regulate a range of enzymatic reactions. Second, it affords a large amplification to a small signal. The concentration of epinephrine needed to stimulate glycogenolysis in muscle is $\sim 10^{-10}$ M. This subnanomolar level of hormone can raise $[cAMP]_i$ to $\sim 10^{-6}$ M. Thus, the catalytic cascades amplify the hormone signal 10,000-fold, resulting in the liberation of enough glucose to raise blood glucose levels from ~ 5 to ~ 8 mM. Although the effects of cAMP on the synthesis and degradation of glycogen are confined to muscle and liver, a wide variety of cells use cAMP-mediated activation cascades in the response to a wide variety of hormones.

Protein phosphatases reverse the action of kinases

As discussed, one way that the cell can terminate a cAMP signal is to use a phosphodiesterase to degrade cAMP. In this way, the subsequent steps along the signaling pathway can also be terminated. However, because the downstream effects of cAMP often involve phosphorylation of effector proteins at serine and threonine residues by kinases such as PKA, another powerful way to terminate the action of cAMP is to dephosphorylate these effector proteins. Such dephosphorylation events are mediated by enzymes called serine/threonine phosphoprotein phosphatases.

Four groups of **serine/threonine phosphoprotein phosphatases (PP)** are known, 1, 2a, 2b, and 2c. These enzymes themselves are regulated by phosphorylation at their serine, threonine, and tyrosine residues. The balance between kinase and phosphatase activity plays a major role in the control of signaling events.

PP1 dephosphorylates many proteins phosphorylated by PKA, including those phosphorylated in response to epinephrine (see Chapter 58). Another protein, **phosphoprotein phosphatase inhibitor 1 (I-1)**, can bind to and inhibit PP1. Interestingly, PKA phosphorylates and thus activates I-1 (Fig. 3-7), thereby inhibiting PP1 and preserving the phosphate groups added by PKA in the first place.

PP2a, which is less specific than PP1, appears to be the main phosphatase responsible for reversing the action of other protein serine/threonine kinases. The Ca^{2+}-dependent PP2b, also known as **calcineurin**, is prevalent in the brain, skeletal muscle, and cardiac muscle and is also the target of the immunosuppressive reagents FK-506 and cyclosporine. The importance of PP2c is presently unclear.

In addition to serine/threonine kinases such as PKA, a second group of kinases involved in regulating signaling pathways (discussed later in this chapter) are known as **tyrosine kinases** because they phosphorylate their substrate proteins on tyrosine residues. The enzymes that remove phosphates from these tyrosine residues are much more variable than the serine and threonine phosphatases. The first **phosphotyrosine phosphatase (PTP)** to be characterized was the *cytosolic* enzyme PTP1B from human placenta. PTP1B has a high degree of homology with **CD45**, a *membrane protein* that is both a receptor and a tyrosine phosphatase. cDNA sequence analysis has identified a large number of PTPs that can be divided into two classes: membrane-spanning receptor-like proteins such as CD45 and cytosolic forms such as PTP1B. A number of intracellular PTPs contain so-called Src homology 2 (**SH2**) **domains**, a peptide sequence or motif that interacts with phosphorylated tyrosine groups. Several of the PTPs are themselves regulated by phosphorylation.

cGMP exerts its effect by stimulating a nonselective cation channel in the retina

cGMP is another cyclic nucleotide that is involved in G protein signaling events. In the outer segments of rods and cones in the visual system, the G protein does not couple to an enzyme that *generates* cGMP but, as noted earlier, couples to an enzyme that breaks it down. As discussed further in Chapter 15, light activates a GPCR called **rhodopsin**, which activates the G protein **transducin**, which in turn activates the **cGMP phosphodiesterase** that lowers $[cGMP]_i$. The fall in $[cGMP]_i$ closes cGMP-gated nonselective cation channels that are members of the same family of CNG ion channels that cAMP activates in olfactory signaling (see Chapter 15).

G PROTEIN SECOND MESSENGERS: PRODUCTS OF PHOSPHOINOSITIDE BREAKDOWN

Many messengers bind to receptors that activate phosphoinositide breakdown

Although the phosphatidylinositols (PIs) are minor constituents of cell membranes, they are largely distributed in the internal leaflet of the membrane and play an important role in signal transduction. The inositol sugar moiety of PI molecules (see Fig. 2-2A) can be phosphorylated to yield the two major phosphoinositides that are involved in signal transduction: **phosphatidylinositol 4,5-bisphosphate ($PI_{4,5}P_2$ or PIP_2)** and phosphatidylinositol 3,4,5-trisphosphate ($PI_{3,4,5}P_3$).

Certain membrane-associated receptors act though G proteins (e.g., G_q) that stimulate phospholipase C (PLC) to cleave PIP_2 into **inositol 1,4,5-trisphosphate (IP_3)** and **diacylglycerol (DAG)**, as shown in Figure 3-8A. PLCs are classified into three families (β, γ, δ) that differ in their catalytic properties, cell type–specific expression, and modes of activation. PLCβ is typically activated downstream of certain G proteins (e.g., G_q), whereas PLCγ contains an SH2 domain

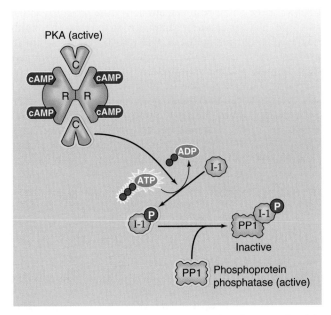

Figure 3-7 Activation of phosphoprotein phosphatase 1 (PP1) by PKA. I-1, inhibitor of PP1.

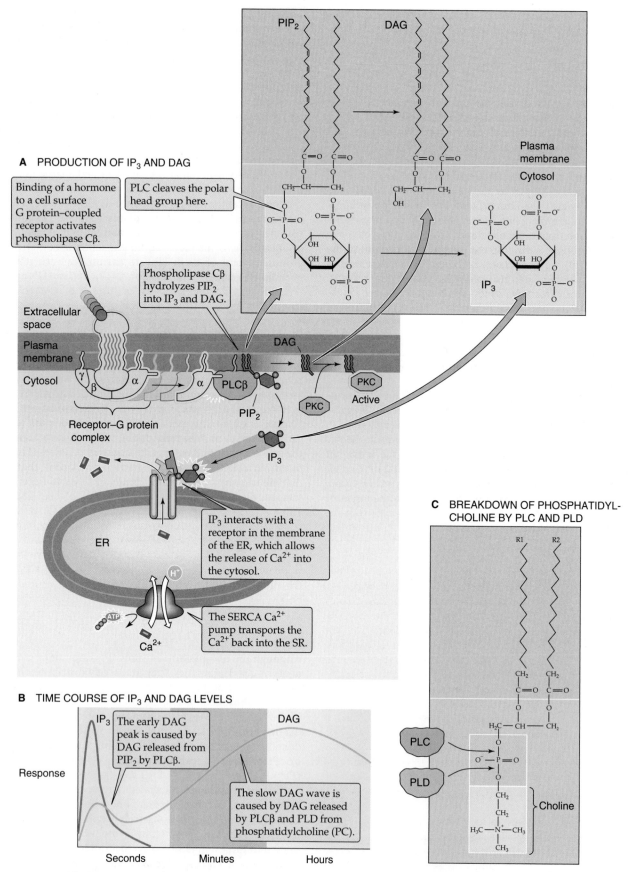

A PRODUCTION OF IP₃ AND DAG

Binding of a hormone to a cell surface G protein–coupled receptor activates phospholipase Cβ.

PLC cleaves the polar head group here.

Phospholipase Cβ hydrolyzes PIP₂ into IP₃ and DAG.

IP₃ interacts with a receptor in the membrane of the ER, which allows the release of Ca²⁺ into the cytosol.

The SERCA Ca²⁺ pump transports the Ca²⁺ back into the SR.

C BREAKDOWN OF PHOSPHATIDYL-CHOLINE BY PLC AND PLD

B TIME COURSE OF IP₃ AND DAG LEVELS

The early DAG peak is caused by DAG released from PIP₂ by PLCβ.

The slow DAG wave is caused by DAG released by PLCβ and PLD from phosphatidylcholine (PC).

Figure 3-8   Second messengers in the DAG/IP₃ pathway. ER, endoplasmic reticulum; SERCA, sarcoplasmic and endoplasmic reticulum Ca²⁺-ATPase.

and is activated downstream of certain tyrosine kinases. Stimulation of PLCβ results in a rapid increase in cytosolic IP$_3$ levels as well as an *early* peak in DAG levels (Fig. 3-8B). Both products are second messengers. DAG remains in the plane of the membrane to activate protein kinase C, which migrates from the cytosol and binds to DAG in the membrane. The water-soluble IP$_3$ travels through the cytosol to stimulate Ca^{2+} release from intracellular stores. It is within this system that Ca^{2+} was first identified as a messenger that mediates the stimulus-response coupling of endocrine cells.

Phosphatidylcholines (PCs), which—unlike PI—are an abundant phospholipid in the cell membrane, are also a source of DAG. The cell can produce DAG from PC by either of two mechanisms (Fig. 3-8C). First, PLC can directly convert PC to phosphocholine and DAG. Second, **phospholipase D (PLD)**, by cleaving the phosphoester bond on the other side of the phosphate, converts PC to choline and phosphatidic acid (PA; also phospho-DAG). This PA can then be converted to DAG by PA-phosphohydrolase. Production of DAG from PC, either directly (by PLC) or indirectly (by PLD), produces the *slow* wave of increasing cytosolic DAG shown in Figure 3-8B. Thus, in some systems, the formation of DAG is biphasic and consists of an early peak that is transient and parallels the formation of IP$_3$, followed by a late phase that is slow in onset but sustained for several minutes.

Factors such as **tumor necrosis factor α (TNF-α)**, **interleukin 1 (IL-1)**, **interleukin 3 (IL-3)**, **interferon α (IFN-α)**, and **colony-stimulating factor** stimulate the production of DAG from PC. Once generated, some DAGs can be further cleaved by DAG lipase to **arachidonic acid**, which can have signaling activity itself or can be metabolized to other signaling molecules, the **eicosanoids**. We cover arachidonic acid metabolism later in this chapter.

Inositol triphosphate liberates Ca^{2+} from intracellular stores

As discussed earlier, IP$_3$ is generated by the metabolism of membrane phospholipids and then travels through the cytosol to release Ca^{2+} from intracellular stores. The **IP$_3$ receptor (ITPR)** is a ligand-gated Ca^{2+} channel located in the membrane of the *endoplasmic* reticulum (Fig. 3-8A). This Ca^{2+} channel is structurally related to the Ca^{2+} release channel (or ryanodine receptor), which is responsible for releasing Ca^{2+} from the *sarcoplasmic* reticulum of muscle and thereby switching on muscle contraction (see Chapter 9). The IP$_3$ receptor is a tetramer composed of subunits of ~260 kDa. At least three genes encode the subunits of the receptor. These genes are subject to alternative splicing, which further increases the potential for receptor diversity. The receptor is a substrate for phosphorylation by protein kinases A and C and calcium-calmodulin (Ca^{2+}-CaM)–dependent protein kinases.

Interaction of IP$_3$ with its receptor results in passive efflux of Ca^{2+} from the endoplasmic reticulum and thus a rapid rise in the free cytosolic Ca^{2+} concentration. The IP$_3$-induced changes in [Ca^{2+}]$_i$ exhibit complex temporal and spatial patterns. The rise in [Ca^{2+}]$_i$ can be brief or persistent and can oscillate repetitively, spread in spirals or waves within a cell,

or spread across groups of cells that are coupled by gap junctions. In at least some systems, the frequency of [Ca^{2+}]$_i$ oscillations seems to be physiologically important. For example, in isolated pancreatic acinar cells, graded increases in the concentration of ACh produce graded increases in the *frequency*—but not the *magnitude*—of repetitive [Ca^{2+}]$_i$ spikes. The mechanisms responsible for [Ca^{2+}]$_i$ oscillations and waves are complex. It appears that both propagation and oscillation depend on positive feedback mechanisms, in which low [Ca^{2+}]$_i$ facilitates Ca^{2+} release, as well as on negative feedback mechanisms, in which high [Ca^{2+}]$_i$ inhibits further Ca^{2+} release.

The dephosphorylation of IP$_3$ terminates the release of Ca^{2+} from intracellular stores; an ATP-fueled Ca^{2+} pump (SERCA; see Chapter 5) then moves the Ca^{2+} back into the endoplasmic reticulum. Some of the IP$_3$ is further phosphorylated to IP$_4$, which may mediate a slower and more prolonged response of the cell or may promote the refilling of intracellular stores. In addition to IP$_3$, **cyclic ADP ribose (cADPR)** can mobilize Ca^{2+} from intracellular stores and augment a process known as calcium-induced Ca^{2+} release. Although the details of these interactions have not been fully elucidated, cADPR appears to bind to the Ca^{2+} release channel (ryanodine receptor) in a Ca^{2+}-CaM–dependent manner.

In addition to the increase in [Ca^{2+}]$_i$ produced by the release of Ca^{2+} from intracellular stores, [Ca^{2+}]$_i$ can also rise as a result of enhanced influx of this ion through Ca^{2+} channels in the plasma membrane. For Ca^{2+} to function as a second messenger, it is critical that [Ca^{2+}]$_i$ be normally maintained at relatively low levels (at or below ~100 nM). Leakage of Ca^{2+} into the cell through Ca^{2+} channels is opposed by the extrusion of Ca^{2+} across the plasma membrane by both an ATP-dependent Ca^{2+} pump and the Na-Ca exchanger (see Chapter 5).

As discussed later, increased [Ca^{2+}]$_i$ exerts its effect by binding to cellular proteins and changing their activity. Some Ca^{2+}-dependent signaling events are so sensitive to Ca^{2+} that a [Ca^{2+}]$_i$ increase of as little as 100 nM can trigger a vast array of cellular responses. These responses include secretion of digestive enzymes by pancreatic acinar cells, release of insulin by β cells, contraction of vascular smooth muscle, conversion of glycogen to glucose in the liver, release of histamine by mast cells, aggregation of platelets, and DNA synthesis and cell division in fibroblasts.

Calcium activates calmodulin-dependent protein kinases

How does an increase in [Ca^{2+}]$_i$ lead to downstream responses in the signal transduction cascade? The effects of changes in [Ca^{2+}]$_i$ are mediated by Ca^{2+}-binding proteins, the most important of which is **calmodulin (CaM)**. CaM is a high-affinity cytoplasmic Ca^{2+}-binding protein of 148 amino acids. Each molecule of CaM cooperatively binds four calcium ions. Ca^{2+} binding induces a major conformational change in CaM that allows it to bind to other proteins (Fig. 3-9). Although CaM does not have intrinsic enzymatic activity, it forms a complex with a number of enzymes and thereby confers a Ca^{2+} dependence on their activity. For example, binding of the Ca^{2+}-CaM complex activates the enzyme that degrades cAMP, cAMP phosphodiesterase.

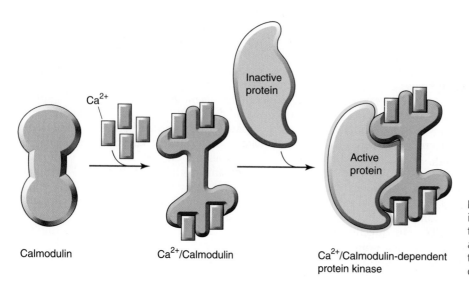

Figure 3-9 Calmodulin. After four intracellular Ca^{2+} ions bind to calmodulin, the Ca^{2+}-CaM complex can bind to and activate another protein. In this example, the activated protein is a Ca^{2+}-CaM–dependent kinase.

Many of the effects of CaM occur as the Ca^{2+}-CaM complex binds to and activates a family of Ca^{2+}-CaM–dependent kinases (**CaM kinases**). These kinases phosphorylate certain serine and threonine residues of a variety of proteins. An important CaM kinase in smooth muscle cells is myosin light chain kinase (MLCK) (see Chapter 9). Another CaM kinase is glycogen phosphorylase kinase (PK), which plays a role in glycogen degradation (see Chapter 58).

MLCK, PK, and some other CaM kinases have a rather narrow substrate specificity. The ubiquitous CaM kinase II, on the other hand, has a broad substrate specificity. Especially high levels of this multifunctional enzyme are present at the synaptic terminals of neurons. One of the actions of CaM kinase II is to phosphorylate and thereby activate the rate-limiting enzyme (tyrosine hydroxylase; see Fig. 13-8C) in the synthesis of catecholamine neurotransmitters. CaM kinase can also phosphorylate itself, which allows it to remain active in the absence of Ca^{2+}.

Diacylglycerols and Ca^{2+} activate protein kinase C

As noted earlier, hydrolysis of PIP_2 by PLC yields not only the IP_3 that leads to Ca^{2+} release from internal stores but also DAG (Fig. 3-8A). The most important function of DAG is to activate **protein kinase C (PKC)**, a serine/threonine kinase. In mammals, the PKC family comprises at least 10 members that differ in their tissue and cellular localization. This family is further subdivided into three groups that all require membrane-associated phosphatidylserine but have different requirements for Ca^{2+} and DAG. The *classical* PKC family members PKCα, PKCβ, and PKCγ require both DAG and Ca^{2+} for activation, whereas the *novel* PKCs (such as PKCδ, PKCε, and PKCη) are independent of Ca^{2+}, and the *atypical* PKCs (PKCζ and PKCλ) appear to be independent of both DAG and Ca^{2+}. As a consequence, the signals generated by the PKC pathway depend on the isoforms of the enzyme that a cell expresses as well as on the levels of Ca^{2+} and DAG at specific locations at the cell membrane.

In its basal state, PKCα is an inactive, soluble cytosolic protein. When Ca^{2+} binds to cytosolic PKC, PKC can interact with DAG, which is located in the inner leaflet of the plasma membrane. This interaction with DAG activates PKCα by raising its affinity for Ca^{2+}. This process is often referred to as translocation of PKC from the cytoplasm to the membrane. In most cells, the Ca^{2+} signal is transient, whereas the resulting physiological responses, such as proliferation and differentiation, often persist substantially longer. Sustained activation of PKCα may be essential for maintaining these responses. Elevated levels of active PKCα are maintained by a slow wave of elevated DAG (Fig. 3-8B), which is due to the hydrolysis of PC by PLC and PLD.

Physiological stimulation of the classical and novel PKCs by DAG can be mimicked by the exogenous application of a class of tumor promoters called **phorbol esters**. These plant products bind to these PKCs, cause them to translocate to the plasma membrane, and thus specifically activate them even in the absence of DAG.

Among the major substrates of PKC are the myristoylated, alanine-rich C kinase substrate (**MARCKS**) proteins. These acidic proteins contain consensus sites for PKC phosphorylation as well as CaM- and actin-binding sites. MARCKS proteins cross-link actin filaments and thus appear to play a role in translating extracellular signals into actin plasticity and changes in cell shape. Unphosphorylated MARCKS proteins are associated with the plasma membrane, and they cross-link actin. Phosphorylation of the MARCKS proteins causes them to translocate into the cytosol, where they are no longer able to cross-link actin. Thus, mitogenic growth factors that activate PKC may produce morphological changes and anchorage-independent cell proliferation, in part by modifying the activity of MARCKS proteins.

PKC can also directly or indirectly modulate transcription factors and thereby enhance the transcription of specific genes (see Chapter 4). Such genomic actions of PKC explain why phorbol esters are tumor promoters.

G PROTEIN SECOND MESSENGERS: ARACHIDONIC ACID METABOLITES

As previously discussed, PLC can hydrolyze PIP$_2$ and thereby release two important signaling molecules, IP$_3$ and DAG. In addition, both PLC and PLD can release DAG from PC. However, other hydrolysis products of membrane phospholipids can also act as signaling molecules. The best characterized of these hydrolysis products is **arachidonic acid (AA)**, which is attached by an ester bond to the second carbon of the glycerol backbone of membrane phospholipids (Fig. 3-10). Phospholipase A$_2$ initiates the cellular actions of AA by releasing this fatty acid from glycerol-based phospholipids. A series of enzymes subsequently convert AA into a family of biologically active metabolites that are collectively called **eicosanoids** (from the Greek *eikosi* for 20) because, like AA, they all have 20 carbon atoms. Three major pathways can convert AA into these eicosanoids (Fig. 3-11). In the first pathway, cyclooxygenase enzymes produce *thromboxanes, prostaglandins,* and *prostacyclins.* In the second pathway, 5-lipoxygenase enzymes produce *leukotrienes* and some hydroxyeicosatetraenoic acid *(HETE)* compounds. In the third pathway, the epoxygenase enzymes, which are members of the cytochrome P-450 class, produce other *HETE* compounds as well as *cis*-epoxyeicosatrienoic acid *(EET)* compounds. These three enzymes catalyze the stereospecific insertion of molecular O$_2$ into various positions in AA. The cyclooxygenases, lipoxygenases, and epoxygenases are selectively distributed in different cell types, further increasing the complexity of eicosanoid biology. Eicosanoids have powerful biological activities, including effects on allergic and inflammatory processes, platelet aggregation, vascular smooth muscle, and gastric acid secretion.

Phospholipase A$_2$ is the primary enzyme responsible for releasing arachidonic acid

The first step in the phospholipase A$_2$ (PLA$_2$) signal transduction cascade is binding of an extracellular agonist to a membrane receptor (Fig. 3-11). These receptors include those for serotonin (5-HT$_2$ receptors), glutamate (mGLUR1 receptors), fibroblast growth factor-ß, IFN-α, and IFN-γ. Once the receptor is occupied by its agonist, it can activate a G protein that belongs to the G$_i$/G$_o$ family. The mechanism by which this activated G protein stimulates PLA$_2$ is not well understood. It does not appear that a G protein α subunit is involved. The G protein ßγ dimer may stimulate PLA$_2$ either directly or through mitogen-activated protein **(MAP) kinase** (see Chapter 4), which phosphorylates PLA$_2$ at a serine residue. The result is rapid hydrolysis of phospholipids that contain AA.

In contrast to the *direct* pathway just mentioned, agonists acting on other receptors may promote AA release indirectly. First, a ligand may bind to a receptor coupled to PLC, which would lead to the release of DAG (Fig. 3-11). As noted earlier, DAG lipase can cleave DAG to yield AA and a monoacylglycerol. Agonists that act through this pathway include dopamine (D$_2$ receptors), adenosine (A$_1$ receptors), norepinephrine (α$_2$-adrenergic receptors), and serotonin (5-HT$_1$ receptors). Second, any agonist that raises [Ca^{2+}]$_i$ can promote AA formation because Ca^{2+} can stimulate some cytosolic forms of PLA$_2$. Third, any signal transduction pathway that activates MAP kinase can also enhance AA release because MAP kinase phosphorylates PLA$_2$.

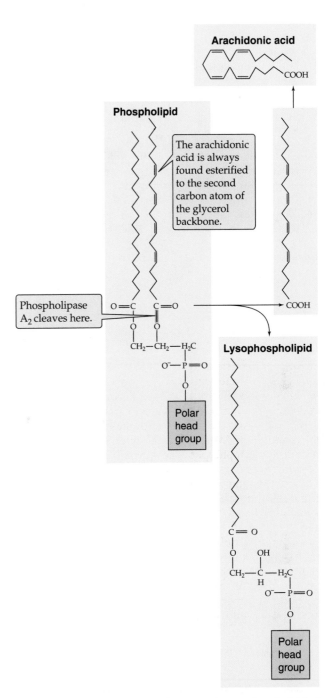

Figure 3-10 Release of AA from membrane phospholipids by PLA$_2$. AA is esterified to membrane phospholipids at the second carbon of the glycerol backbone. PLA$_2$ cleaves the phospholipid at the indicated position and releases AA as well as a lysophospholipid.

Cyclooxygenases, lipoxygenases, and epoxygenases mediate the formation of biologically active eicosanoids

Once it is released from the membrane, AA can diffuse out of the cell, be reincorporated into membrane phospholipids, or be metabolized (Fig. 3-11).

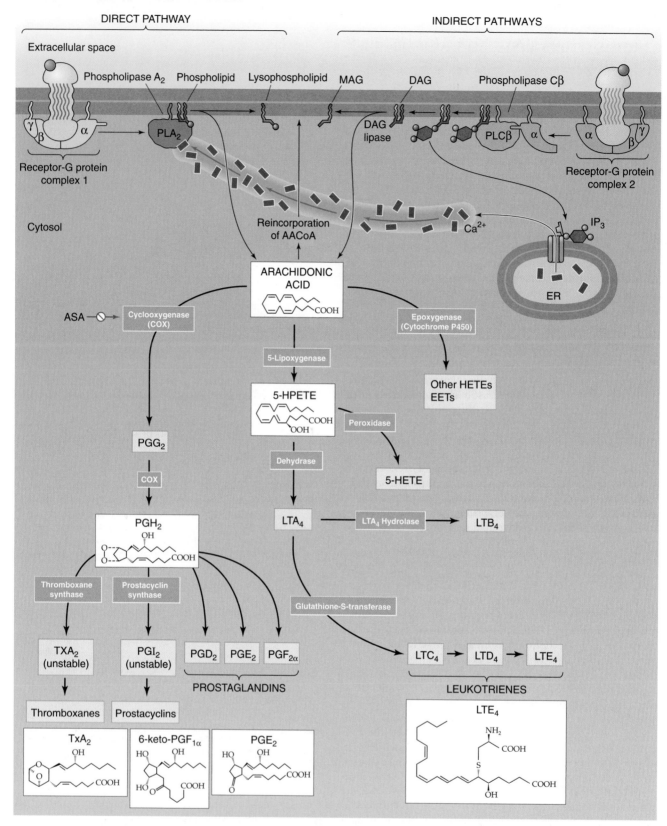

Figure 3-11 AA signaling pathways. In the direct pathway, an agonist binds to a receptor that activates PLA$_2$, which releases AA from a membrane phospholipid (see Fig. 3-10). In one of three indirect pathways, an agonist binds to a different receptor that activates PLC and thereby leads to the formation of DAG and IP$_3$, as in Figure 3-8; DAG lipase then releases the AA from DAG. In a second indirect pathway, the IP$_3$ releases Ca^{2+} from internal stores, which leads to the activation of PLA$_2$ (see the direct pathway). In a third indirect pathway (not shown), mitogen-activated protein kinase stimulates PLA$_2$. Regardless of its source, the AA may follow any of three pathways to form a wide array of eicosanoids. The cyclooxygenase pathway produces thromboxanes, prostacyclins, and prostaglandins. The 5-lipoxygenase pathway produces 5-HETE and the leukotrienes. The epoxygenase pathway leads to the production of other HETEs and EETs. ASA, acetylsalicylic acid; EET, *cis*-epoxyeicosatrienoic acid; ER, endoplasmic reticulum; HETE, hydroxyeicosatetraenoic acid; HPETE, hydroperoxyeicosatetraenoic acid; MAG, monoacylglycerol.

In the first pathway of AA metabolism (Fig. 3-11), **cyclo-oxygenases** catalyze the stepwise conversion of AA into the intermediates prostaglandin G_2 (PGG$_2$) and prostaglandin H_2 (PGH$_2$). PGH$_2$ is the precursor of the other **prostaglandins**, the **prostacyclins** and the **thromboxanes**. As noted in the box titled Inhibition of Cyclooxygenase Isoforms by Aspirin, cyclooxygenase exists in two isoforms, COX-1 and COX-2. In many cells, COX-1 is expressed in a constitutive fashion, whereas COX-2 levels can be induced by specific stimuli. For example, in monocytes stimulated by inflammatory agents such as IL-1β, only levels of COX-2 increase. These observations have led to the concept that expression of COX-1 is important for homeostatic prostaglandin functions such as platelet aggregation and regulation of vascular tone, whereas upregulation of COX-2 is primarily important for mediating prostaglandin-dependent inflammatory responses. However, as selective inhibitors of COX-2 have become available, it has become clear that this is an oversimplification.

In the second pathway of AA metabolism, **5-lipoxygenase** initiates the conversion of AA into biologically active **leukotrienes**. For example, in myeloid cells, 5-lipoxygenase converts AA to 5-HPETE, which is short-lived and rapidly degraded by a peroxidase to the corresponding alcohol 5-HETE. Alternatively, a dehydrase can convert 5-HPETE to an unstable epoxide, LTA$_4$, which can be either further metabolized by LTA$_4$ hydrolase to LTB$_4$ or coupled ("conjugated") to the tripeptide glutathione (see Chapter 46). This conjugation—through the cysteine residue of glutathione—yields LTC$_4$. Enzymes sequentially remove portions of the glutathione moiety to produce LTD$_4$ and LTE$_4$. LTC$_4$, LTD$_4$, and LTE$_4$ are the "cysteinyl" leukotrienes; they participate in allergic and inflammatory responses and make up the mixture previously described as the **slow-reacting substance of anaphylaxis**.

The third pathway of AA metabolism begins with the transformation of AA by **epoxygenase** (a cytochrome P-450 oxidase). Molecular O$_2$ is a substrate in this reaction. The epoxygenase pathway converts AA into two major products, **HETEs** and **EETs**. Members of both groups display a diverse array of biological activities. Moreover, the cells of different tissues (e.g., liver, kidney, eye, and pituitary) use different biosynthetic pathways to generate different epoxygenase products.

Prostaglandins, prostacyclins, and thromboxanes (cyclooxygenase products) are vasoactive, regulate platelet action, and modulate ion transport

The metabolism of PGH$_2$ to generate selected prostanoid derivatives is cell specific. For example, platelets convert PGH$_2$ to **thromboxane A$_2$ (TXA$_2$)**, a short-lived compound that can aggregate platelets, bring about the platelet release reaction, and constrict small blood vessels. In contrast, endothelial cells convert PGH$_2$ to **prostacyclin I$_2$** (also known as PGI$_2$), which *inhibits* platelet aggregation and *dilates* blood vessels. Many cell types convert PGH$_2$ to prostaglandins. Acting locally in a paracrine or autocrine fashion, **prostaglandins** are involved in such processes as platelet aggregation, airway constriction, renin release, and inflammation.

Eicosanoid Nomenclature

The nomenclature of the eicosanoids is not as arcane as it might first appear. The numerical subscript 2 (as in PGH$_2$) or 4 (as in LTA$_4$) refers to the number of double bonds in the eicosanoid backbone. For example, AA has four double bonds, as do the leukotrienes.

For the cyclooxygenase metabolites, the letter (A to I) immediately preceding the 2 refers to the structure of the 5-carbon ring that is formed about halfway along the 20-carbon chain of the eicosanoid. For the leukotrienes, the letters A and B that immediately precede the 4 refer to differences in the eicosanoid backbone. For the cysteinyl leukotrienes, the letter C refers to the full glutathione conjugate (see Fig. 46-8). Removal of glutamate from LTC$_4$ yields LTD$_4$, and removal of glycine from LTD$_4$ yields LTE$_4$, leaving behind only cysteine.

For 5-HPETE and 5-HETE, the fifth carbon atom (counting the carboxyl group as number 1) is derivatized with a hydroperoxy- or hydroxy- group, respectively.

Inhibition of Cyclooxygenase Isoforms by Aspirin

Cyclooxygenase is a bifunctional enzyme that first oxidizes AA to PGG$_2$ through its *cyclooxygenase* activity and then *peroxidizes* this compound to PGH$_2$. Cyclooxygenase exists in two forms, COX-1 and COX-2. X-ray crystallographic studies of **COX-1** reveal that the sites for the two enzymatic activities (i.e., cyclooxygenase and peroxidase) are adjacent but spatially distinct. The cyclooxygenase site is a long hydrophobic channel. **Aspirin** (acetylsalicylic acid) irreversibly inhibits COX-1 by acetylating a serine residue at the top of this channel. Several of the other nonsteroidal anti-inflammatory drugs (NSAIDs) interact, through their carboxyl groups, with other amino acids in the same region.

COX-1 activation plays an important role in intravascular thrombosis as it leads to **thromboxane A$_2$** synthesis by platelets. Inhibition of this process by low-dose aspirin is a mainstay for prevention of coronary thrombosis in patients with atherosclerotic coronary artery disease. However, COX-1 activation is also important for producing cytoprotective **prostacyclins** in the gastric mucosa. It is the loss of these compounds that can lead to the unwanted side effect of gastrointestinal bleeding after chronic aspirin ingestion.

Inflammatory stimuli induce **COX-2** in a number of cell types, and it is inhibition of COX-2 that provides the anti-inflammatory actions of high-dose aspirin (a weak COX-2 inhibitor) and other nonselective cyclooxygenase inhibitors such as **ibuprofen**. Because the two enzymes are only 60% homologous, pharmaceutical companies have now generated compounds that specifically inhibit COX-2, such as **rofecoxib** and **celecoxib**. These work well as anti-inflammatory agents and have a reduced likelihood of causing gastrointestinal bleeding because they do not inhibit COX-1–dependent prostacyclin production. At least one of the selective COX-2 inhibitors has been reported to increase the risk of thrombotic cardiovascular events when it is taken for long periods.

Prostaglandin synthesis has also been implicated in the pathophysiological mechanisms of cardiovascular disease, cancer, and inflammatory diseases. NSAIDs such as aspirin, acetaminophen, ibuprofen, indomethacin, and naproxen directly target cyclooxygenase. NSAID inhibition of cyclooxygenase is a useful tool in the treatment of inflammation and fever and, at least in the case of aspirin, in the prevention of heart disease.

The diverse cellular responses to prostanoids are mediated by a family of G protein–coupled **prostanoid receptors**. This family currently has nine proposed members, including receptors for thromboxane/prostaglandin H_2 (TP), PGI_2 (IP), PGE_2 (EP_{1-4}), PGD_2 (DP and CRTH2), and $PGF_{2\alpha}$ (FP). These prostanoid receptors signal through G_q, G_i, or G_s, depending on cell type. These in turn regulate intracellular adenylyl cyclase and phospholipases.

The leukotrienes (5-lipoxygenase products) play a major role in inflammatory responses

The biological effects of many lipoxygenase metabolites of AA have led to the suggestion that they have a role in allergic and inflammatory diseases (Table 3-3). LTB_4 is produced by inflammatory cells such as neutrophils and macrophages. The cysteinyl leukotrienes including **LTC_4** and **LTE_4** are synthesized by mast cells, basophils, and eosinophils, cells that are commonly associated with allergic inflammatory responses such as **asthma** and **urticaria**.

The **cysteinyl leukotriene receptors** cysLT1 and cysLT2 are GPCRs found on airway smooth muscle cells as well as on eosinophils, mast cells, and lymphocytes. CysLT1, which couples to both pertussis toxin–sensitive and pertussis

toxin–insensitive G proteins, mediates phospholipase-dependent increases in $[Ca^{2+}]_i$. In the airways, these events produce a potent bronchoconstriction, whereas activation of the receptor in mast cells and eosinophils causes release of the proinflammatory cytokines histamine and TNF-α.

In addition to their role in the inflammatory response, the lipoxygenase metabolites can also influence the activity of many ion channels, either directly or by regulating protein kinases. For example, in synaptic nerve endings, lipoxygenase metabolites decrease the excitability of cells by activating K^+ channels. Lipoxygenase products may also regulate secretion. In pancreatic islet cells, free AA generated in response to glucose appears to be part of a negative feedback loop that prevents excess insulin secretion by inhibiting CaM kinase II.

The HETEs and EETs (epoxygenase products) tend to enhance Ca^{2+} release from intracellular stores and to enhance cell proliferation

The epoxygenase pathway leads to the production of HETEs other than 5-HETE as well as EETs. HETEs and EETs have

Table 3-3 Involvement of Leukotrienes in Human Disease

Disease	Evidence
Asthma	Bronchoconstriction from inhaled LTE_4; identification of LTC_4, LTD_4, and LTE_4 in the serum or urine or both of patients with asthma
Psoriasis	LTB_4 and LTE_4 found in fluids from psoriatic lesions
Adult respiratory distress syndrome	Elevated levels of LTB_4 detected in the plasma of patients with ARDS
Allergic rhinitis	Elevated levels of LTB_4 found in nasal fluids
Gout	LTB_4 detected in joint fluid
Rheumatoid arthritis	Elevated LTB_4 found in joint fluids and serum
Inflammatory bowel disease (ulcerative colitis and Crohn disease)	Identification of LTB_4 in gastrointestinal fluids and LTE_4 in urine

Role of Leukotrienes in Disease

Since the original description of the slow-reacting substance of anaphylaxis, which is generated during antigenic challenge of a sensitized lung, leukotrienes have been presumed to play a part in allergic disease of the airways (Table 3-3). The involvement of cells (mast cells, basophils, and eosinophils) that produce cysteinyl leukotrienes (LTC_4 through LTF_4) in these pathobiological processes supports this concept. In addition, the levels of LTC_4, LTD_4, and LTE_4 are increased in lavage fluid from the nares of patients with allergic rhinitis after the application of specific antigens to the nasal airways. Introducing LTC_4 or LTD_4 into the airways as an aerosol (nebulizer concentration of only 10 µM) causes maximal expiratory airflow (a rough measure of airway resistance; see Chapter 27) to decline by ~30%. This bronchoconstrictor effect is 1000-fold more potent than that of histamine, the "reference" agonist. Leukotrienes affect both large and small airways; histamine affects relatively smaller airways. Activation of the cysLT1 receptor in mast cells and eosinophils results in the chemotaxis of these cells to sites of inflammation. Because antagonists of the cysLT1 receptor (e.g., **montelukast sodium**) can partially block these bronchoconstrictive and proinflammatory effects, these agents are useful in the treatment of allergen-induced asthma and rhinitis.

In addition to their involvement in allergic disease, several of the leukotrienes are associated with other inflammatory disorders. Synovial fluid from patients with **rheumatoid arthritis** contains 5-lipoxygenase products. Another example is the skin disease **psoriasis**. In patients with active psoriasis, LTB_4, LTC_4, and LTD_4 have been recovered from skin chambers overlying abraded lesions. Leukotrienes also appear to be involved in inflammatory bowel disease. LTB_4 and other leukotrienes are generated and released in vitro from intestinal mucosa obtained from patients with **ulcerative colitis** or **Crohn disease**.

Table 3-4 Actions of Epoxygenase Products

	Cell/Tissue	Action
HETEs	Stimulated mononuclear leukocytes	↑ Cell proliferation
		↑ Ca^{2+} release from intracellular stores
		↓ TNF production
	β Cells of pancreatic islets	Implicated in the destruction of these cells in type 1 (juvenile-onset) diabetes mellitus
		↓ Release of fibrinolytic factors
		↓ Binding of antithrombin
	Endothelial cells	↑ Cell proliferation
		↑ Migration
	Vascular smooth muscle cells	Formation of atherosclerotic plaque?
		Potent vasoconstrictors
		"Myogenic" vasoconstrictive response of renal and cerebral arteries
	Blood vessels	
EETs	Cells, general	↑ Ca^{2+} release from intracellular stores
		↑ Na-H exchange
		↑ Cell proliferation
		↓ Cyclooxygenase activity
	Endocrine cells	↓ Release of somatostatin, insulin, glucagon
	Toad bladder	↓ Vasopressin-stimulated H_2O permeability
		↓ Renin release
	Blood vessels	Vasodilation
		Angiogenesis
	Endothelium	↑ Tumor cell adhesion
	Platelets	↓ Aggregation

been implicated in a wide variety of processes, some of which are summarized in Table 3-4. For example, in stimulated mononuclear leukocytes, **HETEs** enhance Ca^{2+} release from intracellular stores and promote cell proliferation. In smooth muscle cells, HETEs increase proliferation and migration; these AA metabolites may be one of the primary factors involved in the formation of atherosclerotic plaque. In blood vessels, HETEs can be potent vasoconstrictors. **EETs** enhance the release of Ca^{2+} from intracellular stores, increase Na-H exchange, and stimulate cell proliferation. In blood vessels, EETs primarily induce vasodilation and angiogenesis, although they have vasoconstrictive properties in the smaller pulmonary blood vessels.

Degradation of the eicosanoids terminates their activity

Inactivation of the products of eicosanoids is an important mechanism for terminating their biological action. In the case of cyclooxygenase products, the enzyme 15-hydroxy-prostaglandin dehydrogenase catalyzes the initial reactions that convert biologically active prostaglandins into their inactive 15-keto metabolites. This enzyme also appears to be active in the catabolism of thromboxanes.

As far as the 5-lipoxygenase products are concerned, the specificity and cellular distribution of the enzymes that metabolize leukotrienes parallel the diversity of the enzymes involved in their synthesis. For example, 20-hydrolase-LTB_4, a member of the P-450 family, catalyzes the ω oxidation of LTB_4, thereby terminating its biological activity. LTC_4 is metabolized through two pathways. One oxidizes the LTC_4.

The other pathway first removes the glutamic acid residue of the conjugated glutathione, which yields LTD_4, and then removes the glycine residue, which yields LTE_4, which is readily excreted into the urine.

In the case of epoxygenase (cytochrome P-450) products, it has been difficult to characterize their metabolic breakdown because the reactions are so rapid and complex. Both enzymatic and nonenzymatic hydration reactions convert these molecules to the corresponding vicinyl diols. Some members of this group can form conjugates with reduced glutathione (GSH).

Platelet-activating factor is a lipid mediator unrelated to arachidonic acid

Although it is not a member of the AA family, platelet-activating factor (PAF) is an important lipid signaling molecule. PAF is an *ether* lipid that the cell synthesizes either de novo or by remodeling of a membrane-bound precursor. PAF occurs in a wide variety of organisms and mediates many biological activities. In mammals, PAF is a potent inducer of platelet aggregation and stimulates the chemotaxis and degranulation of neutrophils, thereby facilitating the release of LTB_4 and 5-HETE. PAF is involved in several aspects of allergic reactions; for example, it stimulates histamine release and enhances the secretion of IgE, IgA, and TNF. Endothelial cells are also an important target of PAF; PAF causes a negative shift of V_m in these cells by activating Ca^{2+}-dependent K^+ channels. PAF also enhances vascular permeability and the adhesion of neutrophils and platelets to endothelial cells.

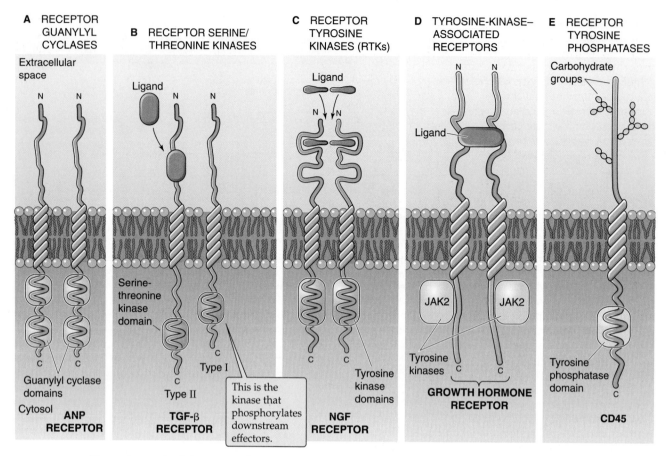

Figure 3-12 Catalytic receptors. **A,** Receptor guanylyl cyclases have an extracellular ligand-binding domain. **B,** Receptor serine/threonine kinases have two subunits. The ligand binds only to the type II subunit. **C,** Receptor tyrosine kinases (RTKs) similar to the NGF receptor dimerize on binding a ligand. **D,** Tyrosine kinase–associated receptors have *no* intrinsic enzyme activity but associate noncovalently with soluble, non-receptor tyrosine kinases. **E,** Receptor tyrosine phosphatases have intrinsic tyrosine phosphatase activity. ANP, atrial natriuretic peptide; JAK, Janus kinase (originally "just another kinase"); NGF, nerve growth factor; TGF-β, transforming growth factor β.

PAF exerts its effects by binding to a specific receptor on the plasma membrane. A major consequence of PAF binding to its GPCR is formation of IP_3 and stimulation of a group of MAP kinases. PAF acetylhydrolase terminates the action of this signaling lipid.

RECEPTORS THAT ARE CATALYTIC

A number of hormones and growth factors bind to cell surface proteins that have—or are associated with—enzymatic activity on the cytoplasmic side of the membrane. Here we discuss five classes of such catalytic receptors (Fig. 3-12):

Receptor guanylyl cyclases catalyze the generation of cGMP from GTP.

Receptor serine/threonine kinases phosphorylate serine or threonine residues on cellular proteins.

Receptor tyrosine kinases (RTKs) phosphorylate tyrosine residues on themselves and other proteins.

Tyrosine kinase–associated receptors interact with cytosolic (i.e., non–membrane bound) tyrosine kinases.

Receptor tyrosine phosphatases cleave phosphate groups from tyrosine groups of cellular proteins.

The receptor guanylyl cyclase transduces the activity of atrial natriuretic peptide, whereas a soluble guanylyl cyclase transduces the activity of nitric oxide

Receptor (Membrane-Bound) Guanylyl Cyclase Some of the best characterized examples of a transmembrane protein with guanylyl cyclase activity (Fig. 3-12A) are the receptors for the natriuretic peptides. These are a family of related small proteins (~28 amino acids) including **atrial natriuretic peptide (ANP)**, B-type or brain natriuretic peptide (BNP), and C-type natriuretic peptide (CNP). For example, in response to atrial stretch, cardiac myocytes release ANP and BNP. ANP and BNP have two major effects. First, they act on vascular smooth muscle to dilate blood vessels (see Chapter 23). Second, they enhance Na^+ excretion into urine, which is termed natriuresis (see Chapter 40). Both activities contribute to lowering of blood pressure and effective circulating blood volume (see Chapter 5).

Natriuretic peptide receptors NPR-A and NPR-B are membrane proteins with a single membrane-spanning segment. The extracellular domain binds the ligand. The intracellular domain has two consensus catalytic domains for guanylyl cyclase activity. Binding of a natriuretic peptide induces a conformational change in the receptor that causes receptor dimerization and activation. Thus, binding of ANP to its receptor causes the conversion of GTP to cGMP and raises intracellular levels of cGMP. In turn, cGMP activates a **cGMP-dependent kinase** (PKG or cGK) that phosphorylates proteins at certain serine and threonine residues. In the renal medullary collecting duct, the cGMP generated in response to ANP may act not only through PKG but also by directly modulating ion channels (see Chapter 35).

Soluble Guanylyl Cyclase In contrast to the receptor for ANP, which is an intrinsic membrane protein with guanylyl cyclase activity, the receptor for **nitric oxide (NO)** is a soluble (i.e., cytosolic) guanylyl cyclase. This soluble guanylyl cyclase (sGC) is totally unrelated to the receptor guanylyl cyclase and contains a heme moiety that binds NO.

NO plays an important role in the control of blood flow and blood pressure. Vascular endothelial cells use the enzyme **NO synthase (NOS)** to cleave arginine into citrulline plus NO in response to stimuli such as ACh, bradykinin, substance P, thrombin, adenine nucleotides, and Ca^{2+}. These agents trigger the entry of Ca^{2+}, which binds to cytosolic CaM and then stimulates NOS. Activation of NOS also requires the cofactors tetrahydrobiopterin and NADPH. The newly synthesized NO rapidly diffuses out of the endothelial cell and crosses the membrane of a neighboring smooth muscle cell. In smooth muscle, NO stimulates its "receptor," soluble guanylyl cyclase, which then converts GTP to cGMP. As a result, $[cGMP]_i$ may increase 50-fold and relax the smooth muscle.

The importance of NO in the control of blood flow had long been exploited unwittingly to treat **angina pectoris**. Angina is the classic chest pain that accompanies inadequate blood flow to the heart muscle, usually as a result of coronary artery atherosclerosis. Nitroglycerin relieves this pain by spontaneously breaking down and releasing NO, which relaxes the smooth muscles of peripheral arterioles, thereby reducing the work of the heart and relieving the associated pain.

In addition to its role as a chemical signal in blood vessels, NO appears to play an important role in the destruction of invading organisms by macrophages and neutrophils. NO also serves as a neurotransmitter and may play a role in learning and memory (see Chapter 13). Some of these actions may involve different forms of NOS.

The importance of the NO signaling pathway was recognized by the awarding of the 1998 Nobel Prize for Physiology or Medicine to R. F. Furchgott, L. J. Ignarro, and F. Murad for their discoveries concerning NO as a signaling molecule in the cardiovascular system.

Some catalytic receptors are serine/threonine kinases

Earlier in this chapter we discussed how activation of various G protein–linked receptors can initiate a cascade that eventually activates kinases (e.g., PKA, PKC) that phosphorylate proteins at serine and threonine residues. In addition, some receptors are *themselves* serine/threonine kinases—such as the one for transforming growth factor β (TGF-β)—and are thus catalytic receptors.

The TGF-β superfamily includes a large group of cytokines, including five TGF-βs, antimüllerian hormone, the inhibins, the activins, bone morphogenic proteins, and other glycoproteins, all of which control cell growth and differentiation. Members of this family participate in embryogenesis, suppress epithelial cell growth, promote wound repair, and influence immune and endocrine functions. Unchecked TGF-β signaling is important in progressive fibrotic disorders (e.g., liver cirrhosis, idiopathic pulmonary fibrosis) that result in replacement of normal organ tissue by deposits of collagen and other matrix components.

The receptors for TGF-β and related factors are glycoproteins with a single membrane-spanning segment and intrinsic serine/threonine kinase activity. Receptor types I and II (Fig. 3-12B) are required for ligand binding and catalytic activity. The **type II receptor** first binds the ligand, followed by the formation of a stable ternary complex of ligand, type II receptor, and type I receptor. Recruitment of the type I receptor into the complex results in phosphorylation of the type I receptor at serine and threonine residues, which in turn activates the kinase activity of the type I receptor and propagates the signal to downstream effectors.

Receptor tyrosine kinases produce phosphotyrosine motifs recognized by SH domains of downstream effectors

In addition to the class of receptors with intrinsic *serine/threonine* kinase activity, other plasma membrane receptors have intrinsic *tyrosine* kinase activity. All **receptor tyrosine kinases** discovered to date phosphorylate themselves in addition to other cellular proteins. Epidermal growth factor (EGF), platelet-derived growth factor (PDGF), vascular endothelial growth factor (VEGF), insulin and insulin-related growth factor type 1 (IGF-1), fibroblast growth factor (FGF), and nerve growth factor (NGF) can all bind to receptors that possess intrinsic tyrosine kinase activity.

Creation of Phosphotyrosine (pY) Motifs Most RTKs are single-pass transmembrane proteins that contain a single intracellular kinase domain (Fig. 3-12C). Binding of a ligand, such as NGF, induces a conformational change in the receptor that facilitates the formation of receptor dimers. Dimerization allows the two cytoplasmic catalytic domains to phosphorylate each other ("autophosphorylation") and thereby activate the receptor complex. The activated receptors also catalyze the addition of phosphate to tyrosine (Y) residues on specific cytoplasmic proteins. The resulting **phosphotyrosine motifs** of the receptor and other protein substrates serve as high-affinity binding sites for a number of intracellular signaling molecules. These interactions lead to the formation of a signaling complex and the activation of downstream effectors. Activation of **insulin** and **IGF-1** receptors occurs by a somewhat different mechanism: the complex analogous to the dimeric NGF receptor exists even before ligand binding, as we will discuss in Chapter 51.

Table 3-5 Tyrosine Phosphopeptides of the PDGF Receptor That Are Recognized by SH2 Domains on Various Proteins

Tyrosine (Y) That Is Phosphorylated in the PDGF Receptor	Phosphotyrosine (PY) Motif Recognized by the SH2-Containing Protein	SH2-Containing Protein
Y579	pYIYVD	Src family kinases
Y708	pYMDMS	p85
Y719	pYVPML	p85
Y739	pYNAPY	GTPase-activating protein
Y1021	pYIIPY	PLCγ

Recognition of pY Motifs by SH2 and SH3 Domains   The phosphotyrosine motifs created by tyrosine kinases serve as high-affinity binding sites for the recruitment of many cytoplasmic or membrane-associated proteins that contain a region such as an SH2 (Src homology 2), SH3 (Src homology 3), or PTB (phosphotyrosine-binding) domains. **SH2** domains are ~100 amino acids in length. They are composed of relatively well conserved residues that form the binding pocket for pY motifs as well as more variable residues that are implicated in binding specificity. These residues that confer binding specificity primarily recognize the three amino acids located on the C-terminal side of the phosphotyrosine. For example, the activated PDGF receptor has five such pY motifs (Table 3-5), each of which interacts with a specific SH2-containing protein.

SH3 domains are ~50 amino acids in length and bind to proline-rich regions in other proteins. Although these interactions are typically constitutive, phosphorylation at distant sites can change protein conformation and thereby regulate the interaction. Like SH2 interactions, SH3 interactions appear to be responsible for targeting of signaling molecules to specific subcellular locations. SH2- or SH3-containing proteins include growth factor receptor-bound protein 2 (GRB2), PLCγ, and the receptor-associated tyrosine kinases of the Src family.

The MAPK Pathway   A common pathway by which activated RTKs transduce their signal to cytosol and even to the nucleus is a cascade of events that increase the activity of the small GTP-binding protein Ras. This **Ras-dependent signaling pathway** involves the following steps (Fig. 3-13):

Step 1: A ligand binds to the extracellular domain of a specific **RTK**, thus causing receptor dimerization.
Step 2: The now-activated RTK phosphorylates itself on tyrosine residues of the cytoplasmic domain (autophosphorylation).
Step 3: **GRB2** (growth factor receptor-bound protein 2), an SH2-containing protein, recognizes pY residues on the activated receptor.
Step 4: Binding of GRB2 recruits **SOS** (son of sevenless), a guanine nucleotide exchange protein.

Step 5: SOS activates **Ras** by causing GTP to replace GDP on Ras.
Step 6: The activated GTP-Ras complex activates other proteins by physically recruiting them to the plasma membrane. In particular, the active GTP-Ras complex interacts with the N-terminal portion of the serine/threonine kinase **Raf-1** (also known as **MAP kinase kinase kinase**), which is the first in a series of sequentially activated protein kinases that ultimately transmits the activation signal.
Step 7: Raf-1 phosphorylates and activates a protein kinase called **MEK** (also known as MAP kinase kinase or MAPKK). MEK is a multifunctional protein kinase that phosphorylates substrates on *both* tyrosine and serine/threonine residues. The JAK system (see next section) also activates MEK.
Step 8: MEK phosphorylates **MAP kinase** (MAPK), also called extracellular signal-regulated kinase (ERK1, ERK2). Activation of MAPK requires dual phosphorylation on neighboring serine and tyrosine residues.
Step 9: MAPK is an important effector molecule in Ras-dependent signal transduction because it phosphorylates many cellular proteins.
Step 10: Activated MAPK also translocates to the nucleus, where it phosphorylates a number of nuclear proteins that are transcription factors. Phosphorylation of a transcription factor by MAPK can enhance or inhibit binding to DNA and thereby enhance or suppress transcription.

Two other signal transduction pathways (cAMP and Ca^{2+}) can modulate the activity of some of the protein intermediates in this MAP kinase cascade, suggesting multiple points of integration for the various signaling systems.

Tyrosine kinase–associated receptors activate loosely associated tyrosine kinases such as Src and JAK

Some of the receptors for cytokines and growth factors that regulate cell proliferation and differentiation do not themselves have *intrinsic* tyrosine kinase activity but can associate with nonreceptor tyrosine kinases (Fig. 3-12D). Receptors in this class include those for several cytokines, including IL-2, IL-3, IL-4, IL-5, IL-6, leukemia inhibitory factor (LIF), granulocyte-macrophage colony-stimulating factor (GM-CSF), and erythropoietin (EPO). The family also includes receptors for growth hormone (GH), prolactin (PRL), leptin, ciliary neurotrophin factor (CNTF), oncostatin M, and IFN-α, IFN-β, and IFN-γ.

The **tyrosine kinase–associated receptors** typically comprise multiple subunits that form homodimers (αα), heterodimers (αβ), or heterotrimers (αβγ). For example, the IL-3 and the GM-CSF receptors are heterodimers (αβ) that share common β subunits with transducing activity. However, none of the cytoplasmic portions of the receptor subunits contains kinase domains or other sequences with recognized catalytic function. Instead, tyrosine kinases of the Src family and Janus family (JAK or Janus kinases) associate noncovalently with the cytoplasmic domains of these receptors. Thus, these are **receptor-associated tyrosine kinases**. Ligand binding to these receptors results in receptor dimerization

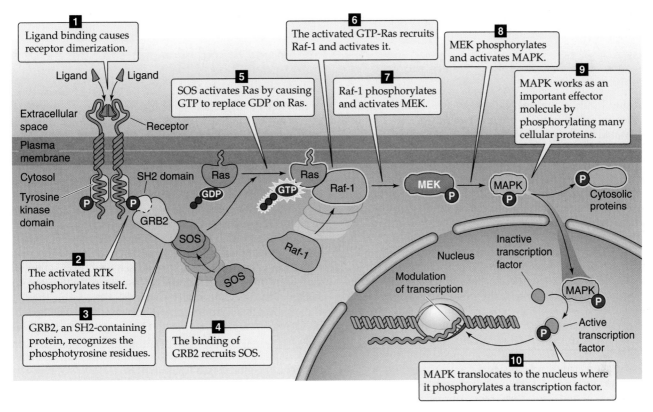

1 Ligand binding causes receptor dimerization.

6 The activated GTP-Ras recruits Raf-1 and activates it.

8 MEK phosphorylates and activates MAPK.

5 SOS activates Ras by causing GTP to replace GDP on Ras.

7 Raf-1 phosphorylates and activates MEK.

9 MAPK works as an important effector molecule by phosphorylating many cellular proteins.

Ligand   Ligand

Extracellular space

Receptor

Plasma membrane

Cytosol

SH2 domain   Ras   Ras   Raf-1   MEK   MAPK   Cytosolic proteins

Tyrosine kinase domain   GDP   GTP

GRB2

SOS   Raf-1   Nucleus   Inactive transcription factor   MAPK

SOS   Modulation of transcription

2 The activated RTK phosphorylates itself.

3 GRB2, an SH2-containing protein, recognizes the phosphotyrosine residues.

4 The binding of GRB2 recruits SOS.

Active transcription factor

10 MAPK translocates to the nucleus where it phosphorylates a transcription factor.

Figure 3-13 Regulation of transcription by the Ras pathway. A ligand, such as a growth factor, binds to a specific RTK, leading to an increase in gene transcription in a 10-step process.

and tyrosine kinase activity. The activated kinase then phosphorylates tyrosines on both itself and the receptor. Thus, tyrosine kinase–associated receptors, together with their tyrosine kinases, function much like the RTKs discussed in the previous section. A key difference is that for the tyrosine kinase–*associated* receptors, the receptors and kinases are encoded by separate genes and the proteins are only loosely associated with one another.

The **Src** family of receptor-associated tyrosine kinases includes at least nine members. Alternative initiation codons and tissue-specific splicing (see Chapter 4) result in at least 14 related gene products.

The conserved regions of Src-related proteins can be divided into five domains: (1) an N-terminal myristilation site, through which the kinase is tethered to the membrane; (2) an SH3 domain, which binds to proline-rich regions of the kinase itself or to other cytosolic proteins; (3) an SH2 domain, which binds phosphorylated tyrosines; (4) the catalytic domain, which has tyrosine kinase activity; and (5) a noncatalytic C terminus. Members of this family are kept in the inactive state by tyrosine phosphorylation at a conserved residue in the C terminus, causing this pY to bind to the amino-terminal SH2 domain of the same molecule, obscuring the intervening kinase domain. Dephosphorylation of the pY residue, after the activation of such phosphatases as RPTPα or SHP-2, releases this inhibition, and the kinase domain can then phosphorylate its intracellular substrates.

Many of the Src family members were first identified in transformed cells or tumors because of mutations that caused them to be constitutively active. When these mutations result in malignant transformation of the cell, the gene in question is designated an **oncogene**; the normal, unaltered physiological counterpart of an oncogene is called a **proto-oncogene**.

The **Janus family** of receptor-associated tyrosine kinases in mammals includes **JAK1, JAK2, and Tyk2**. JAK stands for "just another kinase." Major downstream targets of the JAKs include one or more members of the STAT (signal transducers and activators of transcription) family. When phosphorylated, STATs interact with other STAT family members to form a complex that translocates to the nucleus (see Chapter 4). There, the complex facilitates the transcription of specific genes that are specialized for a rapid response, such as those that are characterized by the **acute-phase response** of inflammation (see Chapter 59). For example, after IL-6 binds to hepatocytes, the STAT pathway is responsible for producing **acute-phase proteins**. During inflammation, these acute-phase proteins function to limit tissue damage by inhibiting the proteases that attack healthy cells as well as diseased ones. The *pattern* of STAT activation provides a mechanism for cytokine individuality. For example, EPO activates STAT5a and STAT5b as part of the early events in erythropoiesis, whereas IL-4 or IL-12 activates STAT4 and STAT6.

Attenuation of the cytokine JAK-STAT signaling cascade involves the production of **inhibitors** that suppress tyrosine phosphorylation and activation of the STATs. For example, IL-6 and LIF both induce expression of the inhibitor SST-1, which contains an SH2 domain and prevents JAK2 or Tyk2 from activating STAT3 in M1 myeloid leukemia cells.

Receptor tyrosine phosphatases are required for lymphocyte activation

Tyrosine residues that are phosphorylated by the tyrosine kinases described in the preceding two sections are *de*phosphorylated by phosphotyrosine phosphatases (PTPs), which can be either cytosolic or membrane bound (i.e., the receptor tyrosine phosphatases). We discussed the cytosolic PTPs earlier. Both classes of *tyrosine* phosphatases have structures very different from the ones that dephosphorylate *serine* and *threonine* residues. Because the tyrosine phosphatases are highly active, pY groups tend to have brief life spans and are relatively few in number in unstimulated cells.

The **CD45** protein, found at the cell surface of T and B lymphocytes, is an example of a receptor tyrosine phosphatase. CD45 makes a single pass through the membrane. Its glycosylated extracellular domain functions as a receptor for antibodies, whereas its cytoplasmic domain has tyrosine phosphatase activity (Fig. 3-12E). During their maturation, lymphocytes express several variants of CD45 characterized by different patterns of alternative splicing and glycosylation. CD45 plays a critical role in signal transduction in lymphocytes. For instance, CD45 dephosphorylates and thereby activates Lck and Fyn (two receptor-associated tyrosine kinases of the Src family) and triggers the phosphorylation of other proteins downstream in the signal transduction cascade. This interaction between receptor tyrosine phosphatases and tyrosine kinase–associated receptors is another example of crosstalk between signaling pathways.

NUCLEAR RECEPTORS

Steroid and thyroid hormones enter the cell and bind to members of the nuclear receptor superfamily in the cytoplasm or nucleus

A number of important signaling molecules produce their effects not by binding to receptors on the cell membrane but by binding to **nuclear receptors** (also called intracellular receptors) that can act as transcription regulators, a concept that we will discuss in more depth in Chapter 4. This family includes receptors for steroid hormones, prostaglandins, vitamin D, thyroid hormones, and retinoic acid (Table 3-6). In addition, this family includes related receptors, known as orphan receptors, whose ligands have yet to be identified. Steroid hormones, vitamin D, and retinoic acid appear to enter the cell by diffusing through the lipid phase of the cell membrane. Thyroid hormones, which are charged amino acid derivatives, may cross the cell membrane either by diffusion or by carrier-mediated transport. Once inside the cell, these substances bind to intracellular receptors. The ligand-bound receptors are activated **transcription factors** that regulate the expression of target genes by binding to specific DNA sequences. In addition, steroid hormones can also have nongenomic effects (see Chapter 47).

The family of nuclear receptors contains at least 32 genes and has been classically divided into two subfamilies based on structural homology. One subfamily consists of receptors for **steroid hormones**, including the glucocorticoids and mineralocorticoids (see Chapter 50), androgens (see Chapter 50), and estrogens and progesterone (see Chapter 55). These receptors function primarily as *homodimers* (Table 3-2). The other group includes receptors for **retinoic acid** (see Chapter 4), **thyroid hormone** (see Chapter 49), and **vitamin D** (see Chapter 52). These receptors appear to act as *heterodimers* (Table 3-2). As we will see in Chapters 4 and 47, other nuclear

---

Oncogenes

The ability of certain viral proteins (**oncogenes**) to transform a cell from a normal to a malignant phenotype was initially thought to occur because these viral proteins acted as transcriptional activators or repressors. However, during the last 20 years, only a few of these viral proteins have been found to work in this manner. The majority of oncogenes harbor mutations that transform them into constitutively active forms of normal cellular signaling proteins called **proto-oncogenes**. Most of these aberrant proteins (i.e., the oncogenes) encode proteins important in a key signal transduction pathway. For example, expression of the viral protein v-erb B is involved in fibrosarcomas, and both v-erb A and v-erb B are associated with leukemias. **v-erb B** resembles a constitutively activated receptor tyrosine kinase (epidermal growth factor receptor), and the retroviral **v-erb A** is derived from a cellular gene encoding a thyroid hormone receptor. Other receptors and signaling molecules implicated in cell transformation include Src, Ras, and platelet-derived growth factor receptor. A mutation in protein tyrosine phosphatase 1C results in abnormal hematopoiesis and an increased incidence of lymphoreticular tumors.

Table 3-6 Nuclear Steroid and Thyroid Receptors

Receptor	Full Name	Dimeric Arrangement
GR	Glucocorticoid receptor	GR/GR
MR	Mineralocorticoid receptor	MR/MR
PR	Progesterone receptor	PR/PR
ER	Estrogen receptor	ER/ER
AR	Androgen receptor	AR/AR
VDR	Vitamin D receptor	VDR/RXR
TR	Thyroid hormone receptor	TR/RXR
RAR	Retinoic acid receptor	RAR/RXR
SXR	Steroid and xenobiotic receptor	SXR/RXR
CAR	Constitutive androstane receptor	CAR/RXR

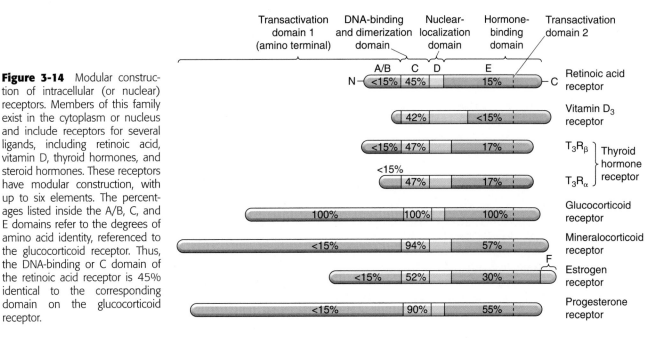

Figure 3-14 Modular construction of intracellular (or nuclear) receptors. Members of this family exist in the cytoplasm or nucleus and include receptors for several ligands, including retinoic acid, vitamin D, thyroid hormones, and steroid hormones. These receptors have modular construction, with up to six elements. The percentages listed inside the A/B, C, and E domains refer to the degrees of amino acid identity, referenced to the glucocorticoid receptor. Thus, the DNA-binding or C domain of the retinoic acid receptor is 45% identical to the corresponding domain on the glucocorticoid receptor.

receptors recognize a wide range of **xenobiotics** and metabolites and respond by modulating the expression of genes that encode transporters and enzymes involved in drug metabolism (see Chapter 46).

The intracellular localization of the different unoccupied receptors varies. The glucocorticoid (GR) and mineralocorticoid (MR) receptors are mainly cytoplasmic, the estrogen (ER) and progesterone (PR) receptors are primarily nuclear, and the thyroid hormone (TR) and retinoic acid (RAR/RXR) receptors are bound to DNA in the nucleus. Cytoplasmic receptors are complexed to chaperone (or "heat shock") proteins. Hormone binding induces a conformational change in these receptors that causes dissociation from the cytoplasmic chaperone and unmasks a nuclear transport signal that allows the hormone-receptor complex to translocate into the nucleus.

All nuclear receptors contain six functionally distinct domains, designated A to F from the N terminus to the C terminus (Fig. 3-14), that are differentially conserved among the various proteins. The N-terminal A/B region differs widely among receptors and contains the first of two transactivation domains. **Transactivation** is the process by which a ligand-induced conformational change of the receptor results in a change in conformation of the DNA, thus initiating transcription. The C region, the most highly conserved among receptor types, contains the DNA-binding domain and is also involved in **dimerization** (Table 3-6). It is composed of two "zinc finger" structures. The D, or hinge, region contains the "nuclear localization signal" and may also contain transactivation sequences. The E domain is responsible for hormone binding. Like the C region, it is involved in dimerization through its "basic zipper" region (see Chapter 4). Finally, like the A/B region, the E region contains a transactivation domain. The small C-terminal F domain is of unknown function.

Activated nuclear receptors bind to sequence elements in the regulatory region of responsive genes and either activate or repress DNA transcription

One of the remarkable features of nuclear receptors is that they bind to specific DNA sequences—called **hormone response elements**—in the regulatory region of responsive genes. The various nuclear receptors display specific cell and tissue distributions. Thus, the battery of genes affected by a particular ligand depends on the complement of receptors in the cell, the ability of these receptors to form homodimers or heterodimers, and the affinity of these receptor-ligand complexes for a particular response element on the DNA.

In addition to their ability to affect transcription by directly binding to specific regulatory elements, several nuclear receptors modulate gene expression by acting as transcriptional repressors (see Chapter 4). For example, the glucocorticoids, acting through their receptor, can attenuate components of the inflammatory response by interacting with or "quenching" the transcription factor activator protein 1 (AP-1) and nuclear factor κB (NF-κB).

REFERENCES

Books and Reviews

Attisano L, Wrana JL: Signal transduction by the TGF-β superfamily. Science 2002; 296:1646-1647.

Clapham DE, Neer EJ: New roles of G protein βγ dimers in transmembrane signalling. Nature 1993; 365:403-406.

Edwards DP: Regulation of signal transduction pathways by estrogen and progesterone. Annu Rev Physiol 2005; 67:335-376.

Exton JH: Phosphoinositide phospholipases and G proteins in hormone action. Annu Rev Physiol 1994; 56:349-369.

Neves SR, Ram PT, Iyengar R: G protein pathways. Science 2002; 296:1636-1639.

Vane JR, Botting RM: Mechanism of action of nonsteroidal anti-inflammatory drugs. Am J Med 1998; 104(Suppl):S2-S8.

Journal Articles

Conklin BR, Bourne HR: Structural elements of Gα subunits that interact with Gβγ, receptors, and effectors. Cell 1993; 73:631-641.

Fraser ID, Tavalin SJ, Lester LB, et al: A novel lipid-anchored A-kinase anchoring protein facilitates cAMP-responsive membrane events. EMBO J 1998; 17:2261-2272.

Hildebrandt JD: Role of subunit diversity in signaling by heterotrimeric G proteins. Biochem Pharmacol 1997; 54:325-339.

Rodig SJ, Meraz MA, White JM, et al: Disruption of the Jak1 gene demonstrates obligatory and nonredundant roles of the Jaks in cytokine-induced biological responses. Cell 1998; 93:373-383.

CHAPTER 4

REGULATION OF GENE EXPRESSION

Peter Igarashi

In this chapter, we discuss general principles of gene structure and expression as well as mechanisms underlying the regulation of tissue-specific and inducible gene expression. We will see that proteins (transcription factors) control gene transcription by interacting with regulatory elements in DNA (e.g., promoters and enhancers). Because many transcription factors are effector molecules in signal transduction pathways, these transcription factors can coordinately regulate gene expression in response to physiological stimuli. Finally, we describe the important roles of chromatin structure and post-transcriptional regulation of gene expression. Because many of the proteins and DNA sequences are known by abbreviations, the Glossary at the end of the chapter identifies these entities.

FROM GENES TO PROTEINS

Gene expression differs among tissues and—in any tissue—may vary in response to external stimuli

The haploid human genome contains 30,000 to 40,000 distinct genes, but only a fraction of that number—10,000 or so—is actively translated into proteins in any individual cell. Cells from different tissues have distinct morphological appearances and functions and respond differently to external stimuli, even though their DNA content is identical. For example, although all cells of the body contain an albumin gene, only liver cells (hepatocytes) can synthesize and secrete albumin into the bloodstream. Conversely, hepatocytes cannot synthesize myosin and some other contractile proteins that skeletal muscle cells produce. The explanation for these observations is that expression of genes is regulated so that some genes are active in hepatocytes and others are silent. In skeletal muscle cells, a different set of genes is active; others, such as those expressed only in the liver, are silent. How is one cell type programmed to express liver-specific genes, whereas another cell type expresses a set of genes that are appropriate for skeletal muscle? This phenomenon is called **tissue-specific gene expression.**

A second issue is that genes in individual cells are generally not expressed at constant, unchanging levels (constitu-tive expression). Rather, their expression levels often vary widely in response to environmental stimuli. For example, when blood glucose levels decrease, α cells in the pancreas secrete the hormone glucagon. Glucagon circulates in the blood until it reaches the liver, where it causes a 15-fold increase in expression of the gene that encodes phospho-enolpyruvate carboxykinase (PEPCK), an enzyme that catalyzes the rate-limiting step in gluconeogenesis (see Chapter 51). Increased gluconeogenesis then contributes to restoration of blood glucose levels toward normal. This simple regulatory loop, which necessitates that the liver cells perceive the presence of glucagon and stimulate PEPCK gene expression, illustrates the phenomenon of **inducible gene expression.**

Genetic information flows from DNA to proteins

The "central dogma of molecular biology" states that genetic information flows unidirectionally from DNA to proteins. Deoxyribonucleic acid (DNA) is a polymer of nucleotides, each containing a nitrogenous base (adenine, T; guanine, G; cytosine, C; or thymine, T) attached to deoxyribose 5′-phosphate. The polymerized nucleotides form a polynucleotide strand in which the sequence of the nitrogenous bases constitutes the genetic information. With few exceptions, all cells in the body share the same genetic information. Hydrogen bond formation between bases (A and T, or G and C) on the two complementary strands of DNA produces a double-helical structure. DNA has two functions. The first is to serve as a self-renewing data repository that maintains a constant source of genetic information for the cell. This role is achieved by DNA replication, which ensures that when cells divide, the progeny cells receive exact copies of the DNA. The second purpose of DNA is to serve as a template for the translation of genetic information into proteins, which are the functional units of the cell. This second purpose is broadly defined as **gene expression.**

Gene expression involves two major processes (Fig. 4-1). The first process—**transcription**—is the synthesis of RNA from a DNA template, mediated by an enzyme called RNA polymerase II. The resultant RNA molecule is identical in sequence to one of the strands of the DNA template except that the base uracil (U) replaces thymine (T). The second

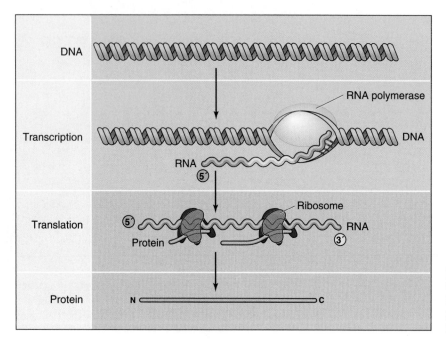

Figure 4-1   Pathway from genes to proteins. Gene expression involves two major processes. First, the DNA is transcribed into RNA by RNA polymerase. Second, the RNA is translated into protein on the ribosomes.

process—**translation**—is the synthesis of protein from RNA. During translation, the genetic code in the sequence of RNA is "read" by transfer RNA (tRNA), and then amino acids carried by the tRNA are covalently linked together to form a polypeptide chain. In eukaryotic cells, transcription occurs in the nucleus, whereas translation occurs on ribosomes located in the cytoplasm. Therefore, an intermediary RNA, called **messenger RNA (mRNA)**, is required to transport the genetic information from the nucleus to the cytoplasm (see Chapter 2). The complete process, proceeding from DNA in the nucleus to protein in the cytoplasm, constitutes gene expression.

The gene consists of a transcription unit

Figure 4-2 depicts the structure of a typical eukaryotic gene. The **gene** consists of a segment of DNA that is transcribed into RNA. It extends from the site of transcription initiation to the site of transcription termination. The region of DNA that is immediately adjacent to and upstream (i.e., in the 5′ direction) from the transcription initiation site is called the **5′ flanking region**. The corresponding domain that is downstream (3′) from the transcription termination site is called the **3′ flanking region**. (Recall that DNA strands have directionality because of the 5′ to 3′ orientation of the phosphodiester bonds in the sugar-phosphate backbone of DNA. By convention, the DNA strand that has the same sequence as the RNA is called the coding strand, and the complementary strand is called the noncoding strand. The 5′ to 3′ orientation refers to the coding strand.) Although the 5′ and 3′ flanking regions are not transcribed into RNA, they frequently contain DNA sequences, called **regulatory elements**, that control gene transcription. The site where transcription of the gene begins, sometimes called the cap site, may have a variant of the nucleotide sequence 5′-ACTT(T/C)TG-3′ (called the cap sequence), where T/C means T *or* C. The A

is the **transcription initiation site**. Transcription proceeds to the **transcription termination site**, which has a less defined sequence and location in eukaryotic genes. Slightly upstream from the termination site is another sequence called the **polyadenylation signal**, which often has the sequence 5′-AATAAA-3′.

The RNA that is initially transcribed from a gene is called the **primary transcript** (Fig. 4-2) or heterogeneous nuclear RNA (hnRNA). Before it can be translated into protein, the primary transcript must be processed into a mature mRNA in the nucleus. Most eukaryotic genes contain **exons**, DNA sequences that are present in the mature mRNA, alternating with **introns**, which are not present in the mRNA. The primary transcript is colinear with the coding strand of the gene and contains the sequences of both the exons and the introns. To produce a mature mRNA that can be translated into protein, the cell must process the primary transcript in four steps.

First, the cell removes the sequences of the introns from the primary transcript by a process called **pre-mRNA splicing**. Splicing involves the joining of the sequences of the exons in the RNA transcript and the removal of the intervening introns. As a result, **mature mRNA** (Fig. 4-2) is shorter and not colinear with the coding strand of the DNA template.

Second, the cell adds an unusual guanosine base, which is methylated at the 7 position, through a 5′-5′ phosphodiester bond to the 5′ end of the transcript. The result is a 5′ methyl **cap**. The presence of the 5′ methyl cap is required for export of the mRNA from the nucleus to the cytoplasm as well as for translation of the mRNA.

The third processing step is cleavage of the RNA transcript about 20 nucleotides downstream from the polyadenylation signal, near the 3′ end of the transcript.

The fourth step is the addition of a string of 100 to 200 adenine bases at the site of the cleavage to form a **poly(A) tail**. This tail contributes to mRNA stability.

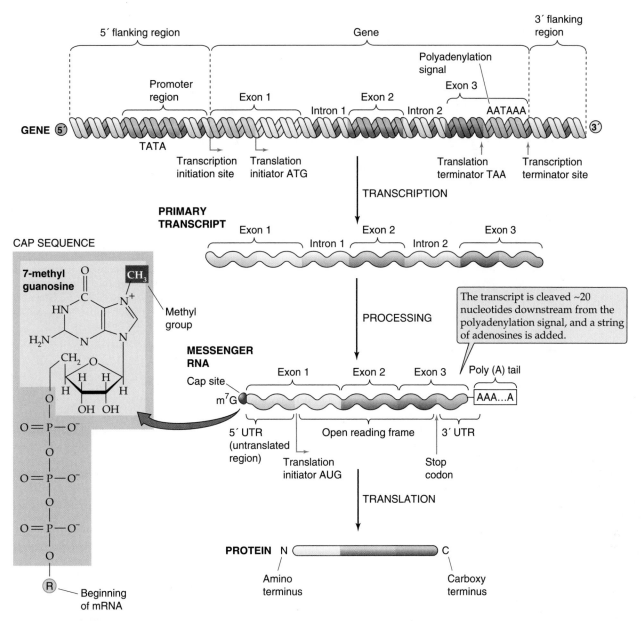

Figure 4-2 Structure of a eukaryotic gene and its products. The figure depicts a gene, a primary RNA transcript, the mature mRNA, and the resulting protein. The 5′ and 3′ numbering of the gene refers to the coding strand. m⁷G, 7-methyl guanosine; ATG, AATAAA, and the like are nucleotide sequences.

The mRNA produced by RNA processing contains a coding region that is translated into protein as well as sequences at the 5′ and 3′ ends that are not translated into protein (the 5′ and 3′ untranslated regions, respectively). Translation of the mRNA on ribosomes always begins at the codon AUG, which encodes methionine, and proceeds until the ribosome encounters one of the three stop codons (UAG, UAA, or UGA). Thus, the 5′ end of the mRNA is the first to be translated and provides the N terminus of the protein; the 3′ end is the last to be translated and contributes the C terminus.

DNA is packaged into chromatin

Although DNA is commonly depicted as linear, chromosomal DNA in the nucleus is actually organized into a higher order structure called chromatin. This packaging is required to fit DNA with a total length of ~1 m into a nucleus with a diameter of 10^{-5} m. **Chromatin** consists of DNA associated with **histones** and other nuclear proteins. The basic building block of chromatin is the **nucleosome** (Fig. 4-3), each of which consists of a protein core and 147 bp of associated DNA. The protein core is an octamer of the histones H2A, H2B, H3, and H4. DNA wraps twice around the core

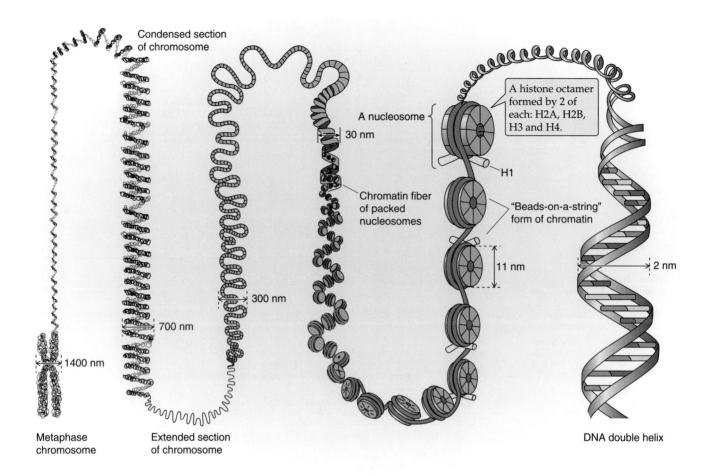

Condensed section
of chromosome

A nucleosome

30 nm

A histone octamer
formed by 2 of
each: H2A, H2B,
H3 and H4.

H1

Chromatin fiber
of packed
nucleosomes

"Beads-on-a-string"
form of chromatin

11 nm

2 nm

300 nm

700 nm

1400 nm

Metaphase
chromosome

Extended section
of chromosome

DNA double helix

Figure 4-3   Chromatin structure.

histones to form a solenoid-like structure. A linker histone, H1, associates with segments of DNA between nucleosomes. Regular arrays of nucleosomes have a beads-on-a-string appearance and constitute the so-called 11-nm fiber of chromatin, which can condense to form the 30-nm fiber.

Transcription from DNA in chromatin requires partial disruption of the regular nucleosome structure and some unwinding of the DNA. The alteration in the interaction between DNA and histones is called **chromatin remodeling**. One mechanism of chromatin remodeling involves histone acetylation (Fig. 4-4). The N termini of core histone proteins contain many lysine residues that impart a highly positive charge. These positively charged domains can bind tightly to the negatively charged DNA through electrostatic interactions. Tight binding between DNA and histones is associated with gene inactivity. However, if the ε-amino groups of the lysine side chains are chemically modified by **acetylation**, the positive charge is neutralized and the interaction with DNA is weakened. This modification is believed to result in a loosening of chromatin structure, which permits transcriptional regulatory proteins to gain access to the DNA. Certain enzymes can acetylate histones (histone acetyltransferases) or deacetylate them (histone deacetylases). **Histone acetyltransferases (HATs)** acetylate histones and thus produce local alterations in chromatin structure that are more favorable for transcription. Conversely, **histone deacetylases (HDACs)** remove the acetyl groups, leading to tighter binding between DNA and histones and inhibition of transcription.

In addition to histone acetylation and deacetylation, another mechanism of chromatin remodeling involves the **SWI/SNF family** of proteins. SWI/SNF (switching mating type/sucrose non-fermenting) are large multiprotein complexes, initially identified in yeast but evolutionarily conserved in all animals. SWI/SNF chromatin-remodeling complexes can inhibit the association between DNA and histones by using the energy of ATP to peel the DNA away from the histones, thereby making this DNA more accessible to transcription factors.

Gene expression may be regulated at multiple steps

Gene expression involves eight steps (Fig. 4-5):

Step 1: **Chromatin remodeling.** Before a gene can be transcribed, some local alteration in chromatin structure must occur so that the enzymes that mediate transcription can gain access to the DNA. Chromatin remodeling may involve histone acetylation or SWI/SNF chromatin remodeling proteins.

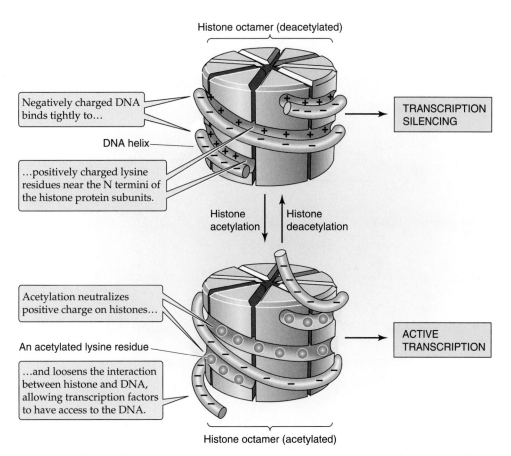

Figure 4-4 Effect of histone acetylation on the interaction between histone proteins and DNA. When the histone octamer is deacetylated *(top)*, positively charged lysine groups on the histone strongly attract a strand of DNA. When the histone octamer becomes acetylated *(bottom)*, the acetyl groups neutralize the positive charge on the histone and allow the DNA strand to loosen.

Step 2: **Initiation of transcription.** In this step, RNA polymerase is recruited to the gene promoter and begins to synthesize RNA that is complementary in sequence to one of the strands of the template DNA. For most eukaryotic genes, initiation of transcription is the critical, rate-limiting step in gene expression.

Step 3: **Transcript elongation.** During transcript elongation, RNA polymerase proceeds down the DNA strand and sequentially adds ribonucleotides to the elongating strand of RNA.

Step 4: **Termination of transcription.** After producing a full-length RNA, the enzyme halts elongation.

Step 5: **RNA processing.** As noted before, RNA processing involves (1) pre-mRNA splicing, (2) addition of a 5′ methylguanosine cap, (3) cleavage of the RNA strand, and (4) polyadenylation.

Step 6: **Nucleocytoplasmic transport.** The next step in gene expression is the export of the mature mRNA through pores in the nuclear envelope (see Chapter 2) into the cytoplasm. Nucleocytoplasmic transport is a regulated process that is important for mRNA quality control.

Step 7: **Translation.** The mRNA is translated into proteins on ribosomes. During translation, the genetic code on the mRNA is read by tRNA, and then amino acids carried by the tRNA are added to the nascent polypeptide chain.

Step 8: **mRNA degradation.** Finally, the mRNA is degraded in the cytoplasm by a combination of endonucleases and exonucleases.

Each of these steps is potentially a target for regulation (Fig. 4-5):

1. Gene expression may be regulated by global as well as by local alterations in chromatin structure.
2. An important, related alteration in chromatin structure is the state of methylation of the DNA.
3. Initiation of transcription can be regulated by transcriptional activators and transcriptional repressors.
4. Transcript elongation may be regulated by premature termination in which the polymerase falls off (or is displaced from) the template DNA strand; such termination results in the synthesis of truncated transcripts.
5. Pre-mRNA splicing may be regulated by alternative splicing, which generates different mRNA species from the same primary transcript.
6. At the step of nucleocytoplasmic transport, the cell prevents expression of aberrant transcripts, such as those with defects in mRNA processing. In addition, aberrant transcripts containing premature stop codons may be degraded in the nucleus through a process called nonsense-mediated decay.
7. Control of translation of mRNA is a regulated step in the expression of certain genes, such as the transferrin receptor.
8. Control of mRNA stability contributes to steady-state levels of mRNA in the cytoplasm and is important for the overall expression of many genes.

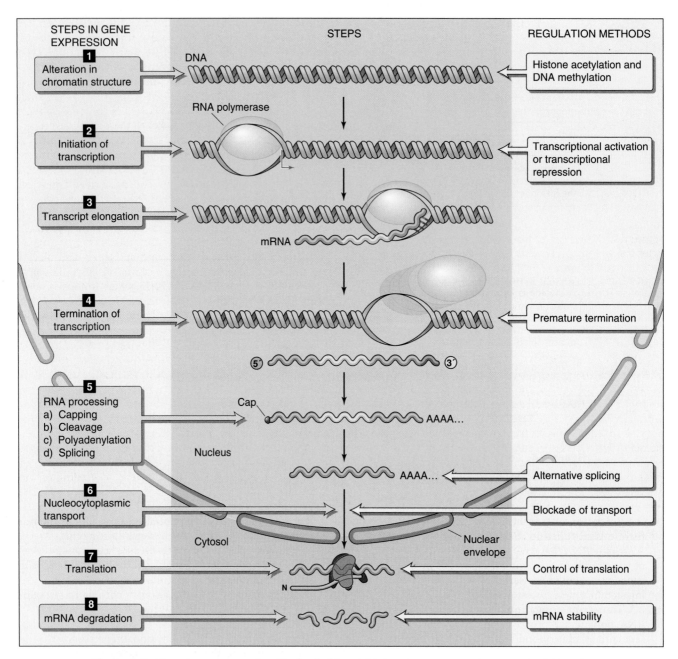

Figure 4-5 Steps in gene expression. Nearly all of the eight steps in gene expression are potential targets for regulation.

Although any of these steps may be critical for regulating a particular gene, transcription initiation is the most frequently regulated (step 2) and is the focus of this chapter. At the end of the chapter, we describe examples of control of gene expression at steps that are subsequent to the initiation of transcription—post-transcriptional regulation.

Transcription factors are proteins that regulate gene transcription

A general principle is that gene transcription is regulated by interactions of specific proteins with specific DNA sequences. The proteins that regulate gene transcription are called **transcription factors**. These proteins are sometimes referred to as ***trans*-acting** factors because they are encoded by genes that reside elsewhere in the genome from the genes that they regulate. Many transcription factors recognize and bind to specific sequences in DNA. The binding sites for these transcription factors are called **regulatory elements**. Because they are located on the same piece of DNA as the genes that they regulate, these regulatory elements are sometimes referred to as ***cis*-acting** factors.

Figure 4-6 illustrates the overall scheme for the regulation of gene expression. Transcription requires proteins (transcription factors) that bind to specific DNA sequences (regulatory elements) located near the genes they regulate (target

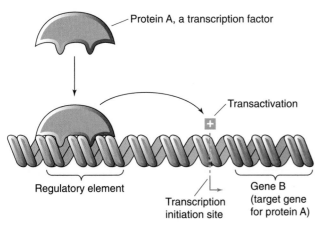

Figure 4-6 Regulation of transcription. Protein A, a transcription factor that is encoded by gene A (not shown), regulates another gene, gene B. Protein A binds to a DNA sequence (a regulatory element) that is upstream from gene B; this DNA sequence is a *cis*-acting element because it is located on the same DNA as gene B. In this example, protein A stimulates (transactivates) the transcription of gene B. Transcription factors also can inhibit transcription.

genes). Once the proteins bind to DNA, they stimulate (or inhibit) transcription of the target gene. A particular transcription factor can regulate the transcription of multiple target genes. In general, regulation of gene expression can occur at the level of either transcription factors or regulatory elements. Examples of regulation at the transcription factor level include variation in the abundance of the proteins, their DNA-binding activities, and their ability to stimulate (or to inhibit) transcription. Examples of regulation at the regulatory element level include alterations in chromatin structure (which influences accessibility to transcription factors) and covalent modifications of DNA, especially methylation.

THE PROMOTER AND REGULATORY ELEMENTS

The basal transcriptional machinery mediates gene transcription

Genes are transcribed by an enzyme called **RNA polymerase**, which catalyzes the synthesis of RNA that is complementary in sequence to a DNA template. Eukaryotes have three distinct RNA polymerases: RNA polymerase I (Pol I) transcribes genes encoding ribosomal RNA. RNA polymerase II (Pol II or RNAPII) transcribes genes into mRNA, which is later translated into protein. Finally, RNA polymerase III (Pol III) transcribes genes that encode tRNA and small nuclear RNA. This discussion is confined to the protein-encoding genes transcribed by Pol II (so-called class II genes).

Pol II is a large protein (molecular mass of 600 kDa) comprising 10 to 12 subunits (the largest of which is structurally related to bacterial RNA polymerase) and is capable of transcribing RNA from synthetic DNA templates in vitro. Although Pol II catalyzes mRNA synthesis, by itself it is incapable of binding to DNA and initiating transcription at specific sites. The recruitment of Pol II and initiation of

transcription requires an assembly of proteins called **general transcription factors**. Six general transcription factors are known, TFIIA, TFIIB, TFIID, TFIIE, TFIIF, and TFIIH, each of which contains multiple subunits. These general transcription factors are essential for the transcription of all class II genes, which distinguishes them from the transcription factors discussed later that are involved in the transcription of specific genes. Together with Pol II, the general transcription factors constitute the **basal transcriptional machinery**, which is also known as the **RNA polymerase holoenzyme** or **preinitiation complex** because its assembly is required before transcription can begin. The basal transcriptional machinery assembles at a region of DNA that is immediately upstream from the gene and includes the transcription initiation site. This region is called the **gene promoter** (Fig. 4-7).

In vitro, the general transcription factors and Pol II assemble in a stepwise, ordered fashion on DNA. The first protein that binds to DNA is **TFIID**, which induces a bend in the DNA and forms a platform for the assembly of the remaining factors. Once TFIID binds to DNA, the other components of the basal transcriptional machinery assemble spontaneously by protein-protein interactions. The next general transcription factor that binds is **TFIIA**, which stabilizes the interaction of TFIID with DNA. Assembly of TFIIA is followed by assembly of **TFIIB**, which interacts with TFIID and also binds DNA. TFIIB then recruits a preassembled complex of **Pol II** and **TFIIF**. Entry of the Pol II–TFIIF complex into the basal transcriptional machinery is followed by binding of **TFIIE** and **TFIIH**. TFIIF and TFIIH may assist in the transition from basal transcriptional machinery to an elongation complex, which may involve unwinding of the DNA that is mediated by the helicase activity of TFIIH. Although this stepwise assembly of Pol II and general transcription factors occurs in vitro, the situation in vivo may be different. In vivo, Pol II has been observed in a multiprotein complex containing general transcription factors and other proteins. This preformed complex may be recruited to DNA to initiate transcription.

The promoter determines the initiation site and direction of transcription

The promoter is a *cis*-acting regulatory element that is required for expression of the gene. In addition to locating the *site* for initiation of transcription, the promoter also determines the *direction* of transcription. Perhaps somewhat surprisingly, no unique sequence defines the gene promoter. Instead, the promoter consists of modules of simple sequences (elements). The most important element in many promoters is the Goldberg-Hogness **TATA box**. Examination of the sequences of a large number of promoters reveals that the TATA box has the consensus sequence 5′-GNGTATA(A/T)A(A/T)-3′, where N is any nucleotide. The TATA box is usually located ~30 bp upstream (5′) from the site of transcription initiation. The general transcription factor TFIID—the first component of the basal transcriptional machinery—recognizes the TATA box, which is thus believed to determine the site of transcription initiation. TFIID itself is composed of **TATA-binding protein (TBP)** and at least 10 **TBP-associated factors (TAFs)**. The TBP

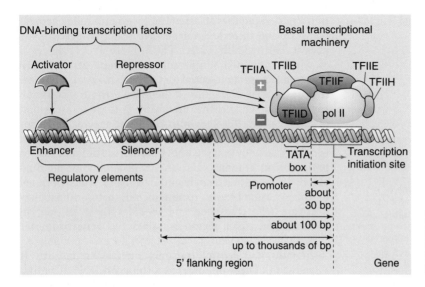

Figure 4-7 Promoter and DNA regulatory elements. The basal transcriptional machinery assembles on the promoter. Transcriptional activators bind to enhancers, and repressors bind to negative regulatory elements.

subunit is a sequence-specific DNA-binding protein that binds to the TATA box. Reconstitution studies indicate that recombinant TBP can replace TFIID in basal transcription, but it fails to support elevated levels of transcription in the presence of transcriptional activators. Thus, TBP-associated factors are involved in the activation of gene transcription (more on this later).

Many eukaryotic genes, especially the ubiquitously expressed "housekeeping" genes, do not contain a TATA box in their promoters. What determines the site of transcription initiation in TATA-less promoters? At least part of the answer appears to be a series of small DNA sequence elements, collectively called the **initiator (Inr)**. Inr functions analogously to the TATA box to position the basal transcriptional machinery in these genes. Interestingly, it appears that TFIID can also bind to the Inr element, so it may function to establish assembly of the basal transcriptional machinery on both TATA-containing and TATA-less gene promoters. However, in TATA-less promoters, the site of transcription initiation appears to be less precisely defined, and often several transcripts that originate at several distinct but neighboring sites are produced.

In addition to the TATA box and Inr, gene promoters contain additional DNA elements that are necessary for initiating transcription. These elements consist of short DNA sequences and are sometimes called **promoter-proximal sequences** because they are located within ~100 bp upstream from the transcription initiation site. Promoter-proximal sequences are a type of regulatory element that is required for the transcription of specific genes. Well-characterized examples include the GC box (5′-GGGCGG-3′) and the CCAAT box (5′-CCAAT-3′) as well as the CACCC box and octamer motif (5′-ATGCAAAT-3′). These DNA elements function as binding sites for additional proteins (transcription factors) that are necessary for initiating transcription of particular genes. The proteins that bind to these sites are believed to help recruit the basal transcriptional machinery to the promoter. Examples include the transcription factor NF-Y, which recognizes the CCAAT box, and Sp1, which recognizes the GC box. The CCAAT box is often located

~50 bp upstream from the TATA box, whereas multiple GC boxes are frequently found in TATA-less gene promoters. Some promoter-proximal sequences are present in genes that are active only in certain cell types. For example, the CACCC box found in gene promoters of β-globin is recognized by the erythroid-specific transcription factor EKLF (erythroid Kruppel-like factor).

Positive and negative regulatory elements modulate gene transcription

Although the promoter is the site where the basal transcriptional machinery binds and initiates transcription, the promoter alone is not generally sufficient to initiate transcription at a physiologically significant rate. High-level gene expression generally requires activation of the basal transcriptional machinery by specific transcription factors, which bind to additional regulatory elements located near the target gene. Two general types of regulatory elements are recognized. First, **positive regulatory elements** or **enhancers** represent DNA-binding sites for proteins that activate transcription; the proteins that bind to these DNA elements are called **activators**. Second, **negative regulatory elements (NREs)** or **silencers** are DNA-binding sites for proteins that inhibit transcription; the proteins that bind to these DNA elements are called **repressors** (Fig. 4-7).

A general property of enhancers and silencers is that they consist of modules of relatively short sequences of DNA, generally 6 to 12 bp. Sometimes they contain distinct sequences, such as direct or inverted repeats, but often they do not. Regulatory elements are generally located in the vicinity of the genes that they regulate. Typically, regulatory elements do not reside within the portion of the gene that encodes protein but rather are located in noncoding regions, most frequently in the 5′ flanking region that is upstream from the promoter. However, some enhancers and silencers are located downstream from the transcription initiation site and are embedded either in introns or in the 3′ flanking region of the gene. In fact, some enhancers and silencers can function at great physical distances from the gene promoter, many hundreds of base pairs away. Moreover, the distance between the enhancer or silencer and the promoter can often be varied experimentally without substantially affecting transcriptional activity. In addition, many regulatory elements work equally well if their orientation is inverted. Thus, in contrast to the gene promoter, enhancers and silencers exhibit position independence and orientation independence. Another property of regulatory elements is that they are active on heterologous promoters; that is, if enhancers and silencers from one gene are placed near a promoter for a different gene, they can stimulate or inhibit transcription of the second gene.

After transcription factors (activators or repressors) bind to regulatory elements (enhancers or silencers), they may interact with the basal transcriptional machinery to alter gene transcription. How do transcription factors that bind to regulatory elements physically distant from the promoter interact with components of the basal transcriptional machinery? Regulatory elements may be located hundreds of base pairs from the promoter. This distance is much too great to permit proteins that are bound at the regulatory element and promoter to come into contact along a two-dimensional linear strand of DNA. One model that has been proposed to explain the long-range effects of transcription factors is the **DNA looping** model. According to this model, the transcription factor binds to the regulatory element, and the basal transcriptional machinery assembles on the gene promoter. Looping out of the intervening DNA permits physical interaction between the transcription factor and the basal transcriptional machinery, which subsequently leads to alterations in gene transcription.

Locus control regions and boundary elements influence transcription within multigene chromosomal domains

In addition to enhancers and silencers, which regulate the expression of *individual* genes, some *cis*-acting regulatory elements are involved in the regulation of chromosomal domains containing multiple genes.

The first of this type of element to be discovered was the **locus control region (LCR)**, also called the locus-activating region or dominant control region. The LCR is a dominant, positive-acting *cis*-element that regulates the expression of several genes within a chromosomal domain. LCRs were first identified at the β-globin gene locus, which encodes the β-type subunits of hemoglobin. Together with α-type subunits, these β-globin–like subunits form embryonic, fetal, and adult hemoglobin (see the box on this topic in Chapter 29). The β-globin gene locus consists of a cluster of five genes (ε, γ_G, γ_A, δ, β) that are distributed over 90 kb on chromosome 11. During ontogeny, the genes exhibit highly regulated patterns of expression in which they are transcribed only in certain tissues and only at precise developmental stages. Thus, embryonic globin (ε) is expressed in the yolk sac, fetal globins (γ_G, γ_A) are expressed in fetal liver, and adult globins (δ, β) are expressed in adult bone marrow. This tightly regulated expression pattern requires a regulatory region that is located far from the structural genes. This region, designated the LCR, extends from 6 to 18 kb upstream from the ε-globin gene. The LCR is essential for high-level expression of the

β-globin–like genes within red blood cell precursors because the promoters and enhancers near the individual genes permit only low-level expression.

The β-globin LCR contains five sites, each with an enhancer-like structure that consists of modules of simple sequence elements that are binding sites for the erythrocyte-specific transcription factors GATA-1 and NF-E2. It is believed that the LCRs perform two functions: one is to alter the chromatin structure of the β-globin gene locus so that it is more accessible to transcription factors, and the second is to serve as a powerful enhancer of transcription of the individual genes. In one model, temporal-dependent expression of β-type globin genes is achieved by sequential interactions involving activator proteins that bind to the LCR and promoters of individual genes (Fig. 4-8).

A potential problem associated with the existence of LCRs that can exert transcriptional effects over long distances is that the LCRs may interfere with the expression of nearby genes. One solution to this problem is provided by **boundary elements**, which function to insulate genes from neighboring regulatory elements. Boundary elements (or matrix-attachment regions) are believed to represent sites of attachment of DNA to the chromosome scaffold, and loops of physically separated DNA are generated that may correspond to discrete functional domains.

Figure 4-8 summarizes our understanding of the arrangement of *cis*-acting regulatory elements and their functions. Each gene has its own promoter where transcription is initiated. Enhancers are positive-acting regulatory elements that may be located either near or distant from the transcription initiation site; silencers are regulatory elements that inhibit gene expression. A cluster of genes within a chromosomal domain may be under the control of an LCR. Finally, boundary elements (or matrix-attachment regions) functionally insulate one chromosomal domain from another.

TRANSCRIPTION FACTORS

DNA-binding transcription factors recognize specific DNA sequences

The preceding discussion has emphasized the structure of the gene and the *cis*-acting elements that regulate gene expression. We now turn to the proteins that interact with these DNA elements and thus regulate gene transcription. Because the basal transcriptional machinery—Pol II and the general transcription factors—is incapable of efficient gene transcription alone, additional proteins are required to stimulate the activity of the enzyme complex. The additional proteins include transcription factors that recognize and bind to specific DNA sequences (enhancers) located near their target genes as well as others that do not bind to DNA.

Examples of **DNA-binding transcription factors** are shown in (Table 4-1). The general mechanism of action of a specific transcription factor is depicted in Figure 4-7. After the basal transcriptional machinery assembles on the gene promoter, it can interact with a transcription factor that binds to a specific DNA element, the enhancer. Looping out

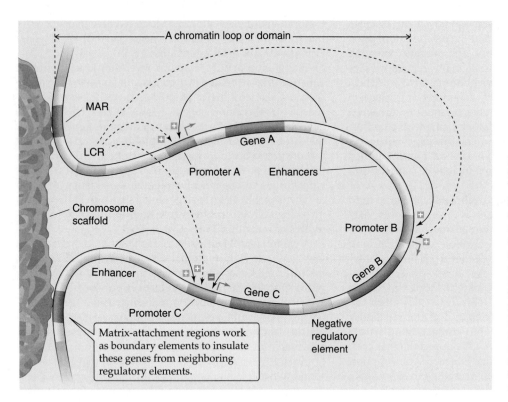

Figure 4-8 *cis*-Acting elements that regulate gene transcription. This model shows a loop of chromatin that contains genes A, B, and C. The matrix-attachment region (MAR) is a boundary element on the DNA. Matrix-attachment regions attach to the chromosome scaffold and thus isolate this loop of chromatin from other chromosomal domains. Contained within this loop are several *cis*-acting elements (i.e., DNA sequences that regulate genes on the same piece of DNA), including promoters, enhancers, negative regulatory elements, and the LCR.

Abnormalities of Regulatory Elements in β-Thalassemias

The best characterized mutations affecting DNA regulatory elements occur at the gene cluster encoding the β-globin–like chains of hemoglobin. Some of these mutations result in thalassemia, whereas others cause hereditary persistence of fetal hemoglobin. The **β-thalassemias** are a heterogeneous group of disorders characterized by anemia caused by a deficiency in production of the β chain of hemoglobin. The anemia can be mild and inconsequential or severe and life-threatening. The thalassemias were among the first diseases to be characterized at the molecular level. As described in the text, the β-globin gene locus consists of five β-globin–like genes that are exclusively expressed in hematopoietic cells and exhibit temporal colinearity. As expected, many patients with β-thalassemia have mutations or deletions that affect the coding region of the β-globin gene. These patients presumably have thalassemia because the β-globin gene product is functionally abnormal or absent. In addition, some patients have a deficiency in β-globin as a result of inadequate levels of expression of the gene. Of particular interest are patients with the Hispanic and Dutch forms of β-thalassemia. These patients have deletions of portions of chromosome 11. However, the deletions do not extend to include the β-globin gene itself. Why, then, do these patients have β-globin deficiency? It turns out that the deletions involve the region 50 to 65 kb upstream from the β-globin gene, which contains the LCR. In these cases, deletion of the LCR results in failure of expression of the β-globin gene, even though the *structural gene* and its *promoter* are completely normal. These results underscore the essential role that the LCR plays in β-globin gene expression.

of the intervening DNA permits physical interaction between the transcription factor and the basal transcriptional machinery, which subsequently leads to stimulation of gene transcription. The specificity with which transcription factors bind to DNA depends on the interactions between the amino acid side chains of the transcription factor and the purine and pyrimidine bases in DNA. Most of these interactions consist of noncovalent hydrogen bonds between amino acids and DNA bases. A peptide capable of a specific pattern of hydrogen bonding can recognize and bind to the reciprocal pattern in the major (and to a lesser extent the minor) groove of DNA. Interaction with the DNA backbone may also occur and involves electrostatic interactions (salt bridge formation) with anionic phosphate groups. The site that a transcription factor recognizes (Table 4-1) is generally short, usually less than a dozen or so base pairs.

DNA-binding transcription factors do not recognize single, unique DNA sequences; rather, they recognize a *family* of closely related sequences. For example, the transcription factor AP-1 (activator protein 1) recognizes the sequences

5′-TGACTCA-3′

5′-TGAGTCA-3′

5′-TGAGTCT-3′

and so on, as well as each of the complementary sequences. That is, some *redundancy* is usually built into the recognition sequence for a transcription factor. An important consequence of these properties is that the recognition site for a transcription factor may occur many times in the genome. For example, if a transcription factor recognizes a 6-bp sequence, the sequence would be expected to occur once every 4^6 (or 4096) base pairs, that is, 7×10^5 times in the

Table 4-1 DNA-Binding Transcription Factors and the DNA Sequences They Recognize

Name	Type	Recognition Site*	Binds as
Sp1	Zinc finger	5'-GGGCGG-3'	Monomer
AP-1 (c-Fos and c-Jun)	Basic zipper	5'-TGASTCA-3'	Dimer
C/EBP	Basic zipper	5'-ATTGCGCAAT-3'	Dimer
Heat shock factor	Basic zipper	5'-NGAAN-3'	Trimer
ATF/CREB	Basic zipper	5'-TGACGTCA-3'	Dimer
c-Myc	Basic helix-loop-helix	5'-CACGTG-3'	Dimer
Oct-1	Helix-turn-helix	5'-ATGCAAAT-3'	Monomer
NF-1	Novel	5'-TTGGCN5GCCAA-3'	Dimer

*N, any nucleotide; S, G, or C; W, A, or T.

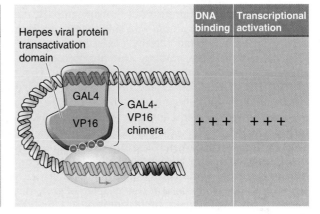

Figure 4-9 Modular design of specific transcription factors. **A,** DNA-binding transcription factors have independent domains for binding to DNA regulatory sequences and for activating transcription. In this example, amino acids 1 through 147 of the GAL4 transcription factor bind to DNA, whereas amino acids 768 through 881 activate transcription. **B,** Replacement of the transactivation domain of GAL4 with that of VP16 results in a chimera that is a functional transcription factor.

human genome. If redundancy is permitted, recognition sites will occur even more frequently. Of course, most of these sites will not be relevant to gene regulation but will instead have occurred simply by chance. This high frequency of recognition sites leads to an important concept: *transcription factors act in combination.* Thus, high-level expression of a gene requires that a combination of multiple transcription factors binds to multiple regulatory elements. Although it is complicated, this system ensures that transcription activation occurs only at appropriate locations. Moreover, this system permits greater fine-tuning of the system, inasmuch as the activity of individual transcription factors can be altered to modulate the overall level of transcription of a gene.

An important general feature of DNA-binding transcription factors is their **modular** construction (Fig. 4-9A). Transcription factors may be divided into discrete domains that bind DNA (**DNA-binding domains**) and domains that acti-

vate transcription (**transactivation domains**). This property was first directly demonstrated for a yeast transcription factor known as GAL4, which activates certain genes when yeast grows in galactose-containing media. GAL4 has two domains. One is a so-called zinc finger domain (discussed later) that mediates sequence-specific binding to DNA. The other domain is enriched in acidic amino acids (i.e., glutamate and aspartate) and is necessary for transcriptional activation. This "acidic blob" domain of GAL4 can be removed and replaced with the transactivation domain from a different transcription factor, VP16 (Fig. 4-9B). The resulting GAL4-VP16 chimera binds to the same DNA sequence as normal GAL4 but mediates transcriptional activation through the VP16 transactivation domain. This type of "domain swapping" experiment indicates that transcription factors have a modular construction in which physically distinct domains mediate binding to DNA and transcriptional activation (or repression).

Transcription factors that bind to DNA can be grouped into families based on tertiary structure

On the basis of sequence conservation as well as structural determinations from x-ray crystallography and nuclear magnetic resonance spectroscopy, DNA-binding transcription factors have been grouped into families. Members of the same family use common structural motifs for binding DNA (Table 4-1). These structures include the zinc finger, basic zipper (bZIP), basic helix-loop-helix (bHLH), helix-turn-helix (HTH), and β sheet. Each of these motifs consists of a particular tertiary protein structure in which a component, usually an α helix, interacts with DNA, especially the major groove of the DNA.

Zinc Finger   The term **zinc finger** describes a loop of protein held together at its base by a zinc ion that tetrahedrally coordinates to either two histidine residues and two cysteine residues or four cysteine residues. Sometimes two zinc ions coordinate to six cysteine groups. Figure 4-10A shows a zinc finger in which Zn^{2+} coordinates to two residues on an α helix and two residues on a β sheet of the protein. The loop (or finger) of protein can protrude into the major groove of DNA, where amino acid side chains can interact with the base pairs and thereby confer the capacity for sequence-specific DNA binding. Zinc fingers consist of 30 amino acids with the consensus sequences $Cys-X_{2-4}-Cys-X_{12}-His-X_{3-5}-His$, where X can be any amino acid. Transcription factors of this family contain at least two zinc fingers and may contain dozens. Three amino acid residues at the tips of each zinc finger contact a DNA subsite that consists of three bases in the major groove of DNA; these residues are responsible for site recognition and binding (Table 4-1). Zinc fingers are found in many mammalian transcription factors, including several that we discuss in this chapter—Egr-1, Wilms tumor protein (WT-1), and stimulating protein 1 (Sp1; Table 4-1)—as well as the steroid hormone receptors.

Basic Zipper   This bZIP family (also known as the leucine zipper family) consists of transcription factors that bind to DNA as dimers (Fig. 4-10B). Members include C/EBPβ (CCAAT/enhancer binding protein β), c-Fos, c-Jun, and CREB (cAMP response element binding protein). Each monomer consist of two domains, a basic region that contacts DNA and a leucine zipper region that mediates dimerization. The basic region contains about 30 amino acids and is enriched in arginine and lysine residues. This region is responsible for sequence-specific binding to DNA through an α helix that inserts into the major groove of DNA. The leucine zipper consists of a region of about 30 amino acids in which every seventh residue is a leucine. Because of this spacing, the leucine residues align on a common face every second turn of an α helix. Two protein subunits that both contain leucine zippers can associate because of hydrophobic interactions between the leucine side chains; they form a tertiary structure called a *coiled coil*. Proteins of this family interact with DNA as *homo*dimers or as structurally related *hetero*dimers. Dimerization is essential for transcriptional activity because mutations of the leucine residues abolish both dimer formation and the ability to bind DNA and

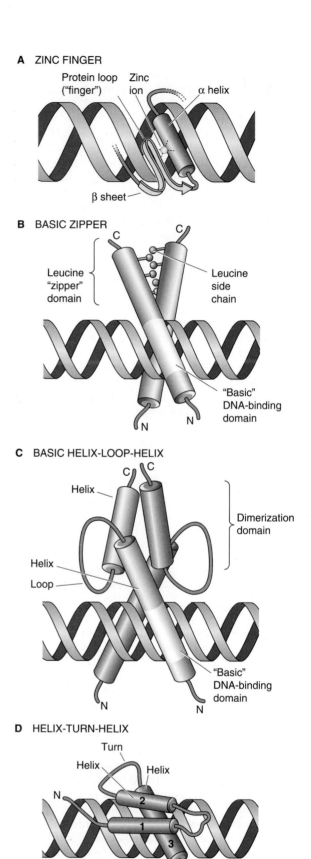

A ZINC FINGER

Protein loop ("finger")   Zinc ion   α helix

β sheet

B BASIC ZIPPER

Leucine "zipper" domain

C   C

Leucine side chain

N   N

"Basic" DNA-binding domain

C BASIC HELIX-LOOP-HELIX

C   C

Helix

Dimerization domain

Helix

Loop

"Basic" DNA-binding domain

N   N

D HELIX-TURN-HELIX

Turn

Helix   Helix

N

2

1

3

C

Figure 4-10   Families of transcription factors.

activate transcription. The crystal structure reveals that these transcription factors resemble scissors in which the blades represent the leucine zipper domains and the handles represent the DNA-binding domains (Fig. 4-10B).

Basic Helix-Loop-Helix Similar to the bZIP family, members of the bHLH family of transcription factors also bind to DNA as dimers. Each monomer has an extended α-helical segment containing the basic region that contacts DNA, linked by a loop to a second α helix that mediates dimer formation (Fig. 4-10C). Thus, the bHLH transcription factor forms by association of four amphipathic α helices (two from each monomer) into a bundle. The basic domains of each monomer protrude into the major grooves on opposite sides of the DNA. bHLH proteins include the MyoD family, which is involved in muscle differentiation, and E proteins (E12 and E47). MyoD and an E protein generally bind to DNA as heterodimers.

Helix-Turn-Helix In prokaryotes such as *Escherichia coli*, the HTH family consists of two α helices that are separated by a β turn. In eukaryotes, a modified HTH structure is represented by the so-called homeodomain (Fig. 4-10D), which is present in some transcription factors that regulate development. The homeodomain consists of a 60–amino acid sequence that forms three α helices. Helices 1 and 2 lie adjacent to one another, and helix 3 is perpendicular and forms the DNA recognition helix. Particular amino acids protrude from the recognition helix and contact bases in the major groove of the DNA. Examples of homeodomain proteins include the Hox proteins, which are involved in mammalian pattern formation; engrailed homologues that are important in nervous system development; and the POU family members Pit-1, Oct-1, and unc-86.

Coactivators and corepressors are transcription factors that do not bind to DNA

Some transcription factors that are required for the activation of gene transcription do not directly bind to DNA. These proteins are called **coactivators**. Coactivators work in concert with DNA-binding transcriptional activators to stimulate gene transcription. They function as adapters or protein intermediaries that form protein-protein interactions between activators bound to enhancers and the basal transcriptional machinery assembled on the gene promoter (Fig. 4-7). Coactivators often contain distinct domains, one that interacts with the transactivation domain of an activator and a second that interacts with components of the basal transcriptional machinery. Transcription factors that interact with repressors and play an analogous role in transcriptional repression are called **corepressors**.

One of the first coactivators found in eukaryotes was the VP16 herpesvirus protein discussed earlier (Fig. 4-9B). VP16 has two domains. The first is a transactivation domain that contains a region of acidic amino acids that in turn interacts with two components of the basal transcriptional machinery, general transcription factors TFIIB and TFIID. The other domain of VP16 interacts with the ubiquitous activator Oct-1, which recognizes a DNA sequence called the octamer motif (Table 4-1). Thus, VP16 activates transcription by bridging an activator and the basal transcriptional machinery.

Coactivators are of two types. The first plays an essential role in the transcriptional activation of many, perhaps all, eukaryotic genes. These coactivators include the TBP-associated factors and Mediator. As discussed previously, **TAFs** were first identified as subunits of the general transcription factor TFIID. Although TAFs are not required for basal transcription, they are essential for *transcriptional activation* by an activator protein, with which they interact directly. For example, the transcriptional activator Sp1 binds to a 250-kDa TAF called TAF_{250}. TAF_{250} binds to a smaller TAF_{110}, which in turn binds to TBP. This sequence establishes an uninterrupted linkage between Sp1 and the TBP component of TFIID that binds to the TATA box in the gene promoter. **Mediator**, a multiprotein complex consisting of 28 to 30 subunits, also appears to be required for activated gene transcription but not basal transcription. Consistent with their essential roles, TAFs and Mediator are present in the basal transcriptional machinery or preinitiation complex.

A second type of coactivator is involved in the transcriptional activation of specific genes. This type of coactivator is not a component of the basal transcriptional machinery. Rather, these coactivators are recruited by a DNA-binding transcriptional activator through protein-protein interactions. An example is the coactivator CBP (CREB-binding protein), which interacts with a DNA-binding transcription factor called CREB (Table 4-1).

Transcriptional activators stimulate transcription by three mechanisms

Once transcriptional activators bind to enhancers (i.e., positive regulatory elements on the DNA) and recruit coactivators, how do they stimulate gene transcription? We discuss three mechanisms by which transactivation might be achieved. These mechanisms are not mutually exclusive, and more than one mechanism may be involved in the transcription of a particular gene.

Recruitment of the Basal Transcriptional Machinery We have already introduced the concept by which looping out of DNA permits proteins that are bound to distant DNA enhancer elements to become physically juxtaposed to proteins that are bound to the gene promoter (Fig. 4-11, pathway 1). The interaction between the DNA-binding transcription factor and general transcription factors, perhaps with coactivators as protein intermediaries, enhances the recruitment of the basal transcriptional machinery to the promoter. Two general transcription factors, TFIID and TFIIB, are targets for recruitment by transcriptional activators. For example, the acidic transactivation domain of VP16 binds to TFIIB, and mutations that prevent the interaction between VP16 and TFIIB also abolish transcriptional activation. Conversely, mutations of TFIIB that eliminate the interaction with an acidic activator also abolish transactivation but have little effect on *basal* transcription.

Chromatin Remodeling A second mechanism by which transcriptional activators may function is alteration of chromatin structure. Transcription factors can bind to HATs

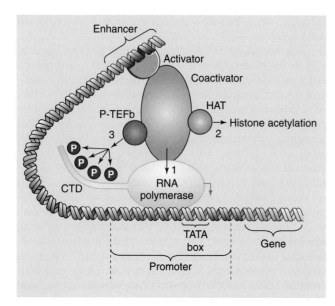

Figure 4-11 Mechanisms of transcriptional activation. The transcriptional activator binds to the enhancer and directly or indirectly (through coactivators) activates transcription by recruiting RNA polymerase to the promoter **1,** recruiting histone acetyltransferases that remodel chromatin **2,** or stimulating the phosphorylation of the C-terminal domain (CTD) of RNA polymerase **3.**

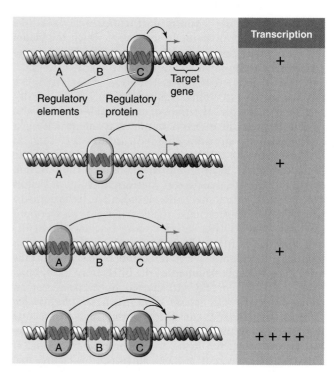

Figure 4-12 Synergism of transcriptional activators. The promoter contains three DNA enhancer elements A, B, and C. Binding of a transcription factor to only one of the enhancer elements (A, B, or C) causes a modest activation of transcription. Simultaneous binding of different transcription factors to each of the three enhancer elements can produce a supra-additive increase in transcription (i.e., synergy).

either directly or indirectly through coactivators (Fig. 4-11, pathway 2). As discussed previously, HATs play an important role in chromatin remodeling before the initiation of gene transcription. By acetylating lysine residues on histones, they inhibit the electrostatic interaction between histones and DNA, which facilitates the binding of additional transcriptional activators and the basal transcriptional machinery. Interestingly, several coactivator proteins that mediate transcriptional activation, such as CBP, possess intrinsic histone acetylase activity. These observations suggest that transcriptional activation is mediated by coactivator proteins that not only bind to components of the basal transcriptional machinery but also promote histone acetylation and thus produce local alterations in chromatin structure that are more favorable for transcription.

Stimulation of RNA Polymerase II A third mechanism by which transcriptional activators function is by stimulating RNA Pol II (Fig. 4-11, pathway 3). The C-terminal domain (CTD) of the largest subunit of Pol II contains 52 repeats of the sequence Tyr-Ser-Pro-Thr-Ser-Pro-Ser, which can be phosphorylated at multiple serine and threonine residues. A cyclin-dependent kinase called positive transcription elongation factor b (P-TEFb) phosphorylates the CTD. Phosphorylation of the CTD occurs coincident with initiation of transcription and is required for chain elongation. Thus, transcriptional activators that interact with P-TEFb may stimulate the conversion of the Pol II holoenzyme from an initiation complex into an **elongation complex.**

Taken together, these three mechanisms of interaction lead to an attractive model for activation of transcription. The transcriptional activator that is bound to an enhancer presents a functional domain (e.g., an acidic domain) that

either directly or through coactivators interacts with histone acetylases and components of the basal transcriptional machinery. These interactions result in chromatin remodeling and facilitate the assembly of the basal transcriptional machinery on the gene promoter. Subsequent interactions—with the CTD of Pol II, for example—may stimulate transcriptional elongation.

Transcriptional activators act in combination

Two or more activators may increase the rate of transcription by an amount that is greater than the sum of each of the activators alone. Almost all naturally occurring promoters contain more than one site for binding of transcriptional activators. A promoter region that contains only a single copy of an enhancer element shows only weak stimulation, whereas a promoter containing multiple copies of an enhancer exhibits substantial activation (Fig. 4-12). Two mechanisms for synergy have been proposed.

In the first, synergy may reflect **cooperative binding to DNA**; that is, binding of one transcription factor to its recognition site enhances binding of a second transcription factor to a different site. This phenomenon occurs with the glucocorticoid receptor (GR), which binds to a site on DNA known as the **glucocorticoid response element** (GRE). Binding of GRs to the multiple GREs is cooperative in that binding of the first receptor promotes binding of additional receptors. Thus, the presence of multiple copies of the GRE greatly stimulates gene expression in comparison to a single copy of the GRE.

In the second case, synergy reflects **cooperative protein-protein interactions** between transcription factors and multiple sites on the basal transcriptional machinery. For example, a transcriptional activator that recruits TFIID could synergize with another activator that recruits TFIIB. Similarly, a transcriptional activator that interacts with a HAT could synergize with another activator that interacts with components of the basal transcriptional machinery. Here, the effect on transcription depends on the cumulative effects of multiple transcription factors, each bound to its cognate recognition site and interacting with chromatin remodeling proteins and the basal transcriptional machinery.

Transcription factors may act in combination by binding to DNA as **homodimers** or **heterodimers**. This synergism is particularly true for members of the bZIP and bHLH families but also for steroid and thyroid hormone receptors. Often, different combinations of monomers have different DNA binding *affinities*. For example, the thyroid hormone receptor (TR) can bind to DNA as a homodimer, but the heterodimer formed from the thyroid receptor and the 9-*cis*-retinoic acid receptor (TR/RXR) has much higher binding affinity. As we saw earlier, the transcription factor MyoD, which is involved in muscle differentiation, requires heterodimerization with the ubiquitous proteins E12 and E47 for maximal DNA binding. Different combinations of monomers may also have different DNA binding *specificities* and thus be targeted to different sites on the DNA. Finally, different combinations of monomers may have different *transactivational properties*. For example, the c-Myc protein can bind to DNA as a homodimer or as a heterodimer with Max, but c-Myc/Max heterodimers have greater transcriptional activity.

Transcriptional repressors act by competition, quenching, or active repression

Cells can regulate transcription not only *positively* through transcriptional activators but also *negatively* through transcriptional repressors. Repression of transcription is important for tissue specificity in that it allows cells to silence certain genes where they should not be expressed. Repression is also important for regulating inducible gene expression by rapidly turning off transcription after removal of the inducing stimulus.

Transcriptional repressors may act by three mechanisms. First, some repressors inhibit the binding of transcriptional activators because they **compete** for DNA-binding sites that are identical to, or overlap with, those for activators. An example is the CCAAT displacement protein (CDP), which binds to the CAAT box in the promoter of the γ-globin gene and thereby prevents binding of the transcriptional activator CP1. This action helps prevent inappropriate expression of the fetal globin gene in adults.

Second, some repressors inhibit the activity of transcriptional activators not by interfering with DNA binding but by a direct protein-protein interaction with activators. This form of repression is termed **quenching**. A classic example in yeast is the GAL80 repressor, which inhibits transcriptional activation by GAL4. By binding to the transactivation domain of GAL4, GAL80 blocks transcriptional activation. Dissociation of GAL80 (which occurs in the presence of galactose) relieves the inhibition of GAL4, which can then induce expression of galactose-metabolizing genes. Transcriptional repression can also be mediated by proteins that prevent transcriptional activators from entering the nucleus. For example, the heat shock protein hsp90 binds to GR and prevents this transcriptional activator from entering the nucleus.

A third class of repressors binds to a silencer (or NRE) and then directly inhibits transcription. This mechanism is referred to as **active repression**. The opposite of transcriptional activators, these proteins contain domains that mediate repression. Repression domains may directly interact with and inhibit the assembly or activity of the basal transcriptional machinery. Alternatively, transcriptional repressors may inhibit transcription through protein-protein interactions with corepressors. Some transcriptional corepressors, such as the N-CoR adapter protein that mediates repression by steroid hormone receptors, can interact with HDAC. By removing the acetyl groups from lysine residues in histones, HDACs promote tighter binding between DNA and histones and inhibit transcription initiation.

The activity of transcription factors may be regulated by post-translational modifications

Cells can regulate the activity of transcription factors by controlling the amount of transcription factor they synthesize. In addition, cells can modulate the activity of preformed transcription factors by three general mechanisms of post-translational modification (Table 4-2).

Phosphorylation The best studied post-translational modification affecting transcription factor activity is phosphorylation, which increases or decreases (1) transport of the transcription factor from the cytoplasm into the nucleus, (2) the affinity with which the transcription factor binds to DNA, and (3) transcriptional activation.

For transcription factors that reside in the cytoplasm under basal conditions, migration from the cytoplasm into the nucleus is a necessary step. Many proteins that are transported into the nucleus contain a sequence that is relatively enriched in basic amino acid residues (i.e., arginine and lysine). This sequence, the **nuclear localization signal**, is required for transport of the protein into the nucleus. Phosphorylation at sites within or near the nuclear localization signal can dramatically change the rate of nuclear translocation. Phosphorylation can also modulate import into the nucleus by regulating the binding of transcription factors to cytoplasmic anchors. In the case of the transcription factor NF-κB (Fig. 4-13A), binding to the cytoplasmic anchor IκB conceals the nuclear localization signal on the p50 and p65 subunits of NF-κB from the nuclear translocation machinery. Only after these two other subunits dissociate from the phosphorylated IκB is the transcription factor dimer free to enter the nucleus.

Phosphorylation can also regulate transcription factor activity by altering the *affinity* of the transcription factor for its target recognition sequences on DNA. As a result,

Table 4-2 Post-translational Modifications of Transcription Factors

Modification	Modifying Group	Modified Amino Acid	Transcription Factor (Example)	Effects (Example)
Phosphorylation	-PO₄	Ser/Thr, Tyr	p53, HIF-1α, GR, Sp1, PPAR-α, β-catenin, STAT1, CREB, NFAT	Altered affinity for coactivators Promotes ubiquitination Altered protein-protein or protein-DNA interactions
Site-specific proteolysis	None	None	SREBP-1, Notch, NF-κB, ATF6	Generation of an active transcription factor from an inactive precursor
Acetylation	-COCH₃	Lys	Sp3, p53, MEF2, STAT3	Regulation of protein stability DNA binding Protein-protein interactions
Methylation	-CH3	Arg, Lys	PGC-1α, STAT1, CBP	Inhibition of protein-protein interactions
Glycosylation	GlcNAc	Ser/Thr	Elf-1, c-Myc, Sp1, ER	Stimulation of transcriptional activity Nuclear transport Protein stability
Ubiquitination	Ubiquitin	Lys	SREBP-1, c-Myc, VP16, β-catenin, p53, Smad2	Targeting for proteasomal degradation (polyubiquitination) Transcriptional activation (monoubiquitination)
Sumoylation	SUMO	Lys	ER, SF-1, AR	Inhibition of transcriptional activity
Hydroxylation	-OH	Pro, Asn	HIF-1α	Altered affinity for coactivators Altered protein-protein interactions
Nitrosylation	-NO	Cys	NF-κB, Sp1, HIF-1α	Inhibition of DNA binding or protein degradation

AR, androgen receptor; ATF6, activating transcription factor 6; ER, estrogen receptor; GlcNaC, N-acetylglucosamine; GR, glucocorticoid receptor; PGC-1α, PPAR-γ cofactor 1α; SF-1, steroidogenic factor 1; SUMO, small ubiquitin-related modifier.

phosphorylation increases or decreases DNA-binding activity. For example, phosphorylation of SRF (serum response factor), a transcription factor that activates the c-*fos* gene in response to growth factors, enhances DNA binding. In contrast, phosphorylation of the transcription factor c-Jun by casein kinase II inhibits binding to DNA.

Phosphorylation can greatly influence the *transactivation properties* of transcription factors. c-Jun is an example in which transcriptional activity is increased by the phosphorylation of serine residues located within the transactivation domain near the N terminus of the protein. Phosphorylation of a transcriptional activator may stimulate its activity by increasing its binding affinity for a coactivator. Phosphorylation can also *inhibit* transcriptional activation by reducing transcriptional activation or stimulating active transcriptional repression.

Effects of phosphorylation on nuclear translocation, DNA binding, and transactivation are not mutually exclusive. Moreover, in addition to phosphorylation by protein kinases, dephosphorylation by protein phosphatases may also regulate transcriptional activity.

Site-Specific Proteolysis Many transcription factors undergo proteolytic cleavage at specific amino acid residues, particularly in response to exogenous signals. Site-specific proteolysis often converts an inactive precursor protein into an active transcriptional regulator. One example is NF-κB. Although phosphorylation can regulate NF-κB by controlling its binding to IκB (Fig. 4-13A), proteolysis can also regulate NF-κB (Fig. 4-13B). A 105-kDa precursor of the 50-kDa subunit of NF-κB (p50), which we mentioned earlier, binds to and thereby retains the 65-kDa subunit of NF-κB (p65) in the cytoplasm. Proteolysis of this larger precursor yields the 50-kDa subunit that together with the 65-kDa subunit constitutes the active NF-κB transcription factor.

Another form of site-specific proteolysis, which creates active transcription factors from inactive membrane-tethered precursors, is called **regulated intramembranous proteolysis (RIP)**. The best characterized example is the **sterol regulatory element binding protein (SREBP)**, a membrane protein that normally resides in the endoplasmic reticulum. In response to depletion of cellular cholesterol, SREBP undergoes RIP, which releases an N-terminal fragment

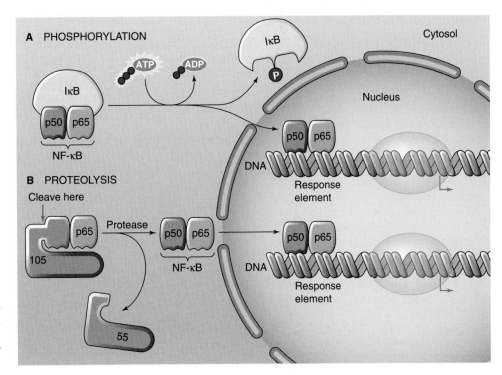

Figure 4-13 Regulation of transcription factors by post-translational modification. **A,** The phosphorylation of the cytoplasmic anchor IκB releases the p50 and p65 subunits of NF-κB, allowing them to translocate into the nucleus. **B,** Proteolytic cleavage of a 105-kDa precursor releases the p50 subunit of NF-κB. Together with the p65 subunit, the p50 subunit can now translocate to the nucleus.

containing a bHLH motif. The proteolytic fragment translocates to the nucleus, where it binds to DNA and activates transcription of genes that encode enzymes involved in cholesterol biosynthesis and the LDL receptor (see Chapter 2).

Other Post-translational Modifications In addition to phosphate groups, a variety of other covalent attachments can affect the activity of transcription factors (Table 4-3). These small molecules—such as acetyl groups, methyl groups, sugars or peptides, hydroxyl groups, or nitro groups—attach to specific amino acid residues in the transcription factor. Post-translational modifications of transcription factors can affect their stability, intracellular localization, dimerization, DNA-binding properties, or interactions with coactivators. For example, **acetylation** of lysine residues in the p53 transcription factor increases binding to DNA and inhibits degradation. **Methylation** of an arginine residue in the coactivator CBP inhibits its interaction with the transcription factor CREB. The **O-glycosylation**, a covalent modification in which sugar groups attach to serine or threonine residues, stimulates NF-κB. **Ubiquitin** is a small peptide that is covalently attached to lysine groups in proteins. Addition of multiple ubiquitin groups (polyubiquitination) frequently results in degradation of the protein by the proteosome (see Chapter 2). However, addition of a single ubiquitin group (monoubiquitination) may stimulate the activity of a transcription factor, perhaps by increasing its affinity for transcriptional elongation factors. Conversely, **sumoylation**, covalent modification of lysine residues with small ubiquitin-like modifiers (SUMO), may inhibit activity by altering the localization of a transcription factor within the nucleus. As we will see in the next section, extracellular signals often trigger

Table 4-3 Examples of Transcription Factors That Regulate Gene Expression in Response to Physiological Stimuli

Physiological Stimulus	Transcription Factor	Target Genes (Example)
Hypoxia	HIF-1α	Vascular endothelial growth factor, erythropoietin, glycolytic enzymes
DNA damage	p53	*CIP1/WAF1, GADD45, PCNA, MDM2*
Cholesterol depletion	SREBP-1	HMG-CoA reductase, fatty acid synthase, LDL receptor
Viruses, oxidants	NF-κB	Tumor necrosis factor α, interleukin 1β, interleukin 2, granulocyte colony-stimulating factor, inducible nitric oxide synthase, intercellular cell adhesion molecule
Heat stress	HSF1	Heat shock proteins, αB-crystallin
Fatty acids	PPAR-α	Lipoprotein lipase, fatty acid transport protein, acyl-CoA synthetase, carnitine palmitoyltransferase I

post-translational modifications to regulate the activity of transcription factors.

The expression of some transcription factors is tissue specific

Some transcription factors are ubiquitous, either because these transcription factors regulate the transcription of genes that are expressed in many different tissues or because they are required for the transcription of many different genes. Examples of ubiquitous transcription factors are the DNA-binding transcription factors Sp1 and NF-Y, which bind to regulatory elements (i.e., GC boxes and CCAAT boxes, respectively) that are present in many gene promoters. Other transcription factors are present only in certain tissues or cell types; these transcription factors are involved in the regulation of tissue-specific gene expression.

Tissue-specific activators bind to enhancers present in the promoters and regulatory regions of genes that are expressed in a tissue-specific manner. Conversely, tissue-specific repressors bind to silencers that prevent transcription of a gene in nonexpressing tissues. Each tissue-specific transcription factor could regulate the expression of multiple genes. Because the short sequences of enhancers and silencers may occur by chance, the combined effect of multiple transcription factors—each binding to distinct regulatory elements near the gene—prevents illegitimate transcription in nonexpressing tissues. In addition to activation by transcriptional activators, tissue-specific gene expression may also be regulated by transcriptional repression. In this case, transcriptional repressors prevent transcription of a gene in nonexpressing tissues. Tissue-specific expression probably also involves permanent silencing of nonexpressed genes through epigenetic modifications, such as DNA methylation, that we discuss later.

Pit-1 is an HTH-type tissue-specific transcription factor that regulates the pituitary-specific expression of genes encoding growth hormone, thyroid-stimulating hormone, and prolactin. MyoD and myogenin are bHLH-type transcription factors that bind to the E box sequence CANNTG of promoters and enhancers of many genes expressed in skeletal muscle, such as myosin heavy chain and muscle creatine kinase. EKLF as well as GATA-1 and NF-E2 mediate the erythroid-specific expression of β-globin genes. The combined effects of HNF-1, HNF-3, HNF-4, C/EBP, and other transcription factors—each of which may individually be present in *several* tissues—mediate the *liver*-specific expression of genes such as albumin and α_1-antitrypsin. Many tissue-specific transcription factors play important roles in embryonic development. For example, myogenin is required for skeletal muscle differentiation, and GATA-1 is required for the development of erythroid cells.

What is responsible for the tissue-specific expression of the transcription factor itself? Although the answer is not known, many tissue-specific transcription factors are themselves under the control of other tissue-specific factors. Thus, a transcriptional cascade involving multiple tissue-specific proteins may regulate tissue-specific gene expression. Ultimately, however, tissue specificity is likely to arise from external signals that direct gene expression down a particular pathway.

REGULATION OF INDUCIBLE GENE EXPRESSION BY SIGNAL TRANSDUCTION PATHWAYS

How do cells activate previously quiescent genes in response to environmental cues? How are such external signals transduced to the cell nucleus to stimulate the transcription of specific genes? Transcription factors may be thought of as effector molecules in signal transduction pathways (see Chapter 3) that modulate gene expression. Several such signaling pathways have been defined. Lipid-soluble steroid and thyroid hormones can enter the cell and interact with specific receptors that are themselves transcription factors. However, most cytokines, hormones, and mitogens cannot diffuse into the cell interior and instead bind to specific receptors that are located on the cell surface. First, we consider three pathways for transducing signals from cell surface receptors into the nucleus: a cAMP-dependent pathway, a Ras-dependent pathway, and the JAK-STAT pathway. Next, we examine the mechanisms by which steroid or thyroid hormones act through nuclear receptors. Finally, we discuss how transcription factors coordinate gene expression in response to physiological stimuli.

cAMP regulates transcription through the transcription factors CREB and CBP

cAMP is an important second messenger in the response to agonists binding to specific cell surface receptors. Increases in $[cAMP]_i$ stimulate the transcription of certain genes, including those that encode a variety of hormones, such as somatostatin (see Chapter 48), the enkephalins (see Chapter 13), glucagon (see Chapter 51), and vasoactive intestinal polypeptide (see Chapter 41). Many genes that are activated in response to cAMP contain within their regulatory regions a common DNA element called **CRE** (cAMP response element) that has the consensus sequence 5'-TGACGTCA-3'. Several different transcription factors bind to CRE, among them **CREB**, a 43-kDa member of the bZIP family. As shown in Figure 4-14, increases in $[cAMP]_i$ stimulate protein kinase A (PKA) by causing dissociation of the PKA regulatory subunit. The catalytic subunit of PKA then translocates into the nucleus, where it phosphorylates CREB and other proteins. Activation of CREB is rapid (30 minutes) and declines gradually during a 24-hour period. This phosphorylation greatly increases the affinity of CREB for the coactivator **CBP**. CBP is a 245-kDa protein that contains two domains, one that binds to phosphorylated CREB and another that activates components of the basal transcriptional machinery. Thus, CBP serves as a "bridge" protein that communicates the transcriptional activation signal from CREB to the basal transcriptional machinery. In addition, because CBP has intrinsic HAT activity, its recruitment by CREB also results in chromatin remodeling that facilitates gene transcription. The result of phosphorylating CREB is a 10- to 20-fold stimulation of CREB's ability to induce the transcription of genes containing a CRE.

How is the transcriptional signal terminated? When $[cAMP]_i$ is high, PKA phosphorylates and activates phosphoprotein phosphatase 1 in the nucleus. When cAMP levels fall, the still-active phosphatase dephosphorylates CREB.

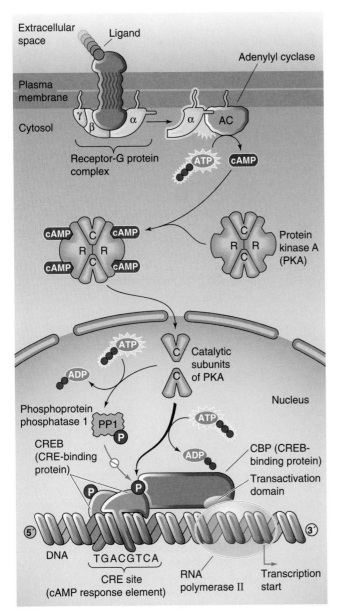

Figure 4-14 Regulation of gene transcription by cAMP. Phosphorylated CREB binds CBP, which has a transactivation domain that stimulates the basal transcriptional machinery. In parallel, phosphorylation activates PP1, which dephosphorylates CREB, terminating the activation of transcription.

Receptor tyrosine kinases regulate transcription through a Ras-dependent cascade of protein kinases

As discussed in Chapter 3, many growth factors bind to cell surface receptors that when activated by the ligand have tyrosine kinase activity. Examples of growth factors that act through such receptor tyrosine kinases (RTKs) are epidermal growth factor (EGF), platelet-derived growth factor (PDGF), insulin, insulin-like growth factor type 1 (IGF-1), fibroblast growth factor (FGF), and nerve growth factor (NGF). The common pathway by which activation of RTKs is transduced into the nucleus is a cascade of events that increase the activity of the small guanosine triphosphate (GTP)–binding

protein Ras. This **Ras-dependent signaling pathway** culminates in the activation of MAP kinase (MAPK), which translocates to the nucleus, where it phosphorylates a number of nuclear proteins that are transcription factors. Phosphorylation of a transcription factor by MAPK can enhance or inhibit binding to DNA and can stimulate either transactivation or transrepression. Transcription factors that are regulated by the Ras-dependent pathway include c-Myc, c-Jun, c-Fos, and Elk-1. Many of these transcription factors regulate the expression of genes that promote cell proliferation.

Tyrosine kinase–associated receptors can regulate transcription through JAK-STAT

A group of cell surface receptors termed tyrosine kinase–associated receptors lack *intrinsic* tyrosine kinase activity. The ligands that bind to these receptors include several cytokines, growth hormone, prolactin, and interferons (IFN-α, IFN-β, and IFN-γ). Although the receptors themselves lack catalytic activity, their cytoplasmic domains are associated with the JAK family of protein tyrosine kinases.

Binding of ligand to certain tyrosine kinase–associated receptors activates a member of the JAK family, which results in phosphorylation of cytoplasmic proteins, among which are believed to be latent cytoplasmic transcription factors called **STATs** (signal transducers and activators of transcription). When phosphorylated on tyrosine residues, the STAT proteins dimerize and thereby become competent to enter the nucleus and induce transcription.

A well-characterized example of the JAK-STAT pathway is the activation of **interferon-responsive genes** by IFN-α and IFN-γ. IFN-α activates the JAK1 and Tyk2 kinases that are associated with its receptor (Fig. 4-15A). Subsequent phosphorylation of two different STAT monomers causes the monomers to dimerize. This STAT heterodimer enters the nucleus, where it combines with a third 48-kDa protein to form a transcription factor that binds to a DNA sequence called the IFN-α–stimulated response element (ISRE). In the case of IFN-γ (Fig. 4-15B), the receptor associates with the JAK1 and JAK2 (rather than Tyk2) kinases, and subsequent phosphorylation of a *single* kind of STAT monomer causes these monomers to dimerize. These STAT homodimers also enter the nucleus, where they bind to the DNA at IFN-γ response elements called γ activation sites (GAS), without requiring the 48-kDa protein.

Nuclear receptors are transcription factors

Steroid and thyroid hormones are examples of ligands that activate gene expression by binding to cellular receptors that are themselves transcription factors. Members of the steroid and thyroid hormone receptor superfamily, also called the nuclear receptor superfamily, are grouped together because they are structurally similar and have similar mechanisms of action. After these hormones enter the cell, they bind to receptors in the cytoplasm or nucleus. Ligand binding converts the receptors into active transcription factors. The transcription factors bind to specific regulatory elements on the DNA, called **hormone response elements**, and activate the transcription of *cis*-linked genes. The family of nuclear receptors includes receptors that bind glucocorticoids (GR),

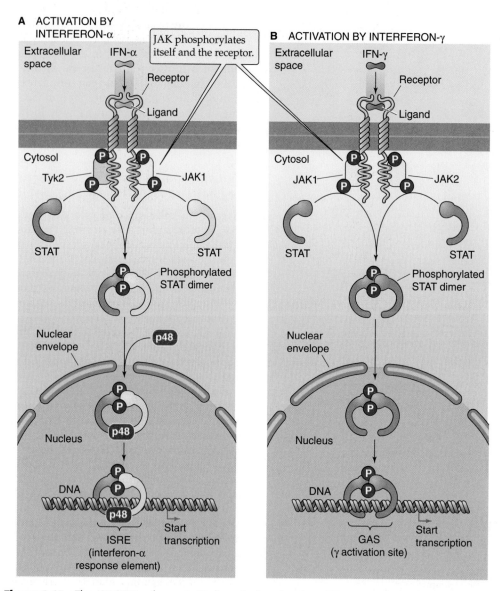

Figure 4-15 The JAK-STAT pathway. **A,** Binding of a ligand such as IFN-α to a tyrosine kinase–associated receptor causes JAK1 and Tyk2 to phosphorylate themselves, the receptor, and two different STAT monomers. The phosphorylation of the STAT monomers leads to the formation of a *hetero*dimer, which translocates to the nucleus and combines with a third protein (p48). The complex binds to the ISRE and activates gene transcription. **B,** Binding of a ligand such as IFN-γ to a tyrosine kinase–associated receptor causes JAK1 and JAK2 to phosphorylate themselves, the receptor, and two identical STAT monomers. The phosphorylation of the STAT monomers leads to the formation of a *homo*dimer, which translocates to the nucleus. The complex binds to the GAS response element and activates gene transcription.

mineralocorticoids (MR), estrogens (ER), progesterone (PR), androgens (AR), thyroid hormone (TR), vitamin D (VDR), retinoic acid (RAR), lipids (peroxisome proliferator–activated receptor, PPAR), and 9-*cis*-retinoic acid (retinoid X receptor, RXR) as well as bile acids (bile acid receptor, FXR) and xenobiotics (steroid and xenobiotic receptor, SXR; constitutive androstane receptor, CAR) (see Chapter 46).

With the exception of the thyroid hormones, the hormones that bind to these receptors are lipophilic molecules that enter cells by diffusion and do not require interaction with cell surface receptors. The thyroid hormones differ in

that they are electrically charged and may cross the cell membrane through transporters (see Chapter 49).

Modular Construction The nuclear receptors have a modular construction consisting of an N-terminal transactivation domain, a DNA-binding domain, and a C-terminal ligand-binding domain. These receptors bind to specific DNA sequences by two *zinc fingers,* each of which contains four cysteine residues rather than the two histidines and two cysteines that are typical of many other zinc finger proteins (Fig. 4-10A). Particularly important for DNA recognition is

Table 4-4 Nuclear Receptors

Receptor	Full Name	Dimeric Arrangement
GR	Glucocorticoid receptor	GR/GR
MR	Mineralocorticoid receptor	MR/MR
PR	Progesterone receptor	PR/PR
ER	Estrogen receptor	ER/ER
AR	Androgen receptor	AR/AR
VDR	Vitamin D receptor	VDR/RXR
TR	Thyroid hormone receptor	TR/RXR
RAR	Retinoic acid receptor	RAR/RXR
PPAR	Peroxisome proliferator–activated receptor	PPAR/RXR
FXR	Bile acid receptor	FXR/RXR
SXR	Steroid and xenobiotic receptor	SXR/RXR
CAR	Constitutive androstane receptor	CAR/RXR

the P box motif in the hormone receptor, a sequence of six amino acids at the C-terminal end of each finger. These P boxes make base pair contacts in the major groove of DNA and determine the DNA-binding specificities of the zinc finger.

Dimerization   GR, MR, PR, ER, and AR bind to DNA as **homodimers** (Table 4-4). The recognition sites for these receptors (except for ER) consist of two 6-bp DNA sequences that are separated by three other base pairs. The 6-bp DNA sequences, commonly called **half-sites**, represent binding sites for each zinc finger monomer.

In contrast, VDR, TR, RAR, and PPAR preferentially bind to DNA as **heterodimers** formed with RXR, the receptor for 9-*cis*-retinoic acid. Thus, the dimers are VDR/RXR, TR/RXR, RAR/RXR, and PPAR/RXR. Interestingly, these heterodimers work even in the absence of the ligand of RXR (i.e., 9-*cis*-retinoic acid). Only the VDR, TR, RAR, or PPAR part of the dimer needs to be occupied by its hormone ligand. These heterodimers recognize a family of DNA sites containing a DNA sequence such as 5′-AGGTCA-3′, followed by a DNA spacer and then by a direct repeat of the previous 6-bp DNA sequence. Moreover, because VDR/RXR, TR/RXR, and RAR/RXR may each recognize the *same* 6-bp sequences, binding specificity also depends on the length of the spacer between the direct repeats. The VDR/RXR, TR/RXR, and RAR/RXR heterodimers preferentially recognize separations of 3 bp, 4 bp, and 5 bp, respectively, between the repeats of 5′-AGGTCA-3′. This relationship forms the basis for the so-called **3-4-5 rule.**

Activation of Transcription   Ligand binding activates nuclear receptors through two main mechanisms: regulation

of subcellular localization and interactions with coactivators. Some nuclear receptors, such as GR, are normally located in the cytoplasm and are maintained in an inactive state by association with a cytoplasmic anchoring protein (Fig. 4-16A). The protein that retains GR in the cytoplasm is a **molecular chaperone**, the 90-kDa heat shock protein **hsp90**. GR must bind to hsp90 to have a high affinity for a glucocorticoid hormone. When glucocorticoids bind to the GR, hsp90 dissociates from the GR and exposes a nuclear localization signal that permits the transport of GR into the nucleus. The receptor must remain hormone bound for receptor dimerization, which is a prerequisite for binding to the GRE on the DNA. Other receptors, such as TR, are normally already present in the nucleus before binding the hormone (Fig. 4-16B). For these receptors, binding of hormone is evidently not essential for dimerization or binding to DNA. However, ligand binding is necessary at a subsequent step for transactivation.

Although nuclear receptors may stimulate gene expression by interacting directly with components of the basal transcriptional machinery, full transcriptional activation requires **coactivators** that interact with the receptor in a ligand-dependent manner. More than 200 coactivators may interact directly or indirectly with nuclear receptors through mechanisms that include the following:

1. *Recruitment of basal transcriptional machinery.* Coactivators that belong to the **SRC** (**steroid receptor coactivator**)/p160 family bind only to the ligand-bound form of the receptor. On binding to the nuclear receptor, SRC/p160 coactivators recruit a second coactivator, CBP, which then promotes recruitment of the basal transcriptional machinery. Nuclear receptors also bind in a ligand-

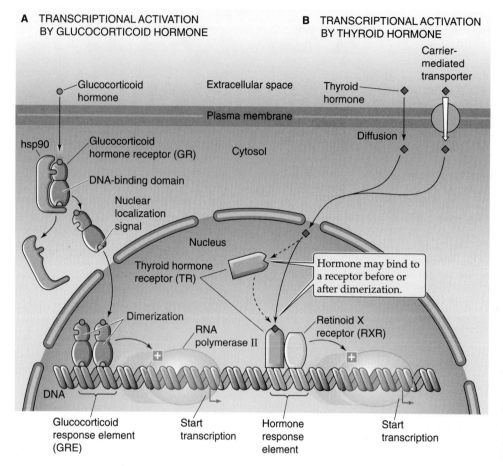

**A TRANSCRIPTIONAL ACTIVATION
BY GLUCOCORTICOID HORMONE**

**B TRANSCRIPTIONAL ACTIVATION
BY THYROID HORMONE**

Carrier-
mediated
transporter

Glucocorticoid
hormone

Extracellular space

Thyroid
hormone

Plasma membrane

hsp90

Glucocorticoid
hormone receptor (GR)

Cytosol

Diffusion

DNA-binding domain

Nuclear
localization
signal

Nucleus

Thyroid hormone
receptor (TR)

Hormone may bind to
a receptor before or
after dimerization.

Dimerization

RNA
polymerase II

Retinoid X
receptor (RXR)

DNA

Glucocorticoid
response element
(GRE)

Start
transcription

Hormone
response
element

Start
transcription

Figure   4-16 Transcriptional activation by glucocorticoid and thyroid hormones. **A,** The binding of a glucocorticoid hormone to a cytoplasmic receptor causes the receptor to dissociate from the chaperone hsp90 (90-kDa heat shock protein). The free hormone-receptor complex can then translocate to the nucleus, where dimerization leads to transactivation. **B,** The binding of thyroid hormone to a receptor in the nucleus leads to transactivation. The active transcription factor is a heterodimer of the thyroid hormone receptor and the retinoid X receptor.

dependent manner to the coactivator TRAP220, a component of Mediator, which is part of the basal transcriptional machinery.

2. *Binding to a chromatin remodeling complex.* Nuclear receptors also interact with Brg1 (Brahma-related gene 1), the central motor component of the chromatin remodeling complex SWI/SNF.

3. *Histone acetylation.* Several coactivators have enzymatic activities that mediate chromatin remodeling. Both SRC-1 and CBP have intrinsic HAT activity.

4. *Histone methylation.* The coactivator CARM1 is a methyltransferase that methylates specific arginine residues in histones, thereby enhancing transcriptional activation.

5. *Ubiquitination.* Nuclear receptors recruit components of the ubiquitin-proteosome pathway (see Chapter 2) to the promoter region of nuclear receptor target genes. Ubiquitination appears to promote transcript elongation.

Repression of Transcription   Nuclear receptors sometimes function as active repressors, perhaps acting by several alternative mechanisms. First, a receptor may form inactive heterodimers with other members of the nuclear receptor family. Second, a receptor may compete with other transcription factors for DNA-binding sites. For example, when the TR—without bound thyroid hormone—interacts with its own DNA response element, the TR acts as a repressor. In addition, the receptor TRa can dimerize with one of the retinoic acid receptors (RXRb) to interfere with binding of

ER to its response element. This competition may be one of the mechanisms that retinoids use to inhibit estrogen-induced alterations in gene expression and growth in mammary tissue. Finally, nuclear receptors can also inhibit gene transcription by interacting with corepressors, such as N-CoR, Sin3A, and Sin3B. These corepressors can recruit HDACs that enhance nucleosome assembly, resulting in transcriptional repression.

Physiological stimuli can modulate transcription factors, which can coordinate complex cellular responses

In response to physiological stimuli, some transcription factors regulate the expression of several genes (Table 4-3). As an example, we discuss how oxygen concentration ($[O_2]$) controls gene expression.

When chronically exposed to low $[O_2]$ (hypoxia), many cells undergo dramatic changes in gene expression. For example, cells switch from oxidative metabolism to glycolysis, which requires the induction of genes encoding glycolytic enzymes. Many tissues activate the gene encoding the vascular endothelial growth factor (VEGF), which stimulates angiogenesis and improves the blood supply to chronically hypoxic tissues. The kidney activates the gene encoding erythropoietin, a hormone that stimulates red cell production in the bone marrow. These changes in gene expression promote survival of the cell or organism in a hypoxic

Role of a Chimeric Transcription Factor in Acute Promyelocytic Leukemia

Correct regulation of gene expression involves both transcription factors and the DNA regulatory elements to which they bind. Abnormalities of either could and do result in abnormal regulation of gene expression, which is often manifested as disease. An example of a transcription factor abnormality is acute promyelocytic leukemia (APL), a hematologic malignant disease in which cells of the granulocyte lineage (promyelocytes) fail to differentiate. Normally, retinoic acid (RA) binds to **retinoic acid receptor α (RARα)**, a member of the steroid-thyroid hormone receptor superfamily. RARα forms heterodimers with **retinoid X receptor (RXR)** and binds to retinoic acid response elements (RAREs) that are present in genes involved in cell differentiation. In the absence of RA, RARα/RXR heterodimers bind to RAREs and recruit the corepressor N-CoR, which in turn recruits HDACs that inhibit gene transcription. Binding of RA to RARα leads to dissociation of N-CoR, which permits binding of the CBP coactivator and activation of RARα-responsive genes that promote cell differentiation. Ninety percent of patients with APL have a translocation affecting chromosomes 15 and 17, t(15;17), that produces a chimeric transcription factor containing the DNA- and hormone-binding domains of RARα, fused to the nuclear protein **PML**. The PML/RARα chimeric protein also binds to RA and forms heterodimers with RXR but has an abnormally high affinity for N-CoR. At physiological levels of RA, N-CoR remains bound to PML/RARα, blocking promyelocytic differentiation. However, high concentrations of RA induce dissociation of N-CoR and permit differentiation. This mechanism explains why high concentrations of exogenous RA can be used to induce clinical remissions in patients with APL.

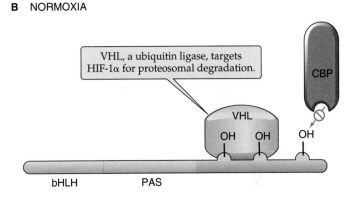

A HYDROXYLATION

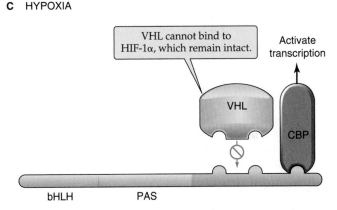

B NORMOXIA

C HYPOXIA

Figure 4-17   Regulation of HIF-1α by oxygen. **A,** In the presence of oxygen, HIF-1α is hydroxylated on proline and asparagine by hydroxylases. **B,** Hydroxylation of HIF-1α promotes its degradation and inhibits its interaction with coactivators. **C,** In hypoxic conditions, dehydroxylation of HIF-1α promotes its stabilization and transcriptional activity.

environment. A key mediator in the response to hypoxia is a transcription factor called **hypoxia-inducible factor 1α (HIF-1α)**.

HIF-1α (Fig. 4-17A) belongs to the bHLH family of transcription factors. In addition, it contains a PAS domain that mediates dimerization. HIF-1α binds to DNA as a heterodimer with HIF-1β. **HIF-1β** is expressed at constant levels in cells, but the abundance of HIF-1α changes markedly in response to changes in [O$_2$]. At a normal [O$_2$] (normoxia), HIF-1α levels are low. Under hypoxic conditions, the abundance of HIF-1α increases. HIF-1α together with HIF-1β binds to an enhancer, called a **hypoxia response element**, that is present in many genes activated during hypoxia, including genes encoding glycolytic enzymes, VEGF, and erythropoietin.

The cell regulates the abundance of HIF-1α by hydroxylation—a post-translational modification—at specific proline and asparagine residues. Oxygen activates the prolyl and asparaginyl hydroxylases (Fig. 4-17A). Proline hydroxylation stimulates the interaction of HIF-1α with VHL, a protein that targets HIF-1α for proteosomal degradation (Fig. 4-17B). Asparagine hydroxylation inhibits the interaction of HIF-1α with the transcriptional coactivator CBP. Because

both of these hydroxylations reduce transcriptional activity, normoxic conditions lower the expression of HIF-1α target genes.

In contrast, under hypoxic conditions, the hydroxylases are inactive, and HIF-1α is not hydroxylated on proline and asparagine residues. HIF-1α accumulates in the nucleus and interacts with CBP, which activates the transcription of downstream target genes, including VEGF and erythropoietin (Fig. 4-17C). The net result is a system in which the expression of multiple hypoxia-inducible genes is coordinately and tightly regulated through post-translational modification of a common transcriptional activator.

REGULATION OF GENE EXPRESSION BY CHANGES IN DNA STRUCTURE

You might recall that at the outset of this chapter we noted that gene expression entails several steps, beginning with alteration of chromatin structure (Fig. 4-1, step 1). Having already discussed the control of transcription (Fig. 4-1, step 2) in the previous three sections, we return in this penultimate section to the first step and consider how changes in chromatin structure and the methylation of both histones and DNA have long-term effects on gene expression. In the last section, we examine several of the later steps in gene expression.

Chromatin exists in two forms

As discussed earlier, DNA in the nucleus is organized into a higher order structure called chromatin, which consists of DNA and associated histones. Chromatin exists in two general forms that can be distinguished cytologically by their different degrees of condensation. **Heterochromatin** is a highly condensed form of chromatin that is transcriptionally inactive. In general, highly organized chromatin structure is associated with *repression* of gene transcription. Heterochromatin contains mostly repetitive DNA sequences and relatively few genes. **Euchromatin** has a more open structure and contains genes that are actively transcribed. Even in the transcriptionally active "open" euchromatin, local chromatin structure may influence the activity of individual genes. We have already seen that transcriptional activators recruit HATs that remodel chromatin and promote binding of additional transcription factors and the basal transcriptional machinery. Conversely, transcriptional repressors recruit HDACs that promote nucleosome assembly and inhibit gene transcription.

Chemical modification of the histones regulates the establishment and maintenance of euchromatin and heterochromatin. Especially important is **methylation**, in which a methyltransferase covalently attaches methyl groups to arginine residues and, most significantly, to specific lysine residues in the core histones. In *euchromatin*, methylation of histone H3 at Lys-4, Lys-36, and Lys-79 correlates with transcriptional *activation*. In *heterochromatin*, demethylation of these residues but methylation of H3 at Lys-9 and Lys-27 and of H4 at Lys-20 correlates with transcriptional *repression*. This pattern of differential methylation in transcriptionally active and inactive chromatin is referred to as a **histone code**.

Methylation of H3 at Lys-9 recruits heterochromatin protein 1 (HP1), which then self-dimerizes to produce higher order structures (Fig. 4-18A). In addition, HP1 recruits HDAC, which promotes nucleosome assembly. Together, these modifications produce a closed chromatin conformation.

Chromatin modifications can have long-term influences on gene expression

The structure of chromatin can have a long-term influence on gene expression. The following are three examples of long-term regulation of gene expression.

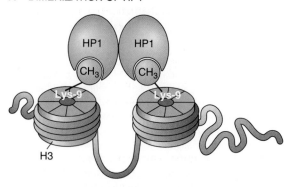

A   DIMERIZATION OF HP1

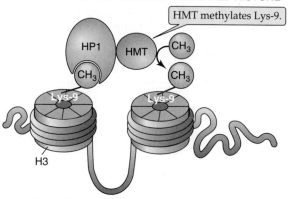

B   RECRUITMENT OF HMT BY METHYLATED HISTONE

HMT methylates Lys-9.

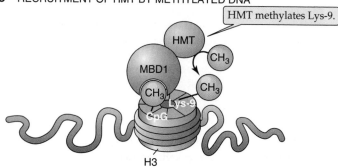

C   RECRUITMENT OF HMT BY METHYLATED DNA

HMT methylates Lys-9.

Figure 4-18   Gene silencing by chromatin modification. **A,** HP1 binds to methylated Lys-9 in histone H3. Because the HP1 self-dimerizes, the result is chromatin condensation. **B,** HP1 recruits a histone methyltransferase (HMT) that promotes further lysine methylation, leading to recruitment of additional HP1, propagating histone methylation. **C,** MBD1 binds to methylated cytosine groups in DNA and can also recruit HMT.

X-inactivation. Females carry two X chromosomes (see Chapter 53), whereas males carry only one copy. To express X-linked genes at the same levels as males, females during development permanently inactivate one of the X chromosomes by globally converting one X chromosome from euchromatin to heterochromatin.

Imprinting. Cells contain two copies of every gene, one inherited from each parent, and usually express each copy identically. In a few cases, however, genes are differentially expressed, depending on whether they are inherited from the mother or the father. This phenomenon is called **genomic imprinting**. For example, the insulin-like growth factor 2 gene (*IGF2;* see Chapter 48) is *paternally* imprinted—only the copy inherited from the father is expressed; the maternal copy is not expressed.

Tissue-specific gene silencing. Many tissue-specific genes are globally inactivated during embryonic development, later to be reactivated only in particular tissues. For example, globin genes are silenced except in erythroid cells. The silencing of genes in nonexpressing tissues is associated with chromatin modifications that are similar to those found in heterochromatin.

X-inactivation, imprinting, and tissue-specific silencing require long-term inactivation of gene expression and the maintenance of this inactivation during DNA replication and cell division. For example, the inactivated X chromosome remains inactivated in the two progeny cells after mitosis. Similarly, genes silenced by imprinting or by tissue-specific silencing remain inactive in progeny cells. The maintenance of gene silencing is an example of **epigenetic regulation of gene expression**—"epigenetic" because the heritable changes do not depend on DNA sequences.

Chromatin modification mediates the epigenetic regulation of gene expression. As is the case for transcriptional *repression* in heterochromatin, the methylation of histone H3 at Lys-9 (H3-K9) is characteristic of silencing by X-inactivation, imprinting, and tissue-specific gene silencing. Cells maintain this H3-K9 methylation during division, possibly by using the HP1 discussed earlier (Fig. 4-18A). After it binds to methylated histones, HP1 recruits a histone methyltransferase (HMT) that methylates other H3-K9 residues (Fig. 4-18B), providing a mechanism for propagating histone methylation. During DNA replication, the HMT recruited to a silenced gene on a parental strand of chromatin adds methyl groups to histones on the daughter strands, which maintains gene silencing in the progeny.

Methylation of DNA is associated with gene inactivation

Methylation of cytosine residues at the N5 position is the only well-documented postsynthetic modification of DNA in higher eukaryotes. Approximately 5% of cytosine residues are methylated in mammalian DNA. Methylation usually occurs on cytosine residues that are immediately upstream from guanosines (i.e., CpG dinucleotides).

Several lines of evidence implicate DNA methylation in the control of gene expression.

1. Although CpG dinucleotides are relatively underrepresented in mammalian genomes, they are frequently clustered near the 5′ ends of genes (forming so-called **CpG islands**). Moreover, methylation of cytosines in these locations is associated with inhibition of gene expression. For example, the inactivated X chromosome in females contains heavily methylated genes.
2. Methylation/demethylation may explain tissue-specific and stage-dependent gene expression. For example, globin genes are methylated in nonexpressing tissues but hypomethylated in erythroid cells. During fetal development, fetal globin genes are demethylated and then become methylated in the adult.

3. Foreign genes that are introduced into cells are transcriptionally inactive if they are methylated but active if demethylated at the 5′ end.
4. Chemical demethylating agents, such as 5-azacytidine, can activate previously inactive genes.

How does DNA methylation cause gene inactivation? One simple mechanism is that methylation inhibits the binding of an essential transcriptional activator. For example, methylation of CpG dinucleotides within the GFAP (glial fibrillary acidic protein) promoter prevents STAT3 binding. A more common mechanism is that methylation produces binding sites for proteins that promote gene inactivation. Cells contain a protein called MeCP2 that binds specifically to methylated CpG dinucleotides as well as to the HDAC. Thus, DNA methylation may silence genes by promoting histone deacetylation. In addition, methylated DNA binds to **methyl-CpG binding protein 1 (MBD1)**, a protein that complexes with HMT (Fig. 4-18C). These last two interactions provide mechanisms coupling DNA methylation to histone modifications that promote heterochromatin formation and gene silencing.

POST-TRANSCRIPTIONAL REGULATION OF GENE EXPRESSION

Although initiation of transcription (Fig. 4-5, step 2) is the most frequently regulated step in gene expression, for certain genes subsequent steps are more important for determining the overall level of expression. These processes are generally classified as **post-transcriptional regulation**. The mechanisms for regulating these steps are less well understood than are those for regulating transcription initiation, but some information comes from the study of model genes. Post-transcriptional processes that we review here are pre-mRNA splicing (step 5) and transcript degradation (step 8).

Alternative splicing generates diversity from single genes

Eukaryotic genes contain introns that must be removed from the primary transcript to create mature mRNA; this process is called **pre-mRNA splicing**. Splicing involves the joining of two sites on the RNA transcript, the **5′ splice-donor site** and the **3′ splice-acceptor site**, and removal of the intervening intron (Fig. 4-19). The first step involves cleavage of the pre-mRNA at the 5′ splice-donor site. Second, joining of the 5′ end of the intron to an adenosine residue located within the intron forms a "lariat" structure. Third, ligation of the 5′ and 3′ splice sites releases the lariat intron. The splicing reaction occurs in the nucleus, mediated by ribonucleoprotein particles (snRNPs) that are composed of proteins and small nuclear RNA (snRNA). Together, the assembly of pre-mRNA and snRNPs forms a large complex called the **spliceosome**.

The location of the 5′ and 3′ splice sites is based, at least in part, on the sequences at the ends of the introns. The 5′ splice-donor site has the consensus sequence 5′-(C/A)AG ↓ GU(G/A)AGU-3′; the vertical arrow represents the boundary between the exon and the intron. The 3′ splice-acceptor

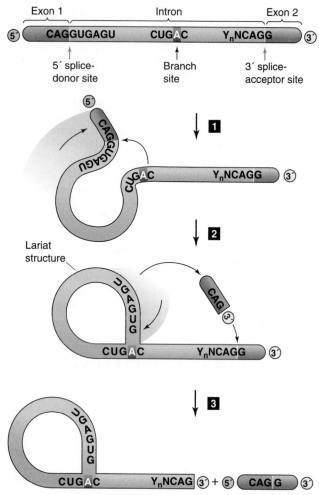

Exon 1 | Intron | Exon 2

5′ splice-donor site   Branch site   3′ splice-acceptor site

Lariat structure

Figure 4-19   Mechanism of pre-mRNA splicing. This example illustrates how a 5′ splice-donor site at one end of exon 1 can link to the 3′ splice-acceptor site at the end of exon 2, thereby splicing out the intervening intron. The process can be divided into three steps: (1) cleavage of the pre-mRNA at the 5′ splice-donor site; (2) joining of the 5′ end of the intron to an adenosine residue that is located within the intron, forming a lariat structure; and (3) ligation of the 5′ and 3′ splice sites and release of the lariat intron.

site has the consensus sequence 5′-Y_nNCAG ↓ G-3′; Y_n represents a polypyrimidine tract (i.e., a long sequence of only C and U), and N represents any nucleotide. An intronic site located more than 17 nucleotides upstream from the 3′ acceptor site (5′-YNCUGAC-3′), called the branch point, is also present and contains the adenosine (red background in Fig. 4-19) that contributes to formation of the lariat structure.

Many genes undergo **alternative splicing**, which refers to differential splicing of the same primary transcript to produce mature transcripts that contain different combinations of exons. If the coding region is affected, the resulting splicing variants will encode proteins with distinct primary structures that may have different physiological functions. Thus, alternative splicing is a mechanism for increasing the diversity of proteins that a single gene can produce. Figure 4-20 summarizes seven patterns of alternative splicing.

Retained Intron   In some cases, the cell may choose whether to splice out a segment of RNA. For example, the γA isoform of rat γ-fibrinogen lacks the seventh intron, whereas the γB isoform retains the intron (Fig. 4-20A). The retained intron encodes a unique 12–amino acid C terminus in γB-fibrinogen.

Alternative 3′ Splice Sites   In this case, the length of an intron is variable because the *downstream* boundary of the intron can be at either of two or more different 3′ splice-acceptor sites (Fig. 4-20B). For example, in rat fibronectin, a single donor site may be spliced to any of three acceptor sites. The presence or absence of the amino acids encoded by the sequence between the different splice-acceptor sites results in fibronectin isoforms with different cell adhesion properties.

Alternative 5′ Splice Sites   Here also, the length of the intron is variable. However, in this case, it is the *upstream* boundary of the intron that can be at either of two or more different 5′ splice-donor sites (Fig. 4-20C). For example, cells can generate mRNA encoding 3-hydroxy-3-methylglutaryl–coenzyme A (HMG-CoA) reductase (see Chapter 46) with different 5′ untranslated regions by splicing from multiple donor sites for the first intron to a single acceptor site.

Cassette Exons   In some cases, the cell may choose either to splice in an exon or group of exons (**cassette exons**) or to not splice them in (Fig. 4-20D). An example is the α-tropomyosin gene, which contains 12 exons. All α-tropomyosin transcripts contain the invariant exons 1, 4 to 6, 8, and 9. All muscle-like cells splice in exon 7, but hepatoma (i.e., liver tumor) cells do not splice in exon 7; they directly link exon 6 to exon 8.

Mutually Exclusive Exons   In yet other cases, the cell may splice in **mutually exclusive exons** (Fig. 4-20E). One of the Na/K/Cl cotransporter genes (*NKCC2*) is an example. Isoforms containing distinct 96-bp exons are differentially expressed in the kidney cortex and medulla. Because the encoded amino acid sequence is predicted to reside in the membrane, the isoforms may have different kinetic properties. The α-tropomyosin gene again is another example. Smooth muscle cells splice in exon 2 but not exon 3. Striated muscle cells and myoblasts splice in exon 3 but not exon 2. Fibroblasts and hepatoma cells do not splice in either of these two exons.

Alternative 5′ Ends   Cells may differentially splice the 5′ end of the gene (Fig. 4-20F) and thereby select different promoters. In the case of the myosin light chain gene (see Chapter 9), which consists of nine exons, one transcript is initiated from a promoter that is located upstream from exon 1, skips exons 2 and 3, and includes exons 4 to 9. The other transcript is initiated instead at a promoter located in the first *intron* and consists of exons 2, 3, and 5 to 9. Because the coding region is affected, the two transcripts encode proteins that differ at their N-terminal ends. These splice variants are found in different cells or different developmental stages. α-Amylase (see Chapter 45) is another example. Transcription can begin from two different sites and produce mRNA

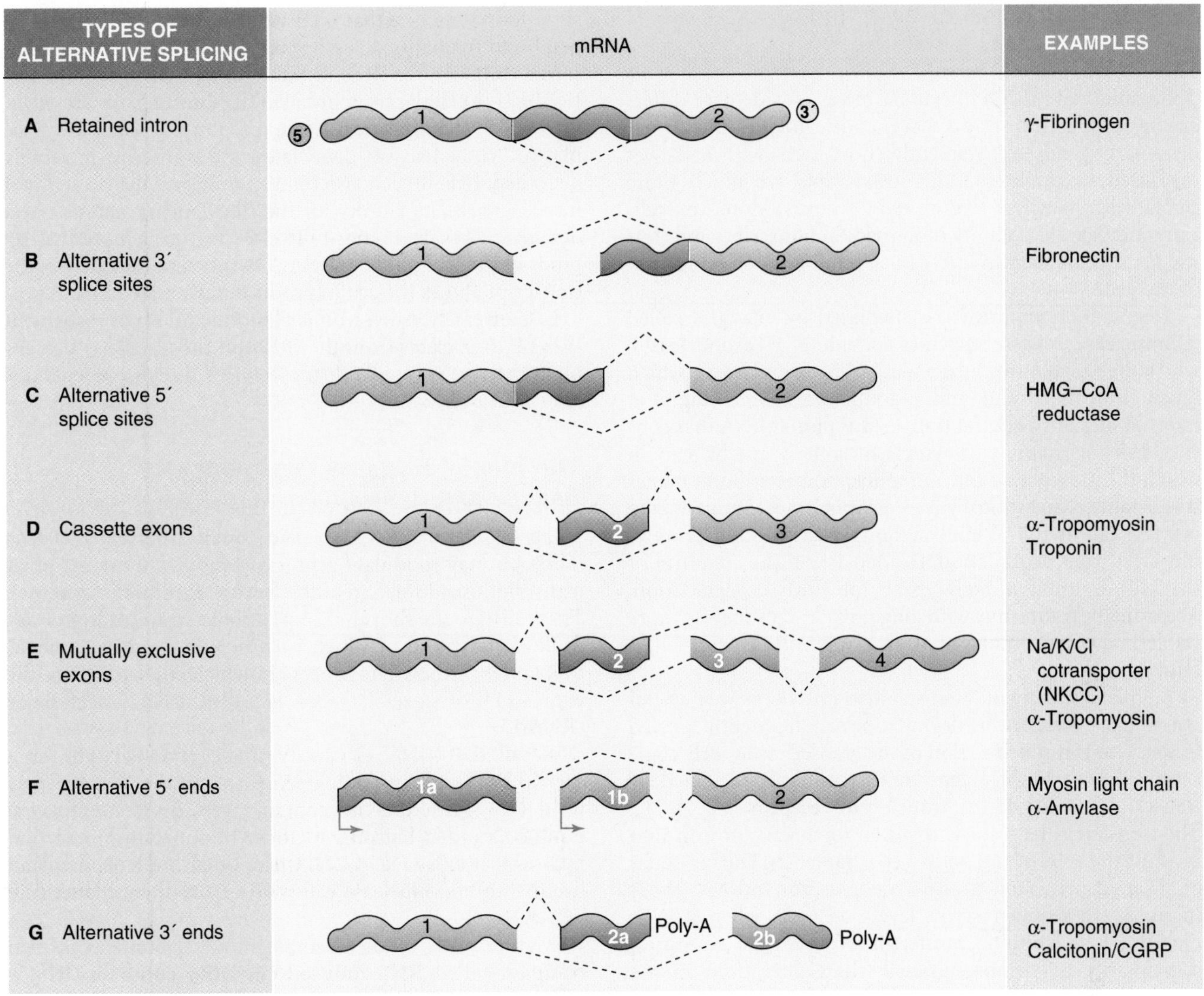

TYPES OF ALTERNATIVE SPLICING	mRNA	EXAMPLES
A Retained intron		γ-Fibrinogen
B Alternative 3′ splice sites		Fibronectin
C Alternative 5′ splice sites		HMG–CoA reductase
D Cassette exons		α-Tropomyosin Troponin
E Mutually exclusive exons		Na/K/Cl cotransporter (NKCC) α-Tropomyosin
F Alternative 5′ ends		Myosin light chain α-Amylase
G Alternative 3′ ends		α-Tropomyosin Calcitonin/CGRP

Figure 4-20   Types of alternative splicing. CGRP, calcitonin gene–related peptide; HMG-CoA, 3-hydroxy-3-methylglutaryl coenzyme A; Poly-A, polyadenylic acid.

that contains different first exons. Because the two mRNAs have different promoters, this alternative splicing permits differential regulation of gene expression in liver and salivary glands.

Alternative 3′ Ends   Finally, cells may differentially splice the transcript near the 3′ end of the gene (Fig. 4-20G) and thereby alter the site of cleavage and polyadenylation. Such splicing may also affect the coding region. Again, α-tropomyosin is an example. Striated muscle cells splice in exon 11, which contains one alternative 3′ untranslated region. Smooth muscle cells splice in exon 12 instead of exon 11. Another example is the calcitonin gene, which encodes both the hormone calcitonin (see Chapter 52) and calcitonin gene–related peptide α (CGRPα). Thyroid C cells produce one splice variant that includes exons 1 to 4 and encodes

calcitonin. Sensory neurons, on the other hand, produce another splice variant that excludes exon 4 but includes exons 5 and 6. It encodes a different protein, CGRPα.

These examples illustrate that some splicing variants are expressed only in certain cell types but not in others. Clearly, control of alternative splicing must involve steps other than initiation of transcription because many splice variants have identical 5′ ends. In some genes, the control elements that are required for alternative splicing have been identified, largely on the basis of deletion mutations that result in aberrant splicing. These control elements can reside in either introns or exons and are located within or near the splice sites. The proteins that interact with such elements remain largely unknown, although some RNA-binding proteins that may be involved in regulation of splicing have been identified.

Regulatory elements in the 3′ untranslated region control mRNA stability

The stability of mRNA in cytoplasm varies widely for different transcripts. Transcripts that encode cytokines and immediate-early genes are frequently short-lived, with half-lives measured in minutes. Other transcripts are much more stable, with half-lives that exceed 24 hours. Moreover, cells can modulate the stability of individual transcripts and thus use this mechanism to affect the overall level of expression of the gene.

Degradation of mRNA is mediated by enzymes called **ribonucleases**. These enzymes include 3′-5′ exonucleases, which digest RNA from the 3′ end; 5′-3′ exonucleases, which digest from the 5′ end; and endonucleases, which digest at internal sites. A structural feature of typical mRNA that contributes to its stability in cytoplasm is the 5′ methyl cap, in which the presence of the 5′-5′ phosphodiester bond makes it resistant to digestion by 5′-3′ exonucleases. Similarly, the poly(A) tail at the 3′ end of the transcript often protects messages from degradation. Deadenylation (i.e., removal of the tail) is often a prerequisite for mRNA degradation. Accordingly, transcripts with long poly(A) tails may be more stable in cytoplasm than are transcripts with short poly(A) tails.

Regulatory elements that stabilize mRNA, as well as elements that accelerate its degradation, are frequently located in the 3′ untranslated region of the transcripts. A well-characterized example of a gene that is primarily regulated by transcript stability is the **transferrin receptor** (Fig. 4-21). The transferrin receptor is required for uptake of iron into most of the cells of the body (see Chapter 2). During states of iron deprivation, transferrin receptor mRNA levels increase, whereas transcript levels decrease when iron is plentiful. Regulation of transferrin receptor gene expression is primarily post-transcriptional; these alterations in the level of transferrin receptor mRNA are achieved through changes in the half-life of the message.

Regulation of transferrin receptor mRNA stability depends on elements that are located in the 3′ untranslated region called **iron response elements (IREs)**. An IRE is a stem-loop structure that is created by intramolecular hydrogen bond formation. The human transferrin receptor transcript contains five IREs in the 3′ untranslated region. The IRE binds a cellular protein called IRE-binding protein (IRE-BP), which stabilizes transferrin receptor mRNA in the cytoplasm. When IRE-BP dissociates, the transcript is rapidly degraded. IRE-BP can also bind to iron, and the presence of iron decreases its affinity for the IRE. During states of iron deficiency, less iron binds to IRE-BP, and thus more IRE-BP binds to the IRE on the mRNA. The increased stability of the transcript allows the cell to produce more transferrin receptors. Conversely, when iron is plentiful and binds to IRE-BP, IRE-BP dissociates from the IRE, and the transferrin receptor transcript is rapidly degraded. This design prevents cellular iron overload.

RNA interference may regulate mRNA stability and translation

Small regulatory RNAs, called **small interfering RNAs (siRNA)**, may modulate gene expression both at the post-transcriptional level and at the level of chromatin structure. These siRNAs are short (~22 bp) double-stranded RNA molecules, one strand of which is complementary in sequence to a target mRNA. The process in which siRNAs silence the expression of specific genes is called **RNA interference (RNAi)**.

Recall that RNA is usually single stranded. However, certain non–protein-coding sequences in the genome may yield RNA transcripts that contain inverted repeats, allowing double-stranded hairpins to form through intramolecular hydrogen bonds (Fig. 4-22). Cleavage of the hairpin structure by an endonuclease called Dicer produces the mature siRNA.

Mature siRNA can assemble into a ribonucleoprotein complex called **RNA-induced silencing complex (RISC)**, which specifically cleaves a target mRNA that is complementary in sequence to one of the strands of the siRNA (Fig. 4-22A). In addition, the binding of an siRNA to a complementary mRNA can inhibit translation of the mRNA into protein (Fig. 4-22B). Finally, siRNAs can assemble into another

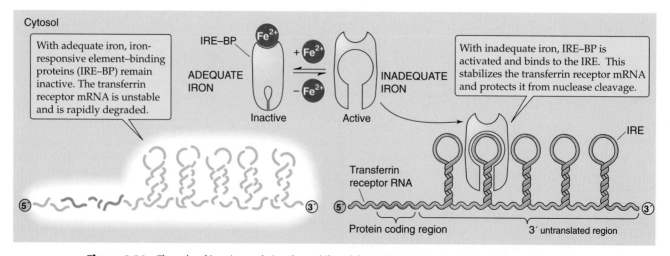

Figure 4-21 The role of iron in regulating the stability of the mRNA for the transferrin receptor. The mRNA that encodes the transferrin receptor has a series of IREs in its 3′ untranslated region.

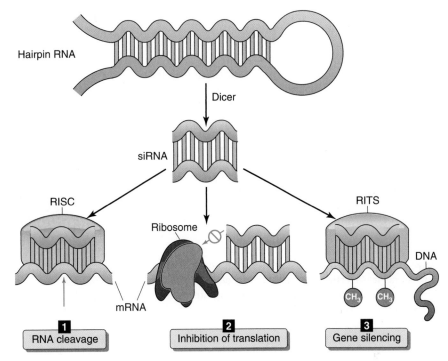

Figure 4-22 Regulation of gene expression by RNA interference. The siRNA is produced from hairpin RNA by Dicer. **1,** Assembly of siRNA in the RISC complex results in cleavage of the target mRNA. **2,** The siRNA can also inhibit mRNA translation. **3,** Assembly of siRNA in the RITS complex promotes DNA methylation and gene silencing.

ribonucleoprotein complex called **RNA-induced transcriptional silencing (RITS)**, which promotes DNA and histone methylation and thus the formation of heterochromatin (Fig. 4-22C).

Hundreds of genes that are potentially regulated by RNAi have been identified, and it is likely that this number will continue to grow. Because the expression of siRNAs is often tissue specific and developmentally regulated, RNAi may be an important mechanism for silencing gene expression during cell differentiation.

REFERENCES

Books and Reviews

Conaway RC, Conaway JW: General initiation factors for RNA polymerase II. Annu Rev Biochem 1993; 63:161-190.

Karin M: Signal transduction from the cell surface to the nucleus through the phosphorylation of transcription factors. Curr Opin Cell Biol 1994; 6:415-424.

Maniatis T, Goodbourn S, Fischer JA: Regulation of inducible and tissue-specific gene expression. Science 1987; 236:1237-1245.

McKeown M: Alternative mRNA splicing. Annu Rev Cell Biol 1992; 8:133-155.

Pabo CO, Sauer RT: Transcription factors: Structural families and principles of DNA recognition. Annu Rev Biochem 1992; 61:1053-1095.

Ptashne M, Gann A: Genes & Signals. Cold Spring Harbor, NY: Cold Spring Harbor Laboratory Press, 2002.

Turner BM: Chromatin and Gene Regulation: Molecular Mechanisms in Epigenetics. Oxford: Blackwell Science, 2001.

Journal Articles

Casey JL, Koeller DM, Ramin VC, et al: Iron regulation of transferrin receptor mRNA levels requires iron-responsive elements and a rapid turnover determinant in the 3′ untranslated region of the mRNA. EMBO J 1989; 8:3693-3699.

Gillies SD, Morrison SL, Oi VT, Tonegawa S: A tissue-specific transcription enhancer element is located in the major intron of a rearranged immunoglobulin heavy chain gene. Cell 1983; 33:717-728.

Koleske AJ, Young RA: An RNA polymerase II holoenzyme responsive to activators. Nature 1994; 368:466-469.

Schindler C, Shuai K, Prezioso VR, Darnell JE Jr: Interferon-dependent tyrosine phosphorylation of a latent cytoplasmic transcription factor. Science 1992; 257:809-813.

van der Ploeg LH, Flavell RA: DNA methylation in the human γδβ-globin locus in erythroid and nonerythroid tissues. Cell 1980; 19:947-958.

GLOSSARY

AP-1 activator protein 1, a Jun/Fos heterodimer that is a transcription factor (Table 4-1).

AR androgen receptor.

ATF-2 activating transcription factor 2, a transcription factor (Table 4-1).

bHLH basic helix-loop-helix family of transcription factors.

Brg1 Brahma-related gene 1, central motor component of SWI/SNF.

bZIP basic zipper family of transcription factors.

CAR constitutive androstane receptor.

CARM1 a coactivator and methyltransferase that methylates histones.

cAMP cyclic adenosine monophosphate.

CBP CREB-binding protein, 245 kDa, a coactivator.

C/EBPβ CCAAT/enhancer binding protein β, a transcription factor (Table 4-1).

c-Fos a transcription factor.

c-Jun a transcription factor.

c-Myc a transcription factor (Table 4-1).

CRE   cAMP response element, a DNA sequence.

CREB   CRE binding protein, 43 kDa.

CREM   cAMP response element modifier, a transcriptional repressor.

CTD   C-terminal domain of the largest subunit of Pol II.

DNA   deoxyribonucleic acid.

E box   sequence of six nucleotides (CANNTG, where N is any nucleotide) recognized by transcription factors MyoD and myogenin.

EGF   epidermal growth factor.

Egr-1   a transcription factor (activator) that binds through zinc fingers to the same DNA site as WT-1 (repressor).

EKLF   erythroid Kruppel-like factor (a transcription factor).

Elk-1   a transcription factor.

ER   estrogen receptor.

FGF   fibroblast growth factor.

FXR   bile acid receptor.

GAL4   a yeast transcription factor that activates certain genes when yeast grows in galactose-containing media.

GAS   interferon γ activation site.

GATA-1   a transcription factor.

GFAP   glial fibrillary acidic protein.

GR   glucocorticoid receptor.

GRB2   growth factor receptor-bound protein 2, a protein that contains SH2 domains that bind to phosphotyrosine residues on an activated receptor tyrosine kinase. GRB2 also contains SH3 domains that bind to proline-rich regions of SOS.

GRE   glucocorticoid response element.

HAT   histone acetyltransferase.

HDAC   histone deacetylase.

HIF-1α and HIF-1β   hypoxia-inducible factors.

HMT   histone methyltransferase.

HNF-1, HNF-3, HNF-4   transcription factors.

hnRNA   heterogeneous nuclear RNA, primary transcript of DNA, unprocessed.

HP1   heterochromatin protein 1.

hsp90   90-kDa heat shock protein, a molecular chaperone.

HTH   helix-turn-helix family of transcription factors.

IFN-α, β, γ   interferons α, β, and γ.

IGF-1 and IGF-2   insulin-related growth factors.

Inr   "initiator," a promoter sequence in both TATA-containing and TATA-less genes.

IRE   iron response element.

ISRE   interferon-stimulated response element.

JAK1, JAK2   Janus kinase, a protein tyrosine kinase.

LCR   locus control region, a site distant from the structural genes.

MAPK or MAP kinase   mitogen-activated protein kinase; also known as ERK-1, ERK-2 for extracellular signal-regulated kinase.

MBD1   methyl-CpG binding protein 1.

MeCP2   binds to methylated CpG dinucleotides on DNA.

MEK   MAP kinase kinase (MAPKK). In the Ras cascade, it is phosphorylated by Raf-1 (MAPKKK) and phosphorylates MAP kinase (MAPK). It is also activated by JAK, part of the receptor-associated tyrosine kinase pathway.

mRNA   messenger RNA.

MR   mineralocorticoid receptor.

MyoD   a bHLH-type transcription factor.

N-CoR   a corepressor of transcription; also known as SMRT.

NF-1   nuclear factor 1, a transcription factor (Table 4-1).

NF-E2   nuclear factor E2, a heterodimeric protein complex composed of p45 and small Maf family proteins considered crucial for the proper differentiation of erythrocytes and megakaryocytes in vivo.

NF-κB   a transcription factor and protein complex responsible for regulating the immune response to infection.

NF-Y   ubiquitous multisubunit CCAAT binding protein composed of three subunits: NF-YA, NF-YB, NF-YC.

NGF   nerve growth factor.

NRE   negative regulatory element.

Oct-1   ubiquitous DNA-binding protein that recognizes a DNA sequence called the octamer motif (Table 4-1).

P box   sequence of six amino acids at the C terminus of a zinc finger.

p62TCF   ternary complex factor, a transcription factor.

PDGF   platelet-derived growth factor.

PEPCK   phosphoenolpyruvate carboxykinase, the enzyme that catalyzes the rate-limiting step in gluconeogenesis.

Pit-1   an HTH-type pituitary-specific transcription factor.

Pol II   RNA polymerase II, the polymerase that transcribes DNA to mRNA.

PPAR   peroxisome proliferator–activated (i.e., lipid) receptor.

PR   progesterone receptor.

P-TEFb   positive transcription elongation factor b, a kinase that phosphorylates the CTD of Pol II.

Raf-1   a serine/threonine kinase, also known as MAP kinase kinase kinase (MAPKKK).

RAR   retinoic acid receptor.

RARE   retinoic acid response element.

Ras   a low-molecular-weight GTP-binding protein.

RIP   regulated intramembraneous proteolysis.

RISC   RNA-induced silencing complex.

RITS   RNA-induced transcriptional silencing.

RNA   ribonucleic acid.

RNAi   RNA interference.

RNAPII   an alternative designation for RNA polymerase II (Pol II).

RTK   receptor tyrosine kinase.

RXR   retinoid X receptor.

SH2   Src homology domain 2, a domain on a protein that binds to phosphotyrosine-containing sites.

SH3   Src homology domain 3, a domain on a protein that binds to proline-rich sequences.

Sin3A, Sin3B   corepressors.

siRNA   small interfering RNA.

snRNA   small nuclear RNA.

snRNP   a complex of proteins and snRNA.

SOS   son of "sevenless" protein, a guanine nucleotide exchange protein that is part of the Ras signaling cascade. It becomes active when it binds to GRB2. It promotes the conversion of inactive GDP-Ras to active GTP-Ras.

Sp1   stimulating protein 1, a transcription factor.

SRC   steroid receptor coactivator.

SREBP   sterol regulatory element binding protein.

SRF   serum response factor, a transcription factor.

STAT   signal transducer and activator of transcription.

SUMO   small ubiquitin-like modifiers.

SWI/SNF   multiprotein complexes initially identified in yeast as "switching mating type/sucrose non-fermenting."

SXR   steroid and xenobiotic receptor.

TAFs   TBP-associated factors.

TATA box   common gene promoter sequence.

TBP   TATA-binding protein.

TFIIA   transcription factor IIA.

TFIIB   transcription factor IIB.

TFIID   transcription factor IID.

TFIIE   transcription factor IIE.

TFIIF   transcription factor IIF.

TFIIH   transcription factor IIH.

TR   thyroid hormone receptor.

TRAP220   a component of Mediator.

tRNA   transfer RNA.

Tyk   a protein tyrosine kinase related to JAK.

UTR   untranslated region of mRNA.

VDR   vitamin D receptor.

VEGF   vascular endothelial growth factor.

VHL   a protein that targets HIF-1α for proteosomal degradation.

VP16   viral protein from herpes simplex virus, a transcription factor.

WT-1   Wilms tumor protein, a transcriptional repressor that binds through zinc fingers to the same DNA site as Egr-1 (activator).

CHAPTER 5

TRANSPORT OF SOLUTES AND WATER

Peter S. Aronson, Walter F. Boron, and Emile L. Boulpaep

The cells of the human body live in a carefully regulated fluid environment. The fluid inside the cells, the **intracellular fluid (ICF)**, occupies what is called the intracellular compartment, and the fluid outside the cells, the **extracellular fluid (ECF)**, occupies the extracellular compartment. The barriers that separate these two compartments are the **cell membranes**. For life to be sustained, the body must rigorously maintain the volume and composition of the intracellular and extracellular compartments. To a large extent, such regulation is the result of transport across the cell membrane. In this chapter, we discuss how cell membranes regulate the distribution of ions and water in the intracellular and extracellular compartments.

THE INTRACELLULAR AND EXTRACELLULAR FLUIDS

Total body water is the sum of the intracellular and extracellular fluid volumes

Total body water is ~60% of total body weight in a young adult human male, approximately 50% of total body weight in a young adult human female (Table 5-1), and 65% to 75% of total body weight in an infant. Total body water accounts for a lower percentage of weight in females because they typically have more adipose tissue, and fat cells have a lower water content than muscle does. Even if gender and age are taken into consideration, the fraction of total body weight contributed by water is not constant for all individuals under all conditions. For example, variability in the amount of adipose tissue can influence the fraction. Because water represents such a large fraction of body weight, acute changes in total body water can be detected simply by monitoring body weight.

The anatomy of the body fluid compartments is illustrated in Figure 5-1. The prototypic 70-kg male has ~42 liters of total body water (60% of 70 kg). Of these 42 liters, ~60% (25 liters) is intracellular and ~40% (17 liters) is extracellular. *Extracellular fluid* is composed of blood plasma, interstitial fluid, and transcellular fluid.

Plasma Volume Of the ~17 liters of ECF, only ~20% (~3 liters) is contained within the cardiac chambers and blood vessels, that is, within the intravascular compartment. The *total* volume of this intravascular compartment is the **blood volume**, ~5.5 liters. The extracellular 3 liters of the blood volume is the plasma volume. The balance, ~2.5 liters, consists of the cellular elements of blood: erythrocytes, leukocytes, and platelets. The fraction of blood volume that is occupied by these cells is called the **hematocrit**. The hematocrit is determined by centrifuging blood that is treated with an anticoagulant and measuring the fraction of the total volume that is occupied by the packed cells.

Interstitial Fluid About 75% (~13 liters) of the ECF is outside the intravascular compartment, where it bathes the nonblood cells of the body. Within this interstitial fluid are two smaller compartments that communicate only slowly with the bulk of the interstitial fluid: dense connective tissue, such as cartilage and tendons, and bone matrix.

The barriers that separate the intravascular and interstitial compartments are the walls of **capillaries**. Water and solutes can move between the interstitium and blood plasma by crossing capillary walls and between the interstitium and cytoplasm by crossing cell membranes.

Transcellular Fluid Finally, ~5% (~1 liter) of ECF is trapped within spaces that are completely surrounded by epithelial cells. This transcellular fluid includes the synovial fluid within joints and the cerebrospinal fluid surrounding the brain and spinal cord. Transcellular fluid does *not* include fluids that are, strictly speaking, outside the body, such as the contents of the gastrointestinal tract or urinary bladder.

Intracellular fluid is rich in K+, whereas the extracellular fluid is rich in Na+ and Cl−

Not only do the various body fluid compartments have very different volumes, they also have radically different compositions, as summarized in Figure 5-1. Table 5-2 is a more comprehensive listing of these values. *Intracellular fluid* is high in K^+ and low in Na^+ and Cl^-; *extracellular fluids* (interstitial and plasma) are high in Na^+ and Cl^- and low in K^+.

Table 5-1 Approximate Water Distribution in Adult Humans*

	Men	Typical Volume (liters)	Women	Typical Volume (liters)
Total body water (TBW)	60% of body weight	42	50% of body weight	35
Intracellular fluid (ICF)	60% of TBW	25	60% of TBW	21
Extracellular fluid (ECF)	40% of TBW	17	40% of TBW	14
Interstitial fluid	75% of ECF	13	75% of ECF	10
Plasma volume (PV)	20% of ECF	3	20% of ECF	3
Blood volume (BV)	PV/(1 − Hct)	5.5	PV/(1 − Hct)	5
Transcellular fluid	5% of ECF	1	5% of ECF	1

*Assuming a body weight of 70 kg for both sexes and a hematocrit (Hct) of 45% for men and 40% for women.

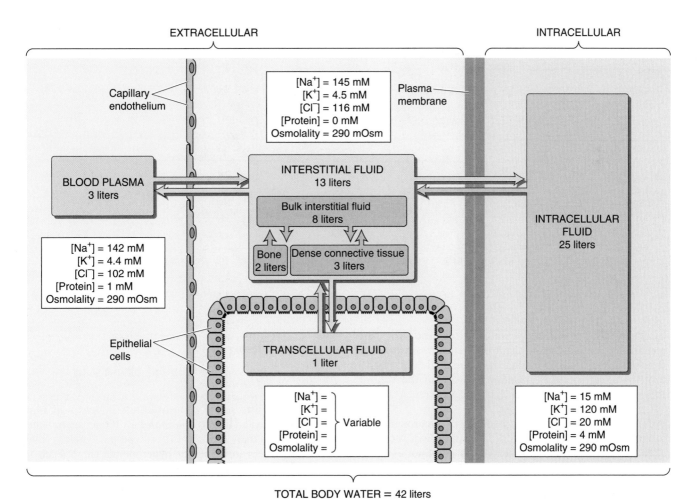

Figure 5-1 The fluid compartments of a prototypic adult human weighing 70 kg. Total body water is divided into four major compartments: intracellular fluid *(green)*, interstitial fluid *(blue)*, blood plasma *(red)*, and transcellular water such as synovial fluid *(tan)*. Color codes for each of these compartments are maintained throughout this book.

The cell maintains a relatively high K^+ concentration ($[K^+]_i$) and low Na^+ concentration ($[Na^+]_i$), not by making its membrane totally impermeable to these ions but by using the Na-K pump to actively extrude Na^+ from the cell and to actively transport K^+ into the cell.

The composition of transcellular fluids differs greatly both from each other and from plasma because they are secreted by different epithelia. The two major constituents of ECF, the plasma and interstitial fluid, have similar composition as far as small solutes are concerned. For most cells, it is the composition of the interstitial fluid enveloping the cells that is the relevant parameter. The major difference between plasma and interstitial fluid is the absence of plasma proteins from the interstitium. These plasma proteins, which

Table 5-2 Approximate Solute Composition of Key Fluid Compartments

Solute	Plasma	Protein-Free Plasma	Interstitium	Cell
Na^+ (mM)	142	153	145	15
K^+ (mM)	4.4	4.7	4.5	120
Ca^{2+} (mM)	1.2 (ionized) 2.4 (total)*	1.3 (ionized)	1.2 (ionized)	0.0001 (ionized)
Mg^{2+} (mM)	0.6 (ionized) 0.9 (total)*	0.6 (ionized)	0.55 (ionized)	1 (ionized) 18 (total)
Cl^- (mM)	102	110	116	20
HCO_3^- (mM)	22†	24	25	16
$H_2PO_4^-$ and HPO_4^{2-} (mM)	0.7 (ionized) 1.4 (total)‡	0.75 (ionized)	0.8 (ionized)	0.7 (free)
Proteins	7 g/dL 1 mmol/L 14 mEq/L	–	1 g/dL	30 g/dL
Glucose (mM)	5.5	5.9	5.9	Very low
pH	7.4	7.4	7.4	~7.2
Osmolality (mosmole/kg H_2O)	291	290	290	290

*Total includes amounts ionized, complexed to small solutes, and protein bound.
†Arterial value. The value in mixed-venous blood would be ~24 mM.
‡As discussed in Chapter 52, levels of total plasma inorganic phosphate are not tightly regulated and vary between 0.8 and 1.5 mM.

cannot equilibrate across the walls of most capillaries, are responsible for the usually slight difference in small-solute concentrations between plasma and interstitial fluid. Plasma proteins affect solute distribution because of the volume they occupy and the electrical charge they carry.

Volume Occupied by Plasma Proteins The proteins and, to a much lesser extent, the lipids in plasma ordinarily occupy ~7% of the total plasma volume. Clinical laboratories report the plasma composition of ions (e.g., Na^+, K^+) in units of milliequivalents (meq) per liter of plasma solution. However, for cells bathed by interstitial fluid, more meaningful units would be **milliequivalents per liter of protein-free plasma solution** because it is only the protein-free portion of plasma—and not the proteins dissolved in this water—that can equilibrate across the capillary wall. For example, we can obtain $[Na^+]$ in protein-free plasma (which clinicians call plasma water) by dividing the laboratory value for plasma $[Na^+]$ by the plasma water content (usually 93%):

$$[Na^+]_{plasma\ water} = \frac{142\ meq/L\ plasma}{0.93}$$
$$= 153\ meq/L\ plasma\ water \tag{5-1}$$

Similarly, for Cl^-,

$$[Cl^-]_{plasma\ water} = \frac{102\ meq/L\ plasma}{0.93}$$
$$= 110\ meq/L\ plasma\ water \tag{5-2}$$

Table 5-2 lists solute concentrations in terms of both liters of *plasma* and liters of *plasma water*. If the plasma water fraction is less than 93% because of hyperproteinemia (high levels of protein in blood) or hyperlipemia (high levels of lipid in blood), the values that the clinical laboratory reports for electrolytes may appear abnormal even though the physiologically important concentration (solute concentration per liter of plasma water) is normal. For example, if a patient's plasma proteins and lipids occupy 20% of plasma volume and consequently plasma water is only 80% of plasma, a correction factor of 0.80 (rather than 0.93) should be used in Equation 5-1. If the clinical laboratory were to report a very low plasma $[Na^+]$ of 122 meq/L plasma, the patient's $[Na^+]$ relevant to interstitial fluid would be 122/0.80 = 153 meq/L plasma water, which is quite normal.

Effect of Protein Charge For noncharged solutes such as glucose, the correction for protein and lipid volume is the only correction needed to predict interstitial concentrations from plasma concentrations. Because plasma proteins carry a net negative charge and because the capillary wall confines them to the plasma, they tend to retain cations in plasma. Thus, the **cation** concentration of the protein-free solution of the interstitium is lower by ~5%. Conversely, because these negatively charged plasma proteins repel anions, the **anion** concentration of the protein-free solution of the interstitium is higher by ~5%. We consider the basis for these 5% corrections in the discussion of the Gibbs-Donnan equilibrium.

Thus, for a monovalent cation such as Na^+, the interstitial concentration is 95% of the $[Na^+]$ of the protein-free plasma water, the value from Equation 5-1:

$$[Na^+]_{interstitium} = 153 \, meq/L \, plasma \, water \times 0.95$$
$$= 145 \, meq/L \, interstitial \, fluid \quad (5\text{-}3)$$

For a monovalent anion such as Cl^-, the interstitial concentration is 105% of the $[Cl^-]$ of the protein-free water of plasma, a value already obtained in Equation 5-2:

$$[Cl^-]_{interstitium} = 110 \, meq/L \, plasma \, water \times 1.05$$
$$= 116 \, meq/L \, interstitial \, fluid \quad (5\text{-}4)$$

Thus, for cations (e.g., Na^+), the two corrections (0.95/0.93) nearly cancel each other. On the other hand, for anions (e.g., Cl^-), the two corrections (1.05/0.93) are cumulative and yield a total correction of ~13%.

All body fluids have approximately the same osmolality, and each fluid has equal numbers of positive and negative charges

Osmolality Despite the differences in solute composition among the intracellular, interstitial, and plasma compartments, they all have approximately the same osmolality. Osmolality describes the total concentration of all particles that are free in a solution. Thus, glucose contributes one particle, whereas fully dissociated NaCl contributes two. Particles bound to macromolecules do not contribute at all to osmolality. In all body fluid compartments, humans have an osmolality—expressed as the number of osmotically active particles per kilogram of water—of ~290 mosmol/kg H_2O (290 mOsm).

Plasma proteins contribute ~14 meq/L (Table 5-2). However, because these proteins usually have many negative charges per molecule, not many particles (~1 mM) are necessary to account for these milliequivalents. Moreover, even though the protein concentration—measured in terms of grams per liter—may be high, the high molecular weight of the average protein means that the protein concentration—measured in terms of moles per liter—is very low. Thus, proteins actually contribute only slightly to the total number of osmotically active particles (~1 mOsm).

Summing the *total* concentrations of all the solutes in the cells and interstitial fluid (including metabolites not listed in Table 5-2), we would see that the *total* solute concentration of the intracellular compartment is higher than that of the interstitium. Because the flow of water across cell membranes is governed by differences in osmolality across the membrane, and because the net flow is normally zero, intracellular and extracellular osmolality must be the same. How, then, do we make sense of this discrepancy? For some ions, a considerable fraction of their total intracellular store is

bound to cellular proteins or complexed to other small solutes. In addition, some of the proteins are themselves attached to other materials that are out of solution. In computing osmolality, we count each particle once, whether it is a free ion, a complex of two ions, or several ions bound to a protein. For example, most of the intracellular Mg^{2+} and phosphate and virtually all the Ca^{2+} are either complexed or bound. Some of the electrolytes in blood plasma are also bound to plasma proteins; however, the bound fraction is generally much lower than the fraction in the cytosol.

Electroneutrality All solutions must respect the principle of bulk electroneutrality: the number of positive charges in the overall solution must be the same as the number of negative charges. If we add up the major cations and anions in the cytosol (Table 5-2), we see that the sum of $[Na^+]_i$ and $[K^+]_i$ greatly exceeds the sum of $[Cl^-]_i$ and $[HCO_3^-]_i$. The excess positive charge reflected by this difference is balanced by the negative charge on intracellular macromolecules (e.g., proteins) as well as smaller anions such as organic phosphates.

There is a similar difference between major cations and anions in blood plasma, where it is often referred to as the **anion gap**. The clinical definition of anion gap is

$$\text{Anion gap}_{plasma} = [Na^+]_{plasma}$$
$$- ([Cl^-]_{plasma} + [HCO_3^-]_{plasma}) \quad (5\text{-}5)$$

Note that plasma $[K^+]$ is ignored. The anion gap, usually 9 to 14 meq/L, is the difference between ignored anions and ignored cations. Among the ignored anions are anionic proteins as well as small anionic metabolites. Levels of anionic metabolites, such as acetoacetate and β-hydroxybutyrate, can become extremely high, for example, in type 1 diabetic patients with very low levels of insulin (see Chapter 51). Thus, the anion gap increases under these conditions.

The differences in ionic composition between the ICF and ECF compartments are extremely important for normal functioning of the body. For example, because the K^+ gradient across cell membranes is a major determinant of electrical excitability, clinical disorders of extracellular $[K^+]$ can cause life-threatening disturbances in the heart rhythm. Disorders of extracellular $[Na^+]$ cause abnormal extracellular osmolality, with water being shifted into or out of brain cells; if uncorrected, such disorders lead to seizures, coma, or death.

These examples of clinical disorders emphasize the absolute necessity of understanding the processes that control the volume and composition of the body fluid compartments. These processes are the ones that move water and solutes between the compartments and between the body and the outside world.

SOLUTE TRANSPORT ACROSS CELL MEMBRANES

In passive, noncoupled transport across a permeable membrane, a solute moves down its electrochemical gradient

We are all familiar with the way that water can flow from one side of a dike to another, provided the water levels between the two sides of the dike are different and the water has an open pathway (a breach in the dike) to move from one side to the other. In much the same way, a substance can passively move across a membrane that separates two compartments when there is both a favorable driving force and an open pathway through which the driving force can exert its effect.

When a pathway exists for transfer of a substance across a membrane, the membrane is said to be **permeable** to that substance. The **driving force** that determines the passive transport of solutes across a membrane is the **electrochemical gradient** or electrochemical potential energy difference acting on the solute between the two compartments. This **electrochemical potential energy difference** includes a contribution from the concentration gradient of the solute—the chemical potential energy difference—and, for charged solutes (e.g., Na^+, Cl^-), a contribution from any difference in voltage that exists between the two compartments—the electrical potential energy difference.

This concept of how force and pathway determine passive movement of solutes is most easily illustrated by the example of passive, noncoupled transport. **Noncoupled transport** of a substance X means that movement of X across the membrane is not directly coupled to the movement of any other solute or to any chemical reaction (e.g., the hydrolysis of ATP). What, then, are the driving forces for the net movement of X? Clearly, if the concentration of X is higher in the outside compartment ($[X]_o$) than in the inside compartment ($[X]_i$), and assuming no voltage difference, the concentration gradient will act as the driving force to bring about the net movement of X across the membrane from outside to inside (Fig. 5-2). If [X] is the same on both sides but there is a voltage difference across the membrane—that is, the electrical potential energy on the outside (Ψ_o) is not the same as on the inside (Ψ_i)—this voltage difference will also drive the net movement of X, provided X is charged. The concentration gradient for X and the voltage difference across the membrane are the two determinants of the electrochemical potential energy difference for X between the two compartments. Because the movement of X by such a noncoupled mechanism is not directly coupled to the movement of other solutes or to any chemical reactions, the electrochemical gradient for X is the only driving force that contributes to the transport of X. Thus, the transport of X by a noncoupled, passive mechanism must always proceed "downhill," in the direction down the electrochemical potential energy difference for X.

Regardless of *how* X moves passively through the membrane—whether X moves through lipid or through a membrane protein—the direction of the overall driving force acting on X determines the direction of net transport. In the example in Figure 5-2, the overall driving force favors net transport from outside to inside (influx). However, X may still move from inside to outside (efflux). Movement of X across the membrane in one direction or the other is known as **unidirectional flux**. The algebraic sum of the two unidirectional fluxes is the **net flux**, or the net transport rate. Net transport occurs only when the unidirectional fluxes are unequal. In Figure 5-2, the overall driving force makes unidirectional influx greater than unidirectional efflux, resulting in net influx.

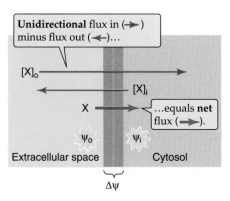

Figure 5-2 Uncoupled transport of a solute across a cell membrane. The net passive movement of a solute (X) depends on both the difference in concentration between the inside of the cell ($[X]_i$) and the outside of the cell ($[X]_o$) and the difference in voltage between the inside of the cell (Ψ_i) and the outside of the cell (Ψ_o).

When no net driving force is acting on X, we say that X is at **equilibrium** across the membrane and there is no net transport of X across the membrane. However, even when X is in equilibrium, there may be and usually are equal and opposite movements of X across the membrane. Net transport takes place only when the net driving force acting on X is displaced from the equilibrium point, and transport proceeds in the direction that would bring X back to equilibrium.

Equilibrium is actually a special case of a **steady state**. In a steady state, by definition, the conditions related to X do not change with time. Thus, a transport system is in a steady state when both the driving forces acting on it and the rate of transport are constant with time. Equilibrium is the particular steady state in which there is no net driving force and thus no net transport.

How can a steady state persist when X is not in equilibrium? Returning to the dike analogy, the downhill flow of water can be constant only if some device, such as a pump, keeps the water levels constant on both sides of the dike. A cell can maintain a nonequilibrium steady state for X only when some device, such as a mechanism for actively transporting X, can compensate for the passive movement of X and prevent the intracellular and extracellular concentrations of X from changing with time. This combination of a pump and a leak maintains both the concentrations of X and the passive flux of X.

At equilibrium, the chemical and electrical potential energy differences across the membrane are equal but opposite

As noted in the preceding section, the driving force for the passive, uncoupled transport of a solute is the electrochemical potential energy difference for that solute across the membrane that separates the inside (i) from the outside (o). We define the electrochemical potential energy difference as

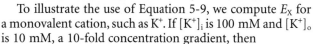

$$\underbrace{\Delta\tilde{\mu}_X}_{\substack{\text{Electrochemical}\\\text{potential energy}\\\text{difference}}} = RT\ln\frac{[X]_i}{[X]_o} + \underbrace{z_X F(\Psi_i - \Psi_o)}_{\substack{\text{Electrical}\\\text{potential energy}\\\text{difference}}}$$

$$\underbrace{RT\ln\frac{[X]_i}{[X]_o}}_{\substack{\text{Chemical}\\\text{potential energy}\\\text{difference}}}$$

(5-6)

where z_X is the valence of X, T is absolute temperature, R is the gas constant, and F is Faraday's constant. The first term on the right-hand side of Equation 5-6, the difference in chemical potential energy, describes the energy change (joules/mole) as X moves across the membrane if we disregard the charge—if any—on X. The second term, the difference in electrical potential energy, describes the energy change as a mole of charged particles (each with a valence of z_X) moves across the membrane. The difference ($\Psi_i - \Psi_o$) is the **voltage difference across the membrane (V_m)**, also known as the **membrane potential**.

By definition, X is at equilibrium when the electrochemical potential energy difference for X across the membrane is zero:

$$\Delta\tilde{\mu}_X = 0 \qquad (5-7)$$

Thus, $\Delta\tilde{\mu}_x$ is the *net driving force* (*units:* joules/mole). When $\Delta\tilde{\mu}_x$ is *not* zero, X is *not* in equilibrium and will obviously tend either to enter the cell or to leave the cell, provided a pathway exists for X to cross the membrane.

It is worthwhile to consider two special cases of the equilibrium state (Equation 5-7). First, when either the chemical or the electrical term in Equation 5-6 is zero, the other must also be zero. For example, when X is uncharged ($z_X = 0$), as in the case of glucose, equilibrium can occur only when [X] is equal on the two sides of the membrane. Alternatively, when X is charged, as in the case of Na^+, but the voltage difference (i.e., V_m) is zero, equilibrium likewise can occur only when [X] is equal on the two sides of the membrane. Second, when neither the chemical nor the electrical term in Equation 5-6 is zero, equilibrium can occur only when the two terms are equal but of opposite sign. Thus, if we set $\Delta\tilde{\mu}_x$ in Equation 5-6 to zero, as necessary for a state of equilibrium,

$$0 = RT\ln\frac{[X]_i}{[X]_o} + z_X F V_m$$

$$-\frac{RT}{z_X F}\ln\frac{[X]_i}{[X]_o} = V_m \qquad (5-8)$$

$$V_m = E_X = -\frac{RT}{z_X F}\ln\frac{[X]_i}{[X]_o}$$

This relationship is the **Nernst equation**, which describes the conditions when an ion is in equilibrium across a membrane. Given values for $[X]_i$ and $[X]_o$, X can be in equilibrium only when the voltage difference across the membrane equals the **equilibrium potential** (E_X), also known as the Nernst potential. Stated somewhat differently, E_X is the value that the membrane voltage *would have to have* for X to be in equilibrium. If we express the logarithm to the base 10, then for the special case in which the temperature is 29.5°C:

$$V_m = E_X = -\frac{(60\,\text{mV})}{z_X}\log_{10}\frac{[X]_i}{[X]_o} \qquad (5-9)$$

At normal body temperature (37°C), the coefficient is ~61.5 mV instead of 60 mV. At 20°C, it is ~58.1 mV.

To illustrate the use of Equation 5-9, we compute E_X for a monovalent cation, such as K^+. If $[K^+]_i$ is 100 mM and $[K^+]_o$ is 10 mM, a 10-fold concentration gradient, then

$$E_K = -\frac{(60\,\text{mV})}{1}\log_{10}\frac{100}{10} = -60\,\text{mV} \qquad (5-10)$$

Thus, a 10-fold gradient of a monovalent ion such as K^+ is equivalent, as a driving force, to a voltage difference of 60 mV. For a divalent ion such as Ca^{2+}, a 10-fold concentration gradient can be balanced as a driving force by a voltage difference of 60 mV/2, or only 30 mV.

($V_m - E_X$) is the net electrochemical driving force acting on an ion

When dealing with an ion (X), it is more convenient to think about the net driving force in voltage (*units:* mV) rather than electrochemical potential energy difference (*units:* joules/mole). If we divide all terms in Equation 5-6 by the product of valence and Faraday's constant ($z_X F$), we obtain

$$\underbrace{\frac{\Delta\mu_X}{z_X F}}_{\substack{\text{Net}\\\text{driving}\\\text{force}}} = \underbrace{\frac{RT}{z_X F}\ln\frac{[X]_i}{[X]_o}}_{-E_X} + \underbrace{(\Psi_i - \Psi_o)}_{V_m} \qquad (5-11)$$

Because the energy terms previously expressed as *joules per mole* were divided by *coulombs per mole* (i.e., $z_X F$)—all three energy terms enclosed in braces are now in units of joules per coulomb or *volts*. The term on the left is the net electrochemical driving force acting on ion X. The first term on the right, as defined in Equation 5-8, is the negative of the Nernst equilibrium potential ($-E_X$). The second term on the right is the membrane voltage (V_m). Thus, a convenient equation expressing the net driving force is

$$\text{Net driving force in volts} = (V_m - E_X) \qquad (5-12)$$

In Table 5-3, we use this equation—along with the values in Table 5-2 for extracellular (i.e., interstitial) and intracellular concentrations and a typical V_m of −60 mV—to compute the net driving force of Na^+, K^+, Ca^{2+}, Cl^-, HCO_3^-, and H^+. When the net driving force is negative, cations will enter the cell and anions will exit. Stated differently, when V_m is more negative than E_X (i.e., the cell is *too negative* for X to be in equilibrium), a cation will tend to enter the cell and an anion will tend to exit.

In simple diffusion, the flux of an uncharged substance through membrane lipid is directly proportional to its concentration difference

The difference in electrochemical potential energy of a solute X across the membrane is a useful parameter because it

Table 5-3 Net Electrochemical Driving Forces Acting on Ions in a Typical Cell*

Extracellular Concentration $[X]_o$	Intracellular Concentration $[X]_i$	Membrane Voltage V_m	Equilibrium Potential (mV) $E_X = -(RT/zF) \ln ([X]_i/[X]_o)$	Electrochemical Driving Force $(V_m - E_X)$
Na⁺ 145 mM	15 mM	−60 mV	+61 mV	−121 mV
K⁺ 4.5 mM	120 mM	−60 mV	−88 mV	+28 mV
Ca²⁺ 1.2 mM	10^{-7} M	−60 mV	+125 mV	−185 mV
Cl⁻ 116 mM	20 mM	−60 mV	−47 mV	−13 mV
HCO₃⁻ 25 mM	16 mM	−60 mV	−12 mV	−48 mV
H⁺ 40 nM pH 7.4	63 nM 7.2	−60 mV	−12 mV	−48 mV

*Calculated at 37°C using -RT/zF = -26.71 mV.

allows us to predict whether X is in equilibrium across the cell membrane (i.e., Is $\Delta\tilde{\mu}_X = 0$?) or, if not, whether X would tend to passively move into the cell or out of the cell. As long as the movement of X is not coupled to the movement of another substance or to some biochemical reaction, the only factor that determines the direction of net transport is the driving force $\Delta\tilde{\mu}_X = 0$. The ability to predict the movement of X is independent of any detailed knowledge of the actual transport pathway mediating its passive transport. In other words, we can understand the overall *energetics* of X transport without knowing anything about the transport mechanism itself, other than knowing that it is passive.

So far, we have discussed only the *direction* of net transport, not the *rate*. How will the rate of X transport vary if we vary the driving force $\Delta\tilde{\mu}_X$? Unlike the issue of direction, determining the rate—that is, the **kinetics**—of transport requires knowing the peculiarities of the actual mechanism that mediates passive X transport.

Most transport systems are so complicated that a straightforward relationship between transport rate and $\Delta\tilde{\mu}_X$ may not exist. Here we examine the simplest case, which is **simple diffusion**. How fast does an uncharged, hydrophobic solute move through a lipid bilayer? Gases (e.g., CO_2), a few endogenous compounds (e.g., steroid hormones), and many drugs (e.g., anesthetics) are both uncharged and hydrophobic. Imagine that such a solute is present on both sides of the membrane but at a higher concentration on the outside (Fig. 5-2). Because X has no electrical charge and because $[X]_o$ is greater than $[X]_i$, the net movement of X will be *into* the cell. How *fast* X moves is described by its **flux** (J_X), namely, the number of moles of X crossing a unit area of membrane (typically 1 cm²) per unit time (typically 1 second). Thus J_X has the units moles/(cm²·s). The better that X can dissolve in the membrane lipid (i.e., the higher the lipid-water **partition coefficient** of X), the more easily X will be able to traverse the membrane-lipid barrier. The flux of X will also be greater if X moves more readily once it is in the membrane (i.e., a higher **diffusion coefficient**) and if the distance that it must traverse is short (i.e., a smaller **membrane**

thickness). We can combine these three factors into a single parameter called the **permeability coefficient** of X (P_X). Finally, the flux of X will be greater as the difference in [X] between the two sides of the membrane increases (a large **gradient**).

These concepts governing the simple diffusion of an electrically neutral substance were quantified by Adolf Fick in the 1800s and applied by others to the special case of a cell membrane. They are embodied in the following equation, which is a simplified version of **Fick's law**:

$$J_X = P_X([X]_o - [X]_i) \qquad (5\text{-}13)$$

As already illustrated in Figure 5-2, we can separate the *net* flux of X into a *unidirectional influx* ($J_X^{o \to i}$) and a *unidirectional efflux* ($J_X^{i \to o}$). The net flux of X into the cell is simply the difference between the unidirectional fluxes:

$$\text{Unidirectional influx: } J_X^{o \to i} = P_X[X]_o$$
$$\text{Unidirectional efflux: } J_X^{i \to o} = P_X[X]_i \qquad (5\text{-}14)$$
$$\text{Net flux: } J_X = P_X([X]_o - [X]_i)$$

Thus, unidirectional influx is proportional to the outside concentration, unidirectional efflux is proportional to the inside concentration, and net flux is proportional to the concentration *difference* (not the *ratio* $[X]_o/[X]_i$, but the *difference* $[X]_o - [X]_i$). In all cases, the proportionality constant is P_X.

A description of the *kinetic* behavior of a transport system (Equation 5-14)—that is, how fast things move—cannot violate the laws of *energetics*, or thermodynamics (Equation 5-6)—that is, the direction in which things move to restore equilibrium. For example, the laws of thermodynamics (Equation 5-6) predict that when the concentration gradient for a neutral substance is zero (i.e., when $[X]_o/[X]_i = 1$), the system is in equilibrium and therefore the net flux must be zero. The law of simple diffusion (Equation 5-14), which is a kinetic description, also predicts that when the concentration gradient for a neutral substance is zero (i.e., $[X]_o - [X]_i = 0$), the flux is zero.

Some substances cross the membrane passively through intrinsic membrane proteins that can form pores, channels, or carriers

Because most ions and hydrophilic solutes of biological interest partition poorly into the lipid bilayer, simple passive diffusion of these solutes through the lipid portion of the membrane is negligible. Noncoupled transport across the plasma membrane generally requires specialized pathways that allow particular substances to cross the lipid bilayer. In all known cases, such pathways are formed from **integral membrane proteins**. Three types of protein pathways through the membrane are recognized:

1. The membrane protein forms a **pore** that is always open (Fig. 5-3A). Physiological examples are the porins in the outer membranes of mitochondria, cytotoxic pore-forming proteins such as the perforin released by lymphocytes, and perhaps the aquaporin water channels. A physical equivalent is a straight, open tube. If you look though this tube, you always see light coming through from the opposite side.
2. The membrane protein forms a **channel** that is alternately open and closed because it is equipped with a movable barrier or gate (Fig. 5-3B). Physiological examples include virtually all ion channels, such as the ones that allow Na^+, Cl^-, K^+, and Ca^{2+} to cross the membrane. The process of opening and closing of the barrier is referred to as **gating**. Thus, a channel is a gated pore, and a pore is a nongated channel. A physical equivalent is a tube with a shutter near one end. As you look through this tube, you see the light flickering as the shutter opens and closes.
3. The membrane protein forms a **carrier** surrounding a conduit that never offers a continuous transmembrane path because it is equipped with at least two gates that are never open at the same time (Fig. 5-3C). Between the two gates is a compartment that can contain one or more binding sites for the solute. If the two gates are both closed, one (or more) of the transiting particles is trapped, or **occluded**, in that compartment. Physiological examples include carriers that move single solutes through the membrane by a process known as facilitated diffusion, which is discussed in the next section. A physical equivalent is a tube with shutters at both ends. As you look through this tube, you never see any light passing through because both shutters are never open simultaneously.

Water-filled pores can allow molecules, some as large as 45 kDa, to cross membranes passively

Some membrane proteins form **pores** that provide an aqueous transmembrane conduit that is always open (Fig. 5-3A). Among the large-size pores are the **porins** (Fig. 5-4) found in the outer membranes of gram-negative bacteria and mitochondria. Mitochondrial porin allows solutes as large as 5 kDa to diffuse passively from the cytosol into the mitochondria's intermembrane space.

One mechanism by which cytotoxic T lymphocytes kill their target cells is by releasing monomers of a pore-forming protein known as **perforin**. Perforin monomers polymerize within the target cell membrane and assemble like staves of a barrel to form large, doughnut-like channels with an internal diameter of 16 nm. The passive flow of ions, water, and other small molecules through these pores kills the target cell. A similar pore plays a crucial role in the defense against bacterial infections. The binding of antibodies to an invading bacterium ("classic" pathway), or simply the presence of native polysaccharides on bacteria ("alternative" pathway), triggers a cascade of reactions known as the **complement cascade**. This cascade culminates in the formation of a doughnut-like structure with an internal diameter of 10 nm. This pore is made up of monomers of C9, the final component of the complement cascade.

The **nuclear pore complex (NPC)**, which regulates traffic into and out of the nucleus (see Chapter 2), is remarkably large. The NPC is made up of at least 30 different proteins and has a molecular mass of 10^8 Da and an outer diameter of ~100 nm. It can transport huge molecules (approaching 10^6 Da) in a complicated process that involves ATP hydrolysis. In addition to this active component of transport, the NPC also has a passive component. Contained within the massive NPC is a simple aqueous pore with an internal diameter of ~9 nm that allows molecules smaller than 45 kDa to move between the cytoplasm and nucleus but almost completely restricts the movement of globular proteins that are larger than ~60 kDa.

The plasma membranes of many types of cells have proteins that form channels just large enough to allow water molecules to pass through. The first water channel to be studied was **aquaporin** 1 (AQP1), a 28-kDa protein. AQP1 belongs to a larger family of aquaporins that has representatives in organisms as diverse as bacteria, plants, and animals. In mammals, the various aquaporin isoforms have different tissue distributions, different mechanisms of regulation, and varying abilities to transport small neutral molecules other than water. In the lipid bilayer, AQP1 (Fig. 5-5) exists as tetramers. Each monomer consists of six membrane-spanning helices as well as two shorter helices that dip into the plane of the membrane. These structures form a permeation pathway for the single-file diffusion of water. For his discovery of the aquaporins, Peter Agre shared the 2003 Nobel Prize in Chemistry.

Gated channels, which alternately open and close, allow ions to cross the membrane passively

Gated **ion channels**, like the aquaporins just discussed, consist of one or more polypeptide subunits with α-helical membrane-spanning segments. These channels have several functional components (Fig. 5-3B). The first is a **gate** that determines whether the channel is open or closed, each state reflecting a different conformation of the membrane protein. Second, the channel generally has one or more **sensors** that can respond to one of several different types of signals: (1) changes in membrane voltage, (2) second-messenger systems

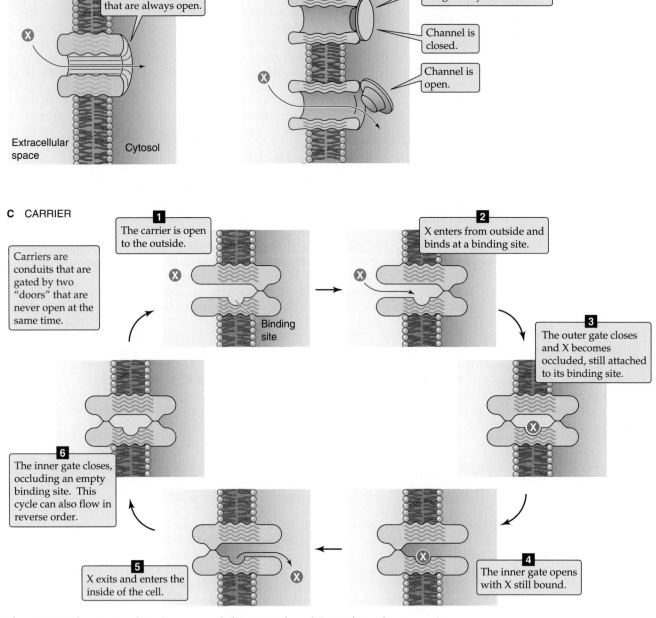

A   PORE (NON-GATED CHANNEL)

Pores are conduits that are always open.

X

Extracellular space

Cytosol

B   CHANNEL (GATED PORE)

Channels are conduits that are gated by a "door."

Channel is closed.

Channel is open.

X

C   CARRIER

Carriers are conduits that are gated by two "doors" that are never open at the same time.

1 The carrier is open to the outside.

X

Binding site

2 X enters from outside and binds at a binding site.

X

3 The outer gate closes and X becomes occluded, still attached to its binding site.

X

6 The inner gate closes, occluding an empty binding site. This cycle can also flow in reverse order.

5 X exits and enters the inside of the cell.

X

4 The inner gate opens with X still bound.

X

Figure 5-3   Three types of passive, noncoupled transport through integral membrane proteins.

that act at the cytoplasmic face of the membrane protein, or (3) ligands, such as neurohumoral agonists, that bind to the extracellular face of the membrane protein. These signals regulate transitions between the open and closed states. A third functional component is a **selectivity filter**, which determines the *classes* of ions (e.g., anions or cations) or the *particular* ions (e.g., Na^+, K^+, Ca^{2+}) that have access to the channel pore. The fourth component is the actual **open-channel pore** (Fig. 5-3B). Each time that a channel assumes the open conformation, it provides a continuous pathway between the two sides of the membrane so that ions can flow

through it passively by diffusion until the channel closes again. During each channel opening, many ions flow through the channel pore, usually a sufficient number to be detected as a small current by sensitive patch-clamping techniques (see Chapter 6).

Na^+ Channels   Because **the electrochemical driving force for Na^+** ($V_m - E_{Na}$) is always strongly *negative* (Table 5-3), a large, inwardly directed net driving force or gradient favors the passive movement of Na^+ into virtually every cell of the body. Therefore, an open Na^+ channel will act as a conduit

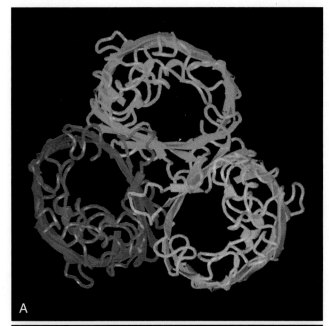

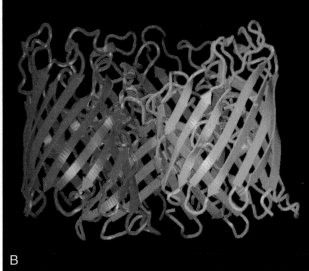

Figure 5-4 Structure of the PhoE porin of *Escherichia coli*. **A,** Top view of a porin trimer that shows the backbones of the polypeptide chains. Each of the three identical monomers, which are shown in different colors, contains 330 amino acids. The center of each monomer is a pore. **B,** Side view of a porin trimer. The extracellular surface is shown at the top. Each monomer consists of a β barrel with 16 antiparallel β sheets (i.e., adjacent polypeptide strands are oriented in opposite directions) surrounding a large cavity that at its narrowest point has an oval cross section (internal diameter, 0.7 × 1.1 nm). The images are based on high-resolution electron microscopy, at a resolution of 3.5 Å (0.35 nm). *(Reproduced from Jap BK, Walian PJ: Structure and functional mechanisms of porins. Physiol Rev 1996; 76:1073-1088.)*

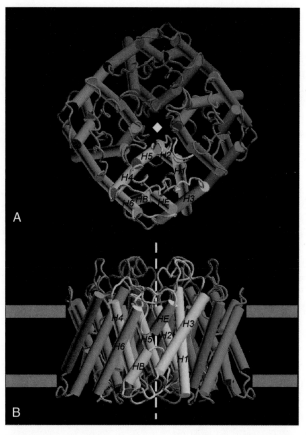

Figure 5-5 Structure of the human AQP1 water channel. **A,** Top view of an aquaporin tetramer. Each of the four identical monomers is made up of 269 amino acids and has a pore at its center. **B,** Side view of aquaporin. The extracellular surface is shown at the top. The images are based on high-resolution electron microscopy at a resolution of 3.8 Å (0.38 nm). *(Reproduced from Murata K, Mitsuoka K, Hirai T, et al: Structural determinants of water permeation through aquaporin-1. Nature 407:599-605, 2000. © 2000 Macmillan Magazines Ltd.)*

for the passive entry of Na⁺. One physiological use for channel-mediated Na⁺ entry is the transmission of information. Thus, voltage-gated Na⁺ channels are responsible for generating the action potential (e.g., "nerve impulse") in many excitable cells. Another physiological use of Na⁺ channels can be found in epithelial cells such as those in certain segments of the renal tubule and intestine. In this case, ENaC Na⁺ channels are largely restricted to the apical surface of the cell, where they allow Na⁺ to enter the epithelial cell from the renal tubule lumen or intestinal lumen. This passive influx is a key step in the movement of Na⁺ across the entire epithelium, from lumen to blood.

K⁺ Channels The **electrochemical driving force for K⁺** $(V_m - E_K)$ is usually fairly close to zero or somewhat *positive* (Table 5-3), so K⁺ is either at equilibrium or tends to move *out* of the cell. In virtually all cells, K⁺ channels play a major role in generating a resting membrane voltage that is inside-negative. Other kinds of K⁺ channels play a key role in excitable cells, where these channels help terminate action potentials.

Ca²⁺ Channels The **electrochemical driving force for Ca²⁺** $(V_m - E_{Ca})$ is always strongly *negative* (Table 5-3), so Ca²⁺ tends to move *into* the cell. When Ca²⁺ channels are open, Ca²⁺ rapidly enters the cell down a steep electrochemical gradient. This inward movement of Ca²⁺ plays a vital role in transmembrane signaling for both excitable and nonexcitable cells as well as in generating action potentials in some excitable cells.

Proton Channels The plasma membranes of many cell types contain Hv1 H⁺ channels. Under normal conditions, the H⁺ driving force generally tends to move H⁺ *into* cells if Hv1 channels are open. However, Hv1 channels tend to be *closed* under normal conditions and activate only when the membrane depolarizes or the cytoplasm acidifies—that is, when the driving force favors the *outward* movement of H⁺. Hv1 channels may therefore help mediate H⁺ extrusion from the cell during states of strong membrane depolarization (e.g., during an action potential) or severe intracellular acidification.

Anion Channels Most cells contain one or more types of anion-selective channels through which the passive, noncoupled transport of Cl⁻—and, to a lesser extent, HCO_3^-—can take place. The electrochemical driving force for Cl⁻ ($V_m - E_{Cl}$) in most cells is modestly *negative* (Table 5-3), so Cl⁻ tends to move *out of* these cells. In certain epithelial cells with Cl⁻ channels on their basolateral membranes, the passive movement of Cl⁻ through these channels plays a role in the transepithelial movement of Cl⁻ from lumen to blood.

Some carriers facilitate the passive diffusion of small solutes such as glucose

Carrier-mediated transport systems transfer a broad range of ions and organic solutes across the plasma membrane. Each carrier protein has a specific affinity for binding one or a small number of solutes and transporting them across the bilayer. The simplest passive carrier-mediated transporter is one that mediates *facilitated diffusion*. Later, we will introduce *cotransporters* (which carry two or more solutes in the same direction) and *exchangers* (which move them in opposite directions).

 All carriers that do not either hydrolyze ATP or couple to an electron transport chain are members of the **solute carrier (SLC) superfamily**, which is organized according to the homology of the deduced amino acid sequences (Table 5-4). Each of the 43 SLC families contains 1 to 27 variants, which share a relatively high amino acid sequence identity (20% to 25%) among the isoforms. Members of an SLC family may differ in molecular mechanism (facilitated diffusion versus exchange), kinetic properties (e.g., solute specificity and affinity), regulation (e.g., phosphorylation), sites of membrane targeting (e.g., plasma membrane versus intracellular organelles), tissues in which they are expressed (e.g., kidney versus brain), or developmental stage at which they are expressed.

Carrier-mediated transport systems behave according to a general kinetic scheme for facilitated diffusion that is outlined in Figure 5-3C. This model illustrates how, in a cycle of six steps, a carrier could passively move a solute X into the cell.

This mechanism can mediate only the downhill, or passive, transport of X. Therefore, it mediates a type of diffusion called **facilitated diffusion**. When [X] is equal on the two sides of the membrane, no *net* transport will take place,

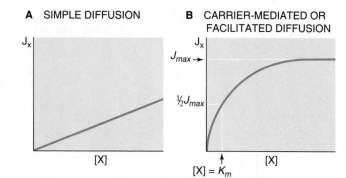

Figure 5-6 Dependence of transport rates on solute concentration. **A,** The net flux of the solute X through the cell membrane is J_X. **B,** The maximal flux of X (J_{max}) occurs when the carriers are saturated. The flux is half of its maximal value ($1/2 J_{max}$) when the concentration of X is equal to the K_m.

although equal and opposite *unidirectional* fluxes of X may still occur.

In a cell membrane, a fixed number of carriers is available to transport X. Furthermore, each carrier has a limited speed with which it can cycle through the steps illustrated in Figure 5-3C. Thus, if the extracellular X concentration is gradually increased, for example, the influx of X will eventually reach a maximal value once all the carriers have become loaded with X. This situation is very different from the one that exists with simple diffusion, that is, the movement of a solute through the lipid phase of the membrane. Influx by simple diffusion increases linearly with increases in $[X]_o$, with no maximal rate of transport. As an example, if X is initially absent on *both* sides of the membrane and we gradually increase [X] on *one* side, the net flux of X (J_X) is described by a straight line that passes through the origin (Fig. 5-6A). However, with carrier-mediated transport, J_X reaches a maximum (J_{max}) when [X] is high enough to occupy all the carriers in the membrane (Fig. 5-6B). Thus, the relationship describing carrier-mediated transport follows the same Michaelis-Menten kinetics as enzymes do:

$$V = \frac{[S] V_{max}}{K_m + [S]} \quad (5\text{-}15)$$

This equation describes how the velocity of an enzymatic reaction (V) depends on the substrate concentration ([S]), the Michaelis constant (K_m), and the maximal velocity (V_{max}). The comparable equation for carrier-mediated transport is identical, except that fluxes replace reaction velocities:

$$J_X = \frac{[X] J_{max}}{K_m + [X]} \quad (5\text{-}16)$$

Thus, K_m is the solute concentration at which J_X is half of the maximal flux (J_{max}). The lower the K_m, the higher the apparent **affinity** of the transporter for the solute.

Historically, the name *carrier* suggested that carrier-mediated transport occurs as the solute binds to a miniature ferryboat that shuttles back and forth across the membrane.

Table 5-4 Some Families in the SLC Superfamily of Solute Carriers

Family	Description	Examples
SLC1 (7)*	Glutamate transporters	EAAT1
SLC2 (14)	Facilitated transport of hexoses	GLUT1, GLUT4
SLC3 (2)	Heavy subunits of heterodimeric amino acid transporters (with SLC7)	
SLC4 (10)	HCO_3^- exchangers and cotransporters	AE1 (Cl-HCO_3 exchanger) NBCe1 (electrogenic Na/HCO_3 cotransporter) NBCn1 (electroneutral Na/HCO_3 cotransporter) NDCBE (Na^+-driven Cl-HCO_3 exchanger)
SLC5 (8)	Na^+/glucose cotransporters	SGLT1 to 5 (glucose)
SLC6 (16)	Na^+- and Cl^--coupled cotransport of "neurotransmitters"	B^0AT1 (Na^+-coupled amino acid) GAT1-3, GBT1 (Na^+- and Cl^--coupled GABA) ATB^{0+} (Na^+- and Cl^--coupled amino acids)
SLC7 (14)	Transporter subunits of heterodimeric amino acid transporters (with SLC3)	
SLC8 (3)	Na-Ca exchangers	NCX1 to 3
SLC9 (9)	Na-H exchangers	NHE1 to 8
SLC10 (6)	Na/bile salt cotransporters	
SLC11 (2)	H^+-driven metal ion cotransporters	DMT1
SLC12 (9)	Cation-coupled Cl^- cotransporters	NKCC1, NKCC2 (Na/K/Cl cotransporter) NCC (Na/Cl cotransporter) KCC1 (K/Cl cotransporter)
SLC13 (5)	Na^+-coupled sulfate and carboxylate cotransporters	NaDC1 (mono-, di-, and tricarboxylates) NaSi (sulfate)
SLC14 (2)	Facilitated transport of urea	UT
SLC15 (4)	H^+-driven oligopeptide cotransporters	PepT1
SLC16 (14)	Monocarboxylate transporters	MCT1 (H^+-coupled monocarboxylate cotransporter) TAT1 (facilitated diffusion of aromatic amino acids)
SLC17 (8)	Type I Na/phosphate cotransporters and vesicular Glu transporters	NaPi-I
SLC18 (3)	Vesicular amine transporters	
SLC19 (3)	Folate/thiamine transporters	
SLC20 (2)	Type III Na/phosphate cotransporters	NaPi-III
SLC21 (11)	Organic anion transporters	OATP PGT

*Number of genes in parentheses.

Table 5-4 The SLC Superfamily of Solute Carriers—cont'd

Family	Description	Examples
SLC22 (18)*	Organic cations, anions, zwitterions	OCT1 to 3 (facilitated diffusion of organic *cations*) OAT1 to 5 (exchange or facilitated diffusion of organic *anions*) URAT (urate exchanger)
SLC23 (4)	Na/ascorbic acid transporters	
SLC26 (10)	Multifunctional anion exchangers	DRA (Cl-HCO_3 exchanger) Pendrin (exchanges HCO_3^-, Cl^-, or I^-) CFEX (exchanges Cl^-, HCO_3^-, oxalate, formate)
SLC28 (3)	Na/nucleoside transporters	
SLC34 (3)	Type II Na/phosphate cotransporters	NaPi-IIa, NaPi-IIc
SLC36 (4)	H^+-coupled amino acid cotransporters	PAT1
SLC38 (6)	Na^+-driven neutral amino acid transporters (system A and N)	SNAT3 (cotransports amino acids with Na^+ in exchange for H^+) System N (cotransports amino acids with Na^+ in exchange for H^+) SNAT1, 2, 4 (system A cotransports amino acids with Na^+)
SLC39 (14)	Metal ion transporters	ZIP1 (uptake of Zn^{2+})
SLC40 (1)	Basolateral Fe transporter (facilitated diffusion)	Ferroportin (MTP1, Fe^{2+})
SLC42 (3)	NH_3 channels	RhAG

*Number of genes in parentheses.

Small polypeptides that act as shuttling carriers exist in nature, as exemplified by the antibiotic valinomycin. Such "ion carriers," or **ionophores**, bind to an ion on one side of the membrane, diffuse across the lipid phase of the membrane, and release the ion on the opposite side of the membrane. Valinomycin is a K^+ ionophore that certain bacteria produce to achieve a selective advantage over their neighbors. However, none of the known carrier-mediated transport pathways in animal cell membranes are ferries.

An example of a membrane protein that mediates facilitated diffusion is the **glucose transporter GLUT1** (Fig. 5-7), a member of the SLC2 family (Table 5-4). The GLUTs have 12 membrane-spanning segments as well as multiple hydrophilic polypeptide loops facing either the ECF or ICF. It could not possibly act as a ferryboat shuttling back and forth across the membrane. Instead, some of the membrane-spanning segments of carrier-mediated transport proteins most likely form a permeation pathway through the lipid bilayer, as illustrated by the amphipathic membrane-spanning segments 7, 8, and 11 in Figure 5-7. These membrane-spanning segments, as well as other portions of the protein, probably also act as the gates and solute-binding sites that allow transport to proceed in the manner outlined in Figure 5-3C.

The SLC2 family includes 12 hexose transporters (GLUTs). Whereas GLUT1 is constitutively expressed on the cell surface, GLUT4 in the basal state is predominantly present in the membranes of intracellular vesicles, which represent a storage pool for the transporters. Because a solute such as glucose permeates the lipid bilayer so poorly, its uptake by the cell depends strictly on the activity of a carrier-mediated transport system for glucose. Insulin increases the rate of carrier-mediated glucose transport into certain cells by recruiting the GLUT4 isoform to the plasma membrane from the storage pool (see Chapter 51).

Two other examples of transporters that mediate facilitated diffusion are the **urea transporter (UT)** family, which are members of the SLC14 family (Table 5-4), and the **organic cation transporter (OCT)** family, which are members of the SLC22 family. Because OCT moves an electrical charge (i.e., carries current), it is said to be **electrogenic.**

Table 5-5 Comparison of Properties of Pores, Channels, and Carriers

	Pores	Channels	Carriers
Example	Water channel (AQP1)	Shaker K^+ channel	Glucose transporter (GLUT1)
Conduit through membrane	Always open	Intermittently open	Never open
Unitary event	None (continuously open)	Opening	Cycle of conformational changes
Particles translocated per "event"	—	$6 \times 10^{4*}$	1-5
Particles translocated per second	up to 2×10^9	10^6 to 10^8 when open	200-50,000

*Assuming a 100-pS channel, a driving force of 100 mV, and an opening time of 1 ms.

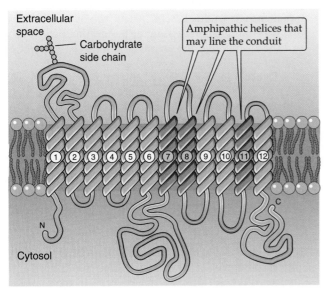

Figure 5-7 Structure of the GLUT family of glucose transporters. The 12 membrane-spanning segments are connected to each other by intracellular and extracellular loops.

Extracellular space
Carbohydrate side chain
Amphipathic helices that may line the conduit
Cytosol

The physical structure of pores, channels, and carriers is quite similar

Pores, ion channels, and carriers all have multiple transmembrane segments surrounding a solute permeation pathway. Moreover, some channels also contain binding sites within their permeation pathways, so transport is saturable with respect to ion concentration. However, pores, channels, and carriers are fundamentally distinct kinetically (Table 5-5). *Pores*, such as the porins, are thought to be continuously open and allow vast numbers of particles to cross the membrane. No evidence suggests that pores have conformational states. *Channels* undergo conformational transitions between closed and open states. When they are open, they are open to both intracellular and extracellular solutions simultaneously. Thus, while the channel is open, it allows multiple ions, perhaps millions, to cross the membrane per open event. Because the length of time that a particular channel remains open varies from one open event to the

next, the number of ions flowing through that channel per open event is not fixed. *Carriers* have a permeation pathway that is virtually never open simultaneously to both intracellular and extracellular solutions. Whereas the fundamental event for a channel is opening, the fundamental event for a carrier is a complete cycle of conformational changes. Because the binding sites in a carrier are limited, each cycle of a carrier can transport only one or a *small, fixed* number of solute particles. Thus, the number of particles per second that can move across the membrane is generally several orders of magnitude lower for a single carrier than for a single channel.

We have seen how carriers can mediate facilitated diffusion of glucose, which is a passive or downhill process. However, carriers can also mediate **coupled** modes of transport. The remainder of this section is devoted to these carriers, which act as pumps, cotransporters, and exchangers.

The Na-K pump, the most important primary active transporter in animal cells, uses the energy of ATP to extrude Na^+ and to take up K^+

Active transport is a process that can transfer a solute uphill across a membrane—that is, against its electrochemical potential energy difference. In **primary active transport**, the driving force needed to cause net transfer of a solute against its electrochemical gradient comes from the favorable energy change that is associated with an exergonic chemical reaction, such as ATP hydrolysis. In **secondary active transport**, the driving force is provided by coupling the *uphill* movement of that solute to the *downhill* movement of one or more other solutes for which a favorable electrochemical potential energy difference exists. A physical example is to use a motor-driven winch to lift a large weight into the air (primary active transport) and then to transfer this large weight to a seesaw, on the other end of which is a lighter child. The potential energy stored in the elevated weight will then lift the child (secondary active transport). For transporters, it is commonly the favorable inwardly directed Na^+ electrochemical gradient, which itself is set up by a *primary* active transporter, that drives the *secondary* active transport of another solute. In this and the next section, we discuss primary active transporters, which are also referred to as **pumps**. The pumps discussed here are all energized by ATP hydrolysis and hence are **ATPases**.

As a prototypic example of a primary active transporter, consider the nearly ubiquitous **Na-K pump** (or Na,K-ATPase, **NKA**). This substance was the first enzyme recognized to be an ion pump, a discovery for which Jens Skou shared the 1997 Nobel Prize in Chemistry. The Na-K pump is located in the plasma membrane and has both α and β subunits (Fig. 5-8A). The α subunit, which has 10 transmembrane segments, is the catalytic subunit that mediates active transport. The β subunit, which has one transmembrane segment, is essential for proper assembly and membrane targeting of the Na-K pump. Four α isoforms and two β isoforms have been described. These isoforms have different tissue and developmental patterns of expression as well as different kinetic properties.

With each forward cycle, the pump couples the extrusion of three Na^+ ions and the uptake of two K^+ ions to the intracellular hydrolysis of one ATP molecule. By themselves, the transport steps of the Na-K pump are energetically uphill; that is, if the pump were not an ATPase, the transporter would run in reverse, with Na^+ leaking into the cell and K^+ leaking out. Indeed, under extreme experimental conditions, the Na-K pump can be reversed and forced to synthesize ATP! However, under physiological conditions, hydrolysis of one ATP molecule releases so much free energy—relative to the aggregate free energy needed to fuel the uphill movement of three Na^+ and two K^+ ions—that the pump is poised far from its equilibrium and brings about the net active exchange of Na^+ for K^+ in the desired directions.

Although animal cells may have other pumps in their plasma membranes, the Na-K pump is the only primary active transport process for Na^+. The Na-K pump is also the most important primary active transport mechanism for K^+. In cells throughout the body, the Na-K pump is responsible for maintaining a low $[Na^+]_i$ and a high $[K^+]_i$ relative to ECF. In most epithelial cells, the Na-K pump is restricted to the basolateral side of the cell.

The Na-K pump exists in two major conformational states: E_1, in which the binding sites for the ions face the inside of the cell; and E_2, in which the binding sites face the outside. The Na-K pump is a member of a large superfamily of pumps known as **E_1-E_2 ATPases** or **P-type ATPases**. It is the ordered cycling between these two states that underlies the action of the pump. Figure 5-8B is a simplified model showing the eight stages of this catalytic cycle of the α subunit:

Stage 1: **ATP-bound E_1•ATP state.** The cycle starts with the ATP-bound E_1 conformation, just after the pump has released its bound K^+ to the ICF. The Na^+-binding sites face the ICF and have high affinities for Na^+.

Stage 2: **Na^+-bound E_1•ATP•3Na^+ state.** Three intracellular Na^+ ions bind.

Stage 3: **Occluded E_1-P•(3Na^+) state.** The ATP previously bound to the pump phosphorylates the pump at an aspartate residue. Simultaneously, ADP leaves. This phosphorylation triggers a minor conformational change in which the E_1 form of the pump now occludes the three bound Na^+ ions within the permeation pathway. In this state, the Na^+ binding sites are inaccessible to both the ICF and ECF.

Stage 4: **Deoccluded E_2-P•3Na^+ state.** A major conformational change shifts the pump from the E_1 to the E_2 conformation and has two effects. First, the pump becomes deoccluded, so that the Na^+-binding sites now communicate with the *extracellular* solution. Second, the Na^+ affinities of these binding sites decrease.

Stage 5: **Empty E_2-P state.** The three bound Na^+ ions dissociate into the external solution, and the protein undergoes a minor conformational change to the empty E_2-P form, which has high affinity for binding of extracellular K^+. However, the pore still communicates with the extracellular solution.

Stage 6: **K^+-bound E_2-P•2K^+ state.** Two K^+ ions bind to the pump.

Stage 7: **Occluded E_2•(2K^+) state.** Hydrolysis of the acylphosphate bond, which links the phosphate group to the aspartate residue, releases the inorganic phosphate into the intracellular solution and causes a minor conformational change. In this E_2•(2K^+) state, the pump occludes the two bound K^+ ions within the permeation pathway so that the K^+-binding sites are inaccessible to both the ECF and ICF.

Stage 8: **Deoccluded E_1•ATP•2K^+ state.** Binding of intracellular ATP causes a major conformational change that shifts the pump from the E_2 back to the E_1 state. This conformational change has two effects. First, the pump becomes deoccluded, so that the K^+-binding sites now communicate with the *intracellular* solution. Second, the K^+ affinities of these binding sites decrease.

Stage 1: **ATP-bound E_1•ATP state.** Dissociation of the two bound K^+ ions into the intracellular solution returns the pump to its original E_1•ATP state, ready to begin another cycle.

Because each cycle of hydrolysis of one ATP molecule is coupled to the extrusion of three Na^+ ions from the cell and the uptake of two K^+ ions, the *stoichiometry* of the pump is three Na^+ to two K^+, and each cycle of the pump is associated with the net extrusion of one positive charge from the cell. Thus, the Na-K pump is *electrogenic*.

Just as glucose flux through the GLUT1 transporter is a saturable function of [glucose], the rate of active transport by the Na-K pump is a saturable function of $[Na^+]_i$ and $[K^+]_o$. The reason is that the number of pumps is finite and each must bind three Na^+ ions and two K^+ ions. The transport rate is also a saturable function of $[ATP]_i$ and therefore depends on the metabolic state of the cell. In cells with high Na-K pump rates, such as renal proximal tubules, a third or more of cellular energy metabolism is devoted to supplying ATP to the Na-K pump.

A hallmark of the Na-K pump is that it is blocked by a class of compounds known as **cardiac glycosides**, examples of which are ouabain and digoxin; digoxin is widely used for a variety of cardiac conditions. These compounds have a high affinity for the extracellular side of the E_2-P state of the pump, which also has a high affinity for extracellular K^+. Thus, the binding of extracellular K^+ competitively antagonizes the binding of cardiac glycosides. An important clinical correlate is that hypokalemia (a low $[K^+]$ in blood plasma) potentiates digitalis toxicity in patients.

A Na–K PUMP

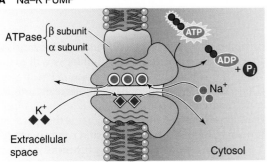

B ENZYMATIC CYCLE OF THE Na–K PUMP

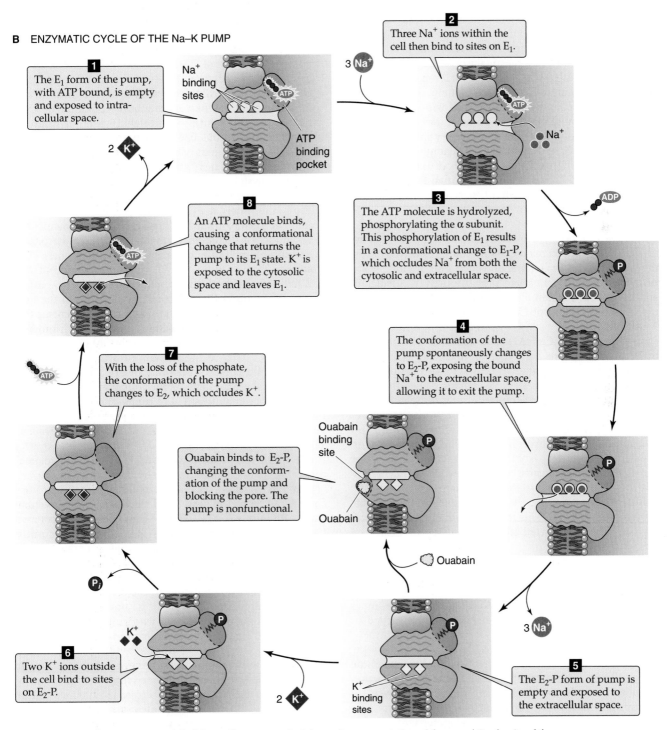

1 The E_1 form of the pump, with ATP bound, is empty and exposed to intra-cellular space.

2 Three Na^+ ions within the cell then bind to sites on E_1.

3 The ATP molecule is hydrolyzed, phosphorylating the α subunit. This phosphorylation of E_1 results in a conformational change to E_1-P, which occludes Na^+ from both the cytosolic and extracellular space.

4 The conformation of the pump spontaneously changes to E_2-P, exposing the bound Na^+ to the extracellular space, allowing it to exit the pump.

5 The E_2-P form of pump is empty and exposed to the extracellular space.

6 Two K^+ ions outside the cell bind to sites on E_2-P.

7 With the loss of the phosphate, the conformation of the pump changes to E_2, which occludes K^+.

8 An ATP molecule binds, causing a conformational change that returns the pump to its E_1 state. K^+ is exposed to the cytosolic space and leaves E_1.

Ouabain binds to E_2-P, changing the conformation of the pump and blocking the pore. The pump is nonfunctional.

Figure 5-8   Model of the sodium pump. **A,** Schematic representation of the α and β subunits of the pump. **B,** The protein cycles through at least eight identifiable stages as it moves 3 Na^+ ions out of the cell and 2 K^+ ions into the cell.

Besides the Na-K pump, other P-type ATPases include the H-K and Ca^{2+} pumps

The family of P-type ATPases—all of which share significant sequence similarity with the α subunit of the Na-K pump—includes several subfamilies.

The H-K Pump Other than the Na-K pump, relatively few primary active transporters are located on the plasma membranes of animal cells. In the parietal cells of the gastric gland, an H-K pump (**HKA**) extrudes H^+ across the apical membrane into the gland lumen. Similar pumps are present in the kidney and intestines. The H-K pump mediates the active extrusion of H^+ and the uptake of K^+, all fueled by ATP hydrolysis, probably in the ratio of two H^+ ions, two K^+ ions, and one ATP molecule. Like the Na-K pump, the H-K pump is composed of α and β subunits, each with multiple isoforms. The α subunit of the H-K pump also undergoes phosphorylation through E_1 and E_2 intermediates during its catalytic cycle (Fig. 5-8B) and, like the α subunit of the Na-K pump, is a member of the P_{2C} subfamily of P-type ATPases. The Na-K and H-K pumps are the only two P-type ATPases with known β subunits, all of which share significant sequence similarity.

Ca^{2+} Pumps Most if not all cells have a primary active transporter at the plasma membrane that extrudes Ca^{2+} from the cell. These pumps are abbreviated **PMCA** (for plasma membrane Ca^{2+}-ATPase), and at least four PMCA isoforms appear in the P_{2B} subfamily of P-type ATPases. These pumps exchange one H^+ for one Ca^{2+} for each molecule of ATP that is hydrolyzed.

Ca^{2+} pumps (or Ca^{2+}-ATPases) also exist on the membrane surrounding such intracellular organelles as the sarcoplasmic reticulum in muscle cells and the endoplasmic reticulum in other cells, where they play a role in the active sequestration of Ca^{2+} into intracellular stores. The **SERCAs** (for sarcoplasmic and endoplasmic reticulum calcium ATPase) appear to transport two H^+ and two Ca^{2+} ions for each molecule of ATP hydrolyzed. The three known SERCAs, which are in the P_{2A} subfamily of P-type ATPases, are expressed in different muscle types (see Table 9-1).

Other Pumps Among the other P-type ATPases is the copper pump ATP7B. This member of the P_{1B} subfamily of P-type ATPases is mutated in Wilson disease (see the box on this topic in Chapter 46).

The F-type and the V-type ATPases transport H^+

F-type or F_oF_1 ATPases The ATP synthase of the inner membrane of mitochondria, also known as an F-type or F_oF_1 ATPase, catalyzes the final step in the ATP synthesis pathway.

The F_oF_1 ATPase of mitochondria (Fig. 5-9A) looks a little like a lollipop held in your hand. The hand-like F_o portion is embedded in the membrane and serves as the pathway for H^+ transport. The F_o portion has at least three different subunits (a, b, and c), for an overall stoichiometry of ab_2c_{10-12}. The lollipop-like F_1 portion is outside the plane of the membrane and points into the mitochondrial matrix. The "stick" consists of a γ subunit, with an attached ϵ subunit. The "candy" portion of F_1, which has the ATPase activity, consists of three alternating pairs of α and β subunits as well as an attached δ subunit. Thus, the overall stoichiometry of F_1 is $\alpha_3\beta_3\gamma\delta\epsilon$. The entire F_oF_1 complex has a molecular mass of ~500 kDa.

A fascinating property of the F_oF_1 ATPase is that parts of it rotate. We can think of the hand, stick, and candy portions of the F_oF_1 ATPase as having three distinct functions. (1) The hand (the c proteins of F_o) acts as a turbine that rotates in the plane of the membrane, driven by the H^+ ions that flow through the turbine—down the H^+ electrochemical gradient—into the mitochondrion. (2) The stick is an axle (γ and ϵ subunits of F_1) that rotates with the turbine. (3) The candy (the α and β subunits of F_1) is a stationary chemical factory—energized by the rotating axle—that synthesizes one ATP molecule for each 120-degree turn of the turbine/axle complex. In addition, the a and b subunits of F_o, and possibly the δ subunit of F_1, form a stator that holds the candy in place while the turbine/axle complex turns. Paul Boyer and John Walker shared part of the 1997 Nobel Prize in Chemistry for elucidating this "rotary catalysis" mechanism.

Under physiological conditions, the mitochondrial F_oF_1 ATPase runs as an ATP synthase (i.e., "backward" for an H^+ pump)—the final step in oxidative phosphorylation—because of a large, inwardly directed H^+ gradient across the inner mitochondrial membrane (Fig. 5-9B). The citric acid cycle captures energy as electrons and transfers these electrons to reduced nicotinamide adenine dinucleotide (NADH) and reduced flavin adenine dinucleotide ($FADH_2$). NADH and $FADH_2$ transfer their high-energy electrons to the **electron transport chain**, which consists of four major complexes on the inner membrane of the mitochondrion (Fig. 5-9B). As this "respiratory chain" transfers the electrons from one electron carrier to another, the electrons gradually lose energy until they finally combine with 2 H^+ and $\frac{1}{2}$ O_2 to form H_2O. Along the way, three of the four major complexes of the respiratory chain (I, III, IV) pump H^+ across the inner membrane into the intermembrane space (i.e., the space between the inner and outer mitochondrial membranes). These "pumps" are *not* ATPases. The net result is that electron transport has established a large out-to-in H^+ gradient across the mitochondrial inner membrane.

The F_oF_1 ATPase—which is complex V in the respiratory chain—can now use this large electrochemical potential energy difference for H^+. The H^+ ions then flow backward (i.e., down their electrochemical gradient) into the mitochondrion through the F_oF_1 ATPase, which generates ATP in the matrix space of the mitochondrion from ADP and inorganic phosphate. The entire process by which electron transport generates an H^+ gradient and the F_oF_1 ATPase harnesses this H^+ gradient to synthesize ATP is known as the chemiosmotic hypothesis. Peter Mitchell, who proposed this hypothesis in 1961, received the Nobel Prize in Chemistry for his work in 1978.

The precise stoichiometry is unknown but may be one ATP molecule synthesized for every three H^+ ions flowing downhill into the mitochondrion (one H^+ for each pair of $\alpha\beta$ subunits of F_1). If the H^+ gradient across the mitochondrial inner membrane reverses, the F_oF_1 ATPase will actually function as an ATPase and use the energy of ATP hydrolysis to pump H^+ out of the mitochondrion. Similar F_oF_1 ATPases are also present in bacteria and chloroplasts.

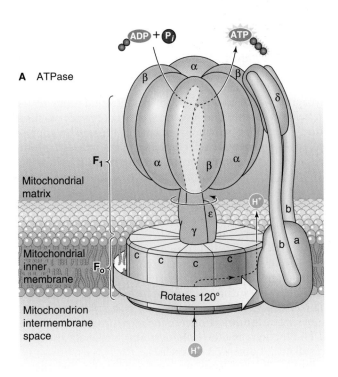

A ATPase

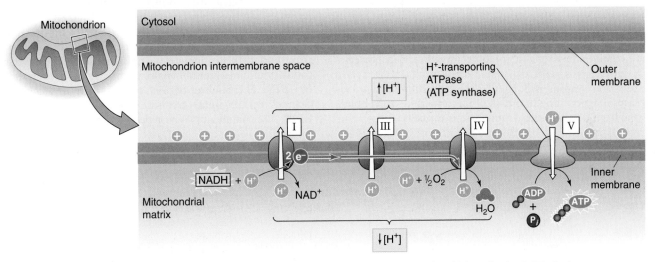

B MODEL OF THE CHEMIOSMOTIC HYPOTHESIS

Figure 5-9 The F_oF_1 ATPase and its role as the ATP synthase in the mitochondrial synthesis of ATP. **A,** A cartoon of the F_oF_1 ATPase. The pump has two functional units, F_o (which historically stood for oligomycin-sensitive factor) and F_1 (which historically stood for factor 1). **F_o** is the transmembrane portion that contains the ion channel through which the H^+ passes. The **F_1** is the ATPase. In one complete cycle, the downhill movement of H^+ ions causes the c subunits of F_o and the axle formed by the subunits of F1 to rotate 360 degrees in three 120-degree steps, causing the α and β subunits to sequentially synthesize and release 3 ATP molecules, for a synthase stoichiometry of ~3 H^+ per ATP. However, the mitochondrion uses ~1 additional H^+ to import inorganic phosphate and to exchange cytosolic ADP for mitochondrial ATP. Thus, a total of ~4 H^+ would be needed per ATP. **B,** Complexes I, III, and IV of the respiratory chain use the energy of 1 NADH to pump H^+ out of the mitochondrial matrix; the consensus is 10 H^+ per NADH. The resulting H^+ gradient causes the mitochondrial F_oF_1 ATPase to run as an ATP synthase. Thus, the mitochondrion synthesizes (10 H^+/NADH) × (1 ATP/4 H^+) = 2.5 ATP/NADH. Similarly, the consensus is that complexes III and IV use the energy of 1 $FADH_2$ to pump 6 H^+ out of the mitochondrial matrix (not shown). Thus, the mitochondrion synthesizes (6 H^+/$FADH_2$) × (1 ATP/4 H^+) = 1.5 ATP/$FADH_2$.

V-type H⁺ Pump The membranes surrounding such intracellular organelles as lysosomes, endosomes, secretory vesicles, storage vesicles, and the Golgi apparatus contain a so-called vacuolar-type (or V-type) H^+-ATPase that pumps H^+ from the cytoplasm to the interior of the organelles. The low pH generated inside these organelles is important for sorting proteins, dissociating ligands from receptors, optimizing the activity of acid hydrolases, and accumulating neurotransmitters in vesicles. The apical membranes of certain renal tubule cells as well as the plasma membranes of certain other cells also have V-type H^+ pumps that extrude H^+ from the cell. These V-type H^+ pumps, unlike the gastric H-K pump, are independent of K^+. Instead, the V-type H^+ pump is similar to the hand-held, lollipop-like structure of the F-type ATPase, with which it shares a significant—although low—level of amino acid homology. For example, the hand of the V-type pump has only six subunits, but each is twice as large as a c subunit in the F-type ATPase.

ATP-binding cassette (ABC) transporters can act as pumps, channels, or regulators

The so-called ABC proteins all have a motif in their amino acid sequence that is an ATP-binding cassette (ABC). In humans, this family includes at least 49 members in seven subfamiles named ABCA through ABCG (Table 5-6). Some are pumps that presumably hydrolyze ATP to provide energy for solute transport. Some may hydrolyze ATP, but they do not couple the liberated energy to perform active transport. In other cases, ATP regulates ABC proteins that function as ion channels or regulators of ion channels or transporters.

ABC1 Subfamily ABC1 (ABCA1) is an important transporter for mediating the efflux of phospholipids and cholesterol from macrophages and certain other cells.

MDR Subfamily The **multidrug resistance transporters (MDRs)** are ATPases and primary active transporters. The MDR proteins are tandem repeats of two structures, each of which has six membrane-spanning segments and a nucleotide-binding domain that binds ATP. MDR1, also called P-glycoprotein, extrudes cationic metabolites and drugs across the cell membrane. The substrates of MDR1 appear to have little in common structurally, except that they are hydrophobic. A wide variety of cells express MDRs, including those of the liver, kidney, and gastrointestinal tract. MDR1 plays an important and clinically antagonistic role in cancer patients in that it pumps a wide range of anticancer drugs out of cancer cells, thereby rendering cells resistant to these drugs.

MRP/CFTR Subfamily Another member of the ABC superfamily that is of physiological interest is the cystic fibrosis transmembrane regulator (CFTR), which is mutated in the hereditary disease **cystic fibrosis** (see the box on this topic in Chapter 43). CFTR is a 170-kDa glycoprotein that is present at the apical membrane of many epithelial cells. CFTR functions as a low-conductance Cl^- channel as well as a regulator of other ion channels.

Like MDR1, CFTR has two membrane-spanning domains (MSD1 and MSD2), each composed of six membrane-spanning segments (Fig. 5-10). Also like MDR1, CFTR has two nucleotide-binding domains (NBD1 and NBD2). Unlike MDR1, however, a large cytoplasmic regulatory (R) domain separates the two halves of CFTR. The regulatory domain contains multiple potential protein kinase A and protein kinase C phosphorylation sites. Phosphorylation of these sites, under the influence of neurohumoral agents that control fluid and electrolyte secretion, promotes activation of CFTR. The binding of ATP to the NBDs also controls channel opening and closing. Thus, ATP regulates the CFTR Cl^- channel by two types of mechanisms: protein

Table 5-6 ABC Transporters

Subfamily*	Alternative Subfamily Name	Examples
ABCA (12)	ABC1	ABCA1 (cholesterol transporter)
ABCB (11)	MDR (multidrug resistance)	ABCB1 (MDR1 or P-glycoprotein 1) ABCB4 (MDR2/3) ABCB11 (bile salt export pump, BSEP)
ABCC (13)	MRP/CFTR	ABCC2 (multidrug resistance–associated protein 2, MRP2) ABCC7 (cystic fibrosis transmembrane regulator, CFTR) ABCC8 (sulfonylurea receptor, SUR1) ABCC9 (SUR2)
ABCD (4)	ALD	ABCD1 (ALD, mediates uptake of fatty acids by peroxisomes)
ABCE (1)	OABP	ABCE1 (RNASELI, blocks RNase L)
ABCF (3)	GCN20	ABCF1 (lacks transmembrane domains)
ABCG (5)	White	ABCG2 (transports sulfated steroids) ABCG5/ABCG8 (heterodimer of "half" ABCs that transport cholesterol)

*Number of genes in parentheses.

phosphorylation and interaction with the nucleotide-binding domains.

Cotransporters, one class of secondary active transporters, are generally driven by the energy of the inwardly directed Na⁺ gradient

Like pumps or primary active transporters, secondary active transporters can move a solute uphill (against its electrochemical gradient). However, unlike the pumps, which fuel the process by hydrolyzing ATP, the secondary active transporters fuel it by coupling the uphill movement of one or more solutes to the downhill movement of other solutes. The two major classes of secondary active transporters are cotransporters (or symporters) and exchangers (or antiporters). Cotransporters are intrinsic membrane proteins that move the "driving" solute (the one whose gradient provides the energy) and the "driven" solutes (which move uphill) in the *same* direction.

Na⁺/Glucose Cotransporter The **Na⁺/glucose cotransporter (SGLT)** is located at the apical membrane of the cells that line the proximal tubule and small intestine (Fig. 5-11A). The SGLTs, which belong to the SLC5 family (Table 5-4), consist of a single subunit, probably with 14 membrane-spanning segments. The SGLT2 and SGLT3 isoforms move one Na⁺ ion with each glucose molecule (i.e., 1:1 stoichiometry of Na⁺ to glucose), whereas the SGLT1 isoform moves two Na⁺ ions with each glucose molecule.

For the Na⁺/glucose cotransporter with 1:1 stoichiometry, the overall driving force is the sum of the electrochemical potential energy difference for Na⁺ and the chemical potential energy difference for glucose. Thus, the highly favorable, inwardly directed Na⁺ electrochemical gradient can drive the uphill accumulation of glucose from the lumen of the kidney tubule or gut into the cell. Figure 5-12 shows how the Na⁺ gradient drives glucose accumulation into membrane vesicles derived from the brush border of renal proximal tubules. Equilibrium is achieved when the electrochemical potential energy difference for Na⁺ in one direction is balanced by the chemical potential energy difference for glucose in the opposite direction:

$$\Delta\tilde{\mu}_{Na} = -\Delta\mu_{glucose} \tag{5-17}$$

We can express $\Delta\tilde{\mu}_{Na}$ in terms of the Na⁺ concentrations and membrane voltage and can express $\Delta\mu_{glucose}$ in terms of the glucose concentrations. If we substitute these expressions into Equation 5-17, we derive the following relationship for the maximal glucose concentration gradient that can be generated by a given electrochemical potential energy difference for Na⁺:

$$\frac{[Glucose]_i}{[Glucose]_o} = \frac{[Na^+]_o}{[Na^+]_i} \times 10^{-V_m/(60\,mV)} \tag{5-18}$$

In an epithelial cell that has a 10-fold Na⁺ concentration gradient and a 60-mV inside-negative voltage across the apical membrane, the Na⁺ electrochemical gradient can gen-

erate a 10×10^1, or 100-fold, glucose concentration gradient across the plasma membrane. In other words, the 10:1 Na⁺ concentration gradient buys a 10-fold glucose gradient, and the V_m of −60 mV buys another 10-fold. However, the leakage of glucose out of the cell by other pathways at the basolateral membrane prevents the Na⁺-glucose cotransporter from coming to equilibrium.

The Na⁺/glucose cotransporter with 2:1 stoichiometry is capable of generating an even larger concentration gradient for glucose across the plasma membrane. Such a cotransporter would be in equilibrium when

$$2\Delta\tilde{\mu}_{Na} = -\Delta\mu_{glucose} \tag{5-19}$$

The maximal glucose gradient is

$$\frac{[Glucose]_i}{[Glucose]_o} = \left(\frac{[Na^+]_o}{[Na^+]_i}\right)^2 \times 10^{-2V_m/(60\,mV)} \tag{5-20}$$

In the same epithelial cell with a 10-fold Na⁺ concentration gradient and a V_m of −60 mV, the Na⁺ electrochemical gradient can generate a glucose concentration gradient of $10^2 \times 10^2$, or 10,000-fold! In other words, the 10:1 Na⁺ concentration gradient—when squared for two Na⁺ ions—buys a 100-fold glucose gradient, and the −60 mV membrane voltage—when multiplied by two for the effective charge on two Na⁺ ions—buys another 100-fold.

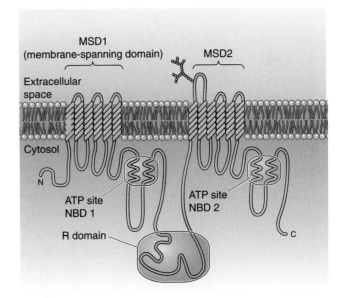

Figure 5-10 Cystic fibrosis transmembrane conductance regulator (CFTR). The CFTR Cl⁻ channel has two membrane-spanning domains (MSD1 and MSD2). A large cytoplasmic regulatory (R) domain separates the two halves of the molecule, each of which has an ATP-binding domain (NBD1 and NBD2). The most common mutation in cystic fibrosis is the deletion of the phenylalanine at position 508 (ΔF508) in the NBD1 domain. *(Model modified from Riordan JR, Rommens JM, Kerem B, et al: Identification of the cystic fibrosis gene: cloning and complementary DNA. Science 1989; 245: 1066-1073.)*

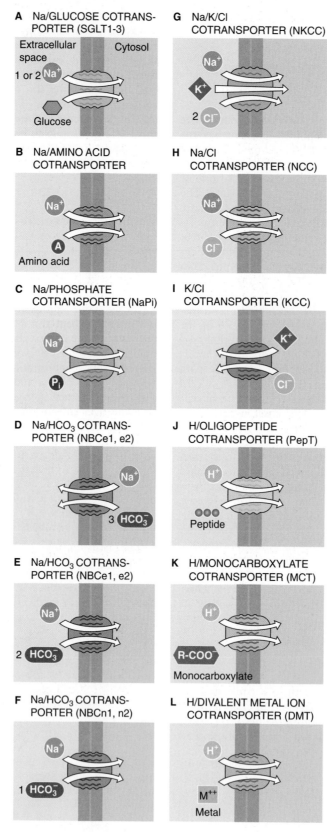

Figure 5-11   Representative cotransporters.

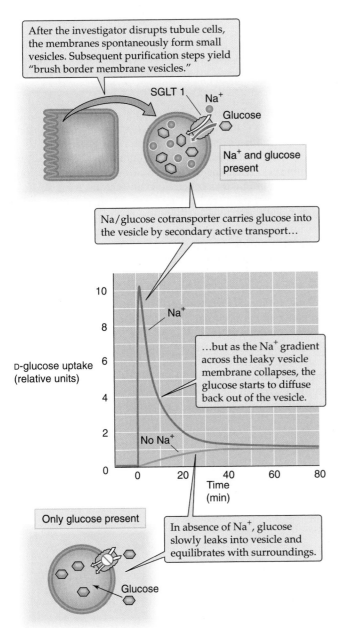

After the investigator disrupts tubule cells, the membranes spontaneously form small vesicles. Subsequent purification steps yield "brush border membrane vesicles."

SGLT 1

Na^+

Glucose

Na^+ and glucose present

Na/glucose cotransporter carries glucose into the vesicle by secondary active transport...

Na^+

No Na^+

D-glucose uptake (relative units)

Time (min)

...but as the Na^+ gradient across the leaky vesicle membrane collapses, the glucose starts to diffuse back out of the vesicle.

Only glucose present

In absence of Na^+, glucose slowly leaks into vesicle and equilibrates with surroundings.

Glucose

Figure 5-12 Na^+-driven glucose uptake into brush border membrane vesicles.

Because the cotransporter protein has specific sites for binding Na^+ and glucose and because the number of transporters is fixed, the rate of transport by SGLT is a saturable function of the glucose and Na^+ concentrations.

Na^+-Driven Cotransporters for Organic Solutes Functionally similar, but structurally distinct from one another, are a variety of Na^+ cotransporters in the proximal tubule and small intestine. **Na^+-driven amino acid transporters** (Fig. 5-11B) belong to both the SLC6 and SLC38 families (Table 5-4). SLC13 includes **Na^+-coupled cotransporters** for **monocarboxylates, dicarboxylates, and tricarboxylates;** SLC5 includes Na^+-coupled cotransporters for monocarboxylates.

Na/HCO₃ Cotransporters The **NBCs** belong to the SLC4 family and are a key group of acid-base transporters. In the basolateral membranes of certain epithelial cells, the **electrogenic NBCs** (NBCe1/e2, *e* for electro*genic*) operate with the Na^+:HCO_3^- stoichiometry of 1:3 (Fig. 5-11D) and—for typical ion and voltage gradients—mediate electrogenic HCO_3^- *efflux*. Here, these NBCs mediate HCO_3^- absorption into the blood. In most other cells, these same two transporters operate with a stoichiometry of 1:2—probably because of the absence of a key protein partner—and mediate the electrogenic HCO_3^- *influx* (Fig. 5-11E). Finally, the electroneutral NBCs (NBCn1/n2, *n* for electro*neutral*) operate with the Na^+:HCO_3^- stoichiometry of 1:1 (Fig. 5-11F) and also mediate HCO_3^- *influx*. In these last two cases, the Na^+ electrochemical gradient drives the uphill accumulation of HCO_3^-, which is important for epithelial HCO_3^- secretion and for the regulation of intracellular pH (pH_i) to relatively alkaline values.

Na^+-Driven Cotransporters for Other Inorganic Anions Important examples include the **inorganic phosphate cotransporters** (**NaPi**; Fig. 5-11C)—which are members of the SLC17, SLC20, and SLC34 families—and sulfate cotransporter (SLC13) (Table 5-4).

Na/K/Cl Cotransporter The three types of cation-coupled Cl^- cotransporters all belong to the SLC12 family. The first is the **Na/K/Cl cotransporter** (**NKCC**), which harnesses the energy of the inwardly directed Na^+ electrochemical gradient to drive the accumulation of Cl^- and K^+ (Fig. 5-11G). One variant of this cotransporter, NKCC1 (SLC12A2), is present in a wide variety of nonepithelial cells as well as in the *basolateral* membranes of some epithelial cells. Another variant of the Na/K/Cl cotransporter, NKCC2 (SLC12A1), is present on the *apical* membrane of cells lining the thick ascending limb of the loop of Henle in the kidney (see Chapter 35). A characteristic of the NKCCs is that they are inhibited by furosemide and bumetanide, which are called loop diuretics because they increase urine flow by inhibiting transport at the loop of Henle. Because of its sensitivity to bumetanide, NKCC is sometimes called the bumetanide-sensitive cotransporter (BSC).

Na/Cl Cotransporter The second type of cation-coupled Cl^- cotransporter is found in the apical membrane of the early distal tubule of the kidney (see Chapter 35). This K^+-*independent* **Na/Cl cotransporter** (**NCC** or SLC12A3) is blocked by thiazide diuretics rather than by loop diuretics (Fig. 5-11H). For this reason, NCC has also been called the thiazide-sensitive cotransporter (TSC).

K/Cl Cotransporter The third type of cation-coupled Cl^- cotransporter is Na^+-*independent* **K/Cl cotransporter** (**KCC**1 to 4 or SLC12A4 to 7). Because the Na-K pump causes K^+ to accumulate inside the cell, the K^+ electrochemical gradient is outwardly directed across the plasma membrane (Fig. 5-11I). In addition, pathways such as the NKCC and the Cl-HCO_3 anion exchanger (see later) bring Cl^- into the cell, so that in most cells the Cl^- electrochemical gradient is also outwardly directed. Thus, the net driving force acting on the K/Cl cotransporter favors the exit of K^+ and Cl^- from the cell.

H⁺-Driven Cotransporters Although the majority of known cotransporters in animal cells are driven by the inward movement of Na⁺, some are instead driven by the downhill, inward movement of H⁺. The **H/oligopeptide cotransporter PepT1** and related proteins are members of the SLC15 family (Table 5-4). PepT1 is electrogenic and responsible for the uptake of small peptides (Fig. 5-11J) from the lumen into the cells of the renal proximal tubule and small intestine (see Chapters 36 and 45). The **H⁺-driven amino acid cotransporters** (e.g., PAT1) are members of the SLC36 family. The **monocarboxylate cotransporters**, such as **MCT1**, are members of the SLC16 family. They mediate the electroneutral, H⁺-coupled flux of lactate, pyruvate, or other monocarboxylates across the cell membranes of most tissues in the body (Fig. 5-11K). In the case of lactate, MCT1 can operate in either the net inward or net outward direction, depending on the lactate and H⁺ gradients across the cell membrane. MCT1 probably moves lactate out of cells that produce lactate by glycolysis but into cells that consume lactate. The **divalent metal ion cotransporter (DMT1)**, a member of the SLC11 family, couples the influx of H⁺ to the influx of ferrous iron (Fe^{2+}) as well as to a variety of other divalent metals, some of which (Cd^{2+}, Pb^{2+}) are toxic to cells (Fig. 5-11L). DMT1 is expressed at high levels in the kidney and proximal portions of the small intestine.

Exchangers, another class of secondary active transporters, exchange ions for one another

The other major class of secondary active transporters is the exchangers, or antiporters. Exchangers are intrinsic membrane proteins that move one or more "driving" solutes in one direction and one or more "driven" solutes in the *opposite* direction. In general, these transporters exchange cations for cations or anions for anions.

Na-Ca Exchanger The nearly ubiquitous **Na-Ca exchangers (NCX)** belong to the SLC8 family (Table 5-4). They most likely mediate the exchange of three Na⁺ ions per Ca^{2+} ion (Fig. 5-13A). NCX is electrogenic and moves net positive charge in the same direction as Na⁺. Under most circumstances, the inwardly directed Na⁺ electrochemical gradient across the plasma membrane drives the uphill extrusion of Ca^{2+} from the cell. Thus, in concert with the plasma membrane Ca^{2+} pump, this transport system helps maintain the steep, inwardly directed electrochemical potential energy difference for Ca^{2+} that is normally present across the plasma membrane of all cells.

NCX uses the inwardly directed Na⁺ electrochemical gradient to drive the secondary active efflux of Ca^{2+}. With a presumed stoichiometry of three Na⁺ per Ca^{2+}, the effectiveness of the Na⁺ electrochemical gradient as a driving force is magnified; thus, NCX is at equilibrium when the Ca^{2+} electrochemical gradient is balanced by three times the Na⁺ electrochemical gradient:

$$\Delta\tilde{\mu}_{Ca} = 3\Delta\tilde{\mu}_{Na} \tag{5-21}$$

Alternatively,

$$\frac{[Ca^{2+}]_o}{[Ca^{2+}]_i} = \left(\frac{[Na^+]_o}{[Na^+]_i}\right)^3 \cdot 10^{-V_m/60\,mV} \tag{5-22}$$

In a cell with a 10-fold Na⁺ concentration gradient and a V_m of −60 mV, the electrochemical potential energy difference for Na⁺ can buy a Ca^{2+} concentration gradient of $10^3 \times 10^1$, or 10,000-fold, which is the Ca^{2+} gradient across most cell membranes. Thus, the effect of the 10-fold inward Na⁺ concentration gradient is cubed and can account for a 10^3-fold Ca^{2+} concentration gradient across the plasma membrane. In addition, the stoichiometry of three Na⁺ per Ca^{2+} produces a net inflow of one positive charge per transport cycle. Thus, the 60-mV inside-negative V_m acts as the equivalent driving force to another 10-fold concentration gradient.

Na-H Exchanger The **Na-H exchangers (NHE)**, which belong to the SLC9 family (Table 5-4), mediate the 1:1 exchange of extracellular Na⁺ for intracellular H⁺ across the plasma membrane (Fig. 5-13B). One or more of the nine known NHEs are present on the plasma membrane of almost every cell in the body. Through operation of NHEs, the inwardly directed Na⁺ electrochemical gradient drives the uphill extrusion of H⁺ from the cell and raises pH_i. The ubiquitous NHE1, which is present in nonepithelial cells as

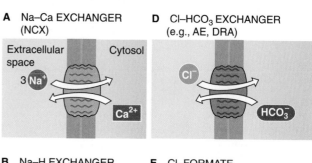

A Na–Ca EXCHANGER (NCX)

B Na–H EXCHANGER (NHE)

C Na-DRIVEN Cl–HCO₃ EXCHANGER (NDCBE)

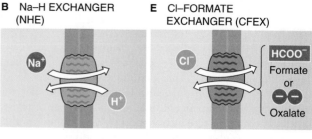

D Cl–HCO₃ EXCHANGER (e.g., AE, DRA)

E Cl–FORMATE EXCHANGER (CFEX)

F ORGANIC ANION TRANSPORTER (OAT)

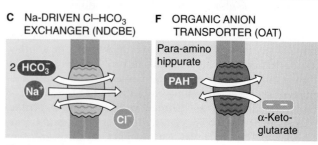

Figure 5-13 Representative exchangers.

well as on the basolateral membranes of epithelia, plays a major role in pH$_i$ regulation and cell volume. NHE3 is present at the apical membranes of several epithelia, where it plays a major role in acid secretion (see Chapter 39) or Na$^+$ absorption.

Another cation exchange process that involves H$^+$ is the organic cation–H$^+$ exchanger that secretes cationic metabolites and drugs across the apical membrane of renal proximal tubule cells and hepatocytes.

Na$^+$-Driven Cl-HCO$_3$ Exchanger   A second Na$^+$-coupled exchanger that is important for pH$_i$ regulation is the **Na$^+$-driven Cl-HCO$_3$ exchanger (NDCBE)**, which is a member of the SLC4 family (Table 5-4). This electroneutral transporter couples the movement of one Na$^+$ ion and the equivalent of two HCO$_3^-$ ions in one direction to the movement of one Cl$^-$ ion in the opposite direction (Fig. 5-13C). NDCBE uses the inwardly directed Na$^+$ electrochemical gradient to drive the uphill entry of HCO$_3^-$ into the cell. Thus, like the NHEs, NDCBE helps keep pH$_i$ relatively alkaline.

Cl-HCO$_3$ Exchanger   A third group of exchangers that are involved in acid-base transport are the Cl-HCO$_3$ exchangers (Fig. 5-13D) that function independently of Na$^+$. These may be members of either the SLC4 or the SLC26 families (Table 5-4). Virtually all cells in the body express one of the three electroneutral SLC4 of Cl-HCO$_3$ exchangers, also known as **anion exchangers (AE1–AE3)**. AE1 is important for transporting HCO$_3^-$ into the red blood cell in the lung and out of the red blood cell in peripheral tissues (see Chapter 29). In other cells, where the inwardly directed Cl$^-$ gradient almost always drives HCO$_3^-$ out of the cell, AE2 and AE3 play important roles in pH$_i$ regulation by tending to acidify the cell. Moreover, the uptake of Cl$^-$ often plays a role in cell volume regulation.

Several members of the **SLC26 family** can function as Cl-HCO$_3$ exchangers and thereby play important roles in epithelial Cl$^-$ and HCO$_3^-$ transport. Because the stoichiometry need not be 1 : 1, SLC26 transport can be electrogenic. As described next, even SLC26 proteins that exchange Cl$^-$ for HCO$_3^-$ also transport a wide variety of *other* anions.

Other Anion Exchangers   A characteristic of the SLC26 family is their multifunctionality. For example, **CFEX**—present in the apical membranes of renal proximal tubule cells—can mediate **Cl-formate exchange** and **Cl-oxalate exchange** (Fig. 5-13E). These activities appear to be important for the secondary active uptake of Cl$^-$. **Pendrin** not only mediates Cl-HCO$_3$ exchange but may also transport I$^-$, which may be important in the thyroid gland (see Chapter 49).

Anion exchangers other than those in the SLC4 and SLC26 families also play important roles. The **organic anion transporting polypeptides (OATP)** are members of the SLC21 family. In the liver, OATPs mediate the uptake of bile acids, bilirubin, and the test substrate bromosulphthalein. Another member of the SLC21 family is the **prostaglandin transporter (PGT)**, which mediates the uptake of prostanoids (e.g., prostaglandins E$_2$ and F$_{2\alpha}$ and thromboxane B$_2$).

The **organic anion transporters (OAT)** are members of the diverse SLC22 family. The OATs—by exchange or facili-

tated diffusion—mediate the uptake of endogenous organic anions (Fig. 5-13F) as well as drugs, including penicillin and the test substrate *p*-aminohippurate. **URAT1**, another SLC22 member, is an exchanger that mediates urate transport in the renal proximal tubule. Surprisingly, the OCT transporters that mediate the facilitated diffusion of organic *cations* are also members of SLC22.

REGULATION OF INTRACELLULAR ION CONCENTRATIONS

Figure 5-14 illustrates the tools at the disposal of a prototypic cell for managing its intracellular composition. Cells in different tissues—and even different cell types within the same tissue—have different complements of channels and transporters. Epithelial cells and neurons may segregate specific channels and transporters to different parts of the cell (e.g., apical versus basolateral membrane or axon versus soma/dendrite). Thus, different cells may have somewhat different intracellular ionic compositions.

The Na-K pump keeps [Na$^+$] inside the cell low and [K$^+$] high

The most striking and important gradients across the cell membrane are those for Na$^+$ and K$^+$. **Sodium** is the predominant cation in ECF, where it is present at a concentration of ~145 mM (Fig. 5-14). Na$^+$ is relatively excluded from the intracellular space, where it is present at only a fraction of the extracellular concentration. This Na$^+$ gradient is maintained primarily by active extrusion of Na$^+$ from the cell by the Na-K pump (Fig. 5-14, no. 1). In contrast, **potassium** is present at a concentration of only ~4.5 mM in ECF, but it is the predominant cation in the intracellular space, where it is accumulated ~25- to 30-fold above the outside concentration. Again, this gradient is the direct result of primary active uptake of K$^+$ into the cell by the Na-K pump. When the Na-K pump is inhibited with ouabain, [Na$^+$]$_i$ rises and [K$^+$]$_i$ falls.

In addition to generating concentration gradients for Na$^+$ and K$^+$, the Na-K pump plays an important role in generating the inside-negative membrane voltage, which is ~60 mV in a typical cell. The Na-K pump accomplishes this task in two ways. First, because the Na-K pump transports three Na$^+$ ions out of the cell for every two K$^+$ ions, the pump itself is **electrogenic**. This electrogenicity causes a net outward current of positive charge across the plasma membrane and tends to generate an inside-negative V_m. However, the pump current itself usually makes only a small contribution to the negative V_m. Second, and quantitatively much more important, the active K$^+$ accumulation by the Na-K pump creates a concentration gradient that favors the exit of K$^+$ from the cell through K$^+$ channels (Fig. 5-14, no. 2). The tendency of K$^+$ to *exit* through these channels, with unmatched negative charges left behind, is the main cause of the inside-negative membrane voltage. When K$^+$ channels are blocked with an inhibitor such as Ba^{2+}, V_m becomes considerably less negative (i.e., the cell depolarizes). In most cells, the principal pathway for current flow across the plasma membrane (i.e., the principal ionic conductance) is through K$^+$ channels. We discuss the generation of membrane voltage in Chapter 6.

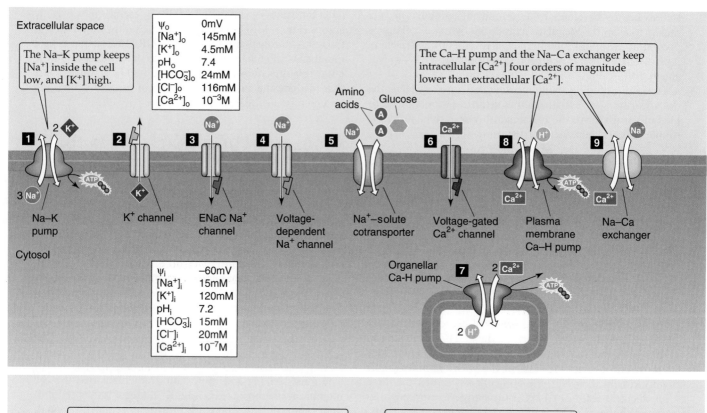

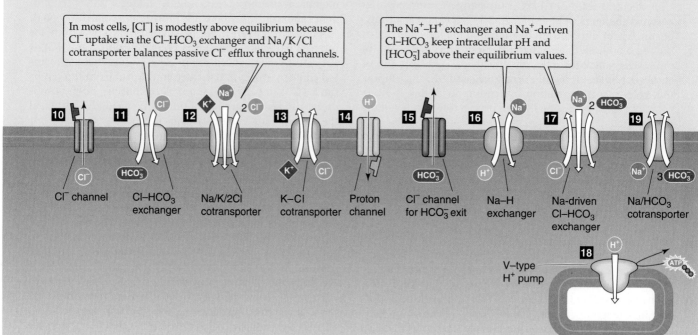

Figure 5-14   Ion gradients, channels, and transporters in a typical cell.

The inside-negative V_m, together with the large concentration gradient for Na^+, summates to create a large, inwardly directed Na^+ electrochemical gradient that strongly favors passive Na^+ entry. Given the large amount of energy that is devoted to generation of this favorable driving force for Na^+ entry, one might expect that the cell would permit Na^+ to move into the cell only through pathways serving important physiological purposes. The simple passive entry of Na^+ through channels—without harnessing of this Na^+ entry for some physiological purpose—would complete a futile cycle that culminates in active Na^+ extrusion. It would make little teleologic sense for the cell to use up considerable energy stores to extrude Na^+ only to let it passively diffuse back in with no effect. Rather, cells harness the energy of Na^+ entry for three major purposes:

1. In certain **epithelial cells**, amiloride-sensitive Na^+ channels (ENaC) are largely restricted to the *apical* or luminal surface of the cell (Fig. 5-14, no. 3), and the Na-K pumps are restricted to the *basolateral* surface of the cell. In this way, *transepithelial* Na^+ transport takes place rather a futile cycling of Na^+ back and forth across a single plasma membrane.
2. In **excitable cells**, passive Na^+ entry occurs through voltage-dependent Na^+ channels (Fig. 5-14, no. 4) and plays a critical role in generation of the action potential. In such cells, Na^+ is cycled at high energy cost across the plasma membrane for the important physiological purpose of information transfer.
3. Virtually **every cell** in the body uses the electrochemical Na^+ gradient across the plasma membrane to drive the secondary active transport of nutrients and ions (Fig. 5-14, no. 5).

The Ca^{2+} pump and the Na-Ca exchanger keep intracellular $[Ca^{2+}]$ four orders of magnitude lower than extracellular $[Ca^{2+}]$

Whereas the concentration of Ca^{2+} in the extracellular space is ~ 1 mM (10^{-3} M), that in the ICF is only ~ 100 nM (10^{-7} M), a concentration gradient of 10^4-fold. Because of the inside-negative membrane voltage of a typical cell and the large chemical gradient for Ca^{2+}, the inwardly directed electrochemical gradient for Ca^{2+} across the plasma membrane is enormous, far larger than that for any other ion. Many cells have a variety of Ca^{2+} channels through which Ca^{2+} can enter the cell (Fig. 5-14, no. 6). In general, Ca^{2+} channels are gated by voltage (see Chapter 7) or by humoral agents (see Chapter 13) so that rapid Ca^{2+} entry into the cell occurs only in short bursts. However, given the existence of pathways for passive Ca^{2+} transport *into* cells, we may ask what transport mechanisms keep $[Ca^{2+}]_i$ low and thus maintain the enormous Ca^{2+} electrochemical gradient across the plasma membrane.

Ca^{2+} Pumps (SERCA) in Organelle Membranes Ca^{2+} pumps (ATPases) are present on the membranes that surround various intracellular organelles, such as the sarcoplasmic reticulum and endoplasmic reticulum (Fig. 5-14, no. 7). These pumps actively sequester cytosolic Ca^{2+} in intracellular stores. These stores of Ca^{2+} can later be released into the cytoplasm in bursts as part of a signal transduction process in response to membrane depolarization or humoral agents. Even though Ca^{2+} sequestration in intracellular stores is an important mechanism for regulating $[Ca^{2+}]_i$ in the short term, there is a limit to how much Ca^{2+} a cell can store. Therefore, in the steady state, Ca^{2+} extrusion across the cell membrane must balance the passive influx of Ca^{2+}.

Ca^{2+} Pump (PMCA) on the Plasma Membrane The plasma membranes of most cells contain a Ca^{2+} pump that plays a major role in extruding Ca^{2+} from the cell (Fig. 5-14, no. 8). It would seem that rising levels of intracellular Ca^{2+} would stimulate the Ca^{2+} pump to extrude Ca^{2+} and thereby return $[Ca^{2+}]_i$ toward normal. Actually, the pump *itself* is incapable of this type of feedback control; because it has such a high K_m for $[Ca^{2+}]_i$, the pump is virtually inactive at physiological $[Ca^{2+}]_i$. However, as $[Ca^{2+}]_i$ rises, the Ca^{2+} binds to a protein known as **calmodulin** (CaM, see Chapter 3), which has a high affinity for Ca^{2+}. The newly formed Ca^{2+}-CaM binds to the Ca^{2+} pump, lowers the pump's K_m for $[Ca^{2+}]_i$ into the physiological range, and thus stimulates Ca^{2+} extrusion. As $[Ca^{2+}]_i$ falls, Ca^{2+}-CaM levels inside the cell also fall so that Ca^{2+}-CaM dissociates from the Ca^{2+} pump, thereby returning the pump to its inactive state. At resting $[Ca^{2+}]_i$ levels of ~ 100 nM, the Ca^{2+} pump is the major route of Ca^{2+} extrusion.

Na-Ca Exchanger (NCX) on the Plasma Membrane NCX (Fig. 5-14, no. 9) plays a key role in extruding Ca^{2+} only when $[Ca^{2+}]_i$ rises substantially above normal levels. Thus, NCX is especially important in restoring low $[Ca^{2+}]_i$ when large influxes of Ca^{2+} occur. This property is most notable in excitable cells such as neurons and cardiac muscle, which may be challenged with vast Ca^{2+} influxes through voltage-gated Ca^{2+} channels during action potentials.

In most cells, $[Cl^-]$ is modestly above equilibrium because Cl^- uptake by the Cl-HCO_3 exchanger and Na/K/Cl cotransporter balances passive Cl^- efflux through channels

The $[Cl^-]$ in all cells is below the $[Cl^-]$ in the extracellular space. Virtually all cells have **anion-selective channels** (Fig. 5-14, no. 10) through which Cl^- can permeate passively. In a typical cell with a 60-mV inside-negative membrane voltage, $[Cl^-]_i$ would be a tenth that of $[Cl^-]_o$ if Cl^- were passively distributed across the plasma membrane. Such is the case for skeletal muscle. However, for most cell types, $[Cl^-]_i$ is approximately twice as high as that predicted for passive distribution alone, which indicates the presence of transport pathways that mediate the active uptake of Cl^- into the cell. Probably the most common pathway for Cl^- uptake is the **Cl-HCO_3 exchanger** (Fig. 5-14, no. 11). Because $[HCO_3^-]_i$ is several-fold higher than if it were passively distributed across the cell membrane, the outwardly directed electrochemical potential energy difference for HCO_3^- can act as a driving force for the uphill entry of Cl^- through Cl-HCO_3 exchange. Another pathway that can mediate uphill Cl^- transport into the cell is the **Na/K/Cl cotransporter** (Fig. 5-14, no. 12), which is stimulated by low $[Cl^-]_i$.

Given the presence of these transport pathways mediating Cl^- uptake, why is $[Cl^-]_i$ only ~2-fold above that predicted for passive distribution? The answer is that the passive Cl^- efflux through anion-selective channels in the plasma membrane opposes Cl^- uptake mechanisms. Another factor that tends to keep Cl^- low in some cells is the **K/Cl cotransporter.** KCC (Fig. 5-14, no. 13), driven by the outward K^+ gradient, tends to move K^+ and Cl^- out of cells. Thus, the K^+ gradient promotes Cl^- efflux both by generating the inside-negative V_m that drives Cl^- out of the cell through channels and by driving K/Cl cotransport.

The Na-H exchanger and Na^+-driven HCO_3^- transporters keep the intracellular pH and $[HCO_3^-]$ above their equilibrium values

H^+, HCO_3^-, and CO_2 within a particular compartment are generally in equilibrium with one another. Extracellular pH is normally ~7.4, $[HCO_3^-]_o$ is 24 mM, and P_{CO_2} is ~40 mm Hg. In a typical cell, intracellular pH is ~7.2. Because $[CO_2]$ is usually the same on both sides of the cell membrane, $[HCO_3^-]_i$ can be calculated to be ~15 mM. Even though the ICF is slightly more acidic than the ECF, pH_i is actually much more alkaline than it would be if H^+ and HCO_3^- were passively distributed across the cell membrane. H^+ can enter the cell passively and HCO_3^- can exit the cell passively, although both processes occur at a rather low rate. H^+ can permeate certain **cation channels** and perhaps H^+-selective channels (Fig. 5-14, no. 14), and HCO_3^- moves fairly easily through most **Cl^- channels** (Fig. 5-14, no. 15). Because a membrane voltage of -60 mV is equivalent as a driving force to a 10-fold concentration gradient of a monovalent ion, one would expect $[H^+]$ to be 10-fold higher within the cell than in the ECF, which corresponds to a pH_i that is 1 pH unit more acidic than pH_o. Similarly, one would expect $[HCO_3^-]_i$ to be only one tenth of $[HCO_3^-]_o$. The observation that pH_i and $[HCO_3^-]_i$ are maintained higher than predicted for passive distribution across the plasma membrane indicates that cells must actively extrude H^+ or take up HCO_3^-.

The transport of acid out of the cell or base into the cell is collectively termed acid extrusion. In most cells, the **acid extruders** are secondary active transporters that are energized by the electrochemical Na^+ gradient across the cell membrane. The most important acid extruders are the **Na-H** (Fig. 5-14, no. 16) and the **Na^+-driven Cl-HCO₃ exchangers** (Fig. 5-14, no. 17), as well as the **Na/HCO₃ cotransporters** with Na^+:HCO_3^- stoichiometries of 1:2 and 1:1. These transport systems are generally sensitive to changes in pH_i; they are stimulated when the cell is acidified and inhibited when the cell is alkalinized. Thus, these transporters maintain pH_i in a range that is optimal for cell functioning. Less commonly, certain epithelial cells that are specialized for acid secretion use **V-type H^+ pumps** (Fig. 5-14, no. 18) or **H-K pumps** on their apical membranes to extrude acid. These epithelia include the renal collecting duct and the stomach. As noted earlier, virtually all cells have V-type H^+ pumps on the membranes surrounding such intracellular organelles as lysosomes, endosomes, and Golgi.

Because most cells have powerful acid extrusion systems, one might ask why the pH_i is not far more alkaline than ~7.2. Part of the answer is that transport processes that act as **acid**

loaders balance acid extrusion. Passive leakage of H^+ and HCO_3^- through *channels,* as noted earlier, tends to acidify the cell. Cells also have *transporters* that generally move HCO_3^- out of cells. The most common is the Cl-HCO₃ exchanger (Fig. 5-14, no. 11). Another is the electrogenic NBC with the Na^+:HCO_3^- stoichiometry of 1:3 (Fig. 5-14, no. 19), which moves HCO_3^- out of the cell across the basolateral membrane of renal proximal tubules.

WATER TRANSPORT AND THE REGULATION OF CELL VOLUME

Water transport is driven by osmotic and hydrostatic pressure differences across membranes

Transport of water across biological membranes is always passive. No water pumps have ever been described. To a certain extent, single water molecules can dissolve in lipid bilayers and thus move across cell membranes at a low but finite rate by simple diffusion. The ease with which H_2O diffuses through the lipid bilayer depends on the lipid composition of the bilayer. Membranes with low fluidity (see Chapter 2), that is, those whose phospholipids have long saturated fatty acid chains with few double bonds (i.e., few kinks), exhibit lower H_2O permeability. The addition of other lipids that decrease fluidity (e.g., cholesterol) may further reduce H_2O permeability. Therefore, it is not surprising that the plasma membranes of many types of cells have specialized water channels—the aquaporins—that serve as passive conduits for water transport. The presence of aquaporins greatly increases membrane water permeability. In some cells, such as erythrocytes or the renal proximal tubule, AQP1 is always present in the membrane. The collecting duct cells of the kidney regulate the H_2O permeability of their apical membranes by inserting AQP2 water channels into their apical membranes under the control of arginine vasopressin.

Water transport across a membrane is always a linear, nonsaturable function of its net driving force. The direction of net passive transport of an uncharged solute is always down its chemical potential energy difference. For water, we must consider two passive driving forces. The first is the familiar chemical potential energy difference ($\Delta\mu_{H_2O}$), which depends on the difference in **water concentration** on the two sides of the membrane. The second is the energy difference, per mole of water, that results from the difference in **hydrostatic pressure** ($\Delta\mu_{H_2O, pressure}$) across the membrane. Thus, the relevant energy difference across the membrane is the sum of the chemical and pressure potential energy differences:

$$\Delta\mu_{H_2O,total} = \Delta\mu_{H_2O} + \Delta\mu_{H_2O,pressure}$$

$$\underbrace{\Delta\mu_{H_2O,total}}_{\text{Total energy difference}} = RT \ln \underbrace{\frac{[H_2O]_i}{[H_2O]_o}}_{\text{Chemical part}} + \underbrace{\bar{V}_W (P_i - P_o)}_{\text{Pressure part}} \quad (5\text{-}23)$$

P is the hydrostatic pressure and $\bar{V}_w$ is the partial molar volume of water (i.e., volume occupied by 1 mole of water).

Because the product of pressure and volume is work, the second term in Equation 5-23 is work per mole. Dealing with water concentrations is cumbersome and imprecise because $[H_2O]$ is very high (i.e., ~56 M) and does not change substantially in the dilute solutions that physiologists are interested in. Therefore, it is more practical to work with the inverse of $[H_2O]$, namely, the concentration of osmotically active solutes, or **osmolality**. The units of osmolality are osmoles per kilogram H_2O, or Osm. In dilute solutions, the H_2O gradient across the cell membrane is roughly proportional to the difference in osmolalities across the membrane:

$$\ln\frac{[H_2O]_i}{[H_2O]_o} \cong \bar{V}_W(\text{Osm}_o - \text{Osm}_i) \qquad (5\text{-}24)$$

Osmolality is the total concentration of all osmotically active solutes in the indicated compartment (e.g., $Na^+ + Cl^- + K^+ + ...$). Substituting Equation 5-24 into Equation 5-23 yields a more useful expression for the total energy difference across the membrane:

$$\underbrace{\Delta\mu_{H_2O,\text{total}}}_{\substack{\text{Emergy} \\ \text{mole}}} \cong \underbrace{\bar{V}_W}_{\substack{\text{Volume} \\ \text{mole}}}\; [\underbrace{RT(\text{Osm}_o - \text{Osm}_i) + (P_i - P_o)}_{\text{Pressure}}] \qquad (5\text{-}25)$$

In this equation, the terms inside the brackets have the units of pressure (force/area) and thus describe the *driving force* for water movement from the inside to the outside of the cell. This driving force determines the flux of water across the membrane:

$$J_V = L_p[RT(\text{Osm}_o - \text{Osm}_i) + (P_i - P_o)] \qquad (5\text{-}26)$$

J_V is positive when water flows out of the cell and has the units liters/($cm^2 \cdot s$). The proportionality constant L_p is the **hydraulic conductivity**.

Water is in equilibrium across the membrane when the net driving force for water transport is nil. If we set $\Delta\mu_{H_2O,\text{total}}$ to zero in Equation 5-25:

$$RT(\text{Osm}_i - \text{Osm}_o) = (P_i - P_o)$$
$$\underbrace{(\pi_i - \pi_o)}_{\substack{\text{Osmotic} \\ \text{pressure difference} \\ \Delta\pi}} = \underbrace{(P_i - P_o)}_{\substack{\text{Hydrostatic pressure} \\ \text{difference} \\ \Delta P}} \qquad (5\text{-}27)$$

The term on the left is referred to as the **osmotic pressure difference** ($\Delta\pi$). Thus, at equilibrium, the osmotic pressure difference is equal to the hydrostatic pressure difference (ΔP). An osmotic pressure difference of 1 mosmol/kg H_2O (or 1 mOsm) is equivalent to a hydrostatic pressure difference of 19.3 mm Hg at normal body temperature.

The plasma membranes of animal cells are not so rigid (unlike the walls of plant cells) and cannot tolerate any significant hydrostatic pressure difference without deforming. Therefore, the hydrostatic pressure difference *across a cell membrane* is virtually always near zero and is therefore not a significant driving force for water transport.

Movement of water in and out of cells is driven by osmotic gradients only, that is, by differences in osmolality across the membrane. For example, if the osmolality is greater outside the cell than inside, water will flow out of the cell and the cell will shrink. Such a movement of water driven by osmotic gradients is called **osmosis**. Water is at equilibrium across *cell membranes* only when the osmolality inside and outside the cell is the same.

Hydrostatic pressure differences are an important driving force for driving fluid out across the *walls of capillaries* (see Chapter 20). Small solutes permeate freely across most capillaries. Thus, any difference in *osmotic* pressure as a result of these small solutes does not exert a driving force for water flow across that capillary. The situation is quite different for plasma proteins, which are too large to penetrate the capillary wall freely. As a result, the presence of a greater concentration of plasma proteins in the intravascular compartment than in interstitial fluid sets up a difference in osmotic pressure that tends to pull fluid back into the capillary. This difference is called the **colloid osmotic pressure** or **oncotic pressure**. Water is at equilibrium across the wall of a *capillary* when the colloid osmotic and hydrostatic pressure differences are equal. When the hydrostatic pressure difference exceeds the colloid osmotic pressure difference, the resulting movement of water out of the capillary is called **ultrafiltration**.

Because of the presence of impermeant, negatively charged proteins within the cell, Donnan forces will lead to cell swelling

NaCl, the most abundant salt in ECF, is largely excluded from the intracellular compartment by the direct and indirect actions of the Na-K pump. This relative exclusion of NaCl from the intracellular space is vital for maintaining normal cell water content (i.e., cell volume). In the absence of Na-K pumps, cells tend to swell even when both the intracellular and extracellular osmolalities are normal and identical. This statement may appear to contradict the principle that there can be no water flux without a difference in osmolality across the cell membrane (Equation 5-26). To understand this apparent paradox, consider a simplified model that illustrates the key role played by **negatively charged, impermeant macromolecules** (i.e., proteins) inside the cell (Fig. 5-15).

Imagine that a semipermeable membrane separates a left compartment (analogous to the *extra*cellular space) and a right compartment (analogous to the *intra*cellular space). The two compartments are rigid and have equal volumes throughout the experiment. The right compartment is fitted with a pressure gauge. The membrane is nondeformable and permeable to Na^+, Cl^-, and water, but it is not permeable to a negatively charged macromolecule (Y). For the sake of simplicity, assume that each Y carries 150 negative charges and is restricted to the intracellular solution. Figure 5-15A illustrates the ionic conditions at the beginning of the experiment. At this initial condition, the system is far out of equilibrium; although $[Na^+]$ is the same on both sides of the membrane, $[Cl^-]$ and $[Y^{-150}]$ have opposing concentration gradients of 150 mM.

What will happen now? The system will tend toward equilibrium. Cl^- will move down its concentration gradient into the cell. This entry of negatively charged particles will gener-

A INITIAL CONDITION

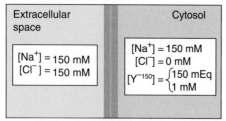

B INTERMEDIATE STATE
(after 10 mM NaCl has moved to cytosol)

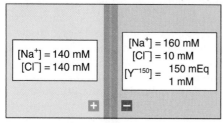

C FINAL EQUILIBRIUM

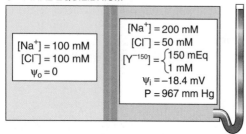

Figure 5-15 Gibbs-Donnan equilibrium. A semipermeable membrane separates two compartments that have rigid walls and equal volumes. The membrane is permeable to Na^+, Cl^-, and water but not to the macromolecule Y, which carries 150 negative charges. The calculations of ψ_i and P assume a temperature of 37°C.

ate an inside-negative membrane voltage, which in turn will attract Na^+ and cause Na^+ to move into the cell. In the final equilibrium condition, both Na^+ and Cl^- will be distributed so that the concentration of each is balanced against the same V_m, which is given by the Nernst equation (Equation 5-8):

$$V_m = -\frac{RT}{F} \ln \frac{[Na^+]_i}{[Na^+]_o} \qquad (5\text{-}28)$$

$$V_m = -\frac{RT}{(-1)F} \ln \frac{[Cl^-]_i}{[Cl^-]_o} \qquad (5\text{-}29)$$

Because V_m must be the same in the two cases, we combine the two equations, obtaining

$$-\ln \frac{[Na^+]_i}{[Na^+]_o} = \ln \frac{[Cl^-]_i}{[Cl^-]_o}$$

$$\frac{[Na^+]_o}{[Na^+]_i} = \frac{[Cl^-]_i}{[Cl^-]_o} = r \qquad (5\text{-}30)$$

where r is the Donnan ratio because this equilibrium state is a **Gibbs-Donnan equilibrium** (often shortened to Donnan equilibrium). All the values for ionic concentrations in Equa-

tion 5-30 are *new* values. As Na^+ entered the cell, not only did $[Na^+]_i$ rise but $[Na^+]_o$ also fell, by identical amounts. The same is true for Cl^-. How much did the Na^+ and Cl^- concentrations have to change before the system achieved equilibrium? An important constraint on the system as it approaches equilibrium is that in each compartment, the total number of positive charges must balance the total number of negative charges (bulk electroneutrality) at all times. Imagine an *intermediate* state, between the initial condition and the final equilibrium state, in which 10 mM of Na^+ and 10 mM of Cl^- have moved into the cell (Fig. 5-15B). This condition is still far from equilibrium because the Na^+ ratio in Equation 5-30 is 0.875, whereas the Cl^- ratio is only 0.071; thus, these ratios are not equal. Therefore, Na^+ and Cl^- continue to move into the cell until the Na^+ ratio and the Cl^- ratio are both 0.5, the Donnan r ratio (Fig. 5-15C). This ratio corresponds to Nernst potentials of −18.4 mV for both Na^+ and Cl^-.

However, although the ions are in equilibrium, far more osmotically active particles are now on the inside than on the outside. Ignoring the osmotic effect of Y^{-150}, the sum of $[Na^+]$ and $[Cl^-]$ on the inside is 250 mM, whereas it is only 200 mM on the outside. Because of this 50-mOsm gradient (ΔOsm) across the membrane, water cannot be at equilibrium and will therefore move into the cell. In our example, the right (inside) compartment is surrounded by a rigid wall so that only a minuscule amount of water needs to enter the cell to generate a hydrostatic pressure of 967 mm Hg to oppose the additional net entry of water. This equilibrium hydrostatic pressure difference (ΔP) opposes the osmotic pressure difference ($\Delta \pi$):

$$
\begin{aligned}
\Delta P &= \Delta \pi \\
&= RT\Delta Osm \\
&= RT[([Na^+]_i + [Cl^-]_i) - ([Na^+]_o + [Cl^-]_o)] \\
&= RT(50\,mM) \qquad\qquad (5\text{-}31) \\
&= 967\,mm\,Hg \\
&= 1.3\,atm
\end{aligned}
$$

Thus, in the rigid "cell" of our example, achieving Gibbs-Donnan equilibrium would require developing within the model cell a hydrostatic pressure that is 1.3 atm greater than the pressure in the left compartment (outside).

The Na-K pump maintains cell volume by doing osmotic work that counteracts the passive Donnan forces

Unlike in the preceding example, the plasma membranes of animal cells are not rigid but deformable, so that transmembrane hydrostatic pressure gradients cannot exist. Thus, in animal cells, the distribution of ions toward the Donnan equilibrium condition would, it appears, inevitably lead to progressive water entry, cell swelling, and ultimately bursting. Although the Donnan equilibrium model is artificial (e.g., ignoring all ions other than Na^+, Cl^-, and Y^{-150}), it nevertheless illustrates a point that is important for real cells: the negative charge on impermeant intracellular solutes (e.g., proteins and organic phosphates) will lead to bursting unless the cell does "osmotic work" to counteract the passive

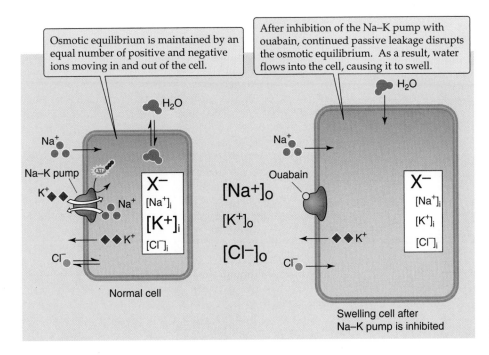

Osmotic equilibrium is maintained by an equal number of positive and negative ions moving in and out of the cell.

After inhibition of the Na–K pump with ouabain, continued passive leakage disrupts the osmotic equilibrium. As a result, water flows into the cell, causing it to swell.

Normal cell

Swelling cell after Na–K pump is inhibited

Figure 5-16   Role of the Na-K pump in maintaining cell volume.

Donnan-like swelling. The net effect of this osmotic work is to largely exclude NaCl from the cell and thereby make the cell functionally impermeable to NaCl. In a sense, NaCl acts as a functionally impermeant solute in the extracellular space that offsets the osmotic effects of intracellular negative charges. This state of affairs is not an equilibrium but a *steady state* maintained by active transport.

To illustrate the role of active transport, consider a somewhat more realistic model of a cell (Fig. 5-16). Under "normal" conditions, $[Na^+]_i$, $[K^+]_i$, and $[Cl^-]_i$ are constant because (1) the active extrusion of three Na^+ ions in exchange for two K^+ ions is balanced by the passive influx of three Na^+ ions and the passive efflux of two K^+ ions and (2) the net flux of Cl^- is zero (i.e., we assume that Cl^- is in equilibrium). When the Na-K pump is inhibited, the passive entry of three Na^+ ions exceeds the net passive efflux of two K^+ ions and thereby results in a gain of one intracellular cation and an immediate, small depolarization (i.e., cell becomes less negative inside). In addition, as intracellular $[K^+]$ slowly declines after inhibition of the Na-K pump, the cell depolarizes even further because the outward K^+ gradient is the predominant determinant of the membrane voltage. The inside-negative V_m is the driving force that is largely responsible for excluding Cl^- from the cell, and depolarization of the cell causes Cl^- to enter through anion channels. Cl^- influx results in the gain of one intracellular anion. The net gain of one intracellular cation and one anion increases the number of osmotically active particles and in so doing creates the inward osmotic gradient that leads to cell swelling. Thus, in the normal environment in which cells are bathed, the action of the Na-K pump is required to prevent the cell swelling that would otherwise occur.

A real cell, of course, is far more complex than the idealized cell in Figure 5-16, having myriad interrelated channels and transporters (Fig. 5-14). These other pathways, together with the Na-K pump, have the net effect of excluding NaCl and other solutes from the cell. Because the solute gradients that drive transport through these other pathways

ultimately depend on the Na-K pump, inhibiting the Na-K pump will de-energize these other pathways and lead to cell swelling.

Cell volume changes trigger rapid changes in ion channels or transporters, returning volume toward normal

The joint efforts of the Na-K pump and other transport pathways are necessary for maintaining normal cell volume. What happens if cell volume is acutely challenged? A subset of "other pathways" respond to the cell volume change by transferring solutes across the membrane, thereby returning the volume toward normal.

Response to Cell Shrinkage   If we increase extracellular osmolality by adding an impermeant solute such as mannitol (Fig. 5-17A), the extracellular solution becomes **hyperosmolal** and exerts an osmotic force that draws water out of the cell. The cell continues to shrink until the osmolality inside and out becomes the same. Many types of cells respond to this shrinkage by activating solute uptake processes to increase cell solute and water content. This response is known as a **regulatory volume increase (RVI)**. Depending on the cell type, cell shrinkage activates different types of solute uptake mechanisms. In many types of cells, shrinkage activates the ubiquitous NHE1 isoform of the *Na-H exchanger*. In addition to mediating increased uptake of Na^+, extrusion of H^+ alkalinizes the cell and consequently activates *Cl-HCO₃ exchange*. The net effect is thus the entry of Na^+ and Cl^-. The resulting increase in intracellular osmoles then draws water into the cell to restore cell volume toward normal. Alternatively, the RVI response may be mediated by activation of the NKCC1 isoform of the *Na/K/Cl cotransporter*.

Response to Cell Swelling   If extracellular osmolality is decreased by the addition of water (Fig. 5-17B), the extracellular solution becomes **hypo-osmolal** and exerts a lesser

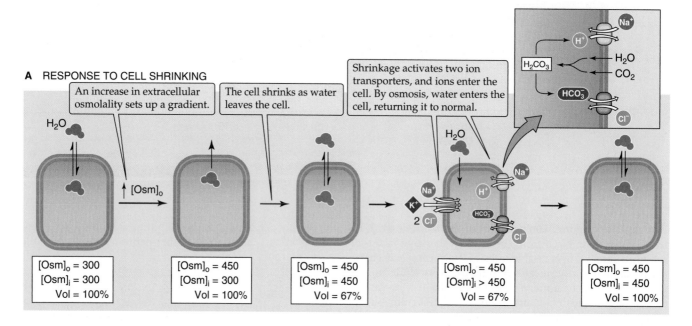

A RESPONSE TO CELL SHRINKING

An increase in extracellular osmolality sets up a gradient.

The cell shrinks as water leaves the cell.

Shrinkage activates two ion transporters, and ions enter the cell. By osmosis, water enters the cell, returning it to normal.

$[Osm]_o = 300$
$[Osm]_i = 300$
Vol = 100%

$[Osm]_o = 450$
$[Osm]_i = 300$
Vol = 100%

$[Osm]_o = 450$
$[Osm]_i = 450$
Vol = 67%

$[Osm]_o = 450$
$[Osm]_i > 450$
Vol = 67%

$[Osm]_o = 450$
$[Osm]_i = 450$
Vol = 100%

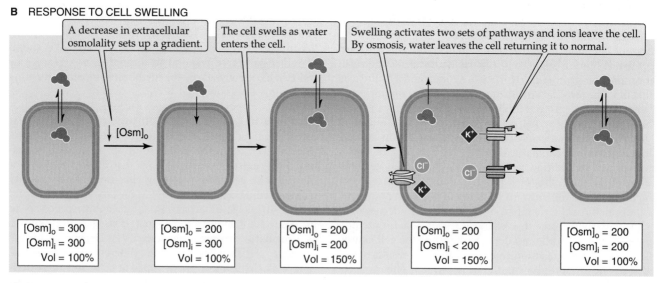

B RESPONSE TO CELL SWELLING

A decrease in extracellular osmolality sets up a gradient.

The cell swells as water enters the cell.

Swelling activates two sets of pathways and ions leave the cell. By osmosis, water leaves the cell returning it to normal.

$[Osm]_o = 300$
$[Osm]_i = 300$
Vol = 100%

$[Osm]_o = 200$
$[Osm]_i = 300$
Vol = 100%

$[Osm]_o = 200$
$[Osm]_i = 200$
Vol = 150%

$[Osm]_o = 200$
$[Osm]_i < 200$
Vol = 150%

$[Osm]_o = 200$
$[Osm]_i = 200$
Vol = 100%

Figure 5-17 Short-term regulation of cell volume.

Disorders of Extracellular Osmolality

Regulatory adjustments in cell volume can be extremely important clinically. In major disorders of extracellular osmolality, the principal signs and symptoms arise from abnormal brain function, which can be fatal. For example, it is all too common for the elderly or infirm, unable to maintain proper fluid intake because of excessive heat or disability, to be brought to the emergency department in a state of severe dehydration. The hyperosmolality that results from dehydration can lead to brain shrinkage, which in extreme cases can cause intracerebral hemorrhage from tearing of blood vessels. If the brain cells compensate for this hyperosmolality by the long-term mechanisms discussed (e.g., manufacturing of idiogenic osmoles), cell shrinkage may be minimized. However, consider the consequence if an unsuspecting physician, unaware of the nuances of cell volume regulation, rapidly corrects the elevated extracellular hyperosmolality back down to normal. Rapid water entry into the brain cells will cause cerebral edema (i.e., brain swelling) and may result in death from herniation of the brainstem through the tentorium. For this reason, severe disturbances in ECF osmolality must usually be corrected slowly.

osmotic force so that water moves into the cell. The cell continues to swell until the osmolality inside and out becomes the same. Many cell types respond to this swelling by activating solute efflux pathways to decrease cell solute and water content and thereby return cell volume toward normal. This response is known as a **regulatory volume decrease (RVD)**. Depending on the cell type, swelling activates different types of solute efflux mechanisms. In many types of cells, swelling activates Cl^- or K^+ channels (or both). Because the electrochemical gradients for these two ions are generally directed outward across the plasma membrane, activating these channels causes a net efflux of K^+ and Cl^-, which lowers the intracellular solute content and causes water to flow out of the cell. The result is restoration of cell volume toward normal. Alternatively, the RVD response may be initiated by activating the *K/Cl cotransporter*.

In the normal steady state, the transport mechanisms that are responsible for RVI and RVD are usually not fully quiescent. Not only does cell shrinkage activate the transport pathways involved in RVI (i.e., solute loaders), it also appears to inhibit at least some of the transport pathways involved in RVD (i.e., solute extruders). The opposite is true of cell swelling. In all cases, it is the Na-K pump that ultimately generates the ion gradients that drive the movements of NaCl and KCl that regulate cell volume in response to changes in extracellular osmolality.

Cells respond to long-term hyperosmolality by accumulating new intracellular organic solutes

Whereas the acute response (seconds to minutes) to hyperosmolality (i.e., RVI) involves the uptake of salts, chronic adaptation (hours to days) to hyperosmolality involves accumulating organic solutes (*osmolytes*) within the cell. Examples of such intracellularly accumulated osmolytes include two relatively impermeant alcohol derivatives of common sugars (i.e., sorbitol and inositol) as well as two amines (betaine and taurine). Generation of organic solutes (*idiogenic osmoles*) within the cell plays a major role in raising intracellular osmolality and restoring cell volume during chronic adaptation to hyperosmolality—a response that is particularly true in brain cells. Sorbitol is produced from glucose by a reaction that is catalyzed by the enzyme **aldose reductase**. Cell shrinkage is a powerful stimulus for the synthesis of aldose reductase.

In addition to synthesizing organic solutes, cells can also transport them into the cytosol from the outside. For example, cells use distinct Na^+-coupled cotransport systems to accumulate inositol, betaine, and taurine. In some types of cells, shrinkage induces greatly enhanced expression of these transporters, thereby leading to the accumulation of these intracellular solutes.

The gradient in tonicity—or effective osmolality—determines the osmotic flow of water across a cell membrane

Total body water is distributed among blood plasma, the interstitial, intracellular, and transcellular fluids. The mechanisms by which water exchanges between interstitial fluid and ICF, and between interstitial fluid and plasma, rely on the principles that we have just discussed.

Water Exchange Across Cell Membranes Because cell membranes are not rigid, hydrostatic pressure differences never arise between cell water and interstitial fluid. Increasing the *hydrostatic* pressure in the interstitial space will cause the cell to compress so that the intracellular hydrostatic pressure increases to a similar extent. Thus, water does not enter the cell under these conditions. However, increasing the interstitial *osmotic* pressure, thus generating a $\Delta\pi$, is quite a different matter. If we suddenly increase ECF osmolality by adding an *impermeant* solute such as mannitol, the resulting osmotic gradient across the cell membrane causes water to move out of the cell. If the cell does not have an RVI mechanism or if the RVI mechanism is blocked, cell volume will remain reduced indefinitely.

On the other hand, consider what would happen if we suddenly increase ECF osmolality by adding a *permeant* solute such as urea. Urea can rapidly penetrate cell membranes by facilitated diffusion through members of the UT family of transporters; however, cells have no mechanism for extruding urea. Because urea penetrates the membrane more slowly than water does, the initial effect of applying urea is to shrink the cell (Fig. 5-18). However, as urea gradually equilibrates across the cell membrane and abolishes the initially imposed osmotic gradient, the cell reswells to its initial volume. Thus, sustained changes in cell volume do not occur with a change in the extracellular concentration of a permeant solute.

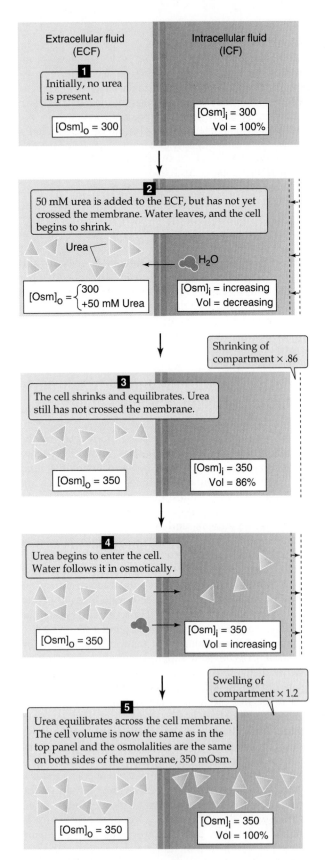

Figure 5-18 Effect of urea on the volume of a single cell bathed in an infinite volume of extracellular fluid. We assume that the cell membrane is permeable only to water during the initial moments in steps 2 and 3. Later, during steps 4 and 5, we assume that the membrane is permeable to both water and urea.

The difference between the effects of mannitol and urea on the final cell volume illustrates the need to distinguish between total osmolality and **effective osmolality** (also known as **tonicity**). In terms of clinically measured solutes, total and effective osmolality of the ECF can be approximated as

$$\text{Total osmolality (mOsm)} \cong 2 \cdot [Na^+] + \frac{\text{Glucose (mg/dL)}}{18} + \frac{\text{BUN (mg/dL)}}{2.8}$$

$$\text{Tonicity or effective osmolality (mOsm)} \cong 2 \cdot [Na^+] + \frac{\text{Glucose (mg/dL)}}{18} \quad \text{(5-32)}$$

BUN stands for blood urea nitrogen, that is, the concentration of the nitrogen that is contained in the plasma as urea. In Equation 5-32, the clinical laboratory reports $[Na^+]$ in milliequivalents per liter. Because the laboratory reports the glucose and BUN concentrations in terms of milligrams per deciliter, we divide glucose by one tenth of the molecular weight of glucose and BUN by one tenth of the summed atomic weights of the two nitrogen atoms in urea. The computed tonicity does not include BUN because—as we saw earlier—urea easily equilibrates across most cell membranes. On the other hand, the computed tonicity includes both Na^+ and glucose. It includes Na^+ because Na^+ is *functionally impermeant* owing to its extrusion by the Na-K pump. Tonicity includes glucose because this solute does not appreciably accumulate in most cells as a result of metabolism. In some clinical situations, the infusion of impermeant solutes, such as radiographic contrast agents or mannitol, can also contribute to tonicity of the ECF.

Osmolality describes the number of osmotically active solutes in a single solution. If we regard a plasma osmolality of 290 mOsm as being normal, solutions having an osmolality of 290 mOsm are **isosmolal**, solutions with osmolalities above 290 mOsm are hyperosmolal, and those with osmolalities below 290 mOsm are hypo-osmolal. On the other hand, when we use the terms *isotonic, hypertonic,* and *hypotonic,* we are comparing one solution with another solution (e.g., ICF) across a well-defined membrane (e.g., a cell membrane). A solution is **isotonic** when its *effective* osmolality is the same as that of the reference solution, which for our purposes is the ICF. A **hypertonic** solution is one that has a higher effective osmolality than the reference solution, and a **hypotonic** solution has a lower effective osmolality.

Shifts of water between the intracellular and interstitial compartments result from alterations in *effective* ECF osmolality, or *tonicity.* Clinically, such changes in tonicity are usually caused by decreases in $[Na^+]$ in the plasma and ECF (hyponatremia), increases in $[Na^+]$ (hypernatremia), or increases in glucose concentration (hyperglycemia). Changes in the concentration of a highly permeant solute such as urea, which accumulates in patients with kidney failure, have no effect on tonicity.

Water Exchange Across the Capillary Wall The barrier separating the blood plasma and interstitial compartments, the capillary wall, is—to a first approximation—freely permeable to solutes that are smaller than plasma proteins. Thus, the only *net* osmotic force that acts across the capillary wall is that caused by the asymmetric distribution of proteins in plasma versus interstitial fluid. Several terms may be used for the osmotic force that is generated by these impermeant plasma proteins, such as protein osmotic pressure, colloid osmotic pressure, and oncotic pressure. These terms are synonymous and can be represented by the symbol $\pi_{oncotic}$. The **oncotic pressure difference** ($\Delta\pi_{oncotic}$), which tends to pull water from the interstitium to the plasma, is opposed by the hydrostatic pressure difference across the capillary wall (ΔP), which drives fluid from plasma into the interstitium. All net movements of water across the capillary wall are accompanied by the small solutes dissolved in this water, at their ECF concentrations; that is, the pathways taken by the water across the capillary wall are so large that small solutes are not *sieved* out.

To summarize, fluid shifts between plasma and the interstitium respond only to changes in the balance between ΔP and $\Delta\pi_{oncotic}$. Small solutes such as Na^+, which freely cross the capillary wall, do not contribute significantly to osmotic driving forces across this barrier and move along with the water in which they are dissolved. We will return to this subject when we discuss the physiology of capillaries in Chapter 20.

Adding isotonic saline, pure water, or pure NaCl to the ECF will increase ECF volume but will have divergent effects on ICF volume and ECF osmolality

Adding various combinations of NaCl and **solute-free water** to the ECF will alter the volume and composition of the body fluid compartments. Three examples illustrate the effects seen with intravenous therapy. In Figure 5-19A, we start with a total body water of 42 liters (60% of a 70-kg person), subdivided into an ICF volume of 25 liters (60% of total body water) and an ECF volume of 17 liters (40% of total body water). These numerical values are the same as those in Figure 5-1 and Table 5-1.

Infusion of Isotonic Saline Consider the case in which we infuse or ingest 1.5 liters of isotonic saline, which is a 0.9% solution of NaCl in water (Fig. 5-19B). This solution has an effective osmolality of 290 mOsm in the ECF. This 1.5 liters is initially distributed throughout the ECF and raises ECF volume by 1.5 liters. Because the effective osmolality of the ECF is unaltered, no change occurs in the effective osmotic gradient across the cell membranes, and the added water moves neither into nor out of the ICF. This outcome is, of course, in accord with the definition of an *isotonic* solution. Thus, we see that adding isotonic saline to the body is an efficient way to expand the ECF without affecting the ICF. Similarly, if it were possible to remove isotonic saline from the body, we would see that this measure would efficiently contract the ECF and again have no effect on the ICF.

Infusion of "Solute-Free" Water Now consider a case in which we either ingest 1.5 liters of pure water or infuse 1.5 liters of an isotonic (5%) glucose solution (Fig. 5-19C). Infusing the glucose solution intravenously is equivalent, in the long run, to infusing pure water because the glucose is metabolized to CO_2 and water, with no solutes left behind in the ECF. Infusing pure water would be unwise inasmuch as it would cause the cells near the point of infusion to burst.

How do the effects of adding 1.5 liters of pure water compare with those of the previous example? At first, the 1.5 liters of pure water will be rapidly distributed throughout the ECF and increase its volume from 17 to 18.5 liters (Fig. 5-19C, Early). This added water will also dilute the preexisting solutes in the ECF, thereby lowering ECF osmolality to 290 mOsm × 17/18.5 = 266 mOsm. Because intracellular osmolality remains at 290 mOsm at this imaginary, intermediate stage, a large osmotic gradient is created that favors the entry of water from the ECF into the ICF. Water will move into the ICF and consequently lower the osmolality of the ICF and simultaneously raise the osmolality of the ECF until osmotic equilibrium is restored (Fig. 5-19C, Final). Because the added water is distributed between the ICF and ECF according to the initial ICF/ECF ratio of 60%/40%, the final ECF volume is 17.6 liters (i.e., 17 liters expanded by 40% of 1.5 liters). Thus, infusion of solute-free water is a relatively *ineffective* means of expanding the ECF. More of the added water has ended up intracellularly (60% of 1.5 liters = 0.9 L of expansion). The major effect of the water has been to dilute the osmolality of body fluids. The initial total body solute content was 290 mOsm × 42 L = 12,180 milliosmoles. This same solute has now been diluted in 42 + 1.5 or 43.5 liters, so the final osmolality is 12,180/43.5 = 280 mOsm.

Ingestion of Pure NaCl Salt The preceding two "experiments" illustrate two extremely important principles that govern fluid and electrolyte homeostasis, namely, that adding or removing Na^+ will mainly affect ECF volume (Fig. 5-19B), whereas adding or removing solute-free water will mainly affect the *osmolality* of body fluids (Fig. 5-19C). The first point can be further appreciated by considering a third case, one in which we add the same amount of NaCl that is contained in 1.5 liters of isotonic (i.e., 0.9%) saline: 1.5 L × 290 mOsm = 435 mosmol. However, we will not add any water. At first, these 435 milliosmoles of NaCl will rapidly distribute throughout the 17 liters of ECF and increase the osmolality of the ECF (Fig. 5-19D, Early). The initial, total osmolal content of the ECF was 290 mOsm × 17 L = 4930 mosmol. Because we added 435 milliosmoles, we now have 5365 milliosmoles in the ECF. Thus, the ECF osmolality is 5365/17 = 316 mOsm. The resulting hyperosmolality draws water out of the ICF into the ECF until osmotic equilibrium is re-established. What is the final osmolality? The total number of milliosmoles dissolved in total body water is the original 12,180 milliosmoles plus the added 435 milliosmoles, for a total of 12,615 milliosmoles. Because these milliosmoles are dissolved in 42 liters of total body water, the final osmolality of the ICF and ECF is 12,615/42 = 300 mOsm. In the new equilibrium state, the ECF volume has increased by 0.9 liter even though no water at all was added to the body. Because the added ECF volume has come from the ICF, the ICF shrinks by 0.9 liter. This example further illustrates the principle that the total body content of Na^+ is the major determinant of ECF volume.

Whole-body Na⁺ content determines ECF volume, whereas whole-body water content determines osmolality

Changes in ECF volume are important because they are accompanied by proportional changes in the volume of

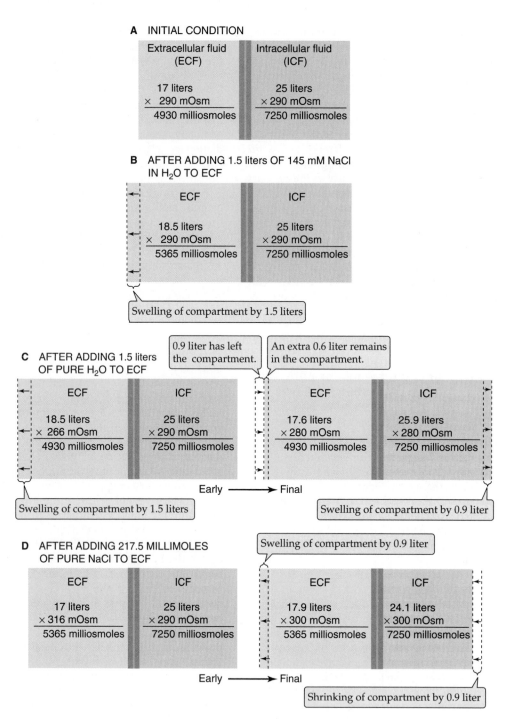

Figure 5-19 Effect on body fluid compartments of infusing different solutions.

blood plasma, which in turn affects the adequacy with which the circulatory system can perfuse vital organs with blood. The blood volume that is necessary to achieve adequate perfusion of key organs is sometimes referred to as the **effective circulating volume**. Because the body generally stabilizes osmolality, an increase in extracellular Na^+ content will increase ECF volume:

$$\underbrace{\text{Extracellular Na}^+ \text{ content}}_{\text{millimoles}} = \underbrace{[Na^+]_o}_{\text{millimoles/liter}} \times \underbrace{\text{ECF volume}}_{\text{liters}}$$

$$\cong \left(\frac{\text{Osmolality}}{2}\right) \times \underbrace{\text{ECF volume}}_{\text{liters}}$$

(5-33)

Because cells contain very little Na^+, extracellular Na^+ content is nearly the same as **total body Na^+** content.

We will see in Chapter 40 how the body regulates effective circulating volume; increases in effective circulating volume, which reflect increases in ECF volume or total body Na^+ *content*, stimulate the renal excretion of Na^+. In contrast, the plasma Na^+ *concentration* does *not* regulate renal excretion of Na^+. It makes sense that regulation of Na^+ excretion is not sensitive to the plasma Na^+ concentration because the concentration is not an indicator of ECF volume.

As discussed, when we hold osmolality constant, Na^+ content determines ECF volume. What would happen if we held constant the Na^+ content, which is a major part of total body osmoles? An increase in **total body water** would decrease **osmolality**.

$$\underbrace{\text{Total body osmoles}}_{\text{milliosmoles}} = \underbrace{[\text{Osmolality}]}_{\text{milliosmoles/liter}} \times \underbrace{\text{Total body water}}_{\text{liters}}$$

$$(5\text{-}34)$$

Thus, a net gain or loss of solute-free water has a major impact on the *osmolality* and *[Na^+]* of the ECF. Moreover, because a large part (~60%) of the added solute-free water distributes into the ICF, a gain or loss of solute-free water affects ICF more than ECF. We will see in Chapter 40 how the body regulates osmolality; a small decrease in osmolality triggers osmoreceptors to diminish thirst (resulting in diminished intake of solute-free water) and increase renal water excretion. In emergency states of very low ECF and effective circulating volume, some crosstalk occurs between the volume and osmolality control systems. As a result, the body not only will try to conserve Na^+ but will also seek water (by triggering thirst) and conserve water (by concentrating the urine). Although water (in comparison to saline) is not a very good expander of plasma and ECF volume, it is better than nothing.

TRANSPORT OF SOLUTES AND WATER ACROSS EPITHELIA

Thus far we have examined how cells transport solutes and water across their membranes and thereby control their intracellular composition. We now turn our attention to how the body controls the milieu intérieur, namely, the ECF that bathes the cells. Just as the cell membrane is the barrier between the ICF and ECF, epithelia are the barriers that separate the ECF from the outside world. In this subchapter, we examine the fundamental principles of how epithelial cells transport solutes and water across epithelial barriers.

An epithelium is an uninterrupted sheet of cells that are joined together by junctional complexes (see Chapter 2). These junctions serve as a selectively permeable barrier between the solutions on either side of the epithelium and demarcate the boundary between the apical and basolateral regions of the cell membrane. The apical and basolateral membranes are remarkably different in their transport function. This polarization allows the epithelial cell to transport water and selected solutes from one compartment to another. In other words, the epithelium is capable of vectorial trans-port. In many cases, transport of solutes across an epithelium is an active process.

Membranes may be called by different names in different epithelia. The **apical membrane** can be known as the brush border, the mucosal membrane, or the luminal membrane. The **basolateral membrane** is also known as the serosal or peritubular membrane.

The epithelial cell generally has different electrochemical gradients across its apical and basolateral membranes

Imagine an artificial situation in which an epithelium separates two identical solutions. Furthermore, imagine that there is no difference in voltage across the epithelium and no difference in hydrostatic pressure. Under these circumstances, the driving forces for the *passive movement* of solutes or water across the epithelium would be nil. Because the apical and basolateral membranes of the cell share the same cytosol, the electrochemical gradients across the apical and basolateral membranes would be identical.

However, this example is virtually never realistic for two reasons. First, because the composition of the "outside world" is not the same as that of ECF, transepithelial concentration differences occur. Second, transepithelial voltage is not zero. Thus, the electrochemical gradients across the apical and basolateral membranes of an epithelial cell are generally very different.

Electrophysiological methods provide two major types of information about ion transport by epithelial cells. First, electrophysiological techniques can define the electrical driving forces that act on ions either across the entire epithelium or across the individual apical and basolateral cell membranes. Second, these electrical measurements can define the overall electrical resistance of the epithelium or the electrical resistance of the individual apical and basolateral cell membranes.

The voltage difference between the solutions on either side of the epithelium is the **transepithelial voltage** (V_{te}). We can measure V_{te} by placing one microelectrode in the lumen of the organ or duct of which the epithelium is the wall and a second reference electrode in the blood or interstitial space (Fig. 5-20A). If we instead insert the first microelectrode directly into an epithelial cell (Fig. 5-20A), the voltage difference between this cell and the reference electrode in blood or the interstitial space measures the **basolateral cell membrane voltage** (V_{bl}). Finally, if we compare the intracellular electrode with a reference electrode in the lumen (Fig. 5-20A), the voltage difference is the **apical cell membrane voltage** (V_a). Obviously, the sum of V_a and V_{bl} is equal to the transepithelial voltage (Fig. 5-20B). It is also possible to insert ion-sensitive microelectrodes into the lumen or the epithelial cells and thereby determine the local activity of ions such as Na^+, K^+, H^+, Ca^{2+}, and Cl^-.

By using the same voltage electrodes that we introduced in the preceding paragraph, we can pass electrical current across either the whole epithelium or the individual apical and basolateral membranes. From Ohm's law, it is thus possible to calculate the **electrical resistance** of the entire wall of the epithelium, or transepithelial resistance (R_{te}); that of the apical membrane, or apical resistance (R_a); or that of the basolateral membrane, or basolateral resistance (R_{bl}).

A EPITHELIAL VOLTAGES

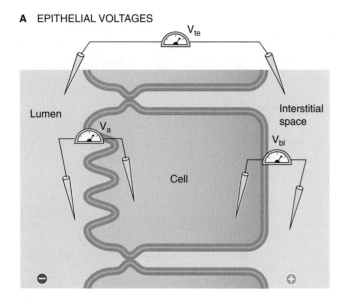

B ELECTRICAL PROFILE ACROSS AN EPITHELIAL CELL

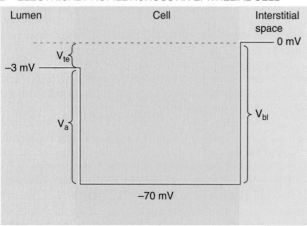

Figure 5-20 Measurement of voltages in an epithelium. **A,** The transepithelial voltage difference between electrodes placed in the lumen and interstitial space (or blood) is V_{te}. The basolateral voltage difference between electrodes placed in the cell and interstitial space is V_{bl}. The apical voltage difference between electrodes placed in the lumen and cell is V_a. **B,** Relative to the reference voltage of zero in the interstitial space, the voltage inside the cell in this example is −70 mV, and the voltage in the lumen is −3 mV. These values are typical of a cell in the renal proximal tubule or a small intestine.

Tight and leaky epithelia differ in the permeabilities of their tight junctions

One measure of how tightly an epithelium separates one compartment from another is its resistance to the flow of electrical current. The range of transepithelial electrical resistance is quite large. For example, 1 cm^2 of a rat proximal tubule has a resistance of only 6 Ω, whereas 1 cm^2 of a rabbit urinary bladder has a resistance of 70,000 Ω. Why is the range of R_{te} values so great? The cells of these epithelia do not differ greatly in either their apical or basolateral mem-

brane resistances. Instead, the epithelia with low electrical resistances have a low-resistance pathway located in their tight junctions. Epithelia are thus classified as either "tight" (high electrical resistance) or "leaky," depending on the relative resistance of their tight junctions. In other words, the tight junctions of leaky epithelia are relatively more permeant to the diffusion of ions than the tight junctions of tight epithelia.

Now that we have introduced the concept that solutes and water can move between epithelial cells through tight junctions, we can define two distinct pathways by which substances can cross epithelia. First, a substance can cross through the cell by sequentially passing across the apical and then the basolateral membranes, or vice versa. This route is called the **transcellular pathway**. Second, a substance can bypass the cell entirely and cross the epithelium through the tight junctions and lateral intercellular spaces. This route is called the **paracellular pathway**.

As might be expected, leaky epithelia are not so good at maintaining large transepithelial ion or osmotic gradients. In general, **leaky epithelia** perform bulk transepithelial transport of solutes and water in a nearly isosmotic fashion (i.e., the transported fluid has about the same osmolality as the fluid from which it came). Examples include the small intestine and the proximal tubule of the kidney. As a general rule, **tight epithelia** generate or maintain large transepithelial ion concentration or osmotic gradients. Examples include the distal nephron of the kidney, the large intestine, and the tightest of all epithelia, the urinary bladder (whose function is to be an absolutely impermeable storage vessel).

In addition to tight junctions, epithelia share a number of basic properties First, the Na-K pump is located exclusively on the basolateral membrane (Fig. 5-21). The only known exception is the choroid plexus, where the Na-K pump is located on the apical membrane.

Second, most of the K$^+$ that is taken up by the Na$^+$ pump generally recycles back out across the basolateral membrane through K$^+$ channels (Fig. 5-21). A consequence of the abundance of these K$^+$ channels is that the K$^+$ gradient predominantly determines V_{bl}, which is usually 50 to 60 mV, inside negative.

Third, as in other cells, [Na$^+$]$_i$, typically 10 to 30 mM, is much lower in an epithelial cell than in the ECF. This low [Na$^+$]$_i$ is a consequence of the active extrusion of Na$^+$ by the Na-K pump. The large, inwardly directed Na$^+$ electrochemical gradient serves as a driving force for Na$^+$ entry through apical Na$^+$ channels and for the secondary active transport of other solutes across the apical membrane (e.g., by Na$^+$/glucose cotransport, Na-H exchange, Na/K/Cl cotransport) or basolateral membrane (e.g., by Na-Ca exchange).

Epithelial cells can absorb or secrete different solutes by inserting specific channels or transporters at either the apical or basolateral membrane

By placing different transporters at the apical and basolateral membranes, epithelia can accomplish net transepithelial transport of different solutes in either the absorptive or secretory direction. For example, the renal proximal tubule moves glucose from the tubule lumen to the blood by using the Na$^+$/glucose cotransporter (SGLT) to move glucose into

A Na⁺ ABSORPTION ("USSING MODEL")

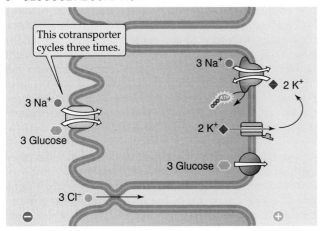

Na⁺ enters across apical membrane via channels, but is pumped out across basolateral membrane.

The K⁺ pumped into cell recycles back out.

3 Na⁺

Epithelial cell

Apical membrane

Basolateral membrane

Tight junction

Exterior milieu (lumen)

3 Cl⁻

Interstitial space

3 Na⁺

2 K⁺

ATP

2 K⁺

The lumen is negative compared with interstitium.

B K⁺ SECRETION

3 Na⁺

3 Na⁺

2 K⁺

ATP

K⁺

K⁺

2 Cl⁻

C GLUCOSE ABSORPTION

This cotransporter cycles three times.

3 Na⁺

3 Glucose

3 Cl⁻

3 Na⁺

2 K⁺

ATP

2 K⁺

3 Glucose

D Cl⁻ SECRETION

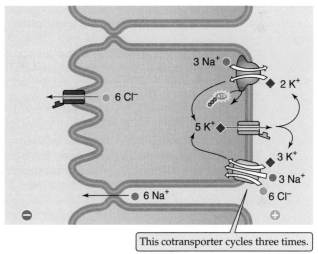

6 Cl⁻

3 Na⁺

2 K⁺

ATP

5 K⁺

3 K⁺

3 Na⁺

6 Na⁺

6 Cl⁻

This cotransporter cycles three times.

Figure 5-21 Models of epithelial solute transport.

the cell across the apical membrane, but it uses facilitated diffusion of glucose (GLUT) to move glucose out of the cell across the basolateral membrane. Clearly, the proximal tubule cell could not use the same Na⁺/glucose cotransporter at both the apical and basolateral membranes because the electrochemical Na⁺ gradient is similar across both membranes.

We will now look at four examples to illustrate how epithelia can absorb or secrete various solutes by using the transporters discussed earlier in this chapter.

Na⁺ Absorption Consider the model in Figure 5-21A, which is similar to that first proposed by Hans Ussing and coworkers to explain NaCl absorption across the frog skin. The basolateral Na-K pump pumps Na⁺ out of the cell, thereby lowering [Na⁺]ᵢ and generating an inward Na⁺ electrochemical gradient across the apical membrane. This apical Na⁺ gradient in turn provides the driving force for Na⁺ to enter the cell passively across the apical membrane through

ENaC Na⁺ channels. The Na⁺ that enters the cell in this way is pumped out across the basolateral membrane in exchange for K⁺, which recycles back out across the basolateral membrane. Note that the Na-K pump generates a current of positive charge across the cell from lumen to interstitium. This current, in turn, creates a lumen-negative transepithelial voltage that can then provide a driving force for passive Cl⁻ absorption across the tight junctions—through the so-called paracellular pathway. The net result is NaCl absorption. This process is the mechanism for NaCl reabsorption in the collecting tubule of the kidney.

K⁺ Secretion With slight alterations, the same basic cell model can perform K⁺ secretion as well as Na⁺ absorption (Fig. 5-21B). Adding K⁺ channels to the apical membrane allows some of the K⁺ that is taken up by the Na-K pump across the basolateral membrane to be secreted across the apical membrane. This mechanism is the basis of K⁺ secretion in the collecting tubule of the kidney. Such a model accurately predicts that drugs such as amiloride, which blocks apical ENaC Na^+ channels in these cells, will inhibit K^+ secretion as well as Na^+ reabsorption.

Glucose Absorption   The small intestine and proximal tubule absorb nutrients that are present in the luminal compartment by secondary active cotransport of Na^+ with organic solutes. An example is Na^+ cotransport with glucose by SGLT (Fig. 5-21C). The inwardly directed electrochemical Na^+ gradient across the apical membrane, generated by the Na-K pump, now drives the entry of both Na^+ and glucose. Glucose, which has accumulated in the cell against its concentration gradient, exits passively across the basolateral membrane by a carrier-mediated transporter (GLUT) that is not coupled to Na^+. Again, the flow of positive current across the cell generates a lumen-negative transepithelial voltage that can drive passive Cl^- absorption across the tight junctions. The net effect is to absorb both NaCl and glucose.

Cl^- Secretion   If the cell places the Na^+-coupled Cl^- entry mechanism on the basolateral membrane, the same basic cell model can mediate NaCl *secretion* into the lumen (Fig. 5-21D). The inwardly directed Na^+ electrochemical gradient now drives secondary active Cl^- uptake across the basolateral membrane by the Na/K/Cl cotransporter NKCC1. Cl^- accumulated in the cell in this way can then exit across the apical membrane passively through Cl^- channels such as CFTR. Notice that negative charges now move across the cell from interstitium to lumen and generate a lumen-negative voltage that can drive passive Na^+ secretion across the tight junctions (paracellular pathway). The net process is NaCl secretion, even though the primary active transporter, the Na-K pump, is pumping Na^+ from the cell to the interstitium. Secretory cells in the intestine and pulmonary airway epithelium use this mechanism for secreting NaCl.

Water transport across epithelia passively follows solute transport

In general, water moves passively across an epithelium in response to osmotic gradients. An epithelium that secretes salt will secrete fluid, and one that absorbs salt will absorb fluid. The finite permeability of the bare lipid bilayer to water and the presence of aquaporins in most cell membranes ensure that osmotic equilibration for most cells is rapid. In addition, particularly in leaky epithelia, tight junctions provide a pathway for water movement between the epithelial cells. However, epithelial water permeability (hydraulic conductivity) varies widely because of differences in membrane lipid composition and in abundance of aquaporins. The presence of aquaporins in the plasma membrane may be either constitutive or highly regulated.

Absorption of a Hyperosmotic Fluid   If the epithelium absorbs more salt than its isotonic equivalent volume of water, the absorbate is hyperosmotic. An example is the thick ascending limb of the loop of Henle in the kidney, which reabsorbs a large amount of salt but relatively little water. As a result, dilute fluid is left behind in the lumen, and the renal interstitium is rendered hyperosmotic.

Absorption of an Isosmotic Fluid   In certain epithelia, such as the renal proximal tubule and small intestine, net water movement occurs with no detectable osmotic gradients across the epithelium (Fig. 5-22). Moreover, the reabsorbed fluid appears to be isosmotic with respect to luminal fluid. Of course, fluid absorption could not really occur without the requisite solute driving force across the epithelium. Two explanations, which are not exclusive, have been offered.

First, the water permeability of epithelia performing isosmotic water reabsorption might be extremely high because of the high constitutive expression of aquaporins in the apical and basolateral membranes. Thus, modest transepithelial osmotic gradients (perhaps only 1 to 2 mOsm), which are the product of solute absorption, are sufficient to drive water transport at the rates observed. Measurements cannot distinguish such small osmotic gradients from no gradient at all.

Second, the lateral intercellular spaces between the epithelial cells (lateral interspaces; see Fig. 5-22, option 1) as well as the spaces between the infoldings of the basal membrane (basal labyrinth; see Fig. 5-22, option 2) might be modestly hyperosmotic as a consequence of the accumulation of absorbed solutes in a localized region. The resulting localized osmotic gradient would pull water into the lateral interspaces from the cell (across the lateral portion of the basolateral membrane) or from the lumen (across the tight junction). Similarly, a localized osmotic gradient would pull water into the basal labyrinth from the cell (across the basal portion of the basolateral membrane). By the time that the fluid emerges from these spaces and reaches the interstitium, it would have become nearly isosmotic.

Absorption of a Hypo-osmotic Fluid   If both sides of an epithelium are bathed by isosmotic solutions, it is not possible to concentrate the fluid in the lumen. You might think that you could accomplish the task by absorbing a hypo-osmotic fluid. However, this would require absorbing more water than solute, which would require water transport to "lead" rather than to follow solute transport. Indeed, active transport of water does not occur, and water cannot move against an osmotic gradient. Hypo-osmotic fluid absorption does indeed occur in the body but requires that the osmolality of the basolateral compartment exceed that of the apical compartment. As we will see in Chapter 38, the medullary collecting duct uses this approach to concentrate the urine. The collecting duct absorbs a hypo-osmotic fluid because (1) the interstitial fluid in the renal medulla is hyperosmotic and (2) the water permeability of the renal collecting duct is high due to the insertion of AQP2—under hormonal control—into the apical membrane.

Epithelia can regulate transport by controlling transport proteins, tight junctions, and the supply of the transported substances

A large range of physiological stimuli regulate the rates at which specific epithelia transport specific solutes. Virtually all known intracellular signaling cascades (see Chapter 3) have been implicated in mediating these regulatory effects.

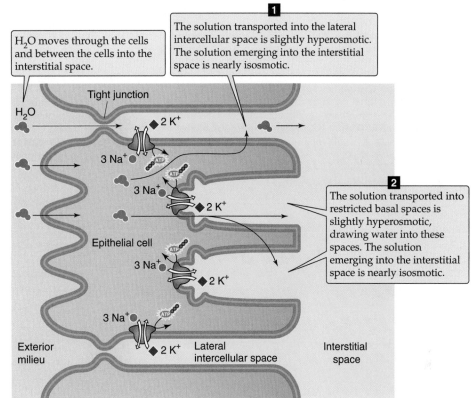

1 The solution transported into the lateral intercellular space is slightly hyperosmotic. The solution emerging into the interstitial space is nearly isosmotic.

H₂O moves through the cells and between the cells into the interstitial space.

2 The solution transported into restricted basal spaces is slightly hyperosmotic, drawing water into these spaces. The solution emerging into the interstitial space is nearly isosmotic.

Tight junction

H_2O

$2 K^+$

$3 Na^+$

$3 Na^+$

$2 K^+$

Epithelial cell

$3 Na^+$

$2 K^+$

$3 Na^+$

$2 K^+$

Exterior milieu

Lateral intercellular space

Interstitial space

Figure 5-22 Model of isotonic water transport in a leaky epithelium. Na-K pumps present on the lateral and basal membrane pump Na^+ into two restricted spaces: the lateral intercellular space and restricted spaces formed by infoldings of the basal membrane. The locally high osmolality in the lateral intercellular space pulls water from the lumen and the cell. Similarly, the locally high osmolality in the restricted basal spaces pulls water from the cell. The solution that emerges from these two restricted spaces—and enters the interstitial space—is only slightly hypertonic (virtually isotonic) compared with the luminal solution.

Ultimately, these cascades must affect the rates at which specific solutes move through transporters or channels.

Increased Synthesis (or Degradation) of Transport Proteins One approach for modifying transport activity is to change the number of transport molecules in the cell. For example, the hormone aldosterone directly or indirectly increases the transcription rate of genes that encode Na-K pump subunits, thereby increasing Na-K pump synthesis in the distal nephron of the kidney.

Recruitment of Transport Proteins to the Cell Membrane Cells can also change the functional activity of transporters by storing some of them in an intracellular organelle "pool" and then inserting them into the cell membrane. For example, histamine causes cytoplasmic "tubulovesicles" containing H-K pumps (the pool) to fuse with the apical membrane of gastric parietal cells, thereby initiating gastric acid secretion.

Post-translational Modification of Preexisting Transport Proteins Another approach for modulating the transporter rate is to change the activity of preexisting transport proteins. For example, increases in the level of intracellular cyclic adenosine monophosphate (cAMP) enhance the phosphorylation of apical membrane Cl^- channels that are involved in NaCl secretion by intestinal and airway epithelia. The cystic fibrosis gene product (CFTR) is a Cl^- channel whose function is regulated by phosphorylation. A defect in the regulation of apical membrane Cl^- channels is the primary physiological abnormality in cystic fibrosis.

Changes in the Paracellular Pathway The passive movement of solutes across the tight junction can contribute to either "forward" transepithelial movement of the solute or backleak of the solute, depending on the solute gradients. Thus, the epithelium can modulate net transport by changing the permeability of the paracellular pathway. For example, the Na^+ permeability of the tight junctions of the proximal tubule increases when ECF volume increases. This increase in the permeability of the paracellular pathway may lower net Na^+ reabsorption because of increased backleak of absorbed Na^+ from the lateral interspace, across the tight junction, and into the lumen.

Luminal Supply of Transported Species Changes in the concentration of transported solutes can have profound effects on rates of net solute transport. As fluid moves along the renal proximal tubule, for example, the very process of glucose absorption depletes glucose from the lumen, thereby slowing further glucose absorption. Increasing the rate at which fresh, high-glucose fluid enters the proximal tubule lumen raises the glucose concentration at the site of glucose uptake and thus increases the rate of glucose absorption.

REFERENCES

Books and Reviews
Alper SL: The band 3–related anion exchanger (AE) gene family. Annu Rev Physiol 1991; 53:549-564.
Boyer PD: The ATP synthase—a splendid molecular machine. Annu Rev Biochem 1997; 66:717-749.

Frizzell RA (guest editor of special issue): Physiology of cystic fibrosis. Physiol Rev 1999; 79.

Gadsby DC, Dousmanis AG, Nairn AC: ATP hydrolysis cycles the gating of CFTR Cl⁻ channels. Acta Physiol Scand Suppl 1998; 43:247-256.

Kaplan MR, Mount DB, Delpire E, et al: Molecular mechanisms of NaCl cotransport. Annu Rev Physiol 1996; 58:649-668.

Lang F, Busch GL, Ritter M, et al: Functional significance of cell volume regulatory mechanisms. Physiol Rev 1998; 78:247-306.

Palacin M, Estevez R, Bertran J, Zorzano A: Molecular biology of mammalian plasma membrane amino acid transporters. Physiol Rev 1998; 78:969-1054.

Steel A, Hediger MA: The molecular physiology of sodium- and proton-coupled solute transporters. News Physiol Sci 1998; 13:123-131.

Journal Articles

Canessa CM, Schild L, Buell G, et al: Amiloride-sensitive epithelial Na⁺ channel is made of three homologous subunits. Nature 1994; 367:463-467.

Hediger MA, Coady MJ, Ikeda IS, Wright EM: Expression cloning and cDNA sequencing of the Na⁺/glucose transporter. Nature 1987; 330:379-381.

Preston GM, Agre P: Isolation of the cDNA for erythrocyte integral membrane protein of 28 kilodaltons: Member of an ancient channel family. Proc Natl Acad Sci USA 1991; 88:1110-1114.

Skou JC: The influence of some cations on an adenosine triphosphatase from peripheral nerves. Biochim Biophys Acta 1957; 23:394-401.

CHAPTER 6

ELECTROPHYSIOLOGY OF THE CELL MEMBRANE

Edward G. Moczydlowski

Physics is concerned with the fundamental nature of matter and energy, whereas the goal of medical physiology is to understand the workings of living tissue. Despite their different perspectives, physics and physiology share common historical roots in the early investigations of charge and electricity. In the late 1700s, Luigi Galvani, a professor of anatomy in Bologna, Italy, used the leg muscles of a dissected frog to assay the presence of electrical charge stored in various ingenious devices that were the predecessors of modern capacitors and batteries. He observed that frog legs vigorously contracted when electrical stimulation was applied either directly to the leg muscle or to the nerves leading to the muscle (Fig. 6-1). Such early physiological experiments contributed to the development of electromagnetic theory in physics and electrophysiological theory in biology.

The phenomenon of "animal electricity" is central to the understanding of physiological processes. Throughout this book, we will describe many basic functions of tissues and organs in terms of electrical signals mediated by cell membranes. Whereas electrical currents in a metal wire are conducted by the flow of electrons, electrical currents across cell membranes are carried by the major inorganic ions of physiological fluids: Ca^{2+}, Na^+, K^+, Cl^-, and HCO_3^-. Many concepts and terms used in cellular electrophysiology are the same as those used to describe electrical circuits. At the molecular level, electrical current across cell membranes flows through three unique classes of integral membrane proteins (see Chapter 2): ion channels, electrogenic ion transporters, and electrogenic ion pumps. The flow of ions through specific types of channels is the basis of electrical signals that underlie neuronal activity and animal behavior. Opening and closing of such channels is the fundamental process behind electrical phenomena such as the nerve impulse, the heartbeat, and sensory perception. Channel proteins are also intimately involved in hormone secretion, ionic homeostasis, osmoregulation, and regulation of muscle contractility.

This chapter begins with a review of basic principles of electricity and introduces the essentials of electrophysiology. We also discuss the molecular biology of ion channels and provide an overview of channel structure and function.

IONIC BASIS OF MEMBRANE POTENTIALS

Principles of electrostatics explain why aqueous pores formed by channel proteins are needed for ion diffusion across cell membranes

The plasma membranes of most living cells are electrically polarized, as indicated by the presence of a transmembrane voltage—or a **membrane potential**—in the range of 0.1 V. In Chapter 5, we discussed how the energy stored in this miniature battery can drive a variety of transmembrane transport processes. Electrically excitable cells such as brain neurons and heart myocytes also use this energy for signaling purposes. The brief electrical impulses produced by such cells are called **action potentials**. To explain these electrophysiological phenomena, we begin with a basic review of electrical energy.

Atoms consist of negatively (−) and positively (+) charged elementary particles, such as electrons (e^-) and protons (H^+), as well as electrically neutral particles (neutrons). Charges of the same sign repel each other, and those of opposite sign attract. Charge is measured in units of **coulombs** (C). The **unitary charge** of one electron or proton is denoted by e_0 and is equal to 1.6022×10^{-19} C. Ions in solution have a charge valence (z) that is an integral number of elementary charges; for example, $z = +2$ for Ca^{2+}, $z = +1$ for K^+, and $z = -1$ for Cl^-. The charge of a single ion (q_0), measured in coulombs, is the product of its valence and the elementary charge:

$$q_0 = ze_0 \qquad \text{(6-1)}$$

In an aqueous solution or a bulk volume of matter, the number of positive and negative charges is always equal. Charge is also conserved in any chemical reaction.

The attractive electrostatic force between two ions that have valences of z_1 and z_2 can be obtained from Coulomb's law. This force (**F**) is proportional to the product of these valences and inversely proportional to the square of the distance (r) between the two. The force is also inversely proportional to a dimensionless term called the **dielectric constant** (ε):

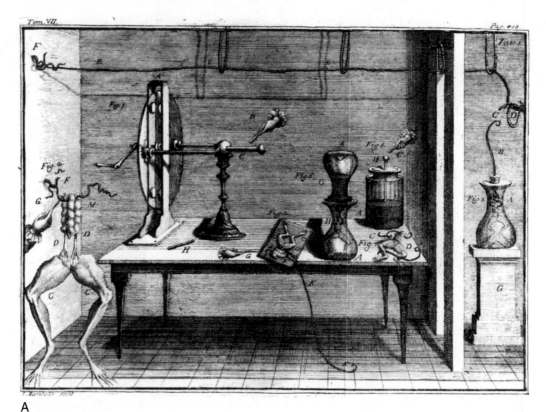

A

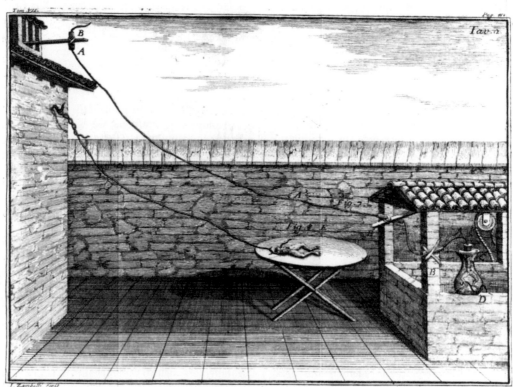

B

$$F \propto \frac{z_1 \cdot z_2}{\varepsilon r^2} \qquad (6\text{-}2)$$

Because the dielectric constant of water is ~40-fold greater than that of the hydrocarbon interior of the cell membrane, the electrostatic force between ions is reduced by a factor of ~40 in water compared with membrane lipid.

If we were to move the Na^+ ion from the extracellular to the intracellular fluid without the aid of any proteins, the Na^+ would have to cross the membrane by "dissolving" in the lipids of the bilayer. However, the energy required to transfer the Na^+ ion from water (high ε) to the interior of a phospholipid membrane (low ε) is ~36 kcal/mol. This value is 60-fold higher than molecular thermal energy at room temperature. Thus, the probability that an ion would dissolve in the bilayer (i.e., partition from an aqueous solution into the lipid interior of a cell membrane) is essentially zero. This analysis explains why inorganic ions cannot readily cross a phospholipid membrane without the aid of other molecules such as specialized transporters or channel proteins, which provide a favorable polar environment for the ion as it moves across the membrane (Fig. 6-2).

Membrane potentials can be measured by use of microelectrodes and voltage-sensitive dyes

The voltage difference across the cell membrane, or the **membrane potential** (V_m), is the difference between the electrical potential in the cytoplasm (Ψ_i) and the electrical potential in the extracellular space (Ψ_o). Figure 6-3A shows how to measure V_m with an intracellular electrode. The sharp tip of a microelectrode is gently inserted into the cell and measures the transmembrane potential with respect to the electrical potential of the extracellular solution, defined as ground (i.e., $\Psi_o = 0$). If the cell membrane is not damaged by electrode impalement and the impaled membrane seals tightly around the glass, this technique provides an accurate measurement of V_m. Such a voltage measurement is called an **intracellular recording**.

For an amphibian or mammalian skeletal muscle cell, resting V_m is typically about −90 mV, meaning that the interior of the resting cell is ~90 mV more negative than the exterior. There is a simple relationship between the electrical potential difference across a membrane and another parameter, the **electrical field** (E):

$$E = \frac{V_m \leftarrow \text{ Electrical potential difference}}{a \leftarrow \text{ Distance across the membrane}} \quad (6\text{-}3)$$

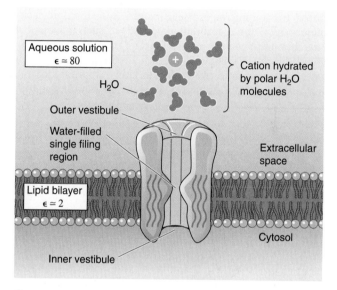

Figure 6-2   Formation of an aqueous pore by an ion channel. The dielectric constant of water ($\varepsilon = 80$) is ~40-fold higher than the dielectric constant of the lipid bilayer ($\varepsilon = 2$).

Figure 6-1   Early electrophysiological experiments of Galvani. **A,** Electrical stimulation of a dissected frog with diverse sources of electricity. On the center of the table is a board with a dissected frog that has been prepared for an experiment (Fig. Ω). A hand with a charged metal rod (G) is about to touch the sacral nerves (D), contracting the limbs (C). A metal wire (F) penetrates the spinal cord; a second metal wire (K) grounds the first wire to the floor. On the left side of the table (Fig. 1) is a large "electrical machine" with a rotating disk (A), a conductor (C), and a hand holding a metal rod (B) that is about to be charged. On the extreme left of the room (Fig. 2), a dissected frog is suspended from an iron wire that penetrates the spinal cord (F); the wire is attached to the wall by a hook. A hand with a charged metal rod (G) is touching the wire, stimulating the sacral nerves (D) and causing the legs (C) to twitch. Outside the room on the extreme right side (Fig. 3) is a frog in a glass jar (A). Emerging from the glass jar is an iron wire (B) that is attached at one end to a hook on the frog and ends in a hook (C) in the air. A silk loop (D) near this hook connects to a long conductor (F) that runs near the ceiling to a hook in the wall at the extreme left of the main room. At the far right/front of the table in the main room (Fig. 4) is a dissected frog with one conductor connected to a nerve (C) and another connected to a muscle (D). Just behind this frog (Fig. 5) is a "Leiden jar" (A) containing small lead shot used by hunters. A hand with a charged metal rod (C) is about to touch a conductor (B) emerging from the jar. To the left of the Leiden jar (Fig. 6) is an inverted jar (A) with lead shot (C). This jar sits on top of a similar jar (B) containing a suspended, dissected frog and is connected by a conductor to the lead shot in the upper jar. The legs of the frog are grounded to lead shot near the bottom of the jar. **B,** Electrical stimulation of the leg muscles of a dissected frog by "natural electricity" (i.e., lightning). In one experiment (Fig. 7), an iron wire (A) runs from near the roof, through several insulating glass tubes (B), to a flask (C) that contains a freshly dissected frog. A second wire (D) grounds the frog's legs to the water in the well. In a second experiment (Fig. 8), a noninsulated wire extends from an iron hook fastened to the wall and to the spinal cord of a frog (E), which is on a table coated with oil. (*From Galvani L: De viribus electricitatis in motu musculari commentarius Aloysii Galvani, Bononiae. New Haven, CT: Yale University, Harvey Cushing/John Hay Whitney Medical Library, 1791.*)

Accordingly, for a V_m of -0.1 V and a membrane thickness of $a = 4$ nm (i.e., 40×10^{-8} cm), the magnitude of the electrical field is ~250,000 V/cm. Thus, despite the small transmembrane *voltage,* cell membranes actually sustain a very large electrical *field.* Later, we discuss how this electrical field influences the activity of a particular class of membrane signaling proteins called voltage-sensitive ion channels (see Chapter 7).

Skeletal muscle cells, cardiac cells, and neurons typically have resting membrane potentials of approximately -60 to -90 mV; smooth muscle cells have membrane potentials in the range of -55 mV; and the V_m of the human erythrocyte is only about -9 mV. However, certain bacteria and plant cells have transmembrane voltages as large as -200 mV. For very small cells such as erythrocytes, small intracellular organelles such as mitochondria, and fine processes such as the synaptic endings of neurons, V_m cannot be directly measured with a microelectrode. Instead, spectroscopic techniques allow the membrane potentials of such inaccessible membranes to be measured indirectly (Fig. 6-3B). This technique involves labeling of the cell or membrane with an appropriate organic dye molecule and monitoring of the absorption or fluorescence of the dye. The optical signal of

the dye molecule can be independently calibrated as a function of V_m. Whether V_m is measured directly by a microelectrode or indirectly by a spectroscopic technique, virtually all biological membranes have a nonzero membrane potential. This transmembrane voltage is an important determinant of any physiological transport process that involves the movement of charge.

Measurements of V_m have shown that many types of cells are electrically excitable. Examples of excitable cells are neurons, muscle fibers, heart cells, and secretory cells of the pancreas. In such cells, V_m exhibits characteristic time-dependent changes in response to electrical or chemical stimulation. When the cell body, or soma, of a neuron is electrically stimulated, electrical and optical methods for measuring V_m detect an almost identical response at the cell body (Fig. 6-3C). The optical method provides the additional insight that the V_m changes are similar but delayed in the more distant neuronal processes that are inaccessible to a microelectrode (Fig. 6-3D). When the cell is not undergoing such active responses, V_m usually remains at a steady value that is called the **resting potential.** In the next section, we discuss the origin of the membrane potential and lay the groundwork for understanding its active responses.

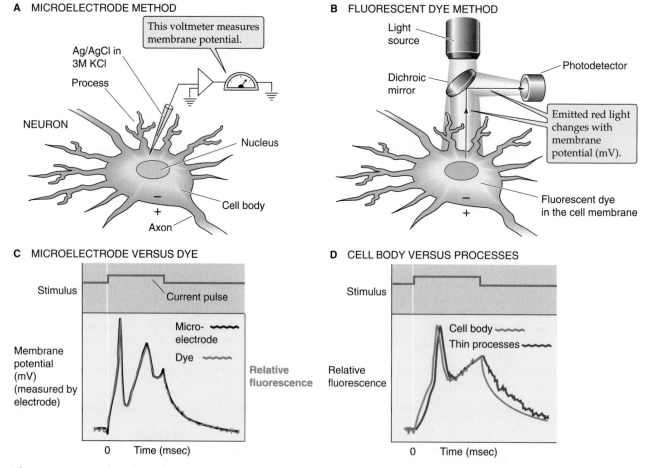

Figure 6-3 Recording of membrane potential. (**C** and **D,** Data modified from Grinvald A: Real-time optical mapping of neuronal activity: From single growth cones to the intact mammalian brain. Annu Rev Neurosci 1985; 8:263-305. © Annual Reviews www.annualreviews. org.)

Membrane potential is generated by ion gradients

In Chapter 5, we introduced the concept that some integral membrane proteins are electrogenic transporters in that they generate an electrical current that sets up an electrical potential across the membrane. One class of electrogenic transporters includes the adenosine triphosphate (ATP)–dependent *ion pumps*. These proteins use the energy of ATP hydrolysis to produce and to maintain concentration gradients of ions across cell membranes. In animal cells, the Na-K pump and Ca^{2+} pump are responsible for maintaining normal gradients of Na^+, K^+, and Ca^{2+}. The reactions catalyzed by these ion transport enzymes are electrogenic because they lead to separation of charge across the membrane. For example, enzymatic turnover of the Na-K pump results in the translocation of three Na^+ ions out of the cell and two K^+ ions into the cell, with a net movement of one positive charge out of the cell. In addition to electrogenic pumps, cells may express *secondary active transporters* that are electrogenic, such as the Na^+/glucose cotransporter (see Chapter 5).

It may seem that the inside negative V_m originates from the continuous pumping of positive charges out of the cell by the electrogenic Na-K pump. The resting potential of large cells—whose surface-to-volume ratio is so large that ion gradients run down slowly—is maintained for a long time even when metabolic poisons block ATP-dependent energy metabolism. This finding implies that an ATP-dependent pump is not the immediate energy source underlying the membrane potential. Indeed, the squid giant axon normally has a resting potential of −60 mV. When the Na-K pump in the giant axon membrane is specifically inhibited with a cardiac glycoside (see Chapter 5), the immediate positive shift in V_m is only 1.4 mV. Thus, in most cases, the direct contribution of the Na-K pump to the resting V_m is very small.

In contrast, many experiments have shown that cell membrane potentials depend on ionic **concentration gradients**. In a classic experiment, Paul Horowicz and Alan Hodgkin measured the V_m of a frog muscle fiber with an intracellular microelectrode. The muscle fiber was bathed in a modified physiological solution in which SO_4^{2-} replaced Cl^-, a manipulation that eliminates the contribution of anions to V_m. In the presence of normal extracellular concentrations of K^+ and Na^+ for amphibians ($[K^+]_o = 2.5$ mM and $[Na^+]_o = 120$ mM), the frog muscle fiber has a resting V_m of approximately −94 mV. As $[K^+]_o$ is increased above 2.5 mM by substitution of K^+ for Na^+, V_m shifts in the positive direction. As $[K^+]_o$ is decreased below 2.5 mM, V_m becomes more negative (Fig. 6-4). For $[K^+]_o$ values greater than 10 mM, the V_m measured in Figure 6-4 is approximately a linear function of the *logarithm* of $[K^+]_o$. Numerous experiments of this kind have demonstrated that the *immediate* energy source of the membrane potential is not the active pumping of ions but rather the potential energy stored in the ion concentration gradients themselves. Of course, it is the ion pumps—and the secondary active transporters that derive their energy from these pumps—that are responsible for generating and maintaining these ion gradients.

One way to investigate the role of ion gradients in determining V_m is to study this phenomenon in an in vitro (cell-

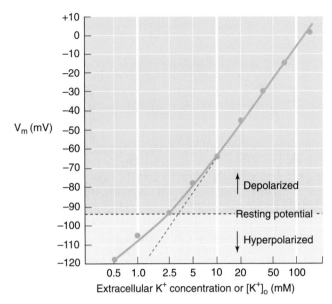

Figure 6-4 Dependence of resting potential on extracellular K^+ concentration in a frog muscle fiber. The slope of the linear part of the curve is 58 mV for a 10-fold increase in $[K^+]_o$. Note that the horizontal axis for $[K^+]_o$ is plotted using a logarithmic scale. *(Data from Hodgkin AL, Horowicz P: The influence of potassium and chloride ions on the membrane potential of single muscle fibers. J Physiol [Lond] 1959; 148:127-160.)*

free) system. Many investigators have used an artificial model of a cell membrane called a **planar lipid bilayer**. This system consists of a partition with a hole ~200 μm in diameter that separates two chambers filled with aqueous solutions (Fig. 6-5). It is possible to paint a planar lipid bilayer having a thickness of only ~4 nm across the hole, thereby sealing the partition. By incorporating membrane proteins and other molecules into planar bilayers, one can study the essential characteristics of their function in isolation from the complex metabolism of living cells. Transmembrane voltage can be measured across a planar bilayer with a voltmeter connected to a pair of Ag/AgCl electrodes that are in electrical contact with the solution on each side of the membrane through salt bridges. This experimental arrangement is much like an intracellular voltage recording, except that both sides of the membrane are completely accessible to manipulation.

The ionic composition of the two chambers on opposite sides of the bilayer can be adjusted to simulate cellular concentration gradients. Suppose that we put 4 mM KCl on the left side of the bilayer and 155 mM KCl on the right side to mimic, respectively, the external and internal concentrations of K^+ for a mammalian muscle cell. To eliminate the osmotic flow of water between the two compartments (see Chapter 5), we also add a sufficient amount of a nonelectrolyte (e.g., mannitol) to the side with 4 mM KCl. We can make the membrane selectively permeable to K^+ by introducing purified K^+ channels or K^+ ionophores into the membrane. Assuming that the K^+ channels are in an open state and are impermeable to Cl^-, the right ("internal") compartment quickly becomes electrically negative with respect to the left ("external") compartment because positive charge (i.e., K^+) diffuses from high to low concentration. However, as the

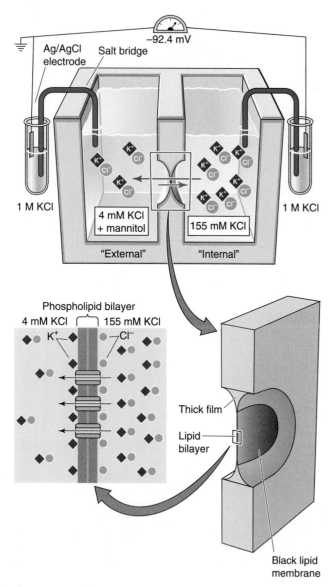

Figure 6-5 Diffusion potential across a planar lipid bilayer containing a K⁺-selective channel.

For mammalian cells, nernst potentials for ions typically range from −100 mV for K⁺ to +100 mV for Ca²⁺

The model system of a planar bilayer (impermeable membrane), unequal salt solutions (ionic gradient), and an ion-selective channel (conductance pathway) contains the minimal components essential for generating a membrane potential. The hydrophobic membrane bilayer is a formidable barrier to inorganic ions and is also a poor conductor of electricity. Poor conductors are said to have a high **resistance** to electrical current, in this case, ionic current. On the other hand, ion channels act as molecular conductors of ions. They introduce a **conductance pathway** into the membrane and lower its resistance.

In the planar bilayer experiment of Figure 6-5, V_m originates from the diffusion of K⁺ down its concentration gradient. Membrane potentials that arise by this mechanism are called **diffusion potentials**. At equilibrium, the diffusion potential of an ion is the same as the equilibrium potential (E_X) given by the **Nernst equation** previously introduced as Equation 5-8.

$$E_X = -\frac{RT}{z_X F}\ln\frac{[X]_i}{[X]_o} \qquad (6\text{-}4)$$

The Nernst equation predicts the equilibrium membrane potential for any concentration gradient of a particular ion across a membrane. E_X is often simply referred to as the **Nernst potential**. The Nernst potentials for K⁺, Na⁺, Ca²⁺, and Cl⁻, respectively, are written as E_K, E_{Na}, E_{Ca}, and E_{Cl}.

The linear portion of the plot of V_m versus the logarithm of $[K^+]_o$ for a frog muscle cell (Fig. 6-4) has a **slope** that is ∼58.1 mV for a 10-fold change in $[K^+]_o$, as predicted by the Nernst equation. Indeed, if we insert the appropriate values for R and F into Equation 6-4, select a temperature of 20°C, and convert the logarithm base e (ln) to the logarithm base 10 ($\log_{10}$), we obtain a coefficient of −58.1 mV, and the Nernst equation becomes

$$E_K = (-58.1\,\text{mV})\log_{10}\frac{[K^+]_i}{[K^+]_o} \qquad (6\text{-}5)$$

For a negative ion such as Cl⁻, where $z = -1$, the sign of the slope is positive:

$$E_{Cl} = (+58.1\,\text{mV})\log_{10}\frac{[Cl^-]_i}{[Cl^-]_o} \qquad (6\text{-}6)$$

For Ca²⁺ ($z = +2$), the slope is half of −58.1 mV, or approximately −30 mV. Note that a Nernst slope of 58.1 mV is the value for a univalent ion at 20°C. For mammalian cells at 37°C, this value is 61.5 mV.

At $[K^+]_o$ values above ∼10 mM, the magnitude of V_m and the slope of the plot in Figure 6-4 are virtually the same as those predicted by the Nernst equation (Equation 6-5), suggesting that the resting V_m of the muscle cell is almost equal to the K⁺ diffusion potential. When V_m follows the Nernst

negative voltage develops in the right compartment, the negativity opposes further K⁺ efflux from the right compartment. Eventually, the voltage difference across the membrane becomes so negative as to halt further net K⁺ movement. At this point, the system is in **equilibrium**, and the transmembrane voltage reaches a value of 92.4 mV, right-side negative. In the process of generating the transmembrane voltage, a separation of charge has occurred in such a way that the excess *positive* charge on the left side (low [K⁺]) balances the same excess *negative* charge on the right side (high [K⁺]). Thus, the stable voltage difference (−92.4 mV) arises from the separation of K⁺ ions from their counterions (in this case Cl⁻) across the bilayer membrane.

TABLE 6-1 Ion Concentration Gradients in Mammalian Cells

Ion (X)	$[X]_{out}$ (mM)	$[X]_{in}$ (mM)	$[X]_{out}/[X]_{in}$	V_x^* (mV)
Skeletal muscle				
K^+	4.5	155	0.026	−95
Na^+	145	12	12	+67
Ca^{2+}	1.0	10^{-4}	10,000	+123
Cl^-	116	4.2	29	−89
HCO_3^-	24	12	2	−19
Most other cells				
K^+	4.5	120	0.038	−88
Na^+	145.4	15	9.67	+61
Ca^{2+}	1.0	10^{-4}	10,000	+123
Cl^-	116	20	5.8	−47
HCO_3^-	24	15	1.6	−13

*Nernst equilibrium potential for ion X at 37°C.

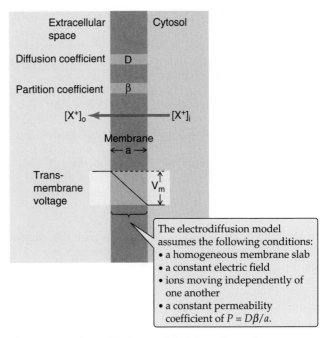

Figure 6-6 Electrodiffusion model of the cell membrane.

equation for K^+, the membrane is said to behave like a potassium electrode because ion-specific electrodes monitor ion concentrations according to the Nernst equation.

Table 6-1 lists the expected Nernst potentials for K^+, Na^+, Ca^{2+}, Cl^-, and HCO_3^- as calculated from the known concentration gradients of these physiologically important inorganic ions for mammalian skeletal muscle and a typical non-muscle cell. For a mammalian muscle cell with a V_m of −80 mV, E_K is ~15 mV more negative than V_m, whereas E_{Na} and E_{Ca} are about +67 and +123 mV, respectively, far more positive than V_m. E_{Cl} is ~9 mV more negative than V_m in muscle cells but slightly more positive than the typical V_m of −60 mV in most other cells.

What determines whether the cell membrane potential follows the Nernst equation for K^+ or Cl^- rather than that for Na^+ or Ca^{2+}? As we shall see in the next two sections, the membrane potential is determined by the relative permeabilities of the cell membrane to the various ions.

Currents carried by ions across membranes depend on the concentration of ions on both sides of the membrane, the membrane potential, and the permeability of the membrane to each ion

Years before ion channel proteins were discovered, physiologists devised a simple but powerful way to predict the membrane potential, even if several different kinds of permeable ions are present at the same time. The first step, which we discuss in this section, is to compute an ionic current, that

is, the movement of a single ion species through the membrane. The second step, which we describe in the following section, is to obtain V_m by summating the currents carried by each species of ion present, assuming that each species moves independently of the others.

The process of ion permeation through the membrane is called **electrodiffusion** because both electrical and concentration gradients are responsible for the ionic current. To a first approximation, the permeation of ions through most channel proteins behaves as though the flow of these ions follows a model based on the Nernst-Planck electrodiffusion theory, which was first applied to the diffusion of ions in simple solutions. This theory leads to an important equation in medical physiology called the constant-field equation, which predicts how V_m will respond to changes in ion concentration gradients or membrane permeability. Before introducing this equation, we first consider some important underlying concepts and assumptions.

Without knowing the molecular basis for ion movement through the membrane, we can treat the membrane as a "black box" characterized by a few fundamental parameters (Fig. 6-6). We must assume that the rate of ion movement through the membrane depends on (1) the external and internal concentrations of the ion X ($[X]_o$ and $[X]_i$, respectively), (2) the transmembrane voltage (V_m), and (3) a permeability coefficient for the ion X (P_X). In addition, we make four major assumptions about how the ion X behaves in the membrane:

The membrane is a homogeneous medium with a thickness a.

The voltage difference varies linearly with distance across the membrane (Fig. 6-6). This assumption is equivalent to stating that the *electrical field*—that is, the change in voltage with distance—is constant throughout the thickness of the membrane. This requirement is therefore called the **constant-field assumption**.

The movement of an ion through the membrane is independent of the movement of any other ions. This assumption is called the **independence principle**.

The permeability coefficient P_X is a constant (i.e., it does not vary with the chemical or electrical driving forces). P_X (*units:* cm/s) is defined as $P_X = D_X\beta/a$. D_X is the diffusion coefficient for the ion in the membrane, β is the membrane/water partition coefficient for the ion, and a is the thickness of the membrane. Thus, P_X describes the ability of an ion to dissolve in the membrane (as described by β) and to diffuse from one side to the other (as described by D_X) over the distance a.

With these assumptions, we can calculate the current carried by a single ion X (I_X) through the membrane by using the basic physical laws that govern (1) the movement of molecules in solution (Fick's law of diffusion; see Equation 5-13), (2) the movement of charged particles in an **electrical field** (electrophoresis), and (3) the direct proportionality of current to voltage (Ohm's law). The result is the **Goldman-Hodgkin-Katz (GHK)** *current* equation, named after the pioneering electrophysiologists who applied the constant-field assumption to Nernst-Planck electrodiffusion:

$$I_X = \frac{z^2 F^2 V_m P_X}{RT}\left(\frac{[X]_i - [X]_o e^{(-zFV_m/RT)}}{1 - e^{(-zFV_m/RT)}}\right) \quad \text{(6-7)}$$

I_X, or the rate of ions moving through the membrane, has the same units as electrical current: amperes (coulombs per second). Thus, the GHK current equation relates the current of ion X through the membrane to the internal and external concentrations of X, the transmembrane voltage, and the

permeability of the membrane to X. The GHK equation thus allows us to predict how the current carried by X depends on V_m. This **current-voltage (*I-V*) relationship** is important for understanding how ionic currents flow into and out of cells.

Figure 6-7A shows how the K^+ current (I_K) depends on V_m, as predicted by Equation 6-7 for the normal internal (155 mM) and external (4.5 mM) concentrations of K^+. By convention, a current of ions flowing into the cell (**inward current**) is defined in electrophysiology as a negative-going current, and a current flowing out of the cell (**outward current**) is defined as a positive current. (As in physics, the direction of current is always the direction of movement of positive charge. This convention means that an inward flow of Cl^- is an outward current.) For the case of 155 mM K^+ inside the cell and 4.5 mM K^+ outside the cell, an inward current is predicted at voltages that are more negative than −95 mV, and an outward current is predicted at voltages that are more positive than −95 mV (Fig. 6-7A). The value of −95 mV is called the **reversal potential** (V_{rev}) because it is precisely at this voltage that the direction of current reverses (i.e., the net current equals zero). If we set I_K equal to zero in Equation 6-7 and solve for V_{rev}, we find that the GHK current equation reduces to the Nernst equation for K^+ (Equation 6-5). Thus, the GHK current equation for an ion X predicts a reversal potential (V_{rev}) equal to the Nernst potential (E_X) for that ion; that is, the current is zero when the ion is in electrochemical equilibrium. At V_m values more negative than V_{rev}, the net driving force on a cation is inward; at voltages that are more positive than V_{rev}, the net driving force is outward.

Figure 6-7B shows the analogous *I-V* relationship predicted by Equation 6-7 for physiological concentrations of Na^+. In this case, the Na^+ current (I_{Na}) is inward at V_m values

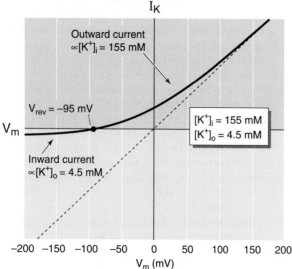

A POTASSIUM CURRENT

I_K

Outward current ∝$[K^+]_i$ = 155 mM

V_{rev} = −95 mV

V_m

Inward current ∝$[K^+]_o$ = 4.5 mM

$[K^+]_i$ = 155 mM
$[K^+]_o$ = 4.5 mM

−200 −150 −100 −50 0 50 100 150 200
V_m (mV)

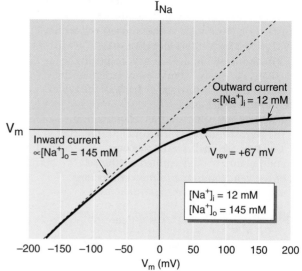

B SODIUM CURRENT

I_{Na}

Outward current ∝$[Na^+]_i$ = 12 mM

V_m

Inward current ∝$[Na^+]_o$ = 145 mM

V_{rev} = +67 mV

$[Na^+]_i$ = 12 mM
$[Na^+]_o$ = 145 mM

−200 −150 −100 −50 0 50 100 150 200
V_m (mV)

Figure 6-7 Current-voltage relationships predicted by the GHK current equation. **A,** The curve is the K^+ current predicted from the GHK equation (Equation 7)—assuming that the membrane is perfectly selective for K^+—for a $[K^+]_i$ of 155 mM and a $[K^+]_o$ of 4.5 mM. The *dashed line* represents the current that can be expected if both $[K^+]_i$ and $[K^+]_o$ were 155 mM (Ohm's law). **B,** The curve is the Na^+ current predicted from the GHK equation—assuming that the membrane is perfectly selective for Na^+—for a $[Na^+]_i$ of 12 mM and a $[Na^+]_o$ of 145 mM. The *dashed line* represents the current that can be expected if both $[Na^+]_i$ and $[Na^+]_o$ were 145 mM.

more negative than V_{rev} (+67 mV) and outward at voltages that are more positive than this reversal potential. Here again, V_{rev} is the same as the Nernst potential, in this case, E_{Na}.

Membrane potential depends on ionic concentration gradients and permeabilities

In the preceding section, we discussed how to use the GHK current equation to predict the current carried by any *single* ion, such as K^+ or Na^+. If the membrane is permeable to the monovalent ions K^+, Na^+, and Cl^-—and only to these ions—the **total ionic current** carried by these ions across the membrane is the sum of the individual ionic currents:

$$I_{total} = I_K + I_{Na} + I_{Cl} \qquad (6\text{-}8)$$

The individual ionic currents given by Equation 6-7 can be substituted into the right-hand side of Equation 6-8. Note that for the sake of simplicity, we have not considered currents carried by electrogenic pumps or other ion transporters; we could have added extra "current" terms for such electrogenic transporters. At the resting membrane potential (i.e., V_m is equal to V_{rev}), the sum of all ion currents is zero (i.e., $I_{total} = 0$). When we set I_{total} to zero in the expanded Equation 6-8 and solve for V_{rev}, we get an expression known as the **GHK *voltage* equation** or the **constant-field equation**:

$$V_{rev} = \frac{RT}{F} \ln\left(\frac{P_K[K^+]_o + P_{Na}[Na^+]_o + P_{Cl}[Cl^-]_i}{P_K[K^+]_i + P_{Na}[Na^+]_i + P_{Cl}[Cl^-]_o} \right) \qquad (6\text{-}9)$$

Because we derived Equation 6-9 for the case of $I_{total} = 0$, it is valid only when zero net current is flowing across the membrane. This zero net current flow is the steady-state condition that exists for the cellular *resting* potential, that is, when V_m equals V_{rev}. The logarithmic term of Equation 6-9 indicates that resting V_m depends on the concentration gradients and the permeabilities of the various ions. However, resting V_m depends primarily on the concentrations of the most permeant ion.

The principles underlying Equation 6-9 show why the plot of V_m versus $[K^+]_o$ in Figure 6-4, which summarizes data obtained from a frog muscle cell, bends away from the idealized Nernst slope at very low values of $[K^+]_o$. Imagine that we expose a mammalian muscle cell to a range of $[K^+]_o$ values, always substituting extracellular K^+ for Na^+, or vice versa, so that the sum of $[K^+]_o$ and $[Na^+]_o$ is kept fixed at its physiological value of 4.5 + 145 = 149.5 mM. To simplify matters, we assume that the membrane permeability to Cl^- is very small (i.e., $P_{Cl} \cong 0$). We can also rearrange Equation 6-9 by dividing the numerator and denominator by P_K and representing the ratio P_{Na}/P_K as α. At 37°C, this simplified equation becomes

$$V_{rev} = (61.5\,\text{mV}) \times \log_{10}\left(\frac{[K^+]_o + \alpha[Na^+]_o}{[K^+]_i + \alpha[Na^+]_i} \right) \qquad (6\text{-}10)$$

Figure 6-8 shows that when α is zero—that is, when the membrane is impermeable to Na^+—Equation 6-10 reduces to the Nernst equation for K^+ (Equation 6-4), and the plot

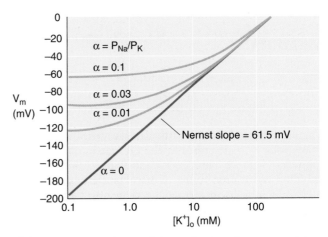

Figure 6-8 Dependence of the resting membrane potential on $[K^+]_o$ and on the P_{Na}/P_K ratio, α. The *blue line* describes an instance in which there is no Na^+ permeability (i.e., $P_{Na}/P_K = 0$). The three *orange curves* describe the V_m predicted by Equation 6-10 for three values of α greater than zero and assumed values of $[Na^+]_o$, $[Na^+]_i$, and $[K^+]_i$ for skeletal muscles, as listed in Table 6-1. The deviation of these orange curves from linearity is greater at low values of $[K^+]_o$, where the $[Na^+]_o$ is relatively larger.

of V_m versus the logarithm of $[K^+]_o$ is linear. If we choose an α of 0.01, however, the plot bends away from the ideal at low $[K^+]_o$ values. This bend reflects the introduction of a slight permeability to Na^+. As we increase this P_{Na} further by increasing α to 0.03 and 0.1, the curvature becomes even more pronounced. Thus, as predicted by Equation 6-10, increasing the permeability of Na^+ relative to K^+ tends to shift V_m in a positive direction, toward E_{Na}. In some skeletal muscle cells, an α of 0.01 best explains the experimental data.

The constant-field equation (Equation 6-9) and simplified relationships derived from it (e.g., Equation 6-10) show that steady-state V_m depends on the concentrations of all permeant ions, weighted according to their relative permeabilities. Another very useful application of the constant-field equation is determination of the ionic selectivity of channels. If the I-V relationship of a particular channel is determined in the presence of known gradients of two different ions, one can solve Equation 6-10 to obtain the permeability ratio, α, of the two ions from the measured value of the reversal potential, V_{rev}.

In general, the resting potential of most vertebrate cells is dominated by high permeability to K^+, which accounts for the observation that the resting V_m is typically close to E_K. The resting permeability to Na^+ and Ca^{2+} is normally very low. Skeletal muscle cells, cardiac cells, and neurons typically have resting membrane potentials ranging from −60 to −90 mV. As discussed in Chapter 7, excitable cells generate action potentials by transiently increasing Na^+ or Ca^{2+} permeability and thus driving V_m in a positive direction toward E_{Na} or E_{Ca}. A few cells, such as vertebrate skeletal muscle fibers, have high permeability to Cl^-, which therefore contributes to the resting V_m. This high permeability also explains why the Cl^- equilibrium potential in skeletal muscle is essentially equivalent to the resting potential (Table 6-1).

ELECTRICAL MODEL OF A CELL MEMBRANE

The cell membrane model includes various ionic conductances and electromotive forces in parallel with a capacitor

The current carried by a particular ion varies with membrane voltage, as described by the I-V relationship for that ion (e.g., Fig. 6-7). This observation suggests that the contribution of each ion to the electrical properties of the cell membrane may be represented by elements of an electrical circuit. The various ionic gradients across the membrane provide a form of stored electrical energy, much like that of a battery. In physics, the voltage source of a battery is known as an **emf** (electromotive force). The equilibrium potential of a given ion can be considered an emf for that ion. Each of these batteries produces its own ionic **current** across the membrane, and the sum of these individual ionic currents is the total ionic current (Equation 6-8). According to **Ohm's law**, the emf or voltage (V) and current (I) are directly related to each other by the **resistance** (R)—or inversely to the reciprocal of resistance, **conductance** (G):

$$V = IR \quad \text{Ohm's law}$$
$$= I/G \quad \quad \text{(6-11)}$$

Thus, the slopes of the lines in Figure 6-7 represent conductances because $I = GV$. In a membrane, we can represent each ionic permeability pathway with an electrical conductance. Ions with high permeability or conductance move through a low-resistance pathway; ions with low permeability move through a high-resistance pathway. For cell membranes, V_m is measured in millivolts, membrane current (I_m) is given in amps per square centimeter of membrane area, and membrane resistance (R_m) has the units of ohms × square centimeter. Membrane conductance (G_m), the reciprocal of membrane resistance, is thus measured in units of ohms^{-1} per square centimeter, which is equivalent to siemens per square centimeter.

Currents of Na^+, K^+, Ca^{2+}, and Cl^- generally flow across the cell membrane through distinct pathways. At the molecular level, these pathways correspond to specific types of ion channel proteins (Fig. 6-9A). It is helpful to model the electrical behavior of cell membranes by a circuit diagram (Fig. 6-9B). The electrical current carried by each ion flows through a separate parallel branch of the circuit that is under the control of a **variable resistor** and an emf. For instance, the variable resistor for K^+ represents the conductance provided by K^+ channels in the membrane (G_K). The emf for K^+ corresponds to E_K. Similar parallel branches of the circuit in Figure 6-9B represent the other physiologically important ions. Each ion provides a component of the total conductance of the membrane, so $G_K + G_{Na} + G_{Ca} + G_{Cl}$ sum to G_m.

The GHK voltage equation (Equation 6-9) predicts steady-state V_m, provided the underlying assumptions are valid. We can also predict steady-state V_m (i.e., when the net current across the membrane is zero) with another, more

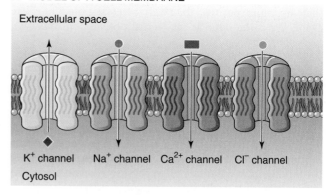

A MODEL OF A CELL MEMBRANE

Extracellular space

K^+ channel Na^+ channel Ca^{2+} channel Cl^- channel

Cytosol

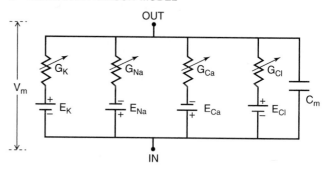

B EQUIVALENT CIRCUIT MODEL

OUT

V_m G_K G_{Na} G_{Ca} G_{Cl} C_m

E_K E_{Na} E_{Ca} E_{Cl}

IN

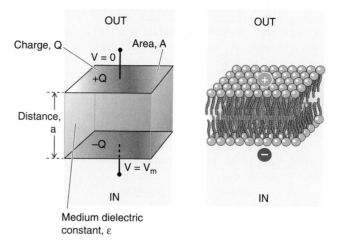

C PARALLEL–PLATE CAPACITOR   LIPID MEMBRANE

OUT   OUT

Charge, Q   Area, A
V = 0
+Q

Distance, a

−Q

V = V_m

IN   IN

Medium dielectric constant, ε

Figure 6-9 Electrical properties of model cell membranes. **A,** Four different ion channels are arranged in parallel in the cell membrane. **B,** The model represents each channel in **A** with a variable resistor. The model represents the Nernst potential for each ion as a battery in series with each variable resistor. Also shown is the membrane capacitance, which is parallel with each of the channels. **C,** On the left is an idealized capacitor, which is formed by two parallel plates, each with an area A and separated by a distance d. On the right is a capacitor that is formed by a piece of lipid membrane. The two *plates* are, in fact, the electrolyte solutions on either side of the membrane.

general equation that assumes channels behave like separate ohmic conductances:

$$V_m = \frac{G_K}{G_m} E_K + \frac{G_{Na}}{G_m} E_{Na} + \frac{G_{Ca}}{G_m} E_{Ca} + \frac{G_{Cl}}{G_m} E_{Cl} \ldots \quad (6\text{-}12)$$

Thus, V_m is the sum of equilibrium potentials (E_X), each weighted by the ion's fractional conductance (e.g., G_X/G_m).

One more parallel element, a **capacitor**, is needed to complete our model of the cell membrane as an electrical circuit. A capacitor is a device that is capable of storing separated charge. Because the lipid bilayer can maintain a separation of charge (i.e., a voltage) across its ~4-nm width, it effectively functions as a capacitor. In physics, a capacitor that is formed by two parallel plates separated by a distance a can be represented by the diagram in Figure 6-9C. When the capacitor is charged, one of the plates bears a charge of $+Q$ and the other plate has a charge of $-Q$. Such a capacitor maintains a potential difference (V) between the plates. **Capacitance (C)** is the magnitude of the charge stored per unit potential difference:

$$C = \frac{Q}{V} \quad (6\text{-}13)$$

Capacitance is measured in units of farads (F); 1 farad = 1 coulomb/volt. For the particular geometry of the parallel-plate capacitor in Figure 6-9C, capacitance is directly proportional to the surface area (A) of one side of a plate, to the dielectric constant of the medium between the two plates (ε), and to the permittivity constant (ε_o), and it is inversely proportional to the distance (a) separating the plates.

$$C = \frac{A \varepsilon \varepsilon_0}{a} \quad (6\text{-}14)$$

Because of its similar geometry, the cell membrane has a capacitance that is analogous to that of the parallel-plate capacitor. The capacitance of 1 cm^2 of most cell membranes is ~1 μF; that is, most membranes have a specific capacitance of 1 μF/cm^2. We can use Equation 6-14 to estimate the thickness of the membrane. If we assume that the average dielectric constant of a biological membrane is $\varepsilon = 5$ (slightly greater than the value of 2 for pure hydrocarbon), Equation 6-14 gives a value of 4.4 nm for a—that is, the thickness of the membrane. This value is quite close to estimates of membrane thickness that have been obtained by other physical techniques.

The separation of relatively few charges across the bilayer capacitance maintains the membrane potential

We can also use the capacitance of the cell membrane to estimate the amount of charge that the membrane actually separates in generating a typical membrane potential. For example, consider a spherical cell with a diameter of 10 μm and a [K$^+$]$_i$ of 100 mM. This cell needs to lose only 0.004% of its K$^+$ to charge the capacitance of the membrane to a voltage of −61.5 mV. This small loss of K$^+$ is clearly insignifi-cant in comparison with a cell's total ionic composition and does not significantly perturb concentration gradients. In general, cell membrane potentials are sustained by a very small separation of charge.

Because of the existence of membrane capacitance, total membrane current has two components (Fig. 6-9), one carried by ions through channels, and the other carried by ions as they charge the membrane capacitance.

Ionic current is directly proportional to the electrochemical driving force (Ohm's law)

Figure 6-10 compares the equilibrium potentials for Na$^+$, K$^+$, Ca^{2+}, and Cl$^-$ with a resting V_m of −80 mV. In our discussion of Figure 6-7, we saw that I_K or I_{Na} becomes zero when V_m equals the reversal potential, which is the same as the E_X or emf for that ion. When V_m is more negative than E_X, the current is negative or inward, whereas when V_m is more positive than E_X, the current is positive or outward. Thus, the ionic current depends on the difference between the actual V_m and E_X. In fact, the ionic current through a given conductance pathway is proportional to the difference ($V_m - E_X$), and the proportionality constant is the ionic conductance (G_X):

$$I_X = G_X(V_m - E_X) \quad (6\text{-}15)$$

This equation simply restates Ohm's law (Equation 6-11). The term ($V_m - E_X$) is often referred to as the **driving force**

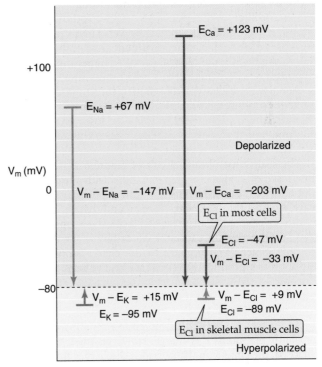

Figure 6-10 Electrochemical driving forces acting on various ions. For each ion, we represent both the equilibrium potential (e.g., E_{Na} = +67 mV) as a horizontal bar and the net driving force for the ion (e.g., $V_m - E_{Na}$ = −147 mV) as an arrow assuming a resting potential (V_m) of −80 mV. The values for the equilibrium potentials are those for mammalian skeletal muscle in Table 6-1 as well as a typical value for E_{Cl} in a non-muscle cell.

in electrophysiology. In our electrical model of the cell membrane (Fig. 6-9), this driving force is represented by the difference between V_m and the emf of the battery. The larger the driving force, the larger the observed current. Returning to the I-V relationship for K^+ in Figure 6-7A, when V_m is more positive than E_K, the driving force is positive, producing an outward (i.e., positive) current. Conversely, at V_m values more negative than E_K, the negative driving force produces an inward current.

In Figure 6-10, the arrows represent the magnitudes and directions of the driving forces for the various ions. For a typical value of the resting potential (−80 mV), the driving force on Ca^{2+} is the largest of the four ions, followed by the driving force on Na^+. In both cases, V_m is more negative than the equilibrium potential and thus draws the positive ion *into* the cell. The driving force on K^+ is small. V_m is more positive than E_K and thus pushes K^+ out of the cell. In muscle, V_m is slightly more positive than E_{Cl} and thus draws the anion inward. In most other cells, however, V_m is more negative than E_{Cl} and pushes the Cl^- out.

Capacitative current is proportional to the rate of voltage change

The idea that ionic channels can be thought of as conductance elements (G_X) and that ionic current (I_X) is proportional to driving force ($V_m - E_X$) provides a framework for understanding the electrical behavior of cell membranes. Current carried by inorganic ions flows through open channels according to the principles of electrodiffusion and Ohm's law, as explained above. However, when V_m is changing—as it does during an action potential—another current due to the membrane capacitance also shapes the electrical responses of cells. This current, which flows only while V_m is changing, is called the capacitative current. How does a capacitor produce a current? When voltage across a capacitor changes, the capacitor either gains or loses charge. This movement of charge onto or off the capacitor is an electrical (i.e., the capacitative) current.

The simple membrane circuit of Figure 6-11A, which is composed of a capacitor (C_m) in parallel with a resistor (R_m) and a switch, can help illustrate how capacitative currents arise. Assume that the switch is open and that the capacitor is initially charged to a voltage of V_0, causing a separation of charge (Q) across the capacitor. According to the definition of capacitance (Equation 6-13), the charge stored by the capacitor is a product of capacitance and voltage.

$$Q = C_m V_0 \qquad (6\text{-}16)$$

As long as the switch in the circuit remains open, the capacitor maintains this charge. However, when the switch is closed, the charge on the capacitor discharges through the resistor, and the voltage difference between the circuit points labeled "In" and "Out" decays from V_0 to a final value of zero (Fig. 6-11B). This voltage decay follows an exponential time course. The time required for the voltage to fall to 37% of its initial value is a characteristic parameter called the **time constant** (τ), which has units of time:

$$\tau = R_m \cdot C_m \qquad (6\text{-}17)$$

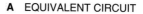

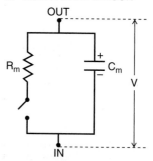

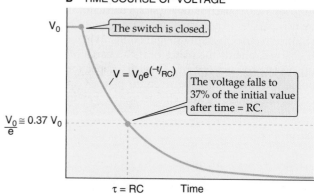

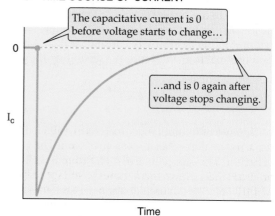

A   EQUIVALENT CIRCUIT

B   TIME COURSE OF VOLTAGE

V_0 ⟵ The switch is closed.

$V = V_0 e^{(-t/RC)}$

The voltage falls to 37% of the initial value after time = RC.

$\dfrac{V_0}{e} \cong 0.37\,V_0$

$\tau = RC$ Time

C   TIME COURSE OF CURRENT

The capacitative current is 0 before voltage starts to change…

0

…and is 0 again after voltage stops changing.

I_C

Time

Figure 6-11   Capacitative current through a resistance-capacitance (RC) circuit.

Thus, the time course of the decay in voltage is

$$V = V_0 e^{-t/RC} \qquad (6\text{-}18)$$

Figure 6-11C shows that the **capacitative current** (I_C) is zero before the switch is closed, when the voltage is stable at V_0. When we close the switch, charge begins to flow rapidly off the capacitor, and the magnitude of I_C is maximal. As the charge on the capacitor gradually falls, the rate at which charge flows off the capacitor gradually falls as well until I_C is zero at "infinite" time. Note, however, that V and I_C relax with the same time constant.

In Figure 6-11, current and voltage change freely. Figure 6-12 shows two related examples in which either current or

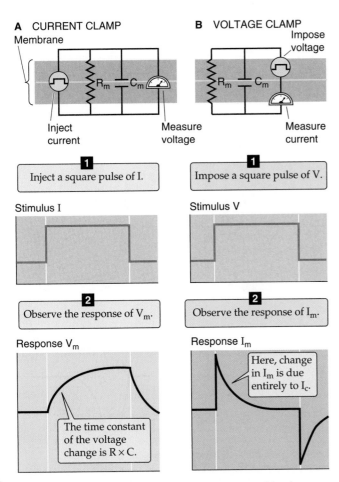

A CURRENT CLAMP

Membrane

Inject current   Measure voltage

1 Inject a square pulse of I.

Stimulus I

2 Observe the response of V_m.

Response V_m

The time constant of the voltage change is R × C.

B VOLTAGE CLAMP

Impose voltage

Measure current

1 Impose a square pulse of V.

Stimulus V

2 Observe the response of I_m.

Response I_m

Here, change in I_m is due entirely to I_C.

Figure 6-12 Voltage and current responses caused by the presence of a membrane capacitance.

voltage is abruptly changed to a fixed value, held constant for a certain time, and returned to the original value. This pattern is called a square pulse. In Figure 6-12A, we control, or "clamp," the current and allow the voltage to follow. When we inject a square pulse of current across the membrane, the voltage changes to a new value with a rounded time course determined by the *RC* value of the membrane. In Figure 6-12B, we clamp voltage and allow the current to follow. When we suddenly change voltage to a new value, a transient capacitative current flows as charge flows onto the capacitor. The capacitative current is maximal at the beginning of the square pulse, when charge flows most rapidly onto the capacitor, and then falls off exponentially with a time constant of *RC*. When we suddenly decrease the voltage to its original value, I_C flows in the direction opposite that observed at the beginning of the pulse. Thus, I_C appears as brief spikes at the beginning and end of the voltage pulse.

A voltage clamp measures currents across cell membranes

Electrophysiologists use a technique called **voltage clamping** to deduce the properties of ion channels. In this method, specialized electronics are used to inject current into the cell to set the membrane voltage to a value that is different from

the resting potential. The device then measures the total current required to clamp V_m to this value. A typical method of voltage clamping involves impaling a cell with two sharp electrodes, one for monitoring V_m and one for injecting the current. Figure 6-13A illustrates how the technique can be used with a *Xenopus* (i.e., frog) oocyte. When the voltage-sensing electrode detects a difference from the intended voltage, called the command voltage, a feedback amplifier rapidly injects opposing current to maintain a constant V_m. The magnitude of the injected current needed to keep V_m constant is equal, but opposite in sign, to the membrane current and is thus an accurate measurement of the **total membrane current (I_m)**.

I_m is the sum of the individual currents through each of the parallel branches of the circuit in Figure 6-9B. For a simple case in which only one type of ionic current (I_X) flows through the membrane, I_m is simply the sum of the capacitative current and the ionic current:

$$I_m = \underbrace{I_C}_{\substack{\text{Capacitative} \\ \text{current}}} + \underbrace{I_X}_{\substack{\text{Ionic} \\ \text{current}}}$$

$$= I_C + G_X(V_m - E_X)$$

(6-19)

Equation 6-19 suggests a powerful way to analyze how ionic conductance (G_X) changes with time. For instance, if we abruptly change V_m to another value and then hold V_m constant (i.e., we *clamp* the voltage), the capacitative current flows for only a brief time at the voltage transition and disappears by the time that V_m reaches its new steady value (Fig. 6-12B). Therefore, after I_C has decayed to zero, any additional changes in I_m must be due to changes in I_X. Because V_m is clamped and the ion concentrations do not change (i.e., E_X is constant), only one parameter on the right side of Equation 6-19 is left free to vary, G_X. In other words, we can directly monitor changes in G_X because this conductance parameter is directly proportional to I_m when V_m is constant (i.e., clamped).

Figure 6-13B shows examples of records from a typical voltage-clamp experiment on an oocyte expressing voltage-gated Na^+ channels. In this experiment, a cell membrane is initially clamped at a resting potential of −80 mV. V_m is then stepped to −120 mV for 10 ms (a step of −40 mV) and finally returned to −80 mV. Such a negative-going V_m change is called a **hyperpolarization**. With this protocol, only brief spikes of current are observed at the beginning and end of the voltage step and are due to the charging of membrane capacitance. No current flows in between these two spikes.

What happens if we rapidly change V_m in the opposite direction by shifting the voltage from −80 to −40 mV (a step of +40 mV)? Such a positive-going change in V_m from a reference voltage is called a **depolarization**. In addition to the expected transient *capacitative* current, a large, inward, time-dependent current flows. This current is an *ionic* current and is due to the opening and closing kinetics of a particular class of channels called voltage-gated Na^+ channels, which open only when V_m is made sufficiently positive. We can remove the contribution of the capacitative current to the total current by subtracting the inverse of the rapid transient current recorded during the hyperpolarizing pulse of the

A OOCYTE TWO-ELECTRODE VOLTAGE CLAMP

B VOLTAGE CLAMP METHOD OF MEASURING IONIC CURRENT

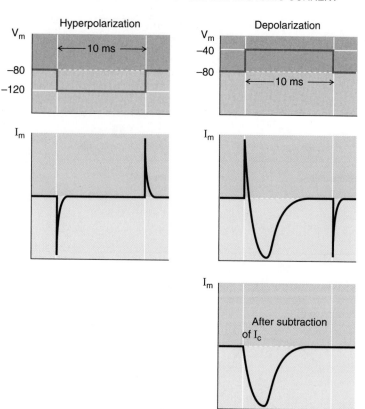

Figure 6-13 Two-electrode voltage clamp. **A,** Two microelectrodes impale a *Xenopus* oocyte. One electrode monitors membrane potential (V_m) and the other passes enough current (I_m) through the membrane to clamp V_m to a predetermined command voltage ($V_{command}$). **B,** In the left panel, the membrane is clamped for 10 ms to a hyperpolarized potential (40 mV more negative). Because a hyperpolarization does not activate channels, no ionic currents flow. Only transient capacitative currents flow after the beginning and end of the pulse. In the right panel, the membrane is clamped for 10 ms to a depolarized potential (40 mV more positive). Because the depolarization opens voltage-gated Na^+ channels, a large inward Na^+ current flows, in addition to the transient capacitative current. Adding the transient capacitative currents in the left panel to the total current in the right panel, thereby canceling the transient capacitative currents (I_c), yields the pure Na^+ current shown at the bottom in the right panel.

same magnitude. The remaining slower current is inward (i.e., downward) and represents I_{Na}, which is directly proportional to G_{Na} (Equation 6-19).

The ionic current in Figure 6-13B (lower right panel) is called a **macroscopic current** because it is due to the activity of a large population of channels sampled from a whole cell. Why did we observe Na^+ current only when we shifted V_m in a positive direction from the resting potential? As described later, such Na^+ channels are actually members of a large family of voltage-sensitive ion channels that are activated by *depolarization*. A current activated by depolarization is commonly observed when an electrically excitable cell, such as a neuron, is voltage clamped under conditions in which Na^+ is the sole extracellular cation.

A modern electrophysiological method called **whole-cell voltage clamping** involves the use of a single microelectrode both to monitor V_m and to pass current into the cell. In this method, a glass micropipette electrode with a smooth, fire-polished tip that is ~1 μm in diameter is pressed onto the surface of a cell (Fig. 6-14A). One then applies slight suction to the inside of the pipette, forming a high-resistance seal between the circular rim of the pipette tip and the cell membrane. The piece of sealed membrane is called a **patch**, and the pipette is called a **patch pipette**. Subsequent application of stronger suction causes the patch to rupture, creating a continuous, low-resistance pathway between the inside of the cell and the pipette. In this configuration, **whole-cell currents** can be recorded (Fig. 6-14B). Because single cells can be dissociated from many different tissues and studied in culture, this method has proved very powerful for analyzing the physiological roles of various types of ion channels and their regulation at the cellular level. The approach for recording whole-cell currents with a patch pipette was introduced by Erwin Neher and Bert Sakmann, who received the Nobel Prize in Physiology or Medicine in 1991.

The patch-clamp technique resolves unitary currents through single-channel molecules

Voltage-clamp studies of ionic currents at the whole-cell (i.e., macroscopic) level led to the question of how many channels are involved in the production of a macroscopic

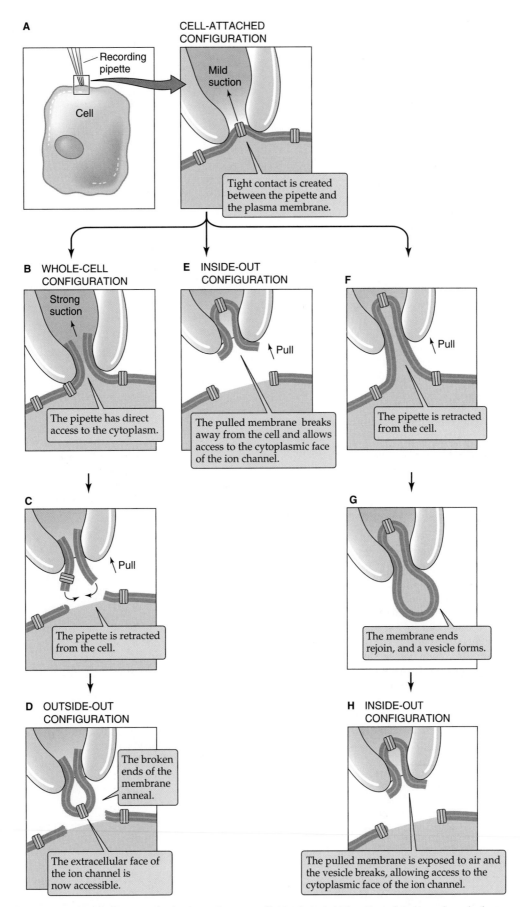

Figure 6-14 Patch-clamp methods. *(Data from Hamill OP, Marty A, Neher E, et al: Improved patch-clamp techniques for high-resolution current recording from cells and cell-free membrane patches. Pflugers Arch 1981; 391:85-100.)*

current. Electrophysiologists realized that if the area of a voltage-clamped membrane was reduced to a very small fraction of the cell surface area, it might be possible to observe the activity of a single channel.

This goal was realized when Neher and Sakmann developed the **patch-clamp technique**. Applying suction to a patch pipette creates a high-resistance seal between the glass and the cell membrane, as described in the preceding section for whole-cell voltage clamping. However, instead of rupturing the enclosed membrane patch as in the whole-cell approach, the tiny membrane area within the patch is kept intact so that one can record current from channels within the patch. A current recording made with the patch pipette attached to a cell is called a **cell-attached recording** (Fig. 6-14A). After a cell-attached patch is established, it is also possible to withdraw the pipette from the cell membrane to produce an **inside-out patch configuration** by either of two methods (Fig. 6-14E or Fig. 6-14F-H). In this configuration, the *intracellular* surface of the patch membrane faces the bath solution. One can also arrive at the opposite orientation of the patch of membrane by starting in the cell-attached configuration (Fig. 6-14A), rupturing the cell-attached patch to produce a whole-cell configuration (Fig. 6-14B), and then pulling the pipette away from the cell (Fig. 6-14C). When the membranes reseal, the result is an **outside-out patch configuration** in which the *extracellular* patch surface faces the bath solution (Fig. 6-14D).

The different patch configurations summarized in Figure 6-14 are useful for studying drug-channel interactions, receptor-mediated processes, and biochemical regulatory mechanisms that take place at either the inner or external surface of cell membranes.

Single-channel currents sum to produce macroscopic membrane currents

Figure 6-15 illustrates the results of a patch-clamp experiment that is analogous to the macroscopic experiment on the right-hand side of Figure 6-13B. Under the diagram of the voltage step in Figure 6-15A are eight current records, each of which is the response to an identical step of depolarization lasting 45 ms. The smallest, nearly rectangular transitions of current correspond to the opening and closing of a single Na^+ channel. When two or three channels in the patch are open simultaneously, the measured current level is an integral multiple of the single-channel or "unitary" transition.

The opening and closing process of ion channels is called **gating**. Patch-clamp experiments have demonstrated that

---

Figure 6-15 Outside-out patch recordings of Na^+ channels. **A,** Eight single-current responses—in the same patch on a myotube (a cultured skeletal muscle cell)—to a depolarizing step in voltage (cytosolic side of patch negative). **B,** Average current. The record in black shows the average of many single traces, such as those in **A.** The blue record shows the average current when tetrodotoxin blocks the Na^+ channels. (*Data from Weiss RE, Horn R: Single-channel studies of TTX-sensitive and TTX-resistant sodium channels in developing rat muscle reveal different open channel properties. Ann NY Acad Sci 1986; 479:152-161.*)

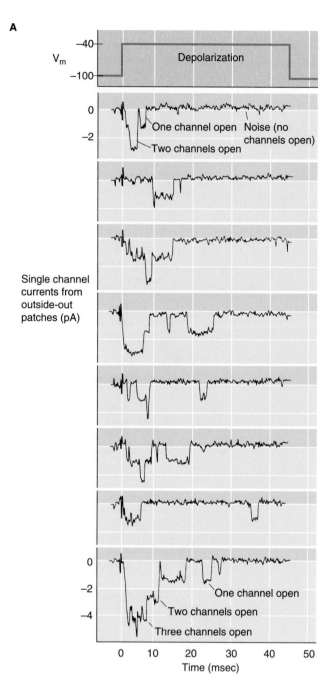

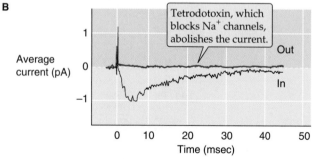

macroscopic ionic currents represent the gating of single channels that have discrete unitary currents. Averaging consecutive, microscopic Na⁺ current records produces a time-dependent current (Fig. 6-15B) that has the same shape as the macroscopic I_m shown in Figure 6-13B. If one does the experiment in the same way but blocks Na⁺ channels with tetrodotoxin, the averaged current is equivalent to the zero current level, indicating that Na⁺ channels are the only channels present within the membrane patch.

Measuring the current from a single channel in a patch at different clamp voltages reveals that the size of the discrete current steps depends on voltage (Fig. 6-16A). Plotting the **unitary current (*i*)** of single channels versus the voltage at which they were measured yields a single-channel *I-V* relationship (Fig. 6-16B) that is similar to the one we discussed earlier for macroscopic currents (Fig. 6-7). This single-channel *I-V* relationship reverses direction at a certain potential (V_{rev}), just like a macroscopic current does. If a channel is permeable to only one type of ion present in the solution, the V_{rev} equals the equilibrium potential for that ion (E_X). However, if the channel is permeable to more than one ion, the single-channel reversal potential depends on the relative permeabilities of the various ions, as described by the GHK voltage equation (Equation 6-9).

The slope of a single-channel *I-V* relationship is a measure of the conductance of a single channel, the **unitary conductance (*g*)**. Every type of ion channel has a characteristic value of *g* under a defined set of ionic conditions. The single-channel conductance of most known channel proteins is in the range of 1 to 500 picosiemens (pS), where 1 pS is equal to 10^{-12} ohm⁻¹.

How do we know that the unitary current in fact corresponds to just a single channel? One good indication is that such conductance measurements are close to the theoretical value expected for ion diffusion through a cylindrical, water-filled pore that is long enough to span a phospholipid membrane and that has a diameter large enough to accept an ion. The unitary conductance of typical channels corresponds to rates of ion movement in the range of 10^6 to 10^8 ions per second per channel at 100 mV of driving force. These rates of ion transport through single channels are many orders of magnitude greater than typical rates of ion transport by ion pumps (~500 ions/s) or by the fastest ion cotransporters and exchangers (~50,000 ions/s). The high ionic flux through channels places them in a unique class of transport proteins whose unitary activity can be resolved by patch-clamp current recordings.

Single channels can fluctuate between open and closed states

When a channel has opened from the **closed state** (zero current) to its full unitary conductance value, the channel is said to be in the **open state**. Channel gating thus represents the transition between closed and open states. A single-channel record is actually a record of the conformational changes of a single protein molecule as monitored by the duration of opening and closing events.

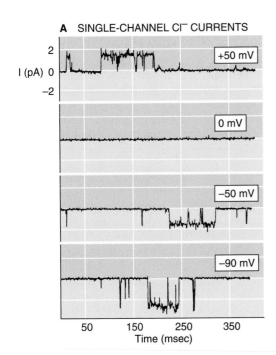

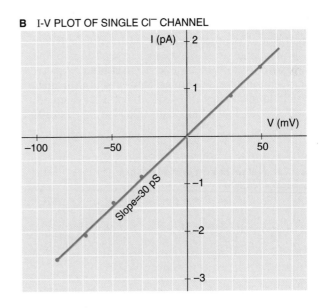

Figure 6-16 Voltage dependence of currents through single Cl⁻ channels in outside-out patches. **A,** The channel is a γ-aminobutyric acid A (GABA_A) receptor channel, which is a Cl⁻ channel activated by GABA. Identical solutions, containing 145 mM Cl⁻, were present on both sides of the patch. **B,** The magnitudes of the single-channel current transitions (y-axis) vary linearly with voltage (x-axis). *(Data from Bormann J, Hamill OP, Sakmann B: Mechanism of anion permeation through channels gated by glycine and γ-aminobutyric acid in mouse cultured spinal neurones. J Physiol [Lond] 1987; 385:243-286.)*

Examination of the consecutive records of a patch recording, such as that in Figure 6-15A, shows that the gating of a single channel is a probabilistic process. On average, there is a certain probability that a channel will open at any given time, but such openings occur randomly. For example, the average record in Figure 6-15B indicates that the probability that the channels will open is highest ~4 ms after the start of the depolarization.

The process of channel gating can be represented by kinetic models that are similar to the following hypothetical two-state scheme.

$$C \underset{k_c}{\overset{k_o}{\rightleftharpoons}} O \qquad (6\text{-}20)$$

This scheme indicates that a channel can reversibly change its conformation between closed (C) and open (O) states according to first-order reactions that are determined by an opening rate constant (k_o) and a closing rate constant (k_c). The **probability of channel opening (P_o)** is the fraction of total time that the channel is in the open state.

We already have seen in Figure 6-15 that the *average* of many single-channel records from a given patch produces a time course that is similar to a macroscopic current recorded from the same cell. The same is true for the *sum* of the individual single-channel current records. This conclusion leads to an important principle: macroscopic ionic current is equal to the product of the **number of channels (N)** within the membrane area, the unitary current of single channels, and the probability of channel opening:

$$I = NP_o i \qquad (6\text{-}21)$$

Comparison of the magnitude of macroscopic currents recorded from large areas of voltage-clamped membrane with the magnitude of unitary current measured by patch techniques indicates that the surface density of ion channels typically falls into the range of 1 to 1000 channels per square micrometer of cell membrane, depending on the channel and cell type.

MOLECULAR PHYSIOLOGY OF ION CHANNELS

Classes of ion channels can be distinguished on the basis of electrophysiology, pharmacological and physiological ligands, intracellular messengers, and sequence homology

Mammalian cells express a remarkable array of ion channels. One way of making sense of this diversity is to classify channels according to their functional characteristics. Among these characteristics are electrophysiological behavior, inhibition or stimulation by various pharmacological agents, activation by extracellular agonists, and modulation by intracellular regulatory molecules. In addition, we can classify channels by structural characteristics, such as amino acid sequence homology and the kinds of subunits of which they are composed.

Electrophysiology This approach consists of analyzing ionic currents by voltage-clamp techniques and then characterizing channels on the basis of ionic selectivity, dependence of gating on membrane potential, and kinetics of opening and closing.

One of the most striking differences among channels is their **selectivity** for various ions. Indeed, channels are generally named according to which ion they are most permeable to—for example, Na^+ channels, Ca^{2+} channels, K^+ channels, and Cl^- channels.

Another major electrophysiological characteristic of channels is their **voltage dependence**. In electrically excitable cells (e.g., nerve, skeletal muscle, heart), a major class of channels becomes activated—and often inactivated—as a steep function of V_m. For example, the Na^+ channel in nerve and muscle cells is increasingly more activated as V_m becomes more positive (see Chapter 7). Such voltage-gated channels are generally highly selective for Na^+, Ca^{2+}, or K^+.

Channels are also distinguished by the kinetics of **gating** behavior. For example, imagine two channels, each with an open probability (P_o) of 0.5. One channel might exhibit openings and closures with a duration of 1 second each on average, whereas the other may have the same P_o with openings and closures of 1 ms each on average. Complex gating patterns of some channels are characterized by bursts of many brief openings, followed by longer silent periods.

Pharmacological Ligands Currents that are virtually indistinguishable by electrophysiological criteria can sometimes be distinguished pharmacologically. For example, subtypes of voltage-gated Na^+ channels can be distinguished by their sensitivity to the peptide toxin μ-conotoxin, which is produced by *Conus geographus*, a member of a family of venomous marine mollusks called Cone snails. This toxin strongly inhibits the Na^+ channels of adult rat skeletal muscle but has little effect on the Na^+ channels of neurons and cardiac myocytes. Another conotoxin (ω-conotoxin) from another snail specifically inhibits voltage-gated Ca^{2+} channels in the spinal cord. A synthetic version of this conotoxin (ziconotide) is available for treatment of neuropathic pain in patients.

Physiological Ligands Some channels are characterized by their unique ability to be activated by the binding of a particular molecule termed an **agonist**. For example, at the vertebrate neuromuscular junction, a channel called the nicotinic acetylcholine (ACh) receptor opens in response to the binding of ACh released from a presynaptic nerve terminal. Other agonist-gated channels are activated directly by neurotransmitters such as glutamate, serotonin (5-hydroxytryptamine [5-HT]), γ-aminobutyric acid (GABA), and glycine.

Intracellular Messengers Channels can be categorized by their physiological regulation by intracellular messengers. For example, increases in $[Ca^{2+}]_i$ stimulate some ionic currents, in particular K^+ and Cl^- currents. Channels underlying such currents are known as Ca^{2+}-gated K^+ channels and Ca^{2+}-gated Cl^- channels, respectively. Another example is seen in the plasma membrane of light-sensitive rod cells of the retina, in which a particular type of channel is directly activated by intracellular cyclic guanosine monophosphate.

The four functional criteria—electrophysiology, pharmacology, extracellular agonists, and intracellular regulators—for characterizing channels are not mutually exclusive. For example, one of the major types of Ca^{2+}-activated K^+ channels is also voltage-gated.

Sequence Homology The diversity of channels implied by functional criteria ultimately requires a molecular biological approach to channel classification. Such an approach began in the 1970s and 1980s with the biochemical purification of channel proteins. Membrane biochemists originally used rich, natural sources of ion channels, such as the electrical organs of the torpedo ray and *Electrophorus* eel, to isolate channel proteins such as the nicotinic ACh receptor (see Chapter 8) and the voltage-gated Na^+ channel, respectively. Amino acid sequencing of purified channel proteins provided the information needed to prepare oligonucleotide probes for isolating the coding sequences of channels from cDNA clones, in turn derived from mRNA. Genes coding for many different types of ion channel proteins have been cloned in this way. This work has confirmed that the diversity of channels foreshadowed by physiological assays corresponds to an enormous diversity at the molecular level.

When annotation of the human genome is completed, a definitive catalogue of ion channels of significance to medical physiology will eventually be available. On the basis of the data bank of mammalian channel protein sequences, we recognize at least 24 distinct families of channel proteins (Table 6-2). Despite rapid progress in the cloning of channels, detailed knowledge of the three-dimensional structures of channels is emerging more slowly because of the difficulty in crystallizing membrane proteins for x-ray crystallographic analysis. However, molecular information gleaned from sequence analysis and structural information on several channel proteins has revealed a number of important themes that we discuss in the remainder of this chapter.

Many channels are formed by a radially symmetric arrangement of subunits or domains around a central pore

The essential function of a channel is to facilitate the passive flow of ions across the hydrophobic membrane bilayer according to the electrochemical gradient. This task requires the channel protein to form an aqueous pore. The ionophore gramicidin is a small peptide that forms a unique helix dimer that spans the membrane; the hollow cylindrical region inside the helix is the channel pore. Another interesting type of channel structure is that of the **porin** channel proteins (see Chapter 5), which are present in the outer membranes of mitochondria and gram-negative bacteria. This protein forms a large pore through the center of a barrel-like structure; the 16 staves of the barrel are formed by 16 strands of the protein, each of which are in a β-sheet conformation. However, the structural motifs of a hole through a helix (gramicidin) or a hole through a 16-stranded β barrel (porin) appear to be exceptions rather than the rule.

For the majority of eukaryotic channels, the aqueous pores are located at the center of an oligomeric rosette-like

arrangement of homologous subunits in the plane of the membrane (Fig. 6-17). Each of these subunits, in turn, is a polypeptide that weaves through the membrane several times. In some cases, the channel is not a true homo-oligomer or hetero-oligomer but rather a pseudo-oligomer: the subunits are replaced by a single polypeptide composed of repetitive homologous domains. The rosette-like arrangement of these domains surrounds a central pore. In the case of gap junction channels and ACh receptor channels, which we discuss in the following two sections, it has been possible to use cryoelectron microscopy to construct images of the channel from membrane preparations in which the proteins exist in a densely packed two-dimensional crystalline array. This technique has provided low-resolution pictures that show how the polypeptide chains of the channel proteins weave through the membrane.

Gap junction channels are made up of two connexons, each of which has six identical subunits called connexins

Gap junctions are protein channels that connect two cells with a large, unselective pore (~1.5 nm in diameter) that allows ions and small molecules as large as 1 kDa to pass between cells. These channels have been found in virtually all mammalian cells with only a few exceptions, such as adult skeletal muscle and erythrocytes. For example, gap junctions interconnect hepatocytes of the liver, cardiac muscle fibers of the heart and smooth muscle of the gut, β cells of the pancreas, and epithelial cells in the cornea of the eye, to name just a few. Gap junctions provide pathways for chemical communication and electrical coupling between cells. The basic structure deduced for a gap junction from the liver is shown in Figure 6-18A. The gap junction comprises two apposed hexameric structures called **connexons**, one contributed by each cell. These connexons contact each other to bridge a gap of ~3 nm between the two cell membranes. Each connexon has six identical subunits surrounding a central pore, so-called radial hexameric symmetry. Each of these subunits is an integral membrane protein called **connexin** (Cx) that has a molecular mass of 26 to 46 kDa. The aqueous pore formed at the center of the six connexin subunits has a diameter that is estimated to be 1.2 to 2 nm. At the cytoplasmic end of the connexon, the pore appears to open to a wider funnel-shaped entrance.

A given connexon hexamer in a particular cell membrane may be formed from a single connexin (homomeric) or a mixture of different connexin proteins (heteromeric). The apposition of two identical connexon hexamers forms a **homotypic channel**; the apposition of dissimilar connexon hexamers forms a **heterotypic channel**. Such structural variation in the assembly of connexons provides for greater diversity of function and regulation.

In one mode of regulation, increases in $[Ca^{2+}]_i$ can cause gap junctions to close. For Ca^{2+}-dependent gating, it is possible to visualize a structural change in the conformation of the connexon. In the absence of Ca^{2+}, the pore is in an open configuration and the connexin subunits are tilted 7 to 8 degrees from an axis perpendicular to the plane of the membrane. After the addition of Ca^{2+}, the pore closes and the

Text continued on p. 172

Table 6-2 Major Families of Human Ion Channel Proteins

Channel Family	Description	Human Gene Symbols (Number of Genes) Protein Names	Noted Physiological Functions	Known Human Genetic and Autoimmune Diseases	Notes for Topology Figure
1. Connexin channels	Hexameric gap junction channels	GJA (7) GJB (7) GJC (3) GJD (3)	Cell-cell communication Electrical coupling and cytoplasmic diffusion of molecules between interconnected cells	Charcot-Marie-Tooth disease Erythrokeratodermia variabilis Nonsyndromic sensorineural hearing loss	4 TMs (Fig. 6-21A)
2. K$^+$ channels (canonical members of VGL voltage-gated-like channel superfamily)	Homo- or heterotetrameric voltage-gated (K$_V$ channels)	$KCNA$ (8) Shaker related or Kv1 $KCNB$ (2) Shab related or Kv2 $KCNC$ (4) Shaw related or Kv3 $KCND$ (3) Shal related or Kv4 $KCNF$ (1) modulatory $KCNG$ (4) modulatory $KCNH$ (8) eag related $KCNQ$ (5) KQT related $KCNS$ (3) modulatory $KCNV$ (2)	Electrical signaling Repolarization of action potentials Frequency encoding of action potentials ($KCNH2$ = cardiac HERG channel) $KCNQ1$ = cardiac $KVLQT1$ channel)	Familial periodic cerebellar ataxia Cardiac LQT1 ($KCNQ1$ mutations) Romano-Ward syndrome Jervall-Lange-Nielsen syndrome (deafness) Benign familial neonatal epilepsy Cardiac LQT2 ($KCNH2/HERG$ mutations)	6 TMs (Fig. 6-21B)
	Tetrameric small and intermediate conductance Ca^{2+}-activated K$^+$ channels	$KCNN$ (4) SK$_{Ca}$ and IK$_{Ca}$	Repolarization of action potentials Slow phase of AP after-hyperpolarization Regulates AP inter-spike interval and firing frequency Activated by Ca^{2+}-calmodulin Voltage-insensitive		6 TMs (Fig. 6-21C)
	Tetrameric large conductance K$_{Ca}$ channel family	$KCNMA$(1) Slo1 or BK$_{Ca}$ $KCNT1$ (1) Slo2.1 or Slick $KCNT2$ (1) Slo2.2 or Slack $KCNU$(1) Slo3	Slo1 (BK$_{Ca}$) is a voltage- and Ca^{2+}-activated K$^+$ channel BK$_{Ca}$ mediates fast component of AP after hyperpolarization Feedback regulation of contractile tone of smooth muscle Feedback regulation release of neurotransmitters at nerve terminals and auditory hair cells Slo2.1 (Slick) and Slo2.2 (Slack) have low intrinsic voltage dependence and are both synergistically activated by internal Na$^+$ and Cl$^-$ Slo3 is sensitive to internal pH and is exclusively expressed in spermatocytes and mature spermatozoa	Generalized epilepsy and paroxysmal dyskinesia (Slo1)	7 TMs Fig. 6-21D

	Structure	Gene (subfamily)	Function	Disease	TMs (Figure)
Homo- or hetero-tetrameric inward rectifier		KCNJ (15) Kir	Genesis and regulation of resting membrane potential; regulation of electrical excitability; release of insulin in pancreas and coupling of metabolism to excitability (K_{ATP}) Includes ROMK1 in kidney, IRK, GIRK muscarinicR-coupled K-channel in heart, KATP channels in pancreas and many other tissues; activated by PIP_2	Bartter's syndrome Familial persistent hyperinulinaemic hypoglycemia of infancy	2 TMs (Fig. 6-21E)
Dimeric tandem two-pore		KCNK (15) K_{2P}	Genesis and regulation of resting membrane potential Regulation of AP firing frequency Sensory perception of touch, stretch, and temperature May be involved in mechanism of general anesthesia Activated by heat, internal pH, PIP_2, fatty acids, G proteins General anesthetics		4 TMs (Fig. 6-21F)
3. Hyperpolarization-activated cyclic nucleotide-gated cation channels (VGL superfamily member)	Tetrameric cation-selective HCN channels	HCN (4)	Na^+/K^+ selective, cAMP-activated, cGMP-activated, I_f current in heart, I_h current in neurons; generation of AP automaticity in heart and CNS neurons Mediates depolarizing current that triggers the next AP in rhythmically firing cells		6 TMs (Fig. 6-21G)
4. cyclic nucleotide gated cation channels (VGL superfamily member)	Tetrameric CNG channels	CNGA (4) CNGB (2)	Cation non-selective channels permeable to Na^+, K^+ and Ca^{2+} Sensory transduction mechanism in vision and olfaction cGMP and cAMP-gated cation-selective channels in rods, cones, and olfactory receptor neurons	Retinitis pigmentosa	6 TMs (Fig. 6-21H)
5. Transient receptor potential cation channels (VGL superfamily member)	Tetrameric TRP channels	TRPA (1) TRPC (7) TRPM (8) TRPV (6) MCOLN (3) PKD (3)	Cation non-selective channels permeable to Na^+, K^+, and Ca^{2+} Involved in polymodal sensory transduction of pain, itch, thermosensation, various chemicals, osmotic and mechanical stress TRPV family is also called the vanilloid receptor family that includes the capsaicin receptor	Proteinuric kidney diseases of focal and segmental glomerulosclerosis Hypomagnesia with secondary hypocalcemia Polycystic kidney disease; mucolipidosis type IV	6 TMs (Fig. 6-21I)

Continued

Table 6-2 Major Families of Human Ion Channel Proteins—cont'd

Channel Family	Description	Human Gene Symbols (Number of Genes) Protein Names	Noted Physiological Functions	Known Human Genetic and Autoimmune Diseases	Notes for Topology Figure
6. Voltage-gated Na⁺ channels (VGL superfamily member)	Pseudo-tetrameric Na⁺ channels	*SCN* (10) Na$_V$	Na⁺ selective, voltage-activated channels that mediate the depolarizing upstroke of propagating APs in neurons and muscle. Blocked by local anesthetics	Hyperkalemic periodic paralysis, paramyotonia congenita, K⁺-aggravated myotonia, cardiac long QT syndrome (LQT3). Generalized epilepsy with febrile seizures	6 TMs × 4 (Fig. 6-21J)
7. Voltage-gated Ca²⁺ channels (VGL superfamily member)	Pseudo-tetrameric Ca²⁺ channels	*CACNA* (10) Ca$_V$ *NALCN* (1) Na⁺ leak	CACNA genes encode Ca²⁺ selective, voltage-activated channels that mediate prolonged depolarizing phase of APs in muscle and neurons. Entry of Ca²⁺ via Ca$_V$ triggers release of transmitter and hormone secretion; molecular target of Ca-blocker drugs. NALCN gene encodes a voltage-insensitive Na⁺ channel that mediates a resting Na⁺ leak current in neurons	Hypokalemic periodic paralysis. Malignant hyperthermia. Episodic ataxia type-2. Familial hemiplegic migraine. Spinocerebellar ataxia type-6. Lambert-Eaton syndrome	6 TMs × 4 (Fig. 6-21K)
8. Ligand-gated ion channels Pentameric Cys-loop-receptor superfamily	Pentameric nicotinic, cholinergic receptor cation channels	*CHRNA* (9) α *CHRNB* (4) β *CHRND* (1) δ *CHRNE* (1) ε *CHRNG* (1) γ	Na⁺, K⁺ nonselective cation channels activated by binding of ACh. Depolarizing post-synaptic potentials. Excitatory EPSPs. Site action of nicotine	Slow channel syndrome. Fast channel syndrome. Nocturnal frontal lobe epilepsy. Myasthenia gravis	4 TMs (Fig. 6-21L)
	Pentameric serotonin 5-HT$_3$ ionotropic receptor cation channels	*HTR3A* (1) *HTR3B* (1) *HTR3C* (1) *HTR3D* (1) *HTR3E* (1)	Na⁺, K⁺ non-selective cation channels activated by binding of 5HT. Depolarizing post-synaptic potentials. Excitatory EPSPs		4 TMs (Fig. 6-21L)
	Pentameric GABA$_A$ ionotropic receptor	*GABRA* (6) *GABRB* (3) *GABRD* (1) *GABRE* (1) *GABRG* (3) *GABRP* (1) *GABRQ* (1) *GABRR* (3)	Cl⁻-selective anion channels activated by binding of GABA. Mediates hyperpolarizing postsynaptic potentials. Inhibitory IPSPs. Site of action of benzodiazepines and barbiturates		4 TMs (Fig. 6-21L)

		Gene	Function	Disease	TMs
9. Glutamate-activated cation channels	Pentameric glycine ionotropic receptor	GLRA (4), GLRB (1)	Cl⁻-selective anion channels activated by binding of glycine. Inhibitory IPSPs	Startle disease	4 TMs (Fig. 6-21L)
	Tetrameric AMPA-kainate receptor cation-selective channels	GRIK (5), GRIA (4)	Na⁺, K⁺ non-selective cation channels activated by binding of glutamate. Depolarizing postsynaptic potentials. Excitatory EPSPs. Involved in long-term potentiation of neuronal memory	Rasmussen's encephalitis	3 TMs (Fig. 6-21M)
	Tetrameric NMDA receptor cation selective channels	GRIN (7)	Na⁺, K⁺, Ca²⁺ nonselective cation channels activated by binding of glutamate excitatory EPSP. Involved in long-term potentiation model of neuronal memory		3 TMs (Fig. 6-21M)
10. Purinergic ligand-gated cation channel	Multimeric P2X receptor cation channels (functional channel is believed to be a trimer)	P2RX (6)	ATP-activated cation channels permeable to Na⁺, K⁺, Ca²⁺. Involved in excitatory synaptic transmission and regulation of blood clotting. Channel activated by synaptic co-release of ATP in catecholamine-containing synaptic vesicles		2 TMs (Fig. 6-21N)
11. Epithelial Na⁺ channel-degenerins	Heterotrimeric ENaC epithelial amiloride-sensitive Na⁺ channel. Homotrimeric ASIC acid sensing cation channel	SCNN1A (1) α, SCNN1B (1) β subunit, SCNN1D (1) δ subunit, SCNN1G (1) γ subunit, ACCN (5)	SCNN1 genes encode amiloride-sensitive Na⁺ selective channels mediating Na⁺ transport across tight epithelia. ACCN genes encode ASIC cation channels activated by external H⁺ that are involved in pain sensation in sensory neurons following acidosis	Liddle's syndrome hypertension Pseudohypoaldosteronism type-1	2 TMs (Fig. 6-21O)

Continued

Table 6-2 Major Families of Human Ion Channel Proteins—cont'd

Channel Family	Description	Human Gene Symbols (Number of Genes) Protein Names	Noted Physiological Functions	Known Human Genetic and Autoimmune Diseases	Notes for Topology Figure
12. Cystic fibrosis transmembrane regulator	CFTR Channel protein contains two internally homologous domains	CFTR (1)	Cl⁻-selective channel coupled to cAMP regulation Important Cl⁻ transport pathway in secretory and absorptive epithelia Regulated by ATP binding and hydrolysis at two intracellular NBD binding domains	Cystic fibrosis	12 TMs (Fig. 6-21P)
13. ClC Cl⁻ channels	Dimeric ClC Cl⁻ channels	CLCA (4) CLCN (9)	Cl⁻-selective voltage-sensitive anion channels in muscle, neurons and many other tissues Regulation of electrical excitability in skeletal muscle Mediates Cl⁻ transport in epithelia Regulatory volume decrease	Becker and Thompson myotonia congenital Nephrolithiasis Bartter's syndrome type III Dent's disease	14 α helices (Fig. 6-21Q)
14. IP₃-activated Ca²⁺ Channel	Tetrameric IP₃ receptor channel	ITPR (3)	Intracellular cation channel permeable to Na⁺, K⁺ and Ca²⁺ Activated by binding of IP₃ and Ca²⁺ Coupled to receptor activation of PLC and hydrolysis of PIP2 Regulated by binding of ATP Mediates excitation-contraction coupling in smooth muscle and participates in intracellular Ca²⁺ release and signaling in many cells		6 TMs (Fig. 6-21R)
15. RYR Ca²⁺ release channel	Tetrameric ryanodine receptor Ca²⁺-release channel	RYR (3)	Intracellular cation channel permeable to Ca²⁺ Intracellular Ca²⁺-release channel activated by mechanical coupling to Caᵥ channel in skeletal muscle or by plasma membrane Ca²⁺ entry in heart and smooth muscle	Malignant hyperthermia central core disease	4 TMs (Fig. 6-21S)

16. ORAI store-operated Ca²⁺ channels	Multimeric ORAI Ca²⁺-selective channels	*ORAI* (3) (Also known as I$_{CRAC}$ for Ca²⁺-release activated Ca²⁺ current or SOC channel for store-operated Ca²⁺ entry)	ORAI is a plasma membrane Ca²⁺ channel predominantly found in non-excitable cells, such as epithelia and lymphocytes. ORAI is activated via PLC-coupled pathways leading to IP3-activated Ca²⁺ release from ER. Ca²⁺ depletion in ER activates an ER membrane protein (STIM) that activates *ORAI* resulting in entry of extracellular Ca²⁺. Functions in lymphocyte activation and epithelial secretion	Severe combined immunodeficiency syndrome (SCID)	4 TMs (Fig. 6-21T)

Data from:

Bosanac I, Michikawa T, Mikoshiba K, Ikura M: Structural insights into the regulatory mechanism of IP3 receptor. Biochim Biophys Acta 2004; 1742: 89-102.

Chen TY: Structure and function of ClC channels. Annu Rev Physiol 2005; 67: 809-839.

Clapham DE, Runnels LW, Strübing C: The TRP ion channel family. Nature Rev Neurosci 2001; 2:387-396.

Dorwart M, Thibodeau P, Thomas P: Cystic fibrosis: recent structural insights. J Cyst Fibros 2004; 2:91-94.

Dutzler R: The structural basis of ClC chloride channel function. Trends Neurosci 2004; 27: 315-320.

Dutzler R, Campbell ER, Cadene M, et al: X-ray structure of a ClC chloride channel at 3.0 Å reveals the molecular basis of anion selectivity. Nature 2002; 415:287-294.

Foskett JK, White C, Cheung K-H, Mak DD: Inositol trishosphate receptor Ca²⁺ release channels. Physiol Rev 2007; 87:593-658.

Hamilton SL: Ryanodine receptors. Cell Calcium 2005; 38:253-260.

Jasti J, Furukawa H, Gonzales EB, Gouaux E: Structure of acid-sensing ion channel 1 at 1.9 Å resolution and low pH. Nature 2007; 449:316-324.

Khakh BS, North RA: P2X receptors as cell-surface ATP sensors in health and disease. Nature 2006; 442:527-532.

Kellenberger S, Schild L: Epithelial sodium channel/degenerin family of ion channels: a variety of functions for a shared structure. Physiol Rev 2002; 82:735-767.

Kim D: Fatty-acid sensitive two-pore domain K⁺ channels. Trends Pharm Sci 2003; 24:648-654.

Lewis RS: The molecular choreography of a storeoperated calcium channel. Nature 2007; 446:284-287.

Lu B, Su Y, Das S, et al: The neuronal channel NALCN contributes resting sodium permeability and is required for normal respiratory rhythm. Cell 2007; 129:371-383.

Maylie J, Bond CT, Herson PS, et al: Small conductance Ca²⁺-activated K⁺ channels and calmodulin. J Physiol (London) 2003; 554.2:255-261.

Mese G, Richard G, White TW: Gap junctions: basic structure and function. J Invest Dermatol 2007; 127:2516-2524.

Nilius B, Droogmans G: Amazing chloride channels: an overview. Acta Physiol Scand 2003; 177:119-147.

Nilius B, Owsianik G, Voets T, Peters JA: Transient receptor potential channels in disease. Physiol Rev 2007; 87:165-217.

Pederson SF, Owsianik G, Nilius B: TRP channels: and overview. Cell Calcium 2005; 38:233-252.

Riordan JR: Assembly of functional CFTR chloride channels. Annu Rev Physiol 2005; 67:701-718.

Rooslid TP, Le K-T, Choe S:04. Cytoplasmic gatekeepers of K⁺ channel flux: a structural perspective. Trends Biochem Sci 2004; 29:39-45.

Salkoff L, Butler A, Ferreira G, et a: High-conductance potassium channels of the SLO family. Nature Rev Neurosci 2006; 5:921-931.

Stocker M: Ca⁽²⁺⁾-activated K⁺ channels: molecular determinants and function of the SK family. Nat Rev Neurosci 2004; 5:758-770.

Taylor CW, da Fonseca PCA, Morris EP: IP3 receptors: the search for structure. Trends Biochem Sci 2004; 29:210-219.

Vial C, Roberts JA, Evans RJ: Molecular properties of ATP-gated P2X receptor ion channels. Trends Pharm Sci 2004; 25:487-493.

Williams AJ, West DJ, Sitsapesan R: Light at the end of the Ca⁽²⁺⁾-release channel tunnel: structures and mechanisms involved in ion translocation in ryanodine receptor channels. Q Rev Biophys 2001; 34:61-104.

Wollmuth LP, Sobolevsky AI: Structure and gating of the glutamate receptor ion channel. Trends Neurosci 2004; 27:321-328.

Yu FH, Catterall WA: The VGL-chanome: a protein superfamily specialized for electrical signaling and ionic homeostasis. Science STKE 2004 re15.

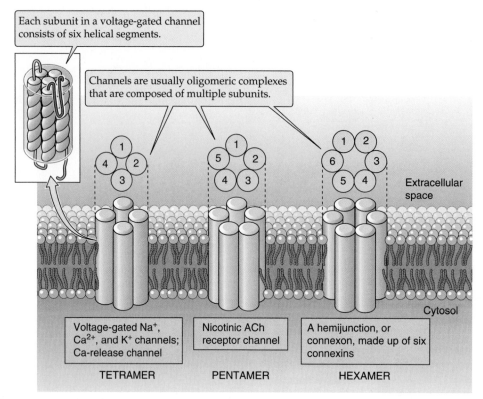

Figure 6-17 Structure of ion channels. Most ion channels consist of four to six subunits that are arranged like a rosette in the plane of the membrane. The channel can be made up of (1) identical, distinct subunits (homo-oligomer); (2) distinct subunits that are homologous but not identical (hetero-oligomer); or (3) repetitive subunit-like domains within a single polypeptide (pseudo-oligomer). In any case, these subunits surround the central pore of the ion channel. Note that each subunit is itself made up of several transmembrane segments.

subunits move to a more parallel alignment (Fig. 6-18B). The gating of the gap junction channel may thus correspond to a conformational change that involves concerted tilting of the six connexin subunits to widen (open) or to constrict (close) the pore.

The gating properties of gap junctions can be studied by measuring electrical currents through gap junctions, using two patch electrodes simultaneously placed in a pair of coupled cells (Fig. 6-18C). When the two cells are clamped at different values of V_m, so that current flows from one cell to the other through the gap junctions, the current measured in either cell fluctuates as a result of the opening and closing of individual gap junction channels. Because the amount of current that enters one cell is the same as the amount of current that leaves the other cell, the current fluctuations in the two cells are mirror images of one another. Studies of this type have shown that increases in $[Ca^{2+}]_i$ or decreases in intracellular pH generally favor the closing of gap junction

channels. In addition, gating of gap junction channels can be regulated by the voltage difference between the coupled cells as well as by phosphorylation.

Nicotinic acetylcholine receptor channels are $\alpha_2\beta\gamma\delta$ pentamers made up of four homologous subunits

In contrast to the gap junction channel, which is a hexamer made up of six identical subunits, the nicotinic ACh receptor is a pentameric channel comprising four different homologous subunits. The α subunit is represented twice; therefore, the pentamer has a subunit composition of $\alpha_2\beta\gamma\delta$. The nicotinic ACh receptor channel is located in a specialized region of the skeletal muscle membrane, at the postsynaptic nerve terminal. The receptor responds to ACh released from the nerve terminals by opening and allowing cations to flow through its pore (see Chapter 8). Images of the ACh receptor

Figure 6-18 Gap junction channels. In **C,** the left panel shows the preparation of the two cells, each of which is voltage clamped by means of a patch pipette in the whole-cell configuration (see Fig. 6-14). Because Cell 1 is clamped to −40 mV and Cell 2 is clamped to −80 mV, current flows through the gap junctions from Cell 1 to Cell 2. The right panel shows that the current recorded by the electrode in Cell 1 is the mirror image of the current recorded in Cell 2. The fluctuating current transitions represent the openings and closings of individual gap junction channels. (Data from Veenstra RD, DeHaan RL: Measurement of single channel currents from cardiac gap junctions. Science 1986; 233:972-974.)

A GAP-JUNCTION CHANNELS IN APPOSING MEMBRANES

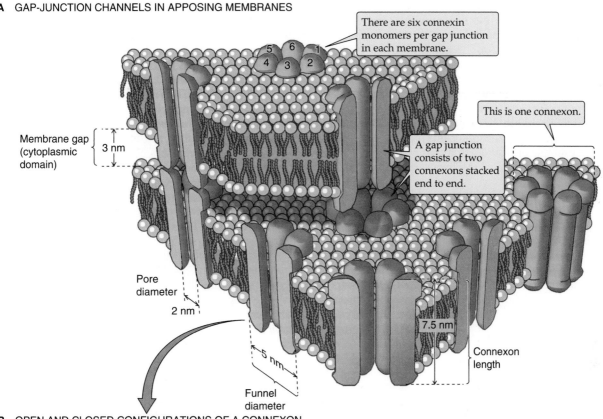

There are six connexin monomers per gap junction in each membrane.

This is one connexon.

A gap junction consists of two connexons stacked end to end.

Membrane gap (cytoplasmic domain)

3 nm

Pore diameter

2 nm

5 nm

7.5 nm

Connexon length

Funnel diameter

B OPEN AND CLOSED CONFIGURATIONS OF A CONNEXON

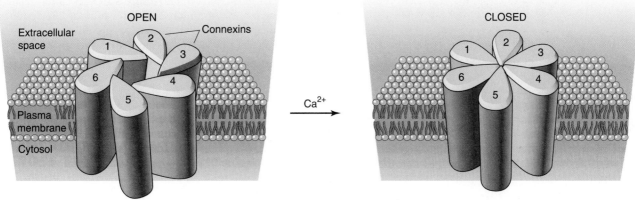

OPEN

Extracellular space

Connexins

Plasma membrane

Cytosol

Ca²⁺

CLOSED

C ELECTRICAL COUPLING OF TWO CELLS CONNECTED BY GAP JUNCTIONS

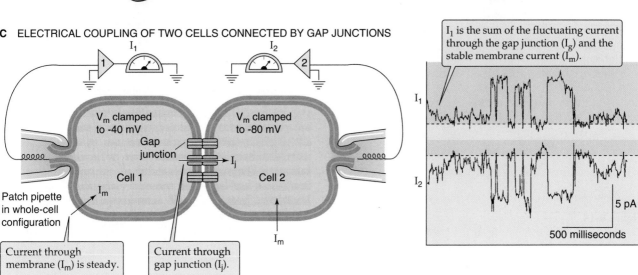

I_1

I_2

V_m clamped to -40 mV

Gap junction

I_j

V_m clamped to -80 mV

Cell 1

Cell 2

I_m

I_m

Patch pipette in whole-cell configuration

Current through membrane (I_m) is steady.

Current through gap junction (I_j).

I_1 is the sum of the fluctuating current through the gap junction (I_g) and the stable membrane current (I_m).

I_1

I_2

5 pA

500 milliseconds

show a pentameric radial symmetry that corresponds to a rosette-like arrangement of the five subunits (Fig. 6-19). When viewed from the extracellular face of the membrane, a hole with a diameter of 2 to 2.5 nm is observed in the center of the rosette and corresponds to the extracellular entrance to the cation-selective channel. The structural changes induced by ACh binding that control opening and closing of the channel appear to occur in a central region of the protein that lies within the plane of the lipid bilayer. We discuss the structure and function of this particular class of channels, an example of **ligand-gated channels** (or agonist-gated channels), in more detail in Chapter 8.

An evolutionary tree called a dendrogram illustrates the relatedness of ion channels

A comparison of amino acid sequences of channels and the nucleotide sequences of genes that encode them provides insight into the molecular evolution of these proteins. The current human genome database contains at least 256 different genes encoding channel proteins. Like other proteins,

specific isoforms of channels are differentially expressed in different parts of cells in various tissues and at certain stages of development. In particular, many different kinds of channels are expressed in the brain. In the central nervous system, the great diversity of ion channels provides a means of specifically and precisely regulating the complex electrical activity of a huge number of neurons that are connected in numerous functional pathways.

As an example of the diversity and species interrelatedness of a channel family, consider the connexins. Figure 6-20A compares 14 sequences of homologous proteins that are members of the connexin family. Like many other proteins, connexins are encoded by a family of related genes that evolved by gene duplication and divergence. In the connexin family, various subtypes are named according to their protein molecular masses. Thus, rat Cx32 refers to a rat connexin with a protein molecular mass of ~32 kDa. The various connexins differ primarily in the length of the intracellular C-terminal domain.

By aligning connexin sequences according to identical amino acids and computing the relative similarity of each pair of connexin sequences, it is possible to reconstruct a hypothetical family tree of evolutionary relationships. Such a tree is called a **dendrogram**. The one in Figure 6-20A includes 9 rat, 2 human, 1 chicken, and 2 frog (*Xenopus*) connexins. The branch lengths of the tree correspond to relative evolutionary distances as measured by sequence divergence. Clusters of sequences in the tree represent highly related groups of proteins. The connexin tree indicates that the Cx32 genes from rats and humans are very closely related, differing by only 4 amino acids of a total of 284 residues. Thus, these Cx32 proteins probably represent the same functional genes in these two species—**orthologous genes**. The closely related Cx43 genes from the rat and human are also likely to be orthologues.

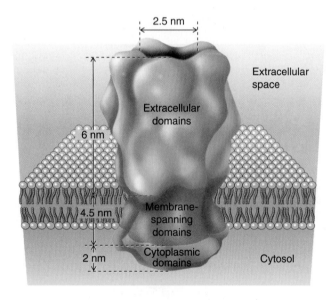

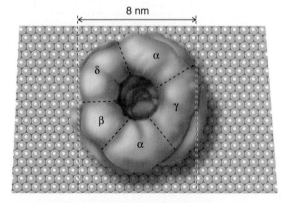

Figure 6-19   Three-dimensional image of the nicotinic ACh receptor channel. *(Data from Toyoshima C, Unwin N: Ion channel of acetylcholine receptor reconstructed from images of postsynaptic membranes. Nature 1988; 336:247-250.)*

Charcot-Marie-Tooth Disease

Many human genetic diseases have been identified in which the primary defect has been mapped to mutations of ion channel proteins. For example, Charcot-Marie-Tooth disease is a rare form of hereditary neuropathy that involves the progressive degeneration of peripheral nerves. Patients with this inherited disease have been found to have various mutations in the human gene for one of the gap junction proteins, connexin 32 (Cx32), which is located on the X chromosome. Cx32 appears to be involved in forming gap junctions between the folds of Schwann cell membranes. These **Schwann cells** wrap around the axons of peripheral nerves and form a layer of insulating material called **myelin**, which is critical for the conduction of nerve impulses. Apparently, mutations in Cx32 interfere with the normal function of these cells and result in the disruption of myelin and axonal degeneration. Some of these mutations have been identified at the amino acid level by gene sequencing. Many other human diseases involve either a genetic defect of a particular channel protein or an autoimmune response directed against a channel protein (Table 6-2).

A VARIOUS SPECIES

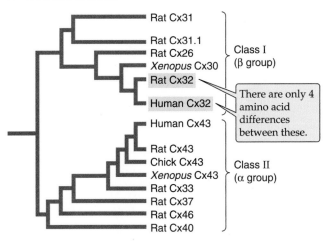

B HUMAN

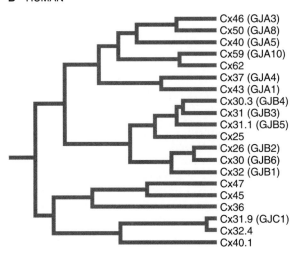

Figure 6-20 Family tree of hypothetical evolutionary relationships among connexin sequences of gap junction channels. In **A**, The dendrogram is based on amino acid sequence differences among 14 connexins in various species. The summed length of the horizontal line segments connecting two connexins is a measure of the degree of difference between the two connexins. In **B**, the dendrogram is based strictly on human sequences. (**A**, Data from Dermietzel R, Spray DC: Gap junctions in the brain: Where, what type, how many and why? *Trends Neurosci* 1993; 16:186-192. **B**, Data from White TW: Nonredundant gap junction functions. *News Physiol Sci* 2003; 18:95-99.)

A sequence analysis restricted to only *human* connexin genes reveals three families (Fig. 6-20B): CJA, CJB, and CJC. Members of a family of channel proteins often exhibit different patterns of tissue expression. For example, Cx32 is expressed in the liver, Schwann cells, and oligodendrocytes, whereas Cx43 is expressed in heart and many other tissues.

The functional properties of cloned channel genes are generally consistent with the classification of channel subtypes based on molecular evolution. For example, ion channels that share the property of being voltage gated also share sequence homology of their voltage-sensing domain. We discuss voltage-gated channels in Chapter 7.

Hydrophobic domains of channel proteins can predict how these proteins weave through the membrane

From sequence information of many ion channels, a number of common structural principles emerge. Like other integral membrane proteins (see Chapter 2), channel proteins generally have several segments of hydrophobic amino acids, each long enough (~20 amino acids) to span the lipid bilayer as an α helix. If the channel has N membrane-spanning segments, it also has $N + 1$ hydrophilic domains of variable length that connect or terminate the membrane spans. Putative transmembrane segments are normally identified by hydropathy analysis (see Table 2-1), which identifies long segments of hydrophobic amino acid residues. In some cases, supporting biochemical evidence indicates that such domains are actually embedded in the membrane. By analogy to a few membrane proteins of known three-dimensional structure, such as the bacterial photosynthetic reaction center, it is generally presumed that such hydrophobic transmembrane domains have an α-helical conformation. The intervening hydrophilic segments that link the transmembrane regions together are presumed to form extracellular and intracellular protein domains that contact the aqueous solution.

The primary sequences of channel proteins are often schematically represented by hypothetical folding diagrams, such as that shown in Figure 6-21A for Cx32, one of the connexins that we have already discussed. Cx32 is a polypeptide of 284 amino acids that contains four identifiable hydrophobic transmembrane segments. In connexins, these transmembrane segments are known as M1, M2, M3, and M4. Biochemical evidence indicates that the N-terminal and C-terminal hydrophilic segments of connexin are located on the cytoplasmic side of the membrane and that the M3 domain is involved in forming part of the gap junction pore. Mutations in Cx32 can lead to a rare hereditary neuropathy known as Charcot-Marie-Tooth disease (see the box on this disease).

Protein superfamilies, subfamilies, and subtypes are the structural bases of channel diversity

Table 6-2 summarizes the basic functional and structural aspects of currently recognized families of the pore-forming subunits of human ion channel proteins. The table (1) groups these channels into structurally related protein families; (2) describes their properties; (3) lists the assigned human gene symbols, number of genes, and protein names; (4) summarizes noted physiological functions; (5) lists human diseases associated with the corresponding ion channels; and (6) provides a reference to Figure 6-21 that indicates the hypothetical membrane topology. Because the membrane topology diagrams in Figure 6-21 are based primarily on hydropathy analysis, they should be considered "best-guess" representations unless the structure has been confirmed by direct approaches (e.g., inward rectifier K^+ channels and ClC chloride channels). We briefly summarize major aspects of the molecular physiology of human ion channel families, in the order of their presentation in Table 6-2. More detailed functional information on many of these channels is discussed in numerous chapters of this text.

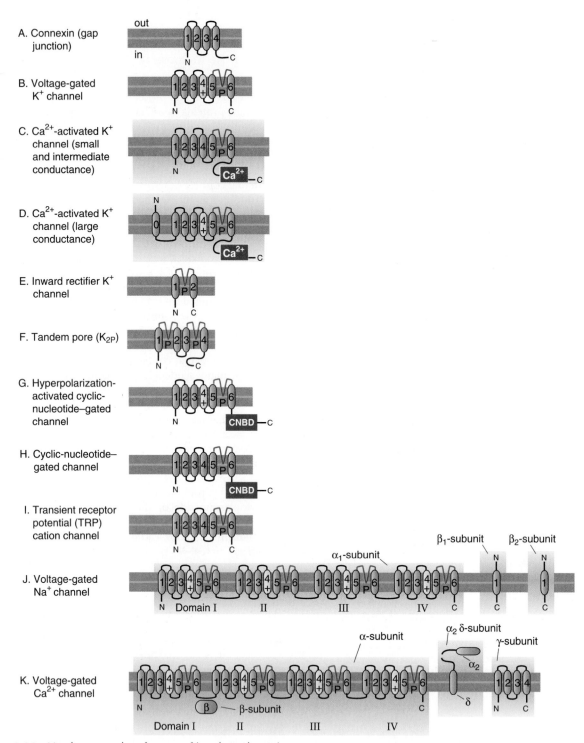

Figure 6-21 Membrane topology features of ion channel proteins.

Connexins We discussed these channels earlier in the section on gap junctions, in Figures 6-18 and 6-20, and in the box on Charcot-Marie-Tooth disease.

K⁺ Channels These channels form the largest and most diverse family of ion channels and share a common K⁺-selective pore domain containing two transmembrane segments (TMs). The family includes five distinct subfamilies, all of which we will discuss in Chapter 7: (1) Kv voltage-gated K⁺

channels, (2) small- and intermediate-conductance Ca^{2+}-activated K⁺ channels (SK_{Ca} and IK_{Ca}), (3) large-conductance Ca^{2+}- and voltage-activated K⁺ channels (BK_{Ca}), (4) inward rectifier K⁺ channels (Kir), and (5) dimeric tandem two-pore K⁺ channels (K2P). For the first two subfamilies, the pore-forming complex consists of four subunits, each of which contains six TMs denoted S1 to S6 (Fig. 6-21B and 6-21C). BK_{Ca} channels are similar to Kv channels but have an additional S0 TM (Fig. 6-21D). The Kir channels consist of four subunits, each

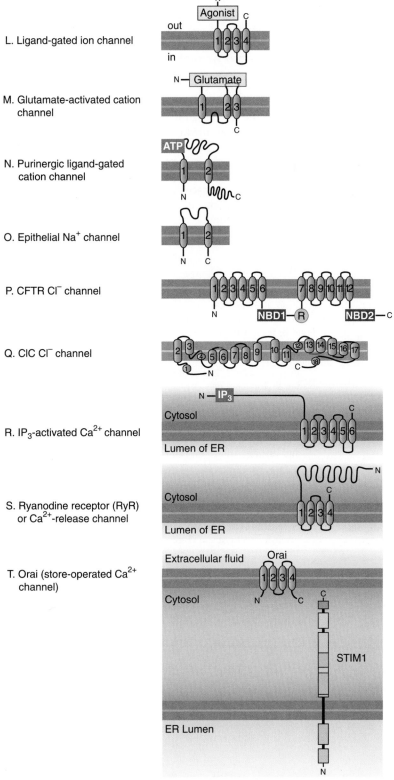

L. Ligand-gated ion channel

M. Glutamate-activated cation channel

N. Purinergic ligand-gated cation channel

O. Epithelial Na⁺ channel

P. CFTR Cl⁻ channel

Q. ClC Cl⁻ channel

R. IP₃-activated Ca²⁺ channel

S. Ryanodine receptor (RyR) or Ca²⁺-release channel

T. Orai (store-operated Ca²⁺ channel)

Figure 6-21, cont'd

of which contains two TMs analogous to S5 and S6 in the Kv channels (Fig. 6-21E). The K2P channels appear to be a tandem duplication of Kir channels (Fig. 6-21F).

HCN, CNG, and TRP Channels Hyperpolarization-activated, cyclic nucleotide–gated cation channels (**HCN** channels, Fig. 6-21G) play a critical role in electrical automaticity of the heart (see Chapter 21) and rhythmically firing neurons of the brain. **CNG** channels form a family of cation-selective channels that are directly activated by intracellular cyclic guanosine monophosphate (cGMP) or cyclic adenosine monophosphate (cAMP). These channels play an important role in visual and olfactory sensory transduction. The CNGs have the same basic S1 through S6 motif as K^+ channels, but they contain a unique cyclic nucleotide–binding domain at the C terminus (Fig. 6-21H). Transient receptor potential cation channels (**TRP** channels, Fig. 6-21I) are divided into at least six subfamilies: TRPA (for **a**nkyrin like), TRPC (for **c**anonical), TRPM (for **m**elastatin), TRPML (for **m**ucolipin), TRPP (for **p**olycystin 2), and TRPV (for **v**anilloid). One TRPV is activated by capsaicin, the "hot" ingredient of chili peppers; a TRPM responds to menthol, the "cool"-tasting substance in eucalyptus leaves. The capsaicin receptor TRP channel appears to function in pain and temperature sensation.

Voltage-Gated Na^+ Channels   The pore-forming subunits of voltage-gated Na^+ channels (**Nav**, see Chapter 7) comprise four domains (I, II, III, and IV), each of which contains the S1 to S6 structural motif (Fig. 6-21J) that is homologous to Kv K^+ channel monomers. Because domains I to IV of Nav channels are organized as four tandem repeats within the membrane, these domains are referred to as **pseudosubunits**. The Nav channels are associated with a unique family of auxiliary β-subunits, which are known to modify the gating behavior and membrane localization of the channel-forming α-subunit.

Voltage-Gated Ca^{2+} Channels   The pore-forming subunits of voltage-gated Ca^{2+} channels (**Cav**, see Chapter 7) are analogous to those for the Nav channels. Like Nav channels, Cav channels (Fig. 6-21K) are multisubunit complexes consisting of **accessory proteins** in addition to the channel-forming subunits.

Ligand-Gated Channels   The agonist-activated channels are also represented by three large and diverse gene families. The **pentameric Cys-loop receptor family** (Fig. 6-21L) includes cation- or Cl^--selective ion channels that are activated by binding of ACh (see Chapter 8), serotonin, GABA, and glycine (see Chapter 13). **Glutamate-activated cation channels** (Fig. 6-21M) include two subfamilies of excitatory AMPA-kainate and NMDA receptors (see Chapter 13). **Purinergic ligand-gated cation channels** (Fig. 6-21N) are activated by binding of extracellular ATP and other nucleotides (see Chapters 20 and 34).

Other Ion Channels   Amiloride-sensitive Na^+ channels (**ENaC**) are prominent in Na^+-transporting epithelia (Fig.

6-21O). The **cystic fibrosis transmembrane conductance regulator** (**CFTR**, see Chapter 5) is a Cl^- channel (Fig. 6-21P) that is a member of the ABC protein family. The unrelated ClC family of Cl^- channels are dimeric (Fig. 6-21Q). Table 6-2 includes two types of Ca^{2+} release channels. **ITPR** (see Chapter 3) is present in the endoplasmic reticulum membrane and is gated by the intracellular messenger inositol 1,4,5-trisphosphate (Fig. 6-21R). **RYR** (see Chapter 9) is located in the sarcoplasmic reticulum membrane of muscle and plays a critical role in the release of Ca^{2+} during muscle contraction (Fig. 6-21S). Finally, a recently discovered family of Ca^{2+}-selective channel proteins known as **ORAI** store-operated Ca^{2+} channels (Fig. 6-21T) has been found to play a role in entry of extracellular Ca^{2+} across the plasma membrane linked to IP_3 metabolism and depletion of intracellular Ca^{2+} from the endoplasmic reticulum of non-excitable cells (see p. 257).

REFERENCES

Books and Reviews

Ashcroft FM: Ion Channels and Disease: Channelopathies. New York: Academic Press, 2000.

Hille B: Ionic Channels of Excitable Membranes, 3rd ed. Sunderland, MA: Sinauer Associates, 2001.

Kim D: Fatty acid–sensitive two-pore domain K^+ channels. Trends Pharm Sci 2003; 24:648-654.

Neher E: Ion channels for communication between and within cells. Science 1992; 256:498-502.

Sakmann B, Neher E (eds): Single Channel Recording, 2nd ed. New York: Plenum Press, 1995.

Wei CJ, Xu X, Lo CW: Connexins and cell signaling in development and disease. Annu Rev Cell Dev Biol 2004; 20:811-838.

Journal Articles

Hamill OP, Marty A, Neher E, et al: Improved patch-clamp techniques for high resolution current recording from cells and cell-free membrane patches. Pflugers Arch 1981; 391:85-100.

Ho K, Nichols CG, Lederer J, et al: Cloning and expression of an inwardly rectifying ATP-regulated potassium channel. Nature 1993; 362:31-38.

Sigworth FJ, Neher E: Single Na-channel currents observed in cultured rat muscle cells. Nature 1980; 287:447-449.

Ressot C, Bruzzone R: Connexin channels in Schwann cells and the development of the X-linked form of Charcot-Marie-Tooth disease. Brain Res Rev 2000; 32:192-202.

CHAPTER 7

ELECTRICAL EXCITABILITY AND ACTION POTENTIALS

Edward G. Moczydlowski

Cellular communication in the nervous system is based on electrical and chemical signaling events that are mediated by ion channels. Certain types of cells, including neurons and myocytes, have a remarkable property called **electrical excitability**. In cells with this property, depolarization of the membrane above a certain **threshold** voltage triggers a spontaneous all-or-none response called an **action potential**. This action potential is a transient, regenerative electrical impulse in which the membrane potential (V_m) rapidly rises to a peak that is ~100 mV more positive than the normal, negative resting voltage (V_{rest}). Such signals, also called spikes, can propagate for long distances along nerve or muscle fibers. Conduction of action potentials allows information from sensory organs to be transmitted along afferent nerves leading to the brain. Conversely, the brain exerts voluntary and involuntary control over muscles and other effector organs by efferent nerves leading away from it.

In the first part of this chapter, we examine the biophysical and molecular basis of action potentials and the mechanisms that underlie their genesis and propagation. The second part deals with the structure and function of voltage-gated ion channel proteins. Finally, we examine the conduction properties of neurons—called cable properties—and how they determine the spread of action potentials along the axon.

MECHANISMS OF NERVE AND MUSCLE ACTION POTENTIALS

An action potential is a transient depolarization triggered by a depolarization beyond a threshold

The change in membrane potential that occurs during an action potential can be accurately measured by recording V_m with an intracellular microelectrode. Figure 7-1A is a diagram illustrating various features of a typical action potential recorded from an electrically stimulated nerve or muscle cell. If the depolarizing stimulus causes V_m to become more positive than a threshold voltage, the depolarization triggers an action potential. The initial depolarizing (positive-going)

phase of an action potential consists of a rapid and smooth increase in V_m from the negative resting potential to a maximum positive value that typically lies between +10 and +40 mV. This sharp rise in V_m to the peak voltage of the action potential is then followed by a slower repolarizing (negative-going) phase. The part of the action potential that lies above 0 mV is called the **overshoot**. As we will see, the time course and shape of the repolarization phase vary considerably among different excitable tissues and cells. The repolarization phase may lead directly back to V_{rest}, or it may undershoot and give rise to a voltage minimum that is more negative than V_{rest} before relaxing back to V_{rest}. Such an undershoot is an example of an **afterhyperpolarization**.

The threshold, amplitude, time course, and duration of the action potential depend on the following factors:

1. the gating (opening and closing) and permeability properties of specific types of ion channels—these properties depend on both V_m and time;
2. the intracellular and extracellular concentrations of the ions that pass through these channels, such as Na^+, K^+, Ca^{2+}, and Cl^-; and
3. membrane properties such as capacitance, resistance, and the geometry of the cell.

The shape of the action potential in a given cell reflects the specialized functions of that cell. For example, the brief action potentials of a nerve axon permit rapid signaling, whereas the prolonged, repetitive action potentials of cardiac and certain types of smooth muscle cells mediate the slow, rhythmic contractions of these tissues. Figure 7-1B compares action potentials recorded from an invertebrate nerve fiber (unmyelinated squid axon), a vertebrate nerve fiber (myelinated rabbit axon), a skeletal muscle fiber, and a cardiac atrial myocyte. This comparison illustrates the diversity in the duration and shape of the repolarizing phase of action potentials. The shape of the action potential is subject to hormonal modulation in certain cell types. As one example, the peptide hormone endothelin, produced by vascular endothelial cells, shortens the duration of the action potential when it is applied to a guinea pig atrial myocyte. Modulation of the shape and frequency of action potentials occurs

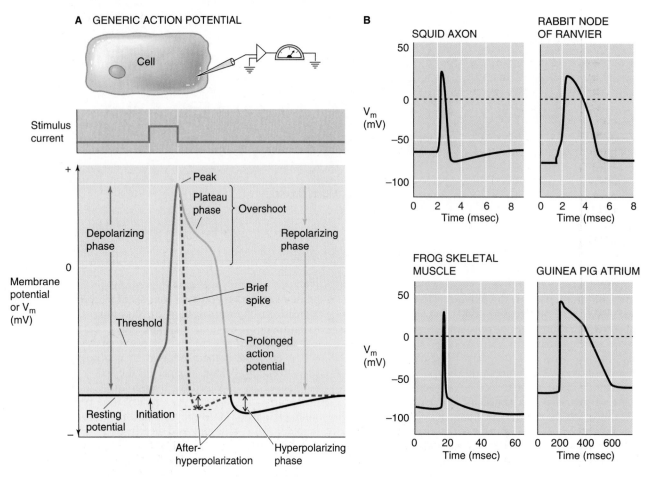

Figure 7-1 The action potential.

by various biochemical regulatory mechanisms that affect the function of ion channels.

In contrast to an action potential, a graded response is proportional to stimulus intensity and decays with distance along the axon

Not all electrical activity in nerve or muscle cells is characterized by an all-or-none response. As shown earlier in Figure 6-12A, when we apply a small square pulse of hyperpolarizing current to a cell membrane, V_m gradually becomes more negative and then stabilizes (Fig. 7-2A). In such an experiment, the observed change in V_m approximates an exponential time course, with a time constant (see Chapter 6) that is determined by the product of membrane resistance and capacitance ($\tau = RC$). Figure 7-2A also shows that progressively greater hyperpolarizing currents produce progressively larger V_m responses, but the time constant is always the same. The size of the **graded voltage change** (i.e., the steady-state ΔV_m) is proportional to the strength of the stimulus (i.e., the current), in accord with Ohm's law.

If instead of imposing a hyperpolarizing stimulus we impose a small *depolarizing* stimulus, V_m changes to the same extent and with the same time course as we described for the hyperpolarizing stimulus, but in the opposite direction (Fig. 7-2A). The size of ΔV_m is also proportional to the size of the depolarizing stimulus—up to a point. If the membrane is

excitable, a square wave depolarization above the threshold triggers an action potential, or voltage spike. Smaller or **subthreshold depolarizations** will not elicit an action potential. *Hyperpolarizations* are always ineffective. Thus, both hyperpolarizations and subthreshold depolarizations behave like graded voltage changes. That is, the magnitude of a cell's voltage change increases proportionally with the size of the stimulus. Such graded responses can be seen in the response of certain cells to synaptic transmitters, to sensory stimuli (e.g., light), or, in the laboratory, to the injection of current into cells through a microelectrode.

Why do excitable cells exhibit threshold behavior? As V_m becomes progressively more and more positive, the **gating** process (i.e., transitions from closed to open states) of certain types of voltage-gated ion channels becomes activated. When V_m passes the threshold, opening of these voltage-gated channels initiates the runaway depolarization that characterizes the rising phase of the action potential. Thus, the firing of an action potential is a binary, all-or-none event; that is, the spike has a constant, nongraded voltage peak that occurs only if the depolarizing stimulus exceeds the threshold.

Thus far we have seen that graded responses and action potentials differ markedly from one another if we examine the cell at one particular site. However, graded responses and action potentials also behave very differently in the way that they spread along the membrane from the site of origin. Figure 7-2B illustrates how a graded hyperpolarizing

A RESPONSE TO GRADED CURRENT STIMULI

Stimulus current   Response

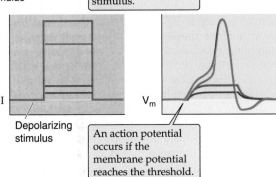

Hyperpolarizing stimulus

Electrotonic potentials are proportional to the stimulus.

Depolarizing stimulus

An action potential occurs if the membrane potential reaches the threshold.

B RESPONSE TO STIMULI AS A FUNCTION OF DISTANCE

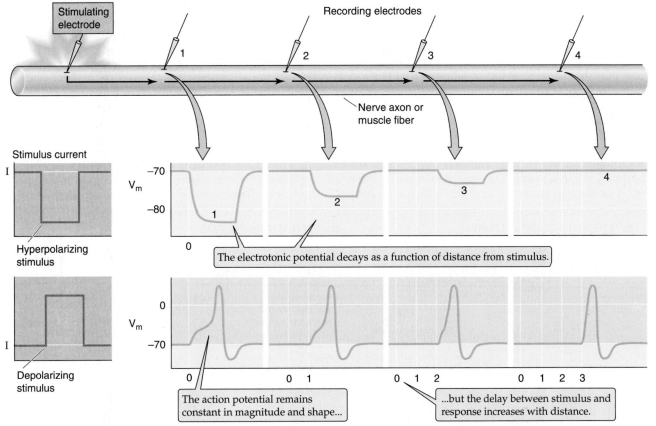

Stimulating electrode

Recording electrodes

Nerve axon or muscle fiber

Stimulus current

Hyperpolarizing stimulus

The electrotonic potential decays as a function of distance from stimulus.

Depolarizing stimulus

The action potential remains constant in magnitude and shape...

...but the delay between stimulus and response increases with distance.

Figure 7-2 Basic properties of action potentials. **A,** The upper panels show four graded hyperpolarizing stimuli and the V_m responses. The lower panels show four graded depolarizing stimuli and the V_m responses. Note that the two largest stimuli evoke identical action potentials. **B,** A stimulating electrode injects current at the extreme left of the cell. Four recording electrodes monitor V_m at equidistant sites to the right. If the stimulus is hyperpolarizing, the graded V_m responses decay with distance from the stimulus site. If the stimulus is depolarizing and large enough to evoke an action potential, a full action potential appears at each of the recording sites. However, the action potential arrives at the most distant sites with increasing delay.

response spreads along the axon of a neuron or along a skeletal muscle fiber. As the graded response spreads, its magnitude decays exponentially with the distance from the site of stimulation because of loss of energy to the medium. This decay is called **electrotonic conduction**. We see the same kind of electrotonic spread for a subthreshold, depolarizing stimulus. The electrotonic spread of graded responses is governed by the same physical principles that determine the spread of electrical current in an electrical cable. We briefly discuss **cable theory** at the end of this chapter.

Propagation of an action potential signal is very different from the spread of a graded signal. In a healthy axon or muscle fiber, action potentials propagate at a constant velocity (up to ~130 m/s), without change in amplitude or shape. The amplitude of a propagating action potential does not diminish with distance, as would a graded, subthreshold response, because excitation of voltage-gated channels in adjacent regions of the excitable membrane progressively regenerates the original response. Because the action potential in a given nerve fiber propagates at a constant velocity, the time delay between the stimulus and the peak of the action potential increases linearly with distance from the point of stimulus.

Excitation of a nerve or muscle depends on the product (strength × duration) of the stimulus and on the refractory period

In the preceding section, the importance of the *magnitude* (intensity) of the depolarizing stimulus emerged as a critical factor for firing of an action potential. However, the *duration* of the stimulus pulse is also important. A large stimulus is effective in triggering an action potential even at short duration, and a small stimulus may be effective at long duration (Fig. 7-3A). This strength-duration relationship arises because the same minimum electrical charge necessary to excite an action potential can come from a current that is either brief but large or prolonged but small. It is the *product*

of strength and duration that determines excitability, and thus these two parameters are inversely related in their effectiveness. However, regardless of the stimulus strength, successful stimulation requires a minimum duration (vertical asymptote in Fig. 7-3A). Conversely, regardless of the stimulus duration, successful stimulation requires a minimum strength (horizontal asymptote in Fig. 7-3A).

An important feature of excitable cells is their ability to fire repetitive action potentials. Once a cell fires an action potential, how quickly can it fire a second? If we were to impose a current step that produced a graded response, we could immediately add a second current step while the first persisted. As long as V_m did not exceed the threshold, the result would be a simple algebraic and instantaneous summation of the two graded responses. The situation for action potentials is quite different. First, action potentials never summate. Second, after one action potential fires, a finite time must elapse before it is possible to trigger a second. The time after initiation of an action potential when it is impossible or difficult to produce a second spike is the **refractory period** (Fig. 7-3B). The **absolute refractory period** lasts from initiation of the spike to a time after the peak when repolarization is almost complete. During this time, a second action potential cannot be elicited, regardless of the stimulus strength or duration. After this period, a second action potential can be evoked during the **relative refractory period**, but the minimal stimulus necessary for activation is stronger or longer than predicted by the strength-duration curve for the first action potential. The two phases of the refractory period arise from the gating properties of particular Na+ and K+ channels and the overlapping time course of their currents.

The action potential arises from changes in membrane conductance to Na+ and K+

Approximately 200 years after Luigi Galvani (1737–1798) discovered "animal electricity," the electrochemical basis of the nerve action potential was finally elucidated by the com-

A   STRENGTH-DURATION CURVE

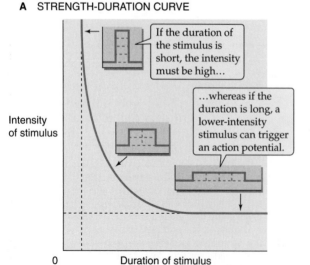

B   REFRACTORY PERIODS

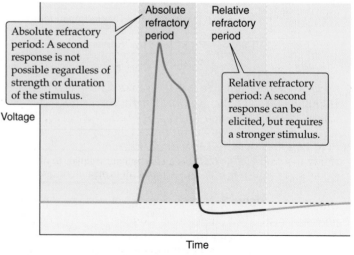

Figure 7-3   Nerve and muscle excitability. The curve in **A** represents the combination of the minimum stimulus intensity and duration that is required to reach threshold and to evoke an action potential.

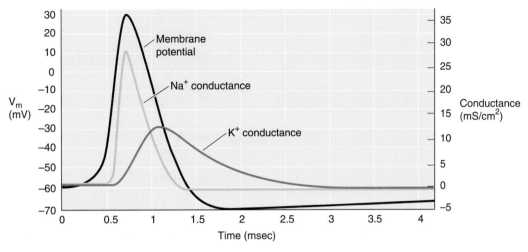

Figure 7-4 Changes in ionic conductance that underlie the action potential. *(Data from Hodgkin AL, Huxley AF: A quantitative description of membrane current and its application to conduction and excitation in nerve. J Physiol [Lond] 1952; 117:500-544.)*

bined application of modern electrical recording techniques and the theory of electrodiffusion (see Chapter 6). We now understand that the nerve action potential is a phenomenon involving voltage-dependent currents of Na^+ and K^+ that flow through distinct molecular pathways called Na^+ channels and K^+ channels. In 1963, the Nobel Prize in Physiology or Medicine was awarded to A. L. Hodgkin and A. F. Huxley for their quantitative description of these ionic currents in the squid giant axon in studies involving two-electrode voltage-clamp recordings. Invertebrate axons are unmyelinated, and axons in certain squid nerves have an unusually large diameter (500 to 1000 μm), which allows both external and internal ionic concentrations to be manipulated experimentally. The basic concepts underlying the Hodgkin-Huxley analysis have since been extended to a wide variety of voltage-dependent ionic currents.

The squid axon generates a very brief action potential signal without a significant plateau phase (Fig. 7-4). Ionic permeability changes underlying this impulse can be interpreted with a form of the constant-field equation (see Equation 6-9) that includes only Na^+ and K^+:

$$V_{rev} = \frac{RT}{F} \ln\left(\frac{P_K[K^+]_o + P_{Na}[Na^+]_o}{P_K[K^+]_i + P_{Na}[Na^+]_i} \right) \quad (7-1)$$

According to Equation 7-1, the negative resting potential (about −60 mV) of the axon membrane corresponds to a K^+/Na^+ permeability ratio (P_K/P_{Na}) of ~14:1. The change in V_m to a value near +40 mV at the peak of the action potential must involve a transient and selective increase in the permeability to either Na^+ or Ca^{2+} because the equilibrium potential of these cations lies in the positive voltage range (see Fig. 6-10). Experimentally, if $[Na^+]_o$ is reduced by replacing it with a nonelectrolyte such as sucrose, the nerve action potential decreases in amplitude. Complementary experiments measuring radioactive tracer fluxes of Na^+ and K^+ also demonstrate that action potentials are accompanied by a small influx of Na^+ and an efflux of K^+. These and related findings showed that the waveform of the squid action potential is produced by separate permeability pathways for Na^+ and K^+.

The time course of the action potential (Fig. 7-4) can be dissected into an initial, transient increase in Na^+ conductance (and thus permeability), followed by a similar but delayed increase in K^+ conductance. As one would predict from our discussion of Equation 6-12, a transient increase in Na^+ conductance—relative to K^+—would shift V_m toward the positive Na^+ equilibrium potential (E_{Na}); the subsequent increase in K^+ conductance would restore the original negative resting potential, which approaches the K^+ equilibrium potential (E_K). We can thus attribute the depolarizing and repolarizing phases of the action potential to a transient reversal of the large resting conductance of K^+ relative to Na^+.

The Na^+ and K^+ currents that flow during the action potential are time and voltage dependent

The assumption of independent permeability pathways—or distinct channels for Na^+ and K^+—has been verified by ionic substitution and pharmacological experiments. Figure 7-5 illustrates the use of inhibitors to pharmacologically dissect Na^+ and K^+ currents (I_{Na} and I_K) from the total membrane current (I_m) in a typical excitable membrane preparation, such as a myelinated vertebrate nerve fiber bathed in a normal physiological solution. In a myelinated nerve, these currents flow through small segments of the axon that are *not* covered with myelin; these segments are called nodes of Ranvier. As we shall see, pharmacological dissection of Na^+ and K^+ currents allows us to determine how they vary with time and how they depend on V_m.

Time Dependence of Na^+ and K^+ Currents Stepwise *hyperpolarization* of the nerve membrane (from a "holding potential" of −80 to −140 mV) by a voltage-clamp technique produces a transient capacitative current (see Chapter 6) but

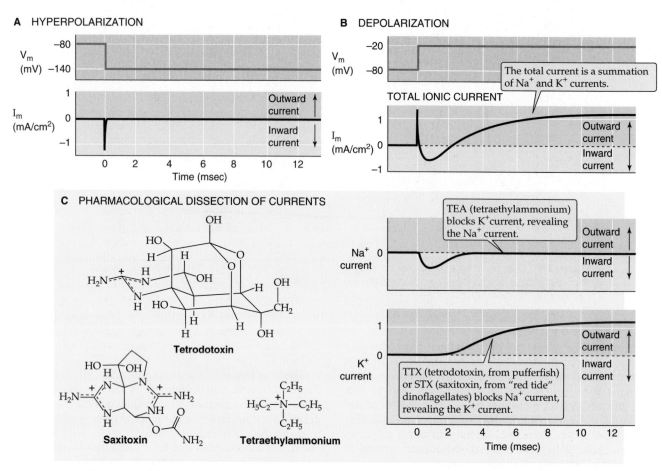

Figure 7-5   Dissection of Na⁺ and K⁺ currents by voltage-clamp analysis and pharmacology. **A,** In a typical voltage-clamp experiment, a sudden *hyper*polarization from −80 to −140 mV results in a transient capacitative current but no ionic currents. **B,** In a voltage-clamp experiment, a sudden *de*polarization from −80 to −20 mV results in a transient capacitative current followed first by an inward ionic current and then by an outward ionic current. **C,** Blockade of the outward current by TEA leaves only the inward current, which is carried by Na⁺. Conversely, a blockade of the inward current by TTX or STX leaves only the outward current, which is carried by K⁺.

little or no ionic current (Fig. 7-5A). However, a step *depolarization* of equivalent magnitude produces a capacitative transient current that is followed by a large, time-dependent ionic current (Fig. 7-5B). This ionic current first flows inward, reaches a maximum in the inward direction, and then reverses to the outward direction. The initial inward current corresponds to a movement of cations into the axon. After the reversal of I_m, the outward current corresponds to an outward movement of cations. Ion substitution experiments—in which selected ions are removed from either the outside or the inside of the cell—have shown that the inward current corresponds to Na⁺ current and the outward current corresponds to K⁺ current. Applying a particular organic cation, tetraethylammonium (TEA), to an axon prevents the outward I_K and reveals the isolated inward I_{Na} (Fig. 7-5C, top I_m record). Conversely, adding either tetrodotoxin (TTX) or saxitoxin (STX)—which we discuss later—abolishes the inward I_{Na} and reveals the isolated outward I_K (Fig. 7-5C, bottom I_m record). TEA, TTX, and STX are cationic molecules that act as specific ion channel blockers. Millimolar concentrations of TEA block the outer entrance of certain neuronal K⁺ channels, and nanomolar concentrations of TTX (or STX) block the outer entrance of neuronal Na⁺ channels. Biophysical evidence suggests that these particular molecules act by binding in the outer vestibule of their respective channels, thus occluding the channel pore to permeant ions. Thus, the terms *channel block* and *blocking agent* are often used to describe their effect.

Voltage Dependence of Na⁺ and K⁺ Currents   The ability to use specific inhibitors to resolve separate pathways for Na⁺ and K⁺ current in excitable membranes makes it possible to characterize how these ionic currents depend on V_m. Figure 7-6A illustrates an idealized family of records of total membrane current (I_m) recorded from a myelinated nerve axon. In each case, V_m was initially clamped to −60 mV and then rapidly shifted to a more positive value. The five traces in Figure 7-6A show the current evoked by depolarizations to −45, −30, 0, +30, and +60 mV. By repeating the same experiment in the presence of TEA or TTX, one can obtain the unique time course and voltage dependence of I_{Na} and I_K.

The time course of I_{Na} obtained in the presence of TEA to block K^+ channels is distinctly biphasic (Fig. 7-6B). Immediately after a depolarizing voltage step to a V_m of −30 mV, for example, the inward I_{Na} (downward-going) reaches a "peak" value and then returns to zero. The initial phase of this time course (before the peak) is called **activation**, and the later phase (after the peak) is called **inactivation**.

In contrast to I_{Na}, a depolarizing voltage step to a V_m of +60 mV, for example, causes the outward I_K to activate with a definite lag time that gives rise to a sigmoidal time course (Fig. 7-6C). Moreover, I_K takes longer to reach its maximal value (peak). Notice that the K^+ current is sustained even at the end of the depolarizing pulse. Thus, I_K does not show significant inactivation during the same rapid time scale as does I_{Na}.

If we plot the peak Na^+ and K^+ currents obtained at each of the clamped voltages in Figure 7-6B and C versus the clamped voltages, we obtain the two *I-V* relationships shown in Figure 7-6D. Because the currents in Figure 7-6B and C represent the activity of many individual ion channels, the plots in Figure 7-6D are **macroscopic current-voltage relationships**. The *I-V* relationship for K^+ is the more straightforward of the two. If we step V_m from −60 mV to increasingly more positive values, the peak I_K is outward and increases with voltage in a monotonic fashion, as expected from Ohm's law ($\Delta I = \Delta V/R$). Because such nerve K^+ channels pass current in the outward direction and activate with a time delay (Fig. 7-6C) under physiological conditions, the term **delayed rectifier K^+** current (or delayed, outwardly rectifying K^+ channel) has been coined. We discuss this delayed outward rectifying K^+ current and the K^+ channel responsible for it in more detail later.

The voltage dependence of the peak Na^+ current is biphasic. Stepping V_m from −60 mV to more positive values at first causes I_{Na} to become increasingly negative (i.e., inward) and then to reach a peak. This portion of the Na^+ *I-V* relationship is sometimes referred to as the negative resistance region because the negative slope corresponds to an anomalous or negative resistance value according to Ohm's law ($\Delta I = \Delta V/R$). At more positive values of V_m, the peak I_{Na} reverses direction and becomes more positive, with a nearly linear or ohmic dependence on voltage.

Macroscopic Na^+ and K^+ currents result from the opening and closing of many channels

The complex macroscopic *I-V* relationships of the Na^+ and K^+ currents (Fig. 7-6D) reflect the single-channel conductance and gating of Na^+ and K^+ channels. The pore of an open channel is expected to have a linear or ohmic *I-V* relationship:

$$i_X = g_X(V_m - E_X) \qquad (7\text{-}2)$$

Here, i_x is the single-channel current and g_x is the single-channel conductance. We already introduced a similar relationship as Equation 6-15. Figure 7-7A illustrates the predicted linear behavior of single-channel currents as a function of V_m for hypothetical Na^+ and K^+ channels. Assuming a Na^+ reversal potential (E_{Na}) of +50 mV, the Na^+ current is zero at a V_m of +50 mV. Similarly, with an E_K of −80 mV,

the K^+ current is zero at a V_m of −80 mV. Assuming a unitary conductance of 20 pS for each channel, the two *I-V* relationships have the same slope. Note that these idealized single-channel *I-V* plots for Na^+ and K^+ approximate the shape of the macroscopic peak *I-V* relationships of Figure 7-6D for the positive V_m range (i.e., in the right upper quadrant of Fig. 7-6D). In this V_m range, both the Na^+ and K^+ channels through which the currents flow are maximally activated at the peaks of their respective time courses. Thus, the macroscopic peak *I-V* relationships (Fig. 7-6D) are nearly linear in this range, just as they would be for idealized, fully open channels (Fig. 7-7A).

However, in the negative voltage range, the macroscopic peak *I-V* relationships for Na^+ and K^+ in Figure 7-6D deviate from the linear (or ohmic) behavior in Figure 7-7A. Why, as the voltage is made more negative, does the inward Na^+ current fail to increase further and even decrease (negative resistance)? Similarly, why, as the voltage becomes more negative, does the outward K^+ current fall to zero long before the voltage reaches an E_K of −80 mV? The answer is that the probability that the Na^+ and K^+ channels are "open" (P_o)—and therefore able to conduct current—depends on voltage. We introduced the concept of open probability in Chapter 6. To see why V_m might affect P_o, we consider a simplified model.

Assume that a channel protein molecule may exist in either of two conformational states, closed (C) and open (O), and that these two conformational states are in equilibrium with one another:

$$C \rightleftharpoons O$$

The equilibrium constant K_{eq} for this reaction is the ratio of the concentrations of open to closed channels, which can also be expressed as the ratio of the probability that the channel is open (P_o) to the probability that the channel is closed (P_c):

$$K_{eq} = \frac{[\text{Open}]}{[\text{Closed}]} = \frac{P_o}{P_c} \qquad (7\text{-}3)$$

In the case of voltage-gated channel proteins, V_m changes affect K_{eq} and thus the distribution of channels between the open and closed states. The probability of a channel's being open depends on V_m, according to a Boltzmann distribution (Fig. 7-7B).

If the valence (z) of the voltage-sensing part of the channel protein (i.e., the "gating charge") is positive, the probability of channel opening should increase from 0 to 1 in a sigmoid fashion as V_m becomes more positive. Figure 7-7B shows the behavior of P_o for hypothetical Na^+ and K^+ channels that simulate Na^+ and K^+ channels in real cells.

To summarize, Figure 7-7A shows that once a single channel is open, the current flowing through the open channel is linearly related to V_m. Figure 7-7B shows that the likelihood that the channel is open depends on V_m in a sigmoid fashion. The actual macroscopic current (I_X) depends on the number of channels (N) in the area of membrane being sampled, the open probability, and the single-channel current, as we already pointed out in Equation 6-21:

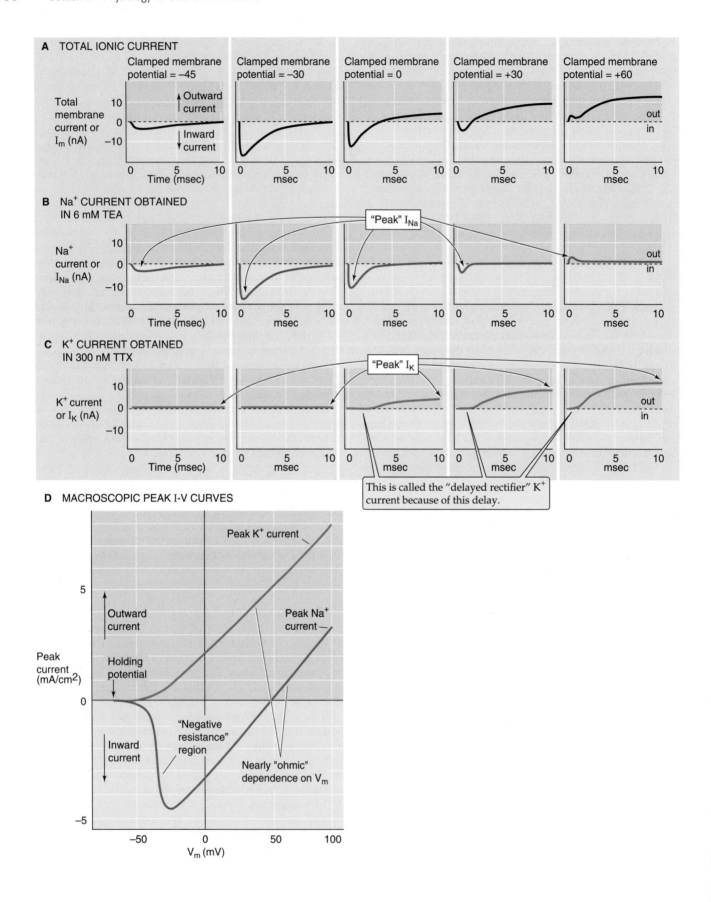

Figure 7-6 Voltage dependence of ionic currents. **A,** The *top panels* show the time course of the total ionic current. This is a voltage-clamp experiment on a frog node of Ranvier. Sudden shifting of V_m from a holding potential of −60 mV to −45, −30, 0, +30, and +60 mV elicits ionic currents that depend on V_m. **B,** These results are comparable to those in **A,** except that TEA abolished the outward K$^+$ currents, leaving the Na$^+$ current. Notice that the peak Na$^+$ current varies with V_m. **C,** These results are comparable to those in **A,** except that TTX abolished the inward Na$^+$ currents, leaving the K$^+$ current. Notice that the peak K$^+$ current varies with V_m. **D,** The *blue curve* is a plot of peak Na$^+$ currents from experiments that are similar to those in **B.** The *green curve* is a plot of peak K$^+$ currents from experiments that are similar to those in **C.** Notice that both the Na$^+$ and K$^+$ currents are linear or ohmic in the positive voltage range. In a more negative V_m range, the Na$^+$ current exhibits negative resistance, that is, the magnitude of the current becomes more negative rather than more positive as V_m increases in the positive direction. (**A-C,** *Data from Hille B: Common mode of action of three agents that decrease the transient change in sodium permeability in nerves. Nature 1966; 210:1220-1222; and Hille B: The selective inhibition of delayed potassium currents in nerve by tetraethylammonium ions. J Gen Physiol 1967; 50:1287-1302.* **D,** *Data from Cole KS, Moore JW: Ionic current measurements in the squid giant axon membrane. J Gen Physiol 1960; 44:123-167.*)

$$I_X = NP_o i_X \qquad (7-4)$$

Thus, we can use Equation 7-4 to compute the macroscopic currents (*I*) contributed by our hypothetical Na$^+$ and K$^+$ channels. We merely multiply the number of channels (which we assume to be 100 for both cations), the open probability for Na$^+$ and K$^+$ channels in Figure 7-7B, and the single-channel currents for Na$^+$ and K$^+$ in Figure 7-7A. If we compare the resulting hypothetical I_{Na} and I_K curves in Figure 7-7C, which are based on a simple theory, with actual data on macroscopic *I-V* relationships (Fig. 7-6D), we see that this model provides a reasonable description of voltage-sensitive ionic currents.

The Hodgkin-Huxley model predicts macroscopic currents and the shape of the action potential

Even before the concepts of single channels and channel proteins emerged, Hodgkin and Huxley in 1952 formulated voltage-dependent and time-dependent parameters to predict the ionic currents that underlie the action potential of the squid giant axon. Hodgkin and Huxley defined a series of three dimensionless parameters, *n*, *m*, and *h*, each of which can have a value between 0 and 1. The activation parameter *n* describes the probability that the K$^+$ channels are open (Fig. 7-8A). The activation parameter *m* describes the probability that the Na$^+$ channels are open (Fig. 7-8B, blue curve). Because Hodgkin and Huxley observed that the Na$^+$ current **inactivates**, they introduced the inactivation parameter *h* to describe this process (Fig. 7-8B, violet curve).

Hodgkin and Huxley developed an equation for total membrane current (I_m) and used it to predict the shape of the action potential in the squid giant axon. Figure 7-8C shows their *predicted* action potential, which is triggered by a brief depolarization. Figure 7-8D shows an actual recording. The close agreement between the Hodgkin-Huxley (HH) theory and experiment indicates that this model provides a reasonable description of nerve excitation. The fundamental observation of Hodgkin and Huxley was that a rapid increase in Na$^+$ conductance causes the upswing or depolarizing phase of the action potential as V_m approaches E_{Na}, whereas inactivation of Na$^+$ conductance and delayed activation of K$^+$ conductance underlie the repolarization of V_m to its resting value near E_K. The importance of the HH

model in electrophysiology is that it was the first analysis to accurately describe the time course and voltage dependence of ionic currents that occur during an action potential.

In addition to delineating the basis of the action potential waveform, the HH model also explains threshold behavior and the refractory period. For an action potential to fire, an external stimulus must depolarize the membrane above threshold to activate a sufficient number of Na$^+$ channels. The external stimulus can come from an electrode, a synaptic event, or propagation of a depolarizing wave along the cell membrane. What determines whether a stimulus will be sufficient to reach the threshold V_m for firing of an action potential? The number of Na$^+$ channels activated by the stimulus is determined by the voltage dependence of the *activation* process (i.e., *m* parameter). Opposing the local depolarization that is produced by the current flowing through these Na$^+$ channels are current losses that occur because of passive spread of the current through intracellular and extracellular fluid (see the later discussion of cable theory). Also opposing depolarization is the hyperpolarizing effect of currents through any open K$^+$ or Cl$^-$ channels in the membrane. Thus, the **threshold** is the level of depolarization at which the depolarizing effect of the open Na$^+$ channels becomes sufficiently self-reinforcing to overcome these opposing influences. Once threshold is reached, further activation of Na$^+$ channels rapidly drives V_m toward E_{Na}.

The basis of the **absolute refractory period**, the time during which a second action potential cannot occur under any circumstances, is *Na$^+$ channel inactivation*. In other words, it is impossible to recruit a sufficient number of Na$^+$ channels to generate a second spike unless previously activated Na$^+$ channels have recovered from inactivation (i.e., *h* parameter), a process that takes several milliseconds. The **relative refractory period**, during which a stronger than normal stimulus is required to elicit a second action potential, depends largely on delayed *K$^+$ channel opening* (i.e., *n* parameter). In other words, for a certain period after the peak of the action potential, the increased K$^+$ conductance tends to hyperpolarize the membrane, so a stronger depolarizing stimulus is required to activate the population of Na$^+$ channels that in the meantime have recovered from inactivation.

Another key feature of the HH model is that it implies that V_m activates a channel by inducing the movement of an electrically charged gating particle or voltage sensor across the membrane. Physically, this gating could occur by the

A   SINGLE-CHANNEL I-V RELATIONSHIPS

Single-channel current i(pA)

$g_K = 20$ pS, $E_K = -80$ mV

E_K

E_{Na} Na⁺

K⁺

−100   −50   0   50   100   mV

Unitary current:
$i_x = g_x (V_m - E_x)$

$g_{Na} = 20$ pS, $E_{Na} = +50$ mV

**B   VOLTAGE DEPENDENCE OF
SINGLE-CHANNEL OPEN PROBABILITIES**

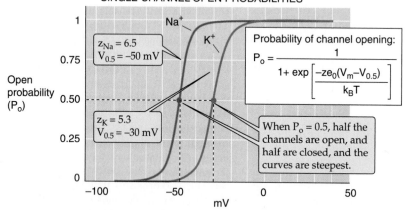

Open probability (P_o)

Na⁺   K⁺

$z_{Na} = 6.5$
$V_{0.5} = -50$ mV

Probability of channel opening:
$$P_o = \cfrac{1}{1 + \exp\left[\cfrac{-ze_0(V_m - V_{0.5})}{k_B T}\right]}$$

$z_K = 5.3$
$V_{0.5} = -30$ mV

When $P_o = 0.5$, half the channels are open, and half are closed, and the curves are steepest.

C   RECONSTRUCTED I-V RELATIONSHIPS

Macroscopic current I(nA)

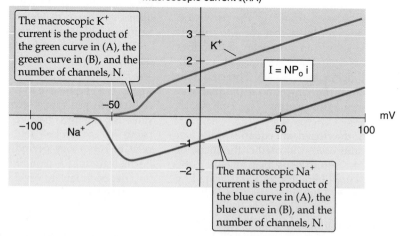

The macroscopic K⁺ current is the product of the green curve in (A), the green curve in (B), and the number of channels, N.

K⁺

$I = NP_o\, i$

Na⁺

The macroscopic Na⁺ current is the product of the blue curve in (A), the blue curve in (B), and the number of channels, N.

Figure 7-7   The microscopic basis of macroscopic *I-V* relationships. **A,** The *blue line* represents the *I-V* relationship of an idealized, open Na⁺ channel. The *green line* represents the *I-V* relationship of an idealized, open K⁺ channel. Because the channels are assumed to always be fully open (i.e., the conductance does not change with voltage), the current through them is linear or ohmic. **B,** The *blue curve* shows the open probability of Na⁺ channels. The equation in the inset will generate this curve if the values $z_{Na} = 6.5$ and $V_{0.5}$ = −50 mV are inserted. The *green curve* shows the open probability of K⁺ channels. The equation in the *inset* will generate this curve if the values $z_K = 5.3$ and $V_{0.5}$ = −30 mV are inserted. **C,** We can obtain a reasonable estimate for the macroscopic Na⁺ current and the macroscopic K⁺ current by multiplying the single-channel current in **A,** the P_o in **B,** and the number of channels (*N*). We assume that there are 100 Na⁺ and 100 K⁺ channels.

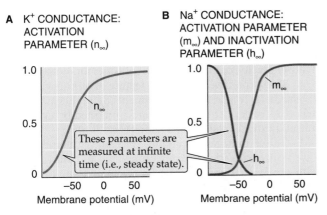

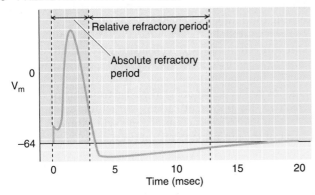

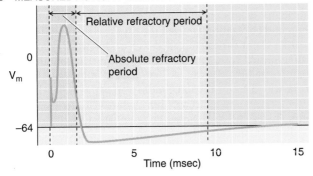

Figure 7-8 Voltage-dependent parameters of the Hodgkin-Huxley model and their use in predicting the shape of the action potential. **A,** The *n* parameter describes the probability that each of four particles in the K⁺ channel is in the proper state for channel opening. It is believed that these four "particles" are the gates of the four K⁺-channel subunits. The parameter plotted here is the value of *n* at infinite time. **B,** The *m* parameter describes the probability that each of three particles in the Na⁺ channel is in the proper state for channel opening. The *h* parameter describes the probability that an inactivation particle is *not* in the proper state for inactivating the Na⁺ channel. Thus, a high *h* favors the open state of the channel. The parameters plotted here are the values of *m* and *h* at infinite time. **C,** Hodgkin and Huxley used data similar to those in **A** and **B** to compute the time course of an action potential in the squid giant axon. **D,** The actual data are very similar to the computed action potential in **C.** *(Data from Hodgkin AL, Huxley AF: A quantitative description of membrane current and its application to conduction and excitation in nerve. J Physiol 1952; 117:500-544.)*

movement of a charged portion of the channel protein through all or part of the transmembrane electrical field or by the reorientation of an electrical dipole (a neutral structure with positive and negative polarity) within the electrical field of the membrane. Thus, the HH model correctly predicted that activation of a voltage-gated Na⁺ channel or K⁺ channel should be accompanied by a small movement of gating charge, which should produce a **gating current**. This prediction was satisfied in 1973 when Armstrong and Bezanilla recorded a very small, rapid outward current that is activated by depolarization in a voltage-clamped squid axon in which the ionic current of the Na⁺ channels is completely blocked by TTX (Fig. 7-5C, bottom I_m record). This tiny, transient gating current is almost finished by the time that the slower K⁺ current begins to flow. The properties of such gating currents account for the voltage dependence of channel activation kinetics. Although the key features of the HH theory are correct, modern patch-clamp studies of single Na⁺ and K⁺ channels have revealed that the kinetics of channel gating are much more complicated than originally assumed. Such complexity is to be expected inasmuch as the conformational dynamics of large protein molecules cannot generally be adequately described by simple models that incorporate only a few discrete states.

PHYSIOLOGY OF VOLTAGE-GATED CHANNELS AND THEIR RELATIVES

A large superfamily of structurally related membrane proteins includes voltage-gated and related channels

In Chapter 6, we previewed families of channels that include voltage-gated Na⁺ channels, Ca²⁺ channels, and K⁺ channels. These voltage-gated channels are part of a larger superfamily of channel proteins called the **voltage-gated–like (VGL) ion channel superfamily**, which includes additional voltage-gated channels, as well as genetically related channels that are not strictly activated by voltage. Figure 7-9 shows a dendrogram with four branches corresponding to four distinct families belonging to the VGL superfamily. In this section, we discuss how structural relationships among these proteins determine their physiological functions.

Initial progress toward biochemical characterization of the voltage-gated ion channels responsible for the action potential began with the discovery of naturally occurring, specific, high-affinity neurotoxins such as TTX and STX and their use as biochemical probes. Tritium-labeled derivatives of TTX and STX were prepared chemically and used in radioligand-binding assays to directly measure the number of voltage-gated Na⁺ channels in excitable tissues.

The electroplax organ of the electric eel (*Electrophorus electricus*) proved to be a convenient source of tissue for the first successful biochemical purification of the Na⁺ channel protein by Agnew and coworkers in 1978. These Na⁺ channels consist of a large glycosylated α subunit of ~200 kDa that contains the TTX binding site. Reconstitution experiments revealed that this subunit—by itself—mediates ionic selectivity for Na⁺, voltage-dependent gating and pharmacological sensitivity to various neurotoxins. Thus, the α subunit

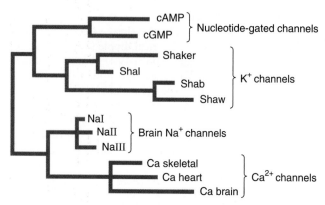

Figure 7-9 Family tree of hypothetical evolutionary relationships among voltage-gated cation channels based on sequences of the S4 segments. This dendrogram of the superfamily of voltage-gated channels shows four distinct branches or families. Only a few examples of each are depicted. The family of nucleotide-gated channels is represented by mammalian channels that are gated by cAMP and cGMP. The family of K$^+$ channels is presented by four types of *Drosophila* channels. The family of Na$^+$ channels is represented by three types of Na$^+$ channels from mammalian brain. Finally, the family of Ca^{2+} channels is represented by mammalian channels from skeletal muscle, heart, and brain. *(Data from Strong M, Chandy KG, Gutman GA: Molecular evolution of voltage-sensitive ion channel genes: On the origin of electrical excitability. Mol Biol Evol 1993; 10:221-242.)*

is the channel-forming protein. Similar biochemical purification procedures on rat skeletal muscle and brain led to the identification of analogous mammalian Na$^+$ channel α subunits, which are protein products of related genes.

In addition to the α subunit, the functional complex of the rat skeletal muscle Na$^+$ channel also contains a 38-kDa subunit, and the rat brain Na$^+$ channel contains both a 33- and a 36-kDa subunit. These smaller subunits of mammalian Na$^+$ channels are called **β subunits** and appear to play a role in modulating channel gating or channel expression. In mammals, four genes encode auxiliary β subunits—termed β$_1$–β$_4$—that preferentially associate with different α subunits in different tissues.

Molecular biological studies of voltage-gated channels began in 1984 with the cloning of the *Electrophorus* **Na$^+$ channel** α subunit by the laboratory of Shosaku Numa. These investigators used antibodies raised against the purified α subunit to screen a cDNA library, and they isolated the cDNA encoding the electroplax Na$^+$ channel. In addition, direct sequencing of channel peptides provided partial amino acid sequence information. Similar strategies led to the purification and cloning of voltage-gated **Ca^{2+} channel** proteins from skeletal muscle and brain tissue. The primary sequence of the α$_1$ subunit of the Ca^{2+} channel is structurally homologous to the α subunit of the Na$^+$ channel.

In contrast to the biochemical approach used for Na$^+$ and Ca^{2+} channels, the initial breakthrough in the molecular biology of **K$^+$ channels** came with the study of *Shaker* mutants of the fruit fly *Drosophila*. These mutants are called Shaker because their bodies literally shake under the influence of ether anesthesia. This phenotype is due to defective voltage-gated K$^+$ channels. The laboratory of L. Y. Jan and Y. N. Jan, and those of O. Pongs and M. Tanouye, used molecu-

lar genetic techniques to identify and clone the first K$^+$ channel genes in 1987.

The hydropathy (see Chapter 2) plots for voltage-gated K$^+$ channels (Fig. 7-10A) typically reveal six distinct peaks of hydrophobicity, corresponding to transmembrane segments S1 to S6—a conserved structural feature of all voltage-gated K$^+$ channels. Transmembrane segments S1 to S6 have an α-helical secondary structure and are connected by cytoplasmic and extracellular linker regions (Fig. 7-10B).

Extensive mutagenesis studies on cloned channel genes have associated various channel functions and binding sites with particular domains. The **S4 segment** (Fig. 7-10) has four to seven arginine or lysine residues that occur at every third S4 residue in voltage-gated K$^+$, Na$^+$, and Ca^{2+} channels. Functional evidence indicates that these positively charged residues of the S4 segment have a major role in the **voltage-sensing mechanism** of channel activation.

The extracellular linker region between the S5 and S6 segments is termed the **P region** (for pore region) and contains residues that form the binding sites for toxins and external blocking molecules such as TEA. The P region also contains residues that are critical determinants of the ionic selectivity for permeant cations. Structural evidence indicates that the S6 transmembrane segment forms the internal aspect of the ion conduction pathway.

Since the discovery and recognition of diverse genes belonging to the voltage-gated channel superfamily, structural-biological studies have substantially advanced our understanding of the three-dimensional structure of certain channel proteins. In 1998, a major breakthrough in the structure of ion channel proteins occurred when MacKinnon and colleagues reported the crystal structure of a bacterial K$^+$ channel protein called KcsA. This work revealed the three-dimensional structure of a protein that contained segments analogous to the S5-P-S6 part of voltage-gated channels, which forms the ion conduction pathway. For his work on the structural biology of ion channels, Roderick MacKinnon shared the 2003 Nobel Prize in Chemistry.

In 2005, another breakthrough by the MacKinnon laboratory revealed the entire structure of a mammalian voltage-gated K$^+$ channel containing both the S1–S4 voltage-sensing domain and the S5-P-S6 pore domain (see Fig. 7-11 and the box on page 191).

Figure 7-12 shows a comparison of the predicted membrane-folding diagrams of three families of voltage-gated channels: Na$^+$, Ca^{2+}, and K$^+$ channels. The channel-forming subunit of each type of channel is called the α subunit for Na$^+$ and K$^+$ channels and the α$_1$ subunit for Ca^{2+} channels. Other identified accessory subunits are designated β$_1$ and β$_2$ for Na$^+$ channels; α$_2$, β, γ, and δ for Ca^{2+} channels; and β for K$^+$ channels.

The α and α$_1$ subunits of this protein superfamily all contain the common S1-S6 structural motif composed of the S1-S4 voltage-sensing domain and the S5-P-S6 pore domain that we described earlier for K$^+$ channels. The α subunit of Na$^+$ channels (Fig. 7-12A) and the α$_1$ subunit of Ca^{2+} channels (Fig. 7-12B) consist of four internally homologous repeats—domains I, II, III, and IV—each containing an S1-S6 motif. K$^+$ channels (Fig. 7-12C) are likely to be an evolutionary precursor of the voltage-gated channel families inasmuch as their pore-forming α subunit contains only one S1-S6

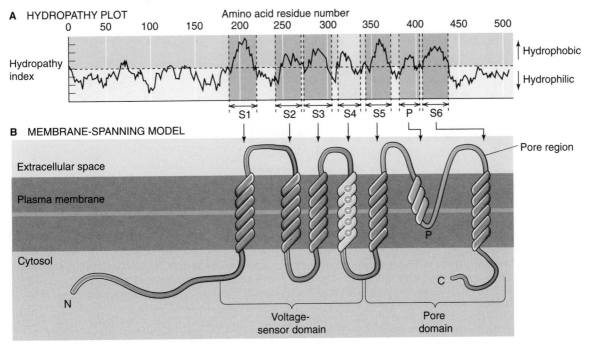

A HYDROPATHY PLOT

Amino acid residue number

Hydropathy index

Hydrophobic

Hydrophilic

S1 S2 S3 S4 S5 P S6

B MEMBRANE-SPANNING MODEL

Extracellular space

Plasma membrane

Cytosol

Pore region

P

C

N

Voltage-sensor domain

Pore domain

Figure 7-10 Membrane topology of a single subunit of a voltage-gated K$^+$ channel. **A,** This voltage-dependent K$^+$ channel, a member of the Shaker family (Kv1.1), has six transmembrane segments (S1 to S6) with a high hydropathy index. Each of these six segments (highlighted in *green* or *yellow*) is presumed to traverse the membrane completely. In addition, the channel also has a smaller region (highlighted in *red*) with a somewhat lower hydropathy index, termed the P region. **B,** This model is based on the hydropathy data in **A.** The six membrane-spanning segments are assumed to be α helices. The S4 segment (highlighted in *yellow*) has a large number of positively charged lysine and arginine residues and is part of the voltage-sensing domain that comprises the entire S1–S4 region. S5 and S6—as well as the intervening P region—comprise the pore domain (see the box on page 191), which lines the pore of the channel. *(Data from Shen NV, Pfaffinger PJ: Conservation of K$^+$ channel properties in gene subfamilies. In Peracchia C [ed]: Handbook of Membrane Channels: Molecular and Cellular Physiology, pp 5-16. New York: Academic Press, 1994.)*

Crystal Structure of a Mammalian K$^+$ Channel

In 2005, the MacKinnon laboratory solved the crystal structure of a rat voltage-gated K$^+$ channel called Kv1.2, which is homologous to the *Drosophila* Shaker channel. This structure, which shows the channel in an open state, reveals that the S1-S4 domain containing the voltage-sensing S4 element is spatially separated from the K$^+$ pore domain (S5-P-S6). The tetrameric Kv1.2 channel has a pinwheel shape when it is viewed from the extracellular surface (Fig. 7-11A). The central square portion of the Kv1.2 pinwheel is the pore—formed by the assembly of four S5-P-S6 domains, one from each monomer—and closely resembles the *entire* bacterial KcsA channel. The four wings of the pinwheel correspond to the four S1-S4 voltage sensor domains. The four Kv1.2 monomers (yellow, green, blue, and red in Figure 7-11A) form an interlinked assembly in which the S1-S4 voltage-sensing domain of any given monomer lies closest to the S5-P-S6 domain of an adjacent monomer.

A lateral view of Kv1.2 shows an intracellular T1 domain formed by the four N-terminal segments of the channel (Fig. 7-11B). The T1 domain of Kv channels is also called the

tetramerization domain because it helps assemble and maintain the tetrameric structure of the channel. This view also shows four separately attached intracellular β subunits. These β subunits of Kv channels are part of a separate gene family of soluble accessory proteins with structural homology to oxidoreductase enzymes. Certain variants of both the T1 domain and β subunits may contain an N-terminal inactivation peptide that produces the rapid N-type inactivation (ball-and-chain mechanism) of some Kv channels by plugging the intracellular entrance to the pore.

Figure 7-11C shows a lateral view of a single Kv1.2 monomer in an open configuration as well as a single β subunit. On depolarization, the S4 segment presumably moves within the membrane toward the extracellular side of the membrane. This mechanical movement of the S4 segment shifts an α-helical S4-S5 linker, causing a bending of the S6 transmembrane α helix from a linear configuration in the closed state to a curved configuration in the open state of the channel shown. Thus, voltage-dependent channel activation is an electromechanical coupling mechanism.

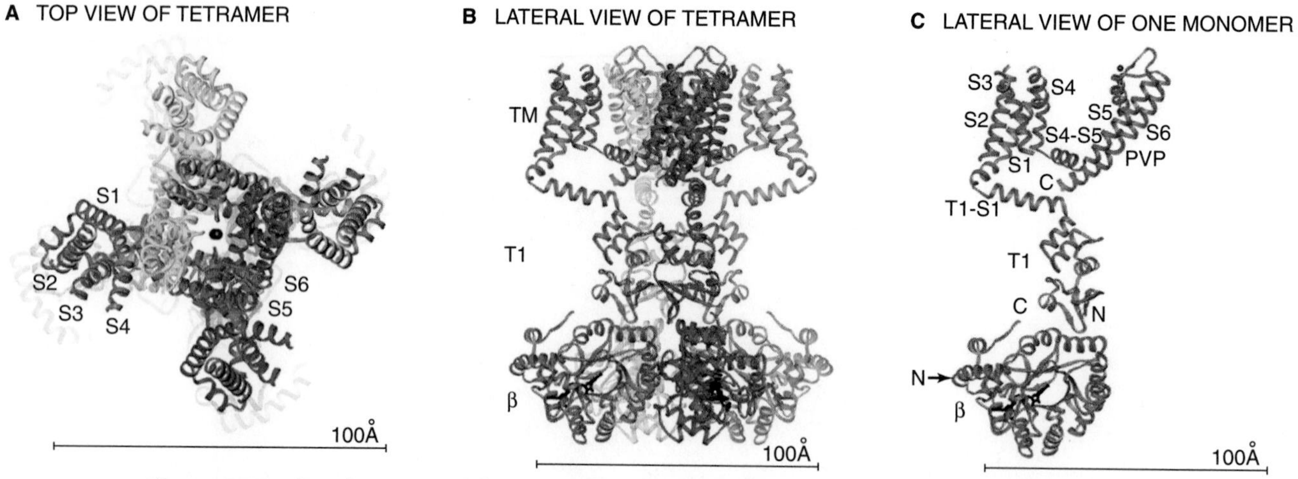

A TOP VIEW OF TETRAMER   **B** LATERAL VIEW OF TETRAMER   **C** LATERAL VIEW OF ONE MONOMER

Figure 7-11 Crystal structure of the mammalian K+ channel, Kv1.2, at a resolution of 2.9 Å. **A,** Four α subunits of the channel, each in a unique color viewed from the extracellular side; a K+ ion is shown in the central open pore. **B,** Side view of the four α and four β subunits of the channel, each in a unique color with extracellular solution on the top and intracellular solution on the bottom. The transmembrane domain (TM) of each α subunit is preceded by an NH_2 terminus (T1 domain). The T1 domain is located over the intracellular entryway to the pore but allows access of K+ ions to the pore through "side portals." The T1 domain is also a docking platform for the oxidoreductase β subunit. Each β subunit is colored according to the α subunit it contacts. **C** shows a side view of one α subunit and adjacent β subunit. Transmembrane segments are labeled S1 to S6. Tetramers of segments S5, pore helix, and S6 constitute the conduction pore in the shape of an inverted "teepee." The selectivity filter lies in the wide portion (extracellular end) of the teepee. Helices S1 to S4 constitute the voltage sensors that are connected by a linker helix (S4-S5) to the pore. The PVP sequence (Pro-Val-Pro) on S6 is critical for gating. *(From Long SB, Campbell EB, MacKinnon R: Crystal structure of a mammalian voltage-dependent Shaker family K+ channel. Science 2005; 309:897-903.)*

motif. Voltage-gated K+ channels are homo-oligomers of four α subunits, a tetramer (Fig. 7-11). Because Na+ and Ca2+ channels are composed of four internally homologous repeats of S1-S6, all α subunits of these families function as either tetrameric (K+ channels) or pseudotetrameric (Na+ and Ca2+ channels) units. Molecular evolution of the pseudotetrameric structure of Na+ and Ca2+ channels is believed to have occurred by consecutive gene duplication of a primordial gene containing the basic S1-S6 motif.

Na+ channels generate the rapid initial depolarization of the action potential

Because the equilibrium potential for Na+ and Ca2+ is in the positive voltage range for normal cellular ionic gradients, channels that are selectively permeable to these ions mediate electrical depolarization. However, prolonged cellular depolarization is an adverse condition inasmuch as it results in sustained contraction and rigor of muscle fibers, cardiac dysfunction, and abnormally elevated levels of intracellular Ca2+, which leads to cell death. Thus, it is critical that Na+ and Ca2+ channels normally reside in a closed conformation at the resting membrane potential. Their opening is an intrinsically transient process that is determined by the kinetics of channel activation and inactivation.

The primary role of voltage-gated Na+ channels is to produce the initial depolarizing phase of fast action potentials in neurons and skeletal and cardiac muscle. The selectivity of Na+ channels for Na+ is much higher than that for other alkali cations. The permeability ratio of Na+ relative to

K+ (P_{Na}/P_K) lies in the range of 11 to 20 under physiological conditions. Voltage-gated Na+ channels are virtually impermeable to Ca2+ and other divalent cations under normal physiological conditions.

Although Na+ channels do not significantly conduct Ca2+ ions across the cell membrane, the voltage dependence of Na+ channel gating is nevertheless dependent on the extracellular Ca2+ concentration ($[Ca^{2+}]_o$). If $[Ca^{2+}]_o$ is progressively increased above the normal physiological level, the voltage activation range of Na+ channels progressively shifts to a more positive range. In Figure 7-13, this change is represented as a shift in the P_o versus V_m relationship. Similarly, if $[Ca^{2+}]_o$ is decreased, the voltage activation range is shifted to more negative voltages. This phenomenon has important clinical implications because a negative shift corresponds to a **reduced voltage threshold** for action potential firing and results in hyperexcitability and spontaneous muscle twitching. Similarly, a positive voltage shift of Na+ channel gating corresponds to decreased electrical excitability (i.e., the threshold is now farther away from resting V_m), resulting in muscle weakness. Thus, metabolic disorders that result in abnormal plasma [Ca2+], such as hypoparathyroidism (low [Ca2+]) and hyperparathyroidism (high [Ca2+]), can cause marked neurologic and neuromuscular symptoms. The mechanism of this voltage shift in Na+ channel gating by extracellular divalent cations such as Ca2+ is thought to involve an alteration in the transmembrane electrical field that is sensed by the channel protein. Presumably, this effect is caused by Ca2+ binding or electrostatic screening of negative charges at the membrane surface.

A Na⁺ CHANNEL

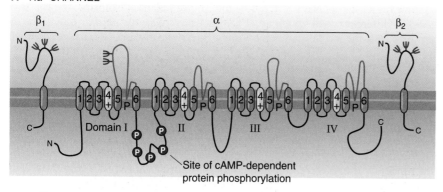
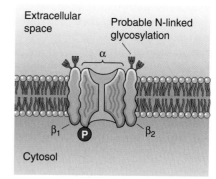

B Ca²⁺ CHANNEL

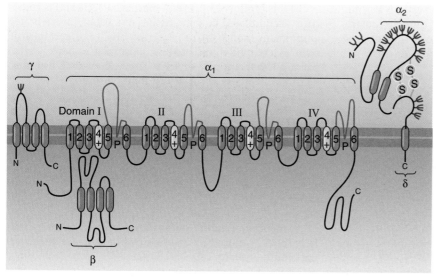
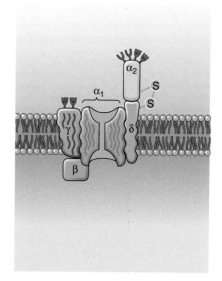

C K⁺ CHANNEL

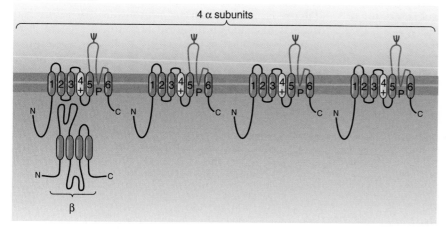
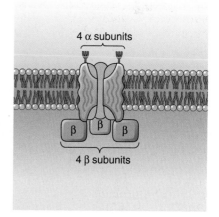

Figure 7-12   Subunit structure and membrane-folding models of voltage-gated channels. **A,** A voltage-gated Na⁺ channel is made up of a pseudo-oligomeric α subunit as well as membrane-spanning β₁ and β₂ subunits. Note that the domains I to IV of the α subunit are homologous to a single subunit of a voltage-gated K⁺ channel (see **C**). **B,** A voltage-gated Ca²⁺ channel is made up of a pseudo-oligomeric α₁ subunit as well as an extracellular α₂ subunit, a cytoplasmic β subunit, and membrane-spanning γ and δ subunits. Note that the domains I to IV of the α subunit are homologous to a single subunit of a voltage-gated K⁺ channel (see **C**). **C,** A voltage-gated K⁺ channel is made up of four α subunits as well as a cytoplasmic β subunit. *(Data from Isom LL, De Jongh KS, Catterall WA: Auxiliary subunits of voltage-gated ion channels. Neuron 1994; 12:1183-1194.)*

Humans have at least ten homologous genes that encode the pore-forming α subunit of Na⁺ channels (Table 7-1). The isoforms encoded by these genes are expressed in different excitable tissues and can be partially discriminated on the basis of their sensitivity to TTX. Four of the isoforms (Nav1.1, 1.2, 1.3, and 1.6) are differentially expressed in various regions of the brain. One isoform (Nav1.4) is the major isoform in skeletal muscle. This muscle Na⁺ channel is also uniquely sensitive to blockade by a peptide toxin called **μ-conotoxin** from a venomous marine snail. Natural mutations in the human gene for this Na⁺ channel result in a variety of human genetic diseases, such as hyperkalemic periodic paralysis, and in several types of myotonia (see the box titled Na⁺ Channel Genetic Defects). Heart ventricular muscle expresses a TTX-insensitive isoform (Nav1.5) that also appears in skeletal muscle after denervation. Various natural mutations in the heart Na⁺ channel cause irregularities in heartbeat characterized by a particular type of long QT syndrome. Neurons from the dorsal root ganglia express Nav1.6, 1.7, 1.8, and 1.9 Na⁺ channel isoforms, the last two of which are TTX insensitive. Various natural mutations in human Nav1.7 underlie genetic diseases characterized either by enhanced sensitivity to pain or deficiency in the perception of pain, indicating a role for Nav1.7 in nociception.

Na⁺ channels are blocked by neurotoxins and local anesthetics

Studies of the mechanism of action of neurotoxins have provided important insight into channel function and structure. The guanidinium **toxins** TTX and STX (Fig. 7-5C) are specific blocking agents of Na⁺ channels that act on the extracellular side of the cell membrane.

TTX is produced by certain marine bacteria and is apparently accumulated in some tissues of various invertebrates, amphibians, and fish. The internal organs of certain fish, such as the puffer fish that is consumed in Japan, often contain lethal amounts of TTX. The flesh of such fish must be carefully prepared to prevent food poisoning.

STX is produced by specific species of marine dinoflagellates that are responsible for "red tide" in the ocean as well as by freshwater cyanobacteria, which can poison ponds and rivers. It is the agent responsible for paralytic shellfish poisoning, which is caused by human ingestion of toxic shellfish that have accumulated STX-producing plankton. Death from TTX and STX intoxication, which ultimately results from respiratory paralysis, can be prevented by the timely administration of mechanical respiration.

As mentioned earlier, the snail peptide μ-conotoxin similarly blocks muscle Na⁺ channels by binding near the external binding site for TTX and STX.

TTX, STX, and μ-conotoxin are important pharmacological probes because they can be used to functionally discriminate among several distinct isoforms of Na⁺ channels (Table 7-1). Other important neurotoxins that act on Na⁺ channels include batrachotoxin (a steroidal alkaloid from

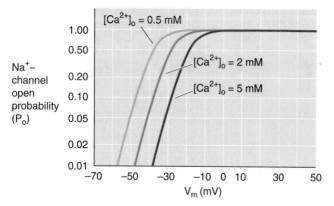

Figure 7-13 Effect of extracellular Ca^{2+} concentration on Na⁺ channel activation. High $[Ca^{2+}]_o$ shifts the P_o versus V_m to more positive voltages (e.g., less excitable). Thus, *hypo*calcemia leads to *hyper*excitability.

TABLE 7-1 Na⁺ Channel α Subunits

Channel Protein	Human Gene	Tissue	Sensitivity to TTX (molar)
Nav1.1	SCN1A	Central nervous system, heart	10^{-9}
Nav1.2	SCN2A	Central nervous system	10^{-9}
Nav1.3	SCN3A	Central nervous system, heart	10^{-9}
Nav1.4	SCN4A	Skeletal muscle	10^{-9}
Nav1.5	SCN5A	Heart, denervated skeletal muscle	Insensitive, 10^{-6}
Nav1.6	SCN8A	Central and peripheral nervous system	10^{-9}
Nav1.7	SCN9A	Peripheral nervous system	10^{-9}
Nav1.8	SCN10A	Peripheral and sensory neurons	Insensitive, 10^{-6}
Nav1.9	SCN11A	Peripheral nervous system	Insensitive, 10^{-6}

certain tropical frogs and birds), various plant alkaloids (veratridine, grayanotoxin, aconitine), natural plant insecticides (pyrethrins), brevetoxins (cyclic polyethers from dinoflagellates), and two distinct classes (α and β) of peptide scorpion toxins. Members of this diverse group of neurotoxins act primarily by altering the gating kinetics of Na^+ channels by promoting both a longer duration of channel opening and channel opening under voltage conditions in which Na^+ channels are normally closed or inactivated.

Local anesthetics are a large group of synthetic drugs that are generally characterized by an aromatic moiety linked to a tertiary amine substituent through an ester or amide linkage (Fig. 7-14A). Drug development of local anesthetics began with the recognition by Carl Koller in 1884 that the plant alkaloid **cocaine** numbs sensation in the tongue, in addition to producing psychoactive effects by its actions on the central nervous system (CNS). Attempts to synthesize safer alternatives to cocaine led to **procaine**, which mimics the local anesthetic effect of cocaine without the CNS effects.

Local anesthetics that are used clinically, such as procaine, **lidocaine**, and **tetracaine**, reversibly block nerve impulse generation and propagation by inhibiting voltage-gated Na^+ channels. The action of these drugs is "use dependent," which means that inhibition of Na^+ current progresses in a time-dependent manner with increasing repetitive stimulation or firing of action potentials (Fig. 7-14B). **Use dependence** occurs because the drug binds most effectively only after the Na^+ channel has already opened. This use-dependent action of the drug further enhances inhibition of nerve impulses at sites where repetitive firing of action potentials takes place. Local anesthetics are used to control pain during dental procedures, many types of minor surgery, and labor in childbirth.

Ca^{2+} channels contribute to action potentials in some cells and also function in electrical and chemical coupling mechanisms

Ca^{2+} channels play important roles in the depolarization phase of certain action potentials, in coupling electrical excitation to secretion or muscle contraction, and in other signal transduction processes. Because $[Ca^{2+}]_o$ is ~1.2 mM, whereas $[Ca^{2+}]_i$ is only ~10^{-7} M, a huge gradient favors the passive influx of Ca^{2+} into cells. At the relatively high $[Ca^{2+}]_o$ that prevails under physiological conditions, voltage-gated Ca^{2+} channels are highly selective for Ca^{2+}, with permeability to Ca^{2+} being ~1000-fold greater than permeability to Na^+. Other alkaline earth divalent cations such as Sr^{2+} and Ba^{2+} also readily permeate through Ca^{2+} channels and are often used as substitute ions for recording the activity of Ca^{2+} channels in electrophysiological studies. However, if $[Ca^{2+}]_o$ is reduced to a *nonphysiological* level of less than 10^{-6} M with the use of chelating agents, Ca^{2+} channels can also conduct large currents of monovalent alkali cations, such as Na^+ and K^+. Thus, in terms of its intrinsic ionic selectivity, the Ca^{2+} channel is functionally similar to the Na^+ channel, except that high-affinity binding of Ca^{2+} in the pore effectively prevents permeation of all other physiological ions except Ca^{2+}.

The mechanism of this extraordinary selectivity behavior is based on ion-ion interactions within the pore. For the Ca^{2+}

Na^+ Channel Genetic Defects

Several human genetic diseases have been traced to inheritable defects in the genes for skeletal and cardiac muscle Na^+ channels. The skeletal muscle gene *SCN4A* is located on human chromosome 17, and the cardiac muscle gene *SCN5A* is located on chromosome 3. One of the muscle disorders is called **hyperkalemic periodic paralysis** because muscle weakness is triggered by an elevation in serum $[K^+]$ that may occur after vigorous exercise or ingestion of foods rich in K^+. A second muscle disorder is called **paramyotonia congenita**. This form of periodic paralysis may be induced in afflicted individuals by exposure to cold temperature and results in symptoms of myotonia (muscle stiffness) associated with abnormal repetitive firing of muscle action potentials. **Long QT syndrome** is an inherited defect in heart rhythm that can lead to sudden death from cardiac arrhythmia. A deletion of three amino acids, ΔKPQ, in the linker region between repetitive domains III and IV of the heart Na^+ channel is one type of mutation that causes this disease. We will see later in the box titled Human Heart Defects Linked to Mutations of K^+ Channels that defects in cardiac K^+ channels can also cause a long QT syndrome. As shown in Figure 7-15, a number of mutations responsible for skeletal muscle diseases have also been identified and mapped within the folding diagram of the muscle Na^+ channel α subunit. These mutations generally occur in one of the putative membrane-spanning segments (S3, S4, S5, and S6). Two paramyotonia congenita mutations have also been located in the intracellular linker segment between repeats III and IV; this linker plays an important role in Na^+ channel inactivation. Electrophysiological analysis of some of these mutations suggests that abnormal kinetics of Na^+ channel gating is the underlying cause of the profound symptoms associated with these diseases. For example, the occasional failure of the mutant heart Na^+ channel to inactivate results in long bursts of openings and abnormal prolongation of the action potential.

---

channel to conduct current, at least two Ca^{2+} ions must bind simultaneously close to sites within the channel. Interactions between individual ions within the narrow region of the channel pore appear to control ion selectivity and the ionic flux. Variations on this general mechanism, referred to as **multi-ion conduction**, have also been described for many other classes of ion channels, notably K^+ channels. Multi-ion conduction generally appears to play an important role in determining the permeation properties of channels that have a high degree of ionic selectivity, such as Ca^{2+} channels and K^+ channels.

One of the major functions of voltage-gated Ca^{2+} channels is to contribute to the depolarizing phase of **action potentials** in certain cell types. The gating of voltage-gated Ca^{2+} channels is slower than that of Na^+ channels. Whereas Na^+ channels are most important in initiating action potentials and generating rapidly propagating spikes in axons, Ca^{2+} channels often give rise to a more sustained depolarizing current, which is the basis for the long-lived action potentials

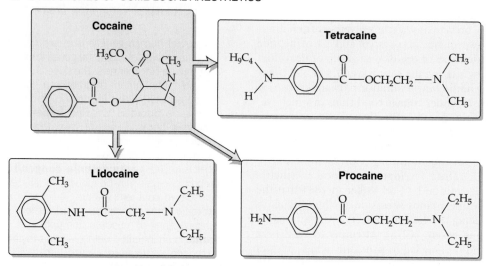

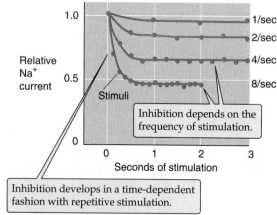

Figure 7-14   Effect of local anesthetics. **A,** The three clinically useful local anesthetics shown here are synthetic analogues of the plant alkaloid cocaine. **B,** In the presence of lidocaine, the relative Na$^+$ current decays with time during repetitive stimulation. However, the inhibition becomes more pronounced as the rate of stimulation increases from 1/s to 8/s. (*Data from Hille B: Local anesthetics: Hydrophilic and hydrophobic pathways for the drug-receptor reaction. J Gen Physiol 1977; 69:497-515.*)

observed in cardiac cells, smooth muscle cells, secretory cells, and many types of neurons.

The exquisite selectivity of Ca^{2+} channels under physiological conditions endows them with special roles in **cellular regulation**. If a depolarizing electrical stimulus or a signal transduction cascade activates these Ca^{2+} channels, the subsequent influx of Ca^{2+} raises $[Ca^{2+}]_i$, and Ca^{2+} can thereby serve as an important second messenger in regulating the activity of a multitude of intracellular proteins and enzymes. Thus, in serving as a major gateway for Ca^{2+} influx across the plasma membrane, Ca^{2+} channels have not only an electrical function in membrane depolarization but also an important biochemical function in signal transduction.

Ca^{2+} channels also play a pivotal role in a special subset of signal transduction processes known as excitation-contraction coupling and excitation-secretion coupling. **Excitation-contraction (EC) coupling** refers to the process by which an electrical depolarization at the cell membrane leads to cell contraction, such as the contraction of a skeletal muscle fiber. In EC coupling of skeletal muscle, one class of plasma membrane Ca^{2+} channel that is located in the transverse tubule membrane of skeletal muscle serves as the voltage sensor and forms a direct structural linkage to intracellular Ca^{2+} release channels that are located in the sarcoplasmic reticulum membrane. In contrast, Ca^{2+} channels play a different role in EC coupling in cardiac muscle, where Ca^{2+} channels in the plasma membrane mediate an initial influx of Ca^{2+}. The resultant increase in $[Ca^{2+}]_i$ triggers an additional release of Ca^{2+} stored in the sarcoplasmic reticulum by a process known as Ca^{2+}-induced Ca^{2+} release (see Chapter 9).

Excitation-secretion coupling is the process by which depolarization of the plasma membrane causes release of

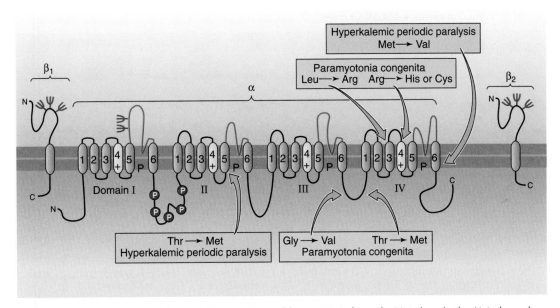

Figure 7-15   Some naturally occurring mutations of human Na⁺ channels. Mutations in the Na⁺ channel of human skeletal muscle can cause at least two genetic diseases. Hyperkalemic periodic paralysis can be caused by mutations in membrane-spanning segment S5 of domain II and S6 of domain IV. Paramyotonia congenita can be caused by mutations in membrane-spanning segment S3 of domain IV and S4 of domain IV and also by mutations in the intracellular segment that links domains III and IV. *(Data from Catterall WA: Cellular and molecular biology of voltage-gated sodium channels. Physiol Rev 1992; 72:S15-S48.)*

neurotransmitters in the nervous system and the secretion of hormones in the endocrine system. Such processes require an increase in $[Ca^{2+}]_i$ through the plasma membrane to trigger exocytosis of synaptic and secretory vesicles. Thus, in providing a primary signal for the initiation of cellular contraction and neurotransmitter/hormone release, Ca^{2+} channels are a fundamental locus of control.

Because Ca^{2+} channels must fulfill diverse roles, higher vertebrates use a family of genes that encode structurally homologous but functionally diverse Ca^{2+} channels. Mammals have at least 10 distinct genes for the channel-forming α_1 subunit of Ca^{2+} channels (Table 7-2). Biochemical and cloning work has also identified four accessory subunits of Ca^{2+} channels: α_2, δ, β, and γ (Fig. 7-12B). The α_2 and δ subunits are the products of a single gene; after translation, proteolytic cleavage of the polypeptide yields α_2 and δ. Coexpression studies have shown that these accessory subunits can greatly influence the kinetics, voltage sensitivity, and peak currents that are exhibited by various α_1 channel subunits. This structural complexity and diversity at the genetic level are mirrored by a diversity of Ca^{2+} currents that have been differentiated in various cell types on the basis of their functional characteristics.

Ca²⁺ channels are characterized as L-, T-, P/Q-, N-, and R-type channels on the basis of kinetic properties and inhibitor sensitivity

An example of the functional diversity of Ca^{2+} channels is illustrated in Figure 7-16, which shows two different types of voltage-gated Ca^{2+} channels that have been identified in

cardiac ventricular cells by the patch-clamp technique. If the cell-attached patch, initially clamped at −50 mV, is suddenly depolarized to +10 mV, currents appear from a large-conductance (18 to 25 pS), slowly inactivating Ca^{2+} channel (Fig. 7-16A). However, if the same patch is initially clamped at −70 mV and depolarized to only −20 mV, currents appear instead from a small-conductance (8 pS), rapidly inactivating Ca^{2+} channel (Fig. 7-16B). These two types of Ca^{2+} channels are respectively named **L-type** (for long-lived) and **T-type** (for transient) channels. T-type channels are activated at a lower voltage threshold (more negative than −30 mV) than are other types of Ca^{2+} channels and are also inactivated over a more negative voltage range. These characteristics of T-type channels permit them to function briefly in the initiation of action potentials and to play a role in the repetitive firing of cardiac cells and neurons. Other types of Ca^{2+} channels, including L-, N-, P/Q-, and R-type channels, which are activated at a higher voltage threshold (more positive than −30 mV), mediate the long-lived plateau phase of slow action potentials and provide a more substantial influx of Ca^{2+} for contractile and secretory responses. N-, P/Q-, and R-type Ca^{2+} channels appear to mediate the entry of Ca^{2+} into certain types of presynaptic nerve terminals and thus play an important role in facilitating the release of neurotransmitters.

In addition to discrimination on the basis of gating behavior, Ca^{2+} channel isoforms can also be distinguished by their sensitivity to different drugs and toxins (Table 7-2). **Ca²⁺ channel blockers** are an important group of therapeutic agents. Figure 7-17 shows the structures of representatives of three different classes of Ca^{2+} channel blockers: 1,4-dihy-

TABLE 7-2 Properties and Classification of Ca²⁺ Channel α Subunits

Property	CHANNEL				
	L	T	N	P/Q	R
Kinetics	Long duration	Transient	Intermediate-long duration	Intermediate-long duration	Intermediate
Voltage activation	High threshold (>−30 mV)	Low threshold (<−30 mV)	High threshold (>−30 mV)	High threshold (>−30 mV)	High threshold (>−30 mV)
Pharmacology	Blocked by DHPs	Less sensitive to DHPs	Insensitive to DHPs, blocked by ω-conotoxin GVIA	Insensitive to DHPs, blocked by ω-agatoxin IVA	Insensitive to DHPs, ω-conotoxin GVIA, and ω-agatoxin IVA
Location	Heart, skeletal muscle, neurons, vascular smooth muscle, uterus, neuroendocrine cells	Sinoatrial node of heart, brain neurons	Presynaptic terminals, dendrites, and cell bodies of neurons	Cerebellar Purkinje and granule cells, cell bodies of central neurons	Cerebellar granule cells, neurons
Function	EC coupling in skeletal muscle, link membrane depolarization to intracellular Ca signaling	Repetitive firing of action potentials in heart and many neurons	Exocytotic neurotransmitter release	Exocytotic neurotransmitter release	Exocytotic neurotransmitter release
Channel protein (gene)	Cav1.1 (*CACNA1S*) Cav1.2 (*CACNA1C*) Cav1.3 (*CACNA1D*) Cav1.4 (*CACNA1F*)	Cav3.1 (*CACNA1G*) Cav3.2 (*CACNA1H*) Cav3.3 (*CACNA1I*)	Cav2.2 (*CACNA1B*)	Cav2.1 (*CACNA1A*)	Cav2.3 (*CACNA1E*)

DHP, 1,4-dihydropyridine.

dropyridines (DHPs), phenylalkylamines, and benzothiazepines. These synthetic compounds are used in the treatment of cardiovascular disorders such as angina pectoris (see Chapter 24) and hypertension and also are being evaluated for their potential in treatment of various diseases of the CNS.

DHPs such as nitrendipine selectively block L-type Ca²⁺ channels. Phenylalkylamines (e.g., verapamil) and benzothiazepines (e.g., diltiazem) also inhibit L-type Ca²⁺ channels; however, these other two classes of drugs act at sites that are distinct from the site that binds DHPs. Particular DHP derivatives, such as Bay K8644, actually *enhance* rather than inhibit Ca²⁺ channel currents. DHPs can have the contrasting effects of either inhibitors (antagonists) or activators (agonists) because they act not by plugging the channel pore directly but by binding to a site composed of transmembrane helices S5 and S6 in domain III and S6 in domain IV. Drug binding in this region probably induces various conformational changes in channel structure and thereby perturbs Ca²⁺ permeation and gating behavior.

Other molecules that are useful in discriminating Ca²⁺ channel isoforms are present in the venom of the marine snail *Conus geographus* and the funnel web spider *Agelenopsis aperta*. The snail produces a peptide called ω-conotoxin GVIA, which selectively blocks N-type Ca²⁺ channels; the spider produces the peptide ω-agatoxin IVA, which selectively blocks P/Q-type Ca²⁺ channels. In contrast, an R-type neuronal Ca²⁺ channel is resistant to these two peptide toxins.

The summary of the basic properties of L-, T-, N-, P/Q-, and R-type Ca²⁺ channels contained in Table 7-2 indicates their presumed correspondence to 10 known genes that encode α₁ subunits.

K⁺ channels determine resting potential and regulate the frequency and termination of action potentials

K⁺ channels are the largest and most diverse family of voltage-gated ion channels. Humans have at least 78 distinct genes

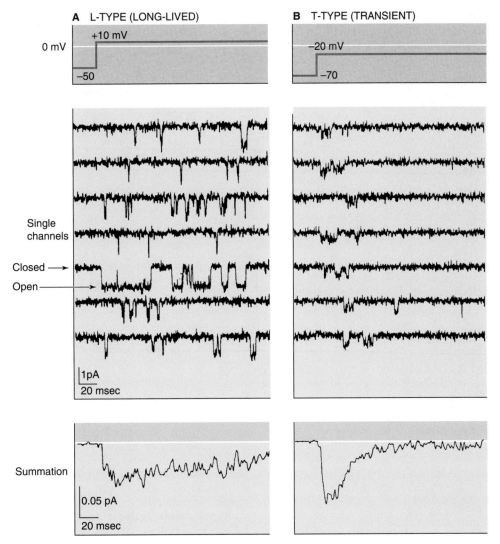

A L-TYPE (LONG-LIVED)

0 mV

+10 mV

−50

Single channels

Closed →

Open →

1 pA

20 msec

Summation

0.05 pA

20 msec

B T-TYPE (TRANSIENT)

−20 mV

−70

Figure 7-16 Current records from two types of Ca²⁺ channel. **A,** This is an experiment on guinea pig ventricular myocytes in which cell-attached patches were used. The authors studied the currents that are carried by Ba²⁺ through these L-type Ca²⁺ channels because they conduct Ba²⁺ even better than Ca²⁺. Shown in the middle panel are seven single-channel current records that were obtained during and after a shift of the cytosolic voltage from −50 to +10 mV. Note that the channel activity (i.e., downward deflections) begins only after depolarization and continues more or less at the same level throughout the depolarization. The lower panel shows the average of many records that are similar to those shown in the middle panel. **B,** The experiments summarized for these T-type Ca²⁺ channels were identical in design to those shown in **A,** except that the depolarizing step shifted cytosolic voltage from −70 to −20 mV. Note that once again, the channel activity begins only after depolarization *(middle panel)*. However, the channel activity is transient; it wanes during a sustained depolarization, as confirmed by the average current shown in the lower panel. *(Data from Nilius B, Hess P, Lansman JB, Tsien RW: A novel type of cardiac calcium channel in ventricular cells. Nature 1985; 316:443-446.)*

encoding K⁺ channels with the complete S1 to S6 motif. Ion conduction through most types of K⁺ channels is very selective for K⁺ according to the permeability sequence K⁺ > Rb⁺ > NH₄⁺ ≫ Cs⁺ > Li⁺, Na⁺, Ca²⁺. Under normal physiological conditions, the permeability ratio P_K/P_{Na} is greater than 100 and Na⁺ can block some K⁺ channels. Some K⁺ channels can pass Na⁺ current in the complete absence of K⁺. This finding is analogous to the behavior of Ca²⁺ channels, which can pass Na⁺ and K⁺ currents in the absence of Ca²⁺.

Given such strong K⁺ selectivity and an equilibrium potential near −80 mV, the primary role of K⁺ channels in excitable cells is inhibitory. K⁺ channels oppose the action of excitatory Na⁺ and Ca²⁺ channels and stabilize the resting, nonexcited state. Whereas some K⁺ channels are major determinants of the resting potential, the voltage dependence and kinetics of other K⁺ channels in excitable cells have specialized functions, such as mediating the repolarization and shaping of action potentials, controlling firing frequency, and

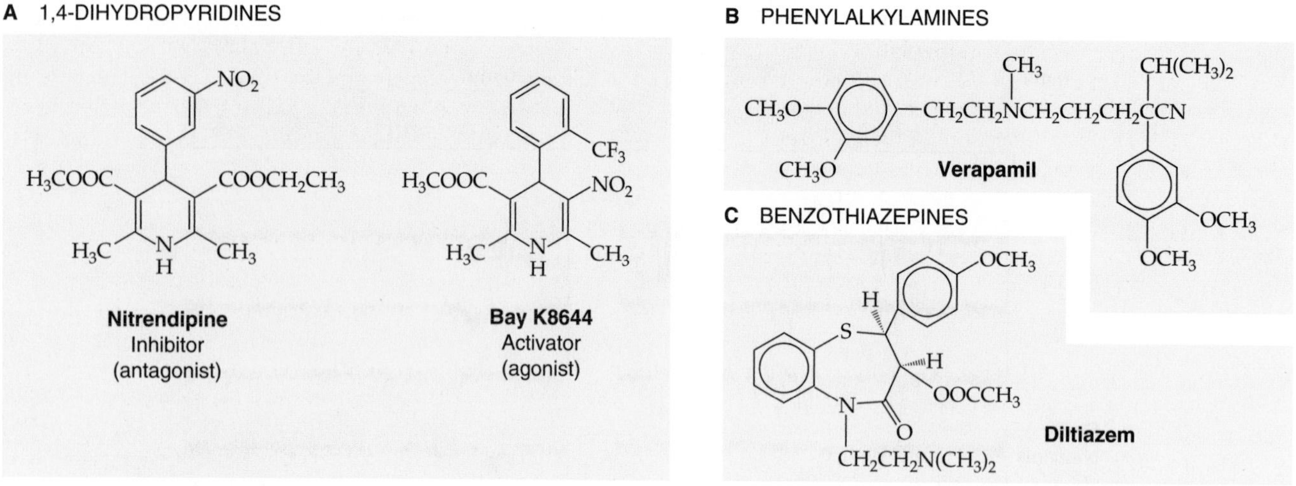

A 1,4-DIHYDROPYRIDINES

Nitrendipine
Inhibitor
(antagonist)

Bay K8644
Activator
(agonist)

B PHENYLALKYLAMINES

Verapamil

C BENZOTHIAZEPINES

Diltiazem

Figure 7-17 Antagonists and agonists of L-type Ca^{2+} channels. **A,** 1,4-Dihydropyridines. One, nitrendipine, is an antagonist; another, Bay K8644, is an agonist. **B,** Phenylalkylamines. Verapamil is an antagonist. **C,** Benzothiazepines. Diltiazem is an antagonist.

Ca^{2+} Channel and Autoimmune Genetic Defects

Ca^{2+} channels have been linked to a large variety of genetic diseases. In mice, an interesting mutation results in **muscular dysgenesis**, or failure of normal skeletal muscle to develop. These mice lack a functional Ca^{2+} channel α_1 subunit in their skeletal muscle. They die shortly after birth, but their cultured muscle cells provide an assay system to investigate the mechanism of EC coupling. Contraction of such defective muscle cells can be rescued by expression of cloned genes for either the skeletal Cav1.1 (*CACNA1S* gene) or the cardiac Cav1.2 (*CACNA1C* gene) L-type Ca^{2+} channels. As discussed in Chapter 9, a physiologically distinguishing feature of EC coupling in normal skeletal versus cardiac muscle is that skeletal muscle does not require extracellular Ca^{2+}, whereas cardiac muscle does. Indeed, when the rescue is accomplished with skeletal Cav1.1, contraction does not require extracellular Ca^{2+}; when the rescue is accomplished with cardiac α_{1C}, contraction *does* require extracellular Ca^{2+}. Such studies have provided strong support for the concept that EC coupling in skeletal muscle takes place by direct coupling of Cav1.1 to the Ca^{2+} release channels of the sarcoplasmic reticulum; in cardiac muscle, EC coupling occurs as Ca^{2+} entering through α_{1C}-containing channels induces the release of Ca^{2+} from internal stores. Mutagenesis experiments with chimeric α_1 subunits containing artificially spliced segments of the cardiac and skeletal channel isoforms have shown that the intracellular linker region between repeats II and III is the domain of the α_1 subunit that determines the skeletal versus the cardiac type of EC coupling.

A human pathologic condition called **Lambert-Eaton syndrome** has been characterized as an impairment of presynaptic Ca^{2+} channels at motor nerve terminals. Lambert-Eaton syndrome is an autoimmune disorder that is most often seen in patients with certain types of cancer, such as small cell lung carcinoma. Patients afflicted with this condition produce antibodies against presynaptic Ca^{2+} channels that somehow reduce the number of such channels able to function in the depolarization-induced influx of Ca^{2+} for neurotransmitter release.

Hypokalemic periodic paralysis (not to be confused with hyperkalemic periodic paralysis, discussed earlier in the box titled Na^+ Channel Genetic Defects) is an autosomal dominant muscle disease of humans. Affected family members have a point mutation in the *CACNA1S* gene encoding the skeletal Cav1.1, located in transmembrane segment S4 of domain II. This finding explains the basis for a human disorder involving defective EC coupling of skeletal muscle. Certain other rare human genetic diseases result in neurologic symptoms of migraine (severe headache) and ataxia (a movement disorder). One of these diseases, **familial hemiplegic migraine**, is caused by point mutations at various locations in the human *CACNA1A* gene encoding Cav2.1. These locations include the S4 region of domain I, the P region of domain II, and the S6 helices of domains I and IV. Another such genetic disease caused by mutations in the human *CACNA1A* gene encoding Cav2.1 is called **episodic ataxia type 2**, a condition associated with the occurrence of ataxia originating from the cerebellum. Discovery of the genetic origin of such diseases has led to the realization that delicate perturbations of Ca^{2+} channel activity can have profound consequences on proper function of the human nervous system.

defining the bursting behavior of rhythmic firing. Such functions are broadly important in regulating the strength and frequency of all types of muscle contraction, in terminating transmitter release at nerve terminals, and in attenuating the strength of synaptic connections. Finally, in epithelia, K^+ channels also function in K^+ absorption and secretion.

Before molecular cloning revealed the structural relationships among the various kinds of K^+ channels, electrophysiologists classified K^+ currents according to their functional properties and gating behavior. They grouped the macroscopic K^+ currents into four major types:

1. delayed outward rectifiers;
2. transient outward rectifiers (A-type currents);
3. Ca^{2+}-activated K^+ currents; and
4. inward rectifiers.

These four fundamental K^+ currents are the macroscopic manifestation of five distinct families of genes (Table 6.2):

1. Kv channels (voltage-gated K^+ channels related to the Shaker family);
2. Small conductance K_{Ca} channels (Ca^{2+}-activated K^+ channels), including, SK_{Ca} and IK_{Ca} channels;
3. Large-conductance K_{Ca} channels (Ca^{2+}-activated K^+ channels, including BK_{Ca} and Na^+-activated K^+ channels);
4. Kir channels (inward rectifier K^+ channels); and
5. K2P channels (two-pore K^+ channels).

In the next three sections, we discuss the various families of K^+ channels and their associated macroscopic currents.

The Kv (or shaker-related) family of K^+ channels mediates both the delayed outward rectifier current and the transient A-type current

The K^+ current in the HH voltage-clamp analysis of the squid giant axon is an example of a **delayed outward rectifier**. Figure 7-18A shows that this current activates with a sigmoidal lag phase (i.e., it is *delayed* in time, as in Fig. 7-6C). Figure 7-18B is an *I-V* plot of peak currents obtained in experiments such as that in Figure 7-18A; it shows that the outward current rises steeply at positive voltages (i.e., it is an *outward* rectifier).

A second variety of K^+ current that is also outwardly rectifying is the **transient A-type** K^+ current. This current was first characterized in mollusk neurons, but similar currents are common in the vertebrate nervous system. A-type currents are activated and inactivated over a relatively rapid time scale. Because their voltage activation range is typically more negative than that of other K^+ currents, they are activated in the negative V_m range that prevails during the afterhyperpolarizing phase of action potentials. In neurons that spike repetitively, this A-type current can be very important in determining the interval between successive spikes and thus the timing of repetitive action potentials. For example, if the A-type current is small, V_m rises relatively quickly toward the threshold, and consequently the interspike interval is short and the firing frequency is high (Fig. 7-18C).

However, if the A-type current is large, V_m rises slowly toward the threshold, and therefore the interspike interval is long and the firing frequency is low (Fig. 7-18D). Because the nervous system often encodes information as a frequency-modulated signal, these A-type currents play a critical role.

The channels responsible for both the delayed outward rectifier and the transient A-type currents belong to the **Kv channel family** (where *v* stands for voltage-gated). The prototypic protein subunit of these channels is the Shaker channel of *Drosophila*. All channels belonging to this family contain the conserved S1-S6 core that is characteristic of the Shaker channel (Fig. 7-10) but may differ extensively in the length and sequence of their intracellular N-terminal and C-terminal domains. The voltage-sensing element in the S4 segment underlies activation by depolarization; the S4 segment actually moves outward across the membrane with depolarizing voltage, thus increasing the probability of the channel's being open (see the box titled Crystal Structure of a Mammalian K^+ Channel).

The Kv channel family has multiple subclasses (see Table 6-2). Individual members of this Kv channel family, whether in *Drosophila* or humans, exhibit profound differences in gating kinetics that are analogous to delayed rectifier (slow activation) or A-type (rapid inactivation) currents. For example, Figure 7-18E shows the macroscopic currents of four subtypes of rat brain Kv1 (or Shaker) channels heterologously expressed in frog oocytes. All of these Kv1 channel subtypes (Kv1.1 to Kv1.4) exhibit sigmoidal activation kinetics when they are examined on a brief time scale—in the millisecond range (left side of Fig. 7-18E). That is, these channels display some degree of "delayed" activation. Different Kv channels exhibit different rates of activation. Thus, these currents can modulate action potential duration by either keeping it *short* (e.g., in nerve and skeletal muscle) when the delayed rectifier turns on quickly or keeping it *long* (e.g., in heart) when the delayed rectifier turns on slowly.

Kv1 channels also differ markedly in their *inactivation* kinetics when they are observed over a long time scale—in the range of seconds (right side of Fig. 7-18E). Kv1.1 exhibits little time-dependent inactivation (i.e., the current is sustained throughout the stimulus). On the other hand, the Kv1.4 channel completely inactivates in less than 1 second. Kv1.2 and Kv1.3 show intermediate behavior.

How are Kv channels inactivated? The structural basis for one particular type of K^+ channel inactivation, known as **N-type inactivation**, is a stretch of ~20 amino acid residues at the N terminus of some fast-inactivating Kv channels. This domain acts like a ball to block or to plug the internal mouth of the channel after it opens, thereby resulting in inactivation (Fig. 7-18F). Thus, this process is also known as the **ball-and-chain mechanism** of K^+ channel inactivation. Particular kinds of β subunits that are physically associated with some isoforms of Kv channels have structural elements that mimic this N-terminal ball domain and rapidly inactivate K^+ channel α subunits that lack their own inactivation ball domain (Fig. 7-11).

Various delayed rectifier K^+ channels are blocked by either internal or external application of quaternary ammonium ions such as **TEA**. We already have described an example of how TEA can inhibit the outward rectifier K^+ current (Fig. 7-5C) in pharmacological dissection of the currents underly-

A DELAYED ACTIVATION OF Kv CHANNELS

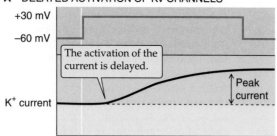

+30 mV

−60 mV

The activation of the current is delayed.

K⁺ current

Peak current

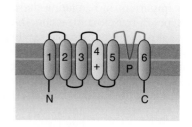

1 2 3 4+ 5 P 6

N   C

B OUTWARD RECTIFICATION OF Kv CHANNELS

Peak K current (I_K)

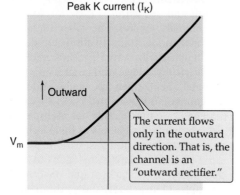

Outward

V_m

The current flows only in the outward direction. That is, the channel is an "outward rectifier."

C A-TYPE OUTWARD RECTIFIER: SMALL CURRENT

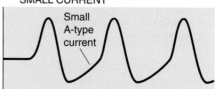

Small A-type current

D A-TYPE OUTWARD RECTIFIER: LARGE CURRENT

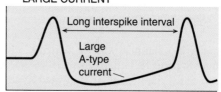

Long interspike interval

Large A-type current

E DIFFERENCES IN GATING KINETICS AMONG Kv-TYPE DELAYED OUTWARD RECTIFIERS

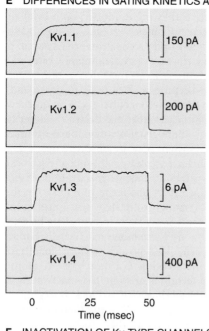

Kv1.1   150 pA

Kv1.2   200 pA

Kv1.3   6 pA

Kv1.4   400 pA

0   25   50
Time (msec)

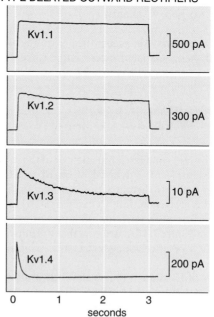

Kv1.1   500 pA

Kv1.2   300 pA

Kv1.3   10 pA

Kv1.4   200 pA

0   1   2   3
seconds

F INACTIVATION OF Kv-TYPE CHANNELS

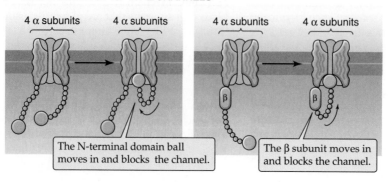

4 α subunits   4 α subunits   4 α subunits   4 α subunits

β   β

The N-terminal domain ball moves in and blocks the channel.

The β subunit moves in and blocks the channel.

ing the action potential. Many transient A-type K^+ currents are inhibited by another organic cation, **4-aminopyridine**. Two distinct families of peptide toxins—**charybdotoxins** of scorpion venom and **dendrotoxins** of mamba snake venom—can discriminate particular subtypes of Kv and K_{Ca} channels, depending on the particular amino acids present in the P region.

Two families of K_{Ca} K^+ channels mediate Ca^{2+}-activated K^+ currents

Ca^{2+}-activated K^+ channels—K_{Ca} channels—appear to be present in the plasma membrane of cells in many different tissues. In patch-clamp experiments, they are easily recog-

---

Human Heart Defects Linked to Mutations of K^+ Channels

A congenital cardiac abnormality in some people results in lengthening of the QT interval of the electrocardiographic signal—long QT syndrome—which corresponds to a prolonged cardiac action potential. Affected children and young adults can exhibit an arrhythmic disturbance of the ventricular heartbeat that results in sudden death. As we have already seen in the box titled Na$^+$ Channel Genetic Defects, one form of a long QT syndrome involves defects in cardiac Na$^+$ channels. However, several forms of this syndrome are caused by mutations in cardiac K$^+$ channel proteins. Some families have mutations in the *KCNQ1* gene encoding KvLQT1, a 581-residue protein belonging to the Kv family of voltage-gated K$^+$ channels. Another form of this disease involves mutations in the *KCNH2* gene encoding HERG, which is related to the ether-a-go-go *Drosophila* mutant, a more distant relative of the Kv channels. Both KvLQT1 and HERG K$^+$ channels participate in repolarization of the cardiac action potential. Such defective repolarization can lead to premature heartbeats or asynchronous ventricular contraction, with subsequent death. The KvLQT1 K$^+$ channel also physically associates with another small membrane protein called minK. Mutations in minK also cause a form of long QT syndrome. K$^+$ channels are also crucial for proper function of the auditory system. Thus, congenital deafness is commonly associated with mutations in some of these K$^+$ channels.

---

nized because the opening probability of individual channels increases at positive values of V_m (Fig. 7-19A). P_o also increases with increasing $[Ca^{2+}]$ on the *intracellular* surface of the membrane patch (Fig. 7-19B). Figure 7-19C shows how increasing $[Ca^{2+}]_i$ causes a negative shift in the P_o versus V_m plot for these channels. A particular type of K_{Ca} channel called the maxi-K_{Ca} or BK (for "big" K^+) channel is noted for its large unitary conductance (~300 pS) and distinctive gating activity.

In principle, K_{Ca} channels provide a stabilizing mechanism to counteract repetitive excitation and intracellular Ca^{2+} loading. K_{Ca} channels mediate the afterhyperpolarizing phase of action potentials (Fig. 7-1A) in cell bodies of various neurons. They have also been implicated in terminating bursts of action potentials in bursting neuronal pacemaker cells. Thus, the gradual increase in $[Ca^{2+}]_i$ that occurs during repetitive firing triggers the opening of K_{Ca} channels, which results in hyperpolarization and a quiescent interburst period that lasts until intracellular Ca^{2+} accumulation is reversed by the action of Ca^{2+} pumps. K_{Ca} channels are also present at high density in many types of smooth muscle cells, where they appear to contribute to the relaxation of tension by providing a hyperpolarizing counterbalance to Ca^{2+}-dependent contraction. In a number of nonexcitable cells, K_{Ca} channels are activated during cell swelling and contribute to regulatory volume decrease (see Chapter 5).

Drosophila genetics also led the way to identification of the first of several genes that encode members of the **K_{Ca} channel family**. Electrophysiological studies of the *Slowpoke* mutation in flies showed that this mutation eliminated a fast, Ca^{2+}-activated K^+ current that is present in larval muscle and neurons. Subsequent cloning and sequencing of the *Slowpoke* gene product revealed a channel-forming subunit that has an S1-S6 core domain similar to that of the Kv family, but it also contains a unique C-terminal domain of ~850 residues (Fig. 7-19). Because BK$_{Ca}$ channels—like Kv channels—have a voltage-sensing domain that is analogous to S4, they are also activated by positive voltage. Structure-function studies on this class of K^+ channel indicate that the unique C-terminal domain contains the Ca^{2+}-binding sites that function in channel activation.

In addition to the BK$_{Ca}$ family, another K^+ channel gene family includes intermediate- and small-conductance Ca^{2+}-activated K^+ channels, respectively termed IK$_{Ca}$ and SK$_{Ca}$. Unlike BK$_{Ca}$ channels, the closely related IK$_{Ca}$ and SK$_{Ca}$ chan-

---

Figure 7-18 Outwardly rectifying K^+ channels. **A,** Note that in a voltage-clamp experiment, a depolarizing step in V_m activates the current, but with a delay. **B,** The current-voltage relationship is shown for a delayed outward rectifying K^+ channel, as in **A. C,** This A-type K^+ current is active at relatively negative values of V_m and tends to hyperpolarize the cell. In a spontaneously spiking neuron, a low level of the A-type current allows V_m to rise relatively quickly toward the threshold, which produces a relatively short interspike interval and thus a high firing rate. **D,** In a spontaneously spiking neuron, a high level of the A-type current causes V_m to rise relatively slowly toward the threshold, which produces a relatively long interspike interval and thus a low firing rate. **E,** These experiments were performed on four different types of K^+ channels (Kv1.1, 1.2, 1.3, and 1.4) from mammalian brain and expressed in *Xenopus* oocytes. Shown are the results of voltage-clamp experiments in which V_m was stepped from −80 mV to 0 mV. The left panel, at high time resolution, shows that some of these channels activate more slowly than others. The right panel, at a longer time scale, shows that inactivation gradually speeds up from Kv1.1 to Kv1.4. **F,** The left panel shows N-type inactivation, so called because the N or amino terminus of the protein is essential for inactivation. Each of the four subunits is thought to have an N-terminal "ball" tethered by a "chain" that can swing into place to block the pore. The right panel shows a variant in which certain β subunits can provide the ball-and-chain for Kv channel α subunits that themselves lack this capability at their N termini. *(Data from Stühmer W, Ruppersberg JP, Schroter KH, et al: Molecular basis of functional diversity of voltage-gated potassium channels in mammalian brain. EMBO J 1989; 8:3235-3244.)*

A VOLTAGE DEPENDENCE

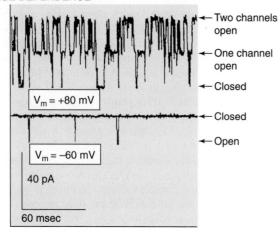

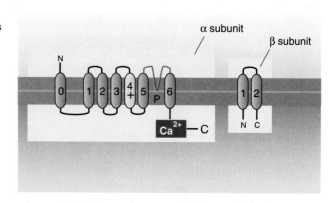

B CALCIUM DEPENDENCE

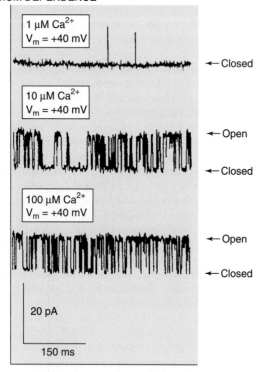

C COMBINED EFFECTS OF CHANGING V_m AND $[Ca^{2+}]_i$

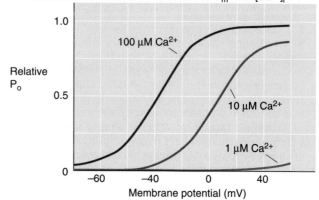

Figure 7-19 Ca^{2+}-activated K^+ channels (K_{Ca}). **A,** Shown is an experiment on K_{Ca} channels that are expressed in *Xenopus* oocytes and studied by use of a patch pipette in an inside-out configuration. When V_m is held at −60 mV, there is very little channel activity. On the other hand, when V_m is +80 mV, both channels in the patch are open most of the time. **B,** The experiment is the same as in **A** except that V_m is always held at +40 mV and the $[Ca^{2+}]$ on the cytosolic side of the patch varies from 1 to 10 to 100 μM. Note that channel activity increases with increasing $[Ca^{2+}]_i$. **C,** Combined effects of changing V_m and $[Ca^{2+}]_i$. Shown is a plot of relative open probability (P_o) of the K_{Ca} channels versus V_m at three different levels of Ca^{2+}. The data come from experiments such as those shown in **B**. *(Data from Butler A, Tsunoda S, McCobb DP, et al: mSlo, a complex mouse gene encoding "maxi" calcium-activated potassium channels. Science 1993; 261:221-224.)*

nels are voltage *insensitive* and are activated by the Ca^{2+}-binding protein calmodulin (see Chapter 3). In some cells, IK_{Ca} and SK_{Ca} channels participate in action potential repolarization and afterhyperpolarization, thus regulating action potential firing frequency. Certain types of these channels function in the activation of lymphocytes.

The Kir K⁺ channels mediate inward rectifier K⁺ currents, and K2P channels may sense stress

In contrast to delayed rectifiers and A-type currents—which are *outwardly* rectifying K⁺ currents—the inward rectifier K⁺ current (also known as the anomalous rectifier) actually conducts more K⁺ current in the *inward* direction than in the outward direction. Such inwardly rectifying, steady-state K⁺ currents have been recorded in many types of cells, including heart, skeletal muscle, and epithelia. Physiologically, these channels help clamp the resting membrane potential close to the K⁺ equilibrium potential and prevent excessive loss of intracellular K⁺ during repetitive activity and long-duration action potentials. In epithelial cells, these inwardly rectifying K⁺ currents are important because they stabilize V_m in the face of electrogenic ion transporters that tend to depolarize the cell (see Chapter 3).

In contrast to the Kv and K_{Ca} channel families, the channel-forming subunits of the inward rectifier (Kir) K⁺ channel family are smaller proteins (~400 to 500 residues) that do not contain a complete S1-S6 core domain. However, they do have a conserved region that is similar to the S5-P-S6 segment of Kv channels (Fig. 7-20A; see the box titled Crystal Structure of a Mammalian K⁺ Channel). The conserved P region is the most basic structural element that is common to all K⁺ channels. The lack of an S1-S4 voltage-sensing domain in inward rectifier channels accounts for the observation that unlike Kv channels, Kir K⁺ channels are not steeply activated by voltage.

Figure 7-20B shows a series of single-channel currents that were obtained from a Kir channel, with equal concentrations of K⁺ on both sides of the membrane as well as Mg^{2+} on the cytosolic side. Under these conditions, the channel conducts K⁺ current only in the inward direction. An *I-V* plot (Fig. 7-20C) derived from data such as these shows typical inward rectification of the unitary current. At negative values of V_m, the inward current decreases linearly as voltage becomes more positive, and no outward current is present at positive values of V_m. However, when Mg^{2+} is omitted from the cytosolic side of the membrane, the channel now exhibits a linear or **ohmic** *I-V* **curve** even over the positive range of V_m values. Thus, the inward rectification is due to **intracellular block** of the channel by Mg^{2+}. Inhibition of outward K⁺ current in the presence of intracellular Mg^{2+} results from voltage-dependent binding of this divalent metal ion. Positive internal voltage favors the binding of Mg^{2+} to the inner mouth of this channel (Fig. 7-20D), as would be expected if the Mg^{2+} binding site is located within the transmembrane electrical field. Because Mg^{2+} is impermeant, it essentially blocks outward K⁺ current. However, negative values of V_m pull the Mg^{2+} out of the channel. Moreover, incoming K⁺ tends to displace any remaining Mg^{2+}. Thus, the Kir channel

favors K⁺ influx over efflux. Intracellular polyamines such as spermine and spermidine—which, like Mg^{2+}, carry a positive charge—also produce inward rectification of inward rectifier channels. These organic cations are important channel-modulating factors that also determine the current-voltage behavior of this particular class of ion channels.

The Kir family of K⁺ channels exhibits various modes of regulation. One Kir subfamily (the G protein–activated, inwardly rectifying K⁺ channels or **GIRKs**) is regulated by the βγ subunits of heterotrimeric **G proteins** (see Chapter 3). For example, stimulation of the vagus nerve slows the heartbeat because the vagal neurotransmitter acetylcholine binds to postsynaptic muscarinic receptors in the heart that are coupled to G proteins. The binding of acetylcholine to its receptor causes the release of G protein βγ subunits, which diffuse to a site on neighboring GIRK channels to activate their opening. The resulting increase in outward K⁺ current hyperpolarizes the cardiac cell, thereby slowing the rate at which V_m approaches the threshold for firing action potentials and lowering the heart rate. GIRK channels are also activated by the membrane phospholipid PIP_2. Thus, G protein–coupled receptors that activate phospholipase C lead to the release of PIP_2, thereby activating GIRK channels.

The members of another subfamily of Kir K⁺ channels, the **K_{ATP} channels**, are directly regulated by adenine nucleotides. K_{ATP} channels are present in the plasma membrane of many cell types, including skeletal muscle, heart, neurons, insulin-secreting β cell of the pancreas, and renal tubule. These channels are inhibited by intracellular adenosine triphosphate (ATP) and activated by adenosine diphosphate (ADP) in a complex fashion. They are believed to provide a direct link between cellular metabolism on the one hand and membrane excitability and K⁺ transport on the other. For example, if cellular ATP levels fall because of oxygen deprivation, such channels could theoretically open and hyperpolarize the cell to suppress firing of action potentials and further reduce energy expenditure. In the pancreatic β cell, an increase in glucose metabolism increases the ATP/ADP ratio. This increased ratio inhibits enough K_{ATP} channels to cause a small depolarization, which in turn activates voltage-gated Ca^{2+} channels and results in insulin secretion (see Chapter 51).

K_{ATP} channels are the target of a group of synthetic drugs called **sulfonylureas** that include tolbutamide and glibenclamide. Sulfonylureas are used in the treatment of type 2 (or non–insulin-dependent) diabetes mellitus because they inhibit pancreatic K_{ATP} channels and stimulate insulin release. Newer and chemically diverse synthetic drugs called K⁺ channel openers (e.g., pinacidil and cromakalim) activate K_{ATP} channels. The therapeutic potential of K⁺ channel openers is being explored in light of their ability to relax various types of smooth muscle. The ability of sulfonylurea drugs to inhibit K_{ATP} channels depends on an accessory subunit called SUR (for sulfonylurea receptor). This protein is a member of the ATP-binding cassette family of proteins (see Chapter 5), which includes two nucleotide-binding domains.

The newest family of K⁺ channels is that of the two-pore or K2P channels, which consist of a tandem repeat of the

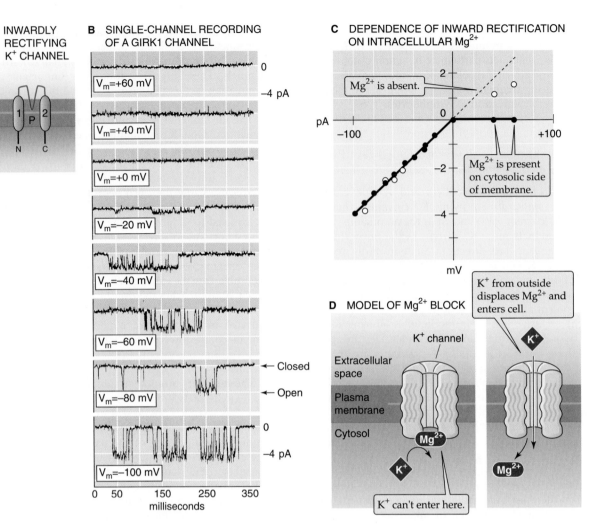

Figure 7-20 Inwardly rectifying K⁺ channels. **A,** This family of channels has only two membrane-spanning segments that correspond to the S5-P-S6 domain of the voltage-gated K⁺ channels. **B,** The GIRK1 channels were expressed in *Xenopus* oocytes and studied by use of a patch pipette in the inside-out configuration. V_m was clamped to values between −100 mV and +60 mV, and [Mg²⁺] was 2.5 mM on the cytosolic side. Note that channel activity increases at more negative voltages but is virtually inactive at positive voltages. **C,** The *I-V* plot shows that there is inward rectification only in the presence of Mg²⁺ on the cytosolic side. In the absence of Mg²⁺, the *I-V* relationship is nearly linear or ohmic. **D,** As shown in the left panel, cytosolic Mg²⁺ occludes the channel pore and prevents the *exit* of K⁺. However, even in the presence of Mg²⁺, K⁺ can move into the cell by displacing the Mg²⁺. *(Data from Kubo Y, Reuveny E, Slesinger PA, et al: Primary structure and functional expression of a rat G protein–coupled muscarinic potassium channel. Nature 1993; 364:802-806.)*

basic Kir topology (see Fig. 6-21F). Because the monomeric subunit of K2P channels contains two linked S5-P-S6 pore domains of the basic Shaker Kv channel, the functional K2P channel is likely to be a dimer of the monomer subunit, which is itself a pseudodimer. K2P channels have been implicated in genesis of the resting membrane potential. K⁺ channels encoded by the 15 human genes for K2P channels may be activated by various chemical and physical signals including PIP₂, membrane stretch, heat, intracellular pH, and general anesthetics. These channels are thought to be involved in a wide range of sensory and neuronal functions.

PROPAGATION OF ACTION POTENTIALS

The propagation of electrical signals in the nervous system involves local current loops

The extraordinary functional diversity of ion channel proteins provides a large array of mechanisms by which the membrane potential of a cell can be changed to evoke an electrical signal or biochemical response. However, channels alone do not control the spread of electrical current. Like electricity in a copper wire, the passive spread of current in biological tissue depends on the nature of the conducting

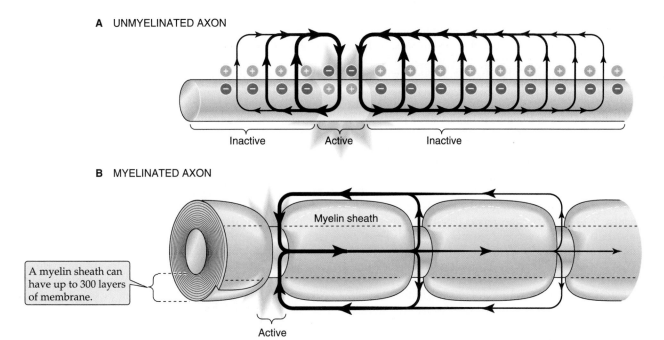

A UNMYELINATED AXON

Inactive   Active   Inactive

B MYELINATED AXON

Myelin sheath

A myelin sheath can have up to 300 layers of membrane.

Active

Figure 7-21 Local current loops during action-potential propagation. **A,** In an unmyelinated axon, the ionic currents flow at one instant in time as a result of the action potential ("active" zone). In the "inactive" zones that are adjacent to the active zone, the outward currents lead to a depolarization. If the membrane is not in an absolute refractory period and if the depolarization is large enough to reach threshold, the immediately adjacent inactive zones will become active and fire their own action potential. In the more distant inactive zones, the outward current is not intense enough to cause V_m to reach threshold. Thus, the magnitudes of the outward currents decrease smoothly with increasing distance from the active zone. **B,** In this example, the "active" zone consists of a single node of Ranvier. In a myelinated axon, the ionic current flows only through the nodes, where there is no myelin and the density of Na^+ channels is very high. Ionic current does not flow through the internodal membrane because of the high resistance of myelin. As a result, the current flowing down the axon is conserved, and the current density at the nodes is very high. This high current density results in the generation of an action potential at the node. Thus, the regenerative action potential propagates in a "saltatory" manner by jumping from node to node. Note that the action potential is actually conducted through the internodal region by capacitative current due to charge displacement across the membrane arising from the resistance-capacitance properties of the membrane (see Fig. 6-11).

and insulating medium. Important factors include geometry (i.e., cell shape and tissue anatomy), electrical resistance of the aqueous solutions and cell membrane, and membrane capacitance. Furthermore, the electrotonic spread of electrical signals is not limited to excitable cells.

Efficient propagation of a change in V_m is essential for the *local* integration of electrical signals at the level of a single cell and for the *global* transmission of signals across large distances in the body. As we discussed earlier in this chapter (Fig. 7-2), *action potentials* propagate in a regenerative manner without loss of amplitude as long as the depolarization spreads to an adjacent region of excitable membrane and does so with sufficient strength to depolarize the membrane above its threshold. However, many types of *nonregenerative,* subthreshold potentials also occur and spread for short distances along cell membranes. These **graded responses**, which we also discussed earlier, contrast with the all-or-nothing nature of action potentials. Such nonregenerative signals include **receptor potentials** generated during the transduction of sensory stimuli and **synaptic potentials** generated by the opening of agonist-activated channels.

With a graded response, the greater the stimulus, the greater the voltage response. For example, the greater the intensity of light that is shined on a mammalian photorecep-

tor cell in the retina, the greater the hyperpolarization produced by the cell. Similarly, the greater the concentration of acetylcholine that is applied at a postsynaptic neuromuscular junction, the greater the resulting depolarization (i.e., synaptic potential). Of course, if this depolarization exceeds the threshold in an excitable cell, an all-or-nothing action potential is initiated. The generation of a physiological response from a graded potential change critically depends on its **electrotonic** spread to other regions of the cell. Like the subthreshold voltage responses produced by injection of a current into a cell through a microelectrode, the electrotonic spread of graded responses declines with distance from the site of initiation. Graded signals dissipate over distances of a few millimeters and thus have only local effects; propagated action potentials can travel long distances through nerve axons.

Electrotonic spread of voltage changes along the cell occurs by the flow of electrical current that is carried by ions in the intracellular and extracellular medium along pathways of the least electrical resistance. Both depolarizations and hyperpolarizations of a small area of membrane produce **local circuit currents**. Figure 7-21A illustrates how the transient voltage change that occurs during an action potential at a particular active site results in local current flow. The cytosol of the active region, where the membrane is depolarized, has a slight excess of positive charge compared with the adjacent inactive regions of the cytosol, which have a slight excess of negative charge. This charge imbalance within the cytosol causes currents of ions to flow from the electrically excited region to adjacent regions of the cytoplasm. Because current always flows in a complete circuit along pathways of least resistance, the current spreads longitudinally from positive to negative regions along the cytoplasm, moves outward across membrane conductance pathways ("leak channels"), and flows along the extracellular medium back to the site of origin, thereby closing the current loop. Because of this flow of current (i.e., positive charge), the region of membrane immediately adjacent to the active region becomes more depolarized, and V_m eventually reaches threshold. Thus, an action potential is generated in this adjacent region as well. Nerve and muscle fibers conduct impulses in both directions if an inactive fiber is excited at a central location, as in this example. However, if an action potential is initiated at one end of a nerve fiber, it will travel only to the opposite end and stop because the refractory period prevents backward movement of the impulse. Likewise, currents generated by subthreshold responses migrate equally in both directions.

Myelin improves the efficiency with which axons conduct action potentials

The flow of electrical current along a cylindrical nerve axon has often been compared with electrical flow through an undersea cable. Similar principles apply to both types of conducting fiber. An underwater cable is designed to carry an electrical current for long distances with little current loss; therefore, it is constructed of a highly conductive (low resistance) metal in its core and a thick plastic insulation wrapped around the core to prevent loss of current to the surrounding seawater. In contrast, the axoplasm of a nerve fiber has much higher resistance than a copper wire, and the nerve membrane is inherently electrically leaky because of background channel conductance. Therefore, in a biological fiber such as a nerve or muscle cell, some current is passively lost into the surrounding medium, and the amplitude of the signal rapidly dissipates over a short distance.

Animal nervous systems use two basic strategies to improve the conduction properties of nerve fibers: (1) increasing the diameter of the axon, thus decreasing the internal resistance of the cable; and (2) myelination, which increases the electrical insulation around the cable. As **axon diameter** increases, the conduction velocity of action potentials increases because the internal resistance of the axoplasm is inversely related to the internal cross-sectional area of the axon. Unmyelinated nerve fibers of the invertebrate squid giant axon (as large as ~1000 μm in diameter) are a good example of this type of size adaptation. These nerve axons mediate the escape response of the squid from its predators and can propagate action potentials at a velocity of ~25 m/s.

In vertebrates, **myelination** of smaller diameter (~1 to 5 μm) nerve axons serves to improve the efficiency of impulse propagation, especially over the long distances that nerves traverse between the brain and the extremities. Axons are literally embedded in myelin, which consists of concentrically wound wrappings of the membranes of glial cells (see

Chapter 11). The thickness of the myelin sheath may amount to 20% to 40% of the diameter of a nerve fiber, and the sheath may consist of as many as 300 membrane layers. The glial cells that produce myelin are called Schwann cells in the periphery and oligodendrocytes in the brain. Because resistors in series add directly and capacitors in series add as the sum of the reciprocal, the insulating resistance of a myelinated fiber with 300 membrane layers is increased by a factor of 300 and the capacitance is decreased to 1/300 that of a single membrane. This large increase in membrane resistance minimizes loss of current across the leaky axonal membrane and forces the current to flow longitudinally along the inside of the fiber.

In myelinated peripheral nerves, the myelin sheath is interrupted at regular intervals, forming short (~1 μm) uncovered regions called **nodes of Ranvier**. The length of the myelinated axon segments between adjacent unmyelinated nodes ranges from 0.2 to 2 mm. In mammalian axons, the density of voltage-gated Na⁺ channels is very high in the nodal membrane. The unique anatomy of myelinated axons results in a mode of impulse propagation known as **saltatory conduction**. Current flow that is initiated at an excited node flows directly to adjacent nodes with little loss of transmembrane current through the internode region (Fig. 7-21B). In other words, the high membrane resistance in the internode region effectively forces the current to travel from node to node.

The high efficiency of impulse conduction in such axons allows several adjacent nodes in the same fiber to fire an action potential virtually simultaneously as it is being propagated. Thus, saltatory conduction in a myelinated nerve can reach a very high velocity, up to 130 m/s. The action potential velocity in a myelinated nerve fiber can thus be several-fold greater than that in a giant unmyelinated axon, even though the axon diameter in the myelinated fiber may be more than two orders of magnitude smaller. During conduction of an action potential in a myelinated axon, the intracellular regions between nodes also depolarize. However, no transmembrane current flows in these internodal regions, and therefore no dissipation of ion gradients occurs. The nodal localization of Na⁺ channels conserves ionic concentration gradients that must be maintained at the expense of ATP hydrolysis by the Na-K pump.

The cable properties of the membrane and cytoplasm determine the velocity of signal propagation

Following the analogy of a nerve fiber as an underwater cable, **cable theory** allows one to model the pathways of electrical current flow along biomembranes. The approach is to use circuit diagrams that were first employed to describe the properties of electrical cables. Figure 7-22A illustrates the equivalent circuit diagram of a cylindrical electrical cable or membrane that is filled and bathed in a conductive electrolyte solution. The membrane itself is represented by discrete elements, each with a transverse membrane resistance (r_m) and capacitance (c_m) connected in parallel (a representation we used earlier, in Fig. 6-11A). Consecutive membrane elements are connected in series by discrete resistors, each of which represents the electrical resistance of a finite length of

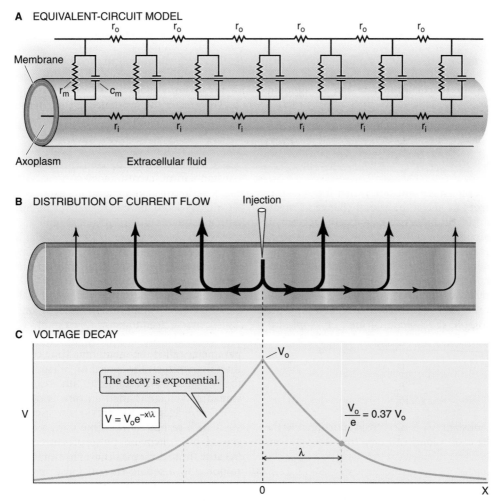

Figure 7-22 Passive cable properties of an axon. **A,** The axon is represented as a hollow, cylindrical "cable" that is filled with an electrolyte solution. All of the electrical properties of the axon are represented by discrete elements that are expressed in terms of the length of the axon. r_i is the resistance of the internal medium. Similarly, r_o is the resistance of the external medium. r_m and c_m are the membrane resistance and capacitance per discrete element of axon length. **B,** When current is injected into the axon, the current flows away from the injection site in both directions. The current density smoothly decays with increasing distance from the site of injection. **C,** Because the current density decreases with distance from the site of current injection in **B,** the electrotonic potential (V) also decays exponentially with distance in both directions. V_o is the maximum change in V_m that is at the site of current injection.

the external medium (r_o) or internal medium (r_i). The parameters r_m, c_m, r_o, and r_i refer to a unit length of axon (Table 7-3).

How do the various electrical components of the cable model influence the electrotonic spread of current along an axon? To answer this question, we inject a steady electrical current into an axon with a microelectrode to produce a constant voltage (V_0) at a particular point ($x = 0$) along the length of the axon (Fig. 7-22B). This injection of current results in the longitudinal spread of current in both directions from point $x = 0$. The voltage (V) at various points along the axon decays exponentially with distance (x) from the point of current injection (Fig. 7-22C), according to the following equation:

$$V = V_0 e^{-x/\lambda} \qquad (7\text{-}5)$$

The parameter λ has units of *distance* and is referred to as the **length constant** or the **space constant**. One length constant away from the point of current injection, V is $1/e$, or ~37% of the maximum value of V_0. The decaying *currents* that spread away from the location of a current-passing electrode are called **electrotonic currents**. Similarly, the spread of subthreshold *voltage* changes away from a site of origin is referred to as electrotonic spread, unlike the regenerative propagation of action potentials.

The length constant depends on the three resistance elements in Figure 7-22A:

$$\lambda = \sqrt{\frac{r_m}{r_o + r_i}} \qquad (7\text{-}6)$$

We can simplify this expression by noting that internal resistance is much larger than external resistance, so the contribution of r_o to the denominator can be ignored. Thus,

$$\lambda = \sqrt{\frac{r_m}{r_i}} \qquad (7\text{-}7)$$

The significance of the length constant is that it determines how far the electrotonic spread of a local change in membrane potential is able to influence neighboring regions of membrane. The longer the length constant, the farther down the axon a voltage change spreads.

How does the diameter of an axon affect the length constant? To answer this question, we must replace r_m and r_i (expressed in terms of axon length) in Equation 7-7 with the **specific resistances** R_m and R_i (expressed in terms of the area of axon membrane or cross-sectional area of axoplasm). Making the substitutions according to the definitions in Table 7-3, we have

$$\lambda = \sqrt{\frac{aR_m}{2R_i}} \qquad (7\text{-}8)$$

Thus, the length constant (λ) is directly proportional to the square root of the axon radius (a). Equation 7-8 confirms

TABLE 7-3   Cable Parameters

Parameter	Units	Definition or Relationship
r_m	$\Omega \times cm$	Membrane resistance (per unit length of axon)
r_o	Ω/cm	Extracellular resistance (per unit length of axon)
r_i	Ω/cm	Intracellular resistance (per unit length of axon)
c_m	$\mu F/cm$	Membrane capacitance (per unit length of axon)
$R_m = r_m \times 2\pi a$	$\Omega \times cm^2$	Specific membrane resistance (per unit area of membrane)
$R_i = r_i \times \pi a^2$	$\Omega \times cm$	Specific internal resistance (per unit cross-sectional area of axoplasm)
$C_m = c_m/(2\pi a)$	$\mu F/cm^2$	Specific membrane capacitance (per unit area of membrane)

a, radius of the axon; Ω, ohm; F, farad.

basic intuitive notions about what makes an efficiently conducting electrical cable:

1. The greater the specific membrane resistance (R_m) and cable radius, the greater the length constant and the less the loss of signal.
2. The greater the resistance of the internal conductor (R_i), the smaller the length constant and the greater the loss of signal.

These relationships also confirm measurements of length constants in different biological preparations. For example, the length constant of a squid axon with a diameter of ~1 mm is ~13 mm, whereas that of a mammalian nerve fiber with a diameter of ~1 μm is ~0.2 mm.

So far, we have been discussing the *spatial* spread of voltage changes that are stable in *time*. In other words, we assumed that the amount of injected current was steady. What happens if the current is not steady? For example, what happens at the beginning of a stimulus when we (or a physiological receptor) first turn the current "on"? To answer these questions, we need to know how rapidly V_m changes in time at a particular site, which is described by a second cable parameter called the membrane **time constant** (τ_m). Rather than determining the spread of voltage changes in space, as the length constant does, the time constant influences the spread of voltage changes in *time* and thus the *velocity* of signal propagation. We previously discussed the time constant with respect to the time course of the change in V_m caused by a stepwise pulse of current (see Fig. 6-12A). Because the membrane behaves like an RC circuit, the voltage response to a square current pulse across a small piece of membrane follows an exponential time course with a time constant that is equal to the product of membrane resistance and capacitance:

$$\tau_m = R_m \cdot C_m \qquad (7\text{-}9)$$

We introduced this expression earlier as Equation 6-17. The shorter the time constant, the more quickly a neighboring region of membrane will be brought to threshold and the sooner the region will fire an action potential. Thus, the shorter the time constant, the faster the speed of impulse propagation, and vice versa. In contrast, conduction velocity is directly proportional to the length constant. The greater the length constant, the farther a signal can spread before decaying below threshold and the greater the area of membrane that the stimulus can excite. These relationships explain why, in terms of relative conduction velocity, a high-resistance, low-capacitance *myelinated* axon has a distinct advantage over an *unmyelinated* axon of the same diameter for all but the smallest axons (<1 μm in diameter; see Chapter 12).

In summary, the cable parameters of length constant and time constant determine the way in which graded potentials and action potentials propagate over space and time in biological tissue. These parameters are in turn a function of material properties that include resistance, capacitance, and geometric considerations. The dependence of impulse conduction velocity on fiber diameter has been studied experimentally and analyzed theoretically for unmyelinated and myelinated nerve axons. For *unmyelinated* axons, conduction velocity increases roughly with the square root of the axon's diameter, just as the length constant increases with the square root of the axon's diameter or radius (Equation 7-8). In contrast, the conduction velocity of *myelinated* fibers is a linear function of diameter and increases ~6 m/s per 1-μm increase in outer diameter. Thus, a mammalian myelinated axon with an outer diameter of ~4 μm has roughly the same impulse velocity as a squid giant axon with a diameter of 500 μm! However, for myelinated fibers with a very small diameter (<1 μm), the adverse effect of high internal resistance of the axoplasm predominates, and conduction is slower than in unmyelinated axons of the same outer diameter. For outer diameters that are greater than ~1 μm, the increased membrane resistance and reduced capacitance caused by myelination result in much faster conduction velocities.

The physiological importance of myelin in action potential propagation is most dramatically illustrated in the pathology that underlies human demyelinating diseases such as **multiple sclerosis**. As discussed more fully in Chapter 11, multiple sclerosis is an autoimmune disorder in which the myelin sheath surrounding CNS axons is progressively lost (see Chapter 12 for the box on Demyelinating Diseases). Gradual demyelination is responsible for an array of neurological symptoms that involve various degrees of paralysis and altered or lost sensation. As myelin is eliminated, the loss of membrane resistance and increased capacitance mean that propagated action potentials may ultimately fail to reach the next node of Ranvier and thus result in nerve blockage.

REFERENCES

Books and Reviews

Ackerman MJ, Clapham DE: Ion channels—basic science and clinical disease. N Engl J Med 1997; 336:1575-1586.

Catterall WA: Cellular and molecular biology of voltage-gated sodium channels. Physiol Rev 1992; 72 (Suppl):S15-S48.

Chandy KG, Gutman GA: Voltage-gated K$^+$ channel genes. In North RA (ed): Handbook of Receptors and Channels: Ligand and Voltage-Gated Ion Channels, pp 1-71. Boca Raton, FL: CRC Press, 1995.

Hille B: Ionic Channels of Excitable Membranes, 3rd ed. Sunderland, MA: Sinauer Associates, 2001.

Pallotta BS, Wagoner PK: Voltage-dependent potassium channels since Hodgkin and Huxley. Physiol Rev 1992; 72 (Suppl): S49-S67.

Tsien RW, Wheeler DB: Voltage-gated calcium channels. In Carafoli E, Klee CB (eds): Calcium as a Cellular Regulator, pp 171-199. New York: Oxford University Press, 1999.

Journal Articles

Cole KS, Moore JW: Ionic current measurements in the squid giant axon membrane. J Gen Physiol 1960; 44:123-167.

Hille B: The selective inhibition of delayed potassium currents in nerve by tetraethylammonium ions. J Gen Physiol 1967; 50:1287-1302.

Ho K, Nichols CG, Lederer WJ, et al: Cloning and expression of an inwardly rectifying ATP-regulated potassium channel. Nature 1993; 362:31-38.

Hodgkin AL, Huxley AF: A quantitative description of membrane current and its application to conduction and excitation in nerve. J Physiol (Lond) 1952; 117:500-544.

Kim YI, Neher E: IgG from patients with Lambert-Eaton syndrome blocks voltage-dependent calcium channels. Science 1988; 239:405-408.

Kubo Y, Reuveny E, Slesinger PA, et al: Primary structure and functional expression of a rat G protein–coupled muscarinic potassium channel. Nature 1993; 364:802-806.

Long SB, Campbell EB, MacKinnon R: 2005 Voltage sensor of Kv1.2: Structural basis of electromechanical coupling. Science Express July 7, 2005.

Ptacek LJ, Gouw L, Kwiecinski H, et al: Sodium channel mutations in paramyotonia congenita and hyperkalemic periodic paralysis. Ann Neurol 1993; 33:300-307.

CHAPTER 8

SYNAPTIC TRANSMISSION AND THE NEUROMUSCULAR JUNCTION

Edward G. Moczydlowski

The ionic gradients that cells maintain across their membranes provide a form of stored electrochemical energy that cells can use for electrical signaling. The combination of a resting membrane potential of −60 to −90 mV and a diverse array of voltage-gated ion channels allows excitable cells to generate action potentials that propagate over long distances along the surface membrane of a *single* nerve axon or muscle fiber. However, another class of mechanisms is necessary to transmit such electrical information from cell to cell throughout the myriad neuronal networks that link the brain with sensory and effector organs. Electrical signals must pass across the specialized gap region between two apposing cell membranes that is called a **synapse**. The process underlying this cell-to-cell transfer of electrical signals is termed **synaptic transmission**. Communication between cells at a synapse can be either electrical or chemical. Electrical synapses provide direct electrical continuity between cells by means of gap junctions, whereas chemical synapses link two cells together by a chemical **neurotransmitter** that is released from one cell and diffuses to another.

In this chapter we discuss the general properties of synaptic transmission and then focus mainly on synaptic transmission between a motor neuron and a skeletal muscle fiber. This interface between the motor neuron and the muscle cell is called the neuromuscular junction. In Chapter 13, the focus is on synaptic transmission between neurons in the central nervous system (CNS).

MECHANISMS OF SYNAPTIC TRANSMISSION

Electrical continuity between cells is established by electrical or chemical synapses

Once the concept of bioelectricity had taken hold among physiologists of the 19th century, it became clear that the question of how electrical signals flow between cells posed a fundamental biological problem. Imagine that two cells lie side by side without any specialized device for communication between them. Furthermore, imagine that a flat, 20-μm^2 membrane area of the first or **presynaptic** cell is separated—

by 15 nm—from a similar area of the second or **postsynaptic** cell. In his classic book on electrophysiology, Katz calculated that a voltage signal at the presynaptic membrane would suffer 10,000-fold attenuation in the postsynaptic membrane. A similar calculation based on the geometry and cable properties of a typical nerve-muscle synapse suggests that an action potential arriving at a nerve terminal could depolarize the postsynaptic membrane by only 1 μV after crossing the synaptic gap—an attenuation of 10^5. Clearly, the evolution of complex multicellular organisms required the development of special synaptic mechanisms for electrical signaling to serve as a workable means of intercellular communication.

Two competing hypotheses emerged in the 19th century to explain how closely apposed cells could communicate electrically. One school of thought proposed that cells are directly linked by microscopic connecting bridges that enable electrical signals to flow directly. Other pioneering physiologists used pharmacological observations to infer that cell-to-cell transmission was chemical in nature. Ultimate resolution of this question awaited both the development of electron microscopic techniques, which permitted visualization of the intimate contact region between cells, and further studies in neurochemistry, which identified the small, organic molecules that are responsible for neurotransmission. By 1960, accumulated evidence led to the general recognition that cells use *both* direct electrical and indirect chemical modes of transmission to communicate with one another.

The essential structural element of intercellular communication, the synapse, is a specialized point of contact between the membranes of two different but connected, cells. Electrical and chemical synapses have unique morphological features, distinguishable by electron microscopy. One major distinction is the distance of separation between the two apposing cell membranes. At **electrical synapses**, the adjacent cell membranes are separated by ~3 nm and appear to be nearly sealed together by a plate-like structure that is a fraction of a micrometer in diameter. Freeze-fracture images of the intramembrane plane in this region reveal a cluster of closely packed intramembranous particles that represent a **gap junction**. As described in Chapter 6, a gap junction corresponds to planar arrays of connexons, each of which is made up of six connexin monomers (see Fig. 6-18). The multiple connexons from apposing cells physically connect the two cells together through multiple aqueous channels.

In contrast to the gap junction, the apposing cell membranes of the **chemical synapse** are separated by a much larger distance of ~30 nm at a neuronal chemical synapse and up to 50 nm at the vertebrate nerve-muscle synapse. An additional characteristic of a chemical synapse is the presence of numerous synaptic vesicles on the side of the synapse that initiates the signal transmission, termed the *presynaptic* side. These vesicles are sealed, spherical membrane-bound structures that range in diameter from 40 to 200 nm and contain a high concentration of chemical neurotransmitter.

The contrasting morphological characteristics of electrical and chemical synapses underline the contrasting mechanisms by which they function (Table 8-1). Electrical synapses pass voltage changes directly from one cell to another across the low-resistance continuity that is provided by the connexon channels. On the other hand, chemical synapses link two cells by the diffusion of a chemical transmitter across the large gap separating them. Key steps in chemical neurotransmission include release of transmitter from synaptic vesicles into the synaptic space, diffusion of transmitter across the cleft of the synapse, and activation of the postsynaptic cell by binding of transmitter to a specific receptor protein on the postsynaptic cell membrane.

Direct evidence for the existence of chemical synapses actually predated the experimental confirmation of electrical synapses. The foundations of synaptic physiology can be traced to early studies of the autonomic nervous system. Early in the 1900s, researchers noted that adrenal gland extracts, which contain epinephrine, elicited physiological effects (e.g., an increase in heart rate) that were similar to those elicited by stimulation of sympathetic nerve fibers. In 1904, Elliot proposed that sympathetic nerves might release a substance analogous to epinephrine that would function in chemical transmission between a nerve and its target organ. Similar studies suggested that the vagus nerve, which is parasympathetic, produces a related substance that is responsible for depression of the heartbeat.

A classic experiment performed by Loewi in 1921 is widely cited as the first definitive evidence for chemical neurotransmission. Loewi used an ingenious bioassay to test for the release of a chemical substance by the vagus nerve. He repeatedly stimulated the vagus nerve of a cannulated frog heart and observed a slowing of the heartbeat. At the same time, he collected the artificial saline that emerged from the ventricle of this overstimulated heart. When he later applied the collected fluid from the vagus-stimulated heart to a different heart, he observed that this perfusate slowed the second heart in a manner that was identical to direct vagal stimulation. He also later identified the active compound in the perfusion fluid, originally called *Vagusstoff,* as acetylcholine (ACh).

Efforts by Dale and coworkers to understand the basis of neurotransmission between motor nerves and skeletal muscle culminated in the identification of ACh as the endogenous excitatory neurotransmitter. Thus, the inherent complexity of chemical synaptic transmission was evident from these earliest investigations, which indicated that the same neurotransmitter (ACh) could have an inhibitory action at one synapse (vagus nerve–heart) and an excitatory action at another synapse (motor nerve–skeletal muscle). For their work on nerve transmission across chemical synapses, Otto Loewi and Sir Henry Dale received the Nobel Prize in Medicine in 1936.

Electrical synapses directly link the cytoplasm of adjacent cells

Whereas overwhelming support for chemical synaptic transmission accumulated in the first half of the 20th century, the first direct evidence for electrical transmission came much later from electrophysiological recordings of a crayfish nerve preparation. In 1959, Furshpan and Potter used two pairs of stimulating and recording electrodes to show that depolarization of a presynaptic nerve fiber (the crayfish abdominal nerve) resulted in excitation of a postsynaptic nerve cell (the motor nerve to the tail muscle) with virtually no time delay. In contrast, chemical synapses exhibit a characteristic delay of ~1 ms in the postsynaptic voltage signal after excitation of the presynaptic cell. The demonstration of an electrical synapse between two nerve membranes highlighted an important functional difference between electrical and chemical synapses—immediate signal propagation (electrical) versus briefly delayed communication (chemical) through the junction.

An electrical synapse is a true structural connection formed by connexon channels of gap junctions that link the cytoplasm of two cells (Fig. 8-1). These channels thus provide a low-resistance path for electrotonic current flow and allow voltage signals to flow with little attenuation and no delay between two or more coupled cells. Many types of gap junctions pass electrical current with equal efficiency in both directions (**reciprocal synapses**). In other words, the current passing through the gap junction is ohmic; it varies linearly

TABLE 8-1 Summary of Properties of Electrical and Chemical Synapses

	ELECTRICAL	CHEMICAL Ionotropic	Metabotropic
Agonist	None	e.g., ACh	e.g., ACh
Membrane protein	Connexon	Receptor/channel	Receptor/G protein
Speed of transmission	Instantaneous	~1 ms delay	Seconds to minutes

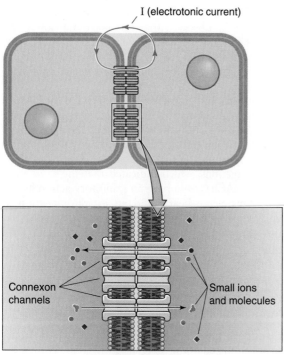

I (electrotonic current)

Connexon channels

Small ions and molecules

Cell-cell gap junction

Figure 8-1 An electrical synapse. An electrical synapse consists of one or more gap junction channels permeable to small ions and molecules.

with the transjunctional voltage (i.e., the V_m difference between the two cells). However, the crayfish synapse described by Furshpan and Potter allows depolarizing current to pass readily only in one direction, from the presynaptic cell to the postsynaptic cell. Such electrical synapses are called **rectifying synapses** to indicate that the underlying junctional conductance is voltage dependent. Studies of cloned and expressed connexins have shown that the voltage dependence of electrical synapses arises from unique gating properties of different connexin isoforms. Some isoforms are voltage dependent; others are voltage independent. Intrinsic rectification can also be altered by the formation of a gap junction that is composed of two hemichannels, each made up of a different connexin monomer. Such hybrid connexins are called heterotypic channels.

Chemical synapses use neurotransmitters to provide electrical continuity between adjacent cells

By their very nature, chemical synapses are inherently rectifying or polarized. They propagate current in one direction: from the presynaptic cell that releases the transmitter to the postsynaptic cell that contains the receptors that recognize and bind the transmitter. However, the essentially vectorial nature of chemical synaptic transmission belies the possibility that the postsynaptic cell can influence synapse formation or transmitter release by the presynaptic cell. Studies of synapse development and regulation have shown that postsynaptic cells also play an active role in synapse formation. In the CNS, postsynaptic cells may also produce retrograde

signaling molecules, such as nitric oxide, that diffuse back into the presynaptic terminal and modulate the strength of the synaptic connection (see Chapter 13). Furthermore, the presynaptic membrane at some synapses contains receptors that may either inhibit or facilitate the release of transmitter by biochemical mechanisms. Thus, chemical synapses should be considered a unidirectional pathway for signal propagation that can be modulated by bidirectional chemical communication between two interacting cells.

The process of chemical transmission can be summarized by the following series of steps (Fig. 8-2):

Step 1: Neurotransmitter molecules are packaged into synaptic vesicles. Specific transport proteins in the vesicle membrane use the energy of an H^+ gradient to energize uptake of the neurotransmitter in the vesicle.

Step 2: An action potential, which involves voltage-gated Na^+ and K^+ channels (see Chapter 7), arrives at the presynaptic nerve terminal.

Step 3: Depolarization opens voltage-gated Ca^{2+} channels, which allows Ca^{2+} to enter the presynaptic terminal.

Step 4: The increase in intracellular Ca^{2+} concentration ($[Ca^{2+}]_i$) triggers the fusion of synaptic vesicles with the presynaptic membrane. As a result, packets (quanta) of transmitter molecules are released into the synaptic cleft.

Step 5: The transmitter molecules diffuse across the synaptic cleft and bind to specific receptors on the membrane of the postsynaptic cell.

Step 6: The binding of transmitter activates the receptor, which in turn activates the postsynaptic cell.

Step 7: The process is terminated by (1) enzymatic destruction of the transmitter (e.g., hydrolysis of ACh by acetylcholinesterase), (2) uptake of transmitter into the presynaptic nerve terminal or into other cells by Na^+-dependent transport systems, or (3) diffusion of the transmitter molecules away from the synapse.

The molecular nature of chemical synapses permits enormous diversity in functional specialization and regulation. Functional diversity occurs at the level of the transmitter substance, receptor protein, postsynaptic response, and subsequent electrical and biochemical processes. Many different small molecules are known—or proposed—to serve as neurotransmitters (see Chapter 13). These molecules include both small organic molecules, such as norepinephrine, ACh, serotonin (5-hydroxytryptamine [5-HT]), glutamate, γ-aminobutyric acid (GABA), and glycine, and peptides such as endorphins and enkephalins.

Neurotransmitters can activate ionotropic or metabotropic receptors

Neurotransmitter receptors transduce information by two molecular mechanisms: some are ligand-gated ion channels and others are G protein–coupled receptors (see Chapter 3). Several neurotransmitter molecules, such as glutamate and ACh, serve as ligands (agonists) for both types of receptors. In the particular case of glutamate, glutamate receptors that are ion channels are known as **ionotropic receptors**, and glutamate receptors coupled to G proteins are called **metabo-**

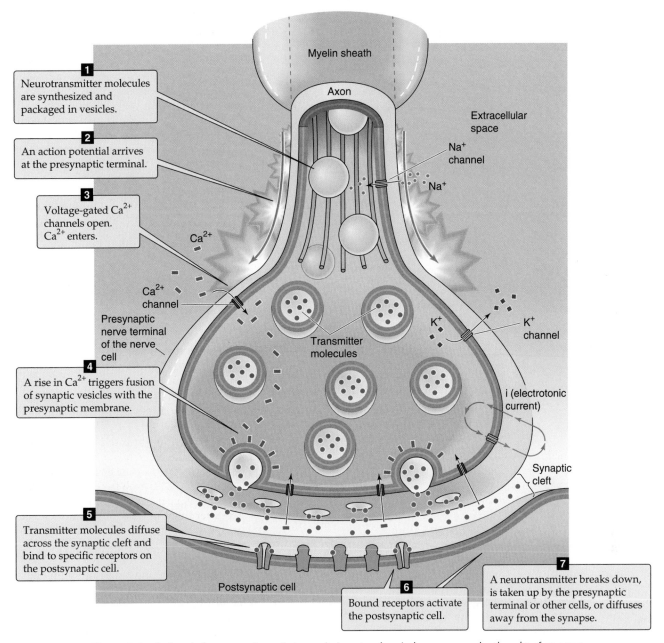

1 Neurotransmitter molecules are synthesized and packaged in vesicles.

2 An action potential arrives at the presynaptic terminal.

3 Voltage-gated Ca^{2+} channels open. Ca^{2+} enters.

4 A rise in Ca^{2+} triggers fusion of synaptic vesicles with the presynaptic membrane.

5 Transmitter molecules diffuse across the synaptic cleft and bind to specific receptors on the postsynaptic cell.

6 Bound receptors activate the postsynaptic cell.

7 A neurotransmitter breaks down, is taken up by the presynaptic terminal or other cells, or diffuses away from the synapse.

Myelin sheath

Axon

Extracellular space

Na$^+$ channel

Na$^+$

Ca^{2+}

Ca^{2+} channel

Presynaptic nerve terminal of the nerve cell

Transmitter molecules

K$^+$

K$^+$ channel

i (electrotonic current)

Synaptic cleft

Postsynaptic cell

Figure 8-2 A chemical synapse. Synaptic transmission at a chemical synapse can be thought of as occurring in seven steps.

tropic receptors. This nomenclature is often used to describe the two major functional classes of receptors for transmitters other than glutamate.

Ionotropic and metabotropic receptors determine the ultimate functional response to transmitter release. Activation of an ionotropic receptor causes rapid opening of ion channels. This channel activation in turn results in depolarization or hyperpolarization of the postsynaptic membrane, the choice depending on the ionic selectivity of the conductance change. Activation of a metabotropic G protein–linked receptor results in the production of active α and βγ subunits, which initiate a wide variety of cellular responses by direct interaction with either ion channel proteins or other

second-messenger effector proteins (see Chapter 3). By their very nature, ionotropic receptors mediate fast ionic synaptic responses that occur on a millisecond time scale, whereas metabotropic receptors mediate slow, biochemically mediated synaptic responses in the range of seconds to minutes.

Figure 8-3 compares the basic processes mediated by two prototypic ACh receptors (AChRs): (1) the ACh-activated ion channel at the neuromuscular junction of skeletal muscle, an ionotropic receptor also known as the **nicotinic** AChR (Fig. 8-3A), and (2) the G protein–linked AChR at the atrial parasympathetic synapse of the heart, a metabotropic receptor also known as the **muscarinic** AChR (Fig. 8-3B). The nicotinic versus muscarinic distinction was a classic *pharma-*

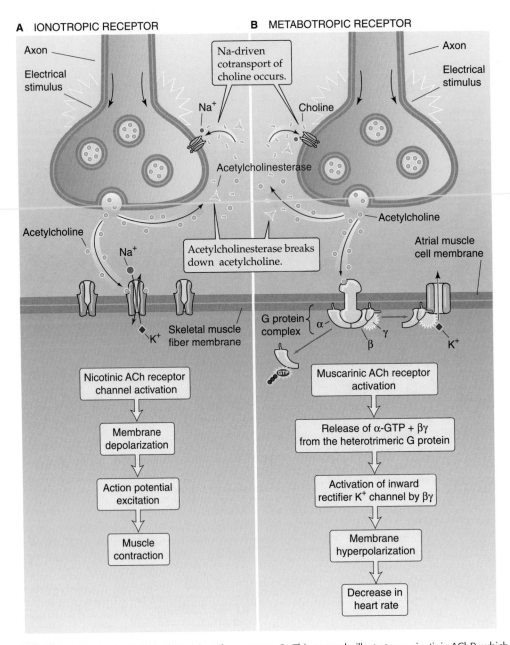

A IONOTROPIC RECEPTOR

B METABOTROPIC RECEPTOR

Axon

Electrical stimulus

Na-driven cotransport of choline occurs.

Na⁺

Choline

Axon

Electrical stimulus

Acetylcholinesterase

Acetylcholine

Acetylcholine

Na⁺

Acetylcholinesterase breaks down acetylcholine.

Atrial muscle cell membrane

K⁺

Skeletal muscle fiber membrane

G protein complex

α

β

γ

GTP

K⁺

Nicotinic ACh receptor channel activation

↓

Membrane depolarization

↓

Action potential excitation

↓

Muscle contraction

Muscarinic ACh receptor activation

↓

Release of α-GTP + βγ from the heterotrimeric G protein

↓

Activation of inward rectifier K⁺ channel by βγ

↓

Membrane hyperpolarization

↓

Decrease in heart rate

Figure 8-3 Ionotropic and metabotropic ACh receptors. **A,** This example illustrates a nicotinic AChR, which is a ligand-gated channel on the postsynaptic membrane. In a skeletal muscle, the end result is muscle contraction. **B,** This example illustrates a muscarinic AChR, which is coupled to a heterotrimeric G protein. In a cardiac muscle, the end result is decreased heart rate. Note that the presynaptic release of ACh is similar here and in **A**.

cological classification based on whether the AChR is activated by nicotine or muscarine, two natural products that behave like agonists. In the case of the ionotropic (nicotinic) receptor, opening of the AChR channel results in a transient increase in permeability to Na⁺ and K⁺, which directly produces a brief depolarization that activates the muscle fiber. In the case of the metabotropic (muscarinic) receptor, activation of the G protein–coupled receptor opens an inward

rectifier K⁺ channel, or GIRK (see Chapter 7), through βγ subunits released from an activated heterotrimeric G protein. Enhanced opening of these GIRKs produces membrane hyperpolarization and leads to inhibition of cardiac excitation (see Chapter 21). These two functionally distinct mechanisms are the molecular basis for the seemingly conflicting observations of early physiologists that ACh (*Vagusstoff*) activates skeletal muscle but inhibits heart muscle.

SYNAPTIC TRANSMISSION AT THE NEUROMUSCULAR JUNCTION

Neuromuscular junctions are specialized synapses between motor neurons and skeletal muscle

The chemical synapse between peripheral motor nerve terminals and skeletal muscle fibers is the most intensely studied synaptic connection in the nervous system. Even though the detailed morphology and the specific molecular components (e.g., neurotransmitters and receptors) differ considerably among different types of synapses, the basic electrophysiological principles of the neuromuscular junction are applicable to many other types of chemical synapses, including neuronal synaptic connections in the brain, to which we will return in Chapter 13. In this chapter, we focus on the neuromuscular junction in discussing the basic principles of synaptic transmission.

Motor neurons with cell bodies in the spinal cord have long axons that branch extensively near the point of contact with the target muscle (Fig. 8-4). These axon processes each innervate a separate fiber of skeletal muscle. The whole assembly of muscle fibers innervated by the axon from one motor neuron is called a **motor unit.**

Typically, an axon makes a single point of synaptic contact with a skeletal muscle fiber, midway along the length of the muscle fiber. This specialized synaptic region is called the **neuromuscular junction** or the **end plate** (Fig. 8-4). An individual end plate consists of a small tree-like patch of unmyelinated nerve processes that are referred to as terminal arborizations. The bulb-shaped endings that finally contact the muscle fiber are called **boutons.** Schwann cells are intimately associated with the nerve terminal and form a cap over the face of the nerve membrane that is located away from the muscle membrane. The postsynaptic membrane of the skeletal muscle fiber lying directly under the nerve terminal is characterized by extensive invaginations known as **postjunctional folds.** These membrane infoldings greatly increase the surface area of the muscle plasma membrane in the postsynaptic region. The intervening space of the **synaptic cleft,** which is ~50 nm wide, is filled with a meshwork of proteins and proteoglycans that are part of the extracellular matrix. A particular region of the muscle basement membrane called the synaptic basal lamina contains various proteins (e.g., collagen, laminin, agrin) that mediate adhesion of the neuromuscular junction and play important roles in synapse development and regeneration. The synaptic basal lamina also contains a high concentration of the enzyme **acetylcholinesterase (AChE),** which ultimately terminates synaptic transmission by rapidly hydrolyzing free ACh to choline and acetate.

Electron micrographs of the bouton region demonstrate the presence of numerous spherical synaptic vesicles, each with a diameter of 50 to 60 nm. The cell bodies of motor neurons in the spinal cord produce these vesicles, and the microtubule-mediated process of fast axonal transport (see Chapter 2) translocates them to the nerve terminal. The quantal nature of transmitter release (described later in more detail) reflects the fusion of individual synaptic vesicles with the plasma membrane of the presynaptic terminal. Each synaptic vesicle contains 6000 to 10,000 molecules of ACh. The ACh concentration in synaptic vesicles is ~150 mM. ACh is synthesized in the nerve terminal—outside the vesicle—from choline and acetyl coenzyme A by the enzyme **choline acetyltransferase.** The ACh moves into the synaptic vesicle through a specific ACh-H exchanger, which couples the inward transport of ACh to the efflux of H^+. Energetically, this process is driven by the vesicular proton electrochemical gradient (positive voltage and low pH inside), which in turn is produced by a vacuolar-type H^+ pump fueled by ATP (see Chapter 5). The nerve terminal also contains numerous mitochondria that produce the ATP required to fuel energy metabolism.

The process of fusion of synaptic vesicles and release of ACh occurs at differentiated regions of the presynaptic membrane called **active zones.** In electron micrographs, active zones appear as dense spots over which synaptic vesicles are closely clustered in apposition to the membrane. High-resolution images of active zones reveal a double, linear array of synaptic vesicles and intramembranous particles. These zones are oriented directly over secondary *post*synaptic clefts that lie between adjacent postjunctional folds. Molecular localization studies have shown that the density of ionotropic (nicotinic) AChRs is very high at the crests of postjunctional folds. Examination of the detailed microarchitecture of the neuromuscular synapse thus reveals a highly specialized structure for delivery of neurotransmitter molecules to a precise location on the postsynaptic membrane.

Acetylcholine activates nicotinic acetylcholine receptors to produce an excitatory end-plate current

Electrophysiological experiments on muscle fibers have characterized the electrical nature of the postsynaptic response at the muscle end plate. Figure 8-5 illustrates results obtained from a classic experiment performed by Fatt and Katz in 1951. Their work is the first description of how stimulation of the motor nerve affects the membrane potential (V_m) at the postsynaptic region (i.e., muscle cell) of the neuromuscular junction. Nerve stimulation normally drives the V_m of the muscle above threshold and elicits an action potential (see Chapter 7). However, Fatt and Katz were interested not in seeing the action potential but in studying the small, graded electrical responses that are produced as ACh binds to receptors on the muscle cell membrane. Therefore, Fatt and Katz greatly reduced the response of the AChRs by blocking most of them with a carefully selected concentration of *d*-tubocurarine, which we discuss later. They inserted a KCl-filled microelectrode into the end-plate region of a frog sartorius muscle fiber. This arrangement allowed them to measure tiny changes in V_m at one particular spot of the muscle cell.

When Fatt and Katz electrically excited the motor nerve axon, they observed a transient depolarization in the muscle membrane after a delay of a few milliseconds. The delay represents the time required for the release of ACh, its diffusion across the synapse, and activation of postsynaptic AChRs. The positive voltage change follows a biphasic time course: V_m rapidly rises to a peak and then more slowly

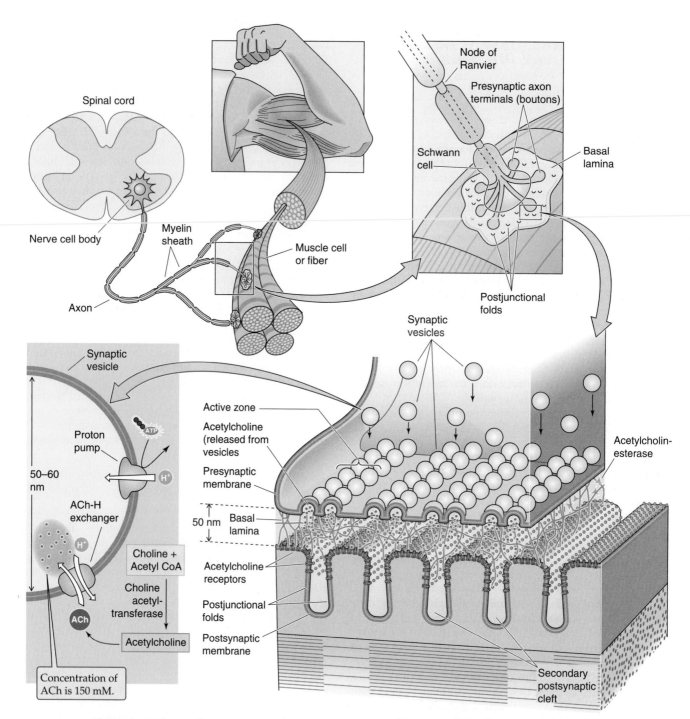

Figure 8-4 The vertebrate neuromuscular junction or motor end plate. A motor neuron, with its cell body in the ventral horn of the spinal cord, sends out an axon that progressively bifurcates to innervate several muscle fibers (a motor unit). The neuron contacts a muscle fiber at exactly one spot called a neuromuscular junction or motor end plate. The end plate consists of an arborization of the nerve into many presynaptic terminals, or boutons, as well as the specializations of the postsynaptic membrane. A high-magnification view of a bouton shows that the synaptic vesicles containing the neurotransmitter ACh cluster and line up at the active zone of the presynaptic membrane. The active zones on the presynaptic membrane are directly opposite the secondary postsynaptic clefts that are created by infoldings of the postsynaptic membrane (postjunctional folds). Depolarization of the bouton causes the vesicles to fuse with the presynaptic membrane and to release their contents into the synaptic cleft. The ACh molecules must diffuse at least 50 nm before reaching nicotinic AChRs. Note the high density of AChRs at the crests of the postjunctional folds. The activity of the released ACh is terminated mainly by an acetylcholinesterase. The bouton reloads its discharged synaptic vesicles by resynthesizing ACh and transporting this ACh into the vesicle through an ACh-H exchanger.

relaxes back to the resting value, consistent with an exponential time course. This signal, known as the **end-plate potential (EPP)**, is an example of an **excitatory postsynaptic potential**. It is produced by the transient opening of AChR channels, which are selectively permeable to monovalent cations such as Na^+ and K^+. The increase in Na^+ conductance drives V_m to a more positive value in the vicinity of the end-plate region. In this experiment, curare blockade allows only a small number of AChR channels to open, so that the EPP does not reach the threshold to produce an action potential. If the experiment is repeated by inserting the microelectrode at various distances from the end plate, the amplitude of the potential change is successively diminished and its peak is increasingly delayed. This decrement with distance occurs because the EPP originates at the end-plate region and spreads away from this site according to the passive cable properties of the muscle fiber. Thus, the EPP in Figure 8-5 is an example of a propagated, graded response. However, without the curare blockade, more AChR channels would open and a larger EPP would ensue, which would drive V_m above threshold and consequently trigger a regenerating action potential (see Chapter 7).

What ions pass through the AChR channels during generation of the EPP? This question can be answered by the same voltage-clamp technique that was used to study the basis of the action potential (see Fig. 7-5B). Figure 8-6A illustrates the experimental preparation for a two-electrode voltage-clamp experiment in which the motor nerve is stimulated while the muscle fiber in the region of its end plate is voltage clamped to a chosen V_m. The recorded current, which is proportional to the conductance change at the muscle end plate, is called the **end-plate current (EPC)**. The EPC has a characteristic time course that rises to a peak within 2 ms after stimulation of the motor nerve and falls exponentially back to zero (Fig. 8-6B). The time course of the EPC corresponds to the opening and closing of a population of AChR channels, governed by the rapid binding and disappearance of ACh as it diffuses to the postsynaptic membrane and is hydrolyzed by AChE.

As shown in Figure 8-6B, when the muscle fiber is clamped to a "holding potential" of −120 mV, we observe a large inward current (i.e., the EPC). This inward current decreases in magnitude as V_m is made more positive, and the current reverses direction to become an outward current at positive values of V_m. A plot of the peak current versus the clamped V_m shows that the reversal potential for the EPC is close to 0 mV (Fig. 8-6C). Because the EPC specifically corresponds to current through AChR channels, this reversal potential reflects the ionic selectivity of these channels when extracellular Na^+ and K^+ concentrations ([Na^+]$_o$ and [K^+]$_o$) are normal.

By varying the concentrations of the extracellular ions while monitoring the shift in the reversal potential of the EPC, researchers found that the AChR channel is permeable to Na^+, K^+, and Ca^{2+} but not to anions such as Cl^-. Because of its low extracellular concentration, the current attributable to Ca^{2+} is small under physiological conditions and its contribution can be ignored. By plugging the values for the various cations into the Goldman-Hodgkin-Katz voltage equation (see Equation 6-9), one can obtain the permeability of the AChR channel to various alkali monovalent ions, rela-

tive to Na^+ permeability. The result is the following sequence of relative permeability: 0.87 (Li^+), 1.00 (Na^+), 1.11 (K^+), and 1.42 (Cs^+). This weak ionic selectivity stands in marked contrast to typical voltage-gated Na^+ channels, which have P_{Na}/P_K ratios of ~20, and voltage-gated K^+ channels, which have P_K/P_{Na} ratios greater than 100. On this basis, the ionotropic

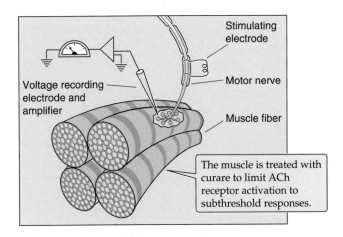

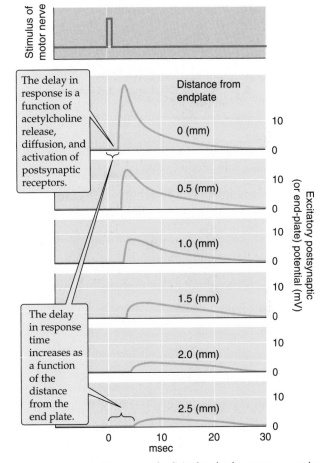

Figure 8-5 End-plate potentials elicited at the frog neuromuscular junction by stimulation of the motor neuron. The magnitude of the excitatory postsynaptic potential is greatest near the end plate and decays farther away. *(Data from Fatt P, Katz B: An analysis of the end-plate potential recorded with an intracellular electrode. J Physiol 1951; 115:320-370.)*

A   EXPERIMENTAL PREPARATION

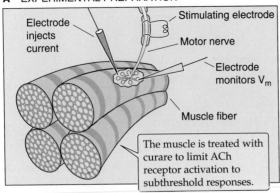

The muscle is treated with curare to limit ACh receptor activation to subthreshold responses.

B   END-PLATE CURRENTS OBTAINED AT VARIOUS HOLDING POTENTIALS

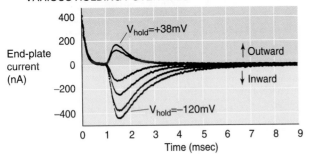

C   I-V RELATIONSHIP FOR PEAK END-PLATE CURRENT

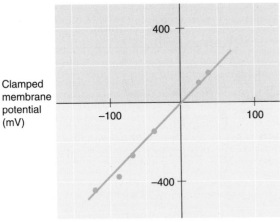

Figure 8-6   End-plate currents obtained at different membrane potentials in a voltage-clamp experiment. **A,** Two-electrode voltage clamp is used to measure the EPC in a frog muscle fiber. The tips of the two microelectrodes are in the muscle fiber. **B,** The six records represent EPCs that were obtained while the motor nerve was stimulated and the postsynaptic membrane was clamped to V_m values of −120, −91, −68, −37, +24, and +38 mV. Notice that the peak current reverses from inward to outward as the holding potential shifts from −37 to +24 mV. **C,** The reversal potential is near 0 mV because the nicotinic AChR has a poor selectivity for Na$^+$ versus K$^+$. *(Data from Magleby KL, Stevens CF: The effect of voltage on the time course of end-plate current. J Physiol 1975; 223:151-171.)*

(nicotinic) AChR channel at the muscle end plate is often classified as **a nonselective cation channel**. Nevertheless, the weak ionic selectivity of the AChR is well suited to its basic function of raising V_m above the threshold of about −50 mV, which is necessary for firing of an action potential. When the nicotinic AChR channel at the muscle end plate opens, the normally high resting permeability of the muscle plasma membrane for K$^+$ relative to Na$^+$ falls so that Na$^+$ and K$^+$ become equally permeant and V_m shifts to a value between E_K (approximately −80 mV) and E_{Na} (approximately +50 mV).

As we shall see in Chapter 13, which focuses on synaptic transmission in the CNS, similar principles hold for generation of postsynaptic currents by other types of agonist-gated channels. For example, the receptor-gated channels for serotonin and glutamate are cation selective and give rise to *depolarizing* **excitatory postsynaptic potentials**. In contrast, the receptor-gated channels for glycine and GABA are anion selective and drive V_m in the hyperpolarizing direction, toward the equilibrium potential for Cl$^−$. These *hyperpolarizing* postsynaptic responses are called **inhibitory postsynaptic potentials**.

The nicotinic acetylcholine receptor is a member of the pentameric Cys-loop receptor family of ligand-gated ion channels

The molecular nature of the nicotinic AChR channel was revealed by studies that included protein purification, amino acid sequencing of isolated subunits, and molecular cloning. Purification of the receptor was aided by the recognition that the electric organs of certain fish are a particularly rich source of the nicotinic AChR. In the electric eel and torpedo ray, the electric organs are embryologically derived from skeletal muscle. The torpedo ray can deliver large electrical discharges by summating the simultaneous depolarizations of a stack of many disk-like cells called electrocytes. These cells have the skeletal muscle isoform of the nicotinic AChR, which is activated by ACh released from presynaptic terminals.

The purified torpedo AChR consists of four subunits (α, β, γ, and δ) in a pentameric stoichiometry of 2α:1β:1γ:1δ (Fig. 8-7). Each subunit has a molecular mass of ~50 kDa and is homologous to the other subunits. The primary sequences of nicotinic AChR subunits are ~90% identical between the torpedo ray and human.

The α, β, γ, and δ subunits each have four distinct hydrophobic regions known as M1 to M4, which correspond to membrane-spanning segments. For each of the subunits, the M2 transmembrane segment lines the aqueous pore through which Na$^+$ and K$^+$ cross the membrane.

The pentameric complex has two agonist binding sites. One ACh binding site is formed at the interface of the extracellular domain of one α subunit and the extracellular domain of the γ subunit. The other site is located between the extracellular domain of the other α subunit and the extracellular domain of the δ subunit.

AChRs of normal adult *muscle fibers* are present in high density in the junctional folds of the postsynaptic membrane. However, in developing muscle fibers of the mammalian embryo and in denervated fibers of adult skeletal

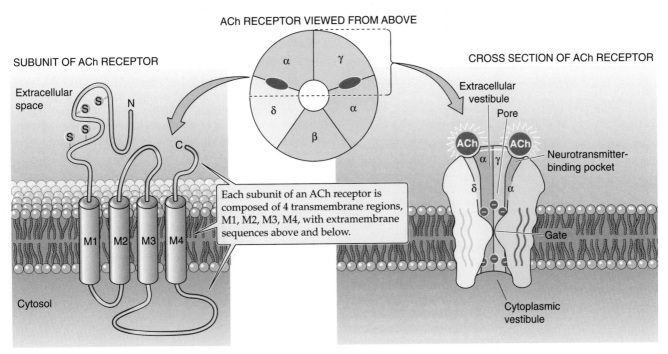

Figure 8-7 Structure of the nicotinic AChR. The nicotinic AChR is a heteropentamer with the subunit composition of $\alpha_2\beta\gamma\delta$. These subunits are homologous to one another, and each has four membrane-spanning segments (M1 to M4).

muscle, AChRs are also widely distributed in the membrane outside the end-plate region. The two types of AChRs, called junctional and nonjunctional receptors, have different functional properties. The unitary conductance of nonjunctional receptors is ~50% larger and the single-channel lifetime is longer in duration than that of junctional receptors. The basis for this phenomenon is a difference in subunit composition. The *nonjunctional* (or fetal) receptors are a pentameric complex with a subunit composition of $\alpha_2\beta\gamma\delta$ in mammals, just as in the electric organ of the torpedo ray. For the *junctional* AChR in adult skeletal muscle, substitution of an ϵ subunit for the fetal γ subunit results in a complex with the composition $\alpha_2\beta\epsilon\delta$.

The functional properties of the two types of receptors have been studied by coexpressing the cloned subunits in *Xenopus* oocytes. Figure 8-8A shows patch-clamp recordings of single ACh-activated channels in oocytes that had been injected with mRNA encoding either α, β, γ, δ or α, β, ϵ, δ. Measurements of currents at different voltages yielded single-channel *I-V* curves (Fig. 8-8B) showing that the channel formed with the ϵ subunit had a unitary conductance of 59 pS, whereas that formed with the γ subunit had a conductance of 40 pS. The mean lifetime of single-channel openings at 0 mV was 1.6 ms for ϵ-type and 4.4 ms for γ-type receptors, closely corresponding to values found in native fetal and adult muscle, respectively. The different functional properties of junctional and nonjunctional nicotinic AChRs presumably reflect their specialized roles in synaptic transmission versus development and synapse formation.

Humans have nine genes that encode homologous α subunits of nicotinic ACh-activated receptors (see Fig. 6-21L).

The α subunit of the skeletal muscle receptor (α_1) is encoded by the *CHRNA1* gene. The eight other α subunits (α_2 to α_9), which are expressed in neuronal tissues, are encoded by genes *CHRNA2* to *CHRNA9*. Only the protein products of genes α_1, α_7, and α_8 bind a venom protein called α-bungarotoxin, a venom protein from a snake called the Taiwanese banded krait. In addition, at least four β subunits exist, encoded by human genes *CHRNB1* to *CHRNB4* (see Fig. 6-21). Besides the β subunit of the skeletal muscle AChR—which is called β_1—there are three neuronal homologues (β_2, β_3, β_4). Heteromeric association of different combinations of these subunits could potentially produce a large number of functional receptor isoforms. Although the exact physiological role of nicotinic AChR channels in various *neuronal* pathways remains to be established, AChRs in the brain play a role in addiction to the nicotine contained in tobacco.

Besides nicotinic AChRs, three other related classes of agonist-activated channels are recognized, including ionotropic receptor channels that are activated by **serotonin** (5-HT_3 receptor), glycine (GlyR), and **GABA** ($GABA_A$ receptor). As mentioned previously, AChR and 5-HT_3 receptor channels are both permeable to cations and thus produce excitatory currents, whereas glycine-activated and $GABA_A$ channels are permeable to anions such as Cl^- and produce inhibitory currents. Figure 8-9 shows examples of macroscopic and unitary Cl^- currents mediated by glycine-activated and $GABA_A$ channels. Cloned genes encoding subunits of these receptor channels encode proteins that are homologous to AChR subunits. Their primary amino acid sequences share a common arrangement of M1, M2, M3, and M4 transmembrane segments, as described earlier for the nicotinic AChR (Fig. 8-7). These proteins all belong to the **pen-**

A SINGLE-CHANNEL CURRENTS

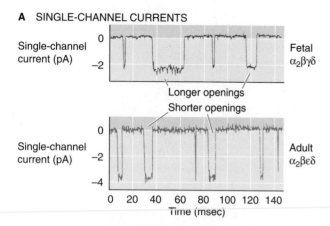

B I-V RELATIONSHIPS

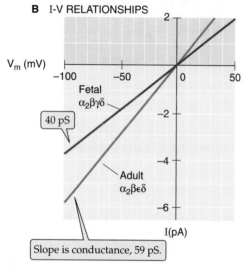

Figure 8-8 Properties of fetal and adult AChRs from skeletal muscle. **A,** The results of patch-clamp experiments, with the patch pipettes in the outside-out configuration and the patch exposed to 0.5 μM ACh, are summarized. In the upper panel, the investigators expressed the fetal acetylcholine receptor channel (AChR), which has the subunit composition $\alpha_2\beta\gamma\delta$, in *Xenopus* oocytes. In the lower panel, the investigators expressed the adult AChR, which has the subunit composition $\alpha_2\beta\epsilon\delta$. Notice that the mean open times are greater for the fetal form, whereas the unitary currents are greater for the adult form. **B,** The two lines summarize data that are similar to those obtained in **A**. The single-channel conductance of the adult form (59 pS) is higher than that of the fetal form (40 pS). *(Data from Mishina M, Takai T, Imoto K, et al: Molecular distinction between fetal and adult forms of muscle acetylcholine receptor. Nature 1986; 321:406-411.)*

tameric **Cys-loop receptor family** of ligand-gated ion channels (see Fig. 6-21), so named because they contain a highly conserved pair of disulfide-bonded cysteine residues. Sequence analysis of these genes indicates that they evolved from a common ancestor. The basis for cation versus anion selectivity appears to reside solely within the M2 segment. Mutation of only three residues within the M2 segment of a cation-selective α subunit of a neuronal nicotinic AChR is sufficient to convert it to an anion-selective channel activated by ACh.

Activation of acetylcholine receptor channels requires binding of two acetylcholine molecules

The EPC is the sum of many single-channel currents, each representing the opening of a single AChR channel at the neuromuscular junction. Earlier we described the random opening and closing of an idealized channel in a two-state model in which the channel could be either closed or open (see Chapter 7):

$$C \rightleftharpoons O \qquad (8\text{-}1)$$

In the case of an *agonist*-activated channel, such as the AChR channel, binding of an agonist to the channel in its closed state favors channel opening. This gating process may be represented by the following kinetic model:

$$C \rightleftharpoons AC \rightleftharpoons AO \qquad (8\text{-}2)$$

Closed channel	Closed channel	Open channel
No agonist	Agonist bound	Agonist bound

In this two-step scheme, the closed state (C) of the channel must bind one molecule of the agonist ACh to form a closed, agonist-bound channel (AC) before it can convert to an open, agonist-bound channel (AO). However, studies of the dependence of the probability of channel opening on agonist concentration indicate that binding of *two* molecules of ACh is required for channel opening. This feature of nicotinic receptor gating is described by the following modification of Equation 8-2:

$$C \rightleftharpoons A_1C \rightleftharpoons A_2C \rightleftharpoons A_2O \qquad (8\text{-}3)$$

1 agonist	2 agonists	Open

Understanding the kinetics of channel opening can be very important for clarifying the mechanism by which certain channel inhibitors work. For example, a competitive inhibitor could prevent binding of the agonist ACh. However, many noncompetitive antagonists of the AChR channel, including some local anesthetics, act by entering the lumen of the channel and blocking the flow of ionic current. Figure 8-10A shows the results of a patch-clamp experiment in which a single AChR channel opened and closed in response to its agonist, ACh. After the addition of QX-222, an analogue of the local anesthetic agent lidocaine (see Chapter 7), to the extracellular side, the channel exhibits a rapidly flickering behavior. This flickering represents a series of brief interruptions of the open state by numerous closures (Fig. 8-10B). This type of flickering block is caused by rapid binding and unbinding of the anesthetic drug to a site in the mouth of the *open* channel. When the drug binds, it blocks the channel to the flow of ions (A_2B). Conversely, when the drug dissociates, the channel becomes unblocked (A_2O):

$$C \rightleftharpoons A_1C \rightleftharpoons A_2C \rightleftharpoons A_2O \rightleftharpoons A_2B \qquad (8\text{-}4)$$

Blocked

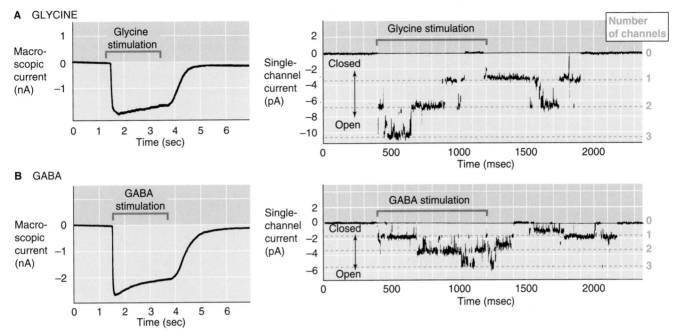

Figure 8-9   Currents activated by glycine and GABA. **A,** These experiments were performed on cultured mouse spinal cord neurons by patch-clamp techniques. The left panel shows the macroscopic Cl⁻ current, which is measured in the whole-cell configuration and carried by glycine receptor (GlyR) channels when exposed to glycine. The right panel shows single-channel currents that are recorded in the outside-out patch configuration. In both scenarios, the holding potential was −70 mV. **B,** The left panel shows the macroscopic Cl⁻ current that is carried by GABA$_A$ receptor channels when exposed to GABA. The right panel shows single-channel currents. *(Data from Bormann J, Hamill OP, Sakmann B: Mechanism of anion permeation through channels gated by glycine and γ-aminobutyric acid in mouse spinal neurones. J Physiol 1987; 385:243-286.)*

Channel blockers are often used as molecular tools to study the mechanism of ion permeation. For example, in combination with site-directed mutagenesis, QX-222 was helpful in locating amino acid residues on the M2 transmembrane segment that form part of the blocker binding site, thus identifying residues that line the aqueous pore.

Miniature end-plate potentials reveal the quantal nature of transmitter release from the presynaptic terminals

Under physiological conditions, an action potential in a *presynaptic* motor nerve axon produces a depolarizing *postsynaptic* EPP that peaks at ~40 mV more positive than the resting V_m. This large signal results from the release of ACh from only about 200 synaptic vesicles, each containing 6000 to 10,000 molecules of ACh. The neuromuscular junction is clearly designed for excess capacity inasmuch as a single end plate is composed of numerous synaptic contacts (~1000 at the frog muscle end plate), each with an active zone that is lined with dozens of mature synaptic vesicles. Thus, a large inventory of ready vesicles (>10⁴), together with the ability to synthesize ACh and to package it into new vesicles, allows the neuromuscular junction to maintain a high rate of successful transmission without significant loss of function as a result of presynaptic depletion of vesicles or ACh.

The original notion of a vesicular mode of transmitter delivery is based on classic observations of EPPs under con-

ditions of reduced ACh release. In 1950, Fatt and Katz observed an interesting kind of electrophysiological "noise" in their continuous, high-resolution recordings of V_m with a microelectrode inserted at the end-plate region of a frog muscle fiber. Their recordings from resting muscle fibers that were not subjected to nerve stimulation revealed the occurrence of tiny depolarizations of ~0.4 mV that appeared at random intervals. These small depolarizations were blocked by curare, an antagonist of AChR channels, and they increased in size and duration with the application of neostigmine, an inhibitor of AChE. Because the spontaneous V_m fluctuations also exhibited a time course similar to that of the normal EPP, they were named **miniature end-plate potentials** (also known as MEPPs or minis). These observations suggested that even in the absence of nerve stimulation, there is a certain low probability of transmitter release at the presynaptic terminal, resulting in the opening of a small number of AChRs in the postsynaptic membrane. An examination of the size of individual MEPPs suggested that they occur in discrete multiples of a unitary amplitude. This finding led to the notion that ACh release is *quantized,* with the quantum event corresponding to ACh release from one synaptic vesicle.

Another way of studying the quantal release of ACh is to stimulate the presynaptic motor neuron and to monitor V_m at the end plate under conditions when the probability of ACh release is greatly decreased. How can we decrease the probability of ACh release? The amplitude of the EPP that is

A CONTROL

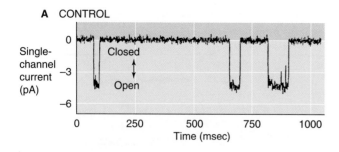

B LIDOCAINE ANALOGUE

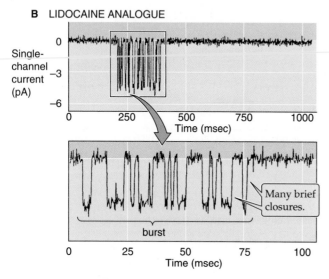

Figure 8-10   The effect of a local anesthetic on the AChR. **A,** Single-channel recording of nicotinic AChR expressed in a *Xenopus* oocyte. The patch was in the outside-out configuration, and the holding potential was −150 mV. The continuous presence of 1 μM ACh caused brief channel openings. **B,** This experiment is similar to that in **A** except that in addition to the ACh, the lidocaine analogue QX-222 (20 μM) was present at the extracellular surface of the receptor channel. Note that the channel opening is accompanied by rapid flickering caused by many brief channel closures. The time scale of the lower panel is expanded 10-fold. *(Data from Leonard RJ, Labarca CG, Charnet P, et al: Evidence that the M2 membrane-spanning region lines the ion channel pore of the nicotinic receptor. Science 1988; 242:1578-1581.)*

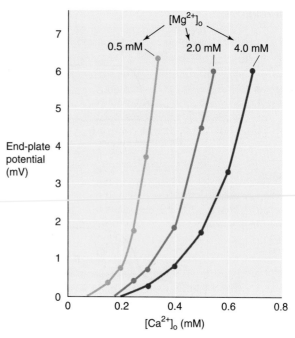

Figure 8-11   The effect of extracellular Ca^{2+} and Mg^{2+} on EPPs. The data obtained by stimulating the motor neuron and monitoring the evoked subthreshold EPP show that the EPP is stimulated by increasing levels of Ca^{2+} but inhibited by increasing levels of Mg^{2+}. *(Data from Dodge FA Jr, Rahaminoff R: Cooperative action of calcium ions in transmitter release at the neuromuscular junction. J Physiol 1967; 193:419-432.)*

evoked in response to nerve stimulation is decreased by lowering $[Ca^{2+}]_o$ and increasing $[Mg^{2+}]_o$. A low $[Ca^{2+}]_o$ decreases Ca^{2+} entry into the presynaptic terminal (Fig. 8-2, step 3). A high $[Mg^{2+}]_o$ partially blocks the presynaptic Ca^{2+} channels and thus also decreases Ca^{2+} entry. Therefore, the consequence of either decreased $[Ca^{2+}]_o$ or increased $[Mg^{2+}]_o$ is a fall in $[Ca^{2+}]_i$ in the presynaptic terminal, which reduces transmitter release and thus the amplitude of the EPP (Fig. 8-11). Del Castillo and Katz exploited this suppression of transmitter release under conditions of low $[Ca^{2+}]_o$ and high $[Mg^{2+}]_o$ to observe the V_m changes caused by the quantal release of transmitter. Figure 8-12A shows seven superimposed records of MEPPs that were recorded from a frog muscle fiber during seven repetitive trials of nerve stimulation under conditions of reduced $[Ca^{2+}]_o$ and elevated $[Mg^{2+}]_o$. The records are aligned at the position of the nerve stimulus artifact. The amplitudes of the peak responses occur in discrete multiples of ~0.4 mV. Among the seven

records were one "nonresponse," two responses of ~0.4 mV, three responses of ~0.8 mV, and one response of ~1.2 mV. One of the recordings also revealed a spontaneous MEPP with a quantal amplitude of ~0.4 mV that appeared later in the trace. Del Castillo and Katz proposed that the macroscopic EPP is the sum of many unitary events, each having a magnitude of ~0.4 mV. Microscopic observation of numerous vesicles in the synaptic terminal naturally led to the supposition that a single vesicle releases a relatively fixed amount of ACh and thereby produces a unitary MEPP. According to this view, the quantized MEPPs thus correspond to the fusion of discrete numbers of synaptic vesicles: 0, 1, 2, 3, and so on.

For elucidating the mechanism of synaptic transmission at the neuromuscular junction, Bernard Katz shared the 1970 Nobel Prize in Physiology or Medicine.

Direct sensing of extracellular transmitter also shows quantal release of transmitter

Instead of using the postsynaptic AChR as a biological detector of quantum release, one can use a microscopic electrochemical sensor to measure neurotransmitter levels directly. Figure 8-13 shows results from an experiment in which a fine carbon fiber electrode was placed very close to the presynaptic terminal membrane of a leech neuron that uses serotonin as its only neurotransmitter. The carbon fiber is an electrochemical detector of serotonin (Fig. 8-13A); the current measured by this electrode corresponds to four electrons per serotonin molecule oxidized at the tip. Stimulation

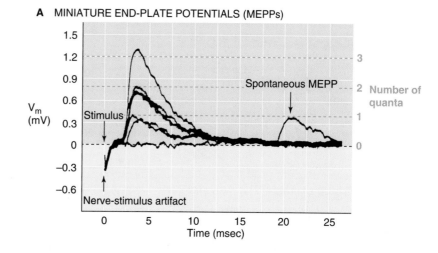

A MINIATURE END-PLATE POTENTIALS (MEPPs)

Figure 8-12 Evoked and spontaneous MEPPs. **A,** The investigators recorded V_m in frog skeletal muscle fibers that were exposed to extracellular solutions having a $[Ca^{2+}]$ of 0.5 mM and a $[Mg^{2+}]$ of 5 mM. These values minimize transmitter release, and therefore it was possible to resolve the smallest possible MEPP, which corresponds to the release of a single synaptic vesicle (i.e., 1 quantum). The investigators stimulated the motor neuron seven consecutive times and recorded the evoked MEPPs. In one trial, the stimulus evoked no response (0 quanta). In two trials, the peak MEPP was about 0.4 mV (1 quantum). In three others, the peak response was about 0.8 mV (2 quanta). Finally, in one, the peak was about 1.2 mV (3 quanta). In one case, a MEPP of the smallest magnitude appeared spontaneously. **B,** The histogram summarizes data from 198 trials on a cat neuromuscular junction in the presence of 12.5 mM extracellular Mg^{2+}. The data are in bins with a width of 0.1 mV. The distribution has eight peaks. The first represents stimuli that evoked no responses. The other seven represent stimuli that evoked MEPPs that were roughly integral multiples of the smallest MEPP. The curve overlying each cluster of bins is a gaussian or "normal" function and facilitates calculation of the average MEPP for each cluster of bins. The peak values of these gaussians follow a Poisson distribution. *(Data from Magleby KL: Neuromuscular transmission. In Engel AG, Franzini-Armstrong C [eds]: Myology, Basic and Clinical, 2nd ed, pp 442-463. New York, McGraw-Hill, 1994.)*

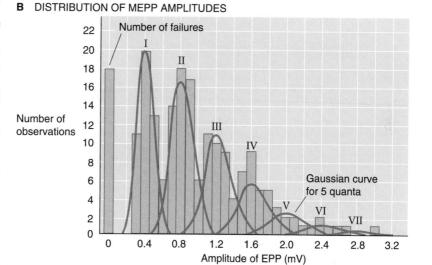

B DISTRIBUTION OF MEPP AMPLITUDES

of the leech neuron to produce an action potential also elicits an oxidation current, as measured by the carbon fiber, that corresponds to the release of serotonin. At a $[Ca^{2+}]_o$ of 5 mM, the current is large and composed of many small spikes (Fig. 8-13B, top). On the other hand, reducing $[Ca^{2+}]_o$ to 1 mM—presumably reducing Ca^{2+} influx into the nerve terminal and thus reducing the number of quanta released—reveals individual spikes of serotonin release. The release spikes come in two sizes, small and large (Fig. 8-13B, bottom), corresponding to two separate classes of synaptic vesicles that are evident on electron micrographs. Injection of the cell with tetanus toxin, which blocks the release of synaptic vesicles, abolishes the serotonin release spikes. Thus, the spikes represent genuine events of synaptic exocytosis.

The nearly immediate appearance of the small release spikes after electrical stimulation of the cell shows that this type of vesicular release is extremely rapid. From the height and duration of the small and large spikes in Figure 8-13B, one can estimate the amount of electrical charge and thus the number of serotonin molecules oxidized at the carbon

fiber per spike. A unitary *small* event corresponds to the release of ~4700 serotonin molecules, whereas a unitary *large* event corresponds to the release of 15,000 to 300,000 serotonin molecules. Thus, the amount of serotonin released by the small synaptic vesicles of the leech neuron is about half the number of ACh molecules contained in a synaptic vesicle at the frog neuromuscular junction. These and other observations of the synaptic function of nerve-muscle and nerve-nerve synapses have led to the conclusion that *chemical neurotransmission operates by a fundamentally similar mechanism* at many types of synapses in different animal species (see Chapter 13).

Short-term or long-term changes in the relative efficiency of neurotransmitter release can increase or decrease the *strength* of a particular synapse and thereby give rise to an alteration in behavior. Three types of synaptic modulation occur at the neuromuscular junction, and they differ in how they affect the quantal release of neurotransmitter.

Facilitation is a *short-lived* enhancement of the EPP in response to a *brief* increase in the frequency of nerve stimula-

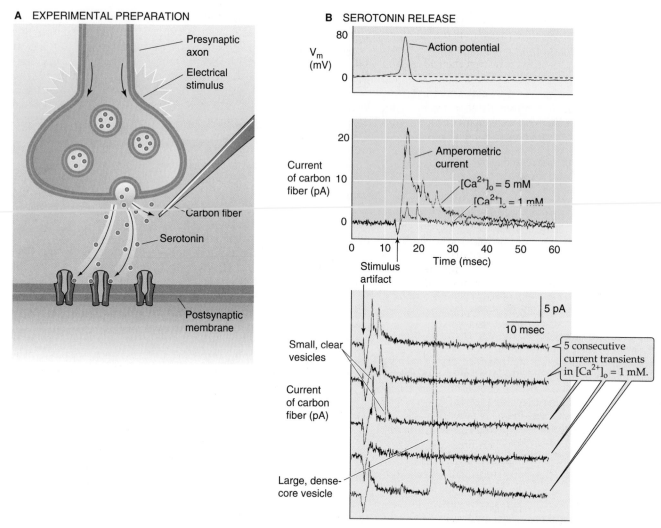

Figure 8-13 Detection of serotonin that is released from synaptic vesicles. **A,** The serotonin that is released from a synaptic terminal of a leech neuron can be detected electrochemically by use of a carbon fiber microelectrode. The current carried by the carbon fiber increases with the amount of serotonin that is released, reflecting the oxidation of serotonin molecules on the surface of the carbon fiber. **B,** The *top panel* shows the action potential recorded from the stimulated motor neuron. The *middle panel* shows the evoked serotonin release (measured as a current) at both a $[Ca^{2+}]_o$ of 5 mM (high level of serotonin release) and a $[Ca^{2+}]_o$ of 1 mM (lower level or release). The *bottom panel* shows five consecutive trials at a $[Ca^{2+}]_o$ of 1 mM and illustrates that the release of serotonin can occur in either small quanta or very large quanta. These two sizes of quanta correspond to small clear vesicles and large dense-core vesicles, both of which can be observed by electron microscopy. *(Data from Bruns D, Jahn R: Real-time measurement of transmitter release from single synaptic vesicles. Nature 1995; 377:62-65.)*

tion. One way that facilitation may occur is by a transient increase in the mean number of quanta per nerve stimulus.

Potentiation (or post-tetanic potentiation) is a *long-lived* and pronounced increase in transmitter release that occurs after a *long* period of high-frequency nerve stimulation. This effect can last for minutes after the conditioning stimulus. Potentiation may be caused by a period of intense nerve firing, which increases $[Ca^{2+}]_i$ in the presynaptic terminal and thus increases the probability of exocytosis.

Synaptic **depression** is a *transient* decrease in the efficiency of transmitter release and, consequently, a reduction in the EPP in response to a period of frequent nerve stimulation. Depression may result from temporary depletion of transmitter-loaded vesicles from the presynaptic terminal,

that is, a reduction in the number of available quanta. Thus, these three temporal changes in synaptic strength and efficiency appear to reflect changes at different steps of synaptic transmission. Similar modulation of synaptic strength in the CNS provides a mechanistic paradigm to understand how individual nerve terminals may "learn" (see Chapter 13).

Synaptic vesicles package, store, and deliver neurotransmitters

The physiology of synaptic vesicles in the nervous system is a variation on the universal theme used by endocrine-like cells in animals from the most primitive invertebrates up to mammals (see Chapter 3). Many of the proteins involved in synaptic vesicle movement and turnover are related to those involved in the intracellular membrane trafficking processes that take place in almost all eukaryotic cells. This trafficking involves vesicular translocation from the endoplasmic reticulum to the Golgi network and fusion with the plasma membrane. Genetic analysis of the yeast secretory pathway has identified various gene products that are homologous to those associated with synaptic vesicles of higher vertebrates. Thus, the processes underlying synaptic function are inherently quite similar to cellular exocytosis and endocytosis.

As shown in Figure 8-14, **nascent synaptic vesicles** are produced in the neuronal cell body by a process similar to the **secretory pathway**. Thus, the membrane proteins of synaptic vesicles are synthesized in the rough endoplasmic reticulum and are then directed to the Golgi network, where processing, maturation, and sorting occur. Nascent synaptic vesicles—which are, in fact, secretory vesicles—are then transported to the nerve terminal by **fast axonal transport** mediated by the microtubule system, which also carries mitochondria to the terminal (see Chapter 2).

Vesicles destined to contain *peptide* neurotransmitters travel down the axon with the presynthesized peptides or peptide precursors already inside. On arrival at the nerve terminal (Fig. 8-14), the vesicles—now called **dense-core secretory granules** (100 to 200 nm in diameter)—become randomly distributed in the cytoplasm of the terminal as discussed in more detail in Chapter 13.

Vesicles destined to contain *non-peptide* neurotransmitters (e.g., ACh) travel down the axon with no transmitter inside. On arrival at the nerve terminal (Fig. 8-14), the vesicles take up the non-peptide neurotransmitter that is synthesized locally in the nerve terminal. These non-peptide synaptic vesicles, which are *clear* and 40 to 50 nm in diameter, then attach to the actin-based cytoskeletal network. At this point, the mature clear synaptic vesicles are functionally ready for Ca²⁺-dependent transmitter release and become docked at specific release sites in the **active zones** of the presynaptic membrane. After exocytotic fusion of the clear synaptic vesicles, endocytosis through clathrin-coated vesicles (see Chapter 2) recovers membrane components and recycles them to an endosome compartment in the terminal. Synaptic vesicles may then be re-formed within the terminal for reuse in neurotransmission, or they may be transported back to the cell body for turnover and degradation.

The purification of synaptic vesicles has made it possible to analyze their composition, which has facilitated the molecular characterization of many proteins that are intrinsic to synaptic vesicle function. Figure 8-15 summarizes a number of the major classes of synaptic vesicle proteins.

The uptake of non-peptide neurotransmitters is accomplished by the combination of a vacuolar-type H⁺-ATPase and a neurotransmitter transport protein. The **vacuolar-type H⁺ pump** is a large, multisubunit complex that catalyzes the inward movement of H⁺ into the vesicle, coupled to the hydrolysis of cytosolic ATP to ADP and inorganic phosphate (see Chapter 5). The resulting pH and voltage gradients across the vesicle membrane energize the uptake of neurotransmitters into the vesicle by a unique family of **neurotransmitter transport proteins** that exchange neurotransmitters in the cytosol for H⁺ in the vesicle. This family of transporters includes members specific for ACh, monoamines (e.g., serotonin), catecholamines (e.g., norepinephrine), glutamate, and GABA/glycine.

Another cloned synaptic vesicle protein named **SV2** (for synaptic vesicle protein 2) structurally resembles a transport protein. However, a transport substrate for SV2 has not been identified, and its function is unknown.

Synaptobrevin is a 19-kDa synaptic vesicle protein containing one transmembrane segment. Synaptobrevin, which is a v-SNARE (see Chapter 2), is essential for transmitter

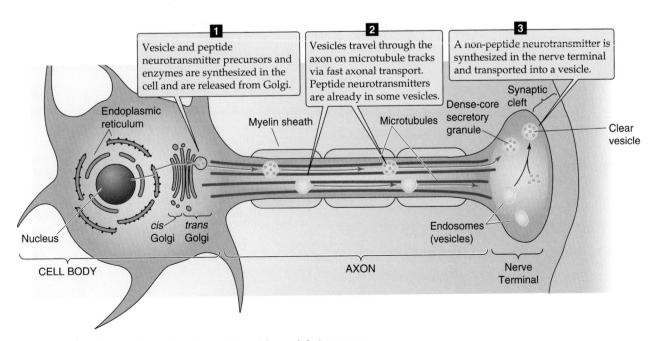

Figure 8-14 Synthesis and recycling of synaptic vesicles and their content.

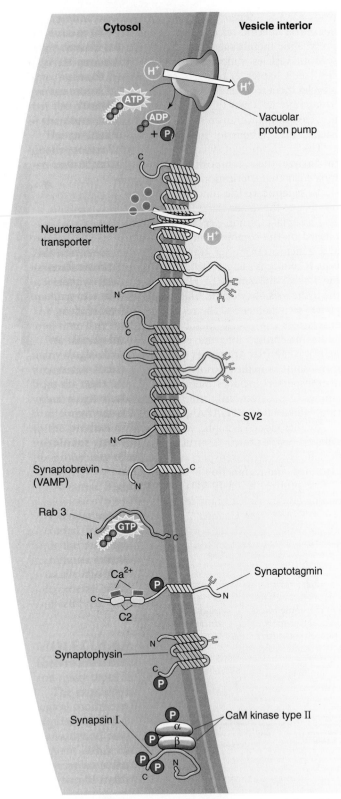

Figure 8-15 Membrane-associated proteins of synaptic vesicles.

release. As discussed in the next section, synaptobrevin on the *vesicle* membrane forms a complex with two proteins on the *presynaptic* membrane and helps drive vesicle fusion. Tetanus toxin or botulinum toxins B, D, F, and G are endoproteinases that digest synaptobrevin and are potent inhibitors of synaptic vesicle exocytosis.

Rab3 is a member of a large family of low-molecular-weight GTP-binding proteins that appears to be universally involved in cellular membrane trafficking (see Chapter 2) through the binding and hydrolysis of GTP. **Synaptotagmin** is the synaptic vesicle Ca^{2+} receptor, a protein with two external repetitive domains that are homologous to the C2 domain of protein kinase C. The C2 domains appear to mediate binding of Ca^{2+}, a process that also depends on the presence of acidic phospholipids. Synaptotagmin senses a local rise in $[Ca^{2+}]_i$ and triggers the exocytosis of docked vesicles.

Another major constituent, **synaptophysin**, is an integral membrane protein with four transmembrane segments that exhibits channel-forming activity in planar bilayers. It may be involved in the formation of a fusion pore during exocytosis. The **synapsins** are a group of synaptic vesicle proteins that are phosphorylated by both cAMP-dependent and calmodulin-dependent protein kinases. Interactions of synapsins with cytoskeletal proteins and their inhibition by phosphorylation have led to the notion that synapsins normally mediate the attachment of synaptic vesicles to the actin cytoskeleton. With an increase in $[Ca^{2+}]_i$ and subsequent phosphorylation, the synapsin detaches and permits vesicles to move to active sites at the synaptic membrane.

Neurotransmitter release occurs by exocytosis of synaptic vesicles

Although the mechanism by which synaptic vesicles fuse with the plasma membrane and release their contents is far from fully understood, we have working models (Fig. 8-16) for the function of various key components and steps involved in synaptic vesicle release. These models are based on a variety of in vitro experiments. The use of specific toxins that act at nerve synapses and elegant functional studies of genetic mutants in *Drosophila, C. elegans,* and gene knockout mice have provided important information on the role of various components.

We have already introduced the key proteins located in the synaptic vesicle. Of these, we now focus on the v-SNARE synaptobrevin and the Ca^{2+} sensor synaptotagmin. In addition, several other proteins—located in the target area of the presynaptic membrane of the nerve terminal—play an important role in the fusion process. **Syntaxin** is anchored in the presynaptic membrane by a single membrane-spanning segment. **SNAP-25** is tethered to the presynaptic membrane by palmitoyl side chains. Both syntaxin and SNAP-25 are t-SNARES (see Chapter 2). *Botulinum toxins A and E,* which are endoproteinases, specifically cleave SNAP-25; another endoproteinase, *botulinum toxin C1,* specifically cleaves syntaxin. These toxins block the fusion of synaptic vesicles.

According to the model shown in Figure 8-16, docking of the vesicle to the presynaptic membrane occurs as n-Sec-1 dissociates from syntaxin. The free ends of synaptobrevin, syntaxin, and SNAP-25 begin to coil around each other. The

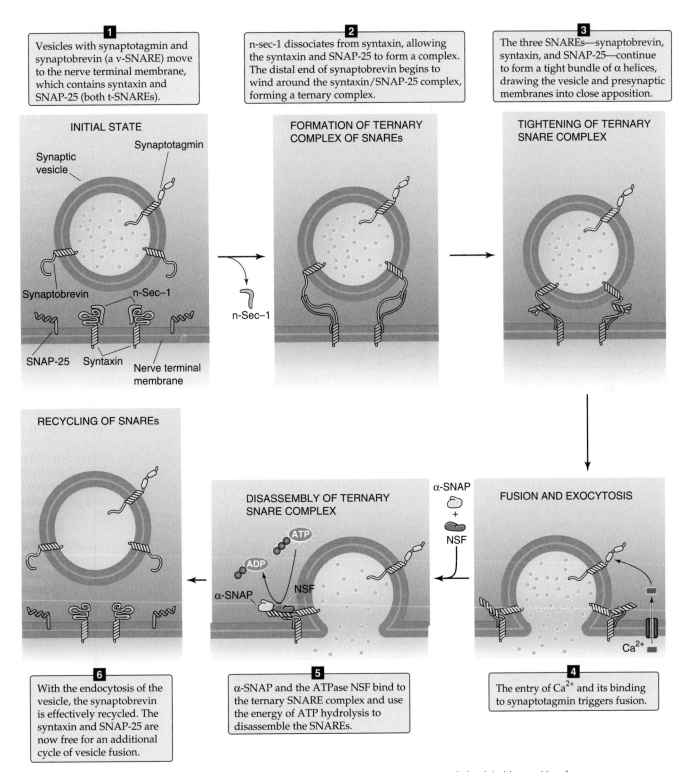

1 Vesicles with synaptotagmin and synaptobrevin (a v-SNARE) move to the nerve terminal membrane, which contains syntaxin and SNAP-25 (both t-SNAREs).

2 n-sec-1 dissociates from syntaxin, allowing the syntaxin and SNAP-25 to form a complex. The distal end of synaptobrevin begins to wind around the syntaxin/SNAP-25 complex, forming a ternary complex.

3 The three SNAREs—synaptobrevin, syntaxin, and SNAP-25—continue to form a tight bundle of α helices, drawing the vesicle and presynaptic membranes into close apposition.

INITIAL STATE

Synaptotagmin

Synaptic vesicle

Synaptobrevin

n-Sec–1

SNAP-25   Syntaxin

Nerve terminal membrane

FORMATION OF TERNARY COMPLEX OF SNAREs

n-Sec–1

TIGHTENING OF TERNARY SNARE COMPLEX

RECYCLING OF SNAREs

DISASSEMBLY OF TERNARY SNARE COMPLEX

ATP

ADP

α-SNAP   NSF

α-SNAP

+

NSF

FUSION AND EXOCYTOSIS

Ca²⁺

6 With the endocytosis of the vesicle, the synaptobrevin is effectively recycled. The syntaxin and SNAP-25 are now free for an additional cycle of vesicle fusion.

5 α-SNAP and the ATPase NSF bind to the ternary SNARE complex and use the energy of ATP hydrolysis to disassemble the SNAREs.

4 The entry of Ca²⁺ and its binding to synaptotagmin triggers fusion.

Figure 8-16 Model of synaptic vesicle fusion and exocytosis. NSF, *N*-ethylmaleimide-sensitive factor; SNAP-25, synaptosome-associated protein 25 kDa; α-SNAP, soluble NSF attachment protein; SNARE, SNAP receptor.

result is a ternary complex, an extraordinarily stable rod-shaped structure of α helices. As the energetically favorable coiling of the three SNAREs continues, the vesicle membrane is pulled ever closer to the presynaptic membrane. Ca^{2+} enters through voltage-gated Ca^{2+} channels located in register with the active zone of the presynaptic membrane. A local

increase in $[Ca^{2+}]_i$ triggers the final event, fusion and exocytosis. The synaptic vesicle protein synaptotagmin is believed to be the actual sensor of increased $[Ca^{2+}]_i$ because knockout mice and *Drosophila* mutants lacking the appropriate isoform of this protein have impaired Ca^{2+}-dependent transmitter release. The soluble α-SNAP binds to the ternary complex formed by the intertwined SNAREs and promotes the binding of NSF (an ATPase), which uses the energy of ATP hydrolysis to disassemble the three tightly wound SNAREs. The now-free synaptobrevin presumably undergoes endocytosis, whereas the syntaxin and SNAP-25 on the presynaptic membrane are available for the next round of vesicle fusion.

The model just presented leaves unanswered some important questions. For example, what is the structure of the fusion pore detected by electrophysiological measurements as a primary event in membrane fusion? Also, the model does not fully explain the basis for the rapid catalysis of fusion by Ca^{2+}. Neuroscientists are very interested in the details of synaptic vesicle fusion because this exocytotic process might be a target for controlling synaptic strength and may thus play a role in the synaptic plasticity that is responsible for changes in animal behavior.

Re-uptake or cleavage of the neurotransmitter terminates its action

Effective transmission across chemical synapses requires not only release of the neurotransmitter and activation of the receptor on the postsynaptic membrane but also rapid and efficient mechanisms for removal of the transmitter. At synapses where ACh is released, this removal is accomplished by enzymatic destruction of the neurotransmitter. However, the more general mechanism in the nervous system involves re-uptake of the neurotransmitter mediated by specific, high-affinity transport systems located in the presynaptic plasma membrane and surrounding glial cells. These secondary active transport systems use the normal ionic gradients of Na^+, K^+, H^+, or Cl^- to achieve concentrative uptake of transmitter. Vertebrates have two distinct families of neurotransmitter transport proteins. The first family is characterized by a common motif of 12 membrane-spanning segments and includes transporters with specificity for catecholamines, serotonin, GABA, glycine, and choline. Energy coupling of transport in this class of systems is generally based on cotransport of the substrate with Na^+ and Cl^-. The second family is represented by transporters for the excitatory amino acids glutamate and aspartate; in these systems, substrate transport generally couples to cotransport of Na^+ and H^+ and to exchange of K^+.

At the neuromuscular junction and other cholinergic synapses, immediate termination of the action of ACh is accomplished enzymatically by the action of AChE. Although AChE is primarily found at the neuromuscular junction, AChE activity can be detected throughout the nervous system. The enzyme occurs in a variety of physical forms. The **globular** or **G forms** exist as monomers, dimers, or tetramers of a common, ~72-kDa glycoprotein catalytic subunit. These molecules can be found either in soluble form or bound to cell membranes through a GPI linkage (see Chapter 2) in which a post-translational modification attaches the C terminus of the protein to a glycolipid moiety. The **asymmetric** or **A forms** consist of one to three tetramers of the globular enzyme coupled through disulfide bond linkage to a collagen-like structural protein. The largest asymmetric form, which has 12 catalytic subunits attached to the collagen-like tail, is the major species located at the neuromuscular junc-

tion. The triple-helical, collagen-like tail attaches the asymmetric AChE complex to extracellular matrix components of the synaptic basal lamina. The various physical forms of AChE are a result of the alternative splicing that occurs in the transcription of a single AChE gene.

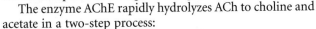

The enzyme AChE rapidly hydrolyzes ACh to choline and acetate in a two-step process:

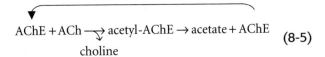

$$AChE + ACh \longrightarrow acetyl\text{-}AChE \rightarrow acetate + AChE \qquad (8\text{-}5)$$
$$\qquad\qquad choline$$

In the first step of the reaction, the enzyme cleaves choline from ACh, which results in the formation of an intermediate in which the acetate group is covalently coupled to a serine group on the enzyme. The second step is the hydrolysis and release of this acetate as well as the free enzyme. The nerve terminal recovers the extracellular choline through a high-affinity, Na^+-coupled uptake system and uses it for the synthesis of ACh.

TOXINS AND DRUGS AFFECTING SYNAPTIC TRANSMISSION

Much of our knowledge of the synaptic physiology of the neuromuscular junction and the identities of its various molecular components have been derived from experiments using specific pharmacological agents and toxins that permit functional dissection of the system. Figure 8-17 illustrates the relative synaptic location and corresponding pharmacology of AChE as well as several ion channels and proteins involved in exocytosis.

Guanidinium neurotoxins such as tetrodotoxin prevent depolarization of the nerve terminal, whereas dendrotoxins inhibit repolarization

The action potential is the first step in transmission: a nerve action potential arriving at the terminal initiates the entire process. As discussed in Chapter 7, the depolarizing phase of the action potential is mediated by voltage-dependent Na^+ channels that are specifically blocked by nanomolar concentrations of the small guanidinium neurotoxins **tetrodotoxin** and **saxitoxin** (see Fig. 7-5C).

The mamba snake toxin **dendrotoxin** (see Chapter 7) has an effect that is precisely opposite that of tetrodotoxin: it facilitates the release of ACh that is evoked by nerve stimulation. Dendrotoxins are a family of ~59-residue proteins with three disulfide bonds that block certain isoforms of voltage-gated K^+ channels by binding to an extracellular site in the P-region domain with high affinity. These toxins reveal the important role of K^+ channels in terminating the process of transmitter release. Blockade of presynaptic K^+ channels by dendrotoxin inhibits repolarization of the presynaptic membrane, thereby prolonging the duration of the action potential and facilitating the release of transmitter in response to the entry of extra Ca^{2+} into the nerve terminal.

Diseases of the Human Acetylcholine Receptor: Myasthenia Gravis and a Congenital Myasthenic Syndrome

The term *myasthenia* means muscle weakness (from the Greek *mys* and *asthenia*) and is usually used clinically to denote weakness in the absence of primary muscle disease, neuropathy, or CNS disorder. **Myasthenia gravis**, one specific type of myasthenia and the most common adult form, afflicts 25 to 125 of every 1 million people. It can occur at any age but has a bimodal distribution, with peak incidences occurring among people in their 20s and 60s. Those afflicted at an early age tend to be women with hyperplasia of the thymus; those who are older are more likely to be men with coexisting cancer of the thymus gland. The cells of the thymus possess nicotinic AChRs, and the disease arises as a result of antibodies directed against these receptors. The antibodies then lead to skeletal muscle weakness caused in part by competitive antagonism of AChRs. Symptoms include fatigue and weakness of skeletal muscle. Two major forms of the disease are recognized: one that involves weakness of only the extraocular muscles and another that results in generalized weakness of all skeletal muscles. In either case, myasthenia gravis is typified by fluctuating symptoms, with weakness greatest toward the end of the day or after exertion. In severe cases, paralysis of the respiratory muscles can lead to death. Treatment directed at enhancing cholinergic transmission, alone or combined with thymectomy or immunosuppression, is highly effective in most patients.

Progress toward achieving an understanding of the cause of myasthenia gravis was first made when electrophysiological analysis of involved muscle revealed that the amplitude of the miniature EPP was decreased, although the frequency of quantal events was normal. This finding suggested either a defect in the postsynaptic response to ACh or a reduced concentration of ACh in the synaptic vesicles. A major breakthrough occurred in 1973, when Patrick and Lindstrom found that symptoms similar to those of humans with myasthenia developed in rabbits immunized with AChR protein purified from the electric eel. This finding was shortly followed by the demonstration of anti-AChR antibodies in human patients with myasthenia gravis and a severe reduction in the surface density of AChR in the junctional folds. These anti-AChR antibodies are directed against one or more subunits of the receptor, where they bind and activate complement and accelerate destruction of the receptors. The most common target of these antibodies is a region of the AChR α subunit called MIR (main immunogenic region).

Myasthenia gravis is now recognized to be an acquired autoimmune disorder in which the spontaneous production of anti-AChR antibodies results in progressive loss of muscle AChRs and degeneration of postjunctional folds. Treatment is aimed at either reducing the potency of the immunological attack or enhancing cholinergic activity within the synapse. Reduction of the potency of the immunological attack is achieved by the use of immunosuppressants (most commonly corticosteroids) or plasmapheresis (removal of antibodies from the patient's serum). Some patients with myasthenia gravis have a thymoma (a tumor of the thymus gland) that is often readily seen on routine chest radiographs. In these patients, removal of the thymoma leads to clinical improvement in nearly 75% of the cases. Enhancement of cholinergic activity is achieved through the use of AChE inhibitors; pyridostigmine is the most widely used agent. The dosage of these drugs must be carefully monitored to prevent *over*exposure of the remaining AChRs to ACh. Overexposure can lead to overstimulation of the postsynaptic receptors, prolonged depolarization of the postsynaptic membrane, inactivation of neighboring Na^+ channels, and thus synaptic blockade.

Another condition characterized by progressive muscle weakness and fatigue is the **Lambert-Eaton syndrome** (see the box titled Ca^{2+} Channel and Autoimmune Genetic Defects in Chapter 7). Lambert-Eaton syndrome is caused by antibodies that attack the presynaptic Ca^{2+} channel and can be distinguished from myasthenia gravis in several ways. First, it primarily attacks the limb muscles, not the ocular and bulbar muscles. Second, repetitive stimulation of a particular muscle leads to enhanced amplitude of the postsynaptic action potential, whereas in patients with myasthenia, repetitive stimulation leads to progressive lessening of the action potential. Thus, repeated muscle stimulation leads to increasing contractile strength in patients with Lambert-Eaton syndrome and to decreasing strength in patients with myasthenia.

The term **congenital myasthenic syndrome** refers to a variety of inherited disorders, present at birth, that affect neuromuscular transmission in a variety of ways. Because specific cases can involve AChE deficiency, abnormal presynaptic release of ACh, or defective AChR function (without the presence of antireceptor antibodies), the signs and symptoms can also vary widely. In 1995, an unusual example of a congenital myasthenic syndrome disorder was traced to a mutation in the ε subunit of the human AChR. Single-channel recordings from biopsy samples of muscle fibers of a young myasthenic patient revealed a profound alteration in AChR kinetics. The burst duration of AChR openings was greatly prolonged in comparison with that of normal human AChR channels. The molecular defect is a point mutation of Thr to Pro at position 264 in the adult ε subunit of the AChR. This amino acid residue corresponds to an evolutionarily conserved position in the M2 membrane-spanning segment, which is involved in formation of the channel pore. Thus, a human mutation in the pore region of the AChR protein results in failure of the channel to close normally, thereby causing excessive depolarization and pathological consequences at the muscle end plate.

This mutation is only one of at least 53 mutations in 55 different kinships that have been identified in the AChR. Some of the other mutations result in electrophysiological changes similar to those described earlier. Thus, failure of neuromuscular transmission may be induced by multiple mechanisms, and even those related to the AChR can have many causes.

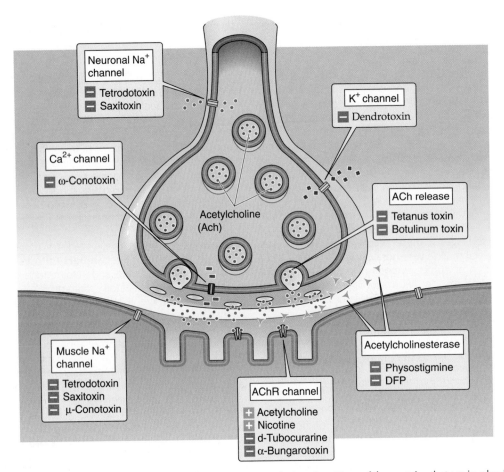

Figure 8-17 Pharmacology of the vertebrate neuromuscular junction. Many of the proteins that are involved in synaptic transmission at the mammalian neuromuscular junction are the targets of naturally occurring or synthetic drugs. The antagonists are shown as minus signs highlighted in *red*. The agonists are shown as plus signs highlighted in *green*.

ω-Conotoxin blocks Ca²⁺ channels that mediate Ca²⁺ influx into nerve terminals, inhibiting synaptic transmission

The exocytotic fusion of mature synaptic vesicles positioned at presynaptic active zones and the subsequent release of ACh require the entry of Ca^{2+} into the nerve terminal. Ca^{2+} enters the presynaptic terminal through voltage-gated Ca^{2+} channels that are activated by the depolarization of an incoming action potential. One type of voltage-gated Ca^{2+} channel, the N-type isoform, has been localized to the region of the active zone of the frog neuromuscular junction. Voltage-clamp experiments demonstrate that a class of molluscan peptide toxins called ω-**conotoxins** (see Chapter 7) block N-type Ca^{2+} currents in a virtually irreversible fashion. Exposure of a frog nerve-muscle preparation to ω-conotoxin thus inhibits the release of neurotransmitter. This effect is manifested as an abolition of muscle EPP when the preparation is stimulated through the nerve. The ω-conotoxins are 24 to 29 residues long and contain three disulfide bonds. Imaging with confocal laser scanning microscopy has shown that ω-conotoxin binds at highest density to voltage-dependent Ca^{2+} channels in the presynaptic nerve terminal, directly across the synaptic cleft from AChR channels. This observation implies that Ca^{2+} channels are located precisely at the active zones of synaptic vesicle fusion. This arrangement provides for focal entry and short-range diffusion of Ca^{2+} entering the nerve terminal to the exact sites involved in promoting Ca^{2+}-dependent transmitter release.

Bacterial toxins such as tetanus and botulinum toxins cleave proteins involved in exocytosis, preventing fusion of synaptic vesicles

Another class of neurotoxins that specifically inhibits neurotransmitter release includes the tetanus and botulinum toxins. These large protein toxins (~150 kDa) are respectively produced by the bacteria *Clostridium tetani* and *Clostridium botulinum* (see the box titled Clostridial Catastrophes). *C. tetani* is the causative agent of tetanus ("lockjaw"), which is characterized by a general increase in muscle tension and muscle rigidity, beginning most often with the muscles of mastication. The reason for this paradoxical enhancement of muscle action is that the toxins have their greatest effect on *inhibition* of synaptic transmission by inhibitory neurons in the spinal cord, neurons that would normally *inhibit* muscle

TABLE 8-2 Neurotoxins That Block Fusion of Synaptic Vesicles

Toxin	Target
Tetanus	Synaptobrevin
Botulinum B, D, F, G	Synaptobrevin
Botulinum A/E	SNAP-25
Botulinum C1	Syntaxin

contraction. *C. botulinum* causes botulism, which is characterized by weakness and paralysis of skeletal muscle as well as by a variety of symptoms that are related to inhibition of cholinergic nerve endings in the autonomic nervous system.

In humans, infection by these bacteria can lead to death because the toxins that they synthesize are potent inhibitors of neurotransmitter release. This inhibition occurs because both tetanus and botulinum toxin proteins have zinc-dependent endoproteinase activity (Table 8-2). These toxins enter nerve terminals and specifically cleave three different proteins required for synaptic vesicle exocytosis. **Tetanus toxin** and **botulinum toxins** B, D, F, and G cleave synaptobrevin, an integral membrane protein of the synaptic vesicle membrane. Botulinum toxins C1 and A/E, respectively, cleave syntaxin and SNAP-25, two proteins associated with the presynaptic membrane. These neurotoxins also have useful medical and cosmetic applications. For example, botulinum toxin is used to treat certain disorders characterized by muscle spasms. Injection of a small amount of botulinum toxin into the eye muscles of a patient with strabismus (a condition in which both eyes cannot focus on the same object because of abnormal hyperactivity of particular eye muscles) is able to suppress aberrant muscle spasms and to restore normal vision. A commercial preparation of botulinum toxin known as Botox has also gained popularity for the temporary treatment of facial wrinkles that occur in human aging.

Both agonists and antagonists of the nicotinic acetylcholine receptor can prevent synaptic transmission

The ionotropic (nicotinic) AChR channel located in the postsynaptic muscle membrane (Fig. 8-17) also has a rich and diverse pharmacology that can be exploited for clinical applications as well as for elucidating many functional aspects of the neuromuscular junction. Figure 8-18 shows the chemical structures of two classes of agents that act on the nicotinic AChR. These agents are classified as agonists or antagonists according to whether they activate opening of the channel or prevent its activation. Many **agonists** have a structure similar to that of the natural neurotransmitter ACh. In general, such agonists activate the opening of AChR channels with the same unitary conductance as those activated by ACh, but with different kinetics of channel opening

Clostridial Catastrophes

Botulism, although hardly one of the most common causes of food poisoning today, is still the illness that many people think of when food-borne disorders are discussed. The neurotoxin of *Clostridium botulinum* is potent, and only a small amount of contamination can lead to death. The most common source of botulism is homemade foods. The spores of this organism can survive boiling temperatures for a number of hours, and if the cooked food is allowed to stand at room temperature for more than 16 hours, the clostridial spores can germinate and produce toxin. Symptoms of the illness may appear several hours to more than a week after ingestion, although most cases occur within 18 to 36 hours. Patients begin to complain of symptoms attributable to inhibition of synaptic vesicle release in the autonomic nervous system (see Chapter 14), such as dry mouth, double vision, and difficulty in swallowing and speaking, and later begin to experience gastrointestinal complications, including vomiting, pain, and diarrhea. Symptoms attributable to inhibition of synaptic vesicle release at the neuromuscular junction, such as weakness and paralysis of the limbs, may soon follow; ultimately, paralysis of the respiratory muscles (see Chapter 27) can be fatal. Prompt intervention with mechanical ventilation has reduced the mortality from botulism dramatically, and the figure today stands at about 20%. Almost all deaths occur among the first victims of a contaminated ingestion because the disease is not quickly recognized; those who fall victim later, when the diagnosis is much easier, do much better.

Vaccination has reduced the number of cases of **tetanus** reported in the United States to only about 100 each year, almost all occurring in inadequately vaccinated individuals. The disease is caused by a neurotoxin (tetanospasmin) produced by *Clostridium tetani*. The organism gains entry to its host through a cut or puncture wound. The toxin then travels along the peripheral nerves to the spinal cord, the major site of its attack. There, the toxin inhibits synaptic vesicle release by interneurons that normally inhibit firing of the motor neurons that, in turn, activate skeletal muscle. Thus, because the toxin suppresses inhibition of the normal reflex arc, muscle contraction leads to profound spasms, most characteristically of the jaw muscles but potentially affecting any muscle in the body. Symptoms can commence on the day of the injury or as long as 2 months later. Complications include respiratory arrest, aspiration pneumonia, rib fractures caused by the severe spasms, and a host of other pulmonary and cardiac manifestations.

and closing. The synthetic drugs **carbamylcholine** (or carbachol) and **succinylcholine** contain the choline moiety of ACh that is required for receptor activation. Carbamylcholine is a carbamyl ester of choline; succinylcholine (or succinyldicholine) is a dimer of ACh linked together through the acetyl methyl group. Both of these agents are resistant to hydrolysis by muscle AChE, but succinylcholine is susceptible to hydrolysis by plasma and liver esterases. This property allows prolonged activation of AChRs.

Succinylcholine is used to produce sustained muscle relaxation or "flaccid paralysis," which is useful in certain

AGONISTS

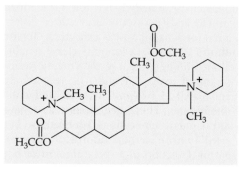

Figure 8-18   Agonists and antagonists of the nicotinic AChR.

types of surgery in which it is important to prevent excitation and contraction of skeletal muscles. This paralytic action occurs because succinylcholine prolongs the opening of AChR channels and thereby depolarizes the muscle membrane in the vicinity of the end plate. Such depolarization results in initial repetitive muscle excitation and tremors, followed by relaxation secondary to **inactivation of Na⁺ channels** in the vicinity of the end plate. This effect prevents the spread of muscle action potentials beyond the end-plate region. On a longer time scale, such agents also lead to **desensitization of the AChR** to agonist, which further inhibits neuromuscular transmission.

Another important agent acting on AChRs is **nicotine**, a natural constituent of tobacco that is responsible for the stimulant action and at least some of the addictive effects of smoking. The selective ability of nicotine to activate AChR channels is the basis of the classification scheme of nicotinic AChRs versus muscarinic AChRs (Fig. 8-3). Nicotine is not an agonist of the muscarinic or G protein–linked receptors, which instead are activated by the mushroom alkaloid muscarine. Although nicotine is able to activate the AChR at the

neuromuscular junction, the physiological effects of smoking are primarily manifested in the CNS and autonomic ganglia, where other neuronal isoforms of nicotinic AChRs are located.

A classic example of a nicotinic AChR **antagonist** is *d*-tubocurarine (Fig. 8-18), the active ingredient of curare, a poison extracted from plants of the genus *Strychnos*. The indigenous tribes of the Amazon region used curare to poison arrows for hunting. *d*-**Tubocurarine** is a competitive inhibitor of ACh binding to two activation sites on the α subunits of the AChR. This action leads to flaccid paralysis of skeletal muscle from inhibition of the nicotinic AChR. However, curare does not cause depolarization. A hallmark of the action of *d*-tubocurarine is that it can be reversed by an increase in concentration of the natural agonist ACh by binding competition. A large increase in local ACh concentration can be produced indirectly by an inhibitor of AChE such as neostigmine (see later).

Figure 8-18 also shows the structure of **pancuronium**, which is a synthetic bis-quaternary ammonium steroid derivative. This drug is also useful for the production of neuromuscular blockade in surgery, and it is actually a more potent, selective competitive antagonist of the muscle nicotinic AChR than *d*-tubocurarine is.

Another class of nicotinic AChR inhibitors is a family of ~8-kDa proteins present in the venom of Elapidae snakes (e.g., cobras). These toxins include α-bungarotoxin (α-Bgt) and homologous α toxins, which bind very strongly to nicotinic receptors. The specific binding of α-Bgt to the nicotinic AChR of skeletal muscle is virtually irreversible. When α-Bgt binds to the nicotinic AChR, it obstructs the agonist binding site and prevents activation of the receptor by ACh. The radioiodinated derivative ^{125}I-labeled α-Bgt has been widely used as a ligand for purifying the nicotinic AChR from various tissues. Fluorescent derivatives of α-Bgt can also be used as specific labels for localizing AChRs at the muscle end plate. The same snake venom (*Bungarus multicinctus*) that contains α-Bgt also contains a homologous protein toxin called κ-bungarotoxin (κ-Bgt). This toxin has little effect on nicotinic AChR channels at the neuromuscular junction, but it does inhibit AChR channels in neuronal tissue. The differential effect of α-Bgt and κ-Bgt on muscle and neuronal currents activated by both ACh and nicotine led to the recognition that different classes of nicotinic receptors exist in the CNS versus skeletal muscle. The basis for these isoforms is the differential expression of multiple genes for homologous nicotinic AChR subunits.

Inhibitors of acetylcholinesterase prolong and magnify the end-plate potential

A variety of specific inhibitors of anticholinesterase have been helpful in defining the contribution of AChE to responses at the muscle end plate. Inhibition of AChE generally increases the amplitude and prolongs the duration of the postsynaptic response to ACh; thus, the enzyme plays an important role in limiting the excitatory action of ACh under normal physiological conditions. In the absence of ACh breakdown by AChE, the prolonged decay of the EPP reflects the underlying kinetics of activated receptors and slow depletion of the agonist in the vicinity of the junctional folds by diffusion of ACh.

The plant alkaloid **physostigmine** (also known as eserine) is the prototypic anticholinesterase (Fig. 8-19). **Neostigmine** (also called prostigmine), a synthetic anti-AChE drug that is partially analogous to physostigmine, is used to treat myasthenia gravis. As discussed earlier in the box about diseases of the human acetylcholine receptor, this disease is caused by the autoimmune destruction and loss of nicotinic AChRs at the muscle end plate. As shown in Equation 8-5, the acetyl-AChE must undergo hydrolysis to recycle AChE for its next round of catalysis. Physostigmine and neostigmine produce a carbamoylated form of AChE that is inactive. The slow hydrolysis of the carbamoylated enzyme relieves esterase inhibition.

Another important class of synthetic AChE inhibitors consists of **organophosphorus compounds**, which are *irreversible* inhibitors. These inhibitors are typified by diisopropylfluorophosphate (**DFP**; Fig. 8-19). Such compounds react with the serine residue of AChE and form an essentially irreversible covalent modification of the enzyme. Such agents rank high among the most potent and lethal of toxic chemi-

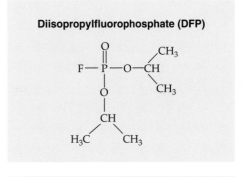

Figure 8-19   Structures of AChE inhibitors.

cals. Their devastating effect is due to excessive enhancement of cholinergic neurotransmission, mediated by both muscarinic and nicotinic receptor pathways throughout the body. For example, exposure to toxic organophosphorus agents results in the flaccid paralysis of respiratory muscles because of initial muscle stimulation followed by depolarization blockade. The lethality of these compounds dramatically underlines the essential role of AChE in terminating cholinergic neurotransmission. Chemical warfare agents (i.e., "nerve gas" such as sarin) are volatile forms of these compounds. Related compounds, such as Malathion (Fig. 8-19), which are relatively selective for insects, are widely used as agricultural insecticides.

A natural organophosphorus neurotoxin is produced by *Anabena flos-aquae*, a toxic cyanobacterium (blue-green alga). Known as **anatoxin-a(s)**, this toxin is a potent inhibitor of AChE and is responsible for the poisoning of dogs and farm animals that drink from contaminated ponds. Another interesting class of natural inhibitors includes the **fasciculins**, a family of small protein toxins present in mamba snake venom that inhibit AChE with very high affinity and specificity.

REFERENCES

Books and Reviews

Engel AG, Ohno K, Sine SM: Congenital myasthenic syndromes: A diverse array of molecular targets. J Neurocytol 2003; 32:1017-1037.

Jahn R: Principles of exocytosis and membrane fusion. Ann N Y Acad Sci 2004; 1014:170-178.

Katz B: Nerve, Muscle, and Synapse. New York: McGraw-Hill, 1966.

Lichman JW, Sanes JR: Watching the neuromuscular junction. J Neurocytol 2003; 32:767-775.

Südhof TC: The synaptic vesicle cycle. Annu Rev Neurosci 2004; 27:509-547.

Van der Kloot W, Molgó J: Quantal acetylcholine release at the vertebrate neuromuscular junction. Physiol Rev 1994; 74:899-989.

Journal Articles

Brejc K, van Dijk WJ, Klaassen RV, et al: Crystal structure of an ACh-binding protein reveals the ligand-binding domain of nicotinic receptors. Nature 2001; 411:269-276.

Del Castillo J, Katz B: Interaction at end-plate receptors between different choline derivatives. Proc R Soc Lond B Biol Sci 1957; 146:369-381.

Fatt P, Katz B: Spontaneous subthreshold activity at motor nerve endings. J Physiol 1952; 117:109-128.

Furshpan EJ, Potter DD: Transmission at the giant motor synapse of the crayfish. J Physiol 1959; 145:289-325.

Magleby KL, Stevens CF: A quantitative description of end-plate currents. J Physiol 1972; 233:173-197.

Noda M, Takahashi H, Tanabe T, et al: Structural homology of *Torpedo californica* acetylcholine receptor subunits. Nature 1983; 302:528.

Ohno K, Hutchinson DO, Milone M, et al: Congenital myasthenic syndrome caused by prolonged acetylcholine receptor channel openings due to a mutation in the M2 domain of the epsilon subunit. Proc Natl Acad Sci USA 1995; 92:758-762.

CHAPTER 9

CELLULAR PHYSIOLOGY OF SKELETAL, CARDIAC, AND SMOOTH MUSCLE

Edward G. Moczydlowski and Michael Apkon

The primary function of muscle is to generate force or movement in response to a physiological stimulus. The human body contains three fundamentally different types of muscle adapted to specialized functions. Skeletal muscle is responsible for the voluntary movement of bones that underlie locomotion and work production. Skeletal muscle also controls the breathing cycle of the lungs through contraction of the diaphragm and functions as a pump assisting return of the venous blood supply to the heart. Cardiac muscle is specific to the heart as the biomechanical pump driving the delivery of blood to the lungs and tissues. Smooth muscle provides mechanical control of organ systems such as the digestive, urinary, and reproductive tracts as well as the blood vessels of the circulatory system and the airway passages of the respiratory system.

Contraction of muscles is initiated either by a chemical neurotransmitter or paracrine factor or by direct electrical excitation. All muscles transduce chemical energy released by hydrolysis of ATP into mechanical work. The unique physiological role of each of the three basic muscle types dictates inherent differences in the rate and duration of contraction, metabolism, fatigability, and ability to regulate contractile strength. For example, both skeletal and cardiac muscle must be capable of rapid force development and shortening. However, skeletal muscle must be able to maintain contractile force for relatively long periods. Cardiac muscle contracts only briefly with each heartbeat but must sustain this rhythmic activity for a lifetime. Smooth muscle, like skeletal muscle, must be able to regulate contraction over a wide range of force development and elastic changes in the size of organs such as the urinary bladder and uterus. In some tissues (e.g., sphincters), smooth muscle sustains contraction without fatigue for very long periods. Despite these differences, the trigger for muscle contraction is the same for all three types of muscle: a rise in the free cytosolic Ca^{2+} concentration ($[Ca^{2+}]_i$).

This chapter describes the fundamental physiology of muscle excitation, the coupling of excitation to contraction, the molecular mechanism of contraction, the regulation of contraction, and the related issues of muscle diversity. We describe general molecular mechanisms shared by all muscle cells and contrast the unique features of skeletal, cardiac, and smooth muscle. Because molecular mechanisms specific to cardiac myocytes are best understood in the unique context of the heart as a pump, we discuss details of cardiac muscle physiology at greater depth in Chapters 22 and 23.

SKELETAL MUSCLE

Contraction of skeletal muscle is initiated by motor neurons that innervate motor units

The smallest contractile unit of skeletal muscle is a multinucleated, elongated cell called a **muscle fiber** or **myofiber** (Fig. 9-1). A bundle of linearly aligned muscle fibers forms a **fascicle**. In turn, bundles of fascicles form a muscle, such as the biceps. The whole muscle is contained within an external sheath extending from the tendons called the **epimysium**. Fascicles within the muscle are enveloped by a sheath called the **perimysium**. Single muscle fibers within individual fascicles are surrounded by a sheath called the **endomysium**. The highly organized architecture of skeletal muscle fibers and connective tissue allows skeletal muscle to generate considerable mechanical force in a vectorial manner. Beneath the endomysium surrounding each muscle fiber is the plasma membrane of the muscle cell called the **sarcolemma**. An individual skeletal muscle cell contains a densely arranged parallel array of cylindrical elements called **myofibrils**. Each myofibril is essentially an end-to-end chain of regular repeating units—or **sarcomeres**—that consist of smaller interdigitating filaments called **myofilaments**, which contain both thin filaments and thick filaments.

As discussed in Chapter 8, a motor nerve axon contacts each muscle fiber to form a synapse near the middle of the fiber called the **neuromuscular junction**. The specialized region of sarcolemma in closest contact with the presynaptic nerve terminal is called the **motor end plate**. Although skeletal muscle fibers can be artificially excited by direct electrical stimulation, physiological excitation of skeletal muscle always involves chemical activation by release of acetylcholine (ACh) from the motor nerve terminal. Binding of ACh to the nicotinic receptor gives rise to a graded depolarizing **end-plate potential**. An end-plate potential of sufficient

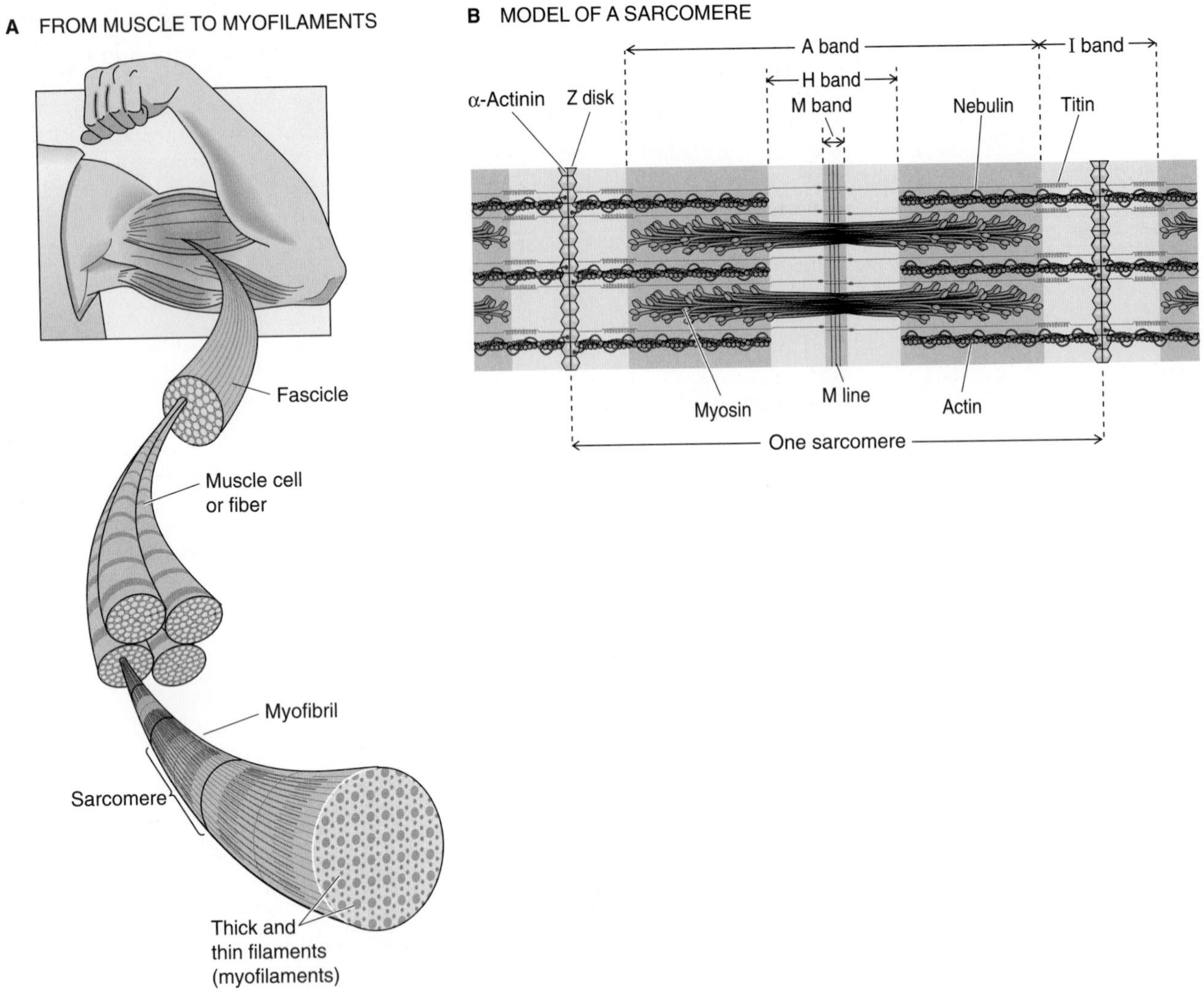

A FROM MUSCLE TO MYOFILAMENTS

Fascicle

Muscle cell
or fiber

Myofibril

Sarcomere

Thick and
thin filaments
(myofilaments)

B MODEL OF A SARCOMERE

α-Actinin   Z disk

A band

H band
M band

Nebulin   Titin

I band

Myosin

M line

Actin

One sarcomere

Figure 9-1   Structure of skeletal muscle.

magnitude triggers a propagating action potential in the region of sarcolemma adjacent to the end plate by raising the membrane potential to the firing threshold.

All skeletal muscle is under voluntary or reflex control by **motor neurons** of the somatic motor system. Somatic motor neurons are efferent neurons with cell bodies located in the central nervous system (CNS). A single muscle cell responds to only a single motor neuron whose cell body—except for cranial nerves—resides in the ventral horn of the spinal cord. However, the axon of a motor neuron typically branches near its termination to innervate a few or many individual muscle cells. The group of muscle fibers innervated by all of the collateral branches of a single motor neuron is referred to as a **motor unit**. A whole muscle can produce a wide range of forces and a graded range of shortening by varying the number of motor units excited within the muscle. The **innervation ratio** of a whole skeletal muscle is defined as the number of muscle fibers innervated by a single motor neuron. Muscles with a small innervation ratio control fine movements involving small forces. For example, fine, high-precision movements of the extraocular muscles that control positioning movements of the eye are achieved through an

innervation ratio of as little as ~3 muscle fibers per neuron. Conversely, muscles with a large innervation ratio control coarse movement requiring development of large forces. Postural control by the soleus muscle uses an innervation ratio of ~200. The gastrocnemius muscle, which is capable of developing large forces required in athletic activities such as jumping, has innervation ratios that vary from ~100 to ~1000.

Action potentials propagate from the sarcolemma to the interior of muscle fibers along the transverse tubule network

Although the ultimate intracellular signal that triggers and sustains contraction of skeletal, cardiac, or smooth muscle cells is a rise in $[Ca^{2+}]_i$, the three types of muscle cells differ substantially in the detailed mechanism by which a depolarization of the sarcolemmal membrane results in a rise in $[Ca^{2+}]_i$. Ca^{2+} can enter the cytoplasm from the extracellular space through voltage-gated ion channels, or alternatively, Ca^{2+} can be released into the cytoplasm from the intracellular Ca^{2+} storage reservoir of the sarcoplasmic reticulum. Thus, both extracellular and intracellular sources may contribute to the increase in $[Ca^{2+}]_i$. However, the relative importance of these two sources of Ca^{2+} varies among the different muscle types. The process by which electrical "excitation" of the surface membrane triggers an increase of $[Ca^{2+}]_i$ in muscle is known as **excitation-contraction coupling** or EC coupling.

Action potentials originating at the surface membrane of skeletal and cardiac muscle fibers propagate into the interior of the cell through specialized membrane invaginations. In skeletal and cardiac muscle, these invaginations take the form of radially projecting tubes of membrane called **transverse tubules** or **T tubules** (Fig. 9-2A). T tubules penetrate the muscle fiber and surround the myofibrils at two points in each sarcomere: at the junctions of the A and I bands. A cross section through the A-I junction shows a complex, branching array of T tubules penetrating to the center of the muscle cell and surrounding the individual myofibrils. Along

its length, the tubule associates with two **cisternae**, which are specialized regions of the **sarcoplasmic reticulum (SR)**. The SR of muscle cells is a specialized version of the endoplasmic reticulum of noncontractile cells and serves as a storage organelle for intracellular Ca^{2+}. The combination of the T-tubule membrane and its two neighboring cisternae is called a **triad**; this structure plays a crucial role in the coupling of excitation to contraction in skeletal and cardiac muscle. *Smooth* muscle, in contrast, has more rudimentary and shallow invaginations called **caveolae** (Fig. 9-2B).

Depolarization of the T-tubule membrane results in Ca^{2+} release from the sarcoplasmic reticulum at the triad

The propagation of the action potential into the T tubules depolarizes the triad region of the T tubules, activating **L-type Ca^{2+} channels** (see Chapter 7). These voltage-gated

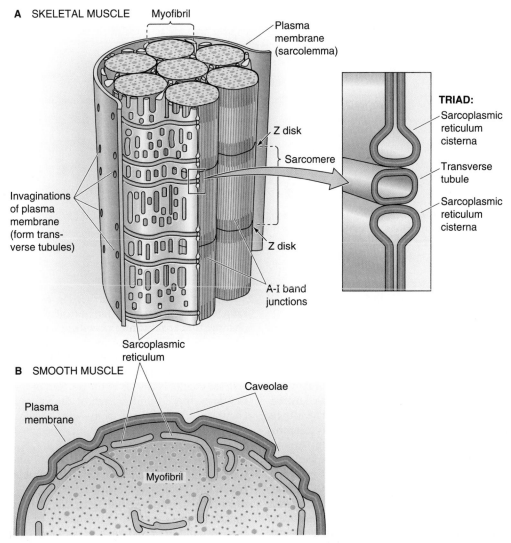

Figure 9-2 Plasma membrane invaginations. **A,** The transverse tubules (T tubules) are extensions of the plasma membrane, penetrating the muscle cell at two points in each sarcomere: the junctions of the A and I bands. **B,** Smooth muscle cells have rudimentary invaginations of the plasma membrane, called caveolae, contacting the sarcoplasmic reticulum.

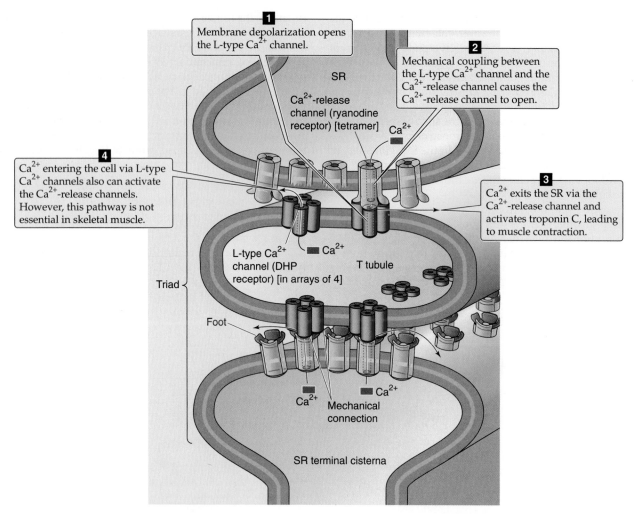

Figure 9-3 EC coupling in skeletal muscle. A tetrad of four L-type Ca^{2+} channels on the T tubules faces a single Ca^{2+}-release channel of the SR, so that each L-type Ca^{2+} channel interacts with the foot of one of the four subunits of the Ca^{2+}-release channel. Note that half of the Ca^{2+}-release channels lack associations with L-type Ca^{2+} channels. DHP, dihydropyridine.

channels cluster in groups of four called tetrads (Fig. 9-3) and have a pivotal role as the **voltage sensor** in EC coupling. Electron microscopy reveals a checkerboard pattern of projections arising from the T-tubule membrane and extending toward the cisternae of the SR; these projections probably represent the cytoplasmic face of these L-type Ca^{2+} channels. Functional complexes of L-type Ca^{2+} channels contain the α_1-subunit of the voltage-gated Ca^{2+} channel as well as the accessory α_2-δ, β, and γ subunits (see Fig. 7-12B). The L-type Ca^{2+} channel is also often referred to as the **DHP receptor** because it is inhibited by a class of antihypertensive and antiarrhythmic drugs known as dihydropyridines. Depolarization of the T-tubule membrane produces conformational changes in each of the four voltage-activated L-type Ca^{2+} channels of the tetrad, resulting in two major effects. First, the conformational changes allow Ca^{2+} to enter through the four channel pores. Second, and more important in skeletal muscle, the conformational changes in the four L-type Ca^{2+} channels induce a conformational change in each of the four subunits of another channel—the Ca^{2+}-release channel—that is located in the SR membrane.

The **Ca^{2+}-release channel** (see Fig. 6-21S) has a homotetrameric structure quite different from that of the L-type Ca^{2+} channel that constitutes the voltage sensor for EC coupling. The Ca^{2+}-release channel in the SR is also known as the **ryanodine receptor** because it is inhibited by a class of drugs that include the plant alkaloids *ryanodine* and *caffeine*. Ca^{2+}-release channels cluster in the portion of the SR membrane that faces the T tubules. Each of the four subunits of these channels has a large extension—also known as a foot. These feet project as a regular array into the cytosol. The foot of each of the four Ca^{2+}-release channel subunits is complementary to the cytoplasmic projection of one of the four L-type Ca^{2+} channels in a tetrad on the T tubule (Fig. 9-3). The physical proximity of these two proteins as well as the ability of both DHP and ryanodine to block muscle contraction suggests that physical and mechanical interaction between these two different Ca^{2+} channels underlies EC coupling. The precise mechanism of interaction between these proteins is not entirely understood, although it is not solely electrical in nature inasmuch as ionic conductance of the Ca^{2+}-release channel is not strongly voltage dependent. A large cytoplasmic projection on the α_1 subunit of the L-type Ca^{2+} channel appears to be necessary for interaction between the two Ca^{2+} channels on opposing T-tubule and SR membranes. Thus, it is likely that direct *mechanical* coupling exists between this projection and the Ca^{2+}-release channel. On this basis, the mechanism of EC coupling in skeletal muscle is termed an electromechanical coupling mechanism.

After depolarization of the L-type Ca^{2+} channel on the T-tubule membrane and mechanical activation of the Ca^{2+}-release channel in the SR, Ca^{2+} stored in the SR rapidly leaves through the Ca^{2+}-release channel. The resultant rapid increase in $[Ca^{2+}]_i$ activates troponin C, initiating formation of cross-bridges between myofilaments, as described later. EC coupling in skeletal muscle thus includes the entire process we have just described, beginning with the depolarization of the T-tubule membrane to the initiation of the cross-bridge cycle of contraction.

Although we have stressed that EC coupling in skeletal muscle primarily involves direct *mechanical* coupling between the L-type Ca^{2+} channel in the T-tubule membrane and the Ca^{2+}-release channel of the SR, a second mechanism for activating the Ca^{2+}-release channel may also contribute.

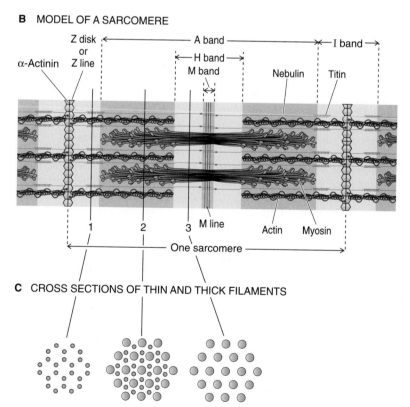

A ELECTRON MICROGRAPH OF SARCOMERE

A band

I band   H band

One sarcomere

B MODEL OF A SARCOMERE

α-Actinin   Z disk or Z line   A band   I band

H band   M band   Nebulin   Titin

1   2   3   M line   Actin   Myosin

One sarcomere

C CROSS SECTIONS OF THIN AND THICK FILAMENTS

Figure 9-4 Structure of the sarcomere.

Intracellular Ca^{2+} can directly activate the Ca^{2+}-release channel in the SR—a process known as **Ca^{2+}-induced Ca^{2+} release (CICR)**. The source of the elevated $[Ca^{2+}]_i$ for CICR is the Ca^{2+} released from the SR, as well as the Ca^{2+} that enters the cell via L-type Ca^{2+} channels during action potentials. However, this influx of external Ca^{2+} from the lumen of T tubules is not required for contraction of mammalian *skeletal muscle*. Indeed, skeletal muscle contraction persists even when Ca^{2+} is absent from the extracellular fluid of the muscle fiber. As described below, Ca^{2+} influx through L-type Ca^{2+} channels nevertheless plays an essential role in EC coupling in *cardiac* muscle.

Striations of skeletal muscle fibers correspond to ordered arrays of thick and thin filaments within myofibrils

There are two types of myofilaments: thick filaments composed primarily of a protein called myosin and thin filaments largely composed of a protein called **actin** (see Chapter 2). The **sarcomere** is defined as the repeating unit between adjacent Z disks or Z lines (Fig. 9-4A and B). A myofibril is thus a linear array of sarcomeres stacked end to end. The highly organized sarcomeres within skeletal and cardiac muscle are responsible for the striped or striated appearance of muscle fibers of these tissues as visualized by various microscopic imaging techniques. Thus, both skeletal muscle and cardiac muscle are referred to as **striated muscle**. In contrast, smooth muscle lacks striations because actin and myosin have a less regular pattern of organization in these myocytes.

In striated muscle, **thin filaments** are 5 to 8 nm in diameter and 1 μm in length. Thin filaments are tethered together at one end, where they project from a dense disk known as the **Z disk** (Fig. 9-4B). The Z disk is oriented perpendicular to the axis of the myofibril and has the diameter of the myofibril. Thin filaments project from both faces of the Z disk. Not only do Z disks tether the thin filaments of a single myofibril together, but connections between the Z disks also tether each myofibril to its neighbors and align the sarcomeres.

The **thick filaments** are 10 nm in diameter and, in striated muscle, 1.6 μm in length (Fig. 9-4B). They lie between and partially interdigitate with the thin filaments. This partial interdigitation results in alternating light and dark bands along the axis of the myofibril. The light bands, which represent regions of the thin filament that do not overlap with thick filaments, are known as **I bands** because they are *isotropic* to polarized light as demonstrated by polarization microscopy. The Z disk is visible as a dark perpendicular line at the center of the I band. The dark bands, which represent the myosin filaments, are known as **A bands** because they are anisotropic to polarized light. During contraction, the A bands are unchanged in length, whereas the I bands shorten.

When the A band is viewed in cross section where the thick and thin filaments overlap, six thin filaments (actin) surround each thick filament (myosin) in a tightly packed hexagonal array (Fig. 9-4C). Within the A bands, the pivoting heads of the thick myosin filaments, the molecular motors, establish cross-bridges to the thin actin filaments. As discussed later, the ATP-dependent cycle of making and breaking cross-bridges causes the actin filament to be drawn over the myosin filament and thereby results in muscle contraction.

Thin and thick filaments are supramolecular assemblies of protein subunits

Thin Filaments The backbone of the thin filament is a double-stranded α-helical polymer of **actin** molecules (Fig. 9-5A). Each helical turn of a single strand of filamentous actin or F-actin consists of 13 individual actin monomers and is ~70 nm long. F-actin is associated with two important regulatory, actin-binding proteins: tropomyosin and troponin.

Individual **tropomyosin** molecules consist of two identical α helices that coil around each other and sit near the two grooves that are formed by the two helical actin strands. Head-to-tail contact between neighboring tropomyosin molecules results in two nearly continuous helical filaments that shadow the actin double helix. The length of a single tropomyosin molecule corresponds to about seven actin monomers (i.e., a half turn of the actin helix). As we describe later, the role of tropomyosin is to regulate the binding of myosin head groups to actin.

Troponin is a heterotrimer consisting of (1) **troponin T** (TnT or TNNT), which binds to a single molecule of tropomyosin; (2) **troponin C** (TnC or TNNC), which binds Ca^{2+}; and (3) **troponin I** (TnI or TNNI), which binds to actin and inhibits contraction. Troponin C is closely related to another Ca^{2+}-binding protein, calmodulin (CaM; see Chapter 3). Thus, each troponin heterotrimer interacts with a single tropomyosin molecule, which in turn interacts with seven actin monomers. The troponin complex also interacts directly with the actin filaments. The coordinated interaction among troponin, tropomyosin, and actin allows actin-myosin interactions to be regulated by changes in $[Ca^{2+}]_i$.

Thick Filaments Like actin thin filaments, thick filaments are also an intertwined complex of proteins (Fig. 9-5B). A thick filament is a bipolar assembly of multiple **myosin II** molecules. Each myosin II molecule is a hexamer (actually two trimers) composed of two intertwined *heavy chains*, two *alkali* (or *essential*) *light chains*, and two *regulatory light chains*. The two **heavy chains** have three regions: a rod, a hinge, and a head region. The *rod* portions are α helices that wrap around each other. At the *hinge* regions, the molecule flares open to form two globular *heads*, which are the cross-bridges between the thick and thin filaments of the sarcomere. The heads of the heavy chains—also called S1 fragments—each possess a site for binding actin as well as a site for binding and hydrolyzing ATP. The head portion of each myosin forms a complex with two light chains, one regulatory and one alkali. The **alkali light chain** plays an essential role in stabilizing the myosin head region. The **regulatory light chain**, as its name implies, regulates the ATPase activity of myosin. The activity of the myosin regulatory light chain is in turn regulated through phosphorylation by Ca^{2+}-dependent and Ca^{2+}-independent kinases. Figure 9-5C summarizes the interaction between a

A   THIN FILAMENT

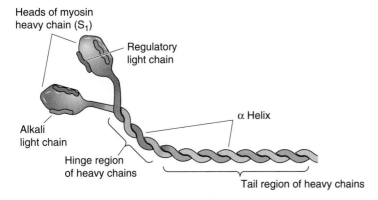

B   MYOSIN MOLECULE

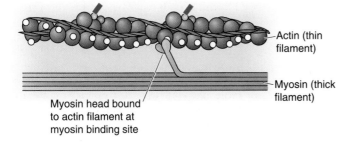

C   INTERACTION OF THIN AND THICK FILAMENTS

Figure 9-5   Structure of thin and thick filaments.

thin filament and a single pair of myosin head groups from a thick filament.

Running alongside the thick filaments of skeletal muscle is a large protein called titin. **Titin** is the largest known protein, with a linear sequence of ~25,000 amino acids (~3000 kDa). Titin is tethered from the M line in the middle of the A band to each of the neighboring Z disks. The M line also serves as the attachment site for myosin molecules within the thick filament. Titin appears to be involved in the elastic behavior of muscle by maintaining the resting length of muscle during relaxation. **Nebulin** is another large protein (600 to 900 kDa) of muscle that runs from the Z disk along the actin thin filaments.

An increase in [Ca²⁺]ᵢ triggers contraction by removing the inhibition of cross-bridge cycling

Underlying muscle contraction is a cycle in which myosin II heads bind to actin, these cross-bridges become distorted, and finally the myosin heads detach from actin. Energy for this cycling comes from the hydrolysis of ATP. However, if unregulated, the cycling would continue until the myocyte is depleted of ATP. It is not surprising, then, that skeletal,

cardiac, and smooth muscle have particular mechanisms for regulating cross-bridge cycling. In all three cell types, an increase in $[Ca^{2+}]_i$ initiates and allows cross-bridge cycling to continue. During this excitatory increase, $[Ca^{2+}]_i$ may rise from its resting level of less than 10^{-7} M to greater than 10^{-5} M. The subsequent decrease in $[Ca^{2+}]_i$ is the signal to cease cross-bridge cycling and to relax. The tightly regulated decrease in $[Ca^{2+}]_i$ is achieved by transport processes that remove Ca^{2+} from the **sarcoplasm**, the term used for the cytoplasm of a muscle fiber.

Regardless of the muscle type, Ca^{2+} exerts its effect by binding to *regulatory* proteins rather than directly interacting with contractile proteins. In the absence of Ca^{2+}, these regulatory proteins act in concert to inhibit actin-myosin interactions, thus inhibiting the contractile process. When Ca^{2+} binds to one or more of these proteins, a conformational change takes place in the regulatory complex that releases the inhibition of contraction.

In skeletal muscle, the **troponin C** (TNNC2 subtype) has two pairs of Ca^{2+}-binding sites. Two high-affinity sites—located on the C-lobe of TNNC2—are aways occupied by Ca^{2+} or Mg^{2+} under physiological conditions. On the other hand, two *low-affinity* sites—located on the N-lobe of

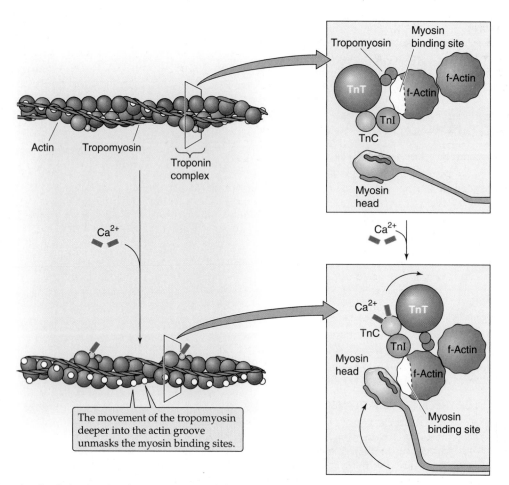

Figure 9-6 The role of Ca^{2+} in triggering the contraction of skeletal and cardiac muscle.

TNNC2—bind and release Ca^{2+} as $[Ca^{2+}]_i$ rises and falls in the sarcoplasm, thereby regulating the binding of actin to myosin (Fig. 9-6). Binding of Ca^{2+} to these low-affinity sites induces a conformational change in the troponin complex that has two effects. The first effect is that the C terminus of the inhibitory **troponin I** moves away from the actin/tropomyosin filament, thereby permitting the tropomyosin molecule to move. According to one hypothesis, the other effect, transmitted through **troponin T**, is to push tropomyosin away from the myosin binding site on the actin and into the actin groove. With the steric hindrance removed, the myosin head is able to interact with actin and to engage in cross-bridge cycling.

During the cross-bridge cycle, contractile proteins convert the energy of ATP hydrolysis into mechanical energy

The cross-bridge cycle that we introduced in the preceding section occurs in five steps (Fig. 9-7). Initially, the myosin head is attached to an actin filament after the "power stroke" from the previous cycle and after the actomyosin complex has released ADP. In the absence of ATP, the system could remain locked in the rigid conformation of the ADP-bound actomyosin complex for an indefinitely long period limited only by protein decomposition. Such a state of extreme muscle rigidity called **rigor mortis** develops in a corpse soon after death from lack of ATP after cessation of metabolism.

In this rigid state, the myosin head is fixed at a 45-degree angle with respect to the actin and myosin filaments.

Step 1: **ATP binding.** ATP binding to the head of the myosin heavy chain (MHC) reduces the affinity of myosin for actin, causing the myosin head to release from the actin filament. If all cross-bridges in a muscle were in this state, the muscle would be fully relaxed.

Step 2: **ATP hydrolysis.** The breakdown of ATP to ADP and inorganic phosphate (P_i) occurs on the myosin head; the products of hydrolysis are retained on the myosin. As a result of hydrolysis, the myosin head pivots around the hinge into a "cocked" position (perpendicular or at a 90-degree angle to the thick and thin filaments). This rotation causes the tip of the myosin to move ~11 nm along the actin filament so that it now lines up with a new actin monomer two monomers farther along the actin filament (see the box titled Measuring the Force of a Single Cross-Bridge Cycle). Once again, if all cross-bridges in a muscle were in this state, the muscle would be fully relaxed.

Step 3: **Cross-bridge formation.** The cocked myosin head now binds to its new position on the actin filament. This binding reflects the increased affinity of the myosin-ADP-P_i complex for actin.

Step 4: **Release of P_i from the myosin.** Dissociation of P_i from the myosin head triggers the power stroke, a conformational change in which the myosin head bends ~45

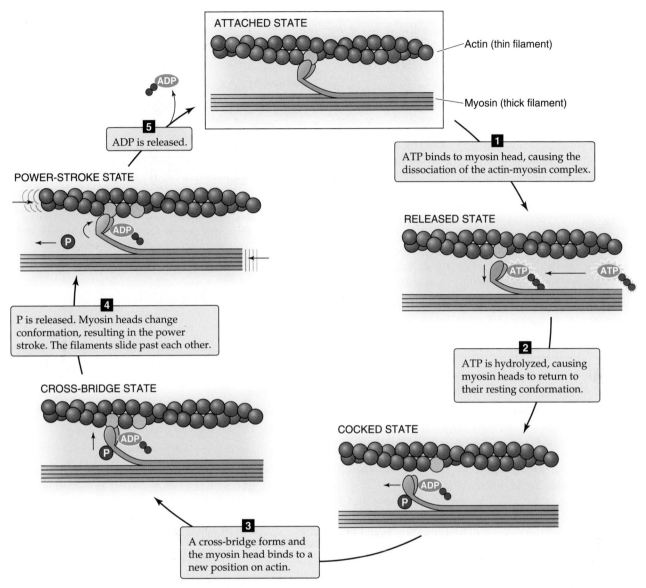

Figure 9-7 The cross-bridge cycle in skeletal and cardiac muscle. Each cycle advances the myosin head by two actin monomers, or ~11 nm.

degrees about the hinge and pulls the actin filament ~11 nm toward the tail of the myosin molecule. This conformational change causes the actin filament to be drawn along the myosin filament, thereby generating force and motion.

Step 5: **ADP release.** Dissociation of ADP from myosin completes the cycle, and the actomyosin complex is left in a rigid state. The myosin head remains in the same position and at a 45-degree angle with respect to the thick and thin filaments. The ADP–free myosin complex remains bound to actin until another ATP molecule binds and initiates another cycle.

The ADP–free myosin complex ("attached state" in Fig. 9-7) would quickly bind ATP at the concentrations of ATP normally found within cells. If unrestrained, this cross-bridge cycling would continue until the cytoplasm is depleted of ATP. At that time, the muscle would remain in the stiff attached state because release of the cross-bridges from actin requires binding of ATP to myosin.

These steps show that $[ATP]_i$ does not regulate the cross-bridge cycle of actin-myosin interaction. Skeletal and cardiac muscle control the cycle of contraction at the third step by preventing cross-bridge formation until the tropomyosin moves out of the way in response to an increase in $[Ca^{2+}]_i$.

Because ATP stores are small, the cell must regenerate the ATP needed for muscle contraction

Each round of the cross-bridge cycle consumes one molecule of ATP. In skeletal muscle, the entire cellular store of ATP is sufficient to allow only a few seconds of continuous maximal contraction. Therefore, the muscle cell must resynthesize ATP from ADP at a rate comparable to the rate of ATP consumption. Skeletal muscle has specialized energy stores that permit rapid regeneration of ATP. The most readily available pool of this energy is the high-energy phosphate bond of **phosphocreatine**. The enzyme **creatine kinase** transfers the high-energy phosphate of phosphocreatine to ADP, thereby rephosphorylating ADP to ATP. The phosphocreatine content of skeletal muscle is adequate to replenish the ATP pool several times, but it is still inadequate to sustain the energy needs of contracting muscle for more than 10 seconds.

In comparison with the energy stored as phosphocreatine, glycogen is a far more abundant energy source within skeletal muscle. **Glycogen** that has been previously stored by muscle can be enzymatically degraded to pyruvic acid. Degradation of glycogen to pyruvate is rapid and liberates energy that the cell invests in phosphorylating ADP to yield ATP. Pyruvate is further metabolized along with other foodstuffs by *oxidative metabolism,* which during the long term is the primary mechanism for the regeneration of ATP (see Chapter 58). The rate of ATP generation by oxidative metabolism is limited by the rate of oxygen delivery to the muscle. However, glycolytic formation of pyruvate occurs independently of oxygen, as does the conversion of pyruvate to lactate. The pathway of *anaerobic metabolism* of muscle glycogen ensures that energy stores are sufficient to sustain muscle activity for nearly a minute even when oxygen is unavailable. In Chapter 60, we will discuss the aerobic and anaerobic metabolism of exercising muscle in more depth.

Termination of contraction requires re-uptake of Ca^{2+} into the sarcoplasmic reticulum

After the action potential in the skeletal muscle has subsided, Ca^{2+} must be removed from the cytoplasm for contraction to actually cease and for relaxation to occur. Removal of Ca^{2+} from the sarcoplasm occurs by two mechanisms. Ca^{2+} may be extruded across the cell plasma membrane or sequestered within intracellular compartments (Fig. 9-8).

The cell may extrude Ca^{2+} by use of either the Na-Ca exchanger (NCX or SLC8) or the Ca^{2+} pump at the plasma membrane (PMCA). Extrusion across the cell membrane, however, would eventually totally deplete the cell of Ca^{2+} and is therefore a minor mechanism for Ca^{2+} removal from the cytoplasm. Instead, Ca^{2+} re-uptake into the SR is the most important mechanism by which the cell returns $[Ca^{2+}]_i$ to resting levels. Ca^{2+} re-uptake by the SR is mediated by a sarcoplasmic and endoplasmic reticulum Ca^{2+}-ATPase (SERCA)–type Ca^{2+} pump (see Chapter 5).

High $[Ca^{2+}]$ within the SR lumen inhibits the activity of SERCA. This inhibition of SR Ca^{2+} pump activity is delayed by Ca^{2+}-binding proteins within the SR lumen. These Ca^{2+}-binding proteins buffer the $[Ca^{2+}]$ increase in the SR during Ca^{2+} re-uptake and thus markedly increase the Ca^{2+} capacity of the SR. The principal Ca^{2+}-binding protein in skeletal muscle, **calsequestrin**, is also present in cardiac and some smooth muscle. **Calreticulin** is a ubiquitous Ca^{2+}-binding protein that is found in particularly high concentrations within the SR of smooth muscle. These proteins have a tremendous capacity to bind Ca^{2+}, with up to 50 binding sites per protein molecule.

Ca^{2+}-binding proteins are not located diffusely within the SR. Rather, calsequestrin is highly localized to the region of the SR immediately beneath the triad junction. Calsequestrin appears to bind directly at the triad, where it forms a complex with the Ca^{2+}-release channel and with two other triad proteins, junctin and triadin. Here, calsequestrin is

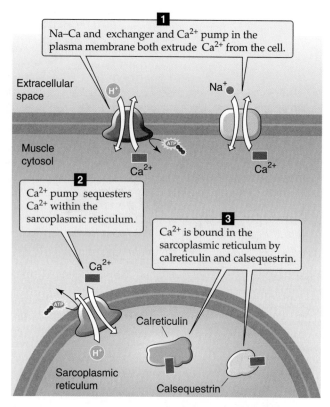

Figure 9-8 Mechanisms of Ca^{2+} removal from the cytoplasm.

poised not only to aid muscle relaxation by buffering Ca^{2+} within the SR lumen but also to unload its Ca^{2+} in the vicinity of the Ca^{2+}-release channel and thus facilitate EC coupling. It has been hypothesized that EC coupling promotes Ca^{2+} release from calsequestrin, making Ca^{2+} available for exit from the SR.

Muscle contractions produce force or shortening and, in the extreme, can be studied under either isometric or isotonic conditions

The total force generated by a muscle is the sum of the forces generated by many independently cycling actin-myosin cross-bridges. The number of simultaneously cycling cross-bridges depends substantially on the initial length of the muscle fiber and on the pattern or frequency of muscle cell stimulation. When muscle is stimulated to contract, it exerts a force tending to pull the attachment points at either end toward each other. This force is referred to as the **tension** developed by the muscle.

Two mechanical—and artificial—arrangements can be used to study muscle contraction. In one, the attachment points are immobile, thereby fixing the muscle *length.* Here, stimulation causes an increase in tension, but no shortening. Because these contractions occur at constant length, they are referred to as **isometric contractions** (Fig. 9-9A). In the second arrangement, one of the two attachment points is mobile, and a force—or load—tends to pull this mobile point away from the fixed one. Here, stimulation causes shortening, provided the tension developed by the muscle is

Malignant Hyperthermia

Malignant hyperthermia (MH) is a genetic disorder affecting between 1 in 10,000 and 1 in 50,000 individuals. Affected individuals are at risk for a potentially life-threatening syndrome on exposure to any of the various inhalation anesthetic agents, particularly halothane. Administration of succinylcholine can also trigger or exaggerate MH. This drug is a short-acting inotropic (nicotinic) ACh receptor antagonist that acts by first opening the ACh receptor channel and then blocking it, thereby resulting in a burst of muscle activity, followed by paralysis. Onset of the syndrome in the setting of the operating room is typified by the development of tachypnea (rapid breathing), low plasma $[O_2]$, high plasma $[CO_2]$, tachycardia (rapid heart rate), and *hyperthermia* (rising body temperature) as well as by rigidity, sweating, and dramatic swings in blood pressure. The patient's temperature may rise as rapidly as 1°C every 5 minutes. The onset of MH is usually during anesthesia, but it can occur up to several hours later. If untreated, the patient will develop respiratory and lactic acidosis, muscle rigidity, and a breakdown of muscle tissue that leads to the release of K^+ and thus profound hyperkalemia. These episodes reflect a progressively severe hypermetabolic state in the muscle tissues. Fortunately, our evolving understanding of the physiological process of MH has led to the development of a therapeutic regimen that has greatly improved the once-dismal prognosis.

The major features of the syndrome—hyperthermia, muscle rigidity, and an increased metabolic rate—led early investigators to suggest that MH is a disease of abnormal regulation of muscle contraction. According to this hypothesis, uncontrolled muscle contraction—somehow triggered by the administration of halothane and succinylcholine—causes excessive ATP hydrolysis to provide energy for contraction. The increased rate of ATP hydrolysis leads to an increased metabolic rate as muscle tries to replenish and to sustain its ATP stores. Hyperthermia develops because of the heat liberated by the hydrolysis of ATP.

Further support for this hypothesis came from the observation that more tension developed in muscle fibers obtained by biopsy from susceptible individuals than in fibers from normal individuals when the fibers were exposed to halothane. In muscle fibers from both humans and a strain of swine susceptible to MH, Ca^{2+}-induced Ca^{2+} release from the SR is enhanced compared with fibers from unaffected subjects. Furthermore, caffeine, which causes the Ca^{2+}-release channels to open, induced greater contractions in fibers from susceptible subjects. Taken together, these observations suggested the possibility that MH results from an abnormality in the Ca^{2+}-release channel in the SR membrane.

In both humans and animals, inheritance of MH follows a mendelian autosomal dominant pattern. Cloning of the gene (*RYR1*) encoding the Ca^{2+}-release channel (ryanodine receptor) allowed genetic linkage analysis to demonstrate that human MH is closely linked in some families to the *RYR1* gene on chromosome 19. In swine, MH results from a single amino acid substitution in *RYR1* (Cys for Arg at position 614). An analogous substitution is present in some human kindreds as well. This substitution increases the probability that the Ca^{2+}-release channel will be open. In other families, MH has been associated with other genetic abnormalities in the *RYR1* gene. In still others, MH does not appear to be genetically linked to the *RYR1* gene. It is possible that defects in other steps along the excitation-contraction cascade can result in abnormal regulation of muscle contraction and the MH phenotype. For example, when they are under anesthesia, patients with some forms of muscular dystrophy may have metabolic crises that resemble MH.

MH also occurs in domestic livestock. The incidence of MH is particularly high in swine, and episodes are triggered by a variety of physical and environmental stresses (porcine stress syndrome). MH in animals has significant economic importance in view of the potential loss from fatal episodes and the devaluation of meat as a result of muscle destruction during nonfatal episodes.

In humans, a condition similar to MH may occur in patients treated with neuroleptic agents such as the phenothiazines or haloperidol. It is called the *neuroleptic malignant syndrome* and appears to result from abnormally high neuronal input to the muscle cells.

Therapy for MH now involves administration of the drug dantrolene, cessation of anesthesia, and aggressive efforts aimed at cooling the body. **Dantrolene** is an effective therapeutic agent because it blocks EC coupling between T tubules and the SR, thus interrupting the otherwise uncontrolled progression of muscle contractions. The drug can be given acutely in an effort to abort an ongoing attack, or in a person known to be at risk, it can be given before the initiation of anesthesia to prevent onset of the syndrome. Therapy also includes intravenous hydration and the judicious use of diuretics to keep the urine flowing; this lessens damage to the kidneys from the release of breakdown products, such as myoglobin from the damaged muscles. Sodium bicarbonate is given to counter the lactic acidosis, and patients may be mechanically hyperventilated to blow off the excess CO_2.

Despite the intensive protocol just outlined, MH is still associated with high mortality. The relatives of a patient with a documented history of one episode of MH should be carefully screened to see whether they, too, carry the inherited trait; many of the affected relatives may demonstrate baseline elevations in muscle enzyme levels in their blood (e.g., an increase in creatine kinase levels).

---

greater than the opposing load. Because these shortenings occur at constant load, they are referred to as **isotonic contractions** (see Fig. 9-9B). Both isometric and isotonic contractions can be examined at different initial muscle lengths. Moreover, they can be measured during individual muscle twitches that are evoked by single muscle action potentials as well as during other patterns of stimulation.

Muscle length influences tension development by determining the degree of overlap between actin and myosin filaments

The iso*metric* force of contractions depends on the initial length of the muscle fiber. Unstimulated muscle may be elongated somewhat by applying tension and stretching it.

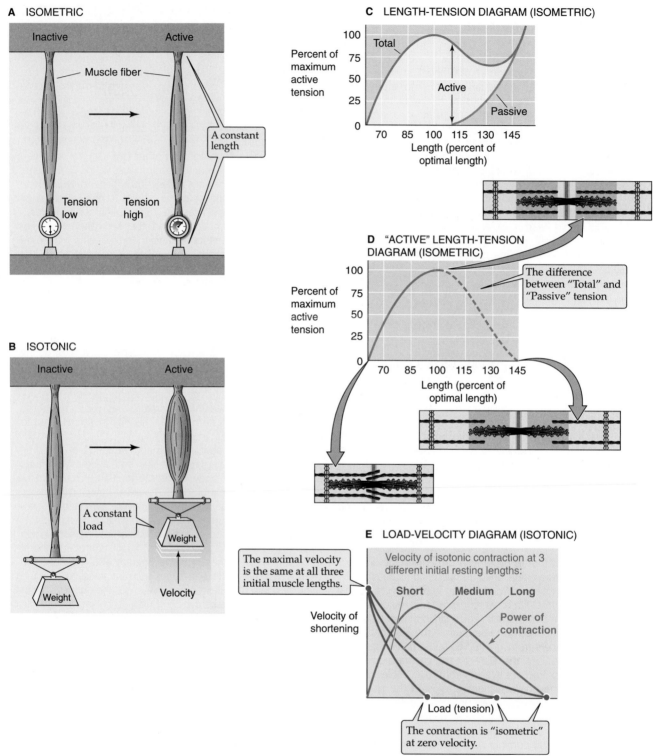

A ISOMETRIC

Inactive   Active

Muscle fiber

A constant length

Tension low   Tension high

B ISOTONIC

Inactive   Active

A constant load

Weight

Weight   Velocity

C LENGTH-TENSION DIAGRAM (ISOMETRIC)

Percent of maximum active tension

Total

Active

Passive

Length (percent of optimal length)

D "ACTIVE" LENGTH-TENSION DIAGRAM (ISOMETRIC)

Percent of maximum active tension

The difference between "Total" and "Passive" tension

Length (percent of optimal length)

E LOAD-VELOCITY DIAGRAM (ISOTONIC)

The maximal velocity is the same at all three initial muscle lengths.

Velocity of isotonic contraction at 3 different initial resting lengths:

Short   Medium   Long

Power of contraction

Velocity of shortening

Load (tension)

The contraction is "isometric" at zero velocity.

Figure 9-9   Isometric and isotonic contraction. **A,** Experimental preparation for study of muscle contraction under *isometric* conditions. **B,** Experimental preparation for study of muscle contraction under *isotonic* conditions. **C,** The passive curve represents the tension that is measured at various muscle lengths before muscle contraction. The total curve represents the tension that is measured at various muscle lengths during muscle contraction. Muscle length is expressed as the percent of "optimal" length, that is, the length at which active isometric tension is maximal. **D,** The active tension is the difference between the total and the passive tensions in **C**. **E,** Each of the three *blue curves* shows that the velocity of muscle shortening is faster if the muscle lifts a lighter weight—it is easier to lift a feather (left side of each curve/low load) than to lift a barbell (right side of each curve/high load). The three *blue curves* also show that for any given velocity of shortening, a longer muscle can develop a greater tension than can a shorter muscle.

Measuring the Force of a Single Cross-Bridge Cycle

The force of a single cross-bridge cycle has been measured directly. Finer, Simmons, and Spudich used **optical tweezers** to manipulate a single actin filament and to place it in proximity to a myosin molecule immobilized on a bead (Fig. 9-10). With the use of video-enhanced microscopy, these investigators were able to detect movements of the actin filament as small as 1 nm. The optical tweezers could also exert an adjustable force opposing movement of the actin filament. When the tweezers applied only a small opposing force and the experiment was conducted in the presence of ATP, they observed that the actin moved over the myosin bead in step-like displacements of 11 nm. This observation, made under "microscopically isotonic" conditions, suggests that the quantal displacement of a single cross-bridge cycle is ~11 nm. When the tweezers applied a force sufficiently large to immobilize the actin filament, the investigators observed step-like impulses of force that averaged ~5 pN. This observation, made under "microscopically isometric" conditions, suggests that the quantal force developed during a single cross-bridge cycle is ~5 pN. Interestingly, these isometric force impulses lasted longer when the ATP concentration was lower. This last finding is consistent with the notion that ATP binding to myosin must occur to allow detachment of the cross-bridges (step 1 in the cycle in Fig. 9-7).

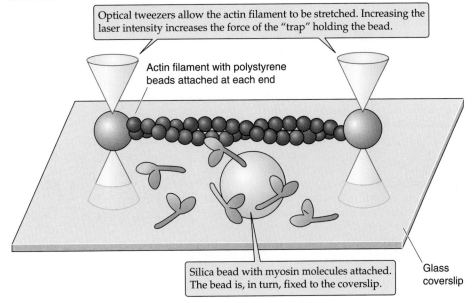

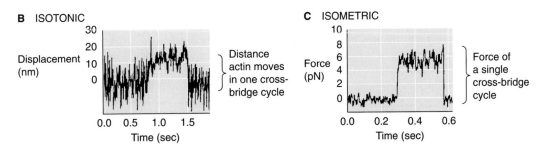

Figure 9-10 Microscopic measurements of cross-bridge force and displacement. **A,** An actin filament is attached at each end to a polystyrene bead. The optical tweezers, a finely focused beam of laser light, can trap the bead at its focal point and physically move it. By adjusting the laser intensity, the experimenter can alter the strength of the trap (i.e., the force with which the bead is held). In this experiment, two optical tweezers were used to suspend the actin filament above a coverglass. Attached to this coverglass is a silica bead, and myosin molecules are bound to the bead. **B,** In an isotonic experiment, the force between the actin filament and the fixed myosin/silica bead is kept constant by use of a stable laser intensity. The experimenter measures, as a function of time, the displacement of the polystyrene bead away from the center of the trap. Thus, in one cross-bridge cycle, the myosin-actin interaction pulls the polystyrene bead ~11 nm away from the center of the trap. **C,** In an isometric experiment, the experimenter measures, as a function of time, the extra force that needs to be applied (i.e., increase in laser intensity) to keep the polystyrene bead at a fixed position near the center of the trap. Thus, in one cross-bridge cycle, the myosin-actin interaction exerts a force of ~5 pN. (*Data from Finer JT, Mehta AD, Spudich JA: Characterization of single actin-myosin interactions. Biophys J 1995; 68:291s-296s.*)

The tension measured before muscle contraction is referred to as **passive tension** (Fig. 9-9C). Because muscle gets stiffer as it is distended, it takes increasing amounts of passive tension to progressively elongate the muscle cell. If at any fixed length (i.e., isometric conditions) the muscle is stimulated to contract, an additional **active tension** develops because of cross-bridge cycling. The total measured tension is thus the sum of the passive and active tensions. This incremental or *active* tension—the difference between total tension and passive tension—is quite small when the muscle is less than ~70% of its normal resting length (Fig. 9-9D). As muscle length increases toward its normal length, active tension increases. Active tension is maximal at a length—usually called L_0—that is near the normal muscle length. Active tension decreases with further lengthening; thus, active tension is again small when the muscle is stretched beyond 150% of its normal resting length. Although the relationship between muscle length and tension has been best characterized for skeletal muscle, the tension of cardiac and smooth muscle also appears to depend on length in a similar manner.

This length-tension relationship is a direct result of the anatomy of the thick and thin filaments within individual sarcomeres (Fig. 9-9D). As muscle length increases, the ends of the actin filaments arising from neighboring Z disks are pulled away from each other. When length is increased beyond 150% of its resting sarcomere length, the ends of the actin filaments are pulled beyond the ends of the myosin filaments. Under this condition, no interaction occurs between actin and myosin filaments and hence no development of active tension. As muscle length shortens from this point, actin and myosin filaments begin to overlap and tension can develop; the amount of tension developed corresponds to the degree of overlap between the actin and the myosin filaments. As the muscle shortens further, opposing actin filaments slide over one another and the ends of the myosin filaments and—with extreme degrees of shortening—eventually butt up against the opposing Z disks. Under these conditions, the spatial relationship between actin and myosin is distorted and active tension falls. The maximal degree of overlap between actin and myosin filaments, and hence maximal active tension, corresponds to a sarcomere length that is near its normal resting length.

At higher loads, the velocity of shortening is lower because more cross-bridges are simultaneously active

Under iso*tonic* conditions, the velocity of shortening decreases as the applied load opposing contraction of the muscle fiber increases. This point is obvious; anyone can lift a single French fry much faster than a sack of potatoes. As shown for any of the three blue curves in Figure 9-9E—each of which represents a different initial length of muscle—the relationship between velocity and load is hyperbolic. Thus, the smaller the load applied to the muscle, the greater its velocity of shortening. Conversely, the greater the load, the lower the velocity of shortening.

The load (or tension)–velocity relationship is perhaps best understood by considering the situation at maximum load for a resting muscle length (i.e., *isometric* conditions). This situation is represented by the upper blue curve in Figure 9-9E. At any time, all the available cross-bridges are engaged in resisting the opposing force. None are left over to make the muscle shorten. If the number of engaged cross-bridges were decreased, the muscle would lengthen. At a slightly smaller load but at the same isotonic muscle length, fewer cross-bridges need to be engaged to resist the opposing load. Thus, extra cross-bridges are available to ratchet the thick myosin filaments over the thin actin filaments, but at a very low velocity. At a still lower load, even more cross-bridges are available for ratcheting the myosin over the actin, and the velocity increases further. At very low loads, it is reasonable to expect that as the myosin filament slides along the actin filament, only a tiny fraction of the actin monomers need to interact with myosin heads to overcome the load. Under these conditions of vanishingly small loads, the speed with which the thick and thin filaments slide over each other is limited only by the time that it takes for the ATP-consuming cross-bridge cycle to occur. With increasing velocity, the probability of actin-myosin interactions decreases. Thus, fewer cross-bridges are simultaneously active at higher shortening velocities, and less tension develops.

Note that the upper blue curve in Figure 9-9E applies to a particular initial length of the muscle, that is, the *resting* length. We already saw in Figure 9-9C that the total isometric tension (i.e., the maximal load that the muscle can sustain at zero velocity) increases with initial muscle length. This principle is confirmed in Figure 9-9E: the longer the initial length, the larger the maximal load under zero-velocity conditions (i.e., the three different intercepts with the abscissa). In contrast to this maximal *load*, which depends very much on length, maximal *velocity* is independent of length, as shown by the common intercept of the family of curves with the ordinate. The explanation for this effect, as we have already noted, is that maximal velocity (at no load) depends on the maximal rate of cross-bridge turnover, not on the initial overlap of the thin and thick filaments.

The velocity-tension curve reveals an interesting relationship between muscle power and applied load. Muscle does measurable mechanical work only when it displaces a load. This mechanical **work** (W) is the product of load (F) and displacement (Δx). **Power** (P) is the rate at which work is performed, or work per unit time (Δt):

$$P = \frac{W}{\Delta t} = \frac{F \cdot \Delta x}{\Delta t} \qquad (9\text{-}1)$$

Because velocity (v) is $\Delta x / \Delta t$, it follows that

$$P = F \cdot v \qquad (9\text{-}2)$$

For a given load (F), we can calculate the power by reading the velocity (v) from the uppermost of the three blue load-velocity relationships in Figure 9-9E. Power is maximal at intermediate loads (where both F and v are moderate) and falls to zero at maximum load (where $v = 0$) and at zero load (where $F = 0$).

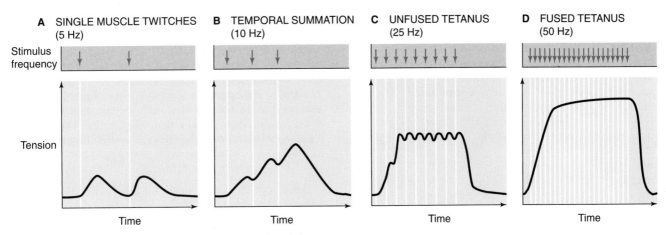

Figure 9-11 Frequency summation of skeletal muscle twitches.

In a single skeletal muscle fiber, the force developed may be increased by summing multiple twitches in time

At sufficiently low stimulation frequencies, the tension developed falls to the resting level between individual twitches (Fig. 9-11A). Single skeletal muscle twitches last between 25 and 200 ms, depending on the type of muscle. Although each twitch is elicited by a single muscle action potential, the duration of contraction is long compared with the duration of the exciting action potential, which lasts only several milliseconds. Because the muscle twitch far exceeds the duration of the action potential, it is possible to initiate a second *action potential* before a first *contraction* has fully subsided. When this situation occurs, the second action potential stimulates a twitch that is superimposed on the residual tension of the first twitch, thereby achieving greater isometric tension than the first (compare Fig. 9-11A and B). This effect is known as **summation.**

If multiple action potentials occur close enough in time, the multiple twitches can summate and thus greatly increase the tension developed. Summation is more effective at increasing tension when the action potentials are grouped more closely in time, as in Figure 9-11C. In other words, tension is higher when action potentials are evoked at higher frequency. Because this type of tension enhancement depends on the frequency of muscle stimulation, it is referred to as **frequency summation.**

When the stimulation frequency is increased sufficiently, the individual twitches occur so close together in time that they fuse (Fig. 9-11D) and cause the muscle tension to remain at a steady plateau. The state in which the individual twitches are no longer distinguishable from each other is referred to as **tetanus.** Tetanus arises when the time between successive action potentials is insufficient to return enough Ca^{2+} to the SR to lower $[Ca^{2+}]_i$ below a level that initiates relaxation. In fact, a sustained increase in $[Ca^{2+}]_i$ persists until the tetanic stimulus ceases. At stimulation frequencies above the **fusion frequency** that causes tetanus, muscle fiber tension increases very little.

In a whole skeletal muscle, the force developed may be increased by summing the contractions of multiple fibers

In addition to determining the frequency with which it stimulates a single muscle fiber, the CNS can control muscle force by determining the number of individual muscle fibers that it stimulates at a given time. As each additional motor neuron cell body within the spinal cord is excited, those muscle fibers that are part of the *motor unit* of that motor neuron are added to the contracting pool of fibers (Fig. 9-12). This effect is known as **multiple-fiber summation.** In general, smaller motor neurons serve motor units consisting of fewer individual muscle fibers. Because a given excitatory stimulus will generate a larger excitatory postsynaptic potential (see Chapter 8) in motor neurons with smaller cell bodies, the small motor units are recruited even with minimal neuronal stimulation. As neuronal stimulation intensifies, larger motor neurons innervating larger motor units are also recruited. The progressive recruitment of first small and then larger and larger motor units is referred to as the **size principle.** The group of all motor neurons innervating a single muscle is called a **motor neuron pool.**

Multiple-fiber summation, sometimes referred to as **spatial summation,** is an important mechanism that allows the force developed by a whole muscle to be relatively constant in time. It is true that the CNS could direct the force to be relatively constant over time merely by driving a fixed number of motor units within the muscle to tetanus, where the force fluctuations are very small (Fig. 9-11D). However, adding tetanic motor units would increase total muscle force by rather large individual increments. Instead, the CNS can activate individual motor units asynchronously so that some units are developing tension while others are relaxing. Thus, whole-muscle force can be relatively constant with time, even when individual fibers are not stimulated to tetanus. Smooth, nontetanic contraction is essential for fine motor control.

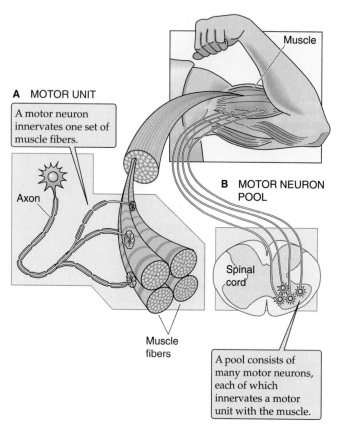

A MOTOR UNIT

A motor neuron innervates one set of muscle fibers.

Muscle

Axon

B MOTOR NEURON POOL

Spinal cord

Muscle fibers

A pool consists of many motor neurons, each of which innervates a motor unit with the muscle.

Figure 9-12 The motor unit and the motor neuron pool.

boring cells as well. Thus, the generation of an action potential is just as critical for initiating contraction in cardiac muscle as it is in skeletal muscle but is triggered by the sinoatrial node and the specialized conduction system of the heart as described in Chapter 21.

Cardiac myocytes receive synaptic input from autonomic neurons, but the sympathetic and parasympathetic divisions of the autonomic nervous system (see Chapter 14) use these synapses to *modulate* rather than to *initiate* cardiac muscle function.

Cardiac contraction requires Ca^{2+} entry through L-type Ca^{2+} channels

Whereas EC coupling in skeletal muscle does not require Ca^{2+} influx through L-type Ca^{2+} channels, cardiac contraction has an *absolute requirement* for Ca^{2+} influx through these channels during the action potential. Because the T-tubule lumen is an extension of the extracellular space, it facilitates the diffusion of Ca^{2+} from bulk extracellular fluid to the site of the L-type Ca^{2+} channels on the T-tubule membrane. Thus, the Ca^{2+} can simultaneously reach superficial and deep regions of the muscle. The increase in $[Ca^{2+}]_i$ resulting from Ca^{2+} influx alone is not, however, sufficient to initiate contraction. Rather, the increase in $[Ca^{2+}]_i$ that is produced by the L-type Ca^{2+} channels is greatly amplified by Ca^{2+}-induced Ca^{2+} release from the SR through the Ca^{2+}-release channels. Indeed, because the Ca^{2+}-release channels remain open for a longer period than do L-type Ca^{2+} channels, the contribution of CICR to the rise in $[Ca^{2+}]_i$ is greater

CARDIAC MUSCLE

Action potentials that propagate between adjacent cardiac myocytes through gap junctions initiate contraction of cardiac muscle

Cardiac muscle and its individual myocytes have a morphological character different from that of skeletal muscle and its cells (Fig. 9-13). Cardiac myocytes are shorter, branched, and interconnected from end to end by structures called **intercalated disks**, which can be observed as dark lines at the level of a light microscope. The intercalated disks connecting the ends of adjoining cardiac myocytes contain **desmosomes** that link adjacent cells mechanically and **gap junctions** (see Chapter 6) that link cells electrically. Cardiac muscle thus acts as mechanical and electrical syncytium of coupled cells, unlike skeletal muscle fibers, which are separate cells bundled together by connective tissue. Like skeletal muscle, cardiac muscle is striated and its sarcomeres contain similar arrays of thin and thick filaments.

Contraction of cardiac muscle cells is not initiated by neurons as in skeletal muscle but by electrical excitation originating from the heart's own **pacemaker**, the sinoatrial node (see Chapter 21), which generates spontaneous and periodic action potentials. When an action potential is initiated in one cell, current flows through the gap junctions and depolarizes neighboring cells. If depolarization causes the membrane potential (V_m) to be more positive than threshold, self-propagating action potentials occur in the neigh-

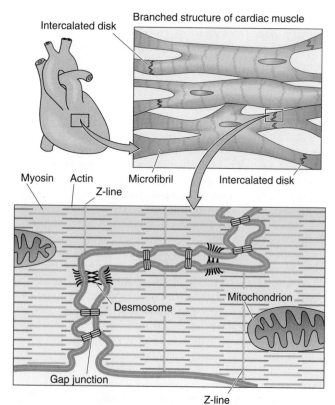

Intercalated disk

Branched structure of cardiac muscle

Myosin   Actin   Microfibril   Intercalated disk

Z-line

Desmosome

Mitochondrion

Gap junction

Z-line

Figure 9-13 Electrical coupling of cardiac myocytes.

than the flux contributed by the L-type Ca^{2+} channels of the T tubules.

It appears that each L-type Ca^{2+} channel controls only one SR Ca^{2+}-release channel. The physical proximity of L-type Ca^{2+} channels of the T-tubule membrane and the Ca^{2+}-release channel in the SR at the triad junctions allows this tight local control. Although Ca^{2+} diffuses in the cytosol away from its SR release site, Ca^{2+} release at one site does not appear to be able to induce Ca^{2+} release from a neighboring SR Ca^{2+}-release channel. Thus, Ca^{2+} release events are not propagated along the myocyte. In fact, the SR Ca^{2+}-release channel does not appear to respond to generalized increases in cytoplasmic $[Ca^{2+}]_i$. Generalized cardiac muscle contractions occur as a result of the spatial and temporal summation of individual CICR events.

Cross-bridge cycling and termination of cardiac muscle contraction are similar to the events in skeletal muscle

Cardiac muscle is generally similar to skeletal muscle in the interaction of the actin and myosin during cross-bridge cycling, the resynthesis of ATP, and the termination of contraction. However, there are a few important differences. For example, the regulatory protein **troponin C** (Fig. 9-6) of cardiac muscle, which is of the TNNC1 subtype, has just a single, active low-affinity Ca^{2+} binding site, rather than the two high-affinity and two low-affinity sites of TNNC2 in skeletal muscle. In addition, the termination of cardiac contraction has an additional feature compared with skeletal muscle. In cardiac muscle, SR Ca^{2+} pump activity is inhibited by the regulatory protein **phospholamban**. When phospholamban is phosphorylated by cAMP-dependent protein kinase (PKA), its ability to inhibit the SR Ca^{2+} pump is lost. Thus, activators of PKA, such as the neurotransmitter epinephrine, may enhance the rate of cardiac myocyte relaxation (see Chapter 22).

In cardiac muscle, increasing the entry of Ca^{2+} enhances the contractile force

Whereas frequency summation and multiple-fiber summation are important mechanisms for regulating the strength of skeletal muscle contractions, these mechanisms would not be consistent with the physiological demands of cardiac muscle. Because cardiac muscle must contract only once with each heartbeat and must fully relax between each contraction, frequency summation is precluded. Furthermore, the extensive electrical coupling between cardiac myocytes, as well as the requirement that cardiac muscle contract homogeneously, eliminates the potential for multiple-fiber summation. Therefore, the strength of cardiac muscle contraction must be regulated by modulating the contractile force generated during each individual muscle twitch. This type of regulation is an important part of the adaptive response to exercise and is mediated by norepinephrine, a neurotransmitter released by the sympathetic nervous system.

Because an increase in $[Ca^{2+}]_i$ activates contraction by removing the inhibitory influence of the regulatory proteins, it is reasonable to consider that contractile function may be regulated either by modulating the magnitude of the rise in $[Ca^{2+}]_i$ or by altering the Ca^{2+} sensitivity of the regulatory proteins. In fact, both these mechanisms are important in controlling the force of cardiac muscle contraction.

In cardiac muscle, a significant proportion of the activator Ca^{2+} enters the cell through voltage-gated Ca^{2+} channels that open during the cardiac action potential. Most of this Ca^{2+} influx occurs through L-type Ca^{2+} channels. How does norepinephrine increase the contractile force of the heart? This hormone acts through the β-type adrenergic receptor to increase the generation of cAMP, to activate PKA (see Chapter 3), and in turn to phosphorylate the L-type Ca^{2+} channels, thereby increasing the passive influx of Ca^{2+}. An increased $[Ca^{2+}]_i$ leads to an increase in contractile force. The cAMP pathway also appears to increase the Ca^{2+} sensitivity of the contractile apparatus by phosphorylating one or more of the regulatory proteins. Thus, cAMP causes an increase in the force generated for any given $[Ca^{2+}]_i$.

Reciprocal control over Ca^{2+} entry is provided by cGMP-dependent phosphorylation of the L-type Ca^{2+} channels. ACh, acting through muscarinic ACh receptors, raises intracellular cGMP concentrations. In turn, the cGMP-dependent phosphorylation of L-type Ca^{2+} channels, at sites distinct from those phosphorylated by the cAMP-dependent kinase, causes a decrease in Ca^{2+} influx during the cardiac action potential and thus a decrease in the force of contraction.

Ca^{2+} entry may also be regulated indirectly by modulating other ion channels so that they either change their Ca^{2+} permeability or alter the duration of the action potential. Norepinephrine, for example, may increase the Ca^{2+} permeability of voltage-gated Na^+ channels. Receptor transduction mechanisms that inhibit voltage-gated K^+ currents may prolong the cardiac action potential and thereby increase net Ca^{2+} influx through L-type Ca^{2+} channels without modulating the Ca^{2+} channels themselves.

SMOOTH MUSCLE

Smooth muscles may contract in response to either neuromuscular synaptic transmission or electrical coupling

Like skeletal muscle, smooth muscle receives synaptic input from the nervous system. However, the synaptic input to smooth muscle differs from that of skeletal muscle in two ways. First, the neurons are part of the autonomic nervous system rather than the somatic nervous system (see Chapter 14). Second, the neuron makes multiple contacts with a smooth muscle cell. At each contact point, the axon diameter expands to form a series of swellings called **varicosities** that contain the presynaptic components for vesicular release of transmitter. Each varicosity is close to the postsynaptic membrane of the smooth muscle cell, but there is relatively little specialization of the postsynaptic membrane. Rather than being closely clustered at the neuromuscular junction, as in skeletal muscle, the neurotransmitter receptors in smooth muscle are spread more widely across the postsynaptic membrane.

The mechanisms of intercellular communication among smooth muscle cells are more diverse than those of skeletal or cardiac muscle. In some organs, smooth muscle is innervated in a manner similar to skeletal muscle in that each smooth muscle cell receives synaptic input. However, a difference is that a smooth muscle cell may receive input from more than one neuron. Moreover, there is little electrical coupling among these smooth muscle cells (i.e., few gap junctions). As a result, each smooth muscle cell may contract independently of its neighbor. Because this type of smooth muscle behaves like multiple, independent cells or groups of cells, it is called **multiunit smooth muscle** (Fig. 9-14A). Note that the "multi" in multiunit refers to the muscle fibers acting independently of one another as multiple units. Multiunit smooth muscles are capable of finer control. Indeed, multiunit smooth muscle is found in the iris and ciliary body of the eye, the piloerector muscles of the skin, and some blood vessels.

In contrast to multiunit smooth muscle, the smooth muscle cells of most organs have extensive intercellular communication in the manner of cardiac muscle cells. In this type of smooth muscle, gap junctions permit electrical communication between neighboring cells. This communication allows coordinated contraction of many cells. Because these cells contract as a single unit, this type of smooth muscle is called **unitary smooth muscle** (Fig. 9-14B). Unitary smooth muscle is the predominant smooth muscle type within the walls of visceral organs such as the gastrointestinal tract, the uterus, and many blood vessels. For this reason, unitary smooth muscle is often referred to as **visceral smooth muscle**. Among unitary smooth muscles, variation in the strength of intercellular coupling from organ to organ leads to variation in the spatial extent of a single unit. For example, in the bladder, extensive coupling among cells defines large functional units, which allows the muscular wall of the bladder to contract in synchrony. On the other hand, the smooth muscle cells of blood vessels couple to form smaller, independently functioning units that are more akin to multiunit smooth muscle. In fact, electrical coupling of smooth muscle units exhibits a tissue-specific continuum from multiunit to unitary coupling.

Action potentials of smooth muscles may be brief or prolonged

Whereas both skeletal muscle and cardiac muscle produce action potentials that initiate contraction, smooth muscle cells produce a wide range of V_m variations that can either initiate or modulate contraction. Action potentials that are similar to those seen in skeletal muscle are observed in unitary smooth muscle and in some multiunit muscle. Like cardiac muscle cells, some smooth muscle cells exhibit prolonged action potentials that are characterized by a prominent plateau. Still other smooth muscle cells cannot generate action potentials at all. In these cells, V_m changes in a graded fashion (see Chapter 7) rather than in the all-or-none manner of action potentials. The stimuli that produce a **graded response** of V_m include many circulating and local humoral factors as well as mechanical stimuli, such as stretching of the cell. These graded V_m changes may be either hyperpolarizing or depolarizing; they sum temporally as well as spatially. If the summation of graded depolarizations brings V_m above threshold—in a smooth muscle cell capable of producing an action potential—an action potential will then ensue.

Action potentials are usually seen in unitary (visceral) smooth muscle. These action potentials typically have a slower upstroke and longer duration (up to ~100 ms) than do skeletal muscle action potentials (~2 ms). The action potential in a smooth muscle cell can be a simple spike, a spike followed by a plateau, or a series of spikes on top of slow waves of V_m (Fig. 9-15A). In any case, the upstroke or depolarizing phase of the action potential reflects opening of voltage-gated Ca^{2+} channels. The inward Ca^{2+} current further depolarizes the cell and thereby causes still more voltage-gated Ca^{2+} channels to open. Thus, some smooth muscle cells can undergo the same type of regenerative depolarization that is seen in skeletal muscle. However, the rate of rise of the action potential in smooth muscle is lower because Ca^{2+} channels open more slowly than do Na^+ channels in skeletal and cardiac muscle (see Chapter 7). Repolarization of the smooth muscle cell is also relatively slow. Two

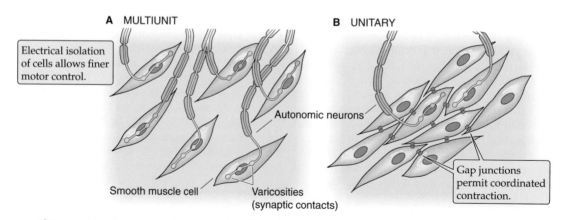

Figure 9-14 Smooth muscle organization. **A,** Each smooth muscle cell receives its own synaptic input. **B,** Only a few of the smooth muscle cells receive direct synaptic input.

A   TYPES OF SMOOTH-MUSCLE ACTION POTENTIALS

B   GENERATION OF SLOW WAVES

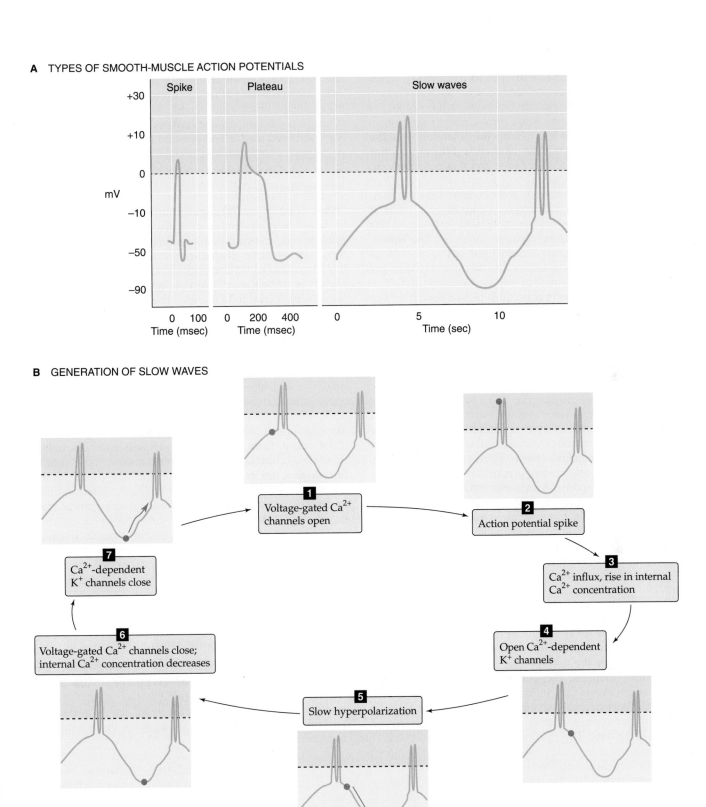

Figure 9-15   Action potentials and slow waves in smooth muscle.

explanations may be offered for this slower repolarization. First, voltage-gated Ca^{2+} channels, which are responsible for the depolarization phase of the action potential, inactivate slowly. Second, the repolarization phase of the action potential reflects the delayed activation of voltage-gated K^+ channels and, in some cases, Ca^{2+}-activated K^+ channels.

Some smooth muscle cells have fast, voltage-gated Na^+ channels. However, even when these channels are present, they do not appear to be necessary for generating an action potential. Their main role may be to allow more rapid activation of voltage-gated Ca^{2+} channels and thus contribute to a faster rate of depolarization.

In some unitary smooth muscle, repolarization is so delayed that the action potential contour displays a prominent plateau. These plateau potentials may be several hundred milliseconds in duration, as in cardiac muscle. Plateau action potentials occur in smooth muscle of the genitourinary tract, including the ureters, bladder, and uterus. The long V_m plateau allows the entry of Ca^{2+} to continue for a longer period and thus allows $[Ca^{2+}]_i$ to remain high for a longer period, thereby prolonging the contraction.

Some smooth muscle cells can initiate spontaneous electrical activity

Although smooth muscle cells undergo changes in V_m in response to neural, hormonal, or mechanical stimulation, many smooth muscle cells are capable of initiating spontaneous electrical activity. In some cells, this spontaneous activity results from pacemaker currents. These currents result from time- and voltage-dependent properties of ion currents that produce either a spontaneous increase in inward, or depolarizing, currents (e.g., voltage-gated Ca^{2+} currents) or a spontaneous decrease in outward, or hyperpolarizing, currents (e.g., voltage-gated K^+ currents). The pacemaker currents cause the cell to depolarize until V_m reaches threshold, triggering an action potential.

In other smooth muscle cells, this spontaneous electrical activity results in regular, repetitive oscillations in V_m. These V_m oscillations occur at a frequency of several oscillations per minute and are referred to as **slow waves** (Fig. 9-15B). One hypothesis for the origin of slow-wave potentials suggests that voltage-gated Ca^{2+} channels—active at the resting V_m—depolarize the cell enough to activate more voltage-gated Ca^{2+} channels. This activation results in progressive depolarization and Ca^{2+} influx. The increase in $[Ca^{2+}]_i$ activates Ca^{2+}-dependent K^+ channels, which leads to progressive hyperpolarization and termination of the depolarization phase of the wave. These periodic depolarizations and $[Ca^{2+}]_i$ increases cause periodic, tonic contractions of the smooth muscle. When the amplitude of the slow V_m waves is sufficient to depolarize the cell to threshold, the ensuing action potentials lead to further Ca^{2+} influx and phasic contractions.

Other hypotheses to explain spontaneous electrical and mechanical activity in smooth muscle cells are based on oscillatory changes in other intracellular ions or molecules. For example, increased $[Ca^{2+}]_i$ during an action potential might stimulate Na-Ca exchange and lead to a cyclic increase in $[Na^+]_i$ and thus an increase in the rate of Na^+ extrusion by the electrogenic Na-K pump. Alternatively, the inositol 1,4,5-trisphosphate (IP_3) receptor channel (see Chapter 3) might spontaneously open and release Ca^{2+}. The effect on $[Ca^{2+}]_i$ would be self-reinforcing because of Ca^{2+}-activated Ca^{2+} release through the IP_3 receptor. At high $[Ca^{2+}]_i$, this channel is inhibited and the Ca^{2+} release event is terminated, followed by re-uptake of Ca^{2+} into the SR. The $[Ca^{2+}]_i$ increases may themselves lead to periodic electrical activity by stimulating Ca^{2+}-activated inward and outward currents.

Some smooth muscles contract without action potentials

Whereas action potential generation is essential for initiating contraction of skeletal and cardiac muscle, many smooth muscle cells contract despite being unable to generate an action potential. As discussed previously, V_m oscillations can lead to tonic contractions in the absence of action potentials. Action potentials usually do not occur in **multiunit** smooth muscle. For example, in the smooth muscle that regulates the iris, excitatory neurotransmitters such as norepinephrine and ACh cause a local depolarization, the **junctional potential**, which is similar to the end-plate potential in skeletal muscle. Junctional potentials spread electrotonically (i.e., in a graded fashion) throughout the muscle fiber, thereby altering V_m and triggering the entry of Ca^{2+} through voltage-gated slow (L-type) Ca^{2+} channels. Changes in V_m—by an unknown mechanism—may also modulate the activity of the enzyme phospholipase C, which cleaves phosphoinositides to release the intracellular second messengers diacylglycerol (DAG) and IP_3 (see Chapter 3). Both these second messengers are modulators of contractile force. In the absence of action potentials, some unitary smooth muscle, including some vascular smooth muscle, also contracts as a result of graded V_m changes.

Some smooth muscle cells contract without any change in V_m. For example, a neurotransmitter can bind to a receptor, activate a G protein, and lead to the generation of IP_3, which in turn leads to the release of Ca^{2+} from the SR.

In smooth muscle, both extracellular and intracellular Ca^{2+} activate contraction

Smooth muscle cells use three major pathways—which are not mutually exclusive—for producing the rise in $[Ca^{2+}]_i$ that triggers contraction (Fig. 9-16): (1) Ca^{2+} entry through voltage-gated channels in response to cell depolarization, (2) Ca^{2+} release from the SR, and (3) Ca^{2+} entry through voltage-independent channels.

Ca^{2+} Entry Through Voltage-Gated Channels Smooth muscle cells respond to stimulation with graded depolarizations or action potentials. In either case, depolarization may produce an influx of Ca^{2+} through voltage-gated L-type Ca^{2+} channels.

Ca^{2+} Release from the SR Sarcoplasmic Ca^{2+} release may occur by either of two mechanisms: Ca^{2+}-induced Ca^{2+} release or IP_3-mediated Ca^{2+} release. As we have already seen, CICR plays a key role in EC coupling in cardiac muscle, in

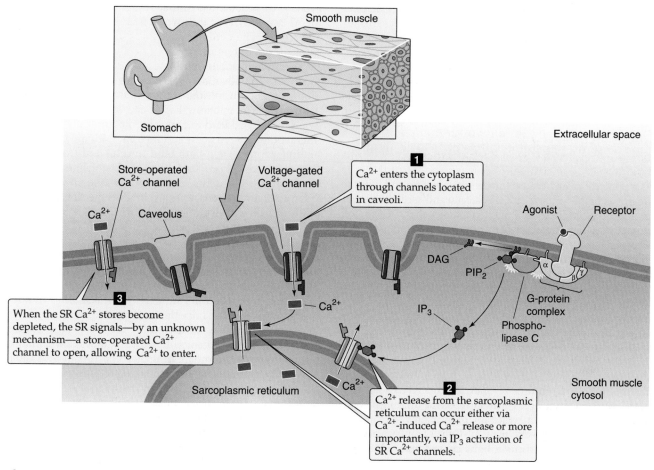

Figure 9-16 EC coupling in smooth muscle.

which the L-type Ca^{2+} channels are highly ordered and close to the Ca^{2+}-release channels in the SR. Thus, Ca^{2+} influx through L-type Ca^{2+} channels can trigger CICR. In smooth muscle, the relationship between the plasma membrane and the SR is not as regularly organized as it is in striated muscle. Nevertheless, electron-dense couplings have been observed bridging the 8- to 10-nm gap between the cell membranes and elements of the SR in smooth muscle. Although CICR occurs in smooth muscle cells under some conditions, it requires $[Ca^{2+}]_i$ levels that are higher than those that typically occur under physiological conditions, and its role remains unclear.

A more important mechanism for Ca^{2+} release from the SR of smooth muscle is the IP_3 pathway. The existence of this pathway is supported by the observation that some extracellular agonists can elicit smooth muscle contraction with minimal depolarization and negligible Ca^{2+} influx. Furthermore, even for agonists such as serotonin and norepinephrine, which activate a Ca^{2+}-influx pathway, the observed increase in $[Ca^{2+}]_i$ is out of proportion to that expected from Ca^{2+} influx alone. Thus, another pathway must exist for increasing $[Ca^{2+}]_i$. Some agonists cause smooth muscle contraction by triggering the production of IP_3, which binds to a specific receptor on the membrane of the smooth muscle SR (see Chapter 3). The IP_3 receptor is a ligand-gated Ca^{2+}

channel. Thus, a receptor in the plasma membrane can—via IP_3—indirectly induce Ca^{2+} release from the SR and hence contraction.

Ca^{2+} Entry Through Voltage-Independent Channels We have just noted that extracellular ligands binding to G-protein–coupled receptors can lead to the release of Ca^{2+} from the SR. The eventual depletion of Ca^{2+} stores in the SR somehow leads to the activation of **store-operated Ca^{2+} channels (SOCs)**, which mediate Ca^{2+} influx across the cell membrane. The Ca^{2+} entering through these channels allows $[Ca^{2+}]_i$ to remain elevated even after SR depletion and also appears to replenish SR Ca^{2+} stores. SOCs play an important role in a variety of cell types. In lymphocytes—although perhaps not in smooth muscle—a fall in $[Ca^{2+}]$ inside the endoplasmic reticulum (ER) activates a protein called STIM1 in the ER membrane (see Fig. 6-21T). STIM1, by direct mechanical linkage, then activates a plasma-membrane Ca^{2+} channel called Orai, which in turn mediates an uptake of Ca^{2+}. Electrophysiologists refer to the Ca^{2+}-release–activated Ca^{2+} current as I_{CRAC}. Missense mutations in the human Orai1 gene eliminate I_{CRAC} in lymphocytes—where I_{CRAC} plays a vital role in lymphocyte activation—and result in a severe combined immunodeficiency syndrome (SCID).

Both the Ca^{2+} release from the SR and the entry of Ca^{2+} via SOCs are voltage *independent*. These two mechanisms provide the Ca^{2+} that underlies one form of **pharmaco-mechanical coupling**. Thus, drugs, excitatory neurotransmitters, and hormones can induce smooth muscle contraction that is independent of action-potential generation, as discussed in the previous section.

The cross-bridge cycle in smooth muscle is controlled by phosphorylation of myosin light chain by myosin light chain kinase

As we noted earlier, because smooth muscle actin and myosin are not as highly organized as in skeletal and cardiac muscle, smooth muscle does not exhibit striations characteristic of striated muscle. The actin filaments of smooth muscle are oriented mainly parallel or oblique to the long axis of the cell. Multiple actin filaments appear to join at specialized locations in the cell called **dense bodies**. Dense bodies are found immediately beneath the cell membrane as well as within the interior of the myocyte. Thick filaments are interspersed among the thin filaments in smooth muscle and are far less abundant than in skeletal or cardiac muscle.

In comparison to skeletal and cardiac muscle, an entirely different mechanism controls cross-bridge turnover in smooth muscle. Here, an increase in $[Ca^{2+}]_i$ initiates a slow chain of events that ultimately increases the ATPase activity of the myosin (Fig. 9-17). The first step is the binding of four Ca^{2+} ions to **calmodulin**, which is closely related to troponin C of striated muscle. Next, the Ca^{2+}-CaM complex activates an enzyme known as **myosin light chain kinase (MLCK)**, which in turn phosphorylates the regulatory light chain that is associated with the myosin II molecule. Phosphorylation of the light chain alters the conformation of the myosin head, which greatly increases its ATPase activity and allows it to interact with actin and to act as a molecular motor. Thus, in smooth muscle, CaM rather than troponin C is the Ca^{2+}-binding protein responsible for transducing the contraction-triggering increases in $[Ca^{2+}]_i$. Note that in smooth muscle, contraction cannot begin until MLCK increases the ATPase activity of myosin, which is a time-consuming process. In skeletal and cardiac muscle, on the other hand, the ATPase activity of the myosin head is constitutively high, and cross-bridge cycling can begin as soon as the tropomyosin is moved out of the way.

The mechanism just outlined activates the *thick* filaments in smooth muscle. Other mechanisms act on the thin filaments of smooth muscle to remove the tonic inhibition to actin-myosin interactions that are caused by steric hindrance. Two proteins, caldesmon and calponin, tonically inhibit the interaction between actin and myosin. Both are Ca^{2+}-CaM–binding proteins, and both bind to actin and tropomyosin. **Calponin**, which is found in a fixed stoichiometry with tropomyosin and actin (one calponin–one tropomyosin–seven actin monomers), tonically inhibits the ATPase activity of myosin. As we saw earlier, the increase in $[Ca^{2+}]_i$ that triggers smooth muscle contraction activates Ca^{2+}-CaM. Besides activating MLCK, this Ca^{2+}-CaM complex has two effects on calponin. First, Ca^{2+}-CaM binds to calponin. Second, Ca^{2+}-CaM activates Ca^{2+}-CaM–dependent protein kinase, which phosphorylates calponin. Both effects reduce calponin's inhibition of myosin's ATPase activity. **Caldesmon** is another regulatory protein of smooth muscle that appears to act like calponin by tonically inhibiting the actin-activated ATPase activity of myosin in smooth muscle. Caldesmon contains binding domains for actin, myosin, tropomyosin, and Ca^{2+}-CaM. It appears to block the interaction of actin with myosin; however, the exact mechanism is controversial.

Although the steps of cross-bridge cycling in smooth muscle are similar to those in skeletal and cardiac muscle (Fig. 9-7), smooth muscle controls the initiation of the cross-bridge cycle differently—at step 2 in Figure 9-7, where Ca^{2+} confers ATPase activity to the myosin head, as discussed before. Recall that the ATPase activity of striated muscle is always high and Ca^{2+} regulates the access of the myosin head to the actin. Another difference between smooth and striated muscle is that the frequency of cross-bridge cycling in smooth muscle is less than one tenth that in skeletal muscle. This variation reflects differences in the properties of myosin isoforms that are expressed in various cell types. Even though cross-bridge cycling occurs less frequently in smooth muscle, force generation may be as great or greater, perhaps because

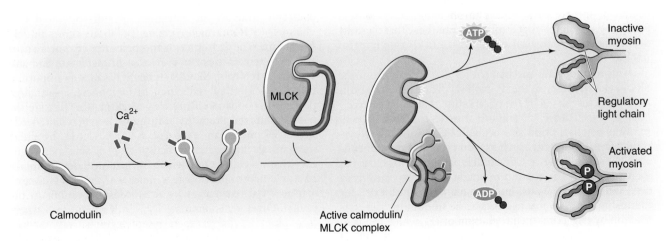

Figure 9-17 The role of Ca^{2+} in triggering the contraction of smooth muscle.

the cross-bridges remain intact for a longer period with each cycle. It is likely that this longer period during which the cross-bridges are intact reflects a lower rate of ADP release from the smooth muscle isoform of myosin.

Termination of smooth muscle contraction requires dephosphorylation of myosin light chain

Because Ca^{2+} triggers smooth muscle contraction by inducing phosphorylation of the myosin regulatory light chain, merely restoring $[Ca^{2+}]_i$ to its low resting value may not allow muscle relaxation. Rather, relaxation of smooth muscle requires myosin light chain (MLC) dephosphorylation, which is accomplished by **myosin light chain phosphatase**. This phosphatase is a heterotrimer consisting of subunits with molecular masses of 130, 20, and 37 kDa. The 130-kDa subunit confers specificity by binding to myosin; the 37-kDa protein is the catalytic subunit responsible for the dephosphorylating activity.

Smooth muscle contraction may also occur independently of increases in $[Ca^{2+}]_i$

Whereas many excitatory stimuli rely on increases in $[Ca^{2+}]_i$ to evoke contraction, some stimuli appear to cause contraction without a measurable increase in $[Ca^{2+}]_i$. One mechanism by which excitatory stimuli might induce Ca^{2+}-independent contractions is by modulating the activity of contractile or regulatory proteins directly. Thus, the amount of force developed at any given $[Ca^{2+}]_i$ may vary. This force/$[Ca^{2+}]_i$ ratio may be increased or decreased and is generally higher during pharmacomechanical activation than during depolarization-activated contractions. Because phosphorylation of the MLC is a major determinant of contractile force in smooth muscle, Ca^{2+}-independent contractions may result either from an increase in the rate of MLC phosphorylation by MLCK or from a decrease in the rate of MLC dephosphorylation by MLC phosphatase. One second-messenger system that can decrease the activity of phosphatases is protein kinase C (PKC; see Chapter 3). Some excitatory stimuli are therefore capable of initiating smooth muscle contraction by inducing IP_3-mediated release of Ca^{2+} from intracellular stores as well as by producing PKC-mediated decreases in MLC phosphatase activity. These pathways are further examples of **pharmacomechanical coupling**.

In smooth muscle, contractile force is enhanced by increasing the entry of Ca^{2+} as well as by increasing the Ca^{2+} sensitivity of the contractile apparatus

Unlike skeletal muscle, in which force development results from the summation of individual muscle *twitches*, individual smooth muscle cells can maintain a sustained contraction that can be graded in strength over a wide range. Contractile force in smooth muscle largely depends on the relative balance between the phosphorylation and dephosphorylation of MLCs. The rate of MLC phosphorylation is regulated by the Ca^{2+}-CaM complex, which in turn depends

on *levels of intracellular Ca^{2+}*. Smooth muscle cells can regulate $[Ca^{2+}]_i$ over a wider range than in skeletal and cardiac muscle for several reasons. First, some smooth muscle cells do not generate action potentials. Rather, their membrane potential varies slowly in response to neurotransmitters or hormones. This graded response of V_m allows finer regulation of Ca^{2+} influx through voltage-gated channels. Second, release of Ca^{2+} from intracellular stores may be modulated through neurotransmitter-induced generation of intracellular second messengers such as IP_3. This modulation allows finer control of Ca^{2+} release than occurs in the SR Ca^{2+}-release channel by L-type Ca^{2+} channels in skeletal and cardiac muscle.

A second level of control over contractile force occurs by regulating the *Ca^{2+} sensitivity* of proteins that regulate contraction. For example, inhibiting *myosin light chain phosphatase* alters the balance between phosphorylation and dephosphorylation, in effect allowing a greater contraction at a lower $[Ca^{2+}]_i$. Some neurotransmitters act by inhibiting the phosphatase, which appears to occur through activation of G-protein–coupled receptors. Another mechanism for governing the Ca^{2+} sensitivity of proteins that regulate contraction is alteration of the Ca^{2+} sensitivity of the *myosin light chain kinase*. For example, MLCK itself is phosphorylated at specific sites by several protein kinases, including PKA, PKC, and Ca^{2+}-CaM–dependent kinases. Phosphorylation by any of these kinases decreases the sensitivity of MLCK to activation by the Ca^{2+}-CaM complex.

Smooth muscle maintains high force at low energy consumption

Smooth muscle is often called on to maintain high force for long periods. If smooth muscle consumed ATP at rates similar to striated muscle, metabolic demands would be considerable and the muscle would be prone to fatigue. Unlike striated muscle, however, smooth muscle is able to maintain high force at a low rate of ATP hydrolysis. This low-energy consumption/high-tension state is referred to as the **latch state**. The latch state in smooth muscle is unique because high tension can be maintained despite a decrease in the degree of muscle activation by excitatory stimuli. As a result, force is maintained at a lower level of MLCK phosphorylation.

The mechanism underlying the latch state is not entirely known, although it appears to be due in large part to changes in the kinetics of actin-myosin cross-bridge formation and detachment. These changes may be a direct result of a decrease in the rate at which dephosphorylated cross-bridges detach. Tension is directly related to the number of attached cross-bridges. Furthermore, the proportion of myosin heads cross-bridged to actin is related to the ratio of attachment rates to detachment rates. Therefore, it is reasonable to expect that a decrease in the detachment rate would allow a greater number of cross-bridges to be maintained and would result in a lower rate of cross-bridge cycling and ATP hydrolysis. Thus, smooth muscle appears to be able to slow down cross-bridge cycling just before detachment, a feat that can be accomplished in skeletal muscle (Fig. 9-7) only at low ATP levels (as in *rigor mortis*).

TABLE 9-1   Isoform Expression of Contractile and Regulatory Proteins

	Skeletal Slow (I)	Skeletal Fast Oxidative (IIa)	Skeletal Fast Fatigable (IIb)	Cardiac	Smooth
Myosin heavy chain	MHC-I	MHC-IIa	MHC-IIb, -IIx	αMHC and βMHC	MHC-SM1, -SM2 (multiple isoforms)
Myosin light chain	MLC-1aS, -1bS	MLC-1f, -3f	MLC-1f, -3f	MLC-1v, -1a	MLC-17a, -17b
SR Ca^{2+}-ATPase	SERCA2a	SERCA1	SERCA1	SERCA2a	SERCA2a, 2b (b > > > a)
Phospholamban	Present	Absent	Absent	Present	Present
Calsequestrin	"Fast" and "cardiac"	"Fast"	"Fast"	"Cardiac"	? "Cardiac" ? "Fast"
Ca^{2+} release mechanisms	RYR1 (Ca^{2+}-release channel or "ryanodine" receptor)	RYR1	RYR1	RYR2	IP_3R (3 isoforms) RYR3
Ca^{2+} sensor	Troponin C_1 (TNNC1)	Troponin C_2 (TNNC2)	Troponin C_2 (TNNC2)	Troponin C_1 (TNNC1)	Calmodulin (multiple isoforms)

DIVERSITY AMONG MUSCLES

As we have seen, each muscle type (skeletal, cardiac, and smooth) is distinguishable on the basis of its unique histology, EC coupling mechanisms, and regulation of contractile function. However, even within each of the three categories, muscle in different locations must serve markedly different purposes, with different demands for strength, speed, and fatigability. This diversity is possible because of differences in the expression of specific isoforms for various contractile and regulatory proteins (Table 9-1).

Skeletal muscle is composed of slow-twitch and fast-twitch fibers

Some skeletal muscles must be resistant to fatigue and be able to maintain tension for relatively long periods, although they need not contract rapidly. Examples are muscles that maintain body posture, such as the soleus muscle of the lower part of the leg. In contrast, some muscles need to contract rapidly, yet infrequently. Examples are the extraocular muscles, which must contract rapidly to redirect the eye as an object of visual interest moves about.

Individual muscle fibers are classified as *slow twitch (type I)* or *fast twitch (type II)*, depending on their rate of force development. These fiber types are also distinguished by their histologic appearance and their ability to resist fatigue.

Slow-twitch fibers (Table 9-2) are generally thinner and have a denser capillary network surrounding them. These **type I** fibers also appear red because of a large amount of the oxygen-binding protein **myoglobin** (see Chapter 29) within the cytoplasm. This rich capillary network together with myoglobin facilitates oxygen transport to the slow-twitch fibers, which mostly rely on oxidative metabolism for

energy. The metabolic machinery of the slow-twitch fiber also favors oxidative metabolism because it has low glycogen content and glycolytic enzyme activity but a rich mitochondrial and oxidative enzyme content. Oxidative metabolism is slow but efficient, making these fibers resistant to fatigue.

Fast-twitch fibers differ among themselves with respect to fatigability. Some fast-twitch fibers are fatigue resistant; they rely on oxidative metabolism (**type IIa**) and are quite similar to slow-twitch fibers with respect to myoglobin content (indeed, they are red) and metabolic machinery. One important difference is that fast-twitch oxidative fibers contain abundant glycogen and have a greater number of mitochondria than slow-twitch fibers do. These features ensure adequate ATP generation to compensate for the increased rate of ATP hydrolysis in fast-twitch fibers.

Other fast-twitch fibers are not capable of sufficient oxidative metabolism to sustain contraction. Because these fibers must rely on the energy that is stored within glycogen (and phosphocreatine), they are more easily fatigable. Fatigable fast-twitch fibers (**type IIb**) have fewer mitochondria and lower concentrations of myoglobin and oxidative enzymes. Because of their low myoglobin content, type IIb muscle fibers are white. They are, however, richer in glycolytic enzyme activity than other fiber types are.

In reality, slow- and fast-twitch fibers represent the extremes of a continuum of muscle fiber characteristics. Moreover, each whole muscle is composed of fibers of each twitch type, although one of the fiber types predominates in any given muscle. The differences between fiber types derive in large part from differences in isoform expression of the various contractile and regulatory proteins (Table 9-1).

Differences in the rate of contraction, for example, may be directly correlated with the maximal rate of myosin ATPase activity. The human genome database lists at least 15 MHC genes, with their respective splice variants. Individual isoform expression varies among muscle types and is devel-

TABLE 9-2 Properties of Fast- and Slow-Twitch Muscle Fibers

	Slow Twitch	Fast Twitch	Fast Twitch
Synonym	Type I	Type IIa	Type IIb
Fatigue	Resistant	Resistant	Fatigable
Color	Red (myoglobin)	Red (myoglobin)	White (low myoglobin)
Metabolism	Oxidative	Oxidative	Glycolytic
Mitochondria	High	Higher	Fewer
Glycogen	Low	Abundant	High

opmentally regulated. At least four isoforms of the MHC protein are expressed in skeletal muscle (MHC-I, MHC-IIa, MHC-IIb, MHC-IIx/d). For the most part, a muscle fiber type expresses a single MHC isoform, the ATPase activity of which appears to correspond to the rate of contraction in that fiber type. Whereas most fibers express one of these isoforms, some fibers express a combination of two different isoforms. These hybrid cells have rates of contraction that are intermediate between the two pure fiber types.

Differences in the rates and strength of contraction may also result from differences in **myosin light chain** isoform expression or from isoform differences among other components of the EC coupling process. Three skeletal muscle isoforms have been identified. MLC-1as and MLC-1bs are expressed in slow-twitch fibers, whereas MLC-1f and MLC-3f are expressed in fast-twitch fibers.

Isoform differences also exist for the **SR Ca^{2+} pump** (i.e., the SERCA), calsequestrin, the Ca^{2+}-release channel, and troponin C. Furthermore, some proteins, such as phospholamban, are expressed in one fiber type (slow twitch) and not the other.

One particularly interesting feature of muscle differentiation is that fiber-type determination is not static. Through exercise training or changes in patterns of neuronal stimulation, alterations in contractile and regulatory protein isoform expression may occur. For example, it is possible for a greater proportion of fast-twitch fibers to develop in a specific muscle with repetitive training. It is even possible to induce cardiac-specific isoforms in skeletal muscle, given appropriate stimulation patterns.

The properties of cardiac cells vary with location in the heart

Just as skeletal muscle consists of multiple fiber types, so too does heart muscle. The electrophysiological and mechanical properties of cardiac muscle vary with their location (i.e., atria versus conducting system versus ventricle). Moreover, even among cells within one anatomical location, functional differences may exist between muscle cells near the surface of the heart (*epicardial cells*) and those lining the interior of the same chambers (*endocardial cells*). As in skeletal muscle, many of these differences reflect differences in isoform

expression of the various contractile and regulatory proteins. Although some of the protein isoforms expressed in cardiac tissue are identical to those expressed in skeletal muscle, many of the proteins have cardiac-specific isoforms (Table 9-1). The MHC in heart, for example, exists in two isoforms, α and β, which may be expressed alone or in combination.

Smooth muscle cells may differ markedly among tissues and may adapt their properties with time even in a single tissue

When one considers that smooth muscle has a broad range of functions, including regulating the diameter of blood vessels, propelling food through the gastrointestinal tract, regulating the diameter of airways, and delivering a newborn infant from the uterus, it is not surprising that smooth muscle is a particularly diverse type of muscle. In addition to being distinguished as unitary or multiunit muscle, smooth muscle in different organs diverges with respect to nerve and hormonal control, electrical activity, and characteristics of contraction.

Even among smooth muscle cells within the same sort of tissue, important functional differences may exist. For example, vascular smooth muscle cells within the walls of two arterioles that perfuse different organs may vary in their contractile response to various stimuli. Differences may even exist between vascular smooth muscle cells at two different points along one arterial pathway.

The phenotype of smooth muscle within a given organ may change with shifting demands. The uterus, for example, is composed of smooth muscle—the myometrium—that undergoes remarkable transformation during gestation as it prepares for parturition (see Chapter 56). In addition to hypertrophy, greater coupling develops between smooth muscle cells through the increased formation of gap junctions. The cells also undergo changes in their expression of contractile protein isoforms. Changes in the expression of ion channels and hormone receptors facilitate rhythmic electrical activity. This activity is coordinated across the myometrium by propagation of action potentials and increases in $[Ca^{2+}]_i$ through the gap junctions. These rhythmic, coordinated contractions develop spontaneously, but they are strongly influenced by the hormone oxytocin, levels of which increase just before and during labor and just after parturition.

These differences in smooth muscle function among various tissues or even over the lifetime of a single cell probably reflect differences in protein composition. Indeed, in comparison to striated muscle, smooth muscle cells express a wider variety of isoforms of contractile and regulatory proteins (Table 9-1). This variety is a result of both multiple genes and alternative splicing (see Chapter 4). This richness in diversity is likely to have important consequences for smooth muscle cell function, although the precise relationship between the structure and function of these protein isoforms is not yet clear.

Smooth muscle cells express a wide variety of neurotransmitter and hormone receptors

Perhaps one of the most impressive sources of diversity among smooth muscle cells relates to differences in response to neurotransmitters, environmental factors, and circulating hormones. Smooth muscle cells differ widely with respect to the types of cell surface receptors that mediate the effects of these various mediators. In general, smooth muscle cells each express a variety of such receptors, and receptor stimulation may lead to either contraction or relaxation. Many substances act through different receptor subtypes in different cells, and these receptor subtypes may act through different mechanisms. For example, whereas some neurotransmitter/hormone receptors may be ligand-gated ion channels, others act through heterotrimeric G proteins that either act directly on targets or act through intracellular second messengers such as cAMP, cGMP, or IP_3 and DAG.

The list of neurotransmitters, hormones, and environmental factors regulating the function of vascular smooth muscle cells alone is vast (see Chapter 23). A few of these vasoactive substances include epinephrine, norepinephrine, serotonin, angiotensin, vasopressin, neuropeptide Y, nitric oxide, endothelin, and oxygen. Identical stimuli, however, may result in remarkably different physiological responses by smooth muscle in different locations. For example, systemic arterial smooth muscle cells relax when the oxygen concentration around them decreases, whereas pulmonary arterial smooth muscle contracts when local oxygen decreases (see Chapter 31).

A summary comparison between muscle types is presented in Table 9-3.

TABLE 9-3 Summary of Comparisons Between Muscle Types

	Skeletal	Cardiac	Smooth
Mechanism of excitation	Neuromuscular transmission	Pacemaker potentials Electrotonic depolarization through gap junctions	Synaptic transmission Hormone-activated receptors Electrical coupling Pacemaker potentials
Electrical activity of muscle cell	Action potential spikes	Action potential plateaus	Action potential spikes, plateaus Graded membrane potential changes Slow waves
Ca^{2+} sensor	Troponin	Troponin	Calmodulin
Excitation-contraction coupling	L-type Ca^{2+} channel (DHP receptor) in T-tubule membrane coupling to Ca^{2+}-release channel (ryanodine receptor) in SR	Ca^{2+} entry through L-type Ca^{2+} channel (DHP receptor) triggers Ca^{2+}-induced Ca^{2+} release from SR	Ca^{2+} entry through voltage-gated Ca^{2+} channels Ca^{2+}- and IP_3-mediated Ca^{2+} release from SR Ca^{2+} entry through store-operated Ca^{2+} channels
Terminates contraction	Breakdown of ACh by acetylcholinesterase	Action potential repolarization	Myosin light chain phosphatase
Twitch duration	20-200 ms	200-400 ms	200 ms—sustained
Regulation of force	Frequency and multifiber summation	Regulation of calcium entry	Balance between MLCK phosphorylation and dephosphorylation Latch state
Metabolism	Oxidative, glycolytic	Oxidative	Oxidative

REFERENCES

Books and Reviews

Farah CS, Reinach FC: The troponin complex and regulation of muscle contraction. FASEB J 1995; 9:755-767.

Franzini-Armstrong C, Protasi F: Ryanodine receptors of striated muscles: A complex channel capable of multiple interactions. Physiol Rev 1997; 77:699-729.

Holda J, Klishin A, Sedova M, et al: Capacitative calcium entry. News Physiol Sci 1998; 13:157-163.

Horowitz A, Menice CB, Laporte R, Morgan KG: Mechanisms of smooth muscle contraction. Physiol Rev 1996; 76:967-1003.

Parekh AB, Penner R: Store depletion and calcium influx. Physiol Rev 1997; 77:901-930.

Striggow F, Ehrlich BE: Ligand-gated calcium channels inside and out. Curr Opin Cell Biol 1996; 8:490-495.

Journal Articles

Cannell MB, Cheng H, Lederer WJ: The control of calcium release in heart muscle. Science 1995; 268:1045-1049.

Finer JT, Simmons RM, Spudich JA: Single myosin molecule mechanics: Piconewton forces and nanometre steps. Nature 1994; 368:113-119.

Gordon AM, Huxley AF, Julian FJ: The variation in isometric tension with sarcomere length in vertebrate muscle. J Physiol 1966; 184:170-192.

Mickelson JR, Louis CF: Malignant hyperthermia: Excitation-contraction coupling, Ca^{2+}-release channel, and cell Ca^{2+} regulation defects. Physiol Rev 1996; 76:537-592.

THE NERVOUS SYSTEM

CHAPTER 10

ORGANIZATION OF THE NERVOUS SYSTEM

Bruce R. Ransom

The human brain is the most complex tissue in the body. It mediates behavior ranging from simple movements and sensory perception to learning and memory. It is the organ of the mind. Many of the brain's functions are poorly understood. In fact, the most prominent function of the human brain, its capacity to think, is hardly understood at all. Our lack of knowledge about fundamental aspects of brain function stands in marked contrast to the level of comprehension that we have about the primary functions of other organ systems, such as the heart, lungs, and kidneys. Nevertheless, tremendous strides have been made in the past few decades. While philosophers ponder the paradox of a person thinking about thinking, physiologists are trying to learn about learning.

In this part of the book, we present the physiology of the nervous system in a manner that is intended to be complementary to texts on neurobiology and neuroanatomy. In this chapter, we review the basic cellular, developmental, and gross anatomy of the nervous system. In Chapter 11, we discuss the fluid environment of the neurons in the brain, how this environment interacts with the rest of the extracellular fluid of the body, and the role of glial cells. Chapters 12 and 13 focus on the broad physiological principles that underlie how the brain's cellular elements operate. Another major goal of this section is to provide more detailed information on those parts of the nervous system that play key roles in the physiology of other systems in the body. Thus, in Chapter 14, we discuss the autonomic nervous system, which controls "viscera" such as the heart, lungs, and gastrointestinal tract. Finally, in Chapters 15 and 16, we discuss the special senses and simple neuronal circuits.

The nervous system can be divided into central, peripheral, and autonomic nervous systems

The manner in which the nervous system is subdivided is somewhat arbitrary. All elements of the nervous system work closely together in a way that has no clear boundaries. Nevertheless, the traditional definitions of the subdivisions provide a useful framework for talking about the brain and its connections and are important if only for that reason.

The **central nervous system (CNS)** consists of the brain and spinal cord (Table 10-1). It is covered by three "membranes"—the meninges. The outer membrane is the dura mater; the middle is the arachnoid; and the delicate inner membrane is called the pia mater. Within the CNS, some neurons that share similar functions are grouped into aggregations called **nuclei**.

The **peripheral nervous system (PNS)** consists of those parts of the nervous system that lie outside the dura mater (Table 10-1). These elements include sensory receptors for various kinds of stimuli, the peripheral portions of spinal and cranial nerves, and all the peripheral portions of the autonomic nervous system (see the next paragraph). The **sensory** nerves that carry messages from the periphery to the CNS are termed **afferent nerves** (Latin, *ad + ferens,* or carrying toward). Conversely, the peripheral **motor** nerves that carry messages from the CNS to peripheral tissues are called **efferent nerves** (Latin, *ex + ferens,* or carrying away). **Peripheral ganglia** are groups of nerve cells concentrated into small knots or clumps that are located outside the CNS.

The **autonomic nervous system (ANS)** is that portion of the nervous system that regulates and controls visceral functions, including heart rate, blood pressure, digestion, temperature regulation, and reproductive function. Although the ANS is a functionally distinct system, it is anatomically composed of parts of the CNS and PNS (Table 10-1). Visceral control is achieved by reflex arcs that consist of visceral afferent (i.e., sensory) neurons that send messages from the periphery to the CNS, control centers in the CNS that receive this input, and visceral motor output. Moreover, visceral afferent fibers typically travel together with visceral efferent fibers.

Each area of the nervous system has unique nerve cells and a different function

Nervous tissue is composed of neurons and neuroglial cells. **Neurons** vary greatly in their structure throughout the nervous system, but they all share certain features that tailor them for the unique purpose of electrical communication (see Chapter 12). Neuroglial cells, often simply called **glia**, are not primary signaling cells and have variable structures that are suited for their diverse functions (see Chapter 11).

The human brain contains $\sim 10^{11}$ neurons and several times as many glial cells. Each of these neurons may interact

TABLE 10-1 Subdivisions of the Nervous System

Subdivision	Components	Special Features
Central	Brain (including CN II and retina) and spinal cord	Oligodendrocytes provide myelin Axons cannot regenerate
Peripheral	Peripheral ganglia (including cell bodies); sensory receptors; peripheral portions of spinal and cranial nerves (except CN II), both afferent and efferent	Schwann cells provide myelin Axons can regenerate
Autonomic	Selected portions of the CNS and PNS	Functionally distinct system

CN, cranial nerve.

with thousands of other neurons, which helps explain the awesome complexity of the nervous system.

No evidence suggests that the human brain contains receptors, ion channels, or cells that are unique to humans and not seen in other mammals. The unparalleled capabilities of the human brain are presumed to result from its unique patterns of connectivity and its large size.

The brain's diverse functions are the result of tremendous regional specialization. Different brain areas are composed of neurons that have special shapes, physiological properties, and connections. One part of the brain, therefore, cannot substitute functionally for another part that has failed. Any compensation of neural function by a patient with a brain lesion (e.g., a stroke) reflects enhancement of existing circuits or recruitment of latent circuits. A corollary is that damage to a specific part of the brain causes predictable symptoms that can enable a clinician to establish the anatomical location of the problem, a key step in diagnosis of neurological diseases.

CELLS OF THE NERVOUS SYSTEM

The neuron doctrine first asserted that the nervous system is composed of many individual signaling units—the neurons

In 1838, Schleiden and Schwann proposed that the nucleated cell is the fundamental unit of structure and function in both plants and animals. They reached this conclusion by microscopic observation of plant and animal tissues that had been stained to reveal their cellular composition. However, the brain proved to be more difficult to stain than other tissues, and until 1885, when Camillo Golgi introduced his silver impregnation method, "the black reaction," there was no clear indication that the brain is composed of individual cells. The histologist Santiago Ramón y Cajal worked relent-

lessly with the silver-staining method and eventually concluded that not only is nervous tissue composed of individual cells but the anatomy of these cells also confers a functional polarization to the passage of nervous signals; the tapering branches near the cell body are the receptive end of the cell, and the long-axis cylinder conveys signals away from the cell. In the absence of any reliable physiological evidence, Cajal was nevertheless able to correctly anticipate how complex cell aggregates in the brain communicate with each other.

The pathologist Heinrich von Waldeyer referred to the individual cells in the brain as neurons. He wrote a monograph in 1891 that assembled the evidence in favor of the cellular composition of nervous tissue, a theory that became known as the neuron doctrine. It is ironic that Golgi, whose staining technique made these advances possible, never accepted the neuron doctrine, and he argued vehemently against it when he received his Nobel Prize along with Cajal in 1906. The ultimate proof of the neuron doctrine was established by electron microscopic observations that definitively demonstrated that neurons are entirely separate from one another, even though their processes come into very close contact.

Nerve cells have four specialized regions: cell body, dendrites, axon, and presynaptic terminals

Neurons are specialized for sending and receiving signals, a purpose reflected in their unique shapes and physiological adaptations. The structure of a typical neuron can generally be divided into four distinct domains: (1) the cell body, also called the soma or perikaryon; (2) the dendrites; (3) the axon; and (4) the presynaptic terminals (Fig. 10-1).

Cell Body As the name *perikaryon* implies, the cell body is the portion of the cell surrounding the nucleus. It contains much of the cell's complement of endoplasmic reticular membranes as well as the Golgi complex. The cell body appears to be responsible for many of the neuronal housekeeping functions, including the synthesis and processing of proteins.

Dendrites Dendrites are tapering processes of variable complexity that arise from the cell body. The dendrites and cell body are the main areas for receiving information. Thus, their membranes are endowed with **receptors** that bind and respond to the neurotransmitters released by neighboring cells. The chemical message is translated by membrane receptors into an electrical or a biochemical event that influences the state of excitability of the receiving neuron. The cytoplasm of the dendrites contains dense networks of microtubules as well as extensions of the endoplasmic reticulum.

Axon Perhaps the most remarkable feature of the neuron, the axon is a projection that arises from the cell body, like the dendrites. Its point of origin is a tapered region known as the **axon hillock**. Just distal to the cone-shaped hillock is an untapered, unmyelinated region known as the **initial segment**. This area is also called the spike initiation zone because it is where an action potential (see Chapter 7) nor-

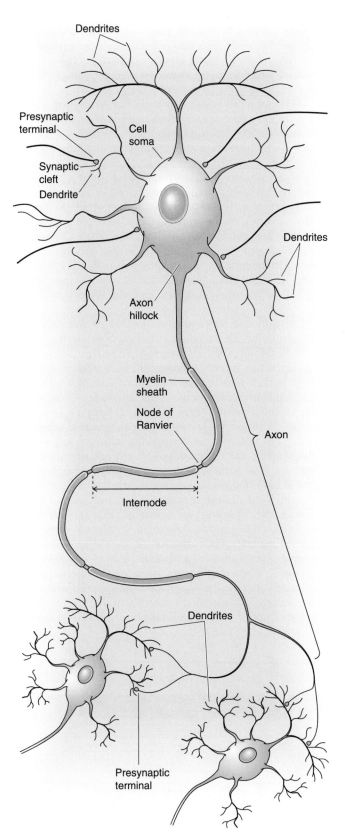

Dendrites

Presynaptic terminal

Cell soma

Synaptic cleft

Dendrite

Dendrites

Axon hillock

Myelin sheath

Node of Ranvier

Axon

Internode

Dendrites

Presynaptic terminal

Figure 10-1 Structure of a typical neuron.

mally arises as the result of the electrical events that have occurred in the cell body and dendrites. In contrast to the dendrites, the axon is thin, does not taper, and can extend for more than a meter. Because of its length, the typical axon contains much more cytoplasm than does the cell body, up to 1000 times as much. The neuron uses special metabolic mechanisms to sustain this unique structural component. The cytoplasm of the axon, the axoplasm, is packed with parallel arrays of microtubules and microfilaments that provide structural stability and a means to rapidly convey materials back and forth between the cell body and the axon terminus.

Axons are the message-sending portion of the neuron. The axon carries the neuron's signal, the action potential, to a specific target, such as another neuron or a muscle. Some axons have a special electrical insulation, called **myelin**, that consists of the coiled cell membranes of glial cells that wrap themselves around the nerve axon (see Chapter 11). If the axon is *not* covered with myelin, the action potential travels down the axon by continuous propagation. On the other hand, if the axon is myelinated, the action potential jumps from one node of Ranvier (the space between adjacent myelin segments) to another in a process called saltatory conduction (see Chapter 7). This adaptation greatly speeds impulse conduction.

Presynaptic Terminals   At its target, the axon terminates in multiple endings—the presynaptic terminals—usually designed for rapid conversion of the neuron's electrical signal into a chemical signal. When the action potential reaches the presynaptic terminal, it causes the release of chemical signaling molecules in a complex process called synaptic transmission (see Chapters 8 and 13).

The junction formed between the presynaptic terminal and its target is called a chemical synapse. **Synapse** is derived from the Greek for "joining together" or "junction"; this word and concept were introduced in 1897 by the neurophysiologist Charles Sherrington, whose contributions led to a share of the 1932 Nobel Prize in Medicine or Physiology. A synapse comprises the presynaptic terminal, the membrane of the target cell (postsynaptic membrane), and the space between the two (synaptic cleft). In synapses between two neurons, the presynaptic terminals primarily contact dendrites and the cell body. The area of the postsynaptic membrane is frequently amplified to increase the surface that is available for receptors. This amplification can occur either through infolding of the plasma membrane or through the formation of small projections called **dendritic spines**.

The molecules released by the presynaptic terminals diffuse across the synaptic cleft and bind to receptors on the postsynaptic membrane. The receptors then convert the chemical signal of the transmitter molecules—either directly or indirectly—back into an electrical signal.

In many ways, neurons can be thought of as highly specialized *endocrine cells*. They package and store hormones and hormone-like molecules, which they release rapidly into the extracellular space by exocytosis (see Chapter 2) in response to an external stimulus, in this case a nerve action potential. However, instead of entering the bloodstream to exert *systemic* effects, the substances secreted by neurons act over the very short distance of a synapse to communicate *locally* with a single neighboring cell (see Chapter 5).

In a different sense, neurons can be thought of as *polarized cells* with some of the properties of epithelial cells. Like epithelial cells, neurons have different populations of membrane proteins at each of the distinct domains of the neuronal plasma membrane, an arrangement that reflects the individual physiological responsibilities of these domains. Thus, the design of the nervous system permits information transfer across synapses in a selective and coordinated way that serves the needs of the organism and summates to produce complex behavior.

The cytoskeleton helps compartmentalize the neuron and also provides the tracks along which material travels between different parts of the neuron

Neurons are compartmentalized in both structure and function. *Dendrites* are tapered, have limited length, and contain neurotransmitter receptor proteins in their membranes. *Axons* can be very long and have a high density of Na^+ channels. *Dendrites* and the *cell body* contain mRNA, ribosomes, and a Golgi apparatus. These structures are absent in axons.

How does this compartmentalization come about? The answer is not certain, but **microtubule-associated proteins (MAPs)** appear to play an important role. (Note that these MAPs are totally unrelated to the mitogen-activated protein [MAP] kinase introduced in Chapter 4.) Two major classes of MAPs are found in the brain: high-molecular-weight proteins such as MAP-1 and MAP-2 and lower molecular weight tau proteins. Both classes of MAPs associate with microtubules and help link them to other cell components. MAP-2 is found only in cell bodies and dendrites. Dephosphorylated tau proteins are confined entirely to axons. In cultured neurons, suppressing the expression of tau protein prevents formation of the axon without altering formation of the dendrites.

Microtubules may also help create the remarkable morphological and functional divisions in neurons. In axons, microtubules assemble with their plus ends pointed away from the cell body; this orientation polarizes the flow of material into and out of the axon. The cytoskeletal "order" provided in part by the microtubules and the MAPs helps define what should or should not be in the axonal cytoplasm. In dendrites, the microtubules do not have a consistent orientation, which gives the dendrites a greater structural and functional similarity to the cell body.

The neuron cell body is the main manufacturing site for the membrane proteins and membranous organelles that are necessary for the structural integrity and function of its processes. Axons have no protein synthetic ability, whereas dendrites have some free ribosomes and may be able to engage in limited protein production. The transport of proteins from the cell body all the way to the end of long axons is a challenging task. The neuron also has a second task: moving various material in the opposite direction, from presynaptic terminals at the end of the axon to the cell body. The neuron solves these problems by using two distinct mechanisms for moving material to the presynaptic terminals in an "anterograde" direction and a third mechanism for transport in the opposite or "retrograde" direction (Table 10-2).

Fast Axoplasmic Transport   If the flow of materials from the soma to the distant axon terminus were left to the whims of simple diffusion, their delivery would be far too slow to be of practical use. It could take months for needed proteins to diffuse to the end of an axon, and the presynaptic terminals are high-volume consumers of these molecules. To overcome this difficulty, neurons exploit a rapid, pony express–style system of conveyance known as **fast axoplasmic transport** (Table 10-2). Membranous organelles, including vesicles and mitochondria, are the principal freight of fast axoplasmic transport. The proteins, lipids, and polysaccharides that move at fast rates in axons do so because they have caught a ride with a membranous organelle (i.e., sequestered inside the organelle, or bound to or inserted into the organellar membrane). The peptide and protein contents of dense-core secretory granules, which are found in the presynaptic axonal terminals, are synthesized as standard secretory proteins (see Chapter 2). Thus, they are cotranslationally inserted across the membranes of the rough endoplasmic reticulum and subsequently processed in the cisternae of the Golgi complex. They are shipped to the axon in the lumens of Golgi-derived carrier vesicles (Table 10-2).

TABLE 10-2 Features of Axoplasmic Transport

Transport Type	Speed (mm/day)	Mechanism	Material Transported
Fast anterograde	~400	Saltatory movement along microtubules by the motor molecule kinesin (ATP dependent)	Mitochondria Vesicles containing peptide and other neurotransmitters, some degradative enzymes
Fast retrograde	~200–300	Saltatory movement along microtubules by the motor molecule dynein (ATP dependent)	Degraded vesicular membrane Absorbed exogenous material (toxins, viruses, growth factors)
Slow anterograde	~0.2–8	Not clear; possibly by molecular motors	Cytoskeletal elements (e.g., neurofilament and microtubule subunits) Soluble proteins of intermediary metabolism Actin

Organelles and vesicles, and their macromolecule payloads, move along **microtubules** with the help of a microtubule-dependent motor protein called **kinesin** (Fig. 10-2A). The kinesin motor is itself an ATPase that produces vectorial movement of its payload along the microtubule (see Chapter 2). This system can move vesicles down the axon at rates of up to 400 mm/day; variations in cargo speed simply reflect more frequent pauses during the journey. Kinesins always move toward the plus end of microtubules (i.e., away from the cell body), and transport function is lost if the microtubules are disrupted. The nervous system has many forms of kinesin that recognize and transport different cargo. It is not known how the motor proteins recognize and attach to their intended payloads.

Fast Retrograde Transport   Axons move material back toward the cell body with a different motor protein called **dynein** (Fig. 10-2B). Like kinesin, dynein (see Chapter 2) also moves along microtubule tracks and is an ATPase (Table 10-2). However, dynein moves along microtubules in the opposite direction of kinesin (Fig. 10-2C). Retrograde transport provides a mechanism for target-derived growth factors, like nerve growth factor, to reach the nucleus of a neuron where it can influence survival. How this signal is transmitted up the axon has been a persistent question. It may be endocytosed at the axon's terminal and transported to the cell body in a "signaling endosome." The loss of ATP production, as occurs with blockade of oxidative metabolism, causes fast axonal transport in both the anterograde and retrograde directions to fail.

Slow Axoplasmic Transport   Axons also have a need for hundreds of other proteins, including cytoskeletal proteins and soluble proteins that are used as enzymes for intermediary metabolism. These proteins are delivered by a slow anterograde axoplasmic transport mechanism that moves material at a mere 0.2 to 8 mm/day, the nervous system's equivalent of snail mail. The slowest moving proteins are neurofilament and microtubule subunits (0.2 to 1 mm/day). The mechanism of slow axoplasmic transport is not well understood, but motor molecules appear to be involved. In fact, the difference between slow and fast axonal transport may primarily be the number of transport *interruptions* during the long axonal journey.

Neurons can be classified on the basis of their axonal projection, their dendritic geometry, and the number of processes emanating from the cell body

The trillions of nerve cells in the CNS have great structural diversity. Typically, neurons are classified on the basis of where their axons go (i.e., where they "project"), the geometry of their dendrites, and the number of processes that emanate from the cell body (Fig. 10-3). The real significance of these schemes is that they have functional implications.

Axonal Projection   Neurons with long axons that connect with other parts of the nervous system are called **projection neurons** (or principal neurons or Golgi type I cells). Each of these cells has a clearly defined axon that arises from the axon hillock located on the cell body or proximal dendrite and extends away from the cell body, sometimes for remarkable distances. Some neurons in the cortex, for example, project to the distal part of the spinal cord, a stretch of nearly a meter. All the other processes that a projection neuron has are dendrites. The other type of neuron that is defined in this way has all of its processes confined to one region of the brain. These neurons are called **interneurons** (or intrinsic neurons or Golgi type II cells). Some of these cells have very short axons, whereas others seem to lack a conventional axon altogether and may be referred to as *anaxonal*. The anaxonal neuron in the retina is called an amacrine (from the Greek for "no large/long fiber") cell.

Dendritic Geometry   A roughly pyramid-shaped set of dendritic branches characterizes **pyramidal cells**, whereas a radial pattern of dendritic branches defines **stellate cells**. This classification often includes mention of the presence or absence of dendritic spines, those small, protuberant projections that are sites for synaptic contact. All pyramidal cells appear to have spines, but stellate cells may have them (spiny) or not (aspiny).

Number of Processes   Neurons can also be classified by the number of processes that extend from their cell bodies. The dorsal root ganglion cell is the classic **unipolar** neuron. The naming of the processes of primary sensory neurons, like the dorsal root ganglion cell, is often ambiguous. The process that extends into the CNS from this unipolar neuron is easily recognized as an axon because it carries information *away* from the cell body. On the other hand, the process that extends to sensory receptors in the skin and elsewhere is less easily defined. It is a typical axon in the sense that it can conduct an action potential, has myelin, and is characterized by an axonal cytoskeleton. However, it conveys information *toward* the cell body, which is usually the function of a dendrite. **Bipolar** neurons, such as the retinal bipolar cell, have two processes extending from opposite sides of the cell body. Most neurons in the brain are **multipolar**. Cells with many dendritic processes are designed to receive large numbers of synapses.

Most neurons in the brain can be categorized by two or more of these schemes. For example, the large neurons in the cortical area devoted to movement (i.e., the motor cortex) are multipolar, pyramidal, projection neurons. Similarly, a retinal bipolar cell is both an interneuron and a bipolar cell.

Glial cells provide a physiological environment for neurons

Glial cells are defined in part by what they lack: axons, action potentials, and synaptic potentials. They are much more numerous than neurons and are diverse in structure and function. The main types of CNS glial cells are oligodendrocytes, astrocytes, and microglial cells. In the PNS, the main types of glial cells are satellite cells in autonomic and sensory ganglia, Schwann cells, and enteric glial cells. Glial function is discussed in Chapter 11. Oligodendrocytes form the myelin sheaths of CNS axons, and Schwann cells myelinate periph-

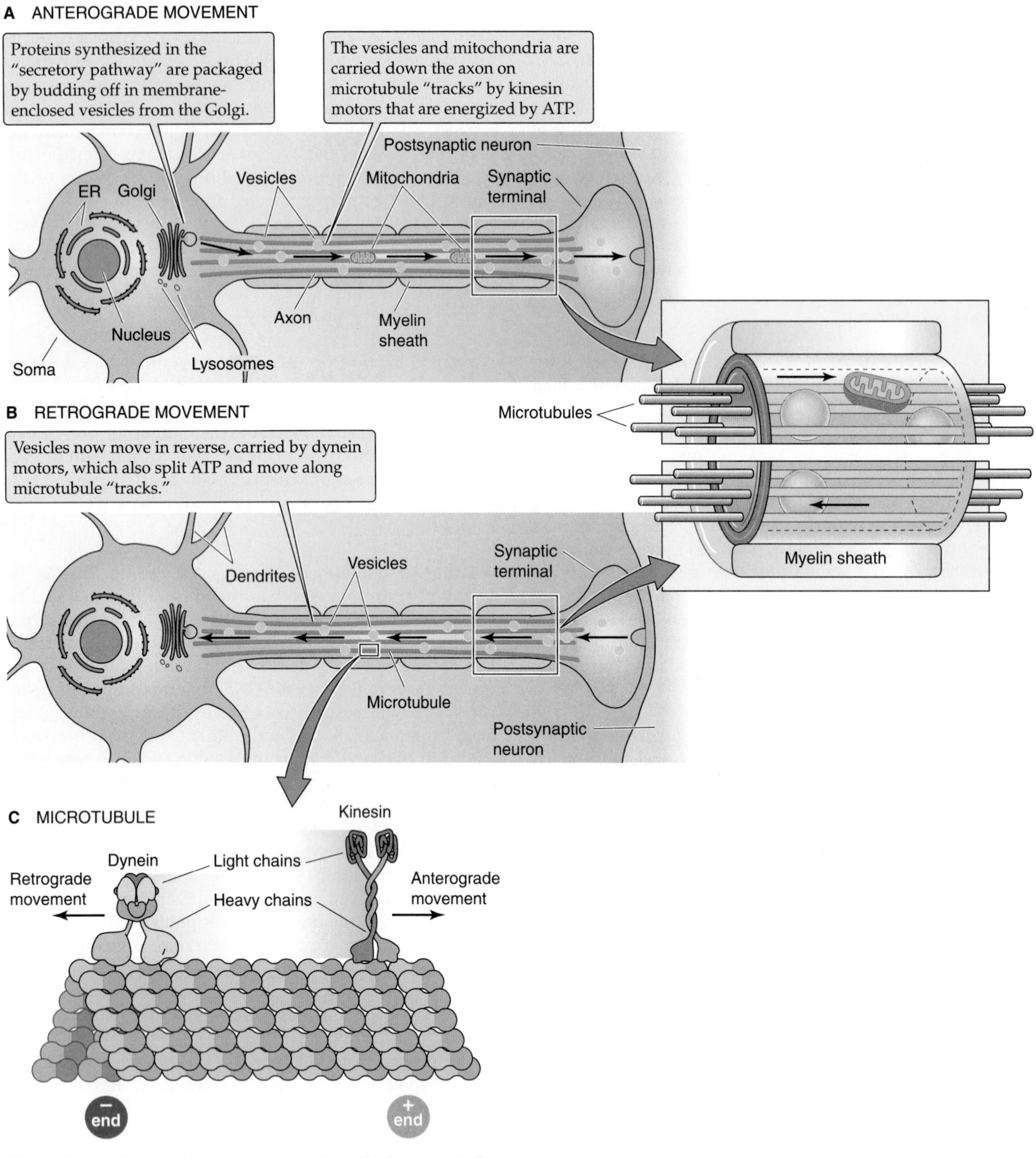

A ANTEROGRADE MOVEMENT

Proteins synthesized in the "secretory pathway" are packaged by budding off in membrane-enclosed vesicles from the Golgi.

The vesicles and mitochondria are carried down the axon on microtubule "tracks" by kinesin motors that are energized by ATP.

Postsynaptic neuron

ER Golgi   Vesicles   Mitochondria   Synaptic terminal

Nucleus

Soma   Lysosomes   Axon   Myelin sheath

Microtubules

B RETROGRADE MOVEMENT

Vesicles now move in reverse, carried by dynein motors, which also split ATP and move along microtubule "tracks."

Dendrites   Vesicles   Synaptic terminal

Microtubule

Postsynaptic neuron

Myelin sheath

C MICROTUBULE

Kinesin

Dynein   Light chains

Retrograde movement   Heavy chains   Anterograde movement

− end   + end

Figure 10-2   Fast axoplasmic transport. ER, endoplasmic reticulum.

eral nerves. Glial cells are involved in nearly every function of the brain and are far more than simply "nerve glue," a literal translation of the name neuroglia (from the Greek *neuron,* nerve, and *glia,* glue).

In depictions of the nervous system, the presence of glial cells is sometimes minimized or neglected altogether. Glia fills in almost all the space around neurons, with a narrow extracellular space left between neurons and glial cells that has an average width of only ~0.02 μm. The composition of the extracellular fluid, which has a major impact on brain function, as well as the function of glial cells is taken up in detail in Chapter 11.

Basis for classification	Example	Functional implication	Structure
1. Axonal projection			
Goes to a distant brain area	Projection neuron or Principal neuron or Golgi type I cell (cortical motor neuron)	Affects different brain areas	Dorsal root ganglion cell 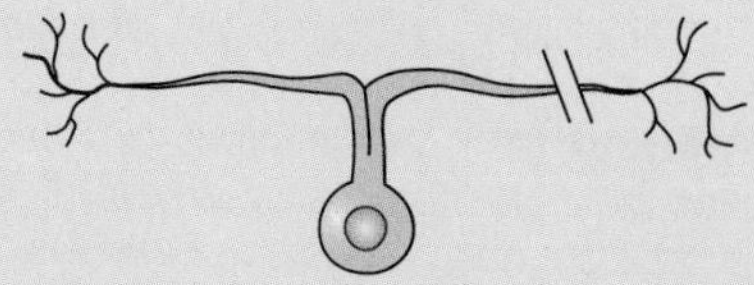
Stays in a local brain area	Intrinsic neuron or Interneuron or Golgi type II cell (cortical inhibitory neuron)	Affects only nearby neurons	Retinal bipolar cell 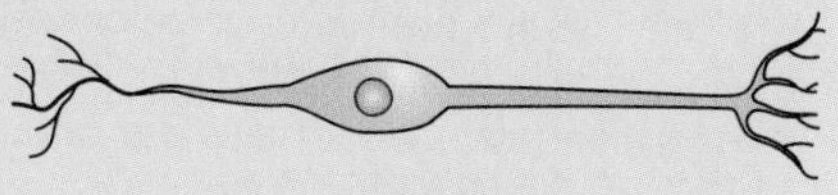
2. Dendritic pattern			
Pyramid-shaped spread of dendrites	Pyramidal cell (hippocampal pyramidal neuron)	Large area for receiving synaptic input; determines the pattern of incoming axons that can interact with the cell (i.e., pyramid-shaped)	Pyramidal cell 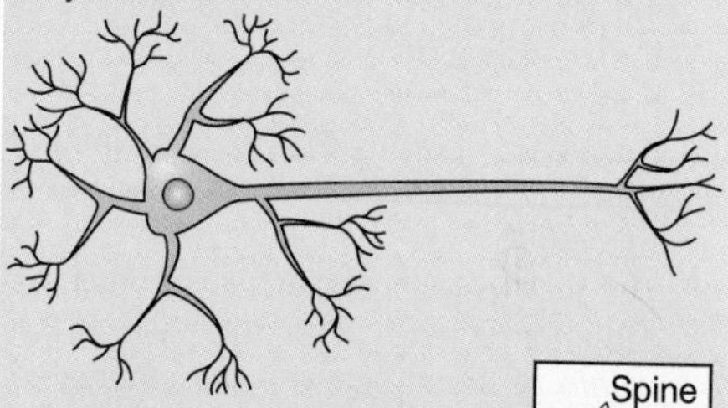
Radial-shaped spread of dendrites	Stellate cell (cortical stellate cell)	Large area for receiving synaptic input; determines pattern of incoming axons that can interact with the cell (i.e., star-shaped)	Stellate cell 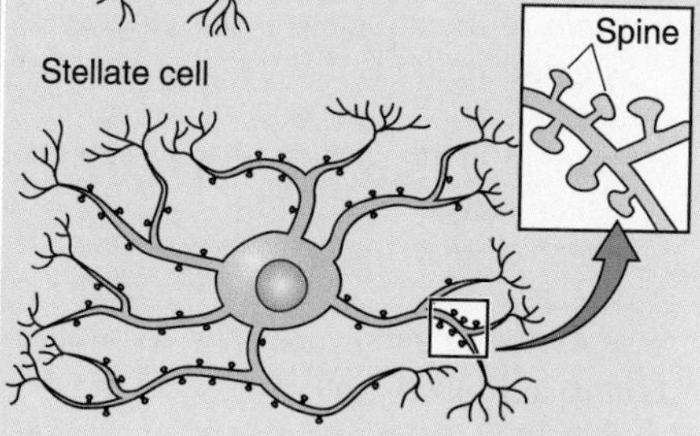 / Spine
3. Number of processes			
One process exits the cell body	Unipolar neuron (dorsal root ganglion cell)	Small area for receiving synaptic input: highly specialized function	Unipolar 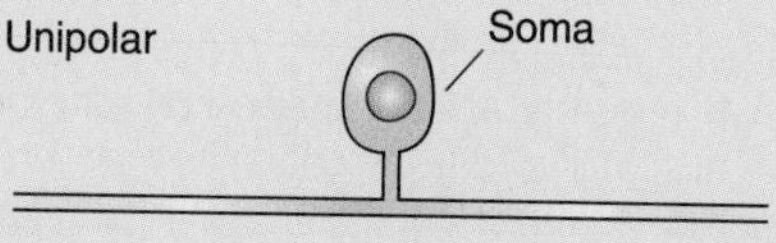 / Soma
Two processes exit the cell body	Bipolar neuron (retinal bipolar cell)	Small area for receiving synaptic input: highly specialized function	Bipolar 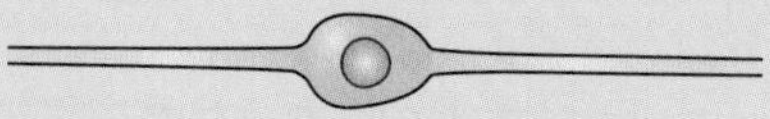
Many processes exit the cell body	Multipolar neuron (spinal motor neuron)	Large area for receiving synaptic input; determines the pattern of incoming axons that can interact with the cell	Multipolar 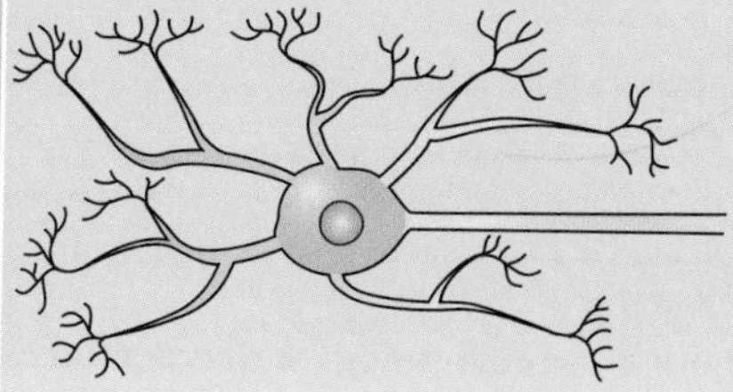

Figure 10-3 Classification of neurons based on their structure.

Definitions of Neural Modalities

The type of information, or neural **modality**, that a neuron transmits is classically categorized by three terms that refer to different attributes of the neuron.

1. The first category defines the *direction* of information flow.
   Afferent (sensory): neurons that transmit information into the CNS from sensory cells or sensory receptors outside the nervous system. Examples are the dorsal root ganglion cell and neurons in the sensory nucleus of the fifth cranial nerve.
   Efferent (motor): neurons that transmit information out of the CNS to muscles or secretory cells. Examples are spinal motor neurons and motor neurons in the ANS.
2. The second category defines the *anatomical distribution* of the information flow.
   Visceral: neurons that transmit information to or from internal organs or regions that arise embryologically from the branchial arch (e.g., chemoreceptors of the carotid body).
   Somatic: neurons that transmit information to or from all nonvisceral parts of the body, including skin and muscle.
3. The third category, which is somewhat arbitrary, defines the information flow on the basis of the *embryological origin* of the structure being innervated.
   Special: neurons that transmit information to or from a "special" subset of visceral or somatic structures. For example, in the case of **special visceral** neurons, information travels to or from structures derived from the branchial arch region of the embryo (e.g., pharyngeal muscles). In the case of **special somatic** neurons, which handle only sensory information, the neurons arise from the organs of special sense (e.g., retina, taste receptors, cochlea).
   General: neurons that transmit information to or from visceral or somatic structures that are not in the special group.

Each axon in the body conveys information of only a single modality. In this classification scheme, a motor neuron in the spinal cord is described as a general somatic efferent neuron. A motor neuron in the brain stem that innervates branchial arch–derived chewing muscles is described as a special visceral efferent neuron. Because each of these three categories defines two options, you might expect a total of eight distinct neural modalities. In practice, however, only seven neural modalities exist. The term *special somatic efferent* neuron is not used.

DEVELOPMENT OF NEURONS AND GLIAL CELLS

Neurons differentiate from the neuroectoderm

Although the embryology of the nervous system may seem like an odd place to begin studying the physiology of the brain, there are a number of reasons to start here. Knowledge of the embryology of the nervous system greatly facilitates comprehension of its complex organization. Events in the development of the nervous system highlight how different neuronal cell types evolve from a single type of precursor cell and how these neurons establish astonishingly specific connections. Finally, the characteristics of brain cell proliferation as well as the growth of neuronal processes during development provide insight into the consequences of brain injury.

The vertebrate embryo consists of three primitive tissue layers at the stage of gastrulation: endoderm, mesoderm, and ectoderm (Fig. 10-4). The entire nervous system arises from ectoderm, which also gives rise to the skin. Underlying the ectoderm is a specialized cord of mesodermal cells called the notochord. Cells of the notochord somehow direct or "induce" the overlying ectoderm, or **neuroectoderm**, to form the neural tube in a complex process called neurulation.

The first step in neurulation is formation of the neural plate at about the beginning of the third fetal week. Initially, the neural plate is only a single layer of neuroectoderm cells. Rapid proliferation of these cells, especially at the lateral margins, creates a neural groove bordered by neural folds. Continued cell division enlarges the neural folds, and they eventually fuse dorsally to form the neural tube. The neural tube is open at both ends, the anterior and posterior neuropores. The neural tube ultimately gives rise to the brain and spinal cord. The lumen of the neural tube, the neural canal, becomes the four **ventricles** of the brain and the central canal of the spinal cord. Congenital malformations of the brain commonly arise from developmental defects in the neural tube.

The **neural crest** derives from symmetric lateral portions of the neural plate. Neural crest cells migrate to sites in the body where they form the vast majority of the PNS and most of the peripheral cells of the ANS, including the sympathetic ganglia and the chromaffin cells of the adrenal medulla. On the sensory side, these neural crest derivatives include unipolar neurons whose cell bodies are in the dorsal root ganglia, as well as the equivalent sensory cells of cranial nerves V, VII, IX, and X. Neural crest cells also give rise to several nonneuronal structures, including Schwann cells, satellite glial cells in spinal and cranial ganglia, and pigment cells of the skin.

The human brain begins to exhibit some regional specialization around the fourth gestational week (Fig. 10-5A, B). By then, it is possible to discern an anterior part called the **prosencephalon**, a midsection called the **mesencephalon**, and a posterior part called the **rhombencephalon**. Rapid brain growth ensues, and important new regions emerge in just another week (Fig. 10-5C). Distinct regions called *brain vesicles*, which are destined to become separate parts of the adult brain, are set apart as swellings in the rostral-caudal plane (Fig. 10-5B, C). The prosencephalon is now divisible into the **telencephalon**, which will give rise to the basal ganglia and cerebral cortex, and the **diencephalon**, which becomes the thalamus, subthalamus, hypothalamus, and neurohypophysis (the posterior or neural portion of the pituitary). Similarly, the rhombencephalon can now be divided into the **metencephalon**, which will give rise to the

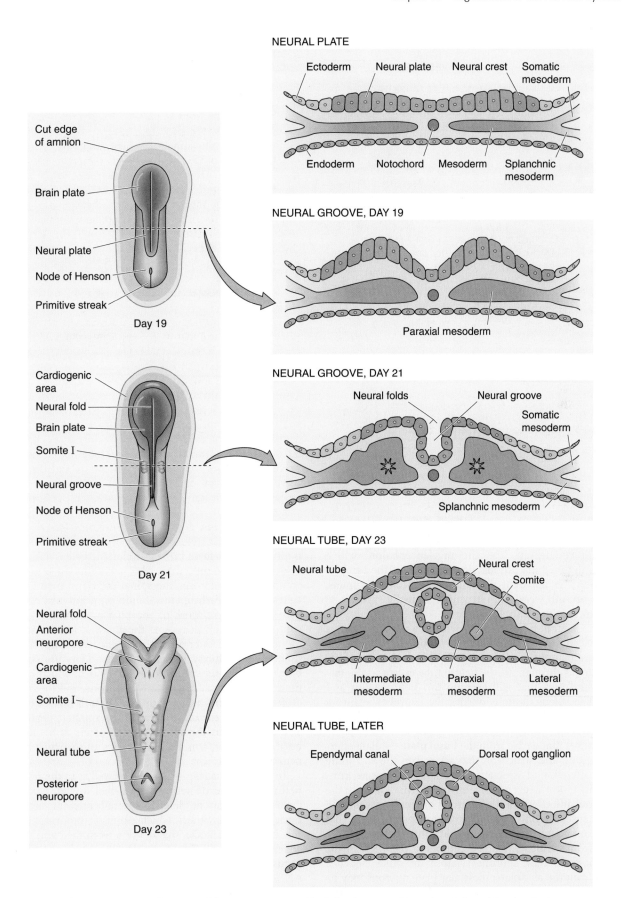

Figure 10-4   Development of the nervous system. The left column provides a dorsal view of the developing nervous system at three different time points. The right column shows cross sections of the dorsal portion of the embryo at five different stages, three of which correspond to the dorsal views shown at the left.

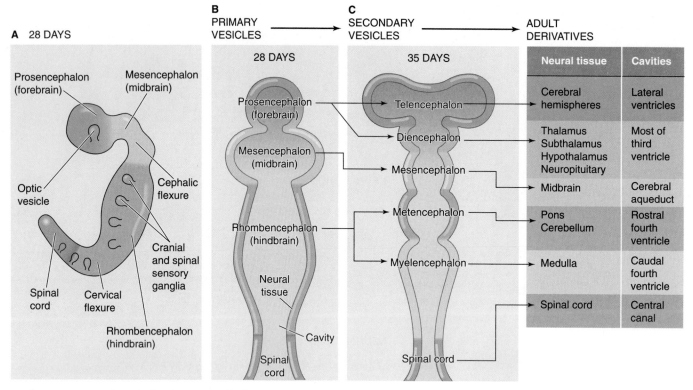

Figure 10-5   Embryonic development of the brain.

pons and cerebellum, and the **myelencephalon**, which becomes the medulla. Robust development of the cerebral cortex becomes apparent in mammals, especially humans, after the seventh week. This structure gradually expands so that it enwraps the rostral structures.

As the neural tube thickens with cell proliferation, a groove called the **sulcus limitans** forms on the inner, lateral wall of the neural tube (Fig. 10-6A). This anatomical landmark extends throughout the neural tube except in the farthest rostral area that will become the diencephalon and cortex. The sulcus limitans divides the neural tube into a ventral area called the basal plate and a dorsal area called the alar plate.

Structures that derive from the **basal plate** mediate efferent functions, and structures that arise from the **alar plate** mediate afferent and associative functions. Efferent neurons are mainly motor neurons that convey information from the CNS to outside effectors (i.e., muscles or secretory cells). In a strict sense, the only true *afferent* neurons are those that derive from neural crest cells and that convey sensory information from various kinds of receptors to the CNS. In the CNS, these afferent neurons synapse on other neurons derived from the alar plate; these alar plate neurons may be referred to as afferent because they receive sensory information and pass it along to other parts of the CNS. However, it

is also appropriate to call these alar plate–derived neurons associative.

The development of the spinal cord and medulla illustrates how this early anatomical division into alar and basal plates helps make sense of the final organization of these complex regions. Neurons of the alar and basal plates proliferate, migrate, and aggregate into discrete groups that have functional specificity. In the spinal cord (Fig. 10-6B, C), the basal plate develops into the ventral horn, which contains the cell bodies of somatic motor neurons, and the intermediolateral column, which contains the cell bodies of autonomic motor neurons. Both regions contain interneurons. The alar plate in the spinal cord develops into the dorsal horn, which contains the cell bodies onto which sensory neurons synapse.

In the medulla (Fig. 10-6D, E), as well as in the rest of the brain, aggregates of neurons are called **nuclei**. Nuclei that develop from the alar plate are generally afferent, such as the nucleus tractus solitarii, which plays an important sensory role in the ANS. Nuclei that develop from the basal plate are generally efferent, such as the dorsal motor nucleus of the vagus nerve, which plays an important *motor* role in the ANS. The choroid plexus that invaginates into the lumen of the central canal is responsible for secreting cerebrospinal fluid (see Chapter 11).

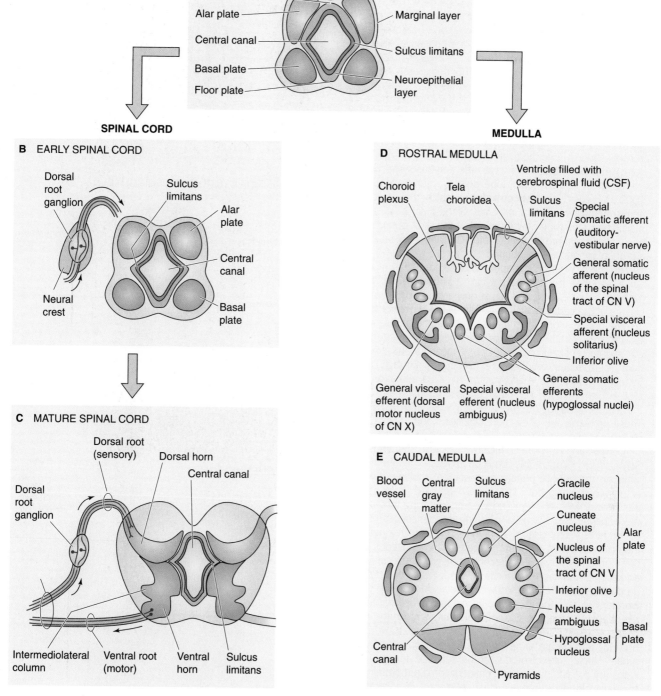

Figure 10-6 Development of the spinal cord and medulla. **A,** In this cross section through the neural tube, the sulcus limitans is the landmark that separates the ventral basal plate from the dorsal alar plate. The basal plate will form efferent (or motor-type) structures, whereas the alar plate will form afferent and associative (or sensory-type) functions. **B,** The true afferent neurons are those in the dorsal root ganglion, which derive from neural crest cells. These afferents will contact the neurons in the alar plate, which will become associative. **C,** The basal plate has developed into the ventral horn and intermediolateral column (motor), whereas the alar plate has developed into the dorsal horn (associative). **D,** The basal plate has developed into nuclei with motor functions, whereas the alar plate has developed into nuclei with sensory functions. The roof of the rostral medulla becomes the fourth ventricle. **E,** This cross section shows the same gross separation between motor and associative-sensory functions as is seen with the rostral medulla and the spinal cord.

Abnormalities of Neural Tube Closure

Closure of the neural tube in humans normally occurs between 26 and 28 days of gestation. A disturbance in this process results in a midline congenital abnormality called a **dysraphism** (from the Greek *dys,* abnormal, + *rhaphē,* seam or suture). The defect can be so devastating that it is incompatible with life or, alternatively, have so little consequence that it goes unnoticed throughout life. These midline embryonic abnormalities also involve the primitive mesoderm and ectoderm associated with the neural tube. Therefore, the vertebral bodies or skull (derived from mesoderm) and the overlying skin (derived from ectoderm) may be affected along with the nervous system.

The most serious neural tube defect, occurring in 1 of 1000 deliveries, is **anencephaly**, in which the cerebral hemispheres are absent and the rest of the brain is severely malformed. Overlying malformations of the skull, brain coverings, and scalp are present (Table 10-3). Affected fetuses are often spontaneously aborted.

The most common dysraphisms affect formation of the spinal vertebral bodies and are called **spina bifida**. The problem may be slight and cause only a minor problem in closure of the vertebral arch, called spina bifida occulta (Fig. 10-7A). This malformation affects ~10% of the population, usually at the fifth lumbar or first sacral vertebra, and generally causes no significant sequelae. If the dura and arachnoid membranes herniate (i.e., protrude) through the vertebral defect, the malformation is called spina bifida cystica (Fig. 10-7B); if the spinal cord also herniates through the defect, it is called myelomeningocele (Fig. 10-7C). These problems are often more significant and may cause severe neurological disability.

Genetic and nongenetic factors can cause dysraphism. Some severe forms of this condition appear to be inherited, although the genetic pattern suggests that multiple genes are involved. Nongenetic factors may also play a role, as in the case of folic acid deficiency. Mothers taking folic acid (see Chapter 56) before and during the periconceptional period have a decreased risk of having a fetus with a neural tube closure defect. Current medical recommendations are that women *contemplating* becoming pregnant receive folic acid supplementation, and it has been suggested that bread products should be enriched with folic acid to ensure that women will have the protective advantage of this vitamin if they become pregnant. Other factors that increase the risk of these defects are maternal heat exposure (e.g., from a hot tub) and certain drugs such as the anticonvulsant valproate. Neural tube disorders can be detected during pregnancy by measuring the concentration of α-fetoprotein in maternal blood or amniotic fluid. α-Fetoprotein is synthesized by the fetal liver and, for unclear reasons, increases in concentration abnormally with failure of neural tube closure.

A   SPINA BIFIDA OCCULTA

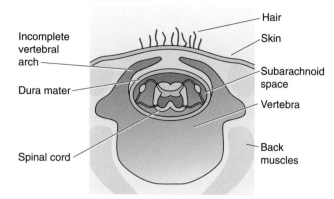

B   SPINA BIFIDA CYSTICA OR MENINGOCELE

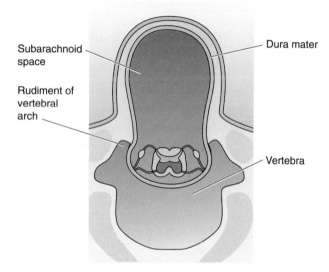

C   MYELOMENINGOCELE

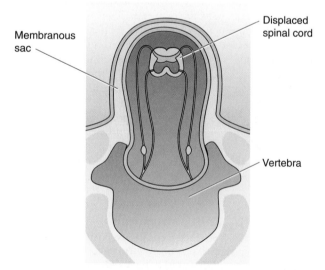

Figure 10-7   Variations of spina bifida. **A,** An incomplete vertebral arch with no herniation. **B,** The dura and arachnoid membranes herniate through the vertebral defect. **C,** The spinal cord and meninges herniate through the vertebral defect.

TABLE 10-3 Defects of Neural Tube Closure

Malformation	Characteristics
Brain Defects	
Anencephaly	Absence of the brain, with massive defects in the skull, meninges, and scalp
Cephalocele	Partial brain herniation through skull defect (cranium bifidum)
Meningocele	Meningeal herniation through skull or spine defect
Spina Bifida Defects	
Spina bifida occulta	Vertebral arch defect only
Spina bifida cystica	Herniation of the dura and arachnoid through a vertebral defect
Myelomeningocele	Herniation of the spinal cord and meninges through a vertebral defect

Neurons and glial cells originate from cells in the proliferating germinal matrix near the ventricles

The trillions of neurons and glial cells that populate the brain arise from rapidly dividing stem cells called **neuroepithelial cells** located near the ventricles (which derive from the neural canal) of the embryonic CNS. This germinal area (Fig. 10-8A) is divided into two regions, the **ventricular zone (VZ)** and the **subventricular zone (SVZ)**. Most of the neurons in the human brain are generated during the first 120 days of embryogenesis. Growth factors such as epidermal growth factor and platelet-derived growth factor and hormones such as growth hormone influence the rate of cell division of the **neuroepithelial cells**. The signals that direct one immature neuron to become a cortical pyramidal cell and another to become a retinal ganglion cell are not understood. Neuroepithelial cells generate different classes of neural precursor cells that develop into different mature cell types. In the developing brain, **radial cells** (Fig. 10-8), so called because their processes extend from the ventricular surface to the brain's outer surface, appear very early in neurogenesis and generate most of the projection neurons in forebrain cortex. Inhibitory interneurons, in contrast, arise from neural precursor cells located in the SVZ. Neurons are probably not fully differentiated when first created and their mature characteristics may depend on their interactions with the chemical environment or other cells in a specific anatomical region of the nervous system.

The VZ appears to produce separate **progenitor cells** that produce only neurons, oligodendrocytes, astrocytes, and ependymal cells (Fig. 10-8B). The VZ does not contribute to the population of Schwann cells, which derive from neural crest tissue, or to microglial cells, which arise from the mesodermal cells that briefly invade the brain during early postnatal development. Recent work shows that the embryonic and perinatal VZ and SVZ may give rise to the adult SVZ, which is in part responsible for limited adult neurogenesis.

Neuronal progenitor cells appear earliest and produce nearly the entire complement of adult neurons during early embryonic life. Glial cells arise later in development. Neurons are confined to specific locations of the brain, whereas glial cells are more evenly distributed.

Many more neurons are created during fetal development than are present in the adult brain. Most neurons, having migrated to a final location in the brain and differentiated, are lost through a process called programmed cell death, or **apoptosis** (Greek for "falling off"). Apoptosis is a unique form of cell death that requires protein synthesis and can be triggered by removal of specific trophic influences, such as the action of a growth factor. In contrast to necrotic cell death, which rapidly leads to loss of cell membrane integrity after some insult causes a toxic increase in $[Ca^{2+}]_i$, apoptosis evolves more slowly. For example, in the retina, ~60% of the ganglion cells and thus ~60% of the retinal axons are lost in the first 2 weeks of extrauterine life as a result of programmed retinal ganglion cell death. This process of sculpting the final form of a neuronal system by discarding neurons through programmed death is a common theme in developmental biology.

The number of glial cells in different areas of the brain appears to be determined by signals from nearby neurons or axons. For example, in the optic nerve, the final number of glia in the nerve is closely determined by the number of axons. When programmed cell death is prevented by expression of the *bcl-2* gene in transgenic animals, the number of axons in the optic nerve is dramatically increased, as well as the number of astrocytes and oligodendrocytes. Thus, glial cell–axon ratios remain relatively constant. The axon-dependent signal or signals responsible for these adjustments in glial cell number are not known, but the process appears to operate by influencing both glial cell survival and proliferation.

Neurons migrate to their correct anatomical position in the brain with the help of adhesion molecules

During embryogenesis, the long processes of radial cells create an organized, cellular scaffolding on which neurons can migrate to their final position in the brain shortly after they appear. Migrating neurons contact radial cells (Fig. 10-8B) and move along their processes toward their final positions in the developing cortex. Thus, the prearranged positions of these radial processes determine the direction of neuronal migration. The importance of the radial framework for assisting neuronal migration is illustrated by the failure of neurons to populate the cortex normally when the radial processes are interrupted by hemorrhage in the fetal brain.

The navigation mechanisms used by migrating cells in the nervous system and elsewhere in the body are only partially understood. Proteins that promote selective cellular aggregation are called **cell-cell adhesion molecules** (CAMs; see Chapter 2) and include the Ca^{2+}-dependent cadherins and Ca^{2+}-independent neural cell adhesion molecules (N-CAMs). These molecules are expressed by developing cells in an organized, sequential manner. Cells that express the appropriate

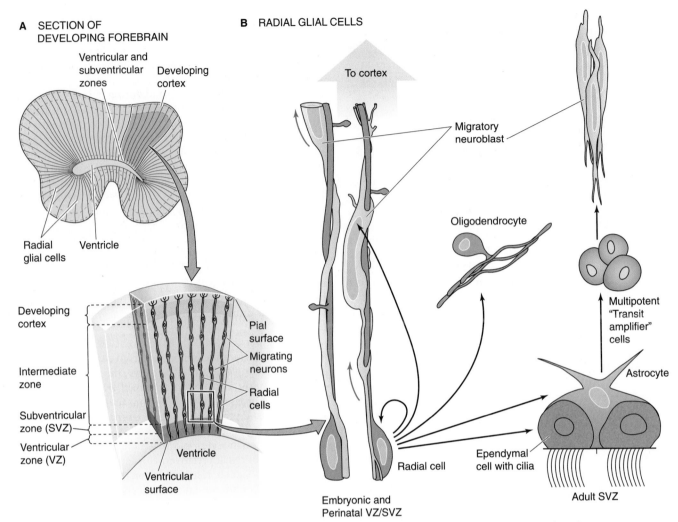

A SECTION OF DEVELOPING FOREBRAIN

Ventricular and subventricular zones

Developing cortex

Radial glial cells

Ventricle

Developing cortex

Intermediate zone

Subventricular zone (SVZ)

Ventricular zone (VZ)

Pial surface

Migrating neurons

Radial cells

Ventricle

Ventricular surface

B RADIAL GLIAL CELLS

To cortex

Migratory neuroblast

Oligodendrocyte

Multipotent "Transit amplifier" cells

Astrocyte

Radial cell

Ependymal cell with cilia

Embryonic and Perinatal VZ/SVZ

Adult SVZ

Figure 10-8 Arrangement of radial cells and migrating neurons. **A,** The *upper portion* is a coronal section of developing occipital cerebral lobe of fetal monkey brain. The *lower portion* is a magnified view. The ventricular zone contains the germinal cells that give rise to the neurons as well as to the cell bodies of the radial cells. These radial cells extend from the ventricular surface to the pial surface, which overlies the developing cortex. **B,** The more magnified view on the left shows the cell bodies of two radial cells as well as their processes that extend upward toward the cortex. Also shown are two migratory neuroblasts moving from the ventricular zone toward the cortex along the fibers of the radial cells. The black arrows indicate possible pathways of proliferation and differentiation. *(Data from Rakic P: Mode of cell migration to the superficial layers of fetal monkey neocortex. J Comp Neurol 1972; 145:61-84; and Tramontin AD, Garcia-Verdugo JM, Lim DA, Alvarez-Buylla A: Postnatal development of radial glia and the ventricular zone (VZ): a continuum of the neural stem cell compartment. Cerebral Cortex 2003; 13:580-587.)*

adhesion molecules have a strong tendency to adhere to one another. These Velcro-like molecules can assemble cells in a highly ordered fashion; experimentally, disrupted germ cells can properly reorganize themselves into a three-layered structure that replicates the normal embryonic pattern.

Another mechanism that assists migrating cells is the presence of **extracellular matrix** molecules such as laminin and fibronectin. These glycoproteins are selectively secreted by both neurons and astrocytes and form a kind of extracellular roadway with which migrating cells can interact. Growing axons express at their surface **cell matrix adhesion molecules** called integrins that bind laminin and fibronectin (see Chapter 2). As a result, growing axons move together in fascicles.

Perhaps the least understood mechanism related to cell migration is **chemotaxis**, the ability of a cell to follow a chemical signal emitted from a target cell. The tips of developing axons, called growth cones, appear to follow such chemical cues as they grow toward their specific targets. For example, a molecule called netrin, secreted by midline cells, attracts developing axons destined to cross the midline. On the other hand, molecules like slit repel axons by interacting with specific receptors on the growth cone. Such signals steer axon growth cones, perhaps by localized changes in intracellular $[Ca^{2+}]$, leading to the strategic insertion of new patches of membrane on the surface of the growth cone.

Neurons do not regenerate

Neurons Most human neurons arise in about the first 4 months of intrauterine life. After birth, neurons do not divide, and if a neuron is lost for any reason, it is generally

Axonal Degeneration and Regeneration

Axons have their own mitochondria and produce the ATP that they need to maintain the steep ion gradients necessary for excitability and survival. In this sense, they are metabolically independent of the cell body. However, they cannot make proteins and are unable to sustain themselves if separated from the cell body (Fig. 10-2). If an axon is cut, in either the PNS or the CNS, a characteristic series of changes takes place (Fig. 10-9):

Step 1: **Degeneration of the synaptic terminals distal to the lesion.** Synaptic transmission occurring at the axon terminal fails within hours because this complex process is dependent on material provided by axonal transport. Visible changes in the degenerating terminal are seen a few days after the lesion. The terminal retracts from the postsynaptic target.

Step 2: **Wallerian degeneration.** The lesion divides the axon into proximal and distal segments. The distal segment degenerates slowly during a period of several weeks in a process named after its discoverer, Augustus Waller. Eventually, the entire distal segment is destroyed and removed.

Step 3: **Myelin degeneration.** If the affected axon is myelinated, the myelin degenerates. The myelinating cell (i.e., the Schwann cell in the PNS and the oligodendrocyte in the CNS) usually survives this process. Schwann cells are immediately induced to divide, and they begin to synthesize trophic factors that may be important for regeneration.

Step 4: **Scavenging of debris.** Microglia in the CNS and macrophages and Schwann cells in the PNS scavenge the debris created by the breakdown of the axon and its myelin. This step is more rapid in the PNS than in the CNS.

Step 5: **Chromatolysis.** After axonal injury, most neuron cell bodies swell and undergo a characteristic rearrangement of organelles called chromatolysis. The nucleus also swells and moves to an eccentric position. The endoplasmic reticulum, normally close to the nucleus, reassembles around the periphery of the cell body. Chromatolysis is reversible if the neuron survives and is able to re-establish its distal process and contact the appropriate target.

Step 6: **Retrograde transneuronal degeneration.** Neurons that are synaptically connected to injured neurons may themselves be injured, a condition called transneuronal or trans-synaptic degeneration. If the neuron that synapses on the injured cell undergoes degeneration, it is called retrograde degeneration.

Step 7: **Anterograde transneuronal degeneration.** If a neuron that received synaptic contacts from an injured cell degenerates, it is called anterograde degeneration. The magnitude of these transneuronal effects (retrograde and anterograde degeneration) is quite variable.

---

not replaced, which is the main reason for the relatively limited recovery from serious brain and spinal cord injuries. It has been argued that this lack of regenerative ability is a design principle to ensure that learned behavior and memories are preserved in stable populations of neurons throughout life. A notable exception to this rule is olfactory bulb neurons, which are continually renewed throughout adult life by a population of stem cells or neuronal progenitor cells. As noted earlier, cells in the adult SVZ have the capacity to generate neurons and may do so to a limited extent throughout life. Learning how to induce these cells to make functional new CNS neurons after severe neural injury is the holy grail of regeneration research.

Glia   Unlike neurons, glial cells can be replaced if they are lost or injured in an adult. Such repopulation depends on progenitor cells committed to the glial cell lineage. Either the progenitor cells reside in a latent state (or are slowly turning over) in adult brains or true multipotential stem cells are activated by specific conditions, such as brain injury, to produce de novo glial progenitors. The most typical reaction of mammalian brains to a wide range of injuries is the formation of an **astrocytic glial scar**. This scar is produced primarily by an enlargement of individual astrocytes, a process called *hypertrophy,* and increased expression of a particular cytoskeleton protein, glial acidic fibrillary protein. Only a small degree of astrocytic *proliferation* (i.e., an increase

in cell number) accompanies this reaction. **Microglial cells,** which derive from cells related to the monocyte-macrophage lineage in blood and not from neuroepithelium, also react strongly to brain injury and are the main cells that proliferate at the injury site.

Axons   Another reason that relatively little recovery follows severe brain and spinal cord injury is that axons within the CNS do not regenerate effectively. This lack of axon regeneration in the CNS is in sharp contrast to the behavior of axons in the PNS, which can regrow and reconnect to appropriate end organs, either muscle or sensory receptors. For example, if the median nerve of the forearm is crushed by blunt trauma, the distal axon segments die off in a process called wallerian degeneration (see the box titled Axonal Degeneration and Regeneration) because the sustaining relationship with their proximal cell bodies is lost. These PNS axons can slowly regenerate and connect to muscles and sensory receptors in the hand. It is believed that the inability of CNS axons to regenerate is the fault of the local environment more than it is an intrinsic property of these axons. For example, on their surface, oligodendrocytes and myelin carry molecules, such as myelin-associated glycoprotein, that inhibit axon growth. Experiments have shown that if severed CNS axons are given the opportunity to regrow in the same environment that surrounds axons in the PNS, they are capable of regrowth and can make functional connections

A NORMAL NEURON   **B** DEGENERATING NEURON

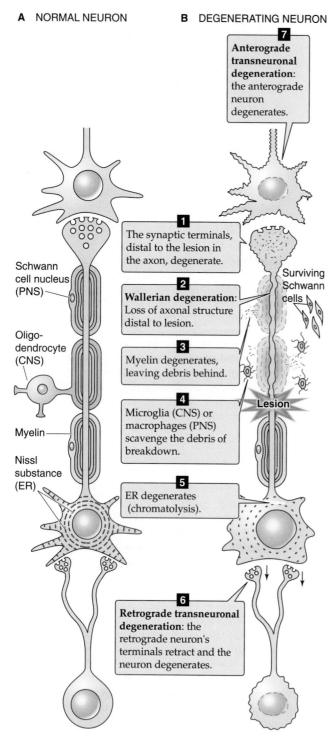

7 **Anterograde transneuronal degeneration:** the anterograde neuron degenerates.

Schwann cell nucleus (PNS)

Oligo-dendrocyte (CNS)

Myelin

Nissl substance (ER)

1 The synaptic terminals, distal to the lesion in the axon, degenerate.

2 **Wallerian degeneration:** Loss of axonal structure distal to lesion.

3 Myelin degenerates, leaving debris behind.

4 Microglia (CNS) or macrophages (PNS) scavenge the debris of breakdown.

5 ER degenerates (chromatolysis).

6 **Retrograde transneuronal degeneration:** the retrograde neuron's terminals retract and the neuron degenerates.

Surviving Schwann cells

Lesion

Figure 10-9 Nerve degeneration. **A,** Normal neuron. **B,** Degenerating neuron. ER, endoplasmic reticulum.

with CNS targets. The remarkable ability of damaged peripheral nerves to regenerate, even in mammals, has encouraged hope that CNS axons might, under the right conditions, be able to perform this same feat. It would mean that victims of spinal cord injury might walk again.

SUBDIVISIONS OF THE NERVOUS SYSTEM

A rudimentary knowledge of the anatomy of the nervous system is a prerequisite to discussion of its physiology. This section provides an overview of nervous system anatomy that builds on what has already been discussed about its embryological development. We in turn consider the CNS, PNS, and ANS (Table 10-1).

The directional terms used to describe brain structures can be somewhat confusing because the human nervous system, unlike that of lower vertebrates, bends during development. Thus, the dorsal surface of the cerebral cortex is also superior, whereas the dorsal surface of the spinal cord is also posterior (Fig. 10-10A).

The CNS consists of the telencephalon, cerebellum, diencephalon, midbrain, pons, medulla, and spinal cord

The CNS can be conveniently divided into five major areas: (1) telencephalon, (2) cerebellum, (3) diencephalon, (4) brainstem (consisting of the midbrain, pons, and medulla), and (5) spinal cord (Fig. 10-10B). Each of these areas has symmetric right and left sides.

Telencephalon One of the crowning glories of evolution is the human **cerebral cortex**, the most conspicuous part of the paired cerebral hemispheres. The human cerebral cortex has a surface area of ~2200 cm^2 and is estimated to contain 1.5 to 2×10^{10} neurons. The number of synaptic contacts between these cells is $\sim 3 \times 10^{14}$. The cortical surface area of mammals increases massively from mouse to monkey to humans in a ratio of 1:100:1000. The capacity for information processing by this neuronal machine is staggering and includes a remarkable range of functions: thinking, learning, memory, and consciousness.

The cortex is topographically organized in two ways. First, certain areas of the cortex mediate specific functions. For example, the area that mediates motor control is a well-defined strip of cortex located in the frontal lobe (Fig. 10-10C). Second, within a portion of cortex that manages a specific function (e.g., motor control, somatic sensation, hearing, or vision), the parts of the body spatially map onto this cortex in an orderly way. We discuss this principle of **somatotopy** in Chapter 16.

Another part of the telencephalon is the great mass of axons that stream into and out of the cerebral cortex and connect it with other regions. The volume of axons needed to interconnect cortical neurons increases as a power function of cortical surface area, which increases so dramatically from mice to humans. Thus, the *relative* volume of white matter to gray matter is 5-fold greater in humans versus mice. The final part of the telencephalon includes the **basal ganglia**, which comprise the striatum (caudate nucleus and putamen) and globus pallidus. These structures have indirect connections with motor portions of the cerebral cortex and are involved in motor control.

A   AXES OF THE CNS

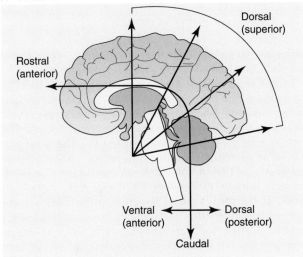

B   MAJOR COMPONENTS OF THE CNS

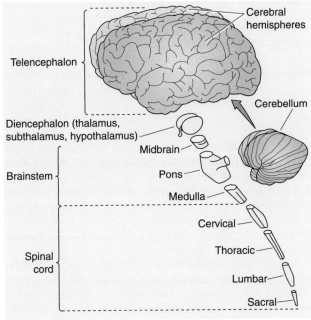

C   SURFACE ANATOMY OF THE CEREBRAL CORTEX

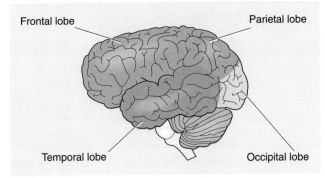

Figure 10-10   Gross anatomy of the CNS.

Cerebellum   This brain region lies immediately dorsal to the brainstem. Although the cerebellum represents only ~10% of the CNS by volume, it contains ~50% of all CNS neurons. The exceedingly large number of input connections to the cerebellum conveys information from nearly every type of receptor in the nervous system, including visual and auditory input. Combined, these afferent fibers outnumber the efferent projections by an estimated ratio of 40:1.

Functionally and by virtue of its connections, the cerebellum can be divided into three parts. Phylogenetically, the vestibulocerebellum (also called the archicerebellum) is the oldest of these three parts, followed by the spinocerebellum (also called the paleocerebellum) and then by the cerebrocerebellum (also called the neocerebellum).

The **vestibulocerebellum** is closely related to the vestibular system, whose sensors are located in the inner ear and whose way stations are located in the pons and medulla. It helps maintain the body's balance. The **spinocerebellum** receives strong input from muscle stretch receptors through connections in the spinal cord and brainstem. It helps regulate muscle tone. The **cerebrocerebellum**, the largest part of the human cerebellum, receives a massive number of projections from sensorimotor portions of the cerebral cortex through neurons in the pons. It coordinates motor behavior. Much of the cerebellum's output reaches the contralateral (i.e., on the opposite side of the body) motor cortex by way of the thalamus. Other efferent projections reach neurons in all three parts of the brainstem.

Diencephalon   This brain region consists of the thalamus, the subthalamus, and the hypothalamus, each with a very different function. The **thalamus** is the main integrating station for sensory information that is bound for the cerebral cortex, where it will reach the level of conscious perception. Along with the **subthalamus**, the thalamus also receives projections from the basal ganglia that are important for motor function. Input to the thalamus from the cerebellum (specifically, the cerebrocerebellum) is important for normal motor control. Patients with **Parkinson disease**, a severe movement disorder, gradually lose the ability to make voluntary movements; in some of these patients, it is possible to improve movement by stimulating certain areas of the thalamus or subthalamus. Control of arousal and certain aspects of memory function also reside in discrete areas of the thalamus.

The **hypothalamus** is the CNS structure that most affects the ANS. It performs this function through strong, direct connections with autonomic nuclei in the brainstem and spinal cord. It also acts as part of the endocrine system in two major ways. First, specialized neurons located within specific nuclei in the hypothalamus synthesize certain hormones (e.g., arginine vasopressin and oxytocin) and transport them down their axons to the posterior pituitary gland, where the hormones are secreted into the blood. Second, other specialized neurons in other nuclei synthesize "releasing hormones" (e.g., gonadotropin-releasing hormone) and release them into a plexus of veins, called a portal system, that carries the releasing hormones to cells in the anterior pituitary. There, the releasing hormones stimulate certain cells (e.g., gonadotrophs) to secrete hormones (e.g., follicle-stimulating hormone or luteinizing hormone) into the bloodstream. We discuss these principles in Chapter 47. The hypothalamus also has specialized centers that play important roles in controlling body temperature and hunger (see Chapters 58 and 59), thirst (see Chapter 40), and the cardiovascular system. It is the main control center of the ANS.

Brainstem (Midbrain, Pons, and Medulla)   This region lies immediately above, or rostral to, the spinal cord. Like the spinal cord, the midbrain, pons, and medulla have a segmental organization, receive sensory (afferent) information, and send out motor (efferent) signals through paired nerves that are called **cranial nerves**. The midbrain, pons, and medulla also contain important control centers for the ANS (see Chapter 14). In addition to motor neurons, autonomic neurons, and sensory neurons present at each level, the caudal brainstem serves as a conduit for a large volume of axons traveling from higher CNS centers to the spinal cord (descending pathways) and vice versa (ascending pathways). In addition, this portion of the brainstem contains a loosely organized interconnected collection of neurons and fibers called the **reticular formation**. This neuronal network has diffuse connections with the cortex and other brain regions and affects the level of consciousness or arousal.

The **midbrain** has somatic motor neurons that control eye movement. These neurons reside in the nuclei for CN III and CN IV. Other midbrain neurons are part of a system, along with the cerebellum and cortex, for motor control. The midbrain also contains groups of neurons that are involved in relaying signals related to hearing and vision.

Just caudal to the midbrain is the **pons**, which contains the somatic motor neurons that control mastication (nucleus for CN V), eye movement (nucleus for CN VI), and facial muscles (nucleus for CN VII). The pons also receives somatic sensory information from the face, scalp, mouth, and nose (portion of the nucleus for CN V). It is also involved in processing information that is related to hearing and equilibrium (nucleus for CN VIII). Neurons in the ventral pons receive input from the cortex, and these neurons in turn form a massive direct connection with the cerebellum (see earlier) that is crucial for coordinating motor movements.

The most caudal portion of the brainstem is the **medulla**. The organization of the medulla is most similar to that of the spinal cord. The medulla contains somatic motor neurons that innervate the muscles of the neck (nucleus of CN XI) and tongue (nucleus of CN XII). Along with the pons, the medulla is involved in controlling blood pressure, heart rate, respiration, and digestion (nuclei of CN IX and X). The medulla is the first CNS way station for information traveling from the special senses of hearing and equilibrium.

Spinal Cord   Continuous with the caudal portion of the medulla is the spinal cord. The spinal cord runs from the base of the skull to the body of the first lumbar vertebra. Thus, it does not run the full length of the vertebral column in adults.

The spinal cord consists of 31 segments that each have a motor and sensory nerve root. (The sensory nerve root of the first cervical segment is very small and can be missing.) These nerve roots combine to form 31 bilaterally symmetric pairs of spinal nerves. The spinal roots, nerves, and ganglia are part of the PNS (see later).

Sensory information from the skin, muscle, and visceral organs enters the spinal cord through fascicles of axons called dorsal roots (Fig. 10-11A). The point of entry is called the dorsal root entry zone. Dorsal root axons have their cell bodies of origin in the spinal ganglia (i.e., **dorsal root ganglia**) associated with that spinal segment.

Ventral roots contain strictly efferent fibers (Fig. 10-11B). These fibers arise from motor neurons (i.e., general somatic efferent neurons) whose cell bodies are located in the ventral (or anterior) *gray* horns of the spinal cord (gray because they contain mainly cell bodies without myelin) and from preganglionic autonomic neurons (i.e., general visceral efferent neurons) whose cell bodies are located in the intermediolateral gray horns (i.e., between the dorsal and ventral gray horns) of the cord. Most of the efferent fibers are somatic efferents that innervate skeletal muscle to mediate voluntary movement. The other fibers are visceral efferents that synapse with postganglionic autonomic neurons, which in turn innervate visceral smooth muscle or glandular tissue.

Each segment of the spinal cord contains groups of associative neurons in its dorsal gray horns. Some but not all incoming sensory fibers synapse on these associative neurons, which in turn contribute axons to fiber paths that both mediate synaptic interactions within the spinal cord and convey information to more rostral areas of the CNS by way of several conspicuous **ascending tracts** of axons (Fig. 10-11C). Similarly, **descending tracts** of axons from the cerebral cortex and brainstem control the motor neurons whose cell bodies are in the ventral horn, thus leading to coordinated voluntary or posture-stabilizing movements. The most important of these descending tracts is called the lateral **corticospinal tract**; ~90% of its cell bodies of origin are in the contralateral cerebral cortex. These ascending and descending tracts are located in the *white* portion of the spinal cord (white because it contains mostly myelinated axons). The spatial organization of spinal cord neurons and fiber tracts is complex but orderly and varies somewhat among the 31 segments.

If sensory fibers enter the spinal cord and synapse directly on motor neurons in that same segment, this connection underlies a simple **segmental reflex** or interaction. If the incoming fibers synapse with neurons in other spinal segments, they can participate in an **intersegmental reflex** or interaction. Finally, if the incoming signals travel rostrally to the brainstem before they synapse, they constitute a **suprasegmental interaction**.

The peripheral nervous system comprises the cranial and spinal nerves, their associated sensory ganglia, and various sensory receptors

The PNS serves four main purposes: (1) it transduces physical or chemical stimuli both from the external environment and from within the body into raw sensory information through receptors; (2) it conveys sensory information to the CNS along axon pathways; (3) it conveys motor signals from the CNS along axon pathways to target organs, primarily skeletal and smooth muscle; and (4) it converts the motor signals to chemical signals at synapses on target tissues in the periphery. Figure 10-11B summarizes these four functions for a simple reflex arc in which a painful stimulus to the foot

A SPINAL CORD AND NERVE ROOTS

Posterior median septum
Dorsal root entry zone
Posterior funiculus
Anterior gray horn
Posterior intermediate septum
Posterior gray horn
Lateral funiculus
Anterior funiculus

Root filaments { Dorsal / Ventral
Dorsal root ganglion
Mixed spinal nerve
Anterior median fissure
Pia mater
Arachnoid
Dura mater
Root sleeve

B A SPINAL REFLEX ARC

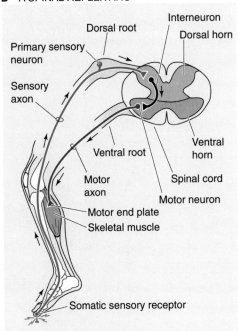

Dorsal root
Interneuron
Dorsal horn
Primary sensory neuron
Sensory axon
Motor axon
Ventral root
Motor neuron
Ventral horn
Spinal cord
Motor end plate
Skeletal muscle
Somatic sensory receptor

C ASCENDING AND DESCENDING TRACTS

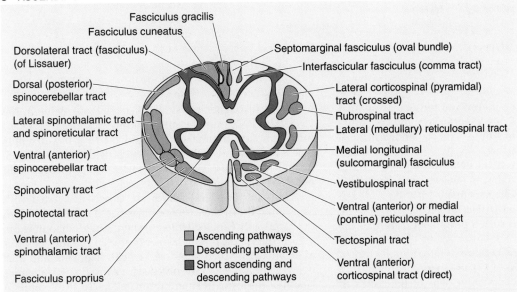

Fasciculus gracilis
Fasciculus cuneatus
Dorsolateral tract (fasciculus) (of Lissauer)
Dorsal (posterior) spinocerebellar tract
Lateral spinothalamic tract and spinoreticular tract
Ventral (anterior) spinocerebellar tract
Spinoolivary tract
Spinotectal tract
Ventral (anterior) spinothalamic tract
Fasciculus proprius

Septomarginal fasciculus (oval bundle)
Interfascicular fasciculus (comma tract)
Lateral corticospinal (pyramidal) tract (crossed)
Rubrospinal tract
Lateral (medullary) reticulospinal tract
Medial longitudinal (sulcomarginal) fasciculus
Vestibulospinal tract
Ventral (anterior) or medial (pontine) reticulospinal tract
Tectospinal tract
Ventral (anterior) corticospinal tract (direct)

☐ Ascending pathways
☐ Descending pathways
☐ Short ascending and descending pathways

Figure 10-11   Spinal cord. **A,** Each spinal segment has dorsal and ventral nerve roots that carry sensory and motor nerve fibers, respectively. **B,** The simple "flexor" reflex arc is an illustration of the four functions of the PNS: (1) a receptor transduces a painful stimulus into an action potential, (2) a primary sensory neuron conveys the information to the CNS, (3) the CNS conveys information to the target organ by a motor neuron, and (4) the electrical signals are converted to signals at the motor end plate. **C,** Ascending pathways, which carry information to more rostral areas of the CNS, are shown on the left. Descending pathways, which carry information in the opposite direction, are shown on the right.

results in retraction of the foot from the source of the pain.

Like the CNS, the PNS can be divided into *somatic* and *autonomic* parts. The somatic division includes the sensory neurons and axons that innervate the skin, joints, and muscle as well as the motor axons that innervate skeletal muscle.

The somatic division of the PNS primarily deals with the body's *external environment,* either to gather information about this environment or to interact with it through voluntary motor behavior. The ANS, discussed in the next section and in Chapter 14, is a functionally distinct part of both the CNS and PNS (Table 10-1). The autonomic portion

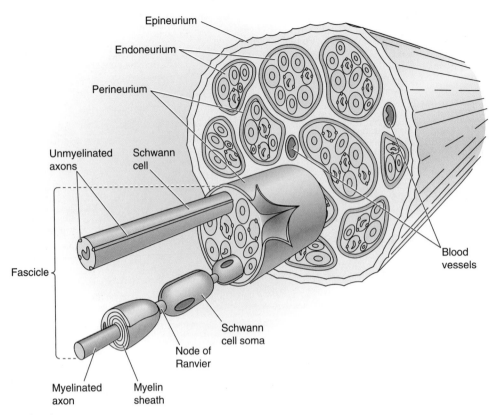

Figure 10-12   Peripheral nerve.

of the PNS consists of the motor and sensory axons that innervate smooth muscle, the exocrine glands, and other viscera. This division mainly deals with the body's *internal environment*.

Three important aspects of the PNS are discussed in other chapters. Sensory transduction is reviewed in Chapter 15, synaptic transmission in Chapters 8 and 13, and peripheral neuronal circuits in Chapter 16. Here, we focus primarily on the system of axons that is such a prominent feature of the PNS.

Axons in the PNS are organized into bundles called **peripheral nerves** (Fig. 10-12). These nerves contain, in a large nerve such as the sciatic nerve, tens of thousands of axons. Individual axons are surrounded by loose connective tissue called the **endoneurium**. Within the nerve, axons are bundled together in small groups called fascicles, each one covered by a connective tissue sheath known as the **perineurium**. The perineurium contributes structural stability to the nerve. Fascicles are grouped together and surrounded by a matrix of connective tissue called the **epineurium**. Fascicles within a nerve anastomose with neighboring fascicles. Axons shift from one fascicle to another along the length of the nerve, but they tend to remain in roughly the same general area within the nerve over long distances. The interlocking meshwork of fascicles adds further mechanical strength to the nerve. Axons range in diameter from less than 1 to 20 μm. Because axons are extremely fragile, adaptations that enhance mechanical stability are very important. The PNS is designed

to be much tougher, physically, than nervous tissue in the CNS. The PNS must be mechanically flexible, tolerant of minor physical trauma, and sustainable by a blood supply that is less dependable than the one providing for the CNS. A spinal cord transplanted to the lower part of the leg would not survive the running of a 100-meter dash.

Axons in peripheral nerves are closely associated with Schwann cells. In the case of a myelinated axon, a Schwann cell forms a myelinated wrap around a single adjacent axon, a single internodal myelin segment between 250 and 1000 μm in length. Many such internodal myelin segments, and thus many Schwann cells, are necessary to myelinate the entire length of the axon. In an unmyelinated nerve, the cytoplasm of a Schwann cell envelops but does not wrap around axons. Unmyelinated axons outnumber myelinated axons by about 2:1 in typical human nerves. Diseases that affect the PNS can disrupt nerve function by causing either loss of myelin or axonal injury.

The functional organization of a peripheral nerve is best illustrated by a typical thoracic spinal nerve and its branches. Every spinal nerve is formed by the dorsal and ventral roots joining together and emerging from the spinal cord at that segmental level (Fig. 10-11). The dorsal roots coalesce and display a spindle-shaped swelling called the spinal or dorsal root ganglion, which contains the cell bodies of the sensory axons in the dorsal roots. Individual neurons are called dorsal root ganglion cells or spinal ganglion cells and are typical unipolar neurons that give rise to a single process that

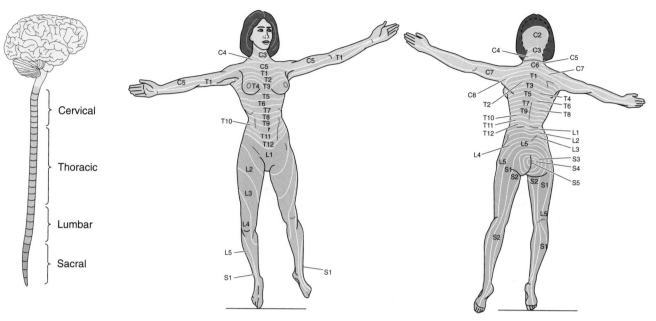

Figure 10-13   Dermatomes. A dermatome is the area of cutaneous sensory innervation that a single spinal segment provides.

bifurcates in a T-like manner into a peripheral and central branch (Fig. 10-3). The central branch carries sensory information into the CNS and the peripheral branch terminates as a sensory ending. The peripheral process, which brings information toward the cell body, meets one definition of a dendrite; however, it has all the physiological and morphological features of a peripheral axon.

Spinal nerves divide into several branches that distribute motor and sensory axons to the parts of the body associated with that segment. Axons conveying autonomic motor or autonomic sensory signals also travel in these branches. These branches are said to be "mixed" because they contain both efferent and afferent axons. Further nerve division occurs as axons travel to supply their targets, such as the skin, muscle, or blood vessels. In the case of thoracic spinal nerves, the subdivision is orderly and has a similar pattern for most of the nerves. In the cervical and lumbosacral areas, however, the spinal nerves from different segments of the spinal cord intermingle to form a **nerve plexus**. The subsequent course of the nerves in the upper and lower extremities is complex. The pattern of cutaneous innervation of the body is shown in Figure 10-13. The area of cutaneous innervation provided by a single dorsal root and its ganglion is called a **dermatome**. Severing a single dorsal root does not produce anesthesia in that dermatome because of overlap between the cutaneous innervation provided by adjacent dorsal roots. The sole exception to this rule is the C2 root, sectioning of which causes a patch of analgesia on the back of the head; neither C3 nor the trigeminal nerve innervates skin in this area. Also note that no dermatomes are shown for the first cervical and the coccygeal segments because they are small

or may be missing (in the case of the first cervical segment).

The autonomic nervous system innervates effectors that are not under voluntary control

The nervous system regulates some physiological mechanisms in a way that is independent or *autonomous* of voluntary control. Control of body temperature is an example of a fundamental process that most individuals cannot consciously regulate. Other examples include blood pressure and heart rate. The absence of voluntary control means that the ANS has little cortical representation.

The ANS has three divisions: sympathetic, parasympathetic, and enteric. The sympathetic and parasympathetic divisions have both CNS and PNS parts. The enteric division is entirely in the PNS. The **parasympathetic** and **sympathetic** efferent systems are composed of two neurons. The cell body of the first neuron is located in the CNS and that of the second in the PNS. The sympathetic and parasympathetic divisions innervate most visceral organs and have a yin-yang functional relationship. The **enteric** division regulates the rhythmic contraction of intestinal smooth muscle and also regulates the secretory functions of intestinal epithelial cells. It receives afferent input from the gut wall and is subject to modulation by the two other divisions of the ANS.

All the divisions have both efferent and afferent connections, although the efferent actions of the ANS are usually emphasized. We consider the ANS in detail in Chapter 14.

Peripheral Nerve Disease

The symptoms of peripheral nerve disease, or **neuropathy**, are numbness (i.e., a sensory deficit) and weakness (i.e., a motor deficit). Such symptoms may arise from disturbances in many parts of the nervous system. How, then, can one tell whether a problem is the result of disease in the PNS?

Motor axons directly innervate and have "trophic" effects on skeletal muscle. If the axon is cut or dies, this trophic influence is lost and the muscle undergoes denervation atrophy. In addition, individual muscle fibers may twitch spontaneously (**fibrillation**). The cause of fibrillation is still debated, but it may be related to the observation that acetylcholine receptors spread beyond the neuromuscular junction and become "supersensitive" to their agonist. If true, these observations imply continuing exposure to acetylcholine, even if it is in smaller quantities. Schwann cells at denervated junctions may be the source of acetylcholine. When a motor axon is first damaged but has not yet lost continuity with the muscle fibers that it innervates, these muscle cells may twitch in unison. These small twitches can be seen under the skin and are called **fasciculations**. They are probably due to spontaneous action potentials in dying or injured motor neurons or their axons.

When the PNS is affected by a diffuse or generalized disease (e.g., the result of a metabolic problem or toxin), all peripheral nerves are involved, but symptoms arise first in the longest nerves of the body (i.e., those traveling from the spinal cord to the feet). This predilection for affecting the longest nerves often causes a "stocking pattern" defect in sensation and sometimes in strength. If both the feet and hands are affected, the process is called a "stocking and glove" defect. With progression of the disease, the level of involvement moves centripetally (i.e., up the leg, toward the trunk), and the sensory or motor dysfunction comes to involve more proximal portions of the legs and arms. One of the most common causes of this diffuse pattern of PNS involvement is the sensorimotor polyneuropathy associated with diabetes. Other causes include chronic renal failure (uremia), thiamine deficiency (often seen with alcohol abuse), and heavy metal poisoning.

If a patient exhibits weakness or sensory loss that is associated with muscle fibrillation and atrophy and a stocking or stocking and glove pattern of sensory disturbance, a PNS problem is likely. Patients with peripheral neuropathy may also complain of tingling sensations (**paresthesias**) or pain in areas of the body supplied by the diseased nerves.

REFERENCES

Books and Reviews

Abrous DN, Koehl M, Le Moal M: Adult neurogenesis: From precursors to network and physiology. Physiol Rev 2005; 85: 523-569.

Gage FH: Stem cells of the central nervous system. Curr Opin Neurobiol 1998; 8:671-676.

Hirokawa N: Kinesin and dynein superfamily proteins and the mechanism of organelle transport. Science 1998; 279:519-526.

Kandel ER, Schwartz JH, Jessell TM: Principles of Neural Science, 4th ed. New York: McGraw-Hill, 2000.

Journal Articles

Burne JF, Staple JK, Raff MC: Glial cells are increased proportionally in transgenic optic nerves with increased numbers of axons. J Neurosci 1996; 16:2064-2073.

Chiasson BJ, Tropepe V, Morshead CM, van der Kooy D: Adult mammalian forebrain ependymal and subependymal cells demonstrate proliferative potential, but only subependymal cells have neural stem cell characteristics. J Neurosci 1999; 19:4462-4471.

Colbert CM, Johnston D: Axonal action-potential initiation and Na$^+$ channel densities in the soma and axon initial segment of subicular pyramidal neurons. J Neurosci 1996; 16:6676-6686.

CHAPTER 11

THE NEURONAL MICROENVIRONMENT

Bruce R. Ransom

Extracellular fluid in the brain provides a highly regulated environment for central nervous system neurons

Everything that surrounds individual neurons can be considered part of the **neuronal microenvironment**. Technically, therefore, the neuronal microenvironment includes the extracellular fluid (ECF), capillaries, glial cells, and adjacent neurons. Although the term often is restricted to just the immediate ECF, the ECF cannot be meaningfully discussed in isolation because of its extensive interaction with brain capillaries, glial cells, and cerebrospinal fluid (CSF). How the microenvironment interacts with neurons and how the brain (used here synonymously with *central nervous system,* or *CNS*) stabilizes it to provide constancy for neuronal function are the subjects of this discussion.

The concentrations of solutes in **brain extracellular fluid** (BECF) fluctuate with neural activity, and conversely, changes in ECF composition can influence nerve cell behavior. Not surprisingly, therefore, the brain carefully controls the composition of this important compartment. It does so in three major ways. First, the brain uses the blood-brain barrier to protect the BECF from fluctuations in blood composition. Second, the CSF, which is synthesized by choroid plexus epithelial cells, strongly influences the composition of the BECF. Third, the surrounding glial cells "condition" the BECF.

The brain is physically and metabolically fragile

The ratio of brain weight to body weight in humans is the highest in the animal kingdom. The average adult brain weight is ~1400 g in men and ~1300 g in women, approximately the same weight as the liver (see Chapter 46). This large and vital structure, which has the consistency of thick pudding, is protected from mechanical injury by a surrounding layer of bone and by the CSF in which it floats.

The brain is also *metabolically* fragile. This fragility arises from its high rate of energy consumption, absence of significant stored fuel in the form of glycogen (~5% of the amount in the liver), and rapid development of cellular damage when ATP is depleted. However, the brain is not the greediest of the body's organs; both the heart and kidney cortex have higher metabolic rates. Nevertheless, although it constitutes only 2% of the body by weight, the brain receives ~15% of resting blood flow and accounts for ~20% and 50%, respectively, of total resting oxygen and glucose utilization. The brain's high metabolic demands arise from the need of its neurons to maintain the steep ion gradients on which neuronal excitability depends. In addition, neurons rapidly turn over their actin cytoskeleton. Neuroglial cells, the other major cells in the brain, also maintain steep transmembrane ion gradients. More than half of the energy consumed by the brain is directed to maintain ion gradients, primarily through operation of the Na-K pump (see Chapter 5). An interruption of the continuous supply of oxygen or glucose to the brain results in rapid depletion of energy stores and disruption of ion gradients. Because of falling ATP levels in the brain, consciousness is lost within 10 seconds of a blockade in cerebral blood flow. Irreversible nerve cell injury can occur after only 5 minutes of interrupted blood flow.

CEREBROSPINAL FLUID

CSF is a colorless, watery liquid. It fills the ventricles of the brain and forms a thin layer around the outside of the brain and spinal cord in the subarachnoid space. CSF is secreted within the brain by a highly vascularized epithelial structure called the **choroid plexus** and circulates to sites in the subarachnoid space where it enters the venous blood system. The composition of CSF is highly regulated, and because CSF is in slow diffusional equilibrium with BECF, it helps regulate the composition of BECF. The choroid plexus can be thought of as the brain's "kidney" in that it stabilizes the composition of CSF, just as the kidney stabilizes the composition of blood plasma.

CSF fills the ventricles and subarachnoid space

The **ventricles** of the brain are four small compartments located within the brain (Fig. 11-1A). Each ventricle contains a choroid plexus and is filled with CSF. The ventricles are linked together by channels, or foramina, that allow CSF to

A VENTRICLES OF THE BRAIN

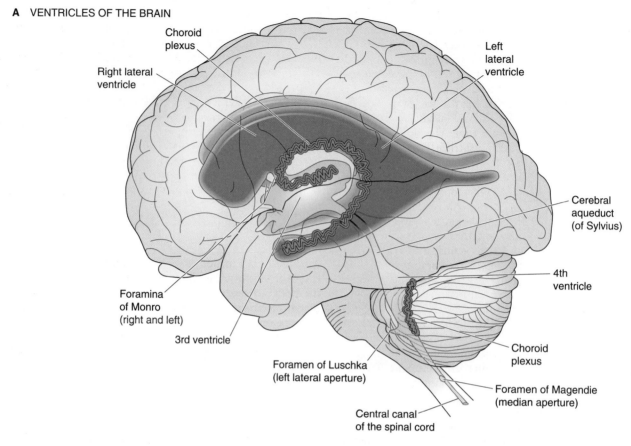

Choroid
plexus

Right lateral
ventricle

Left
lateral
ventricle

Cerebral
aqueduct
(of Sylvius)

4th
ventricle

Choroid
plexus

Foramen of Magendie
(median aperture)

Foramina
of Monro
(right and left)

3rd ventricle

Foramen of Luschka
(left lateral aperture)

Central canal
of the spinal cord

B CSF CIRCULATION

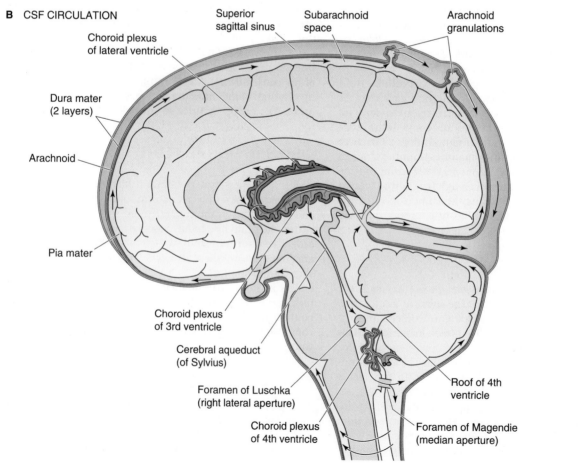

Choroid plexus
of lateral ventricle

Superior
sagittal sinus

Subarachnoid
space

Arachnoid
granulations

Dura mater
(2 layers)

Arachnoid

Pia mater

Choroid plexus
of 3rd ventricle

Cerebral aqueduct
(of Sylvius)

Foramen of Luschka
(right lateral aperture)

Choroid plexus
of 4th ventricle

Roof of 4th
ventricle

Foramen of Magendie
(median aperture)

move easily between them. The two **lateral ventricles** are the largest and are symmetrically located within the cerebral hemispheres. The choroid plexus of each lateral ventricle is located along the inner radius of this horseshoe-shaped structure (Fig. 11-1B). The two lateral ventricles each communicate with the **third ventricle**, which is located in the midline between the thalami, through the two interventricular **foramina of Monro**. The choroid plexus of the third ventricle lies along the ventricle roof. The third ventricle communicates with the fourth ventricle by the **cerebral aqueduct of Sylvius**. The **fourth ventricle** is the most caudal ventricle and is located in the brainstem. It is bounded by the cerebellum superiorly and by the pons and medulla inferiorly. The choroid plexus of the fourth ventricle lies along only a portion of this ventricle's tent-shaped roof. The fourth ventricle is continuous with the central canal of the spinal cord. CSF escapes from the fourth ventricle and flows into the subarachnoid space through three foramina: the two laterally placed **foramina of Luschka** and the midline opening in the roof of the fourth ventricle, called the **foramen of Magendie**. We shall see later how CSF circulates throughout the subarachnoid space of the brain and spinal cord.

The brain and spinal cord are covered by two membranous tissue layers called the **leptomeninges**, which are in turn surrounded by a third, tougher layer. The innermost of these three layers is the pia mater; the middle is the arachnoid mater (or arachnoid membrane); and the outermost layer is the dura mater (Fig. 11-2). Between the arachnoid mater and pia mater (i.e., the leptomeninges) is the **subarachnoid space**, which is filled with CSF that escaped from the fourth ventricle. The CSF in the subarachnoid space completely surrounds the brain and spinal cord. In adults, the subarachnoid space and the ventricles with which they are continuous contain ~150 mL of CSF, 30 mL in the ventricles and 120 mL in the subarachnoid spaces of the brain and spinal cord.

The **pia mater** (Latin for "tender mother") is a thin layer of connective tissue cells that is very closely applied to the surface of the brain and covers blood vessels as they plunge through the arachnoid into the brain. A nearly complete layer of astrocytic endfeet—the **glia limitans**—abuts the pia from the brain side and is separated from the pia by a basement membrane. The pia adheres so tightly to the associated glia limitans in some areas that they seem to be continuous with each other; this combined structure is sometimes called the pial-glial membrane or layer. This layer does *not* restrict diffusion of substances between the BECF and the CSF.

The **arachnoid membrane** (Greek for "cobweb-like") is composed of layers of cells, resembling those that make up the pia, linked together by *tight junctions*. The arachnoid isolates the CSF in the subarachnoid space from blood in the overlying vessels of the dura mater. The cells that constitute the arachnoid and the pia are continuous in the trabeculae

that span the subarachnoid space. These arachnoid and pial layers are relatively avascular; thus, the leptomeningeal cells that form them probably derive nutrition from the CSF that they enclose as well as from the ECF that surrounds them. The leptomeningeal cells can phagocytose foreign material in the subarachnoid space.

The **dura mater** is a thick, inelastic membrane that forms an outer protective envelope around the brain. The dura has two layers that split to form the intracranial venous sinuses. Blood vessels in the dura mater are outside the blood-brain barrier (see later), and substances could easily diffuse from dural capillaries into the nearby CSF if it were not for the blood-CSF barrier created by the arachnoid.

The brain floats in CSF, which acts as a shock absorber

An important function of CSF is to buffer the brain from mechanical injury. The CSF that surrounds the brain reduces the effective weight of the brain from ~1400 g to less than 50 g. This buoyancy is a consequence of the difference in the specific gravities of brain tissue (1.040) and CSF (1.007). The mechanical buffering that the CSF provides greatly diminishes the risk of acceleration-deceleration injuries in the same way that wearing a bicycle helmet reduces the risk of head injury. As you strike a tree, the foam insulation of the helmet gradually compresses and reduces the velocity of your head. Thus, the deceleration of your head is not nearly as severe as the deceleration of the outer shell of your helmet. The importance of this fluid suspension system is underscored by the consequences of reduced CSF pressure, which sometimes happens transiently after the diagnostic procedure of removal of CSF from the spinal subarachnoid space (see the box titled Lumbar Puncture). Patients with reduced CSF pressure experience severe pain when they try to sit up or to stand because the brain is no longer cushioned by shock-absorbing fluid and small gravity-induced movements put strain on pain-sensitive structures. Fortunately, the CSF leak that can result from lumbar puncture is only temporary; the puncture hole easily heals itself, with prompt resolution of all symptoms.

The choroid plexuses secrete CSF into the ventricles, and the arachnoid granulations absorb it

Most of the CSF is produced by the **choroid plexuses**, which are present in four locations (Fig. 11-1): the two lateral ventricles, the third ventricle, and the fourth ventricle. The capillaries within the brain appear to form a small amount of CSF. Total CSF production is ~500 mL/day. Therefore, the entire volume of CSF, ~150 mL, is replaced or "turns over" about three times each day.

Figure 11-1 The brain ventricles and the cerebrospinal fluid. **A,** This is a transparent view, looking from the left side of the brain. The two lateral ventricles communicate with the third ventricle, which in turn communicates with the fourth ventricle. **B,** Each ventricle contains a choroid plexus, which secretes CSF. The CSF escapes from the fourth ventricle and into the subarachnoid space through the two lateral foramina of Luschka and the single foramen of Magendie.

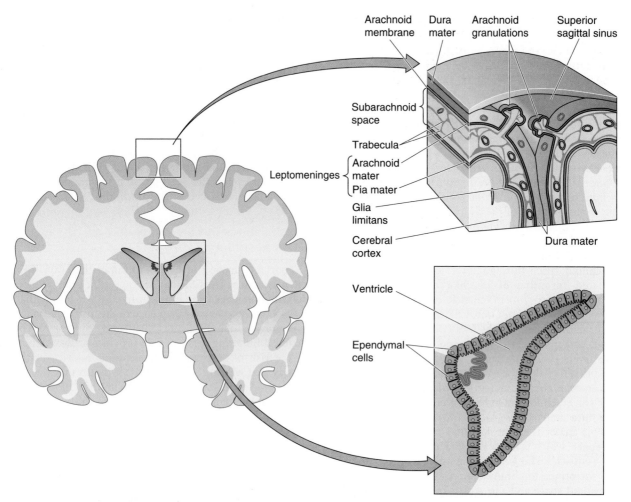

Figure 11-2 The meninges and ependymal cells. The figure represents a coronal section through the anterior portion of the brain. The *upper inset* shows the three layers of meninges: the dura mater, which here is split into two layers to accommodate the superior sagittal sinus (filled with venous blood); the arachnoid mater, which is formed by cells that are interconnected by tight junctions; and the pia mater, which closely adheres to a layer composed of astrocyte endfeet that are covered by a basement membrane (glia limitans). The *lower inset* shows ependymal cells lining the interior of the frontal horn of the left ventricle. Both the subarachnoid space and the cavities of the ventricles are filled with CSF.

Secretion of new CSF creates a slight pressure gradient, which drives the circulation of CSF from its ventricular sites of origin into the subarachnoid space through three openings in the fourth ventricle, as discussed earlier. CSF percolates throughout the subarachnoid space and is finally absorbed into venous blood in the superior sagittal sinus, which lies between the two cerebral hemispheres (Fig. 11-2). The sites of absorption are specialized evaginations of the arachnoid membrane into the venous sinus (Fig. 11-3A). These absorptive sites are called pacchionian granulations or simply **arachnoid granulations** when they are large (up to 1 cm in diameter) and **arachnoid villi** if their size is microscopic. These structures act as pressure-sensitive, one-way valves for bulk CSF clearance; CSF can cross into venous blood, but venous blood cannot enter CSF. The actual mechanism of CSF absorption may involve transcytosis (see Chapter 20), the formation of giant fluid-containing vacuoles that cross from the CSF side of the arachnoid epithelial cells to the blood side (Fig. 11-3A).

CSF may also be absorbed into spinal veins from herniations of arachnoid cells into these venous structures. Net CSF movement into venous blood is promoted by the pressure of the CSF, which is higher than that of the venous blood. When intracranial pressure (equivalent to CSF pressure) exceeds ~70 mm H$_2$O, absorption commences and increases with intracranial pressure (Fig. 11-3B). In contrast to CSF absorption, CSF formation is not sensitive to intracranial pressure. This arrangement helps stabilize intracranial pressure.

If intracranial pressure increases, CSF absorption selectively increases as well so that absorption exceeds formation (Fig. 11-3B). This response results in a lower CSF volume and a tendency to counteract the increased intracranial pressure. However, if absorption of CSF is impaired even at an initially normal intracranial pressure, CSF volume increases and causes an increase in intracranial pressure. Such an increase in intracranial pressure can lead to a disturbance in brain function.

Lumbar Puncture

One of the most important diagnostic tests in neurology is the sampling of CSF by lumbar puncture. Critical information about the composition of CSF and about intracranial pressure can be obtained from this procedure. The anatomist Vesalius noted in 1543 that the ventricles are filled with a clear fluid, but the diagnostic technique of placing a needle into the lumbar subarachnoid space to obtain CSF was not introduced until 1891 by the neurologist Heinrich Quincke. The method of lumbar puncture is dictated by spine anatomy. In adults, the spinal cord ends at the interspace between L1 and L2 (see Chapter 10). A hollow needle for sampling of CSF can be safely inserted into the subarachnoid space at the level of the L3-L4 interspace, well below the end of the spinal cord.

Once the needle is in the subarachnoid space, the physician attaches it to a manometer to measure pressure. With the patient lying on the side, normal pressure varies from 100 to 180 mm H_2O, or 7 to 13 mm Hg. With the subject in this position and in the absence of a block to the free circulation of CSF, lumbar CSF pressure roughly corresponds to intracranial pressure. The physician can demonstrate direct communication of the pressure in the intracranial compartment to the lumbar subarachnoid space by gently compressing the external jugular veins in the neck for 10 seconds. This maneuver, called the **Queckenstedt test**, rapidly increases intracranial pressure because it increases the volume of intracranial venous blood. It quickly leads to an increase in lumbar pressure, which just as rapidly dissipates when the jugular pressure is removed.

CSF pressure can become elevated because of a pathological mass within the cranium, such as a tumor or collection of blood, or because the brain is swollen as a result of injury or infection (see the later box titled Cerebral Edema). If a "mass lesion" (i.e., any pathological process that occupies intracranial space) is large or critically placed, it can displace the brain and cause interference with the free circulation of CSF. For example, an expanding mass in the cerebellum can force the inferior part of the cerebellum into the foramen magnum and block flow of CSF into the spinal subarachnoid space. Under these conditions, performance of lumbar puncture can precipitate a neurological catastrophe. If a needle is placed in the lumbar subarachnoid space and fluid is removed for diagnostic examination or leaks out after the needle is removed, the ensuing decrease in pressure in the lumbar space creates a pressure gradient across the foramen magnum and potentially forces the brain down into the spinal canal. This disaster is called *herniation*. For this reason, a computed tomographic scan or magnetic resonance image of the head is usually obtained before a lumbar puncture is attempted; the imaging study can rule out the possibility of a large intracranial lesion that might raise intracranial pressure and increase the risk of herniation when the subarachnoid space is punctured and CSF withdrawn. The Queckenstedt test must also be avoided when an intracranial mass is suspected because it could enhance the pressure gradient and hasten herniation.

A   MECHANISM OF CSF ABSORPTION

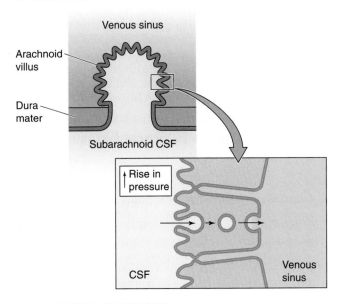

B   RATE OF CSF ABSORPTION

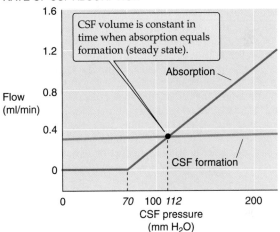

Figure 11-3 Absorption of CSF. **A,** Arachnoid villi—or the larger arachnoid granulations (not shown)—are specialized evaginations of the arachnoid membrane through the dura mater and into the lumen of the venous sinus. The absorption of CSF may involve transcytosis. Note that arachnoid villi and granulations serve as one-way valves; fluid cannot move from the vein to the subarachnoid space. **B,** The rate of CSF formation is virtually insensitive to changes in the pressure of the CSF. On the other hand, the absorption of CSF increases steeply at CSF pressures above ~70 mm H_2O.

The epithelial cells of the choroid plexus secrete the CSF

Each of the four choroid plexuses is formed during embryological development by invagination of the tela choroidea into the ventricular cavity (Fig. 11-4). The tela choroidea consists of a layer of ependymal cells covered by the pia mater and its associated blood vessels. The choroid epithelial cells (Fig. 11-4, first inset) are specialized ependymal cells and therefore contiguous with the ependymal lining of the ventricles at the margins of the choroid plexus. Choroid epithelial cells are cuboidal and have an apical border with microvilli and cilia that project into the ventricle (i.e., into the CSF). The plexus receives its blood supply from the anterior and posterior choroidal arteries; blood flow to the plexuses—per unit mass of tissue—is ~10-fold greater than the average cerebral blood flow. Sympathetic and parasympathetic nerves innervate each plexus, and sympathetic input appears to inhibit CSF formation. A high density of relatively

---

Normal-Pressure Hydrocephalus

Impaired CSF absorption is one mechanism proposed to explain a clinical form of ventricular enlargement called **normal-pressure hydrocephalus**. This condition is somewhat misnamed because the intracranial pressure is often intermittently elevated. Damage to the arachnoid villi can occur most commonly from infection or inflammation of the meninges or from the presence of an irritating substance, such as blood in the CSF after a subarachnoid hemorrhage. A spinal tap reveals normal pressure readings, but computed tomography or magnetic resonance imaging of the head shows enlargement of all four ventricles. Patients with normal-pressure hydrocephalus typically have progressive dementia, urinary incontinence, and gait disturbance, probably caused by stretching of axon pathways that course around the enlarged ventricles. A flexible plastic tube can be placed in one of the lateral ventricles to shunt CSF to venous blood or to the peritoneal cavity, thereby reducing CSF pressure. This procedure may reduce ventricular size and decrease neurological symptoms. The "shunting" procedure is also used for patients with obstructive hydrocephalus. In this condition, CSF outflow from the ventricles is blocked, typically at the aqueduct of Sylvius.

---

leaky capillaries is present within each plexus; as discussed later, these capillaries are outside the blood-brain barrier. The choroid epithelial cells are bound to one another by tight junctions that completely encircle each cell, an arrangement that makes the epithelium an effective barrier to free diffusion. Thus, although the choroid capillaries are outside the blood-brain barrier, the choroid epithelium insulates the ECF around these capillaries (which has a composition more similar to that of arterial blood) from the CSF. Moreover, the thin neck that connects the choroid plexus to the rest of the brain isolates the ECF near the leaky choroidal capillaries from the highly protected BECF in the rest of the brain.

The composition of CSF differs considerably from that of plasma; thus, CSF is not just an ultrafiltrate of plasma (Table 11-1). For example, CSF has lower concentrations of K^+ and amino acids than plasma does, and it contains almost no protein. Moreover, the choroid plexuses rigidly maintain the concentration of ions in CSF in the face of large swings in ion concentration in plasma. This ion homeostasis includes K^+, H^+/HCO_3^-, Mg^{2+}, Ca^{2+}, and, to a lesser extent, Na^+ and Cl^-. All these ions can affect neural function, hence the need for tight homeostatic control. The neuronal microenvironment is so well protected from the blood by the choroid plexuses and the rest of the blood-brain barrier that essential **micronutrients**, such as vitamins and trace elements that are needed in very small amounts, must be selectively transported into the brain. Some of these micronutrients are transported into the brain primarily by the choroid plexus and others primarily by the endothelial cells of the blood vessels. In comparison, the brain continuously metabolizes relatively large amounts of "macronutrients," such as glucose and some amino acids.

CSF forms in two sequential stages. First, ultrafiltration of plasma occurs across the fenestrated capillary wall (see

---

TABLE 11-1 Composition of Cerebrospinal Fluid

Solute	Plasma (mM of protein-free plasma)	CSF (mM)	CSF/Plasma Ratio
Na^+	153	147	0.96
K^+	4.7	2.9	0.62
Ca^{2+}	1.3 (ionized)	1.1 (ionized)	0.85
Mg^{2+}	0.6 (ionized)	1.1 (ionized)	1.8
Cl^-	110	113	1.03
HCO_3^-	24	22	0.92
$H_2PO_4^-$ and HPO_4^{2-}	0.75 (ionized)	0.9	1.2
pH	7.40	7.33	
Amino acids	2.6	0.7	0.27
Proteins	7 g/dL	0.03 g/dL	0.004
Osmolality (mOsm)	290	290	1.00

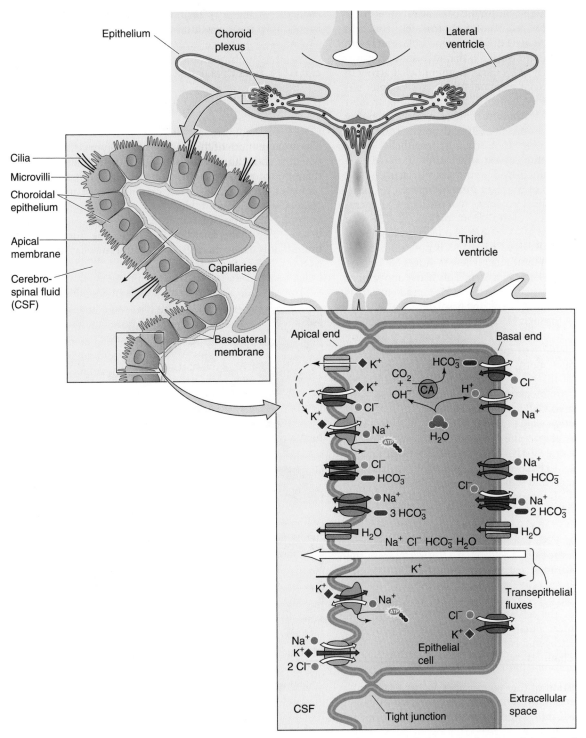

Figure 11-4 Secretion of CSF by the choroid plexus. The *top panel* shows the location of the choroid plexuses in the two lateral ventricles and the third ventricle. The *middle panel* shows the organization of a single fold of choroidal epithelial cells, with the basolateral membranes of the epithelial cells overlying capillaries and the apical membranes facing the CSF. The *bottom panel* shows a single choroid epithelial cell and several of the transporters and channels that are believed to play a role in the isosmotic secretion of CSF. CA, carbonic anhydrase.

Chapter 20) into the ECF beneath the basolateral membrane of the choroid epithelial cell. Second, choroid epithelial cells secrete fluid into the ventricle. CSF production occurs with a net transfer of NaCl and NaHCO$_3$ that drives water movement isosmotically (Fig. 11-4, large transepithelial arrow in the right inset). The renal proximal tubule (see Chapter 35) and small intestine (see Chapter 5) also perform near-isosmotic transport, but in the direction of *absorption* rather than *secretion*. In addition, the choroid plexus conditions CSF by absorbing K$^+$ (Fig. 11-4, small transepithelial arrow in the right inset) and certain other substances (e.g., a metabolite of serotonin, 5-hydroxyindoleacetic acid).

The upper portion of the right inset of Figure 11-4 summarizes the ion transport processes that mediate CSF secretion. The net secretion of Na$^+$ from plasma to CSF is a two-step process. The Na-K pump in the choroid plexus, unlike in other epithelia (see Chapter 5), is unusual in being located on the *apical* membrane, where it moves Na$^+$ out of the cell into the CSF—the first step. This active movement of Na$^+$ out of the cell generates an inward Na$^+$ gradient across the *basolateral* membrane, energizing basolateral Na$^+$ entry—the second step—through Na-H exchange and Na$^+$-coupled HCO$_3^-$ transport. In the case of Na-H exchange, the limiting factor is the availability of intracellular H$^+$, which carbonic anhydrase generates, along with HCO$_3^-$, from CO$_2$ and H$_2$O. Thus, blocking of the Na-K pump with ouabain halts CSF formation, whereas blocking of carbonic anhydrase with acetazolamide slows CSF formation.

The net secretion of Cl$^-$, like that of Na$^+$, is a two-step process. The first step is the intracellular accumulation of Cl$^-$ by the basolateral Cl-HCO$_3$ exchanger. Note that the net effect of parallel Cl-HCO$_3$ exchange and Na-H exchange is NaCl uptake. The second step is efflux of Cl$^-$ across the apical border into the CSF through either a Cl$^-$ channel or a K/Cl cotransporter.

HCO$_3^-$ secretion into CSF is important for neutralizing acid produced by CNS cells. At the basolateral membrane, the epithelial cell probably takes up HCO$_3^-$ directly from the plasma filtrate through electroneutral Na/HCO$_3$ cotransporters (see Fig. 5-11F) and the Na$^+$-driven Cl-HCO$_3$ exchanger (see Fig. 5-13C). As noted before, HCO$_3^-$ can also accumulate inside the cell after CO$_2$ entry. The apical step, movement of intracellular HCO$_3^-$ into the CSF, probably occurs by an electrogenic Na/HCO$_3$ cotransporter (see Fig. 5-11D) and Cl$^-$ channels (which are generally permeable to HCO$_3^-$).

The lower portion of the right inset of Figure 11-4 summarizes K$^+$ absorption from the CSF. The epithelial cell takes up K$^+$ by the Na-K pump and the Na/K/Cl cotransporter at the apical membrane (see Fig. 5-11G). Most of the K$^+$ recycles back to the CSF, but a small amount exits across the basolateral membrane and enters the blood. The concentration of K$^+$ in freshly secreted CSF is ~3.3 mM. Even with very large changes in plasma [K$^+$], the [K$^+$] in CSF changes very little. The value of [K$^+$] in CSF is significantly lower in the subarachnoid space than in choroid secretions, which suggests that brain capillary endothelial cells remove extracellular K$^+$ from the brain.

Water transport across the choroid epithelium is driven by a small osmotic gradient favoring CSF formation. This water movement is facilitated by expression of the water channel aquaporin 1 on both the apical and basal membranes as in renal proximal tubule (see Chapter 35).

BRAIN EXTRACELLULAR SPACE

Neurons, glia, and capillaries are packed tightly together in the CNS

The average width of the space between brain cells is ~20 nm, which is about three orders of magnitude smaller than the diameter of either a neuron or glial cell body (Fig. 11-5). However, because the surface membranes of neurons and glial cells are highly folded (i.e., have a large surface-to-volume ratio), the BECF in toto has a sizable volume fraction, ~20%, of the total brain volume. The fraction of the brain that is occupied by BECF varies somewhat in different

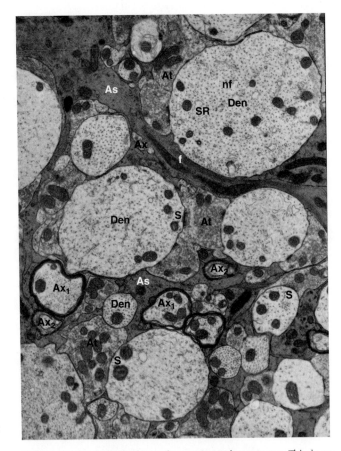

Figure 11-5 Tight packing of neurons and astrocytes. This is an electron micrograph of a section of the spinal cord from an adult rat showing the intermingling and close apposition of neurons and glial cells, mainly astrocytes. Neurons and glial cells are separated by narrow clefts that are ~20 nm wide and not visible at this magnification. The BECF in this space creates a tortuous path for the extracellular diffusion of solutes. Astrocyte processes are colored. As, astrocytes; At, en passant synapses; Ax, unmyelinated axons, Ax$_1$ and Ax$_2$, myelinated axons; Den, dendrites; f, astrocytic fibrils; nf, neurofilaments; S, synapses; SR, smooth endoplasmic reticulum. *(Modified from Peters A, Palay SL, Webster H: The Fine Structure of the Nervous System. Philadelphia: WB Saunders, 1976.)*

areas of the CNS. Moreover, because brain cells can increase volume rapidly during intense neural activity, the BECF fraction can reversibly decrease within seconds from ~20% to ~17% of brain volume.

Even though the space between brain cells is extremely small, diffusion of ions and other solutes within this thin BECF space is reasonably high. However, a particle that diffuses through the BECF from one side of a neuron to the other must take a circuitous route that is described by a parameter called **tortuosity**. For a normal width of the cell-to-cell spacing, this tortuosity reduces the rate of diffusion by ~60% compared with movement in free solution. Decreases in cell-to-cell spacing can further slow diffusion. For example, brain cells, especially glial cells, swell under certain pathological conditions and sometimes with intense neural activity. Cell swelling is associated with a reduction in BECF because water moves from the BECF into cells. The intense cell swelling associated with acute anoxia, for example, can reduce BECF volume from ~20% to ~5% of total brain volume. By definition, this reduced extracellular volume translates to reduced cell-to-cell spacing, further slowing the extracellular movement of solutes between the blood and brain cells (see the box titled Cerebral Edema).

The BECF is the route by which important molecules such as oxygen, glucose, and amino acids reach brain cells and by which the products of metabolism, including CO_2 and catabolized neurotransmitters, leave the brain. The BECF also permits molecules that are released by brain cells to diffuse to adjacent cells. Neurotransmitter molecules released at synaptic sites, for example, can spill over from the synaptic cleft and contact nearby glial cells and neurons, in addition to their target postsynaptic cell. Glial cells express neurotransmitter receptors, and neurons have **extrajunctional receptors**; therefore, these cells are capable of receiving "messages" sent through the BECF. Numerous trophic molecules secreted by brain cells diffuse in the BECF to their targets. Intercellular communication by way of the BECF is especially well suited for the transmission of tonic signals that are ideal for longer term modulation of the behavior of aggregates of neurons and glial cells. The chronic presence of variable amounts of neurotransmitters in the BECF supports this idea.

The CSF communicates freely with the BECF, thereby stabilizing the composition of the neuronal microenvironment

CSF in the ventricles and the subarachnoid space can exchange freely with BECF across two borders, the pia mater and ependymal cells. The **pial-glial membrane** (Fig. 11-2, upper inset) has paracellular gaps (see Chapter 2) through which substances can equilibrate between the subarachnoid space and BECF. **Ependymal cells** (Fig. 11-2, lower inset) are special glial cells that line the walls of the ventricles and form the cellular boundary between the CSF and the BECF. These cells form gap junctions between themselves that mediate intercellular communication, but they do not create a tight epithelium (see Chapter 5). Thus, macromolecules and ions

---

Cerebral Edema

Almost any type of insult to the brain causes cell swelling. This swelling is frequently accompanied by a *net accumulation of water* within the brain that is referred to as **cerebral edema**. Cell swelling in the absence of net water accumulation in the brain does *not* constitute cerebral edema. For example, intense neural activity causes a rapid shift of fluid from the BECF to the intracellular space, with no net change in brain water content. In cerebral edema, the extra water comes from the blood, as shown in Figure 11-6.

The mechanisms by which glial cells and neurons swell are not completely understood. Neuron cell bodies and dendrites, but not axons, swell when they are exposed to high concentrations of the neurotransmitter **glutamate**. This transmitter, along with others, is released to the BECF in an uncontrolled fashion with brain injury. Activation of ionotropic glutamate receptors (see Chapter 13) allows Na^+ to enter neurons, and water and Cl^- follow passively. Glial cells, both astrocytes and oligodendrocytes, swell vigorously under pathological conditions. One mechanism of glial swelling is an increase in $[K^+]_o$, which is a common ionic disturbance in a variety of brain pathological processes. This elevated $[K^+]_o$ causes a net uptake of K^+, accompanied by the passive influx of Cl^- and water.

Cerebral edema can be life-threatening when it is severe. The problem is a mechanical one. The skull is an inelastic container housing three relatively noncompressible substances: brain, CSF, and blood. A significant increase in the volume of CSF, blood, or brain rapidly causes increased pressure within the skull (Fig. 11-3). If the cerebral edema is *generalized*, it can be tolerated until intracerebral pressure exceeds arterial blood pressure, at which point blood flow to the brain stops, with disastrous consequences. Fortunately, sensors in the medulla detect the increased intracerebral pressure and can partially compensate (Cushing reflex), to a point, by increasing arterial pressure (see Chapter 24). *Focal* cerebral edema (i.e., edema involving an isolated portion of the brain) causes problems by displacing nearby brain tissue. This abnormality may result in distortion of normal anatomical relationships, with selective pressure on critical structures such as the brainstem.

Clinical evidence of cerebral edema results directly from the increased intracranial pressure and includes headache, vomiting, altered consciousness, and focal neurological problems such as stretching and dysfunction of the sixth cranial nerve.

Hyperventilation is the most effective means of combating the acute increase in intracranial pressure associated with severe cerebral edema. Hyperventilation causes a prompt respiratory alkalosis (see Chapter 28) that is rapidly translated to an increase in the pH surrounding vascular smooth muscle, thereby triggering vasoconstriction and reduced cerebral blood flow (see Chapter 24). Thus, total intracranial blood content falls, with a rapid subsequent drop in intracranial pressure. Alternatively, the brain can be partially dehydrated by adding osmoles to the blood in the form of intravenously administered mannitol (see Chapter 5).

A CELLULAR UPTAKE OF WATER FROM BLOOD

B RISE IN INTRACRANIAL PRESSURE WITH VOLUME

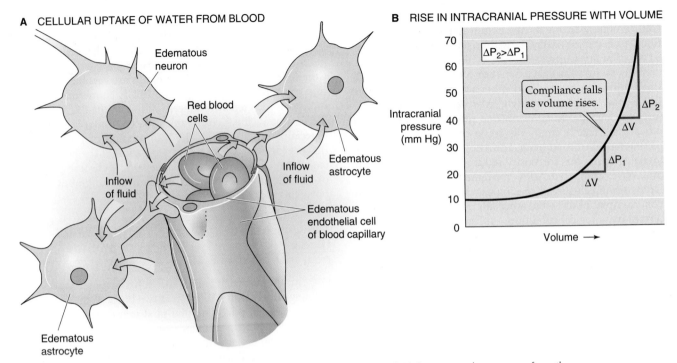

Figure 11-6   Cerebral edema. **A,** In cerebral edema, the brain fluid that accumulates comes from the vascular compartment. Cell swelling due to the mere shift of fluid from the extracellular to the intracellular fluid is *not* cerebral edema. **B,** Although small increases in intracranial volume have little effect on pressure, additional increases in volume cause potentially life-threatening increases in pressure. Note that compliance (i.e., $\Delta V/\Delta P$) falls at increasing volumes.

can also easily pass through this cellular layer through paracellular openings (some notable exceptions to this rule are considered later) and equilibrate between the CSF in the ventricle and the BECF.

Because CSF and BECF can readily exchange with one another, it is not surprising that they have a similar chemical composition. For example, $[K^+]$ is ~3.3 mM in freshly secreted CSF and ~3 mM in both the CSF of the subarachnoid space (Table 11-1) and BECF. The $[K^+]$ of blood is ~4.5 mM. However, because of the extent and vast complexity of the extracellular space, changes in the composition of CSF are reflected slowly in the BECF and probably incompletely.

CSF is an efficient waste management system because of its high rate of production, its circulation over the surface of the brain, and the free exchange between CSF and BECF. Products of metabolism and other substances released by cells, perhaps for signaling purposes, can diffuse into the chemically stable CSF and ultimately be removed on a continuous basis either by bulk resorption into the venous sinuses or by active transport across the choroid plexus into the blood. For example, choroid plexus actively absorbs the breakdown products of the neurotransmitters serotonin (i.e., 5-hydroxyindoleacetic acid) and dopamine (i.e., homovanillic acid).

The ion fluxes that accompany neural activity cause large changes in extracellular ion concentration

As discussed in Chapter 7, ionic currents through cell membranes underlie the synaptic and action potentials by which

neurons communicate. These currents lead to changes in the ion concentrations of the BECF. It is estimated that even a single action potential can transiently lower $[Na^+]_o$ by ~0.75 mM and increase $[K^+]_o$ by a similar amount. Repetitive neuronal activity causes larger perturbations in these extracellular ion concentrations. Because ambient $[K^+]_o$ is much lower than $[Na^+]_o$, activity-induced changes in $[K^+]_o$ are proportionately larger and are of special interest because of the important effect that $[K^+]_o$ has on membrane potential (V_m). For example, K^+ accumulation in the vicinity of active neurons depolarizes nearby glial cells. In this way, neurons signal to glial cells the pattern and extent of their activity. Even small changes in $[K^+]_o$ can alter metabolism and ionic transport in glial cells and may be used for signaling. Changes in the extracellular concentrations of certain common amino acids, such as glutamate and glycine, can also affect neuronal V_m and synaptic function by acting at specific receptor sites. If the nervous system is to function reliably, its signaling elements must have a regulated environment. Glial cells and neurons both function to prevent excessive extracellular accumulation of K^+ and neurotransmitters.

THE BLOOD-BRAIN BARRIER

The blood-brain barrier prevents some blood constituents from entering the brain extracellular space

The unique protective mechanism called the blood-brain barrier was first demonstrated by Ehrlich in 1885. He injected aniline dyes intravenously and discovered that the soft tissues of the body, except for the brain, were uniformly stained. Even though aniline dyes, such as trypan blue, extensively bind to serum albumin, the dye-albumin complex passes across capillaries in most areas of the body, but not the brain. This ability to exclude certain substances from crossing CNS blood vessels into the brain tissue is due to the **blood-brain barrier**. We now recognize that a blood-brain barrier is present in all vertebrates and many invertebrates as well.

The need for a blood-brain barrier can be understood by considering that blood is not a suitable environment for neurons. Blood is a complex medium that contains a large variety of solutes, some of which can vary greatly in concentration, depending on factors such as diet, metabolism, illness, and age. For example, the concentration of many amino acids increases significantly after a protein-rich meal. Some of these amino acids act as neurotransmitters within the brain, and if these molecules could move freely from the blood into the neuronal microenvironment, they would nonselectively activate receptors and disturb normal neurotransmission. Similarly, strenuous exercise can increase plasma concentrations of K^+ and H^+ substantially. If these ionic changes were communicated directly to the microenvironment of neurons, they could disrupt ongoing neural activity. Running a foot race might temporarily lower your IQ. Increases in $[K^+]_o$ would depolarize neurons and thus increase their likelihood of firing and releasing transmitter. H^+ can nonspecifically modulate neuronal excitability and influence the action of certain neurotransmitters. A broad range of blood constituents—including hormones, other ions, and inflammatory mediators such as cytokines—can influence the behavior of neurons or glial cells, which can express receptors for these molecules. For the brain to function efficiently, it must be spared such influences.

The choroid plexus and several restricted areas of the brain lack a blood-brain barrier; that is, they are supplied by leaky capillaries. Intra-arterially injected dyes can pass into the brain extracellular space at these sites through gaps between endothelial cells. The BECF in the vicinity of these leaky capillaries is similar to blood plasma more than to normal BECF. The small brain areas that lack a blood-brain barrier are called the **circumventricular organs** because they surround the ventricular system; these areas include the *area postrema, posterior pituitary, median eminence, organum vasculosum laminae terminalis, subfornical organ, subcommissural organ, and pineal gland* (Fig. 11-7). The ependymal cells that overlie the leaky capillaries in some of these regions (e.g., the choroid plexus) are linked together by tight junctions that form a barrier between the local BECF and the CSF, which must be insulated from the variability of blood composition. Whereas dyes with molecular weights up to 5000 can normally pass from CSF across the ependymal cell layer into the BECF, they do not pass across the specialized ependymal layer at the median eminence, area postrema, and infundibular recess. At these points, the localized BECF-CSF barrier is similar to the one in the choroid plexus. These specialized ependymal cells often have long processes that extend to capillaries within the portal circulation of the pituitary. Although the function of these cells is not known, it has been suggested that they may form a special route for neurohumoral signaling; molecules secreted by hypothalamic cells into the third ventricle could be taken up by these

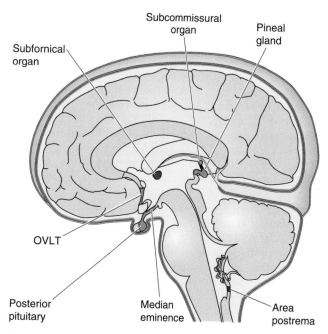

Figure 11-7 Leaky regions of the blood-brain barrier: the circumventricular organs. The capillaries of the brain are leaky in several areas: the area postrema, the posterior pituitary, the subfornical organ, the median eminence, the pineal gland, and the organum vasculosum laminae terminalis (OVLT). In these regions, the neurons are directly exposed to the solutes of the blood plasma. A midline sagittal section is shown.

cells and transmitted to the general circulation or to cells in the pituitary.

Neurons within the circumventricular organs are directly exposed to blood solutes and macromolecules; this arrangement is believed to be part of a neuroendocrine control system for maintaining such parameters as osmolality (see Chapter 40) and appropriate hormone levels, among other things. Humoral signals are integrated by connections of circumventricular organ neurons to endocrine, autonomic, and behavioral centers within the CNS. In the median eminence, neurons discharge "releasing hormones," which diffuse into leaky capillaries for carriage through the pituitary portal system to the anterior pituitary. The lack of a blood-brain barrier in the posterior pituitary is necessary to allow hormones that are released there to enter the general circulation (see Chapter 47). In the organum vasculosum laminae terminalis, leakiness is important in the action of cytokines from the periphery, which act as signals to temperature control centers that are involved in fever (see Chapter 59).

Continuous tight junctions link brain capillary endothelial cells

The blood-brain barrier should be thought of as a physical barrier to diffusion from blood to brain ECF and as a selective set of regulatory transport mechanisms that determine how certain organic solutes move between the blood and brain. Thus, the blood-brain barrier contributes to stabilization and protection of the neuronal microenvironment by facilitating the entry of needed substances, removing waste metabolites, and excluding toxic or disruptive substances.

The structure of brain capillaries differs from that of capillaries in other organs. Capillaries from other organs generally have small, simple openings—or clefts—between their endothelial cells (Fig. 11-8A). In some of these other organs, windows, or fenestrae, provide a pathway that bypasses the cytoplasm of capillary endothelial cells. Thus, in most capillaries outside the CNS, solutes can easily diffuse through the clefts and fenestrae. The physical barrier to solute diffusion in *brain* capillaries (Fig. 11-8B) is provided by the capillary endothelial cells, which are fused to each other by continuous **tight junctions** (or *zonula occludens*; see Chapter 2). The tight junctions prevent water-soluble ions and molecules from passing from the blood into the brain through the paracellular route. Not surprisingly, the electrical resistance of the cerebral capillaries is 100 to 200 times higher than that of most other systemic capillaries.

Elsewhere in the systemic circulation, molecules may traverse the endothelial cell by the process of **transcytosis** (see Chapter 20). In cerebral capillaries, transcytosis is uncommon, and brain endothelial cells have fewer endocytic vesicles than do systemic capillaries. However, brain endothelial cells have many more **mitochondria** than systemic endothelial cells do, which may reflect the high metabolic demands imposed on brain endothelial cells by active transport.

Other interesting features of brain capillaries are the thick **basement membrane** that underlies the endothelial cells, the presence of occasional **pericytes** within the basement membrane sheath, and the **astrocytic endfeet** (or processes) that provide a nearly continuous covering of the capillaries and other blood vessels. Astrocytes may play a crucial role in forming tight junctions between endothelial cells; experiments have shown that these glial cells can induce the formation of tight junctions between endothelial cells derived from capillaries outside the CNS. The close apposition of the astrocyte endfoot to the capillary also could facilitate transport of substances between these cells and blood.

Uncharged and lipid-soluble molecules more readily pass the blood-brain barrier

The capacity of the brain capillaries to exclude large molecules is strongly related to the molecular mass of the molecule and its hydrated diameter (Table 11-2). With a mass of 61 kDa, prealbumin is 14 times as concentrated in blood as in CSF (essentially equivalent to BECF for purposes of this comparison), whereas fibrinogen, which has a molecular mass of 340 kDa, is ~5000 times more concentrated in blood than in CSF. Diffusion of a solute is also generally limited by ionization at physiological pH, by low lipid solubility, and by binding to plasma proteins. For example, gases such as CO_2 and O_2 and drugs such as ethanol, caffeine, nicotine, heroin, and methadone readily cross the blood-brain barrier. However, ions such as K^+ or Mg^{2+} and protein-bound metabolites such as bilirubin have restricted access to the brain. Finally, the blood-brain barrier is permeable to water because of the presence of water channels in the endothelial cells. Thus, water moves across the blood-brain barrier in response to changes in plasma osmolarity. When dehydration raises

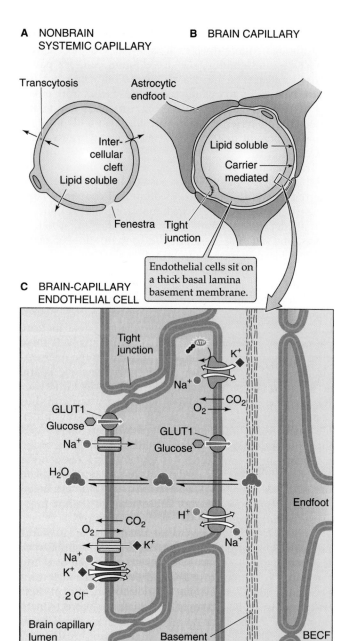

Figure 11-8 The blood-brain barrier function of brain capillaries. **A,** Capillaries from most other organs often have interendothelial clefts or fenestrae, which makes them relatively leaky. **B,** Brain capillaries are not leaky and have reduced transcytosis. **C,** Continuous tight junctions connect the endothelial cells in the brain, making the capillaries relatively tight.

the osmolality of blood plasma (see the box titled Disorders of Extracellular Osmolality in Chapter 5), the increased osmolality of the CSF and BECF can affect the behavior of brain cells.

Cerebral capillaries also express enzymes that can affect the movement of substances from blood to brain and vice versa. Peptidases, acid hydrolases, monoamine oxidase, and other enzymes are present in CNS endothelial cells and can

TABLE 11-2 Comparison of Proteins in Blood Plasma versus Cerebrospinal Fluid

Protein	Molecular Mass (kDa)	Hydrodynamic Radius (nM)	Plasma/CSF Ratio*
Prealbumin	61	3.3	14
Albumin	69	3.6	240
Transferrin	81	3.7	140
Ceruloplasmin	152	4.7	370
IgG	150	5.3	800
IgA	150	5.7	1350
α_2-Macroglobulin	798	9.4	1100
Fibrinogen	340	11.0	4940
IgM	800	12.1	1170
β-Lipoprotein	2240	12.4	6210

*The greater the plasma/CSF ratio, the more the blood-brain barrier excludes the protein from the CSF.

degrade a range of biologically active molecules, including enkephalins, substance P, proteins, and norepinephrine. Orally administered dopamine is not an effective treatment of Parkinson disease (see Chapter 13), a condition in which CNS dopamine is depleted, because dopamine is rapidly broken down by monoamine oxidase in the capillaries. Fortunately, the dopamine precursor compound L-dopa is effective for this condition. Neutral amino acid transporters in capillary endothelial cells move L-dopa to the BECF, where presynaptic terminals take up the L-dopa and convert it to dopamine in a reaction that is catalyzed by dopa decarboxylase.

Transport by capillary endothelial cells contributes to the blood-brain barrier

Two classes of substances can pass readily between blood and brain. The first consists of the small, highly lipid soluble molecules discussed in the preceding section. The second group consists of water-soluble compounds—either critical nutrients entering or metabolites exiting the brain—that traverse the blood-brain barrier by specific transporters. Examples include glucose, several amino acids and neurotransmitters, nucleic acid precursors, and several organic acids. Two major transporter groups provide these functions: the SLC superfamily and ABC transporters (see Chapter 5). As is the case for other epithelial cells, capillary endothelial cells selectively express these and other membrane proteins on either the luminal or basal surface.

Although the choroid plexuses secrete most of the CSF, brain endothelial cells produce some interstitial fluid with a composition similar to that of CSF. Transporters such as those shown in Figure 11-8C are responsible for this CSF-like secretion as well as for the local control of [K⁺] and pH in the BECF.

GLIAL CELLS

Glial cells constitute half the volume of the brain and outnumber neurons

The three major types of glial cells in the CNS are astrocytes, oligodendrocytes, and microglial cells (Table 11-3). As discussed in Chapter 10, the peripheral nervous system (PNS) contains other, distinctive types of glial cells, including satellite cells, Schwann cells, and enteric glia. Glial cells represent about half the volume of the brain and are more numerous than neurons. Unlike neurons, which have little capacity to replace themselves when lost, neuroglial (or simply glial) cells can proliferate throughout life. An injury to the nervous system is the usual stimulus for proliferation.

Historically, glial cells were viewed as a type of CNS connective tissue whose main function was to provide support for the true functional cells of the brain, the neurons. This firmly entrenched concept remained virtually unquestioned for the better part of a century after the early description of these cells by Virchow in 1858. Knowledge about glial cells has accumulated slowly because these cells have proved far more difficult to study than neurons. Because glial cells do not exhibit easily recorded action potentials or synaptic potentials, these cells were sometimes referred to as silent cells. However, glial cells are now recognized as intimate partners with neurons in virtually every function of the brain.

TABLE 11-3 Glial Types

Glial Cell Type	System	Location	GFAP
Astrocytes			
Fibrous	CNS	White matter	Positive
Protoplasmic	CNS	Gray matter	Weakly positive
Radial glial cells	CNS	Throughout brain during development	Positive
Müller cells	CNS	Retina	Positive
Bergmann glia	CNS	Cerebellum	Positive
Ependymal cells	CNS	Ventricular lining	Positive
Oligodendrocytes	CNS	Mainly white matter	Negative
Microglial cells	CNS	Throughout the brain	Negative
Satellite cells	PNS	Sensory and autonomic ganglia	Weakly positive
Schwann cells	PNS	Peripheral axons	Negative
Enteric glial cells	ENS	Gut wall	Positive

ENS, enteric nervous system; GFAP, glial fibrillary acidic protein; PNS, peripheral nervous system.

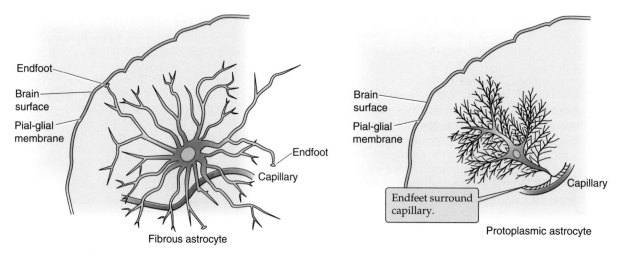

Figure 11-9   Astrocytes. The endfeet of both fibrous and protoplasmic astrocytes abut the pia mater and the capillaries.

Astrocytes supply fuel to neurons in the form of lactic acid

Astrocytes have great numbers of extremely elaborate processes that closely approach both blood vessels and neurons. This arrangement led to the idea that astrocytes transport substances between the blood and neurons. This notion may be true, but it has not been proved. Throughout the brain, astrocytes envelop neurons, and both cells bathe in a common BECF. Therefore, astrocytes are ideally positioned to modify and to control the immediate environment of neurons. Most astrocytes in the brain are traditionally subdivided into fibrous and protoplasmic types. **Fibrous astrocytes** (found mainly in white matter) have long, thin, and well-defined processes; **protoplasmic astrocytes** (found mainly in gray matter) have shorter, frilly processes (Fig. 11-9). Astrocytes are evenly spaced. In cortical regions, the dense processes of an individual astrocyte define its spatial domain, into which adjacent astrocytes do not encroach. The cytoskeleton of these and other types of astrocytes contains an identifying intermediate filament (see Chapter 2) that is composed of a unique protein called **glial fibrillar acidic protein (GFAP)**. The basic physiological properties of both types of astrocyte are similar, but specialized features, such as the expression of neurotransmitter receptors, vary among astrocytes from different brain regions.

During development, another type of astrocyte called the **radial glial cell** (see Chapter 10) is also present. As discussed in Chapter 10, these cells create an organized "scaffolding" by spanning the developing forebrain from the ventricle to the pial surface. Astrocytes in the retina and cerebellum are similar in appearance to radial glial cells. Like astrocytes elsewhere, these cells contain the intermediate filament

GFAP. Retinal astrocytes, called **Müller cells**, are oriented so that they span the entire width of the retina. **Bergmann glial cells** in the cerebellum have processes that run parallel to the processes of Purkinje cells.

Astrocytes store virtually all the **glycogen** present in the adult brain. They also contain all the enzymes needed for metabolizing glycogen. The brain's high metabolic needs are primarily met by glucose transferred from blood because the brain's glucose supply in the form of glycogen is very limited. In the absence of glucose from blood, astrocytic glycogen could sustain the brain for only 5 to 10 minutes. As implied, astrocytes can share with neurons the energy stored in glycogen, but *not* by the direct release of glucose into the BECF. Instead, astrocytes break glycogen down to glucose and even further to lactate, which is transferred to nearby neurons, where it can be aerobically metabolized (Fig. 11-10). The extent to which this metabolic interaction takes place under normal conditions is not known, but it may be important during periods of intense neuronal activity, when the demand for glucose exceeds the supply from blood.

Astrocytes can also provide fuel to neurons in the form of lactate derived directly from glucose, independent of glycogen. Glucose entering the brain from blood first encounters the astrocytic endfoot. Although it can diffuse past this point to neurons, glucose may be preferentially taken up by astrocytes and shuttled through astrocytic glycolysis to lactic acid, a significant portion of which is excreted into the BECF surrounding neurons. Several observations support the notion that astrocytes provide lactate to neurons. First, astrocytes have higher *anaerobic* metabolic rates and export much more lactate than do neurons. Second, neurons and their axons function normally when glucose is replaced by lactate, and some neurons seem to prefer lactate to glucose as fuel.

Note that when they are aerobically metabolized, the two molecules of lactate derived from the breakdown of one molecule of glucose provide nearly as much ATP as the complete oxidation of glucose itself (28 versus 30 molecules of ATP; see Table 58-4 on p. 1231). The advantage of this scheme for neuronal function is that it provides a form of **substrate buffering**, a second energy reservoir that is available to neurons. The availability of *glucose* in the neuronal microenvironment depends on moment-to-moment supply from the blood and varies as a result of changes in neural activity. The concentration of extracellular *lactate*, however, is buffered against such variability by the surrounding astrocytes, which continuously shuttle lactate to the BECF through the metabolism of glucose or by breaking down glycogen.

Astrocytes are predominantly permeable to K⁺ and also help regulate [K⁺]ₒ

The membrane potential of glial cells is more negative than that of neurons. For example, astrocytes have a V_m of about −85 mV, whereas the resting neuronal V_m is about −65 mV. Because the equilibrium potential for K⁺ is about −90 mV in both neurons and glia, the more negative V_m in astrocytes indicates that glial membranes have higher K⁺ selectivity than neuronal membranes do (see Chapter 6). Although glial cells express a variety of K⁺ channels, inwardly rectifying K⁺ channels seem to be important in setting the resting potential. These channels are voltage gated and are open at membrane potentials that are more negative than about −80 mV, close to the observed resting potential of astrocytes. Astrocytes express many other voltage-gated ion channels that were once thought to be restricted to neurons. The significance of voltage-gated Na⁺ and Ca²⁺ channels in glial cells is

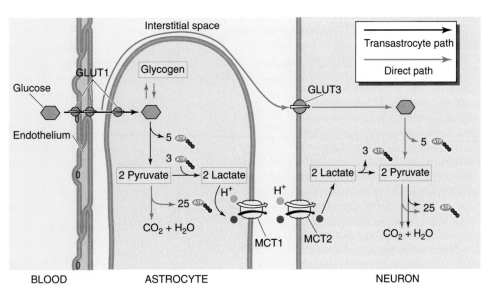

Figure 11-10 Role of astrocytes in providing lactate as fuel for neurons. Neurons have two fuel sources. They can obtain glucose directly from the blood plasma, or they can obtain lactate from astrocytes. In the direct path, the oxidation of one glucose molecule provides 30 ATP molecules to the neuron. In the transastrocyte path, conversion of two lactates to two pyruvates, and then the subsequent oxidation of the pyruvate, provides 28 molecules of ATP to the neuron. GLUT1 and GLUT3, glucose transporters; MCT1 and MCT3, monocarboxylate cotransporters.

unknown. Because the ratio of Na^+ to K^+ channels is low in adult astrocytes, these cells are not capable of regenerative electrical responses such as the action potential.

One consequence of the higher K^+ selectivity of astrocytes is that the V_m of astrocytes is far more sensitive than that of neurons to changes in $[K^+]_o$. For example, when $[K^+]_o$ is raised from 4 to 20 mM, astrocytes depolarize by ~25 mV versus only ~5 mV for neurons. This relative insensitivity of neuronal resting potential to changes in $[K^+]_o$ in the "physiological" range may have emerged as an adaptive feature that stabilizes the resting potential of *neurons* in the face of the transient increases in $[K^+]_o$ that accompany neuronal activity. In contrast, natural stimulation, such as viewing visual targets of different shapes or orientations, can cause depolarizations of up to 10 mV in *astrocytes* of the visual cortex. The accumulation of extracellular K^+ that is secondary to neural activity may serve as a signal—to glial cells—that is proportional to the extent of the activity. For example, small increases in $[K^+]_o$ cause astrocytes to increase their glucose metabolism and to provide more lactate for active neurons. In addition, the depolarization that is triggered by the increased $[K^+]_o$ leads to the influx of HCO_3^- into astrocytes by the electrogenic Na/HCO_3 cotransporter (see Chapter 5); this influx of bicarbonate in turn causes a fall in extracellular pH that may diminish neuronal excitability.

Not only do astrocytes respond to changes in $[K^+]_o$, they also help regulate it (Fig. 11-11A). The need for homeostatic control of $[K^+]_o$ is clear because changes in brain $[K^+]_o$ can influence transmitter release, cerebral blood flow, cell volume, glucose metabolism, and neuronal activity. Active neurons lose K^+ into the BECF, and the resulting increased $[K^+]_o$ tends to act as a positive feedback signal that increases excitability by further depolarizing neurons. This potentially unstable situation is combated by efficient mechanisms that expedite

A MECHANISMS OF K^+ UPTAKE BY ASTROCYTES

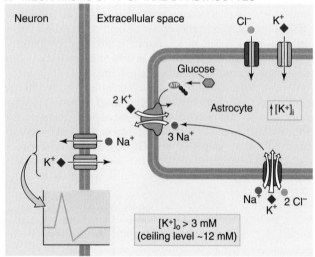

B SPATIAL BUFFERING

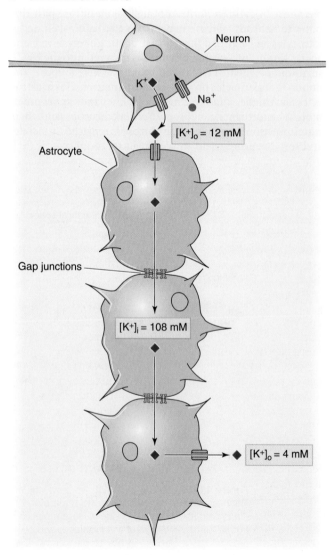

Figure 11-11 K^+ handling by astrocytes. ECS, extracellular space.

K^+ removal and limit its accumulation to a maximum level of 10 to 12 mM, the so-called ceiling level. $[K^+]_o$ would rise far above this ceiling with intense neural activity if K^+ clearance depended solely on passive redistribution of K^+ in the BECF. Neurons and blood vessels can contribute to K^+ homeostasis, but glial mechanisms are probably most important. Astrocytes can take up K^+ in response to elevated $[K^+]_o$ by three major mechanisms: the Na-K pump, the Na/K/Cl cotransporter, and the uptake of K^+ and Cl^- through channels. Conversely, when neural activity decreases, K^+ and Cl^- leave the astrocytes through ion channels.

Gap junctions couple astrocytes to one another, allowing diffusion of small solutes

The anatomical substrate for cell-cell coupling among astrocytes is the **gap junction**, which is composed of membrane proteins called connexins that form large aqueous pores connecting the cytoplasm of two adjacent cells (see Chapter 6). Coupling between astrocytes is strong because hundreds of gap junction channels may be present between two astrocytes. Astrocytes may also be weakly coupled to oligodendrocytes. Ions and organic molecules that are up to 1 kDa in size, regardless of charge, can diffuse from one cell into another through these large channels. Thus, a broad range of biologically important molecules, including nucleotides, sugars, amino acids, small peptides, cAMP, Ca^{2+}, and inositol 1,4,5-trisphosphate (IP_3), have access to this pathway.

Gap junctions may coordinate the metabolic and electrical activities of cell populations, amplify the consequences of signal transduction, and control intrinsic proliferative capacity. The strong coupling among astrocytes ensures that all cells in the aggregate have similar intracellular concentrations of ions and small molecules and similar membrane potentials. Thus, the network of astrocytes functionally behaves like a **syncytium**, much like the myocytes in the heart (see Chapter 21). In ways that are not yet clear, gap junctional communication can be important for the control of cellular proliferation. The most common brain cell-derived tumors in the CNS arise from astrocytes. Malignant astrocyte tumors, like malignant neoplasms derived from other cells that are normally coupled (e.g., liver cells), lack gap junctions.

The coupling among astrocytes may also play an important role in controlling $[K^+]_o$ by a mechanism known as **spatial buffering**. The selective K^+ permeability of glia, together with their low-resistance cell-cell connections, permits them to transport K^+ from focal areas of high $[K^+]_o$, where a portion of the glial syncytium would be depolarized, to areas of normal $[K^+]_o$, where the glial syncytium would be more normally polarized (Fig. 11-11B). Redistribution of K^+ proceeds by way of a current loop in which K^+ enters glial cells at the point of high $[K^+]_o$ and leaves them at sites of normal $[K^+]_o$, with the extracellular flow of Na^+ completing this circuit. At a site of high neuronal activity, $[K^+]_o$ might rise to 12 mM, which would produce a very large depolarization of an isolated, uncoupled astrocyte. However, because of the electrical coupling among astrocytes, the V_m of the affected astrocyte remains more negative than the E_K predicted for a $[K^+]_o$ of 12 mM. Thus, K^+ would tend to passively enter coupled astrocytes through channels at sites of high

$[K^+]_o$. As discussed in the preceding section, K^+ may also enter the astrocyte by transporters.

Astrocytes synthesize neurotransmitters, take them up from the extracellular space, and have neurotransmitter receptors

Astrocytes synthesize at least 20 neuroactive compounds, including both glutamate and γ-aminobutyric acid (GABA). Neurons can manufacture glutamate from glucose or from the immediate precursor molecule glutamine (Fig. 11-12). The glutamine pathway appears to be the primary one in the synthesis of synaptically released glutamate. Glutamine, however, is manufactured only in astrocytes by use of the astrocyte-specific enzyme **glutamine synthetase** to convert glutamate to glutamine. Astrocytes release this glutamine into the BECF through the SNAT3 and 5 transporters (SLC38 family; see Table 5-4) for uptake by neurons through SNAT1 and 2. Consistent with its role in the synthesis of glutamate for neurotransmission, glutamine synthetase is localized to astrocytic processes surrounding glutamatergic synapses. In the presynaptic terminals of neurons, glutaminase converts the glutamine to glutamate, for release into the synaptic cleft by the presynaptic terminal. Finally, astrocytes take up much of the synaptically released glutamate to complete this **glutamate-glutamine cycle**. Disruption of this metabolic interaction between astrocytes and neurons can depress glutamate-dependent synaptic transmission.

Glutamine derived from astrocytes is also important for synthesis of the brain's most prevalent inhibitory neurotransmitter, GABA. In the neuron, the enzyme **glutamic acid decarboxylase** converts glutamate (generated from glutamine) to GABA (see Fig. 13-8A). Because astrocytes play such an important role in the synthesis of synaptic transmitters, these glial cells are in a position to modulate synaptic efficacy.

Astrocytes have **high-affinity uptake systems** for the excitatory transmitter glutamate and the inhibitory transmitter GABA. In the case of glutamate uptake, mediated by EAAT1 and EAAT2 (SLC1 family; see Table 5-4), astrocytes appear to play the dominant role compared with neurons or other glial cells. Glutamate moves into cells accompanied by two Na^+ ions and an H^+ ion, with one K^+ ion moving in the opposite direction (Fig. 11-12). Because a net positive charge moves into the cell, glutamate uptake causes membrane depolarization. The presynaptic cytoplasm may contain glutamate at a concentration as high as 10 mM, and vesicles may contain as much as 100 mM glutamate. Nevertheless, the glutamate uptake systems can maintain extracellular glutamate at concentrations as low as ~1 μM, which is crucial for normal brain function.

Neurotransmitter uptake systems are important because they help terminate the action of synaptically released neurotransmitters. Astrocyte processes frequently surround synaptic junctions and are therefore ideally placed for this function. Under pathological conditions in which transmembrane ion gradients break down, high-affinity uptake systems may work in reverse and release transmitters, such as glutamate, into the BECF.

Astrocytes express a wide variety of ionotropic and metabotropic **neurotransmitter receptors** that are similar

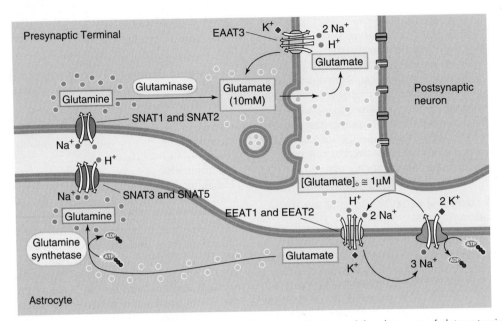

Figure 11-12 Role of astrocytes in the glutamate-glutamine cycle. Most of the glutamate of glutamatergic neurons is generated from glutamine, which the neurons themselves cannot make. However, astrocytes take up some of the glutamate that is released at synapses (or produced by metabolism) and convert it into glutamine. The glutamine then enters the neuron, where it is converted back to glutamate. This glutamate also serves as the source for γ-aminobutyric acid in inhibitory neurons.

or identical to those present on neuronal membranes. As in neurons, activation of these receptors can open ion channels or generate second messengers. In most astrocytes, glutamate produces depolarization by increasing Na^+ permeability, whereas GABA hyperpolarizes cells by opening Cl^- channels, similar to the situation in neurons (see Chapter 13). Transmitter substances released by neurons at synapses can diffuse in the BECF to activate nearby receptors on astrocytes, thus providing, at least theoretically, a form of neuronal-glial signaling.

Astrocytes apparently can actively enhance or depress neuronal discharge and synaptic transmission by releasing neurotransmitters that they have taken up or synthesized. The release mechanisms are diverse and include stimulation by certain neurotransmitters, a fall in $[Ca^{2+}]_o$, or depolarization by elevated $[K^+]_o$. Applying glutamate to cultured astrocytes increases $[Ca^{2+}]_i$, which may oscillate. Moreover, these increases in $[Ca^{2+}]_i$ can travel in waves from astrocyte to astrocyte through gap junctions or through a propagated front of extracellular ATP release that activates astrocytic purinergic receptors, thereby increasing $[Ca^{2+}]_i$ and releasing more ATP. These $[Ca^{2+}]_i$ waves—perhaps by triggering the release of a neurotransmitter from the astrocyte—can lead to changes in the activity of nearby neurons. This interaction represents another form of glial-neuronal communication.

Astrocytes secrete trophic factors that promote neuronal survival and synaptogenesis

Astrocytes, and other glial cell types, are a source of important trophic factors and cytokines, including brain-derived neurotrophic factor, glial-derived neurotrophic factor, basic fibroblast growth factor, and ciliary neurotrophic factor. Moreover, both neurons and glial cells express receptors for these molecules, which are crucial for neuronal survival, function, and repair. The expression of these substances and their cognate receptors can vary during development and with injury to the nervous system.

The development of fully functional excitatory synapses in the brain requires the presence of astrocytes, which act at least in part by secreting proteins called **thrombospondins**. Indeed, synapses in the developing CNS do not form in substantial numbers before the appearance of astrocytes. In the absence of astrocytes, only ~20% of the normal number of synapses form.

Astrocytic endfeet modulate cerebral blood flow

Astrocytic endfeet surround not only capillaries but also small arteries. Neuronal activity can lead to astrocytic $[Ca^{2+}]_i$ waves, as previously described, that spread to the astrocytic endfeet or to isolated increases in endfoot $[Ca^{2+}]_i$. In either case, the result is a rapid increase in blood vessel diameter and thus in local blood flow. A major mechanism of this vasodilation is the stimulation of phospholipase A_2 in the astrocyte, the formation of arachidonic acid, and the liberation through cyclooxygenase 1 (see Fig. 3-11) of a potent vasodilator that acts on vascular smooth muscle. This is one mechanism of neuron-vascular coupling—a local increase in neuronal activity that leads to a local increase in blood flow. Radiologists exploit this physiological principle in a form of **functional magnetic resonance imaging (fMRI)** called blood oxygen level–dependent (BOLD) MRI, which uses blood flow as an index of neuronal activity.

Excitatory Amino Acids and Neurotoxicity

The dicarboxylic amino acid glutamate is the most prevalent excitatory neurotransmitter in the brain (see Chapter 13). Although glutamate is present at millimolar levels inside neurons, the BECF has only micromolar levels of glutamate, except at sites of synaptic release (Fig. 11-12). Excessive accumulation of glutamate in the BECF—induced by ischemia, anoxia, hypoglycemia, or trauma—can lead to neuronal injury. Astrocytes are intimately involved in the metabolism of glutamate and its safe disposition after synaptic release.

In anoxia and ischemia, the sharp drop in cellular levels of ATP inhibits the Na-K pump, thereby rapidly leading to large increases in $[K^+]_o$ and $[Na^+]_i$. These changes result in membrane depolarization, with an initial burst of glutamate release from vesicles in presynaptic terminals. Vesicular release, however, requires cytoplasmic ATP and probably halts rapidly. The ability of astrocytes to remove glutamate from the BECF is impeded by the elevated $[K^+]_o$, elevated $[Na^+]_i$, and membrane depolarization. In fact, the unfavorable ion gradients can cause the transporter to run in reverse and dump glutamate into the BECF. The action of rising levels of extracellular glutamate on *postsynaptic* and astrocytic receptors reinforces the developing ionic derangements by opening channels permeable to Na^+ and K^+. This vicious cycle at the level of the astrocyte can rapidly cause extracellular glutamate to reach levels that are toxic to neurons—**excitotoxicity**.

Astrocytic modulation of blood flow is complex, and increases in $[Ca^{2+}]_i$ in endfeet can sometimes lead to vasoconstriction.

Oligodendrocytes and Schwann cells make and sustain myelin

The primary function of oligodendrocytes as well as of their PNS equivalent, the Schwann cell, is to provide and to maintain myelin sheaths on axons of the central and peripheral nervous systems, respectively. As discussed in Chapter 7, myelin is the insulating "electrical tape" of the nervous system (see Fig. 7-21B). **Oligodendrocytes** are present in all areas of the CNS, although their morphological appearance is highly variable and depends on their location within the brain. In regions of the brain that are dominated by myelinated nerve tracts, called white matter, the oligodendrocytes responsible for myelination have a distinctive appearance (Fig. 11-13A). Such an oligodendrocyte has 15 to 30 processes, each of which connects a myelin sheath to the oligodendrocyte's cell body. Each myelin sheath, which is up to 250 μm wide, wraps many times around the long axis of one axon. The small exposed area of axon between adjacent myelin sheaths is called the **node of Ranvier** (see Chapter 10). In gray matter, oligodendrocytes do not produce myelin and exist as perineuronal satellite cells.

During the myelination process, the leading edge of one of the processes of the oligodendrocyte cytoplasm wraps around the axon many times (Fig. 11-13A, upper axon).

TABLE 11-4 Proteins in Myelin

Protein	CNS (% of total myelin proteins)	PNS (% of total myelin proteins)
MBP	30	<18
PLP	50	<0.01
MAG	<1	<50.1
CNP	<4	<50.4
P0	<0.01	>50
P2	<1	1-15
PMP22	<0.01	5-10
MOG	<0.05	<0.01

CNP, cyclic nucleotide phosphodiesterase; MAG, myelin-associated glycoprotein; MBP, myelin basic protein; MOG, myelin oligodendrocyte glycoprotein; PLP, proteolipid protein; PMP22, peripheral myelin protein 22.

The cytoplasm is then squeezed out of the many cell layers surrounding the axon in a process called **compaction**. This process creates layer on layer of tightly compressed membranes that is called **myelin**. The myelin sheaths remain continuous with the parent glial cells, which nourish them.

In the PNS, a single **Schwann cell** provides a single myelin segment to a single axon of a myelinated nerve (Fig. 11-13B). This situation stands in contrast to that in the CNS, where one oligodendrocyte myelinates many axons. The process of myelination that occurs in the PNS is analogous to that outlined for oligodendrocytes. Axons of unmyelinated nerves are also associated with Schwann cells. In this case, the axons indent the surface of the Schwann cell and are completely surrounded by Schwann cell cytoplasm (Fig. 11-14).

Myelin has a biochemical composition different from that of the oligodendrocyte or Schwann cell plasma membrane from which it arose. Although PNS myelin and CNS myelin look similar, some of the constituent proteins are different (Table 11-4). For example, proteolipid protein is the most common protein in CNS myelin (~50% of total protein) but is absent in PNS myelin. Conversely, P0 is found almost exclusively in PNS myelin.

Myelination greatly enhances conduction of the action potential down the axon because it allows the regenerative electrical event to skip from one node to the next rather than gradually spreading down the whole extent of the axon. This process is called **saltatory conduction** (see Chapter 7). Besides being responsible for CNS myelin, oligodendrocytes play another key role in saltatory conduction: they induce the clustering of Na^+ channels at the nodes (see Fig. 12-5C on p. 318), which is essential for saltatory conduction.

It is well known that severed axons in the PNS can regenerate with restoration of lost function. Regrowth of these damaged axons is coordinated by the Schwann cells in the distal portion of the cut nerve. Severed axons in the CNS do

A OLIGODENDROCYTE

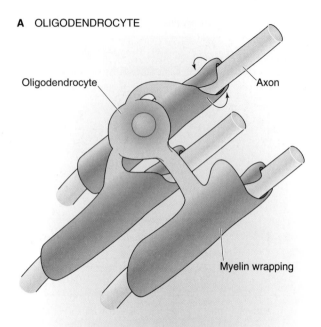

B SCHWANN CELL

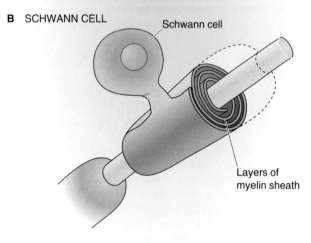

Figure 11-13 Myelination of axons by oligodendrocytes and Schwann cells.

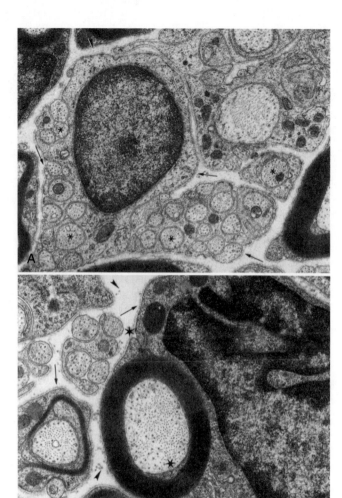

Figure 11-14 Ensheathed versus myelinated axons. **A,** Ensheathed axons. This transmission electron micrograph shows a Schwann cell surrounding several *unmyelinated* peripheral axons, some of which are marked with an *asterisk*. The *arrows* point to the basal lamina. The *arrowhead* points to collagen fibrils. **B,** Myelinated axons. This transmission electron micrograph shows a Schwann cell (nucleus on right side of picture) surrounding a peripheral axon with several layers of myelin. The *lower star* shows the beginning of the spiraling myelin sheath; the *upper star* indicates the termination of the spiral and a small region of noncompacted cytosol. The final magnification is ~14,000 in both panels. *(Reproduced from Bunge RP, Fernandez-Valle C: In Kettemann H, Ransom RR [eds]: Neuroglia, pp. 44-57. New York: Oxford University Press, 1995; courtesy of Mary Bartlett Bunge.)*

not show functional regrowth, in part because of the growth-retarding nature of CNS myelin (see Chapter 10).

Oligodendrocytes are involved in pH regulation and iron metabolism in the brain

Oligodendrocytes and myelin contain most of the enzyme carbonic anhydrase within the brain. The appearance of this enzyme during development closely parallels the maturation of these cells and the formation of myelin. Carbonic anhydrase rapidly catalyzes the reversible hydration of CO_2 and may thus allow the CO_2/HCO_3^- buffer system to be maximally effective in dissipating pH gradients in the brain. The pH regulation in the brain is important because it influences neuronal excitability. The classic example of the brain's sensitivity to pH is the reduced seizure threshold caused by the respiratory alkalosis secondary to hyperventilation (see Chapter 28).

Oligodendrocytes are the cells in the brain most involved with iron metabolism. They contain the iron storage protein ferritin and the iron transport protein transferrin. Iron is necessary as a cofactor for certain enzymes and may catalyze the formation of free radicals under pathological circumstances, such as disruption of blood flow to the brain.

Oligodendrocytes, like astrocytes, have a wide variety of neurotransmitter receptors. Unmyelinated axons can release glutamate when they conduct action potentials, and in principle, this glutamate could signal nearby oligodendrocytes. Ischemia readily injures oligodendrocytes, in part by releas-

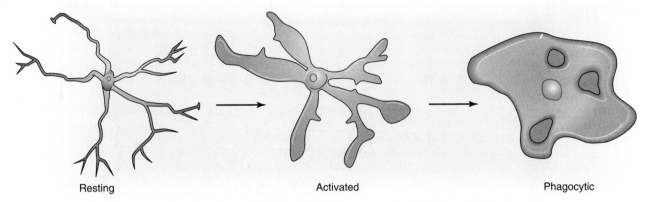

Resting   Activated   Phagocytic

Figure 11-15   Microglial cells. Resting microglial cells become activated by injury to the brain, which causes them to proliferate and to become phagocytic.

ing toxic levels of glutamate. Even white matter, therefore, can suffer excitotoxicity.

Microglial cells are the macrophages of the CNS

Microglial cells are of mesodermal origin and derive from cells related to the monocyte-macrophage lineage. Microglia represent ~20% of the total glial cells within the mature CNS. These cells are rapidly activated by injury to the brain, which causes them to proliferate, to change shape, and to become phagocytic (Fig. 11-15). When activated, they are capable of releasing substances that are toxic to neurons, including free radicals and nitric oxide. It is believed that microglia are involved in most brain diseases, not as initiators but as highly reactive cells that shape the brain's response to any insult.

Microglia are also the most effective antigen-presenting cells within the brain. Activated T lymphocytes are able to breech the blood-brain barrier and enter the brain. To become mediators of tissue-specific disease or to destroy an invading infectious agent, T lymphocytes must recognize specific antigenic targets. Such recognition is accomplished through the process of antigen presentation, which is a function of the microglia.

REFERENCES

Books and Reviews

Brown PD, Davis SL, Speake T, Millar ID: Molecular mechanisms of cerebrospinal fluid production. Neuroscience 2004; 129:957-970.

Kettenmann H, Ransom BR (eds): Neuroglia, 2nd ed. New York: Oxford University Press, 2005.

Nedergaard M, Ransom BR, Goldman SA: New roles for astrocytes: Redefining the functional architecture of the brain. TINS 2003; 26:523-530.

Ohtsuki S: New aspects of the blood-brain-barrier transporters; its physiological roles in the central nervous system. Biol Pharm Bull 2004; 27:1489-1496.

Ullian EM, Christopherson KS, Barres BA: Role for glia in synaptogenesis. Glia 2004; 47:209-216.

Journal Articles

Christopherson KS, Ullian EM, Stokes CC, et al: Thrombospondins are astrocyte-secreted proteins that promote CNS synaptogenesis. Cell 2005; 120:421-433.

Kaplan MR, Meyer-Franke A, Lambert S, et al: Induction of sodium channel clustering by oligodendrocytes. Nature 1997; 386: 724-728.

Newman EA, Zahs KR: Modulation of neuronal activity by glial cells in the retina. J Neurosci 1998; 18:4022-4028.

Takano T, Tian GF, Peng W, et al: Astrocyte-mediated control of cerebral blood flow. Nat Neursci 2006; 9:260-267.

Wender R, Brown AM, Fern R, et al: Astrocytic glycogen influences axon function and survival during glucose deprivation in central white matter. J Neurosci 2000; 20:6804-6810.

CHAPTER 12

PHYSIOLOGY OF NEURONS

Barry W. Connors

Neurons receive, combine, transform, store, and send information

Neurons have arguably the most complex job of any cell in the body. Consequently, they have an elaborate morphology and physiology. Each neuron is an intricate computing device. A single neuron may receive chemical input from tens of thousands of other neurons. It then combines these myriad signals into a much simpler set of electrical changes across its cellular membrane. The neuron subsequently transforms these ionic transmembrane changes according to rules determined by its particular shape and electrical properties and transmits a *single new message* through its axon, which itself may contact and inform hundreds of other neurons. Under the right circumstances, neurons also possess the property of *memory;* some of the information coursing its synapses may be stored for periods as long as years.

This general scheme of neuronal function applies to most neurons in the vertebrate nervous system. However, the scheme is endlessly variable. For example, each region of the brain has several major classes of neurons, and each of these classes has a physiology adapted to perform specific and unique functions. In this chapter, the general principles of neuronal function are outlined, and the almost unlimited variability contained within the general schema is discussed.

Neural information flows from dendrite to soma to axon to synapse

Numerous dendrites converge on a central soma, or cell body, from which a single axon emerges and branches multiple times (see Fig. 10-1). Each branch culminates at a presynaptic terminal that contacts another cell. In most neurons, dendrites are the principal synaptic input sites, although synapses may also be found on the soma, on the axon hillock (the region of the soma neighboring the axon), or even directly on the axons. In some primary sensory neurons, the dendrites themselves are transducers of environmental energy. Regardless of their source, signals—in the form of voltage changes across the membrane—typically flow from dendrites to soma to axon and finally to synapses on the next set of cells.

Excitatory input to a neuron usually generates an inward flow of positive charge (i.e., an inward current) across the dendritic membrane. Because the interior of a resting neuron is polarized negatively with respect to the external environment, this inward current, which makes the membrane voltage more positive (i.e., less negative), is said to **depolarize** the cell. Conversely, inhibitory input to a neuron usually generates an outward current and, thus, hyperpolarization.

If the neuron receives its input from a neighboring cell through a chemical synapse, neurotransmitters trigger currents by activating ion channels. If the cell is a sensory neuron, environmental stimuli (e.g., chemicals, light, mechanical deformation) activate ion channels and produce a flow of current. The change in membrane potential (V_m) caused by the flow of charge is called a **postsynaptic potential (PSP)** if it is generated at the postsynaptic membrane by a neurotransmitter and a **receptor potential** if it is generated at a sensory nerve ending by an external stimulus. In the case of synaptic transmission, the postsynaptic V_m changes may be either positive or negative. If the neurotransmitter is excitatory and produces a *depolarizing* PSP, we refer to the PSP as an **excitatory postsynaptic potential (EPSP)** (see Chapter 8). On the other hand, if the neurotransmitter is inhibitory and produces a *hyperpolarizing* PSP, the PSP is an **inhibitory postsynaptic potential (IPSP)**. In all cases, the stimulus produces a V_m change that may be *graded* from small to large, depending on the strength or quantity of input stimuli (see Chapter 7). Stronger sensory stimuli generate larger receptor potentials; similarly, more synapses activated together generate larger PSPs. A graded response is one form of neural coding whereby the size and duration of the input are encoded as the size and duration of the change in the dendritic V_m.

The synaptic (or receptor) potentials generated at the ends of a dendrite are communicated to the soma, but not usually without substantial attenuation of the signal (Fig. 12-1A). Extended cellular processes such as dendrites behave like leaky electrical cables (see Chapter 7). As a consequence, dendritic potentials usually decline in amplitude before reaching the soma. As an EPSP reaches the soma, it may also

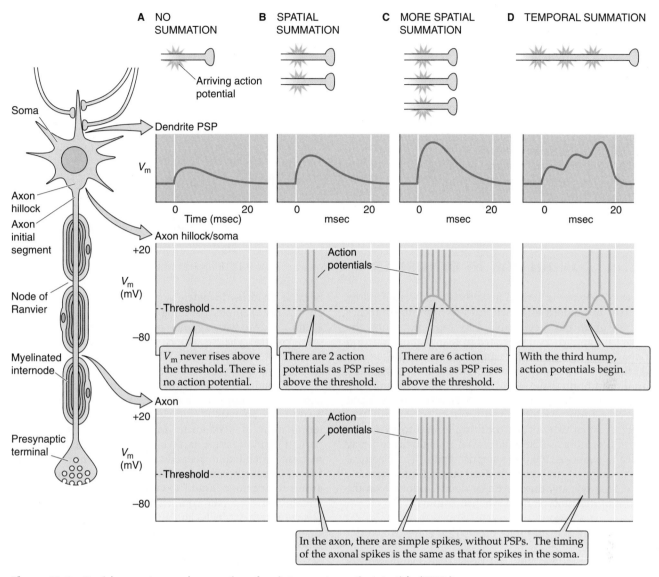

A NO SUMMATION

B SPATIAL SUMMATION

C MORE SPATIAL SUMMATION

D TEMPORAL SUMMATION

Arriving action potential

Dendrite PSP

V_m

Time (msec)

Axon hillock/soma

V_m (mV)

Threshold

Action potentials

V_m never rises above the threshold. There is no action potential.

There are 2 action potentials as PSP rises above the threshold.

There are 6 action potentials as PSP rises above the threshold.

With the third hump, action potentials begin.

Axon

V_m (mV)

Threshold

Action potentials

In the axon, there are simple spikes, without PSPs. The timing of the axonal spikes is the same as that for spikes in the soma.

Soma

Axon hillock

Axon initial segment

Node of Ranvier

Myelinated internode

Presynaptic terminal

Figure 12-1 Spatial versus temporal summation of excitatory postsynaptic potentials (EPSPs).

combine with EPSPs arriving by other dendrites on the cell; this behavior is a type of **spatial summation** and can lead to EPSPs that are substantially larger than those generated by any single synapse (Fig. 12-1B, C). **Temporal summation** occurs when EPSPs arrive rapidly in succession; when the first EPSP has not yet dissipated, a subsequent EPSP tends to add its amplitude to the residual of the preceding EPSP (Fig. 12-1D).

The tendency for synaptic and receptor potentials to diminish with distance along a dendrite puts significant limitations on their signaling abilities. If nothing else happened, these depolarizing potentials would simply dwindle back to the resting membrane potential as they spread through the soma and down into the axon. At best, this passive signal might be carried a few millimeters, clearly inadequate for wiggling a toe when the axon of the motor neuron stretching from the spinal cord to the foot might be 1000 mm long. Some amplification is therefore necessary for certain inputs to generate effective signals to and from the

central nervous system (CNS). Amplification is provided in the form of regenerating **action potentials**. If the V_m change in the soma is large enough to reach the threshold voltage (see Chapter 7), the depolarization may trigger one or more action potentials between the soma and axon, as shown in Figure 12-1B to D. Action potentials are large, rapid fluctuations in V_m. As described in Chapter 7, an action potential is an efficient, rapid, and reliable way to carry a signal over long distances. However, notice that generation of action potentials entails another transformation of neuronal information: the neuron converts the graded-voltage code of the dendrites (i.e., the PSPs) to a temporal code of action potentials in the axon.

Action potentials are fixed in amplitude, not graded, and have uniform shape. So how is information encoded by action potentials? This question has no simple answer and is still hotly debated. Because one axonal spike looks like another (with slight exceptions), neurons can vary only the number of spikes and their timing. For a single axon, information may be encoded by the average rate of action potential firing, the total number of action potentials, their temporal pattern, or some combination of these mechanisms. Figure 12-1 illustrates that as the synaptic potential in the soma increases in size, the resultant action potentials occur more frequently, and the burst of action potentials in the axon lasts longer. Notice also that by the time the signal has propagated well down the axon, the transformation has become complete—the graded potential has waned and vanished, whereas the action potentials have retained their size, number, and temporal pattern. The final output of the neuron is entirely encoded in these action potentials. When action potentials reach axonal terminals, they may trigger the release of a neurotransmitter at the next set of synapses, and the cycle begins again.

SIGNAL CONDUCTION IN DENDRITES

The word *dendrite* is derived from the Greek word *dendron* for "tree," and indeed some dendrites resemble the branches or roots of an oak tree. Inspired by trees, no doubt, the anatomist Camillo Golgi suggested in 1886 that the function of dendrites is to collect nutrients for the neuron. The truth is analogous but more interesting: dendrites arborize through a volume of brain tissue so that they can collect *information* in the form of synaptic input. The dendrites of different types of neurons exhibit a great diversity of shapes. Dendrites are often extensive, accounting for up to 99% of a neuron's membrane. The dendrites of a single neuron may receive as many as 200,000 synaptic inputs. The electrical and biochemical properties of dendrites are quite variable from cell to cell, and they have a profound influence on the transfer of information from synapse to soma.

Dendrites attenuate synaptic potentials

Dendrites tend to be long and thin. Their cytoplasm has relatively low electrical resistivity, and their membrane has relatively high resistivity. These are the properties of a *leaky electrical cable*, which is the premise for **cable theory** (see Chapter 7). Leaky cables are like leaky garden hoses; if ionic current (or water) enters at one end, the fraction of it that exits at the other end depends on the number of channels (or holes) in the cable (hose). A good hose has no holes and all the water makes it through, but most dendrites have a considerable number of channels that serve as leaks for ionic current (see Fig. 7-22).

Cable theory predicts how much current flows down the length of the dendrite through the cytoplasm and how much of it leaks out of the dendrite across the membrane. As summarized in Table 7-3, we can express the leakiness of the membrane by the resistance per unit area of dendritic membrane (**specific membrane resistance**, R_m), which can vary widely among neurons. The intracellular resistance per cross-sectional area of dendrite (**specific resistivity of the cytoplasm**, R_i) is also important in determining current flow inasmuch as a very resistive cytoplasm forces more current to flow out across the membrane rather than down the axis of the dendrite. Another important factor is cable diameter; thick dendrites let more current flow toward the soma than

thin dendrites do. Figure 7-22C illustrates the consequences of a point source of steady current flowing into a leaky, uniform, infinitely long cable made of purely passive membrane. The transmembrane voltage generated by the current falls off exponentially with distance from the site of current injection. The steepness with which the voltage falls off is defined by the length constant (λ; see Chapter 7), which is the distance over which a steady voltage decays by a factor of $1/e$ (~37%). Estimates of the parameter values vary widely, but for brain neurons at rest, reasonable numbers are ~50,000 $\Omega \cdot cm^2$ for R_m and 200 $\Omega \cdot cm$ for R_i. If the radius of the dendrite (*a*) is 1 μm (10^{-4} cm), we can estimate the length constant of a dendrite by applying Equation 7-8.

$$\lambda = \sqrt{\frac{a \cdot R_m}{2R_i}} = \sqrt{\frac{(10^{-4}\,cm)(5 \times 10^4\,\Omega cm^2)}{2(200\Omega cm)}} \quad \text{(12-1)}$$
$$= 0.1118\,cm = 1118\,\mu m$$

Because dendrite diameters vary greatly, λ should also vary greatly. For example, assuming the same cellular properties, a thin dendrite with a radius of 0.1 μm would have a λ of only 354 μm, whereas a thick one with a radius of 5 μm would have a λ of 2500 μm. Thus, the graded signal spreads farther in a thick dendrite.

Real dendrites are certainly not infinitely long, uniform, and unbranched, nor do they have passive membranes. Thus, quantitative analysis of realistic dendrites is complex. Sharp termination of a dendrite *decreases* attenuation because current cannot escape farther down the cable. Branching *increases* attenuation because current has more paths to follow. Gradually expanding to an increased diameter progressively increases λ and thus *decreases* attenuation. Real membranes are never completely passive because all have voltage-gated channels, and therefore their R_m values can change as a function of voltage. Finally, in the working brain, cable properties are not constant but may vary dynamically with ongoing brain activity. For example, as the general level of synaptic input to a neuron rises (which might happen when a brain region is actively engaged in a task), more membrane channels will open and thus R_m will drop as a function of time, with consequent shortening of dendritic length constants. However, all these caveats do not alter the fundamental *qualitative* conclusion: *voltage signals are attenuated as they travel down a dendrite*.

So far, we have described only how a dendrite might attenuate a *sustained* voltage change. Indeed, the usual definition of length constant applies only to a *steady-state* voltage shift. An important complication is that the signal attenuation along a cable depends on the *frequency* components of that signal—how rapidly voltage changes over time. When V_m varies over time, some current is lost to membrane capacitance (see Chapter 6), and less current is carried along the dendrite downstream from the source of the current. Because action potentials and EPSPs entail rapid changes in V_m, with the fastest of them rising and falling within a few milliseconds, they are attenuated much more strongly than the steady-state λ implies. If V_m varies in time, we can define a λ that depends on signal frequency (λ_{AC}, where AC stands for alternating current). When signal frequency is zero (i.e., V_m is steady), $\lambda = \lambda_{AC}$. However, as frequency increases, λ_{AC}

may fall sharply. Thus, *dendrites attenuate high-frequency (i.e., rapidly changing) signals more than low-frequency or steady signals.* Another way to express this concept is that most dendrites tend to be **low-pass filters** in that they let slowly changing signals pass more easily than rapidly changing ones.

Figure 12-2A shows how an EPSP propagates along two different dendrites with very different length constants: when the dendrites have a longer λ, a larger signal arrives at the axon hillock. How do leaky dendrites manage to communicate a useful synaptic signal to the soma? The problem is solved in two ways. The first solution deals with the passive properties of the dendrite membrane. The length (l) of dendrites tends to be relatively small in comparison to their λ; thus, none extend more than one or two steady-state length constants (i.e., the l/λ ratio is smaller than 1). One way that

dendrites achieve a small l/λ ratio is to have a combination of diameter and R_m that gives them a large λ. Another way is that dendrites are not infinitely long cables but "terminated" cables. Figure 12-2B shows that a signal is attenuated more in an infinitely long cable (curve *a*) than in a terminated cable whose length (l) is equal to λ (curve *b*). The attenuation of a purely passive cable would be even less if the terminated cable had a λ 10-fold greater than l (curve *c*). Recall that in our example in Figure 12-2A, such a 10-fold difference in λ underlies the difference in the amplitudes of the EPSPs arriving at the axon hillock.

The second solution to the attenuation problem is to endow dendrites with voltage-gated ion channels (see Chapter 7) that enhance the signal more than would be expected in a purely "passive" system (curve *d*). We discuss the properties of such "active" cables in the next section.

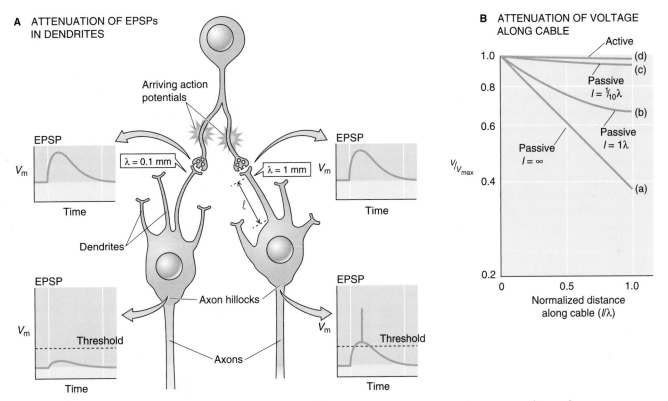

Figure 12-2 Effect of λ on propagation of an EPSP to two different axons. **A,** The neuron at the top fires an action potential that reaches the left and right neurons below, each at a single synapse. The EPSPs are identical. However, the left neuron has a thin dendrite and therefore a small length constant ($\lambda = 0.1$ mm). As a result, the signal is almost completely attenuated by the time it reaches the axon hillock, and there is no action potential. In the right neuron, the dendrite is thicker and therefore has a larger length constant ($\lambda = 1$ mm). As a result, the signal that reaches the axon hillock is large enough to trigger an action potential. **B,** The graph shows four theoretical plots of the decay of voltage (logarithmic plot) along a dendritic cable. The voltage is expressed as a fraction of maximal voltage. The length along the cable is normalized for the length constant (λ). Thus, an l/λ of 1.0 corresponds to one length constant along the dendrite. Curve *a*: If the cable is infinitely long and passive, the voltage decays exponentially with increasing length, so that the semilog plot is linear. Curve *b*: If the cable is terminated at a length that is equal to one length constant, then voltage decays less steeply. Curve *c*: If the cable is terminated at a length that is equal to 10% of the length constant, the voltage decays even less steeply. Curve *d*: If the membrane is not passive but has a slow voltage-gated conductance, the dendritic attenuation will be much smaller. *(Data from Jack JJB, Noble D, Tsien RW: Electrical Current Flow in Excitable Cells. Oxford: Oxford University Press, 1975.)*

Dendritic membranes have voltage-gated ion channels

All mammalian dendrites have voltage-gated ion channels that influence their signaling properties. Dendritic characteristics vary from cell to cell, and the principles of dendritic signaling are studied intensively. Most dendrites have a relatively low density of voltage-gated channels (see Chapter 7) that may amplify, or boost, synaptic signals by adding additional inward current as the signals propagate from distal dendrites toward the soma. We have already introduced the principle of an **active cable** in curve *d* of Figure 12-2B. If the membrane has voltage-gated channels that are able to carry more inward current (usually Na^+ or Ca^{2+}) under depolarized conditions, a sufficiently strong EPSP would drive V_m into the activation range of the voltage-gated channels. These voltage-gated channels would open, and their additional inward current would add to that generated initially by the synaptic channels. Thus, the synaptic signal would fall off much less steeply than in a passive dendrite. Voltage-gated channels can be distributed all along the dendrite and thus amplify the signal along the entire dendritic length, or they can be clustered at particular sites. In either case, voltage-gated channels can boost the synaptic signal considerably, even if the densities of channels are far too low to generate action potentials.

An even more dramatic solution, used by a few dendrites, is to have such a high density of voltage-gated ion channels that they can produce *action potentials*, just as axons can. One of the best documented examples is the Purkinje cell, which is the large output neuron of the cerebellum. As Rodolfo Llinás and colleagues have shown, when the dendrites of Purkinje cells are stimulated strongly, they can generate large, sharp action potentials that are mediated by voltage-gated Ca^{2+} channels (Fig. 12-3). Such Ca^{2+} spikes can sometimes propagate toward—or even into—the soma, but

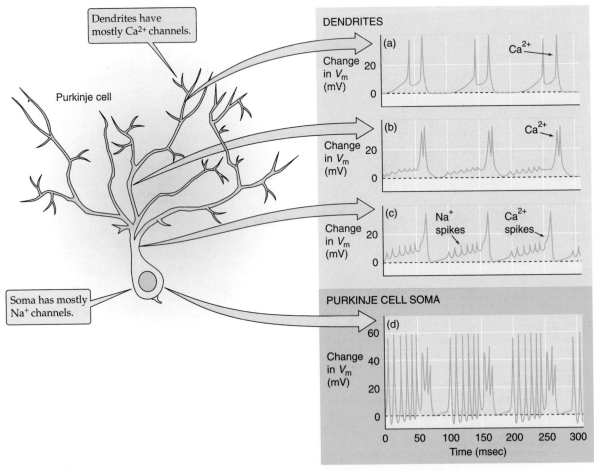

Figure 12-3 Ca^{2+} action potentials (in dendrites of Purkinje cells). Usually, dendrites do not fire action potentials; however, in these Purkinje cells of the cerebellum (*left panel*), the high density of voltage-gated Ca^{2+} channels in the dendrites allows the generation of *slow* dendritic Ca^{2+} spikes (records *a, b,* and *c* on the *right*), which propagate all the way to the axon soma. In the axon soma, these Ca^{2+} action potentials trigger fast Na^+ action potentials (record *d* on the *right*). Moreover, the fast Na^+ spikes back propagate into the dendritic tree but are attenuated. Thus, these fast Na^+ spikes appear as small spikes in the proximal dendrites (record *c*) and even smaller blips in the midlevel dendrites (record *b*). (*Data from Llinás R, Sugimori M: Electrophysiological properties of in vitro Purkinje cell dendrites in mammalian cerebellar slices. J Physiol 1981; 305:197-213.*)

these Ca²⁺ action potentials do not continue down the axon. Instead, they may trigger fast Na⁺-dependent action potentials that are generated by voltage-gated Na⁺ channels in the soma and initial segment. The Na⁺ spikes carry the signal along the axon in the conventional way, and those in the soma are considerably quicker and larger than the dendritic Ca²⁺ spikes. The faster Na⁺ spikes do not propagate too far backward into the dendritic tree because the rapid time course of the Na⁺ spike is strongly attenuated by the inherent filtering properties of the dendrites (i.e., the λ_{AC} is smaller for the rapid frequencies of the Na⁺ action potentials than for the slower Ca²⁺ action potentials). The dendrites of certain other neurons of the CNS, including some pyramidal cells of the cerebral cortex, can also generate spikes that are dependent on Ca²⁺, Na⁺, or both.

Dendritic action potentials, when they exist at all, tend to be slower and weaker than those in axons. The reason is probably that one of the functions of dendrites is to collect and to integrate information from a large number of synapses (often thousands). If each synapse were capable of triggering an action potential, there would be little opportunity for most of the input to have a meaningful influence on a neuron's output. The cell's dynamic range would be truncated; that is, a very small number of active synapses would bring the neuron to its maximum firing rate. However, if dendrites are only weakly excitable, the problem of signal attenuation along dendritic cables can be solved while still allowing the cell to generate an output (i.e., the axonal firing rate) that is indicative of the proportion of its synapses that are active.

Another advantage of voltage-gated channels in dendrites may be the selective boosting of high-frequency synaptic input. Recall that passive dendrites attenuate signals of high frequency more than those of low frequency. However, if dendrites possess the appropriate voltage-gated channels, they will be better able to communicate high-frequency synaptic input.

CONTROL OF SPIKING PATTERNS IN THE SOMA

Electrical signals from dendrites converge and summate at the soma. Although action potentials themselves often appear first at the nearby axon hillock and initial segment of the axon, the large variety of ion channels in the soma and proximal dendritic membranes is critically important in determining and modulating the temporal patterns of action potentials that ultimately course down the axon.

Neurons can transform a simple input into a variety of output patterns

Neurophysiologists have sampled the electrical properties of many different types of neurons in the nervous system, and one general conclusion seems safe: no two types behave the same. The variability begins with the **shape and height** of individual action potentials. Most neurons within the CNS generate action potentials in the conventional way, as described in Chapter 7 (see Fig. 7-4). Fast, voltage-gated Na⁺ channels generate a strong inward current that depolarizes

the membrane from rest, usually in the range of −60 to −80 mV, to a peak that is usually between +10 and +40 mV. This depolarization represents the upstroke of the action potential. The Na⁺ channels then quickly inactivate and close, and certain K⁺ channels (often voltage-gated, delayed outward rectifier channels) open and thus cause V_m to fall and terminate the spike. However, many neurons have somewhat different spike-generating mechanisms and produce spikes with a range of shapes. Although a fast Na⁺ current invariably drives the fast upstroke of neuronal action potentials, an additional fast Ca²⁺ current can frequently occur and, if it is large enough, broaden the spike duration. The greatest variability occurs in the repolarization phase. Many neurons are repolarized by other voltage-gated K⁺ currents in addition to the delayed outward rectifier K⁺ current, and some also have a K⁺ current carried by channels that are rapidly activated by the combination of membrane depolarization and a rise in [Ca²⁺]ᵢ (see Chapter 7).

More dramatic variations occur in the **repetitive spiking patterns** of neurons, observed when the duration of a stimulus is long. One way to illustrate this principle is to apply a simple, continuous stimulus (a current pulse, for example) to each neuron and to measure its output (the number and pattern of action potentials fired at its soma). The current pulse is the equivalent of a steady, strong input of excitatory synaptic currents. The transformation from stimulus input to spiking output can take many different forms. Some examples are shown in Figure 12-4, which illustrates recordings from three types of neurons in the cerebral cortex. In response to a sustained current stimulus, some cells generate a rapid train of action potentials that *do not adapt* (Fig. 12-4A); that is, the spikes occur at a regular interval throughout the current pulse. Other cells fire rapidly at first but then *adapt strongly* (Fig. 12-4B); that is, the spikes gradually become less frequent during the current pulse. Some cells fire a burst of action potentials and then stop firing altogether, and still others generate *rhythmic bursts* of action potentials that continue as long as the stimulus (Fig. 12-4C). These varied behaviors are not arbitrary but are characteristic of each neuron type, and they are as distinctive as each cell's morphology. They are also an intrinsic property of each neuron; that is, a neuron's fundamental firing pattern is determined by the membrane properties of the cell and does not require fluctuations in synaptic input. Of course, synaptic input may also impose particular firing patterns on a neuron. When a neuron is operating in situ, its firing patterns are determined by the interaction of its intrinsic membrane properties and synaptic input.

Rhythmically bursting cells are particularly interesting and occur in a variety of places in the brain. As described in Chapter 16, they may participate in the central circuits that generate rhythmic motor output for behavior such as locomotion and respiration. Cells that secrete peptide neurohormones, such as the magnocellular neurons of the hypothalamus, are also often characterized by rhythmic bursting behavior. These cells release either arginine vasopressin or oxytocin and help control water retention and lactation, respectively (see Chapters 40 and 56). Rhythmic bursting is a more effective stimulus for the synaptic release of peptides than are tonic patterns of action potential. It may be that the bursting patterns and the Ca²⁺ currents that help

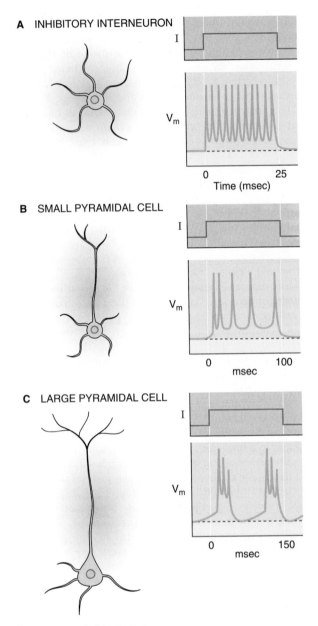

A INHIBITORY INTERNEURON

I

V_m

0   25
Time (msec)

B SMALL PYRAMIDAL CELL

I

V_m

0   100
msec

C LARGE PYRAMIDAL CELL

I

V_m

0   150
msec

Figure 12-4 Spiking patterns.

again; others chop the ongoing stimulus into a more rhythmic output; and still other cells transform the input very little. The mechanisms for this range of transformations include both synaptic circuitry and the diverse membrane properties of each cell type. The different properties allow some cells to be particularly well tuned to specific features of the stimulus—its onset, duration, or amplitude modulation—and they can then communicate this signal to the appropriate auditory nuclei for more complex processing.

Intrinsic firing patterns are determined by a variety of ion currents with relatively slow kinetics

What determines the variety of spiking patterns in each type of neuron, and why do neurons differ in their intrinsic patterns? The key is a large set of ion channel types that have variable and often relatively *slow* kinetics compared with the *quick* Na$^+$ and K$^+$ channels that shape the spike. For a discussion of the properties of such channels, see Chapter 7. Each neuron expresses a different complement of these slow channels and has a unique spatial arrangement of them on its dendrites, soma, and axon initial segment. The channels are gated primarily by membrane voltage and [Ca^{2+}]$_i$, and a neuron's ultimate spiking pattern is determined by the net effects of the slow currents that it generates. We illustrate three examples of systems that have been studied in detail.

1. A neuron with only fast, voltage-gated Na$^+$ channels and delayed rectifier K$^+$ channels will generate repetitive spikes when it is presented with a long stimulus. The pattern of those spikes will be quite regular over time, as for the cerebral cortical interneuron that we have already seen in Figure 12-4A.

2. If the neuron also has another set of K$^+$ channels that activate only very slowly, the spiking pattern becomes more time dependent: the spiking frequency may initially be very high, but it adapts to progressively lower rates as a slow K$^+$ current turns on to counteract the stimulus, as shown for the small pyramidal cell in Figure 12-4B. The strength and rate of adaptation depend strongly on the number and properties of the fast and slow K$^+$ channels.

3. A neuron, by exploiting the interplay between two or more voltage-gated currents, can generate spontaneous rhythmic bursting—as in the case of the large pyramidal neuron in Figure 12-4C—even without ongoing synaptic activity to drive it.

AXONAL CONDUCTION

Axons are specialized for rapid, reliable, and efficient transmission of electrical signals

At first glance, the job of the axon seems mundane compared with the complex computational functions of synapses, dendrites, and somata. After all, the axon has the relatively simple job of carrying the computed signal—a sequence of action potentials—from one place in the brain to another without changing it significantly. Some axons are thin, unmyelinated,

drive them can elicit the relatively high [Ca^{2+}]$_i$ necessary to trigger the exocytosis of peptide-containing vesicles (see Chapter 8). One additional role of rhythmically bursting neurons is to help drive the synchronous oscillations of neural activity in forebrain circuits (i.e., thalamus and cortex) during certain behavioral states, particularly sleep.

Although it has been difficult to prove, the diverse electrical properties of neurons are probably adapted to each cell's particular functions. For example, in the first stage of auditory processing in the brain, cranial nerve VIII axons from the cochlea innervate several types of neurons in the cochlear nucleus of the brainstem. The axons provide similar synaptic drive to each type of neuron, yet the output from each neuron type is distinctly different. Some are tuned to precise timing and respond only to the *onset* of the stimulus and ignore anything else; some respond, pause, and respond

and slow; these properties are sufficient to achieve their functions. However, the axon can be exquisitely optimized, with myelin and nodes of Ranvier, for fast and reliable saltatory conduction of action potentials over very long distances (see Chapter 7). Consider the sensory endings in the skin of your foot, which must send their signals to your lumbar spinal cord 1 meter away (see Fig. 10-11B). The axon of such a sensory cell transmits its message in just a few tens of milliseconds! As we see in our discussion of spinal reflexes in Chapter 16, axons of similar length carry signals in the opposite direction, from your spinal cord to the muscles within your feet, and they do it even faster than the sensory axons. Axons within the CNS can also be very long; examples include the corticospinal axons that originate in the cerebral cortex and terminate in the lumbar spinal cord. Alternatively, many central axons are quite short, only tens of micrometers in length, and they transmit their messages locally between neurons. The spinal interneuron between a sensory neuron and a motor neuron (see Fig. 10-11B) is an example. Some axons target their signal precisely, from one soma to only a few other cells, whereas others may branch profusely to target thousands of postsynaptic cells.

Different parts of the brain have different signaling needs, and their axons are adapted to the local requirements. Nevertheless, the primary function of all axons is to carry electrical signals, in the form of action potentials, from one place to other places and to do so rapidly, efficiently, and reliably. Without myelinated axons, the large, complex brains necessary to control warm, fast mammalian bodies could not exist. For *un*myelinated axons to conduct action potentials sufficiently fast for many purposes, their diameters would have to be so large that the axons alone would take up far too much space and use impossibly large amounts of energy.

Action potentials are usually initiated at the initial segment

The soma, axon hillock, and initial segment of the axon together serve as a kind of focal point in most neurons. The many graded synaptic potentials carried by numerous dendrites converge at the soma and generate one electrical signal. During the 1950s, Sir John Eccles and colleagues used glass microelectrodes to probe the details of this process in spinal motor neurons. Because it appeared that the threshold for action potentials in the initial segment was only ~10 mV above the resting potential, whereas the threshold in the soma was closer to 30 mV above resting potential, they concluded that the neuron's action potentials would be first triggered at the initial segment. Direct evidence now indicates that spikes may begin at the initial segment, at least for some neurons. EPSPs evoked in the dendrites propagate down to and through the soma and trigger an action potential in the initial segment (Fig. 12-5A). The action potential then propagates in two directions: forward (**orthodromically**) into the axon, with no loss of amplitude, and backward into the soma and dendrites, with strong attenuation, as we saw earlier in Figure 12-3. Orthodromic propagation carries the signal to the next set of neurons. The function of backward propagation is not completely understood. It is possible that backwardly propagating spikes trigger bio-

chemical changes in the neuron's dendrites and synapses, and they may have a role in synaptic plasticity.

The axon achieves a uniquely *low* threshold in its initial segment (Fig. 12-5B) by packing voltage-gated Na^+ channels *at a remarkably high density* (in comparison to the soma and dendrites) *in the initial segment* (Fig. 12-5C). The Na^+ channel density in the axon initial segment is ~2000 channels/μm^2, ~1000-fold higher than in the membrane of the soma and dendrites.

Conduction velocity of a myelinated axon increases linearly with diameter

The larger the diameter of an axon, the faster its conduction velocity, other things remaining equal. However, conduction velocity is usually far greater in myelinated axons than it is in unmyelinated axons (see Chapter 7). Thus, a myelinated axon 10 μm in diameter conducts impulses at about the same velocity as an unmyelinated axon ~500 μm in diameter. Myelination confers not only substantial speed advantages but also advantages in efficiency. Almost 2500 of the 10-μm myelinated axons can pack into the volume occupied by one 500-μm axon!

Unmyelinated axons still have a role in vertebrates. At diameters below ~1 μm, unmyelinated axons in the peripheral nervous system (PNS) conduct more rapidly than myelinated ones do. In a testament to evolutionary frugality, the thinnest axons of the peripheral sensory nerves, called **C fibers**, are ~1 μm wide or less, and all are unmyelinated. Axons larger than ~1 μm in diameter are all myelinated (Table 12-1). Every axon has its biological price: the largest axons obviously take up the most room and are the most expensive to synthesize and to maintain metabolically. The largest, swiftest axons are therefore used sparingly. They are used only to carry sensory information about the most rapidly changing stimuli over the longest distances (e.g., stretch receptors in muscle, mechanoreceptors in tendons and skin), or they are used to control finely coordinated contractions of muscles. The thinnest, slowest C fibers are mainly sensory axons related to chronic pain and temperature, for which the speed of the message is not as critical.

The relationship between form and function for axons in the CNS is less obvious than it is in the periphery, in part because it is more difficult to identify each axon's function. Interestingly, in the brain and spinal cord, the critical diameter for the myelination transition may be smaller than in the periphery. Many central myelinated axons are as thin as 0.2 μm. At the other extreme, very few myelinated central axons are larger than 4 μm in diameter.

The myelinated axon membrane has a variety of ion channels that may contribute to its normal and pathological function. Of primary importance is the *voltage-gated Na^+* channel, which provides the rapidly activating and inactivating inward current that yields the action potential. Nine isoforms of the α subunit of the voltage-gated Na^+ channel exist (see Table 7-1). In normal central axons, it is specifically $Na_v1.6$ channels that populate the nodes of Ranvier at a density of 1000 to 2000 channels/μm^2 (Fig. 12-5). The same axonal membrane in the internodal regions, under the myelin, has fewer than 25 channels/μm^2 (versus between 2 and 200 channels/ μm^2 in unmyelinated axons). The dramatically different dis-

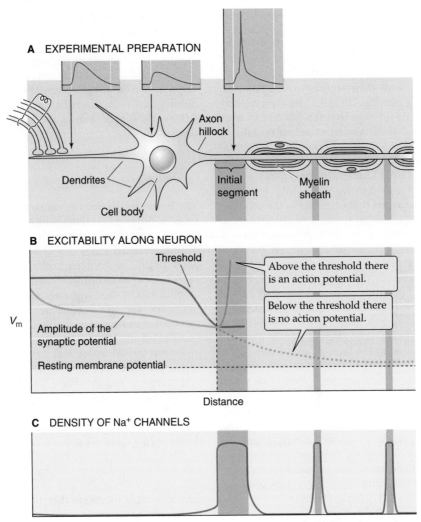

Figure 12-5   Simultaneous recording of action potentials from different parts of a neuron. **A,** In this hypothetical experiment, an excitatory synapse on a dendrite is stimulated, and the response near that dendrite is recorded in the soma and at the initial segment. The EPSP attenuates in the soma and the initial segment, but the EPSP is large enough to trigger an action potential at the initial segment. **B,** The threshold is high (−35 mV) in regions of the neuron that have few Na⁺ channels but starts to fall rather steeply in the hillock and initial segment. Typically, a stimulus of sufficient strength triggers an action potential at the initial segment. **C,** The density of Na⁺ channels is high only at the initial segment and at each node of Ranvier.

tribution of channels between nodal and internodal membrane has important implications for conduction along pathologically demyelinated axons (see later). K⁺ channels are relatively less important in myelinated axons than they are in most other excitable membranes. Very few of these channels are present in the nodal membrane, and fast K⁺ currents contribute little to repolarization of the action potential in mature myelinated axons. This diminished role for K⁺ channels may be a cost-cutting adaptation because the absence of K⁺ currents decreases the metabolic expense of a single action potential by ~40%. However, some K⁺ channels are located in the axonal membrane under the myelin, particularly in the paranodal region. The function of these K⁺ channels is unclear; they may set the resting V_m of the internodes and help stabilize the firing properties of the axon.

Demyelinated axons conduct action potentials slowly, unreliably, or not at all

Numerous clinical disorders selectively damage or destroy myelin sheaths and leave the axonal membranes intact but bare. These **demyelinating diseases** may affect either peripheral or central axons and can lead to severely impaired conduction (Fig. 12-6). The most common demyelinating disease of the CNS is **multiple sclerosis** (see the box titled Demyelinating Diseases), a progressive disorder characterized by distributed zones of demyelination in the brain and spinal cord. Among the demyelinating diseases of peripheral nerves is *Landry-Guillain-Barré syndrome*, which is an inflammatory disorder that may rapidly incapacitate but often ends in substantial recovery. The specific clinical signs

TABLE 12-1 Classes of Peripheral Sensory and Motor Axons, by Size and Conduction Velocity

Erlanger and Gasser's Classification*	Aα	Aβ	Aγ	Aδ	B	C
Function	Sensory afferents from proprioceptors of skeletal muscle Motor neurons to skeletal muscle	Sensory afferents from mechanoreceptors of skin	Motor fibers to intrafusal fibers of muscle spindles	Sensory afferents from pain and temperature receptors	Preganglionic neurons of the autonomic nervous system	Sensory afferents from pain, temperature, and itch receptors
Diameter (μm)	13-20	6-12	3-6	1-5	<3	0.2-1.5
Conduction velocity of action potential (m/s)	80-120	35-75	12-30	5-30	3-15	0.5-2.5
Alternative classification of sensory axons from muscle and tendon†	Ia (sensory from muscle spindle fibers) Ib (sensory from Golgi tendon organs)	II		III		IV

*This A-C classification was introduced by Joseph Erlanger and Herbert Gasser, who shared the 1944 Nobel Prize in Medicine or Physiology for describing the relationship of axon diameter, conduction velocity, and function in a complex peripheral nerve.

†This I-IV classification was introduced by other investigators. It applies only to sensory axons and only to those from muscle and tendon.
Modified from Bear MF, Connors BW, Paradiso MP: Neuroscience: Exploring the Brain, 2nd ed. Baltimore: Lippincott Williams & Wilkins, 2001.

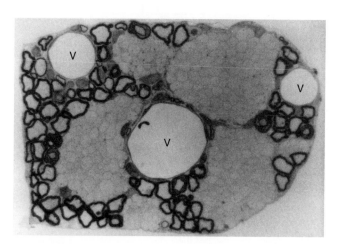

Figure 12-6 Demyelination in the CNS. A cross section of a spinal root from a dystrophic mouse shows amyelinated bundles of axons (thin borders) that are surrounded by myelinated fibers (thick borders). V, lumen of blood vessel. *(From Rosenbluth J: In Waxman SG, Kocsis JD, Stys PK [eds]: The Axon: Structure, Function, and Pathophysiology. New York: Oxford University Press, 1995.)*

of these disorders vary and depend on the particular sets of axons affected.

In a normal, myelinated axon, the action currents generated at a node can effectively charge the adjacent node and bring it to threshold within ~20 μs (Fig. 12-7A) because

myelin serves to increase the resistance and to reduce the capacitance of the pathways between the axoplasm and the extracellular fluid (see Chapter 7). The current flowing across each node is actually 5-fold to 7-fold higher than necessary to initiate an action potential at the adjacent node. Removal of the insulating myelin, however, means that the same nodal action current is distributed across a much longer, leakier, higher capacitance stretch of axonal membrane (Fig. 12-7B). Several consequences are possible. Compared with normal conduction, conduction in a demyelinated axon may continue, but at a *lower velocity,* if the demyelination is not too severe (Fig. 12-7B, record 1). In experimental studies, the internodal conduction time through demyelinated fibers can be as slow as 500 μs, 25 times longer than normal. The ability of axons to transmit *high-frequency* trains of impulses may also be impaired (record 2). Extensive demyelination of an axon causes *total blockade* of conduction (record 3). Clinical studies indicate that the blockade of action potentials is more closely related to symptoms than is the simple slowing of conduction. Demyelinated axons can also become the source of spontaneous, **ectopically generated action potentials** because of changes in their intrinsic excitability (record 4) or mechanosensitivity (record 5). Moreover, the signal from one demyelinated axon can excite an adjacent demyelinated axon and induce **crosstalk** (Fig. 12-7C), which may cause action potentials to be conducted in both directions in the adjacent axon.

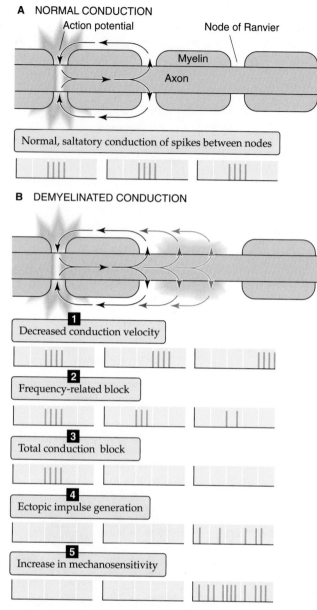

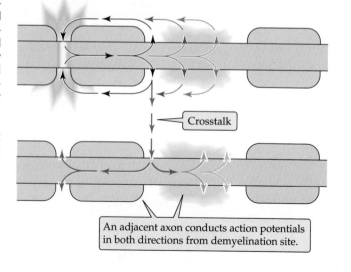

Figure 12-7 Demyelination. **A,** Four action potentials at the leftmost node of Ranvier are conducted—unchanged in amplitude and frequency—to the nodes that are farther to the right. **B,** Action potentials propagate from a normally myelinated region into a demyelinated area. The axial action current that was generated at the last healthy node is distributed across a long region of bare or partially myelinated axonal membrane, with its decreased resistivity and increased capacitance. Thus, the current density at the two affected nodes is greatly reduced. This panel shows five consequences of demyelination: (1) decreased velocity, which is manifested as longer delays for the arrival of the train of spikes; (2) frequency-related block, which does not pass high-frequency trains—as a result, some of the spikes are missing distally; (3) total blockade; (4) ectopic impulse generation—even though there is no input in the proximal portion of the axon, action potentials arise spontaneously beyond the lesion; and (5) increased mechanosensitivity—ectopic action potentials arise by mechanical stimulation. **C,** If the demyelination affects two adjacent axons, action potentials in one (the top axon in this case) cause action potentials to propagate in both directions in the adjacent axon.

Demyelinating Diseases

Multiple sclerosis (MS), the most common demyelinating disease of the CNS, affects more than 350,000 Americans alone. MS is an autoimmune disease directed against the myelin or oligodendrocytes and is thus a purely CNS disease. The trigger is unclear. Some have proposed a viral antigen (including canine distemper virus), but many other theories abound, none of which has been clearly proved. The viral antigen theory is based at least in part on classic studies that concluded that MS has a greater incidence in temperate regions than in the tropics and that one's risk depends on where one spent one's childhood, not adulthood. According to this view, the "incubation" period, or the delay between exposure to an as yet unspecified environmental factor and onset of the first attack, is 10 to 25 years. However, some contemporary neurologists doubt the statistical significance of the temperate/tropic data. No good evidence has been presented for a viral etiology yet. MS is twice as common in women than in men. Susceptibility to MS has also been linked to a number of genetic alleles of the HLA system.

The signs and symptoms of MS are protean, but common features include the following:

1. An optic neuritis may cause decreased visual acuity.
2. An internuclear ophthalmoplegia results in an inability of the eyes to adduct on lateral conjugate gaze, reflecting a lesion in the medial longitudinal fasciculus, a white matter tract. The result is double vision.
3. The Lhermitte sign is an electrical sensation that shoots down the back and into the legs when the neck is flexed.

Elevated IgG levels are typically found in the cerebrospinal fluid, and electrophoresis reveals oligoclonal bands in the IgG region. Magnetic resonance imaging can demonstrate the lesions in MS. Evoked potential studies, which measure nerve fiber conduction in various sensory pathways, are abnormal in almost all established cases and in about two thirds of suspected cases of MS.

MS is defined clinically as a disease that involves demyelination of the CNS with episodes separated in both time and space—at least two episodes of demyelination involving at least two separated regions of the CNS. Remissions and relapses are characteristic of many patients with MS. Thus, episodes of demyelination may be separated by intervals during which the symptoms and signs improve or even completely resolve. It is only the minority of patients who inexorably progress to the point of disability.

An exacerbation is due to the occurrence of active inflammation of a white matter tract in the CNS. A remission then occurs when the inflammation subsides and the axons that have now been demyelinated recover some of their function and are able to conduct action potentials through the area of myelin damage. However, the pathologically demyelinated fibers are not normal. Among the molecular changes that occur, Nav1.2 channels may replace Nav1.6 channels in demyelinated axons. Conduction is often barely adequate under normal circumstances and may become inadequate under stressful situations, such as illness, emotional stress, and exhaustion. Under these circumstances, symptoms will reappear. Such reappearance of symptoms must be distinguished clinically from a new exacerbation. In the reappearance of symptoms, it is an old area of damage that has become dysfunctional. In the new exacerbation, it is a new area of damage caused by new inflammation. The treatments of these two causes of symptoms are very different.

The reasons for remissions and exacerbations are not entirely clear. One explanation focuses on the impaired conduction in the pathologically demyelinated fibers. If conduction is just barely adequate under normal circumstances, it may become inadequate under certain stressful situations, such as illness, emotional stress, and exhaustion; only then will symptoms become evident. A change in temperature is a classic example of circumstances changing conduction. Conduction through demyelinated axons is exquisitely sensitive to temperature, but the direction of the effect is counterintuitive: conduction is "safer" at low temperature. Lower temperatures slow the gating kinetics of Na^+ channels, thereby lengthening the duration of the action potentials and slowing conduction velocity. A decrease of just 2°C increases the duration of an action potential by ~20%. The augmented currents of the broader spike are better able to charge the increased capacitance of the axonal membrane of a demyelinated region, thus making it more likely that the threshold for continued conduction will be reached. When the body temperature of a patient with MS is elevated, for example, by fever or immersion in a hot bath, conduction is compromised and neurological deficits may appear. Conversely, the slightly increased impulse duration gained by cooling of the body may be sufficient to restore conduction through a demyelinated region. Thus, MS patients may experience improved nerve function in cold versus hot environments. These temperature effects on symptoms are explained nicely by the physiology of neural conduction and probably account for evanescent changes in symptoms in many patients. However, the temperature effects do not explain exacerbations and remissions, which are due to appearance and disappearance of inflammation.

Certain drugs can also prolong the duration of action potentials and facilitate conduction through demyelinated axons. Demyelination may expose the voltage-gated K^+ channels, which are normally hidden under the myelin. Activation of outwardly rectifying K^+ channels can further impair spike production in demyelinated axons. However, the K^+ channels also become accessible to pharmacological agents, such as the class of K^+ channel blockers called aminopyridines. Because fast K^+ channels may contribute to the repolarization phase of an action potential, blocking of these K^+ channels can prolong the spike and facilitate its propagation through demyelinated regions. Clinical trials of aminopyridines showed some symptomatic relief in patients with MS, but the drugs have not proved effective enough for routine use.

At present, standard treatment of MS exacerbations includes immunosuppressive agents. The most common is interferon beta, which is one of the class of interferons that have antiviral, antiproliferative, and immune-modulating activity. This drug reduces the number and severity of exacerbations in patients with mild or moderate relapsing and remitting MS and may also help patients with chronic progressive MS. Many new drugs are currently under investigation to help prevent the autoimmune attack, to reduce the damage during an attack, or to improve function in already demyelinated regions.

Another demyelinating disease of the CNS is progressive multifocal leukoencephalopathy, a fatal illness common in

Continued

Demyelinating Diseases—cont'd

patients with acquired immunodeficiency disease and caused by opportunistic infection of the oligodendroglia (myelin-producing cells) by a strain of human papovavirus. Another disorder, central pontine myelinolysis, is caused by too rapid correction of hyponatremia; the sudden osmotic fluctuations appear to produce demyelination.

The most common demyelinating disease of the PNS is Landry-Guillain-Barré syndrome. After a respiratory or other viral infection, an ascending neurological syndrome develops that is characterized by the onset of weakness, leading to paralysis of the legs and subsequent involvement of the hands and arms. In severe cases, the paralysis involves the nerves feeding the brainstem, and patients may lose the ability to swallow or even to breathe, which requires mechanical ventilation for a time.

This initial stage of Landry-Guillain-Barré syndrome reaches a plateau in several weeks and then gradually resolves. Most patients recover completely as long as the physician recognizes the syndrome and initiates supportive treatment. Untreated, this syndrome is often fatal.

The pathological lesions of Landry-Guillain-Barré syndrome consist of lymphocytic infiltration of the myelin sheath produced by Schwann cells in the PNS. The result is segmental demyelination. These patients generally recover fully because the PNS has the ability to remyelinate itself. Axons of the CNS do not remyelinate to any significant extent, which explains why complete recovery in patients with MS is not as common as in these patients.

REFERENCES

Books and Reviews

Ashcroft FM: Ion Channels and Disease. New York: Academic Press, 1999.

Connors BW, Gutnick MJ: Intrinsic firing patterns of diverse neocortical neurons. Trends Neurosci 1990; 13:99-104.

Johnston D, Wu SM-S: Foundations of Cellular Neurophysiology. Cambridge, MA: MIT Press, 1994.

London M, Häusser M: Dendritic computation. Annu Rev Neurosci 2005; 28:503-532.

Waxman SG, Craner MJ, Black JA: Na⁺ channel expression along axons in multiple sclerosis and its models. Trends Pharmacol Sci 2004; 25:584-591.

Zamvil SS, Steinman L. Diverse targets for intervention during inflammatory and neurodegenerative phases of multiple sclerosis. Neuron 2003; 38:685-688.

Journal Articles

Huguenard JR, Hamill OP, Prince DA: Sodium channels in dendrites of rat cortical pyramidal neurons. Proc Natl Acad Sci USA 1989; 86:2473-2477.

Khaliq ZM, Raman IM: Axonal propagation of simple and complex spikes in cerebellar Purkinje neurons. J Neurosci 2005; 25: 454-463.

Larkum ME, Zhu JJ, Sakmann B: Dendritic mechanisms underlying the coupling of the dendritic with the axonal action potential initiation zone of adult rat layer 5 pyramidal neurons. J Physiol 2001; 533:447-466.

Llinás R, Nicholson C: Electrophysiological properties of dendrites and somata in alligator Purkinje cells. J Neurophysiol 1971; 34:534-551.

Magee JC, Johnston D: Synaptic activation of voltage-gated channels in the dendrites of hippocampal pyramidal neurons. Science 1995; 268:301-304.

Swensen AM, Bean BP: Ionic mechanisms of burst firing in dissociated Purkinje neurons. J Neurosci 2003; 23:9650-9663.

CHAPTER 13

SYNAPTIC TRANSMISSION IN
THE NERVOUS SYSTEM

Barry W. Connors

After meticulous study of spinal reflexes, Charles Sherrington deduced that neurons somehow communicate information, one to the next, by a mechanism that is fundamentally different from the way that they conduct signals along their axons. Sherrington had merged his physiological conclusions with the anatomical observations (Fig. 13-1) of his contemporary, the preeminent neuroanatomist Santiago Ramón y Cajal. Cajal had proposed that neurons are distinct entities, fundamental units of the nervous system, that are *discontinuous* with each other. Discontinuous neurons must nevertheless communicate, and Sherrington in 1897 proposed that the **synapse**, a specialized apposition between cells, mediates the signals. The word *synapse* implies "contiguity, not continuity" between neurons, as Cajal himself explained it. When the fine structure of synapses was finally revealed with the electron microscope in the 1950s, the vision of Cajal and Sherrington was amply sustained. Neurons come very close together at chemical synapses, but their membranes and cytoplasm remain distinct. At electrical synapses, which are less common than chemical synapses, the membranes remain distinct, but ions and other small solutes can diffuse through the gap junctions, a form of continuity (see Chapter 8).

NEURONAL SYNAPSES

The molecular mechanisms of neuronal synapses are similar but not identical to those of the neuromuscular junction

Chemical synapses use diffusible **transmitter molecules** to communicate messages between two cells. The first chemical synapse to be understood in detail was the neuromuscular junction (the nerve-muscle synapse) in vertebrate skeletal muscle, which is described in Chapter 8. In this chapter, we are concerned with the properties of the synapses that occur *between neurons*. We now know that all synapses share certain basic biochemical and physiological mechanisms, and thus many basic insights gained from the neuromuscular junction are also applicable to synapses in the brain. However, neuronal synapses differ from neuromuscular junctions in

many important ways; they also differ widely among themselves, and it is the diverse properties of synapses that help make each part of the brain unique.

It is useful to begin by reviewing some of the mechanisms that are common to all chemical synapses (see Figs. 8-2 and 8-3). Synaptic transmission at chemical synapses occurs in seven steps:

Step 1: Neurotransmitter molecules are packaged into membranous vesicles, and the vesicles are concentrated and docked at the presynaptic terminal.

Step 2: The presynaptic membrane depolarizes, usually as the result of an action potential.

Step 3: The depolarization causes voltage-gated Ca^{2+} channels to open and allows Ca^{2+} ions to flow into the terminal.

Step 4: The resulting increase in intracellular $[Ca^{2+}]$ triggers fusion of vesicles with the presynaptic membrane (see Chapter 8). The Ca^{2+} dependence of fusion may be conferred by a neuron-specific protein component of the fusion apparatus called synaptotagmin. The actual fusion events are incredibly fast; each individual exocytosis requires only a fraction of a millisecond to be completed.

Step 5: The transmitter is released into the extracellular space in quantized amounts and diffuses passively across the synaptic cleft.

Step 6: Some of the transmitter molecules bind to receptors in the postsynaptic membrane, and the activated receptors trigger some postsynaptic event, usually the opening of an ion channel or the activation of a G protein–coupled signal cascade.

Step 7: Transmitter molecules diffuse away from postsynaptic receptors and are eventually cleared away by continued diffusion, enzymatic degradation, or active uptake into cells. In addition, the presynaptic machinery retrieves the membrane of the exocytosed synaptic vesicle, perhaps by endocytosis from the cell surface.

The molecular machinery of synapses is closely related to components that are universal in eukaryotic cells (see Chapter 2). A large set of proteins is involved in the docking

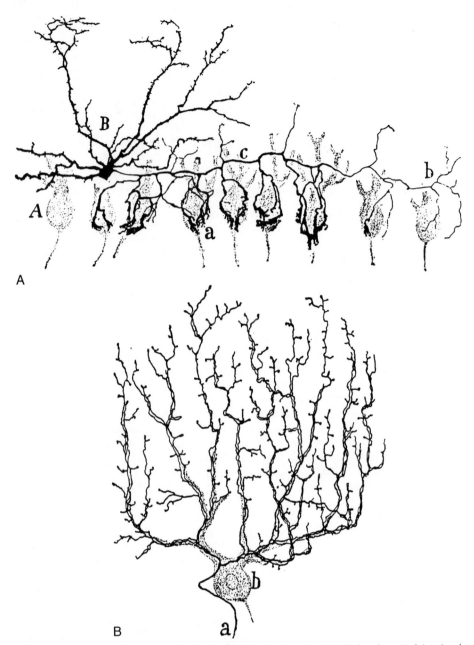

Figure 13-1   Synapses of the mammalian brain. Drawings by Ramón y Cajal taken from Golgi-stained cortex of the cerebellum. **A,** Basket cell (B) from the mouse, making synaptic contacts onto the somata of numerous postsynaptic Purkinje cells (A). The axon (c) of the basket cell branches several times to make baskets (a and b) that synapse onto the somata of Purkinje cells (axosomatic synapse). Ramón y Cajal used the osmic method to stain the Purkinje cell and the Golgi method to stain the basket cell. **B,** A single climbing fiber (a) from a human, making numerous synaptic contacts onto the dendrites of a single Purkinje cell (b). This is an example of axodendritic synapses. Ramón y Cajal used the Golgi method to stain the climbing fiber. *(From Ramón y Cajal S: Histology of the Nervous System of Man and Vertebrates. Swanson N, Swanson LW, trans. New York: Oxford University Press, 1995.)*

and fusion of vesicles, and the proteins present in nerve terminals are amazingly similar to the ones mediating fusion and secretion in yeast. Docking and fusion of synaptic vesicles are discussed in Chapter 8. Ligand-gated ion channels and G protein–coupled receptors (GPCRs), the receptors on the postsynaptic membrane, are also present in all eukaryotic cells and mediate processes as disparate as the recognition of nutrients and poisons as well as the identification of other

members of the species. Even most of the neurotransmitters themselves are simple molecules, identical or very similar to those used in general cellular metabolism. Clearly, the evolutionary roots of synaptic transmission are much older than nervous systems themselves.

Within nervous systems, however, myriad variations on the basic molecular building blocks yield synapses with wide-ranging properties. Neuronal synapses vary widely in

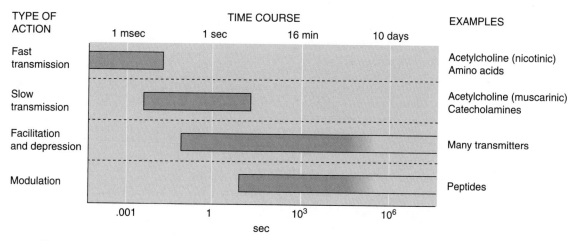

Figure 13-2 Time courses of synaptic events in the nervous system. Different transmitter systems in the brain generate responses that vary widely in how long they last in the postsynaptic cell. Note that the time axis is logarithmic. (*Data from Shepherd GM: Neurobiology, 3rd ed. New York: Oxford University Press, 1994.*)

the size of the synaptic contact, the identity of the neurotransmitter, the nature of the postsynaptic receptors, the efficiency of synaptic transmission, the mechanism used for terminating transmitter action, and the degree and modes of synaptic plasticity. Thus, the properties of neuronal synapses can be tuned to achieve the diverse functions of the brain.

A major difference between the neuromuscular junction and most neuronal synapses is the type of neurotransmitter used. All skeletal neuromuscular junctions use acetylcholine (ACh). In contrast, neuronal synapses use many transmitters. The most ubiquitous are amino acids: glutamate and aspartate excite, whereas γ-aminobutyric acid (GABA) and glycine inhibit. Other transmitters include simple amines, such as ACh, norepinephrine, serotonin, and histamine, as well as a wide array of peptides.

Even more varied than the neuronal transmitters are their receptors. Whereas skeletal muscle manufactures a few modest variants of its ACh receptors, the nervous system typically has several major receptor variants for each neurotransmitter. Knowledge about the wide range of transmitters and receptors is essential to understanding of the chemical activity of the brain as well as the drugs that influence brain activity. For one thing, the many transmitter systems in the brain generate responses with widely varying durations that range from a few milliseconds to days (Fig. 13-2).

Presynaptic terminals may contact neurons at the dendrite, soma, or axon and may contain both clear vesicles and dense-core granules

Chemical synapses between neurons are generally small, often less than 1 µm in diameter, which means that their detailed structure can be seen only with an electron microscope (Fig. 13-3); under the light microscope, brain synapses are usually visible only as swellings along or at the termination of the axons (Fig. 13-1). These swellings are actually the silhouettes of the **bouton terminals**—the presynaptic terminals. Most presynaptic terminals arise from axons, and they

can form synapses on virtually any part of a neuron. The contact site and direction of communication determine the way in which a synapse is named: **axodendritic**, **axosomatic**, and **axoaxonic** synapses (Fig. 13-4). These synapses are the most common types in the nervous system. In many cases, synapses occur on small outpockets of the dendritic membrane called **spines** and are termed **axospinous** synapses. However, not all synapses arise from axons, and **dendrodendritic**, **somatosomatic**, and even **somatodendritic** synapses may be found in the mammalian brain.

Despite their differences in size, site, and shape, all synapses share one basic function: they *deliver a small amount of chemical transmitter onto a circumscribed patch of postsynaptic membrane*. To accomplish this task, they use certain common anatomical features, most of them familiar from discussions of the neuromuscular junction (see Chapter 8).

Synapses are polarized, which means that their two apposed sides have different structures. This polarity reflects the fact that most synapses transmit information in one direction but not in the other (we will see that some rare exceptions do exist). The presynaptic side contains numerous clear **vesicles**, 40 to 50 nm in diameter, that appear empty when viewed by transmission electron microscopy. Synaptic termini may also contain large (100 to 200 nm in diameter), **dense-core secretory granules** that are morphologically quite similar to the secretory granules of endocrine cells. These granules contain neuropeptides, that is, peptides or small proteins that act as neurotransmitters and for which receptors exist in the postsynaptic membranes. Many of these neuropeptides are identical to substances secreted by "traditional" endocrine cells. Endocrine hormones such as adrenocorticotropic hormone, vasoactive intestinal polypeptide, and cholecystokinin are found in dense-core secretory granules present in the terminals of certain central and peripheral neurons.

The clear synaptic vesicles (i.e., not the dense-core granules) are anchored and shifted about by a dense network of cytoskeletal proteins. Some vesicles are clustered close to the part of the presynaptic membrane that apposes the synaptic

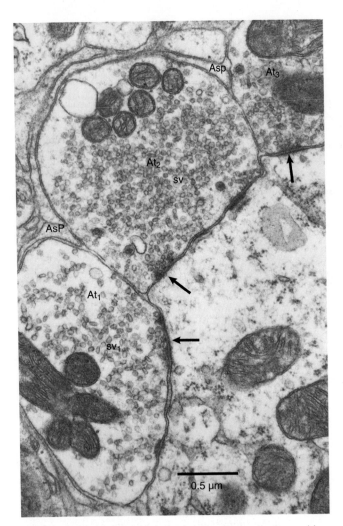

Figure 13-3 Electron micrograph of synapses in the cochlear nucleus. Three presynaptic terminals are filled with vesicles and make contact with the same postsynaptic dendrite. Postsynaptic densities (marking active zones) are indicated by *arrows. (From Peters A, Palay SL, Webster HD: The Fine Structure of the Nervous System: The Neurons and Supporting Cells. Philadelphia: WB Saunders, 1976.)*

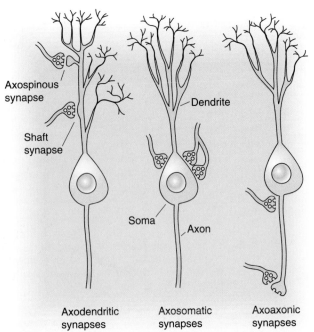

Figure 13-4 The most common synaptic arrangements in the CNS.

contact; these vesicle attachment sites are called **active zones**. Synaptic vesicles are lined up several deep along the active zones, which are probably the regions of actual exocytosis. The number of active zones per synapse varies greatly (active zones are marked with arrows in the synapses of Fig. 13-3). Most synapses in the central nervous system (CNS) have relatively few active zones, often only 1 but occasionally as many as 10 or 20 (versus the hundreds in the neuromuscular junction). If we could view the presynaptic face of an active zone from the perspective of a synaptic vesicle, we would see filaments and particles projecting from the presynaptic membrane, often forming a regular hexagonal arrangement called a **presynaptic grid**. Specific points along the grid are thought to be the vesicle release sites.

Unlike the clear synaptic vesicles containing non-peptide transmitters, dense-core secretory granules are distributed randomly throughout the cytoplasm of the synaptic terminus. They are not concentrated at the presynaptic density,

and they do not appear to release their contents at the active zone. Although the molecular pathways that control exocytosis of the neuronal dense-core granules are still being elucidated, it appears that a rise in $[Ca^{2+}]_i$ is a primary stimulus.

The postsynaptic membrane contains transmitter receptors and numerous proteins clustered in the postsynaptic density

The postsynaptic membrane lies parallel to the presynaptic membrane, and they are separated by a narrow **synaptic cleft** (~30 nm thick) that is filled with extracellular fluid. Transmitter molecules released from the presynaptic terminal must diffuse across the cleft to reach postsynaptic receptors. The most characteristic anatomical feature of the postsynaptic side is the **postsynaptic density**, a strip of granular material visible under the electron microscope on the cytoplasmic face of the membrane (Fig. 13-3). The most important molecular feature of the postsynaptic side is the cluster of transmitter receptors embedded within the postsynaptic membrane. The positions of the receptors are revealed by staining methods that use specific antibodies, toxins, or ligands coupled to some visible tag molecule.

In more than 90% of all excitatory synapses in the CNS, the postsynaptic site is a **dendritic spine**. The ubiquity of spines implies that they serve prominent functions, but their small size (usually less than 1 μm long) makes their function extremely difficult to study. Spines come in a variety of shapes, and their density varies from one dendrite to another (Fig. 13-5); indeed, some central neurons have no spines. The postsynaptic density of spines (as for all central synapses) contains more than 30 proteins in high concentration, including transmitter receptors, protein kinases, a host of

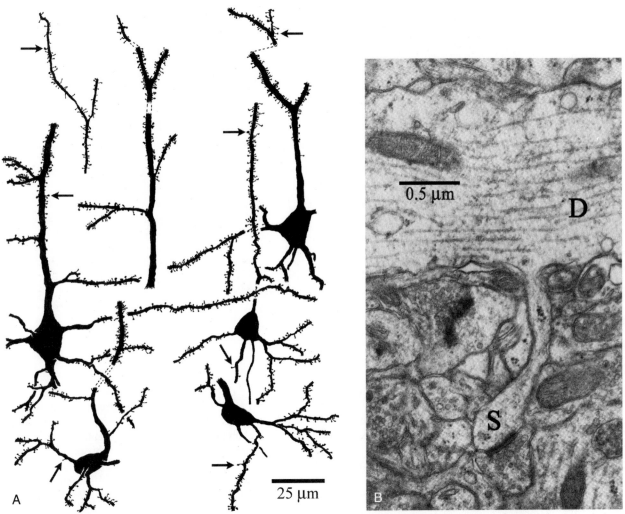

Figure 13-5   Dendritic spines. **A,** Drawings of various dendrites in the neocortex, taken from Golgi-stained material. The numerous protrusions are "spines." **B,** Electron micrograph of an axospinous synapse in the neocortex. Note that the dendritic spine protrudes from the dendritic shaft, making contact with a presynaptic terminal. *(From Feldman ML: In Peters A, Jones EG [eds]: Cerebral Cortex: Cellular Components of the Cerebral Cortex, vol 1, pp 123-200. New York: Plenum, 1984.)*

structural proteins, and proteins that are involved in endocytosis and glycolysis.

Numerous functions for spines have been proposed. It may be that spines increase the opportunity for a dendrite to form synapses with nearby axons. Many hypotheses have focused on the possibility that spines isolate individual synapses from the rest of a cell. This isolation may be electrical or chemical; the narrow spine neck may reduce current flow or the diffusion of chemicals from the spine head into the dendritic shaft. It is unlikely that the electrical resistance of the spine neck is important because given the small conductance generated by a single synapse, neck diameter would have a minimal effect on current flow. However, activation of some excitatory synapses allows substantial amounts of Ca^{2+} to enter the postsynaptic cell. Spines may compartmentalize this Ca^{2+}, thus allowing it to rise to higher levels or preventing it from influencing other synapses on the cell. Because increases in postsynaptic $[Ca^{2+}]_i$ are an essential

trigger for many forms of long-term synaptic plasticity, an attractive but unproven possibility is that dendritic spines play an important role in learning mechanisms.

Some transmitters are used by diffusely distributed systems of neurons to modulate the general excitability of the brain

The brain carries out many sensory, motor, and cognitive functions that require fast, specific, spatially organized neural connections and operations. Consider the detailed neural mapping that allows you to read this sentence or the precise timing required to play the piano. These functions require *spatially focused* networks (Fig. 13-6A).

Other functions, such as falling asleep, waking up, becoming attentive, or changing mood, involve more general alterations of the brain. Several systems of neurons regulate the general excitability of the CNS. Each of these **modulatory**

A SPATIALLY FOCUSED

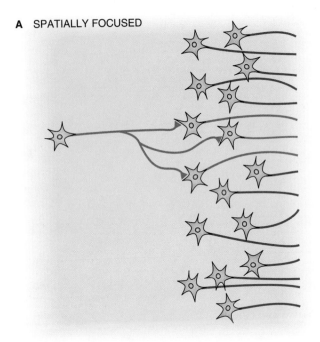

B WIDELY DIVERGENT

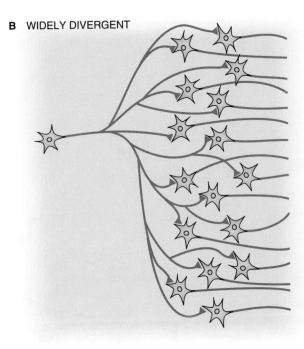

Figure 13-6 Synaptic connections.

systems uses a different neurotransmitter, and the axons of each make widely dispersed, diffuse, almost meandering synaptic connections to carry a simple message to vast regions of the brain. This arrangement can be achieved by a *widely divergent* network (Fig. 13-6B). The functions of the different systems are not well understood, but each appears to be essential for certain aspects of arousal, motor control, memory, mood, motivation, and metabolic state. The modulatory systems are of central importance to clinical medicine. Both the activity of psychoactive drugs and the pathological processes of most psychiatric disorders seem to involve alterations in one or more of the modulatory systems.

The brain has several modulatory systems with diffuse central connections. Although they differ in structure and function, they have certain similarities:

1. Typically, a small set of neurons (several thousand) forms the center of the system.
2. Neurons of the diffuse systems arise from the central core of the brain, most of them from the brainstem.
3. Each neuron can influence many others because each one has an axon that may contact more than 100,000 postsynaptic neurons spread widely across the brain.
4. The synapses made by some of these systems seem designed to release transmitter molecules into the extracellular fluid so that they can diffuse to many neurons rather than be confined to the vicinity of a single synaptic cleft.

The main modulatory systems of the brain are distinct anatomically and biochemically. Separate systems use norepinephrine, serotonin (5-hydroxytryptamine [5-HT]), dopamine, ACh, or histamine as their neurotransmitter.

They all tend to involve numerous **metabotropic transmitter receptors**. Unlike ionotropic receptors, which are themselves channels, metabotropic receptors are coupled to enzymes such as adenylyl cyclase or phospholipase C through G proteins (see Chapter 8). For example, the brain has 10 to 100 times more metabotropic (i.e., muscarinic) ACh receptors than ionotropic (i.e., nicotinic) ACh receptors. We briefly describe the anatomy and possible functions of each major system (Fig. 13-7).

Norepinephrine is used by neurons of the tiny **locus coeruleus** (from the Latin for "blue spot" because of the pigment in its cells), located bilaterally in the brainstem (Fig. 13-7A). Each human locus coeruleus has ~12,000 neurons. Axons from the locus coeruleus innervate just about every part of the brain: the entire cerebral cortex, the thalamus and hypothalamus, the olfactory bulb, the cerebellum, the midbrain, and the spinal cord. Just one of its neurons can make more than 250,000 synapses, and that cell can have one axon branch in the *cerebral* cortex and another in the *cerebellar* cortex! Locus coeruleus cells seem to be involved in the regulation of attention, arousal, and sleep-wake cycles as well as in learning and memory, anxiety and pain, mood, and brain metabolism. Recordings from awake rats and monkeys in behavioral studies show that locus coeruleus neurons are best activated by new, unexpected, nonpainful sensory stimuli in the animal's environment. They are least active when the animals are not vigilant, just sitting around quietly digesting a meal. The locus coeruleus may participate in general arousal of the brain during interesting events in the outside world.

Serotonin-containing neurons are mostly clustered within the nine **raphe nuclei** (Fig. 13-7B). Raphe means "ridge" or "seam" in Greek, and indeed the raphe nuclei lie to either side of the midline of the brainstem. Each nucleus

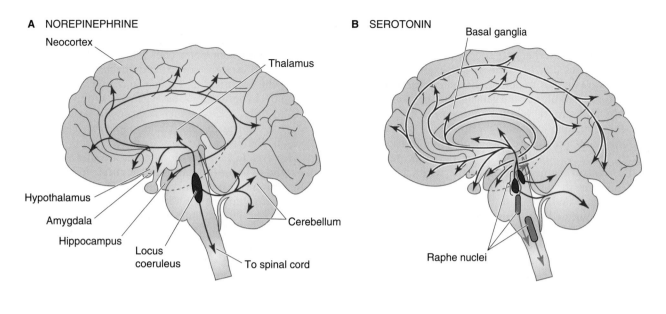

Figure 13-7 Four diffusely connected systems of central neurons using modulatory transmitters. **A,** Neurons containing norepinephrine are located in the locus coeruleus and innervate nearly every part of the CNS. **B,** Neurons containing serotonin are located in two groups of raphe nuclei and project to most of the brain. **C,** Neurons containing dopamine are located in the substantia nigra (and these project to the striatum) and the ventral tegmental area of the midbrain (and these project to the prefrontal cortex and parts of the limbic system). **D,** Neurons containing ACh are located in the basal forebrain complex, which includes the septal nuclei and nucleus basalis; the neurons project to the hippocampus and the neocortex. Other ACh-containing neurons originate in the pontomesencephalotegmental cholinergic complex and project to the dorsal thalamus and part of the forebrain.

projects to different regions of the brain, and together they innervate most of the CNS in the same diffuse way as the locus coeruleus neurons. Similar to neurons of the locus coeruleus, cells of the raphe nuclei fire most rapidly during wakefulness, when an animal is aroused and active. Raphe neurons are quietest during certain stages of sleep. The locus coeruleus and the raphe nuclei are part of a venerable concept called the **ascending reticular activating system**, which implicates the reticular "core" of the brainstem in processes that arouse and awaken the forebrain. Raphe neurons seem

to be intimately involved in the control of sleep-wake cycles as well as the different stages of sleep. Serotonergic raphe neurons have also been implicated in the control of mood and certain types of emotional behavior. Many hallucinogenic drugs, such as LSD, apparently exert their effects through interaction with serotonergic systems. Serotonin may also be involved in clinical depression; some of the most effective drugs now used to treat depression (e.g., fluoxetine [Prozac]) are potent blockers of serotonin re-uptake and thus prolong its action in the brain.

Although **dopamine**-containing neurons are scattered throughout the CNS, two closely related groups of dopaminergic cells have characteristics of the diffuse modulatory systems (Fig. 13-7C). One of these groups is the **substantia nigra** in the midbrain. Its cells project axons to the striatum, a part of the basal ganglia, and they somehow facilitate the initiation of voluntary movement. Degeneration of the dopamine-containing cells in the substantia nigra produces the progressively worsening motor disorders of Parkinson disease. Another set of dopaminergic neurons lies in the **ventral tegmental area** of the midbrain; these neurons innervate the part of the forebrain that includes the prefrontal cortex and parts of the limbic system. They have been implicated in neural systems that mediate reinforcement or reward as well as in aspects of drug addiction and psychiatric disorders, most notably schizophrenia. Members of the class of antipsychotic drugs called neuroleptics are antagonists of certain dopamine receptors.

Acetylcholine is the familiar transmitter of the neuromuscular junction and the autonomic nervous system. Within the brain are two major diffuse modulatory cholinergic systems: the **basal forebrain complex** (which innervates the hippocampus and all of the neocortex) and the **pontomesencephalotegmental cholinergic complex** (which innervates the dorsal thalamus and parts of the forebrain) (Fig. 13-7D). The functions of these systems are poorly understood, but interest has been fueled by evidence that they are involved in the regulation of general brain excitability during arousal and sleep-wake cycles as well as perhaps in learning and memory formation.

Collectively, the diffuse modulatory systems may be viewed as general regulators of brain function, much like the autonomic nervous system (see Chapter 14) regulates the organ systems of the body. Because their axons spread so widely within the CNS, the few modulatory neurons can have an inordinately strong influence on behavior.

Electrical synapses serve specialized functions in the mammalian nervous system

Many cells are coupled to one another through gap junctions. The large and relatively unselective gap junction channels (see Chapter 6) allow ion currents to flow in both directions (in most types of gap junctions) or unidirectionally (in rare types). It follows from Ohm's law that if two cells are coupled by gap junctions and they have different membrane voltages, current will flow from one cell into the other (see Fig. 6-18C). If the first cell generates an action potential, current will flow through the gap junction channels and depolarize the second cell; this type of current flow, for example, is the basis for conduction of excitation across cardiac muscle. Such an arrangement has all the earmarks of a synapse, and indeed, when gap junctions interconnect neurons, we describe them as electrical synapses.

Electrical synapses would seem to have many advantages over chemical synapses: they are extremely fast and limited only by the time constants of the systems involved, they use relatively little metabolic energy or molecular machinery,

they are highly reliable, and they can be bidirectional. Indeed, electrical synapses have now been observed in nearly every part of the mammalian CNS. They interconnect inhibitory neurons of the cerebral cortex and thalamus, excitatory neurons of the brainstem and retina, and a variety of other neurons in the hypothalamus, basal ganglia, and spinal cord. At all of these sites, Cx36—which is expressed exclusively in CNS neurons—forms the electrical synapse (see Fig. 6-18). Glial cells in the brain express several other types of connexins. However, in all of the aforementioned sites, electrical synapses tend to be outnumbered by chemical synapses. Gap junctions universally interconnect the photoreceptors of the retina, the astrocytic glia (see Chapter 11) of all parts of the CNS, and most cells early in development.

Why are chemical synapses, as complex and relatively slow as they are, more prevalent than electrical synapses in the mature brain? Comparative studies suggest several reasons for the predominance of chemical synapses among mammalian neurons. The first is **amplification**. Electrical synapses do not amplify the signal passed from one cell to the next; they can only diminish it. Therefore, if a presynaptic cell is small relative to its coupled postsynaptic cell, the current that it can generate through an electrical synapse will also be small, and thus "synaptic strength" will be low. By contrast, a small bolus of neurotransmitter from a chemical synapse can trigger an amplifying cascade of molecular events that can cause a relatively large postsynaptic change.

A second advantage of chemical synapses is their ability to generate inhibition. **Inhibition** is difficult (although not impossible in specialized cases) to achieve in electrical synapses. Chemical synapses perform this function with ease, by simply opening channels that are selective for ions with relatively negative equilibrium potential.

A third advantage of chemical synapses is that they can transmit information over a **broad time domain**. By using different transmitters, receptors, second messengers, and effectors, chemical synapses can produce a wide array of postsynaptic effects with time courses ranging from a few milliseconds to minutes and even hours. The effects of electrical synapses are generally limited to the time course of the presynaptic event.

A fourth advantage of chemical synapses is that they are champions of **plasticity**; their strength can be a strong function of recent neural activity, and they can therefore play a role in learning and memory, which are essential to the success of vertebrate species. Electrical synapses may also be plastic, but this has not been well studied yet.

It might also be noted that the few perceived advantages of electrical synapses may be more apparent than real. Bidirectionality is clearly not useful in many neural circuits, and the difference in speed of transmission may be too small to matter in most cases. Electrical synapses serve important but specialized functions in the nervous system. They seem to be most prevalent in neural circuits in which speed or high degrees of synchrony are at a premium: quick-escape systems, the fine coordination of rapid eye movements, or the synchronization of neurons generating rhythmic activity. Gap junctions are also effective in diffusely spreading current through large networks of cells, which appears to be their function in photoreceptors and glia.

NEUROTRANSMITTER SYSTEMS OF THE BRAIN

The mammalian nervous system uses dozens of different neurotransmitters that act on more than 100 types of receptors; these receptors stimulate numerous second-messenger systems, which in turn regulate several dozen ion channels and enzymes. We call these pathways of synaptic signaling the *transmitter systems*. It is not enough to know the identity of a transmitter to predict its effect—you also need to know the nature of the components that it interacts with, and these components may vary from one part of the brain to another and even between parts of a single neuron. The components of the transmitter systems are extremely complex. This sub-chapter introduces the intricate and vital web of neurotransmitters. The clinical importance of the subject is difficult to overstate. It is likely that most drugs that alter mental function do so by interacting with neurotransmitter systems in the brain. Disorders of neurotransmitter systems are also implicated in many devastating brain disorders, such as schizophrenia, depression, epilepsy, Parkinson disease, the damage of stroke, and drug addiction.

Most of the brain's transmitters are common biochemicals

Most neurotransmitters are similar or identical to the standard chemicals of life, the same substances that all cells use for metabolism. Transmitter molecules can be large or small. The small ones, such as the **amino acids** glutamate, aspartate, GABA, and glycine, are also simple foods (Fig. 13-8A). Cells use amino acids as an energy source and to build essential proteins, but they have co-opted these common molecules for essential and widespread messenger functions in the brain. Another important class of small neurotransmitters is the amines, including the **monoamines** (e.g., ACh, serotonin, and histamine) listed in Figure 13-8B and the **catecholamines** (e.g., dopamine, norepinephrine, and epinephrine) listed in Figure 13-8C. Neurons synthesize these small transmitters by adding only a few chemical steps to the glucose and amino acid pathways that are present in every cell. **Purine derivatives** can also be important transmitters. For example, a key molecule of cell metabolism that has recently achieved neurotransmitter status is adenosine triphosphate (ATP), which is the major chemical intermediate of energy metabolism and is present in many synaptic vesicles. It is also released from various synapses in the central and peripheral nervous systems. ATP appears to be the transmitter responsible for sympathetic vasoconstriction in small arteries and arterioles, for example. ATP acts on a variety of nucleotide receptors, both ionotropic and metabotropic. Adenosine is also a transmitter in the CNS.

The large-molecule transmitters, which constitute a much more numerous group, are proteins or small bits of protein called **neuroactive peptides**. A few of the better studied neuropeptides are shown in Figure 13-9. Many were originally identified in non-neural tissues, such as the gut or endocrine glands, and were only later found in nerve terminals of the brain or peripheral nervous system. They vary in size from two–amino acid peptides to large polypeptides. Among the

neuroactive peptides are the endorphins (*endo*genous substances with m*orphine*-like actions), which include small peptides called enkephalins. The term *opioids* includes all substances with a morphine-like pharmacology—the endorphins (endogenous) as well as morphine and heroin (exogenous).

The synthesis of most neuropeptides begins like that of any other secretory protein (see Chapter 2), with the ribosome-directed assembly of a large **prehormone**. The prehormone is then cleaved to form a smaller **prohormone** in the Golgi apparatus and further reduced into small active neuropeptides that are packaged into vesicles. Thus, the synthesis of neuropeptides differs significantly from that of the small transmitters.

In summary, then, the neurotransmitters consist of a dozen or so small molecules plus 50 to 100 peptides of various size. The small transmitters are, as a rule, each stored and released by separate sets of neurons. The peptides, however, are usually stored and released from the same neurons as one of the small transmitters (Table 13-1), an arrangement called **co-localization** of neurotransmitters. Thus, GABA may be paired with somatostatin in some synapses, serotonin and enkephalin in others, and so on. The co-localized transmitters may be released together, but of course each acts on its own receptors.

One of the unique substances proposed as a transmitter is a gaseous molecule, the labile free radical **nitric oxide (NO)**. **Carbon monoxide** has also been suggested to be a transmitter, although evidence thus far is meager. NO is synthesized from L-arginine by many cells of the body (see Chapter 3), and it has powerful biological effects. As a neurotransmitter, NO may have unique functions. It seems to be released from both presynaptic and what we normally think of as *post*synaptic neurons. Because NO is *not* packaged into vesicles, its release does not require an increase in $[Ca^{2+}]_i$, although its synthesis does. NO may sometimes act as a retrograde messenger, that is, from postsynaptic to presynaptic structures. Because NO is small and membrane permeable, it can diffuse about much more freely than other transmitter molecules, even penetrating through one cell to affect another beyond it. On the other hand, NO is evanescent, and it breaks down rapidly. The functions of gaseous transmitters are now being vigorously studied and hotly debated.

The **endocannabinoids** are another unusual group of putative neurotransmitters. They include the endogenous lipophilic molecules anandamide (from *ananda*, the Sanskrit word for "internal bliss") and arachidonyl glycerol (2-AG). These substances are called endocannabinoids because they mimic Δ^9-tetrahydrocannabinol (THC), the active ingredient in marijuana, by binding to and activating specific G protein–coupled "cannabinoid" receptors. Remarkably, the brain has more cannabinoid receptors than any other GPCR type. Certain activated neurons synthesize and release endocannabinoids, which diffuse readily to presynaptic terminals, and modulate the further release of conventional transmitters such as GABA and glutamate. Their normal role in the brain is currently unknown. However, activation of cannabinoid receptors with low doses of THC leads to euphoria, relaxed sensations, decreased pain, and increased hunger; it can also impair problem-solving ability, short-term memory,

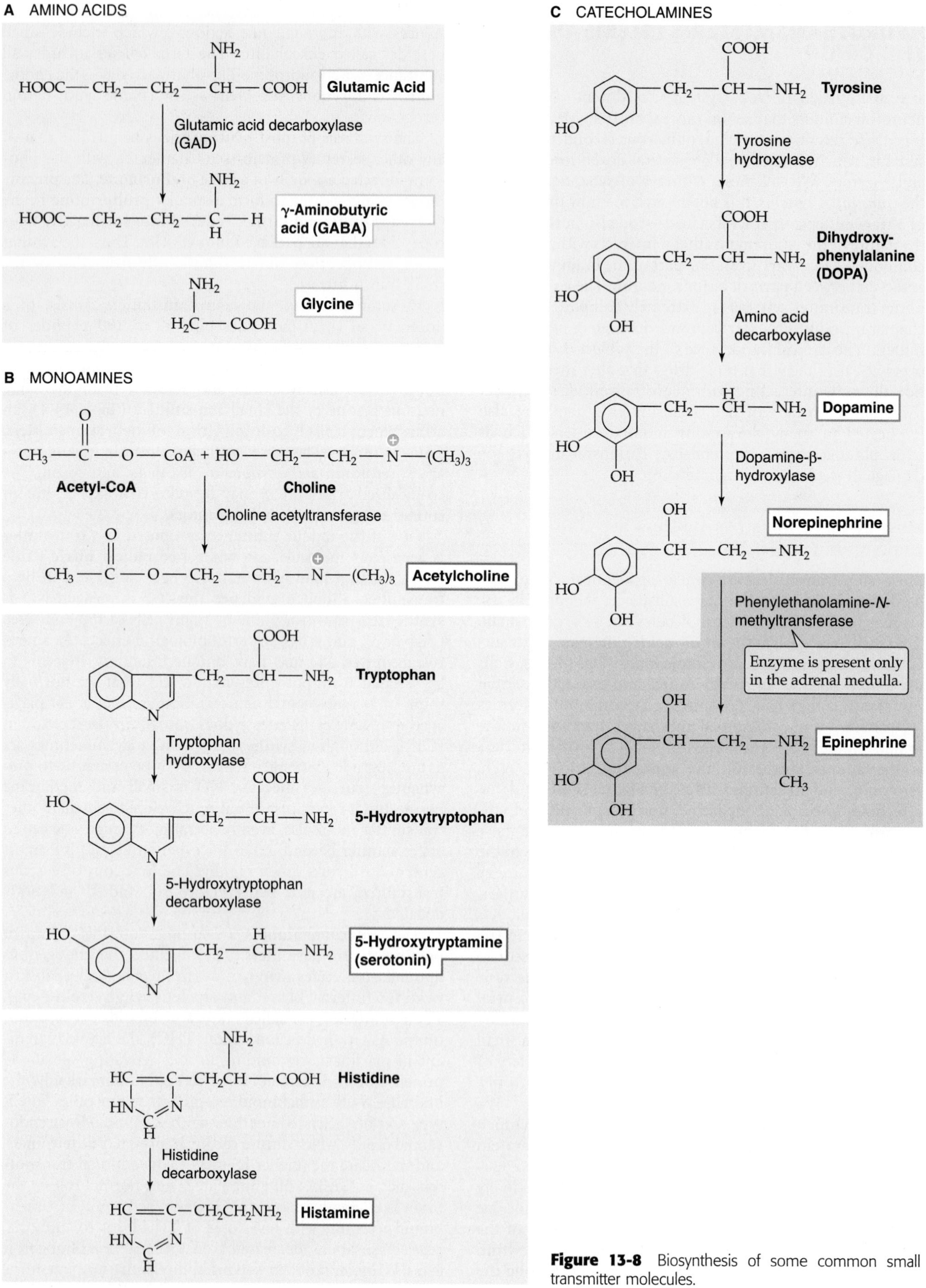

A AMINO ACIDS

B MONOAMINES

C CATECHOLAMINES

Figure 13-8 Biosynthesis of some common small transmitter molecules.

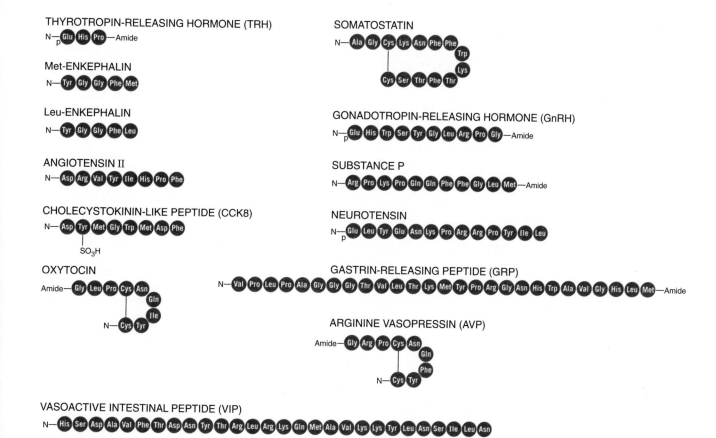

Figure 13-9 Structure of some neuroactive peptides. All peptides are presented with their NH$_2$ termini (i.e., the first to be synthesized) to the left, as is now customary for proteins in general. However, note that for many of the peptide hormones, the amino acid residues were numbered before this convention was established. The *p* on the amino-terminal glutamate on some of these peptides stands for pyroglutamate.

and motor skills. High doses can alter personality and sometimes trigger hallucinations. THC and related drugs have shown some promise for treatment of the nausea and vomiting of cancer patients undergoing chemotherapy, suppression of chronic pain, and stimulation of appetite in some AIDS patients.

Most of the chemicals we call neurotransmitters also exist in non-neural parts of the body. Each chemical may serve dual purposes in that it can mediate communication in the nervous system but do something similar or even entirely different elsewhere. Amino acids, of course, are used to make protein everywhere. NO is a local hormone that relaxes the smooth muscle in blood vessels (see Chapter 20). Surprisingly, the cells with the highest ACh levels are in the cornea of the eye, although corneal cells lack specific receptors for ACh. It is not clear what ACh does for corneal cells, but it almost certainly is not acting as a transmitter. One of the most interesting nonmessenger functions of transmitter molecules is their role in the development of the brain, even

before synapses have appeared. At these early stages of development, transmitters may regulate cell proliferation, migration, and differentiation, somehow helping to form the brain before they help operate it.

Synaptic transmitters can stimulate, inhibit, or modulate the postsynaptic neuron

Each neuromuscular junction has a simple and stereotyped job: when an action potential fires in the motor neuron, the junction must reliably excite its muscle cell to fire an action potential and contract. Decisions about muscle contractions (where, when, and how much) are made within the CNS, and the neuromuscular junction exists simply to communicate that decision to the muscle unambiguously. To perform this function, neuromuscular transmission has evolved to be very strong so that it is fail-safe under even the most extreme of physiological conditions.

TABLE 13-1 Examples of Neuroactive Peptides That Co-localize with Small-Molecule Neurotransmitters

Small Molecule	Peptide*
Acetylcholine	Enkephalin Vasoactive intestinal polypeptide Calcitonin gene–related peptide Substance P Somatostatin and enkephalin Gonadotropin-releasing hormone Neurotensin Galanin
Dopamine	Cholecystokinin Enkephalin Neurotensin
Epinephrine	Enkephalin Neuropeptide Y Neurotensin Substance P
GABA	Cholecystokinin Enkephalin Somatostatin Neuropeptide Y Substance P Vasoactive intestinal polypeptide
Glutamate	Substance P
Glycine	Neurotensin
Norepinephrine	Enkephalin Neuropeptide Y Neurotensin Somatostatin Vasopressin
Serotonin	Cholecystokinin Enkephalin Substance P and thyrotropin-releasing hormone Thyrotropin-releasing hormone

*Each row gives a peptide or combination of peptides that co-localize with the small molecule on the left.

Data from Hall ZW: An Introduction to Molecular Neurobiology. Sunderland, MA: Sinauer, 1992.

Synapses between neurons usually have a more subtle role in communication, and they use a variety of mechanisms to accomplish their more complex tasks. Like neuromuscular junctions, some neuron-neuron synapses (**excitatory**) can rapidly excite. However, other synapses (**inhibitory**) can cause profound inhibition by decreasing postsynaptic excitability directly (postsynaptic inhibition). In a third broad class of synapse (**modulatory**), the synapse often has little or no direct effect of its own but instead regulates or modifies the effect of other excitatory or inhibitory synapses by acting on either presynaptic or postsynaptic membranes. These three basic types of neural synapses are exemplified by their

input to the *pyramidal neuron* of the cerebral cortex. In the example shown in Figure 13-10, a pyramidal neuron in the visual cortex receives an excitatory synaptic input from the thalamus (with use of glutamate as the neurotransmitter), an inhibitory synaptic input from an interneuron (with use of GABA as the neurotransmitter), and a modulatory input from the locus coeruleus (with use of norepinephrine as the neurotransmitter).

Excitatory Synapses Pyramidal cells receive excitatory synapses from many sources, including the axons of the thalamus. Most fast *excitatory synapses* in the brain use **glutamate** or **aspartate** as their transmitter, and the thalamus-to-cortex synapses are no exception (Fig. 13-10). Both amino acids have similar effects on the postsynaptic excitatory amino acid receptors, and it has proved difficult to determine which excitatory amino acid is used in which synapse. For convenience, these types of synapses are often presumptuously referred to as **glutamatergic**. These excitatory amino acids bind to a group of fast, ligand-gated cation channels. When they are activated by synaptic glutamate, glutamate-gated channels generate an **excitatory postsynaptic potential** (EPSP) that is very similar to the one produced by ACh at the neuromuscular junction (see Chapter 8), except that it is much smaller than the EPSP in muscle. In the example shown in Figure 13-11 (left side), glutamate produces the EPSP by activating a nonselective cation channel that has about the same conductance for Na^+ and K^+. Thus, the **reversal potential** (see Chapter 6) of the EPSP is 0 mV, about midway between the equilibrium potential for Na^+ (E_{Na}) and that for K^+ (E_K). An EPSP from the activation of a *single* glutamatergic synapse peaks at 0.01 to a few millivolts (depending on many factors, including the size of the postsynaptic cell and the size of the synapse), whereas one neuromuscular EPSP reaches a peak of ~40 mV—a difference of 40- to 4000-fold. Obviously, most glutamatergic synapses are not designed to be fail-safe. It takes the summation of EPSPs from many such synapses to depolarize a postsynaptic neuron to the threshold for triggering of an action potential.

Inhibitory Synapses Skeletal muscle cells in vertebrates have only excitatory synapses. On the other hand, virtually all central neurons have numerous excitatory *and inhibitory* synapses. Thus, the excitability of most neurons is governed by the dynamic balance of excitation and inhibition at any moment. The inhibitory transmitters **GABA** and **glycine** are the transmitters at the large majority of inhibitory synapses. Indeed, the inhibitory synapse between the interneuron and the pyramidal cell in Figure 13-10 uses GABA. Both GABA and glycine bind to receptors that gate Cl^--selective channels (see Chapter 8). Cl^- conductance usually has an inhibitory influence because the equilibrium potential for Cl^- (E_{Cl}) in neurons is near or slightly negative to the resting potential of the neuron. Thus, the reversal potential for the Cl^--mediated **inhibitory postsynaptic potential** (IPSP) is the same as the E_{Cl}. If Cl^- conductance increases, the membrane potential (V_m) has a tendency to move toward E_{Cl} (Fig. 13-11, right side). The effect is inhibitory because it tends to oppose other factors (mainly EPSPs) that might otherwise move the V_m to the threshold for an action potential.

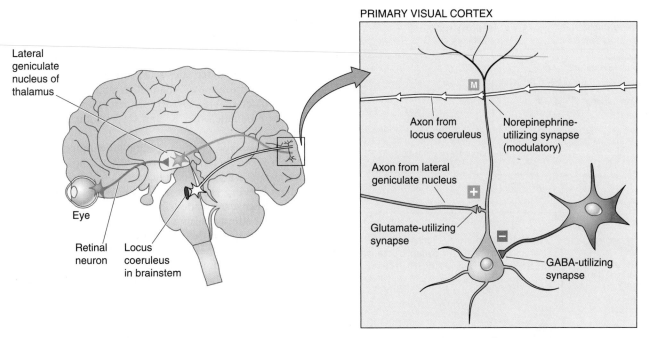

PRIMARY VISUAL CORTEX

Figure 13-10 Synaptic circuitry of the visual cortex. Visual pathways that originate in the retina activate neurons in the lateral geniculate nucleus of the thalamus. These glutamate-containing neurons in turn synapse on cortical pyramidal neurons and produce some *excitation*. Also within the primary visual cortex, a GABA-containing neuron mediates localized *inhibition*. Small cells in the locus coeruleus, a brainstem nucleus, make widely divergent connections onto cortical neurons and release norepinephrine and thus produce *modulation*.

Modulatory Synapses The nervous system is influenced by many forms of *synaptic modulation,* and their mechanisms are covered in more detail later. As an example, consider the axons arising from the *locus coeruleus,* which synapse widely on pyramidal cells in the cerebral cortex (Figs. 13-7A and 13-10). These axons release the transmitter **norepinephrine**, a classic modulator with multiple effects. Norepinephrine acts on β-adrenergic receptors in the pyramidal cell membrane (it may also act on α receptors at the same time). Unlike the actions of the fast amino acid forms of synaptic transmission, this effect of norepinephrine by itself has little or no obvious influence on the activity of a resting neuron. However, a cell exposed to norepinephrine will react more powerfully when it is stimulated by a strong excitatory input (usually by glutamatergic synapses), as shown in Figure 13-12. Thus, norepinephrine *modulates* the cell's response to other inputs.

The molecular mechanisms of **neuromodulators** are complex and diverse, but all begin with a GPCR that activates an intracellular signal cascade (see Chapter 3). Binding of norepinephrine to the β-adrenergic receptor stimulates the intracellular enzyme adenylyl cyclase, which increases intracellular levels of cyclic adenosine monophosphate (cAMP, the second messenger), which in turn stimulates other enzymes to increase their rates of phosphorylation. Within the cortical neuron, phosphorylation of one or more types of K$^+$ channel decreases the probability of the channels being open (see Chapter 6). Fewer open K$^+$ channels mean higher membrane resistance, greater excitability, and less adaptation of spike firing rates during prolonged stimuli. This K$^+$ channel pathway is but one of the many mechanisms by which norepinephrine can affect cells. Other effects are generated when norepinephrine activates other subtypes of adrenergic receptors and thus different second-messenger systems coupled to different channels or enzymes. Modulatory transmitters allow the nervous system tremendous potential and flexibility to vary its state of excitability.

G proteins may affect ion channels directly or indirectly through second messengers

GPCRs exist in every cell (see Chapter 3). In the preceding section we described one example, the receptor for norepinephrine and its second messenger–mediated effect on certain K$^+$ channels. However, norepinephrine alone has at least five major receptor types—two α receptors and three β receptors—that act on numerous effectors. In fact, each transmitter has multiple GPCRs, and their effects are complex and interactive and engage almost all aspects of cell function through several intracellular messenger systems. The various GPCRs can recognize a wide range of transmitter types, from small molecules to peptides.

Activated G proteins can trigger a wide array of responses at synapses by either of the two general pathways introduced in Chapter 3: (1) the G protein may modulate the gating of an ion channel directly or by a very short second-messenger pathway, and (2) the G protein may activate one of several enzyme systems that involve second messengers and subsequent signal cascades.

The first—and simplest—G protein cascade involves a direct receptor–G protein–channel linkage and is sometimes called the **membrane-delimited pathway**. In this case, the G

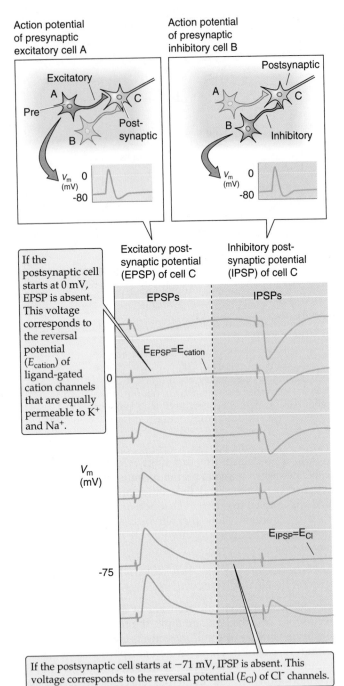

Action potential of presynaptic excitatory cell A

Action potential of presynaptic inhibitory cell B

Excitatory
A
C
Pre
Post-
synaptic
B

V_m 0
(mV)
-80

Postsynaptic
A
C
B
Inhibitory

V_m 0
(mV)
-80

If the postsynaptic cell starts at 0 mV, EPSP is absent. This voltage corresponds to the reversal potential (E_{cation}) of ligand-gated cation channels that are equally permeable to K^+ and Na^+.

Excitatory post-synaptic potential (EPSP) of cell C

Inhibitory post-synaptic potential (IPSP) of cell C

EPSPs

IPSPs

$E_{EPSP}=E_{cation}$

0

V_m
(mV)

$E_{IPSP}=E_{Cl}$

-75

If the postsynaptic cell starts at −71 mV, IPSP is absent. This voltage corresponds to the reversal potential (E_{Cl}) of Cl^- channels.

Figure 13-11 Voltage dependence of EPSPs and IPSPs of the nervous system. An excitatory presynaptic neuron (cell A) and an inhibitory presynaptic neuron (cell B) both synapse on a third neuron (cell C). In this experiment, the investigators injected enough constant current into cell C to initially set the V_m to each of the six values shown in the figure. For each record, the experimenter first stimulated the stimulatory presynaptic neuron to produce an EPSP in the postsynaptic neuron and then stimulated the inhibitory presynaptic neuron to produce an IPSP. These EPSPs and IPSPs reflect the activities of multiple synapses onto cell C. The reversal potential for the EPSP is ~0 mV (i.e., stimulating the stimulatory presynaptic neuron has no effect) because Na^+ and K^+ conduct through the channel equally well. The reversal potential for the IPSP is at about −71 mV (i.e., stimulating the inhibitory presynaptic neuron has no effect). This value is E_{Cl}, indicating that the IPSP is mediated by a Cl^- channel.

protein may be the only messenger between the receptor and the effector. A variety of neurotransmitter–G protein–channel systems use this pathway. For example, in heart muscle, ACh binds to a certain type of muscarinic ACh receptor (M_2) that activates a G protein, the βγ subunits of which in turn cause a K^+ channel to open. (We discuss this example later in Fig. 13-13B.) Other receptors in various cells can modulate other K^+ and Ca^{2+} channels in a similar way.

One advantage of the membrane-delimited pathway is that it is relatively fast, beginning within 30 to 100 ms—not quite as fast as a ligand-gated channel, which uses no intermediary between receptor and channel, but faster than the many-messenger cascades described next. The membrane-delimited pathway is also localized in comparison to the other cascades. Because the G protein cannot diffuse very far within the membrane, only channels nearby can be affected. This type of coupling also allows flexibility because many types of receptors can be coupled to a variety of channels by use of the appropriate G protein intermediate.

The other general type of G protein signaling involves enzyme systems and second messengers, often diffusing through the cytoplasm, to influence an ion channel. The terminology deserves some clarification. Traditionally, the small, diffusible intracellular chemicals (e.g., cAMP, inositol 1,4,5-trisphosphate [IP_3]) that help carry the message between a transmitter receptor and a channel are called *second messengers*. The transmitter itself is counted as the first messenger, but notice that by this logic the receptor is not a messenger at all, even though it transfers a signal from the neurotransmitter to a G protein. The G protein is also not counted as a messenger, nor are the various enzymes that may come before and after the traditional "second messenger" in any signal cascade. Different cascades involve different numbers of messengers, but obviously, most have many more than two! Alas, the terminology is entrenched, although when we speak of second messengers, one should remember that a multiple-messenger cascade is almost always involved. As an added complication, two or more cascades, each with different types of messengers, may sometimes be activated by one type of receptor (an example of *divergence*, see later).

In Chapter 3, we discussed three of these longer, and slower, G protein signal cascades: (1) the adenylyl cyclase pathway, (2) the phospholipase C pathway, and (3) the phospholipase A_2 pathway. Each is activated by a different set of receptors, each uses a different G protein, and each generates different intracellular messengers. Some of these messengers dissolve in the watery cytoplasm, whereas others diffuse within the fatty lipid bilayer. The final link in most of the messenger cascades is a **kinase**.

In a well-known example, cAMP binds to cAMP-dependent protein kinase (protein kinase A), which then phosphorylates amino acids on K^+ or Ca^{2+} channels in the membrane. The addition of phosphate groups to the channel protein changes its conformation slightly, which may strongly influence its probability of being open (see Chapter 6). In Chapter 21, we discuss the stimulation of the β-adrenergic receptor by norepinephrine, which ultimately results in a stronger heartbeat through phosphorylation and opening of myocardial voltage-gated Ca^{2+} channels. By contrast, in the

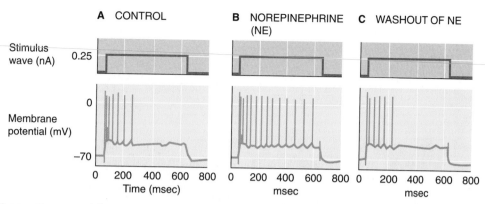

Figure 13-12 Modulatory effect of norepinephrine. **A,** Injecting a neuron from the hippocampus with a sustained depolarizing current pulse leads to a "phasic" action potential response: frequent spiking at the beginning but adaptation as the depolarizing current pulse is maintained. **B,** The application of norepinephrine causes the spiking that is elicited by the depolarizing current pulse to be sustained longer ("tonic"). **C,** The cell returns to its control state as in **A**. (*Data from Madison DV, Nicoll RA: Actions of noradrenaline recorded intracellularly in rat hippocampal CA1 pyramidal neurones, in vitro. J Physiol 1986; 372:221-244.*)

pyramidal cell of the hippocampus, stimulation of β-adrenergic receptors also results in an increase in cAMP, but it has no influence on the cell's Ca^{2+} channels. Instead, it inhibits some of its K^+ channels. As a result, the cell can fire more action potentials during prolonged stimuli (Fig. 13-12).

If transmitter-stimulated kinases were allowed to madly phosphorylate without some method of reversing the process, all proteins would quickly become saturated with phosphates and further regulation would become impossible. Protein phosphatases save the day. They act rapidly to remove phosphate groups (see Chapter 3), and thus the degree of channel phosphorylation at any moment depends on the dynamic balance of phosphorylation and dephosphorylation.

Signaling cascades allow amplification, regulation, and a long duration of transmitter responses

At this point you may be wondering about the perversity of such complex, interconnected, indirect messenger cascades. Do these long chains of command have any benefit? Why not use simple, fast ligand-gated channels (Fig. 13-13A) for all transmitter purposes? In fact, complex messenger cascades seem to have advantages.

One important advantage is *amplification*. When it is activated, one ligand-gated channel is just that: one ion channel in one place. However, activate one GPCR and you potentially influence many channels. Signal amplification can occur at several places in the cascade (see Chapter 3), and a few transmitter molecules can generate a sizable cellular effect. One stimulated receptor can activate perhaps 10 to 20 G proteins, each of which can activate a channel by a membrane-delimited pathway such as the βγ pathway (Fig. 13-13B). Alternatively, the α subunit of one G protein can activate an adenylyl cyclase, which can make many cAMP molecules, and the cAMP molecules can spread to activate

many kinases; each kinase can then phosphorylate many channels (Fig. 13-13C). If all cascade components were tied together in a clump, signaling would be severely limited. The use of small messengers that can diffuse quickly also allows signaling at a distance, over a wide stretch of cell membrane. Signaling cascades also provide many sites for further *regulation* as well as interaction between cascades. Finally, signal cascades can generate *long-lasting chemical changes* in cells, which may form the basis for, among other things, a lifetime of memories.

Neurotransmitters may have both convergent and divergent effects

Two of the most common neurotransmitters in the brain are glutamate and GABA. Either molecule can bind to any of several kinds of receptors, and each of these receptors can mediate a different effect. This ability of one transmitter to activate more than one type of receptor is sometimes called divergence.

Divergence is a rule among neurotransmitters. Every well-studied transmitter can activate multiple receptor subtypes, and recent experience indicates that the number of receptors will continue to escalate as the powerful methods of molecular biology continue to be applied to each system. Divergence means that one transmitter can affect different neurons (or even different parts of the same neuron) in very different ways. It also means that *if* a transmitter affects different neurons in different ways, it *could* be because each neuron has a different type of receptor. However, among transmitter systems that use second messengers, divergence may also occur at points beyond the level of the receptor. For example, norepinephrine can turn on or turn off a variety of ion channels in different cells (Fig. 13-14A). Some of these effects occur because norepinephrine activates different receptors, but some of these receptors may each activate more than one second messenger, *or* a single second

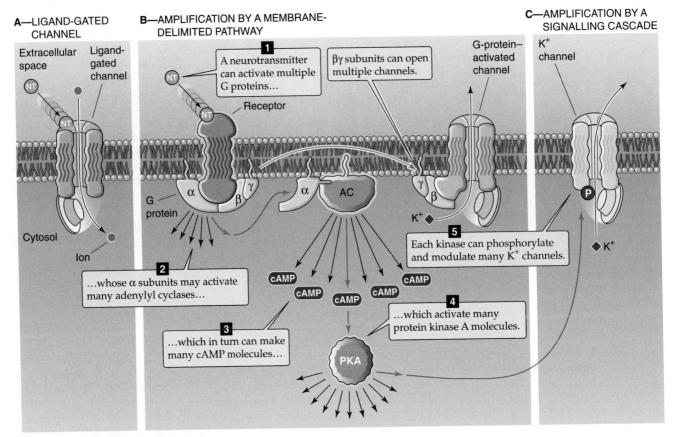

A—LIGAND-GATED CHANNEL

B—AMPLIFICATION BY A MEMBRANE-DELIMITED PATHWAY

C—AMPLIFICATION BY A SIGNALLING CASCADE

Figure 13-13 Amplification. **A,** The neurotransmitter (NT) binds directly to a channel, thereby activating it. **B,** The neurotransmitter binds to a receptor that in turn activates 10 to 20 G proteins. In this example, the βγ subunits directly activate K^+ channels. In addition, each activated α subunit activates an adenylyl cyclase molecule, each of which produces many cAMP molecules that activate protein kinase A (PKA). **C,** Each activated PKA can phosphorylate and thereby modulate many channels. AC, adenylyl cyclase.

messenger (e.g., cAMP) may activate a kinase that influences numerous different channels. Divergence may occur at any stage in the cascade of transmitter effects.

Neurotransmitters can also exhibit **convergence** of effects. This property means that multiple transmitters, each activating its own receptor type, converge on a single type of ion channel in a single cell. For example, some pyramidal cells of the hippocampus have $GABA_B$, $5\text{-}HT_{1A}$, A1 (specific for adenosine), and SS (specific for somatostatin) receptors, all of which activate the same K^+ channel (Fig. 13-14B). Furthermore, in the same cells, norepinephrine, ACh, 5-HT, corticotropin-releasing hormone, and histamine all converge on and depress the slow Ca^{2+}-activated K^+ channels. Analogous to divergence, the molecular site of convergence may occur at a common second-messenger system, or different second messengers may converge on the same ion channel.

Divergence and convergence can occur simultaneously within neurotransmitter systems. Many of them have chemical feedback regulation built in as well.

FAST, AMINO ACID–MEDIATED SYNAPSES IN THE CENTRAL NERVOUS SYSTEM

Fast, amino acid–mediated synapses account for most of the neural activity that we associate with specific information processing in the brain: events directly responsible for sensory perception, motor control, and cognition, for example. Glutamate-mediated excitation and GABA-mediated inhibition have been intensively studied. In physiological terms, these are also the best understood of the brain's synapses, and this section describes their function.

As a rule, postsynaptic events are more easily measured than are presynaptic events; thus, we know more about them. Of course, by measuring postsynaptic events, we also have a window onto the functions of the presynaptic terminal, and in fact this is usually the best view we can get of presynaptic functions. For this reason, we begin our description with the downstream, postsynaptic side of the synapse and then work backward to the presynaptic side.

A DIVERGENT TRANSMITTER ACTIONS

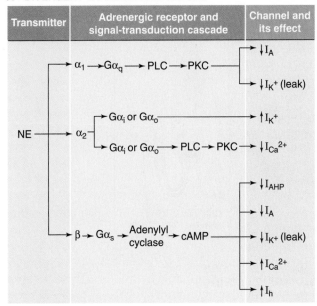

B CONVERGENT TRANSMITTER ACTIONS

Figure 13-14 Divergence and convergence of transmitter effects on channels. **A,** One transmitter, norepinephrine in this case, can activate multiple receptors, which stimulate different G protein/ second messengers, which in turn either stimulate or depress the gating of many types of ion channels. I_{AHP} stands for afterhyperpolarization current, which is mediated by a Ca^{2+}-activated K^+ channel. I_h stands for hyperpolarization-activated cation current. **B,** Multiple transmitters bind to their specific receptors and, by the same or different second-messenger systems, influence the same set of ion channels. ACh, acetylcholine; DA, dopamine; Enk, enkephalin; 5-HT, 5-hydroxytryptamine (serotonin); NE, norepinephrine; SS, somatostatin; SSTR, somatostatin receptor.

Most excitatory postsynaptic potentials in the brain are mediated by two types of glutamate-gated channels

Most glutamate-mediated synapses generate an EPSP with two distinct components, one much faster than the other. Both are triggered by the same presynaptic terminal releasing a single bolus of transmitter, but the two EPSP components are generated by different types of ion channels that are gated by distinct postsynaptic receptors—a case of trans-

mitter divergence. The behavior of these channels helps understand the characteristics of the EPSP.

Glutamate can act on four major classes of receptors: one is a GPCR or *metabotropic* receptor, and three of them are ion channels or *ionotropic* receptors. As noted earlier, **metabotropic receptors** (mGluRs—the *m* stands for metabotropic) have seven membrane-spanning segments and are linked to heterotrimeric G proteins (Fig. 13-15A). At least eight metabotropic receptors have been identified, and comparisons of their primary structure have been used to infer the evolutionary relationships among receptor subunits (Fig. 13-15B). The mGluRs form three groups that differ in their sequence similarity, pharmacology, and associated signal transduction systems.

The three classes of **ionotropic glutamate receptors** are the AMPA, NMDA, and kainate receptors (Table 13-2). By definition, each is activated by binding glutamate, but their pharmacology differs. The receptor names are derived from their relatively specific agonists: **AMPA** stands for α-amino-3-hydroxy-5-methyl-4-isoxazole propionic acid. The AMPA receptor is sometimes called the quisqualate receptor, after another of its agonists, or even the quisqualate/AMPA receptor. NMDA stands for *N*-methyl-D-aspartate. The **kainate** receptor is named for one of its agonists, kainic acid, and it can also be activated by domoic acid. The three ionotropic glutamate receptors can also be distinguished by their selective antagonists. *AMPA* and kainate receptors, but not NMDA receptors, are blocked by drugs such as **CNQX** (6-cyano-7-nitroquinoxaline-2,3-dione). Moreover, AMPA receptors can be specifically antagonized by 2,3-benzodiazepine derivatives, such as GYKI53655. *NMDA* receptors, but not AMPA and kainate receptors, are blocked by **APV** (2-amino-5-phosphonovaleric acid). Selective antagonists of kainate receptors have also been discovered.

At least 22 ionotropic glutamate receptor cDNAs—plus a variety of splice variants—have been cloned. Each of these cDNAs represents a monomer (see Fig 6-21M on p. 177) with a large extracellular region, followed by a transmembrane segment, a loop that partially enters the membrane from the cytosolic side, and then two more transmembrane segments (Fig. 13-15C). The loop appears to line the channel pore. On the basis of kinetic and structural studies, the channel appears to consist of a tetramer of four subunits. Comparisons of primary structures can be used to infer evolutionary relationships among receptor monomeric subunits. Figure 13-15D shows a hypothesized phylogenetic tree for the three classes of ionotropic glutamate receptors, with the major subtypes clustered together. Note that the various NMDA receptor subunits (e.g., NMDAR1, NMDAR2A to NMDAR2D) that combine to make the NMDA receptors are more closely related to each other than to the subunits (e.g., KA1, KA2, GluR5 to GluR7) that combine to make the kainate receptors or to the subunits (e.g., GluR1 to GluR4) that combine to make the AMPA receptors. The *metabotropic* and *ionotropic* glutamate receptors have separate family trees because, although both receptor types bind glutamate, they are so different in structure that it is highly probable they evolved from different ancestral protein lines.

As noted earlier, most glutamate-mediated synapses generate an EPSP with two temporal components (Fig. 13-16A, C). The two phases of the glutamate-mediated EPSP have

A METABOTROPIC GLUTAMATE RECEPTORS

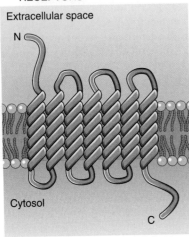

C IONOTROPIC GLUTAMATE RECEPTORS

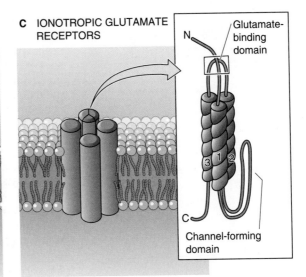

B FAMILY TREE OF METABOTROPIC GLUTAMATE RECEPTORS

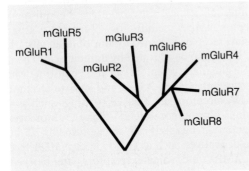

D FAMILY TREE OF IONOTROPIC GLUTAMATE RECEPTORS

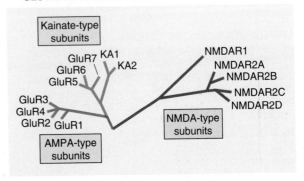

Figure 13-15 Comparison of ionotropic and metabotropic glutamate receptors. In **C,** the *inset* shows a prototypical subunit, with a large extracellular N-terminal region, a membrane-spanning segment, a short loop that partially re-enters the membrane from the cytosolic side, and two more membrane-spanning segments. The glutamate-binding domain consists of parts of both the N-terminal region and the loop connecting membrane-spanning segments 2 and 3. Four of these subunits appear to come together to form a single channel/receptor with a central pore. *AMPA,* α-amino-3-hydroxy-5-methyl-4-isoxazole propionic acid; *NMDA,* N-methyl-D-aspartate.

TABLE 13-2 Ionotropic Glutamate Receptors

Class of Receptor	Agonist	Antagonist	Kinetics	Permeability
AMPA	α-Amino-3-hydroxy-5-methyl-4-isoxazole propionic acid	CNQX (6-cyano-7-nitroquinoxaline-2,3-dione) GYKI53655 (2,3-benzodiazepine derivatives)	Fast	Na$^+$, K$^+$ (Ca^{2+} in a few cases)
NMDA	N-Methyl-D-aspartate	APV (2-amino-5-phosphonovaleric acid)	Slow	Na$^+$, K$^+$, Ca^{2+}
Kainate	Kainic acid Domoic acid	CNQX UBP296 ((*RS*)-1-(2-amino-2-carboxyethyl)-3-(2-carboxybenzyl) pyrimidine-2,4-dione)	Fast	Na$^+$, K$^+$

A EPSP AT –80 mV

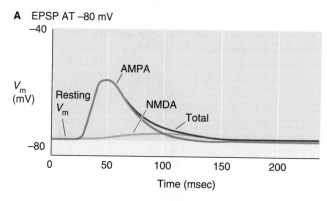

C EPSP AT –40 mV

B ONLY AMPA RECEPTOR CHANNEL OPEN

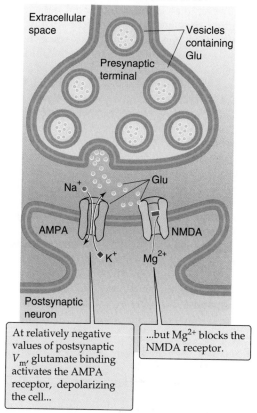

At relatively negative values of postsynaptic V_m, glutamate binding activates the AMPA receptor, depolarizing the cell...

...but Mg^{2+} blocks the NMDA receptor.

D AMPA AND NMDA RECEPTOR CHANNELS OPEN

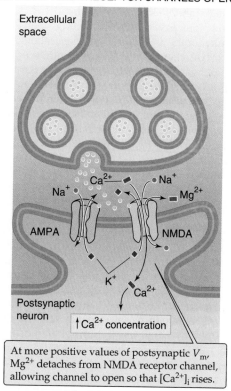

↑Ca^{2+} concentration

At more positive values of postsynaptic V_m, Mg^{2+} detaches from NMDA receptor channel, allowing channel to open so that $[Ca^{2+}]_i$ rises.

Figure 13-16 Glutamate-gated channels. **A,** At most glutamate-mediated synapses, the EPSP *(red curve)* is the sum of two components: (1) a rapid component that is mediated by an AMPA receptor channel *(green curve)* and (2) a slow component that is mediated by an NMDA receptor channel *(orange curve)*. In this example, in which the postsynaptic V_m is relatively negative, the contribution of the NMDA receptor channel is very small. **B,** At a relatively negative initial V_m in the postsynaptic cell, as in **A,** the NMDA receptor channel does not open. The AMPA receptor channel, which is independent of postsynaptic V_m, opens. The result is a fast depolarization. **C,** In this example, in which the postsynaptic V_m is relatively positive, the contribution of the NMDA receptor channel is fairly large. **D,** At a relatively positive initial V_m in the postsynaptic cell, as in **C,** glutamate activates both the AMPA and the NMDA receptor channels. The recruitment of the NMDA receptor channels is important because unlike most AMPA receptor channels, they allow the entry of Ca^{2+} and have slower kinetics.

different pharmacological profiles, kinetics, voltage dependencies, ion dependencies, and permeabilities, and most important, they serve distinct functions in the brain. Pharmacological analysis reveals that the faster phase is mediated by an AMPA-type glutamate receptor and the slower phase by an NMDA-type glutamate receptor. These glutamate-gated channels have been extensively studied with single-channel recording methods. Both AMPA and NMDA receptors have nearly equal permeability to Na^+ and K^+, but they differ in several ways.

AMPA-gated channels are found in most excitatory synapses in the brain, and they mediate fast excitation, with most receptor channels normally letting very little Ca^{2+} into cells. Their single-channel conductance is relatively low, ~15 pS, and they show little voltage dependence.

NMDA-gated channels have more complex behavior. They have higher conductance, ~50 pS, and much slower kinetics. The ion selectivity of NMDA channels is the key to their functions: permeability to Na^+ and K^+ causes depolarization and thus excitation of a cell, but their high permeability to Ca^{2+} allows them to influence $[Ca^{2+}]_i$ significantly. It is difficult to overstate the importance of intracellular $[Ca^{2+}]$. Ca^{2+} can activate many enzymes, regulate the opening of a variety of channels, and affect the expression of genes. Excess Ca^{2+} can even precipitate the death of a cell.

The gating of NMDA channels is unusual: at normal resting voltage (about −70 mV), the channel is clogged by Mg^{2+}, and few ions pass through it; the Mg^{2+} pops out only when the membrane is depolarized above about −60 mV. Thus, the NMDA channel is **voltage dependent** in addition to being ligand gated; both glutamate and a relatively positive V_m are necessary for the channel to open. How do the NMDA-gated channels open? NMDA-gated channels coexist with AMPA-gated channels in many synapses of the brain. When the postsynaptic cell is at a relatively negative resting potential (Fig. 13-16A, B), the glutamate released from a synaptic terminal can open the AMPA-gated channel, which is voltage independent, but not the NMDA-gated channel. However, when the postsynaptic cell is more depolarized because of the action of other synapses (Fig. 13-16C, D), the larger depolarization of the postsynaptic membrane now allows the NMDA-gated channel to open by relieving its Mg^{2+} block. Indeed, under natural conditions, the slower NMDA channels open only after the membrane has been sufficiently depolarized by the action of the faster AMPA channels from many simultaneously active synapses.

The physiological function of **kainate-gated channels** is still a mystery, although recent evidence suggests that they may contribute in a small way to some glutamate-mediated EPSPs. The kainate receptor channels also exist on *presynaptic* GABAergic terminals, where they regulate release of the inhibitory transmitter (i.e., GABA).

Most inhibitory postsynaptic potentials in the brain are mediated by the GABA_A receptor, which is activated by several classes of drugs

GABA mediates the large majority of synaptic inhibition in the CNS, and glycine mediates most of the rest. Both the GABA_A receptor and the glycine receptor are ionotropic receptors that are, in fact, Cl^--selective channels. Note that GABA can also activate the relatively common GABA_B receptor, which is a GPCR or *metabotropic* receptor that is linked to either the opening of K^+ channels or the suppression of Ca^{2+} channels. Finally, GABA can activate the ionotropic GABA_C receptor, which is rare in the brain.

Synaptic inhibition must be tightly regulated in the brain. Too much inhibition causes loss of consciousness and coma, whereas too little leads to a seizure. The need to control inhibition may explain why the GABA_A receptor channel has, in addition to its GABA binding site, several other sites where chemicals can bind and thus dramatically modulate the function of the GABA_A receptor channel. For example, two

classes of drugs, **benzodiazepines** (one of which is the tranquilizer diazepam [Valium]) and **barbiturates** (e.g., the sedative phenobarbital), each binds to its own specific site on the outside face of the GABA_A receptor channel. By themselves, these drugs do very little to the channel's activity. However, when GABA is around, benzodiazepines increase the *frequency* of channel opening, whereas barbiturates increase the *duration* of channel opening. In addition, the benzodiazepines can increase Cl^- conductance of the GABA_A receptor channel. Figure 13-17A to D shows the effects of barbiturates on both the IPSP and the single-channel currents. The result, for both the benzodiazepines and the barbiturates, is more inhibitory Cl^- current, stronger IPSPs, and the behavioral consequences of enhanced inhibition.

Surely, however, the GABA_A receptor did not evolve specialized binding sites just for the benefit of our modern drugs. This sort of logic has motivated research to find endogenous ligands, or natural chemicals that bind to the benzodiazepine and barbiturate sites and serve as regulators of inhibition. Figure 13-17E shows some of the binding sites on the GABA_A receptor. Among the potential natural modulators of the GABA_A receptor may be various metabolites of the steroid hormones progesterone, corticosterone, and testosterone. Some of these hormones increase the lifetime or opening frequency of GABA-activated single-channel currents and may thus enhance inhibition. The steroid effect is unlike the usual genomic mechanisms of steroid hormones (see Chapter 4). Instead, steroids modulate the GABA_A receptor in a manner similar to barbiturates— directly, through binding sites that are distinct from the other drug binding sites on the GABA_A receptor. Thus, these steroids are not the natural agonists of the benzodiazepine and barbiturate binding sites. The GABA_A receptor is also subject to modulation by the effects of phosphorylation triggered by second-messenger signaling pathways within neurons.

The ionotropic receptors for acetylcholine, serotonin, GABA, and glycine belong to the superfamily of ligand-gated/pentameric channels

We now know the amino acid sequences of many ligand-gated ion channels in the brain, including the receptors for ACh, serotonin, GABA, and glycine. Even though they are gated by such different ligands and have such different permeabilities, virtually all have the same overall structure: five protein subunits, with each subunit being made up of four membrane-spanning segments (as shown for the GABA_A receptor channel in Fig. 13-17E and inset). For example, inhibitory GABA_A and glycine receptors have structures very similar to those of excitatory nicotinic ACh receptors, even though the first two are selective for anions and the last is selective for cations. For both the glycine and nicotinic ACh receptors, the transmitters bind only to the α subunits; for the GABA_A receptor, the transmitter can bind to either the α or the β subunit.

The primary structures of the many subunit types are remarkably similar, particularly within the amino acid sequences of the hydrophobic membrane-spanning segments. One such stretch, called the **M2 domain**, tends to

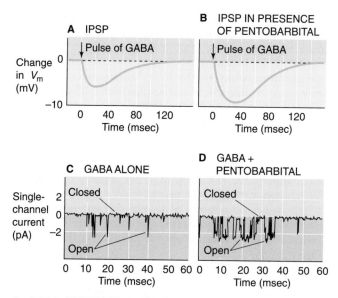

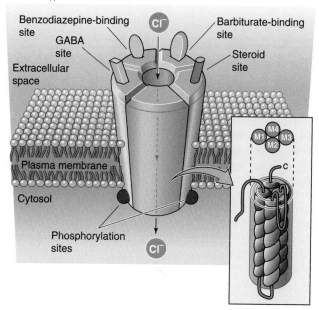

E GABA_A RECEPTOR CHANNEL

Figure 13-17 Physiology and structure of the GABA_A receptor channel. **A,** When a pulse of GABA is released from a synapse, it elicits a small IPSP. **B,** In the presence of a low dose of pentobarbital, the pulse of synaptic GABA elicits a much larger IPSP. Thus, the barbiturate enhances inhibition. **C,** At the single-channel level, GABA by itself elicits brief channel openings. **D,** A barbiturate (50 μM pentobarbital, in this case) does not by itself activate the GABA_A receptor channel but increases the channel open time when GABA is present. **E,** The channel receptor is a heteropentamer. It not only has a pore for Cl⁻ but also separate binding sites for GABA and several classes of channel modulators. The *inset* shows the presumed structure of one of the five monomers. The M2 domain of each of the five subunits presumably lines the central channel pore. *(Data in **C** and **D** from Puia G, Santi MR, Vicini S, et al: Neurosteroids act on recombinant human GABA_A receptors. Neuron 1990; 4:759-765.)*

have repeating sequences of the polar amino acids threonine and serine. Each of the five subunits that constitute a channel contributes one such polar M2 domain, and the set of five combine to form the water-lined pore through which ions can flow (Fig. 13-17E). For the channels gated by GABA and glycine, selectivity for Cl⁻ may be determined by positively charged arginines and lysines near the mouth of the pore.

Not quite *all* ligand-gated channels belong to the same superfamily. We have already seen that the family of ionotropic glutamate receptors is distinct from the family of ligand-gated/pentameric channels. Extensive evidence also indicates that ATP is a synaptic transmitter between certain neurons and at neuron–smooth muscle cell synapses, with rapid actions similar to those of glutamate and ACh. One of the "purinoceptors," called P_{2X}, is an ATP-gated cation channel with relatively high Ca²⁺ permeability. The sequence of this receptor bears little resemblance to either the ionotropic glutamate receptor family or the ligand-gated/pentameric channel superfamily. Instead, each subunit appears to have only two membrane-spanning segments. Functionally, the ATP-gated channel closely resembles the nicotinic ACh receptor; structurally, it is much more akin to the channel family that includes voltage-gated Na⁺ and K⁺ channels (see Chapter 7) and to mechanosensitive channels. This similarity appears to be a case of convergent evolution among ion channels.

Most neuronal synapses release a very small number of transmitter quanta with each action potential

A single neuromuscular junction has ~1000 active zones (see Chapter 8). A single presynaptic impulse releases 100 to 200 quanta of transmitter molecules (i.e., ACh), which generates an EPSP of more than 40 mV in the muscle cell. This is excitation with a vengeance because the total number of quanta is far more than necessary to cause the muscle cell to fire an action potential and generate a brief contraction. Evolution has designed a neuromuscular junction that works every time, with a large margin of excess for safety. Synapses in the brain are quite different. A typical glutamatergic synapse, which has as few as one active zone, generates EPSPs of only 10 to 1000 μV. In most neurons, one EPSP is rarely enough to cause a postsynaptic cell to fire an action potential.

The basis for the small effect of central synapses has been explored by quantal analysis, with refinements of methods originally applied to the neuromuscular junction. In this approach, a single presynaptic axon is stimulated repeatedly while the postsynaptic response is recorded under voltage-clamp conditions. The frequency distribution of amplitudes of excitatory postsynaptic currents (EPSCs) is analyzed, as described for the neuromuscular junction. Recall that according to standard quantal theory:

$$m = np \qquad (13\text{-}1)$$

Here, *m* is the total number of quanta released, *n* is the maximal number of releasable quanta (perhaps equivalent to the number of active zones), and *p* is the average probability of release. Measurement of these parameters is very difficult. Only in rare cases in central neurons is it possible to find amplitude distributions of EPSCs with clearly separate peaks that may correspond to quantal increments of transmitter. In most cases, EPSC distributions are smooth and broad, which makes quantal analysis difficult to interpret. The analysis is hampered because EPSCs are small, it is extremely difficult to identify each small synapse, the dendrites electrically filter the recorded synaptic signals, noise arises from numerous sources (including the ion channels themselves), and synapses exhibit considerable variability. Nevertheless, what is clear is that most synaptic terminals in the CNS release only a small number of transmitter molecules per impulse, often just those contained in a single quantum (i.e., 1000 to 5000 glutamate molecules). Furthermore, the probability of release of that single quantum is often substantially less than 1; in other words, a presynaptic action potential often results in the release of no transmitter at all. When a quantum of transmitter molecules is released, only a limited number of postsynaptic receptors is available for the transmitter to bind to, usually not more than 100. In addition, because not all the receptors open their channels during each response, only 10 to 40 channels contribute current to each postsynaptic response, compared with the thousands of channels opening in concert during each neuromuscular EPSP.

Because most glutamatergic synapses in the brain contribute such a weak excitatory effect, it may require the nearly simultaneous action of many synapses (and the summation of their EPSPs) to bring the postsynaptic membrane potential above the threshold for an action potential. *The threshold number of synapses varies greatly among neurons, but it is roughly in the range of 10 to 100.*

Some exceptions to the rule of small synaptic strengths in the CNS may be noted. One of the strongest connections in the CNS is the one between the climbing fibers and Purkinje cells of the cerebellum (Fig. 13-1B). **Climbing fibers** are glutamatergic axons arising from cells in the inferior olivary nucleus, and they are a critical input to the cerebellum. Climbing fibers and Purkinje cells have a dedicated, one-to-one relationship. The climbing fiber branches extensively and winds intimately around each **Purkinje cell**, making numerous synaptic contacts. When the climbing fiber fires, it generates a massive EPSP (~40 mV, similar to the neuromuscular EPSP) that evokes a burst of spikes in the Purkinje cell. Like the neuromuscular junction, the climbing fiber–Purkinje cell relationship seems to be designed to deliver a suprathreshold response every time it is activated. It achieves this strength in the standard way: each climbing fiber makes ~200 synaptic contacts with each Purkinje cell.

When multiple transmitters co-localize to the same synapse, the exocytosis of large vesicles requires high-frequency stimulation

As we mentioned previously, some presynaptic terminals have two or more transmitters co-localized within them. In these cases, the small transmitters are packaged into relatively small vesicles (~40 nm in diameter), whereas neuropeptides are in larger dense-core vesicles (100 to 200 nm in diameter), as noted earlier. This dual-packaging scheme allows the neuron some control over the relative release of its two types of transmitters (Fig. 13-18A). In general, **low-frequency stimulation** of the presynaptic terminal triggers the release of only the small transmitter (Fig. 13-18B); co-release of both transmitters requires bursts of **high-frequency stimulation** (Fig. 13-18C). This frequency sensitivity may result from the size and spatial profile of presynaptic $[Ca^{2+}]_i$ levels achieved by the different patterns of stimulation. Presynaptic Ca^{2+} channels are located close to the vesicle fusion sites. Low frequencies of activation yield only localized elevations of $[Ca^{2+}]_i$, an amount sufficient to trigger the exocytosis of small vesicles near active zones. Larger peptide-filled vesicles are farther from active zones, and high-frequency stimulation may be necessary to achieve higher, more distributed elevations of $[Ca^{2+}]_i$. With this arrangement, it is obvious that the synaptic effect (resulting from the mixture of transmitters released) depends strongly on the way that the synapse is activated.

PLASTICITY OF CENTRAL SYNAPSES

Use-dependent changes in synaptic strength underlie many forms of learning

Arguably the greatest achievement of a brain is its ability to learn and to store the experience and events of the past so that it is better adapted to deal with the future. Memory is the ability to store and to recall learned changes, and nervous systems without memory are extremely handicapped. Studies of the biological bases for learning and memory have been intense. Although they are far from understood, certain principles have become clear. First, no single mechanism can explain all forms of memory. Even within a single organism, a variety of types of memory exist—and undoubtedly a variety of mechanisms underlie them. Second, evidence is strong that synapses are the physical site of many if not all forms of memory storage in the brain. As the major points of interaction between neurons, synapses are well placed to alter the processing capabilities of a neural circuit in interesting and useful ways. Third, the **synaptic strength** (i.e., the mean amplitude of the postsynaptic response) of many synapses may depend on their previous activity. The sensitivity of a synapse to its past activity can lead to a long-term change in its future effectiveness, which is all we need to build memory into a neural circuit.

Some forms of memory last just a few seconds or minutes, only to be lost or replaced by new memories. **Working memory** is an example. It is the continual series of fleeting memories that we use during the course of a day to remember facts and events, what was just spoken to us, where we put the phone down, whether we are coming or going—things that are useful for the moment but need not be stored longer. Other forms of memory may last for hours to decades and strongly resist disruption and replacement. Such **long-term memory** allows the accumulation of knowledge over a lifetime. Some memories may be formed after only a single trial (recall a particularly dramatic but unique event in your life), whereas others form only with repeated practice (examples include speaking a language or playing the piano). Detailed descriptions of the many types of memory are beyond the scope of this chapter, but it seems obvious that

B   LOW-FREQUENCY STIMULATION

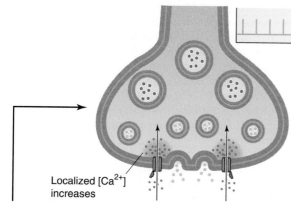

Localized [Ca²⁺]
increases

A   PRESYNAPTIC TERMINAL AT REST

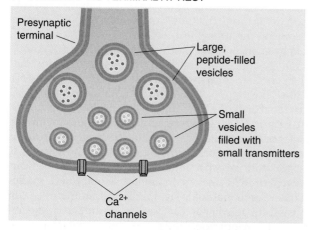

Presynaptic
terminal

Large,
peptide-filled
vesicles

Small
vesicles
filled with
small transmitters

Ca²⁺
channels

C   HIGH-FREQUENCY STIMULATION

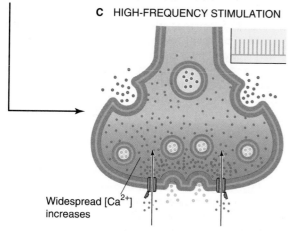

Widespread [Ca²⁺]
increases

Figure 13-18   Selective release of co-localized small transmitters and neuroactive peptides. **A,** The presynaptic terminal at rest is filled with small vesicles (containing small transmitter molecules) and large, dense-core vesicles (containing neuroactive peptides). **B,** Fusion of small vesicles containing small transmitters. **C,** Fusion of large, dense-core vesicles.

A   RESPONSE TO HIGH-FREQUENCY STIMULATION

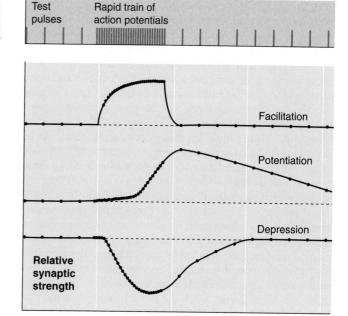

Test
pulses

Rapid train of
action potentials

Facilitation

Potentiation

Depression

Relative synaptic strength

B   RESPONSE TO LOW-FREQUENCY STIMULATION

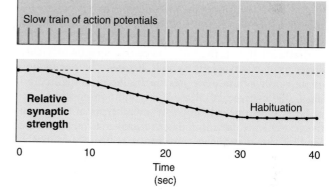

Slow train of action potentials

Relative synaptic strength

Habituation

Time
(sec)

Figure 13-19   Facilitation, potentiation, depression, and habituation. *(Data from Levitan IB, Kaczmarek LK: The Neuron: Cell and Molecular Biology, 2nd ed. New York: Oxford University Press, 1997.)*

cult to demonstrate that specific forms of memory use particular types of synaptic plasticity, and correlation of memory with synaptic plasticity remains a coveted goal of current research.

Short-term synaptic plasticity usually reflects presynaptic changes

Repetitive stimulation of neuronal synapses often yields brief periods of increased or decreased synaptic strength (Fig. 13-19). The usual nomenclature for the short-term increases in strength is **facilitation** (which lasts tens to hundreds of milliseconds), **augmentation** (lasting several seconds), and **potentiation** (lasting tens of seconds to several minutes and outlasting the period of high-frequency stimulation). Not all of them are expressed at every type of synapse. In general, the longer lasting modifications require longer

no single synaptic mechanism would suffice to generate all of them. Neurophysiologists have identified many types of **synaptic plasticity**, the term for activity-dependent changes in the effectiveness of synapses, and some of their mechanisms are well understood. However, it has been very diffi-

periods of conditioning stimuli. Short-term *decreases* in synaptic strength include **depression**, which can occur during high-frequency stimulation, and **habituation**, which is a slowly progressing decrease that occurs during relatively low-frequency activation.

Three potential explanations may be offered for short-term *increases* in synaptic strength. First, the presynaptic terminal may release more transmitter for each action potential. Second, the postsynaptic receptors may be more responsive to transmitter because of a change in their number or sensitivity. Third, both of these explanations may occur simultaneously. Studies involving a variety of synapses suggest that the first explanation is most often true. In these cases, quantal analysis usually shows that synapses become stronger because more neurotransmitter is released during each presynaptic action potential; postsynaptic mechanisms generally do not play a role. This form of plasticity seems to depend on the influx of presynaptic Ca^{2+} during the conditioning tetanus. Katz and Miledi first proposed that synaptic strength is increased because of residual Ca^{2+} left in the terminal after a conditioning train of stimuli at the neuromuscular junction. Recent work supports this hypothesis. The idea is that (1) a tetanic stimulus leads to a substantial increase in presynaptic $[Ca^{2+}]_i$; (2) it takes a relatively long time for presynaptic $[Ca^{2+}]_i$ to decline to baseline, and prolonged stimulation requires prolonged recovery times; and (3) presynaptic action potentials arriving after the conditioning tetanus generate a Ca^{2+} influx that sums with the residual $[Ca^{2+}]_i$ from the preceding tetanus to yield a larger than normal peak $[Ca^{2+}]_i$. Because the dependence of transmitter release on presynaptic $[Ca^{2+}]_i$ is highly nonlinear, the increase in release after conditioning stimuli can be large. It also seems likely that several types of Ca^{2+}-sensitive proteins are present in the presynaptic terminal; the Ca^{2+} binding site that triggers exocytosis is distinct from Ca^{2+} binding sites that regulate short-term increases in transmitter release.

The physiology of a short-term *decrease* in synaptic strength, namely, habituation, has been studied in the marine invertebrate *Aplysia*. The animal reflexively withdraws its gill in response to a stimulus to its skin. Vincent Castellucci and Eric Kandel found that withdrawal becomes less vigorous—that is, the animal habituates—when the stimulus is presented repeatedly. The basis for this behavioral habituation is, at least in part, a decrease in the strength of synapses made by skin sensory neurons onto gill withdrawal motor neurons. Using quantal analysis, Castellucci and Kandel showed that synaptic habituation is due to fewer transmitter quanta being released per action potential. Thus, as with the short-term enhancements of synaptic strength, this example of habituation is due to presynaptic modifications.

Long-term potentiation in the hippocampus may last for days or weeks

In 1973, Timothy Bliss and Terje Lømo described a form of synaptic enhancement that lasted for days or even weeks. This phenomenon, now called **long-term potentiation (LTP)**, occurred in excitatory synapses of the mammalian cerebral cortex. LTP was generated by trains of high-frequency stimulation applied to the presynaptic axons, and it was expressed as an increase in the size of EPSPs. Several properties of LTP, including its longevity and its location in cortical synapses, made it immediately attractive as a candidate for the cellular basis of certain forms of vertebrate learning. Years of intensive research have revealed many details of the molecular mechanisms of LTP. They have also provided some evidence, albeit still indirect, that LTP is involved in learning. Numerous mechanistically distinct types of LTP exist; here we discuss only the best-studied example.

LTP is easily demonstrated in several synaptic relays within the **hippocampus**, a part of the cerebral cortex that has often been considered essential for the formation of certain long-term memories. The best studied of these synapses is between the Schaffer collateral axons of CA3 pyramidal neurons (forming the presynaptic terminals) and CA1 pyramidal neurons (the postsynaptic neurons). In a typical experiment, the strength of synapses to the CA1 neuron is tested by giving a single shock about once every 10 seconds. Stimuli are applied separately to two sets of Schaffer collateral fibers that form two different sets of synapses (Fig. 13-20A). If we stimulate a "control" Schaffer collateral once every 10 seconds, the amplitude of the EPSPs recorded in the postsynaptic CA1 neuron remains rather constant during many tens of minutes (Fig. 13-20B). However, if we *pair* the presynaptic test shocks occurring once every 10 seconds to the "test" pathway with simultaneous postsynaptic depolarization of the CA1 neuron, the amplitude of the EPSP gradually increases several-fold (Fig. 13-20C), indicative of LTP. In this case, the trigger for LTP was the *pairing* of a low-frequency presynaptic input and a strong postsynaptic depolarization. We already saw that Bliss and Lømo originally induced LTP by pairing the low-frequency presynaptic input with brief bursts of tetanic stimulation (50 to 100 stimuli at a frequency of ~100 Hz).

The induction of LTP has several interesting features that enhance its candidacy as a memory mechanism. First, it is **input specific**, which means that only the activated set of synapses onto a particular cell will be potentiated, whereas unactivated synapses to that same neuron remain unpotentiated. Second, induction of LTP requires coincident activity of the presynaptic terminals plus significant depolarization of the postsynaptic membrane. We saw this effect in Figure 13-20C, which showed that inducing LTP required coincident synaptic input and depolarization. Because single hippocampal synapses are quite weak, the requirement for substantial postsynaptic activation means that LTP is best induced in an in vivo situation by **cooperativity**—enough presynaptic axons must cooperate, or fire coincidentally, to strongly activate the postsynaptic cell. The cooperative property of LTP can be used to form associations between synaptic inputs. Imagine that two sets of weak inputs onto one cell are, by themselves, too weak to induce LTP. Perhaps each encodes some sensory feature of an object: the sight (input 1) and sound (input 2) of your pet cat. If the two firing together are strong enough to induce LTP, both sets of synaptic input will tend to strengthen, and the features that they encode (the sight and sound of the cat) will become associated in their enhanced ability to fire the postsynaptic cell. In contrast, for example, the sight of your cat and the sound of

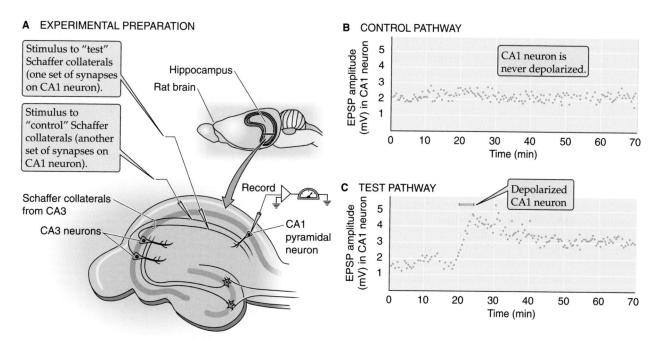

Figure 13-20 Causing long-term potentiation by pairing presynaptic and postsynaptic stimuli. **A,** Pyramidal CA3 neurons in the hippocampus send axons (Schaffer collaterals) to synapse on pyramidal CA1 neurons. In the case of the "control" stimulus, the stimulating electrode stimulates collaterals that activate one set of synapses on the postsynaptic CA1 neuron. In this case, the CA1 neuron receives only *presynaptic* stimuli. In the case of the "test" stimulus, a second electrode stimulates a different set of collaterals that activate a different set of synapses on that *same* CA1 neuron. However, in this case, the presynaptic stimuli will be paired with a *postsynaptic* depolarization that is delivered by a third microelectrode. Aside from pairing or not pairing the presynaptic stimuli with a postsynaptic stimulus, the test and control pathways are equivalent. The third microelectrode records the EPSPs from the CA1 neuron in both the test and control experiments. **B,** In this case, the control Schaffer collaterals are stimulated. Each test pulse is represented by a point on the graph. However, because the CA1 neuron is not depolarized, the amplitude of the EPSPs remains constant (i.e., there is no LTP). **C,** In this case, the test Schaffer collaterals are stimulated. When the CA1 neuron is also depolarized, the amplitude of the EPSPs greatly increases (i.e., LTP has been induced). *(Data from Gustafsson B, Wigstrom H, Abraham WC, Huang YY: Long-term potentiation in the hippocampus using depolarizing current pulses as the conditioning stimulus to single-volley synaptic potentials. J Neurosci 1987; 7:774-780.)*

your telephone will rarely occur together, and their neural equivalents will not become associated.

The molecular mechanisms of one form of LTP in the CA1 region of hippocampus have been partially elucidated. The synapse uses glutamate as its transmitter, and both AMPA and NMDA receptors are activated to generate an EPSP. Induction of this type of LTP depends absolutely on an increase in *post*synaptic $[Ca^{2+}]_i$ levels beyond a critical level and lasting for about 1 to 2 seconds. (Recall that the *short*-term forms of enhancement required a *pre*synaptic increase in $[Ca^{2+}]_i$; see the preceding section.) Under most conditions, postsynaptic $[Ca^{2+}]_i$ levels rise during a tetanic stimulus because of the activation of NMDA receptors, the only type of glutamate-activated channel that is usually permeable to Ca^{2+} (Fig. 13-16). Recall also that the NMDA-type glutamate receptor channel is voltage dependent; to open, it requires V_m to be relatively positive. The cooperativity requirement of LTP is really a requirement for the activation of NMDA receptors so that Ca^{2+} can enter—if the postsynaptic V_m is too negative (as it is when synaptic activation is weak), NMDA channels remain mostly closed. If activation is strong (as it is when multiple inputs cooperate or when tetanus occurs), V_m becomes positive enough to allow NMDA

channels to open. The stimulus-induced rise in postsynaptic $[Ca^{2+}]_i$ is thought to activate at least one essential kinase: **calcium-calmodulin–dependent protein kinase II.** Blocking of this kinase with drugs prevents induction of LTP. Several other types of kinases have been implicated, but the evidence that these mediate—as opposed to modulate—LTP is equivocal.

The molecular pathways leading to the expression and maintenance of LTP are more obscure after the Ca^{2+}-induced activation of kinases. Evidence has been presented both for and against postsynaptic and presynaptic changes explaining the increase in synaptic strength. For the most commonly studied, NMDA receptor–dependent form of LTP described here, there is compelling evidence for a *postsynaptic* mechanism involving an increased number, and perhaps effectiveness, of AMPA receptors. There is also evidence for a *presynaptic* mechanism whereby the release of transmitter might be enhanced, although the molecular details of this possibility are obscure. Sometimes, postsynaptic AMPA receptors appear to be functionally "silent" until LTP mechanisms activate them or insert them into the membrane. Note that the presynaptic hypothesis requires the presence of some rapidly diffusing retrograde messenger that can carry a signal from the postsynaptic side (where rising $[Ca^{2+}]_i$ is clearly a trigger for LTP) back to the presynaptic terminal. There are currently no convincing chemical candidates for the identity of such a retrograde messenger.

There are multiple forms of long-term depression

It is theoretically reasonable to suspect that memory systems have mechanisms not only to increase synaptic strength but to decrease it as well. In fact, **long-term depression (LTD)** can be induced in the same synapses within the hippocampus that generate the $[Ca^{2+}]_i$-dependent LTP described in the preceding section. The critical feature that determines whether the synapses will strengthen or weaken is simply the frequency of stimulation that they receive. For example, several hundred stimuli delivered at 50 Hz produce LTP; the same number delivered at 10 Hz has little effect, and at 1 Hz they produce LTD. One set of synapses can be strengthened or weakened repeatedly, which suggests that each process (LTP and LTD) acts on the same molecular component of the synapses. LTD induced in this way shows the same input specificity as LTP—only the stimulated synapses onto a cell are depressed.

There are multiple forms of LTD, each with distinct molecular mechanisms. One type depends on activation of mGluRs; another apparently requires activation of cannabinoid receptors. We describe the type of LTD that has been studied most extensively. The induction requirements of this form of hippocampal LTD are paradoxically similar to those of LTP: LTD induced by low-frequency stimulation depends on the activation of NMDA receptors, and it requires an increase in postsynaptic $[Ca^{2+}]_i$. The key determinant for whether a tetanic stimulus induces LTP or LTD may be the level to which postsynaptic $[Ca^{2+}]_i$ rises. A simple model that illustrates the induction mechanisms of LTD and LTP is shown in Figure 13-21. Synaptic activation releases glutamate, which activates NMDA receptors, which in turn allow Ca^{2+} to enter the postsynaptic cell. In the case of high-frequency stimulation, postsynaptic $[Ca^{2+}]_i$ rises to very high levels; if stimulation is of low frequency, the rise in postsynaptic $[Ca^{2+}]_i$ is more modest. High levels of $[Ca^{2+}]_i$ lead to a net activation of protein *kinases,* whereas modest levels of $[Ca^{2+}]_i$ preferentially activate protein *phosphatases.* The

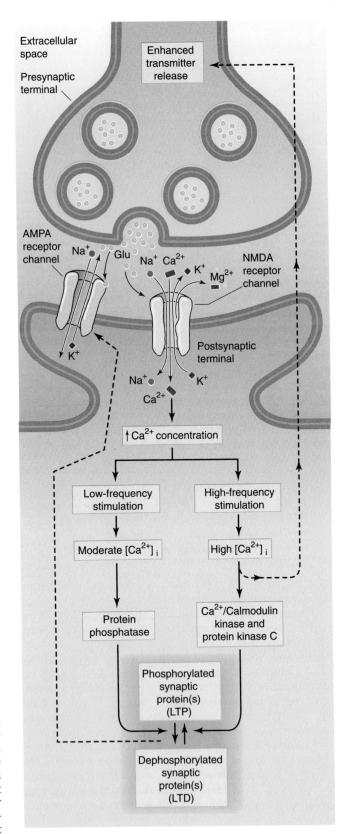

Figure 13-21 Proposed molecular mechanism for long-term potentiation and long-term depression. Glutamate release from the presynaptic terminal activates NMDA receptor channels, which allow Ca^{2+} to enter the postsynaptic cell. The glutamate also activates AMPA receptor channels. Whether the ultimate effect is LTP or LTD appears to depend on the extent to which $[Ca^{2+}]_i$ rises. High levels of $[Ca^{2+}]_i$—produced by high-frequency stimulation—lead to a net activation of protein kinases and thus phosphorylation of one or more synaptic proteins that regulate synaptic strength. One hypothetical pathway has the phosphorylated/dephosphorylated synaptic proteins modulating the AMPA receptor channel. The result is LTP. The postsynaptic neuron also seems to be able to stimulate the presynaptic terminal. A moderate increase in $[Ca^{2+}]_i$—produced by low-frequency stimulation—preferentially activates protein phosphatases, which presumably dephosphorylate the same synaptic proteins as in the previous example. The result is LTD.

kinases and phosphatases in turn act on a synaptic protein or phosphoprotein that somehow regulates synaptic strength. There is good evidence that LTP-inducing stimuli phosphorylate specific residues on AMPA receptors and conversely that LTD-inducing stimuli dephosphorylate other residues on AMPA receptors. These post-translational changes are, however, only part of the story of long-term synaptic plasticity. LTP increases—and LTD decreases—the numbers of AMPA receptors in the postsynaptic membrane by modulating receptor trafficking into and out of the surface membrane. Longer lasting LTP- and LTD-induced changes seem to involve mechanisms that depend on protein synthesis, including structural changes in synapses and spines.

Note that the simple scheme shown in Figure 13-21 leaves unidentified many of the steps between the rise in postsynaptic $[Ca^{2+}]_i$ and the change in synaptic strength; most of the molecular details remain to be determined. However, if the model is correct, it means that synaptic strength (and, by implication, some memory) is under the dynamic control of cellular processes that determine postsynaptic $[Ca^{2+}]_i$. Once again in physiology, $[Ca^{2+}]_i$ has been assigned a pivotal role in a vital process.

Long-term depression in the cerebellum may be important for motor learning

A variety of other types of LTP and LTD have been described in other synapses and even within the same synapses of the CA1 region in the hippocampus. Clearly, multiple means and mechanisms may be used to strengthen and to weaken synapses in the brain over a range of time courses. We briefly describe one other well-studied type of synaptic modification in the mammalian brain, LTD in the cerebellum.

The cerebellum is a large brain structure that is important in motor control and strongly implicated in motor learning. The cortex of the cerebellum is a thin, multiply folded sheet of cells with an intricate but highly repetitious neural structure. The principal cell of the cerebellum is the **Purkinje cell**, a large neuron that uses GABA as its transmitter and whose axon forms the sole output of the cerebellar cortex. Purkinje cells receive two types of excitatory synaptic input: (1) each Purkinje cell receives powerful synaptic contact from just a single climbing fiber, which comes from a cell in the inferior olivary nucleus (Fig. 13-1B); and (2) each Purkinje cell also receives a synapse from ~150,000 **parallel fibers**, which originate from the tiny granule cells of the cerebellum itself. This remarkable conjunction of synaptic inputs is the basis for a theory of motor learning that was proposed by David Marr and James Albus in 1970. They predicted that the parallel fiber synapses should change their strength only if they are active at the same time as the climbing fiber onto the same cell. This idea received important experimental support from the laboratory of Masao Ito.

Ito and colleagues monitored EPSPs in a Purkinje cell while stimulating some of its inputs from parallel fibers and its one climbing fiber input. They found that the EPSPs generated by the parallel fibers became smaller when both the parallel fibers *and* the cell's climbing fiber were coactivated at low frequencies. Stimulating either input alone did not cause any change. Cerebellar LTD can last at least several hours. As with the hippocampal LTP and LTD described

before, cerebellar LTD showed input specificity: only those parallel fibers coactivated with the climbing fiber were depressed, whereas other synapses onto the cell were unchanged.

The mechanism of cerebellar LTD has some similarities to that of LTD in the hippocampus, but it is also distinctly different. Parallel fiber synapses weaken because of reduced effectiveness—a reduction in either number or sensitivity—of *postsynaptic* AMPA-type glutamate receptors. As in the hippocampus, induction of cerebellar LTD requires an increase in postsynaptic $[Ca^{2+}]_i$. However, unlike in the hippocampus, no NMDA-type glutamate receptors are present in the mature cerebellum to mediate Ca^{2+} flux. Instead, Ca^{2+} can enter Purkinje cells through voltage-gated Ca^{2+} channels that are opened during the exceptionally powerful EPSP that the climbing fiber generates. In addition to a rise in postsynaptic $[Ca^{2+}]_i$, cerebellar LTD induction seems to require the activation of metabotropic glutamate receptors and protein kinase C by the parallel fibers. Increases in postsynaptic $[Na^+]_i$ and NO have also been implicated in LTD induction. At present, the relationships between these putative induction factors and the molecular pathways leading to the expression of cerebellar LTD are obscure.

As we pointed out for the hippocampus, most efficient memory systems need mechanisms for both weakening and strengthening of their synapses. It turns out that parallel fiber synapses of the cerebellum can be induced to generate LTP as well as LTD by stimulating them at relatively low (2 to 8 Hz) frequencies. Cerebellar LTP, unlike hippocampal LTP, requires presynaptic but not postsynaptic increases in $[Ca^{2+}]_i$. Potentiation seems to be a result of increased transmitter release from the presynaptic terminal.

REFERENCES

Books and Reviews

Boehning D, Snyder SH: Novel neural modulators. Annu Rev Neurosci 2003; 26:105-131.

Carlisle HJ, Kennedy MB: Spine architecture and synaptic plasticity. Trends Neurosci 2005; 28:182-187.

Collingridge GL, Isaac JT, Wang YT: Receptor trafficking and synaptic plasticity. Nat Rev Neurosci 2004; 5:952-962.

Connors BW, Long MA: Electrical synapses in the mammalian brain. Annu Rev Neurosci 2004; 27:393-418.

Cooper JR, Bloom FE, Roth RH: The Biochemical Basis of Neuropharmacology, 8th ed. New York: Oxford University Press, 2002.

Cowan WM, Südhof TC, Stevens CF: Synapses. Baltimore: Johns Hopkins University Press, 2001.

MacDonald RL, Olsen RW: GABA$_A$ receptor channels. Annu Rev Neurosci 1994; 17:569-602.

Malenka RC, Bear MF: LTP and LTD: An embarrassment of riches. Neuron 2004; 44:5-21.

Mayer ML, Armstrong N: Structure and function of glutamate receptor ion channels. Annu Rev Physiol 2004; 66:161-181.

Mody I, Pearce RA: Diversity of inhibitory neurotransmission through GABA$_A$ receptors. Trends Neurosci 2004; 27:569-575.

Piomelli D. The molecular logic of endocannabinoid signalling. Nat Rev Neurosci 2003; 4:873-884.

Südhof TC: The synaptic vesicle cycle. Annu Rev Neurosci 2004; 27:509-547.

Zucker RS, Regehr WG: Short-term synaptic plasticity. Annu Rev Physiol 2002; 64:355-405.

Journal Articles

Bliss TV, Lomo T: Long-lasting potentiation of synaptic transmission in the dentate area of the anaesthetized rabbit following stimulation of the perforant path. J Physiol 1973; 232:331-356.

Dudek SM, Bear MF: Bidirectional long-term modification of synaptic effectiveness in the adult and immature hippocampus. J Neurosci 1993; 13:2910-2918.

Heuser J, Reese T: Evidence for recycling of synaptic vesicle membrane during transmitter release at the frog neuromuscular junction. J Cell Biol 1973; 57:315-344.

Kamiya H, Zucker RS: Residual Ca^{2+} and short-term synaptic plasticity. Nature 1994; 371:603-606.

Katz B, Miledi R: The role of calcium in neuromuscular facilitation. J Physiol (Lond) 1968; 195:481-492.

Rosenmund C, Stern-Bach Y, Stevens CF: The tetrameric structure of a glutamate receptor channel. Science 1998; 280:1596-1599.

Sabatini BL, Regehr WG: Timing of neurotransmission at fast synapses in the mammalian brain. Nature 1996; 384:170-172.

Shi SH, Hayashi Y, Petralia RS, et al: Rapid spine delivery and redistribution of AMPA receptors after synaptic nmDA receptor activation. Science 1999; 284:1811-1816.

Vignes M, Collingridge GL: The synaptic activation of kainate receptors. Nature 1997; 388:179-182.

Wilson RI, Nicoll RA: Endogenous cannabinoids mediate retrograde signalling at hippocampal synapses. Nature 2001; 410:588-592.

CHAPTER 14

THE AUTONOMIC NERVOUS SYSTEM

George B. Richerson

When we are awake, we are constantly aware of sensory input from our external environment, and we consciously plan how to react to it. When we are asleep, the nervous system has a variety of mechanisms to dissociate cortical function from sensory input and somatic motor output. Among these mechanisms are closing the eyes, blocking the transmission of sensory impulses to the cortex as they pass through the thalamus, and effecting a nearly complete paralysis of skeletal muscles during rapid eye movement (REM) sleep to keep us from physically acting out our dreams.

The conscious and discontinuous nature of cortical brain function stands in sharp contrast with those parts of the nervous system that are responsible for control of our internal environment. These "autonomic" processes never stop attending to the wide range of metabolic, cardiopulmonary, and other visceral requirements of our body. Autonomic control continues whether we are awake and attentive, preoccupied with other activities, or asleep. While we are awake, we are unaware of most visceral sensory input, and we avoid any conscious effort to act on it unless it induces distress. In most cases, we have no awareness of motor commands to the viscera, and most individuals can exert voluntary control over motor output to the viscera only in minor ways. Consciousness and memory are frequently considered the most important functions of the human nervous system, but it is the visceral control system—including the **autonomic nervous system** (ANS)—that makes life and higher cortical function possible.

We have a greater understanding of the physiology of the ANS than of many other parts of the nervous system, largely because it is reasonably easy to isolate peripheral neurons and to study them. As a result of its accessibility, the ANS has served as a key model system for the elucidation of many principles of neuronal and synaptic function.

ORGANIZATION OF THE VISCERAL CONTROL SYSTEM

The autonomic nervous system has sympathetic, parasympathetic, and enteric divisions

Output from the central nervous system (CNS) travels along two anatomically and functionally distinct pathways: the somatic motor neurons, which innervate striated skeletal muscle; and the **autonomic motor neurons**, which innervate smooth muscle, cardiac muscle, secretory epithelia, and glands. All viscera are richly supplied by efferent axons from the ANS that constantly adjust organ function.

The autonomic (from the Greek for "self-governing," functioning independently of the will) nervous system was first defined by Langley in 1898 as including the local nervous system of the gut and the efferent neurons innervating glands and involuntary muscle. Thus, this definition of the ANS includes only *efferent* neurons and *enteric* neurons. Since that time, it has become clear that the efferent ANS cannot easily be dissociated from visceral *afferents* as well as from those parts of the CNS that control the viscera and other autonomic functions. This larger visceral control system monitors afferents from the viscera and the rest of the body, compares this input with current and anticipated needs, and controls output to the body's organ systems.

The ANS has three divisions: sympathetic, parasympathetic, and enteric. The **sympathetic** and **parasympathetic divisions** of the ANS are the two major efferent pathways controlling targets other than skeletal muscle (Fig. 14-1). Each arises in the CNS, and each innervates target tissue by a two-synapse pathway. The cell bodies of the first neurons lie within the CNS. These **preganglionic neurons** are found in columns of cells in the brainstem and spinal cord and send axons out of the CNS to make synapses with **postganglionic neurons** in peripheral ganglia interposed between the CNS and their target cells. Axons from these postganglionic neurons then project to their targets. The sympathetic and parasympathetic divisions can act independently of each other. However, in general, they work synergistically to control visceral activity and often act in opposite ways, like an accelerator and brake to regulate visceral function. An increase in output of the sympathetic division occurs under conditions of stress, anxiety, physical activity, fear, or excitement; parasympathetic output increases during sedentary activity, eating, or other "vegetative" behavior.

The **enteric division** of the ANS is a system of afferent neurons, interneurons, and motor neurons that form networks of neurons called **plexuses** (from the Latin "to braid") that surround the gastrointestinal tract. It can function as a separate and independent nervous system, but it is normally controlled by the CNS through sympathetic and parasympathetic fibers.

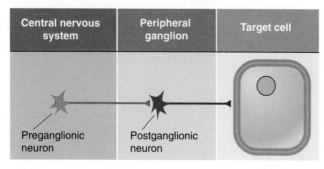

Central nervous system	Peripheral ganglion	Target cell

Figure 14-1 Organization of the sympathetic and parasympathetic divisions of the ANS.

Sympathetic preganglionic neurons originate from spinal segments T1 to L3 and synapse with postganglionic neurons in paravertebral or prevertebral ganglia

Preganglionic Neurons The cell bodies of preganglionic sympathetic motor neurons are located in the thoracic and upper lumbar spinal cord between levels T1 and L3. At these spinal levels, autonomic neurons lie in the **intermediolateral cell column**, or lateral horn, between the dorsal and ventral horns (Fig. 14-2). Axons from preganglionic sympathetic neurons exit the spinal cord through the ventral roots along with axons from *somatic* motor neurons. After entering the spinal nerves, sympathetic efferents diverge from somatic motor axons to enter the white **rami communicantes**. These rami, or branches, are white because most preganglionic sympathetic axons are myelinated.

Paravertebral Ganglia Axons from preganglionic neurons enter the nearest sympathetic paravertebral ganglion through a white ramus. These ganglia lie adjacent to the vertebral column. Although preganglionic sympathetic fibers emerge only from levels T1 to L3, the chain of sympathetic ganglia extends all the way from the upper part of the neck to the coccyx, where the left and right sympathetic chains merge in the midline and form the coccygeal ganglion. In general, one ganglion is positioned at the level of each spinal root, but adjacent ganglia are fused in some cases. The most rostral ganglion, the **superior cervical ganglion**, arises from fusion of C1 to C4 and supplies the head and neck. The next two ganglia are the **middle cervical ganglion**, which arises from fusion of C5 and C6, and the **inferior cervical ganglion** (C7 and C8), which is usually fused with the first thoracic ganglion to form the **stellate ganglion**. Together, the middle cervical and stellate ganglia, along with the upper thoracic ganglia, innervate the heart, lungs, and bronchi. The remaining paravertebral ganglia supply organs and portions of the body wall in a segmental fashion.

After entering a paravertebral ganglion, a preganglionic sympathetic axon has one or more of three fates. It may synapse within that segmental paravertebral ganglion, travel up or down the sympathetic chain to synapse within a neighboring paravertebral ganglion, or enter the greater or lesser splanchnic nerve to synapse within one of the ganglia of the *pre*vertebral plexus.

Prevertebral Ganglia The **prevertebral plexus** lies in front of the aorta and along its major arterial branches and includes the prevertebral ganglia and interconnected fibers (Fig. 14-3). The major prevertebral ganglia are named according to the arteries that they are adjacent to and include the celiac, superior mesenteric, aorticorenal, and inferior mesenteric ganglia. Portions of the prevertebral plexus extend down the major arteries and contain other named and unnamed ganglia and plexuses of nerve fibers, altogether making up a dense and extensive network of sympathetic neuron cell bodies and nerve fibers.

Each *pre*ganglionic sympathetic fiber synapses on many *post*ganglionic sympathetic neurons that are located within one or several nearby paravertebral or prevertebral ganglia. It has been estimated that each preganglionic sympathetic neuron branches and synapses on as many as 200 postganglionic neurons, thus enabling the sympathetic output to have more widespread effects. However, any impulse arriving at its target end organ has only crossed a single synapse between the preganglionic and postganglionic sympathetic neurons.

Postganglionic Neurons The cell bodies of postganglionic sympathetic neurons that are located within *para*vertebral ganglia send out their axons through the nearest **gray rami communicantes**, which rejoin the spinal nerves (Fig. 14-2). These rami are gray because most postganglionic axons are unmyelinated. Because preganglionic sympathetic neurons are located only in the thoracic and upper lumbar spinal segments (T1 to L3), *white* rami are found only at these levels (Fig. 14-4, left). However, because *each* sympathetic ganglion sends out postganglionic axons, *gray* rami are present at all spinal levels from C2 or C3 to the coccyx. Postganglionic sympathetic axons from paravertebral and prevertebral ganglia travel to their target organs within other nerves or by traveling along blood vessels to reach their target organ. Because the paravertebral and prevertebral sympathetic ganglia lie near the spinal cord and thus relatively far from their target organs, the postganglionic axons of the sympathetic division tend to be long. On their way to reach their targets, some postganglionic sympathetic axons travel through *para*sympathetic terminal ganglia or cranial nerve ganglia without synapsing.

Parasympathetic preganglionic neurons originate from the brainstem and sacral spinal cord and synapse with postganglionic neurons in "terminal" ganglia that are located near target organs

The cell bodies of preganglionic parasympathetic neurons are located in the medulla, pons, and midbrain and in the S2 through S4 level of the spinal cord (Fig. 14-4, right). Thus, unlike the sympathetic—or **thoracolumbar**—division, whose preganglionic cell bodies are in the thoracic and lumbar spinal cord, the parasympathetic—or **craniosacral**—division's preganglionic cell bodies are cranial and sacral. The preganglionic parasympathetic fibers originating in the brain distribute with four cranial nerves: the oculomotor nerve (CN III), the facial nerve (CN VII), the glossopharyngeal nerve (CN IX), and the vagus nerve (CN X). The

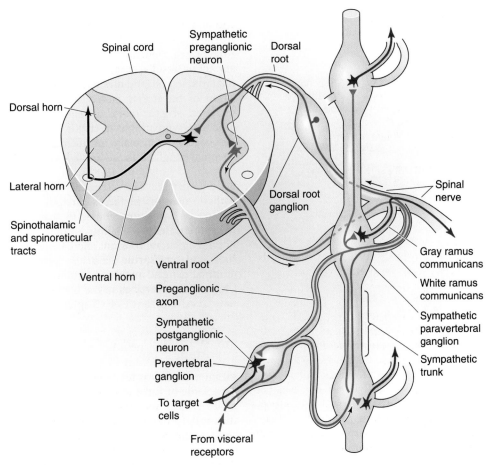

Figure 14-2 Anatomy of the sympathetic division of the ANS. The figure shows a cross section of the thoracic spinal cord and the nearby paravertebral ganglia as well as a prevertebral ganglion. Sympathetic preganglionic neurons are shown in *red* and postganglionic neurons in *dark blue-violet*. Afferent (sensory) pathways are in *blue*. Interneurons are shown in *black*.

preganglionic parasympathetic fibers originating in S2 through S4 distribute with the pelvic splanchnic nerves.

Postganglionic parasympathetic neurons are located in **terminal ganglia** that are more peripherally located and more widely distributed than are the sympathetic ganglia. Terminal ganglia often lie within the walls of their target organs. Thus, in contrast to the sympathetic division, postganglionic fibers of the parasympathetic division are short. In some cases, individual postganglionic parasympathetic neurons are found in isolation or in scattered cell groups rather than in encapsulated ganglia.

Cranial Nerves III, VII, and IX The preganglionic parasympathetic neurons that are distributed with CN III, VII, and IX originate in three groups of nuclei.

1. The **Edinger-Westphal nucleus** is a subnucleus of the oculomotor complex in the midbrain (Fig. 14-5). Parasympathetic neurons in this nucleus travel in the **oculomotor nerve** (CN III) and synapse onto postganglionic neurons in the ciliary ganglion (Fig. 14-4, right). The postganglionic fibers project to two smooth muscles of the eye: the constrictor muscle of the pupil and the ciliary

muscle, which controls the shape of the lens (see Fig. 15-6A).

2. The *superior* **salivatory nucleus** is in the rostral medulla (Fig. 14-5) and contains parasympathetic neurons that project, through a branch of the **facial nerve** (CN VII), to the pterygopalatine ganglion (Fig. 14-4, right). The postganglionic fibers supply the lacrimal glands, which produce tears. Another branch of the facial nerve carries preganglionic fibers to the submandibular ganglion. The postganglionic fibers supply two salivary glands, the submandibular and sublingual glands.

3. The *inferior* **salivatory nucleus** and the rostral part of the **nucleus ambiguus** in the rostral medulla (Fig. 14-5) contain parasympathetic neurons that project through the **glossopharyngeal nerve** (CN IX) to the otic ganglion (Fig. 14-4, right). The postganglionic fibers supply a third salivary gland, the parotid gland.

Cranial Nerve X Most parasympathetic output occurs through the **vagus nerve** (CN X). Cell bodies of vagal preganglionic parasympathetic neurons are found in the medulla within the **nucleus ambiguus** and the **dorsal motor nucleus of the vagus** (Fig. 14-5). This nerve supplies

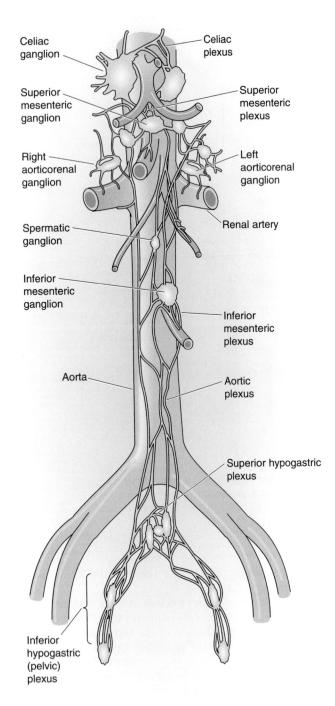

Figure 14-3 Anatomy of the sympathetic *prevertebral* plexus. The ganglia and each associated plexus are named after the artery with which they are associated.

parasympathetic innervation to all the viscera of the thorax and abdomen, including the gastrointestinal tract between the pharynx and distal end of the colon (Fig. 14-4, right). Among other effects, electrical stimulation of the nucleus ambiguus results in activation of striated muscle in the pharynx, larynx, and esophagus and slows the heart. Stimulation of the dorsal motor nucleus of the vagus initiates secretion of gastric acid, insulin, and glucagon. Preganglionic parasympathetic fibers of the vagus nerve join the esophageal, pulmonary, and cardiac plexuses and travel to terminal ganglia that are located within their target organs.

Sacral Nerves The cell bodies of preganglionic parasympathetic neurons in the sacral spinal cord (S2 to S4) are located in a position similar to that of the preganglionic *sympathetic* neurons—although they do not form a distinct intermediolateral column. Their axons leave through ventral roots and travel with the pelvic splanchnic nerves to their terminal ganglia in the descending colon and rectum (see Chapter 41) as well as to the bladder (see Chapter 33) and reproductive organs (see Chapters 54 and 55).

The visceral control system also has an important afferent limb

All internal organs are densely innervated by visceral afferents. Some of these receptors monitor nociceptive (painful) input. Others are sensitive to a variety of mechanical and chemical (physiological) stimuli, including stretch of the heart, blood vessels, and hollow viscera, as well as P_{CO_2}, P_{O_2}, pH, blood glucose, and temperature of the skin and internal organs. Many visceral nociceptive fibers travel in sympathetic nerves (blue projections in Fig. 14-2). Most axons from physiological receptors travel with parasympathetic fibers. As is the case with somatic afferents (see Chapter 10), the cell bodies of visceral afferent fibers are located within the dorsal root ganglia or cranial nerve ganglia (e.g., nodose and petrosal ganglia). Ninety percent of these visceral afferents are unmyelinated.

The largest concentration of visceral afferent axons can be found in the **vagus nerve**, which carries non-nociceptive afferent input to the CNS from all viscera of the thorax and abdomen. Most fibers in the vagus nerve are *afferents*, even though all parasympathetic preganglionic output (i.e., *efferents*) to the abdominal and thoracic viscera also travels in the vagus nerve. Vagal afferents, whose cell bodies are located in the nodose ganglion, carry information about the distention of hollow organs (e.g., blood vessels, cardiac chambers, stomach, bronchioles), blood gases (e.g., P_{O_2}, P_{CO_2}, pH), and body chemistry (e.g., glucose concentration) to the medulla.

Figure 14-4 Organization of the sympathetic and parasympathetic divisions of the ANS. The *left panel* shows the sympathetic division. The cell bodies of sympathetic preganglionic neurons *(red)* are in the intermediolateral column of the thoracic and lumbar spinal cord (T1-L3). Their axons project to paravertebral ganglia (the sympathetic chain) and prevertebral ganglia. Postganglionic neurons *(blue)* therefore have long projections to their targets. The *right panel* shows the parasympathetic division. The cell bodies of parasympathetic preganglionic neurons *(orange)* are either in the brain (midbrain, pons medulla) or in the sacral spinal cord (S2-S4). Their axons project to ganglia very near (or even inside) the end organs. Postganglionic neurons *(green)* therefore have short projections to their targets.

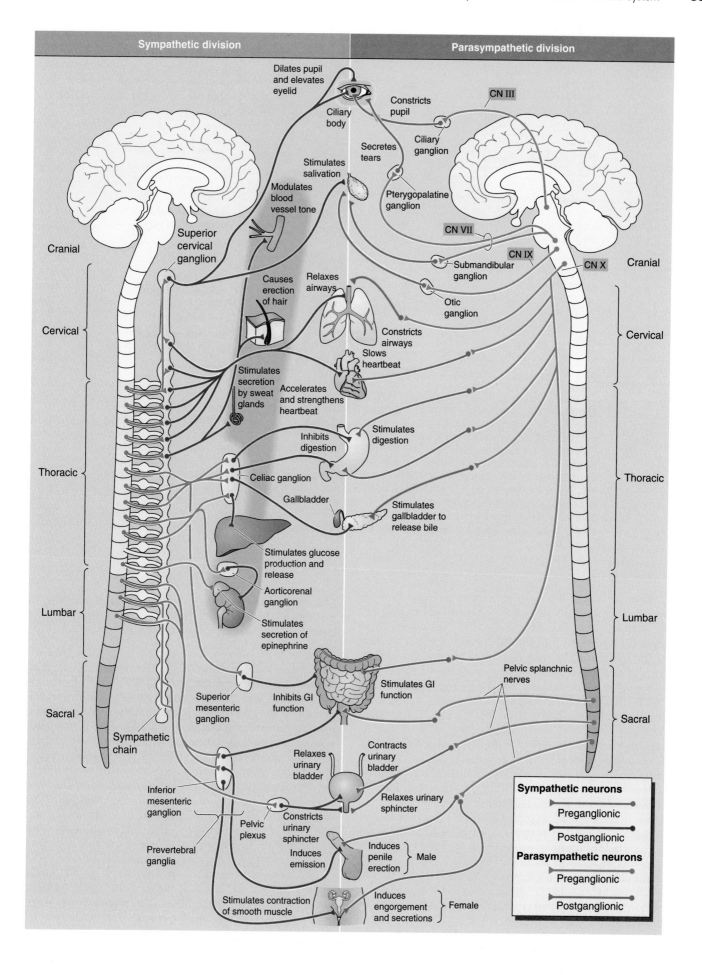

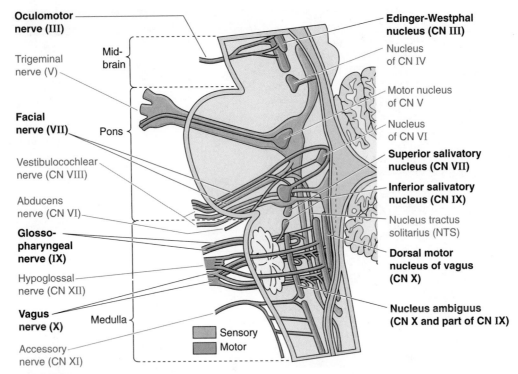

Figure 14-5 Supraspinal nuclei containing neurons that are part of the ANS. These nuclei contain the cell bodies of the preganglionic parasympathetic neurons (i.e., efferent). The Edinger-Westphal nucleus contains cell bodies of preganglionic fibers that travel with CN III to the ciliary ganglion. The superior salivatory nucleus contains cell bodies of preganglionic fibers that travel with CN VII to the pterygopalatine and submandibular ganglia. The inferior salivatory nucleus contains cell bodies of preganglionic fibers that travel with CN IX to the otic ganglion. The rostral portion of the nucleus ambiguus contains preganglionic cell bodies that distribute with CN IX; the rest of the nucleus ambiguus and the dorsal motor nucleus of the vagus contain cell bodies of preganglionic fibers that travel with CN X to a host of terminal ganglia in the viscera of the thorax and abdomen. NTS, which is not part of the ANS, receives visceral afferents and is part of the larger visceral control system. The figure also illustrates other cranial nerves that are not involved in controlling the ANS (gray labels).

Internal organs also have nociceptive receptors that are sensitive to excessive stretch, noxious chemical irritants, and very large decreases in pH. In the CNS, this visceral pain input is mapped (see Chapter 16) *viscerotopically* at the level of the spinal cord because most visceral nociceptive fibers travel with the sympathetic fibers and enter the spinal cord at a specific segmental level along with a spinal nerve (Fig. 14-2). This viscerotopic mapping is also present in the brainstem but not at the level of the cerebral cortex. Thus, awareness of visceral pain is not usually localized to a specific organ but is instead "referred" to the dermatome (see Chapter 10) that is innervated by the same spinal nerve. This **referred pain** results from lack of precision in the central organization of visceral pain pathways. Thus, you know that the pain is associated with a particular spinal nerve, but you do not know where the pain is coming from (i.e., from the skin or a visceral organ). For example, nociceptive input from the left ventricle of the heart is referred to the left T1 to T5 dermatomes and leads to discomfort in the left arm and left side of the chest, whereas nociceptive input from the diaphragm is referred to the C3 to C5 dermatomes and is interpreted as pain in the shoulder. This visceral pain is often felt as a vague burning or pressure sensation.

The enteric division is a self-contained nervous system that surrounds the gastrointestinal tract and receives sympathetic and parasympathetic input

The enteric nervous system (ENS) is a collection of nerve plexuses that surround the gastrointestinal tract, including the pancreas and biliary system. Although it is entirely peripheral, the ENS receives input from the sympathetic and parasympathetic divisions of the ANS. The ENS is estimated to contain more than 100 million neurons, including afferent neurons, interneurons, and efferent postganglionic parasympathetic neurons. Enteric neurons contain many different neurotransmitters and neuromodulators. Thus, not only does the total number of neurons in the enteric division exceed that of the spinal cord, but the neurochemical complexity of the ENS also approaches that of the CNS. The anatomy of the ENS as well as its role in controlling gastrointestinal function is discussed in Chapter 41.

The plexuses of the ENS are a system of ganglia sandwiched between the layers of the gut and connected by a dense meshwork of nerve fibers. The **myenteric** or Auerbach's plexus (Fig. 14-6) lies between the external longitudi-

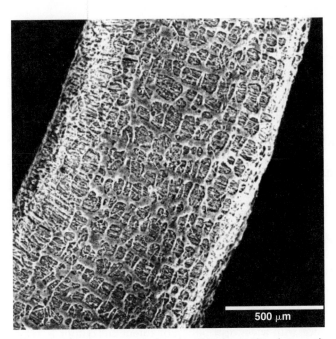

Figure 14-6 The myenteric (Auerbach's) plexus. The photograph is a scanning electron micrograph of the myenteric plexus of the mouse large intestine. The external longitudinal muscle of the intestine was removed so that the view is of the plexus (the highly interconnected meshwork of neuron cell bodies, axons, and dendrites on the surface) spreading over the deeper circular layer of muscle. *(From Burnstock G: Autonomic neuromuscular junctions: Current developments and future directions. J Anat 1986; 146:1-30.)*

nal and the deeper circular smooth muscle layers; the **submucosal** or Meissner's plexus lies between the circular muscle and the most internal layer of smooth muscle, the muscularis mucosae (see Fig. 41-3A). In the intestinal wall, the myenteric plexus is involved primarily in the control of motility, whereas the submucosal plexus is involved in the control of ion and fluid transport. Both the myenteric and the submucosal plexuses receive *pre*ganglionic *parasympathetic* innervation from the vagus nerve (or sacral nerves in the case of the distal portion of colon and rectum). Thus, in one sense, the enteric division is homologous to a large and complex parasympathetic terminal ganglion. The other major input to the ENS is from *post*ganglionic *sympathetic* neurons. Thus, the ENS can be thought of as "postganglionic" with respect to the parasympathetic division and "post-postganglionic" with respect to the sympathetic division. Input from both the sympathetic and parasympathetic divisions modulates the activity of the ENS, but the ENS can by and large function normally without extrinsic input. The isolated ENS can respond appropriately to local stimuli and control most aspects of gut function, including initiating peristaltic activity in response to gastric distention, controlling secretory and absorptive functions, and triggering biliary contractions.

PHOX2B: Master Gene of the Visceral Control System

During development, a complex genetic program expressed in each progenitor cell determines cell fate—ensuring that the cell migrates to the correct location and differentiates into the correct mature cell type. The genes that encode some transcription factors (see Chapter 4) turn on at a specific time during development and trigger normal migration or differentiation of specific cell types. Phox2b is a transcription factor required for development of nearly all neurons within the visceral control system and almost no other class of neuron.

Phox2b is expressed early in development in all neurons of the mammalian visceral control system—including preganglionic and postganglionic parasympathetic neurons, postganglionic (but not preganglionic) sympathetic neurons, enteric neurons, all visceral afferents, and neurons of the nucleus tractus solitarii (NTS), on which they synapse. No other cells express Phox2b, except for neurons of the locus coeruleus in the pons (which plays an important role in cardiovascular control) and certain cranial nerve nuclei (most of which are important for respiratory output and for feeding). Knockout of the mouse *Phox2b* gene leads to loss of development of all these neurons and is fatal. In humans, heterozygous mutations in *PHOX2B* cause **congenital central hypoventilation syndrome (CCHS)**, a congenital form of Ondine's curse (see Chapter 32). Infants with this condition have problems with breathing while they sleep, probably because of a deficiency in detection of O_2 or CO_2 in their blood by peripheral chemoreceptors or defective integration of this information by the NTS. A subset of patients with *PHOX2B* mutations also have Hirschprung disease (see Chapter 41), in which the ENS does not develop normally in a portion of the colon. This combination of CCHS and Hirschprung disease is called **Haddad syndrome**. Some CCHS patients also develop tumors of derivatives of the sympathetic nervous system called neuroblastomas.

As a rule, the neural circuits that carry out individual tasks or behaviors (e.g., locomotion, sleep, vision) are formed by several classes of neurons that follow unrelated developmental pathways before they assemble into a circuit. So far, the visceral control system is unique in that most of its constituent neuronal types differentiate under the control of the same, highly specific transcription factor, Phox2b. *PHOX2B* can thus be considered the "master gene" of the visceral control system.

SYNAPTIC PHYSIOLOGY OF THE AUTONOMIC NERVOUS SYSTEM

The sympathetic and parasympathetic divisions have opposite effects on most visceral targets

All innervation of skeletal muscle in humans is excitatory. In contrast, many visceral targets receive both inhibitory and excitatory synapses. These antagonistic synapses arise from the two opposing divisions of the ANS, the sympathetic and the parasympathetic.

TABLE 14-1   Properties of the Sympathetic and Parasympathetic Divisions

	Sympathetic Preganglionic	Sympathetic Postganglionic	Parasympathetic Preganglionic	Parasympathetic Postganglionic
Location of neuron cell bodies	Intermediolateral cell column in the spinal cord (T1-L3)	Prevertebral and paravertebral ganglia	Brainstem and sacral spinal cord (S2-S4)	Terminal ganglia in or near target organ
Myelination	Yes	No	Yes	No
Primary neurotransmitter	Acetylcholine	Norepinephrine	Acetylcholine	Acetylcholine
Primary postsynaptic receptor	Nicotinic	Adrenergic	Nicotinic	Muscarinic

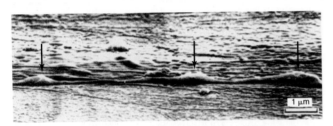

Figure 14-7 Synapses of autonomic neurons with their target organs. Many axons of postganglionic neurons make multiple points of contact (varicosities) with their targets. In this scanning electron micrograph of the axon of a postganglionic sympathetic neuron from a guinea pig grown in tissue culture, the *arrows* indicate varicosities. *(From Burnstock G: Autonomic neuromuscular junctions: Current developments and future directions. J Anat 1986; 146:1-30.)*

In organs that are stimulated during physical activity, the sympathetic division is excitatory and the parasympathetic division is inhibitory. For example, sympathetic input increases the heart rate, whereas parasympathetic input decreases it. In organs whose activity increases while the body is at rest, the opposite is true. For example, the parasympathetic division stimulates peristalsis of the gut, whereas the sympathetic division inhibits it.

Although antagonistic effects of the sympathetic and parasympathetic divisions of the ANS are the general rule for most end organs, exceptions exist. For example, the salivary glands are stimulated by both divisions, although stimulation by the sympathetic division has characteristics different from parasympathetic stimulation (see Chapter 43). In addition, some organs receive innervation from only one of these two divisions of the ANS. For example, sweat glands, piloerector muscles, and most peripheral blood vessels receive input from only the sympathetic division.

Synapses of the ANS are specialized for their function. Rather than possessing synaptic terminals that are typical of somatic motor axons, many postganglionic autonomic neurons have bulbous expansions, or **varicosities**, that are distributed along their axons within their target organ (Fig. 14-7). It was once believed that these varicosities indicated that neurotransmitter release sites of the ANS did not form close contact with end organs and that neurotransmitters needed to diffuse long distances across the extracellular space to reach their targets. However, we now recognize that

many varicosities form synapses with their targets, with a synaptic cleft extending ~50 nm across. At each varicosity, autonomic axons form an "en passant" synapse with their end-organ target. This arrangement results in an increase in the number of targets that a single axonal branch can influence, with wider distribution of autonomic output.

All preganglionic neurons—both sympathetic and parasympathetic—release acetylcholine and stimulate N_2 nicotinic receptors on postganglionic neurons

At synapses between postganglionic neurons and target cells, the two major divisions of the ANS use different neurotransmitters and receptors (Table 14-1). However, in both the sympathetic and parasympathetic divisions, synaptic transmission between preganglionic and postganglionic neurons (termed ganglionic transmission because the synapse is located in a ganglion) is mediated by **acetylcholine (ACh)** acting on nicotinic receptors (Fig. 14-8). Nicotinic receptors are ligand-gated channels (i.e., ionotropic receptors) with a pentameric structure (see Chapter 8). Table 14-2 summarizes some of the properties of nicotinic receptors. The nicotinic receptors on postganglionic autonomic neurons are a molecular subtype (N_2) different from that found at the neuromuscular junction (N_1). Both are ligand-gated ion channels activated by ACh or nicotine. However, whereas the N_1 receptors at the neuromuscular junction (see Chapter 8) are stimulated by decamethonium and preferentially blocked by *d*-tubocurarine, the autonomic N_2 receptors are stimulated by tetramethylammonium but resistant to *d*-tubocurarine. When activated, N_1 and N_2 receptors are both permeable to Na^+ and K^+. Thus, nicotinic transmission triggered by stimulation of preganglionic neurons leads to rapid depolarization of postganglionic neurons.

All postganglionic parasympathetic neurons release acetylcholine and stimulate muscarinic receptors on visceral targets

All postganglionic *para*sympathetic neurons act through muscarinic ACh receptors on the postsynaptic membrane of the target cell (Fig. 14-8). Activation of this receptor can either stimulate or inhibit function of the target cell. Cellular responses induced by muscarinic receptor stimulation are

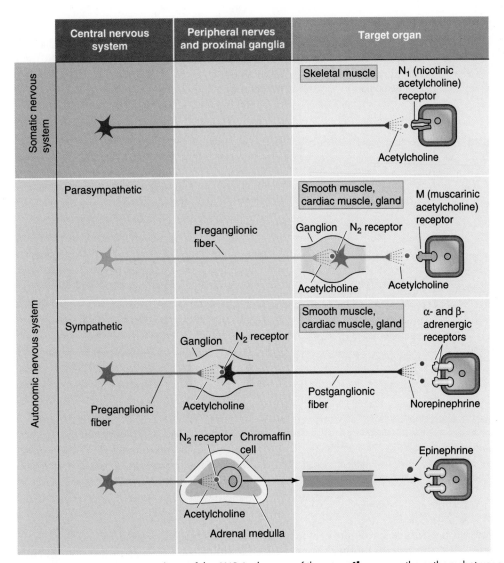

Figure 14-8 Major neurotransmitters of the ANS. In the case of the **somatic** neuron, the pathway between the CNS and effector cell is monosynaptic. The neuron releases ACh, which binds to N_1-type nicotinic receptors on the postsynaptic membrane (i.e., skeletal muscle cell). In the case of both the parasympathetic and sympathetic divisions, the preganglionic neuron releases ACh, which acts at N_2-type nicotinic receptors on the postsynaptic membrane of the postganglionic neuron. In the case of the postganglionic parasympathetic neuron, the neurotransmitter is ACh, but the postsynaptic receptor is a muscarinic receptor (i.e., GPCR) of one of five subtypes (M_1 to M_5). In the case of most postganglionic sympathetic neurons, the neurotransmitter is norepinephrine. The postsynaptic receptor is an adrenergic receptor (i.e., GPCR) of one of two major subtypes (α and β).

more varied than are those induced by nicotinic receptors. Muscarinic receptors are G protein–coupled receptors (GPCRs; see p. 52)—also known as metabotropic receptors—that (1) stimulate the hydrolysis of phosphoinositide and thus increase $[Ca^{2+}]_i$ and activate protein kinase C, (2) inhibit adenylyl cyclase and thus decrease cyclic adenosine monophosphate (cAMP) levels, or (3) directly modulate K^+ channels through the G protein $\beta\gamma$ complex. Because they are mediated by second messengers, muscarinic responses, unlike the rapid responses evoked by nicotine receptors, are slow and prolonged.

Muscarinic receptors exist in five different pharmacological subtypes (M_1 to M_5) that are encoded by five different genes. All five subtypes are highly homologous to each other but very different from the nicotinic receptors, which are ligand-gated ion channels. Subtypes M_1 to M_5 are each stimulated by ACh and muscarine and are blocked by atropine. These muscarinic subtypes have a heterogeneous distribution among tissues, and in many cases a given cell may express more than one subtype. Although a wide variety of *antagonists* inhibit the muscarinic receptors, none is completely selective for a specific subtype. However, it is possible

TABLE 14-2 Signaling Pathways for Nicotinic, Muscarinic, Adrenergic, and Dopaminergic Receptors

Receptor Type	Agonists*	Antagonists	G Protein	Linked Enzyme	Second Messenger
N_1 nicotinic ACh	ACh (nicotine, decamethonium)	d-Tubocurarine, α-bungarotoxin	—	—	—
N_2 nicotinic ACh	ACh (nicotine, TMA)	Hexamethonium	—	—	—
M_1, M_3, M_5 muscarinic ACh	ACh (muscarine)	Atropine, pirenzepine (M_1)	$G\alpha_q$	PLC	IP_3 and DAG
M_2, M_4 muscarinic ACh	ACh (muscarine)	Atropine, methoctramine (M_2)	$G\alpha_i$ and $G\alpha_o$	Adenylyl cyclase	↓ $[cAMP]_i$
α_1-Adrenergic	NE ≥ Epi (phenylephrine)	Phentolamine	$G\alpha_q$	PLC	IP_3 and DAG
α_2-Adrenergic	NE ≥ Epi (clonidine)	Yohimbine	$G\alpha_i$	Adenylyl cylase	↓ $[cAMP]_i$
β_1-Adrenergic	Epi > NE (dobutamine, isoproterenol)	Metoprolol	$G\alpha_s$	Adenylyl cyclase	↑ $[cAMP]_i$
β_2-Adrenergic	Epi > NE (terbutaline, isoproterenol)	Butoxamine	$G\alpha_s$	Adenylyl cyclase	↑ $[cAMP]_i$
β_3-Adrenergic	Epi > NE (isoproterenol)	SR-59230A	$G\alpha_s$	Adenylyl cyclase	↑ $[cAMP]_i$
D_1	Dopamine		$G\alpha_s$	Adenylyl cyclase	↑ $[cAMP]_i$
D_2	Dopamine		$G\alpha_i$	Adenylyl cyclase	↓ $[cAMP]_i$

*Selective agonists are in parentheses.

ACh, acetylcholine; cAMP, cyclic adenosine monophosphate; DAG, diacylglycerol; Epi, epinephrine; IP_3, inositol 1,4,5-trisphosphate; NE, norepinephrine; PLC, phospholipase C; TMA, tetramethylammonium.

to classify a receptor on the basis of its affinity profile for a battery of antagonists. Selective *agonists* for the different isoforms have not been available.

A molecular characteristic of the muscarinic receptors is that the third cytoplasmic loop (i.e., between the fifth and sixth membrane-spanning segments) is different in M_1, M_3, and M_5 on the one hand and M_2 and M_4 on the other. This loop appears to play a role in coupling of the receptor to the G protein downstream in the signal transduction cascade. In general M_1, M_3, and M_5 preferentially couple to $G\alpha_q$ and then to phospholipase C, with release of IP_3 and diacylglycerol. On the other hand, M_2 and M_4 preferentially couple to $G\alpha_i$ or $G\alpha_o$ to inhibit adenylyl cyclase and thus decrease $[cAMP]_i$ (see Chapter 3).

Most postganglionic sympathetic neurons release norepinephrine onto visceral targets

Most postganglionic sympathetic neurons release **norepinephrine** (Fig. 14-8), which acts on target cells through adrenergic receptors. The sympathetic innervation of sweat glands is an exception to this rule. Sweat glands are innervated by sympathetic neurons that release ACh and act through muscarinic receptors. The adrenergic receptors are all GPCRs and are highly homologous to the muscarinic receptors (see Chapter 24). Two major types of adrenergic

receptor are recognized, α and β, each of which exists in multiple subtypes (e.g., α_1, α_2, β_1, β_2, and β_3). In addition, there are heterogeneous α_1 and α_2 receptors, with three cloned subtypes of each. Table 14-2 lists the signaling pathways that are generally linked to these receptors. For example, β_1 receptors in the heart activate the G_s heterotrimeric G protein and stimulate adenylyl cyclase, which antagonizes the effects of muscarinic receptors.

Adrenergic receptor subtypes have a tissue-specific distribution. α_1 Receptors predominate on blood vessels, α_2 on presynaptic terminals, β_1 in the heart, β_2 in high concentration in the bronchial muscle of the lungs, and β_3 in fat cells. This distribution has permitted the development of many clinically useful agents that are selective for different subtypes and tissues. For example, α_1 agonists are effective as nasal decongestants, and α_2 antagonists have been used to treat impotence. β_1 Agonists increase cardiac output in congestive heart failure, whereas β_1 antagonists are useful antihypertensive agents. β_2 Agonists are used as bronchodilators in patients with asthma and chronic lung disease.

The adrenal medulla (see Chapter 50) is a special adaptation of the sympathetic division, homologous to a sympathetic ganglion (Fig. 14-8). It is innervated by preganglionic sympathetic neurons, and the postsynaptic target cells, which are called **chromaffin cells**, are analogous to postganglionic sympathetic neurons. Thus, chromaffin cells have nicotinic ACh receptors. However, rather than possessing axons that release norepinephrine onto a specific target organ, the chromaffin cells reside near blood vessels and release **epinephrine** into the bloodstream. This neuroendocrine component of sympathetic output enhances the ability of the sympathetic division to broadcast its output throughout the body. Norepinephrine and epinephrine both activate all five subtypes of adrenergic receptor, but with different affinities (Table 14-2). In general, the α receptors have a greater affinity for norepinephrine, whereas the β receptors have a greater affinity for epinephrine.

Postganglionic sympathetic and parasympathetic neurons often have muscarinic as well as nicotinic receptors

The simplified scheme described in the preceding discussion is very useful for understanding the function of the ANS. However, two additional layers of complexity are superimposed on this scheme. First, some postganglionic neurons, both sympathetic and parasympathetic, have *muscarinic* in addition to nicotinic receptors. Second, at all levels of the ANS, certain neurotransmitters and postsynaptic receptors are neither cholinergic nor adrenergic. We discuss the first exception in this section and the second in the following section.

If we stimulate the release of ACh from preganglionic neurons or apply ACh to an autonomic ganglion, many postganglionic neurons exhibit both nicotinic and muscarinic responses. Because *nicotinic receptors* (N_2) are ligand-gated ion channels, nicotinic neurotransmission causes a fast, monophasic excitatory postsynaptic potential (EPSP). In contrast, because *muscarinic receptors* are GPCRs, neurotransmission by this route leads to a slower electrical response that can be either inhibitory or excitatory. Thus, depending on the ganglion, the result is a multiphasic postsynaptic response that can be a combination of a fast EPSP through a nicotinic receptor plus either a slow EPSP or a slow inhibitory postsynaptic potential (IPSP) through a muscarinic receptor. Figure 14-9A shows a fast EPSP followed by a slow EPSP.

A well-characterized effect of muscarinic neurotransmission in autonomic ganglia is inhibition of a specific K^+ current called the **M current**. The M current is widely distributed in visceral end organs, autonomic ganglia, and the CNS. In the baseline state, the K^+ channel that underlies the M current is active, thereby producing slight hyperpolarization. In the example shown in Figure 14-9B, with the stabilizing M current present, electrical stimulation of the neuron causes only a single spike. If we now add muscarine to the neuron, activation of the muscarinic receptor turns off the hyperpolarizing M current and thus leads to a small depolarization. If we repeat the electrical stimulation in the continued presence of muscarine (Fig. 14-9C), repetitive spikes appear because loss of the stabilizing influence of the M current increases the excitability of the neuron. The slow, modulatory effects of muscarinic responses greatly enhance the ability of the ANS to control visceral activity beyond what could be accomplished with only fast nicotinic EPSPs.

Nonclassic transmitters can be released at each level of the ANS

In the 1930s, Sir Henry Dale first proposed that sympathetic nerves release a transmitter similar to epinephrine (now known to be norepinephrine) and parasympathetic nerves release ACh. For many years, attention was focused on these two neurotransmitters, primarily because they mediate large and fast postsynaptic responses that can be easily studied. In addition, a variety of antagonists are available to block cholinergic and adrenergic receptors and thereby permit clear characterization of the roles of these receptors in the control of visceral function. More recently, it has become evident that some neurotransmission in the ANS involves neither adrenergic nor cholinergic pathways. Moreover, many neuronal synapses use more than a single neurotransmitter. Such **cotransmission** is now known to be common in the ANS. As many as eight different neurotransmitters may be found within some neurons, a phenomenon known as **co-localization** (see Table 13-1). Thus, ACh and norepinephrine play important but not exclusive roles in autonomic control.

The distribution and function of nonadrenergic, noncholinergic transmitters are only partially understood. However, these transmitters are found at every level of autonomic control (Table 14-3), where they can cause a wide range of postsynaptic responses. These nonclassic transmitters may cause slow synaptic potentials or may modulate the response to other inputs (as in the case of the M current) without having obvious direct effects. In other cases, nonclassic transmitters have no known effects and may be acting in ways that have not been determined.

Although co-localization of neurotransmitters is recognized as a common property of neurons, it is not clear what controls the release of each of the many neurotransmitters. In some cases, the proportion of neurotransmitters released depends on the level of neuronal activity (see Chapter 13). For example, medullary raphe neurons project to the intermediolateral cell column in the spinal cord, where they co-release serotonin, thyrotropin-releasing hormone, and substance P onto sympathetic preganglionic neurons. The proportions of released neurotransmitters are controlled by neuronal firing frequency: at low firing rates, 5-hydroxytryptamine is released alone; at intermediate firing rates, thyrotropin-releasing hormone is also released; and at high firing rates, all three neurotransmitters are released. This frequency-dependent modulation of synaptic transmission provides a mechanism for enhancing the versatility of the ANS.

Two of the most unusual nonclassic neurotransmitters, adenosine triphosphate and nitric oxide, were first identified in the autonomic nervous system

It was not until the 1970s that a nonadrenergic, noncholinergic class of *sympathetic* or *parasympathetic* neurons was first proposed by Geoffrey Burnstock and colleagues, who suggested that adenosine triphosphate (ATP) might act as the neurotransmitter. This idea, that a molecule used as an intracellular energy substrate could also be a synaptic

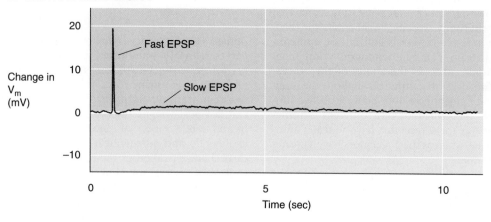

A FAST AND SLOW EPSPs

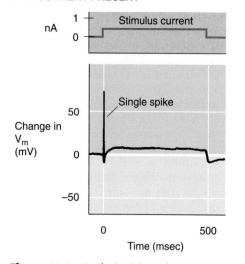

B M CURRENT PRESENT

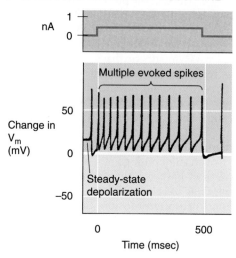

C M CURRENT INHIBITED BY MUSCARINE

Figure 14-9 Dual nicotinic and muscarinic neurotransmission between sympathetic preganglionic and postganglionic neurons. **A,** Stimulation of a frog preganglionic sympathetic neuron releases ACh, which triggers a fast EPSP (due to activation of *nicotinic* receptors on the postganglionic sympathetic neuron), followed by a slow EPSP (due to activation of *muscarinic* receptors on the postganglionic neuron). **B,** The M current (mediated by a K^+ channel) normally hyperpolarizes this rat sympathetic postganglionic neuron, thereby inhibiting trains of action potentials. Thus, injection of current elicits only a single action potential. **C,** In the same experiment as that in **B,** the addition of muscarine stimulates a muscarinic receptor (i.e., GPCR) and triggers a signal transduction cascade that blocks the M current. One result is a steady-state depolarization of the cell. In addition, injection of current now elicits a train of action potentials. (**A,** Data from Adams PR, Brown DA: Synaptic inhibition of the M-current: Slow excitatory post-synaptic potential mechanism in bullfrog sympathetic neurones. J Physiol 1982; 332:263-272. **B** and **C,** Data from Brown DA, Constanti A: Intracellular observations on the effects of muscarinic agonists on rat sympathetic neurones. Br J Pharmacol 1980; 70:593-608.)

transmitter, was initially difficult to prove. However, it is now clear that neurons use a variety of classes of molecules for intercellular communication (see Chapter 13). Two of the most surprising examples of nonclassic transmitters, nitric oxide (NO) and ATP, were first identified and studied as neurotransmitters in the ANS, but they are now known to be more widely used throughout the nervous system.

Adenosine Triphosphate ATP is co-localized with norepinephrine in postganglionic sympathetic vasoconstrictor neurons. It is contained in synaptic vesicles, is released on electrical stimulation, and induces vascular constriction when it is applied directly to vascular smooth muscle. The effect of ATP results from activation of P_2 **purinoceptors** on smooth muscle, which include ligand-gated ion channels (P_{2X}) and GPCRs (P_{2Y} and P_{2U}). P_{2X} receptors are present on autonomic neurons and smooth muscle cells of blood vessels, the urinary bladder, and other visceral targets. P_{2X} receptor channels have a relatively high Ca^{2+} permeability (see Chapter 13). In smooth muscle, ATP-induced depolarization can also activate voltage-gated Ca^{2+} channels (see Chapter 7) and thus lead to an elevation in $[Ca^{2+}]_i$ and a rapid phase of contraction (Fig. 14-10). Norepinephrine, by binding to α_1-adrenergic receptors, acts through a heterotrimeric G protein (see Chapter 3) to facilitate the release of Ca^{2+} from intracellular stores and thereby produce a slower phase of contrac-

TABLE 14-3 Neurotransmitters Present Within the Autonomic Nervous System

	CNS Neurons	Preganglionic Autonomic	Postganglionic Autonomic	Visceral Afferent	Ganglion Interneurons	Enteric Neurons
Acetylcholine		X	X			
Monoamines						
Norepinephrine	X		X			X
Epinephrine						
5-Hydroxytryptamine	X					X
Dopamine					X	X
Amino acids						
Glutamate	X					
Glycine	X					
GABA						X
Neuropeptides						
Substance P	X	X		X	X	X
Thyrotropin-releasing hormone	X			X		X
Enkephalins	X					X
Neuropeptide Y	X		X			X
Neurotensin	X					X
Neurophysin II	X					X
Oxytocin	X					X
Somatostatin	X		X			X
Calcitonin gene–related peptide						X
Galanin		X	X			X
Vasoactive intestinal polypeptide			X			X
Opioids?			X			X
Tachykinins (substance P, neurokinin A, neuropeptide K, neuropeptide γ)						
Cholecystokinin						
Gastrin-releasing peptide						
Dynorphin						
Nonclassical			X			X
Nitric oxide			X			X
ATP						

tion. Finally, the release of neuropeptide Y may, after prolonged and intense stimulation, elicit a third component of contraction.

Nitric Oxide   In the 1970s, it was also discovered that the vascular endothelium produces a substance that induces relaxation of vascular smooth muscle. First called endothelium-derived relaxation factor, it was identified as the free radical NO in 1987. NO is an unusual molecule for intercellular communication because it is a short-lived gas. It is produced locally from L-arginine by the enzyme nitric oxide synthase (NOS; see Chapter 3). The NO then diffuses a short distance to a neighboring cell, where its effects are primarily mediated by the activation of guanylyl cyclase.

NOS is found in the preganglionic and postganglionic neurons of both the sympathetic and parasympathetic divisions as well as in vascular endothelial cells. It is not specific for any type of neuron inasmuch as it is found in both norepinephrine- and ACh-containing cells as well as in neurons containing a variety of neuropeptides. Figure 14-11 shows how a parasympathetic neuron may simultaneously release NO, ACh, and vasoactive intestinal polypeptide, each acting in concert to lower [Ca^{2+}]$_i$ and to relax vascular smooth muscle. Why NO is so ubiquitous and when its release is important are not known. However, evidence now indicates that abnormalities of the NO system are involved in the pathophysiological processes of adult respiratory distress syndrome, high-altitude pulmonary edema, stroke, and other diseases. Understanding of its physiological and pathophysiological roles has led to the introduction of clinical treatments that modulate the NO system. Examples include the use of gaseous NO for treatment of pulmonary edema, NO generators such as nitroglycerin for treatment of angina, and cGMP phosphodiesterase inhibitors such as sildenafil (Viagra) for treatment of erectile dysfunction.

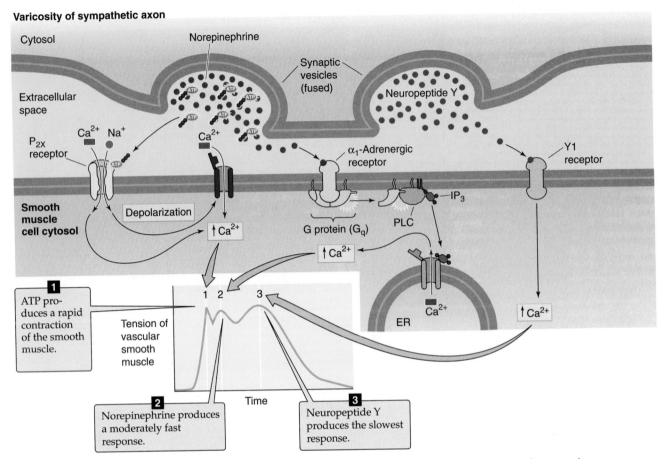

Figure 14-10 Cotransmission with ATP, norepinephrine, and neuropeptide Y in the ANS. In this example, stimulation of a postganglionic sympathetic neuron causes three phases of contraction of a vascular smooth muscle cell. Each phase corresponds to the release of a different neurotransmitter or group of transmitters. In phase 1, ATP binds to a P_{2X} purinoceptor (a ligand-gated cation channel) on the smooth muscle cell, leading to depolarization, activation of voltage-gated Ca^{2+} channels, increased $[Ca^{2+}]_i$, and the rapid phase of contraction. In phase 2, norepinephrine binds to an α_1-adrenergic receptor, which—through a G_q/PLC/IP_3 cascade, leads to Ca^{2+} release from internal stores and the second phase of contraction. In phase 3, when it is present, neuropeptide Y binds to a Y_1 receptor and somehow causes an increase in $[Ca^{2+}]_i$ and thus produces the slowest phase of contraction. ER, endoplasmic reticulum; IP_3, inositol 1,4,5-trisphosphate; PLC, phospolipase C.

CNS CONTROL OF THE VISCERA

Sympathetic output can be massive and nonspecific, as in the fight-or-flight response, or selective for specific target organs

In 1915, Walter Cannon proposed that the entire sympathetic division is activated together and has a uniform effect on all target organs. In response to fear, exercise, and other types of stress, the sympathetic division produces a massive and coordinated output to all end organs simultaneously, and parasympathetic output ceases. This type of sympathetic output is used to ready the body for life-threatening situations—the so-called **fight-or-flight** response. Thus, when a person is presented a fearful or menacing stimulus, the sympathetic division coordinates all body functions to respond appropriately to the stressful situation. This response includes increases in heart rate, cardiac contractility, blood pressure, and ventilation of the lungs; bronchial dilatation; sweating; piloerection; liberation of glucose into the blood; inhibition of insulin secretion; reduction in blood clotting time; mobilization of blood cells by contraction of the spleen; and decreased gastrointestinal activity. This mass response is a primitive mechanism for survival. In some people, such a response can be triggered spontaneously or with minimal provocation; each individual episode is then called a panic attack.

The fight-or-flight response is an important mechanism for survival, but under normal nonstressful conditions, output of the sympathetic division can also be more discrete and organ specific. In contrast to Cannon's original proposal, the sympathetic division does not actually produce uniform effects on all visceral targets. Different postganglionic sympathetic neurons have different electrophysiological proper-

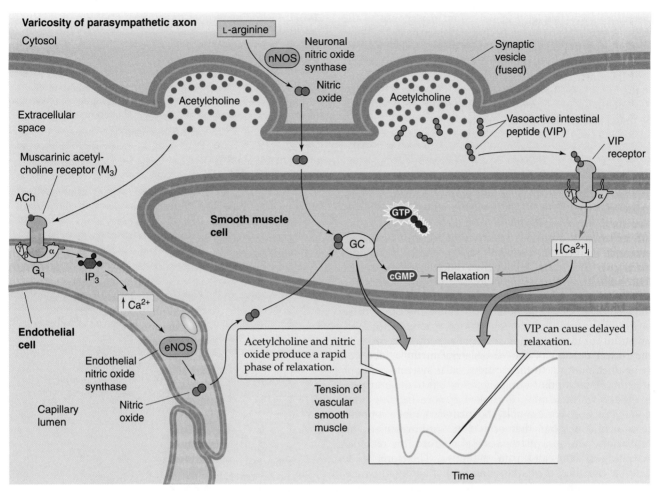

Figure 14-11   Action of NO in the ANS. Stimulation of a postganglionic parasympathetic neuron can cause more than one phase of relaxation of a vascular smooth muscle cell, corresponding to the release of a different neurotransmitter or group of transmitters. The first phase in this example is mediated by both NO and ACh. The neuron releases NO, which diffuses to the smooth muscle cell. In addition, ACh binds to M_3 muscarinic receptors (i.e., GPCR) on endothelial cells, leading to production of NO, which also diffuses to the smooth muscle cell. Both sources of NO activate guanylyl cyclase and raise $[cGMP]_i$ in the smooth muscle cell and contribute to the first phase of relaxation. In the second phase, which tends to occur more with prolonged or intense stimulation, the neuropeptide VIP (or a related peptide) binds to receptors on the smooth muscle cell and causes a delayed relaxation through an increase in $[cAMP]_i$ or a decrease in $[Ca^{2+}]_i$. cGMP, cyclic guanosine monophosphate; GC, guanylyl cyclase; VIP, vasoactive intestinal polypeptide.

ties and, in addition to norepinephrine, release other neurotransmitters. This specific distribution of neuroactive chemicals among neurons is called chemical coding. For example, depolarization of guinea pig postganglionic sympathetic neurons in the *lumbar* sympathetic chain ganglia causes a *brief* burst of action potentials in 95% of the neurons and release of norepinephrine together with ATP and neuropeptide Y. These neurons are thought to innervate arteries and to induce vasoconstriction (Fig. 14-10). In contrast, depolarization of postganglionic sympathetic neurons in the *inferior mesenteric ganglion* causes sustained firing in 80% of the neurons and release of norepinephrine together with somatostatin. These neurons appear to control gut motility and secretion. Thus, sympathetic neurons have cellular properties that are substantially variable. This variability

permits the sympathetic division to produce different effects on targets with different functions.

Parasympathetic neurons participate in many simple involuntary reflexes

As opposed to the sympathetic division, neurons in the parasympathetic division function only in a discrete, organ-specific, and reflexive manner. Together with specific visceral afferents and a small number of interneurons, parasympathetic neurons mediate simple reflexes involving target organs. For example, the output for the baroreceptor reflex (see Chapter 23) is mediated by preganglionic parasympathetic neurons in the dorsal motor nucleus of the vagus. Other examples include urination in response to bladder distention (see Chapter 33); salivation in response to the sight or smell of food (see Chapter 43); vagovagal reflexes (see Chapter 41) in the gastrointestinal tract, such as contraction of the colon in response to food in the stomach; and bronchoconstriction in response to activation of receptors in the lungs (see Chapter 32). The pupillary light reflex is an example of an involuntary parasympathetic reflex that can be tested at the bedside (see Chapter 15).

A variety of brainstem nuclei provide basic control of the autonomic nervous system

In addition to nuclei that contain parasympathetic preganglionic neurons (Fig. 14-5), a variety of other brainstem structures are also involved in visceral control. These structures include the nucleus tractus solitarii, area postrema, ventrolateral medulla, medullary raphe, reticular formation, locus coeruleus, and parabrachial nucleus. These nuclei within the lower part of the brainstem mediate autonomic reflexes, control specific autonomic functions, or modulate the general level of autonomic tone. In some cases, these nuclei play a well-defined role in one specific autonomic function. For example, stimulation of a group of neurons in the rostral portion of the ventrolateral medulla increases sympathetic output to the cardiovascular system—without affecting respiration or sympathetic output to other targets. In other cases, these nuclei are linked to more than one autonomic function. For example, the medullary raphe contains serotonergic neurons that project to cardiovascular and respiratory neurons, gastrointestinal neurons, the reticular activating system, and pain pathways. Therefore, these neurons can affect the background level of autonomic tone. The specific functions of some nuclei are not known, and their involvement in autonomic control is inferred from their anatomical connections, a correlation between neuron activity and activity in autonomic nerves, or the effect of lesions.

One of the most important lower brainstem structures is the **nucleus tractus solitarii (NTS)** in the medulla. The NTS contains second-order sensory neurons that receive all peripheral chemoreceptor (see Chapter 32) and baroreceptor input (see Chapter 23) as well as non-nociceptive afferent input from every organ of the thorax and abdomen. Visceral afferents from the vagus nerve make their first synapse within the NTS, where they combine with other afferent impulses derived from the glossopharyngeal (CN IX), facial (CN VII), and trigeminal (CN V) nerves. These visceral afferents form a large bundle of nerve fibers—the **tractus solitarius**—that the NTS surrounds. Afferent input is distributed to the NTS in a viscerotopic manner, with major subnuclei devoted to respiratory, cardiovascular, gustatory, and gastrointestinal input. The NTS also receives input and sends output to many other CNS regions (Table 14-4), including the brainstem nuclei described earlier as well as the hypothalamus and the forebrain. These widespread interconnections allow the NTS to influence and to be influenced by a wide variety of CNS functions. Thus, the NTS is the major lower brainstem command center for visceral control. It integrates multiple input from visceral afferents and exerts control over autonomic output, thereby participating in autonomic reflexes that maintain the homeostasis of many basic visceral functions.

TABLE 14-4 Connections to and from the Nucleus Tractus Solitarii

Receives input from
Vagus nerve (peripheral chemoreceptor/aortic bodies and aortic baroreceptor, as well as non-nociceptive afferent input from every organ of the thorax and abdomen)
Glossopharyngeal nerve (taste and peripheral chemoreceptors/carotid bodies, carotid baroreceptor)
Facial nerve (taste)
Trigeminal nerve (teeth, sinuses)
Ventrolateral medulla
Medullary raphe
Area postrema
Periaqueductal gray
Parabrachial nucleus
Hypothalamus
Cerebral cortex

Sends output to
Intermediolateral cell column (preganglionic sympathetic neurons) and sacral parasympathetic neurons
Phrenic motor nucleus and other respiratory output pathways
Dorsal motor nucleus of the vagus (preganglionic parasympathetic neurons from the vagus nerve)
Nucleus ambiguus (preganglionic parasympathetic neurons from the vagus nerve)
Ventrolateral medulla
Medullary raphe
Area postrema
Parabrachial nuclei
Reticular formation
Forebrain nuclei
Hypothalamus

The forebrain can modulate autonomic output, and reciprocally, visceral sensory input integrated in the brainstem can influence or even overwhelm the forebrain

Only a subset of the nervous system is necessary to maintain autonomic body homeostasis under most conditions. The necessary structures include (1) the brainstem nuclei discussed in the preceding section, (2) the brainstem nuclei that contain the parasympathetic preganglionic neurons, (3) the spinal cord, and (4) the peripheral ANS. These components are capable of acting autonomously, even without input from higher (i.e., rostral) forebrain regions. However, forebrain regions do play a role in coordinating and modulating activity in the lower centers. Many rostral CNS centers influence autonomic output; these centers include the hypothalamus, amygdala, prefrontal cortex, entorhinal cortex, insula, and other forebrain nuclei.

The **hypothalamus**, especially the paraventricular nucleus, is the most important brain region for coordination of autonomic output. The hypothalamus projects to the parabrachial nucleus, medullary raphe, NTS, central gray matter, locus coeruleus, dorsal motor nucleus of the vagus, nucleus

TABLE 14-5 Interactions Between Cortical and Autonomic Function

Examples of descending cortical control of autonomic output
Fear: initiates fight-or-flight response
Panic attacks: initiate spontaneous fight-or-flight response
Emotional stress (e.g., first day in gross anatomy laboratory) or painful stimuli: lead to massive vasodilation and hypotension, i.e., vasovagal syncope (fainting)
Seizures: can induce sudden cardiac death from massive sympathetic output and arrhythmias
Chronic stress: can lead to peptic ulcers from increased gastric acid secretion
Sleep deprivation: in rats leads to death from loss of thermoregulation and cardiovascular control
Cognitive activity: can initiate sexual arousal
Nervousness (e.g., before an examination) can lead to diarrhea

Examples in which visceral afferents overwhelm cortical function (i.e., nothing else seems to matter)
Hunger
Nausea
Dyspnea
Visceral pain
Bladder and bowel distention
Hypothermia, hyperthermia

ambiguus, and intermediolateral cell column of the spinal cord. Thus, the hypothalamus can initiate and coordinate an integrated response to the body's needs, including modulation of autonomic output as well as control of neuroendocrine function by the pituitary gland (see Chapter 47). The hypothalamus coordinates autonomic function with feeding, thermoregulation, circadian rhythms, water balance, emotions, sexual drive, reproduction, motivation, and other brain functions and thus plays a dominant role in the integration of higher cortical and limbic systems with autonomic control. The hypothalamus can also initiate the fight-or-flight response.

The hypothalamus often mediates interactions between the forebrain and the brainstem. However, a number of forebrain regions also have direct connections to brainstem nuclei involved in autonomic control. Most of these forebrain regions are part of the **limbic system** rather than the neocortex. The paucity of direct neocortical connections probably explains why individuals trained to control autonomic output by biofeedback can generally produce only relatively minor effects on overall autonomic activity rather than regulate output to specific organs. Most individuals are incapable of even limited cortical control over the ANS. However, even though we may have only minimal *conscious* control of autonomic output, cortical processes can strongly modulate the ANS. Emotions, mood, anxiety, stress, and fear can all alter autonomic output (Table 14-5). The pathways for these effects are unknown, but they could be mediated by direct connections or through the hypothalamus.

Not only does forebrain function influence the ANS, visceral activity also influences forebrain function. Visceral afferents reach the neocortex. However, because these afferents are not represented viscerotopically, they cannot be well localized. Nevertheless, visceral afferents can have profound effects on cortical function. Visceral input can modulate the excitability of cortical neurons (see the box titled Vagus Nerve Stimulation in the Treatment of Epilepsy) and, in some cases, can result in such overpowering sensory stimuli that it is not possible to focus cortical activity on any other purpose (Table 14-5).

CNS control centers oversee visceral feedback loops and orchestrate a feedforward response to meet anticipated needs

The ANS maintains physiological parameters within an optimal range by means of **feedback loops** made up of sensors, afferent fibers, central autonomic control centers (discussed in the preceding section), and effector systems. These feedback loops achieve homeostasis by monitoring input from visceral receptors and adjusting the output of both the sympathetic and parasympathetic divisions to specific organs so that they maintain activity at a set-point determined by involuntary CNS control centers. As we have already noted, the sympathetic and parasympathetic divisions usually act in opposite ways to make these adjustments. Blood pressure control is an example of a visceral feedback loop in which the CNS monitors current blood pressure through afferents from baroreceptors, compares it with an internally determined set-point, and appropriately adjusts output to the heart, blood vessels, adrenal gland, and other targets. An increase in blood pressure (see Chapter 23) causes a reflex decrease in sympathetic output to the heart and an increase in parasympathetic output.

Instead of merely responding through feedback loops, the ANS also anticipates the future needs of the individual. For example, when a person begins to exercise, sympathetic output increases before the increase in metabolic need to prevent an exercise debt from occurring (see Chapter 60). Because of this anticipatory response, alveolar ventilation rises to such an extent that blood levels of CO_2 (a byproduct of exercise) actually drop at the onset of exercise. This response is the opposite of what would be expected if the ANS worked purely through feedback loops, in which case an obligatory increase in CO_2 levels would have preceded the increase in respiratory output (see Chapter 32). Similarly, a trained athlete's heart rate begins to increase several seconds before the starting gun fires to signal the beginning of a 100-meter dash. This anticipation of future activity, or **feedforward** stimulation during exercise, is a key component of the regulation of homeostasis during stress because it prevents large changes in physiological parameters that could be detrimental to optimal function. This type of response probably resulted in an evolutionary advantage that permitted the body to respond rapidly and more efficiently to a threat of danger. A system relying solely on feedback could produce a response that is delayed or out of phase with respect to the stimulus. The central neuronal pathways responsible for this anticipatory or feedforward response are not known.

Vagus Nerve Stimulation in the Treatment of Epilepsy

It is often not appreciated just how much effect the ANS can have on cortical function. Table 14-5 lists several examples in which strong input from visceral afferents can overwhelm cortical function, to the point that concentrating on anything else is nearly impossible. As we have already noted, not only does the vagus nerve contain parasympathetic preganglionic *motor* fibers, it also contains a wide variety of *sensory* fibers from viscera in the thorax and abdomen. Discovery of the influence of vagal afferent input on seizures has led to development of the vagus nerve stimulator, which is used clinically. The surgically implanted device electrically stimulates the vagus nerve for 30 seconds every 5 minutes, 24 hours per day. In addition, when patients feel a seizure coming on (an aura), they can activate the device with a hand-held magnet to deliver extra pulses. Clinical studies have shown that this treatment reduces the number of seizures by about half in about one in four patients. It remains to be determined whether a subgroup of patients may be particularly responsive to this treatment. Side effects include hoarseness, coughing, and breathlessness. That this approach works at all indicates how important visceral input is to cortical function. Vagal input can influence many rostral brain structures, but it is not yet clear whether stimulation of peripheral chemoreceptor afferents, pulmonary afferents, or other visceral afferent pathways is important for the anticonvulsant effect. If the specific pathways could be identified, it might be possible to selectively stimulate these pathways or to activate them pharmacologically to produce an anticonvulsant effect with fewer side effects.

The autonomic nervous system has multiple levels of reflex loops

The human nervous system is built in a hierarchy that mirrors phylogenetic evolution (see Chapter 10). Each of the successively more primitive components is capable of independent, organized, and adaptive behavior. In turn, the activity of each of the more primitive levels is modulated by rostral, more phylogenetically advanced components.

The **enteric nervous system** of humans is homologous to the most primitive nervous system, the neural net of jellyfish. In both cases, the component neurons control motility and nutrient absorption and respond appropriately to external stimuli.

The **autonomic ganglia** are homologous to ganglionic nervous systems, such as those of annelid worms. Autonomic ganglia were previously considered a simple relay station for signals from the CNS to the periphery, but it is now clear that they integrate afferent input from the viscera and have substantial independent control mechanisms. The largest of the sympathetic ganglia, the superior cervical ganglion, contains about 1 million neurons. In addition to postganglionic cell bodies, autonomic ganglia also contain interneurons. Axons from interneurons, sensory receptors located in the end organs, and preganglionic neurons converge with postganglionic neuron dendrites to form a dense network of

Crosstalk Between Autonomic Functions Can Be Pathological

Visceral control of each of the body's organs occurs relatively independently of the others. However, some overlap in control systems can be noted for different components of the ANS. For example, stimulation of the baroreceptors causes inhibition of respiration. Conversely, the decrease in thoracic pressure that occurs during inspiration normally triggers a reflex decrease in heart rate. Many neurons in the brainstem and spinal cord have a firing pattern that is modulated in time with both the heartbeat and respiratory activity. This spillover may be responsible for the frequent observation of **sinus arrhythmia** on electrocardiograms of normal patients, whereby the heart rate is irregular because of an exaggeration of the normal influence of respiration on heart rate. These phenomena have no clear evolutionary advantage. Instead, they may simply be due to an error in separating closely related physiological control mechanisms.

In some cases, overlap between physiological control mechanisms can have serious consequences. For example, control of micturition overlaps with cardiorespiratory control. An increase in bladder pressure can lead to apnea and hypertension. Conversely, each breath is accompanied by an increase in neural outflow to the bladder. In patients with obstruction of urinary outflow, as can be seen in men with enlarged prostates, the bladder can become severely distended. If this obstruction is relieved suddenly by insertion of a catheter and the bladder is drained too rapidly, blood pressure can drop precipitously. In extreme cases, the hypotension causes syncope (fainting) or a stroke. A similar phenomenon can occur in some people with less provocation. During emptying of a relatively full bladder, blood pressure can drop precipitously and lead to **postmicturition syncope**, with the patient suddenly falling unconscious on the bathroom floor.

nerve fibers, or a **neuropil**, within the ganglion. This neuropil confers considerable computational capability on the ganglia. As opposed to feedback from skeletal muscle, which occurs only in the CNS, the peripheral synapses of visceral afferents result in substantial integration of autonomic activity at peripheral sites. This integration is enhanced by the variety of neurotransmitters released, for example, by interneurons in autonomic ganglia (Table 14-3). Thus, although fast neurotransmission from preganglionic neurons to postganglionic neurons is an important role of the autonomic ganglia, the ganglia are not simply relays.

The **spinal cord**, which coordinates activity among different root levels, first appeared with the evolution of chordates. The CNS of amphioxus, a primitive chordate, is essentially just a spinal cord. In humans who suffer transection of the low cervical spinal cord—and in whom the outflow of the respiratory system is spared (see Chapter 32)—the caudal spinal cord and lower autonomic ganglia can still continue to maintain homeostasis. However, these individuals are incapable of more complex responses that require reflexes mediated by the cranial nerve afferents and cranial parasympathetic outflow. In many patients, this

Horner Syndrome

One of the keys to neurological diagnosis has always been neuroanatomical localization (Fig. 14-12). A classic condition in which it is important to define neuroanatomy is **Horner syndrome**: the combination of unilateral **ptosis** (drooping eyelid), **miosis** (small pupil), and **anhidrosis** (lack of sweating). Sympathetic neurons innervate the smooth muscle that elevates the eyelid, the pupillary dilator muscle, and the sweat glands of the face. Horner syndrome results from loss of the normal sympathetic innervation on one side of the face. The differential diagnosis of this syndrome is large, but it can be narrowed if the site of involvement of the sympathetic pathways can be identified. Involvement of *first-order sympathetic neurons* can occur at their cell bodies in the hypothalamus or along their axons traveling down to the ipsilateral intermediolateral column of the spinal cord. Thus, a first-order Horner syndrome can be due to ischemia of the lateral medulla (e.g., occlusion of the posterior inferior cerebellar artery, the so-called Wallenberg syndrome). In this case, other brainstem abnormalities will also be present. The *second-order sympathetic neurons,* or *pre*ganglionic neurons, can be affected at their origin in the intermediolateral column or along their axons. Those that supply the eye synapse in the superior cervical ganglion. A second-order Horner syndrome can be the first sign that a Pancoast tumor exists in the apex of the lung and is encroaching on the sympathetic nerves as they travel to the superior cervical ganglion. Finally, *third-order sympathetic neurons,* or *post*ganglionic neurons, can be involved at the ganglion or along their course to the eye. Because they travel within the wall of the carotid artery, these sympathetic nerves can be damaged during a carotid artery "dissection." Dissection is damage to the wall of the artery, often caused by a neck injury. In time, the damage to the vessel can lead to a blood clot that will obstruct blood flow. Thus, a Horner syndrome can be a warning that without treatment, a stroke may be imminent. The key to proper diagnosis is to determine what nearby structures may be involved (the company that it keeps). Two pharmacological tests can also be administered. A dilute 2% to 10% cocaine solution blocks norepinephrine re-uptake into synaptic terminals so that the buildup of norepinephrine near the pupil dilator muscle will dilate the pupil in a healthy person. Cocaine treatment will have less effect on the pupil of a patient with Horner syndrome regardless of where the lesion is because less norepinephrine is in the synaptic cleft. To determine if the Horner syndrome is postganglionic, a solution containing hydroxyamphetamine (Paredrine) can then be given. This drug will cause release of norepinephrine from synaptic terminals if they are present, so it will not cause pupillary dilation in a patient with a third-order Horner syndrome. A combination of a careful neurological examination with these tests will usually allow one to determine where in the sympathetic pathways damage has occurred, thus narrowing the differential diagnosis.

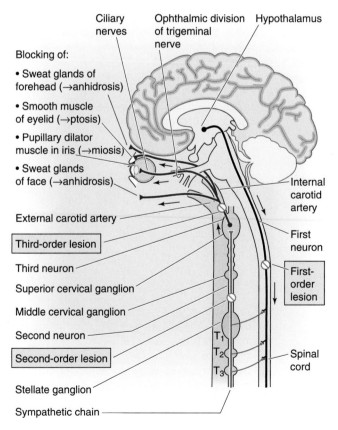

Figure 14-12 Anatomy of the sympathetic innervation to the eyelid, pupil, and facial sweat glands—Horner syndrome. Diagram showing pathways from (1) the hypothalamus to the intermediolateral column in the spinal cord (first-order neuron). (2) A preganglionic sympathetic neuron with the cell body in the intermediolateral column gets a synapse from (1) and sends an axon to the superior cervical ganglion. (3) A postganglionic sympathetic neuron with the cell body in the superior cervical ganglion sends axons to pupillary dilator (smooth) muscles.

situation can lead to maladaptive reflexes such as autonomic hyperreflexia, whereby a full bladder results in hypertension and sweating (see the box on pathological crosstalk).

All vertebrates have a brain that is segmented into three parts (see Chapter 10), the prosencephalon, mesencephalon, and rhombencephalon. With evolution, the more rostral parts took on a more dominant role. The brain of the ammocoete larva of the lamprey is dominated by the **medulla**, which is also the most vital part of the human brain; in contrast to more rostral structures, destruction of the medulla leads to instant death in the absence of life support. The medulla coordinates all visceral control and optimizes it for survival. In humans, normal body homeostasis can continue indefinitely with only a medulla, spinal cord, and peripheral ANS.

In fish, the **midbrain** became the dominant CNS structure in response to the increasing importance of vision. The brain of primitive reptiles is only a brainstem and paleocortex, without a neocortex; the corpus striatum is the dominant structure. Thus, the brainstem is sometimes referred to as the reptilian brain. Finally, the **neocortex** appeared in mammals and became dominant. The phylogenetically advanced portions of the CNS rostral to the medulla—including the hypothalamus, limbic system, and cortex—coordinate activity of the ANS with complex behaviors, motivations, and desires, but they are not required for normal homeostasis.

As a result of this hierarchy, impulses from most visceral afferents never reach the cortex, and we are not usually conscious of them. Instead, they make synapses within the enteric plexuses, autonomic ganglia, spinal cord, and brainstem, and they close reflex loops that regulate visceral output at each of these levels.

REFERENCES

Books and Reviews

Andresen MC, Kunze DL: Nucleus tractus solitarius—gateway to neural circulatory control. Annu Rev Physiol 1994; 56:93-116.

Bennett MR: Transmission at sympathetic varicosities. News Physiol Sci 1998; 13:79-84.

Caulfield MP, Birdsall NJ: International Union of Pharmacology. XVII. Classification of muscarinic acetylcholine receptors. Pharmacol Rev 1998; 50:279-290.

Janig W, McLachlan E: Characteristics of function-specific pathways in the sympathetic nervous system. Trends Neurosci 1992; 15:475-481.

Lundberg JM: Pharmacology of cotransmission in the autonomic nervous system: Integrative aspects on amines, neuropeptides, adenosine triphosphate, amino acids and nitric oxide. Pharmacol Rev 1996; 48:113-178.

Journal Articles

Evans RJ, Derkach V, Surprenant A: ATP mediates fast synaptic transmission in mammalian neurons. Nature 1992; 357:503-505.

Furchgott RF, Zawadzki JV: The obligatory role of endothelial cells in the relaxation of arterial smooth muscle by acetylcholine. Nature 1980; 288:373-376.

Haddad GG, Mazza NM, Defendini R, et al: Congenital failure of automatic control of ventilation, gastrointestinal motility and heart rate. Medicine (Baltimore) 1978; 57:517-526.

Jansen ASP, van Nguyen X, Karpitskiy V, et al: Central command neurons of the sympathetic nervous system: Basis of the fight-or-flight response. Science 1995; 270:644-646.

Palmer RMJ, Ferrige AG, Moncada S: Nitric oxide release accounts for the biological activity of endothelium-derived relaxing factor. Nature 1987; 327:524-526.

Pattyn A, Morin X, Cremer H, et al: The homeobox gene Phox2bx is essential for the development of autonomic neural crest derivatives. Nature 1999; 399:366-370.

CHAPTER 15

SENSORY TRANSDUCTION

Barry W. Connors

Sensory receptors convert environmental energy into neural signals

Sensation is a cognitive process that requires the full powers of the central nervous system (CNS). Sensation begins with the sensory receptors that actually interface with the world, and these receptors use energy from the environment to trigger electrochemical signals that can be transmitted to the brain—a process called **sensory transduction**. Understanding of transduction processes is crucial for several reasons. Without these processes, sensation fails. Moreover, a variety of diseases that specifically affect sensory receptors can impair or abolish sensation without damaging the brain. Transduction also sets the basic limits of perception. It determines the sensitivity, range, speed, versatility, and vigor of a sensory system.

We have a variety of senses, each tuned to particular types of environmental energy. These **sensory modalities** include the familiar ones of seeing, hearing, touching, smelling, and tasting as well as our senses of pain, balance, body position, and movement. In addition, other intricate sensory systems of which we are not conscious monitor the internal milieu and report on the body's chemical and metabolic state. Early in the 19th century, the physiologist Johannes Müller recognized that neurons that are specialized to evaluate a particular type of stimulus energy will produce the appropriate sensation regardless of how they are activated. For example, banging your eye can produce perceptions of light even in the dark, and seizure activity in a region of the cortex devoted to olfaction can evoke repulsive smells even in a rose garden. This property has been called **univariance**; in other words, the sensory receptor and its subsequent neural circuits do not know what stimulated them—they give the same type of response regardless. Specificity for each modality is ensured by the structure and position of the sensory receptor.

Sensory transduction uses adaptations of common molecular signaling mechanisms

Evolution is a conservative enterprise. Good ideas are retained, and with slight modification they are adapted to new purposes. Sensory transduction is a prime example of this principle. The sensory processes that are now understood at the molecular level use systems that are closely related to the ubiquitous signaling molecules in eukaryotic cells. Some modalities (vision, olfaction, some types of taste, and other chemoreception) begin with integral membrane proteins that belong to the superfamily of G protein–coupled receptors (GPCRs; see Chapter 5). The second-messenger pathways use the same substances that are used for so many nonsensory tasks in cells, such as cyclic nucleotides, inositol phosphates, and kinases. Other sensory systems (mechanoreceptors, including the hair cells of audition and the vestibular organs, as well as some taste cells) use modified membrane ion channels in the primary transduction process. Although the structures of most of these channels have not yet been determined, their biophysical properties are generally unremarkable, and they are likely to be related to other, nonsensory ion channels. Indeed, the gating of many ion channels (see Chapter 6) from "nonsensory" cells is sensitive to the physical distortion of the membrane that they lie in, which implies that mechanosensitivity is a widespread (although perhaps epiphenomenal) feature of integral membrane proteins.

To achieve a specificity for certain stimulus energies, many sensory receptors must use specialized cellular structures. These, too, are usually adapted from familiar components. Various receptors are slightly modified epithelial cells. Some situate their transduction sites on modified cilia, whereas others use muscle cells or collagen fibers to channel the appropriate forces to the sensory axon. Many are neurons alone, often just bare axons with no specialization visible by microscopy. Most sensory transduction cells (e.g., oxygen and taste sensors, but not olfactory receptors) lack their own axon to communicate with the CNS. For these cells, the communication system of choice is a relatively standard, Ca^{2+}-dependent system of synaptic transmission onto a primary sensory neuron.

Sensory transduction requires detection and amplification, usually followed by a local receptor potential

Functionally, sensory transducers follow certain general steps. Obviously, they must detect stimulus energy, but they must do so with enough selectivity and speed that stimuli of different types, from different locations, or with different timing are not confused. In most cases, transduction also involves one or more steps of signal amplification so that the sensory cell can reliably communicate small stimuli (e.g., a few stray photons or a smattering of drifting molecules) to a large brain in an environment with much sensory noise. The sensory cell must then convert the amplified signal into an electrical change by altering the gating of some ion channel. This channel gating leads to alterations of the membrane potential (V_m) in the receptor cell—otherwise known as a **receptor potential**. The receptor potential is not an action potential but a graded electrotonic event (see Chapter 7) that can either modulate the activity of other channels (e.g., voltage-gated Na^+ or Ca^{2+} channels) or trigger action potentials in a different portion of the same cell. Very often, the receptor potential regulates the flux of Ca^{2+} into the cell and thus controls the release of some synaptic transmitter molecule onto the sensory afferent neuron.

Ultimately, receptor potentials determine the rate and pattern with which action potentials fire in a sensory neuron. This firing pattern is the signal that is actually communicated to the CNS. Useful information may be encoded in many features of the firing, including its rate, its temporal patterns, its periodicity, its consistency, and its patterns compared with other sensory neurons of the same or even different modalities.

CHEMORECEPTION

Chemoreceptors are ubiquitous, diverse, and evolutionarily ancient

Every cell is bathed in chemicals. Molecules can be food or poison, or they may serve as signals of communication between cells, organs, or individuals. The ability to recognize and to respond to environmental chemicals can allow cells to find nutrients, to avoid harm, to attract a mate, to navigate, or to regulate a physiological process. Chemoreception has basic and universal advantages. It is the oldest form of sensory transduction, and it exists in many forms. Chemoreception does not even require a nervous system. Single-celled organisms such as bacteria can recognize and respond to substances in their environment. In the broadest sense, every cell in the human body is chemosensitive, and chemical signaling between cells is the basis for internal communication through endocrine systems and neurotransmission. In this chapter, we restrict ourselves to chemoreception as a sensory system, the interface between the nervous system and the external and internal chemical milieu.

Chemicals reach the human body by oral or nasal ingestion, contact with the skin, or inhalation, and once there, they diffuse or are carried to the surface membranes of receptor cells through the various aqueous fluids of the body (e.g., mucus, saliva, tears, cerebrospinal fluid, blood plasma). The nervous system constantly monitors these chemical comings and goings with a diverse array of chemosensory receptors. The most familiar of these receptors are the sensory organs of taste (**gustation**) and smell (**olfaction**). However, chemoreception is widespread throughout the body. Chemoreceptors in the skin, mucous membranes, and gut warn against irritating substances, and chemoreceptors in the carotid bodies (see Chapter 32) measure blood levels of O_2, CO_2, and $[H^+]$.

Taste receptors are modified epithelial cells, whereas olfactory receptors are neurons

The tasks of gustatory and olfactory receptors appear similar at first glance. Both recognize the concentration and identity of dissolved molecules, and they communicate this information to the CNS. In fact, the two systems operate in parallel during eating, and the flavors of most foods are strongly dependent on both taste *and* smell. However, the receptor cells of the two systems are quite different. Olfactory receptors are neurons. Each olfactory cell has small dendrites at one end that are specialized to identify chemical stimuli, and at the other end an axon projects directly into the brain. Taste receptor cells are not neurons but rather modified epithelial cells that synapse onto the axons of sensory neurons that communicate with the CNS.

Taste Receptor Cells Taste receptors are located mainly on the dorsal surface of the tongue (Fig. 15-1A), concentrated within small but visible projections called **papillae** (Fig. 15-1B). Papillae are shaped like ridges, pimples, or mushrooms, and each is a few millimeters in diameter. Each papilla in turn has numerous **taste buds** (Fig. 15-1C). One taste bud contains 50 to 150 taste receptor cells, numerous basal and supporting cells that surround the taste cells, plus a set of sensory afferent axons. Most people have 2000 to 5000 taste buds, although exceptional cases range from 500 to 20,000.

The chemically sensitive part of a taste receptor cell is a small apical membrane region near the surface of the tongue. The apical ends have thin extensions called **microvilli** that project into the **taste pore**, a small opening on the surface of the tongue where the taste cells are exposed to the contents of the mouth. Taste cells form synapses with the primary sensory axons near the bottom of the taste bud. However, processing may be more complicated than a simple receptor-to-axon relay. Receptor cells also make both electrical and chemical synapses onto some of the basal cells, some basal cells synapse onto the sensory axons, and some type of information-processing circuit may be present within each taste bud itself.

Cells of the taste bud undergo a constant cycle of growth, death, and regeneration. This process depends on the influence of the sensory nerve because if the nerve is cut, taste buds degenerate.

Olfactory Receptor Cells We smell with receptor cells in the thin **olfactory epithelium**, which is placed high in the nasal cavity (Fig. 15-2A). The olfactory epithelium has three main cell types: **olfactory receptor cells** are the site of transduction; **support cells** are similar to glia and, among other things, help produce mucus; and **basal cells** are the source of new receptor cells (Fig. 15-2B). Olfactory receptors (similar to taste receptors) continually die, regenerate, and grow in a cycle that lasts ~4 to 8 weeks. Olfactory receptor cells are one of the very few types of neurons in the mam-

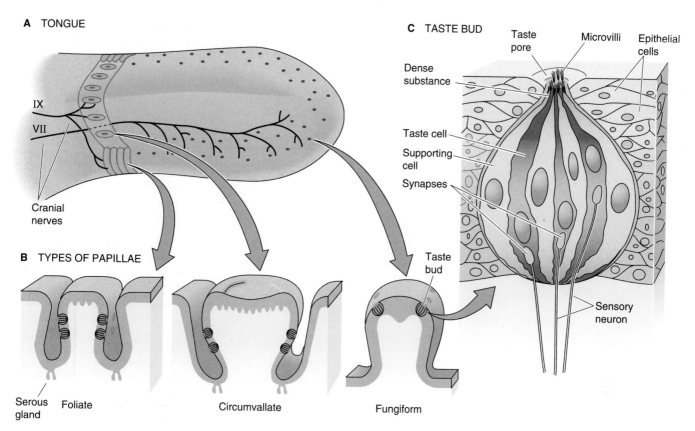

A TONGUE

IX

VII

Cranial
nerves

B TYPES OF PAPILLAE

Serous
gland Foliate

Circumvallate

Fungiform

C TASTE BUD

Dense
substance

Taste cell

Supporting
cell

Synapses

Taste pore   Microvilli   Epithelial cells

Taste
bud

Sensory
neuron

Figure 15-1 Taste receptors.

malian nervous system that are regularly replaced throughout life.

As we breathe or sniff, chemical odorants waft through the many folds of the nasal passages. However, to contact the receptor cells, odorants must first dissolve in and diffuse through a thin mucous layer, which has both a viscous and a watery portion. The normal olfactory epithelium exudes a mucous layer 20 to 50 μm thick. Mucus flows constantly and is normally replaced about every 10 minutes. Mucus is a complex, water-based substance containing dissolved glycosaminoglycans (see Chapter 2); a variety of proteins, including antibodies, odorant-binding proteins, and enzymes; and various salts. The antibodies are critical because olfactory cells offer a direct route for viruses (e.g., rabies) or bacteria to enter the brain. **Odorant-binding proteins** in the mucus probably facilitate the diffusion of odorants toward and away from the receptors. Enzymes may help clear the mucus of odorants and thus speed recovery of the receptors from transient odors.

Both the absolute size and the receptor density of the olfactory epithelium vary greatly among species, and they help determine olfactory acuity. The surface area of the human olfactory epithelium is only ~10 cm², but this limited area is enough to detect some odorants at concentrations as low as a few parts per trillion. The olfactory epithelia of some dogs may be over 170 cm², and dogs have more than 100 times as many receptors in each square centimeter as humans do. The olfactory acuity of some breeds of dog is legendary and far surpasses that of humans. Dogs can often detect the scent of someone who walked by hours before.

Complex flavors are derived from a few basic types of taste receptors, with contributions from sensory receptors of smell, temperature, texture, and pain

Studies of taste discrimination in humans imply that we can distinguish among 4000 to 10,000 different chemicals with our taste buds. However, behavioral evidence suggests that these discriminations represent only five primary taste qualities: **bitter**, **salt**, **sweet**, and **sour** plus a primary quality called **umami** ("delicious" in Japanese). Umami is epitomized by the taste of the amino acid glutamate (monosodium glutamate [MSG] is the familiar culinary form). Unlike an olfactory receptor cell, which apparently expresses only one receptor type (see later), a taste receptor cell may express several.

In many cases, there is an obvious correlation between the chemistry of **tastants** (i.e., chemicals being tasted) and the quality of their taste. Most acids taste sour and most salts taste salty. However, for many other tastants, the linkage between taste and chemical structure is not clear. The familiar sugars (e.g., sucrose and fructose) are satisfyingly sweet, but certain proteins (e.g., monellin) and artificial sweeteners (e.g., saccharin and aspartame, which is made from two amino acids: L-aspartyl-L-phenylalanine methyl ester) are 10,000 to 100,000 times sweeter by weight than these sugars. Bitter substances are also chemically diverse. They include simple ions such as K^+ (KCl actually simultaneously evokes both bitter and salty tastes), larger metal ions such as Mg^{2+}, and complex organic molecules such as quinine.

A   NASAL CAVITY AND OLFACTORY BULB

B   OLFACTORY EPITHELIUM

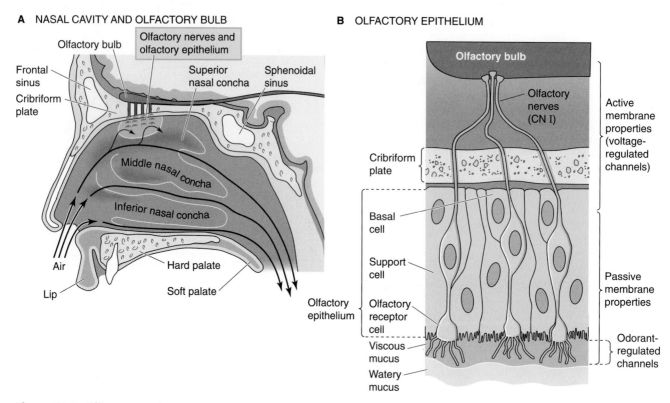

Figure 15-2   Olfactory reception.

If the tongue has only four or five primary taste qualities available to it, how does it discriminate among the myriad complex flavors that embellish our lives? First, the tongue's response to each tastant reflects distinct proportions of each of the primary taste qualities. In this sense, the taste cells are similar to the photoreceptors of our eyes; with only three different types of color-selective photoreceptive cone cells, we can distinguish a huge palette of colors (see later). Second, the flavor of a tastant is determined not only by its taste but also by its smell. Taste and smell operate in parallel, with information converging in the CNS to aid the important discrimination of foods and poisons. For example, without the aid of olfaction, an onion tastes much like an apple—and both are quite bland. Third, the mouth is filled with other types of sensory receptors that are sensitive to texture, temperature, and pain, and these modalities enhance both the identification and enjoyment of foods. A striking example is the experience of spicy food, which is enjoyable to some but painful to others. The spiciness of hot peppers is generated by the chemical **capsaicin**, not because of its activation of taste receptor cells but because of its stimulation of heat-sensitive pain receptors in the mouth (see later).

Taste transduction involves many types of molecular signaling systems

The chemicals that we taste have diverse structures, and taste receptors have evolved a variety of mechanisms for transduction. The taste system has adapted many types of membrane-signaling systems to its purposes. Tastants may pass directly through ion channels (salt), bind to ion channels (sour), or

bind to membrane receptors that activate second-messenger systems, which in turn open or close ion channels (sweet, bitter, and umami). Taste cells have simply used specialized variations of these processes to initiate meaningful signals to the brain.

The receptor potentials of taste cells are usually depolarizing. At least some taste receptor cells can fire action potentials, similar to those of neurons; but if the membrane is sufficiently depolarized by whatever means, voltage-gated Ca^{2+} channels open, and Ca^{2+} enters the cytoplasm and triggers the release of transmitter molecules. The identity of the taste receptor's transmitter or transmitters is unknown.

Some believe that each taste-receptor cell responds to only one of the five basic taste modalities. It is generally accepted that a receptor cell responds to only one out of the group of sweet, bitter, and umami—all of which share a common signal transduction mechanism. Finally, some evidence suggests that each taste-receptor cell is hard-wired to the CNS to convey a particular taste quality. For example, if we express a bitter receptor in sweet taste-receptor cells, a mouse—naturally attracted to sweet tastants—will now be attracted to bitter tastants that now taste sweet.

The complex diversities of taste transduction are not yet fully understood. Many of the details have come from research on the taste cells of catfish, mudpuppies, mice, and rats. Each animal has certain experimental advantages (e.g., very large taste cells), but the differences among species suggest that we may be surprised when it becomes possible to study human mechanisms directly. The following is a summary of the best-understood transduction processes for the five primary taste qualities (Fig. 15-3).

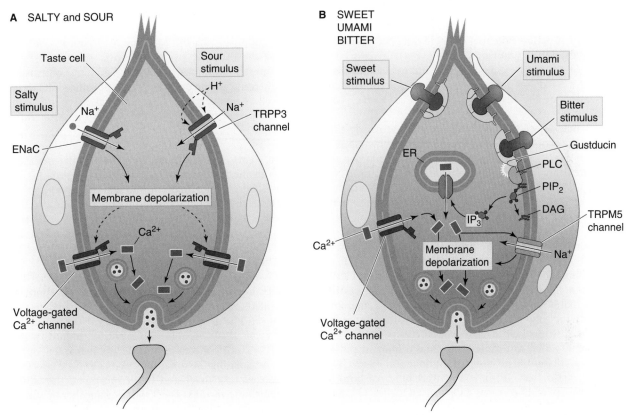

Figure 15-3 Cellular basis of taste transduction. **A,** Salty taste is mediated by an epithelial Na⁺ channel (ENaC) that is sensitive to amiloride. Sour is mediated as extracellular H⁺ activates TRPP3 channels. **B,** Sugars and umami compounds bind to GPCRs consisting of T1R heterodimers. Bitter substances bind to GPCRs consisting of dimers made up of members of the T2R family. DAG, diacylglycerol; ER, endoplasmic reticulum; IP$_3$, inositol 1,4,5-triphosphate; PDE, phosphodiesterase; PIP$_2$, phosphatidyl inositol 4,5-biphosphate; PLC, phospholipase C.

Salt   The most common salty tasting chemical is NaCl, or table salt. The taste of salt is mainly the taste of the cation Na^+, and transduction of $[Na^+]$ in taste cells is relatively simple. Salt-sensitive taste cells have an Na^+-selective channel called ENaC (Fig. 15-3A), common to many epithelial cells, that is blocked by the drug amiloride (see Chapter 35). Unlike the Na^+ channel that generates action potentials in excitable cells, the taste channels are relatively insensitive to voltage and stay open at rest. However, transduction of the $[Na^+]$ in a mouthful of food is somewhat analogous to the behavior of a neuron during the upstroke of an action potential. When $[Na^+]$ rises outside the receptor cell, the gradient for Na^+ across the membrane becomes steeper, Na^+ diffuses down its electrochemical gradient (i.e., it flows into the cell), and the resultant inward current causes the membrane to depolarize to a new voltage. Neurons depolarize during their action potential by increasing Na^+ conductance at a fixed Na^+ gradient (see Fig. 7-4). In contrast, Na^+-sensitive taste cells depolarize by increasing the Na^+ gradient at a fixed Na^+ permeability. The resultant graded depolarization of the taste cell is defined as its receptor potential.

Anions may affect the taste of salts by modulating the saltiness of the cation or by adding a taste of their own. NaCl tastes saltier than Na acetate, perhaps because the larger an anion is, the more it *inhibits* the salty taste of the cation. Na saccharin is sweet because the anion saccharin activates sweetness receptors; it is not salty because Na^+ is present at a very low concentration.

Sour   Sourness is evoked by protons (H^+ ions). The key player is the non-selective cation channel TRPP3 (Fig. 15-3A), a member of the **transient receptor potential (TRP)** family of ion channels (Table 6-2 on p. 167). Decreases in pH—presumably extracellular pH—activate TRPP3, thereby depolarizing the sour-receptor cell. TRPP3 is also known as PKD2L1 because it is a close relative of polycystin 2 (PKD2), a mutation in which can cause autosomal dominant polycystic kidney disease. The taste of carbonation (i.e., CO_2 in drinks) arises as GPI-linked extracellular carbonic-anhydrase IV (p. 654) converts CO_2 to HCO_3^- plus H^+, the latter activating TRPP3.

Sweet   Sweetness is sensed when molecules bind to specific receptor sites on the taste cell membrane and activate a cascade of second messengers (Fig. 15-3B). Two families of taste receptor genes—the T1R family and T2R family—seem to account for sweet, bitter, and umami transduction. These taste receptors are GPCRs, and all use the same basic second-messenger pathway. In the case of sweet transduction, the tastant (e.g., a sugar molecule) binds to a taste receptor that consists of a dimer of T1R2 and T1R3 proteins. The activated receptor then activates a G protein that stimulates phospholipase C, which in turn increases its production of the messenger inositol trisphosphate (IP_3; see Chapter 3). IP_3 triggers the release of Ca^{2+} from internal stores, and the rise in $[Ca^{2+}]_i$ then activates the TRPM5 channel that is specific for taste cells. TRPM5 is a relatively nonselective cation channel that depolarizes the taste cell, triggering the release of neurotransmitter onto the primary gustatory axon (Fig. 15-3B). The sweet receptor complex—the T1R2/T1R3 dimer—is broadly sensitive to sweet-tasting substances. Despite the appearance in Figure 15-3B, sweet-sensing taste cells do not express receptors for either bitter or umami.

Bitter   Bitterness usually warns of poison. Perhaps because poisons are so chemically diverse, we have about 30 different types of bitter receptors to sense them. These are GPCRs in the T2R family. Animals are not very good at distinguishing between different bitter substances because each bitter taste cell expresses the majority of the 30 T2Rs. It may be more important to recognize that something is bitter, and potentially poisonous, than it is to recognize precisely what type of poison it may be. Stimulation of the T2Rs activates a second-messenger pathway that is apparently identical to the one that sweet receptors activate: G proteins, PLC, IP_3, $[Ca^{2+}]_i$ increase, and TRPM5 channel opening. We do not confuse the tastes of sweet and bitter substances because even though they trigger similar signaling systems, each transduction cascade occurs within a specific sweet or bitter taste cell. Moreover, each taste cell makes synaptic contact with a different primary gustatory axon that leads into the CNS.

Amino Acids   Amino acids are critical nutrients that are vital as an energy source and for constructing proteins. Probably as a consequence, many amino acids taste good, although some taste bitter. The **umami** taste, which we know well from Chinese restaurants, is triggered by a mechanism very similar to that for sweet tasting. The umami receptor is a dimer comprising two members of the T1R family, T1R1 and T1R3. Note that the umami and sweet receptors share T1R3. The taste for amino acids seems to depend on T1R1 because mice that lack it are unable to discriminate glutamate and other amino acids, although they retain their ability to detect sweet substances. The umami receptor activates the same signaling mechanisms that sweet and bitter receptors do: G proteins, PLC, IP_3, $[Ca^{2+}]_i$ increase, and TRPM5 channel opening. Again, by isolating the umami receptors in taste cells that do not also express sweet and bitter receptors, the CNS can distinguish the various tastes from one another by somehow knowing which taste cell connects to a particular gustatory axon.

Olfactory transduction involves specific receptors, G protein–coupled signaling, and a cyclic nucleotide–gated ion channel

Our ability to smell chemicals is better developed than our ability to taste them. By one estimate, we can smell more than 400,000 different substances. Interestingly, ~80% of them smell unpleasant. As with taste, it seems likely that smell evolved to serve important protective functions, such as warning us away from harmful substances. With the ability to discriminate so many different smells, you might also expect many different types of transduction mechanisms, as in the taste system. In fact, olfactory receptors probably use only one second-messenger mechanism. Figure 15-4 summarizes the chain of events that leads to an action potential in the olfactory nerve (i.e., CN I):

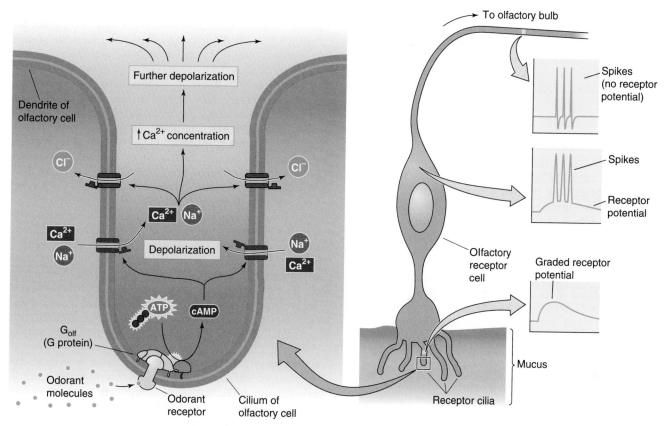

Figure 15-4   Cellular mechanism of odor sensation. ATP, adenosine triphosphate.

Step 1: The odorant binds to a specific **olfactory receptor protein** in the cell membrane of a cilium of an olfactory receptor cell.

Step 2: Receptor activation stimulates a heterotrimeric G protein called G_{olf} (see Chapter 3).

Step 3: The α subunit of G_{olf} in turn activates adenylyl cyclase, which produces cAMP.

Step 4: The cAMP binds to a cAMP-gated cation channel.

Step 5: Opening of this channel increases permeability to Na^+, K^+, and Ca^{2+}.

Step 6: The net inward current leads to membrane depolarization and increased $[Ca^{2+}]_i$.

Step 7: The increased $[Ca^{2+}]_i$ opens Ca^{2+}-activated Cl^- channels. Opening of these channels produces more depolarization because of the relatively high $[Cl^-]_i$ of olfactory receptor neurons.

Step 8: If the receptor potential exceeds the threshold, it triggers action potentials in the soma that travel down the axon and into the brain.

All this molecular machinery, with the exception of the action potential mechanism, is squeezed into the thin cilia of olfactory receptor cells. Moreover, additional modulatory schemes also branch from this basic pathway.

Olfactory receptor cells express a huge family of receptor proteins; in fact, they are the largest family of mammalian genes known! Their discovery in the early 1990s earned Linda Buck and Richard Axel the 2004 Nobel Prize. Rodents have more than 1000 different olfactory receptor genes. Humans have ~350 genes that encode functional receptor proteins. This family of olfactory receptor proteins belongs to the superfamily of GPCRs (see Chapter 3) that also includes the phototransduction protein rhodopsin and the taste receptors for sweet, bitter, and umami described before as well as the receptors for a wide variety of neurotransmitters.

The extracellular surfaces of olfactory receptor proteins have odorant binding sites, each slightly different from the others. Presumably, each receptor protein can bind only certain types of odorants; therefore, some degree of selectivity is conferred to different olfactory receptor cells. Remarkably, each receptor cell seems to express only a single gene of the 1000 different odorant receptor genes in rodents. Thus, 1000 different types of olfactory receptor cells are present, each identified by the one receptor gene that it expresses. Because each odorant may activate a large proportion of the different receptor types, the central olfactory system's task is to decode the patterns of receptor cell activity that signals the identity of each smell.

The structure of the olfactory cAMP-gated channel is closely related to the light-activated channel in photoreceptors of the retina, which is normally gated by an increase in intracellular cyclic guanosine monophosphate ($[cGMP]_i$). The olfactory channel and the photoreceptor channel almost certainly evolved from one ancestral cyclic nucleotide–gated channel, just as the olfactory receptor and photoreceptor proteins probably evolved from an ancestral receptor with seven membrane-spanning segments.

Termination of the olfactory response occurs when odorants diffuse away, scavenger enzymes in the mucous layer break them down, or cAMP in the receptor cell activates other signaling pathways that end the transduction process.

VISUAL TRANSDUCTION

The environment of most species is enveloped by light (Fig. 15-5). Animals have evolved a variety of mechanisms to transduce and to detect light. Their brains analyze visual information to help them locate food, to avoid becoming food, to find a mate, to navigate, and generally to recognize distant objects. Light is an exceptionally useful source of information about the world because it is nearly ubiquitous and can travel far and fast and in straight lines with relatively little dispersion of its energy. The vertebrate eye, which we describe here, has two major components: an **optical** part to gather and focus light and to form an image and a **neural** part (the retina) to convert the optical image into a neural code.

The optical components of the eye collect light and focus it onto the retina

The optical structures of the eye are among the most sophisticated of the specialized non-neural sensory endings, and they are often compared with a camera. As cameras have become more technologically sophisticated, the analogy has improved because the eye has systems to focus automatically, to adjust its sensitivity for widely different light levels, to move to track and to stabilize a target, and even to keep its surface washed and clear (obviously, cameras still have room for improvement). The similarity to a camera breaks down when we consider the retina, which is decidedly not like standard photographic film or electronic light detectors.

Figure 15-6A shows a cross section through the human eye. A ray of light entering the eye passes through several relatively transparent elements to reach the retina; these elements include a thin film of tears and then the cornea, the aqueous humor, the lens, and finally the vitreous humor. **Tears** are a surprisingly complex liquid, based on a plasma ultrafiltrate. They bathe the cornea in a layer that is less than 10 μm thick, keep it wet, and allow O_2 to diffuse from the air to the corneal cells. Tears also contain lysozymes and antibodies to counter infection, a superficial oily layer that greatly slows evaporation and prevents spillage at the lid margins, and a thin mucoid layer to wet the surface of the cornea and to allow the tears to spread smoothly. Tears also help flush away foreign substances. The **cornea** is a thin, transporting epithelium that is devoid of blood vessels and has a cell structure specialized to maintain its high transparency. The **ciliary epithelium**, a part of the ciliary body, constantly secretes **aqueous humor**, a protein-free ultrafiltrate of blood plasma, into the posterior chamber of the eye. The aqueous humor then flows between the iris and the anterior surface of the lens and reaches the **anterior chamber** through the pupil. This aqueous humor keeps the anterior portion of the eye slightly pressurized (~20 mm Hg), which helps maintain the eye's shape. The canals of Schlemm drain the aqueous humor. Excess pressure in the anterior chamber produces a disease called **glaucoma**. In the most common form of glaucoma, blockage of the canals of Schlemm leads to increased intraocular pressure. Pressure damages and kills ganglion cell axons at the optic disc, where they leave the eye and enter the optic nerve. The **lens** is an onion-like structure with closely packed columnar cells that are arranged in concentric shells and encased by a thin, tough, transparent capsule that is composed of epithelial cells. The cells of the lens have a high concentration of proteins called α-crystallins, which help increase the density of the lens and enhance its focusing power. The **posterior chamber**, which is filled with a gelatinous substance called **vitreous humor**, is also kept pressurized by the production of aqueous humor.

The light must be focused to generate a clear optical image on the retina. This is accomplished by the cornea and, to a lesser extent, the lens. Focusing requires the path of the light to be bent, or refracted. Refraction can occur when light passes from a medium in which it travels relatively fast into a medium in which it travels relatively slowly, or vice versa.

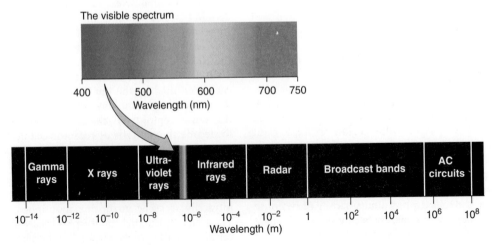

Figure 15-5 The electromagnetic spectrum. AC, alternating current.

A ANATOMY

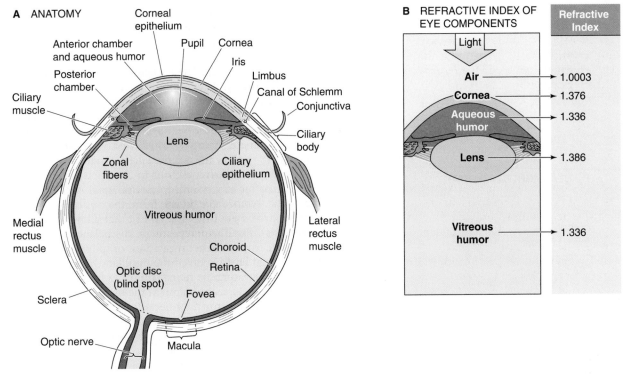

B REFRACTIVE INDEX OF EYE COMPONENTS

	Refractive Index
Air	1.0003
Cornea	1.376
Aqueous humor	1.336
Lens	1.386
Vitreous humor	1.336

Figure 15-6 The eye. **A,** Cross section of the right human eye, viewed from the top. **B,** Bending of light by a structure depends not only on the radius of curvature but also on the difference in the indices of refraction of the two adjoining media.

The **index of refraction** for a substance is essentially a measure of the speed of light within it; for example, light travels faster through air (index of refraction, 1.0003) than through the denser substance of the cornea (index of refraction, 1.376). Two things determine how much a light ray is refracted: the difference in the refractive indices of the two media and the angle between the incident light and the interface between the two media. Simple convex lenses use curved surfaces to control the refraction of light rays so that they converge (or focus) on a distant surface. The focal power (D) of one surface of a spherical lens is

$$\text{Focal power} = \frac{n_2 - n_1}{r} \quad (15\text{-}1)$$

Here, n_1 and n_2 are the refractive indices of the first and second medium and r is the radius of curvature of the lens in meters. The unit of focal power is a *diopter* ($1\ D = 1\ m^{-1}$). Focal power is the reciprocal of focal length. Thus, parallel light rays entering a 1-D lens are focused at 1 m, and those entering a 2-D lens are focused at 0.5 m.

In the case of the eye, most of the focusing takes place at the interface between the air and the tear-covered anterior surface of the cornea because this region is where light encounters the greatest disparity in refractive index on its path to the retina (Fig. 15-6B). With a change of 0.376 in refractive index and a radius of outer curvature of 7.8 mm in a typical human cornea, the focal power is 48.2 D. The curvature on the inner surface of the cornea is reversed, so some focal power is lost as light passes into the aqueous humor. However, the change in refractive index at this surface is only 0.040, so the change is only −5.9 D. The lens

of the eye, with convex curvature on both sides, has a potentially greater focal power than the cornea. However, because of the small difference in refractive index between the substance of the lens and the aqueous and vitreous humors surrounding it, the effective focal power of the lens is lower. The summed focal power of the optics of the relaxed eye is ~60 D, which allows it to focus light from distant objects onto the retina, the center of which is ~24 mm behind the surface of the cornea (Fig. 15-7A). The position of the retinal image is, of course, upside down relative to the object that produced it.

A normal *resting* eye is focused on distant objects, beyond ~7 m. If it were fixed in this position, it would be impossible to see objects that are close up. To focus objects that are closer than 7 m away, the eye needs to increase its focal power, a process called **accommodation**. The eye achieves this goal by changing the shape of the lens. At rest, the lens is suspended around its edge by elastic **zonal fibers** that keep its capsule stretched and relatively flattened. To accommodate, the ciliary muscle fibers contract and release some of the tension in the zonal fibers. Relieved of the radial pull of its fibers, the lens becomes rounder. This increased curvature means increased focal power and a shift of the focal point closer to the eye. There are limits to accommodation, of course, and they are strongly age dependent. Young children have the most pliable lenses and can increase their focal power up to 12 to 14 D. Their **near point**, the closest distance that they are able to focus, is about at the end of their nose.

With age, the lens becomes stiffer and less able to round up and accommodate. By age 30, the near point is ~10 cm, and by the mid-40s, it stretches beyond arm's length. The

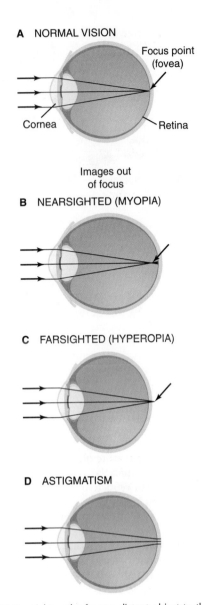

A   NORMAL VISION

Focus point
(fovea)

Cornea ——   —— Retina

Images out
of focus

B   NEARSIGHTED (MYOPIA)

C   FARSIGHTED (HYPEROPIA)

D   ASTIGMATISM

Figure 15-7   Light paths from a distant object to the eye.

diffuse focusing leads to blurring of the image. Most people with astigmatic vision can also wear lenses that compensate for aberrant focusing properties of their eyes.

The **iris** is the colored structure that is visible through the window of the cornea. The iris's hue comes from pigments in its cells, but its function is to create and to adjust the round opening that it encircles—the **pupil**. The pupil is like the aperture of the camera, and the iris is the diaphragm that regulates the amount of light allowed to enter the eye. The iris has sphincter muscles, innervated by postganglionic *parasympathetic* fibers from the ciliary ganglion (Fig. 15-8; see also Fig. 14-4), that allow it to constrict (**miosis**). The iris also has radially oriented muscles, innervated by post-ganglionic *sympathetic* fibers from the superior cervical ganglion (see Figs. 14-4 and 14-12), that allow it to dilate (**mydriasis**). Pupil size depends on the balance of the two autonomic inputs. The regulation of pupillary size by ambient light levels is called the **pupillary light reflex** (Fig. 15-8). Light striking the retina stimulates fibers in the optic nerve (neuron 1) that synapse in the brainstem in the pre-tectal nucleus. Neuron 2 projects to the Edinger-Westphal nuclei on both sides of the brain (see Fig. 14-5), stimulating preganglionic parasympathetic neurons (neuron 3) that project to the ciliary ganglia. These neurons activate post-ganglionic parasympathetic neurons (neuron 4) that constrict both pupils. Thus, control of the pupils in the two eyes is "yoked": an increase in light to only one eye causes its pupil to constrict (the **direct light response**), but it also causes an identical constriction in the other eye, even if that eye saw only constant light levels (the **consensual light response**). Pupillary responses serve two functions: (1) they regulate the total amount of light that enters the eye (over a range of ~16-fold), and (2) they affect the quality of the retinal image in the same way that the aperture affects the depth of focus of a camera (a smaller pupil diameter gives a greater depth of focus).

Other peripheral structures are also essential to proper visual function. The most important are the extraocular muscles that control eye movements and thus the direction of gaze, the tracking of objects, and the coordination of the two eyes to keep their retinal images aligned as the eye, head, and visual world move about. Nuclei in the brainstem also control these tracking functions.

The retina is a small, displaced part of the central nervous system

The retina is a very thin (~200 μm thick in humans) sheet of tissue that lines the back of the eye and contains the light-sensitive cells, the **photoreceptors**. Photoreceptors capture photons, convert their light energy into chemical free energy, and ultimately generate a synaptic signal for relay to other visual neurons in the retina.

The retina is, histologically and embryologically, a part of the CNS. Not only does it transduce light into neural signals, but it also does some remarkably complex processing of visual information before passing it on to other regions of the brain. In addition to the photoreceptor cells, the retina has four additional types of neurons that form an orderly but intricate neural circuit (Fig. 15-9). One type, the **ganglion cell**, generates the sole output of the retina by sending its axons to the thalamus through the optic nerve (CN II).

loss of accommodation with age is called **presbyopia** (from the Greek *presbus* for "old" and *ops* for "eye"); it is the reason that glasses for reading are unavoidable for almost everyone past middle age. Additional refractive flaws may be caused by an eye that is too long or short for its focusing power or by aberrations in the refracting surfaces of the eye. **Myopia**, or nearsightedness, occurs when the eye is too long; distant objects focus in front of the retina and appear blurred (Fig. 15-7B). **Hyperopia** (or hypermetropia), or farsightedness, is a feature of eyes that are too short; even with the lens fully accommodated, a near object focuses behind the retina and appears blurry (Fig. 15-7C). People with myopia can wear concave lenses that move the focal plane of all images back toward the retina. Those with hyperopia can wear convex lenses that move the focal plane forward. **Astigmatism** is caused by uneven curvature of the refractive surfaces of the eye. As a result, a point source of light cannot be brought to a precise focus on the retina (Fig. 15-7D). The resultant

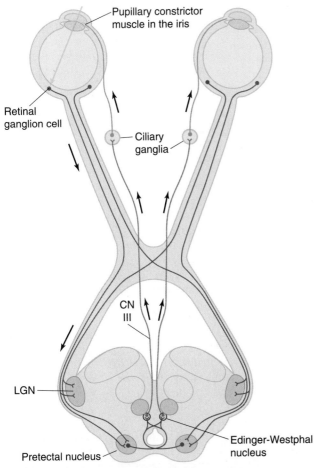

Figure 15-8 The pupillary light reflex. The figure shows the parasympathetic pathways that lead to constriction of the pupils. Pupil diameter depends on the balance between these parasympathetic pathways as well as the sympathetic pathways shown in Figure 14-12. CN III, oculomotor nerve; LGN, lateral geniculate nucleus.

The retina is a highly laminated structure. Through a quirk of evolution, the photoreceptors of the vertebrate eye are on the *outer* surface of the retina, that is, the side facing *away* from the vitreous humor and incoming light. Thus, to reach the transducing cells, light has to first pass through all the retinal neurons. This path causes only minor distortion of image quality because of the thinness and transparency of the neural layers. This seemingly inverted arrangement may actually be an advantage for housekeeping of the eye. Photoreceptors undergo a continuous process of renewal, sloughing off membrane from their outer segments and rebuilding them. They also demand a relatively high energy supply. Because they face the back of the eye, photoreceptors are close to the **pigment epithelium**, which aids the renewal process, and to the blood vessels that supply the retina. These poorly transparent structures (i.e., pigment epithelium and blood vessels) are thus isolated from the light path. In fact, the pigment epithelium also *absorbs* photons that are not first captured by photoreceptors, before they can be reflected and degrade the visual image.

Each human eye has more than 100×10^6 photoreceptors but only 1×10^6 ganglion cells, which implies a high degree of convergence of information as it flows from the transduc-

ing cells to the output cells. Some of this convergence is mediated by a set of interneurons (i.e., cells that make synaptic connections only within the retina) called **bipolar** cells, which directly connect photoreceptors and ganglion cells in a mainly radial direction (Fig. 15-9). The two remaining types of retinal neurons, horizontal cells and amacrine cells, are interneurons that mainly spread horizontally. **Horizontal cells** synapse within the outer layer of the retina and interconnect photoreceptors and bipolar cells to themselves and to each other. Horizontal cells often mediate interactions over a wide area of retina. **Amacrine cells** synapse within the inner layer of the retina and interconnect both bipolar cells and ganglion cells. The circuitry of the retina is much more complex than this picture implies. One hint of this complexity is that its four primary types of neurons are in turn divided into at least 10 to 20 distinct subtypes, each with different physiological and morphological features.

The thinness of the mammalian retina has an interesting biophysical consequence. Because signaling distances are so short, synaptic potentials can spread effectively within its neurons without the help of conventional action potentials. Electrotonic spread of potentials along the dendrites is generally enough. The main exceptions are the ganglion cells, which use action potentials to speed visual information along their axons to the thalamus.

There are two primary types of photoreceptors: rods and cones

The two main types of photoreceptors, rods and cones, are named for their characteristic shapes (Fig. 15-9). The human retina has only one type of rod, which is responsible for our monochromatic dark-adapted vision, and three subtypes of cones, which are responsible for the color-sensitive vision that we experience in brighter environments. Rods outnumber cones by at least 16:1, and each is spread in a distinct pattern across the retina.

In the central area of the primate retina is a small pit 300 to 700 μm in diameter (which accounts for 1 to 2.3 degrees of visual angle) called the **fovea**, which collects light from the center of our gaze (Fig. 15-6). Several adaptations of the fovea allow it to mediate the highest visual acuity in the retina. Neurons of the inner layer of retina are actually displaced laterally to the side of the fovea to minimize light scattering on the way to the receptors. In addition, within the fovea, the ratio of photoreceptors to ganglion cells falls dramatically. Most foveal receptors synapse on only one bipolar cell, which synapses on only one ganglion cell (Fig. 15-10A). Because each ganglion cell is devoted to a very small portion of the visual field, central vision has high resolution. In other words, the **receptive field** of a foveal ganglion cell (i.e., the region of stimulus space that can activate it) is small. At the periphery, the ratio of receptors to ganglion cells is high (Fig. 15-10B); thus, each ganglion cell has a large receptive field. The large receptive field reduces the spatial resolution of the peripheral portion of the retina but increases its sensitivity because more photoreceptors collect light for a ganglion cell. Foveal vision is purely cone mediated, and the sheet of foveal photoreceptors consists of only the smallest cones packed at the highest density (~0.3 μm from the center of one cone to another). Cone density falls to very low levels outside the fovea, and rod density rises.

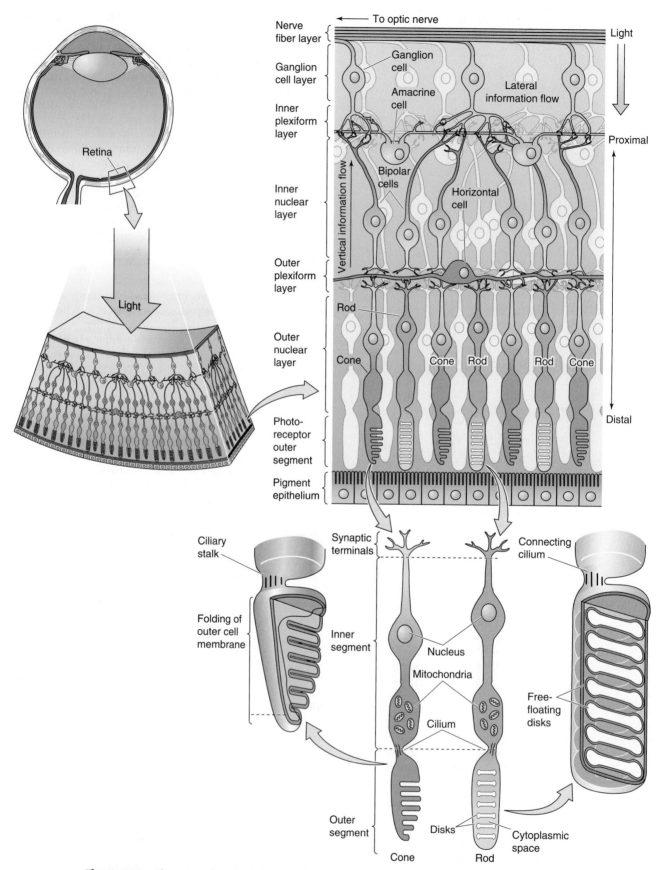

Figure 15-9   The retina—the neural circuits in the retina of a primate. Notice that the incoming light reaches the photoreceptor cells (*rods* and *cones*) only after passing through several thin, transparent layers of other neurons. The pigment epithelium absorbs the light that is not absorbed by the photoreceptor cells and thus minimizes reflections of stray light. The ganglion cells communicate to the thalamus by sending action potentials down their axons. However, the photoreceptor cells and other neurons communicate by graded synaptic potentials that are conducted electrotonically.

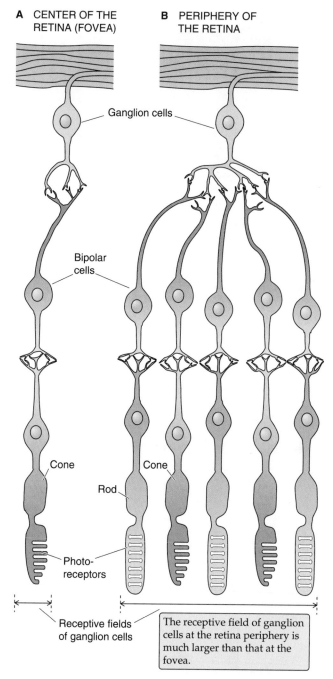

A CENTER OF THE RETINA (FOVEA)

B PERIPHERY OF THE RETINA

Ganglion cells

Bipolar cells

Cone

Rod

Cone

Photo-receptors

Receptive fields of ganglion cells

The receptive field of ganglion cells at the retina periphery is much larger than that at the fovea.

Figure 15-10 Comparison of receptive fields in the fovea and periphery of the retina.

Peripheral vision (i.e., nonfoveal vision, or vision at visual angles more than 10 degrees away from the center of the fovea and thus the center of gaze) is mediated by both rods and cones.

Photoreceptors are elongated cells with synaptic terminals, an inner segment, and an outer segment (Fig. 15-9). The **synaptic terminals** connect to the inner segment by a short axon. The **inner segment** contains the nucleus and metabolic machinery; it synthesizes the photopigments and has a high density of mitochondria. The inner segment also serves an optical function—its high density funnels photons into the outer segment. A thin ciliary stalk connects the inner

segment to the outer segment. The **outer segment** is the transduction site, although it is the last part of the cell to see the light. Structurally, the outer segment is a highly modified cilium. Each rod outer segment has ~1000 tightly packed stacks of *disk membranes,* which are flattened, membrane-bound intracellular organelles that have pinched off from the outer membrane. Cone outer segments have similarly stacked membranes, except that they are infolded and remain continuous with the outer membrane. The disk membranes contain the photopigments—**rhodopsin** in rods and molecules related to rhodopsin in cones. Rhodopsin moves from its synthesis site in the inner segment through the stalk and into the outer segment through small vesicles whose membranes are packed with rhodopsin to be incorporated into the disks.

Photoreceptors hyperpolarize in response to light

The remarkable psychophysical experiments of Hecht and colleagues in 1942 demonstrated that five to seven photons, each acting on only a single rod, are sufficient to evoke a sensation of light in humans. Thus, the rod is performing at the edge of its physical limits because there is no light level smaller than one photon. To detect a single photon requires a prodigious feat of signal amplification. As Denis Baylor has pointed out, "the sensitivity of rod vision is so great that the energy needed to lift a sugar cube one centimeter, if converted to a blue-green light, would suffice to give an intense sensation of a flash to every human who ever existed."

Phototransduction involves a cascade of chemical and electrical events to detect, to amplify, and to signal a response to light. As in many other sensory receptors, photoreceptors use electrical events (receptor potentials) to carry the visual signal from the outer segment to their synapses. Chemical messengers diffusing over such a distance would simply be too slow. The surprising fact about the receptor potential of rods and cones is that it is *hyperpolarizing*. Light causes the cell's V_m to become *more negative* than the resting potential that it maintains in the dark (Fig. 15-11A). At low light intensities, the size of the receptor potential rises linearly with light intensity; but at higher intensities, the response saturates.

Hyperpolarization is an essential step in relaying the visual signal because it directly modulates the rate of transmitter release from the photoreceptor onto its postsynaptic neurons. This synapse is conventional in that it releases more transmitter—in this case glutamate—when its presynaptic terminal is depolarized and less when it is hyperpolarized. Thus, a flash of light causes a *decrease* in transmitter secretion. The upshot is that the vertebrate photoreceptor is most active in the dark.

How is the light-induced hyperpolarization generated? Figure 15-11B shows a method to measure the current flowing across the membrane of the outer segment of a single rod. In the dark, each photoreceptor produces an ionic current that flows steadily into the outer segment and out of the inner segment. This **dark current** is carried mainly by inwardly directed Na^+ ions in the outer segment and by outwardly directed K^+ ions from the inner segment (Fig. 15-11C). Na^+ flows through a nonselective cation channel of the outer segment, which light indirectly regulates, and

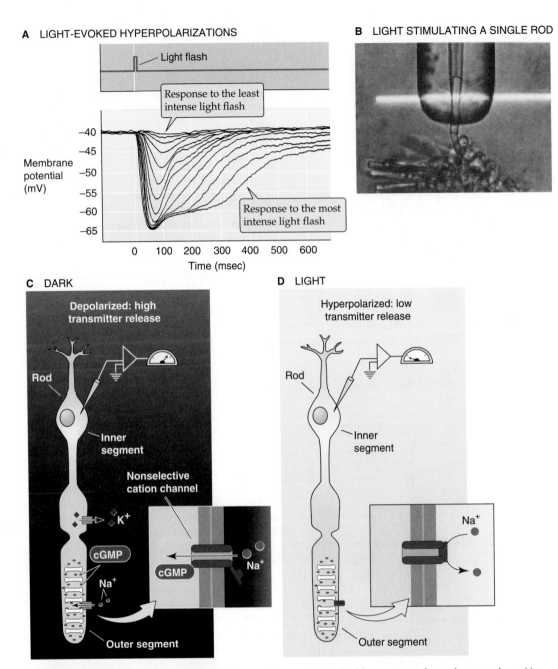

A   LIGHT-EVOKED HYPERPOLARIZATIONS

Light flash

Response to the least intense light flash

Membrane potential (mV)

-40
-45
-50
-55
-60
-65

Response to the most intense light flash

0   100   200   300   400   500   600
Time (msec)

B   LIGHT STIMULATING A SINGLE ROD

C   DARK

Depolarized: high transmitter release

Rod

Inner segment

Nonselective cation channel

cGMP

Na+

K+

cGMP

Na+

Outer segment

D   LIGHT

Hyperpolarized: low transmitter release

Rod

Inner segment

Na+

Outer segment

Figure 15-11   Phototransduction. **A,** The experiment summarized here was performed on a red-sensitive cone from a turtle. A brief flash of light causes a hyperpolarization of the photoreceptor cell. The size of the peak and the duration of the receptor potential increase with the increasing intensity of the flash. At low light intensities, the magnitude of the peak increases linearly with light intensity. At high intensities, the peak response saturates, but the plateau becomes longer. *(Data from Baylor DA, Hodgkin AL, Lamb TD: The electrical response of turtle cones to flashes and steps of light. J Physiol 1974; 242:685-727.)* **B,** A single rod has been sucked into a pipette, allowing the investigators to monitor the current. The horizontal white band is the light used to stimulate the rod. *(Reproduced from Baylor DA, Lamb TD, Yau K-W: Responses of retinal rods to single photons. J Physiol [Lond] 1979; 288:613-634.)* **C,** In the absence of light, Na+ enters the outer segment of the rod through cGMP-gated channels and depolarizes the cell. The electrical circuit for this dark current is completed by K+ leaving the inner segment. The dark current, which depolarizes the cell, leads to constant transmitter release. **D,** In the presence of light, Na+ can no longer enter the cell because cGMP levels are low, and the cGMP-gated channel closes. The photoreceptor cell thus hyperpolarizes, and transmitter release decreases.

K+ flows through a K+ channel in the inner segment, which light does not regulate. Na+ carries ~90% of the dark current in the outer segment, and Ca²⁺, ~10%. In the dark, V_m is about −40 mV. Na-K pumps, primarily located within the inner segments, remove the Na+ and import K+. A Na-Ca exchanger removes Ca²⁺ from the outer segment.

Absorption of photons leads to closure of the nonselective cation channels in the outer segment. The total conductance of the cell membrane decreases. Because the K+ channels of the inner segment remain open, K+ continues to flow out of the cell, and this outward current causes the cell to hyperpolarize (Fig. 15-11D). The number of cation channels that close depends on the number of photons that are absorbed. The range of one rod's sensitivity is 1 to ~1000 photons. Cones are less sensitive, but they are faster than rods; moreover, cone responses do not saturate even at the brightest levels of natural light.

Baylor and colleagues measured the minimum amount of light required to produce a change in receptor current (Fig. 15-11B). They found that absorption of one photon suppresses a surprisingly large current, equivalent to the entry of more than 10^6 Na+ ions, and thus represents an enormous amplification of energy. At the peak of the response, this decrease in Na+ influx represents ~3% of the cell's entire dark current. The single-photon response is also much larger than the background electrical noise in the rod, as it must be to produce the rod's high sensitivity to dim light. Cones respond similarly to single photons, but they are inherently noisier and their response is only ~$\frac{1}{50}$ the size of that in the rod.

Rhodopsin is a G protein–coupled "receptor" for light

How can a single photon stop the flow of 1 million Na+ ions across the membrane of a rod cell? The process begins when the photon is absorbed by rhodopsin, the light receptor molecule. Rhodopsin is one of the most tightly packed proteins in the body, with a density of ~30,000 molecules per square micrometer in the disk membranes. Thus, the packing ratio is 1 protein molecule for every 60 lipid molecules! One rod contains ~10^9 rhodopsin molecules. This staggering density ensures an optimized capture rate for photons passing through a photoreceptor. Even so, only ~10% of the light entering the eye is used by the receptors. The rest is either absorbed by the optical components of the eye or passes between or through the receptors. Rhodopsin has two key components: retinal and the protein opsin. Retinal is the aldehyde of **vitamin A**, or retinol (~500 Da). **Opsin** is a single polypeptide (~41 kDa) with seven membrane-spanning segments (Fig. 15-12A). It is a member of the superfamily of GPCRs (see Chapter 3) that includes many neurotransmitter receptors as well as the odor receptor molecules.

To be transduced, photons are actually absorbed by **retinal**, which is responsible for rhodopsin's color. The tail of retinal can twist into a variety of geometric configurations, one of which is a kinked and unstable version called **11-cis retinal** (Fig. 15-12B). The cis form sits within a pocket (comparable to the ligand binding site of other GPCRs) of the opsin and is covalently bound to it. However, because of its instability, the cis form can exist only in the dark. If 11-cis

retinal absorbs a photon, it isomerizes within 1 picosecond to a straighter and more stable version called **all-trans retinal**. This isomerization in turn triggers a series of conformational changes in the opsin that lead to a form called **metarhodopsin II**, which can activate an attached molecule called transducin. Transducin carries the signal forward in the cascade and causes a reduction in Na+ conductance. Soon after isomerization, all-trans retinal and opsin separate in a process called **bleaching**; this separation causes the color to change from the rosy red (rhodon is Greek for the color "rose") of rhodopsin to the pale yellow of opsin. The photoreceptor cell converts all-trans retinal to retinol (vitamin A), which then translocates to the pigment epithelium and becomes 11-cis retinal. This compound makes its way back to the outer segment, where it recombines with opsin. This cycle of rhodopsin regeneration takes a few minutes.

Transducin is so named because it transduces the light-activated signal from rhodopsin into the photoreceptor membrane's response (Fig. 15-12C). Transducin was the first of the large family of guanosine triphosphate (GTP)–binding proteins (G proteins) to be identified, and its amino acid sequence is very similar to that of other GPCRs (see Chapter 3). When it is activated by metarhodopsin, the α subunit of transducin exchanges a bound guanosine diphosphate (GDP) for a GTP and then diffuses within the plane of the membrane to stimulate a **phosphodiesterase** that hydrolyzes cGMP to 5′-guanylate monophosphate.

cGMP is the diffusible second messenger that links the light-activated events of the disk membranes to the electrical events of the outer membrane. A key discovery by Fesenko and colleagues in 1985 showed that the "light-sensitive" cation channel of rods is actually a cGMP-gated cation channel (see Chapter 6). This cyclic nucleotide–gated channel was the first of its kind to be discovered (we have already discussed a similar channel in olfactory receptors). In the dark, a **constitutively active guanylyl cyclase** that synthesizes cGMP from GTP keeps cGMP levels high within the photoreceptor cytoplasm. This high $[cGMP]_i$ causes the cGMP-gated cation channels to spend much of their time open and accounts for the dark current (Fig. 15-11C). Because light stimulates the phosphodiesterase and thus decreases $[cGMP]_i$, light reduces the number of open cGMP-gated cation channels and thus reduces the dark current. The photoreceptor then hyperpolarizes, transmitter release falls, and a visual signal is passed to retinal neurons.

Strong amplification occurs along the phototransduction pathway. The absorption of 1 photon activates 1 metarhodopsin molecule, which can activate ~700 transducin molecules within ~100 ms. These transducin molecules activate phosphodiesterase, which increases the rate of cGMP hydrolysis by ~100-fold. One photon leads to the hydrolysis of ~1400 cGMP molecules by the peak of the response, thus reducing $[cGMP]$ by ~8% in the cytoplasm around the activated disk. This decrease in $[cGMP]_i$ closes ~230 of the 11,000 cGMP-gated channels that are open in the dark. As a result, the dark current falls by ~2%.

The cGMP-gated channel has additional interesting properties. It responds within milliseconds when $[cGMP]_i$ rises, and it does not desensitize in response to cGMP. The concentration-response curve is very steep at low $[cGMP]_i$

A OPSIN

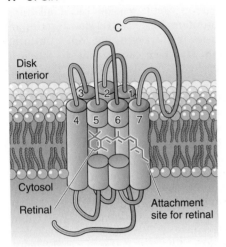

B RETINAL

11-*cis* retinal

Light

All-*trans* retinal

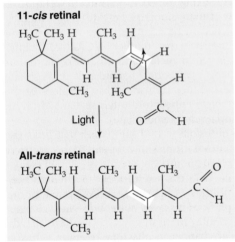

C VISUAL TRANSDUCTION

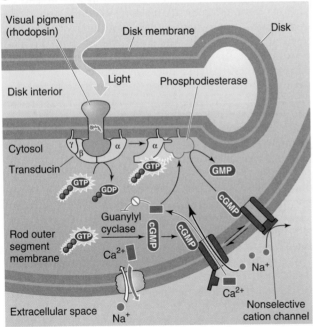

because opening requires the simultaneous binding of three cGMP molecules. Thus, the channel has switch-like behavior at physiological levels of cGMP. Ion conductance through the channel also has steep voltage dependence because Ca^{2+} and Mg^{2+} strongly block the channel (as well as permeate it) within its physiological voltage range. This open-channel block (see Fig. 7-20D) makes the normal single-channel conductance very small, among the smallest of any ion channel; the open channel normally carries a current of only 3×10^{-15} amperes (3 fA)! The current of ion channels is inherently "noisy" as they flicker open and closed. However, the 11,000 channels—each with currents of 3 fA—summate to a rather noise-free dark current of 11,000 channels × 3 fA per channel = 33 pA. In contrast, if 11 channels—each with currents of 3 pA—carried the dark current of 33 pA, the 2% change in this signal (0.66 pA) would be smaller than the noise produced by the opening and closing of a single channel (3 pA). Thus, the small channels give the photoreceptor a high signal-to-noise ratio.

The $[cGMP]_i$ in the photoreceptor cell represents a dynamic balance between the synthesis of cGMP by guanylyl cyclase and the breakdown of cGMP by phosphodiesterase. Ca^{2+}, which enters through the relatively nonselective cGMP-gated channel, synergistically inhibits the guanylyl cyclase and stimulates the phosphodiesterase. These Ca^{2+} sensitivities set up a negative feedback system. In the dark, the incoming Ca^{2+} prevents runaway increases in $[cGMP]_i$. In the light, the ensuing decrease in $[Ca^{2+}]_i$ relieves the inhibition on guanylyl cyclase, inhibits the phosphodiesterase, increases $[cGMP]_i$, and thus poises the system for channel reopening.

The process of termination of the light-activated state of the photoreceptor cell has not been as well defined as the activation process. One mechanism appears to involve the channels themselves. As described in the preceding paragraph, closure of the cGMP-gated channels in the light leads to a fall in $[Ca^{2+}]_i$, which helps replenish cGMP and facilitates channel reopening. Two additional mechanisms involve the proteins rhodopsin kinase and arrestin. **Rhodopsin kinase** phosphorylates light-activated rhodopsin and allows it to be recognized by arrestin. **Arrestin**, an abundant cytosolic protein, binds to the phosphorylated light-activated rhodopsin and helps terminate the activated state of the receptor.

Figure 15-12 Rhodopsin, transducin, and signal transduction at the molecular level. **A,** The opsin molecule is a classic seven-transmembrane receptor that couples to transducin, a G protein. The attachment site of the retinal is amino acid residue 296 in the seventh (i.e., most C-terminal) membrane-spanning segment. **B,** The absorption of a photon by 11-*cis* retinal causes the molecule to isomerize to all-*trans* retinal. **C,** After rhodopsin absorbs a photon of light, it activates many transducins. The activated α subunit of transducin ($G\alpha_t$) in turn activates phosphodiesterase, which hydrolyzes cGMP. The resultant decrease in $[cGMP]_i$ closes cGMP-gated channels and produces a hyperpolarization (receptor potential). GMP, 5'-guanylate monophosphate.

The eye uses a variety of mechanisms to adapt to a wide range of light levels

The human eye can operate effectively over a 10^{10}-fold range of light intensities, which is the equivalent of going from almost total darkness to bright sunlight on snow. However, moving from a bright to a dark environment, or vice versa, requires time for adaptation before the eye can respond optimally. Adaptation is mediated by several mechanisms. One mechanism mentioned earlier is regulation of the size of the pupil by the iris, which can change light sensitivity by ~16-fold. That still leaves the vast majority of the range to account for. During **dark adaptation**, two additional mechanisms with very different time courses are evident, as we can see from a test of the detection threshold for the human eye (Fig. 15-13). The first phase of adaptation is finished within ~10 minutes and is a property of the cones; the second takes at least 30 minutes and is attributed to the rods. A fully dark-adapted retina, relying on rods, can have a light threshold that is as much as 500 times lower than a retina relying on fully dark-adapted cones. In essence, then, the human eye has two retinas in one, a rod retina for low light levels and a cone retina for high light levels. These two systems can operate at the same time; when dark adapted, the rods can respond to the lowest light levels, but cones are available to respond when brighter stimuli appear.

The rapid and slow phases of adaptation that are discussed in the preceding paragraph have both neural and photoreceptor mechanisms. The *neural* mechanisms are relatively fast, operate at relatively low ambient light levels, and involve multiple mechanisms within the neuronal network of the retina. The *photoreceptor* mechanisms involve some of the processes that are described in the previous section. Thus, in bright sunlight, rods become ineffective because most of their rhodopsin remains inactivated, or bleached. After returning to darkness, the rods slowly regenerate rhodopsin and become sensitive once again. However, a component of the cGMP system also regulates photoreceptor sensitivity. In the dark, when baseline $[cGMP]_i$ is relatively high, substantial amounts of Ca^{2+} enter through cGMP-gated channels. The resultant high $[Ca^{2+}]_i$ inhibits guanylyl cyclase and stimulates phosphodiesterase, thereby preventing $[cGMP]_i$ from rising too high. Conversely, when background light levels are high, this same feedback system causes baseline $[cGMP]_i$ to remain high so that $[cGMP]_i$ can fall in response to further increases in light levels. Otherwise, the signal transduction system would become saturated. In other words, the photoreceptor adapts to the increased background light intensity and remains responsive to small changes. Additional adaptation mechanisms regulate the sensitivity of rhodopsin, guanylyl cyclase, and the cGMP-gated channel. Clearly, adaptation involves an intricate network of molecular interaction.

Color vision depends on the different spectral sensitivities of the three types of cones

The human eye responds only to a small region of the electromagnetic spectrum (Fig. 15-5); but within it, we are exquisitely sensitive to the light's wavelength. We see assorted colors in a daytime panorama because objects absorb some wavelengths while reflecting, refracting, or transmitting others. Different sources of light may also affect the colors of a scene; the light from tungsten bulbs is reddish, whereas that of fluorescent bulbs is bluish.

Research on color vision has a long history. In 1801, Thomas Young first outlined the trichromatic theory of color vision, which was championed later in the 19th century by Hermann von Helmholtz. These investigators found that they could reproduce a particular sample hue by mixing the correct intensities of three lights with the primary hues blue, green, and red. They proposed that color vision, with its wide range of distinct, perceived hues, is based on only three different pigments in the eye, each absorbing a different range of wavelengths. Microspectrophotometry of single cones in 1964 amply confirmed this scheme. Thus, although analysis of color by the human brain is sophisticated and complex, it all derives from the responses of only three types of photopigments in cones.

Our sensitivity to the wavelength of light depends on the retina's state of adaptation. When it is dark adapted (also called **scotopic** conditions), the spectral sensitivity curve for human vision is shifted toward shorter wavelengths compared with the curve obtained after light adaptation (**photopic** conditions; Fig. 15-14A). The absolute sensitivity to light can also be several orders of magnitude higher under scotopic conditions (Fig. 15-13). The primary reason for the difference in these curves is that rods are doing the transduction of dim light under dark-adapted conditions, whereas cones transduce in the light-adapted eye. As we would predict, the spectral sensitivity curve for scotopic vision is

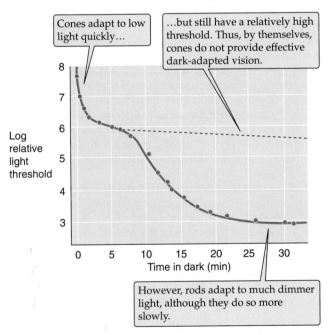

Cones adapt to low light quickly...

...but still have a relatively high threshold. Thus, by themselves, cones do not provide effective dark-adapted vision.

However, rods adapt to much dimmer light, although they do so more slowly.

Figure 15-13 The effect of dark adaptation on the visual threshold. The subject was exposed to light at a level of 1600 millilumens and then switched to the dark. The graph is a plot of the time course of the subject's relative threshold (on a log scale) for detecting a light stimulus. *(Data from Hecht S, Shlaer S, Smith EL, et al: The visual functions of the complete color blind. J Gen Physiol 1948; 31:459-472.)*

A SPECTRAL SENSITIVITY UNDER DARK- AND LIGHT-ADAPTED CONDITIONS

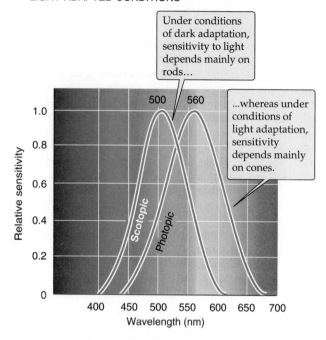

Under conditions of dark adaptation, sensitivity to light depends mainly on rods...

...whereas under conditions of light adaptation, sensitivity depends mainly on cones.

B ABSORBANCE SPECTRA OF THE HUMAN ROD AND CONE RHODOPSINS

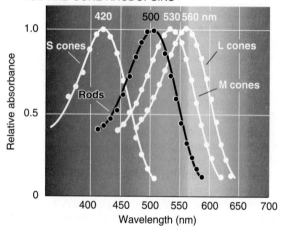

Figure 15-14 Sensitivity of vision and photoreceptors at different wavelengths of light. **A,** The figure shows the results of a psychophysical experiment. Under dark-adapted (scotopic) conditions, the eye is maximally sensitive at ~500 nm. Under light-adapted (photopic) conditions, the human eye is maximally sensitive at ~560 nm. *(Data from Knowles A: The biochemical aspects of vision. In Barlow HB, Mollon JD [eds]: The Senses, pp 82-101. Cambridge: Cambridge University Press, 1982.)* **B,** The spectral sensitivity of rods (obtained with a spectrophotometer) peaks at ~500 nm; that of the three types of cones peaks at ~420 nm for the S (blue), ~530 nm for the M (green), and ~560 nm for the L (red). The absorbance spectrum for each type of cone has been normalized to its peak sensitivity. *(Data from Dartnell HJ, Bowmaker JK, Mollon JD: Microspectrophotometry of human photoreceptors. In Mollon JD, Sharpe LT [eds]: Colour Vision, pp 69-80. London: Academic Press, 1983.)*

quite similar to the absorption spectrum of the rods' rhodopsin, with a peak at 500 nm.

The spectral sensitivity of the light-adapted eye depends on the photopigments in the cones. Humans have three different kinds of cones, and each expresses a photopigment with a different absorbance spectrum. The peaks of their absorbance curves fall at ~420, 530, and 560 nm, which correspond to the violet, yellow-green, and yellow-red regions of the spectrum (Fig. 15-14B). The three cones and their pigments were historically called blue, green, and red, respectively. They are now more commonly called S, M, and L (for short, medium, and long wavelengths); we use this terminology. Because the absolute sensitivity of the short-wavelength cone is only one tenth that of the other two, the spectral sensitivity of photopic human vision is dominated by the two longer wavelength cones (compare the spectral sensitivity functions in Fig. 15-14A with the absorbance spectra of the cones in Fig. 15-14B).

Single cones do not encode the wavelength of a light stimulus. If a cone responds to a photon, it generates the same response regardless of the wavelength of that photon. A glance at Figure 15-14B shows that each type of cone pigment can absorb a wide range of wavelengths. The pigment in a cone is more likely to absorb photons when their wavelength is at its peak absorbance, but light hitting the cone on the fringe of its absorbance range can still generate a large response if the light's intensity is sufficiently high. This property of response **univariance** is the reason that vision in an eye with only one functioning pigment (e.g., scotopic vision using only rods) can only be monochromatic. With a single pigment system, the distinction between different colors and between differences in intensity is confounded. Two different cones (as in most New World monkeys), each with a different but overlapping range of wavelength sensitivity, remove much of the ambiguity in encoding the wavelength of light stimuli. With three overlapping pigments (as in Old World monkeys and humans), light of a single wavelength stimulates each of the three cones to different degrees, and light of any other wavelength stimulates these cones with a distinctly different pattern. Because the nervous system can compare the *relative* stimulation of the three cone types to decode the wavelength, it can also distinguish changes in the intensity (luminance) of the light from changes in its wavelength.

Color capabilities are not constant across the retina. The use of multiple cones is not compatible with fine spatial discrimination because of wavelength-dependent differences in the eye's ability to focus light (**chromatic aberration**) and because very small objects may stimulate only single cones. The fovea has only M and L cones, which limits its color discrimination in comparison to the peripheral portions of the retina but leaves it best adapted to discriminate fine spatial detail.

The four different human visual pigments have a similar structure. The presence of retinal and the mechanisms of its photoisomerization are essentially identical in each. The main difference is the primary structure of the attached protein, the opsin. M and L opsins share 96% of their amino acids. Pairwise comparisons among the other opsins show only 44% or lower sequence similarity, however. Apparently, the different amino acid structures of the opsins affect their

Inherited Defects in Color Vision

Inherited defects in color vision are relatively common, and many are caused by mutations in visual pigment genes. For example, 8% of white males and 1% of white females have some defect in their L or M pigments caused by X-linked recessive mutations. A single abnormal pigment can lead to either **dichromacy** (the absence of one functional pigment) or **anomalous trichromacy** (the absorption spectrum of one pigment shifted relative to normal), often with a consequent inability to distinguish certain colors. Jeremy Nathans and colleagues found that men have only one copy of the L pigment gene; but located right next to it on the X chromosome, they may have one to three copies of the M pigment gene. He proposed that homologous recombination could account for the gene duplication, loss of a gene, or production of the hybrid L-M genes that occur in red-green color blindness. Hybrid L-M pigments have spectral properties intermediate between those of the two normal pigments, probably because their opsins consist of a combination of the traits of the two normal pigments.

Lack of two of the three functional cone pigments leads to **monochromacy**. The number of people who have such true color blindness is very small, less than 0.001% of the population. For example, S-cone monochromacy is a rare X-linked disorder in which both L and M photopigments are missing because of mutations on the X chromosome. The S pigment is on chromosome 7.

charge distributions in the region of the 11-*cis* retinal and shift its absorption spectrum to give the different pigments their specific spectral sensitivities.

VESTIBULAR AND AUDITORY TRANSDUCTION: HAIR CELLS

Balancing on one foot and listening to music both involve sensory systems that have similar transduction mechanisms. Sensation in both the vestibular and auditory systems begins with the inner ear, and both use a highly specialized kind of receptor called the **hair cell**. Common structure and function often suggest a common origin, and indeed, the organs of mammalian hearing and balance both evolved from the **lateral line organs** present in all aquatic vertebrates. The lateral line consists of a series of pits or tubes along the flanks of an animal. Within each indentation are clusters of sensory cells that are similar to hair cells. These cells have microvilli-like structures that project into a gelatinous material that in turn is in contact with the water in which the animal swims. The lateral line is exquisitely sensitive to vibrations or pressure changes in the water in many animals, although it is also sensitive to temperature or electrical fields in some species. Reptiles abandoned the lateral line during their evolution, but they retained the hair-cell–centered sensory structures of the inner ear that evolved from the lateral line.

The vestibular system generates our sense of balance, and the auditory system provides our senses of hearing. **Vestibular sensation** operates constantly while we are awake and communicates to the brain the head's orientation and changes in the head's motion. Such information is essential for generation of muscle contractions that will put our body where we want it to be, to reorient the body when something pushes us aside (vestibular-spinal reflexes), and to move our eyes continually so that the visual world stays fixed on our retinas even though our head may be nodding about (vestibular-ocular reflexes). Vestibular dysfunction can make it impossible to stabilize an image on our moving retinas, and it causes the disconcerting feeling that the world is uncontrollably moving around—**vertigo**. Walking and standing can be difficult or impossible. With time, compensatory adjustments are made as the brain learns to substitute more visual and proprioceptive cues to help guide smooth and accurate movements.

Auditory sensation is often at the forefront of our conscious experience, unlike vestibular information, which we rarely notice unless something goes wrong. Hearing is an exceptionally versatile process that allows us to detect things in our environment, to precisely identify their nature, to localize them well at a distance, and, through language, to communicate with speed, complexity, nuance, and emotion.

Bending the stereovilli of hair cells along one axis causes cation channels to open or to close

Hair cells are mechanoreceptors that are specialized to detect minuscule movement along one particular axis. The hair cell is an epithelial cell; the hair bundles project from the apical end, whereas synaptic contacts occur at the basal end. Hair cells are somewhat different in the vestibular and auditory systems. In this section, we illustrate concepts mainly with the vestibular hair cell (Fig. 15-15A), which comes in two subtypes. Vestibular **type I** cells have a bulbous basal area, surrounded by a calyx-shaped afferent nerve terminal (Fig. 15-15B, left). Vestibular **type II** hair cells are more cylindrical and have several simple, bouton-shaped afferent nerve terminals (Fig. 15-15B, right). As we will see, auditory hair cells also come in two varieties, **inner hair cells** and **outer hair cells**. However, all hair cells sense movement in basically the same way.

As part of their hair bundles, *vestibular* hair cells (Fig. 15-15B) have one large **kinocilium**, which is a true cilium with the characteristic 9 + 2 pattern of microtubules (see Fig. 2-11A). The role of the kinocilium is unknown. In mammals, *auditory* hair cells lose their kinocilium with maturity.

Both vestibular and auditory hair cells have 50 to 150 **stereovilli**, which are filled with actin and are more akin to microvilli. The stereovilli—often called stereocilia, although they lack the typical 9 + 2 pattern of true cilia—are 0.2 to 0.8 μm in diameter and are generally 4 to 10 μm in height. These "hairs" are arranged in a neat array. In the *vestibular* system, the kinocilium stands tallest along one side of the bundle and the stereovilli fall away in height to the opposite side (Fig. 15-15B). Stereovilli are narrower at their base and insert into the apical membrane of the hair cell, where they make a sort of hinge before connecting to a cuticular plate. Within the bundle, stereovilli are connected one to the next, but they can slide with respect to each other as the bundle is deflected side to side. The ends of the stereovilli are inter-

A VESTIBULAR HAIR BUNDLES

B VESTIBULAR HAIR CELLS

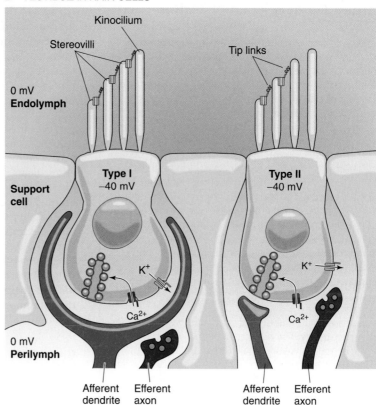

Figure 15-15 Vestibular hair cells. **A,** Scanning electron micrograph of a bullfrog hair cell from the sensory epithelium of the saccule. *(From Corey DP, Assad JA: In Corey DP, Roper SD [eds]: Sensory Transduction. New York: Rockefeller University Press, 1992.)* **B,** Type I and type II cells. *(Data from Philine Wangemann, Kansas State University.)*

connected with very fine strands called **tip links**, which are visible by electron microscopy.

The epithelium of which the hair cells are a part separates perilymph from endolymph. The **perilymph** bathes the basolateral side of the hair cells. In composition (i.e., relatively low [K⁺], high [Na⁺]), perilymph is similar to cerebrospinal fluid. Its voltage is zero—close to that of most other extracellular fluids in the body. The basolateral resting potential of vestibular hair cells and auditory inner hair cells is about −40 mV (Fig. 15-15B). The **endolymph** bathing the stereovilli is singular in composition. It has a very high [K⁺] (150 mM) and a very low [Na⁺] (1 mM), more like cytoplasm than extracellular fluid. It also has a relatively high [HCO₃⁻] (30 mM). The voltage of the vestibular endolymph is ~0 mV relative to perilymph. Across the apical membrane of vestibular hair cells, the *chemical* gradient for K⁺ is small. However, the *electrical* gradient is fairly large, ~40 mV. Thus, a substantial force tends to drive K⁺ into the vestibular hair cell across the apical membrane. Later, we will see that the driving force for K⁺ influx is even higher in the auditory system.

The appropriate stimulus for a hair cell is the bending of its hairs, but not just any deflection will do. Bending of the hair bundle *toward* the longer stereovilli (Fig. 15-16A) excites the cell and causes a depolarizing **receptor potential**. Bending of the hair bundle *away from* the longer stereovilli (Fig. 15-

16B) hyperpolarizes the cell. Only tiny movements are needed. In auditory hair cells, as little as 0.5 nm (which is the diameter of a large atom) gives a detectable response, and the response is saturated at ~150 nm, about the diameter of one stereovillus! In fact, the sensitivity of hair cells is limited only by noise from the brownian motion of surrounding molecules. The cell is also exquisitely selective to direction. If the hairs are bent along the axis 90 degrees to their preferred direction, they are less than one tenth as responsive.

Mechanotransduction in hair cells seems to be accomplished by directly linking the movement of the stereovilli to the gating of apical mechanosensitive cation channels. Electrical measurements, as well as the imaging of intracellular Ca²⁺, imply that the transduction channels are located near the tips of the stereovilli. How is channel gating connected to movement of the hairs? The latency of channel opening is extremely short, less than 40 μs. If one deflects the hairs more rapidly, the channels are activated more quickly. This observation suggests a direct, physical coupling inasmuch as diffusion of a second messenger would take much longer. Corey and Hudspeth have suggested a spring-like molecular linkage between the movement of stereovilli and channel gating. Indirect evidence suggests that the tip links may be the tethers between stereovilli and the channels. Brief exposure to low-Ca²⁺ solutions abolishes transduction, and it also

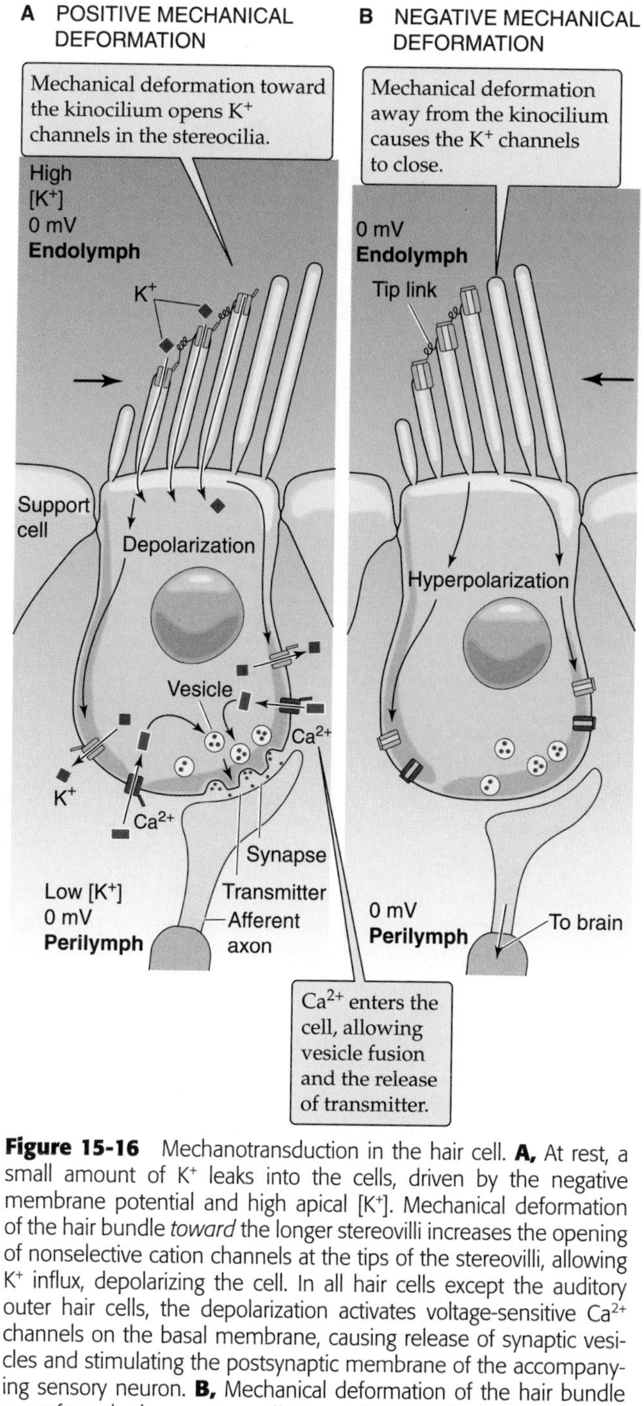

A POSITIVE MECHANICAL DEFORMATION

Mechanical deformation toward the kinocilium opens K⁺ channels in the stereocilia.

High [K⁺]
0 mV
Endolymph

K⁺

Support cell

Depolarization

Vesicle

Ca^{2+}

K⁺

Ca^{2+}

Synapse

Transmitter

Low [K⁺]
0 mV
Perilymph

Afferent axon

Ca^{2+} enters the cell, allowing vesicle fusion and the release of transmitter.

B NEGATIVE MECHANICAL DEFORMATION

Mechanical deformation away from the kinocilium causes the K⁺ channels to close.

0 mV
Endolymph

Tip link

Hyperpolarization

0 mV
Perilymph

To brain

Figure 15-16 Mechanotransduction in the hair cell. **A,** At rest, a small amount of K⁺ leaks into the cells, driven by the negative membrane potential and high apical [K⁺]. Mechanical deformation of the hair bundle *toward* the longer stereovilli increases the opening of nonselective cation channels at the tips of the stereovilli, allowing K⁺ influx, depolarizing the cell. In all hair cells except the auditory outer hair cells, the depolarization activates voltage-sensitive Ca^{2+} channels on the basal membrane, causing release of synaptic vesicles and stimulating the postsynaptic membrane of the accompanying sensory neuron. **B,** Mechanical deformation of the hair bundle *away* from the longer stereovilli causes the nonselective cation channels to close, leading to hyperpolarization.

destroys the tip links without otherwise causing obvious harm to the cells.

The mechanosensitive channels at the tips of the stereovilli are relatively large (~100 pS each) and unselective in that they allow monovalent cations and some divalent cations, including Ca^{2+}, to pass easily. Each hair cell has fewer than 100 channels. Under physiological conditions, K⁺ carries most of the current. When the cell is at rest—hairs straight up—a small but steady leak of depolarizing K⁺ current flows

through the cell. This leak allows the hair cell to respond to both positive and negative deflections of its stereovilli. A positive deflection—toward the tallest stereovilli—further opens the apical channels, leading to *influx* of K⁺ and thus *depolarization*. K⁺ leaves the cell through mechano*insensitive* K⁺ channels on the basolateral side (Fig. 15-16A), along a favorable electrochemical gradient. A negative deflection closes the apical channels and thus leads to *hyperpolarization* (Fig. 15-16B).

The mechanosensitive channel in hair cells seems to be a member of the transient receptor potential (TRP) superfamily of ion channels, specifically the TRPA1 channel expressed at the tips of stereovilli. Knocking down TRPA1 abolishes hair cell transduction. The TRPA1 protein has a long chain of ankyrin repeats leading up to the channel domain. The ankyrin repeats may be part of a "gating spring" that is observed in biophysical studies of channel gating.

A hair cell is not a neuron. Hair cells do not project an axon of their own, and most do not generate action potentials. Instead—in the case of vestibular hair cells and auditory inner hair cells—the membrane near the presynaptic (i.e., basolateral) face of the cell has voltage-gated Ca^{2+} channels that are somewhat active at rest but more active during mechanically induced depolarization (i.e., the receptor potential) of the hair cell. The Ca^{2+} that enters the hair cell through these channels triggers the release of glutamate as well as aspartate in the case of vestibular hair cells. These excitatory transmitters stimulate the postsynaptic terminal of sensory neurons that transmit information to the brain. The greater the transmitter release, the greater the rate of action potential firing in the postsynaptic axon.

In mammals, all hair cells—whether part of the vestibular or auditory system—are contained within bilateral sets of interconnected tubes and chambers called, appropriately enough, the **membranous labyrinth** (Fig. 15-17A, B). The **vestibular** portion has five sensory structures: two **otolithic organs**, which detect gravity (i.e., head position) and linear head movements, and three **semicircular canals**, which detect head rotation. Also contributing to our sense of spatial orientation and motion are proprioceptors and the visual system (see later). The **auditory** portion of the labyrinth is the spiraling **cochlea**, which detects rapid vibrations (sound) transmitted to it from the surrounding air.

The ultimate function of each of these sensory structures is to transmit mechanical energy to their hair cells. In each case, transduction occurs in the manner described earlier. The specificity of the transduction process depends much less on the hair cells than on the structure of the labyrinth organs around them.

The otolithic organs (saccule and utricle) detect the orientation and linear acceleration of the head

The **otolithic organs** are a pair of relatively large chambers—the **saccule** and the **utricle**—near the center of the labyrinth (Fig. 15-17B). These otolithic organs as well as the semicircular canals are (1) lined by epithelial cells, (2) filled with endolymph, (3) surrounded by perilymph, and (4) encased in the temporal bone. Within the epithelium, specialized **vestibular dark cells** secrete K⁺ and are responsible

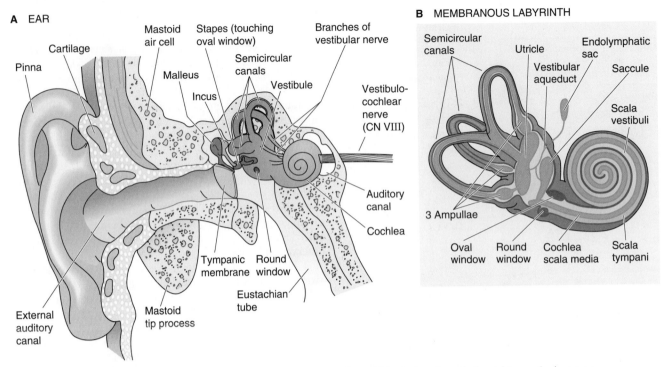

Figure 15-17 The ear, cochlea, and semicircular canals. **A,** This section through the right ear of a human shows the outer, the middle, and the inner ear. **B,** The labyrinth consists of an auditory and a vestibular portion. The auditory portion is the cochlea. The vestibular portion includes the two otolithic organs (the utricle and saccule) and the three semicircular canals.

for the high [K⁺] of the endolymph. The mechanism of K⁺ secretion is similar to that by the stria vascularis in the auditory system (see later).

The saccule and utricle each has a sensory epithelium called the **macula**, which contains the hair cells that lie among a bed of supporting cells. The stereovilli project into the gelatinous **otolithic membrane**, a mass of mucopolysaccharides that is studded with otoliths or **otoconia** (Fig. 15-18A, B). These crystals of calcium carbonate, 1 to 5 μm in diameter, give the otolithic membrane a higher density than the surrounding endolymph. With either a change in the angle of the head or a linear acceleration, the inertia of the otoconia causes the otolithic membrane to move slightly, deflecting the stereovilli.

The macula is vertically oriented (in the sagittal plane) within the **saccule** and horizontally oriented within the **utricle** when the head is tilted down by ~25 degrees, as during walking. In the saccule, the kinocilia point *away from* a curving **reversal line** that divides the macula into two regions (Fig. 15-18A and D). In the utricle, the kinocilia point *toward* the reversal line (Fig. 15-18B and D). The saccule and utricle respond well to changes in head angle and to acceleration of the sort that you experience as a car or an elevator starts or stops. Of course, the head can tilt or experience acceleration in many directions. Indeed, the orientation of hair cells of the saccule and utricle covers a full range of directions. Any tilt or linear acceleration of the head will enhance the stimulation of some hair cells, reduce the stimulation of others, and have no effect on the rest.

Each hair cell synapses on the ending of a primary sensory axon that is part of the **vestibular nerve**, which in turn is a branch of the vestibulocochlear nerve (CN VIII). The cell bodies of these sensory neurons are located in Scarpa's ganglion within the temporal bone. The dendrites project to multiple hair cells, increasing the signal-to-noise ratio. The axons project to the ipsilateral vestibular nucleus in the brainstem. Because the saccule and utricle are paired structures (one on each side of the head), the CNS can simultaneously use information encoded by the full population of otolithic hair cells and unambiguously interpret any angle of tilt or linear acceleration. The push-pull arrangement of increased/decreased activity within each macula (for hair cells of opposite orientation) and between maculae on either side of the head enhances the fidelity of the signal.

The semicircular canals detect the angular acceleration of the head

Semicircular canals (Fig. 15-17B) also sense acceleration, but not the linear acceleration that the otolithic organs prefer. *Angular acceleration* generated by sudden head rotations is the primary stimulus for the semicircular canals. Shake your head side to side or nod it up and down. Each rotation of your head will excite some of your canals and inhibit others.

The semicircular canals stimulate their hair cells differently from the otolithic organs. In each canal, the hair cells are clustered within a sensory epithelium (the **crista ampullaris**) that is located in a bulge along the canal called the **ampulla** (Fig. 15-18C). The hair bundles—all of which have the same orientation—project into a gelatinous, dome-shaped structure called the **cupula**, which spans the lumen

A SACCULE

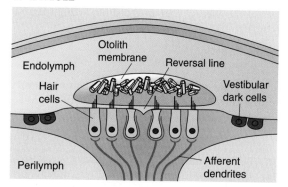

B UTRICLE

C AMPULLA OF A SEMICIRCULAR CANAL

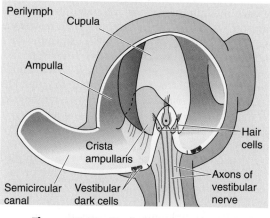

D DIRECTION OF HAIR BUNDLES

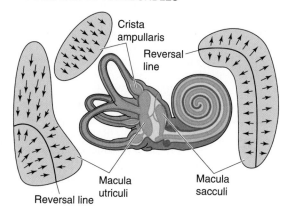

Figure 15-18 Vestibular sensory organs. In **A,** the longer stereovilli point *toward* the reversal line. In **B,** the longer stereovilli point *away from* the reversal line. In **C,** all stereovilli point in the same direction. In **D,** the *arrows* point toward the longer stereovilli (and kinocilia) and thereby indicate the directions of greatest sensitivity for opening of the transduction channels. *(Data from Philine Wangemann, Kansas State University.)*

of the ampulla. The cupula contains no otoconia, and its mucopolysaccharides have the same density as the surrounding endolymph. Thus, the cupula is not sensitive to *linear* acceleration. However, with a sudden rotation of the canal, the endolymph tends to stay behind because of its inertia. The relatively stagnant endolymph exerts a force on the movable cupula, much like wind on a sail. This force bows the cupula, which bends the hairs and (depending on the direction of rotation) either excites or suppresses the release of transmitter from the hair cells onto the sensory axons of the vestibular nerve. This arrangement makes the semicircular canals very sensitive to angular acceleration of the head. If head rotation is maintained at a constant velocity, the friction of endolymph with the canal walls eventually makes the two move together, so that the bending of the cupula gradually extinguishes within seconds. When rotation is then stopped, the inertia of the endolymph causes bending of the cupula in the other direction and thus gives a temporary sensation of counterrotation.

Each side of the head has three semicircular canals that lie in approximately orthogonal planes. The **anterior** canal is tilted ~41 degrees anterolaterally from the sagittal plane, the **posterior** canal is tilted ~56 degrees posterolaterally from

the sagittal plane, and the **lateral** canal is tipped ~25 degrees back from the horizontal plane. Because each canal best senses rotation about a particular axis, the three together give a good representation of all possible angles of head rotation. This complete representation is further ensured because each canal is paired with another on the opposite side of the head. Each member of a pair sits within the same plane and responds to rotation about the same axis. However, whereas rotation excites the hair cells of one canal, it inhibits the canals of its contralateral axis mate. This push-pull arrangement presumably increases the sensitivity of detection.

Outer and middle ears collect and condition air pressure waves for transduction within the inner ear

Sound is a perceptual phenomenon that is produced by periodic longitudinal waves of low pressure (rarefactions) and high pressure (compressions) that propagate through air at a speed of 330 to 340 m/s. Absolute sound intensity is the amplitude of the longitudinal wave, measured in pascal (Pa). Intensities of audible sounds are commonly expressed in **decibel sound pressure level** (dB SPL), which relates the absolute sound intensity (P_T) to a reference pressure (P_{ref}) of 20 µPa, close to the average human threshold at 2000 Hz.

$$\text{dB SPL} = 10 \times \log_{10} \frac{(P_T)^2}{(P_{ref})^2} = 20 \times \log_{10} \frac{P_T}{P_{ref}} \quad \text{(15-2)}$$

The logarithmic scale compresses the wide extent of sound pressures into a convenient range. An increase of 6 dB SPL corresponds to a doubling of the absolute sound pressure level; an increase of 20 dB SPL corresponds to a 10-fold increase.

Sound can be a **pure tone** of a single frequency, measured in hertz (Hz). Sounds produced by musical instruments or the human voice consist of a perceived fundamental frequency (pitch) and overtones. Sound that is **noise** contains no recognizable periodic elements. Pure tones are used clinically for the determination of hearing thresholds (**pure-tone audiogram**). Humans do not perceive as equally loud sounds of the same sound pressure level but different frequency. The psychoacoustic **phon scale** accounts for these differences in perception.

Sound waves vary in frequency, amplitude, and direction; our auditory systems are specialized to discriminate all three. We can also interpret the rapid and intricate temporal patterns of sound frequency and amplitude that constitute words and music. Encoding of sound frequency and amplitude begins with mechanisms in the cochlea, followed by further analysis in the CNS. To distinguish the direction of a sound along the horizontal plane, the brain compares signals from the two ears.

All mammalian ears are strikingly similar in structure. The ear is traditionally divided into outer, middle, and inner components (Fig. 15-17A). We discuss the outer and middle ear here. The **inner ear** consists of the membranous labyrinth, with both its vestibular and auditory components.

Outer Ear Proceeding from outside to inside, the part most visible is the **pinna**, a skin-covered flap of cartilage, and its small extension, the **tragus**. Together, they funnel sound waves into the **external auditory canal**. These structures, which compose the outer ear, focus sound waves on the tympanic membrane. Many animals (e.g., cats) can turn each pinna independently to facilitate hearing without changing head position. The shape of the pinna and tragus tends to emphasize certain sound frequencies over others, depending on their angle of incidence. The external ear parts in humans are essential for localization of sounds in the vertical plane. Sound enters the auditory canal both directly and after being reflected; the sound that we hear is a combination of the two. Depending on a sound's angle of elevation, it is reflected differently off the pinna and tragus. Thus, we hear a sound coming from above our head slightly differently than a sound coming from straight in front of us.

The external auditory canal is lined with skin and penetrates ~2.5 cm into the temporal bone, where it ends blindly at the eardrum (or **tympanic membrane**). Sound causes the tympanic membrane to vibrate, much like the head of a drum.

Middle Ear The air-filled chamber between the tympanic membrane on one side and the **oval window** on the other is

the middle ear (Fig. 15-17A). The **eustachian tube** connects the middle ear to the nasopharynx and makes it possible to equalize the air pressure on opposite sides of the tympanic membrane. The eustachian tube can also provide a path for throat infections and epithelial inflammation to invade the middle ear, leading to otitis media. The primary function of the middle ear is to transfer vibrations of the tympanic membrane to the oval window (Fig. 15-19). The key to accomplishing this task is a chain of three delicate bones called **ossicles**: the **malleus** (or hammer), **incus** (anvil), and **stapes** (stirrup). The ossicles are the smallest bones in the body.

Vibration transfer is not as simple as it might seem because sound starts as a set of pressure waves in the air (within the ear canal) and ends up as pressure waves in a watery cochlear fluid within the inner ear. Air and water have a very different **acoustic impedance**, which is the tendency of each medium to oppose movement brought about by a pressure wave. This impedance mismatch means that sound traveling directly from air to water has insufficient pressure to move the dense water molecules. Instead, without some system of compensation, more than 97% of a sound's energy would be reflected when it met a surface of water. The middle ear serves as an *impedance-matching device* that saves most of the aforementioned energy by two primary methods. First, the tympanic membrane has an area that is ~20-fold larger than that of the oval window, so a given pressure at the air side (the tympanic membrane) is amplified as it is transferred to the water side (the footplate of the stapes). Second, the malleus and incus act as a lever system, again amplifying the pressure of the wave. Rather than being reflected, most of the energy is successfully transferred to the liquids of the inner ear.

Two tiny muscles of the middle ear, the **tensor tympani** and the **stapedius**, insert onto the malleus and the stapes, respectively. These muscles exert some control over the stiffness of the ossicular chain, and their contraction serves to dampen the transfer of sound to the inner ear. They are

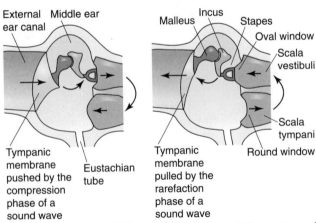

A INWARD MOVEMENT OF TYMPANIC MEMBRANE

External ear canal | Middle ear

Tympanic membrane pushed by the compression phase of a sound wave | Eustachian tube

B OUTWARD MOVEMENT OF TYMPANIC MEMBRANE

Malleus | Incus | Stapes | Oval window | Scala vestibuli

Tympanic membrane pulled by the rarefaction phase of a sound wave | Scala tympani | Round window

Figure 15-19 The middle ear. Displacement of the stapes and the oval window moves fluid in the scala vestibuli, causing opposite fluid movement in the scala tympani and thus an opposite displacement of the round window. (*Data from Philine Wangemann, Kansas State University.*)

reflexively activated when ambient sound levels become high. These reflexes are probably protective and may be particularly important for suppression of self-produced sounds, such as the roar you produce in your head when you speak or chew.

The cochlea is a spiral of three parallel, fluid-filled tubes

The auditory portion of the inner ear is mainly the **cochlea**, a tubular structure that is ~35 mm long and coiled 2.5 times into a snail shape about the size of a large pea (Fig. 15-20). Counting its stereovilli, the cochlea has a million moving parts, making it the most complex mechanical apparatus in the body.

The cut through the cochlea in the lower left panel of Figure 15-20 reveals five cross sections of the spiral. We see that in each cross section, two membranes divide the cochlea into three fluid-filled compartments. On one side is the compartment called the **scala vestibuli** (Fig. 15-20, right panel), which begins at its large end near the oval window—where vibrations enter the inner ear. **Reissner's membrane** separates the scala vestibuli from the middle compartment, the **scala media**. The other boundary of the scala media is the **basilar membrane**, on which rides the **organ of Corti** and

its hair cells. Below the basilar membrane is the **scala tympani**, which terminates at its basal or large end at the round window. Both the oval and round windows look into the middle ear.

Both the scala vestibuli and scala tympani are lined by a network of **fibrocytes** and filled with **perilymph**. Like its counterpart in the vestibular system, this perilymph is akin to cerebrospinal fluid (i.e., low [K$^+$], high [Na$^+$]). Along the lengths of scala vestibuli and scala tympani, the two perilymphs communicate through the leaky interstitial fluid spaces between the fibrocytes. At the apex of the cochlea, the two perilymphs communicate through a small opening called the **helicotrema**. Cochlear perilymph communicates with vestibular perilymph through a wide passage at the base of the scala vestibuli (Fig. 15-17B), and it communicates with the cerebrospinal fluid through the cochlear aqueduct.

The scala media is filled with **endolymph**. Like its vestibular counterpart—with which it communicates through the ductus reuniens (Fig. 15-17B)—auditory endolymph is extremely rich in K$^+$. Unlike vestibular endolymph, which has the same voltage as the perilymph, auditory endolymph has a voltage of +80 mV relative to the perilymph (Fig. 15-20, right panel). This **endocochlear potential**, which is the highest transepithelial voltage in the body, is the main driving

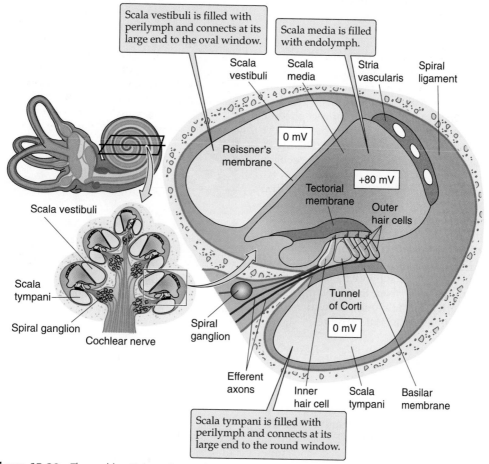

Figure 15-20 The cochlea. Reissner's membrane and the basilar membrane divide the cochlea into three spiraling fluid-filled compartments: the scala vestibuli, the scala media, and the scala tympani. (*Data from Philine Wangemann, Kansas State University.*)

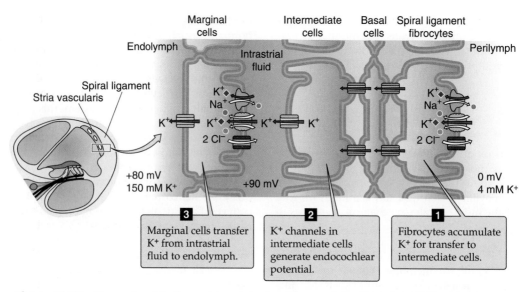

Figure 15-21 K⁺ secretion into the endolymph by the stria vascularis. *(Data from Philine Wangemann, Kansas State University.)*

force for sensory transduction in both inner and outer hair cells. Moreover, loss of the endocochlear potential is a frequent cause of hearing loss. A highly vascularized tissue called the stria vascularis secretes the K⁺ into the scala media, and the K⁺ gradient between endolymph and perilymph generate the endocochlear potential.

The **stria vascularis** is functionally a two-layered epithelium (Fig. 15-21). Marginal cells separate endolymph from a very small intrastrial compartment inside the stria vascularis, and basal cells separate the intrastrial compartment from the interstitial fluid of the spiral ligament, which is contiguous with perilymph. Gap junctions connect one side of the basal cells to intermediate cells and the other side of the basal cells to fibrocytes of the spiral ligament. This architecture is essential for generation of the endocochlear potential.

The fibrocytes are endowed with K⁺ uptake mechanisms that maintain a high [K⁺]ᵢ in the intermediate cells. The KCNJ10 K⁺ channel of the intermediate cells generates the endocochlear potential. The K⁺ equilibrium potential of these cells is extremely negative because of the combination of their very high [K⁺]ᵢ and the very low [K⁺] of the intrastrial fluid. Finally, the marginal cells support the endocochlear potential by mopping up the K⁺ from the intrastrial fluid—keeping the intrastrial [K⁺] very low—and depositing the K⁺ in the endolymph through a KCNQ1 K⁺ channel.

Inner hair cells transduce sound, whereas the active movements of outer hair cells amplify the signal

The business end of the cochlea is the **organ of Corti**, the portion of the basilar membrane that contains the hair cells. The organ of Corti stretches the length of the basilar membrane and has four rows of hair cells: one row of ~3500 **inner hair cells** and three rows with a total of ~16,000 **outer hair cells** (Fig. 15-22). In the *auditory* system, the arrangement of stereovilli is also quite orderly. The hair cells lie within a

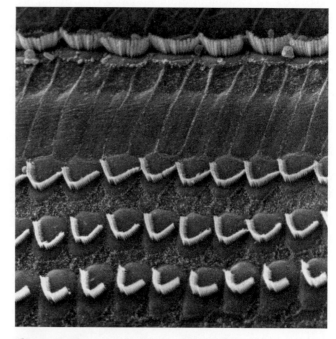

Figure 15-22 Hair cells of the cochlea. A scanning electron microscopic image of outer and inner hair cells of the organ of Corti of a chinchilla after removal of the tectorial membrane. The three rows of outer hair cells are on the bottom, and the single row of inner hair cells is along the top. *(Courtesy of I. Hunter-Duvar, MD, and R. Harrison, PhD, DSc, The Hospital for Sick Children, Toronto, Canada.)*

matrix of supporting cells, with their apical ends facing the endolymph of the scala media (Fig. 15-23A). The stereovilli of *inner* hair cells (Fig. 15-23B) are unique in that they float freely in the endolymph. The stereovilli of the *outer* hair cells (Fig. 15-23C) project into the gelatinous, collagen-containing **tectorial membrane**. The tectorial membrane is firmly

A UPWARD BOWING OF BASILAR MEMBRANE

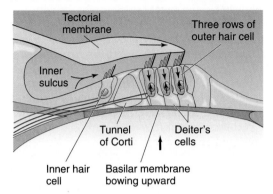

B INNER HAIR CELL **C** OUTER HAIR CELL

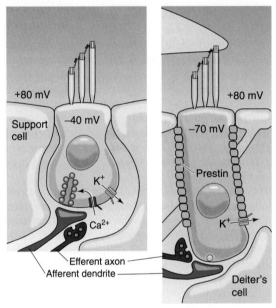

D DOWNWARD BOWING OF BASILAR MEMBRANE

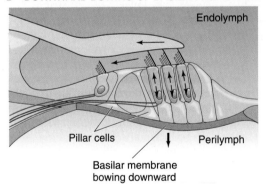

Figure 15-23 Organ of Corti. **A,** Upward movement of basilar membrane tilts hair bundles *toward* longer stereovilli, *opening* transduction channels. **B,** In inner hair cells, depolarization causes enhanced transmitter release. **C,** In outer hair cells, depolarization causes prestin to contract. **D,** Downward movement of basilar membrane tilts hair bundles *away from* longer stereovilli, *closing* transduction channels. *(Data from Philine Wangemann, Kansas State University.)*

attached only along one edge, with a sort of hinge, so that it is free to tilt up and down.

How do air pressure waves actually stimulate the auditory hair cells? Movements of the stapes against the oval window create traveling pressure waves within the cochlear fluids. Consider, for example, what happens as sound pressure falls in the outer ear.

Step 1: **Stapes moves outward.** As a result, the oval window moves *outward*, causing pressure in the scala vestibuli to decrease. Because the perilymph that fills the scala vestibuli and scala tympani is incompressible and the cochlea is encased in rigid bone, the round window moves *inward* (Fig. 15-19B).

Step 2: **Scala vestibuli pressure falls below scala tympani pressure.**

Step 3: **Basilar membrane bows upward.** Because Reissner's membrane is very thin and flexible, the low scala vestibuli pressure pulls up the incompressible scala media, which in turn causes the **basilar membrane** (and the organ of Corti) to bow upward.

Step 4: **Organ of Corti shears toward hinge of tectorial membrane.** The upward bowing of the basilar membrane creates a shear force between the hair bundle of the outer hair cells and the attached tectorial membrane.

Step 5: **Hair bundles of *outer* hair cells tilt toward their longer stereovilli.**

Step 6: **Transduction channels open in *outer* hair cells.** Because K^+ is the major ion, the result is *depolarization* of the outer hair cells (Fig. 15-16A)—**mechanical to electrical transduction**. The transduction-induced changes in membrane potential are called **receptor potentials**. The molecular mechanisms of these V_m changes are basically the same as in vestibular hair cells.

Step 7: **Depolarization contracts the motor protein prestin.** Outer hair cells express very high levels of **prestin** (named for the musical notation *presto*, or fast). The contraction of myriad prestin molecules—each attached to its neighbors—causes the outer hair cell to contract, **electrical to mechanical transduction** or **electromotility**. Conversely, hyperpolarization (during *downward* movements of the basilar membrane) causes outer hair cells to elongate. Indeed, imposing changes in V_m causes cell length to change by as much as ~5%. The change in shape is fast, beginning within 100 μs. The mechanical response of the outer hair cell does not depend on adenosine triphosphate (ATP), microtubule or actin systems, extracellular Ca^{2+}, or changes in cell volume. Prestin is a member of the SLC26 family of anion transporters (see Chapter 5), although it is not clear whether prestin also functions as an anion transporter.

Step 8: **Contraction of outer hair cells accentuates *upward* movement of basilar membrane.** Conversely, outer hair cell *elongation* (during *downward* movements of the basilar membrane) accentuates the *downward* movement of the basilar membrane. Thus, outer hair cells act as a **cochlear amplifier**—sensing and then rapidly accentuating movements of the basilar membrane. The electromotility of outer hair cells is a prerequisite for sensitive hearing and, as we will see later, the ability to discriminate frequencies sharply. In the absence of prestin, the cochlear amplifier ceases to function and animals become deaf.

Step 9: **Endolymph sloshes beneath the tectorial membrane, out of the inner sulcus.** The upward movement of the basilar membrane—accentuated by the cochlear amplifier—forces endolymph to flow out of the **inner sulcus**, beneath the tectorial membrane, toward its tip.

Step 10: *Inner* **hair cell hair bundles bend toward longer stereovilli.** The flow of endolymph now causes the free-floating hair bundles of the inner hair cells to bend.

Step 11: **Transduction channels open in inner hair cells.** As in the outer hair cells, the result is a *depolarization*.

Step 12: **Depolarization opens voltage-gated Ca²⁺ channels.** $[Ca^{2+}]_i$ rises in the inner hair cells.

Step 13: **Synaptic vesicles fuse, releasing glutamate.** The neurotransmitter triggers action potentials in afferent neurons, relaying auditory signals to the brainstem. Note that the response to depolarization is very different in the two types of hair cells. The outer hair cell contracts and thereby amplifies the movement of the basilar membrane. The inner hair cell releases neurotransmitter.

When the stapes reverses direction and moves inward, all of these processes reverse as well. The basilar membrane bows downward. In the outer hair cells, transduction channels close, causing *hyperpolarization* and cell elongation. The accentuated downward movement of the basilar membrane causes endolymph to slosh into the inner sulcus. In inner hair cells, transduction channels close, causing hyperpolarization and reduced neurotransmitter release.

A fascinating clue to the existence of the cochlear amplifier was the early observation that not only does the ear receive sounds, it also generates them! Short click sounds trigger an "echo," a brief vibration of the tympanic membrane that far outlasts the click. A microphone in the auditory canal can detect the echo. On occasion, damaged ears may produce spontaneous "otoacoustic emissions" that can even be loud enough to be heard by a nearby listener.

The cochlea receives sensory and motor innervation from the **auditory or cochlear nerve**, a branch of CN VIII. We discuss the motor innervation later. The cell bodies of the sensory or *afferent* neurons of the cochlear nerve lie within the spiral ganglion, which corkscrews up around the axis of the cochlea (Fig. 15-20, lower left inset). The dendrites of these neurons contact nearby hair cells, whereas the axons project to the cochlear nucleus in the brainstem (see Fig. 16-15). Not surprisingly, ~95% of the roughly 30,000 sensory neurons (i.e., type I cells) of each cochlear nerve innervate the relatively few inner hair cells—the true auditory sensory cells. The remaining 5% of spiral ganglion neurons (i.e., type II cells) innervate the abundant outer hair cells, which are so poorly innervated that they must contribute very little *direct* information about sound to the brain.

The frequency sensitivity of auditory hair cells depends on their position along the basilar membrane of the cochlea

The subjective experience of tonal discrimination is called **pitch**. Young humans can hear sounds with frequencies from ~20 to 20,000 Hz. This range is modest by the standards of most mammals because many hear up to 50,000 Hz, and some, notably whales and bats, can hear sounds with frequencies greater than 100,000 Hz.

A continuous, pure tone produces a wave that travels along the basilar membrane and has different amplitudes at different points along the base-apex axis (Fig. 15-24A). Increases in sound *amplitude* cause an increase in the *rate* of action potentials in these sensory neurons—**rate coding**. The *frequency* of the sound determines *where* along the cochlea the cochlear membranes vibrate most—high frequencies at one end and low at the other—and thus which hair cells are stimulated. This selectivity is the basis for **place coding** in the auditory system, that is, the frequency selectivity of a hair cell depends mainly on its longitudinal position along the cochlear membranes. The cochlea is essentially a spectral analyzer that evaluates a complex sound according to its pure tonal components, with each pure tone stimulating a specific region of the cochlea.

Using optical methods to study cadaver ears, Georg von Békésy found that sounds of a particular frequency generate relatively localized waves in the basilar membrane and that the envelope of these waves changes position according to the frequency of the sound (Fig. 15-24B). Low frequencies generate their maximal amplitudes near the apex. As sound frequency increases, the envelope shifts progressively toward the basal end (i.e., near the oval and round windows). For his work, von Békésy received the 1961 Nobel Prize in Physiology or Medicine.

Two properties of the basilar membrane underlie the low-apical to high-basal gradient of resonance: taper and stiffness (Fig. 15-24C). If we could unwind the *cochlea* and stretch it straight, we would see that it tapers from base to apex. The *basilar membrane* tapers in the opposite direction—wider at the apex, narrower at the base. More important, the narrow basal end is ~100-fold stiffer than its wide and floppy apical end. Thus, the basilar membrane resembles a harp. At one end—the base, near the oval and round windows—it has short, taut strings that vibrate at high frequencies. At the other end—the apex—it has longer, looser strings that vibrate at low frequencies.

Although von Békésy's experiments were illuminating, they were also paradoxical. A variety of experimental data suggested that the tuning of living hair cells is considerably sharper than the broad envelopes of von Békésy's traveling waves on the basilar membrane could possibly produce. Recordings from primary auditory nerve cells are also very sharp, implying that this tuning must occur within the cochlea, not in the CNS. Some enhancement of tuning comes from the structure of the inner hair cells themselves. Those near the base have shorter, stiffer stereovilli, which makes them resonate to higher frequencies than possible with the longer, floppier stereovilli on cells near the apex.

The blue curve in Figure 15-25 approximates von Békésy's envelope of traveling waves for a passive basilar membrane from cadavers. It is important to note that von Békésy used unnaturally loud sounds. With reasonable sound levels, the maximum *passive* displacement of the basilar membrane would be slightly more than 0.1 nm. This distance is less than the pore diameter of an ion channel and also less than the threshold (0.3 to 0.4 nm) for an electrical response from a hair cell. However, measurements from the basilar mem-

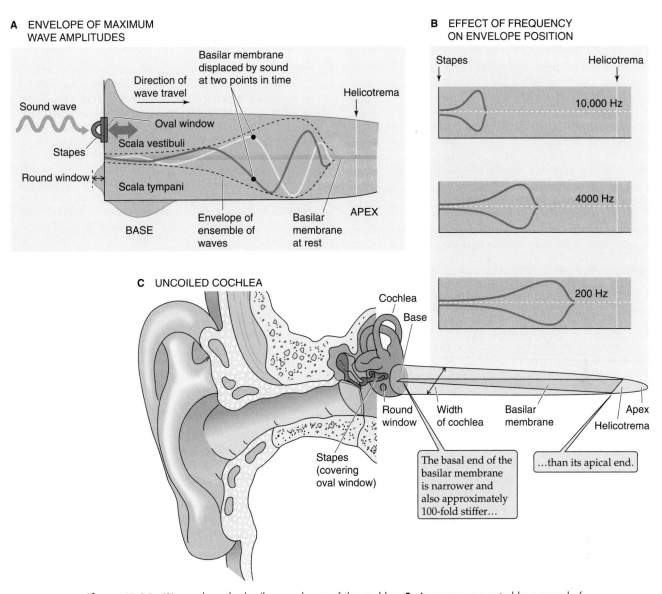

Figure 15-24 Waves along the basilar membrane of the cochlea. **A,** As a wave generated by a sound of a single frequency travels along the basilar membrane, its amplitude changes. The *green* and *yellow curves* represent a sample wave at two different times. The *upper* and *lower broken lines* (i.e., the envelope) encompass all maximum amplitudes of all waves, at all points in time. Thus, a wave can never escape the envelope. The figure exaggerates the amplitudes of the traveling waves ~1 million-fold. **B,** For a pure tone of 10,000 Hz, the envelope is confined to a short region of the basilar membrane near the stapes. For pure tones of 4000 Hz and 200 Hz, the widest part of the envelope moves closer to the helicotrema. **C,** The cochlea narrows in diameter from base to apex, whereas the basilar membrane tapers in the opposite direction.

brane in *living* animals (the orange curve in Fig. 15-25) by very sensitive methods show that movements of the basilar membrane are much more localized and much larger than predicted by von Békésy. The maximal physiological displacement is ~20-fold greater than threshold and ~40-fold greater than that predicted by the passive von Békésy model. Moreover, the physiological displacement decays sharply on either side of the peak, more than 100-fold within ~0.5 mm (recall that the human basilar membrane has a total length of more than 30 mm).

Both the extremely large physiological excursions of the basilar membrane and the exquisitely sharp tuning of the cochlea depend on the **cochlear amplifier** that we introduced earlier. Indeed, selectively damaging outer hair cells—with large doses of certain antibiotics, for example—considerably dulls the sharpness of cochlear tuning and dramatically reduces the amplification.

Tuning of hair cells is also under motor control of neurons that arise in the superior olivary complex in the brainstem and synapse mainly on the outer hair cells and, sparsely, on

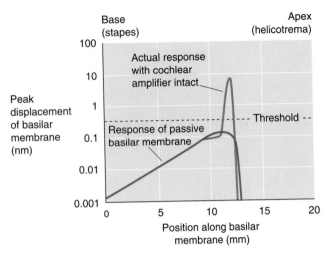

Figure 15-25   Peak movement of basilar membrane. The graph illustrates the displacement of the basilar membrane—in response to a pure tone—as a function of distance along the base-to-apex axis. The *dashed line* indicates the displacement threshold for triggering of an electrical response. (*Data from Ashmore JF: Mammalian hearing and the cellular mechanisms of the cochlear amplifier. In Corey DP, Roper SD [eds]: Sensory Transduction, pp 396-412. New York: Rockefeller University Press, 1992.*)

the afferent axons that innervate the inner hair cells. Stimulation of these olivocochlear efferent fibers suppresses the responsiveness of the cochlea to sound and is thought to provide **auditory focus** by suppressing responsiveness to unwanted sounds—allowing us to hear even in noisy environments. The main efferent neurotransmitter is acetylcholine, which activates ionotropic ACh receptors (see Chapter 6)—nonselective cation channels—and triggers an entry of Ca^{2+}. The influx of Ca^{2+} activates Ca^{2+}-activated K^+ channels, causing a hyperpolarization—effectively an inhibitory postsynaptic potential—that suppresses the electromotility of outer hair cells and action potentials in afferent dendrites. Thus, the efferent axons allow the brain to control the gain of the inner ear.

SOMATIC SENSORY RECEPTORS, PROPRIOCEPTION, AND PAIN

Somatic sensation is the most widespread and diverse of the body's sensory systems (*soma* means "body" in Greek). Its receptors are distributed throughout the body instead of being condensed into small and specialized sensory surfaces, as most other sensory systems are arranged. Somatosensory receptors cover the skin, subcutaneous tissue, skeletal muscles, bones and joints, major internal organs, epithelia, and cardiovascular system. These receptors also vary widely in their specificity. The body has mechanoreceptors to transduce pressure, stretch, vibration, and tissue damage; thermoreceptors to gauge temperature; and chemoreceptors to sense a variety of substances. Somatic sensation (or **somesthesia**) is usually considered to be a combination of at least four sensory modalities: the senses of touch, temperature, body position (proprioception), and pain (nociception).

Cochlear Implants

The most common cause of human deafness is damage to the hair cells of the cochlea. This damage can be caused by genetic factors, a variety of drugs (e.g., some antibiotics, including quinine), chronic exposure to excessively loud sounds, and other types of disease. Even when all hair cells have been destroyed, if the auditory nerve is intact, it is often possible to restore substantial hearing with a cochlear implant.

A cochlear implant is essentially an electronic cochlea. Most of the system resides outside the body. The user wears a headpiece with a microphone, which is connected to a small, battery-powered digital speech processor. This processor sends signals to a miniature radio transmitter next to the scalp, which transmits digitally encoded signals—no wires penetrate the skin—to a receiver/decoder that is surgically implanted in the mastoid bone behind the ear. A very thin and flexible set of wires carries the signals through a tiny hole into the basal end of the cochlea, where an array of 8 to 22 electrodes lies adjacent to the auditory nerve endings (where healthy hair cells would normally be) along the cochlea. Each electrode activates a small portion of the auditory nerve axons.

The cochlear implant exploits the tonotopic arrangement of auditory nerve fibers. By stimulating near the base of the cochlea, it is possible to trigger a perception of high-frequency sounds; stimulation toward the apex evokes low-frequency sounds. The efficacy of the implant can be extraordinary. Users require training of a few months or more, and in many cases, they achieve very good comprehension of spoken speech, even as it comes across on a telephone.

As the technology and safety of cochlear implants have improved, so has their popularity. By 2004, more than 60,000 people were using cochlear implants, ~20,000 of them children. The best candidates for cochlear implants are young children and older children or adults whose deafness was acquired after they learned some speech. Adults whose deafness preceded any experience with speech generally do not fare as well with cochlear implants. Sensory systems, including the auditory system, need to experience normal inputs at a young age to develop properly. When the auditory system is deprived of sounds early in life, it can never develop completely normal function even if sensory inputs are restored during adulthood.

A variety of sensory endings in the skin transduce mechanical, thermal, and chemical stimuli

To meet a wide array of sensory demands, many kinds of specialized receptors are required. Somatic sensory receptors range from simple, bare nerve endings to complex combinations of nerve, muscle, connective tissue, and supporting cells. As we have seen, the other major sensory systems have only one type of sensory receptor or a set of very similar subtypes.

Mechanoreceptors, which are sensitive to physical distortion such as bending or stretching, account for many of the somatic sensory receptors. They exist throughout our bodies and monitor the following: physical contact with the skin, blood pressure in the heart and vessels, stretching of the gut and bladder, and pressure on the teeth. The transduction site of these mechanoreceptors is one or more unmyelinated axon branches. Our progress in understanding the molecular nature of mechanosensory transduction has been relatively slow. Similar to the transduction process in hair cells, cutaneous mechanoreceptive nerve endings probably involve the gating of ion channels. As in hair cells, some of these channels belong to the TRP superfamily. To date, at least seven types of TRP channels, from nearly all of the subfamilies, have been implicated in mechanosensation (in various species and tissues).

The mechanisms by which mechanical force is transferred from cells and their membranes to mechanosensitive channels is unclear. The ion channels may be physically coupled to either extracellular structures (e.g., collagen fibers, like the tip link proteins in hair cells) or cytoskeletal components (e.g., microtubules) that transfer energy from deformation of the cell to the gating mechanism of the channel. It is also possible that some channels may be sensitive to stresses in the lipid bilayer itself and require no other types of anchoring proteins. Mechanically sensitive axons are often surrounded by specialized structures that give them much of their specific sensitivity to different stimuli.

Thermoreceptors respond best to changes in temperature, whereas **chemoreceptors** are sensitive to various kinds of chemical alterations. In the next three sections, we discuss mechanoreceptors, thermoreceptors, and chemoreceptors that are located in the skin.

Mechanoreceptors in the skin provide sensitivity to specific stimuli, such as vibration and steady pressure

Skin protects us from our environment by preventing evaporation of body fluids, invasion by microbes, abrasion, and damage from sunlight. However, skin also provides our most direct contact with the world. The two major types of mammalian skin are *hairy* and *glabrous*. **Glabrous skin** (or hairless) is found on the palms of our hands and fingertips and on the soles of our feet and pads of our toes (Fig. 15-26A). **Hairy skin** makes up most of the rest and differs widely in its hairiness. Both types of skin have an outer layer, the **epidermis**, and an inner layer, the **dermis**, and sensory receptors innervate both. The receptors in the skin are sensitive to many types of stimuli and respond when the skin is vibrated, pressed, pricked, and stroked or when its hairs are bent or pulled. These are quite different kinds of mechanical energy, yet we can feel them all and easily tell them apart. Skin also has exquisite sensitivity; for example, we can reliably feel a dot only 0.006 mm high and 0.04 mm across when it is stroked across a fingertip. The standard Braille dot is 167 times higher!

The sensory endings in the skin take many shapes, and most of them are named after the 19th century European histologists who observed them and made them popular. The largest and best studied mechanoreceptor is **Pacini's corpuscle**, which is up to 2 mm long and almost 1 mm in diameter (Fig. 15-26B). Pacini's corpuscle is located in the subcutaneous tissue of both glabrous and hairy skin. It has

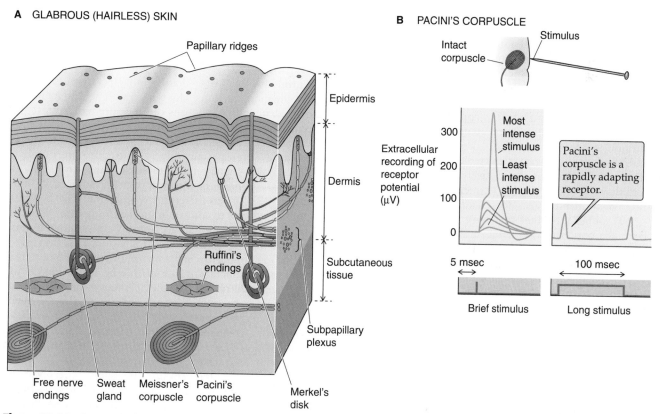

Figure 15-26 Sensors in the skin.

an ovoid capsule with 20 to 70 onion-like, concentric layers of connective tissue and a nerve terminal in the middle. The capsule is responsible for the rapidly adapting nature of the Pacini corpuscle's responses. When the capsule is compressed, energy is transferred to the nerve terminal, its membrane is deformed, and mechanosensitive channels open. Current flowing through the channels generates a depolarizing receptor potential that, if large enough, causes the axon to fire an action potential (Fig. 15-26B, left panel). However, the capsule layers are slick, with viscous fluid between them. If the stimulus pressure is maintained, the layers slip past one another and transfer the stimulus energy away so that the underlying axon terminal is no longer deformed and the receptor potential dissipates (Fig. 15-26B, right panel). When pressure is released, the events reverse themselves and the terminal is depolarized again. In this way, the non-neural covering of Pacini's corpuscle specializes the corpuscle for sensing of vibrations and makes it almost unresponsive to steady pressure. Pacini's corpuscle is most sensitive to vibrations of 200 to 300 Hz, and its threshold increases dramatically below 50 Hz and above ~500 Hz. The sensation evoked by stimulating Pacini's corpuscle is a poorly localized humming feeling.

Werner Lowenstein and colleagues in the 1960s showed the importance of the Pacini corpuscle's capsule to its frequency sensitivity. With fine microdissection, they were able to strip away the capsule from single corpuscles. They found that the resultant naked nerve terminal is much less sensitive to vibrating stimuli and much more sensitive to steady pressure. Clearly, the capsule modifies the sensitivity of the bare mechanoreceptive axon. The encapsulated Pacini's corpuscle is an example of a **rapidly adapting** sensor, whereas the decapsulated nerve ending is an example of a **slowly adapting** sensor.

Several other types of encapsulated mechanoreceptors are located in the dermis, but none has been studied as well as Pacini's corpuscle. **Meissner's corpuscles** (Fig. 15-26A) are located in the ridges of glabrous skin and are about one tenth the size of Pacini's corpuscle. They are rapidly adapting, although less so than Pacini's corpuscles. **Ruffini's corpuscles** resemble diminutive Pacini's corpuscles and, like Pacini's corpuscles, occur in the subcutaneous tissue of both hairy and glabrous skin. Their preferred stimuli might be called "fluttering" vibrations. As relatively *slowly* adapting receptors, they respond best to low frequencies. **Merkel's disks** are also slowly adapting receptors made from a flattened, non-neural epithelial cell that synapses on a nerve terminal. They lie at the border of the dermis and epidermis of glabrous skin. It is not clear whether it is the nerve terminal or epithelial cell that is mechanosensitive. The nerve terminals of **Krause's end bulbs** appear knotted. They innervate the border areas of dry skin and mucous membranes (e.g., around the lips and external genitalia) and are probably rapidly adapting mechanoreceptors.

The **receptive fields** of different types of skin receptors vary greatly in size. Pacini's corpuscles have extremely broad receptive fields (Fig. 15-27A), whereas those of Meissner's corpuscles (Fig. 15-27B) and Merkel's disks are very small. The last two seem to be responsible for the ability of the fingertips to make very fine tactile discriminations. Small receptive fields are an important factor in achieving high spatial resolution. Resolution varies widely, a fact easily demonstrated by measuring the skin's two-point discrimination. Bend a paper clip into a U shape. Vary the distance between the tips and test how easily you can distinguish the touch of one tip versus two on your palm, your fingertips, your lips, your back, and your foot. To avoid bias, a colleague—rather than you—should apply the stimulus. Compare the results with standardized data (Fig. 15-27C).

Two things determine the sensitivity of spatial discrimination in an area of skin. The first is the size of the receptors' receptive fields—if they are small, the two tips of your paper clip are more likely to stimulate different sets of receptors. The second parameter that determines spatial discrimination is the density of the receptors in the skin. Indeed, two-point discrimination of the fingertips is better than that of the palm, even though their receptive fields are the same size. The key to finer discrimination in the fingertips is their higher *density* of receptors. Crowding more receptors into each square millimeter of fingertip has a second advantage: because the CNS receives more information per stimulus, it has a better chance of transducing very small stimuli.

Although we rarely think about it, **hair** is a sensitive part of our somatic sensory system. For some animals, hairs are a major sensory system. Rodents whisk long facial vibrissae (hairs) and feel the texture, distance, and shape of their local environment. Hairs grow from **follicles** embedded in the skin, and each follicle is richly innervated by free, mechanoreceptive nerve endings that either wrap around it or run parallel to it. Bending of the hair causes deformation of the follicle and surrounding tissue, which stretches, bends, or flattens the nerve endings and increases or decreases their firing frequency. Various mechanoreceptors innervate hair follicles, and they may be either slowly or rapidly adapting.

Separate thermoreceptors detect warm and cold

Neurons are sensitive to changes in temperature, as are all of life's chemical reactions. This temperature sensitivity has two consequences: first, neurons can measure temperature; but second, to work properly, most neural circuits need to be kept at a relatively stable temperature. Neurons of the mammalian CNS are especially vulnerable to temperature changes. Whereas skin tissue temperatures can range from 20°C to 40°C without harm or discomfort, brain temperature must be near 37°C to avoid serious dysfunction. The body has complex systems to control brain (i.e., body core) temperature tightly. Even though all neurons are sensitive to temperature, not all neurons are thermoreceptors. Because of specific membrane mechanisms, some neurons are extremely sensitive to temperature and seem to be adapted to the job of sensing it. Although many temperature-sensitive neurons are present in the skin, they are also clustered in the hypothalamus and the spinal cord. The hypothalamic temperature sensors, like their cutaneous counterparts, are important for regulation of the physiological responses that maintain stable body temperature (see Chapter 59).

Perceptions of temperature apparently reflect warmth and cold receptors located in the skin. Thermoreceptors, like mechanoreceptors, are not spread uniformly across the skin. When you map the skin's sensitivity to temperature with a

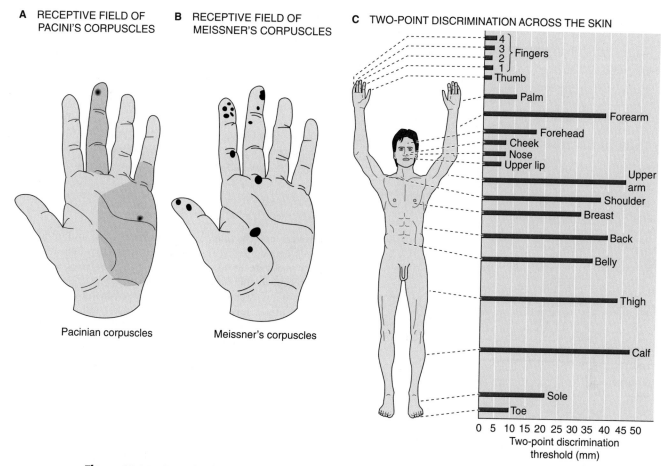

A RECEPTIVE FIELD OF PACINI'S CORPUSCLES

B RECEPTIVE FIELD OF MEISSNER'S CORPUSCLES

C TWO-POINT DISCRIMINATION ACROSS THE SKIN

Pacinian corpuscles

Meissner's corpuscles

4
3
2   Fingers
1
Thumb
Palm
Forearm
Forehead
Cheek
Nose
Upper lip
Upper arm
Shoulder
Breast
Back
Belly
Thigh
Calf
Sole
Toe

0 5 10 15 20 25 30 35 40 45 50
Two-point discrimination
threshold (mm)

Figure 15-27 Receptive fields and spatial discrimination of skin mechanoreceptors. **A,** Each of the two black dots indicates an area of *maximal sensitivity* of a single corpuscle. Each *green area* is the receptive field of a corpuscle (i.e., the corpuscle responds when stimulus strength increases sufficiently anywhere within the area). **B,** Each dot represents the entire receptive field of a single Meissner's corpuscle. Note that the fields are much smaller than in **A**. **C,** The horizontal bars represent the minimum distance at which two points can be perceived as distinct at various locations over the body. Spatial discrimination depends on both receptor density and receptive field size. (**A** and **B,** Data from Vallbo AB, Johansson RS: Properties of cutaneous mechanoreceptors in the human hand related to touch sensation. Hum Neurobiol 1984; 3:3-14. **C,** Data from Weinstein S: Intensive and extensive aspects of tactile sensitivity as a function of body part, sex and laterality. In Kenshalo DR [ed]: The Skin Senses. Springfield, IL: Charles C Thomas, 1968.)

small cold or warm probe, you find spots ~1 mm across that are especially sensitive to *either* hot or cold, but not to both. In addition, some areas of skin in between are relatively insensitive. The spatial dissociation of the hot and cold maps shows that they are separate submodalities, with separate receptors to encode each. Recordings from single sensory fibers have confirmed this conclusion. The responses of thermoreceptors adapt during long stimuli, as many sensory receptors commonly do. Most cutaneous thermoreceptors are probably free nerve endings, without obvious specialization. Their axons are small, either unmyelinated *C fibers* or the smallest-diameter myelinated *Aδ fibers* (see Table 12-1).

We can perceive changes in our average skin temperature of as little as 0.01°C. Within the skin are separate types of thermoreceptors that are sensitive to a range of relatively hot or cold temperatures. Figure 15-28A shows how the steady discharge rate of both types of receptors varies with temperature. **Warmth receptors** begin firing above ~30°C and increase their firing rate until 44°C to 46°C, beyond which

the rate falls off steeply and a sensation of pain begins, presumably mediated by nociceptive endings (see the next section). **Cold receptors** have a much broader temperature response. They are relatively quiet at skin temperatures of ~40°C, but their steady discharge rate increases as the temperature falls to 24°C to 28°C. Further decreases in temperature cause the steady discharge rate of the cold receptors to decrease until the temperature falls to ~10°C. Below that temperature, firing ceases and cold becomes an effective local anesthetic.

In addition to the *tonic* response just described (i.e., the steady discharge rate), cold receptors also have a *phasic* response that enables them to report *changes* in temperature. As shown in Figure 15-28B, when the temperature suddenly shifts from 20.5°C to 15.2°C (both points are to the left of the peak in Fig. 15-28A), the firing rate transiently increases (i.e., the phasic response). However, the new steady-state level is lower, as suggested by the left pair of points in Figure 15-28A. When the temperature suddenly shifts from 35°C to

A STEADY (TONIC) RESPONSES

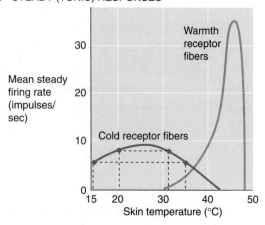

**B TRANSIENT (PHASIC) RESPONSES
OF "COLD" FIBERS**

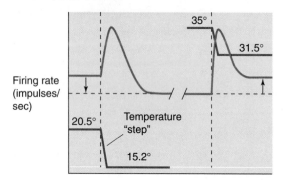

Figure 15-28 Temperature sensitivity of cutaneous thermoreceptors. **A,** The *curves* represent the mean, steady firing rates of neurons from warmth receptors and cold receptors. **B,** These two experiments on cold receptors show effects of cooling steps of nearly identical magnitude but starting from different temperatures (20.5°C and 35°C). In both instances, the transient (phasic) responses are the same: an increase in the firing rate. When the starting temperature is 20.5°C (*to the left of the peak of the blue curve in* **B**), the final firing rate is less than the initial one. However, when the initial temperature is 35°C (*to the right of the peak of the blue curve in* **B**), the final rate is greater than the initial one. (*Data from Somjen GG: Sensory Coding in the Mammalian Nervous System. New York: Appleton-Century-Crofts, 1972.*)

31.5°C (both points are to the right of the peak in Fig. 15-28A), the firing rate in Figure 15-28B transiently increases, and the new steady-state level is higher, as suggested by the right pair of points in Figure 15-28A.

The transduction of relatively warm temperatures is carried out by several types of TRPV channels (specifically TRPV1 to 4). TRPV1 is a vanilloid receptor—it is activated by the vanilloid class of compounds that includes capsaicin, the pungent ingredient that gives spicy foods their burning quality. Aptly enough, chili peppers taste "hot" because they activate some of the same ion channels that heat itself activates! TRPV1 channels have a high temperature threshold (about 43°C) and thus help mediate the painful aspects of thermoreception (see later). Other TRPV channels are activated at more moderate temperatures and presumably provide our sensations of warmth.

Yet another TRP channel, TRPM8, mediates sensations of moderate cold. TRPM8 channels begin to open at temperatures below ~27°C and are maximally activated at 8°C. In a remarkable analogy to the hot-sensitive TRPV1 channel (the capsaicin receptor), the cool-sensitive TRPM8 channel is a menthol receptor. Menthol evokes sensations of cold because it activates the same ion channel that is opened by cold temperatures. In yet another strange twist, the TRPA1 channel that seems to be the hair cell transduction channel (see earlier) is also a painfully cold-sensitive channel in somatic sensory neurons.

Nociceptors are specialized sensory endings that transduce painful stimuli

Physical energy that is informative at low and moderate levels can be destructive at higher intensity. Sensations of pain motivate us to avoid such situations. Nociceptors are the receptors mediating painful feelings to warn us that body tissue is being damaged or is at risk of being damaged (as their Latin roots imply: *nocere,* to hurt, and *recipere,* to receive). The pain-sensing system is entirely separate from the other modalities we have discussed; it has its own peripheral receptors and a complex, dispersed, chemically unique set of central circuits.

Nociceptors vary in their selectivity. **Mechanical** nociceptors respond to strong pressure, in particular, pressure from sharp objects. **Thermal** nociceptors signal either burning heat (above ~45°C, when tissues begin to be destroyed) or unhealthy cold; the heat-sensitive nociceptive neurons express the TRPV1 and TRPV2 channels, whereas the cold-sensitive nociceptors express TRPA1 and TRPM8 channels. **Chemically sensitive,** mechanically insensitive nociceptors respond to a variety of agents, including K^+, extremes of pH, neuroactive substances such as histamine and bradykinin from the body itself, and various irritants from the environment. Finally, **polymodal** nociceptors are single nerve endings that are sensitive to combinations of mechanical, thermal, and chemical stimuli. Nociceptive axons include both fast Aδ fibers and slow, unmyelinated C fibers. Aδ axons mediate sensations of sharp, intense pain; C fibers elicit more persistent feelings of dull, burning pain.

Nociceptors are free nerve endings that are widely distributed throughout the body. They innervate the skin, bone, muscle, most internal organs, blood vessels, and heart. Ironically, they are generally absent from the brain substance itself, although they are in the meninges.

Sensations of pain can be modulated in a variety of ways. Skin, joints, or muscles that have been damaged or inflamed are unusually sensitive to further stimuli. This phenomenon is called **hyperalgesia,** and it can be manifested as a reduced threshold for pain, an increased intensity of painful stimuli, or spontaneous pain. **Primary hyperalgesia** occurs within the area of damaged tissue, but within ~20 minutes after an injury, tissues surrounding a damaged area may become supersensitive by a process called **secondary hyperalgesia.** Hyperalgesia seems to involve processes near peripheral receptors (Fig. 15-29) as well as mechanisms in the CNS. Damaged skin releases a variety of chemical substances from itself, blood cells, and nerve endings. These substances include bradykinin, prostaglandins, serotonin, substance P,

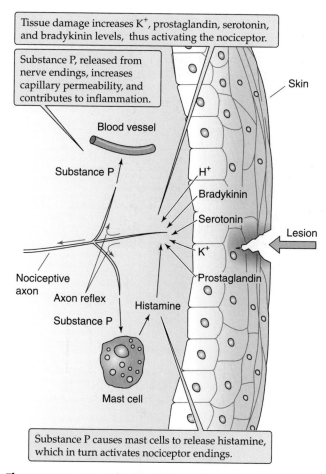

Tissue damage increases K⁺, prostaglandin, serotonin, and bradykinin levels, thus activating the nociceptor.

Substance P, released from nerve endings, increases capillary permeability, and contributes to inflammation.

Blood vessel

Skin

Substance P

H⁺

Bradykinin

Serotonin

Lesion

Nociceptive axon

K⁺

Axon reflex

Prostaglandin

Substance P

Histamine

Mast cell

Substance P causes mast cells to release histamine, which in turn activates nociceptor endings.

Figure 15-29 Hyperalgesia of inflammation.

K⁺, H⁺, and others; they trigger the set of local responses that we know as **inflammation**. As a result, blood vessels become more leaky and cause tissue swelling (or edema) and redness (see Chapter 20 for the box on interstitial edema). Nearby mast cells release the chemical histamine, which directly excites nociceptors. By a mechanism called the **axon reflex**, action potentials can propagate along nociceptive axons from the site of an injury into side branches of the same axon that innervate neighboring regions of skin. The spreading axon branches of the nociceptors themselves may release substances that sensitize nociceptive terminals and make them responsive to previously nonpainful stimuli. Such "silent" nociceptors among our small Aδ and C fibers are normally unresponsive to stimuli—even destructive ones. Only after sensitization do they become responsive to mechanical or chemical stimuli and contribute greatly to hyperalgesia.

The cognitive sensations of pain are under remarkably potent control by the brain, more so than other sensory systems. In some cases, nociceptors may fire wildly, although perceptions of pain are absent; on the other hand, pain may be crippling, although nociceptors are silent. Pain can be modified both by nonpainful sensory input and by neural activity from various nuclei within the brain. For example, pain evoked by activity in nociceptors (Aδ and C fibers) can be reduced by simultaneous activity in low-threshold mechanoreceptors (Aα and Aβ fibers). This phenomenon is a

familiar experience—some of the discomfort of a burn, cut, or bruise can be relieved by gentle massage or rubbing (stimulating mechanoreceptors) around the injured area. In 1965, Melzack and Wall proposed that this phenomenon involves a circuit in the spinal cord that can "gate" the transmission of nociceptive information to the brain; control of the gate could be provided by other sensory information (e.g., tactile stimulation) or by descending control from the brain itself.

A second mechanism for modifying the sensation of pain involves the relatively small peptides called endorphins. In the 1970s, it was discovered that a class of drugs called opioids (including morphine, heroin, and codeine) act by binding tightly and specifically to **opioid receptors** in the brain and, furthermore, that the brain itself manufactures "endogenous morphine-like substances," collectively called endorphins (see Chapter 13).

Muscle spindles sense changes in the length of skeletal muscle fibers, whereas Golgi tendon organs gauge the muscle's force

The somatic sensory receptors described thus far provide information about the *external* environment. However, the body also needs detailed information about itself to know where each of its parts is in space, whether it is moving, and if so, in which direction and how fast. **Proprioception** provides this sense of self and serves two main purposes. First, knowledge of the positions of our limbs as they move helps us judge the identity of external objects. It is much easier to recognize an object if you can actively palpate it than if it is placed passively into your hand so that your skin is stimulated but you are not allowed to personally guide your fingers around it. Second, proprioceptive information is essential for accurately guiding many movements, especially while they are being learned.

Skeletal muscles, which mediate voluntary movement, have two mechanosensitive proprioceptors: the muscle spindles (or stretch receptors) and Golgi tendon organs (Fig. 15-30). Muscle spindles measure the length and rate of stretch of the muscles, whereas the Golgi tendon organs gauge the force generated by a muscle by measuring the tension in its tendon. Together, they provide a full description of the dynamic state of each muscle. The different sensitivities of the spindle and the tendon organ are due partly to their structures but also to their placement: spindles are located in modified muscle fibers called *intrafusal* muscle fibers, which are aligned in *parallel* with the "ordinary" force-generating or *extrafusal* skeletal muscle fibers. On the other hand, Golgi tendon organs are aligned in *series* with the extrafusal fibers.

The **Golgi tendon organ** consists of bare nerve endings of group Ib axons (see Table 12-1). These endings intimately invest an encapsulated collagen matrix and usually sit at the junction between skeletal muscle fibers and the tendon. When tension develops in the muscle as a result of either passive stretch or active contraction, the collagen fibers tend to squeeze and distort the mechanosensitive nerve endings, triggering them to fire action potentials.

The mammalian **muscle spindle** is a complex of modified skeletal muscle fibers (**intrafusal fibers**) combined with both afferent and efferent innervation. The spindle does not con-

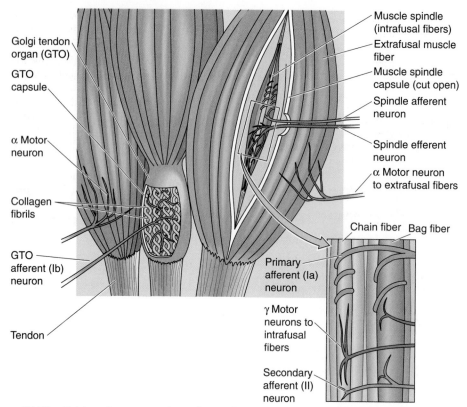

Figure 15-30   Golgi tendon organ and muscle spindle fibers. A muscle contains two kinds of muscle fibers, extrafusal fibers (ordinary muscle fibers that cause contraction) and intrafusal fibers (in parallel with the extrafusal fibers). Some of the extrafusal fibers have Golgi tendon organs located in series between the end of the muscle fiber and the macroscopic tendon. The intrafusal fibers contain muscle spindles, which receive both afferent (sensory) and efferent (motor) innervation. The spindle (*inset*) contains both bag fibers, with nuclei bunched together, and chain fibers, with nuclei in a row.

tribute significant force generation to the muscle but serves a purely sensory function. A simplified summary of the muscle spindle is that it contains two kinds of intrafusal muscle fibers (bag and chain), with two kinds of sensory endings entwined about them (the primary and secondary endings). The different viscoelastic properties of the muscle fibers make them differentially sensitive to the consequences of muscle stretch. Because the primary sensory endings of group Ia axons coil around and strongly innervate individual bag muscle fibers (in addition to chain fibers), they are very sensitive to the dynamics of muscle length (i.e., *changes* in its length). The secondary sensory endings of group II axons mainly innervate the chain fibers and most accurately transduce the static length of the muscle; in other words, they are slowly adapting receptors. The discharge rate of afferent neurons increases when the whole muscle—and therefore the spindle—is stretched.

What is the function of the motor innervation of the muscle spindle? Consider what happens when the α motor neurons stimulate the force-generating extrafusal fibers and the muscle contracts. The spindle, connected in parallel to the extrafusal fibers, quickly tends to go slack, which makes it insensitive to further changes in length. To avoid this situation and to continue to maintain control over the sensitivity of the spindle, γ motor neurons cause the intrafusal muscle

fibers to contract in parallel with the extrafusal fibers. This ability of the spindle's intrafusal fibers to change their length as necessary greatly increases the range of lengths over which the spindle can work. It also means that the sensory responses of the spindle depend not only on the *length* of the whole muscle in which the spindle sits but also on the *contractile state* of its own intrafusal muscle fibers. Presumably, the ambiguity in this code is sorted out centrally by circuits that simultaneously keep track of the spindle's sensory output and the activity of its motor nerve supply.

In addition to the muscle receptors, various mechanoreceptors are found in the connective tissues of **joints**, especially within the capsules and ligaments. Many resemble Ruffini, Golgi, and Pacini end organs; others are free nerve endings. They respond to changes in the angle, direction, and velocity of movement in a joint. Most are rapidly adapting, which means that sensory information about a *moving* joint is rich. Nerves encoding the resting *position* of a joint are few. We are nevertheless quite good at judging the position of a joint, even with our eyes closed. It seems that information from joint receptors is combined with that from muscle spindles and Golgi tendon organs, and probably from cutaneous receptors as well, to estimate joint angle. Removal of one source of information can be compensated by use of the other sources. When an arthritic hip is replaced with a steel and plastic one, patients are still able to tell the angle between their thigh and their pelvis, even though all hip joint mechanoreceptors are long gone.

REFERENCES

Books and Reviews

Copeland BJ, Pillsbury HC 3rd: Cochlear implantation for the treatment of deafness. Annu Rev Med 2004; 55:157-167.

Jordt SE, McKemy DD, Julius D: Lessons from peppers and peppermint: The molecular logic of thermosensation. Curr Opin Neurobiol 2003; 13:487-492.

Kung C: A possible unifying principle for mechanosensation. Nature 2005; 436:647-654.

Lin SY, Corey DP: TRP channels in mechanosensation. Curr Opin Neurobiol 2005; 15:350-357.

Mombaerts P: Genes and ligands for odorant, vomeronasal and taste receptors. Nat Rev Neurosci 2004; 5:263-278.

Santos-Sacchi J: New tunes from Corti's organ: The outer hair cell boogie rules. Curr Opin Neurobiol 2006; 13:459-468.

Journal Articles

Buck L, Axel R: A novel multigene family may encode odorant receptors: A molecular basis for odor recognition. Cell 1991; 65:175-187.

Corey DP, Garcia-Anoveros J, Holt JR, et al: TRPA1 is a candidate for the mechanosensitive transduction channel of vertebrate hair cells. Nature 2004; 432:723-730.

Liberman MC, Gao J, He DZ, et al: Prestin is required for electromotility of the outer hair cell and for the cochlear amplifier. Nature 2002; 419:300-304.

Nelson G, Hoon MA, Chandrashekar J, et al: Mammalian sweet taste receptors. Cell 2001; 106:381-390.

Zhao GQ, Zhang Y, Hoon MA, et al: The receptors for mammalian sweet and umami taste. Cell 2003; 115:255-266.

CHAPTER 16

CIRCUITS OF THE CENTRAL NERVOUS SYSTEM

Barry W. Connors

ELEMENTS OF NEURAL CIRCUITS

Neural circuits process sensory information, generate motor output, and create spontaneous activity

A neuron never works alone. Even in the most primitive nervous systems, all neurons participate in synaptically interconnected networks called **circuits**. In some hydrozoans (small jellyfish), the major neurons lack specialization and are multifunctional. They serve simultaneously as photodetectors, pattern generators for swimming rhythms, and motor neurons. Groups of these cells are monotonously interconnected by two-way electrical synapses into simple ring-like arrangements, and these networks coordinate the rhythmic contraction of the animal's muscles during swimming. This simple neural network also has the flexibility to command defensive changes in swimming patterns when a shadow passes over the animal. Thus, neuronal circuits have profound advantages over unconnected neurons.

In more complex animals, each neuron within a circuit may have very specialized properties. By the interconnection of various specialized neurons, even a simple neuronal circuit may accomplish astonishingly intricate functions. Some neural circuits may be primarily sensory (e.g., the retina) or motor (e.g., the ventral horns of the spinal cord). Many circuits combine features of both, with some neurons dedicated to providing and processing **sensory input**, others to commanding **motor output**, and many neurons (perhaps most!) doing both. Neural circuits may also generate their own intrinsic signals, with no need for any sensory or central input to activate them. The brain does more than just respond reflexively to sensory input, as a moment's introspection will amply demonstrate. Some neural functions—such as walking, running, breathing, chewing, talking, and piano playing—require precise timing, with coordination of rhythmic temporal patterns across hundreds of outputs. These basic rhythms may be generated by neurons and neural circuits called **pacemakers** because of their clock-like capabilities. The patterns and rhythms generated by a pacemaking circuit can almost always be modulated—stopped, started, or altered—by input from sensory or central path-

ways. Neuronal circuits that produce rhythmic motor output are sometimes called **central pattern generators**; we discuss these in a later section.

This chapter introduces the basic principles of neural circuits in the mammalian central nervous system (CNS). We describe a few examples of specific systems in detail to illuminate general principles as well as the diversity of neural solutions to life's complex problems. However, this topic is enormous, and we have necessarily been selective and somewhat arbitrary in our presentation.

Nervous systems have several levels of organization

The function of a nervous system is to generate adaptive behaviors. Because different species face unique problems, we expect brains to differ in their organization and mechanisms. Nevertheless, certain principles apply to most nervous systems. It is useful to define various levels of organization. We can analyze a complex **behavior**—reading the words on this page—in a simple way, with progressively finer detail, down to the level of ion channels, receptors, messengers, and the genes that control them. At the highest level, we recognize neural **subsystems and pathways** (Chapter 10), which in this case include the sensory input from the retina (see Chapter 13) leading to the visual cortex, the central processing regions that make sense of the visual information, and the motor systems that coordinate movement of the eyes and head. Many of these systems can be recognized in the gross anatomy of the brain. Each specific brain region is extensively interconnected with other regions that serve different primary functions. These regions tend to have profuse connections that send information *in both directions* along most sensory/central motor pathways. The advantages of this complexity are obvious; while interpreting visual information, for example, it can be very useful to simultaneously analyze sound and to know where your eyes are pointing and how your body is oriented.

The systems of the brain can be more deeply understood by studying their organization at the cellular level. Within a local brain region, the arrangement of neurons and their synaptic connections is called a **local circuit**. A local circuit

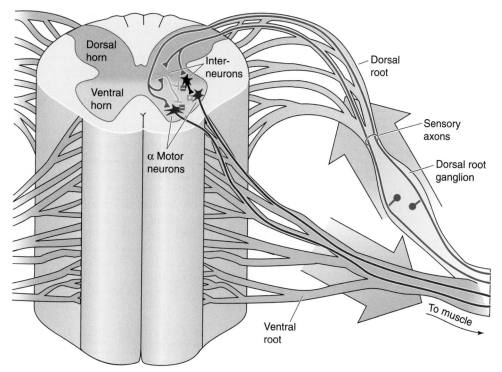

Figure 16-1 Local circuits in the spinal cord. A basic local circuit in the spinal cord consists of inputs (e.g., sensory axons of the dorsal roots), interneurons (both excitatory and inhibitory), and output neurons (e.g., α motor neurons that send their axons through the ventral roots).

typically includes the set of inputs, outputs, and all the interconnected neurons that are essential to functions of the local brain region. Many regions of the brain are composed of a large number of stereotyped local circuits, almost modular in their interchangeability, that are themselves interconnected. Within the local circuits are finer arrangements of neurons and synapses sometimes called **microcircuits**. Microcircuits may be repeated numerous times within a local circuit, and they determine the transformations of information that occur within small areas of dendrites and the collection of synapses impinging on them. At even finer resolution, neural systems can be understood by the properties of their individual neurons (see Chapter 12), **synapses**, membranes, **molecules** (e.g., neurotransmitters and neuromodulators), and ions as well as the **genes** that encode and control the system's molecular biology.

Most local circuits have three elements: input axons, interneurons, and projection (output) neurons

One of the most fascinating things about the nervous system is the wide array of different local circuits that have evolved for different behavioral functions. Despite this diversity, we can define a few general components of local circuits, which we illustrate with two examples from very different parts of the CNS: the ventral horn of the spinal cord and the cerebral neocortex. Some of the functions of these circuits are described in subsequent sections; here, we examine their cellular anatomy.

All local circuits have some form of **input**, which is usually a set of axons that originate elsewhere and terminate in synapses within the local circuit. A major input to the spinal cord (Fig. 16-1) is the afferent sensory axons in the dorsal roots. These axons carry information from somatic sensory receptors in the skin, connective tissue, and muscles (see Chapter 15). However, local circuits in the spinal cord also have many other sources of input, including descending input from the brain and input from the spinal cord itself, both from the contralateral side and from spinal segments above and below. Input to the local circuits of the neocortex (Fig. 16-2) is also easily identified; relay neurons of the thalamus send axons into particular layers of the cortex to bring a range of information about sensation, motor systems, and the body's internal state. By far, the most numerous input to the local circuits of the neocortex comes from the neocortex itself—from adjacent local circuits, distant areas of cortex, and the contralateral hemisphere. These two systems illustrate a basic principle: local circuits receive multiple types of input.

Output is usually achieved with a subset of cells known as *projection neurons*, or *principal neurons*, which send axons to one or more targets. The most obvious spinal output comes from the α motor neurons, which send their axons out through the ventral roots to innervate skeletal muscle fibers. Output axons from the neocortex come mainly from large pyramidal neurons in layer V, which innervate many targets in the brainstem, spinal cord, and other structures, as well as from neurons in layer VI, which make their synapses back onto the cells of the thalamus. However, as was true

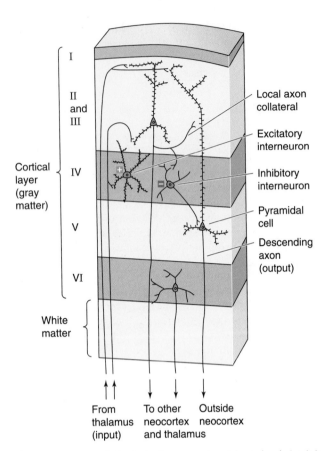

I

II and III

IV — Cortical layer (gray matter)

V

VI

White matter

Local axon collateral

Excitatory interneuron

Inhibitory interneuron

Pyramidal cell

Descending axon (output)

From thalamus (input)

To other neocortex and thalamus

Outside neocortex

Figure 16-2 Local circuits in the neocortex. A basic local circuit in the neocortex consists of inputs (e.g., afferent axons from the thalamus), excitatory and inhibitory interneurons, and output neurons (e.g., pyramidal cells).

with input, most local circuits have multiple output. Thus, spinal neurons innervate other regions of the spinal cord and the brain, whereas neocortical circuits make most of their connections to other neocortical circuits.

Rare, indeed, is the neural circuit that has only input and output cells. **Local processing** is achieved by additional neurons whose axonal connections remain within the local circuit. These neurons are usually called *interneurons*, or *intrinsic neurons*. Interneurons vary widely in structure and function, and a single local circuit may have many different types. Both the spinal cord and neocortex have excitatory and inhibitory interneurons, interneurons that make very specific or widely divergent connections, and interneurons that either receive direct contact from input axons or process only information from other interneurons. In many parts of the brain, interneurons vastly outnumber output neurons. To take an extreme example, the cerebellum has ~10^{11} granule cells—a type of excitatory interneuron—which is more than the total number of all other types of neurons in the entire brain!

Numerous variations on the "principles" of local circuits outlined here may be mentioned. For example, a projection cell may have some of the characteristics of an interneuron, as when a branch of its output axon stays within the local circuit and makes synaptic connections. This branching is

the case for the projection cells of both the neocortex (pyramidal cells) and the spinal cord (α motor neurons). On the other hand, some interneurons may entirely lack an axon and instead make their local synaptic connections through very short neurites or even dendrites. In some rare cases, the source of the input to a local circuit may not be purely synaptic but chemical (as with CO_2-sensitive neurons in the medulla; see Chapter 32) or physical (as with temperature-sensitive neurons in the hypothalamus; see Chapter 59). Although the main neurons within a generic local circuit are wired in *series* (Figs. 16-1 and 16-2), local circuits, often in massive numbers, operate in *parallel* with one another. Furthermore, these circuits usually demonstrate a tremendous amount of *crosstalk*; information from each circuit is shared mutually, and each circuit continually influences its neighbors. Indeed, one of the things that makes analysis of local neural circuits so exceptionally difficult is that they operate in highly interactive, simultaneously interdependent, and expansive networks.

SIMPLE, STEREOTYPED RESPONSES: SPINAL REFLEX CIRCUITS

Passive stretching of a skeletal muscle causes a reflexive contraction of that same muscle and relaxation of the antagonist muscles

Reflexes are among the most basic of neural functions and involve some of the simplest neuronal circuits. A motor *reflex* is a rapid, stereotyped motor response to a particular sensory stimulus. Although the existence of reflexes was long appreciated, it was Sir Charles Sherrington who, beginning in the 1890s, first defined the anatomical and physiological bases for some simple spinal reflexes. So meticulous were Sherrington's observations of reflexes and their timing that they offered him compelling evidence for the existence of synapses, a term he originated.

Reflexes are essential, if rudimentary, elements of behavior. Because of their relative simplicity, more than a century of research has taught us a lot about their biological basis. However, reflexes are also important for understanding of more complex behaviors. Intricate behaviors may sometimes be built up from sequences of simple reflexive responses. In addition, neural circuits that generate reflexes almost always mediate or participate in much more complex behaviors. Here we examine a relatively well understood example of reflex-mediating circuitry.

The CNS commands the body to move about by activating motor neurons, which excite skeletal muscles (Sherrington called motor neurons the final common path). Motor neurons receive synaptic input from many sources within the brain and spinal cord, and the output of large numbers of motor neurons must be closely coordinated to achieve even uncomplicated actions such as walking. However, in some circumstances, motor neurons can be commanded directly by a simple sensory stimulus—muscle stretch—with only the minimum of neural machinery intervening between the sensory cell and motor neuron: one synapse. Understanding of this simplest of reflexes, the

stretch reflex or **myotatic reflex**, first requires knowledge of some anatomy.

Each motor neuron, with its soma in the spinal cord or brainstem, commands a group of skeletal muscle cells; a single motor neuron and the muscle cells that it synapses on are collectively called a **motor unit** (see Chapter 9). Each muscle cell belongs to only one motor unit. The size of motor units varies dramatically and depends on muscle function. In small muscles that generate finely controlled movements, such as the extraocular muscles of the eye, motor units tend to be small and may contain just a few muscle fibers. Large muscles that generate strong forces, such as the gastrocnemius muscle of the leg, tend to have large motor units with as many as several thousand muscle fibers. There are two types of motor neurons (see Table 12-1): α **motor neurons** innervate the main force-generating muscle fibers (the extrafusal fibers), whereas γ **motor neurons** innervate only the fibers of the muscle spindles. The group of all motor neurons innervating a single muscle is called a **motor neuron pool** (see Chapter 9).

When a skeletal muscle is abruptly stretched, a rapid, reflexive contraction of the same muscle often occurs. The contraction increases muscle tension and opposes the stretch. This stretch reflex is particularly strong in physiological extensor muscles—those that resist gravity—and it is sometimes called the myotatic reflex because it is specific for the same muscle that is stretched. The most familiar version is the knee jerk, which is elicited by a light tap on the patellar tendon. The tap deflects the tendon, which then pulls on and briefly stretches the quadriceps femoris muscle. A reflexive contraction of the quadriceps quickly follows (Fig. 16-3). Stretch reflexes are also easily demonstrated in the biceps of the arm and the muscles that close the jaw. Sherrington showed that the stretch reflex depends on the nervous system and requires sensory feedback from the muscle. For example, cutting of the dorsal (sensory) roots to the lumbar spinal cord abolishes the stretch reflex in the quadriceps muscle. The basic circuit for the stretch reflex begins with the primary sensory axons from the **muscle spindles** (see Chapter 15) in the muscle itself. Increasing the length of the muscle stimulates the spindle afferents, particularly the large group Ia axons from the primary sensory endings. In the spinal cord, these group Ia sensory axons terminate monosynaptically onto the α motor neurons that innervate the same (i.e., the homonymous) muscle from which the group Ia axons originated. Thus, stretching of a muscle causes rapid feedback excitation of the same muscle through the minimum possible circuit: one sensory neuron, one synapse, and one motor neuron.

Monosynaptic connections account for much of the rapid component of the stretch reflex, but they are only the beginning of the story. At the same time the stretched muscle is being stimulated to contract, parallel circuits are inhibiting the α motor neurons of its *antagonist* muscles (i.e., those muscles that move a joint in the opposite direction). Thus, as the knee jerk reflex causes contraction of the quadriceps muscle, it simultaneously causes relaxation of its antagonists, including the semitendinosus muscle (Fig. 16-3). To achieve inhibition, branches of the group Ia sensory axons excite specific interneurons that *inhibit* the α motor neurons of the antagonists. This **reciprocal innervation** increases the effec-

tiveness of the stretch reflex by minimizing the antagonistic forces of the antagonist muscles.

Force applied to the Golgi tendon organ during active muscle contraction causes relaxation of the same muscle and contraction of the antagonistic muscles

Skeletal muscle contains another sensory transducer in addition to the stretch receptor: the **Golgi tendon organ** (see Chapter 15). Tendon organs are aligned in series with the muscle; they are exquisitely sensitive to the *tension* within a tendon and thus respond to the force generated by the muscle rather than to muscle length. Tendon organs may respond during passive muscle stretch, but they are stimulated particularly well during active contractions of a muscle. The group Ib sensory axons of the tendon organs excite both excitatory and inhibitory interneurons within the spinal cord (Fig. 16-4). However, in most cases, this interneuron circuitry *inhibits* the muscle in which tension has increased and *excites* the antagonistic muscle; therefore, activity in the tendon organs usually yields effects that are almost the opposite of the stretch reflex. Under other circumstances, particularly in rapid movements, sensory input from Golgi tendon organs actually excites the motor neurons activating the same muscle. In general, reflexes mediated by the Golgi tendon organs serve to control the force within muscles and the stability of particular joints.

Noxious stimuli can evoke complex reflexive movements

Sensations from the skin and connective tissue can also evoke strong spinal reflexes. Imagine walking on a beach and stepping on a sharp piece of shell (Fig. 16-5). Your response is swift and coordinated and does not require thoughtful reflection: you rapidly withdraw the wounded foot by activating the leg flexors and inhibiting the extensors. To keep from falling, you also extend your opposite leg by activating its extensors and inhibiting its flexors. This response is an example of a **flexor reflex**. The original stimulus for the reflex came from fast pain afferent neurons in the skin, primarily the group Aδ axons.

This bilateral flexor reflex response is coordinated by sets of inhibitory and excitatory interneurons within the spinal gray matter. Note that this coordination requires circuitry not only on the side of the cord ipsilateral to the wounded side but also on the contralateral side. That is, while you withdraw the foot that hurts, you must also extend the opposite leg to support your body weight. Flexor reflexes can be activated by most of the various sensory afferents that detect noxious stimuli. Motor output spreads widely up and down the spinal cord, as it must to orchestrate so much of the body's musculature into an effective response. A remarkable feature of flexor reflexes is their specificity. Touching of a hot surface, for example, elicits reflexive withdrawal of the hand in the direction opposite the side of the stimulus, and the strength of the reflex is related to the intensity of the stimulus. Unlike simple stretch reflexes, flexor reflexes coordinate the movement of entire limbs and even pairs of limbs. Such coordination

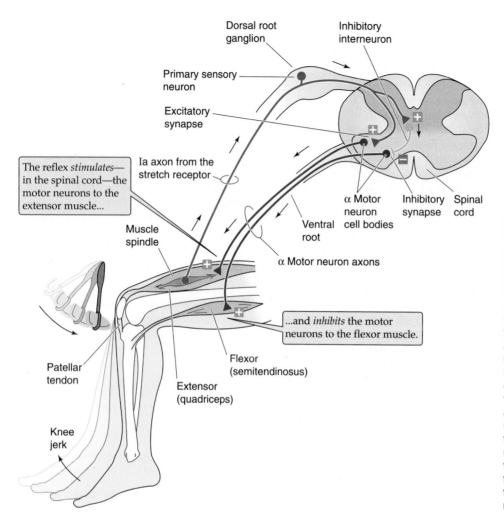

Dorsal root ganglion
Inhibitory interneuron
Primary sensory neuron
Excitatory synapse
Ia axon from the stretch receptor

The reflex *stimulates*—in the spinal cord—the motor neurons to the extensor muscle...

α Motor neuron cell bodies
Inhibitory synapse
Spinal cord
Muscle spindle
Ventral root
α Motor neuron axons
...and *inhibits* the motor neurons to the flexor muscle.
Patellar tendon
Flexor (semitendinosus)
Extensor (quadriceps)
Knee jerk

Figure 16-3 Knee jerk (myotatic) reflex. Tapping of the patellar tendon with a percussion hammer elicits a reflexive knee jerk caused by contraction of the quadriceps muscle: the *stretch reflex*. Stretching of the tendon pulls on the muscle spindle, exciting the primary sensory afferents, which convey their information through group Ia axons. These axons make monosynaptic connections to the α motor neurons that innervate the quadriceps, resulting in the contraction of this muscle. The Ia axons also excite inhibitory interneurons that reciprocally innervate the motor neurons of the antagonist muscle of the quadriceps (the flexor), resulting in relaxation of the semitendinosus muscle. Thus, the reflex relaxation of the antagonistic muscle is polysynaptic.

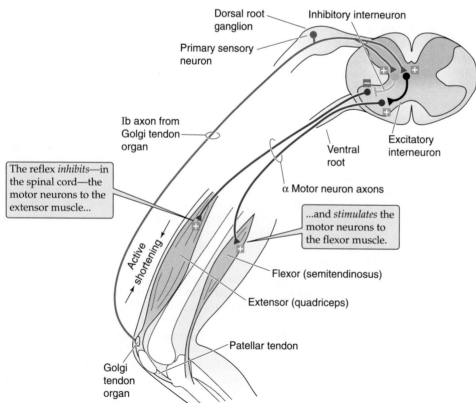

Dorsal root ganglion
Inhibitory interneuron
Primary sensory neuron
Ib axon from Golgi tendon organ

The reflex *inhibits*—in the spinal cord—the motor neurons to the extensor muscle...

Excitatory interneuron
Ventral root
α Motor neuron axons
...and *stimulates* the motor neurons to the flexor muscle.
Active shortening
Flexor (semitendinosus)
Extensor (quadriceps)
Patellar tendon
Golgi tendon organ

Figure 16-4 Golgi tendon organ reflex. Active contraction of the quadriceps muscle elicits a reflexive relaxation of this muscle and contraction of the antagonistic semitendinosus muscle: the *inverse mytotatic reflex*. Contraction of the muscle pulls on the tendon, which squeezes and excites the sensory endings of the Golgi tendon organ, which convey their information through group Ib axons. These axons synapse on both inhibitory and excitatory interneurons in the spinal cord. The inhibitory interneurons innervate α motor neurons to the quadriceps, relaxing this muscle. The excitatory interneurons innervate α motor neurons to the antagonistic semitendinosus muscle, contracting it. Thus, both limbs of the reflex are polysynaptic.

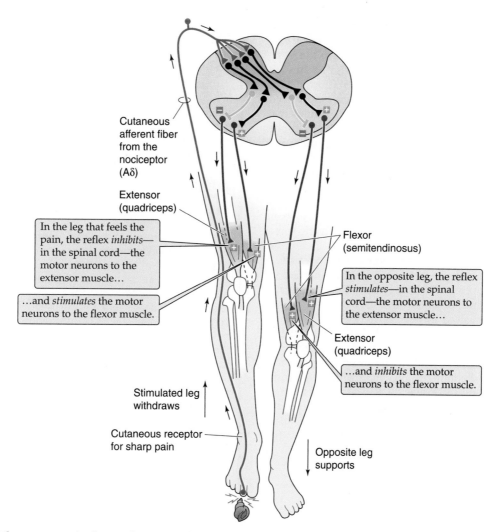

Cutaneous
afferent fiber
from the
nociceptor
(Aδ)

Extensor
(quadriceps)

In the leg that feels the
pain, the reflex *inhibits*—
in the spinal cord—the
motor neurons to the
extensor muscle...

...and *stimulates* the motor
neurons to the flexor muscle.

Flexor
(semitendinosus)

In the opposite leg, the reflex
stimulates—in the spinal
cord—the motor neurons to
the extensor muscle...

Extensor
(quadriceps)

...and *inhibits* the motor
neurons to the flexor muscle.

Stimulated leg
withdraws

Cutaneous receptor
for sharp pain

Opposite leg
supports

Figure 16-5   The flexor reflex. A painful stimulus to the right foot elicits a reflexive flexion of the right knee
and an extension of the left knee: the *flexor reflex*. The noxious stimulus activates nociceptor afferents, which
convey their information through group Aδ axons. These axons synapse on both inhibitory and excitatory
interneurons. The inhibitory interneurons that project to the *right* side of the spinal cord innervate α motor
neurons to the quadriceps and relax this muscle. The excitatory interneurons that project to the *right* side of
the spinal cord innervate α motor neurons to the antagonistic semitendinosus muscle and contract it. The
net effect is a coordinated *flexion* of the right knee. Similarly, the inhibitory interneurons that project to the
left side of the spinal cord innervate α motor neurons to the left semitendinosus muscle and relax this
muscle. The excitatory interneurons that project to the *left* side of the spinal cord innervate α motor neurons
to the left quadriceps and contract it. The net effect is a coordinated *extension* of the left knee.

requires precise and widespread wiring of the spinal
interneurons.

Spinal reflexes are strongly influenced by control centers within the brain

Axons descend from numerous centers within the brainstem
and the cerebral cortex and terminate primarily onto the
spinal interneurons, with some direct input to the motor
neurons. This descending control is essential for all conscious (and much unconscious) command of movement, a
topic beyond the scope of this chapter. Less obvious is that
the descending pathways can alter the strength of reflexes.
For example, to heighten an anxious patient's stretch reflexes,

a neurologist will sometimes ask the patient to perform the
Jendrassik maneuver. The patient clasps his or her hands
together and pulls; while the patient is distracted with that
task, the examiner tests the stretch reflexes of the leg. Another
example of the brain's modulation of a stretch reflex occurs
in catching a falling ball. If a ball were to fall unexpectedly
from the sky and hit your outstretched hand, the force
applied to your arm would cause a rapid *stretch reflex*—contraction in the *stretched* muscles and reciprocal inhibition in
the *antagonist* muscles. The result would be that your hand
slaps the ball back up into the air. However, if you *anticipate*
catching the falling ball, for a short period around the time
of impact (about ±60 ms), both your stretched muscles *and*
the antagonist muscles contract! This maneuver stiffens your

arm just when you need to squeeze that ball to not drop it. Stretch reflexes of the leg also vary dramatically during each step as we walk, thereby facilitating movement of the legs.

Like stretch reflexes, flexor reflexes can also be strongly affected by descending pathways. With mental effort, painful stimuli can be tolerated and withdrawal reflexes suppressed. On the other hand, anticipation of a painful stimulus may heighten the vigor of a withdrawal reflex when the stimulus actually arrives. Most of the brain's influence on spinal circuitry is achieved by control of the many spinal interneurons.

Spinal reflexes are frequently studied in isolation from one another, and textbooks often describe them this way. However, under realistic conditions, many reflex systems operate simultaneously, and motor output from the spinal cord depends on interactions among them as well as on the state of controlling influences descending from the brain. It is now well accepted that reflexes do not simply correct for external perturbations of the body; in addition, they play a key role in the control of all movements.

The neurons involved in reflexes are the same neurons that generate other behaviors. Think again of the flexor response to the sharp shell—the pricked foot is withdrawn while the opposite leg extends. Now imagine that a crab pinches that opposite foot—you respond with the opposite pattern of withdrawal and extension. Repeat this a few times, crabs pinching you left and right, and you have achieved the basic pattern necessary for walking! Indeed, rhythmic locomotor patterns use components of these same spinal reflex circuits, as discussed next.

RHYTHMIC ACTIVITY: CENTRAL PATTERN GENERATORS

Central pattern generators in the spinal cord can create a complex motor program even without sensory feedback

A common feature of motor control is the **motor program**, a set of structured muscle commands that are determined by the nervous system before a movement begins and that can be sent to the muscles with the appropriate timing so that a sequence of movements occurs without any need for sensory feedback. The best evidence for the existence of motor programs is that the brain or spinal cord can command a variety of voluntary and automatic movements, such as walking and breathing (see Chapter 32), even in the complete absence of sensory feedback from the periphery. The existence of motor programs certainly does not mean that sensory information is unimportant; on the contrary, motor behavior without sensory feedback is always different from that with normal feedback. The neural circuits responsible for various motor programs have been defined in a wide range of species. Although the details vary endlessly, certain broad principles emerge, even when vertebrates and invertebrates are compared. Here we focus on **central pattern generators**, well-studied circuits that underlie many of the rhythmic motor activities that are central to animal behavior.

Rhythmic behavior includes walking, running, swimming, breathing, chewing, certain eye movements, shivering,

Motor System Injury

The motor control systems, because of their anatomy, are susceptible to damage from trauma or disease. The nature of a patient's motor deficits often allows the neurologist to diagnose the site of neural damage with great accuracy. When injury occurs to lower parts of the motor system, such as motor neurons or their axons, deficits may be very localized. If the motor nerve to a muscle is damaged, that muscle may develop **paresis** (weakness) or complete **paralysis** (loss of motor function). When motor axons cannot trigger contractions, there can be no reflexes (**areflexia**). Normal muscles are slightly contracted even at rest—they have some *tone*. If their motor nerves are transected, muscles become flaccid (**atonia**) and eventually develop profound **atrophy** (loss of muscle mass) because of the absence of trophic influences from the nerves.

Motor neurons normally receive strong excitatory influences from the upper parts of the motor system, including regions of the spinal cord, the brainstem, and the cerebral cortex. When upper regions of the motor system are injured by stroke, trauma, or demyelinating disease, for example, the signs and symptoms are distinctly different from those caused by lower damage. Complete transection of the spinal cord leads to profound paralysis below the level of the lesion. This is called **paraplegia** when only both legs are selectively affected, **hemiplegia** when one side of the body is affected, and **quadriplegia** when the legs, trunk, and arms are involved. For a few days after an acute injury, there is also areflexia and reduced muscle tone (**hypotonia**), a condition called **spinal shock**. The muscles are limp and cannot be controlled by the brain or by the remaining circuits of the spinal cord. Spinal shock is temporary; after days to months, it is replaced by both an exaggerated muscle tone (**hypertonia**) and heightened stretch reflexes (**hyperreflexia**) with related signs—this combination is called **spasticity**. The mechanisms of spasticity are largely unknown, although the hypertonia is the consequence of tonically overactive stretch reflex circuitry, driven by spinal neurons that have become chronically hyperexcitable.

and even scratching. The central pattern generators driving each of these activities share certain basic properties. At their core is a set of cyclic, coordinated timing signals that are generated by a cluster of interconnected neurons. These basic signals are used to command as many as several hundred muscles, each precisely contracting or relaxing during a particular phase of the cycle; for example, with each walking step, the knee must first be flexed and then extended. Figure 16-6A shows how the extensor and flexor muscles of the left hind limb of a cat contract rhythmically—and out of phase with one another—while the animal walks. Rhythms must also be coordinated with other rhythms; for humans to walk, one leg must move forward while the other thrusts backward, then vice versa, and the arms must swing in time with the legs, but with the opposite phase. For four-footed animals, the rhythms are even more complicated and must be able to accommodate changes in gait (Fig. 16-6B). For coordination to be achieved among the various limbs, sets

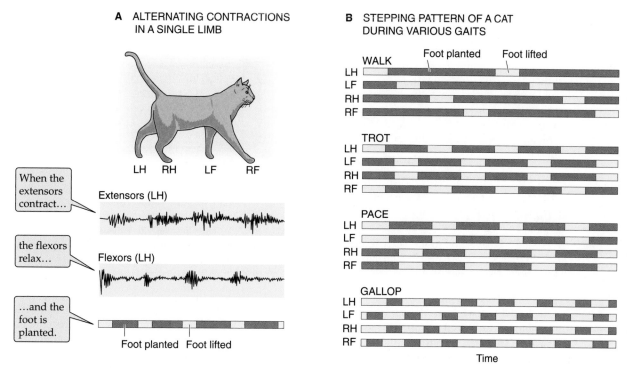

Figure 16-6   Rhythmic patterns during locomotion. **A,** The experimental tracings are electromyograms—extracellular recordings of the electrical activity of muscles—from the extensor and flexor muscles of the left hind limb of a walking cat. The pink bars indicate that the foot is lifted; purple bars indicate that the foot is planted. **B,** The *walk, trot, pace,* and *gallop* not only represent different patterns and frequencies of planting and lifting for a single leg but also different patterns of coordination among the legs. LF, left front; LH, left hind; RF, right front; RH, right hind. *(Data from Pearson K: The control of walking. Sci Am 1976; 2:72-86.)*

of central pattern generators must be interconnected. The motor patterns must also have great flexibility so that they can be altered on a moment's notice—consider the adjustments necessary when one foot strikes an obstacle while walking or the changing motor patterns necessary to go from walking, to trotting, to running, to jumping. Finally, reliable methods must be available for turning the patterns on and off.

The central pattern generators for some rhythmic functions, such as breathing, are in the brainstem (see Chapter 32). Surprisingly, those responsible for locomotion reside in the spinal cord itself. Even with the spinal cord transected so that the lumbar segments are isolated from all higher centers, cats on a treadmill can generate well-coordinated stepping movements. Furthermore, stimulation of sensory afferents or descending tracts can induce the spinal pattern generators in four-footed animals to switch rapidly from walking, to trotting, to galloping patterns by altering not only the frequency of motor commands but also their pattern and coordination. During walking and trotting and pacing, the hind legs *alternate* their movements, but during galloping, they both flex and extend *simultaneously* (compare the leg patterns in Fig. 16-6B). Grillner and colleagues showed that each limb has at least one central pattern generator. If one leg is prevented from stepping, the other continues stepping normally. Under most circumstances, the various spinal pattern generators are coupled to one another, although the nature of

the coupling must change to explain, for example, the switch from trotting to galloping patterns.

Pacemaker cells and synaptic interconnections both contribute to central pattern generation

How do neural circuits generate rhythmic patterns of activity? There is no single answer, and different circuits use different mechanisms. The simplest pattern generators are single neurons whose membrane properties endow them with pacemaker properties that are analogous to those of cardiac muscle cells (see Chapter 21) and smooth muscle cells (see Chapter 9). Even when experimentally isolated from other neurons, pacemaker neurons may be able to generate rhythmic activity by relying only on their intrinsic membrane conductances. It is easy to imagine how intrinsic pacemaker neurons might act as the primary rhythmic driving force for sets of motor neurons that in turn command cyclic behavior. However, within vertebrates, although pacemaker neurons may contribute to some central pattern generators, they do not appear to be solely responsible for generating rhythms. Instead, they are embedded within interconnected circuits, and it is the combination of intrinsic pacemaker properties and synaptic interconnections that generates rhythms.

Neural circuits without pacemaker neurons can also generate rhythmic output. In 1911, Graham Brown proposed a pattern-generating circuit for locomotion. The essence of

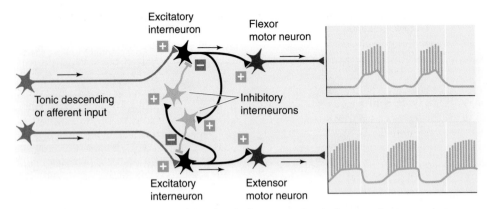

Figure 16-7 Half-center model for alternating rhythm generation in flexor and extensor motor neurons. Stimulation of the upper excitatory interneuron has two effects. First, the stimulated excitatory interneuron excites the motor neuron to the flexor muscle. Second, the stimulated excitatory interneuron excites an inhibitory interneuron, which inhibits the lower pathway. Stimulation of the lower excitatory interneuron has the opposite effects. Thus, when one motor neuron is active, the opposite one is inhibited.

Brown's half-center model is a set of excitatory and inhibitory interneurons arranged to inhibit one another reciprocally (Fig. 16-7). The half-centers are the two halves of the circuit, each commanding one of a pair of antagonist muscles. For the circuit to work, a tonic drive must be applied to the excitatory interneurons; this drive could come from axons originating outside the circuit or from the intrinsic excitability of the neurons themselves. Furthermore, some built-in mechanism must limit the duration of the inhibitory activity so that excitability can cyclically switch from one half-center to the other. Note that feedback from the muscles is not needed for the rhythms to proceed indefinitely. In fact, studies of more than 50 vertebrate and invertebrate motor circuits have confirmed that rhythm generation can continue in the absence of sensory information.

Central pattern generators in the spinal cord take advantage of sensory feedback, interconnections among spinal segments, and interactions with brainstem control centers

The half-center model can produce rhythmic, alternating neural activity, but it is clearly too simplistic to account for most features of locomotor pattern generation. Analysis of vertebrate pattern generators is a daunting task, made difficult by the complexity of the circuits and the behaviors they control. In one of the most detailed investigations, Grillner and colleagues studied a simple model of vertebrate locomotion circuits: the spinal cord of the sea lamprey. Lampreys are among the simplest fish, and they swim with undulating motions of their body by using precisely coordinated waves of body muscle contractions. At each spinal segment, muscle activity alternates—one side contracts as the other relaxes. As in mammals, the rhythmic pattern is generated within the spinal cord, and neurons in the brainstem control the initiation and speed of the patterns. The basic pattern-generating circuit for the lamprey spinal cord is repeated in each of the animal's 100 or so spinal segments.

The lamprey pattern-generating circuit improves on the half-center model in three ways. The first is **sensory feedback**. The lamprey has two kinds of stretch receptor neurons

in the lateral margin of the spinal cord itself. These neurons sense stretching of the cord and body, which occurs as the animal bends during swimming. One type of stretch receptor excites the pattern generator interneurons on that same side and facilitates contraction, whereas the other type inhibits the pattern generator on the contralateral side and suppresses contraction. Because stretching occurs on the side of the cord that is currently relaxed, the effect of both stretch receptors is to terminate activity on the contracted side of the body and to initiate contraction on the relaxed side.

The second improvement of the lamprey circuit over the half-center model is the **interconnection of spinal segments**, which ensures the smooth progression of contractions down the length of the body, so that swimming can be efficient. Specifically, each segment must command its muscles to contract slightly later than the one anterior to it, with a lag of ~1% of a full activity cycle for normal forward swimming. Under some circumstances, the animal can also reverse the sequence of intersegment coordination to allow it to swim backward!

A third improvement over the half-center model is the **reciprocal communication** between the lamprey spinal pattern generators and control centers in the brainstem. Not only does the brainstem use numerous pathways and transmitters to modulate the generators, but the spinal generators also inform the brainstem of their activity.

The features outlined for swimming lampreys are relevant to walking cats and humans. All use spinal pattern generators to produce rhythms. All use sensory feedback to modulate locomotor rhythms (in mammals, feedback from muscle, joint, and cutaneous receptors is all-important). All coordinate the spinal pattern generators across segments, and all maintain reciprocal communication between spinal generators and brainstem control centers.

SPATIAL REPRESENTATIONS: SENSORY AND MOTOR MAPS IN THE BRAIN

We have already seen that the spinal cord can receive sensory input, integrate it, and produce motor output that is totally independent of the brain. The brain also receives this sensory information and uses it to control the motor activity of the spinal reflexes and central pattern generators. How does the brain organize this sensory input and motor output? In many cases, it organizes these functions spatially by use of maps.

In everyday life, we use maps to represent spatial locations. You may use endless ways to construct a map, depending on which features of an area you want to highlight and what sort of transformation you make as you take measurements from the source (the thing being mapped) and place them on the target (the map). Maps of the earth may emphasize topography, the road system, political boundaries, the distributions of air temperature and wind direction, population density, or vegetation. A map is a model of a part of the world—and a very limited model at that. The brain also builds maps, most of which represent very selected aspects of our sensory information about the environment or the motor systems controlling our body. These maps can be spatial, or they can express nonspatial qualities of various sensory modalities (e.g., smell).

The nervous system contains maps of sensory and motor information

Almost all sensory receptors are laid out in planar sheets. In some cases, these receptor sheets are straightforward **spatial maps** of the sensory environment that they encode. For example, the somatic sensory receptors of the skin literally form a map of the body surface. Similarly, a tiny version of the visual scene is projected onto the mosaic of retinal photoreceptors. The topographies of other sensory receptor sheets represent qualities other than spatial features of the sensory stimuli. For example, the position of a hair cell along the basilar membrane in the cochlea determines the range of sound frequencies to which it will respond. Thus, the sheet of hair cells is a **frequency map** of sound rather than a map of the location of sounds in space. Olfactory and taste receptors also do not encode stimulus position; instead, because the receptor specificity varies topographically, the receptor sheets may be **chemical maps** of the types of stimuli. The most interesting thing about sensory receptor maps is that they often project onto many different regions of the CNS. In fact, each sensory surface may be mapped and remapped many times within the brain, the characteristics of each map being unique. In some cases, the brain constructs maps of stimulus features even when these features are not mapped at the level of the receptors themselves. Sound localization is a good example of this property (see the next section). Some neural maps may also combine the features of other neural maps, for example, overlaying visual information with auditory information.

The cerebral cortex has multiple visuotopic maps

Some of the best examples of brain maps are those of the visual fields. Figure 16-8A shows the basic anatomical pathway extending from the retina to the lateral geniculate nucleus of the thalamus and on to the **primary visual cortex** (area V1). Note that area V1 actually maps the visual thalamus, which in turn maps the retina, the first visuotopic map

in the brain. Thus, the V1 map is sometimes referred to as a *retinotopic map*. Figure 16-8B shows how the visual fields are mapped onto cortical area V1. The first thing to notice is that the *left* half of the visual field is represented on the *right* cortex and the *upper* half of the visual field is represented on the *lower* portions of the cortex. This orientation is strictly determined by the system's anatomy. For example, all the retinal axons from the *left* most halves of both eyes (which are stimulated by light from the *right* visual hemifield) project to the *left* half of the brain. Compare the red and blue pathways in Figure 16-8A. During development, each axon must therefore make an unerring decision about which side of the brain to innervate when it reaches the optic chiasm!

The second thing to notice is that scaling of the visual fields onto the visual cortex—often called the **magnification factor**—is not constant. In particular, the central region of the visual fields—the fovea—is greatly magnified on the cortical surface. Behavioral importance ultimately determines mapping in the brain. Primates require vision of particularly high resolution in the center of their gaze; photoreceptors and ganglion cells are thus packed as densely as possible into the central retinal region (see Chapter 15). About half of the primary visual cortex is devoted to input from the relatively small fovea and the retinal area just surrounding it.

Understanding of a visual scene requires us to analyze many of its features simultaneously. An object may have shape, color, motion, location, and context, and the brain can usually organize these features to present a seamless interpretation, or image. The details of this process are only now being worked out, but it appears that the task is accomplished with the help of *numerous* visual areas within the cerebral cortex. Studies of monkey cortex by a variety of electrophysiological and anatomical methods have identified more than 25 areas, most of which are in the vicinity of area V1, that are mainly visual in function. According to recent estimates, humans devote almost half of their neocortex primarily to the processing of visual information. Several features of a visual scene, such as motion, form, and color, are processed in parallel and, to some extent, in separate stages of processing. The neural mechanisms by which these separate features are somehow melded into one image or concept of an object remain unknown, but they depend on strong and reciprocal interconnections between the visual maps in various areas of the brain.

The apparently simple topography of a sensory map looks much more complex and discontinuous when it is examined in detail. Many cortical areas can be described as maps on maps. Such an arrangement is especially striking in the visual system. For example, within area V1 of Old World monkeys and humans, the visuotopic maps of the two eyes remain segregated. In layer IV of the primary visual cortex, this segregation is accomplished by having visual input derived from the left eye alternate every 0.25 to 0.5 mm with visual input from the right. Thus, two sets of information, one from the left eye and one from the right eye, remain separated but adjacent. Viewed edge on, these left-right alternations look like columns (Fig. 16-9A), hence their name: **ocular dominance columns.** Viewed from the surface of the brain, this alternating left-right array of input looks like bands or zebra stripes (Fig. 16-9B).

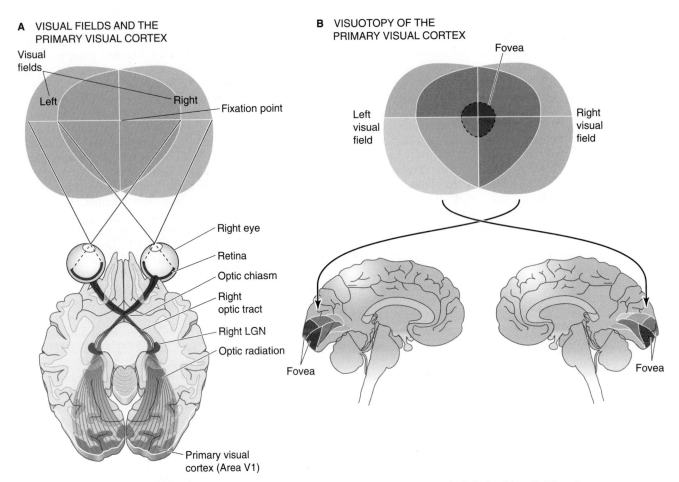

A VISUAL FIELDS AND THE PRIMARY VISUAL CORTEX

Visual fields

Left

Right

Fixation point

Right eye

Retina

Optic chiasm

Right optic tract

Right LGN

Optic radiation

Fovea

Primary visual cortex (Area V1)

B VISUOTOPY OF THE PRIMARY VISUAL CORTEX

Fovea

Left visual field

Right visual field

Fovea

Fovea

Figure 16-8 Visual maps. **A,** The right sides of both retinas (which sense the left visual hemifield) project to the left lateral geniculate, which in turn projects to the left primary visual cortex (area V1). **B,** The upper parts of the visual fields project to lower parts of the contralateral visual cortex, and vice versa. Although the fovea represents only a small part of the visual field, its representation is greatly magnified in the primary visual cortex, reflecting the large number of retinal ganglion cells that are devoted to the fovea. LGN, lateral geniculate nucleus.

Superimposed on the zebra-stripe ocular dominance pattern in layer IV of the primary visual cortex, but quite distinct from these zebra stripes, layers II and III have structures called **blobs**. These blobs are visible when the cortex is stained for the mitochondrial enzyme cytochrome oxidase. Viewed edge on, these blobs look like round pegs (Fig. 16-9A). Viewed from the surface of the brain (Fig. 16-9A, B), the blobs appear as a polka-dot pattern of small dots that are ~0.2 mm in diameter.

Adjacent to the primary visual cortex (V1) is the secondary visual cortex (V2), which has, instead of blobs, a series of thick and thin **stripes** that are separated by pale interstripes. Some other higher order visual areas also have striped patterns. Whereas ocular dominance columns demarcate the left and right eyes, blobs and stripes seem to demarcate clusters of neurons that process and channel different types of visual information between areas V1 and V2 and pass them on to other visual regions of the cortex. For example, neurons within the blobs of area V1 seem to be especially attuned to information about color and project to neurons in the thin stripes of V2. Other neurons throughout area V1 are very sensitive to motion but are insensitive to color. They channel their information mainly to neurons of the thick stripes in V2.

Maps of somatic sensory information magnify some parts of the body more than others

One of the most famous depictions of a neural map came from studies of the human somatosensory cortex by Penfield and colleagues. Penfield stimulated small sites on the cortical surface of locally anesthetized but conscious patients during neurosurgical procedures; from their verbal descriptions of the position of their sensations, he drew a homunculus, a little person representing the **somatotopy**—mapping of the body surface—of the primary somatic sensory cortex (Fig. 16-10A). The basic features of Penfield's map have been confirmed with other methods, including recording from neurons while the body surface is stimulated and modern brain imaging methods, such as positron emission tomography and functional magnetic resonance imaging. The human somatotopic map resembles a trapeze artist hanging upside down—the legs are hooked over the top of the postcentral gyrus and dangling into the medial cortex between the hemi-

A LAYERS OF AREA V1

B SPLIT-OPEN VIEW

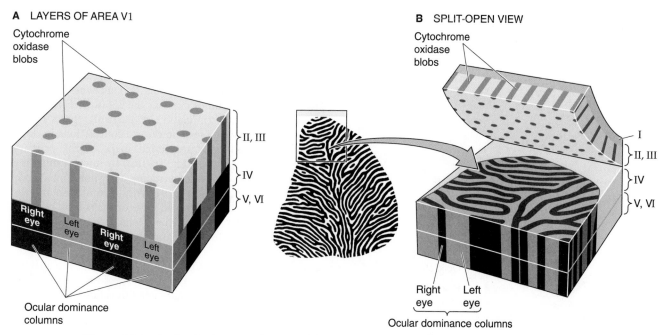

Figure 16-9 Ocular dominance columns and blobs in the primary visual cortex (area V1). **A,** Ocular dominance columns are shown as alternating black (right eye) and gray (left eye) structures in layer IV. The alternating light and dark bands are the result of an autoradiograph taken 2 weeks after injection of one eye with ^{3}H-labeled proline and fucose. The ^{3}H label moved from the optic nerve to neurons in the lateral geniculate and then to the axon terminals in the V1 cortex that are represented in this figure. The blobs are shown as teal-colored pegs in layers II and III. They represent the regular distribution of cytochrome oxidase–rich neurons and are organized in pillar-shaped clusters. **B,** Cutting of the brain parallel to its surface, but between layers III and IV, reveals a polka-dot pattern of blobs in layer II/III and zebra-like stripes in layer IV. *(Data from Hubel D: Eye, Brain and Vision. New York: WH Freeman, 1988.)*

spheres, and the trunk, upper limbs, and head are draped over the lateral aspect of the postcentral gyrus.

Two interesting features should be noticed about the somatotopic map in Figure 16-10A. First, mapping of the body surface is not always continuous. For example, the representation of the hand separates those of the head and face. Second, the map is not scaled like the human body. Instead, it looks like a cartoon character: the mouth, tongue, and fingers are very large, whereas the trunk, arms, and legs are tiny. As was the case for mapping of the visual fields onto the visual cortex, it is clear in Penfield's map that the magnification factor for the body surface is not a constant but varies for different parts of the body. Fingertips are magnified on the cortex much more than the tips of the toes. The relative size of cortex that is devoted to each body part is correlated with the *density* of sensory input received from that part, and 1 mm² of fingertip skin has many more sensory endings than a similar patch on the buttocks. Size on the map is also related to the *importance* of the sensory input from that part of the body; information from the tip of the tongue is more useful than that from the elbow. The mouth representation is probably large because tactile sensations are important in the production of speech, and the lips and tongue are one of the last lines of defense in deciding whether a morsel is a potential piece of food or poison.

The importance of each body part differs among species, and indeed, some species have body parts that others do not.

For example, the sensory nerves from the facial whisker follicles of rodents have a huge representation on the cortex, whereas the digits of the paws receive relatively little. Rodent behavior explains this paradox. Most are nocturnal, and to navigate they actively sweep their whiskers about as they move. By touching their local environment, they can sense shapes, textures, and movement with remarkable acuity. For a rat or mouse, seeing things with its eyes is usually less important than "seeing" things with its whiskers.

As we have already seen for the visual system, other sensory systems usually map their information numerous times. Maps may be carried through many anatomical levels. The somatotopic maps in the cortex begin with the primary somatic sensory axons (see Table 12-1) that enter the spinal cord or the brainstem, each at the spinal segment appropriate to the site of the information that it carries. The sensory axons synapse on second-order neurons, and these cells project their axons into various nuclei of the thalamus and form synapses. Thalamic relay neurons in turn send their axons into the neocortex. The topographical order of the body surface (i.e., *somatotopy*) is maintained at each anatomical stage, and somatotopic maps are located within the spinal cord, the brainstem, and the thalamus as well as in the somatosensory cortex. Within the cortex, the somatic sensory system has several maps of the body, each unique and each concerned with different types of somatotopic information. Multiple maps are the rule in the brain.

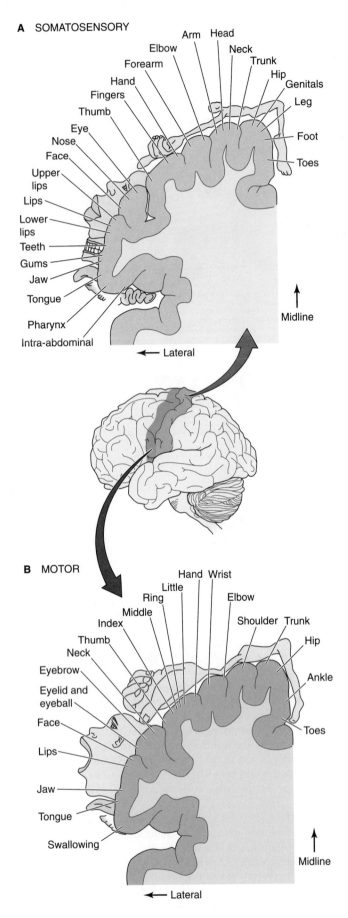

A SOMATOSENSORY

B MOTOR

The cerebral cortex has a motor map that is adjacent to and well aligned with the somatosensory map

Neural maps are not limited to sensory systems; they also appear regularly in brain structures that are considered to be primarily motor. Studies done in the 1860s by Fritsch and Hitzig showed that stimulation of particular parts of the cerebral cortex evokes specific muscle contractions in dogs. Penfield and colleagues generated maps of the primary motor cortex in humans (Fig. 16-10B) by microstimulating and observing the evoked movements. They noted an orderly relationship between the site of cortical stimulation and the body part that moved. Penfield's motor maps look remarkably like his somatosensory maps, which lie in the adjacent cortical gyrus (Fig. 16-10A). Note that the *sensory and motor maps are adjacent and similar* in basic layout (legs represented medially and head laterally), and both have a striking magnification of the head and hand regions. Not surprisingly, there are myriad axonal interconnections between the primary motor and primary somatosensory areas. Functional magnetic resonance imaging of the human motor cortex shows that the motor map for hand movements is not nearly as simple and somatotopic as Penfield's drawings might imply. Movements of individual fingers or the wrist, initiated by the individual, activate specific and widely distributed regions of motor cortex, but these regions also overlap one another. Rather than following an obvious somatotopic progression, it instead appears that neurons in the arm area of the motor cortex form distributed and cooperative networks that control collections of arm muscles. Other regions of the motor cortex also have a distributed organization when they are examined on a fine scale, although Penfield's somatotopic maps still suffice to describe the gross organization of the motor cortex.

In other parts of the brain, *motor and sensory functions may even occupy the same tissue*, and precise alignment of the motor and sensory maps is usually the case. For example, a paired midbrain structure called the *superior colliculus* receives direct, retinotopic connections from the retina as well as input from the visual cortex. Accordingly, a spot of light in the visual field activates a particular patch of neurons in the colliculus. The same patch of collicular neurons can also command, through other brainstem connections, eye and head movements that bring the image of the light spot into the center of the *visual* field so that it is imaged onto the fovea. The *motor map* for orientation of the eyes is in precise register with the visual response map. In addition, the superior colliculus has maps of both *auditory* and *somatosensory* information superimposed on its visual and motor maps; the four aligned maps work in concert to represent points in polysensory space and help control an

---

Figure 16-10 Somatosensory and motor maps. **A,** The plane of section runs through the postcentral gyrus of the cerebral cortex, shown as a blue band on the image of the brain. **B,** The plane of section runs through the precentral gyrus of the cerebral cortex, shown as a violet band on the image of the brain. *(Data from Penfield W, Rasmussen T: The Cerebral Cortex of Man. New York: Macmillan, 1952.)*

animal's orienting responses to prominent stimuli (Fig. 16-11).

Sensory and motor maps are fuzzy and plastic

We have described a sample of the sensory and motor maps in the brain, but we are left to wonder just why neural maps are so ubiquitous, elaborate, and varied. What is the advantage of mapping neural functions in an orderly way? You could imagine other arrangements: spatial information might be widely scattered about on a neural structure, much as the bytes of one large digital file may be scattered across the surface of the hard disk of a computer. Various explanations may be proposed for the phenomenon of orderly mapping in the nervous system, although most remain speculations. Maps may be the most efficient way of generating **nearest-neighbor relationships** between neurons that must be interconnected for proper function. For example, the collicular neurons that participate in sensing stimuli 10 degrees up and 20 degrees to the left and other collicular neurons that command eye movements toward that point undoubtedly need to be strongly interconnected. Orderly collicular mapping enforces togetherness for those cells and minimizes the length of axons necessary to interconnect them. In addition, if brain structures are arranged topographically, neighboring neurons will be most likely to become activated synchronously. Neighboring neurons are very likely to be interconnected in structures such as the cortex, and their synchronous activity serves to reinforce the strength of their interconnections because of the inherent rules governing synaptic plasticity (see Chapter 13).

An additional advantage of mapping is that it may simplify establishment of the proper connections between neurons during **development**. For example, it is easier for an axon from neuron A to find neuron B if distances are short. Maps may thus make it easier to establish interconnections precisely among the neurons that represent the three sensory maps and one motor map in the superior colliculus. Another advantage of maps may be to facilitate the effectiveness of **inhibitory connections**. Perception of the edge of a stimulus (edge detection) is heightened by lateral connections that suppress the activity of neurons representing the space slightly away from the edge. If sensory areas are mapped, it is a simple matter to arrange the inhibitory connections onto nearby neurons and thereby construct an edge-detector circuit.

It is worth clarifying several general points about neural maps. "The map is not the territory, the word is not the thing it describes."* In other words, all maps, including neural maps, are abstract representations of particular experimental measurements. A problem with neural maps is that different experimenters, using different methods, may sometimes generate quite different maps of the same part of the brain. As more and better refined methods become available, our understanding of these maps is evolving. Moreover, the brain itself muddies its maps. Maps of sensory space onto a brain area are not point-to-point representations. On the contrary,

*From Van Vogt AE: The Players of Null-A, p 158. London: Dobson, 1970, as quoted by Dykes and Ruest.

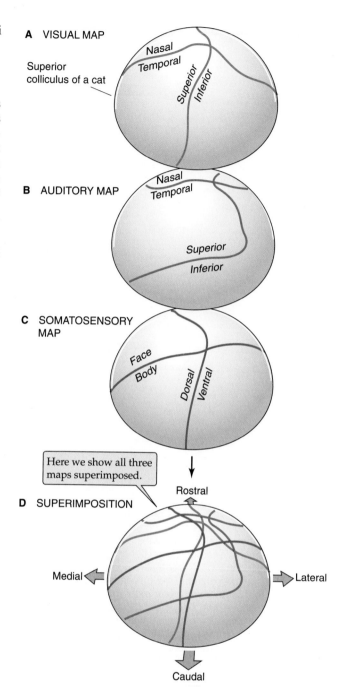

Figure 16-11 Polysensory space in the superior colliculus. In **A,** the illustration shows the representation of visual space that is projected onto the right superior colliculus of a cat. Note that visual space is divided into nasal versus temporal space and superior versus inferior space. In **B** and **C,** the illustrations show comparable auditory and somatosensory maps. In **D,** which shows the superimposition, note the approximate correspondence among the visual *(red),* auditory *(green),* and somatosensory *(blue)* maps, which are superimposed on one another. The motor map for orienting the eyes (not shown) is in almost perfect register with the visual map in **A.** *(Data from Stein BE, Wallace MT, Meredith MA: Neural mechanisms mediating attention and orientation to multisensory cues. In Gazzaniga M [ed]: The Cognitive Neurosciences. Cambridge, MA: MIT Press, 1995.)*

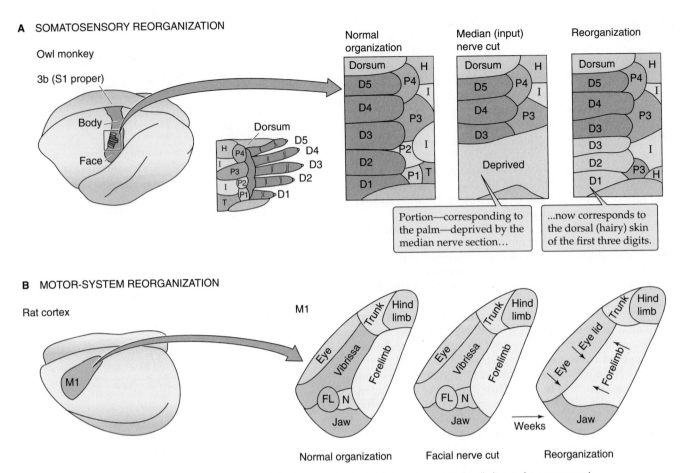

Figure 16-12 Plasticity of maps. **A,** The first panel, labeled "Normal organization," shows the somatotopic organization of the right hand in the left somatosensory cortex of the monkey brain. The colors correspond to different regions of the hand (viewed from the palm side, except for portions labeled "dorsum"). The second panel shows (in *gray*) the territory that is deprived of input by sectioning of the median nerve. The third panel shows that the cortical map is greatly changed several months after nerve section. The nerve was not allowed to regrow, but the previously deprived cortical region now responds to the dorsal skin of D3, D2, and D1. Notice that responses to regions P1, P2, and T have disappeared; region I has encroached; and regions H and P3 have suddenly appeared at a second location. *(Data from Kaas JH: The reorganization of sensory and motor maps in adult mammals. In Gazzaniga M [ed]: The Cognitive Neurosciences. Cambridge, MA: MIT Press, 1995.)* **B,** The first panel, labeled "Normal organization," shows the somatotopic organization of the left motor cortex (M1) of the rat brain. The colors correspond to the muscles that control different regions of the body. The second panel shows (in gray) the territory that normally provides motor output to the facial nerve, which has been severed. The third panel shows that after several weeks, the deprived cortical territory is now remapped. Notice that the deprived territory that once evoked whisker movements now evokes eye, eyelid, and forelimb movements. *(Data from Sanes J, Suner S, Donoghue JP: Dynamic organization of primary motor cortex output to target muscles in adult rats: Long-term patterns of reorganization following motor or mixed peripheral nerve lesions. Exp Brain Res 1990; 79:479-491.)*

a point in sensory space (e.g., a spot of light) activates a relatively large group of neurons in a sensory region of the brain. However, such activation of many neurons is not due to errors of connectivity; the spatial dissemination of activity is part of the mechanism used to encode and to process information. The *strength* of activation is most intense within the center of the activated neuronal group, but the population of more weakly activated neurons may encompass a large portion of an entire brain. This diversity in strength of activation means that a point in sensory space is unlikely to be encoded by the activity of a single neuron, but instead it is represented by the distributed activity in a large popula-

tion of neurons. Such a distributed code has computational advantages, and some redundancy also guards against errors, damage, and loss of information.

Finally, maps may change with time. All sensory and motor maps are clearly dynamic and can be reorganized rapidly and substantially as a function of development, behavioral state, training, or damage to the brain or periphery. Such changes are referred to as **plasticity.** Figure 16-12 illustrates two examples of dramatic changes in neocortical mapping, one sensory and one motor, after damage to peripheral nerves. In both cases, severing of a peripheral nerve causes the part of the map that normally relates to the body part served by this severed nerve to become remapped to another body part. Although the mechanisms of these reorganizations are not yet known, they probably reflect the same types of processes that underlie our ability to learn sensorimotor skills with practice and to adjust and improve after neural damage from trauma or stroke.

TEMPORAL REPRESENTATIONS: TIME-MEASURING CIRCUITS

To localize sound, the brain compares the timing and intensity of input to the ears

Neural circuits are very good at resolving time intervals, in some cases down to microseconds. One of the most demanding tasks of timing is performed by the auditory system as it localizes the source of certain sounds. Sound localization is an important skill, whether you are prey, predator, or pedestrian. Vertebrates use several different strategies for localization of sound, depending on the species, the frequency of the sound, and whether the task is to localize the source in the horizontal (left-right) or vertical (up-down) plane. In this subchapter, we briefly review general strategies of sound localization and then explain the mechanism by which a brainstem circuit measures the relative timing of low-frequency sounds so that the source of the sounds can be localized with precision.

Sound localization along the **vertical plane** (the degree of elevation) depends, in humans at least, on the distinctive shape of the external ear, the *pinna*. Much of the sound that we hear enters the auditory canal directly, and its energy is transferred to the cochlea. However, some sound reflects off the curves and folds of the pinna and tragus before it enters the canal and thus takes slightly longer to reach the cochlea. Notice what happens when the vertical direction of the sound changes. Because of the arcing shape of the pinna, the reflected path of sounds coming from above is shorter than that of sounds from below (Fig. 16-13). The two sets of sounds (the *direct* and, slightly delayed, the *reflected*) combine to create sounds that are slightly different on entering the auditory canal. Because of the interference patterns created by the direct and reflected sounds, the combined sound has spectral properties that are characteristic of the elevation of the sound source. This mechanism of vertical sound localization works well even with one ear at a time, although its precise neural mechanisms are not clear.

Accurate determination of the direction of a sound along the **horizontal plane** (the azimuth) necessitates two working ears. Sounds must first be processed by the cochlea in each ear and then compared by neurons within the CNS to estimate horizontal direction. But what exactly is compared? For sounds that are relatively high in frequency (~2 to 20 kHz), the important measure is the *interaural* (i.e., ear-to-ear) *intensity difference*. Stated simply, the ear facing the sound hears it louder than the ear facing away because the head casts a "sound shadow" (Fig. 16-14A). If the sound is directly to the right or left of the listener, this difference is maximal; if the sound is straight ahead, no difference is heard; and if the sound comes from an oblique direction, intensity differences are intermediate. Note that this system can be fooled.

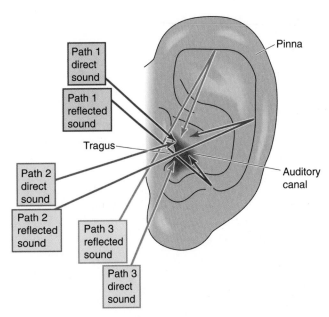

Figure 16-13 Detection of sound in the vertical plane. The detection of sound in the vertical plane requires only one ear. Regardless of the source of a sound, the sound reaches the auditory canal by both direct and reflected pathways. The brain localizes the source of the sound in the vertical plane by detecting differences in the combined sounds from the direct and reflected pathways.

A sound straight ahead gives the same intensity difference (i.e., none) as a sound directly behind.

The interaural intensity difference is not helpful at lower frequencies. Sounds below ~2 kHz have a wavelength that is longer than the width of the head itself. Longer sound waves are diffracted around the head, and differences in *interaural intensity* no longer occur. At low frequencies, the nervous system uses another strategy—it measures *interaural delay* (Fig. 16-14B). Consider a 200-Hz sound coming directly from the right. Its peak-to-peak distance (i.e., the wavelength) is ~172 cm, which is considerably more than the 20-cm width of the head. Each sound wave peak will reach the right ear ~0.6 ms before it reaches the left ear. If the sound comes from a 45-degree angle ahead, the interaural delay is ~0.3 ms; if it comes from straight ahead (or directly behind), the delay is 0 ms. Delays of small fractions of a millisecond are well within the capabilities of certain brainstem auditory neurons to detect. Sounds need not be continuous for the interaural delay to be detected. Sound onset or offset, clicks, or any abrupt changes in the sound give opportunities for interaural time comparisons. Obviously, measurement of interaural delay is subject to the same front-back ambiguity as interaural intensity, and indeed, it is sometimes difficult to distinguish whether a sound is in front of or behind your head.

The brain measures interaural timing by a combination of neural delay lines and coincidence detectors

How does the auditory system measure interaural timing? Surprisingly, to detect very small *time* differences, the nervous system uses a precise arrangement of neurons in

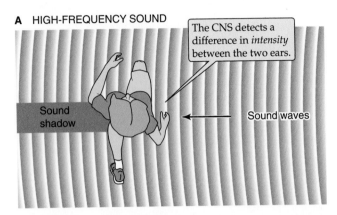

A HIGH-FREQUENCY SOUND

The CNS detects a difference in *intensity* between the two ears.

Sound shadow

Sound waves

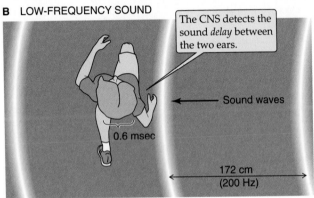

B LOW-FREQUENCY SOUND

The CNS detects the sound *delay* between the two ears.

Sound waves

0.6 msec

172 cm (200 Hz)

Figure 16-14 Sound detection in a horizontal plane. **A,** Two ears are necessary for the detection of sound in a horizontal plane. For frequencies between 2 kHz and 20 kHz, the CNS detects the ear-to-ear *intensity* difference. In this example, the sound comes from the right. The left ear hears a weaker sound because it is in the shadow of the head. **B,** For frequencies below 2 kHz, the CNS detects the ear-to-ear *delay*. In this example, the width of the head is 20 cm, and sound with a frequency of 200 Hz (wavelength of 172 cm) comes from the right. The peak of each sound wave reaches the left ear ~0.6 ms after it reaches the right.

space. Figure 16-15A summarizes the neuroanatomy of the first stages of central auditory processing within the brainstem. Notice that neurons in each of the cochlear nuclei receive information from only the ear on that one side, whereas neurons from the medial superior olivary (MSO) nucleus—and higher CNS centers—receive abundant input from both ears. Because horizontal sound localization requires input from both ears, we may guess that "direction-sensitive neurons" will probably be found somewhere central to the cochlear nuclei. When cochlear nucleus neurons are activated by auditory stimuli, their action potentials tend to fire with a particular phase relationship to the sound stimulus. For example, such a neuron might fire at the peak of every sound wave or at the peak of every fifth sound wave. That is, its firing is *phase locked* to the sound waves, at least for relatively low frequencies. Hence, cochlear neurons preserve the timing information of sound stimuli. Neurons in the MSO nucleus receive synaptic input from axons originating in both cochlear nuclei, so they are well placed to compare the timing (the phase) of sounds arriving at the two ears. Recordings from MSO neurons demonstrate that they

are exquisitely sensitive to interaural time delay, and the optimal delay for superior olivary neurons varies systematically across the nucleus. In other words, the MSO nucleus has a spatial map of *interaural delay*. The olive also has a systematic map of sound *frequency*, so it simultaneously maps two qualities of sound stimuli.

In the brains of birds, and perhaps also in mammals, the tuning of MSO neurons to interaural delay seems to depend on neural circuitry that combines "delay lines" with "coincidence detection," an idea first proposed by Jeffress in 1948. **Delay lines** are the axons from each cochlear nucleus; their length and conduction velocity determine how long it takes sound-activated action potentials to go from a cochlear nucleus to the axon's presynaptic terminals onto MSO neurons (Fig. 16-15B). Axons from both the right and left cochlear nuclei converge and synapse onto a series of neurons in the MSO nucleus. However, each axon (each delay line) may take a different time to conduct its action potential to the same olivary neuron. The difference in conduction delay between the axon from the right side and that from the left side determines the optimal interaural delay for that particular olivary neuron. It is the olivary neuron that acts as the **coincidence detector**: only when action potentials from *both* the left and right ear axons reach the postsynaptic olivary neuron simultaneously (meaning that sound has reached the two ears at a particular interaural delay) is that neuron likely to receive enough excitatory synaptic transmitter to trigger an action potential. If input from the two ears arrives at the neuron out of phase, without coincidence in time, the neuron will not fire. All these postsynaptic superior olivary neurons are fundamentally the same: they fire when there is coincidence between input from the left and right. However, because neurons arrayed across the olive are mapped so that the axons connecting them have different delays, they display coincidence for different interaural delays. Thus, each is **tuned** to a different interaural delay and a different sound locale along the horizontal axis. The orderly arrangement of delay lines across the olive determines each of the neurons' preferred delays (and thus sound location preferences) and leads to the orderly spatial mapping of sound direction.

The neural circuit we just described, which combines axonal delay lines and coincidence detection neurons, may not be the mechanism by which interaural timing is measured in mammalian brains. In the auditory system of gerbils, it appears that synaptic inhibition rather than delay lines generates the sensitivity of superior olivary neurons to interaural delay. It is possible that elements of both delay lines and inhibition are combined to optimize the measurement of timing in mammals.

Neural maps of sound localization are an interesting example of a sensory map that the brain must *compute*. This computed map contrasts with many other sensory maps that are derived more simply, such as by an orderly set of connections between the sensory receptor sheet (e.g., the retinal photoreceptors) and a central brain structure (e.g., the superior colliculus), as described in the preceding subchapter (Fig. 16-8). The cochlea does not have any map for sound location. Instead, the CNS localizes low-frequency sounds by calculating an interaural *time-delay* map, using information from both ears together. Other circuits can build a computed map of interaural *intensity differences*, which can be used for

A SOME MAJOR AUDITORY PATHWAYS

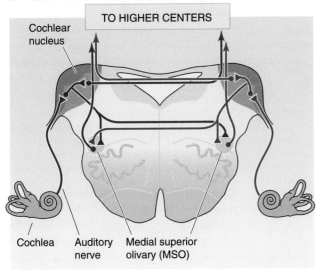

B CALCULATION OF INTERAURAL DELAY BY COINCIDENCE DETECTION

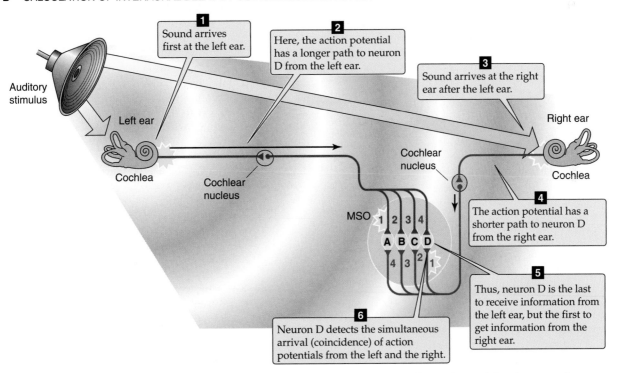

1 Sound arrives first at the left ear.

2 Here, the action potential has a longer path to neuron D from the left ear.

3 Sound arrives at the right ear after the left ear.

4 The action potential has a shorter path to neuron D from the right ear.

5 Thus, neuron D is the last to receive information from the left ear, but the first to get information from the right ear.

6 Neuron D detects the simultaneous arrival (coincidence) of action potentials from the left and the right.

Figure 16-15 CNS processing of sounds. **A,** The figure shows a cross section of the medulla. After a sound stimulus to the cochlea, the cochlear nerve carries an action potential to the cochlear nucleus, which receives information only from the ear on the same side. However, higher auditory centers receive input from both ears. **B,** Neurons in the MSO nucleus are each tuned to a different interaural delay. Only when action potentials from the right and left sides arrive at the MSO neuron simultaneously does the neuron fire an action potential (coincidence detection). In this example, the two action potentials are coincident at MSO neuron D because the brief acoustic delay to the left ear is followed by a long neuronal conduction delay, whereas the long acoustic delay to the right ear is followed by a brief neuronal conduction delay.

localization of high-frequency sounds (Fig. 16-14A). Once these two orderly sensory maps have been computed, they can be remapped onto another part of the brain by a simple system of orderly connections. For instance, the inferior colliculus receives parallel information on both timing delay and intensity difference; it transforms these two sets of information, combines them, and produces a complete map of sound direction. This combination of hierarchic (lower to high centers) and parallel information processing is probably ubiquitous in the CNS and is a general strategy for the analysis of much more complex sensory problems than those described here.

REFERENCES

Books and Reviews

Bear MF, Connors BW, Paradiso MA: Neuroscience: Exploring the Brain, 2nd ed. Baltimore: Lippincott Williams & Wilkins, 2001.

Chklovskii DB, Koulakov AA: Maps in the brain: What can we learn from them? Annu Rev Neurosci 2004; 27:369-392.

Konishi M: Coding of auditory space. Annu Rev Neurosci 2003; 26:31-55.

Palmer AR: Reassessing mechanisms of low-frequency sound localisation. Curr Opin Neurobiol 2004; 14:457-460.

Poppele R, Bosco G: Sophisticated spinal contributions to motor control. Trends Neurosci 2003; 26:269-276.

Sanes JN, Donoghue JP: Plasticity and primary motor cortex. Annu Rev Neurosci 2000; 23:393-415.

Journal Articles

Brand A, Behrend O, Marquardt T, et al: Precise inhibition is essential for microsecond interaural time difference coding. Nature 2002; 417:543-547.

Carr CE, Konishi M: A circuit for detection of interaural time differences in the brainstem of the barn owl. J Neurosci 1990; 10:3227-3246.

Delcomyn F: Neural basis of rhythmic behavior in animals. Science 1980; 210:492-498.

Lacquaniti F, Borghese NA, Carrozzo M: Transient reversal of the stretch reflex in human arm muscles. J Neurophysiol 1991; 49:16-27.

Sanes J, Suner S, Donoghue JP: Dynamic organization of primary motor cortex output to target muscles in adult rats. I. Long-term patterns of reorganization following motor or mixed peripheral nerve lesions. Exp Brain Res 1990; 79:479-491.

THE CARDIOVASCULAR SYSTEM

CHAPTER 17

ORGANIZATION OF THE CARDIOVASCULAR SYSTEM

Emile L. Boulpaep

ELEMENTS OF THE CARDIOVASCULAR SYSTEM

The circulation is an evolutionary consequence of body size

Isolated single cells and small organisms do not have a circulatory system. They can meet their metabolic needs by the simple processes of diffusion and convection of solutes from the *external* to the *internal milieu* (Fig. 17-1A). The requirement for a circulatory system is an evolutionary consequence of the increasing size and complexity of multicellular organisms. Simple diffusion (see Chapter 5) is not adequate to supply nutrients to centrally located cells or to eliminate waste products; in large organisms, the distances separating the central cells from the *external milieu* are too long. A simple closed-end tube (Fig. 17-1B), penetrating from the extracellular compartment and feeding a central cell deep in the core of the organism, would not be sufficient. The concentration of nutrients inside the tube would become very low at its closed end because of both the uptake of these nutrients by the cell and the long path for re-supply leading to the cell. Conversely, the concentration of waste products inside the tube would become very high at the closed end. Such a tube represents a long **unstirred layer**; as a result, the concentration gradients for both nutrients and wastes across the membrane of the central cell are very small.

In complex organisms, a circulatory system provides a steep concentration gradient from the blood to the central cells for nutrients and in the opposite direction for waste products. Maintenance of such steep intracellular-to-extracellular concentration gradients requires a fast convection system that rapidly circulates fluid between surfaces that equilibrate with the *external milieu* (e.g., the lung, gut, and kidney epithelia) and individual central cells deep inside the organism (Fig. 17-1C). In mammals and birds, the exchange of gases with the external milieu is so important that they have evolved a two-pump, dual circulatory system (Fig. 17-1D) that delivers the full output of the "heart" to the lungs (see Chapter 31).

The primary role of the **circulatory system** is the distribution of dissolved gases and other molecules for nutrition, growth, and repair. Secondary roles have also evolved: (1) fast chemical signaling to cells by means of circulating hormones or neurotransmitters, (2) dissipation of heat by delivery of heat from the core to the surface of the body, and (3) mediation of inflammatory and host defense responses against invading microorganisms.

The circulatory system of humans integrates three basic functional parts, or organs: a pump (the **heart**) that circulates a liquid (the **blood**) through a set of containers (the **vessels**). This integrated system is able to adapt to the changing circumstances of normal life. Demand on the circulation fluctuates widely between sleep and wakefulness, between rest and exercise, with acceleration/deceleration, during changes in body position or intrathoracic pressure, during digestion, and under emotional or thermal stress. To meet these variable demands, the entire system requires sophisticated and integrated regulation.

The heart is a dual pump that drives the blood in two serial circuits: the systemic and the pulmonary circulations

A remarkable pump, weighing ~300 g, drives the human circulation. The heart really consists of two pumps, the **left-sided heart**, or main pump, and the **right-sided heart**, or boost pump (Fig. 17-1D). These operate in series and require a delicate equalization of their outputs. The output of each pump is ~5 L/min, but this can easily increase 5-fold during exercise.

During a 75-year lifetime, the two ventricles combined pump 400 million liters of blood (enough to fill a lake 1 km long, 40 m wide, and 10 m deep). The circulating fluid itself is an organ, kept in a liquid state by mechanisms that actively prevent cell-cell adhesion and coagulation. With each heartbeat, the ventricles impart the energy necessary to circulate the blood by generating the pressure head that drives the flow of blood through the **vascular system**. On the basis of its anatomy, we can divide this system of tubes into two main circuits: the **systemic** and the **pulmonary** circulations (Fig. 17-1D). We could also divide the vascular system into a high-pressure part (extending from the contracting left ventricle to the systemic capillaries) and a **low-pressure** part

A UNICELLULAR ORGANISM

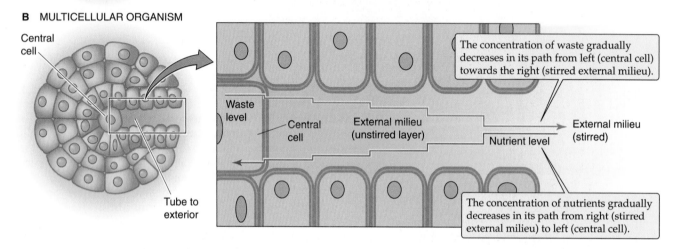

B MULTICELLULAR ORGANISM

C CIRCULATION WITH ONE PUMP

D CIRCULATION WITH TWO PUMPS / TWO CIRCUITS

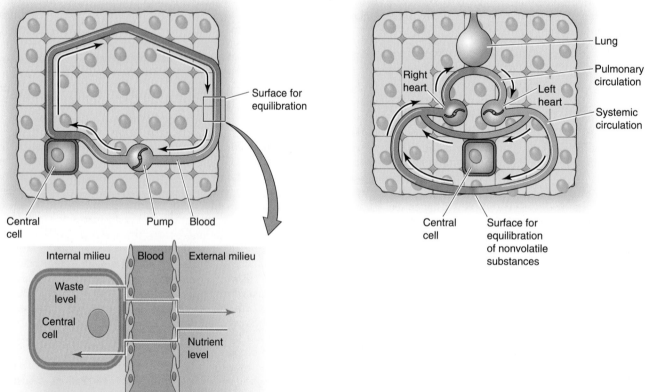

Figure 17-1 Role of the circulatory system in promoting diffusion. In **C,** nutrients and wastes exchange across two barriers: a surface for equilibration between the external milieu and blood, and another surface between blood and the central cell. **Inset,** Blood is the conduit that connects the external milieu (e.g., lumina of lung, gut, and kidney) to the internal milieu (i.e., extracellular fluid bathing central cells). In **D,** the system is far more efficient, using one circuit for exchange of gases with the external milieu and another circuit for exchange of nutrients and nongaseous wastes.

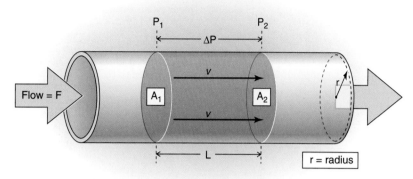

Figure 17-2 Flow through a straight tube. The flow (*F*) between a high-pressure point (*P*₁) and a low-pressure point (*P*₂) is proportional to pressure difference (*ΔP*). *A*₁ and *A*₂ are cross-sectional areas at these two points. A cylindrical bolus of fluid—between the disks at points 1 and 2—moves down the tube with a linear velocity *v*.

(extending from the systemic capillaries, through the right side of the heart, across the pulmonary circulation and left atrium, and into the left ventricle in its relaxed state). The vessels also respond to the changing metabolic demands of the tissues they supply by directing blood flow to (or away from) tissues as demands change. The circulatory system is also self-repairing/self-expanding. Endothelial cells lining vessels mend the surfaces of existing blood vessels and generate new vessels (**angiogenesis**).

Some of the most important life-threatening human diseases are caused by failure of the heart as a pump (e.g., congestive heart failure), failure of the blood as an effective liquid organ (e.g., thrombosis and embolism), or failure of the vasculature either as a competent container (e.g., hemorrhage) or as an efficient distribution system (e.g., atherosclerosis). Moreover, failure of the normal interactions among these three organs can by itself elicit or aggravate many human pathological processes.

HEMODYNAMICS

Blood flow is driven by a constant pressure head across variable resistances

To keep concepts simple, first think of the left side of the heart as a constant pressure generator that maintains a steady mean arterial pressure at its exit (i.e., the aorta). In other words, assume that blood flow throughout the circulation is steady or nonpulsatile (later in the chapter, see discussion of the consequences of normal cyclic variations in flow and pressure that occur as the result of the heartbeat). As a further simplification, assume that the entire systemic circulation is a single, straight tube.

To understand the *steady flow* of blood, driven by a *constant pressure* head, we can apply classical hydrodynamic laws. The most important law is analogous to Ohm's law of electricity:

$$\Delta V = I \cdot R \quad \text{for electricity}$$
$$\Delta P = F \cdot R \quad \text{for liquids} \tag{17-1}$$

That is, the pressure difference (*ΔP*) between an upstream point (pressure *P*₁) and a downstream site (pressure *P*₂) is equal to the product of the flow (*F*) and the resistance (*R*)

between those two points (Fig. 17-2). Ohm's law of hydrodynamics holds at any instant in time, regardless of how simple or how complicated the circuit. This equation also does not require any assumptions about whether the vessels are rigid or compliant, as long as *R* is constant.

In reality, the **pressure difference** (*ΔP*) between the beginning and end points of the human systemic circulation—that is, between the high-pressure side (aorta) and the low-pressure side (vena cava)—turns out to be fairly constant over time. Thus, the heart behaves more like a generator of a constant pressure head than a generator of constant flow, at least within physiological limits. Indeed, **flow** (*F*), the output of the left side of the heart, is quite variable in time and depends greatly on the physiological circumstances (e.g., whether one is active or at rest). Like flow, **resistance** (*R*) varies with time; in addition, it varies with location within the body. The overall resistance of the circulation reflects the contributions of a complex network of vessels in both the systemic and pulmonary circuits.

Blood can take many different pathways *from the left side of the heart to the right side of the heart* (Fig. 17-3): (1) a single capillary bed (e.g., coronary capillaries), (2) two capillary beds in series (e.g., glomerular and peritubular capillaries in the kidney), or (3) two capillary beds in parallel that subsequently merge and feed into a single capillary bed in series (e.g., the parallel splenic and mesenteric circulations, which merge on entering the portal hepatic circulation). In contrast, blood flow *from the right side of the heart to the left side of the heart* can take only a single pathway, across a single capillary bed in the pulmonary circulation. Finally, some blood also courses *from the left side of the heart directly back to the left side of the heart* across shunt pathways, the most important of which is the bronchial circulation.

The overall resistance (*R*ₜₒₜₐₗ) across a circulatory bed results from parallel and serial arrangements of branches and is governed by laws similar to those for the electrical resistance of DC circuits. For multiple resistance elements (*R*₁, *R*₂, *R*₃, . . .) arranged in series:

$$R_{\text{total}} = R_1 + R_2 + R_3 + \ldots \tag{17-2}$$

For multiple elements arranged in parallel:

$$\frac{1}{R_{\text{total}}} = \frac{1}{R_1} + \frac{1}{R_2} + \frac{1}{R_3} + \ldots \tag{17-3}$$

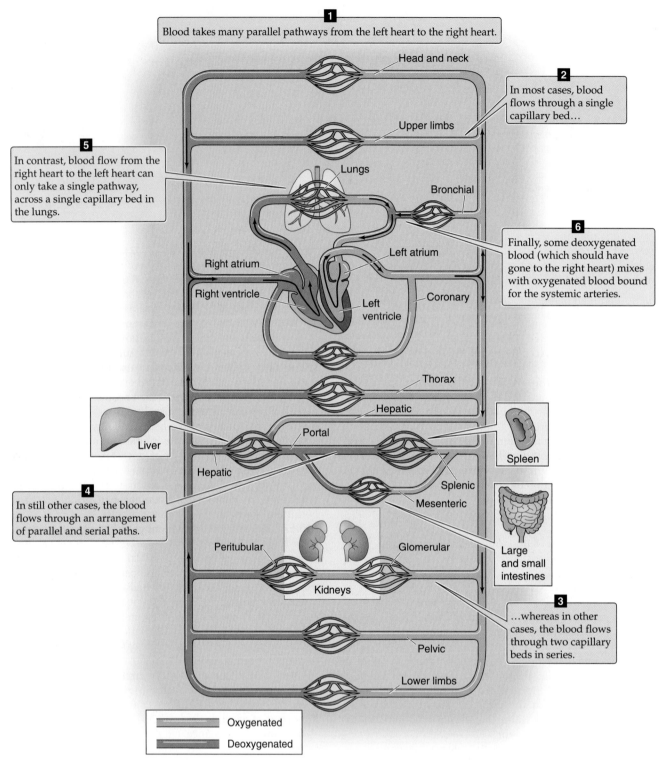

Figure 17-3 Circulatory beds.

Blood pressure is always measured as a pressure difference between two points

Physicists measure pressure in the units of pascals, g/cm², or dynes/cm². However, physiologists most often gauge blood pressure by the height it can drive a column of liquid. This pressure is

$$P = \rho g h \qquad (17\text{-}4)$$

where ρ is the density of the liquid in the column, g is the gravitational constant, and h is the height of the column. Therefore, if we neglect variations in g and know ρ for the fluid in the column (usually water or mercury), we can take

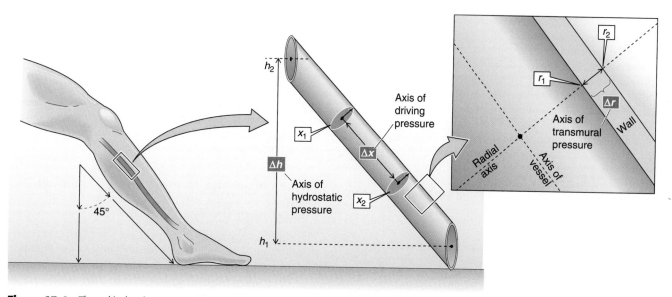

Figure 17-4 Three kinds of pressure differences, and their axes, in a blood vessel.

the height of the liquid column as a measure of blood pressure. Physiologists usually express this pressure in millimeters of mercury (mm Hg) or centimeters of water (cm H_2O). Clinicians use the classical blood pressure gauge (sphygmomanometer) to report arterial blood pressure in millimeters of mercury.

Pressure is never expressed in absolute terms but as a **pressure difference** ΔP relative to some "reference" pressure. We can make this concept intuitively clear by considering pressure as a force F applied to a surface area A.

$$P = F/A \qquad (17\text{-}5)$$

If we apply a force to one side of a free-swinging door, we cannot predict the direction the door will move unless we know what force a colleague may be applying on the opposite side. In other words, we can define a movement or distortion of a mechanical system only by the *difference* between two forces. In electricity, we compare the difference between two voltages. In hemodynamics, we compare the difference between two pressures. When it is not explicitly stated, the reference pressure in human physiology is the atmospheric or barometric pressure (P_B). Because P_B on earth is never zero, a pressure reading obtained at some site within the circulation, and referred to P_B, actually does not express the absolute pressure in that blood vessel but rather the difference between the pressure inside the vessel and P_B.

Because a pressure difference is always between two points—and these two points are separated by some distance (Δx) and have a spatial orientation to one another—we can define a pressure gradient ($\Delta P/\Delta x$) with a spatial orientation. Considering orientation, we can define three different kinds of pressure differences in the circulation:

1. **Driving pressure.** In Figure 17-4, the ΔP between points x_1 and x_2 inside the vessel—along the axis of the vessel—is the axial pressure difference. Because this ΔP causes blood to flow from x_1 to x_2, it is also known as the driving pres-

sure. In the circulation, the driving pressure is the ΔP between the arterial and venous ends of the systemic (or pulmonary) circulation, and it governs blood flow. Indeed, this is the only ΔP we need to consider to understand flow in horizontal rigid tubes (Fig. 17-2).

2. **Transmural pressure.** The ΔP in Figure 17-4 between point r_1 (inside the vessel) and r_2 (just outside the vessel)—along the radial axis—is an example of a radial pressure difference. Although there is normally no pressure difference through the blood along the radial axis, the pressure drops steeply across the vessel wall itself. The ΔP between r_1 and r_2 is the transmural pressure, that is, the difference between the intravascular pressure and the tissue pressure. Because blood vessels are distensible, transmural pressure governs vessel diameter, which is in turn the major determinant of resistance.

3. **Hydrostatic pressure.** Because of the density of blood and gravitational forces, a third pressure difference arises if the vessel does not lie in a horizontal plane, as was the case in Figure 17-2. The ΔP in Figure 17-4 between point h_1 (bottom of a liquid column) and h_2 (top of column)—along the height axis—is the hydrostatic pressure difference $P_1 - P_2$. This ΔP is similar to the P in Equation 17-4 (here, ρ is the density of blood), and it exists even in the absence of any blood flow. If we express increasing altitude in positive units of h, then hydrostatic $\Delta P = -\rho g(h_1 - h_2)$.

Total blood flow, or cardiac output, is the product (heart rate) × (stroke volume)

The flow of blood delivered by the heart, or the total mean flow in the circulation, is the **cardiac output** (CO). The output during a single heartbeat, from either the left or the right ventricle, is the stroke volume (SV). For a given **heart rate** (HR):

$$CO = F = HR \cdot SV \qquad (17\text{-}6)$$

The cardiac output is usually expressed in liters per minute; at rest, it is about 5 L/min in a 70-kg human. Cardiac output depends on body size and is best normalized to body surface area. The cardiac index (L/min/m²) is the cardiac output per square meter of body surface area. The normal adult cardiac index at rest is about 3.0 L/min/m².

The principle of continuity of flow is the principle of conservation of mass applied to flowing fluids. It requires that the volume entering the systemic or pulmonary circuit per unit time be equal to the volume leaving the circuit per unit time, assuming that no fluid has been added or subtracted in either circuit. Therefore, the flow of the right and left sides of the heart (i.e., right and left cardiac outputs) must be equal in the steady state.

Flow in an idealized vessel increases with the fourth power of radius (Poiseuille's equation)

Flow (F) is the displacement of volume (ΔV) per unit time (Δt):

$$F = \frac{\Delta V}{\Delta t} \qquad (17\text{-}7)$$

In Figure 17-2, we could be watching a bolus (the blue cylinder)—with an area A and a length L—move along the tube with a mean velocity $\bar{v}$. During a time interval Δt, the cylinder advances by Δx, so that the volume passing some checkpoint (e.g., at P_2) is ($A \cdot \Delta x$). Thus,

$$F = \frac{\overbrace{\frac{\Delta V}{\Delta t}}^{}}{\underbrace{A \cdot \Delta x}} = A \cdot \frac{\overbrace{\Delta x}^{\bar{v}}}{\Delta t} = A \cdot \bar{v} \qquad (17\text{-}8)$$

This equation holds at any point along the circulation, regardless of how complicated the circulation is or how irregular the cross-sectional area.

In a physically well defined system, it is also possible to *predict* the flow from the geometry of the vessel and the properties of the fluid. In 1840 and 1841, Jean Poiseuille observed the flow of liquids in tubes of small diameter and derived the law associated with his name. In a straight, rigid, cylindrical tube:

$$F = \Delta P \cdot \underbrace{\frac{\pi r^4}{8\eta l}}_{1/R} \qquad (17\text{-}9)$$

This is the Poiseuille-Hagen equation, where F is the flow, ΔP is the driving pressure, r is the inner radius of the tube, l is its length, and η is the viscosity. The Poiseuille equation requires that both driving pressure and the resulting flow be constant.

Three implications of Poiseuille's law are as follows:

1. Flow is directly proportional to the axial pressure difference, ΔP. The proportionality constant—(πr^4)/ ($8\eta l$)—is the reciprocal of resistance (R), as is presented later.

2. Flow is directly proportional to the fourth power of vessel radius.
3. Flow is inversely proportional to both the length of the vessel and the viscosity of the fluid.

Unlike Ohm's law of hydrodynamics ($F = \Delta P/R$), which applies to *all* vessels, no matter how complicated, Poiseuille's equation applies only to rigid, cylindrical tubes. Moreover, later discussion in this chapter reveals that the fluid flowing through the tube must satisfy certain conditions.

Viscous resistance to flow is proportional to the viscosity of blood but does not depend on properties of the blood vessel walls

The simplest approach for expressing vascular resistance is to rearrange Ohm's law of hydrodynamics (see Equation 17-1):

$$R = \frac{\Delta P}{F} \qquad (17\text{-}10)$$

This approach is independent of geometry and is even applicable to very complex circuits, such as the entire peripheral circulation. Moreover, we can conveniently express resistance in units used by physicians for pressure (mm Hg) and flow (mL/s). Thus, the units of total peripheral resistance are mm Hg/(mL/s)—also known as **peripheral resistance units (PRUs)**.

Alternatively, if the flow through the tube fulfills Poiseuille's requirements, we can express "viscous" resistance in terms of the dimensions of the vessel and the *viscous* properties of the circulating fluid. Combining Equation 17-9 and Equation 17-10:

$$R = \frac{8}{\pi} \cdot \frac{\eta l}{r^4} \qquad (17\text{-}11)$$

Thus, *viscous* resistance is proportional to the *viscosity* of the fluid and the length of the tube but inversely proportional to the fourth power of the radius of the blood vessel. Note that this equation makes no statement regarding the properties of the vessel wall per se. The resistance to flow results from the geometry of the fluid—as described by l and r—and the internal friction of the fluid, the **viscosity** (η). Viscosity is a property of the content (i.e., the fluid), unrelated to any property of the container (i.e., the vessel).

The viscosity of blood is a measure of the internal slipperiness between layers of fluid

Viscosity is an expression of the degree of slipperiness between two layers of fluid. Isaac Newton described the interaction as illustrated in Figure 17-5A. Imagine that two parallel planes of fluid, each with an area A, are moving past one another. The velocity of the first is v, and the velocity of the slightly faster moving second plane is $\bar{v} + \Delta v$. The difference in velocity between the moving planes is Δv, and the separation between the two planes is Δx. Thus, the *velocity gradient* in a direction perpendicular to the plane of shear, $\Delta v/\Delta x$ [units: (cm/s)/cm = s⁻¹], is the **shear rate**. The addi-

A DEFINITION OF VISCOSITY

B VISCOUS FLOW IN A CYLINDER

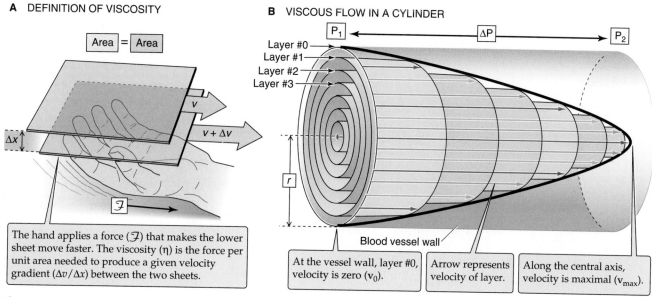

The hand applies a force ($\mathcal{F}$) that makes the lower sheet move faster. The viscosity (η) is the force per unit area needed to produce a given velocity gradient ($\Delta v/\Delta x$) between the two sheets.

At the vessel wall, layer #0, velocity is zero (v_0).

Arrow represents velocity of layer.

Along the central axis, velocity is maximal (v_{max}).

Figure 17-5 Viscosity.

tional *force* that we must apply to the second sheet to make it move faster than the first is the **shear stress**. The greater the area of the sheets, the greater is the force needed to overcome the friction between them. Thus, shear stress is expressed as force per unit area (*F/A*). The *shear stress* required to produce a particular *shear rate* Newton defined as the viscosity:

$$\eta = \frac{\text{shear stress}}{\text{shear rate}} = \frac{F/A}{\Delta v/\Delta x} \qquad (17\text{-}12)$$

Viscosity measures the resistance to sliding when layers of fluid are shearing against each other. The unit of viscosity is a **poise** (P). Whole blood has a viscosity of ~3 centipoise (cP).

If one applies Newton's definition of viscosity to a cylindrical blood vessel, the shearing laminae of the blood are not planar but concentric cylinders (Fig. 17-5B). If we apply a pressure head to the blood in the vessel, each lamina will move parallel to the long axis of the tube. Because of cohesive forces between the inner surface of the vessel wall and the blood, we can assume that an infinitesimally thin layer of blood (Fig. 17-5B, layer 0) close to the wall of the tube cannot move. However, the next concentric cylindrical layer, layer 1, moves in relation to the stationary outer layer 0 but slower than the next inner concentric cylinder, layer 2, and so on. Thus, the velocities increase from the wall to the center of the cylinder. The resulting velocity profile is a parabola with a maximum velocity, v_{max}, at the central axis. The lower the viscosity, the sharper the point of the bullet-shaped velocity profile.

HOW BLOOD FLOWS

As discussed, Poiseuille's relationship (Equation 17-9) is based on solid empirical and theoretical grounds. However, the equation requires the following assumptions:

1. The fluid must be incompressible.
2. The tube must be straight, rigid, cylindrical, and unbranched and have a constant radius.
3. The velocity of the thin fluid layer at the wall must be zero (i.e., no "slippage"). This assumption holds for aqueous solutions but not for some "plastic" fluids.
4. The flow must be laminar. That is, the fluid must move in concentric undisturbed laminae, without the gross exchange of fluid from one concentric shell to another.
5. The flow must be steady (i.e., not pulsatile).
6. The viscosity of the fluid must be constant. First, it must be constant throughout the cross section of the cylinder. Second, it must be constant in the "newtonian" sense; that is, the viscosity must be independent of the magnitude of the shear stress (i.e., force applied) and the shear rate (i.e., velocity gradient produced). In other words, the shear stress at each point is linearly proportional to its shear rate at that point.

To what extent does the circulatory system fulfill the conditions of Poiseuille's equation? The first condition (i.e., incompressible fluid) is well satisfied by blood. If we consider only flow in a vessel segment that is of fairly fixed size (e.g., thoracic aorta), the second assumption (i.e., simple geometry) is also reasonably satisfied. The third requirement (i.e., no slippage) is true for blood in blood vessels. Indeed, if one forms a reservoir out of a piece of vessel (e.g., aorta) and fills it with blood, a meniscus forms with the concave surface facing upward, indicating adherence of blood to the vessel wall.

The fourth and fifth assumptions, which are more complex, are the subject of the next two sections. With regard to the sixth assumption, Chapter 18 addresses the anomalous viscosity of blood.

Blood flow is laminar

From Ohm's law of hydrodynamics ($\Delta P = F \cdot R$), flow should increase linearly with driving pressure if resistance is con-

A PRESSURE-FLOW RELATIONSHIP

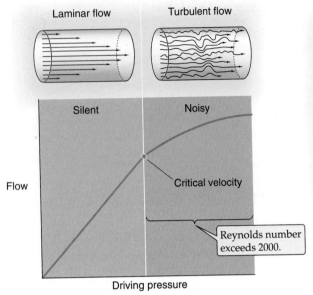

B VELOCITY PROFILES

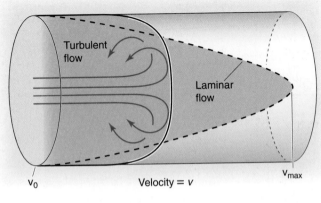

Figure 17-6 Laminar versus turbulent flow.

stant. In cylindrical vessels, flow does indeed increase linearly with ΔP *up to a certain point* (Fig. 17-6A). However, at high flow rates—beyond a critical velocity—flow rises less steeply and is no longer proportional to ΔP but to roughly the square root of ΔP, because R apparently increases. Here, blood flow is no longer laminar but **turbulent**. Because turbulence causes substantial kinetic energy losses, it is energetically wasteful.

The critical parameter that determines when flow becomes turbulent is a dimensionless quantity called **Reynolds number** (*Re*), named after Osborne Reynolds:

$$Re = \frac{2r\bar{v}\rho}{\eta} \qquad (17\text{-}13)$$

Blood flow is laminar when *Re* is below ~2000 and is mostly turbulent when *Re* exceeds ~3000. The terms in the numerator reflect disruptive forces produced by the *inertial momentum* in the fluid. Thus, turbulent blood flow occurs where *r* is large (e.g., aorta) or when $\bar{v}$ is large (e.g., high cardiac output). Turbulent flow can also occur when a local decrease in vessel diameter (e.g., arterial stenosis) causes a local increase in $\bar{v}$. The term in the denominator of Equation 17-13, viscosity, reflects the cohesive forces that tend to keep the layers well organized. Therefore, a low viscosity (e.g., anemia—a low red blood cell count) predisposes to turbulence. When turbulence arises, the parabolic profile of the linear velocity across the radius of a cylinder becomes blunted (Fig. 17-6B).

The distinction between laminar and turbulent flow is clinically very significant. Laminar flow is silent, whereas vortex formation during turbulence sets up **murmurs**. These Korotkoff sounds are useful in assessing arterial blood flow in the traditional auscultatory method for determination of blood pressure. These murmurs are also important for diagnosis of vessel stenosis, vessel shunts, and cardiac valvular

lesions (see the box titled Heart Murmurs and Arterial Bruits). Intense forms of turbulence may be detected not only as loud acoustic murmurs but also as mechanical vibrations or **thrills** that can be felt by touch.

Heart Murmurs and Arterial Bruits

Turbulence as blood flows across diseased heart valves creates murmurs that can be readily detected by auscultation with a stethoscope. The factors causing turbulence are the ones that increase Reynolds number: increases in vessel diameter or blood velocity and decreases in viscosity. Before the advent of sophisticated technology, such as cardiac ultrasonography, clinicians made a fine art of detecting these murmurs in an attempt to diagnose cardiac valvular disease. In general, it was appreciated that normal blood flow across normal heart valves is silent, although murmurs can occur with increased blood flow (e.g., exercise) and are not infrequently heard in young, thin individuals with dynamic circulations. The grading of heart murmurs helps standardize the cardiac examination from observer to observer. Thus, a grade 1 heart murmur is barely audible, grade 2 is one that is slightly more easily heard, and grades 3 and 4 are progressively louder. A grade 5 murmur is the loudest murmur that still requires a stethoscope to be heard. A grade 6 murmur is so loud that it can be heard with the stethoscope off the chest and is often accompanied by a thrill. The location, duration, pitch, and quality of a murmur aid in identifying the underlying valvular disorder.

Blood flowing through diseased arteries can also create a murmur or a thrill. By far the most common cause is atherosclerosis, which narrows the vessel lumen and thus increases velocity. In patients with advanced disease, these murmurs can be heard in virtually every major artery, most easily in the carotid and femoral arteries. Arterial murmurs are usually referred to as bruits.

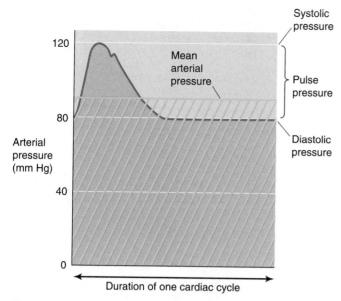

Figure 17-7 Time course of arterial pressure during one cardiac cycle. The area beneath the *blue pressure curve*, divided by the time of one cardiac cycle, is mean arterial pressure (*horizontal yellow line*). The *yellow cross-hatched area* is the same as the blue area.

Pressure and flow oscillate with each heartbeat between maximum systolic and minimum diastolic values

Thus far we have considered blood flow to be steady and driven by a constant pressure generator. That is, we have been working with a *mean* blood flow and a *mean* driving pressure (the difference between the mean arterial and venous pressures). However, we are all aware that the heart is a pump of the "two-stroke" variety, with a filling and an emptying phase. Because both the left and right sides of the heart perform their work in a cyclic fashion, flow is pulsatile in both the systemic and pulmonary circulations.

The mean blood pressure in the large systemic arteries is ~95 mm Hg. This is a single, time-averaged value. In reality, the blood pressure cycles between a maximal **systolic** arterial pressure (~120 mm Hg) that corresponds to the contraction of the ventricle and a minimal **diastolic** arterial pressure (~80 mm Hg) that corresponds to the relaxation of the ventricle (Fig. 17-7). The difference between the systolic pressure and the diastolic pressure is **pulse pressure**. Note that the mean arterial pressure is not the arithmetic mean of systolic and diastolic values, which would be (120 + 80)/2 = 100 mm Hg in our example; rather, it is the area beneath the curve, which describes the pressure in a single cardiac cycle (Fig. 17-7, blue area) divided by the duration of the cycle. A reasonable value for the mean arterial pressure is 95 mm Hg.

Like arterial pressure, flow through arteries also oscillates with each heartbeat. Because both pressure and flow are pulsatile, and because the pressure and flow waves are not perfectly matched in time, we cannot describe the relationship between these two parameters by a simple Ohm's law–like relationship ($\Delta P = F \cdot R$), which is analogous to a simple DC circuit in electricity. Rather, if we were to model pressure and flow in the circulatory system, we would have to use a more complicated approach, analogous to that used to understand AC electrical circuits.

ORIGINS OF PRESSURE IN THE CIRCULATION

Four factors help generate pressure in the circulation: gravity, compliance of the vessels, viscous resistance, and inertia.

Gravity causes a hydrostatic pressure difference when there is a difference in height

Because gravity produces a hydrostatic pressure difference between two points whenever there is a *difference in height* (Δh; Equation 17-4), one must always express pressures relative to some reference *h* level. In cardiovascular physiology, this reference—zero height—is the level of the heart.

Whether the body is recumbent (i.e., horizontal) or upright (i.e., erect) has a tremendous effect on the intravascular pressure. In the horizontal position (Fig. 17-8A), where we assume that the entire body is at the level of the heart, we do not need to add a hydrostatic pressure component to the various intravascular pressures. Thus, the mean pressure in the aorta is 95 mm Hg, and—because it takes a driving pressure of ~5 mm Hg to pump blood into the end of the large arteries—the mean pressure at the end of the large arteries in the foot and head is 90 mm Hg. Similarly, the mean pressure in the large veins draining the foot and head is 5 mm Hg, and—because it takes a driving pressure of ~3 mm Hg to pump blood to the right atrium—the mean pressure in the right atrium is 2 mm Hg.

When a 180-cm tall person is standing (Fig. 17-8B), we must *add* a 130-cm column of blood (the Δh between the heart and large vessels in the foot) to the pressure prevailing in the large arteries and veins of the foot. Because a water column of 130 cm is equivalent to 95 mm Hg, the mean pressure for a large artery in the foot will be 90 + 95 = 185 mm Hg, and the mean pressure for a large vein in the foot will be 5 + 95 = 100 mm Hg. On the other hand, we must *subtract* a 50-cm column of blood from the pressure prevailing in the head. Because a water column of 50 cm is equivalent to 37 mm Hg, the mean pressure for a large artery in the head will be 90 − 37 = 53 mm Hg, and the mean pressure for a large vein in the head will be 5 − 37 = −32 mm Hg. Of course, this "negative" value really means that the pressure in a large vein in the head is 32 mm Hg lower than the reference pressure at the level of the heart.

In this example, we have simplified things somewhat by ignoring the valves that interrupt the blood column. In reality, the veins of the limbs have a series of one-way valves that allow blood to flow only toward the heart. These valves act like a series of relay stations, so that the contraction of skeletal muscle around the veins pushes blood from one valve to another (see Chapter 22). Thus, veins in the foot do not "see" the full hydrostatic column of 95 mm Hg when the leg muscles pump blood away from the foot veins.

Although the absolute arterial and venous pressures are much higher in the foot than in the head, the ΔP that *drives* blood flow is the same in the vascular beds of the foot and

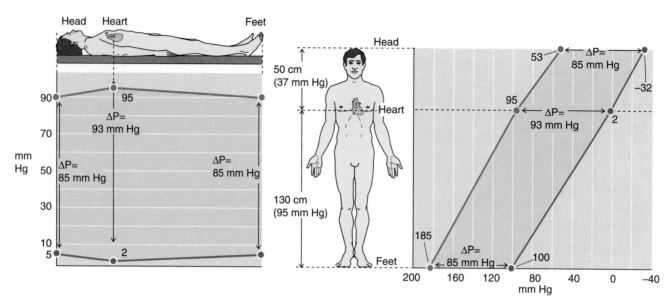

Figure 17-8 Arterial and venous pressures in the horizontal and upright positions. The pressures are different between **A** and **B,** but the driving pressures (ΔP) between arteries and veins (*separation between red and blue lines, violet background*) are the same.

head. Thus, in the horizontal position, the ΔP across the vascular beds in the foot or head is 90 − 5 = 85 mm Hg. In the upright position, the ΔP for the foot is 185 − 100 = 85 mm Hg, and for the head, 53 − (−32) = 85 mm Hg. Thus, gravity does not affect the driving pressure that governs flow. On the other hand, in "dependent" areas of the body (i.e., vessels "below" the heart in a gravitational sense), the hydrostatic pressure does tend to increase the *transmural* pressure (intravascular versus extravascular "tissue" pressure) and thus the diameter of distensible vessels. Because various anatomical barriers separate different tissue compartments, it is assumed that gravity does not appreciably affect this tissue pressure.

Low compliance of a vessel causes the transmural pressure to increase when the vessel blood volume is increased

Until now, we have considered blood vessels to be rigid tubes, which, by definition, have fixed volumes. If we were to try to inject a volume of fluid into a truly rigid tube with closed ends, we could in principle increase the pressure to infinity without increasing the volume of the tube (Fig. 17-9A). At the other extreme, if the wall of the tube were to offer no resistance to deformation (i.e., infinite compliance), we could inject an infinite volume of fluid without increasing the pressure at all (Fig. 17-9B). Blood vessels lie between these two extremes; they are distensible but have a finite compliance (see Chapter 19). Thus, if we were to inject a volume of blood into the vessel, the volume of the vessel would increase by the same amount (ΔV), and the intravascular pressure would also increase (Fig. 17-9C). The ΔP accompanying a given ΔV is greater if the compliance of the

vessel is lower. The relationship between ΔP and ΔV is a *static* property of the vessel wall and holds whether or not there is flow in the vessel. Thus, if we were to infuse blood into a patient's blood vessels, the intravascular pressure would rise throughout the circulation, even if the heart were stopped.

The viscous resistance of blood causes an axial pressure difference when there is flow

As we saw in Ohm's law of hydrodynamics (see Equation 17-1), during steady flow down the axis of a tube (Fig. 17-2), the driving pressure (ΔP) is proportional to both flow and resistance. Viewed differently, if we want to achieve a constant flow, then the greater the resistance, the greater the ΔP that we must apply along the axis of flow. Of the four sources of pressure in the circulatory system, this ΔP due to viscous resistance is the only one that appears in Poiseuille's law (see Equation 17-9).

The inertia of the blood and vessels causes pressure to decrease when the velocity of blood flow increases

For the most part, we have been assuming that the flow of blood as well as its mean linear velocity is steady. However, as we have already noted, blood flow in the circulation is not steady; the heart imparts its energy in a *pulsatile* manner, with each heartbeat. Therefore, $\bar{v}$ in the aorta increases and reaches a maximum during systole and falls off during diastole. As we shall shortly see, these *changes in velocity* lead to compensatory changes in intravascular *pressure*.

The tradeoff between velocity and pressure reflects the conversion between two forms of energy. Although we gen-

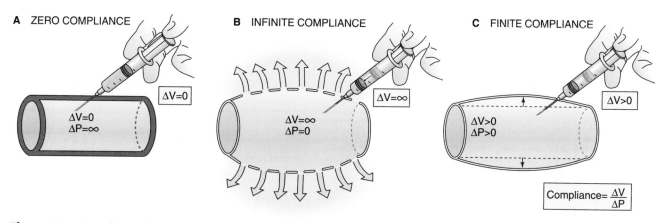

Figure 17-9 Compliance: changes in pressure with vessels of different compliances.

erally state that fluids flow from a higher to a lower *pressure*, it is more accurate to say that fluids flow from a higher to a lower *total energy*. This energy is made up of both the pressure or **potential energy** and the **kinetic energy** ($KE = \frac{1}{2} mv^2$). The impact of the interconversion between these two forms of energy is manifested by the familiar **Bernoulli effect**. As fluid flows along a horizontal tube with a narrow central region, which has half the diameter of the two ends, the pressure in the central region is actually lower than the pressure at the distal end of the tube (Fig. 17-10). How can the fluid paradoxically flow against the *pressure gradient* from the lower pressure central to the higher pressure distal region of the tube? We saw earlier that flow is the product of cross-sectional area and velocity (see Equation 17-8). Because the flow is the same in both portions of the tube, but the cross-sectional area in the center is lower by a factor of 4, the *velocity* in the central region must be 4-fold higher (Fig. 17-10, table at bottom). Although the blood in the central region has a lower potential energy (pressure = 60) than the blood at the distal end of the tube (pressure = 80), it has a 16-fold higher kinetic energy. Thus, the total energy of the fluid in the center exceeds that in the distal region, so that the fluid does indeed flow down the *energy gradient*.

This example illustrates an interconversion between potential energy (pressure) and kinetic energy (velocity) in *space* because velocity changes along the length of a tube even though flow is constant. We will see in Chapter 22 that during ejection of blood from the left ventricle into the aorta, the flow and velocity of blood change with *time* at any point within the aorta. These changes in velocity contribute to the changes in pressure inside the aorta.

The Bernoulli effect has important practical implications for measurement of blood pressure with an open-tipped catheter. The pressure recorded with the open tip facing the flow is higher than the actual pressure by an amount corresponding to the kinetic energy of the oncoming fluid (Fig. 17-11). Conversely, the pressure recorded with the open tip facing away from the flow is lower than the actual pressure by an equal amount. The measured pressure is correct only when the opening is on the side of the catheter, perpendicular to the flow of blood.

HOW TO MEASURE BLOOD PRESSURE, BLOOD FLOW, AND CARDIAC VOLUMES

Blood pressure can be measured directly by puncturing the vessel

One can record blood pressure anywhere along the circulation—inside a heart chamber, inside an artery, within a capillary, or within a vein. Clinicians are generally concerned with the intravascular pressure at a particular site (e.g., in a systemic artery) in reference to the barometric pressure outside the body and not with pressure *differences* between two sites.

The most direct approach for measurement of pressure is to introduce a needle or a catheter into a vessel and position the open tip at a particular site. In the first measurements of blood pressure ever performed, Stephen Hales in 1733 found that a column of blood from a presumably agitated horse rose to fill a brass pipe to a height of 3 meters. It was Poiseuille who measured blood pressure for the first time by connecting a mercury-filled U-tube to arteries through a tube containing a solution of saturated $NaHCO_3$. In modern times, a saline-filled transmission or conduit system connects the blood vessel to a pressure transducer. In its most primitive form, a catheter was connected to a closed chamber, one wall of which was a deformable diaphragm. Nowadays, the pressure transducer is a stiff diaphragm bonded to a strain gauge that converts mechanical strain into a change in electrical resistance, capacitance, or inductance (Fig. 17-12). The opposite face of the diaphragm is open to the atmosphere, so that the blood pressure is referenced to barometric pressure. The overall performance of the system depends largely on the properties of the catheter and the strain gauge. The presence of air bubbles and a long or narrow catheter can decrease the displacement, velocity, and acceleration of the fluid in the catheter. Together, these properties determine overall performance characteristics such as sensitivity, linearity, damping of the pressure wave, and frequency response. To avoid problems with fluid transmission in the catheter, some high-fidelity devices employ a solid-state pressure transducer at the catheter tip.

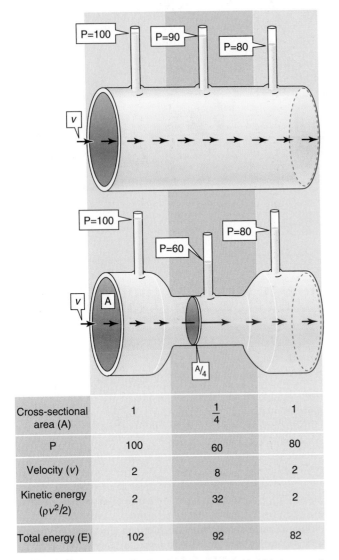

Cross-sectional area (A)	1	$\frac{1}{4}$	1
P	100	60	80
Velocity (v)	2	8	2
Kinetic energy ($\rho v^2/2$)	2	32	2
Total energy (E)	102	92	82

Figure 17-10 Bernoulli effect. For the top tube, which has a uniformly high radius, velocity (v) is uniform and transmural pressure (P) falls linearly with length. The bottom tube has the same upstream and downstream pressures but a constriction in the middle with a cross-sectional area that is only one fourth that of the two ends. Thus, velocity in the narrow portion must be 4-fold higher than it is at the ends. Although the *total energy* of fluid falls linearly along the tube, *pressure* is lower in the middle than at the distal end.

In catheterizations of the **right side of the heart**, the clinician begins by sliding a fluid-filled catheter into an antecubital vein and, while continuously recording pressure, advances the catheter tip into the superior vena cava, through the right atrium and the right ventricle, and past the pulmonary valve into the pulmonary artery. Eventually, the tip reaches and snugly fits into a smaller branch of the pulmonary artery, recording the **pulmonary wedge pressure** (see Chapter 22). The wedge pressure effectively measures the pressure downstream from the catheter tip, that is, the left atrial pressure.

In catheterizations of the **left side of the heart**, the clinician slides a catheter into the brachial artery or femoral artery, obtaining the **systemic arterial blood pressure**. From

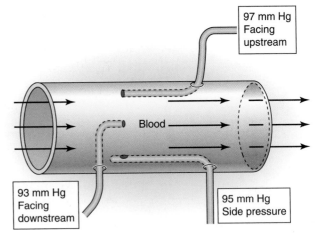

Figure 17-11 Effects of kinetic energy on the measurement of blood pressure with catheters.

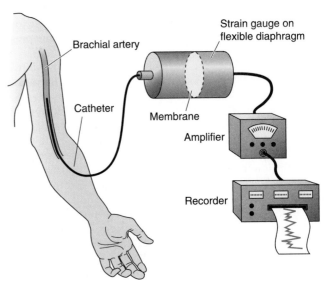

Figure 17-12 Direct method to determine blood pressure.

there, the catheter is advanced into the aorta, the left ventricle, and finally the left atrium.

Clinical measurements of **venous pressure** are typically made by inserting a catheter into the jugular vein. Because of the low pressures, these venous measurements require very sensitive pressure transducers or water manometers.

In the research laboratory, one can measure **capillary pressure** in exposed capillary beds by inserting a micropipette that is pressurized just enough (with a known pressure) to keep fluid from entering or leaving the pipette.

Blood pressure can be measured indirectly by use of a sphygmomanometer

In clinical practice, one may measure arterial pressure indirectly by use of a manual sphygmomanometer (Fig. 17-13). An inextensible cuff containing an inflatable bag is wrapped around the arm (or occasionally the thigh). Inflation of the bag by means of a rubber squeeze-bulb to a pressure level

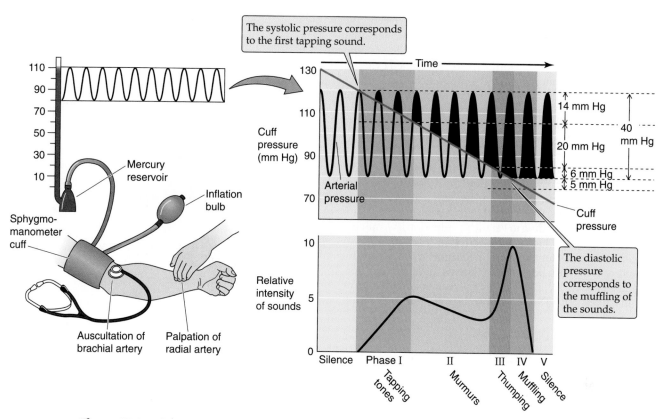

Figure 17-13 Sphygmomanometry. The clinician inflates the cuff to a pressure that is higher than the anticipated systolic pressure and then slowly releases the pressure in the cuff.

above the expected systolic pressure occludes the underlying brachial artery and halts blood flow downstream. The pressure in the cuff, measured by means of a mercury or aneroid manometer, is then allowed to slowly decline (Fig. 17-13, diagonal red line). The physician can use either of two methods to monitor the blood flow downstream of the slowly deflating cuff. In the **palpatory method**, one detects the pulse as an indicator of flow by feeling the radial artery at the wrist. In the **auscultatory method**, the physician detects flow by using a stethoscope to detect the changing character of Korotkoff sounds over the brachial artery in the antecubital space.

The palpatory method permits determination of the systolic pressure, that is, the pressure in the cuff below which it is just possible to detect a radial pulse. Because of limited sensitivity of the finger, palpation probably slightly underestimates systolic pressure. The auscultatory method permits the detection of both systolic and diastolic pressure. The sounds heard during the slow deflation of the cuff can be divided into five phases (Fig. 17-13). During phase I, there is a sharp tapping sound, indicating that a spurt of blood is escaping under the cuff when cuff pressure is just below systolic pressure. The pressure at which these taps are first heard closely represents systolic pressure. In phase II, the sound becomes a blowing or swishing murmur. During phase III, the sound becomes a louder thumping. In phase IV, as the cuff pressure falls toward the diastolic level, the sound becomes muffled and softer. Finally, in phase V, the sound disappears. Although some debate persists about whether the point of muffling or the point of silence is the

correct diastolic pressure, most favor the point of muffling as being more consistent. Actual diastolic pressure may be somewhat overestimated by the point of muffling but underestimated by the point of silence.

Practical problems arise when a sphygmomanometer is used with children or obese adults or when it is used to obtain a measurement on a thigh. Ideally, one would like to use a pressure cuff wide enough to ensure that the pressure inside the cuff is the same as that in the tissue surrounding the artery. In 1967, the American Heart Association recommended that the pneumatic bag within the cuff be 20% wider than the diameter of the limb, extend at least halfway around the limb, and be centered over the artery. More recent studies indicate that accuracy and reliability improve when the pneumatic bag completely encircles the limb, as long as the width of the pneumatic bag is at least the limb diameter.

Blood flow can be measured directly by electromagnetic and ultrasound flowmeters

The spectrum of blood flow measurements in the circulation ranges from determinations of total blood flow (cardiac output) to assessment of flow within an organ or a particular tissue within an organ. Moreover, one can average blood flow measurements over time or record continuously. Examples of continuous recording include recordings of the phasic blood flow that occurs during the cardiac cycle or any other periodic event (e.g., breathing). We discuss both invasive and noninvasive approaches.

Invasive Methods These approaches require direct access to the vessel under study and are thus useful only in research laboratories. The earliest measurements of blood flow involved collecting venous outflow into a graduated cylinder and timing the collection with a stopwatch. This direct approach was limited to short time intervals to minimize blood loss and the resulting changes in hemodynamics. Blood loss could be avoided by ingenious but now antiquated devices that returned the blood to the circulation, in either a manual or a semiautomated fashion.

The most frequently used modern instruments for measurement of blood flow in the research laboratory are **electromagnetic flowmeters** based on the electromagnetic induction principle (Fig. 17-14). The vessel is placed in a magnetic field. According to Faraday's induction law, moving any conductor (including an electrolyte solution, such as blood) at right angles to lines of the magnetic field generates a voltage difference between two points along an axis perpendicular to both the axis of the movement and the axis of the magnetic field. The induced voltage is

$$E = B\bar{v}D \tag{17-14}$$

where B is the density of magnetic flux, $\bar{v}$ is the average linear velocity, and D is the diameter of the moving column of blood.

Ultrasound flowmeters employ a pair of probes, placed at two sites along a vessel. One probe emits an ultrasound signal, and the other records it. The linear velocity of blood in the vessel either induces a change in the frequency of the ultrasound signal (Doppler effect) or alters the transit time of the ultrasound signal. Both the electromagnetic and ultrasound methods measure linear velocity, not flow per se.

Noninvasive Methods The electromagnetic or ultrasonic flowmeters require the surgical isolation of a vessel. However, **ultrasonic methods** are also widely used transcutaneously on surface vessels in humans. This method is based on recording of the backscattering of the ultrasound signal from moving red blood cells. To the extent that the red blood cells move, the reflected sound has a frequency different from that of the emitted sound (Doppler effect). This frequency difference may thus be calibrated to measure flow. **Plethysmographic methods** are noninvasive approaches for measurement of changes in the volume of a limb or even of a whole person (see Chapter 27). Inflation of a pressure cuff enough to occlude veins but not arteries allows blood to continue to flow *into* (but not out of) a limb or an organ, so that the volume increases with time. The record of this rise in volume, as recorded by the plethysmograph, is a measure of blood flow.

With the exception of transcutaneous ultrasonography, the direct methods discussed for measurement of blood flow are largely confined to research laboratories. The next two sections include discussions of two indirect methods that clinicians use to measure mean blood flow.

Cardiac output can be measured indirectly by the Fick method, which is based on the conservation of mass

The Fick method requires that a substance be removed from or added to the blood during its flow through an organ. The

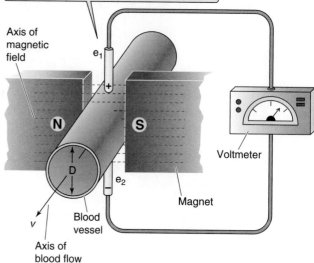

The movement of an electrical conductor (i.e., blood in a vessel) through a magnetic field induces a voltage between two points (e_1 and e_2) along an axis that is mutually perpendicular to both the axis of the magnetic field and the axis of blood flow.

Figure 17-14 Electromagnetic flowmeter.

rate at which X passes a checkpoint in the circulation ($\dot{Q}$) is simply the product of the rate at which blood volume passes the checkpoint (F) and the concentration of X in that blood:

$$\dot{Q} = F \cdot [X]$$

$$\text{Units:} \quad \frac{\text{moles}}{\text{s}} = \frac{\text{liter}}{\text{s}} \cdot \frac{\text{moles}}{\text{liter}} \tag{17-15}$$

The **Fick principle** is a restatement of the law of conservation of mass. The amount of X per unit time that passes a downstream checkpoint ($\dot{Q}_B$) minus the amount of X that passes an upstream checkpoint ($\dot{Q}_A$) must equal the amount of X added or subtracted per unit time ($\dot{Q}_{\text{added/subtracted}}$) between these two checkpoints (Fig. 17-15A):

$$\dot{Q}_{\text{added/subtracted}} = \dot{Q}_B - \dot{Q}_A \tag{17-16}$$

$\dot{Q}_{\text{added/subtracted}}$ is positive for the addition of X. If the volume flow is identical at both checkpoints, combining Equations 17-15 and 17-16 yields

$$\dot{Q}_{\text{added/subtracted}} = F([X]_B - [X]_A) \tag{17-17}$$

We can calculate flow from the amount of X added or subtracted and the concentrations of X at the two checkpoints:

$$F = \frac{\dot{Q}_{\text{added/subtracted}}}{[X]_B - [X]_A} = \frac{\text{moles/min}}{\text{moles/liter}} = \frac{\text{liter}}{\text{min}} \tag{17-18}$$

It is easiest to apply the Fick principle to the blood flow through the lungs, which is the cardiac output (Fig. 17-15B).

A   THE FICK PRINCIPLE

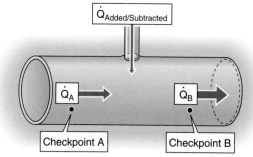

B   MEASUREMENT OF CARDIAC OUTPUT

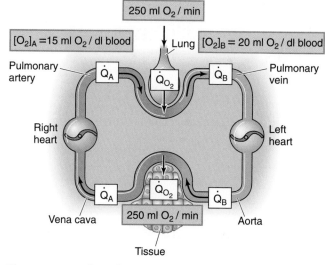

Figure 17-15 The Fick method to determine cardiac output.

The quantity added to the bloodstream is the O_2 uptake ($\dot{Q}_{O_2}$) by the lungs, which we obtain by measuring the subject's O_2 consumption. This value is typically 250 mL of O_2 gas per minute. The upstream checkpoint is the pulmonary artery (*point A*), where the O_2 content ($[O_2]_A$) is typically 15 mL of O_2 per deciliter of blood. The sample for this checkpoint must reflect the O_2 content of mixed venous blood, obtained by means of a catheter within the right atrium or the right ventricle or pulmonary artery. The downstream checkpoint is a pulmonary vein (*point B*), where the O_2 content ($[O_2]_B$) is typically 20 mL of O_2 per deciliter of blood. We can obtain the sample for this checkpoint from any systemic artery. Using these particular values, we calculate a cardiac output of 5 L/min:

$$F = \frac{\dot{Q}_{O_2}}{[O_2]_B - [O_2]_A} = \frac{250\,\text{mL O}_2/\text{min}}{(20-15)\,\text{mL O}_2/\text{dL blood}} \quad \text{(17-19)}$$
$$= 5\,\text{L blood/min}$$

Cardiac output can be measured indirectly by dilution methods

The dye dilution method, inaugurated by G. N. Stewart in 1897 and extended by W. F. Hamilton in 1932, is a variation

of the Fick procedure. One injects a known quantity of a substance (X) into a systemic vein (e.g., antecubital vein) at site A while simultaneously monitoring the concentration downstream at site B (Fig. 17-16A). It is important that the substance not leave the vascular circuit and that it is easy to follow the concentration, by either successive sampling or continuous monitoring. If we inject a single known amount (Q_X) of the indicator, an observer downstream at checkpoint B will see a rising concentration of X, which, after reaching its peak, falls off exponentially. Concentration measurements provide the interval (Δt) between the time the dye makes its first appearance at site B and the time the dye finally disappears there.

If site B is in the pulmonary artery, then the entire *amount* Q_X that we injected into the peripheral vein must pass site B during the interval Δt, carried by the entire cardiac output. We can deduce the average concentration $[\bar{X}]$ during the interval Δt from the concentration-versus-time curve in Figure 17-16B. From the conservation of mass, we know that

$$Q_X = V \cdot [\bar{X}]$$
$$\text{Units: moles} = \text{liter} \cdot \frac{\text{moles}}{\text{liter}} \quad \text{(17-20)}$$

Because the volume of blood (V) that flowed through the pulmonary artery during the interval Δt is, by definition, the product of cardiac output and the time interval (CO · Δt),

$$Q_X = \text{CO} \cdot \Delta t \cdot [\bar{X}]$$
$$\text{Units: moles} = \frac{\text{liter}}{\text{s}} \cdot \text{s} \cdot \frac{\text{moles}}{\text{liter}} \quad \text{(17-21)}$$

Note that the product $\Delta t \cdot \bar{X}$ is the area under the concentration-versus-time curve in Figure 17-16B. Solving for CO, we have

$$\text{CO} = \frac{Q_X}{[\bar{X}] \cdot \Delta t} = \frac{Q_X}{\text{Area}} \quad \text{(17-22)}$$

In practice, cardiologists monitor [X] in the brachial artery. Obviously, only a fraction of the cardiac output passes through a brachial artery; however, this fraction is the same as the fraction of Q_X that passes through the brachial artery. If we were to re-derive Equation 17-22 for the brachial artery, we would end up multiplying both the CO and Q_X terms by this same fraction. Therefore, even though only a small portion of both cardiac output and injected dye passes through any single systemic artery, we can still use Equation 17-22 to compute cardiac output with data from that artery.

Compared with the [X] profile in the pulmonary artery, the [X] profile in the brachial artery is not as tall and is more spread out, so that [$\bar{X}$] is smaller and Δt is longer. However, the product [$\bar{X}$] · Δt in the brachial artery—or any other systemic artery—is the same as in the pulmonary artery. Indocyanine green dye (cardiogreen) is the most common dye employed. Because the liver removes this dye from the circulation, it is possible to repeat the injections, after a sufficient wait, without progressive accumulation of dye in the plasma. Imagine that after we inject 5 mg of the dye, [$\bar{X}$] under the curve is 2 mg/L and Δt is 0.5 min. Thus,

A PRINCIPLE OF DYE DILUTION

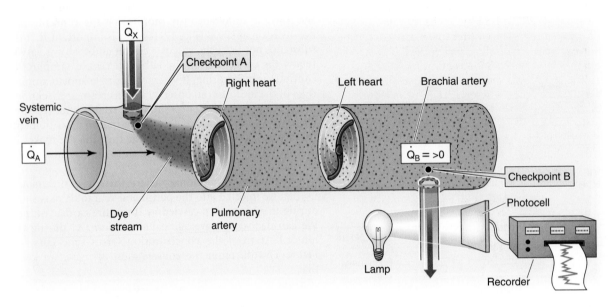

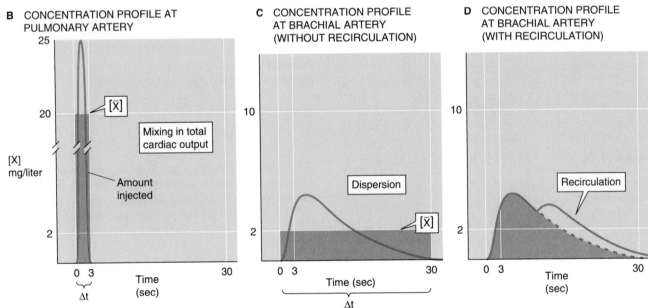

Figure 17-16 Dye dilution method to determine blood flow. In **B, C,** and **D,** the areas underneath the three red curves—as well as the three green areas—are all the same.

$$CO = \frac{5\,mg}{2\,mg/L \times 0.5\,min} = 5\,L/min \qquad (17\text{-}23)$$

A practical problem is that after we inject a marker into a systemic vein, blood moves more quickly through some pulmonary beds than others, so that the marker arrives at checkpoint B at different times. This process, known as dispersion, is the main cause of the flattening of the [X] profile in the brachial artery (Fig. 17-16C) versus the pulmonary artery (Fig. 17-16B). If we injected the dye into the *left atrium* and monitored it in the *systemic veins*, the dispersion would

be far worse because of longer and more varied path lengths in the systemic circulation compared with the pulmonary circulation. In fact, the concentration curve would be so flattened that it would be difficult to resolve the area underneath the [X] profile.

A second practical problem with a closed circulatory system is that before the initial [X] wave has waned, recirculation causes the injected indicator to reappear for a second time in front of the sensor at checkpoint B (Fig. 17-16D). Extrapolation of the exponential decay of the first wave can correct for this problem.

The thermodilution technique is a convenient alternative approach to the dye technique. In this method, one injects a bolus of cold saline, and an indwelling thermistor is used to follow the dilution of these "negative calories" as a change of temperature at the downstream site. In the thermodilution technique, a temperature-versus-time profile replaces the concentration-versus-time profile. During cardiac catheterization, the cardiologist injects a bolus of cold saline into the right atrium and records the temperature change in the pulmonary artery. The distance between upstream injection and downstream recording site is kept short to avoid heat exchange in the pulmonary capillary bed. The advantages of this method are that (1) the injection of cold saline can be repeated without harm, (2) a single venous (versus venous and arterial) puncture allows access to both the upstream and the downstream sites, (3) less dispersion occurs because no capillary beds are involved, and (4) less recirculation occurs because of adequate temperature equilibration in the pulmonary and systemic capillary beds. A potential drawback is incomplete mixing, which may result from the proximity between injection and detection sites.

Regional blood flow can be measured indirectly by "clearance" methods

The methods used to measure regional blood flow are often called clearance methods, although the term here has a meaning somewhat different from its meaning in kidney physiology. Clearance methods are another application of the Fick principle, using the rate of uptake or elimination of a substance by an organ together with a determination of the difference in concentration of the indicator between the arterial inflow and venous outflow (i.e., the **a-v difference**). By analogy with Equation 17-18, we can compute the blood flow through an organ (F) from the rate at which the organ removes the test substance X from the blood ($\dot{Q}_X$) and the concentrations of the substance in arterial blood ($[X]_a$) and venous blood ($[X]_v$):

$$F = \frac{\dot{Q}_X}{[X]_a - [X]_v} = \frac{\text{moles/min}}{\text{moles/liter}} = \text{liters/min} \quad \textbf{(17-24)}$$

One can determine **hepatic blood flow** with use of BSP (bromosulphthalein), a dye that the liver almost completely clears and excretes into the bile (see Chapter 46). Here, $\dot{Q}_X$ is the rate of removal of BSP from the blood, estimated as the rate at which BSP appears in the bile. $[X]_a$ is the concentration of BSP in a systemic artery, and $[X]_v$ is the concentration of BSP in the hepatic vein.

In a similar manner, one can determine **renal blood flow** with use of PAH (p-aminohippurate). The kidneys almost completely remove this compound from the blood and secrete it into the urine (see Chapter 34).

It is possible to determine **coronary blood flow** or **regional blood flow** through skeletal muscle from the tissue clearance of rapidly diffusing inert gases, such as the radioisotopes ^{133}Xe and [85]Kr.

Finally, one can use the rate of disappearance of nitrous oxide (N_2O), a gas that is historically important as the first anesthetic, to compute cerebral blood flow.

A similar although qualitative approach is thallium scanning to assess coronary blood flow. Here one measures the uptake of an isotope by the heart muscle, rather than its clearance (see the box titled Thallium Scanning for Assessment of Coronary Blood Flow).

Ventricular dimensions, ventricular volumes, and volume changes can be measured by angiography and echocardiography

Clinicians can use a variety of approaches to examine the cardiac chambers. **Gated radionuclide imaging** employs compounds of the γ-emitting isotope technetium Tc 99m, which has a half-life of 6 hours. After ^{99m}Tc is injected, a gamma camera provides imaging of the cardiac chambers. ECG gating (i.e., synchronization to a particular spot on the electrocardiogram) allows the apparatus to snap a picture at a specific part of the cardiac cycle and to sum these pictures up over many cycles. Because this method does not provide a high-resolution image, it yields only a *relative* ventricular volume. From the difference between the count at the maximally filled state (end-diastolic volume) and at its minimally filled state (end-systolic volume), the cardiologist can estimate the fraction of ventricular blood that is ejected during systole—**the ejection fraction**—which is an important measure of cardiac function.

Angiography can accurately provide the linear dimensions of the ventricle, allowing the cardiologist to calculate *absolute* ventricular volumes. A catheter is threaded into either the left or the right ventricle, and saline containing a contrast substance (i.e., a chemical opaque to x-rays) is injected into the ventricle. This approach provides a two-dimensional projection of the ventricular volume as a function of time. In magnetic resonance imaging, one obtains a nuclear magnetic resonance (NMR) image of the protons in the water of the heart muscle and blood. However, because standard NMR requires long data acquisition times, it does not provide good time resolution.

Echocardiography, which exploits ultrasonic waves to visualize the heart and great vessels, can be used in two modes. In *M-mode echocardiography* (M is for motion), the technician places a single transducer in a fixed position on the chest wall and obtains a one-dimensional view of heart components. In the upper portion of Figure 17-17A, the ultrasonic beam transects the anterior wall of the right ventricle, the right ventricle, the septum, the left ventricle, the leaflets of the mitral valve, and the posterior wall of the left ventricle. The lower portion of Figure 17-17A shows the positions of the borders between these structures (x-axis) during a single cardiac cycle (y-axis) and thus how the size

A PRINCIPLE OF ECHOCARDIOGRAPHY

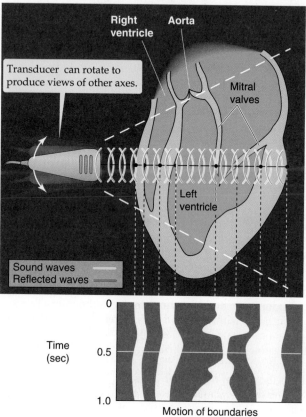

B ASSUMED VENTRICULAR GEOMETRY

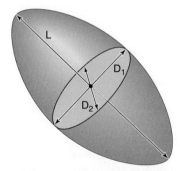

Figure 17-17 M-mode and two-dimensional echocardiography. In **A,** the tracing on the bottom shows the result of an M-mode echocardiogram (i.e., transducer in single position) during one cardiac cycle. The waves represent motion (M) of heart boundaries transected by a stationary ultrasonic beam. In two-dimensional echocardiography *(upper panel),* the probe rapidly rotates between the two extremes *(broken lines),* producing an image of a slice through the heart at one instant in time.

of the left ventricle—along the axis of the beam—changes with time. Of course, the technician can obtain other views by changing the orientation of the beam.

In *two-dimensional echocardiography,* the probe automatically and rapidly pivots, scanning the heart in a single anatomical slice or plane (Fig. 17-17A, area between the two broken lines) and providing a true cross section. This approach is therefore superior to angiography, which provides only a two-dimensional projection. Because cardiac output is the product of heart rate and stroke volume, one can calculate cardiac output from echocardiographic measurements of ventricular end-diastolic and end-systolic volume.

A problem common to angiography and M-mode echocardiography is that it is impossible to compute ventricular volume from a single dimension because the ventricle is not a simple sphere. As is shown in Figure 17-17B, the left ventricle is often assumed to be a *prolate ellipse,* with a long axis L and two short axes D_1 and D_2. To simplify the calculation and to allow ventricular volume to be computed from a single measurement, it is sometimes assumed that D_1 and D_2 are identical and that D_1 is half of L. Unfortunately, use of this algorithm and just a single dimension, as provided by M-mode echocardiography, often yields grossly erroneous volumes. Use of two-dimensional echocardiography to sum information from several parallel slices through the ventricle, or from planes that are at a known angle to one another, can yield more accurate volumes.

In addition to ultrasound methods of angiography, *magnetic resonance angiography* is an application of magnetic resonance tomography to obtain two-dimensional images of slices of ventricular volumes or of blood vessels.

In contrast to standard echocardiography, **Doppler echocardiography** provides information on the velocity, direction, and character of blood flow, just as police radar monitors traffic. In Doppler echocardiography (as with police radar), most information is obtained with the beam parallel to the flow of blood. In the simplest application of Doppler flow measurements, one can continuously monitor the velocity of flowing blood in a blood vessel or part of the heart. On such a record, the x-axis represents time and the y-axis represents the spectrum of *velocities* of the moving red blood cells (i.e., different cells can be moving at different velocities). Flow toward the transducer appears above baseline, whereas flow away from the transducer appears below baseline. The intensity of the record at a single point on the y-axis (encoded by a gray scale or false color) represents the strength of the returning signal, which depends on the *number* of red blood cells moving at that velocity. Thus, Doppler echocardiography is able to distinguish the character of flow: laminar versus turbulent. Alternatively, at one instant in time, the Doppler technician can scan a region of a vessel or the heart, obtaining a two-dimensional, color-encoded map of blood velocities. If we overlay such two-dimensional Doppler data on a two-dimensional echocardiogram, which shows the position of the vessel or cardiac structures, the result is a color, flow-imaging Doppler echocardiogram (Fig. 17-18).

Finally, a magnetic resonance scanner can also be used in two-dimensional phase-contrast mapping to yield quantitative measurements of blood flow velocity.

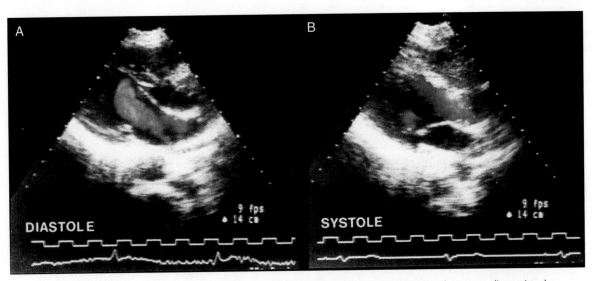

Figure 17-18   The colors, which encode the velocity of blood flow, are superimposed on a two-dimensional echocardiogram, which is shown in a gray scale. In **A,** blood moves through the mitral valve and into the left ventricle during diastole. Because blood is flowing toward the transducer, its velocity is encoded as *red.* In **B,** blood moves out of the ventricle and toward the aortic valve during systole. Because blood is flowing away from the transducer, its velocity is encoded as *blue. (From Feigenbaum H: Echocardiography. In Braunwald E [ed]: Heart Disease: A Textbook of Cardiovascular Medicine, 5th ed. Philadelphia: WB Saunders, 1997.)*

REFERENCES

Books and Reviews

Badeer HS: Hemodynamics for medical students. Adv Physiol Educ 2001; 25:44-52.

Caro CG, Pedley TJ, Schroter RC, Seed WA: The Mechanics of the Circulation. Oxford: Oxford University Press, 1978.

Lassen NA, Henriksen O, Sejrsen P: Indicator methods for measurement of organ and tissue blood flow. In Handbook of Physiology, Section 2: The Cardiovascular System, vol III, pp 21-63. Bethesda, MD: American Physiological Society, 1979.

Levine RA, Gillam LD, Weyman AE: Echocardiography in cardiac research. In Fozzard HA, Haber E, Jennings RB, et al (eds): The Heart and Cardiovascular System, pp 369-452. New York: Raven Press, 1986.

Rowland T, Obert P: Doppler echocardiography for the estimation of cardiac output with exercise. Sports Med 2002; 32:973-986.

Journal Articles

Coulter NA Jr, Pappenheimer JR: Development of turbulence in flowing blood. Am J Physiol 1949; 159:401-408.

Cournand A, Ranges HA: Catheterization of the right auricle. Proc Soc Exp Biol Med 1941; 46:462-466.

Hamilton WF, Moore JW, Kinsman JM, Spurling RG: Studies on the circulation. IV. Further analysis of the injection method and of changes in hemodynamics under physiological and pathological conditions. Am J Physiol 1932; 99:534-551.

Reynolds O: An experimental investigation of the circumstances which determine whether the motion of water shall be direct or sinusoid, and of the law of resistance in parallel channels. Philos Trans R Soc Lond B Biol Sci 1883; 174:935-982.

Thury A, van Langenhove G, Carlier SG, et al: High shear stress after successful balloon angioplasty is associated with restenosis and target lesion revascularization. Am Heart J 2002; 144:136-143.

CHAPTER 18

BLOOD

Emile L. Boulpaep

Blood is a complex fluid consisting of plasma—extracellular fluid rich in proteins—and of formed elements—red blood cells (RBCs), white blood cells (WBCs), and platelets. Total blood volume is ~70 mL/kg body weight in the adult woman and ~80 mL/kg body weight in the adult man (see Table 5-1).

BLOOD COMPOSITION

Whole blood is a suspension of cellular elements in plasma

If you spin down a sample of blood containing an anticoagulant for ~5 minutes at 10,000 g, the bottom fraction contains **formed elements**—RBCs (or erythrocytes), WBCs (leukocytes, which include granulocytes, lymphocytes, and monocytes), and platelets (thrombocytes); the top fraction is blood plasma (Fig. 18-1). The RBCs having the highest density are at the bottom of the tube, whereas most of the WBCs and platelets form a whitish gray layer—the **buffy coat**—between the RBCs and plasma. Only a small amount of WBCs, platelets, and plasma is trapped in the bottom column of RBCs.

The **hematocrit** (see Chapter 5) is the fraction of the total column occupied by RBCs. The normal hematocrit is ~40% for adult women and ~45% for adult men. The hematocrit in the newborn is ~55% and falls to ~35% at 2 months of age, from which time it rises during development to reach adult values at puberty. The hematocrit is a measure of concentration of RBCs, not of total body red cell mass. Expansion of plasma volume in a pregnant woman reduces the hematocrit, whereas her total red cell volume also increases but less than plasma volume (see Chapter 56). Immediately after hemorrhage, the hematocrit may be normal despite the loss of blood volume (see Chapter 25). Total RBC volume is ~28 mL/kg body weight in the adult woman and ~36 mL/kg body weight in the adult man.

Plasma is a pale-white watery solution of electrolytes, plasma proteins, carbohydrates, and lipids. Pink-colored plasma suggests the presence of hemoglobin caused by

hemolysis (lysis of RBCs) and release of hemoglobin into the plasma. A brown-green color may reflect elevated bilirubin levels (see Chapter 46). Plasma can also be cloudy in cryoglobulinemias. The electrolyte composition of plasma differs only slightly from that of interstitial fluid on account of the volume occupied by proteins and their electrical charge (see Table 5-2).

Plasma proteins at a normal concentration of ~7.0 g/dL account for a colloid osmotic pressure or oncotic pressure of ~25 mm Hg (see Chapter 20). Principal plasma proteins are albumin, fibrinogen, globulins, and other coagulation factors. The molecular masses of plasma proteins range up to 970 kDa (Table 18-1). The plasma concentration of **albumin** ranges from 3.5 to 5.5 g/dL, providing the body with a total plasma albumin pool of ~135 g. Albumin is synthesized by the liver at a rate of ~120 mg/kg body weight per day and, because of catabolism, has a half-life in the circulation of ~20 days. Urinary losses of albumin are normally negligible (<20 mg/day; see Chapter 33). Plasma concentration of albumin is typically decreased in hepatic cirrhosis (see Chapter 24). Hepatic synthesis of albumin is strongly enhanced by a low plasma colloid osmotic pressure.

Many plasma proteins are involved in blood coagulation through coagulation cascades, the endpoint of which is the cleavage of **fibrinogen** into fibrin monomers that further assemble into a fibrin polymer. The fibrinogen molecule is a dimer of identical heterotrimers, each composed of Aα, Bβ, and γ chains. Fibrinogen is synthesized only by the liver (see Table 46-3) and circulates in plasma at concentrations of 150 to 300 mg/dL. The acute-phase response (see the box on erythrocyte sedimentation) greatly enhances fibrinogen synthesis. During clotting, the cross-linked polymers of fibrin form strands that trap red and white cells, platelets, and plasma inside the thrombus (i.e., blood clot). Subsequent interaction of myosin and actin in the platelets of the clot allows the clot to shrink to a plug that expels a slightly yellow-tinged fluid. This residual fluid is **serum**, which differs principally from plasma by the absence of fibrinogen and other coagulation factors. However, serum still contains albumin, antibodies, and other proteins. Note that *plasma* can also form a clot, but a plasma clot does not retract because it lacks platelets.

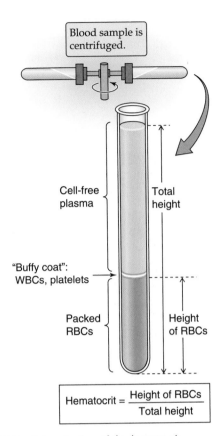

Figure 18-1 Determination of the hematocrit.

$$\text{Hematocrit} = \frac{\text{Height of RBCs}}{\text{Total height}}$$

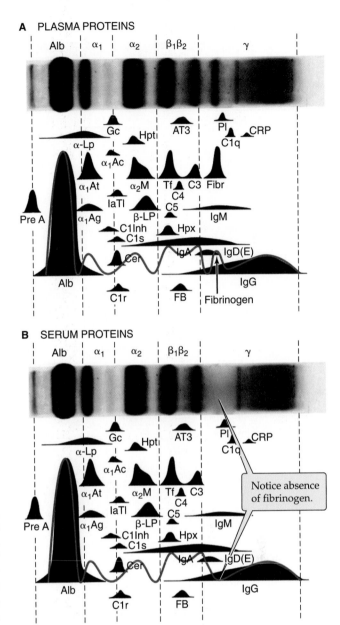

Figure 18-2 Electrophoretic pattern of human plasma proteins (**A**) and (**B**) serum proteins (i.e. without fibrinogens). Normal concentration ranges are as follows: total protein, 6 to 8 g/dL; albumin, 3.1 to 5.4 g/dL; α_1-globulins, 0.1 to 0.4 g/dL; α_2-globulins, 0.4 to 1.1 g/dL; β-globulins, 0.5 to 1.2 g/dL; γ-globulins, 0.7 to 1.7 g/dL.

Subtraction of the albumin and fibrinogen moiety from total protein concentration yields the concentration of all the proteins grouped as **globulins**. Electrophoresis can be used to fractionate plasma proteins. The electrophoretic mobility of a protein depends on its molecular weight (size and shape) as well as its electrical charge. Plasma proteins comprise, in decreasing order of electrophoretic mobility (Fig. 18-2A), albumin, α_1-globulins, α_2-globulins, β-globulins, fibrinogen, and γ-globulins. The three most abundant peaks are albumin, fibrinogen, and γ-globulins. The γ-globulins include the immunoglobulins or antibodies, which can be separated into IgA, IgD, IgE, IgG, and IgM. Immunoglobulins are synthesized by B lymphocytes and plasma cells.

Clinical laboratories most often perform electrophoresis of blood proteins on *serum* instead of plasma (Fig. 18-2B). Table 18-1 shows the major protein components that are readily resolved by electrophoresis. Proteins present in plasma at low concentrations are determined by immunological techniques, such as radioimmunoassay (see Chapter 47) and enzyme-linked immunosorbent assay. Not listed in Table 18-1 are several important carrier proteins present in plasma: transcobalamin (see Chapter 45), ceruloplasmin (see Chapter 46), IGF-binding proteins (see Chapter 48), thyroid-binding globulin (see Chapter 49), corticosteroid-binding globulin and sex hormone–binding globulin (see Chapter 50), and vitamin D–binding protein (see Chapter 52). The liver synthesizes most of the globulins and coagulation factors.

Bone marrow is the source of most blood cells

If you spread a drop of anticoagulated blood thinly on a glass slide, you can detect under the microscope the cellular elements of blood. In such a **peripheral blood smear**, the following mature cell types are easily recognized: erythrocytes, granulocytes (divided in neutrophils, eosinophils, and basophils), lymphocytes, monocytes, and platelets (Fig. 18-3).

Hematopoiesis is the process of generation of all the cell types present in blood. Because of the diversity of cell types generated, hematopoiesis serves multiple roles ranging from the carriage of gases to immune responses and hemostasis. Pluripotent **long-term hematopoietic stem cells (LT-HSCs)**

Table 18-1 Major Plasma Proteins*

Protein Fractions of Human Plasma	Molecular Mass (kDa)	Function
Transthyretin	62	Binds T_3 and T_4 Binds vitamin A
Albumin	69	Oncotic pressure Binds steroids, T_3, bilirubin, bile salts, fatty acids
α_1-Antitrypsin (α_1AT)	54	Protease inhibitor; deficiency causes emphysema
α_2-Macroglobulin	725	Broad-spectrum protease inhibitor Synthesized by liver
Haptoglobin	100	Binds hemoglobin
β-Lipoprotein (LDL)	380	Binds lipid
Transferrin	80	Binds iron
Complement C3	185	Third component of complement system
Fibrinogen	340	Clotting protein; precursor of fibrin
Immunoglobulin A (IgA)	160	Mucosal immunity Synthesized by plasma cells in exocrine glands
Immunoglobulin D (IgD)	170	Synthesized by B lymphocytes
Immunoglobulin E (IgE)	190	Synthesized by B lymphocytes Binds to mast cells or basophils
Immunoglobulin G (IgG)	150	Humoral immunity Synthesized by plasma cells
Immunoglobulin M (IgM)	970	Humoral immunity Synthesized by B lymphocytes

*The proteins are in the approximate order of decreasing electrophoretic mobility.

constitute a population of **adult stem cells** found in bone marrow that are multipotent and able to self-renew. The short-term HSCs (ST-HSCs) give rise to **committed stem cells** or progenitors, which after proliferation are able to differentiate into lineages that in turn give rise to **burst-forming units (BFUs)** or **colony-forming units (CFUs)**, each of which ultimately will produce one or a limited number of mature cell types: erythrocytes, the megakaryocytes that produce platelets, eosinophils, basophils, neutrophils, monocytes-macrophages/dendritic cells, and B or T lymphocytes and natural killer cells (Fig. 18-4). Soluble factors known as **cytokines** guide the development of each lineage. The research of Donald Metcalf demonstrated the importance of a family of hematopoietic cytokines that stimulate colony formation by progenitor cells, the **colony-stimulating factors**. The main colony-stimulating factors are granulocyte-macrophage colony-stimulating factor (GM-CSF), granulocyte colony-stimulating factor (G-CSF), macrophage colony-stimulating factor (M-CSF), interleukins 3 and 5 (IL-3 and IL-5; see Chapter 3), thrombopoietin (TPO), and erythropoietin (EPO; see p. 453).

GM-CSF is a glycoprotein that stimulates proliferation of a common myeloid progenitor and promotes the production of neutrophils, eosinophils, and monocytes-macrophages. Recombinant GM-CSF (sargramostim, Leukine) is used clinically after bone marrow transplantation and in certain acute leukemias.

G-CSF and **M-CSF** are glycoproteins that guide the ultimate development of granulocytes and monocytes-macrophages/dendritic cells, respectively. Recombinant G-CSF (filgrastim, Neupogen) is used therapeutically in neutropenia (e.g., after chemotherapy). M-CSF is also required for osteoclast development (see Chapter 52, particularly Fig. 52-4).

IL-3 (also known as multi-CSF) has a broad effect on multiple lineages. The liver and the kidney constitutively produce this glycoprotein. **IL-5** (colony-stimulating factor, eosinophil), a homodimeric glycoprotein, sustains the terminal differentiation of eosinophilic precursors.

TPO binds to a thrombopoietin receptor called c-Mpl, which is the cellular homologue of the viral oncogene v-*mpl* (murine retrovirus myeloproliferative leukemia virus). On

A NEUTROPHIL

B EOSINOPHIL

C BASOPHIL

D LYMPHOCYTE

E MONOCYTE

F PLATELETS

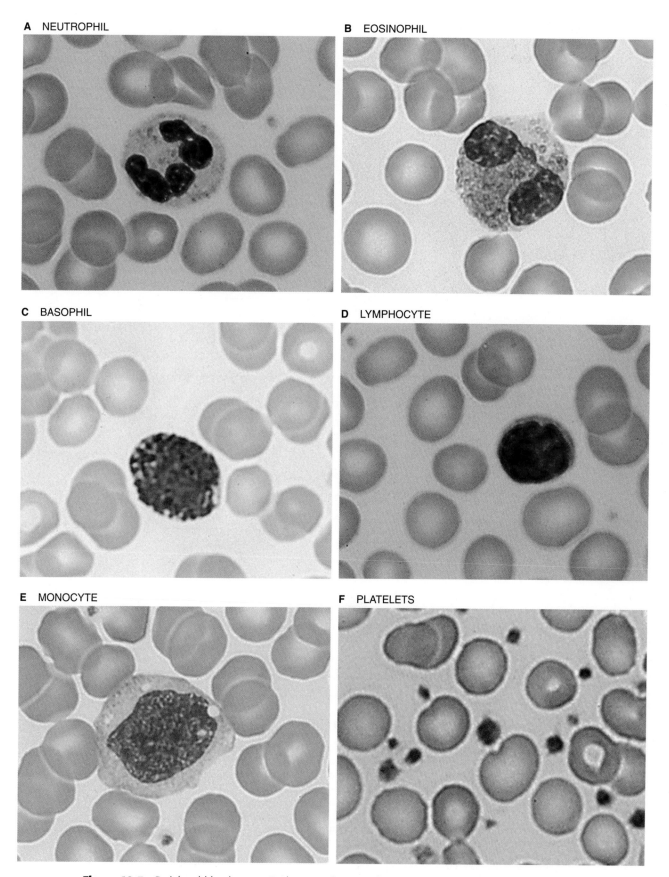

Figure 18-3 Peripheral blood smear. Erythrocytes (average diameter, ~7.5 μm) are present in all panels. The cellular elements are not represented according to their abundance. *(From Goldman L, Ausiello D: Cecil's Textbook of Medicine, 22nd ed. Philadelphia, WB Saunders, 2004.)*

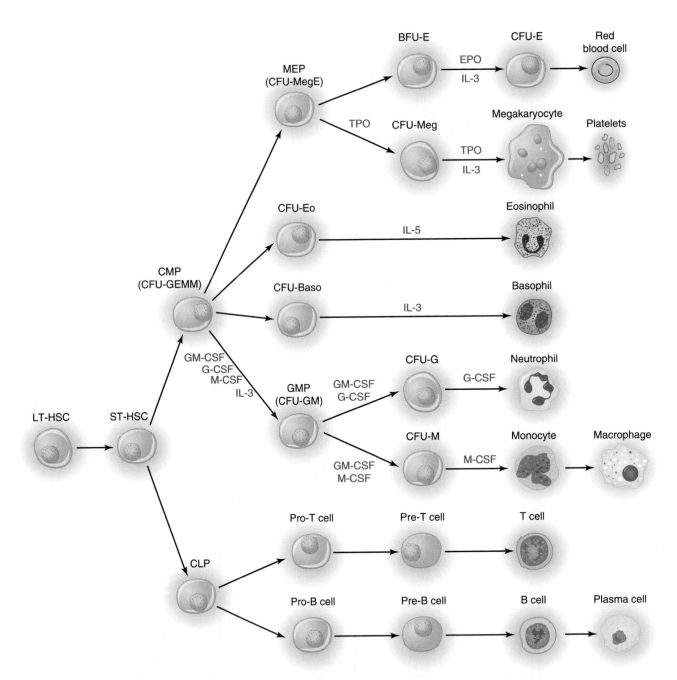

Figure 18-4 Hematopoietic lineages. BFU-E, burst-forming unit–erythroid; CFU, colony-forming unit (with the suffixes -Baso [basophilic], -E [erythroid], -Eo [eosinophil], -G [granulocyte], -GEMM [granulocyte, erythrocyte, monoctye, megakaryocyte], -GM [granulocyte-macrophage], -M [macrophage], -Meg [megakaryocyte], and -MegE [megakaryocyte-erythroid]); CLP, common lymphoid progenitor; CMP, common myeloid progenitor; CSF, colony-stimulating factor (with the prefixes G- [granulocyte], GM- [granulocyte-macrophage], and M- [macrophage]; EPO, erythropoietin; GMP, granulocyte-macrophage progenitor; IL-3 and IL-5, interleukins 3 and 5; LT-HSC, long-term hematopoietic stem cell; MEP, megakaryocyte-erythroid progenitor; ST-HSC, short-term hematopoietic stem cell; TPO, thrombopoietin.

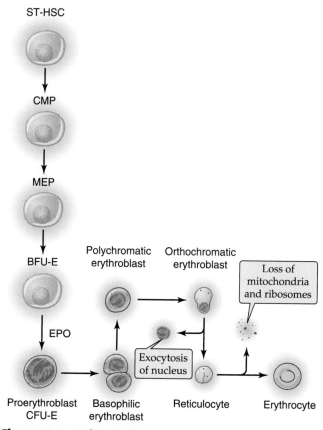

Figure 18-5 Erythropoiesis.

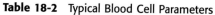

Table 18-2 Typical Blood Cell Parameters

Red cell count (10^6/μL blood)	4.0 (female); 4.5 (male)
Hematocrit (%)	40 (female); 45 (male)
Hemoglobin (g/dL blood)	14.0 (female); 15.5 (male)
Mean red cell volume—MCV (fL/cell)	90
Mean red cell hemoglobin—MCH (pg/cell)	30
Mean cell hemoglobin concentration—MCHC (g/dL RBC)	35
Red cell distribution width—RDW (%)	13
White cell count (10^3/μL blood)	8
Platelet count (10^3/μL blood)	300

Red blood cells are mainly composed of hemoglobin

As evidenced by the magnitude of the hematocrit, RBCs are the most abundant elements in blood. RBCs are non-nucleated biconcave cells with a diameter of ~7.5 μm and a volume of ~90 femtoliters (90×10^{-15} L). Maintaining the shape of the RBC is a cytoskeleton that is anchored to the plasma membrane by glycophorin and the $Cl\text{-}HCO_3$ exchanger AE1 (see Fig. 2-9). The distinctive shape of the RBC provides a much larger surface-to-volume ratio than that of a spherical cell, thereby maximizing diffusion area and minimizing intracellular diffusion distances for gas exchange. The RBC performs three major tasks: (1) carrying of O_2 from the lungs to the systemic tissues, (2) carrying of CO_2 from tissues to the lungs, and (3) assisting in the buffering of acids and bases.

Table 18-2 lists the properties of RBCs that are routinely determined in the clinical laboratory. The most important constituent of the RBC is **hemoglobin**. Globin synthesis begins in the proerythroblast (Fig. 18-5). By the end of the orthochromatic-erythroblast stage, the cell has synthesized all the hemoglobin it will carry. Normal blood hemoglobin content is ~14.0 g/dL in the adult woman and ~15.5 g/dL in the adult man. The hemoglobin concentration in red cell cytosol is extremely high, **~5.5 mM**. The mean cell hemoglobin concentration is ~35 g/dL RBC, or about five times the concentration of proteins in plasma. Enclosure of hemoglobin in red cells has the advantage of minimizing the loss of hemoglobin from the plasma through filtration across the blood capillary walls. The structure and various chemical forms of hemoglobin as well as the carriage of O_2 and CO_2 by hemoglobin are discussed in Chapter 29.

Because the mature RBCs contain no nucleus or other organelles, they can neither synthesize proteins nor engage in oxidative metabolism. The RBC can engage in two meta-

stimulation by TPO, the Mpl receptor induces an increase in number and size of megakaryocytes—the cells that produce platelets—thereby greatly augmenting the number of circulating platelets.

Erythropoietin (EPO), which is homologous to TPO, is produced by the kidney and to a lesser extent by the liver. This cytokine supports erythropoiesis or red cell development (Fig. 18-5). As described earlier, hypoxia increases the abundance of the α subunit of the hypoxia-inducible factor 1 (HIF-1α), enhancing production of erythropoietin mRNA. Although EPO is not absolutely required for early commitment of progenitor cells to the erythroid lineage, it is essential for the differentiation of burst-forming unit–erythroid cells (BFU-E) to CFU-E or **proerythroblasts** (also known as pronormoblasts), which still lack hemoglobin. The further maturation of cells downstream of proerythroblasts does not require EPO. Recombinant EPO has proved effective in the treatment of anemia. Hemoglobin first appears at the stage of **polychromatic erythroblasts** and is clearly evident in **orthochromatic erythroblasts**. The subsequent exocytosis of the nucleus produces **reticulocytes** (Fig. 18-5), whereas the loss of ribosomes and mitochondria yields mature erythrocytes, which enter the circulation. The mature erythrocyte has a life span of ~120 days. Immature reticulocytes may also appear in the circulation when erythropoiesis is heavily activated.

bolic pathways: glycolysis, which consumes 90% of glucose uptake; and the pentose shunt (see Chapter 58), which consumes the remaining 10% of glucose. The cell generates its ATP exclusively by glycolysis. An important constituent of the RBC is **2,3-diphosphoglycerate (2,3-DPG)**. RBCs use DPG mutase to convert 1,3-diphosphoglycerate (1,3-DPG), part of the normal glycolytic pathway (see Chapter 58), into 2,3-DPG. In RBCs, the cytosolic concentration of 2,3-DPG is normally 4 to 5 mM, about the same as the concentration of hemoglobin. 2,3-DPG acts on hemoglobin by reducing the O_2 affinity of hemoglobin (see Chapter 29).

Erythrocytes contain **glutathione** at ~2 mM, more than any other cell of the body outside the hepatocyte (see Chapter 46). A high ratio of reduced glutathione (GSH) to oxidized glutathione (GSSG) protects the RBC against oxidant damage. Glutathione reductase regenerates GSH from GSSG in a reaction that consumes NADPH. The RBC generates all its NADPH from the glycolytic intermediate glucose 6-phosphate through the pentose phosphate pathway (see Fig. 58-1).

RBCs carry two cytoplasmic isoforms of **carbonic anhydrase**, CA I and CA II. These enzymes, which rapidly interconvert CO_2 and HCO_3^-, play a critical role in carrying metabolically produced CO_2 from the systemic tissues to the pulmonary capillaries for elimination in the exhaled air. CA II has one of the fastest known enzymatic turnover rates (see Chapter 29).

CO_2 carriage also depends critically on the **Cl-HCO_3 exchanger AE1** (see Chapters 5 and 29) in the RBC membrane. The transporter was originally known as band 3 protein because of its position on an SDS-polyacrylamide gel of RBC membrane proteins. AE1 is the most abundant membrane protein in RBCs, with ~1 million copies per cell. One AE1 molecule can transport as many as 50,000 ions per second—one of the fastest known transporters. AE1 and most other members of the SLC4 family of HCO_3^- transporters are blocked by a disulfonic stilbene known as DIDS.

The **water channel AQP1** (see Chapter 5) is the second most abundant membrane protein in RBCs, with ~200,000 copies per cell. AQP1 appears to contribute more than half of the CO_2 permeability of the RBC membrane (see Chapter 29).

Leukocytes defend against infections

Table 18-3 summarizes the relative abundance of various leukocytes in the blood. These WBCs are in two major groups, the granulocytes on the one hand and the lymphocytes and monocytes on the other. **Granulocytes** are so named because of their cytoplasmic granules, which on a blood smear stained with Giemsa stain or Wright stain appear red (eosinophils), blue (basophils), or intermediate (neutrophils). The nuclear material is irregularly shaped in the form of the letter S or Z. The name *polymorphonuclear leukocytes* applies to all three types of granulocytes but often is used to refer specifically to neutrophils. The average diameter of a neutrophil is 12 μm, smaller than that of a monocyte (14 to 20 μm) or eosinophil (13 μm), somewhat larger than that of a basophil, and much larger than that of a lymphocyte (6 to 10 μm). Granulocytes have a brief life span in the blood (<12 hours) but on activation can migrate into the tissues.

Table 18-3 Leukocytes*

	Count (10^3/μL blood)	Differential Count (%)
Total leukocytes	7.4	100
Neutrophils	4.4	59 (56% segmented, 3% band)
Lymphocytes	2.5	34
Monocytes	0.3	4
Eosinophils	0.2	3
Basophils	0.04	0.5

*Listed in order of abundance.

Neutrophils   The most abundant leukocytes, neutrophils are identified on the basis of the shape of the nucleus as mature *segmented neutrophils* (56% of leukocytes) and immature *band neutrophils* (3% of leukocytes). Segmented neutrophils have at least two lobes separated by a thin filament, whereas band neutrophils have a nucleus of more uniform thickness. Neutrophils have two types of granules (specific and azurophilic) that contain lysosomal enzymes, peroxidase, collagenase, and other enzymes capable of digesting foreign material. In the presence of a chemotactic attractant, neutrophils approach foreign substances, such as bacteria, to phagocytose them within a phagocytic vacuole. By a process known as degranulation, granules merge with the vacuole and empty their contents into the vacuole. Bacteria are destroyed within the vacuole by the action of hydrogen peroxide (H_2O_2) and superoxide anion radical (O_2^-).

Eosinophils   The granules of eosinophils contain **major basic protein (MBP)**, which is toxic to parasites, as well as other enzymes. These cells are important in the response to parasites and viruses. Eosinophils also play a role in allergic reactions.

Basophils   These cells, the least common granulocytes, are a major source of the cytokine IL-4, which in turn stimulates B lymphocytes to produce IgE antibodies. The granules—which nearly obscure the nucleus—contain histamine, heparin, and peroxidase. Like eosinophils, basophils also play a role in allergic reactions.

Lymphocytes   Like the monocytes discussed next, lymphocytes do not have granules. Although they cannot be distinguished in a blood smear, lymphocytes come in different classes. The lymphocyte precursors originate in the bone marrow, where lineage commitment occurs.

T lymphocytes or T cells, which represent 70% to 80% of peripheral lymphocytes in blood, undergo maturation primarily in the *thymus*. T lymphocytes are responsible for cell-mediated immunity.

B lymphocytes or B cells, which represent 10% to 15% of peripheral lymphocytes in blood, undergo maturation in *bone* marrow and peripheral lymphoid tissue. When B cells interact with antigen in the presence of T cells and macrophages, B cells can transform into **plasma cells**, which abundantly make and secrete antibodies that are directed against specific antigens. Thus, B cells are responsible for humoral immunity.

The remaining lymphocytes in blood include a variety of classes, such as the natural killer cells.

Monocytes Because they migrate from the bone marrow to peripheral tissues, monocytes are not abundant in blood. Rather, monocytes spend most of their long life in peripheral tissues, where they develop into larger macrophages (20 to 40 μm in diameter). The **macrophage** (from the Greek *macros* [large] + *phagein* [eat]) serves two functions: (1) the phagocytosis of pathogens or cellular debris and (2) the presentation of antigens to lymphocytes.

Platelets are nucleus-free fragments

Platelets form in the bone marrow by budding off from large cells called **megakaryocytes**, the maturation of which depends on TPO and IL-3. Each megakaryocyte can produce up to a few thousand platelets. Normal blood contains 150,000 to 450,000 platelets per microliter. A feedback mechanism operates between platelets and megakaryocytes, controlling platelet production. Platelets carry receptors for TPO that are able to bind and remove TPO from the plasma. Thus, a hypoplastic marrow generating few megakaryocytes leads to **thrombocytopenia** (platelet shortage) and thereby little removal of TPO, which in turn stimulates megakaryocyte production and corrects the lack of platelets. Conversely, a hyperplastic marrow creating many megakaryocytes leads to **thrombocytosis** (platelet excess) and thereby greater TPO removal, which ultimately turns off megakaryocyte production.

The life span of platelets is about 10 days. In their unactivated state, these nucleus-free fragments are disk shaped and 2 to 3 μm in diameter (Fig. 18-6). The external coat is rich in platelet receptors, which are glycoproteins. A circumferential band of microtubules composed of tubulin provides an inner skeleton. Actin and myosin contractile filaments are present in the platelet interior. In addition to mitochondria, lysosomes, and peroxisomes, platelets have two types of special organelles: α granules and, less abundantly, dense-core granules. The **α granules** store von Willebrand factor, platelet fibrinogen, and clotting factor V. The fibrinogen inside the platelets actually originates in the liver, which secretes it into the blood plasma, where megakaryocytes and platelets then endocytose the fibrinogen. The **dense-core granules** store ATP, ADP, serotonin, and Ca^{2+}. As discussed later, platelets are essential for hemostasis.

BLOOD VISCOSITY

Poiseuille's equation (see Equation 17-9) is based on several important assumptions. In Chapter 17, we considered the first five, and here we consider the sixth, whether the viscosity of whole blood is constant in a newtonian sense.

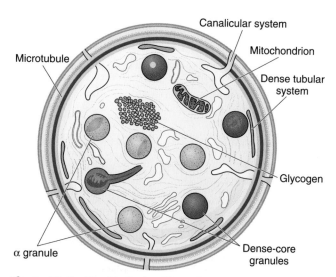

Figure 18-6 Discoid platelet. The surface-connected canalicular system is continuous with the endoplasmic reticulum. *(Redrawn from White JG. In Bloom AL, Forbes CD, Thomas DP, Tuddenham EGD [eds]: Haemostasis and Thrombosis, 3rd ed. New York, Churchill Livingstone, 1994.)*

Whole blood has an anomalous viscosity

Water and saline solutions are homogeneous or newtonian liquids. For these, the relationship between shear stress (force needed to move one lamina faster than its neighbor) and shear rate (velocity gradient between laminae) is linear and passes through the origin (Fig. 18-7, blue line). Viscosity (see Equation 17-12) is the slope of this line. The shear stress to shear rate relationship for a non-newtonian fluid, such as latex house paint, is nonlinear. Blood plasma (Fig. 18-7, yellow line) and serum are nearly newtonian. However, normal *whole blood is non-newtonian*; it has a nonlinear shear stress to shear rate relationship that intersects the y-axis above the origin (Fig. 18-7, red curve). In other words, one has to apply some threshold force (i.e., the yield shear stress) before the fluid will move at all. At lower forces, the fluid is immobile. However, at higher shear rates (such as those achieved physiologically after the velocity of blood flow has increased sufficiently), the relationship between shear stress and shear rate assumes the newtonian ideal, with a slope that corresponds to a viscosity of ~3.2 cP.

The concept of yield shear stress can best be understood by comparing two familiar viscous solutions: honey and mayonnaise. By estimating the effort needed to stir a pot of honey or a jar of mayonnaise with a spoon, one might assume that their apparent viscosity is the same because each solution offers about the same resistance to deformation. However, with use of a more modest deforming force, such as gravity, a striking difference between the two fluids emerges. As one removes the spoon from the pot of honey, gravity causes the honey to drip from the spoon in a continuous stream. In contrast, a glob of mayonnaise stays attached to the spoon. The velocity of the mayonnaise is zero because its yield shear stress is greater than the force of gravity. Honey is a newtonian fluid that behaves similarly at

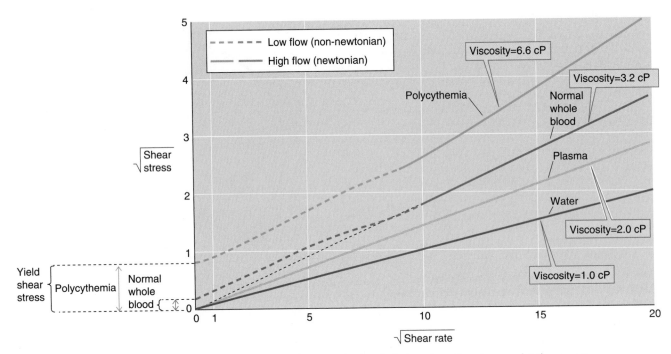

Figure 18-7 Anomalous viscosity of blood. To emphasize deviations from linearity, we plot the square roots of shear stress (Force/Area) and shear rate ($\Delta v/\Delta x$). cP, centipoise.

low and high forces of deformation. Mayonnaise is similar to blood in that its viscosity appears to be infinite at low forces of deformation.

Blood viscosity increases with the hematocrit and the fibrinogen plasma concentration

In practice, the effective viscosity of whole blood depends on several physiological factors: (1) fibrinogen concentration, (2) hematocrit, (3) vessel radius, (4) linear velocity, and (5) temperature. As noted previously, the viscosity of whole blood in the linear (or newtonian) region of Figure 18-7 is ~3.2 cP, assuming a typical fibrinogen concentration of 260 mg/dL, a hematocrit of 40%, and a temperature of 37°C. We will now see how each of these five factors influences the viscosity of blood.

Fibrinogen Fibrinogen, a major protein component of human plasma, is a key element in the coagulation cascade. The main reason for the non-newtonian behavior of blood is the interaction of this fibrinogen with RBCs. Thus, plasma (which contains fibrinogen but not RBCs) is newtonian, as is a suspension of washed RBCs in saline (without fibrinogen). However, the simultaneous presence of fibrinogen and blood cells causes the nonlinear behavior illustrated by the red curve in Figure 18-7. At normal hematocrits, fibrinogen and, perhaps, low-density lipoproteins (see Chapter 46), electrophoretically seen as β-lipoproteins, are the only plasma proteins capable of creating a yield shear stress.

At normal hematocrits, the absence of fibrinogen (in congenital afibrinogenemia) eliminates the yield shear stress altogether. Conversely, hyperfibrinogenemia elevates yield shear stress and, in the extreme, leads to a clustering of RBCs that increases their effective density. This increased effective

density, in turn, causes the RBCs to settle toward the bottom of a vertical tube—easily measured as an increased **erythrocyte sedimentation rate** (see the box). Note that fibrinogen levels tend to increase with age and with smoking.

Erythrocyte Sedimentation Rate

Almost any acute stress to the body (trauma, infection, disease) induces a reaction called the **acute-phase response**. During the course of several hours, in response to inflammatory cytokines, the liver rapidly synthesizes and secretes into the circulatory system a number of proteins that aid in the host response to the threat. Among these proteins is fibrinogen, which causes RBCs to cluster and increases their effective density. When anticoagulated blood from a patient with hyperfibrinogenemia is placed in a glass tube, the RBCs fall more quickly under the influence of gravity than when the blood is from a healthy subject. After 1 hour, this sedimentation leaves a layer of clear plasma on the top of the tube (≤15 mm thick for normal blood and often >40 mm thick in certain inflammatory disorders). This rate of fall is called the erythrocyte sedimentation rate (ESR). Although it is nonspecific because so many different conditions can cause it to increase, the ESR is still widely used by clinicians to assess the presence and severity of inflammation. It is a simple technique, easily performed in a physician's office. As an example of its utility, a patient with an inflammatory process that naturally waxes and wanes, such as lupus erythematosus, may present with nonspecific complaints such as fatigue, weakness, and achiness. An elevated ESR would suggest that these complaints are due to the reactivation of the disease and not just to a poor night's sleep or depression.

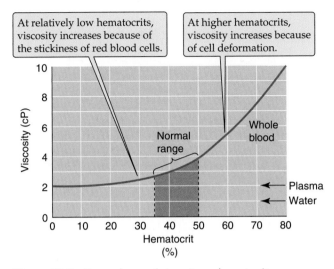

Figure 18-8 Dependence of viscosity on hematocrit.

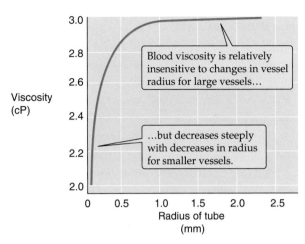

Figure 18-9 Dependence of viscosity on vessel radius.

Hematocrit   Increases in hematocrit elevate blood viscosity by two mechanisms (Fig. 18-8); one prevails at physiological hematocrits, the other at higher hematocrits. Starting from values of 30%, raising of the hematocrit increases the interactions among RBCs—both directly and by proteins such as fibrinogen—and thereby increases viscosity. The reason is that forcing two RBCs more closely together at higher hematocrits makes them more likely to stick to each other. At hematocrits above 60%, the cells are so tightly packed that further increases lead to cell-cell interactions that increasingly deform the RBCs, thereby increasing viscosity. In patients with polycythemia, not only is viscosity high, but the yield stress can be more than 4-fold higher than normal (Fig. 18-7, green curve). Obviously, the combination of a high hematocrit and a high fibrinogen level can be expected to lead to extremely high viscosities.

Vessel Radius   In reasonably large vessels (radius > ~1 mm), blood viscosity is independent of vessel radius (Fig. 18-9). However, the viscosity decreases steeply at lower radii. This Fahraeus-Lindqvist phenomenon has four major causes.

Poiseuille observed not only that RBCs move faster in the center of an arteriole or venule than at the periphery but also that the *concentration* of RBCs is greater at the center. Indeed, very near the wall, he observed a "transparent space" occupied only by plasma (Fig. 18-10A). This axial accumulation of RBCs occurs because the plasma imparts a spin to an erythrocyte caught between two layers of plasma sliding past one another at different velocities (see Fig. 17-5B). This spin causes the cell to move toward the center of the vessel, much like a billiard ball curves when struck off center (Fig. 18-10A, inset of upper panel). One consequence of axial accumulation is that local viscosity is lowest in the cell-poor region near the vessel wall and greatest in the cell-enriched core. The net effect in smaller vessels is that the overall viscosity of the blood is *decreased* because the cell-poor plasma (low intrinsic viscosity) moves to the periphery where the shearing forces are the greatest, whereas the cell-enriched blood (high intrinsic viscosity) is left along the central axis where the shearing forces are least. A second consequence of axial

accumulation is that branch vessels preferentially skim the plasma (plasma skimming) from the main stream of the parent vessel, leading to a lower hematocrit in branch vessels. However, some anatomical sites prevent skimming by means of an arterial cushion (Fig. 18-10A, lower panel).

Poiseuille's equation does not hold in vessels small enough to hold only a few RBCs in their cross section. Hagen's derivation of the equation assumes an infinite number of concentric laminae inside the vessel. In reality, a lamina can be no smaller than the thickness of an erythrocyte, thus severely limiting the number of laminae in small vessels (Fig. 18-10B). If we were to re-derive a Poiseuille-like equation to model a small vessel, it would predict a viscosity that is *lower* than that predicted by Poiseuille's equation for a large vessel.

In vessels (e.g., capillaries) so small that their diameter is about the size of a single erythrocyte, we can no longer speak of the friction between concentric laminae. Instead, in small capillaries, the membrane of the RBC rolls around the cytoplasm in a movement called tank treading, similar to that of the track of a bulldozer (Fig. 18-10C). As two treading erythrocytes shoot down a capillary, they spin the bolus of plasma trapped between them (bolus flow).

In vessels smaller than an erythrocyte, highly deformed—literally bullet-shaped—RBCs squeeze through the capillaries, making the effective viscosity fall even farther below that of the bulk solution (Fig. 18-10D). Under these conditions, a layer of plasma separates the erythrocytes from the capillary wall. The cells automatically "focus" themselves to the centerline of the capillary and maintain a fixed distance between two successive cells.

Velocity of Flow   As for an ideal fluid (see Fig. 17-6A), the dependence of flow on pressure is linear for blood *plasma* (Fig. 18-11, gold curve). However, for *whole blood*, the pressure-flow relationship deviates slightly from linearity at velocities close to zero, and the situation is even worse for polycythemia. These deviations at very low flows have two explanations. First, at low flows, the shear rate is also low, causing the whole blood (like mayonnaise) to behave in a non-newtonian manner (Fig. 18-7) and to have a high apparent viscosity. In fact, as was already seen, one must apply a threshold force to get the blood to move at all. Thus, the red

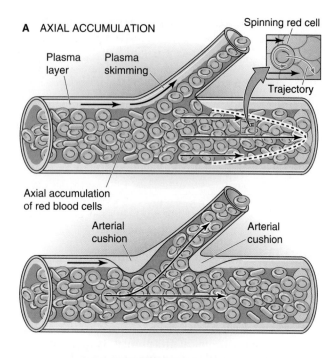

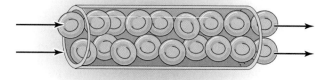

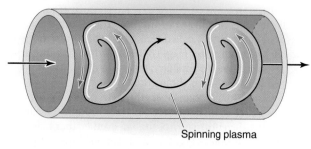

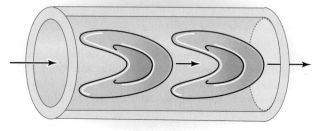

Figure 18-10 Flow of blood in small vessels.

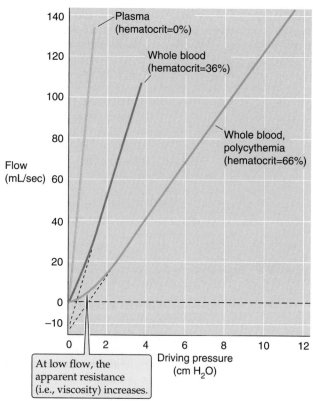

Figure 18-11 Pressure-flow relationships over a range of hematocrits. The slope of the linear portion of each curve is 1/resistance; resistance (or viscosity) increases from plasma to normal whole blood to polycythemic blood.

and green curves in Figure 18-11 have shallower slopes at low flows than at high flows. The second reason for the nonlinear pressure-flow relationship is that the tendency for RBCs to move to the center of the stream—thereby lowering viscosity—requires a modest flow. After this axial accumulation "saturates," however, the relationship becomes linear.

Temperature   Cooling normal whole blood from 37°C to 0°C increases its viscosity ~2.5-fold. However, physiologically, this effect is negligible in humans except during intense cooling of the extremities. On the other hand, in some patients, the presence of **cryoglobulins** in the blood can cause an abnormal rise in viscosity even with less intense cooling of limbs. Cryoglobulins are immunoglobulins that precipitate at a temperature that is less than 37°C but can partially resolubilize on warming. Different cryoglobulins are associated with infections, particularly hepatitis C, as well as with several autoimmune and lymphoproliferative disorders. High blood viscosity from the precipitated cryoglobulins can lead to vessel obstruction and local thrombosis.

HEMOSTASIS AND FIBRINOLYSIS

We have already noted that two essential requirements of the circulatory system are that the blood must be a liquid and that it cannot leak through the walls of the blood vessels. Meeting these two requirements is the job of the fibrinolytic and hemostatic machinery. Blood is normally in a liquid state inside blood vessels because it does not come into contact with negatively charged surfaces (e.g., the collagen beneath endothelial cells) that activate an *intrinsic* coagulation pathway, nor does it contact tissue factors (e.g., released from damaged tissue) that activate an *extrinsic* pathway. Furthermore, thrombolytic pathways keep the coagulation pathways in check. Indeed, plasma contains proteins that can be converted to proteases that digest fibrin and thereby lyse blood clots.

Hemostasis (from the Greek *hemos* [blood] + *stasis* [standing]), or the prevention of hemorrhage, can be achieved by four methods: (1) vasoconstriction, (2) increased tissue pressure, (3) formation of a platelet plug in the case of capillary bleeding, and (4) coagulation or clot formation.

Vasoconstriction contributes to hemostasis because it raises the critical closing pressure—as we discuss in Chapter 19—and thus collapses vessels that have an intravascular pressure below the critical closing pressure. Vessel constriction is also promoted by chemical byproducts of platelet plug formation and of coagulation. For example, activated platelets release the vasoconstrictors thromboxane A_2 (see Chapter 3) and serotonin (see Chapter 13). Moreover, thrombin, a major product of the clotting machinery, triggers the endothelium to generate endothelin 1 (see Chapter 20), the most powerful physiological vasoconstrictor.

Increased tissue pressure contributes to hemostasis because it decreases transmural pressure (see Chapter 17), which is the difference between intravascular pressure and tissue pressure. Transmural pressure is the main determinant of blood vessel radius. Given the fourth-power relationship between flow and blood vessel radius (see Chapter 17), an increase in tissue pressure that causes radius to decrease by a factor of 2 would diminish flow by a factor of 16. We all take advantage of this principle when we press a finger against a small cut to stop the bleeding. A tourniquet increases extravascular pressure and can thus halt an arterial hemorrhage in a limb. Finally, surgeons routinely make use of this principle when applying hemostatic clamps to close off "bleeders."

In this section, we discuss the third and fourth methods of hemostasis, platelet plug formation and coagulation.

Platelets can plug holes in small vessels

In a highly controlled fashion, platelets plug small breaches in the vascular endothelium. Plug formation is a process that includes adhesion, activation, and aggregation.

Adhesion   Platelets normally do not adhere to themselves, to other blood cells, or to endothelial membranes. One preventive factor may be the negative surface charge on both platelets and endothelial cells. In the case of endothelial cells, the negative surface charge reflects the presence of proteoglycans, mainly heparan sulfate. Platelet adhesion occurs in response to an increase in the shearing force (see Chapter 17) at the surface of platelets or endothelial cells and in response to vessel injury or humoral signals.

Platelet adhesion—the binding of platelets to themselves or to other components—is mediated by **platelet receptors**, which are glycoproteins in the platelet membrane. These platelet receptors are integral membrane proteins belonging

to a class of matrix receptors known as integrins (see Chapter 2). They are usually heterodimers linked by disulfide bonds. One ligand naturally present in the blood plasma is **von Willebrand factor (vWF)**, a glycoprotein made by endothelial cells and megakaryocytes. vWF is found in Weibel-Palade bodies of the endothelial cells and in α granules of platelets. High shear, certain cytokines, and hypoxia all trigger the release of vWF from endothelial cells. vWF binds to the platelet receptor known as glycoprotein Ib/Ia (Gp Ib/Ia), which is a dimer of Gp Ib linked to Gp Ia.

A breach of the endothelium exposes platelet receptors to ligands that are components of the subendothelial matrix. These ligands include **collagen**, which binds to Gp Ia/IIa, and **fibronectin** and **laminin** (see Chapter 2), both of which bind to Gp Ic/IIa.

Activation   The binding of these ligands—or of certain other agents (e.g., thrombin) that we will discuss later—triggers a conformational change in the platelet receptors that initiates an intracellular signaling cascade, which leads to an exocytotic event known as the release reaction or platelet activation. The signal transduction cascade involves the activation of phospholipase C (see Chapter 3) and an influx of Ca^{2+}. Activated platelets exocytose the contents of their **dense storage granules**, which include ATP, ADP, serotonin, and Ca^{2+}. Activated platelets also exocytose the contents of their **α granules**, which contain several proteins, including a host of growth factors and three hemostatic factors: vWF (see earlier) and two clotting factors that we will discuss later, clotting factor V and fibrinogen. Activated platelets also use cyclooxygenase (see Chapter 3) to initiate the breakdown of arachidonic acid to thromboxane A_2, which they release. Platelet activation is also associated with marked cytoskeletal and morphological changes as the platelet extends first a broad lamellipodium and then many finger-like filopodia.

Aggregation   Signaling molecules released by activated platelets amplify the platelet activation response. ADP (which binds to P_{2Y12} receptors on platelets), serotonin, and thromboxane A_2 all activate additional platelets, and this recruitment promotes platelet aggregation. Aspirin, an inhibitor of cyclooxygenase, inhibits clotting by reducing the release of thromboxane A_2. Another antiplatelet agent—clopidogrel—acts by inhibiting the P_{2Y12} receptors on the platelet surface. As noted before, vWF released by activated platelets binds to the platelet receptor Gp Ib/Ia, thereby activating even more platelets and forming molecular bridges between platelets. Platelet activation also induces a conformational change in Gp IIb/IIIa, another platelet receptor, endowing it with the capacity to bind fibrinogen. Thus, as a result of the conformational change in Gp IIb/IIIa, the fibrinogen that is always present in blood forms bridges between platelets and thus participates in the formation of a platelet plug. As we will see later, when it is cleaved by thrombin, fibrinogen also plays a critical role in clotting.

A controlled cascade of proteolysis creates a blood clot

A **blood clot** is a semisolid mass composed of both platelets and fibrin and—entrapped in the mesh of fibrin—erythrocytes, leukocytes, and serum. A **thrombus** is also a blood clot, but the term is usually reserved for an *intravascular* clot. Thus, the blood clot formed at the site of a skin wound would usually not be called a thrombus. The relative composition of thrombi varies with the site of **thrombosis** (i.e., thrombus formation). A higher proportion of platelets is present in clots of the arterial circulation, whereas a higher proportion of fibrin is present in clots of the venous circulation.

Platelet plug formation and blood clotting are related but distinct events that may occur in parallel or in the absence of the other. As we will see later, activated platelets can release small amounts of some of the factors (e.g., Ca^{2+}) that play a role in blood clotting. Conversely, as we have already noted, some clotting factors (e.g., thrombin and fibrinogen) play a role in platelet plug formation. Thus, molecular crosstalk between the machinery involved in platelet plug formation and clot formation helps coordinate hemostasis.

The cardiovascular system normally maintains a precarious balance between two pathological states. On the one hand, inadequate clotting would lead to the leakage of blood from the vascular system and, ultimately, to hypovolemia. On the other hand, overactive clotting would lead to thrombosis and, ultimately, to cessation of blood flow. The cardiovascular system achieves this balance between an antithrombotic (anticoagulant) and a prothrombotic (procoagulant) state by a variety of components of the vascular wall and blood. Promoting an antithrombotic state is a normal layer of endothelial cells, which line all luminal surfaces of the vascular system. Promoting a prothrombotic state are events associated with vascular damage: (1) the failure of endothelial cells to produce the proper antithrombotic factors and (2) the physical removal or injury of endothelial cells, which permits the blood to come into contact with thrombogenic factors that lie beneath the endothelium. Also promoting a prothrombotic state is the activation of platelets by any of the ligands that bind to platelet receptors, as discussed earlier. For instance, as platelets flow past artificial mechanical heart valves, the shearing forces can activate the platelets.

According to the classical view, two distinct sequences can precipitate coagulation: the intrinsic pathway and the extrinsic pathway. It is the intrinsic pathway that becomes activated when blood comes into contact with a negatively charged surface—in the laboratory, we can mimic this process by putting blood into a glass test tube. The extrinsic pathway is activated when blood comes in contact with material from damaged cell membranes. In both cases, the precipitating event triggers a chain reaction that converts precursors into activated factors, which in turn catalyze the conversion of other precursors into other activated factors, and so on. Most of these "precursors" are zymogens that give rise to "activated factors" that are serine proteases. Thus, *controlled proteolysis* plays a central role in amplifying the clotting signals. However, the cascades do not occur in the fluid phase of the blood, where the concentration of each of these factors is low. In the case of the intrinsic pathway, the chain reaction occurs mainly at the membrane of activated platelets. In the case of the extrinsic pathway, the reactions occur mainly at a "tissue factor" that is membrane bound. Both pathways

converge on a **common pathway** that culminates in generation of thrombin and, ultimately, "stable" fibrin. Table 18-4 summarizes the names, synonyms, and properties of the procoagulant and anticoagulant factors in various parts of the clotting scheme.

The proteins of the coagulation cascade have a distinct domain structure, including a signal peptide, a propeptide, an EGF-like domain, a kringle domain, and a catalytic domain, whereas some other domains are variable among these proteins. The **signal peptide** domain is required for the translocation of the polypeptide into the endoplasmic reticulum, where the signal peptide is cleaved. The **propeptide** or γ-carboxyglutamic acid–rich domain (Gla domain) is rich in glutamic acid residues that undergo γ-carboxylation under the influence of the γ-carboxylase that is vitamin K dependent. The presence of these γ-carboxyglutamic acid residues is required for Ca^{2+} binding. The **epidermal growth factor–like (EGF-like)** domain may appear multiple times and play a role in forming protein complexes. The **kringle** domain is a loop structure created by several disulfide bonds that also play a role in forming protein complexes and attaching the protease to its target. The **catalytic** domain confers the serine protease function to the coagulation proteins and is homologous to trypsin, chymotrypsin, and other serine proteases.

Intrinsic Pathway (Surface Contact Activation)   The left branch of Figure 18-12 shows the intrinsic pathway, a cascade of protease reactions initiated by factors that are all present within blood. When it is in contact with a negatively charged surface such as glass or the membrane of an activated platelet, a plasma protein called factor XII (Hageman factor) can become **factor XIIa**—the suffix -a indicates that this is the *activated* form of factor XII. A molecule called **high-molecular-weight kininogen (HMWK)**, a product of platelets that may in fact be attached to the platelet membrane, helps anchor factor XII to the charged surface and thus serves as a cofactor. However, this HMWK-assisted conversion of factor XII to factor XIIa is limited in speed. Once a small amount of factor XIIa accumulates, this protease converts prekallikrein to kallikrein, with HMWK as an anchor. In turn, the newly produced **kallikrein** accelerates the conversion of factor XII to factor XIIa—an example of positive feedback. In Chapter 23, we see another example of an interaction between kallikreins and kininogens (e.g., HMWK), in which the proteolytic activity of kallikreins on kininogens leads to the release of small vasodilatory peptides called kinins.

In addition to amplifying its own generation by forming kallikrein, factor XIIa (together with HMWK) also proteolytically cleaves factor XI to factor XIa. In turn, factor XIa (also bound to the charged surface by HMWK) proteolytically cleaves factor IX (Christmas factor) to factor IXa, which is a protease. Factor IXa and two downstream products of the cascade—factors Xa and, most important, thrombin—proteolytically cleave factor VIII to factor VIIIa, a cofactor in the next reaction. Finally, factors IXa and VIIIa together with Ca^{2+} (which may come largely from activated platelets) and negatively charged phospholipids form a trimolecular complex called tenase. **Tenase** then converts factor X (Stuart factor) to factor Xa, yet another protease.

Extrinsic Pathway (Tissue Factor Activation)   The right branch of Figure 18-12 shows the extrinsic pathway, a cascade of protease reactions initiated by factors that are outside the vascular system. Nonvascular cells constitutively express an integral membrane protein called **tissue factor** (tissue thromboplastin, or factor III), which is a receptor for a plasma protein called factor VII. When an injury to the endothelium allows factor VII to come into contact with tissue factor, the tissue factor nonproteolytically activates factor VII to factor VIIa. Subsequently, tissue factor, factor VIIa, and Ca^{2+} form a trimolecular complex analogous to tenase. Like tenase, the trimolecular complex of [tissue factor + factor VIIa + Ca^{2+}] proteolytically cleaves the proenzyme factor X to factor Xa. An interesting feature is that when factor X binds to the trimolecular complex, factor VIIa undergoes a conformational change that prevents it from dissociating from tissue factor.

Regardless of whether factor Xa arises by the intrinsic or extrinsic pathway, the cascade proceeds along the common pathway.

Common Pathway   Factor Xa from either the intrinsic or extrinsic pathway is the first protease of the common pathway

(center of Fig. 18-12). Reminiscent of the conversion of factor VIII to the cofactor VIIIa in the intrinsic pathway, the downstream product thrombin clips factor V to form the cofactor Va. Factor V is highly homologous to factor VIII, and in both cases, the proteolytic activation clips a single protein into two peptides that remain attached to one another. Factors Xa and Va, together with Ca^{2+} and phospholipids, form yet another trimolecular complex called **prothrombinase**. Prothrombinase acts on a plasma protein called prothrombin to form thrombin.

Thrombin is the central protease of the coagulation cascade, responsible for three major kinds of actions:

1. **Activation of downstream components in the clotting cascade.** The main action of thrombin is to catalyze the proteolysis of fibrinogen by cleaving the Aα chain, releasing fibrinopeptide A, and cleaving the Bβ chain, releasing fibrinopeptide B. The release of the fibrinopeptide results in the formation of fibrin monomers that are still soluble. **Fibrin monomers** now composed of α, β, and γ chains then spontaneously polymerize to form a *gel* of **fibrin polymers** that traps blood cells. Thrombin also activates factor XIII to factor XIIIa, which mediates the covalent

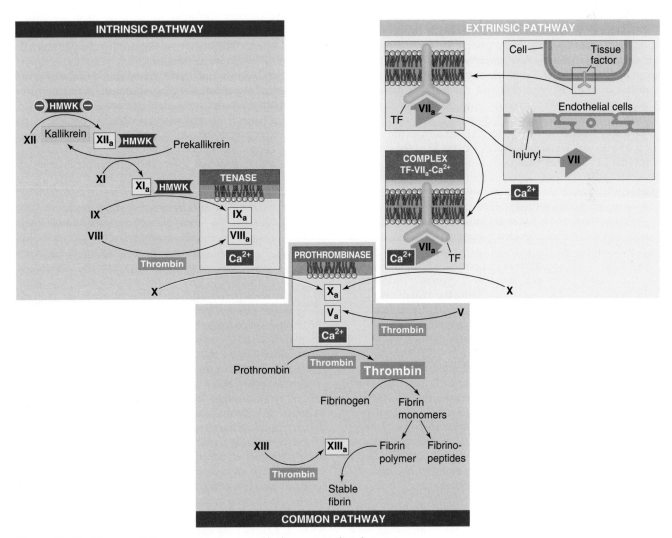

Figure 18-12   The coagulation cascade, showing only the procoagulant factors.

cross-linking of the α and γ chains of fibrin polymers to form a *mesh* called **stable fibrin** that is even less soluble than fibrin polymers.

2. **Positive feedback at several upstream levels of the cascade.** Thrombin can catalyze the formation of new thrombin from prothrombin and can also catalyze the formation of the cofactors Va and VIIIa.

3. **Paracrine actions that influence hemostasis.** First, thrombin causes endothelial cells to release nitric oxide, PGI₂, ADP, vWF, and tissue plasminogen activator (see later). Second, thrombin can activate platelets through PAR-1, a protease-activated receptor that belongs to the family of G protein–coupled receptors (see Chapter 3). Thus, thrombin is a key part of the molecular crosstalk introduced earlier between platelet activation and blood clotting, both of which are required for optimal clot formation. On the one hand, thrombin is a strong catalyst for platelet activation, and on the other hand, activated platelets offer the optimal surface for the intrinsic pathway leading to additional thrombin generation.

Coagulation as a Connected Diagram   The concept of independent intrinsic and extrinsic branches converging on a common pathway is becoming obsolete. In such a "branching tree" (see Chapter 25), multiple branches converge to form larger downstream branches, eventually converging on a single "trunk"—with no crosstalk between branches. However, coagulation is best conceptualized as a "connected diagram" (see Chapter 25) in which the branches may interconnect in both the upstream and downstream directions. One example of interconnections is thrombin's multiple actions just discussed. Another example is the trimolecular complex of [tissue factor + factor VIIa + Ca²⁺] of the extrinsic pathway, which activates factors IX and XI of the intrinsic pathway. In the other direction, factors IXa and Xa of the intrinsic pathway can activate factor VII of the extrinsic pathway. Thus, the intrinsic pathway and extrinsic pathway are strongly interconnected to form a *network*.

What parts of this network are most important for coagulation in vivo? Clinical evidence suggests that coagulation depends largely on the extrinsic pathway. Although tissue factor is normally absent from intravascular cells, inflammation can trigger peripheral blood monocytes and endothelial cells to express tissue factor, increasing the risk of coagulation. Indeed, during sepsis, the tissue factor produced by circulating monocytes initiates intravascular thrombosis.

Anticoagulants keep the clotting network in check

Thus far, our discussion has focused on the coagulation cascade and attendant positive feedback. Just as important are the mechanisms that prevent hemostasis from running out of control. Endothelial cells are the main sources of the agents that help maintain normal blood fluidity. These agents are of two general types, paracrine factors and anticoagulant factors.

Paracrine Factors   Endothelial cells generate prostacyclin (PGI₂; see Chapter 3), which promotes vasodilation (see Chapter 20) and thus blood flow and also inhibits platelet activation and thus clotting. Stimulated by thrombin, endothelial cells also produce nitric oxide (see Chapter 3). Through cGMP, nitric oxide inhibits platelet adhesion and aggregation.

Anticoagulant Factors   As summarized in Figure 18-13, endothelial cells also generate anticoagulant factors that interfere with the clotting cascade that generates fibrin. Table 18-4 lists these factors.

1. **Tissue factor pathway inhibitor (TFPI).** TFPI is a plasma protein that binds to the trimolecular complex [tissue factor + factor VIIa + Ca²⁺] in the extrinsic pathway and blocks the protease activity of factor VIIa. TFPI is GPI linked (see Chapter 2) to the endothelial cell membrane, where it maintains an antithrombotic surface.

2. **Antithrombin III (AT III).** AT III binds to and inhibits factor Xa and thrombin. The sulfated glycosaminoglycans (see Chapter 2) **heparan sulfate** and **heparin** enhance the binding of AT III to factor Xa or to thrombin, thus inhibiting coagulation. Heparan sulfate is present on the external surface of most cells, including endothelial surfaces. Mast cells and basophils release heparin.

3. **Thrombomodulin.** A glycosaminoglycan product of endothelial cells, thrombomodulin can form a complex with thrombin, thereby removing thrombin from the circulation and inhibiting coagulation. In addition, thrombomodulin also binds protein C.

4. **Protein C.** After protein C binds to the thrombomodulin portion of the thrombin-thrombomodulin complex, the thrombin activates protein C. Activated protein C (Ca) is a protease. Together with its cofactor protein S, Ca inactivates the cofactors Va and VIIIa, thus inhibiting coagulation.

5. **Protein S.** This is the cofactor of protein C and is thus an anticoagulant.

Finally, clearance of activated clotting factors by the Kuppfer cells of the liver also keeps hemostasis under control.

Fibrinolysis breaks up clots

As noted earlier, cross-linked stable fibrin traps red and white blood cells as well as platelets in a freshly formed thrombus. Through the interaction of actin and myosin in the platelets, the clot shrinks to a plug and thereby expels serum. After plug formation, fibrinolysis—the breakdown of stable fibrin—breaks up the clot in a more general process known as thrombolysis. As shown in Figure 18-14, the process of fibrinolysis begins with the conversion of plasminogen to plasmin, catalyzed by one of two activators: tissue-type plasminogen activator or urokinase-type plasminogen activator. Table 18-5 summarizes the properties of fibrinolytic factors.

The source of **tissue plasminogen activator (t-PA)**, a serine protease, is endothelial cells. t-PA consists of a single peptide chain with two kringles at the N-terminal portion of the molecule and a protease motif in the C-terminal portion. Kringles are loop structures created by three disulfide bonds and serve to anchor the molecule to its substrate.

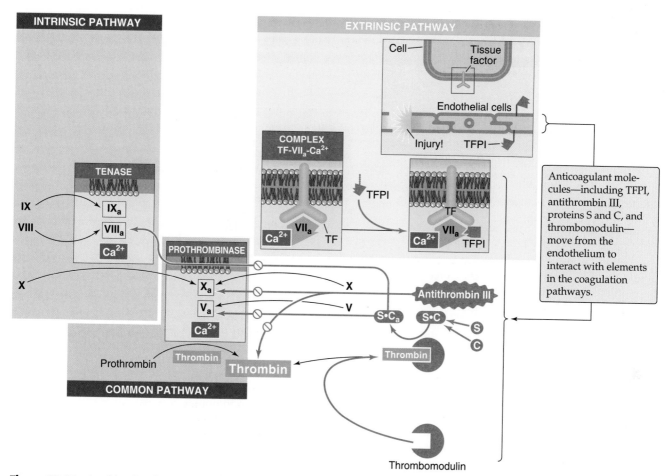

Figure 18-13 An abbreviated version of the coagulation cascade, showing the anticoagulant factors. The anticoagulant pathways are indicated in *red*.

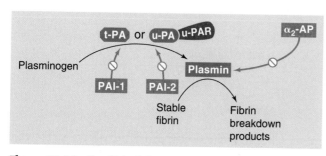

Figure 18-14 The fibrinolytic cascade.

t-PA converts the plasma zymogen plasminogen to the active fibrinolytic protease plasmin. The presence of fibrin greatly accelerates the conversion of plasminogen to plasmin.

Besides t-PA, the other plasminogen activator, **urokinase-type plasminogen activator (u-PA)**, is present in plasma either as a single-chain protein or as the two-chain product of a proteolytic cleavage. Like t-PA, u-PA converts plasminogen to the active protease plasmin. However, this proteolysis requires that u-PA attach to a receptor on the cell surface called urokinase plasminogen activator receptor (u-PAR).

Plasminogen, mainly made by the liver, is a large, single-chain glycoprotein that is composed of an N-terminal heavy chain (A chain) and a C-terminal light chain (B chain). The N-terminal heavy chain contains five kringles, and the C-terminal light chain contains the protease domain. t-PA cleaves plasminogen at the junction between the heavy and light chains, yielding plasmin. However, the two chains in plasmin remain connected by disulfide bonds.

Plasmin is a serine protease that can break down both fibrin and fibrinogen. The five kringles of the heavy chain of plasminogen are still present in plasmin. These anchors attach to lysine residues on fibrin, holding the protease portion of the molecule in place to promote hydrolysis. Plasmin proteolytically cleaves stable fibrin to fibrin breakdown products. Plasmin can also cleave t-PA between the kringle and protease motifs of t-PA. The C terminus of single-chain t-PA nonetheless retains its protease activity.

The cardiovascular system regulates fibrinolysis at several levels, using both enhancing and inhibitory mechanisms. Catecholamines and bradykinin increase the levels of circulating t-PA. Two *serine protease inhibitors* (serpins) reduce the activity of the plasminogen activators: plasminogen activator inhibitor 1 (PAI-1) and plasminogen activator inhibitor 2 (PAI-2). **PAI-1** complexes with and inhibits both single-chain and two-chain t-PA as well as u-PA. PAI-1 is

Table 18-4 Procoagulant and Anticoagulant Factors

Name	Alternate Names	Properties
Procoagulant Factors		
Factor I	Fibrinogen	A plasma globulin
Factor Ia	Fibrin	
Factor II	Prothrombin	A plasma α_2-globulin Synthesis in liver requires vitamin K*
Factor IIa	Thrombin	A serine protease
Factor III (cofactor)	Tissue factor Tissue thromboplastin	An integral membrane glycoprotein; member of type II cytokine receptor family Receptor for factor VIIa Must be present in a phospholipid membrane for procoagulant activity
Factor IV	Ca^{2+}	
Factor V	Labile factor Proaccelerin Accelerator globulin	A plasma protein synthesized by liver and stored in platelets Single-chain protein
Factor Va (cofactor)		Heterodimer held together by a single Ca^{2+} ion Highly homologous to factor VIIIa
Factor VII	Stable factor Serum prothrombin conversion accelerator (SPCA) Proconvertin	A plasma protein Synthesis in liver requires vitamin K*
Factor VIIa		A serine protease
Factor VIII	Antihemophilic factor (AHF) Factor VIII procoagulant component (FVIII:C)	A plasma protein with phospholipid binding domain
Factor VIIIa (cofactor)		Highly homologous to factor Va
Factor IX	Christmas factor Plasma thromboplastin component (PTC)	A plasma protein Synthesis in liver requires vitamin K*
Factor IXa		A protease Disulfide-linked heterodimer
Factor X	Stuart factor	A plasma glycoprotein Synthesis in liver requires vitamin K*
Factor Xa		A protease
Factor XI	Plasma thromboplastin antecedent (PTA)	A plasma protein produced by megakaryocytes and stored in platelets
Factor XIa		A protease Disulfide-linked homodimer
Factor XII	Hageman factor (HAF)	A plasma glycoprotein
Factor XIIa		A protease
Factor XIII	Fibrin stabilizing factor (FSF)	A plasma protein stored in platelets

Table 18-4   Procoagulant and Anticoagulant Factors—cont'd

Name	Alternate Names	Properties
Factor XIIIa		A transglutaminase A tetramer of two A chains and two B chains
HMWK	High-molecular-weight kininogen Fitzgerald factor	A plasma protein stored in platelets Kallikrein clips bradykinin from HMWK
Plasma prekallikrein	Fletcher factor Plasma kallikrein precursor	A plasma protein
Plasma kallikrein		A serine protease Kallikrein clips bradykinin from HMWK
von Willebrand factor	vWf	A plasma glycoprotein made by endothelial cells and megakaryocytes Stabilizes factor VIIIa Promotes platelet adhesion and aggregation
Anticoagulant Factors		
TFPI	Tissue factor pathway inhibitor	Protease inhibitor produced by endothelial cells GPI linked to the cell membrane
Antithrombin III	AT III	A plasma protein Serine protease inhibitor, member of serpin family Inhibits factor Xa and thrombin, and probably also factors XIIa, XIa, and IXa Heparan and heparin enhance the inhibitory action
Thrombomodulin (cofactor)		Glycosaminoglycan on surface of endothelial cell Binds thrombin and promotes activation of protein C
Protein C	Anticoagulant protein C Autoprothrombin IIA	A plasma protein Synthesis in liver requires vitamin K*
Protein Ca		A serine protease Disulfide-linked heterodimer
Protein S (cofactor)		A plasma protein Synthesis in liver requires vitamin K* Cofactor for protein C

*See Chapter 46 for a discussion of vitamin K.

produced mainly by endothelial cells. **PAI-2** mainly inhibits u-PA. PAI-2 is important only in pregnancy as it is produced by the placenta and may contribute to increased risk of thrombosis in pregnancy.

It is of interest that activated protein C, which inhibits coagulation as shown in Figure 18-13, also inhibits PAI-1 and PAI-2, thereby facilitating fibrinolysis. Only one serpin targets plasmin, α_2-**antiplasmin** (α_2-**AP**) made by

liver, kidney, and other tissues. When plasmin is not bound to fibrin (i.e., when the plasmin is in free solution), α_2-AP complexes with and thereby readily inactivates plasmin. However, when plasmin is attached to lysine residues on fibrin, the inhibition by α_2-AP is greatly reduced. In other words, the very presence of a clot (i.e., fibrin) promotes the breakdown of the clot (i.e., fibrinolysis).

Table 18-5 Fibrinolytic Factors

Name	Alternate Names	Properties
Tissue-type plasminogen activator	t-PA	A serine protease that catalyzes hydrolysis of plasminogen at the junction between the N-terminal heavy chain and C-terminal light chain N terminus contains two loop structures called kringles
Urokinase-type plasminogen activator	u-PA	A serine protease
Urokinase-type plasminogen activator receptor	u-PAR	Binds to and required for the activity of u-PA
Plasminogen		Single-chain plasma glycoprotein with large N-terminal and small C-terminal domain N terminus contains five kringles
Plasmin	Fibrinolysin	A serine protease
Plasminogen activator inhibitor 1	PAI-1	A serpin (serine protease inhibitor) In plasma and platelets Forms 1 : 1 complex with t-PA in blood
Plasminogen activator inhibitor 2	PAI-2	A serpin (serine protease inhibitor) Detected only in pregnancy
α_2-Antiplasmin	α_2-AP	A serpin (serine protease inhibitor) Forms 1 : 1 complex with plasmin in blood

REFERENCES

Books and Reviews

Abrams CS: Intracellular signaling in platelets. Curr Opin Hematol 2005; 12:401-405.

Haynes RH: Physical basis of the dependence of blood viscosity on tube radius. Am J Physiol 1960; 198:1193-1200.

Maeda N, Shiga T: Velocity of oxygen transfer and erythrocyte rheology. News Physiol Sci 1994; 9:22-27.

Monroe DM, Hoffman M: What does it take to make the perfect clot? Arterioscler Thromb Vasc Biol 2006; 26:41-48.

Weisel JW: Fibrinogen and fibrin. Adv Protein Chem 2005; 70:247-299.

Journal Articles

Bishop JJ, Nance PR, Popel AS, et al: Effect of erythrocyte aggregation on velocity profiles in venules. Am J Physiol Heart Circ Physiol 2001; 280:H222-H236.

Cinar Y, Senyol AM, Duman K: Blood viscosity and blood pressure: Role of temperature and hyperglycemia. Am J Hypertens 2001; 14:433-438.

Fähraeus R, Lindqvist T: The viscosity of the blood in narrow capillary tubes. Am J Physiol 1931; 96:562-568.

Pennica D, Holmes WE, Kohr WJ, et al: Cloning and expression of human tissue-type plasminogen activator cDNA in E. coli. Nature 1983; 301:214-221.

Pietrangelo A, Panduro A, Chowdhury JR, Shafritz DA: Albumin gene expression is down-regulated by albumin or macromolecule infusion in the rat. J Clin Invest 1992; 89:1755-1760.

CHAPTER 19

ARTERIES AND VEINS

Emile L. Boulpaep

THE ARTERIAL DISTRIBUTION AND VENOUS COLLECTION SYSTEMS

Hemodynamics is the study of the physical laws of blood circulation. It therefore addresses the properties of both the "content" (i.e., blood) and the "container" (i.e., blood vessels). In Chapter 18, we discussed the properties of the blood. This chapter is primarily concerned with the properties of the blood vessels. The circulation is not a system of rigid tubes. Moreover, the anatomy and functions of the various segments of the vasculature differ greatly from one to another. Because the function of the circulation is to carry substances all over the body, the circulatory system branches out into a network of billions of tiny capillaries. We can think of the **arteries** as a *distribution system*, the **microcirculation** as a *diffusion and filtration system*, and the **veins** as a *collection system*.

Physical properties of vessels closely follow the level of branching in the circuit

The aorta branches out into billions of capillaries that ultimately regroup into a single vena cava (Fig. 19-1, panel 1). At each level of arborization of the peripheral circulation, the values of several key parameters vary dramatically:

1. Number of vessels at each level of arborization
2. Radius of a typical individual vessel
3. Aggregate cross-sectional area of all vessels at that level
4. Mean linear velocity of blood flow within an individual vessel
5. Flow (i.e., volume/second) through a single vessel
6. Relative blood volume (i.e., the fraction of the body's total blood volume present in all vessels of a given level)
7. Circulation (i.e., transit) time between two points of the circuit
8. Pressure profile along that portion of the circuit
9. Structure of the vascular walls
10. Elastic properties of the vascular walls

We discuss items 1 to 5 in this section and items 6 to 8 in the following two sections. Items 9 and 10 are the subject of the second subchapter.

The **number of vessels** at a particular level of arborization (Table 19-1) increases enormously from a single aorta to ~10^4 small arteries, ~10^7 arterioles, and finally ~4×10^{10} capillaries. However, only about one fourth of all capillaries are normally open to flow at rest. Finally, all of the blood returns to a single vessel where the superior and inferior venae cavae join.

The **radius of an individual vessel** (r_i; Table 19-1) declines as a result of the arborization, decreasing from 1.1 cm in the aorta to a minimum of ~3 μm in the smallest capillaries. Because the **cross-sectional area** of an individual vessel is proportional to the square of the radius, this parameter decreases even more precipitously.

The aggregate cross-sectional area (Table 19-1) at any level of branching is the sum of the single cross-sectional areas of all parallel vessels at that level of branching. That is, it is the area that you would see if you sliced through all of the vessels at the same level of branching in panel 1 of Figure 19-1.

A fundamental law of vessel branching is that at each branch point, the combined cross-sectional area of daughter vessels exceeds the cross-sectional area of the parent vessel. In this process of bifurcation, the steepest increase in total cross-sectional area occurs in the microcirculation (Fig. 19-1, panel 2). A typical **microcirculation** in the smooth muscle and submucosa of the intestine (Fig. 19-2) encompasses a first-order arteriole, several orders of progressively smaller arterioles, capillaries, several orders of venules into which the capillaries empty, and eventually a first-order venule. In humans, the maximum cross-sectional area occurs not at the level of the capillaries but at the "postcapillary" (i.e., fourth-order) venules. Because of anastomoses among capillaries, capillaries only slightly outnumber fourth-order venules, whereas the cross-sectional unit area of each venule is appreciably greater than the area of a capillary. Assuming that only a quarter of the capillaries are usually open, the peak aggregate cross-sectional area of these postcapillary venules can be ~1000-fold greater than the cross section of the parent artery (e.g., aorta), as shown in panel 2 of Figure 19-1.

The profile of the **mean linear velocity** of flow ($\bar{v}$) along a vascular circuit (Fig. 19-1, panel 3) is roughly a mirror image of the profile of the total cross-sectional area.

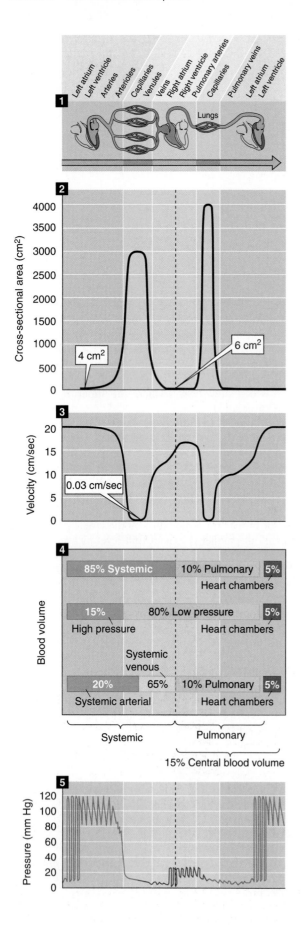

Figure 19-1 Profile of key parameters along the cardiovascular system. Panel 1 *(top)* shows branching of the cardiovascular system, from left side to right side of heart and back to left. Panel 2 shows the variation of aggregate cross-sectional area of all vessels at any level of branching. Panel 3 shows how mean linear velocity of blood varies in typical vessels. Panel 4 shows ways of grouping blood volume in various compartments. Panel 5 shows profile of blood pressure, with superimposed oscillations that represent variations in time.

According to the principle of continuity, which is an application of conservation of mass, **total volume flow** of blood must be the same at any level of arborization. Indeed, as we make multiple vertical slices along the abscissa of panel 1 in Figure 19-1, the aggregate flow for each slice is the same:

$$F_{total} = \underbrace{A_1 \cdot \bar{v}_1}_{\text{Level 1}} = \underbrace{A_2 \cdot \bar{v}_2}_{\text{Level 2}} = \underbrace{A_3 \cdot \bar{v}_3}_{\text{Level 3}} = \dots \qquad \text{(19-1)}$$

As a consequence, $\bar{v}$ must be minimal in the postcapillary venules (~0.03 cm/s), where A_{total} is maximal. Conversely, $\bar{v}$ is maximal in the aorta (~20 to 50 cm/s). Thus, both A_{total} and $\bar{v}$ values range ~1000-fold from the aorta to the capillaries but are inversely related to one another. The vena cava, with a cross-sectional area ~50% larger than that of the aorta, has a mean linear velocity that is about one third less.

Single-vessel flow, in contrast to total flow, ranges by approximately 10 orders of magnitude. In the aorta, the flow is ~83 mL/s, the same as the cardiac output (~5 L/min). When about 25% of the capillaries are open, a *typical* capillary has a mean linear velocity of 0.03 cm/s and a flow of 8×10^{-9} mL/s (8 pL/s)—10 orders of magnitude less than the flow in the aorta. Within the microcirculation, single-vessel flow has considerable range. At one extreme, a first-order arteriole (r_i, ~30 μm) may have a flow of 20×10^{-6} mL/s. At the other, the capillaries that are closed at any given time have zero flow.

Most of the blood volume resides in the systemic veins

The body's **total blood volume** (V) of about 5 L (see Table 5-1) is not uniformly distributed along the x-axis of panel 1 in Figure 19-1. At any level of branching, the total blood volume is the sum of the volumes of all parallel branches. Table 19-2 summarizes—for a hypothetical 70-kg woman—the distribution of total blood volume expressed as both absolute blood volumes and **relative blood volumes** (percentage of total blood volume). Panel 4 in Figure 19-1 summarizes four useful ways of grouping these volumes.

First, we can divide the blood volume into the *systemic* circulation (where ~85% of blood resides), the *pulmonary* circulation (~10%), and the *heart* chambers (~5%). The pulmonary blood volume is quite adjustable (i.e., it can be much higher than 10%) and is carefully regulated.

Second, as can be seen in the next section, we can divide blood volume into what is contained in the *high-pressure* system (~15%), the *low-pressure* system (~80%), and the heart chambers (~5%).

Table 19-1 Key Systemic Vascular Parameters That Vary with Arborization

Parameter	Aorta	Small Arteries*	Arterioles*	Capillaries†	Vena Cava
Number of units (N)	1	8000	2×10^7	1×10^{10} open (4×10^{10} total)	1
Internal radius (r_i)	1.13 cm	0.5 mm	15 µm	3 µm	1.38 cm
Cross-sectional area ($A_i = \pi r_i^2$)	4 cm²	7.9×10^{-3} cm²	7.1×10^{-7} cm²	2.8×10^{-7} cm²	6 cm²
Aggregate cross-sectional area ($A_{total} = N\pi r_i^2$)	4 cm²	63 cm²	141 cm²	2827 cm²‡	6 cm²
Aggregate flow (F_{total})	83 cm³/s (mL/s)	83 cm³/s	83 cm³/s	83 cm³/s	83 cm³/s
Mean linear velocity ($\bar{w} = F_{total}/A_{total}$)	21 cm/s	1.3 cm/s	0.6 cm/s	0.03 cm/s‡	14 cm/s
Single-unit flow ($F_i = F_{total}/N = A_i \cdot \bar{w}$)	83 cm³/s (mL/s)	0.01 cm³/s	4×10^{-6} cm³/s	8×10^{-9} cm³/s‡	83 cm³/s

*The statistics for this column are for a representative generation.
†The values in this column are for the smallest capillaries, at the highest level of branching.
‡Assuming that only 25% of the capillaries are open.

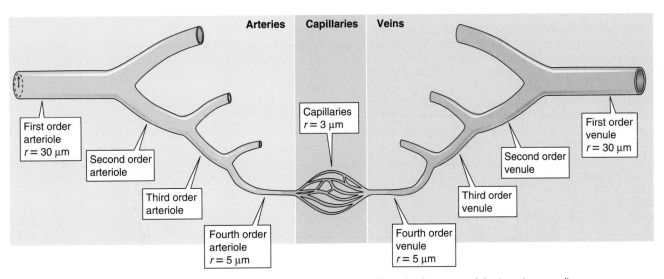

Figure 19-2 Branching in a typical microcirculation, that of the smooth muscle and submucosa of the intestine. *r*, radius.

Third, we can group the blood volumes into those in the *systemic venous system* versus the remainder of the circulation. Of the 85% of the total blood volume that resides in the systemic circulation, about three fourths—or 65% of the total—is on the venous side, particularly in the smaller veins. Thus, the venous system acts as a volume reservoir. Changes in the diameters of veins have a major impact on the amount of blood they contain. For example, an abrupt increase in venous capacity causes pooling of blood in venous segments and may lead to **syncope** (i.e., fainting).

We can also use a fourth approach for grouping of blood volumes—divide the blood into the **central blood volume** (volumes of heart chambers and pulmonary circulation) versus the rest of the circulation. This central blood volume is very adjustable, and it constitutes the filling reservoir for the left side of the heart. Left-sided heart failure can cause the normally careful regulation of the central blood volume to break down.

The **circulation time** is the time required for a bolus of blood to travel either across the entire length of the circula-

Table 19-2 Distribution of Blood Volume*

Region	Absolute Volume (mL)		Relative Volume (%)	
Systemic circulation		4200		84
Aorta and large arteries	300		6.0	
Small arteries	400		8.0	
Capillaries	300		6.0	
Small veins	2300		46.0	
Large veins	900		18	
Pulmonary circulation		440		8.8
Arteries	130		2.6	
Capillaries	110		2.2	
Veins	200		4.0	
Heart (end-diastole)	360	360	7.2	7.2
Total	5000	5000	100	100

*Values are for a 70-kg woman. For a 70-kg man, scale up the absolute values by 10%.

Table 19-3 Mean Pressures in the Systemic and Pulmonary Circulations

Location	Mean Pressure (mm Hg)
Systemic large arteries	95
Systemic arterioles	60
Systemic capillaries	25 (range, 35–15)
Systemic venules	15
Systemic veins	15–3
Pulmonary artery	15
Pulmonary capillaries	10
Pulmonary veins	5

tion or across a particular vascular bed. Total circulation time (the time to go from left to right across panel 1 in Fig. 19-1) is ~1 minute. Circulation time across a single vascular bed (e.g., coronary circulation) may be as short as 10 seconds. Circulation times may be obtained in humans by injection of a substance such as ether into an antecubital vein and measurement of the time to its appearance in the lung (4 to 8 seconds) or by injection of a bitter or sweet substance and measurement of the time to the perception of taste in the tongue (10 to 18 seconds). Although, in the past, circulation time was used clinically as an index of cardiac output, the measurement has little physiological significance. The rationale for determination of circulation time was that a shortening of circulation time could signify an improvement of cardiac output. However, the interpretation is more complicated because circulation time is actually the ratio of blood volume to blood flow:

$$ t = \frac{V}{F} $$

$$ \text{Units: s} = \frac{\text{mL}}{\text{mL/s}} $$

(19-2)

Changes in circulation time may thus reflect changes in volume as well as in flow. For instance, a patient in heart failure may have a decreased cardiac output (i.e., F) or an increased blood volume (i.e., V), both of which would contribute to an elevation of transit time.

The intravascular pressures along the systemic circuit are higher than those along the pulmonary circuit

Panel 5 in Figure 19-1 shows the profile of pressure along the systemic and pulmonary circulations. Pressures are far higher in the systemic than in the pulmonary circulation. Although the cardiac outputs of the left and right sides of

the heart are the same in the steady state, the total resistance of the systemic circulation is far higher than that of the pulmonary circulation (see Chapter 31). This difference explains why the upstream driving pressure averages ~95 mm Hg in the *systemic circulation* but only ~15 mm Hg in the *pulmonary circulation*. Table 19-3 summarizes typical mean values at key locations in the circulation. In both the systemic and pulmonary circulations, the systolic and diastolic pressures decay downstream from the ventricles (Fig. 19-3). The instantaneous pressures vary throughout each cardiac cycle for much of the circulatory system (Fig. 19-1, panel 5). In addition, the systemic venous and pulmonary pressures vary with the respiratory cycle, and venous pressure in the lower limbs varies with the contraction of skeletal muscle.

As noted earlier, the circulation can be divided into a high-pressure and a low-pressure system. The **high-pressure system** extends from the left ventricle in the *contracted state* all the way to the systemic arterioles. The **low-pressure system** extends from the systemic capillaries, through the rest of the systemic circuit, into the right side of the heart, and then through the pulmonary circuit into the left side of the heart in the *relaxed state*. The pulmonary circuit, unlike the systemic circuit, is entirely a low-pressure system; mean arterial pressures normally do not exceed 15 mm Hg, and the capillary pressures do not rise above 10 mm Hg.

Under normal conditions, the steepest pressure drop in the systemic circulation occurs in arterioles, the site of greatest vascular resistance

If we assume for simplicity's sake that the left side of the heart behaves like a constant pressure generator of 95 mm Hg and the right side of the heart behaves like a constant pressure generator of 15 mm Hg, it is the resistance of each vascular segment that determines the profile of pressure fall between the upstream arterial and downstream venous ends of the circulation. In particular, the pressure difference between two points along the axis of the vessel (i.e., the

A SYSTEMIC CIRCULATION

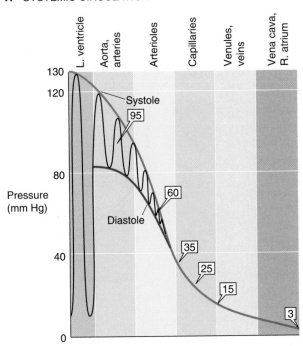

B PULMONARY CIRCULATION

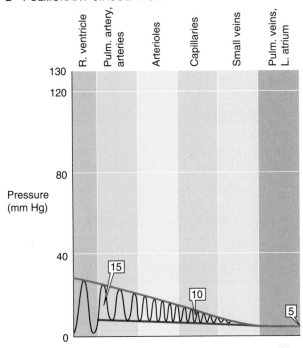

Figure 19-3 Pressure profiles along systemic and pulmonary circulations. In **A** and **B,** the oscillations represent variations in time, not distance. Boxed numbers indicate mean pressures.

driving pressure difference, ΔP) depends on flow and resistance: $\Delta P = F \cdot R$. According to Poiseuille's law, the resistance (R_i) of an individual, unbranched vascular segment is inversely proportional to the fourth power of the radius (see Chapter 17). Thus, the *pressure drop between any two points along the circuit depends critically* on the *diameter of the vessels* between these two points. However, the steepest pressure drop ($\Delta P/\Delta x$) does *not* occur along the capillaries, where vessel diameters are smallest, but rather along the *precapillary arterioles*. Why? The **aggregate resistance** contributed by vessels of a particular order of arborization depends not only on their average radius but also on the *number* of vessels in parallel. The more vessels in parallel, the smaller the aggregate resistance (see Equation 17-3). Although the resistance of a single capillary exceeds that of a single arteriole, capillaries far outnumber arterioles (Table 19-4). The result is that the aggregate resistance is larger in the arterioles, and this is where the steepest ΔP occurs.

Local intravascular pressure depends on the distribution of vascular resistance

We have just seen that the ΔP between an upstream checkpoint and a downstream checkpoint depends on the resistance between these points. What determines the absolute pressure at some location *between* the two checkpoints? To answer this question, we need to know not only the upstream arterial and downstream venous pressures but also the *distribution of resistance* between the two checkpoints. A good example to explain this concept is the distribution of resistance and pressure in the systemic microvasculature. Just how the upstream pressure in the arteriole and the downstream pressure in the venule affect the pressure at the mid-

Table 19-4 Estimates of Total Arteriolar and Capillary Resistances*

	Arterioles	**Capillaries**
Internal radius (r_i)	15 μm	4 μm[†]
Individual resistance (R_i) (units: dyne · s/cm⁵)	~15 × 10⁷	~3000 × 10⁷
Number of units (N)	1 × 10⁷	1 × 10¹⁰
Total resistance ($R_{total} = R_i/N$) (units: dyne · s/cm⁵)	15	3

*Assuming a blood viscosity of 3 cP and a vessel length of 100 μm.
[†]The value of 4 μm is near the average radius of capillaries.

point of the capillary (P_c) depends on the relative size of the upstream and downstream resistances. For the simple circuit illustrated in Figure 19-4A:

$$P_c = \frac{(R_{post}/R_{pre}) \cdot P_a + P_v}{1 + (R_{post}/R_{pre})} \quad (19\text{-}3)$$

P_a is arteriolar pressure, P_v is venular pressure, R_{pre} is precapillary resistance upstream of the capillary bed, and R_{post} is postcapillary resistance downstream of the capillary.

From this equation, we can draw three conclusions about local microvascular pressure. First, even though arteriolar pressure is 60 mm Hg and venular pressure is 15 mm Hg in our example (Table 19-3), capillary pressure is not necessar-

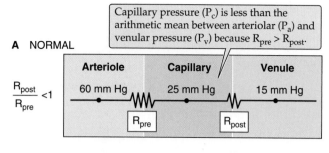

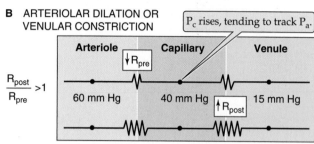

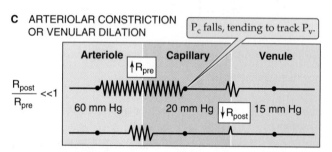

Figure 19-4 Effect of precapillary and postcapillary resistances on capillary pressure.

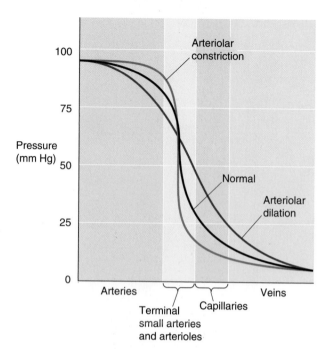

Figure 19-5 Pressure profiles during vasomotion. In this example, we assume that constriction or dilation of terminal arteries and arterioles does not affect the overall driving pressure (ΔP) between aorta and vena cava. This assumption is reasonable in two cases: (1) vasoconstriction or vasodilation is confined to a single parallel vascular bed (e.g., one limb) and does not substantially change total peripheral resistance; and (2) even if total peripheral resistance *does* change, the cardiac pump could still maintain constant systemic arterial and venous pressures.

ily 37.5 mm Hg, the arithmetic mean. According to Equation 19-3, P_c would be the arithmetic mean only if the precapillary and postcapillary resistances were identical (i.e., $R_{post}/R_{pre} = 1$). The finding that P_c is ~25 mm Hg in most vascular beds (Fig. 19-4A) implies that R_{pre} exceeds R_{post} (i.e., $R_{post}/R_{pre} > 1$). Under normal conditions in most microvascular beds, R_{post}/R_{pre} ranges from 0.2 to 0.4.

The second implication of Equation 19-3 is that as long as the *sum* ($R_{pre} + R_{post}$) is constant, reciprocal changes in R_{pre} and R_{post} would not alter the total resistance of the circuit and would therefore leave both P_a and P_v constant. However, as R_{post}/R_{pre} increases, P_c would increase, thereby approaching P_a (Fig. 19-4B). Conversely, as R_{post}/R_{pre} decreases, P_c would decrease, approaching P_v (Fig. 19-4C). This conclusion is also intuitive. If we reduced R_{pre} to zero (but increased R_{post} to keep $R_{post} + R_{pre}$ constant), no pressure drop would occur along the precapillary vessels, and P_c would be the same as P_a. Conversely, if R_{post} were zero, P_c would be the same as P_v.

The third conclusion from Equation 19-3 is that depending on the value of R_{post}/R_{pre}, P_c may be more sensitive to changes in arteriolar than in venular pressure, or vice versa. For example, when the ratio R_{post}/R_{pre} is low (i.e., $R_{pre} > R_{post}$, as in Fig. 19-4A or 19-4C), capillary pressure tends to follow the downstream pressure in large veins. This phenomenon explains why standing may cause the ankles to swell. The

elevated pressure in large leg veins translates to an increased P_c, which, as discussed later, leads to increased transudation of fluid from the capillaries into the interstitial spaces (see Chapter 20). It also explains why elevation of the feet, which lowers the pressure in the large veins, reverses ankle edema.

Vascular resistance varies in time and depends critically on the action of vascular smooth muscle cells. The *major site of control* of vascular resistance in the systemic circulation is the *terminal small arteries (or feed arteries) and arterioles*. Figure 19-5 illustrates the effect of vasoconstriction or vasodilation on the pressure profile. Whereas the overall ΔP between source and endpoint may not vary appreciably during a change in vascular resistance, the *shape* of the local pressure profile may change appreciably. Thus, during arteriolar constriction, the pressure drop between two points along the circuit (i.e., axial pressure gradient, $\Delta P/\Delta x$) is steep and concentrated at the arteriolar site (Fig. 19-5, green curve). During arteriolar dilation, the gradient is shallow and more spread out (Fig. 19-5, violet curve).

Although the effects of vasoconstriction and vasodilation are greatest in the local arterioles (lighter red band in Fig. 19-5), the effects extend both upstream (darker red band) and downstream (purple and blue bands) from the site of vasomotion because the pressure profile along the vessel depends on the resistance profile. Thus, if one vascular element contributes a greater fraction of the total resistance, a greater fraction of the pressure drop will occur along that element.

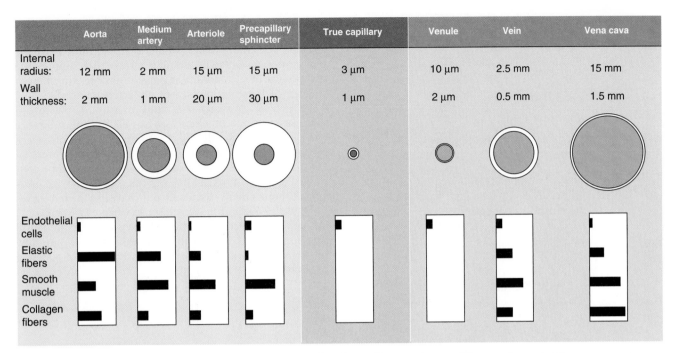

	Aorta	Medium artery	Arteriole	Precapillary sphincter	True capillary	Venule	Vein	Vena cava
Internal radius:	12 mm	2 mm	15 μm	15 μm	3 μm	10 μm	2.5 mm	15 mm
Wall thickness:	2 mm	1 mm	20 μm	30 μm	1 μm	2 μm	0.5 mm	1.5 mm

Figure 19-6 Structure of blood vessels. The values for medium arteries, arterioles, venules, and veins are merely illustrative because the dimensions can range widely. The drawings of the vessels are not to scale.

ELASTIC PROPERTIES OF BLOOD VESSELS

Blood vessels are elastic tubes

The wall of blood vessels consists of three layers: the intima, the media, and the adventitia. Capillaries, which have only an intimal layer of endothelial cells resting on a basal lamina, are the exception. Regardless of the organization of layers, one can distinguish four building blocks that make up the vascular wall: endothelial cells, elastic fibers, collagen fibers, and smooth muscle cells. Figure 19-6 shows how the relative abundance of these components varies throughout the vascular circuit. In addition to these principal components, fibroblasts, nerve endings, and blood cells invade the intima; other extracellular components (e.g., proteoglycans) may also be present.

Endothelial cells form a single, continuous layer that lines all vascular segments. Junctional complexes keep the endothelial cells together in arteries but are less numerous in veins. The organization of the endothelial cell layer in capillaries varies greatly, depending on the organ (see Chapter 20). The glomus bodies in the skin and elsewhere are unusual in that their "endothelial cells" exist in multiple layers of cells called **myoepithelioid cells**. These glomus bodies control small arteriovenous shunts or anastomoses (see Chapter 24).

Elastic fibers are a rubber-like material that accounts for most of the stretch of vessels at normal pressures as well as the stretch of other tissues (e.g., lungs). Elastic fibers have two components: a core of elastin and a covering of microfibrils. The elastin core consists of a highly insoluble polymer of **elastin**, a protein rich in nonpolar amino acids (i.e., glycine, alanine, valine, proline). After being secreted into the

extracellular space, the elastin molecules remain in a random-coil configuration. They covalently cross-link and assemble into a highly elastic network of fibers, capable of stretching more than 100% under physiological conditions. The **microfibrils**, which are composed of glycoproteins and have a diameter of ~10 nm, are similar to those found in the extracellular matrix in other tissues. In arteries, elastic fibers are arranged as concentric, cylindrical lamellae. A network of elastic fibers is abundant everywhere except in the true capillaries, in the venules, and in the aforementioned arteriovenous anastomoses.

Collagen fibers constitute a jacket of far less extensible material than the elastic fibers, like the fabric woven inside the wall of a rubber hose. Collagen can be stretched only 3% to 4% under physiological conditions. The basic unit of the collagen fibers in blood vessels is composed of type I and type III collagen molecules, which are two of the fibrillar collagens. After being secreted, these triple-helical molecules assemble into fibrils that may be 10 to 300 nm in diameter; these in turn aggregate into collagen fibers that may be several microns in diameter and are visible with a light microscope. Collagen fibers are present throughout the circulation except in the capillaries. Collagen and elastic fibers form a network that is arranged more loosely toward the inner surface of the vessel than at the outer surface. Collagen fibers are usually attached to the other components of the vascular wall with some slack, so that they are normally not under tension. Stretching of these other components may take up the slack on the collagen fibers, which may then contribute to the overall tension.

Vascular smooth muscle cells (VSMCs) are also present in all vascular segments except the capillaries. In *elastic* arteries, VSMCs are arranged in spirals with pitch varying from nearly longitudinal to nearly transverse-circular; whereas in

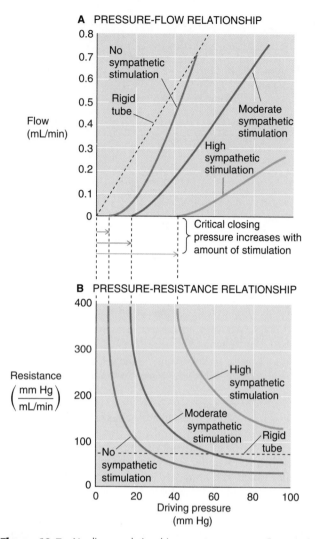

A PRESSURE-FLOW RELATIONSHIP

No sympathetic stimulation

Rigid tube

Moderate sympathetic stimulation

High sympathetic stimulation

Flow (mL/min)

Critical closing pressure increases with amount of stimulation

B PRESSURE-RESISTANCE RELATIONSHIP

Resistance $\left(\dfrac{mm\ Hg}{mL/min}\right)$

High sympathetic stimulation

Moderate sympathetic stimulation

Rigid tube

No sympathetic stimulation

Driving pressure (mm Hg)

Figure 19-7 Nonlinear relationships among pressure, flow, and resistance.

sure gradient) also increases the transmural pressure, causing the vessel to distend. Because radius increases, resistance falls and flow rises more than it would in a rigid tube. Thus, the plot curves upward. The *elastic properties* of vessels are the major cause of such nonlinear pressure-flow relationships in vascular beds exhibiting little or no "active tension."

As *driving* pressure—and thus transmural pressure—increases, vessel radius increases as well, causing resistance (see Chapter 17) to fall (Fig. 19-7B, red curve). Conversely, resistance increases toward infinity when driving pressure falls. In Poiseuille's case, of course, resistance would be constant (Fig. 19-7B, broken line), regardless of the driving pressure. Although many vascular beds behave like the red curves in Figure 19-7A and B, we will see in Chapter 24 that some are highly regulated (i.e., active tension varies with pressure). These special circulations therefore exhibit a pressure-flow relationship that differs substantially from that of a system of elastic tubes.

Contraction of smooth muscle halts blood flow when driving pressure falls below the critical closing pressure

As we have already seen, at low values of driving pressure, resistance rises abruptly toward infinity (Fig. 19-7B, red curve). Viewed differently, flow totally ceases when the pressure falls below about 6 mm Hg, the critical closing pressure (Fig. 19-7A, red curve). The stoppage of flow occurs because of the combined action of elastic fibers and *active tension* from VSMCs. Graded increases in active tension—produced, for example by sympathetic stimulation—shift the pressure-flow relationship to the right and decrease the slope (Fig. 19-7A, blue and green curves), reflecting an increase in resistance over the entire pressure range (Fig. 19-7B, blue and green curves). The critical closing pressure also shifts upward with increasing degrees of vasomotor tone. This phenomenon is important in *hypotensive shock*, where massive vasoconstriction occurs—in an attempt to raise arterial pressure—and critical closing pressures rise to 40 mm Hg or more. As a result, blood flow can stop completely in the limb of a patient in hypotensive shock, despite the persistence of a finite, albeit small, pressure difference between the main artery and vein.

Elastic and collagen fibers determine the distensibility and compliance of vessels

Arteries and veins must withstand very different transmural pressures in vivo (Table 19-3). Moreover, their relative blood volumes respond in strikingly different ways to increases in transmural pressure (Fig. 19-8). Arteries have a low volume capacity but can withstand large transmural pressure differences. In contrast, veins have a large volume capacity (and are thus able to act as blood reservoirs) but can withstand only small transmural pressure differences.

The abundance of structural elements in the vascular walls also differs between arteries and veins (Fig. 19-6). These disparities contribute to differences in the elastic behavior of arteries and veins. We can study the elastic properties of an isolated blood vessel either by recording the "static" volume change produced by pressurizing the vessel

muscular arteries, they are arranged either in concentric rings or as helices with a low pitch. Relaxed VSMCs do not contribute appreciably to the elastic tension of the vascular wall, which is mainly determined by the elastin and collagen fibers. VSMCs exert tension primarily by means of active contraction (see Chapter 9).

Because of the elastic properties of vessels, the pressure-flow relationship of passive vascular beds is nonlinear

Because blood vessels are elastic, we must revise our concept of blood flow, which was based on Poiseuille's law for rigid tubes (see Chapter 17). Poiseuille's law predicts a linear pressure-flow relationship (Fig. 19-7A, broken line). However, in reality, the *pressure-flow relationship is markedly nonlinear* in an in vivo preparation of a vascular bed (Fig. 19-7A, red curve). Starting at the foot of the red curve at a driving pressure of about 6 mm Hg, we see that the curve rises more steeply as the driving pressure increases. The reason is that increase of the driving pressure (i.e., axial pres-

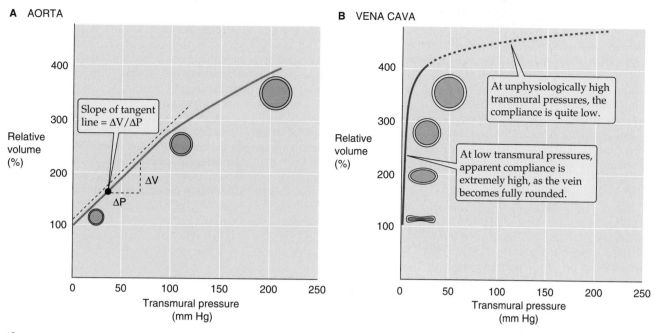

Figure 19-8   Compliance of blood vessels. In **A** and **B,** relative volume of 100% represents fully relaxed volume.

to different levels or, conversely, by recording the "static" pressure change produced by filling the vessel with liquid to different volumes. After the pressure or volume is altered experimentally, it is important to wait until the vessel has finished responding (i.e., it becomes static) before the measurements are recorded.

The **volume distensibility** expresses the elastic properties of blood vessels. Three measurements are useful for assessment of distensibility. First, the **absolute distensibility** is the change in volume for a *macroscopic* step change in pressure, $\Delta V/\Delta P$. Second, because the unstretched size varies among vessels, it is preferable to normalize the volume change to the initial, unstretched volume (V_0) and thus to use a **normalized distensibility** instead:

$$\text{Normalized distensibility} = \frac{(\Delta V/V_0)}{\Delta P} \quad (19\text{-}4)$$

This ratio is a measurement of the fractional change in volume with a given step in pressure. Third, the most useful index of distensibility is **compliance** (*C*), which is the slope of the tangent to any point along the pressure-volume diagram in Figure 19-8:

$$C = \frac{\Delta V}{\Delta P} \quad (19\text{-}5)$$

Here, the ΔV and ΔP values are *minute* displacements. The steeper the slope of a pressure-volume diagram, the greater the compliance (i.e., the easier it is to increase volume). In Figure 19-8, the slope—and thus the compliance—decreases with increasing volumes. For such a non-linear relationship, this variable compliance is the slope of the tangent to the curve at any point. Thus, a compliance reading should always include the transmural pressure or the volume at which it was made. Similar principles apply

to the compliance of airways in the lung (see Chapter 27).

Differences in compliance cause arteries to act as resistors and veins to act as capacitors

As we increase transmural pressure, arteries increase in volume. As they accommodate the volume of blood ejected with every heartbeat, large, muscular systemic arteries (e.g., femoral artery) increase in radius by about 10%. This change for a typical *muscular* artery is much smaller than the distention that one would observe for *elastic* arteries (e.g., aorta), which have fewer layers of smooth muscle and are not under nervous control. The higher compliance of elastic arteries is evident in the pressure-volume diagram in Figure 19-8A—obtained after the smooth muscle is relaxed. The compliance of a relaxed elastic artery is substantial. Increase of the transmural pressure from 0 to 100 mm Hg (near the normal, mean arterial pressure) increases relative volume by ~180%. With further increases in pressure and diameter, compliance decreases only modestly. For example, increase of transmural pressure from 100 to 200 mm Hg increases relative volume by a further ~100 percentage points. Thus, arteries are properly constituted for development and withstanding of high transmural pressures. Because an increase in pressure raises the radius only modestly under physiological conditions, paticularly in muscular arteries, the resistance of the artery (inversely proportional to r^4) does not fall markedly. Because muscular arteries have a rather stable resistance, they are sometimes referred to as **resistance vessels.**

Veins behave very differently. The pressure-volume diagram of a vein (Fig. 19-8B) shows that compliance is extremely high—far higher than for elastic arteries—at least in the low-pressure range. For a relaxed vein, a relatively small increase of transmural pressure from 0 to 10 mm Hg increases volume by ~200%. This high compliance in the low-pressure range is not due to a property of the elastic fibers. Rather, it reflects a change in geometry. At pressures below 6 to 9 mm Hg, the vein's cross section is ellipsoidal. A small rise in pressure causes the vein to become circular, without an increase in perimeter but with a greatly increased cross-sectional area. Thus, in their normal pressure range (Table 19-3), veins can accept relatively large volumes of blood with little buildup of pressure. Because they act as *volume reservoirs*, veins are sometimes referred to as **capacitance vessels**. The true distensibility or compliance of the venous wall—related to the increase in *perimeter* produced by pressures above 10 mm Hg—is rather poor, as shown by the flat slope at higher pressures in Figure 19-8B.

How do veins and elastic arteries compare in response to a sudden increase in volume (ΔV)? When the heart ejects its stroke volume into the aorta, the intravascular pressure increases modestly, from 80 to 120 mm Hg. This change in intravascular pressure—also known as the pulse pressure (see Chapter 17)—is the same as the change in transmural pressure. We have already seen that venous compliance is low in this "arterial" pressure range. Thus, if we were to challenge a vein with a sudden increase in volume (ΔV) in the arterial pressure range, the increase in transmural pressure (ΔP) would be much higher than in an artery of equal size. This is indeed the case when a surgeon uses a saphenous vein segment in a coronary artery bypass graft and anastomoses the vein between two sites on a coronary artery, forming a bypass around an obstructed site.

Changes in the volume of vessels during the cardiac cycle are due to changes in radius rather than length. During ejection of blood during systole, the length of the thoracic aorta may increase by only about 1%.

Laplace's law describes how tension in the vessel wall increases with transmural pressure

Because compliance depends on the elastic properties of the vessel wall, the discussion here focuses on how an external force deforms elastic materials. When the force vanishes, the deformation vanishes, and the material returns to its original state. The simplest mechanical model of a linearly elastic solid is a spring (Fig. 19-9A). The elongation ΔL is proportional to the **force** ($\mathcal{F}$), according to **Hooke's law:**

$$\mathcal{F} = k \cdot \Delta L \qquad (19\text{-}6)$$

k is a constant. If an elastic body requires a larger force to achieve a certain deformation, it is stiffer or less compliant. The largest stress that the material can withstand while remaining elastic is the **elastic limit**. If it is deformed beyond this limit, the material reaches its yield point and, eventually, its breaking point.

Stress is the force per unit cross-sectional area ($\mathcal{F}/A$). Thus, if we pull on an elastic band—stretching it from an initial length L_0 to a final length L—the stress is the force we apply, divided by the area of the band in cross section. **Strain** is the fractional increase in length, that is, $\Delta L/L_0$ or $(L - L_0)/L_0$ (Fig. 19-9B). An equation analogous to Hooke's law describes the relationship between stress and strain:

$$\underbrace{\frac{\mathcal{F}}{A}}_{\text{Stress}} = Y \underbrace{\left(\frac{L - L_0}{L_0} \right)}_{\text{Strain}} \qquad (19\text{-}7)$$

The proportionality factor, Young's **elastic modulus** (Y), is the force per cross-sectional area required to stretch the material to twice its initial length and also the slope of the strain-stress diagram in Figure 19-9B. Thus, the stiffer a material is, the steeper the slope, and the greater the elastic modulus. For example, collagen is more than 1000-fold stiffer than elastin (Table 19-5).

Because the elastic and collagen fibers in blood vessels are not arranged as simple linear springs, the stresses and strains that arise during the pressurization or filling of a vessel occur, at least in principle, along three axes (Fig. 19-10): (1) an elongation of the circumference (θ), (2) an elongation of the axial length (x), and (3) a compression of the thickness of the vessel wall in the direction of the radius (r). In fact, blood vessels actually change little in length during distention, and the thinning of the wall is usually not a major factor. Thus, we can describe the elastic properties of a vessel by considering only what happens along the circumference.

The transmural pressure (ΔP) is the distending force that tends to increase the circumference of the vessel. Opposing this elongation is a force inside the vessel wall. It is convenient to express this wall **tension** (T) as the force that must be applied to bring together the two edges of an imaginary slit, of unit length L, cut in the wall along the longitudinal axis of the vessel (Fig. 19-11). Note that in using tension (units: dynes/cm) rather than stress (units: dynes/cm²), we assume that the thickness of the vessel wall is constant.

Table 19-5 Elastic Moduli (i.e., Stiffness) of Materials

Material	Elastic Modulus (dyne/cm²)*
Smooth muscle	10^4 or 10^5
Elastin	4×10^6
Rubber	4×10^7
Collagen	1×10^{10}
Wood	10^{10} to 10^{12}

*1 mm Hg = 1334 dynes/cm².

A MODEL   **B** STRESS-STRAIN RELATIONSHIP

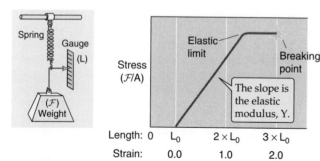

Figure 19-9 · Elastic properties of a spring.

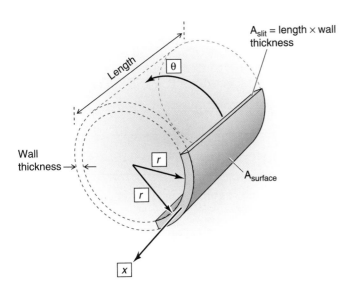

Figure 19-10 Three axes of deformation.

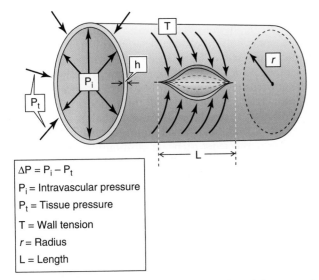

$\Delta P = P_i - P_t$

P_i = Intravascular pressure

P_t = Tissue pressure

T = Wall tension

r = Radius

L = Length

Figure 19-11 Laplace's law. The *circumferential arrows* that attempt to bring together the edges of an imaginary slit along the length of the vessel represent the constricting force of the tension in the wall. The *radial arrows* that push the wall outward represent the distending force. At equilibrium, the two sets of forces balance.

The equilibrium between ΔP and T depends on the vessel radius and is expressed by a law derived independently by Thomas Young and Marquis de Laplace in the early 1800s. For a cylinder,

$$T = \Delta P \cdot r \qquad (19\text{-}8)$$

Thus, for a given transmural pressure, the wall tension in the vessel gets larger as the radius increases.

The vascular wall is adapted to withstand wall tension, not transmural pressure

In Figure 19-8, we plotted the volume of a vessel against transmural pressure, finding that the slope of this relation-

ship is compliance. However, this sort of analysis does not provide us with direct information on the spring-like properties of the materials that make up the vessel wall. With Laplace's law ($T = \Delta P \cdot r$), we can transform the pressure-volume relationship into the same kind of "elastic diagram" that we used in Figure 19-9B to understand the properties of a rubber band.

Figure 19-12A is a re-plot of the pressure-volume diagrams in Figure 19-8. In Figure 19-12B, we reverse the co-ordinate system so that volume is now on the x-axis and pressure on the y-axis. Finally, in Figure 19-12C, we convert volume to radius on the x-axis and use Laplace's law to convert pressure into wall tension on the y-axis. The plots in Figure 19-12C are analogous to a stress-strain diagram for a rubber band (Fig. 19-9B). Thus, stretching the radius of the aorta (solid red curve) causes a considerable rise in wall tension, reflecting the aorta's moderate compliance. The vena cava, on the other hand, fills over a wide range of radii before any wall tension develops, reflecting the shape change that makes it *appear* to be very compliant at the low pressures that are physiological for a vein. However, further stretching of the vein's radius results in a steep rise in wall tension, reflecting the inherently limited compliance of veins.

What does Laplace's law (Equation 19-8) tell us about the wall tension necessary to withstand the pressure inside a blood vessel? On the plot of tension versus radius for the aorta in Figure 19-12C, we have chosen a single point at a radius of 6 mm; because the aorta is relatively stiff, stretching it to this radius produces a wall tension of 120,000 dynes/cm. According to Laplace's law, exactly one *pressure*—200,000 dynes/cm^2 or 150 mm Hg—satisfies this combination of r and T. In Figure 19-12C, this pressure is indicated by the *slope* of the red broken line that connects the origin with our point. In a similar exercise for the vena cava, we assume a radius of ~6.7 mm, which is similar to the one we chose for the aorta; because the vena cava is readily deformed in this range, expanding it to this radius produces a wall tension of only 12,000 dynes/cm (blue broken line). This combination of r and T yields a much lower pressure—18,000 dynes/cm^2, or 13.5 mm Hg. Thus, comparing vessels of *similar size*, Laplace's law tells us that a high wall tension is required to withstand a high pressure.

Comparing two vessels of very *different size* reveals a disparity between wall tension and pressure. A large vein, such as the vena cava, must resist only 10 mm Hg in transmural pressure but is equipped with a fair amount of elastic tissue. A capillary, on the other hand, which must resist a transmural pressure of 25 mm Hg, does not have any elastic tissue at all. Why? The key concept is that what the vessel really has to withstand is not pressure but *wall tension*. According to Laplace's law (Equation 19-8), wall tension is the product of transmural pressure and radius ($\Delta P \cdot r$). Hence, wall tension in a capillary (10 dynes/cm) is much smaller than that in the vena cava (18,000 dynes/cm), even though the capillary is at a higher pressure. Table 19-6 shows that the amount of elastic tissue correlates extremely well with wall tension but very poorly with transmural pressure. The higher the tension that the vessel wall must bear, the greater is its complement of elastic tissue.

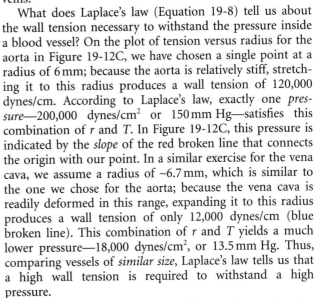

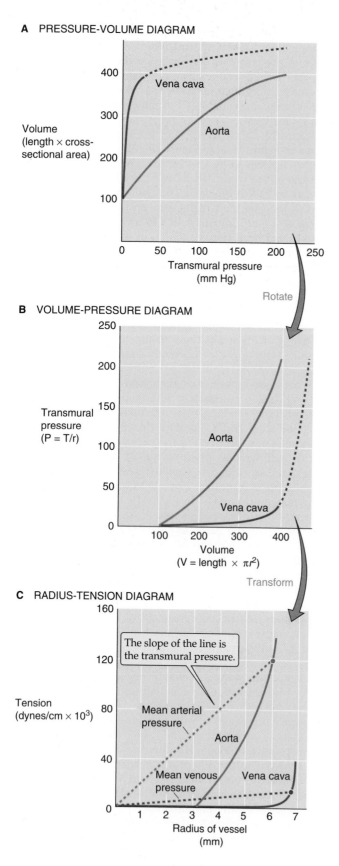

A PRESSURE-VOLUME DIAGRAM

Volume (length × cross-sectional area)

Transmural pressure (mm Hg)

Rotate

B VOLUME-PRESSURE DIAGRAM

Transmural pressure (P = T/r)

Volume (V = length × πr²)

Transform

C RADIUS-TENSION DIAGRAM

Tension (dynes/cm × 10³)

The slope of the line is the transmural pressure.

Mean arterial pressure

Aorta

Mean venous pressure

Vena cava

Radius of vessel (mm)

Figure 19-12 Elastic diagram (tension versus radius) of blood vessels. In **A,** the curves are re-plots of the curves in Figure 19-8. In **B,** the plot is the result of reversing the two axes in **A**. In **C,** the solid *red* and *blue curves* are transformations of the curves in **B**. If we solve for *r,* the *x-axis* of **B** (volume) becomes radius in **C**; if we use Laplace's law ($T = \Delta P \cdot r$) to solve for *T,* the *y-axis* of **B** (transmural pressure) becomes tension in **C**.

Elastin and collagen separately contribute to the wall tension of vessels

The solid red and blue curves in Figure 19-12C are quite different from the linear behavior predicted by Hooke's law (Fig. 19-9B). With increasing stretch, the vessel wall resists additional deformation more; that is, the slope of the relationship becomes steeper. The increasing slope (i.e., increasing elastic modulus) of the radius-tension diagram of a blood vessel is due to the heterogeneity of the elastic material of the vascular wall. Elastic and collagen fibers have different elastic moduli (Table 19-5). We can quantitate the separate contributions of elastic and collagen fibers by "chemical dissection." After selective digestion of elastin with elastase, which unmasks the behavior of collagen fibers, the length-tension relationship is very steep and closer to the linear relationship expected from Hooke's law (Fig. 19-13, orange curve). After selective digestion of collagen fibers with formic acid, which unmasks the behavior of elastic fibers, the length-tension relationship is fairly flat (Fig. 19-13, blue curve). The orange curve (collagen) is steeper than the blue curve (elastin) because collagen is stiffer than elastin (Table 19-5). In a normal vessel (Fig. 19-13, red curve), modest degrees of stretch elongate primarily the elastin fibers along a relatively flat slope. Progressively greater degrees of stretch recruit collagen fibers, resulting in a steeper slope.

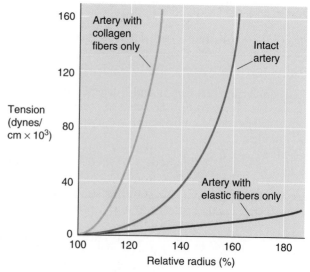

Tension (dynes/cm × 10³)

Artery with collagen fibers only

Intact artery

Artery with elastic fibers only

Relative radius (%)

Figure 19-13 Chemical dissection of elastic moduli of collagen and elastin.

Table 19-6 Comparison of Wall Tensions and Elastic Tissue Content in Various Vessels

	Mean Transmural Pressure ΔP (mm Hg)	Radius (r)	Wall Tension T (dynes/cm)	Elastic Tissue*
Aorta	95	1.13 cm	140,000	+ + + +
Small arteries	90	0.5 cm	60,000	+ + +
Arterioles	60	15 μm	1,200	+
Capillaries	25	3 μm	10	0
Venules	15	10 μm	20	0
Veins	12	>0.02 cm	320	+
Vena cava	10	1.38 cm	18,000	+ +

*The number of plus signs is a relative index of the amount of elastic tissue.

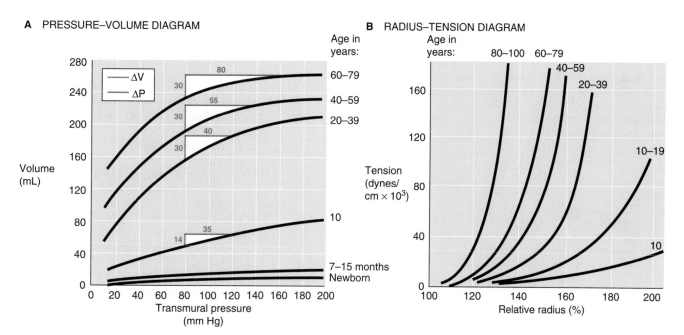

A PRESSURE–VOLUME DIAGRAM

B RADIUS–TENSION DIAGRAM

Figure 19-14 The effect of aging on arteries. In **A** and **B**, a relative radius of 100% represents the fully relaxed value. In **A**, the white triangles show the expected change in transmural pressure (*blue line*) for increase in aortic blood volume (*red line*) produced by each heartbeat—assuming a diastolic pressure of 80 mm Hg.

Aging reduces the distensibility of arteries

With aging, important changes occur in the elastic properties of blood vessels, primarily arteries. We can look at these age relationships for arteries from two perspectives, the pressure-volume curve and the radius-tension curve.

The most obvious difference in aortic pressure-volume curves with increasing age is that the curves shift to progressively higher volumes (Fig. 19-14A), reflecting an increase in diameter. In addition, the compliance of the aorta first rises during growth and development to early adulthood and then falls during later life. After early adulthood, two unfavorable changes occur. First, arteriosclerotic changes reduce the vessel's compliance per se. Thus, during ventricular ejection, a normal-sized increase in aortic volume (ΔV) in a young adult produces a relatively small pulse pressure (ΔP) in the aorta. In contrast, the same change in aortic volume in an elderly individual produces a much larger pulse pressure. Second, because blood pressure frequently rises with age, the older person operates on a flatter portion of the pressure-volume curve, where the compliance is even lower than at lower pressures. Thus, a normal-sized increase in aortic volume produces an even larger pulse pressure.

The second approach for assessment of the effects of age on the elastic properties of blood vessels is to examine the radius-tension diagram (Fig. 19-14B). Because of the progressive, diffuse fibrosis of vessel walls with age, and because of an increase in the amount of collagen, the maximal slope of the radius-tension diagram increases with age. In addition, with age, these curves start to bend upward at lower radii, as the same degree of stretch recruits a larger number of collagen fibers. Underlying this phenomenon is an increased cross-linking among collagen fibers (see Chapter 62) and thus less slack in their connections to other elements in the arterial wall. Thus, even modest elongations challenge the stiffer collagen fibers to stretch.

Active tension from smooth muscle activity adds to the elastic tension of vessels

Although we have been treating blood vessels as though their walls are purely elastic, the **active tension** (see Chapter 9) from VSMCs also contributes to wall tension. Stimulation of VSMCs can reduce the internal radius of muscular feed arteries by 20% to 50%. Laplace's law ($T = \Delta P \cdot r$) tells us that as the VSMC shortens—thereby reducing vessel radius against a constant transmural pressure—there is a decrease in the tension that the muscle must exert to maintain that new, smaller radius.

 For a blood vessel in which both passive elastic components and active smooth muscle components contribute to the total tension, the radius-tension relationship reflects the contributions of each. The red curve in Figure 19-15 shows such a compounded (passive + active) radius-tension diagram for an artery in which the sympathetic neurotransmitter norepinephrine (see Chapter 14) has maximally stimulated the VSMCs. The green curve shows a passive radius-tension relationship for just the elastic component of the tension (after the active component is eliminated by poisoning of the VSMCs with potassium cyanide). Of course, the green curve is the radius-tension diagram on which we have focused the previous figures (e.g., Fig. 19-12C). Subtraction of the green from the red curve in Figure 19-15 yields the *active* length-tension diagram (blue curve) for the vascular smooth muscle.

Elastic tension helps stabilize vessels under vasomotor control

Consider a vessel initially stretched to a radius that is 80% greater than the unstressed radius (i.e., 180 versus 100 on the x-axis of Fig. 19-15). As we inject more fluid into the vessel, the radius increases (i.e., the vessel is more "stressed"). As a result, total wall tension must increase (Fig. 19-15, red curve). The opposite, of course, would happen if we were to withdraw some fluid from the vessel. During such changes in total wall tension, what are the individual contributions of vascular smooth muscle tension and the passive connective tissue tension? In Figure 19-16, we consider two extreme examples, one in which the vessel has only elastic elements and another in which it has only a fixed (i.e., isotonic) active tension.

First, consider a vessel lacking smooth muscle, so that only elastic elements contribute to total wall tension (Fig. 19-16A). If we increase transmural pressure from P (panel 1) to $P + \Delta P$ (panel 2), thereby increasing the radius from r

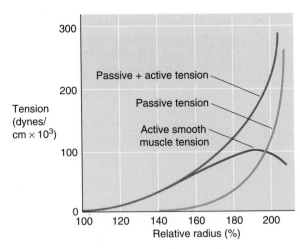

Figure 19-15 Active versus passive tension. The relative radius of 100% is that of an excised vessel maximally stimulated by norepinephrine (*red curve*, total tension) but not "stressed" (i.e., transmural pressure is 0). When the vessel is maximally poisoned with potassium cyanide, the baseline radius is approximately 150% (*green curve*, passive tension), reflecting its relaxed state. The *blue curve* is just the active (i.e., smooth muscle) component of tension.

to $r + \Delta r$, wall tension will automatically increase from T to $T + \Delta T$. This increase in tension allows the vessel to reach a new equilibrium, according to Laplace's law:

$$T + \Delta T = (P + \Delta P) \cdot (r + \Delta r) \qquad (19\text{-}9)$$

Conversely, a decrease in pressure must lead to a decrease in radius and a decrease in tension (panel 3). To achieve either the stable inflation of panel 2 or the stable deflation of panel 3, ΔT cannot be zero. In other words, the passive radius-tension diagram (Fig. 19-15, green curve) cannot have a slope of zero. The vessel wall must have some elasticity.

Second, consider a hypothetical case in which *no elastic fibers* are present and in which the total tension T is kept constant by active elements (i.e., VSMCs) alone. For example, this would be approximately the case for the blue curve in Figure 19-15, between relative radii of 180% and 200%. At the start (Fig. 19-16B, panel 1), we will assume that the smooth muscle tension exactly balances the $P \cdot r$ product. However, when we now increase pressure (panel 2), the automatic adaptation of tension that we saw in the previous example would *not* occur. Indeed, any increase in pressure would make the product $(P + \Delta P) \cdot (r + \Delta r)$ exceed the fixed T of the VSMCs. As a result, the vessel would blow out. Conversely, any decrease in pressure would make the product $(P - \Delta P) \cdot (r - \Delta r)$ fall below the fixed T and lead to full collapse of the vessel (panel 3). This type of instability does in fact occur in **arteriovenous anastomoses**, which are characterized by poor elastic tissue and abundant myoepithelioid cells.

A real vessel, whose wall contains both elastic and smooth muscle elements, can be stable (i.e., neither blown out nor collapsed) over a wide range of radii. The role of elastic tissue in vessels is therefore not only to withstand high transmural pressures but also to stabilize the vessel. Thus, elastic tissue

A STABILITY OF VESSEL WITH ELASTIC WALL TENSION

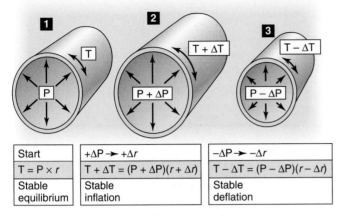

Start	+ΔP → +Δr	−ΔP → −Δr
T = P × r	T + ΔT = (P + ΔP)(r + Δr)	T − ΔT = (P − ΔP)(r − Δr)
Stable equilibrium	Stable inflation	Stable deflation

B INSTABILITY OF VESSEL WITH ONLY A FIXED, ACTIVE WALL TENSION

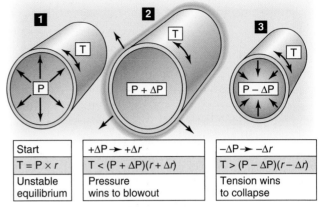

Start	+ΔP → +Δr	−ΔP → −Δr
T = P × r	T < (P + ΔP)(r + Δr)	T > (P − ΔP)(r − Δr)
Unstable equilibrium	Pressure wins to blowout	Tension wins to collapse

Figure 19-16 Mechanical stability of vessels.

ensures a graded response when smooth muscle tone changes. If vessels had only smooth muscle—and no elastic fibers—they would be like those in panels 2 and 3 of Figure 19-16B and tend to be either completely open or completely closed.

An imbalance between passive and active elastic components in blood vessels can be important in disease. For example, when the passive, elastic fibers of a blood vessel are reduced or damaged, vessels tend to become larger (e.g., **aneurysms** or **varicosities**). If the radius exceeds the value compatible with the physical equilibrium governed by Laplace's law, a blowout may occur.

A second pathological example is seen when smooth muscle has undergone maximal stimulation and, conversely, passive elastic elements have regressed. This is the case in **Raynaud disease**, in which exposure to cold leads to extreme constriction of arterioles in the extremities, particularly the fingers. Vessel closure occurs because active smooth muscle tension dominates the radius-tension diagram.

REFERENCES

Books and Reviews

Bakris GL, Bank AJ, Kass DA, et al: Advanced glycation end-product cross-link breakers: A novel approach to cardiovascular pathologies related to the aging process. Am J Hypertens 2004; 17:23S-30S.

Burton AC: Relation of structure to function of the tissues of the wall of blood vessels. Physiol Rev 1954; 34:619-642.

Monos E, Bérczi V, Naádasy G: Local control of veins: Biomechanical, metabolic, and humoral aspects. Physiol Rev 1995; 75:611-666.

Mulvany MJ, Aalkjær C: Structure and function of small arteries. Physiol Rev 1990; 70:921-961.

Zieman SJ, Melenovsky V, Kass DA: Mechanisms, pathophysiology, and therapy of arterial stiffness. Arterioscler Thromb Vasc Biol 2005; 25:932-943.

Journal Articles

Bayliss WM: On the local reactions of the arterial wall to changes in internal pressure. J Physiol Lond 1902; 28:220-231.

Bowditch N (trans): Mécanique céleste by the Marquis de Laplace. Boston: Little, Brown, 1829-1839.

Burton AC: On the physical equilibrium of small blood vessels. Am J Physiol 1947; 164:319-329.

Haluska BA, Jeffriess L, Fathi RB, et al: Pulse pressure vs. total arterial compliance as a marker of arterial health. Eur J Clin Invest 2005; 35:438-443.

Young T: Hydraulic investigations subservient to an intended Croonian lecture on the motion of the blood. Philos Trans R Soc Lond 1808; 98:164-186.

CHAPTER **20**

THE MICROCIRCULATION

Emile L. Boulpaep

The microcirculation serves both nutritional and non-nutritional roles

The primary function of the cardiovascular system is to maintain a suitable environment for the tissues. The microcirculation is the "business end" of the system. The capillary is the principal site for exchange of gases, water, nutrients, and waste products. In most tissues, capillary flow exclusively serves these **nutritional** needs. In a few tissues, however, a large portion of capillary flow is **non-nutritional**. For example, in the glomeruli of the kidneys, capillary flow forms the glomerular filtrate (see Chapter 34). Blood flow through the skin, some of which may shunt through arteriovenous anastomoses, plays a key role in temperature regulation (see Chapter 61). Capillaries also serve other non-nutritional roles, such as signaling (e.g., delivery of hormones) and host defense (e.g., delivery of platelets). In the first part of this chapter, we discuss the nutritional role of capillaries and examine how gases, small water-soluble substances, macromolecules, and water pass across the endothelium. In the last two subchapters, we discuss lymphatics as well as the regulation of the microcirculation.

The morphology and local regulatory mechanisms of the microcirculation are designed to meet the particular needs of each tissue. Because these needs are different, the structure and function of the microcirculation may be quite different from one tissue to the next.

The microcirculation extends from the arterioles to the venules

The microcirculation is defined as the blood vessels from the first-order arteriole to the first-order venule. Although the details vary from organ to organ, the principal components of an idealized microcirculation include a single arteriole and venule, between which extends a network of true capillaries (Fig. 20-1). Sometimes a metarteriole—somewhat larger than a capillary—provides a shortcut through the network. Both the arteriole and the venule have vascular smooth muscle cells (VSMCs). Precapillary sphincters—at the transition between a capillary and either an arteriole or a metarteriole—control the access of blood to particular segments of the network. Sphincter closure or opening creates small local pressure differences that may reverse the direction of blood flow in some segments of the network.

Arteries consist of an inner layer of endothelium, an internal elastic lamina, and a surrounding sheath of at least two continuous layers of innervated VSMCs (see Chapter 19). The inner radius of **terminal arteries** (called feed arteries in muscle) may be as small as 25 μm. **Arterioles** (inner radius, 5 to 25 μm) are similar to arteries but have only a *single* continuous layer of VSMCs, which are innervated. **Metarterioles** are similar to arterioles but of shorter length. Moreover, their VSMCs are discontinuous and are not usually innervated. The **precapillary sphincter** is a small cuff of smooth muscle that usually is not innervated but is very responsive to local tissue conditions. Relaxation or contraction of the precapillary sphincter may modulate tissue blood flow by an order of magnitude or more. Metarterioles and precapillary sphincters are not found in all tissues.

True capillaries (inner radius, 2 to 5 μm) consist of a single layer of endothelial cells surrounded by a basement membrane, a fine network of reticular collagen fibers, and—in some tissues—pericytes. The endothelial cells have a smooth surface and are extremely thin (as little as 200 to 300 nm in height), except at the nucleus. The thickness and density of the capillary **basement membrane** vary among organs. Where large transcapillary pressures occur or other large mechanical forces exist, the basement membrane is thickest. Some endothelial cells have, on both luminal and basal surfaces, numerous **pits** called **caveolae** that are involved in ligand binding. Fluid-phase and receptor-mediated endocytosis can result in 70-nm **caveolin-coated vesicles** (see Chapter 2). In addition, the cytoplasm of capillary endothelial cells is rich in other endocytotic (pinocytotic) **vesicles** that contribute to the transcytosis of water and water-soluble compounds across the endothelial wall. In some cases, the endocytotic vesicles are lined up in a string and even appear linked together to form a **transendothelial channel**.

Linking endothelial cells together are **interendothelial junctions** (Fig. 20-2) where the two cell membranes are ~10 nm apart, although there may be constricted regions where the space or **cleft** between the two cells forms adher-

ing junctions only ~4 nm wide. **Tight junctions** may also be present, in which the apposed cell membranes appear to fuse and **claudins** 1, 3, and 5 (CLDN1, 3, 5) as well as **occludin** seal the gap (see Chapter 2). CLDN5 is quite specific for endothelial cells. Occludin is not found in all endothelia.

Some endothelial cells have membrane-lined, cylindrical conduits—**fenestrations**—that run completely through the cell, from the capillary lumen to the interstitial space. These fenestrations are 50 to 80 nm in diameter and are seen primarily in tissues with large fluid and solute fluxes across the capillary walls (e.g., intestine, choroid plexus, exocrine glands, and renal glomeruli). A thin diaphragm often closes the perforations of the fenestrae (e.g., in intestinal capillaries).

The endothelia of the sinusoidal capillaries in the liver, bone marrow, and spleen have very large fenestrations as well as **gaps** 100 to 1000 nm wide *between* adjacent cells. Vesicles, transendothelial channels, fenestrae, and gaps—as well as structures of intermediate appearance—are part of a spectrum of regulated permeation across the endothelial cells.

Capillaries fall into three groups, based on their degree of leakiness (Fig. 20-3):

1. **Continuous capillary.** This is the most common form of capillary, with interendothelial junctions 10 to 15 nm wide (e.g., skeletal muscle). However, these clefts are absent in the blood-brain barrier (see Chapter 11), whose capillaries have narrow tight junctions.
2. **Fenestrated capillary.** In these capillaries, the endothelial cells are thin and perforated with fenestrations. These

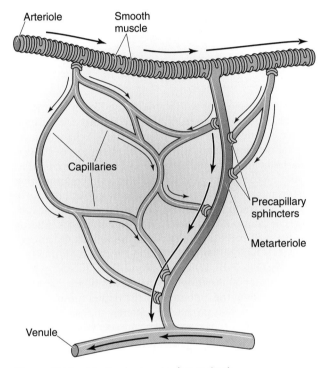

Figure 20-1 Idealized microcirculatory circuit.

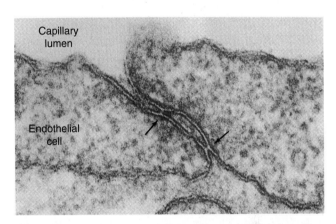

Figure 20-2 Capillary endothelial junctions. This electron micrograph shows the interendothelial junction between two endothelial cells in a muscle capillary. The *arrows* point to tight junctions. (*From Fawcett DW: Bloom and Fawcett. A Textbook of Histology, 12th ed, p 964. New York: Chapman & Hall, 1994.*)

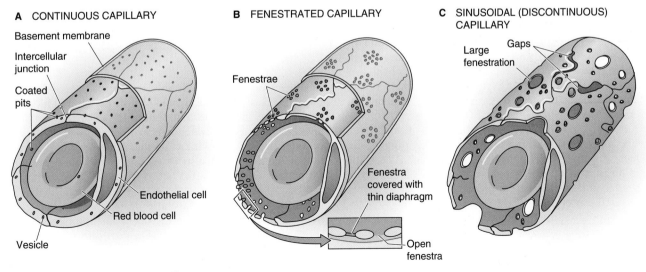

Figure 20-3 Three types of capillaries.

capillaries most often surround epithelia (e.g., small intestine, exocrine glands).

3. **Discontinuous capillary.** In addition to fenestrae, these capillaries have large gaps. Discontinuous capillaries are found in sinusoids (e.g., liver).

At their distal ends, true capillaries merge into **venules** (inner radius, 5 to 25 µm), which carry blood back into low-pressure veins that return blood to the heart. Venules have a discontinuous layer of VSMCs and therefore can control local blood flow. Venules may also exchange some solutes across their walls.

CAPILLARY EXCHANGE OF SOLUTES

The exchange of O_2 and CO_2 across capillaries depends on the diffusional properties of the surrounding tissue

Gases diffuse by a **transcellular route** across the two cell membranes and cytosol of the endothelial cells of the capillary with the same ease that they diffuse through the surrounding tissue. In this section, we focus primarily on the exchange of O_2. Very similar mechanisms exist for the exchange of CO_2, but they run in the opposite direction. Arterial blood has a relatively high O_2 level. As blood traverses a systemic capillary, the principal site of gas exchange, O_2 diffuses across the capillary wall and into the tissue space, which includes the interstitial fluid and the neighboring cells.

The most frequently used model of gas exchange is August Krogh's **tissue cylinder**, a volume of tissue that a single capillary supplies with O_2 (Fig. 20-4A). The cylinder of tissue surrounds a single capillary. According to this model, the properties of the tissue cylinder govern the rate of diffusion of both O_2 and CO_2. The radius of a tissue cylinder in an organ is typically half the average spacing from one capillary to the next, that is, half the mean intercapillary distance. Capillary density and therefore mean intercapillary distance vary greatly among tissues. Among systemic tissues, capillary density is highest in tissues with high O_2 consumption (e.g., myocardium) and lowest in tissues consuming little O_2 (e.g., joint cartilage). Capillary density is extraordinarily high in the lungs (see Chapter 31).

The Krogh model predicts how the concentration or partial pressure of oxygen (P_{O_2}) within the capillary lumen falls along the length of the capillary as O_2 exits for the surrounding tissues (Fig. 20-4A). The P_{O_2} within the capillary at any site along the length of the capillary depends on several factors:

1. The concentration of **free O_2** in the arteriolar blood that feeds the capillary. This dissolved $[O_2]$, which is the same in the plasma and the cytoplasm of the red blood cells, is proportional to the partial pressure of O_2 (see Chapter 29) in the arterioles.
2. The **O_2 content** of the blood. Less than 2% of the total O_2 in arterial blood is dissolved; the rest is bound to hemoglobin inside the red blood cells. Each 100 mL of arterial blood contains ~20 mL of O_2 gas, or 20 volume %—the **O_2 content** (see Table 28-3).

3. The capillary blood flow (F).
4. The **radial diffusion coefficient** (D_r), which governs the diffusion of O_2 out of the capillary lumen. For simplicity, we assume that D_r is the same within the blood, the capillary wall, and the surrounding tissue and that it is the same along the entire length of the capillary.
5. The capillary radius (r_c).
6. The **radius of tissue cylinder** (r_t) that the capillary is supplying with O_2.
7. The **O_2 consumption** by the surrounding tissues ($\dot{Q}_{O_2}$).
8. The **axial distance** (x) along the capillary.

The combination of all these factors accounts for the shape of the concentration profiles within the vessel and the tissue. Although this model appears complicated, it is actually based on many simplifying assumptions.

The O_2 extraction ratio of a whole organ depends primarily on blood flow and metabolic demand

In principle, beginning with a model like Krogh's but more complete, one could sum up the predictions for a single capillary segment and then calculate gas exchange in an entire tissue. However, it is more convenient to pool all the capillaries in an organ and to focus on a single arterial inflow and single venous outflow. The difference in concentration of a substance in the arterial inflow and venous outflow of that organ is the **arteriovenous (a-v) difference** of that substance. For example, if the arterial O_2 *content* ($[O_2]_a$) entering the tissue is 20 mL O_2/dL blood and the venous O_2 content leaving it ($[O_2]_v$) is 15 mL O_2/dL blood, the O_2 a-v difference for that tissue is 5 mL O_2 gas/dL blood.

For a substance like O_2, which *exits* the capillaries, another way of expressing the amount that the tissues remove is the **extraction ratio**. This parameter is merely the a-v difference *normalized* to the arterial content of the substance. Thus, the extraction ratio of oxygen (E_{O_2}) is

$$E_{O_2} = \frac{[O_2]_a - [O_2]_v}{[O_2]_a} \qquad (20\text{-}1)$$

Thus, in our example:

$$E_{O_2} = \frac{20\,\text{mL O}_2/\text{dL} - 15\,\text{mL O}_2/\text{dL}}{20\,\text{mL O}_2/\text{dL}} = \frac{5}{20} = 25\% \qquad (20\text{-}2)$$

In other words, the muscle in this example removes (and burns) 25% of the O_2 presented to it by the arterial blood.

What are the factors that determine O_2 extraction? To answer this question, we return to the hypothetical Krogh cylinder. The same eight factors that influence the P_{O_2} profiles in Figure 20-4A also determine the whole-organ O_2 extraction. Of these factors, the two most important are capillary flow (item 3 in the list) and metabolic demand (item 7). The O_2 extraction ratio decreases with increased flow but increases with increased O_2 consumption. These conclusions make intuitive sense. Greater flow supplies more O_2, so the tissue needs to extract a smaller fraction of the incoming O_2 to satisfy its fixed needs. Conversely, increased metabolic demands require that the tissue extract more of

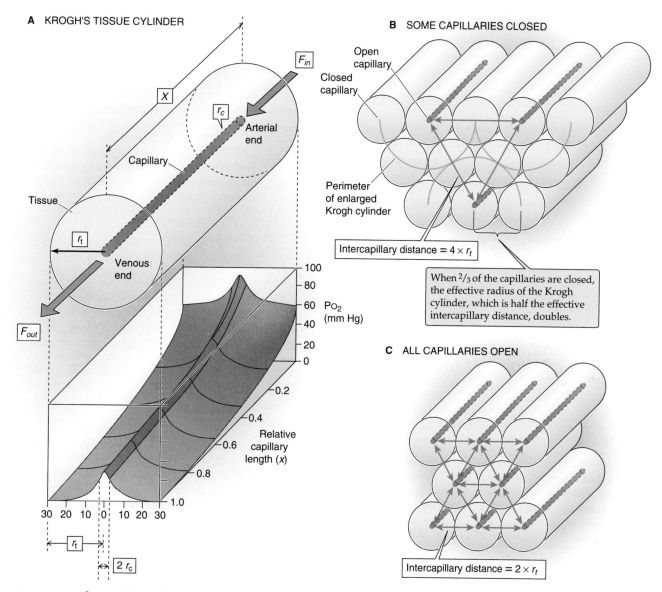

A KROGH'S TISSUE CYLINDER

B SOME CAPILLARIES CLOSED

Open capillary

Closed capillary

Perimeter of enlarged Krogh cylinder

Intercapillary distance = $4 \times r_t$

When $2/3$ of the capillaries are closed, the effective radius of the Krogh cylinder, which is half the effective intercapillary distance, doubles.

C ALL CAPILLARIES OPEN

Intercapillary distance = $2 \times r_t$

Figure 20-4 Delivery and diffusion of O_2 to systemic tissues. In **A,** Krogh's tissue cylinder consists of a single capillary (radius r_c), surrounded by a concentric cylinder of tissue (radius r_t) that the capillary supplies with O_2 and other nutrients. Blood flow into the capillary is F_{in}, and blood flow out of the capillary is F_{out}. The lower panel of **A** shows the profile of partial pressure of O_2 (P_{O_2}) along the longitudinal axis of the capillary and the radial axis of the tissue cylinder.

the incoming O_2. These conclusions are merely a restatement of the Fick principle (see Chapter 17), which we can rewrite as

$$\underbrace{[O_2]_a - [O_2]_v}_{\substack{\text{Related to} \\ \text{extraction ratio}}} = \frac{\dot{Q}_{O_2}}{F} \qquad (20\text{-}3)$$

The term on the left is the a-v difference. The extraction ratio is merely the a-v difference normalized to $[O_2]_a$. Thus, the Fick principle confirms our intuition that the extraction ratio should increase with increasing metabolic demand but decrease with increasing flow.

Another important factor that we have so far ignored is that not all of the capillaries in a tissue may be active at any one time. For example, skeletal muscle contains roughly a half-million capillaries per gram of tissue. However, only ~20% are perfused at rest (Fig. 20-4B). During exercise, when the O_2 consumption of the muscle increases, the resistance vessels and precapillary sphincters dilate to meet the increased demand. This vasodilation increases muscle blood flow and the density of perfused capillaries (Fig. 20-4C). This response is equivalent to decreasing the tissue radius of Krogh's cylinder because each perfused capillary now supplies a smaller region. Other things being equal, reduced diffusion distances cause P_{O_2} in the tissue to increase.

The velocity of blood flow in the capillaries also increases during exercise. All things being equal, this increased velocity would cause P_{O_2} to fall *less steeply* along the capillary lumen. For example, if the velocity were infinite, P_{O_2} would not fall

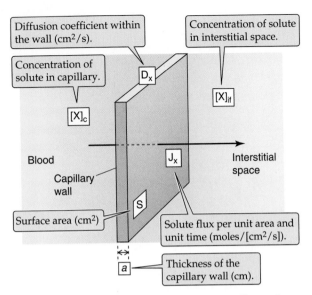

Figure 20-5 Diffusion of a solute across a capillary wall.

at all! In fact, because O_2 consumption rises during exercise, P_{O_2} actually falls *more steeply* along the capillary.

According to Fick's law, the diffusion of small, water-soluble solutes across a capillary wall depends on both the permeability and the concentration gradient

Although the endothelial cell is freely permeable to O_2 and CO_2, it offers a significant barrier to the exchange of lipid-insoluble substances. Hydrophilic solutes that are smaller than albumin can traverse the capillary wall by **diffusion** through a paracellular route (i.e., through the clefts and interendothelial junctions as well as gaps and fenestrae, if these are present).

The amount of solute that crosses a particular surface area of a capillary per unit time is called a **flux**. It seems intuitive that the flux ought to be proportional to the magnitude of the concentration difference across the capillary wall and that it ought to be bigger in leakier capillaries (Fig. 20-5). These ideas are embodied in a form of Fick's law:

$$J_X = P_X \cdot ([X]_c - [X]_{if}) \qquad (20\text{-}4)$$

In Figure 20-5, J_X is the flux of the solute X [units: moles/(cm^2/s)], assuming a positive J_X with flow out of the capillary, into the interstitial fluid. $[X]_c$ and $[X]_{if}$ are the dissolved concentrations of the solute in the capillary and interstitial fluid, respectively. Because the capillary wall thickness a (units: cm) is difficult to determine, we combined the diffusion coefficient D_X (units: cm^2/s) and wall thickness into a single term (D_X/a) called P_X, the **permeability coefficient** (units: cm/s). Thus, P_X expresses the ease with which the solute crosses a capillary by diffusion.

Because, in practice, the surface area (S) of the capillary is often unknown, it is impossible to compute the *flux* of a solute, which is expressed per unit area. Rather, it is more common to compute the *mass flow* $(\dot{Q})$, which is simply the amount of solute transferred per unit time (units: mol/s):

$$\dot{Q} = S \cdot J_X = S \cdot P_X \cdot ([X]_c - [X]_{if}) \qquad (20\text{-}5)$$

The whole-organ extraction ratio for small, hydrophilic solutes provides an estimate of the solute permeability of capillaries

How could we estimate the permeability coefficient for a solute in different capillaries or for different solutes in the same capillary? Unfortunately, it is difficult to determine permeability coefficients in single capillaries. Therefore, investigators use an indirect approach that begins with measurement of the *whole-organ* extraction ratio for the solute X. As we have already seen for O_2 (Equation 20-1), the extraction ratio (E_X) is a normalized a-v difference for X:

$$E_x = \frac{[X]_a - [X]_v}{[X]_a} \qquad (20\text{-}6)$$

Thus, E_X describes the degree to which an organ removes a solute from the circulation. Unlike the situation for O_2, the extraction ratio for small hydrophilic solutes depends not only on total organ blood flow (F) but also on the overall "exchange properties" of all of its capillaries, expressed by the product of permeability and total capillary area $(P_X \cdot S)$. The dependence of E_X on the $P_X \cdot S$ product and F is described by the following equation:

$$E_x = 1 - e^{-(P_X S/F)} \qquad (20\text{-}7)$$

Therefore, by knowing the whole-organ extraction ratio for a solute and blood flow through the organ, we can calculate the product $P_X \cdot S$. The first column of Table 20-1 lists the $P_X \cdot S$ products for a single solute (inulin), determined from Equation 20-7, for a number of different organs. Armed with independent estimates of the capillary surface area (Table 20-1, column 2), we can compute P_X (column 3). P_X increases by a factor of approximately 4 from resting skeletal muscle to heart, reflecting a difference in the density of fluid-filled interendothelial clefts. Because a much greater fraction of the capillaries in the heart are open to blood flow (i.e., S is ~10-fold larger), the $P_X \cdot S$ product for heart is approximately 40-fold higher than for resting skeletal muscle.

The **cerebral vessels** have unique characteristics that constitute the basis of the blood-brain barrier (see Chapter 11). The tight junctions of most brain capillaries do not permit any paracellular flow of hydrophilic solutes; therefore, they exhibit a very low permeability to sucrose or inulin, probably because of the abundant presence of CLDN5 and occludin. In contrast, the *water* permeability of cerebral vessels is similar to that of other organs. Therefore, a large fraction of water exchange in cerebral vessels must occur through the endothelial cells.

Whole-organ $P_X \cdot S$ values are not constant. First, arterioles and precapillary sphincters control the number of capillaries being perfused and thus the available surface area (S). Second, in response to a variety of signaling molecules (e.g., cytokines), endothelial cells can reorganize their cytoskeleton, thereby changing their shape. This deformation widens interendothelial clefts and increases P_X. One example is the increased leakiness that develops during inflammation in

Table 20-1 $P_x \cdot S$ Products for Various Capillary Beds

Tissue	$P_x S$ for Inulin* (10^{-3} cm³/s) (measured)	S, Capillary Surface Area* (cm²) (measured)	P_x, Permeability to Inulin ($\times 10^{-6}$ cm/s) (calculated)
Heart	4.08	800	5.1
Lung	3.80	950	4.0
Small intestine	1.79	460	3.9
Diaphragm	0.76	400	1.9
Ear	0.34	58	5.9
Skeletal muscle at rest	0.09	75	1.2

*All calculations are normalized for 1 g of tissue from rabbits.
   Data from Wittmers LE, Barlett M, Johnson JA: Estimation of the capillary permeability coefficients of inulin in various tissues of the rabbit. Microvasc Res 1976; 11:67-78.

Table 20-2 Permeability Coefficients for Lipid-Insoluble Solutes*

Substance	Radius of Equivalent Sphere† (nm)	Permeability (cm/s)
NaCl	0.14	310×10^{-6}
Urea	0.16	230×10^{-6}
Glucose	0.36	90×10^{-6}
Sucrose	0.44	50×10^{-6}
Raffinose	0.56	40×10^{-6}
Inulin	1.52	5×10^{-6}

*Permeability data are from skeletal muscle of the cat, assuming that the capillary surface area is 70 cm²/g wet tissue.
   †Stokes-Einstein radius.
   Data from Pappenheimer JR: Passage of molecules through capillary walls. Physiol Rev 1953; 33:387-423.

response to the secretion of histamine by mast cells and basophilic granulocytes.

Small polar molecules have a relatively low permeability because they can traverse the capillary wall only by diffusing through water-filled pores (small-pore effect)

Having compared the permeabilities of a single hydrophilic solute (inulin) in several capillary beds, we may address the selectivity of a single capillary wall to several solutes. Table 20-2 shows that the permeability coefficient falls as molecular radius rises. For *lipid-soluble* substances such as CO_2 and O_2, which can diffuse through the *entire* capillary endothelial cell and not just the water-filled pathways, the permeability is much larger than for the solutes in Table 20-2. Early physi-

ologists had modeled endothelial permeability for hydrophilic solutes on the basis of two sets of pores: large pores with diameter of ~10 nm or more and a larger number of **small pores** with an equivalent radius of 3 nm. Small, water-soluble, polar molecules have a relatively low permeability because they can diffuse only by a paracellular path through interendothelial clefts or other water-filled pathways, which constitute only a fraction of the total capillary area. **Discontinuities** or gaps in tight junction strands could form the basis for the small pores. Alternatively, the molecular sieving properties of the small pores may reside in a **fiber matrix** (Fig. 20-6) that consists of either a meshwork of glycoproteins in the paracellular clefts (on the abluminal side of the tight junctions) or the glycocalyx on the surface of the endothelial cell (on the luminal side of the tight junctions). The endothelium-specific calcium-dependent adhesion molecule **VE-cadherin** (CDH5; see Chapter 2) and **platelet/endothelial cell adhesion molecule** (PECAM1 or CD31 antigen) are important glycoprotein components for the postulated fiber matrix in the paracellular clefts. In fact, the small-pore effect is best explained by an arrangement of discontinuities in the tight junctional strands in series with a fiber matrix on either side of the tight junction.

Interendothelial clefts are wider—and fenestrae are more common—at the venular end of the capillary than at its arteriolar end, so that P_x increases along the capillary. Therefore, if the transcapillary concentration difference ($[X]_c - [X]_{if}$) were the same, the solute flux would actually be larger at the venous end of the microcirculation.

Small proteins can also diffuse across interendothelial clefts or through fenestrae. In addition to molecular size, the *electrical charge* of proteins and other macromolecules is a major determinant of their apparent permeability coefficient. In general, the flux of negatively charged proteins is much smaller than that of neutral macromolecules of equivalent size, whereas positively charged macromolecules have the highest apparent permeability coefficient. Fixed negative charges in the endothelial glycocalyx exclude macromolecules with negative charge and favor the transit of macro-

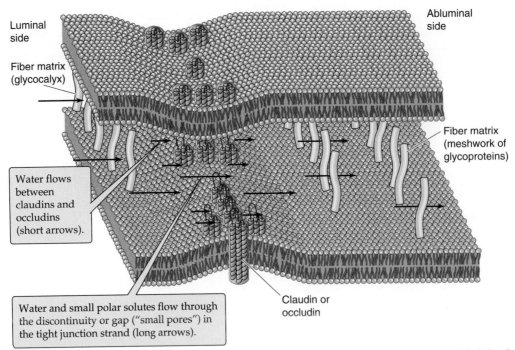

Luminal side

Abluminal side

Fiber matrix (glycocalyx)

Fiber matrix (meshwork of glycoproteins)

Water flows between claudins and occludins (short arrows).

Water and small polar solutes flow through the discontinuity or gap ("small pores") in the tight junction strand (long arrows).

Claudin or occludin

Figure 20-6 Model of endothelial junctional complexes. The figure shows two adjacent endothelial cell membranes at the tight junction, with a portion of the membrane of the upper cell cut away. (Data from Firth JA: Endothelial barriers: From hypothetical pores to membrane proteins. J Anat 2002; 200: 541-548.)

molecules with positive charge. Selective permeability based on the electrical charge of the solute is a striking feature of the filtration of proteins across the glomerular barrier of the nephron (see Chapter 34).

The diffusive movement of solutes is the dominant mode of transcapillary exchange. However, the convective movement of water can also carry solutes. This **solvent drag** is the flux of a dissolved solute that is swept along by the bulk movement of the solvent. Compared with the diffusive flux of a small solute with a high permeability coefficient (e.g., glucose), the contribution of solvent drag is minor.

The exchange of macromolecules across capillaries can occur by transcytosis (large-pore effect)

Macromolecules with a radius exceeding 1 nm (e.g., plasma proteins) can cross the capillary, at a low rate, through wide intercellular clefts, fenestrations, and gaps—when they are present. However, it is caveolae that are predominantly responsible for the large-pore effect that allows transcellular translocation of macromolecules. The **transcytosis** of very large macromolecules by vesicular transport involves (1) equilibration of dissolved macromolecules in the capillary lumen with the fluid phase inside the open vesicle; (2) pinching off of the vesicle; (3) vesicle shuttling to the cytoplasm and probably transient fusion with other vesicles within the cytoplasm, allowing intermixing of the vesicular

Table 20-3 Capillary Permeability to Macromolecules

Macromolecule	Radius of Equivalent Sphere* (nm)	Apparent Permeability (cm/s)
Myoglobin	1.9	0.5×10^{-6}
Plasma albumin†	3.5	0.01×10^{-6}
Ferritin	6.1	~0

*Stokes-Einstein radius.
†Representative value for skeletal muscle.
Data from Pappenheimer JR: Passage of molecules through capillary walls. Physiol Rev 1953; 33:387-423.

content; (4) fusion of vesicles with the opposite plasma membrane; and (5) equilibration with the opposite extracellular fluid phase.

Although one can express the transcytotic movement of macromolecules as a *flux*, the laws of diffusion (Equation 20-4) do not govern transcytosis. Nevertheless, investigators have calculated the "apparent permeability" of typical capillaries to macromolecules (Table 20-3). The resulting "permeability"—which reflects the total movement of the macromolecule, regardless of the pathway—falls off steeply with increases in molecular radius, a feature called **sieving**. This sieving may be the result of steric hindrance when large macromolecules equilibrate across the neck of nascent vesicles or when a network of glycoproteins in the glycocalyx above the vesicle excludes the large macromolecules. In addition, sieving of macromolecules according to molecular size could occur as macromolecules diffuse through infrequent chains of fused vesicles that span the full width of the endothelial cell.

Transcytosis is not as simple as the luminal loading and basal unloading of ferryboats—the cell may process some of the cargo. Although the luminal surface of endothelial cells avidly takes up ferritin (750 kDa), only a tiny portion of endocytosed ferritin translocates to the opposite side of the cell (Table 20-3). The remainder stays for a time in intracellular compartments, where it is finally broken down.

Both transcytosis and chains of fused vesicles are less prominent in brain capillaries. The presence of continuous tight junctions and the low level of transcytosis account for the blood-brain barrier's much lower apparent permeability to macromolecules.

CAPILLARY EXCHANGE OF WATER

Fluid transfer across capillaries is convective and depends on net hydrostatic and osmotic forces (i.e., Starling forces)

The pathway for fluid movement across the capillary wall is a combination of transcellular and paracellular pathways. Endothelial cell membranes express constitutively active **aquaporin 1** (AQP1) water channels (see Chapter 5). It is likely that AQP1 constitutes the principal *transcellular* pathway for water movement. The interendothelial clefts, fenestrae, or gaps may be the anatomical substrate of the *paracellular* pathway.

Whereas the main mechanism for the transfer of gases and other solutes is *diffusion*, the main mechanism for the net transfer of fluid across the capillary membrane is **convection**. As first outlined in 1896 by Ernest Starling, the two driving forces for the convection of fluid—or bulk water movement—across the capillary wall are the transcapillary hydrostatic pressure difference and *effective* osmotic pressure difference, also known as the colloid osmotic pressure or oncotic pressure difference (see Chapter 5).

The **hydrostatic pressure difference** (ΔP) across the capillary wall is the difference between the intravascular pressure (i.e., capillary hydrostatic pressure, P_c) and the extravascular pressure (i.e., interstitial fluid hydrostatic pressure, P_{if}). Note that the term *hydrostatic* includes all sources of intravascular pressure, not only that derived from gravity; it is used here in opposition to *osmotic*.

The **colloid osmotic pressure difference** ($\Delta\pi$) across the capillary wall is the difference between the intravascular colloid osmotic pressure caused by plasma proteins (π_c) and the extravascular colloid osmotic pressure caused by interstitial proteins and proteoglycans (π_{if}). A positive ΔP tends to drive water *out of* the capillary lumen, whereas a positive $\Delta\pi$ attracts water *into* the capillary lumen.

Starling's hypothesis to describe the volume flow (J_V) of fluid across the capillary wall is embodied in the following equation, which is similar to Equation 5-27:

Table 20-4 Terms in Starling Equation

J_V	Volume flux across the capillary wall	cm³ cm⁻² s⁻¹ [cm³/(cm² × s)]
L_p	Hydraulic conductivity*	cm s⁻¹ (mm Hg)⁻¹ [cm/(s × mm Hg)]
P_c	Capillary hydrostatic pressure	mm Hg
P_{if}	Tissue (interstitial fluid) hydrostatic pressure	mm Hg
π_c	Capillary colloid osmotic pressure caused by plasma proteins	mm Hg
π_{if}	Tissue (interstitial fluid) colloid osmotic pressure caused by interstitial proteins and proteoglycans	mm Hg
σ	Average colloid osmotic reflection coefficient	(dimensionless; varies between 0 and 1)
F	Flow of fluid across the capillary wall	cm³/s
S_f	Functional surface area	cm²

*Alternatively, the leakiness of the capillary wall to water may be expressed in terms of water permeability (P_f; units: cm/s). In this case, the hydrostatic and osmotic forces are given in the units of osmolality.

$$J_V = L_p \left[\underbrace{(P_c - P_{if})}_{\substack{\Delta P \\ \text{Hydrostatic} \\ \text{pressure} \\ \text{difference}}} - \sigma \underbrace{(\pi_c - \pi_{if})}_{\substack{\Delta\pi \\ \text{Colloid osmotic} \\ \text{pressure} \\ \text{difference}}} \right] \qquad (20\text{-}8)$$

Net filtration pressure (i.e., net driving force)

Table 20-4 summarizes the terms in this equation. The equation is written so that the flux of water leaving the capillary is positive and that of fluid entering the capillary is negative.

The **hydraulic conductivity** (L_p) is the proportionality constant that relates the net driving force to J_V and expresses the total permeability provided by the ensemble of AQP1 channels and the paracellular pathway.

According to van't Hoff's law, the theoretical colloid osmotic pressure difference ($\Delta\pi_{\text{theory}}$) is proportional to the protein concentration difference ($\Delta[X]$):

$$\Delta\pi_{\text{theory}} = RT\Delta[X] \qquad (20\text{-}9)$$

However, because capillary walls exclude proteins *imperfectly*, the observed colloid osmotic pressure difference

Table 20-5 Effect of Upstream and Downstream Pressure Changes on Capillary Pressure*

	P_a (mm Hg)	P_c (mm Hg)	P_v (mm Hg)
Control	60	25	15
Increased arteriolar pressure	70	27	15
Increased venular pressure	60	33	25

*Constant R_{post}/R_{pre} = 0.3.

($\Delta\pi_{obs}$) is less than the ideal. The ratio $\Delta\pi_{obs}/\Delta\pi_{theory}$ is the **reflection coefficient** (σ) that describes how a semipermeable barrier excludes or "reflects" solute X as water moves across the barrier, driven by hydrostatic or osmotic pressure gradients.

The value of σ can range from 0 to 1. When σ is zero, the moving water perfectly "entrains" the solute, which moves with the water and exerts no osmotic pressure across the barrier. When σ is 1, the barrier completely excludes the solute as the water passes through, and the solute exerts its full or ideal osmotic pressure. To the extent that σ exceeds zero, the membrane sieves out the solute. The σ for plasma proteins is nearly 1.

Because small solutes such as Na^+ and Cl^- freely cross the endothelium, their σ is zero, and they are not included in the Starling equation for the capillary wall (Equation 20-8). Thus, changing the intravascular or interstitial concentrations of such "crystalloids" does *not* create a net effective osmotic driving force across the capillary wall. (Conversely, because plasma membranes have an effective $σ_{NaCl}$ = 1, NaCl gradients *do* shift water between the *intracellular and interstitial* compartments.)

The net driving force in the Starling equation (Equation 20-8), $[(P_c − P_{if}) − σ(\pi_c − \pi_{if})]$, has a special name, the **net filtration pressure**. **Filtration** of fluid from the capillary into the tissue space occurs when the net filtration pressure is positive. In the special case when σ for proteins is 1, the fluid leaving the capillary is protein free; this process is called ultrafiltration. Conversely, **absorption** of fluid from the tissue space into the vascular space occurs when the net filtration pressure is negative. At the arterial end of the capillary, the net filtration pressure is generally positive, so that filtration occurs. At the venous end, the net filtration pressure is generally negative, so that absorption occurs. However, as is discussed later, some organs do not adhere to this general rule.

In the next four sections, we examine each of the four Starling forces that constitute the net filtration pressure: P_c, P_{if}, π_c, and π_{if}.

Capillary blood pressure (P_c) falls from approximately 35 mm Hg at the arteriolar end to approximately 15 mm Hg at the venular end

Capillary blood pressure is also loosely called the capillary *hydrostatic* pressure, to distinguish it from capillary *colloid osmotic* pressure. It is only possible to record P_c in an exposed organ, ideally in a thin tissue (e.g., a mesentery) that allows good transillumination. One impales the lumen of the capil-

lary with a fine micropipette (tip diameter < 5 μm) filled with saline and heparin. The micropipette lumen connects to a manometer, which has a sidearm to a syringe. Immediately after the impalement, blood begins to rise slowly up the pipette. A pressure reading at this time would underestimate the actual P_c because pipette pressure is less than P_c. The syringe makes it possible to apply just enough pressure to the pipette lumen to reach true pressure equilibrium—when fluid flows neither from nor to the pipette. By use of this **null-point** approach, the recorded pressure is the true P_c. In the human skin, P_c is approximately 35 mm Hg at the arteriolar end and approximately 15 mm Hg at the venular end.

When the arteriolar pressure is 60 mm Hg and the venous pressure is 15 mm Hg, the midcapillary pressure is not the mean value of 37.5 mm Hg but only 25 mm Hg (Table 20-5, top row). The explanation for the difference is that normally the precapillary upstream resistance exceeds the postcapillary downstream resistance (R_{post}/R_{pre} is typically 0.3; see Chapter 19). However, the midcapillary pressure is not a constant and uniform value. In Chapter 19, we saw that P_c varies with changes in R_{pre} and R_{post} (see Fig. 19-4). P_c also varies with changes in four other parameters: (1) upstream and downstream pressure, (2) location, (3) time, and (4) gravity.

Arteriolar (P_a) and Venular (P_v) Pressure Because R_{post} is less than R_{pre}, P_c follows P_v more closely than P_a (see Chapter 19). Thus, increasing P_a by 10 mm Hg—at a constant R_{post}/R_{pre} of 0.3—causes P_c to rise by only 2 mm Hg (Table 20-5, middle row). On the other hand, increasing P_v by 10 mm Hg causes P_c to rise by 8 mm Hg (Table 20-5, bottom row).

Location Capillary pressure differs markedly among tissues. For example, the high P_c of glomerular capillaries in the kidney, approximately 50 mm Hg (see Chapter 34), is required for ultrafiltration. The retinal capillaries in the eye must also have a high P_c because they bathe in a vitreous humor that is under a pressure of approximately 20 mm Hg (see Chapter 15). A higher P_c is needed to keep the capillaries patent in the face of the external compressing force. The pulmonary capillaries have unusually *low* P_c values, 5 to 15 mm Hg, minimizing the ultrafiltration that otherwise would lead to the accumulation of edema fluid in the alveolar air spaces (see Chapter 31).

Time Capillary blood pressure varies considerably from moment to moment at any given site, depending on the arteriolar diameter and tone of the precapillary sphincter (i.e., R_{pre}). In individual capillaries, these fluctuations lead to times of net filtration and other times of net fluid absorption.

Gravity   Finally, the effect of gravity on P_c is the same as that discussed for arterial and venous pressure. Thus, a capillary bed below the level of the heart has a higher P_c than a capillary bed at the level of the heart.

Interstitial fluid pressure (P_{if}) is slightly negative, except in encapsulated organs

The interstitium consists of both a solid and a liquid phase. The solid phase is made up of collagen fibers and proteoglycans. In the liquid phase, only a small fraction of interstitial water is totally "free" and capable of moving under the influence of convective forces. Most of the water is trapped in gels (e.g., proteoglycans), in which both water and small solutes move by diffusion. It was once thought that P_{if} in the liquid phase is slightly above barometric pressure throughout the interstitium, but more recent measurements indicate that P_{if} is subatmospheric in many tissues.

Estimation of P_{if} is very difficult because the probe used to make the measurement is far larger than the interstitial space; thus, the measurement itself can alter P_{if}. If one inserts a probe percutaneously and immediately uses a null-point method to measure P_{if} (as outlined earlier for capillary pressure), the values are +1 to +2 mm Hg. However, during the next 4 to 5 hours, the measured value drops to −1 to −2 mm Hg. Arthur Guyton implanted a perforated, hollow plastic sphere under the skin to provide a chronic record of P_{if} (Fig. 20-7). After the wound has healed, the pressure inside the sphere may be as low as −2 to −10 mm Hg after 1 or 2 weeks. Another approach, the wick-in-needle technique, also yields subatmospheric values.

A value of −2 mm Hg is a reasonable average in *loose tissues*, such as the lung and subcutaneous tissue. P_{if} is slightly negative because of fluid removal by the lymphatics (see

later). Inside *rigid enclosed compartments*, such as the bone marrow or brain, P_{if} is positive. It is also positive in *encapsulated organs* such as the kidney, where P_{if} is +1 to +3 mm Hg within the parenchyma. Expansion of high-pressure vessels in the kidney pushes the interstitial fluid against an unyielding fibrous capsule, raising P_{if}. The same principle applies to skeletal muscle, which is surrounded by layers of fascia. In some cases, it is not the interstitial fluid but another specialized compartment that provides the pressure around the capillaries. For renal glomerular capillaries, it is Bowman's space (see Chapter 34)—filled with glomerular filtrate to a pressure of about +10 mm Hg—that is the relevant outside compartment. For pulmonary capillaries, the relevant outside compartment is the alveolus, the pressure of which varies during the respiratory cycle (see Chapter 27).

P_{if} is also sensitive to the addition of fluid to the interstitial compartment. When small amounts of fluid are added to the interstitial compartment, the interstitium behaves like a low-compliance system, so that P_{if} rises steeply for the small amount of added fluid. Adding more fluid disrupts the solid phase of collagen fibers and the gel of proteoglycans, so that large volumes can now accumulate with only small additional pressure increases. In this high-volume range, the interstitial compartment thus behaves like a high-compliance system. This high compliance is especially high in loose subcutaneous tissues, which can accommodate more edema fluid (see the box on interstitial edema) than can muscle.

Capillary colloid osmotic pressure (π_c), which reflects the presence of plasma proteins, is approximately 25 mm Hg

The colloid osmotic pressure difference across the capillary endothelium is due solely to the plasma proteins, such as albumin, globulins, and fibrinogen. Total plasma protein concentration is approximately 7.0 g/dL, which corresponds to approximately 1.5 mM of protein. According to van't Hoff's law (Equation 20-9), these proteins would exert an osmotic pressure of approximately 28 mm Hg if perfectly reflected by the capillary wall ($\sigma = 1$). The σ is indeed close to 1 for the principal plasma proteins—albumin (3.5 to 5.5 g/dL) and the globulins (2.0 to 3.5 g/dL)—so that the actual colloid osmotic pressure ($\sigma\pi_c$) in capillaries is approximately 25 mm Hg. This value is the same as if osmotically active solutes were present at approximately 1.3 mM. Note that because of the very definition of colloid osmotic pressure, we have ignored the osmotic effects of the small solutes in plasma, which have an *osmolality* of 290 mOsm (see Chapter 5).

π_c does vary appreciably along the length of the capillary. Indeed, most capillary beds filter less than 1% of the fluid entering at the arteriolar end. Thus, the loss of protein-free fluid does not measurably concentrate plasma proteins along the capillary and does not appreciably raise π_c.

Because clinical laboratories report plasma protein concentrations in grams per deciliter and not all proteins have the same molecular weight, a plasma protein concentration of 7 g/dL can produce different π_c values, depending on the protein *composition* of the plasma. Because albumin has a much lower molecular weight than γ-globulin, replacement of 1 g of the heavier γ-globulin with 1 g of the lighter albumin

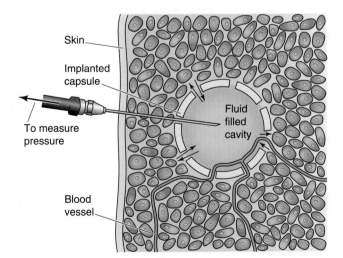

Figure 20-7   Long-term measurement of interstitial fluid pressure with an implanted capsule.

raises π_c. Whereas van't Hoff's law (Equation 20-9) predicts a *linear* relationship between osmotic pressure and concentration, colloid osmotic pressure actually increases more steeply, even when the albumin/globulin ratio is held constant at 1.8 (Fig. 20-8, orange curve). Obviously, the steepness of the curve varies from one plasma protein to the next because all have different molecular weights.

Not only does π_c vary markedly with protein composition and concentration, the reflection coefficient for colloids also varies widely among organs. The lowest values for σ (i.e., greatest leakiness) are in discontinuous capillary beds (e.g., liver); intermediate values are in muscle capillaries, and the highest values ($\sigma = 1$) are in the tight, continuous capillary beds of the brain.

The plasma proteins do more than just act as osmotic agents. Because these proteins also carry negative charges, the **Donnan effect** causes an increase in both the concentrations of cations (see Chapter 5) and the colloid osmotic pressure (see Fig. 5-15) in the capillary lumen.

Interstitial fluid colloid osmotic pressure (π_{if}) varies between 0 and 10 mm Hg among different organs

It is difficult to measure the interstitial fluid colloid osmotic pressure because it is virtually impossible to obtain uncontaminated samples. As a first approximation, we generally assume that π_{if} is the same as the colloid osmotic pressure of *lymph*. The protein content of lymph varies greatly from region to region; for example, it is 1 to 3 g/dL in the legs, 3 to 4 g/dL in the intestine, and 4 to 6 g/dL in the liver. Such lymph data predict that π_{if} ranges from 3 to 15 mm Hg. However, the protein concentration in the interstitial fluid is probably somewhat higher than in the lymph. A total body average value for π_{if} is approximately 3 mm Hg, substantially less than the value of 25 mm Hg for π_c in the capillary lumen.

The π_{if} appears to increase along the axis of the capillary (Table 20-6). The lowest values are near the arteriolar end, where the interstitium receives protein-free fluid from the capillary as the result of filtration. The highest values are near the venular end, where the interstitium loses protein-free fluid to the capillary as the result of absorption.

The Starling principle predicts ultrafiltration at the arteriolar end and absorption at the venular end of most capillary beds

The idealized forces acting on fluid movement across a capillary are shown in Figure 20-9A. With use of the Starling equation and the values in Table 20-6, we can calculate the net transfer of fluid (J_V) at both the arteriolar and venular ends of a typical capillary:

$$J_v = L_p[(P_c - P_{if}) - (\sigma\pi_c - \sigma\pi_{if})]$$
$$\text{Arteriolar end: } J_v = L_p[(35 - (-2)) - (25 - 0.1)]$$
$$= L_p(+12\,\text{mm Hg}) \qquad (20\text{-}10)$$
$$\text{Venular end: } J_v = L_p[(15 - (-2)) - (25 - 3)]$$
$$= L_p(-5\,\text{mm Hg})$$

The net filtration pressure is thus positive (favoring filtration) at the arteriolar end, and it gradually makes the transition to negative (favoring absorption) at the venular end (Fig. 20-9B). At the point where the filtration and reabsorptive forces balance each other, an equilibrium

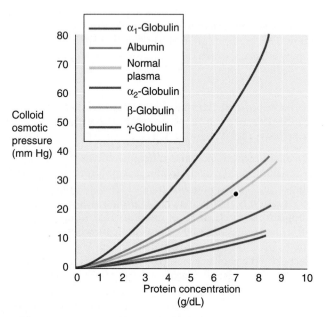

Figure 20-8 Dependence of colloid osmotic pressure on the concentration of plasma proteins. The point on the *orange curve* indicates that normal plasma, a mixture of proteins at a concentration of 7 g/dL, has a colloid osmotic pressure (π_c) of 25 mm Hg.

Table 20-6 Typical Values of Transcapillary Driving Forces for Fluid Movement in Loose, Non-encapsulated Tissue

	Capillary Blood Pressure (P_c)	Interstitial Fluid Pressure (P_{if})	Effective Capillary Colloid Osmotic Pressure ($\sigma\pi_c$)	Effective Interstitial Fluid Colloid Osmotic Pressure ($\sigma\pi_{if}$)	Net Force
Anteriolar end	+35 mm Hg	−2 mm Hg	+25 mm Hg	+0.1 mm Hg*	+12 mm Hg
Venular end	+15 mm Hg	−2 mm Hg	+25 mm Hg	+3 mm Hg	−5 mm Hg

*The low effective colloid osmotic pressure prevails only in the subglycocalyx fluid compartment (see Fig. 20-10B.)

Interstitial Edema

Edema (from the Greek *oidema*, for "swelling") is characterized by an excess of salt and water in the extracellular space, particularly in the interstitium. Edema may be associated with any disease leading to salt retention and expansion of the extracellular fluid volume, in particular, renal, cardiac, and hepatic disease (see Chapter 40). However, interstitial edema can also occur without overall salt and water retention because of microcirculatory alterations that affect the Starling forces. Regardless of the cause, the resulting edema can be either generalized (e.g., widespread swelling of subcutaneous tissue, often first evident in facial puffiness) or localized (e.g., limited to the dependent parts of the body). In this box, we focus on how edema can result from changes in terms that make up the Starling equation.

Hydrostatic Forces
When a person is **standing** for a sustained time, venous pressure and thus capillary pressure (P_c) in the legs increase because of gravity. The result is movement of fluid into the tissue space. In most cases, the lymphatic system can take up the extra interstitial fluid and return it to the vascular space, maintaining proper fluid balance. The return of fluid requires contractions of the leg muscles to compress the veins and lymphatics and to propel the fluid upward through the valves in these vessels and toward the heart. If the standing person does not contract these muscles, the transudation of fluid can exceed the lymphatic return, causing interstitial edema.

An organ that is particularly sensitive to proper fluid balance is the lung. Slight increases in the hydrostatic pressure of the pulmonary capillaries (pulmonary hypertension) can lead to **pulmonary edema**. This condition decreases lung compliance (making lung inflation more difficult; see Chapter 27) and also may severely compromise gas exchange across the pulmonary capillary bed (see Chapter 30). Left-sided heart failure causes blood to back up into the vessels of the lung, raising pulmonary vascular pressures and causing pulmonary edema.

In right-sided heart failure, blood backs up into the systemic veins. As a result, central venous pressure (i.e., the pressure inside the large systemic veins leading to the right side of the heart) rises, causing an increase in the P_c in the lower extremities and abdominal viscera. Fluid transudated from the hepatic and intestinal capillaries may leave the interstitial space and enter the peritoneal cavity, a condition called **ascites**.

Colloid Osmotic Forces
In **nephrotic syndrome**, a manifestation of a number of renal diseases, protein is lost in the urine. The result is a fall in plasma colloid osmotic pressure, a decrease in the ability of the capillaries to retain fluid, and generalized peripheral edema.

In **pregnancy**, synthesis of plasma proteins by the mother does not keep pace with the expanding plasma volume and nutritional demands of the fetus. As a result, maternal plasma protein levels fall. The same occurs in **protein malnutrition**. Although it is less severe than in nephrotic syndrome, the lower capillary colloid osmotic pressure nevertheless leads to edema in the extremities.

The opposite effect is seen in dehydration. A deficit of salt and water causes an *increase* in the plasma protein concentration, increasing the capillary colloid osmotic pressure and thus pulling fluid out of the interstitial space. The result is reduced turgor of the interstitial space. This effect is easily noticed by pinching the skin, which is unable to spring back to its usual firm position.

Properties of the Capillary Wall
Inflammation causes the release of vasodilators, such as histamine and cytokines, into the surrounding tissue. Vasodilation increases the number of open capillaries and therefore the functional surface area (S_f). Cytokines also cause widening of interendothelial clefts and a fall in the reflection coefficient (σ) for proteins. The net effect is enhanced filtration of fluid from capillary lumen to interstitium, so that tissue swelling is one of the hallmarks of inflammation.

Severe head injuries can result in **cerebral edema**, a result of the breakdown of the normally tight endothelial barrier of the cerebral vessels (see Chapter 11). Because the rigid skull prevents expansion of the brain, cerebral edema can lead to occlusion of the cerebral microcirculation.

During ischemia—when blood flow to a tissue is severely reduced or completely stopped—blood vessels deteriorate, causing hydraulic conductivity (L_p) to increase and reflection coefficient to decrease. Once blood flow is reestablished (**reperfusion**), these changes lead to local edema. If the increased leakiness is substantial, large quantities of plasma proteins freely move into the interstitial space, dissipating the colloid osmotic gradient across the capillary wall and aggravating the edema.

Lymphatic Drainage
Lymphatic drainage may become impaired after removal of lymph nodes for cancer surgery or when lymph nodes are obstructed by malignant neoplasms. The reduction in the lymphatic drainage leads to local edema, upstream from the affected nodes.

---

exists, and no net movement of water occurs across the capillary wall.

Net filtration pressure varies—sometimes considerably—among tissues. For example, in the intestinal mucosa, P_c is so much lower than π_c that absorption occurs continually along the entire length of the capillary. On the other hand, in glomerular capillaries, P_c exceeds π_c throughout most of the network, so that filtration may occur along the entire capillary (see Chapter 34). Hydraulic conductivity also can affect the filtration/absorption profile along the capillary. Because the interendothelial clefts become larger toward the

venular end of the capillary, L_p increases along the capillary, from the arteriolar to the venular end.

Ignoring glomerular filtration in the kidney, Landis and Pappenheimer calculated a filtration of ~20 L/day at the arteriolar end of the capillary and an absorption of about 16 to 18 L/day at the venular end, for a net *filtration* of about 2 to 4 L/day from blood to interstitial fluid. This 2 to 4 L of net filtration does not occur uniformly in all capillary beds. The *flow* of fluid across a group of capillaries (F) is the product of the *flux* (J_V) and the functional surface area (S_f): $F = J_V \cdot S_f$. Thus, net filtration of fluid in an organ depends

A INDIVIDUAL HYDROSTATIC AND OSMOTIC PRESSURES

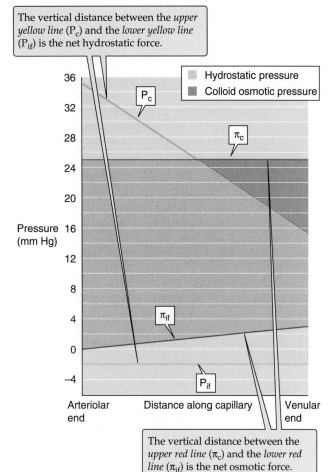

The vertical distance between the *upper yellow line* (P_c) and the *lower yellow line* (P_{if}) is the net hydrostatic force.

The vertical distance between the *upper red line* (π_c) and the *lower red line* (π_{if}) is the net osmotic force.

B NET FILTRATION PRESSURE

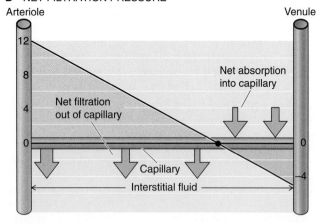

Figure 20-9 Starling forces along a capillary. In **A,** the *yellow lines* are idealized profiles of capillary (P_c) and interstitial (P_{if}) hydrostatic pressures. *Red lines* are idealized capillary (π_c) and interstitial (π_{if}) colloid osmotic pressures. In **B,** the net filtration pressure is ($P_c - P_{if}$) $- \sigma(\pi_c - \pi_{if})$.

not only on the net filtration pressure and the hydraulic conductivity of the capillary wall (terms that contribute to J_V) but also on the surface area of capillaries that happen to be perfused. For example, exercise recruits additional open capillaries in muscle, raising S_f and thereby increasing filtration.

For continuous capillaries, the endothelial barrier for fluid exchange is more complex than considered by Starling

The contribution of Landis and Pappenheimer was to insert experimentally measured values into the Starling equation (Equation 20-8) and to calculate the total body filtration and absorption rates and, by difference, net filtration. Because the estimate of 2 to 4 L for the net filtration rate agreed so well with total lymph flow, the scientific public accepted the entire Landis-Pappenheimer analysis. However, for continuous capillaries, the Landis-Pappenheimer estimates of filtration and absorption are far higher than the modern experimental data. Three major reasons for the discrepancy have emerged. First, Starling's assumptions about the nature of the capillary barrier were overly simplistic. Namely, he assumed that a single barrier separated two well-defined, uniform compartments. Thus, according to Equation 20-8, the dependence of J_V on net filtration pressure ought to be linear, as indicated by the plot in the inset of Figure 20-10A. Second, Landis and Pappenheimer used (1) P_c values that are valid only at the level of the heart (i.e., ignoring gravity), (2) P_c values that are not subject to the vagaries of vasomotion, and (3) unrealistically low values of π_{if} (which would predict a greater absorption).

A revised model has emerged for fluid exchange across continuous endothelia with interendothelial junctions to account for discrepancies between the classical Starling predictions and the modern data. The revised model has two major features. First, the primary barrier for colloid osmotic pressure—that is, the semipermeable "membrane" that reflects proteins but lets water and small solutes pass—is not the *entire* capillary but only the luminal glycocalyx, in particular the glycocalyx overlying the paracellular clefts (Fig. 20-10B). Second, the abluminal surface of the glycocalyx is not in direct contact with the bulk interstitial fluid but is bathed by the **subglycocalyx fluid** at the top of the long paracellular cleft—a third compartment. Thus, the flow across the glycocalyx barrier depends not on P_{if} and π_{if} in the bulk interstitial fluid but on the comparable parameters in the subglycocalyx fluid (P_{sg} and π_{sg}):

$$J_V = L_p[(P_c - P_{sg}) - \sigma(\pi_c - \pi_{sg})] \qquad (20\text{-}11)$$

Let us now examine the predictions of this equation for three states.

1. **During ultrafiltration (i.e., J_V is positive).** Here, the hydrostatic pressure in the subglycocalyx fluid—that is, the fluid in direct contact with the abluminal surface of the glycocalyx—is higher than that in the bulk interstitial fluid (i.e., $P_{sg} > P_{if}$ in Fig. 20-10B). Thus, fluid moves from the subglycocalyx space, along the paracellular cleft, to the bulk interstitial fluid. Moreover, as long as protein-free

A CLASSICAL STARLING MODEL

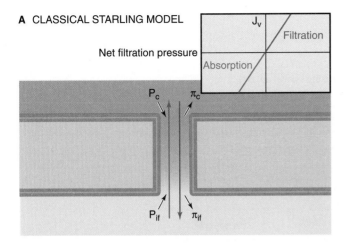

Net filtration pressure

B REVISED MODEL: FILTRATION

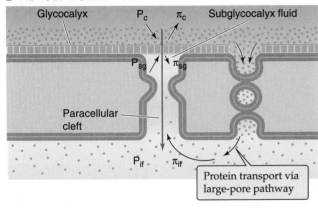

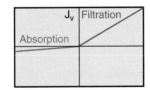

C REVISED MODEL: ABSORPTION

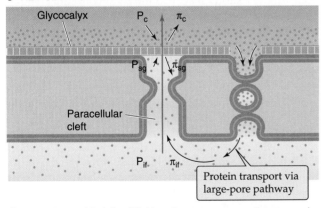

Figure 20-10 Models of fluid exchange across continuous endothelia with interendothelial junctions. P_c, capillary hydrostatic pressure; π_c, capillary colloid osmotic pressures; P_{sg}, subglycocalyx hydrostatic pressure; π_{sg}, subglycocalyx colloid osmotic pressures; P_{if}, interstitial fluid hydrostatic pressure; π_{if}, interstitial fluid colloid osmotic pressures.

ultrafiltrate enters the subglycocalyx space, the colloid osmotic pressure in the subglycocalyx fluid is low ($\pi_{sg} < \pi_{if}$). Both the rise in P_{sg} and the fall in π_{sg} tend to oppose filtration.

Because proteins enter the interstitium through the large-pore pathway, π_{if} in the bulk interstitial compartment is about that of lymph. However, at high rates of ultrafiltration, this π_{if} has no osmotic effect on the glycocalyx barrier because the protein cannot diffuse against the convective flow of fluid from lumen to interstitium. On the other hand, if the ultrafiltration rate is low, interstitial proteins can diffuse from the bulk interstitial space into the paracellular cleft, raising π_{sg} and promoting more ultrafiltration.

2. **Net flow falls to nearly zero (i.e., J_V is ~0).** Here, the parameters in the subglycocalyx fluid (i.e., P_{sg} and π_{sg}) should thus be very close to their values in the bulk interstitial fluid (i.e., P_{if} and π_{if}), and the revised model simplifies to the classical Starling model (Fig. 20-10A).

3. **During absorption (i.e., reversal of flow, where J_V is negative).** Here, water and small solutes move from the subglycocalyx space to the capillary lumen, leaving behind and thereby concentrating the protein in the subglycocalyx space (Fig. 20-10C). The resulting rise of π_{sg} (Equation 20-11) opposes further absorption and, indeed, can quickly bring it to a halt. This effect explains why the plot is nearly flat in the left lower quadrant of the inset between parts B and C in Figure 20-10.

Thus, a more sophisticated understanding of the structure of the endothelial barrier for proteins correctly makes two predictions. First, the fluxes are smaller than predicted by Starling for bulk driving forces because the actual driving force across the glycocalyx barrier (Equation 20-11) is smaller than the net driving force in the Starling equation (Equation 20-8). Second, the magnitude of the flux for a given net driving force is greater for ultrafiltration than for absorption—osmotic asymmetry or rectification.

LYMPHATICS

Lymphatics return excess interstitial fluid to the blood

Lymphatics arise in the interstitium as small thin-walled channels of endothelial cells that then join together to form increasingly larger vessels (Fig. 20-11). The **initial lymphatics** (previously called terminal lymphatics) are similar to capillaries but with many interendothelial junctions that behave like one-way microvalves, also called **primary lymph valves.** Anchoring filaments tether the initial lymphatics to surrounding connective tissue. The walls of the larger **collecting lymphatics** are similar to those of small veins, consisting of endothelium and sparse smooth muscle. The large lymphatic vessels, like the veins, have **secondary lymph valves** that restrict retrograde movement of lymph. Lymph nodes are located along the path of the collecting lymphatics. The large lymphatics ultimately drain into the left and right subclavian veins.

A   EXPANSION PHASE

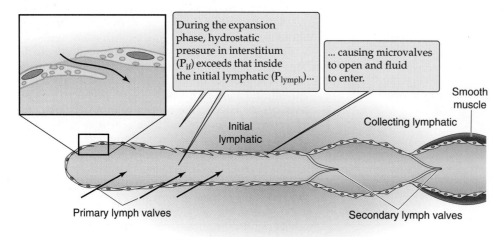

During the expansion phase, hydrostatic pressure in interstitium (P_{if}) exceeds that inside the initial lymphatic (P_{lymph})...

... causing microvalves to open and fluid to enter.

Smooth muscle

Collecting lymphatic

Initial lymphatic

Primary lymph valves

Secondary lymph valves

B   COMPRESSION PHASE

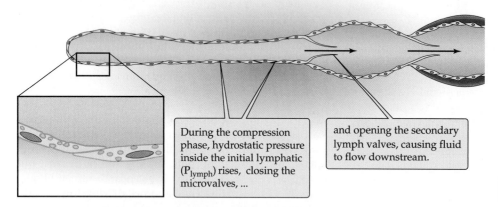

During the compression phase, hydrostatic pressure inside the initial lymphatic (P_{lymph}) rises, closing the microvalves, ...

and opening the secondary lymph valves, causing fluid to flow downstream.

Figure 20-11   Flow of lymph into initial and collecting lymphatics.

At the level of the initial lymphatics, interendothelial junctions have few tight junctions or adhesion molecules connecting neighboring endothelial cells. As a result, flaps of endothelial cells can overlap with each other and act as the microvalve discussed before. Although initial lymphatics may appear collapsed and show no contractile activity, a pressure gradient from the interstitial fluid to the lymphatic lumen deforms the endothelial cells so that the microvalves open and fluid enters the initial lymphatic during the expansion phase (Fig. 20-11A). During this time, the secondary lymph valves are closed.

External pressure (e.g., from skeletal muscle) shuts the microvalves and causes fluid to enter larger lymphatics through the now open secondary lymph valves (Fig. 20-11B).

Most organs contain both initial and collecting lymphatics, but skeletal muscle and intestine have only initial lymphatics within their tissue. Lymphatics are absent from brain. They are most prevalent in the skin and the genitourinary, respiratory, and gastrointestinal tracts.

As we have already seen, filtration at the arteriolar end of capillaries is estimated to exceed absorption at the venular end by 2 to 4 L/day. However, fluid does not normally accumulate in the interstitium because this excess fluid and protein move into the lymphatics. Thus, each day, the lymphatics return to the circulation 2 to 4 L of interstitial fluid, maintaining a steady state. In a model of congenital lymphedema, mice with genetic absence of initial lymphatics have elevated P_{if} and π_{if} as well as interstitial volume expansion (i.e., edema), emphasizing the role of the lymphatics in returning fluid and protein from the interstitial space to the blood.

Flow in Initial Lymphatics   Hydrostatic pressure in the initial lymphatics (P_{lymph}) ranges from −1 mm Hg to +1 mm Hg. Inasmuch as the mean interstitial fluid pressure is somewhat more *negative* than these values, what provides the driving force for interstitial fluid to move into the terminal lymphatics? Transient increases in P_{if} temporarily raise P_{if} above P_{lymph}. Indeed, increases in mean P_{if} cause an increase in lymph flow (Fig. 20-12).

Because the interstitium exhibits a variable compliance, fluid added to the interstitium in its low-compliance range raises the P_{if} substantially, providing the driving force for fluid to enter the lymphatics. In this same range of P_{if} values, lymphatic flow is especially sensitive to increases in P_{if} (steep portion of Fig. 20-12). Thus, lymphatic efflux nicely matches the excess capillary filtration, so that the interstitial fluid

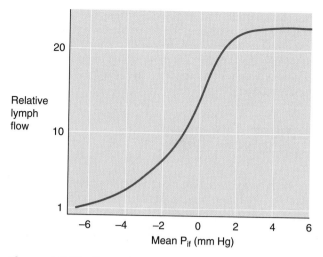

Figure 20-12 Dependence of lymph flow on interstitial pressure.

volume changes very little. The situation is very different if the interstitium is already expanded and in its high-compliance range. In this case, fluid added to the interstitium raises the already elevated P_{if} only moderately (e.g., from +2 to +4 mm Hg). In this range of P_{if} values, lymphatic uptake is not very responsive to increases in P_{if} (flat portion of Fig. 20-12). Thus, in this case, lymphatic return does not compensate well for the excess capillary filtration, so that interstitial fluid volume increases further (i.e., edema begets more edema).

Intermittent compression and relaxation of lymphatics occur during respiration, walking, and intestinal peristalsis. When P_{lymph} in a downstream segment falls below that in an upstream segment, fluid aspiration produces unidirectional flow. This suction may be largely responsible for the sub-atmospheric values of the P_{if} observed in many tissues.

Flow in Collecting Lymphatics Pressures in the collecting lymphatics range from +1 to +10 mm Hg, and they increase progressively with each valve along the vessel. As P_{lymph} rises in the collecting lymphatic vessels, smooth muscle in the lymphatic walls actively contracts by an intrinsic **myogenic** mechanism that also plays a role in blood vessels, as discussed later. Thus, downstream occlusion of a lymphatic vessel increases P_{lymph} and hence the frequency of smooth muscle contractions, whereas an upstream occlusion does the opposite. Because of the presence of one-way valves, smooth muscle contraction drives lymph toward the veins. The rhythmic contraction and relaxation of VSMCs that we will discuss for blood vessels—**vasomotion**—also occurs in lymphatics and is essential for the propulsion of lymph.

In addition to vasomotion, passive processes also propel lymph toward the blood. As is the case for the initial lymphatics, skeletal muscle contraction, respiratory movements, and intestinal contractions all passively compress the collecting lymphatics. This intermittent pumping action moves lymph into the veins.

Transport of Proteins and Cells Proteins that entered interstitial fluid from the capillary cannot return to the cir-

culation because of the adverse chemical gradient across the capillary endothelial wall. The buildup of these macromolecules in the interstitium creates a diffusional gradient from the interstitium to the lymph that complements the convective movement of these macromolecules (along with fluid) into the lymphatic system. In an average person, the lymphatics return 100 to 200 g of proteins to the circulation per day. Even before lymph reaches lymph nodes, it contains leukocytes—which had moved from the blood into the interstitium—but no red blood cells or platelets. Cycles of lymphatic compression and relaxation not only enhance fluid movement but also greatly increase the leukocyte count of lymph.

The circulation of extracellular fluids involves three convective loops: blood, interstitial fluid, and lymph

Extracellular fluid moves in *three convective loops* (Fig. 20-13). The first is the **cardiovascular loop**. Assuming a cardiac output of 5 L/min, the convective flow of blood through the circulation at rest is 7200 L/day. The second is the **transvascular loop**, in which fluid moves out of the capillaries at their arteriolar end and into the capillaries at their venular end. Not counting the kidney, whose glomeruli filter a vast amount of fluid (see Chapter 34), Landis and Pappenheimer estimated that all the other tissues of the body filter ~20 L/day at the arteriolar end of their capillaries and reabsorb 16 to 18 L at the venular end. As noted earlier, both the filtration and absorption values are probably vast overestimates. Nevertheless, the difference between filtration and absorption, 2 to 4 L/day, is a reasonable estimate of the third fluid loop, the **lymphatic loop**.

In addition to convective exchange, a *diffusional exchange* of water and solutes also occurs across the capillaries. The diffusional exchange of **water** occurs at a much higher rate than does convective movement. Using deuterium oxide as a marker, investigators have found that this diffusional exchange is approximately 80,000 L/day across all of the body's systemic capillaries. This value is about an order of magnitude greater than blood flow in the cardiovascular loop and three orders of magnitude larger than the convective flow in the transvascular filtration/absorption loop of the microcirculation. However, the diffusion of water molecules is an *exchange* process that does not contribute appreciably to the *net* movement of water. In other words, every day, 80,000 L of water diffuse out of the capillaries and 80,000 L diffuse back.

With regard to **small solutes** that can diffuse across the capillary endothelium, the traffic is quite different from the convective loops for water. Take glucose as an example. The plasma contains approximately 100 mg/dL glucose, red blood cells have little glucose, and the cardiac output of *plasma* is approximately 2.75 L/min (assuming a hematocrit of 45%). Therefore, each day, the heart pumps approximately 4000 g of glucose. This glucose can enter the interstitium by two mechanisms. First, glucose is dissolved in the water filtered from the arteriolar end of the capillaries. Each day, this filtration process carries 20 L × 100 mg/dL = 20 g of glucose into the interstitium. Second, each day, approximately 20,000 g of glucose enters the interstitium by diffusion. Convection can

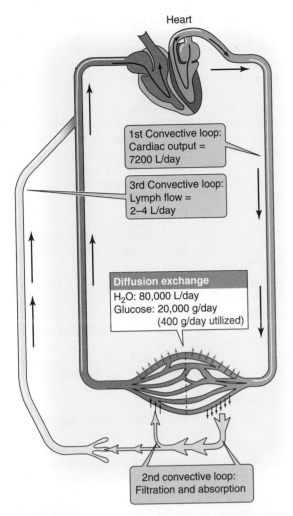

Figure 20-13 Convective loops of extracellular fluid and protein.

Within the figure:

Heart

1st Convective loop:
Cardiac output =
7200 L/day

3rd Convective loop:
Lymph flow =
2–4 L/day

Diffusion exchange
H_2O: 80,000 L/day
Glucose: 20,000 g/day
          (400 g/day utilized)

2nd convective loop:
Filtration and absorption

	Lymph flow (3rd loop)	Entry into capillary (2nd loop)	Exit from capillary (2nd loop)
FLUID	2–4 L/day	16–18 L/day	20 L/day
PROTEIN	95–195 g/day	5 g/day	100–200 g/day
GLUCOSE			20 g/day

supply only a small fraction of the approximately 400 g of glucose that the body consumes each day. Instead, diffusion supplies the majority of the glucose. Nevertheless, the 400 g/day of metabolized glucose is a minuscule fraction of the amount that enters the interstitium by diffusion. Thus, most of the glucose that diffuses into the interstitium diffuses back out again.

Protein traffic provides yet another pattern of circulatory loops. Plasma contains 7 g/dL of proteins, and—assuming a plasma volume of 3 L in a 70-kg human—total plasma protein content is ~210 g. Given a cardiac *plasma* output of 2.75 L/min, the heart pumps ~277,000 g of protein through the circulation every day. Of this protein, 100 to 200 g—nearly the entire plasma content of proteins—moves daily across the capillary walls through the large-pore system by a

transcellular route and to a lesser extent by solvent drag. Because only very small amounts of filtered protein return to the circulation by solvent drag at the venular end of capillaries (~5 g/day), nearly all of the filtered protein (95 to 195 g/day) depends on the convective lymphatic loop for its ultimate recovery.

REGULATION OF THE MICROCIRCULATION

The active contraction of vascular smooth muscle regulates precapillary resistance, which controls capillary blood flow

Smooth muscle tone in arterioles, metarterioles, and precapillary sphincters (see Chapter 19) determines the access resistance to the capillary beds. This resistance upstream of the capillary bed is also known as the afferent or **precapillary resistance** (R_{pre}). The overall resistance of a microcirculatory bed is the sum of R_{pre}, the resistance of the capillary bed itself (R_{cap}), and the efferent or **postcapillary resistance** (R_{post}).

How do these resistances influence the flow of blood (F_{cap}) through a capillary bed? We can answer this question by rearranging the Ohm's law–like expression that we introduced as Equation 17-1:

$$F_{cap} = \frac{\Delta P}{R_{total}} = \frac{P_a - P_v}{R_{pre} + R_{cap} + R_{post}} \tag{20-12}$$

P_a is the pressure just before the beginning of the precapillary resistance, and P_v is the pressure just after the end of the postcapillary resistance. Because the aggregate R_{cap} is small, and R_{post}/R_{pre} is usually approximately 0.3, R_{pre} is usually much greater than $R_{cap} + R_{post}$. Because R_{pre} is the principal determinant of total resistance, capillary flow is roughly inversely proportional to R_{pre}.

Modulating the contractility of VSMCs in *precapillary* vessels is the main mechanism for adjusting perfusion of a particular tissue. VSMCs rely on a different molecular mechanism of contraction than skeletal muscle does, although an increase in $[Ca^{2+}]_i$ is the principal trigger of contraction in both cases. Whereas an increase in $[Ca^{2+}]_i$ in skeletal muscle elicits contraction by interacting with troponin C, an increase in $[Ca^{2+}]_i$ in VSMCs elicits contraction by activating calmodulin (see Chapter 3). The Ca^{2+}-calmodulin complex (Ca^{2+}-CaM) activates myosin light chain kinase (MLCK), which in turn phosphorylates the regulatory myosin light chain (MLC) on each myosin head (see Chapter 9). Phosphorylation of MLC allows the myosin to interact with actin, producing contraction. Relaxation occurs when myosin light chain phosphatase dephosphorylates the MLC. In addition to changes in $[Ca^{2+}]_i$, changes in the activity of MLCK itself can modulate the contraction of VSMCs. Phosphorylation of MLCK by cAMP-dependent protein kinase (PKA) or cGMP-dependent protein kinase (PKG) inactivates the enzyme and thus *prevents* contraction.

Smooth muscle cells can function as a syncytium when they are coupled through gap junctions (unitary smooth muscle), or they can function independently of one another, as do skeletal muscle fibers (multiunit smooth muscle). Most vascular smooth muscle has a multiunit organization. In contrast to skeletal muscle, VSMCs receive multiple excitatory as well as inhibitory inputs. Moreover, these inputs come not only from chemical synapses (i.e., neural control) but also from circulating chemicals (i.e., humoral control). The actual contraction of VSMCs may follow smooth muscle electrical activity in the form of action potentials, slow waves of depolarization, or graded depolarizations without spikes. VSMCs can show spontaneous rhythmic variations in tension leading to periodic changes in vascular resistance and microcirculatory flow in a process called **vasomotion**. These spontaneous, rhythmic, smooth muscle contractions result either from pacemaker currents or from slow waves of depolarization and associated $[Ca^{2+}]_i$ increases in the VSMCs. Humoral agents can also directly trigger contraction of VSMCs through increases in $[Ca^{2+}]_i$, without measurable fluctuations in membrane potential (pharmacomechanical coupling; see Chapter 9).

Table 20-7 summarizes the roles that various membrane proteins (channels, transporters, and receptors) play in controlling the tone of VSMCs. Together with their associated signal transduction pathways, these membrane proteins lead to either contraction (i.e., vasoconstriction) or relaxation (i.e., vasodilation). Although a variety of neurotransmitters and circulating hormones act on smooth muscle through different receptors and transduction pathways, their effects converge on regulating the activity of MLCK.

Tissue metabolites regulate local blood flow in specific vascular beds, independently of the systemic regulation

VSMCs not only control the resistance of arterioles (i.e., R_{pre}) and thus local blood flow, they also control the resistance of small terminal arteries and thereby play an important role in regulating systemic arterial blood pressure. In Chapter 23, we discuss this control of arterial blood pressure (a whole-body function) through VSMCs of small arteries and arterioles, both of which are under the control of *central* mechanisms—the autonomic nervous system and systemic humoral agents (e.g., angiotensin II). However, the subject of this discussion is *local regulatory mechanisms* that use the arterioles to regulate blood flow through specific vascular beds. These local control mechanisms can override any of the neural or systemic humoral influences.

Mechanisms of local control involve (1) myogenic activity and (2) local chemical and humoral factors. **Myogenic regulation** refers to an *intrinsic* mode of control of activity, in which stretch of the VSMC membrane activates stretch-sensitive channels (Table 20-7). The result is a depolarization that affects pacemaker activity, thereby eliciting contraction of the VSMC.

The most prominent **chemical factors** are interstitial P_{O_2}, P_{CO_2}, and pH as well as local concentrations of K^+, lactic acid, adenosine triphosphate (ATP), adenosine diphosphate (ADP), and adenosine (Table 20-8). Total osmolality may also make a contribution. The local regulation of VSMCs by *interstitial* P_{O_2}, P_{CO_2}, and pH is distinct from the regulation of systemic blood pressure by the peripheral chemoreceptors, which respond to changes in *arterial* P_{O_2}, P_{CO_2}, and pH (see Chapter 32) and initiate a complex neural reflex that

modulates VSMC activity (see Chapter 23). In the case of *local* control, chemical changes in interstitial fluid act *directly* on the VSMCs through one of the transduction mechanisms listed in Table 20-7. Changes that typically accompany increased metabolism (e.g., low P_{O_2}, high P_{CO_2}, and low pH) vasodilate vessels in the systemic circulation. Such local changes in P_{O_2}, P_{CO_2}, and pH have opposite effects in the pulmonary circulation (see Chapter 31).

Because blood flow itself can wash out the metabolic intermediates, vasomotion can arise from a local feedback system. For example, if interstitial P_{O_2} falls as a result of increased local O_2 consumption, the ensuing vasodilation will increase O_2 delivery to the metabolizing cells and in turn will tend to cause the local interstitial P_{O_2} to increase. As the P_{O_2} now increases, vascular tone will increase. The timing of release and washout of the chemical factors determines the frequency of the vasomotion. The interstitial fluid volume around the active cells—the volume in which vasoactive metabolites are distributed—also affects this periodicity because it affects the time lag for the concentration of vasoactive substances to rise or to fall. Finally, spontaneous fluctuations in metabolism may confer an additional periodicity to vasomotion.

The endothelium of capillary beds is the source of several vasoactive compounds, including NO, EDHF, and endothelin

The capillary endothelium is the source of several important vasoactive compounds (Table 20-9).

Nitric Oxide (NO) Originally called endothelium-derived relaxing factor, NO is a potent vasodilator. NO also inhibits platelet aggregation, induces platelet disaggregation, and inhibits platelet adhesion. Bradykinin and acetylcholine both stimulate the NOS III (or eNOS) isoform of NO synthase (see Chapter 3) that is constitutively present in endothelial cells. Increases in shear stress—the force acting on the endothelial cell along the axis of blood flow—can also stimulate the enzyme. NOS III, which depends on both Ca^{2+} and calmodulin for its activity, catalyzes the formation of NO from arginine. NO, a lipophilic gas with a short half-life, diffuses locally outside the endothelial cell. Inside the VSMC is the "receptor" for NO, a soluble guanylyl cyclase that converts guanosine triphosphate (GTP) to cyclic guanosine monophosphate (cGMP). cGMP-dependent protein kinase (i.e., PKG) then phosphorylates MLCK and SERCA. Phosphorylation *inhibits* the MLCK, thus leading to a net decrease in the phosphorylation of MLC and a decrease in the interaction between myosin and actin. Phosphorylation *activates* SERCA, thereby decreasing $[Ca^{2+}]_i$. The net result is that NO released by endothelial cells relaxes VSMCs, producing vasodilation.

Physicians have used exogenous organic nitrates (e.g., nitroglycerin) for decades to dilate peripheral vessels for relief of the pain of angina pectoris. These powerful vasodilators exert their activity by breaking down chemically, thereby releasing NO near VSMCs.

Endothelium-Derived Hyperpolarizing Factor (EDHF) In addition to releasing NO, endothelial cells release another

Table 20-7 Molecular Mechanisms Underlying the Contraction and Relaxation of Vascular Smooth Muscle

Contraction (Vasoconstriction)	Relaxation (Vasodilation)
Voltage-gated Ca^{2+} channels, Cav	**Voltage-gated K^+ channels, Kv**
Depolarization $\rightarrow$ voltage-gated Ca^{2+} channels open $\rightarrow$ Ca^{2+} entry $\rightarrow$ $\uparrow[Ca^{2+}]_i$	Depolarization $\rightarrow$ voltage-gated K^+ channels open $\rightarrow$ hyperpolarization $\rightarrow$ Ca^{2+} channels close $\rightarrow$ $\downarrow[Ca^{2+}]_i$
Voltage-gated Na^+ channels, Nav	**Ca^{2+}-dependent K^+ channels**
Depolarization $\rightarrow$ voltage-gated Na^+ channels open $\rightarrow$ more depolarization $\rightarrow$ voltage-gated Ca^{2+} channels open $\rightarrow$ Ca^{2+} entry $\rightarrow$ $\uparrow[Ca^{2+}]_i$	Hyperpolarization $\rightarrow$ voltage-gated Ca^{2+} channels close $\rightarrow$ $\downarrow[Ca^{2+}]_i$
Stretch-activated (SA) nonselective cation channels	**ATP-sensitive K^+ channels, K_{ATP}**
Stretch $\rightarrow$ SA channels open $\rightarrow$ depolarization $\rightarrow$ voltage-gated Ca^{2+} channels open $\rightarrow$ Ca^{2+} entry $\rightarrow$ $\uparrow[Ca^{2+}]_i$	$\downarrow[ATP]_i \rightarrow K_{ATP}$ channels open $\rightarrow$ hyperpolarization $\rightarrow$ Ca^{2+} channels close $\rightarrow$ $\downarrow[Ca^{2+}]_i$
Na-Ca exchanger, NCX	**SR Ca^{2+} pump, SERCA2**
Depolarization $\rightarrow$ voltage-gated Na^+ channels open $\rightarrow$ Na^+ entry $\rightarrow$ $\uparrow[Na^+]_i \rightarrow$ slows Na-Ca^{2+} exchange $\rightarrow$ $\uparrow[Ca^{2+}]_i$	Activation of SERCA2 $\rightarrow$ $\downarrow[Ca^{2+}]_i$
Endothelin receptor, ET_A	**NO receptor, sGC (a soluble guanylyl cyclase)**
ET $\rightarrow$ endothelin receptor $ET_A \rightarrow \uparrow G\alpha_{q/11} \rightarrow \uparrow PLC \rightarrow \uparrow[IP_3]_i \rightarrow$ IP_3 receptor in SR $\rightarrow \uparrow Ca^{2+}$ release $\rightarrow \uparrow[Ca^{2+}]_i$	NO $\rightarrow \uparrow sGC \rightarrow \uparrow[cGMP]_i \rightarrow \uparrow PKG \rightarrow$ $\uparrow$phosphorylation of MLCK $\rightarrow \downarrow$MLCK activity $\rightarrow \downarrow$phosphorylation of MLC $\uparrow$SERCA2 in SR $\rightarrow \downarrow[Ca^{2+}]_i$
Thromboxane receptor, TP	**Prostacyclin (PGI_2) receptor, IP** **Prostaglandin E_2 (PGE_2) receptor, EP_2 and EP_4**
$TXA_2 \rightarrow$ TP receptor: • $\rightarrow Ca^{2+}$ channels open $\rightarrow Ca^{2+}$ entry $\rightarrow \uparrow[Ca^{2+}]_i$ • $\rightarrow \uparrow O_2^- \rightarrow \downarrow$NO	$PGI_2 \rightarrow$ IP receptor *or* $PGE_2 \rightarrow EP_2$ and $EP_4 \rightarrow \uparrow G\alpha_s \rightarrow \uparrow AC \rightarrow \uparrow[cAMP]_i \rightarrow$ $\uparrow PKA \rightarrow \uparrow$phosphorylation of MLCK $\rightarrow \downarrow$MLCK $\rightarrow$ $\downarrow$phosphorylation of MLC
Adrenergic receptor, α_1	**Adrenergic receptor, β_2**
Agonist (e.g., norepinephrine) $\rightarrow$ adrenoreceptor $\alpha_1 \rightarrow$ $\uparrow G\alpha_{q/11} \rightarrow \uparrow PLC \rightarrow \uparrow[IP_3]_i \rightarrow IP_3$ receptor in SR $\rightarrow \uparrow Ca^{2+}$ release $\rightarrow \uparrow[Ca^{2+}]_i$	Agonist (e.g., epinephrine) $\rightarrow$ adrenoreceptor $\beta_2 \rightarrow \uparrow G\alpha_s \rightarrow \uparrow AC \rightarrow$ $\uparrow[cAMP]_i \rightarrow \uparrow PKA \rightarrow \uparrow$phosphorylation of MLCK $\rightarrow \downarrow$MLCK $\rightarrow$ $\downarrow$phosphorylation of MLC
Muscarinic receptor, M_2	**Histamine receptor, H_2**
Agonist (e.g., acetylcholine) $\rightarrow M_2$ receptor $\rightarrow \uparrow G\alpha_{i/o} \rightarrow$ $\downarrow AC \rightarrow \downarrow[cAMP]_i \rightarrow \downarrow PKA \rightarrow \downarrow$phosphorylation of MLCK $\rightarrow$ $\uparrow$MLCK $\rightarrow \uparrow$phosphorylation of MLC	Histamine $\rightarrow H_2$ receptor $\rightarrow \uparrow G\alpha_s \rightarrow \uparrow AC \rightarrow \uparrow[cAMP]_i \rightarrow \uparrow PKA \rightarrow$ $\uparrow$phosphorylation of MLCK $\rightarrow \downarrow$MLCK $\rightarrow \downarrow$phosphorylation of MLC
Purinergic receptor, P_{2X}	**Purinergic receptor, P_{2Y}**
$\uparrow[ATP]_o \rightarrow P_{2X}$ receptor (ligand-gated Ca^{2+} channel = receptor-operated Ca^{2+} channel = ROC) $\rightarrow Ca^{2+}$ entry $\rightarrow \uparrow[Ca^{2+}]_i$	$\uparrow[ATP]_o \rightarrow P_{2Y}$ metabotropic receptor $\rightarrow \uparrow G\alpha_{q/11} \rightarrow \uparrow PLC \rightarrow$ $\uparrow[Ca^{2+}]_i \rightarrow \uparrow NOS \rightarrow$ NO release
Purinergic receptor (adenosine/P1 type), A_1	**Purinergic receptor (adenosine/P1 type), A_1, A_{2A}, A_{2B}**
$\uparrow[Adenosine]_o \rightarrow A_1$ receptor on VSMC in renal afferent arterioles $\rightarrow \uparrow G\alpha_{q/11} \rightarrow \uparrow PLC \rightarrow \uparrow[IP_3]_i \rightarrow IP_3$ receptor in SR $\rightarrow \uparrow Ca^{2+}$ release $\rightarrow \uparrow[Ca^{2+}]_i$	$\uparrow[Adenosine]_o \rightarrow A_1$, A_{2A}, and A_{2B} receptor on *VSMC* $\rightarrow \uparrow G\alpha_s \rightarrow$ $\uparrow AC \rightarrow \uparrow[cAMP]_i \rightarrow \uparrow PKA \rightarrow K_{ATP}$ channels open $\rightarrow$ hyperpolarization $\rightarrow$ voltage-gated Ca^{2+} channels close $\rightarrow \downarrow[Ca^{2+}]_i$ $\uparrow$Phosphorylation of MLCK $\rightarrow \downarrow$MLCK $\rightarrow \downarrow$phosphorylation of MLC $\uparrow[Adenosine]_o \rightarrow A_1$ on *endothelial cell* $\rightarrow \uparrow NOS \rightarrow$ NO release

Table 20-7 Molecular Mechanisms Underlying the Contraction and Relaxation of Vascular Smooth Muscle—cont'd

Contraction (Vasoconstriction)	Relaxation (Vasodilation)
NPY receptor, Y1R	**VIP receptor, VIPR1 and VIPR2**
Neuropeptide Y $\rightarrow$ Y1R $\rightarrow$ $\uparrow G\alpha_{i/o}$ $\rightarrow$ $\downarrow$AC $\rightarrow$ $\downarrow[cAMP]_i$ $\rightarrow$ $\downarrow$PKA $\rightarrow$ $\downarrow$phosphorylation of MLCK $\rightarrow$ $\uparrow$MLCK $\rightarrow$ $\uparrow$phosphorylation of MLC	VIP $\rightarrow$ VIPR1 and VIPR2 receptors $\rightarrow$ $\uparrow G\alpha_s$ $\rightarrow$ $\uparrow$AC $\rightarrow$ $\uparrow[cAMP]_i$ $\rightarrow$ $\uparrow$PKA $\rightarrow$ $\uparrow$phosphorylation of MLCK $\rightarrow$ $\downarrow$MLCK $\rightarrow$ $\downarrow$phosphorylation of MLC Both Ca^{2+}-dependent and voltage-gated K^+ channels open $\rightarrow$ hyperpolarization $\rightarrow$ Ca^{2+} channels close $\rightarrow$ $\downarrow[Ca^{2+}]_i$
Angiotensin receptor, AT₁	**Angiotensin receptor, AT₂**
ANG II $\rightarrow$ AT₁ receptor $\rightarrow$ $\uparrow G\alpha_{q/11}$ $\rightarrow$ $\uparrow$PLC $\rightarrow$ $\uparrow[IP_3]_i$ $\rightarrow$ IP₃ receptor in SR $\rightarrow$ $\uparrow Ca^{2+}$ release $\rightarrow$ $\uparrow[Ca^{2+}]_i$	ANG II $\rightarrow$ AT₂ receptor $\rightarrow$ $\uparrow G\alpha_{q/11}$ $\rightarrow$ $\uparrow$PLC $\rightarrow$ $\uparrow[Ca^{2+}]_i$ $\rightarrow$ $\uparrow$NOS $\rightarrow$ NO release $\rightarrow$ $\uparrow$Bradykinin $\rightarrow$ $\uparrow$NOS III $\rightarrow$ NO release
AVP receptor, V₁ₐR or V₁R	**Natriuretic peptide receptor A, NPR1**
AVP $\rightarrow$ V₁ₐ receptor $\rightarrow$ $G\alpha_q$ $\rightarrow$ $\uparrow$PLC $\rightarrow$ $\uparrow[IP_3]_i$ $\rightarrow$ IP₃ receptor in SR $\rightarrow$ $\uparrow Ca^{2+}$ release $\rightarrow$ $\uparrow[Ca^{2+}]_i$	ANP $\rightarrow$ NPR1 receptor $\rightarrow$ $\uparrow$GC $\rightarrow$ $\uparrow[cGMP]_i$ $\rightarrow$ $\uparrow$PKG $\rightarrow$ $\uparrow$phosphorylation of MLCK $\rightarrow$ $\downarrow$MLCK $\rightarrow$ $\downarrow$phosphorylation of MLC $\uparrow$SERCA2 in SR $\rightarrow$ $\downarrow[Ca^{2+}]_i$
Serotonin (5-hydroxytryptamine) receptor, 5-HT₂ₐ or 5-HT₂ᵦ	**Bradykinin receptor, B2**
5-HT $\rightarrow$ 5-HT₂ₐ or 5-HT₂ᵦ receptor $\rightarrow$ $\uparrow G\alpha_{q/11}$ $\rightarrow$ $\uparrow$PLC $\rightarrow$ $\uparrow[IP_3]_i$ $\rightarrow$ IP₃ receptor in SR $\rightarrow$ $\uparrow Ca^{2+}$ release $\rightarrow$ $\uparrow[Ca^{2+}]_i$	Bradykinin $\rightarrow$ B2R receptor on *endothelial cell* $\rightarrow$ $\uparrow G\alpha_{q/11}$ $\rightarrow$ $\uparrow$PLC $\rightarrow$ $\uparrow[Ca^{2+}]_i$ $\rightarrow$ $\uparrow$eNOS $\rightarrow$ $\uparrow$NO release $\uparrow$PLA₂ $\rightarrow$ $\uparrow$PGI₂ and PGE₂ release

AC, adenylyl cyclase; ANP, atrial natriuretic peptide; AVP, arginine vasopressin; GC, guanylyl cyclase; IP₃, inositol trisphosphate; MLC, myosin light chain; MLCK, myosin light chain kinase; NPY, neuropeptide Y (see Fig. 14-10); NOS, nitric oxide synthase; PKA, protein kinase A (cAMP-stimulated protein kinase); PKG, protein kinase G (cGMP-stimulated protein kinase); PLA₂, phospholipase A₂; PLC, phospholipase C; SR, sarcoplasmic reticulum; VIP, vasoactive intestinal peptide (see Fig. 14-11).

Table 20-8 Local Metabolic Changes That Cause Vasodilation in the Systemic Circulation

Change	Mechanism*
$\downarrow P_{O_2}$	$\downarrow[ATP]_i$, $\uparrow$adenosine release, $\uparrow$PGI₂ release, $\uparrow$NO release
$\uparrow P_{CO_2}$	$\downarrow pH_o$
$\downarrow$pH	$\downarrow pH_o$
$\uparrow[K^+]_o$	Transient hyperpolarization $\rightarrow$ closes voltage-gated Ca^{2+} channels
$\uparrow$[Lactic acid]$_o$	Probably $\downarrow pH_o$
$\downarrow[ATP]_i$	Opens K_{ATP} channels
$\uparrow[ATP]_o$	Activates purinergic receptors P_2
$\uparrow[ADP]_o$	Activates purinergic receptors P_2
$\uparrow[Adenosine]_o$	Activates purinergic receptors P_1

*The subscript *i* refers to intracellular levels, and the subscript *o* refers to interstitial levels.

Table 20-9 Vasoactive Agents Produced by Endothelial Cells

Vasodilators	Vasoconstrictors
Nitric oxide (NO)	Endothelin (ET)
Endothelium-derived hyperpolarizing factor (EDHF)	Endothelium-derived constricting factor 1 (EDCF₁)
Prostacyclin (PGI₂)	Endothelium-derived constricting factor 2 (EDCF₂)

relaxing factor in response to acetylcholine, EDHF. EDHF causes VSMC relaxation by making the membrane potential more negative.

Prostacyclin (PGI₂) Prostacyclin synthase (see Fig. 3-11) metabolizes arachidonic acid to the vasodilator PGI₂. This agent acts by increasing $[cAMP]_i$ and promoting the phosphorylation of MLCK, ultimately decreasing the phosphorylation of myosin light chains. PGI₂ is especially important for dilation of pulmonary vessels at birth (see Chapter 57).

Endothelins (ETs) Endothelial cells produce 21-residue peptides that cause an extremely potent and long-lasting

vasoconstriction in most VSMCs. Many acute and chronic pathological conditions, including hypoxia, promote the release of endothelin, which exists as three isopeptides: ET-1, ET-2, and ET-3. The precursor of **ET-1** is *preproendothelin*, which the endothelial cell converts first to *proendothelin* and then to the mature *endothelin*, which it releases. The ET receptor subtype for vasoconstriction is ET_A. Other endothelin receptors also exist; ET_{B1} mediates vasodilation, ET_{B2} mediates vasoconstriction, and ET_C has as yet no clearly defined function. ET_A receptors predominate in high-pressure parts of the circulation, whereas ET_B receptors predominate in low-pressure parts of the circulation.

The binding of an endothelin to any endothelin receptor subtype ultimately results in an increase in $[Ca^{2+}]_i$. In the *vasoconstriction* response, ET-1 binding to ET_A receptors acts through the phospholipase C pathway to generate inositol trisphosphate, to release Ca^{2+} from intracellular stores, and to raise $[Ca^{2+}]_i$ (see Chapter 3). In a second, delayed phase, which is not well understood, Ca^{2+} entering from the outside contributes to the increase in $[Ca^{2+}]_i$. The increased $[Ca^{2+}]_i$ activates Ca^{2+}-CaM, stimulating MLCK to phosphorylate myosin light chains and culminating in contraction.

Thromboxane A_2 (TXA_2) Endothelial cells and platelets metabolize arachidonic acid through the cyclooxygenase pathway to produce TXA_2 (see Chapter 3). This agent activates TXA_2/prostaglandin H_2 (TP) receptors, leading to opening of L-type Ca channels, thereby increasing $[Ca^{2+}]_i$. In addition, TP activation increases the levels of superoxide anion radical O_2^- in VSMCs. In turn, O_2^- reacts with NO, thereby reducing the vasodilating effect of NO.

Other Endothelial Factors In some systemic arteries of the dog, *anoxia* produces an unexpected effect: an endothelium-dependent *increase* in tension mediated by a putative factor, $EDCF_1$ (endothelium-derived constricting factor). In some dog arteries, rapid *stretch* evokes a contraction that is also endothelium dependent. This putative factor, $EDCF_2$, could be a superoxide anion because superoxide dismutase prevents the contractions.

Autoregulation stabilizes blood flow despite large fluctuations in systemic arterial pressure

As we saw in Chapter 17, the pressure-flow relationship of an idealized, rigid vessel is linear (Fig. 20-14, gray line). In most real (i.e., elastic) vessels, however, increases in pressure cause a dilation that reduces resistance and leads to a steeper-than-linear flow (Fig. 20-14, red curve). However, some vascular beds behave very differently. Despite large changes in the systemic arterial pressure—and thus large changes in the driving pressure—these special vascular beds maintain local blood flow within a narrow range. This phenomenon is called **autoregulation**. These vascular beds behave more or less like rigid tubes at very low and at very high perfusion pressures (Fig. 20-14, blue curve). However, in the physiological pressure range over which autoregulation occurs, changes in perfusion pressure have little effect on flow. Instead, increases in *pressure* lead to increases in *resistance* that keep blood flow within a carefully controlled range.

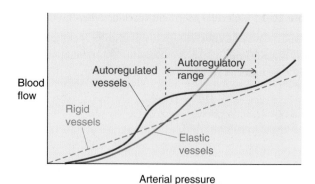

Figure 20-14 Autoregulation of blood flow.

Autoregulatory behavior takes time to develop and is due to an active process. If the perfusion pressure were to increase abruptly, we would see that immediately after the pressure increase, the pressure-flow diagram would look much like the one for the rigid tube in Figure 20-14. However, the vascular arteriolar tone then slowly adjusts itself to produce the characteristic autoregulatory pressure-flow diagram. The contraction of VSMCs that underlies autoregulation is *autonomous*, that is, it is entirely local and independent of neural and endocrine mechanisms. Both myogenic and metabolic mechanisms play an important role in the adjustments of smooth muscle tone during autoregulation. For example, the stretch of VSMCs that accompanies the increased perfusion pressure triggers a myogenic contraction that reduces blood flow. Also, the increase in P_{O_2} (or decrease in P_{CO_2} or increase in pH) that accompanies increased perfusion pressure triggers a metabolic vasoconstriction that reduces blood flow (Table 20-8).

Autoregulation is useful for at least two reasons. First, with an increase in perfusion pressure, autoregulation avoids a waste of perfusion in organs in which the flow is already sufficient. Second, with a decrease in perfusion pressure, autoregulation maintains capillary flow and capillary pressure. Autoregulation is very important under these conditions for organs—particularly the heart, brain, and kidneys—that are very sensitive to ischemia or hypoxia and for organs (again, the kidney) whose job it is to filter the blood.

New blood vessels proliferate in response to growth factors by a process known as angiogenesis

In adults, the anatomy of the microcirculation remains rather constant. Notable exceptions are the growth of new vessels during wound healing, inflammation, and tumor growth and in the endometrium during the menstrual cycle. Increased capillary density is important in physical training and in acclimatization to altitude (see Chapters 60 and 61).

The development of new vessels is called **angiogenesis**. The first step is dissolution of the venular basement membrane at a specific site, followed by activation and proliferation of previously quiescent endothelial cells. The new cells, attracted by growth factors, migrate to form a tube. Eventually, the budding tubes connect with each other, allowing the

Table 20-10 Agents That Affect Vascular Growth

Promoters	Inhibitors
Vascular endothelial growth factor (VEGF)	Endostatin
Fibroblast growth factors (FGFs)	Angiostatin
Angiopoietin 1 (ANGPT1)	Angiopoietin 2 (ANGPT2)

flow of blood and the development of vascular smooth muscle as the new microvascular network establishes itself. Angiogenesis relies on a balance between positive and negative regulation. The body normally produces some factors that promote angiogenesis and others that inhibit it (Table 20-10).

Promoters of Vessel Growth   The principal peptides that induce angiogenesis are two polypeptides: vascular endothelial growth factor (VEGF) and fibroblast growth factor (FGF). Both interact with endothelium-specific receptor tyrosine kinases (see Chapter 3). **VEGF**—related to platelet-derived growth factor (PDGF) and a mitogen for vascular endothelial cells—is produced by fibroblasts and, frequently, by cancer cells. Activated coagulation factor VII (FVIIa; see Chapter 18) promotes VEGF production.

FGF mediates many cellular responses during embryonic, fetal, and postnatal development. At least 22 different fibroblast growth factors exist in humans. FGF-2 (also known as basic fibroblast growth factor or bFGF) has particular angiogenic activity.

VEGF and FGF-2 promote expression of NOS. The resulting NO promotes proliferation and migration of endothelial cells as well as differentiation of vascular tubes.

The targeted delivery of these growth factors is a major obstacle in their therapeutic use. One approach has been to link the growth factor to small beads delivered into the coronary circulation. Clinical trials with local or systemic administration of FGF-2 to patients with ischemic heart disease have shown mixed efficacy. A recombinant, humanized monoclonal antibody against VEGF (Avastin) is being used in patients with advanced non–small cell lung cancer.

Other growth factors have indirect angiogenic effects that are distinct from those of VEGF or FGF. **Angiopoietins** (ANGPT1 and ANGPT2) are proteins that act through a receptor tyrosine kinase (Tie2) expressed almost exclusively in endothelial cells. ANGPT1 is required for *embryonic* vascular development, and ANGPT2—normally an antagonist of ANGPT1 at the Tie2 receptor—is required for *postnatal* angiogenic remodeling. **Angiogenin**, a member of the ribonuclease family, is normally present in plasma, but at levels too low to produce proliferative effects. Plasma angiogenin levels rise in cancer patients. Regulated surface receptors on endothelial cells bind angiogenin, which after endocytosis translocates to the nucleus, where its RNAse activity is essential for its angiogenic effect.

Inhibitors of Vessel Growth   The concept of antiangiogenesis was first advanced by Judah Folkman as a strategy to stop the growth of tumors. He and his colleagues have described two peptides, angiostatin and endostatin, that are inhibitors of angiogenesis.

Angiostatin is a kringle-containing fragment of plasminogen, a key fibrinolytic protein (see Chapter 18). Angiostatin arises by proteolytic cleavage of plasminogen by connective tissue enzymes, such as matrix metalloproteinases and elastase. Angiostatin inhibits angiogenesis by enhancing apoptosis of endothelial cells and inhibiting migration and tube formation, rather than by affecting proliferation. Recombinant angiostatin is being tested in patients with advanced lung cancer.

Endostatin is a peptide breakdown product of collagen XVIII. It is produced by the extracellular matrix of tumors.

We can illustrate the importance of angiogenesis by highlighting three clinical situations in which angiogenesis plays an important role. First, enhancement of vessel growth is important during coronary artery disease, when chronic ischemia of the heart leads to the development of new vessels and thus collateral circulation. Second, angiogenesis enhances the blood supply to a tumor, thereby promoting its growth and opening the principal route by which tumor cells exit the primary tumor during metastasis. Oncologists are exploring the use of angiogenesis inhibitors to treat cancer. Third, angiogenesis may also be important in diabetic retinopathy, where blood vessel proliferation can cause blindness.

REFERENCES

Books and Reviews
Grossman JD, Morgan JP: Cardiovascular effects of endothelin. News Physiol Sci 1997; 12:113-117.

Khurana R, Simons M, Martin JF, Zachary IC: Role of angiogenesis in cardiovascular disease: A critical appraisal. Circulation 2005; 112:1813-1824.

Michel CC: Fluid exchange in the microcirculation. J Physiol 2004; 557:701-702.

Moncada S, Higgs A: The discovery of nitric oxide and its role in vascular biology. Br J Pharmacol 2006; 147:S193-S201.

Segal SS: Regulation of blood flow in the microcirculation. Microcirculation 2005; 12:33-45.

Journal Articles
Adamson RH, Lenz JF, Zhang X, et al: Oncotic pressures opposing filtration across non-fenestrated rat microvessels. J Physiol 2004; 557:889-907.

Buga GM, Gold ME, Fukuto JM, Ignarro LJ: Shear-stress induced release of nitric oxide from endothelial cells grown on beads. Hypertension 1991; 17:187-193.

Furchgott RF, Zawadzki V: The obligatory role of endothelial cells in the relaxation of arterial smooth muscle by acetylcholine. Nature 1988; 336:385-388.

O'Reilly MS, Holmgren L, Shing Y, et al: Angiostatin: A novel angiogenesis inhibitor that mediates the suppression of metastases by a Lewis lung carcinoma. Cell 1994; 79:315-328.

Rees DD, Palmer RMJ, Moncada S: Role of endothelium-derived nitric oxide in the regulation of blood pressure. Proc Natl Acad Sci USA 1989; 86:3375-3378.

CHAPTER 21

CARDIAC ELECTROPHYSIOLOGY AND THE ELECTROCARDIOGRAM

W. Jonathan Lederer

Different cardiac cells serve different and very specialized functions, but all are electrically active. The heart's electrical signal normally originates in a group of cells high in the right atrium that depolarize spontaneously; it then spreads throughout the heart from cell to cell (Fig. 21-1). As this action potential propagates through the heart—sometimes carried by cells that form specialized conducting pathways and sometimes by the very cells that generate the force of contraction—it assumes different appearances within the different cardiac cells (Fig. 21-2). By the speed of the upstroke, we can characterize action potentials as either **slow** (SA and AV nodes) or **fast** (atrial myocytes, Purkinje fibers, and ventricular myocytes).

Because the excitation of cardiac myocytes triggers contraction—a process called *excitation-contraction coupling* (see Chapter 9)—the propagation of action potentials must be carefully timed to synchronize ventricular contraction and thereby optimize the ejection of blood. This chapter focuses on the membrane currents responsible for the generation and transmission of action potentials in heart tissue. We also examine how to record the heart's electrical flow by placement of electrodes on the surface of the body, creating one of the simplest and yet one of the most useful diagnostic tools available to the clinician—the electrocardiogram.

ELECTROPHYSIOLOGY OF CARDIAC CELLS

The cardiac action potential starts in specialized muscle cells of the sinoatrial node and then propagates in an orderly fashion throughout the heart

The cardiac action potential originates in a group of cells called the **sinoatrial (SA) node** (Fig. 21-1), located in the right atrium. These cells depolarize spontaneously and fire off action potentials at a regular, intrinsic rate that is usually between 60 and 100 times per minute for an individual at rest. Both parasympathetic and sympathetic neural input can modulate this intrinsic **pacemaker** activity, or *automaticity* (see Chapter 16).

Because cardiac cells are electrically coupled through gap junctions (Fig. 21-3A), the action potential propagates from cell to cell in the same way that an action potential in nerve conducts along a single, long axon. A spontaneous action potential originating in the SA node will conduct from cell to cell throughout the right atrial muscle and spread to the left atrium. The existence of discrete conducting pathways in the atria is still disputed. About one tenth of a second after its origination, the signal arrives at the **atrioventricular (AV) node** (Fig. 21-1). The impulse does not spread directly from the atria to the ventricles because of the presence of a fibrous **atrioventricular ring**. Instead, the only available pathway is for the impulse to travel from the AV node to the **His-Purkinje fiber system**, a network of specialized conducting cells that carries the signal to the muscle of both ventricles.

The cardiac action potential conducts from cell to cell through gap junctions

The electrical influence of one cardiac cell on another depends on the voltage difference between the cells and on the resistance of the gap junction connection between them. A **gap junction** (see Chapter 8) is an **electrical synapse** (Fig. 21-3A) that permits electrical current to flow between neighboring cells. According to Ohm's law, the current flowing between cell A and the adjacent cell B (I_{AB}) is proportional to the voltage difference between the two cells (ΔV_{AB}) but inversely proportional to the electrical resistance between them (R_{AB}):

$$I_{AB} = \frac{V_A - V_B}{R_{AB}} = \frac{\Delta V_{AB}}{R_{AB}} \qquad (21\text{-}1)$$

When R_{AB} is very small (i.e., when the cells are tightly coupled), the gap junctions are minimal barriers to the flow of depolarizing current.

Imagine that several interconnected cells are initially all at their normal resting potentials (Fig. 21-3B). An action potential propagating from the left of cell A now injects depolarizing current into cell A. As a result, the cell depolarizes to V_A, which is now somewhat positive compared with

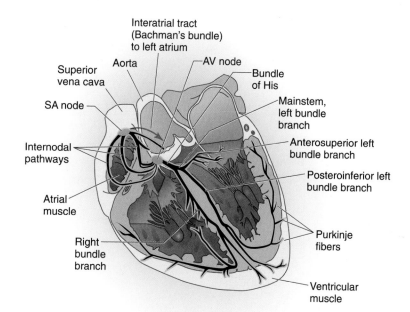

Figure 21-1 Conduction pathways through the heart. A section through the long axis of the heart is shown.

V_B. Thus, a small depolarizing current (i.e., positive charges) will also move from cell A to cell B and depolarize cell B. In turn, current flowing from cell B will then depolarize cell C. By this process, the cells closest to the current source undergo the greatest depolarization.

Imagine that the injected current, coming from the active region of the heart to the left, depolarizes cell A just to its threshold (Fig. 21-3C, red curve) but that cell A has not yet fired an action potential. At this instant, the current passing from cell A to cell B cannot bring cell B to its threshold. Of course, cell A will eventually fire an action potential and, in the process, depolarize enough to inject enough current into cell B to raise cell B to its threshold. Thus, the action potential propagates down the chain of cells, but relatively slowly. On the other hand, if the active region to the left injects *more* current into cell A (Fig. 21-3C, blue curve)—producing a larger depolarization in cell A—the current passing from cell A to cell B will be greater and sufficient to depolarize cell B beyond its voltage threshold for a regenerative action potential. However, at this instant, the current passing from cell B to cell C is still not sufficient to trigger an action potential in cell C. That will have to wait until the active region moves closer to cell C, but the wait is not as long as in the first example (red curve). Thus, the action potential propagates more rapidly in this second example (blue curve).

In principle, we could make the action potential propagate more rapidly down the chain of cells in two ways. First, we could allow more ion channels to open in the active region of the heart, so that depolarizing current is larger (blue curve in Fig. 21-3C). Second, we could lower the threshold for the regenerative action potential ("more negative threshold" in Fig. 21-3C), so that even the small current represented by the red curve is now sufficient to trigger cell B.

Just as in a nerve axon conducting an action potential, the intracellular and extracellular currents in heart muscle must be equal and opposite. In the active region of the heart (to the left of cell A in Fig. 21-3B), cells have reached threshold and their action potentials provide the *source* of current that depolarizes cells that are approaching threshold (e.g., cells A and B). As cell A itself is depolarizing to and beyond threshold, its Na^+ and Ca^{2+} channels are opening, enabling these cations (i.e., positive charge) to enter. The positive charge that enters cell A not only depolarizes cell A but also produces a flow of positive charge to cell B—**intracellular current**. This flow of positive charge discharges the membrane capacitance of cell B, thereby depolarizing cell B and releasing extracellular positive charges that had been associated with the membrane. The movement of this extracellular positive charge from around cell B toward the extracellular region around cell A constitutes the **extracellular current**. The flow of intracellular current from cell A to cell B and the flow of extracellular current from around cell B to around cell A are equal and opposite. It is the flow of this *extracellular* current in the heart that gives rise to an instantaneous electrical vector, which changes with time. Each point on an **electrocardiogram** (ECG) is the sum of the many such electrical vectors, generated by the many cells of the heart.

Cardiac action potentials have as many as five distinctive phases

The initiation time, shape, and duration of the action potential are distinctive for different parts of the heart, reflecting their different functions (Fig. 21-2). These distinctions arise because the myocytes in each region of the heart have a characteristic set of channels and anatomy. Underlying cardiac action potentials are four major time-dependent and voltage-gated membrane currents (Table 21-1):

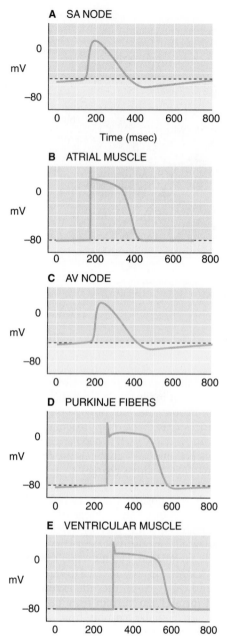

Figure 21-2 Cardiac action potentials. The distinctive shapes of action potentials at five sites along the spread of excitation are shown.

1. The **Na⁺ current** (I_{Na}) is responsible for the rapid **depolarizing** phase of the action potential in atrial and ventricular muscle and in Purkinje fibers.
2. The **Ca²⁺ current** (I_{Ca}) is responsible for the rapid **depolarizing** phase of the action potential in the SA node and AV node; it also triggers contraction in all cardiomyocytes.
3. The **K⁺ current** (I_K) is responsible for the **repolarizing** phase of the action potential in all cardiomyocytes.
4. The **pacemaker current** (I_f) is responsible, in part, for pacemaker activity in SA nodal cells, AV nodal cells, and Purkinje fibers.

Besides these four currents, channels carry numerous other currents in heart muscle. In addition, two *electrogenic* transporters carry current across plasma membranes: the Na-Ca exchanger (NCX1) and the Na-K pump (see Chapter 5).

Traditionally, the changes in membrane potential (V_m) during the cardiac action potential are divided into separate phases, as illustrated in Figure 21-4A for cardiac action potentials from the SA node and in Figure 21-4B for those from ventricular muscle.

Phase 0 is the upstroke of the action potential. If the upstroke is due only to I_{Ca} (Fig. 21-4A), it will be slow. If the upstroke is due to both I_{Ca} and I_{Na} (Fig. 21-4B), it will be fast.

Phase 1 is the rapid repolarization component of the action potential (when it exists). This phase is due to almost total inactivation of I_{Na} or I_{Ca} and may also depend on the activation of a minor K⁺ current not listed previously, called I_{to} (for transient outward current).

Phase 2 is the plateau phase of the action potential, which is prominent in ventricular muscle. It depends on the continued entry of Ca²⁺ or Na⁺ ions through their major channels and on a minor membrane current due to the Na-Ca exchanger NCX1.

Phase 3 is the repolarization component of the action potential. It depends on I_K (Table 21-1).

Phase 4 constitutes the electrical diastolic phase of the action potential. V_m during phase 4 is termed the **diastolic potential**; the most *negative* V_m during phase 4 is the **maximum diastolic potential**. In SA and AV nodal cells, changes in I_K, I_{Ca}, and I_f produce pacemaker activity during phase 4. Purkinje fibers also exhibit pacemaker activity but use only I_f. Atrial and ventricular muscle have no time-dependent currents during phase 4.

The Na⁺ current is the largest current in the heart

The Na⁺ current (I_{Na}; Table 21-1) is the largest current in heart muscle, which may have as many as 200 Na⁺ channels per square micron of membrane. These channels are abundant in ventricular and atrial muscle, in Purkinje fibers, and in specialized conduction pathways of the atria. This current is not present in SA or AV nodal cells.

The channel that underlies I_{Na} is a classic voltage-gated Na⁺ channel, with both α and β₁ subunits (see Chapter 7). The unique cardiac α subunit (Nav1.5) has several phosphorylation sites that make it sensitive to stimulation by cAMP-dependent protein kinase (see Chapter 3).

At the negative resting potentials of the ventricular muscle cells, the Na⁺ channels are closed. However, these channels rapidly activate (in 0.1 to 0.2 ms) in response to local depolarization produced by conducted action potentials and produce a massive inward current that underlies most of the rapid upstroke of the cardiac action potential (phase 0 in Fig. 21-4B). If V_m remains at a positive level, these channels close gradually, in a process known as **inactivation**. This process, which is slower than activation but still fairly rapid (half-time, ~1 ms), is partly responsible for the rapid repolarization of the action potential (phase 1). At the potentials maintained during the plateau of the cardiac action

A   CURRENT FLOW THROUGH GAP JUNCTIONS

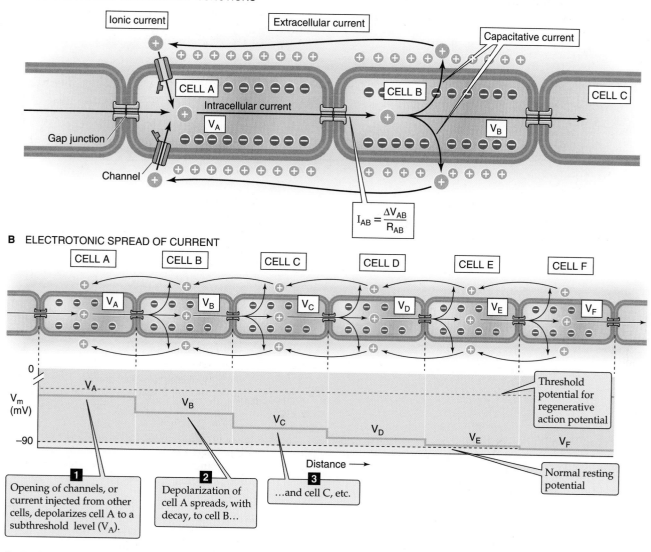

$$I_{AB} = \frac{\Delta V_{AB}}{R_{AB}}$$

B   ELECTROTONIC SPREAD OF CURRENT

1 Opening of channels, or current injected from other cells, depolarizes cell A to a subthreshold level (V_A).

2 Depolarization of cell A spreads, with decay, to cell B...

3 ...and cell C, etc.

Threshold potential for regenerative action potential

Normal resting potential

C   THRESHOLD AND RATE OF PROPAGATION OF ACTION POTENTIAL

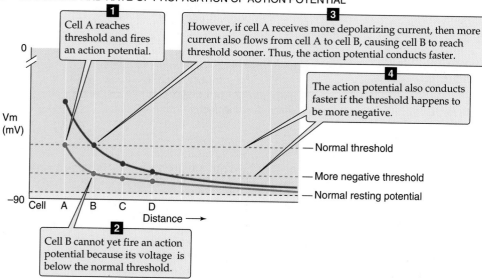

1 Cell A reaches threshold and fires an action potential.

3 However, if cell A receives more depolarizing current, then more current also flows from cell A to cell B, causing cell B to reach threshold sooner. Thus, the action potential conducts faster.

4 The action potential also conducts faster if the threshold happens to be more negative.

— Normal threshold

— More negative threshold

— Normal resting potential

2 Cell B cannot yet fire an action potential because its voltage is below the normal threshold.

Figure 21-3   Conduction in the heart. **A,** An action potential conducting from left to right causes intracellular current to flow from fully depolarized cells on the left, through gap junctions, and into cell A. Depolarization of cell A causes current to flow from cell A to cell B (I_{AB}). Part of I_{AB} discharges the capacitance of cell B (depolarizing cell B), and part flows downstream to cell C. **B,** Subthreshold depolarization of cell A decays with distance. **C,** The speed of conduction increases with greater depolarization of cell A (*blue versus red curves*) or with a more negative threshold.

Table 21-1   Major Cardiac Membrane Currents That Are Time Dependent and Voltage Gated

Current	Name	Channel Protein	Human Gene Symbol	Reversal Potential of Current (mV)	Inhibitors
I_{Na}	Na$^+$ current	Na$_V$1.5 (voltage-gated Na$^+$ channel)	*SCN*	+60	TTX Local anesthetics
I_{Ca}	Ca^{2+} current	Ca$_V$1.2 (L-type Ca^{2+} channel)	*CACNA*	+120	Nifedipine Verapamil
I_K	Repolarizing I_{K_R} Repolarizing I_{K_S} I_{to} G protein–activated ATP-sensitive	HERG + miRP1* KvLQT1 + minK* Kv4.3 (voltage-gated K$^+$ channel) GIRK* Kir + SUR = K$_{ATP}$*	*KCNH2 + KCNE2* *KCNQ1 + KCNE1* *KCND3* *KCNJ* *KCNJ*	−100	Ba^{2+} Cs$^+$ TEA
I_f (Na$^+$ + K$^+$)	Pacemaker current	HCN	*HCN*	−35	Cs$^+$

*These are heteromultimeric channels.

TTX, tetrodotoxin; TEA, tetraethylammonium; HERG, human ether-a-go-go–related gene (related to Kv family of K$^+$ channel genes); GIRK, G protein–activated inwardly rectifying K$^+$ channel; HCN, hyperpolarization activated, cyclic nucleotide gated.

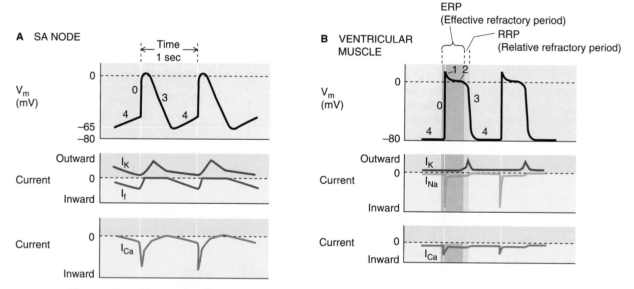

Figure 21-4   Phases of cardiac action potentials. The records in this figure are idealized. I_K, I_{Na}, I_{Ca}, and I_f are currents through K$^+$, Na$^+$, Ca^{2+}, and nonselective cation channels, respectively.

potential—slightly positive to 0 mV during phase 2—a very small but important component of this current remains. The sustained level of I_{Na} helps prolong phase 2.

In cardiac tissues other than the SA and AV nodes, the regenerative spread of the conducted action potential depends in large part on the *magnitude* of I_{Na} (Fig. 21-3C). The depolarization produced by the Na$^+$ current not only activates I_{Na} in neighboring cells but also activates other membrane currents in the same cell, including I_{Ca} and I_K. Local anesthetic **antiarrhythmic drugs**, such as lidocaine, work by partially blocking I_{Na}.

The Ca^{2+} current in the heart passes primarily through L-type Ca^{2+} channels

The Ca^{2+} current (I_{Ca}; Table 21-1) is present in all cardiac myocytes. The L-type Ca^{2+} channel (Ca$_V$1, see Chapter 7) is the dominant one in the heart. T-type Ca^{2+} channels, with different biophysical and pharmacological properties, are also present but in smaller amounts.

In the SA node, the role of I_{Ca}, like that of the other time- and voltage-dependent membrane currents, is to contribute to pacemaker activity. In both the SA and AV nodes, I_{Ca} is the inward current source that is responsible for the upstrokes (phase 0) of the SA and AV nodal action potentials. Because the nodal cells lack the larger I_{Na}, their upstrokes are slower than those in atrial and ventricular muscle (compare A and B of Fig. 21-4). Therefore, the smaller I_{Ca} discharges the membrane capacitance of neighboring cells in the SA and AV nodes less rapidly, so that the speed of the conducted action potential is much slower than that of any other cardiac tissue. This feature in the AV node leads to an **electrical delay** between atrial contraction and ventricular contraction that permits more time for the atria to empty blood into the ventricles.

Although it is smaller, I_{Ca} sums with I_{Na} during the upstroke of the action potentials of the ventricular and atrial muscle and the Purkinje fibers. In this way, it increases the velocity of the conducted action potential in these tissues. Like I_{Na}, I_{Ca} produces virtually no current at very negative potentials because the channels are closed. At more positive values of V_m, the Ca^{2+} channels rapidly *activate* (in ~1 ms) and, by a completely separate and time-dependent process, *inactivate* (half-time, 10 to 20 ms). A small I_{Ca} remains during the phase 2 of the action potential, helping to prolong the plateau. In atrial and ventricular muscle cells, the Ca^{2+} entering through L-type Ca^{2+} channels activates the release of Ca^{2+} from the sarcoplasmic reticulum (SR) by calcium-induced Ca^{2+} release (see Chapter 9). **Blockers of L-type Ca^{2+} channels**—therapeutic agents such as verapamil, diltiazem, and nifedipine—act by inhibiting I_{Ca}.

The repolarizing K⁺ current turns on slowly

Cardiac action potentials last two orders of magnitude longer than action potentials in skeletal muscle because the repolarizing K⁺ current turns on very slowly and—in the case of atrial myocytes, Purkinje fibers, and ventricular myocytes—with a considerable delay. The **repolarizing K⁺ current** (I_K; Table 21-1) is found in all cardiac myocytes and is responsible for repolarizing the membrane at the end of the action potential (phase 3 in Fig. 21-4A, B). Two currents underlie I_K—a relatively rapid component (I_{K_R}) carried by heteromeric HERG/miRP1 channels and a relatively slow component (I_{K_S}) carried by heteromeric KvLQT1/minK channels (see Chapter 7 for the box about heart defects). The I_K membrane current is very small at negative potentials. With depolarization, it slowly activates (20 to 100 ms) but does not inactivate. In SA and AV nodal cells, it contributes to pacemaker activity by deactivating at the diastolic voltage.

In addition to I_K, several other K⁺ currents are present in cardiac tissue.

Early Outward K⁺ Current (A-type Current) Atrial and ventricular muscle cells have some early *t*ransient *o*utward current (I_{to}). This current is activated by depolarization but rapidly inactivates. It contributes to phase 1 repolarization and is analogous to the A-type currents (see Chapter 7) seen in nerves. A Kv4.3 channel mediates the A-type current in heart and certain other cells.

G Protein–Activated K⁺ Current Acetylcholine activates muscarinic receptors and, through the βγ subunits of a G protein, activates an outward K⁺ current mediated by GIRK

K⁺ channels (see Chapter 7). This current is prominent in SA and AV nodal cells, where it decreases pacemaker rate by cell hyperpolarization when it is activated. It also slows the conduction of the action potential through the AV node.

K$_{ATP}$ Current ATP-sensitive K⁺ channels (K$_{ATP}$; see Chapter 7), activated by low intracellular [ATP], are present in abundance and may play a role in electrical regulation of contractile behavior. These channels are heteromultimers of Kir and SUR.

The I_f current is mediated by a nonselective cation channel

The pacemaker current (I_f) is found in SA and AV nodal cells and in Purkinje fibers (Fig. 21-4A, blue curve). The channel underlying this current is a nonspecific cation channel called HCN (for *h*yperpolarization activated, *c*yclic *n*ucleotide gated), which is related to the cyclic nucleotide–gated channels (see Chapter 6). Because the HCN channels conduct both K⁺ and Na⁺, the reversal potential of I_f is around −20 mV, between the Nernst potentials for K⁺ (about −90 mV) and Na⁺ (about +50 mV). The HCN channels have the unusual property (hence the subscript *f*, for "funny" current) that they do not conduct at positive potentials but are activated by *hyperpolarization* at the end of phase 3. The activation is slow (100 ms), and the current does not inactivate. Thus, I_f produces an inward, *depolarizing* current as it slowly activates at the end of phase 3. The I_f current is not the only current that contributes to pacemaker activity; in SA and AV nodal cells, I_{Ca} and I_K also contribute significantly to the phase 4 depolarization.

Different cardiac tissues uniquely combine ionic currents to produce distinctive action potentials

The shape of the action potential differs among different cardiac cells because of the unique combination of various currents—both the voltage-gated/time-dependent currents discussed in the preceding four sections and the "background" currents—present in each cell type. In Chapter 6, we introduced Equation 6-12, which describes V_m in terms of the conductances for the different ions (G_{Na}, G_K, G_{Ca}, G_{Cl}) relative to the total membrane conductance (G_m) and the equilibrium potentials (E_{Na}, E_K, E_{Ca}, E_{Cl}):

$$V_m = \frac{G_K}{G_m} E_K + \frac{G_{Na}}{G_m} E_{Na} + \frac{G_{Ca}}{G_m} E_{Ca} + \frac{G_{Cl}}{G_m} E_{Cl} \dots \quad \textbf{(21-2)}$$

Therefore, as the relative contribution of a particular membrane current becomes dominant, V_m approaches the equilibrium potential for that membrane current (Table 21-2). How fast V_m changes during the action potential depends on the magnitude of each of the currents (see Equation 6-12). Not only does each current *independently* affect the shape of the action potential, but the voltage- and time-dependent currents interact with one another because they affect—and are affected by—V_m. Other important influences on the shape of the cardiac action potential are the membrane capacitance of each cell and the geometry of the conduction pathway (e.g., AV node, bundle of His, ventricular muscle) as the action potential propagates from cell to cell in this functional syncytium through gap junctions. Therefore, it is easy to understand, at a conceptual level, how a particular cell's unique complement of ion channels, the properties of these channels at a particular instant in time, the intracellular ion concentrations, and the cell's geometry can all contribute to the shape of an action potential.

The sinoatrial node is the primary pacemaker of the heart

The Concept of Pacemaker Activity   The normal heart has three intrinsic pacemaking tissues: the SA node, the AV node, and the Purkinje fibers. The term **pacemaker activity** refers to the spontaneous time-dependent depolarization of the cell membrane that leads to an action potential in an otherwise quiescent cell. Any cardiac cell with pacemaker activity can initiate the heartbeat. The pacemaker with the

highest frequency will be the one to trigger an action potential that will propagate throughout the heart. In other words, the fastest pacemaker sets the heart rate and overrides all slower pacemakers. Thus, cardiac pacemakers have a hierarchy among themselves, based on their intrinsic frequency. Two fundamental principles underlie pacemaker activity. The first is that inward or depolarizing membrane currents interact with outward or hyperpolarizing membrane currents to establish regular cycles of spontaneous depolarization and repolarization. The second is that in a particular cell, these currents interact during phase 4 within a narrow range of diastolic potentials: between −70 and −50 mV in SA and AV nodal cells, and between −90 and −65 mV in Purkinje fibers.

Sinoatrial Node   The SA node is found in the right atrium and is the primary site of origin of the electrical signal in the mammalian heart (Table 21-3). It is the smallest electrical region of the heart and constitutes the *fastest normal pacemaker*, with an intrinsic rate of 60 beats per minute or faster in an individual at rest. SA cells are stable oscillators whose currents are always varying with time. The interactions among three time-dependent and voltage-gated membrane currents (I_{Ca}, I_K, and I_f) control the intrinsic rhythmicity of the SA node. The sum of a *decreasing* outward current (I_K; green curve in Fig. 21-4A) and two *increasing* inward currents (I_{Ca} and I_f; red and blue curves in Fig. 21-4A) produces the slow pacemaker depolarization (phase 4) associated with the SA node. The maximum diastolic potential (i.e., the most negative V_m) of the SA nodal cells, which occurs during phase 4 of the action potential, is between −60 and −70 mV. As V_m rises toward the threshold of about −55 mV, I_{Ca} becomes increasingly activated and eventually becomes regenerative, producing the upstroke of the action potential. This depolarization rapidly turns off (i.e., deactivates) I_f, and the whole process begins again.

These membrane currents are under the control of local and circulating agents (e.g., acetylcholine, epinephrine, and norepinephrine) and are also targets for therapeutic agents

Table 21-2   Equilibrium Potentials

Ion	Intracellular Concentration (mM)	Extracellular Concentration (mM)	Equilibrium Potential (mV)
Na$^+$	10	145	+72
K$^+$	120	4.5	−88
Cl$^-$	35	116	−32
H$^+$	pH = 7.1	pH = 7.4	−19
Ca^{2+}	0.0001	1.0	+123

Table 21-3   Electrical Properties of Different Cardiac Tissues

Tissue Name	Function	Principal Time-Dependent and Voltage-Dependent Currents	β-Adrenergic Effect*	Cholinergic Effect†
SA node	Primary pacemaker	I_{Ca}, I_K, I_f	↑ Conduction velocity ↑ Pacemaker rate	↓ Pacemaker rate ↓ Conduction velocity
Atrial muscle	Expel blood from atria	I_{Na}, I_{Ca}, I_K	↑ Strength of contraction	Little effect
AV node	Secondary pacemaker	I_{Ca}, I_K, I_f	↑ Conduction velocity ↑ Pacemaker rate	↓ Pacemaker rate ↓ Conduction velocity
Purkinje fibers	Rapid conduction of action potential Tertiary pacemaker	I_{Na}, I_{Ca}, I_K, I_f	↑ Pacemaker rate	↓ Pacemaker rate
Ventricular muscle	Expel blood from ventricles	I_{Na}, I_{Ca}, I_K	↑ Contractility	Little effect

*For example, epinephrine.
†For example, acetylcholine.

designed to modulate the heart's rhythm (e.g., Ca^{2+} channel blockers and β-adrenergic blockers).

Atrioventricular Node The AV node, located just above the atrioventricular ring, is the secondary site of origin of the electrical signal in the mammalian heart. Normally, the AV node may be excited by an impulse reaching it by way of the specialized atrial conduction pathways (see later). Like that of the SA node, the intrinsic rhythmicity of the AV node depends on the interaction of three time-dependent and voltage-gated currents: I_K, I_{Ca}, and I_f. Electrically, the SA and AV nodes share many properties; they have similar action potentials, pacemaker mechanisms, and drug sensitivities and a similarly slow conduction of action potentials. Because the intrinsic pacemaker rate of the AV node is slower (~40 beats/min) than that of the SA node, it does not set the heart rate; its pacemaker activity is considered secondary. However, if the SA node should fail, the AV node can assume control of the heart and drive it successfully.

Purkinje Fibers The His-Purkinje fiber system originates at the AV node with the bundle of His and splits to form the left and right bundle branches (Fig. 21-1). The right bundle conducts the electrical signal to the right ventricle, and the left bundle conducts the signal to the left ventricle. The anatomy of the left bundle is variable, but this bundle frequently divides into two main branches—the left anterosuperior fascicle (or hemibundle) and the left posteroinferior fascicle.

Purkinje fiber cells have the slowest intrinsic pacemaker rate (20 beats/min or less). Thus, Purkinje fiber cells become functional pacemakers only if the SA and AV pacemakers fail and are considered tertiary pacemakers. On the other hand, the bundle of His and the Purkinje fibers are an effective conduction system within the ventricles because they conduct action potentials more quickly than any other tissue within the heart (Table 21-4).

The action potential of the Purkinje fibers depends on four time- and voltage-dependent membrane currents: I_{Na} (not present in the SA and AV nodal cells), I_{Ca}, I_K, and I_f. The maximum diastolic potential is −80 mV. From that negative V_m, these cells produce a very slow pacemaker depolarization (phase 4) that depends on I_f. Because of their low rate of pacemaker depolarization and therefore the uncertainty of reaching the threshold for triggering of an action potential,

Table 21-4 Conduction Velocity in Different Cardiac Tissues

Tissue	Conduction Velocity (m/s)
SA node	0.05
Atrial pathways	1
AV node	0.05
Bundle of His	1
Purkinje system	4
Ventricular muscle	1

Purkinje fiber cells are unreliable as pacemakers. Normally, the action potential passing through the AV node activates the Purkinje fiber cells, resulting in a rapid upstroke (phase 0), mediated by I_{Na} and I_{Ca}. Because I_{Na} is large, Purkinje fibers conduct action potentials rapidly.

Atrial and ventricular myocytes fire action potentials but do not have pacemaker activity

The resting potential of atrial and ventricular myocytes is substantially more negative (about −80 mV) than the maximum diastolic potential of SA and AV node pacemaker cells (Fig. 21-1).

Atrial Muscle Within each atrium, the action potential spreads among cardiac myocytes by a direct cell-to-cell pathway. The atrial action potential depends on three primary time- and voltage-dependent membrane currents: I_{Na}, I_K, and I_{Ca}. There is no normal spontaneous (i.e., pacemaker) activity in atrial muscle. It has been proposed that atrial muscle has four special conducting bundles (Fig. 21-1). One, **Bachman's bundle** (anterior interatrial myocardial band), is interatrial and conducts the cardiac action potential from the SA node to the left atrium. Three other internodal pathways—the anterior, middle, and posterior internodal pathways—appear to conduct the action potential from the SA node to the AV node. Therefore, the first step in propagation of the cardiac action potential is the depolarization of the atria, following a general axis from right to left and downward (Fig. 21-5, step 1).

If the conduction path through the AV node is blocked, the ventricles will not be activated electrically and will not contract. The spontaneous activity that can arise in the Purkinje fiber cells may provide the necessary electrical signal to activate the ventricles, but this activation occurs normally only at a very low rate, and Purkinje fiber pacemaker activity is fairly unreliable.

Ventricular Muscle After the action potential reaches the AV node, it travels to the His-Purkinje fiber network and out into the ventricular muscle. The only normal electrical access between atrial muscle and the ventricles is the AV node. Because of this single electrical connection between the atria and the ventricles, there is a well-defined and orderly sequence of electrical activity through the rapidly conducting His-Purkinje network to the ventricles. Within the ventricular muscle, the action potential conducts from cell to cell. Steps 2 to 6 in Figure 21-5 summarize the sequence of events in ventricular activation, which is completed in ~100 ms:

Step 2: The septum depolarizes from left to right.
Step 3: The anteroseptal region depolarizes.
Step 4: The myocardium always depolarizes from the endocardium (the cells lining the ventricles) toward the epicardium (cells on the outer surface of the heart). The left ventricle depolarizes at the apex while the Purkinje fibers are still in the process of conducting the action potential toward the base of the left ventricle.
Step 5: Depolarization spreads from the apex toward the base, carried by the Purkinje fibers. This spread to the

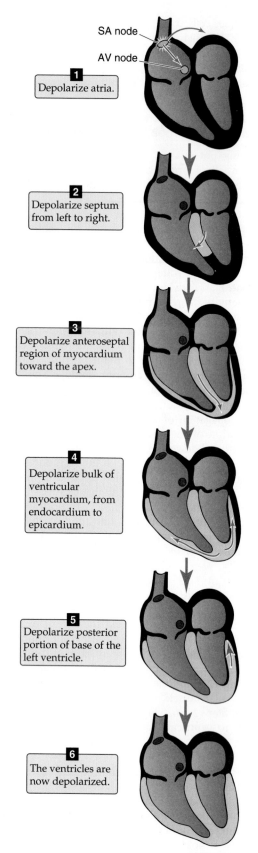

SA node

AV node

1 Depolarize atria.

2 Depolarize septum from left to right.

3 Depolarize anteroseptal region of myocardium toward the apex.

4 Depolarize bulk of ventricular myocardium, from endocardium to epicardium.

5 Depolarize posterior portion of base of the left ventricle.

6 The ventricles are now depolarized.

Figure 21-5 Sequence of depolarization in cardiac tissue.

base begins even as the signal in the apex is still spreading from the endocardium to the epicardium. The last region to depolarize is the posterobasal region of the left ventricle.

Step 6: The ventricles are fully depolarized.

Ventricular muscle has three major time- and voltage-gated membrane currents: I_{Na}, I_{Ca}, and I_K (Fig. 21-4B). Ventricular muscle has no I_f, and healthy ventricular muscle cells show no pacemaker activity. Starting from a resting potential of −80 mV, the rapid upstroke of the ventricular action potential results from the activation of I_{Na} by an external stimulus (e.g., an impulse conducted to the muscle by a Purkinje fiber or by a neighboring ventricular muscle cell). The Ca^{2+} current is of particular importance to ventricular muscle because it provides the Ca^{2+} influx that activates the release of Ca^{2+} from the SR. The rapid repolarization (phase 1), the plateau (phase 2), and the repolarization (phase 3) all appear to be governed by mechanisms similar to those found in the Purkinje fibers. However, the plateau phase is prolonged in ventricular muscle because the inward and outward currents are rather stable during that time (green, orange, and red curves in Fig. 21-4B).

Once a ventricular muscle cell is activated electrically, it is refractory to additional activation. This **effective refractory period** arises because the inward currents (I_{Na} and I_{Ca}) that are responsible for activation are largely inactivated by the membrane depolarization (Fig. 21-4B). The effective refractory period is the same as the *absolute* refractory period in nerve and skeletal muscle. During the effective refractory period, an additional electrical stimulus has no effect on the action potential. At the end of the plateau, the cell begins to repolarize as I_K increases in magnitude. As I_{Ca} and I_{Na} begin to recover from inactivation, the **relative refractory period** begins. During this period, an additional electrical stimulus can produce an action potential, but a smaller one than usual. Refractoriness provides the heart with a measure of electrical safety because it prevents extraneous pacemakers (which may arise pathologically) from triggering **ectopic beats.** An extrasystolic contraction would make the heart a less efficient pump. Refractoriness also prevents tetanus (see Chapter 9), a feature observed in skeletal muscle. Tetanus of the heart would mean perpetual systole and no further contractions.

Acetylcholine and catecholamines modulate pacemaker activity, conduction velocity, and contractility

In principle, the SA node can slow the firing rate of its pacemaker (i.e., negative chronotropic effect) by three mechanisms. First, the steepness of the depolarization during phase 4 can decrease, thereby lengthening the time necessary for V_m to reach threshold (Fig. 21-6A, blue curve). In this way, diastole is longer and the heart rate falls. Second, the maximum diastolic potential can become more negative (Fig. 21-6B, green curve). In this case, beginning at a lower value, V_m requires a longer time to reach the threshold, assuming no change in the steepness of the phase 4 depolarization. Third, the threshold for the action potential can become more positive (Fig. 21-6C, purple curve). Assuming

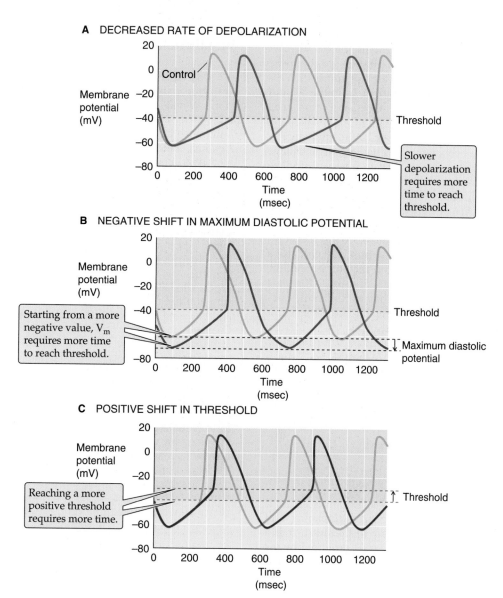

A DECREASED RATE OF DEPOLARIZATION

Membrane potential (mV)

Control

Threshold

Slower depolarization requires more time to reach threshold.

Time (msec)

B NEGATIVE SHIFT IN MAXIMUM DIASTOLIC POTENTIAL

Membrane potential (mV)

Starting from a more negative value, V_m requires more time to reach threshold.

Threshold

Maximum diastolic potential

Time (msec)

C POSITIVE SHIFT IN THRESHOLD

Membrane potential (mV)

Reaching a more positive threshold requires more time.

Threshold

Time (msec)

Figure 21-6 Modulation of pacemaker activity.

no change in either the maximum diastolic potential (i.e., starting point) or the steepness of the phase 4 depolarization, V_m requires a longer time to reach a more positive threshold. Obviously, a combination of these three mechanisms would have an enhanced effect. Conversely, the SA node cells can use each of these three mechanisms in the opposite sense to increase their firing rate (positive chronotropic effect).

Acetylcholine   The vagus nerve, which is parasympathetic (see Chapter 14), releases acetylcholine onto the SA and AV nodes and slows the intrinsic pacemaker activity by all three mechanisms discussed in the preceding paragraph. First, acetylcholine decreases I_f in the SA node (Table 21-1), reducing the steepness of the phase 4 depolarization (Fig. 21-6A). Second, acetylcholine opens GIRK channels, increasing relative K^+ conductance and making the maximum diastolic potential of SA nodal cells more negative (Fig. 21-6B). Third, acetylcholine reduces I_{Ca} in the SA node, thereby reducing

the steepness of the phase 4 depolarization (Fig. 21-6A) and also moving the threshold to more positive values (Fig. 21-6C). All three effects cooperate to lengthen the time for the SA node to depolarize to threshold; the net effect is to lower the heart rate.

The effects of acetylcholine on currents in the AV node are similar to those in the SA node. However, because the pacemaker normally does not reside in the AV node, the physiological effect of acetylcholine on the AV node is to slow **conduction velocity**. The mechanism is an inhibition of I_{Ca} that also makes the threshold more positive for AV nodal cells. Because it is more difficult for one cell to depolarize its neighbors to threshold, conduction velocity falls.

Catecholamines   Sympathetic innervation to the heart is plentiful, releasing mostly norepinephrine. In addition, the adrenal medulla releases epinephrine into the circulation. Catecholamines, which act through β_1-adrenergic receptors, produce an increase in heart rate by two mechanisms. First, catecholamines increase I_f in the nodal cells, thereby increasing the steepness of the phase 4 depolarization (i.e., opposite to the effect in Fig. 21-6A). Second, catecholamines increase I_{Ca} in all myocardial cells. The increase in I_{Ca} in the SA and AV nodal cells steepens the phase 4 depolarization (i.e., opposite to the effect in Fig. 21-6A) and also makes the threshold more negative (i.e., opposite to the effect in Fig. 21-6C). Note that catecholamines do not appear to change the maximum diastolic potential. They do, however, produce shorter action potentials as a result of the actions they have on several specific currents.

In atrial and ventricular muscle, catecholamines cause an increase in the strength of contraction (**positive inotropic effect**) for four reasons. First, the increased I_{Ca} (i.e., Ca^{2+} influx) leads to a greater local increase in $[Ca^{2+}]_i$ and also a greater Ca^{2+}-induced Ca^{2+} release from the SR. Second, the catecholamines increase the sensitivity of the SR Ca^{2+} release channel to cytoplasmic Ca^{2+} (see Chapter 9). Third, catecholamines also enhance Ca^{2+} pumping into the SR by stimulation of the SERCA Ca^{2+} pump (see Chapter 5), thereby increasing Ca^{2+} stores for later release. Fourth, the increased I_{Ca} presents more Ca^{2+} to SERCA, so that SR Ca^{2+} stores increase over time. The four mechanisms make more Ca^{2+} available to troponin C, enabling a more forceful contraction.

THE ELECTROCARDIOGRAM

An electrocardiogram generally includes five waves

The electrocardiogram (ECG) is the standard clinical tool used to measure the electrical activity of the heart. It is a recording of the small *extracellular* signals produced by the movement of action potentials through cardiac myocytes. To obtain a standard 12-lead ECG, one places two **electrodes** on the upper extremities, two on the lower extremities, and six on standard locations across the chest. In various combinations, the electrodes on the extremities generate the six limb leads (three standard and three augmented), and the chest electrodes produce the six precordial leads. In a **lead**, one electrode is treated as the positive side of a voltmeter and one or more electrodes as the negative side. Therefore, a lead records the fluctuation in voltage difference between positive and negative electrodes. By the variation of which electrodes are positive and which are negative, a standard 12-lead ECG is recorded. Each lead looks at the heart from a unique angle and plane, that is, from what is essentially its own unique point of view.

The fluctuations in extracellular voltage recorded by each lead vary from fractions of a millivolt to several millivolts. These fluctuations are called **waves** and are named with the letters of the alphabet (Fig. 21-7). The **P** wave reflects depolarization of the right and left atrial muscle. The **QRS** complex represents depolarization of ventricular muscle. The **T** wave represents repolarization of both ventricles. Finally, the rarely seen **U** wave may reflect repolarization of the papillary muscle. The shape and magnitude of these waves are different in each lead because each lead views the

electrical activity of the heart from a unique position in space. For his discovery of the mechanism of the electrocardiogram, Willem Einthoven was awarded the 1924 Nobel Prize in Physiology or Medicine.

Because the ECG machine uses electrodes attached to the skin to measure the sum of the heart's electrical activity, it requires special amplifiers. The ECG machine also has electrical filters that reduce the electrical noise. Moving limbs, breathing, coughing, shivering, and faulty contact between the skin and an electrode produce artifacts on the recorded ECG.

Because the movement of charge (i.e., the spreading wave of electrical activity in the heart) has both a three-dimensional **direction** and a **magnitude**, the signal measured on an ECG is a **vector**. The system that clinicians use to measure the heart's three-dimensional, time-dependent electrical vector is simple to understand and easy to implement, but it can be challenging to interpret.

A pair of electrocardiogram electrodes defines a lead

To record the complicated time-dependent electrical vector of the heart, the physician or ECG technician constructs a system of leads in two planes that are perpendicular to each

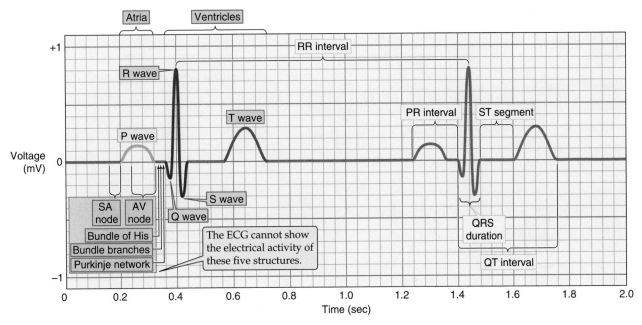

Figure 21-7 Components of the ECG recording.

other. One plane, the **frontal plane**, is defined by the six **limb leads** (Fig. 21-8A). A perpendicular **transverse plane** is defined by the six **precordial leads** (Fig. 21-8B). Each lead is an axis in one of the two planes, onto which the heart projects its electrical activity. The ECG recording from a single lead shows how that lead views the time-dependent changes in voltage of the heart.

Older ECG machines recorded data from the 12 leads one at a time, sequentially. Thus, relatively rare events captured by the recording in one lead might not be reflected in any of the others, which were obtained at different times. Modern ECG machines obtain leads synchronously in groups of 3 or 12. Because the real electrical vector of the heart consists of just one time-dependent vector signal, you might think that a three-lead recording would suffice to localize the vector signal in space. In principle, this is true: only two leads in one plane and one lead in another plane are needed to fully define the original electrical vector of the heart at all moments. However, recording from all 12 leads is extremely useful because a signal of interest may be easier to see in one lead than in another. For example, an acute myocardial infarction involving the inferior (diaphragmatic) portion of the heart might be easily visualized in leads II, III, and aVF but go completely undetected (or produce so-called reciprocal changes) in the other leads.

The Limb Leads   One obtains a 12-lead ECG by having the patient relax in a supine position and connecting four electrodes to the limbs (Fig. 21-8A). Electrically, the torso and limbs are viewed as an equilateral triangle (Einthoven's triangle) with one vertex on the groin and the other two on the shoulder joints (Fig. 21-9A). Because the body is an electrical "volume conductor," an electrical attachment to an arm is electrically equivalent to a connection at the shoulder joint, and an attachment to either leg is equivalent to a connection at the groin. By convention, the left leg represents the groin. The fourth electrode, connected to the right leg, is used for

electrical grounding. The three initial limb leads represent the difference between two of the limb electrodes:

  I (positive connection to left arm, negative connection to right arm). This lead defines an axis in the frontal plane at 0 degrees (Fig. 21-9A, B).

 II (positive to left leg, negative to right arm). This lead defines an axis in the frontal plane at 60 degrees.

III (positive to left leg, negative to left arm). This lead defines an axis in the frontal plane at 120 degrees.

An electronic reconstruction of the three limb connection defines an electrical reference point in the middle of the heart (Fig. 21-9A) that constitutes the negative connection for the augmented "unipolar" limb leads and for the chest leads. The three augmented unipolar limb leads compare one limb electrode to the average of the other two:

aVR (positive connection to *right* arm, negative connection is electronically defined in the middle of the heart). The axis defined by this limb lead in the frontal plane is −150 degrees (Fig. 21-9B). The *a* stands for augmented, and the *V* represents unipolar.

aVL (positive to *left* arm, negative is middle of the heart). The axis defined by this limb lead in the frontal plane is −30 degrees.

aVF (positive to left leg *[foot]*, negative is middle of the heart). The axis defined by this limb lead in the frontal plane is +90 degrees.

Thus, the positive and negative ends of these six leads define axes every 30 degrees in the frontal plane (Fig. 21-9B).

The Precordial Leads   These leads lie in the transverse plane, perpendicular to the plane of the frontal leads. The positive connection is one of six different locations on the

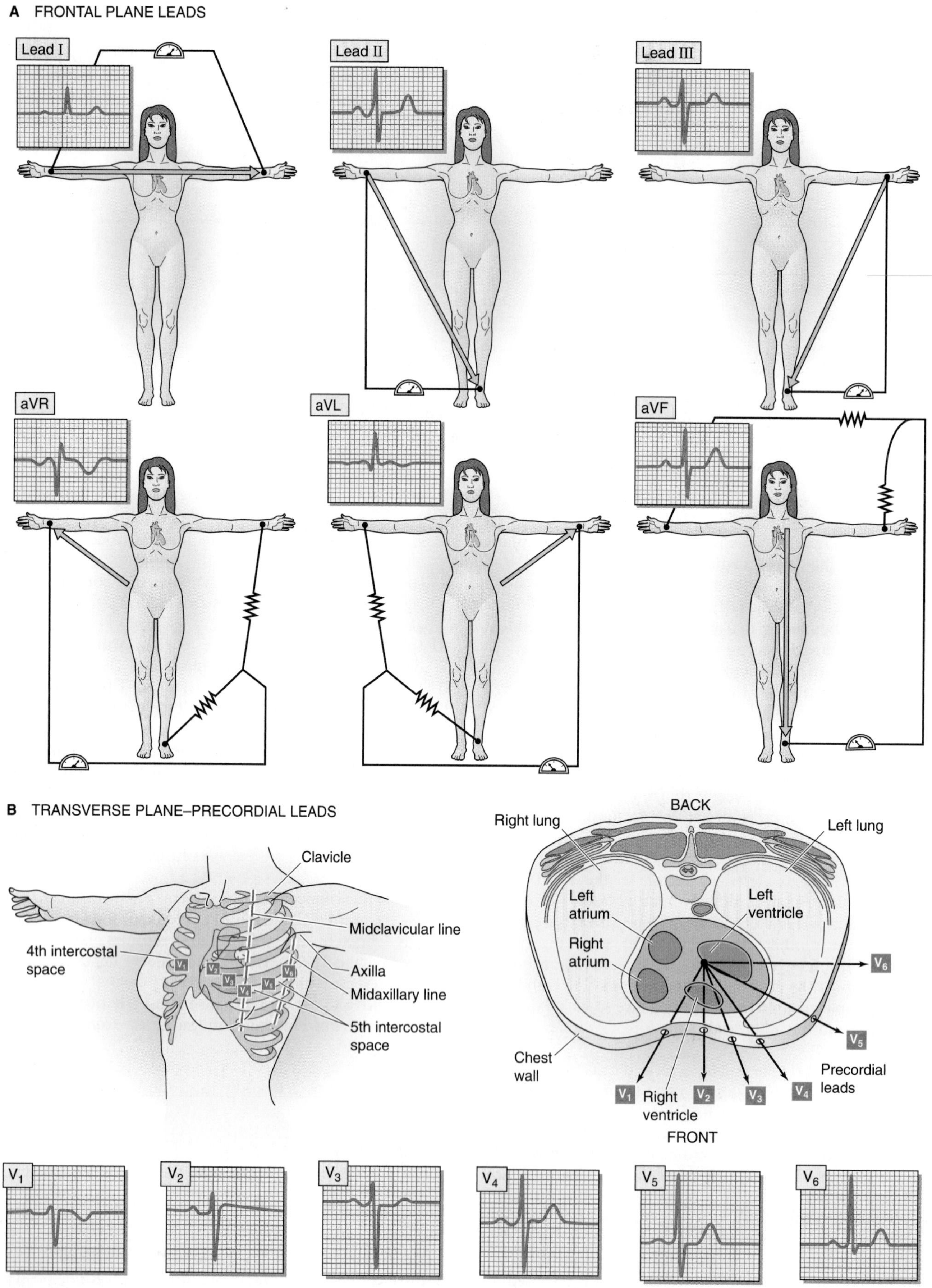

A FRONTAL PLANE LEADS

Lead I

Lead II

Lead III

aVR

aVL

aVF

B TRANSVERSE PLANE–PRECORDIAL LEADS

Clavicle

Midclavicular line

4th intercostal space

Axilla

Midaxillary line

5th intercostal space

BACK

Right lung

Left lung

Left atrium

Left ventricle

Right atrium

Right ventricle

Chest wall

V_1 V_2 V_3 V_4 V_5 V_6

Precordial leads

FRONT

V_1 V_2 V_3 V_4 V_5 V_6

Figure 21-8 The ECG leads.

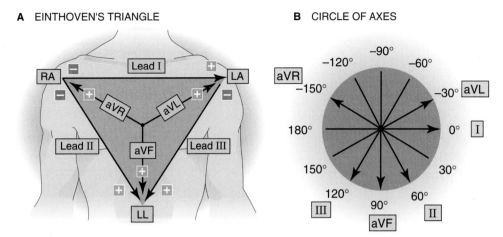

Figure 21-9 Axes of the limb leads. **A,** The frontal plane limb leads behave as if they are located at the shoulders (RA, right arm; LA, left arm) and groin (LL, left leg). Leads I, II, and III are separated from one another by 60 degrees. The augmented leads, referenced to the center of the heart, bisect each of the 60-degree angles formed by leads I, II, and III. **B,** Translating each of the six frontal leads so that they pass through a common point defines a polar coordinate system, providing views of the heart at 30-degree intervals.

chest wall (Fig. 21-8B), and the negative connection is electronically defined in the middle of the heart by averaging of the three limb electrodes. The resultant leads are named V_1 to V_6, where the *V* stands for unipolar:

V_1: fourth intercostal space to the right of the sternum
V_2: fourth intercostal space to the left of the sternum
V_4: fifth intercostal space at the midclavicular line
V_3: halfway between V_2 and V_4
V_6: fifth intercostal space at the midaxillary line
V_5: halfway between V_4 and V_6

It is also possible, on rare occasions, to obtain **special leads** by employing the same negative connection used for the unipolar limb and precordial leads and a positive "probe" connection. Special leads that are used include esophageal leads and an intracardiac lead (e.g., that used to obtain a recording from the His bundle).

A simple two-cell model can explain how a simple electrocardiogram can arise

We can illustrate how the ECG arises from the propagation of action potentials through the functional syncytium of myocytes by examining the electrical activity in two neighboring cardiac cells, A and B, connected by gap junctions (Fig. 21-10A). The depolarization and action potential begin first in cell A (V_A in Fig. 21-10A, green record). The current from cell A then depolarizes cell B through the gap junctions and a brief time later triggers an action potential in cell B (V_B). If we subtract the V_B record from the V_A record, we obtain a record of the intracellular voltage *difference* $V_A - V_B$ (Fig. 21-10B).

We have already seen that according to Ohm's law (Equation 21-1), the *intracellular* current from cell A to cell B (I_{AB}) is proportional to ($V_A - V_B$). The *extracellular* current flowing from the region of cell B to the region of cell A is equal but opposite in direction to the intracellular current flowing

from cell A to cell B. Imagine that an extracellular voltmeter has its negative electrode placed to the left of cell A and its positive electrode to the right of cell B (forming a lead with an axis of 0 degrees). During the upswing in the action potential of cell A, while cell B is still at rest, ($V_A - V_B$) and I_{AB} are both positive, and the voltmeter detects a *positive* difference in voltage (Fig. 21-10C)—analogous to the QRS complex in a real ECG. Later, during the recovery from the action potential in cell A, while cell B is still depolarized, ($V_A - V_B$) and I_{AB} are both negative, and the voltmeter would detect a *negative* difference in voltage. From the extracellular voltage difference in Figure 21-10C, we can conclude that when the wave of depolarization moves *toward* the positive lead, there is a positive deflection in the *extracellular* voltage difference.

If we place the two electrodes at the junction between the two cells, with the positive connection on the bottom and the negative connection on the top, we create a lead with an axis of 90 degrees to the direction of current flow (Fig. 21-10D). Under these conditions, we observe no voltage difference because both extracellular electrodes sense the same voltage at each instant in time. Thus, when a lead is perpendicular to the wave of depolarization, the measured deflection on that lead is **isoelectric**.

If we put our extracellular electrodes in yet a third configuration—with the positive electrode on the left and the negative electrode on the right—we observe a *negative* deflection during the depolarization of cell A because the wave of depolarization is moving *away from* the positive electrode (Fig. 21-10E).

This simple two-cell model demonstrates that the wave of depolarization behaves like a vector, with both magnitude and direction. Two practical methods to determine the direction (or axis) of the vector are presented in the box, Basic Interpretation of the Electrocardiogram.

The QRS equivalent in the extracellular voltage record of our simplistic two-cell analysis is due to a spreading wave of *depolarization*. The T-wave equivalent is negative

A ACTION POTENTIALS OF TWO SEPARATE CELLS

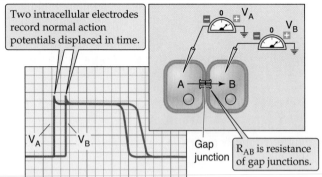

Two intracellular electrodes record normal action potentials displaced in time.

Gap junction

R_{AB} is resistance of gap junctions.

B SUBTRACTED ACTION POTENTIALS

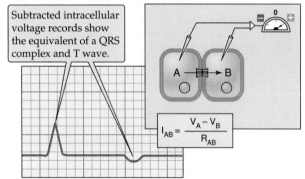

Subtracted intracellular voltage records show the equivalent of a QRS complex and T wave.

$$I_{AB} = \frac{V_A - V_B}{R_{AB}}$$

C DEPOLARIZATION MOVING TOWARD POSITIVE ELECTRODE

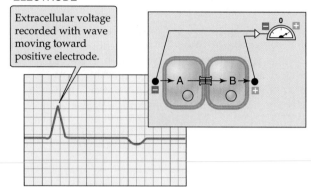

Extracellular voltage recorded with wave moving toward positive electrode.

D DEPOLARIZATION MOVING PERPENDICULAR TO ELECTRODE AXIS

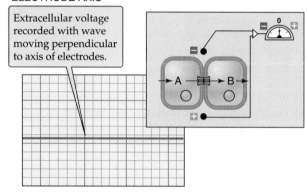

Extracellular voltage recorded with wave moving perpendicular to axis of electrodes.

E DEPOLARIZATION MOVING AWAY FROM POSITIVE ELECTRODE

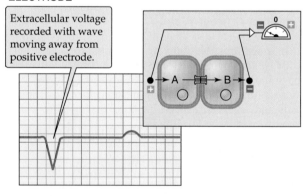

Extracellular voltage recorded with wave moving away from positive electrode.

Figure 21-10 Two-cell model of the ECG.

compared with the QRS equivalent, and it reflects the wave of *repolarization*. If cell A has an action potential that is much longer than cell B (so that positive current again propagates from A to B after the action potential in B is completed), then the T-wave equivalent will be upright, as it is in most ECGs. Thus, on average, the ventricular myocytes that depolarize last are the first to repolarize. In other words, the B cells have shorter action potentials than the A cells.

What happened to the P wave that we see in a real ECG? The P wave reflects the depolarization of the *atrial* myocytes. In our model, we could represent the P wave by introducing a second pair of myocytes (i.e., the atrial cells) and allowing

them to fire their action potentials much earlier than the two ventricular myocytes.

CARDIAC ARRHYTHMIAS

Any change in cardiac rhythm from the normal sinus rhythm is defined as an **arrhythmia**. Although some arrhythmias are pathological and even life-threatening, others are normal and appropriately adaptive, including sinus tachycardia and sinus arrhythmia.

Sinus tachycardia is a heart rate faster than normal, driven by the sinus node. This arrhythmia is seen in

Basic Interpretation of the Electrocardiogram

An ECG provides a direct measurement of the rate, rhythm, and time-dependent electrical vector of the heart. It also provides fundamental information about the origin and conduction of the cardiac action potential within the heart. Because the different parts of the heart activate sequentially, we can attribute the time-dependent changes in the electrical vector of the heart to different regions of the heart. The P wave reflects the atrial depolarization. The QRS complex corresponds to ventricular depolarization. The T wave reflects ventricular repolarization.

ECG paper has a grid of small 1-mm square boxes and larger 5-mm square boxes. The vertical axis is calibrated at 0.1 mV/mm; the horizontal (time) axis, at 0.04 s/mm (small box) or 0.2 s/5 mm (large box). Thus, five large boxes correspond to 1.0 second (Fig. 21-11). Table 21-5 summarizes the steps for interpretation of an ECG.

Rate

We can measure rate in two ways. The direct method is to measure the number of seconds between waves of the same type, for example, the R-R interval. The quotient of 60 divided by the interval in seconds is the heart rate in beats per minute:

$$\text{Rate (beats/min)} = (60 \text{ s/min})/(\text{R-R interval (s/beat)})$$

A quick, alternative method is quite popular (Table 21-6). Measure the number of large boxes that form the R-R interval and remember the series: 300, 150, 100, 75, 60, 50—which corresponds to an interval of 1, 2, 3, 4, 5, or 6 large boxes. Thus,

$$\text{Rate} = 300/(\text{number of large boxes})$$

For example, if 4 large boxes separate the R waves, the heart rate is 75 beats/min.

Rhythm

The determination of rhythm is more complex. One must answer the following questions: Where is the heart's pacemaker? What is the conduction path from the pacemaker to the last cell in the ventricles? Is the pacemaker functioning regularly and at the correct speed? The normal pacemaker is the SA node; the signal then propagates through the AV node and activates the ventricles. When the heart follows this pathway at a normal rate and in this sequence, the rhythm is called a **normal sinus rhythm**.

Careful examination of the intervals, durations, and segments in the ECG tracing can reveal a great deal about the conducted action potential (Fig. 21-7). The **P-wave** duration indicates how long atrial depolarization takes. The **PR interval** indicates how long it takes the action potential to conduct through the AV node before activating the ventricles. The **QRS duration** reveals how long it takes for the wave of depolarization to spread throughout the ventricles. The **QT interval** indicates how long the ventricles remain depolarized and is thus a rough measure of the duration of the overall "ventricular" action potential. The QT segment gets shorter as the heart rate increases, reflecting the shorter action potentials that are observed at high rates. In addition, many other alterations in these waves—and the segments separating them—reflect important physiological and pathophysiological changes in the heart.

Vector (or Axis) of a Wave in the Frontal Plane

Determination of the vector of current flow through the heart is not just an intellectual exercise but can be of great clinical importance. The normal axis of ventricular depolarization in the frontal plane lies between −30 and +90 degrees. However, this axis can change in a number of pathological situations, including hypertrophy of one or both ventricular walls (a common sequela of severe or prolonged hypertension) and conduction blocks in one or several of the ventricular conducting pathways.

We can use two approaches to measure the axis of a wave within the frontal plane (i.e., with use of limb leads). The first is more accurate, but the second is quicker and easier and is usually sufficient for clinical purposes.

The first approach is a **geometric method**. It uses our knowledge of the axes of the different leads and the measured magnitude of the wave projected onto at least two leads in the frontal plane. It involves five steps:

Step 1: **Measure** the height of the wave on the ECG records in two leads, using any arbitrary unit (e.g., number of boxes). A *positive deflection* is one that rises above the baseline, and a *negative deflection* is one that falls below the baseline. In the example in Figure 21-12A, we are estimating the axis of the R wave of the QRS complex. The R wave is +2 units in lead II and −1 unit in lead aVR.

Step 2: **Mark** the height of the measured deflections on the corresponding lead lines on a circle of axes. Any unit of measure will suffice, as long as you use the same unit for both markings. Starting at the center of the circle, mark a *positive deflection* toward the *arrowhead* and a *negative deflection* toward the *tail of the arrow*.

Step 3: **Draw** lines, perpendicular to the lead axes, through each of your two marks.

Step 4: **Connect** the center of the circle of axes (tail of vector) to the intersection of the two perpendicular lines (head of vector). In our example, the intersection is close to the aVF axis.

Step 5: **Estimate** the axis of the vector that corresponds to the R wave, using the "angle" scale of the circle of axes. In this case, the vector is at about 95 degrees, just clockwise to the aVF lead (i.e., 90 degrees).

The second approach is a qualitative **inspection method**. It exploits the varying magnitudes of the wave of interest in recordings from different leads. When the wave is isoelectric (i.e., no deflection, or equal positive and negative deflections), then the electrical vector responsible for that projection must be perpendicular to the isoelectric lead, as we already saw for the two-cell model in Figure 21-10D. The inspection approach requires two steps:

Step 1: **Identify a lead in which the wave of interest is isoelectric** (or nearly isoelectric). In the example in Figure 21-12B, the QRS complex is isoelectric in aVL (−30 degrees). The vector must be perpendicular (or nearly perpendicular) to that lead (i.e., aVL). In our example, the vector must point 90 degrees from −30 degrees and therefore is at either +60 degrees or −120 degrees. Because the leads in the frontal plane define axes every 30 degrees, every lead has another lead to which it is perpendicular.

Continued

Basic Interpretation of the Electrocardiogram—cont'd

Step 2: **Identify a lead in which the wave is largely positive**. In Figure 21-12B, this would be lead II. The vector must lie roughly in the same direction as the orientation of that lead. Because lead II is at +60 degrees, the axis of the vector of the QRS wave must be about +60 degrees and not −120 degrees.

If the wave of interest is not isoelectric in any lead, then find two leads onto which the projections are of similar magnitude and sign. The vector has an axis halfway between those two leads.

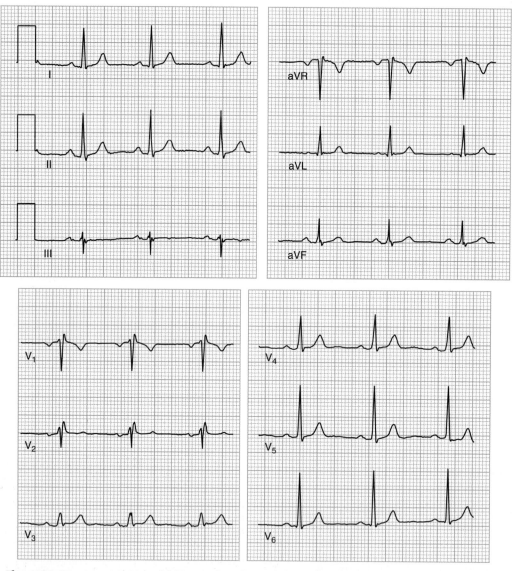

Figure 21-11 A normal 12-lead ECG recording. The recordings were obtained synchronously, three leads at a time (I, II, and III simultaneously; aVR, aVL, and aVF simultaneously; V₁, V₂, and V₃ simultaneously; and V₄, V₅, and V₆ simultaneously). A 1-mV, 200-ms calibration pulse is visible on the left of each of the three rows. The leads are marked on the traces. *(We thank the Division of Cardiology, University of Maryland School of Medicine, for obtaining this ECG recording from the author.)*

Table 21-5 Approach for Reading an ECG

1.	Search for P waves.
2.	Determine the relationship of P waves and QRS complexes.
3.	Identify pacemaker.
4.	Measure the heart rates from different waves (e.g., P-P interval, R-R interval).
5.	Characterize QRS shape (i.e., narrow versus wide).
6.	Examine features of ST segment.
7.	Estimate the mean QRS axis (and the axes of the other waves of interest).
8.	Examine the cardiac rhythm (e.g., look at a 20- to 30-s ECG record from lead II).

Table 21-6 Determination of Heart Rate from the ECG

R-R Interval (in number of large boxes of 0.2 s)	Calculation	Heart Rate (beats per minute)
1	300/1	300
2	300/2	150
3	300/3	100
4	300/4	75
5	300/5	60
6	300/6	50

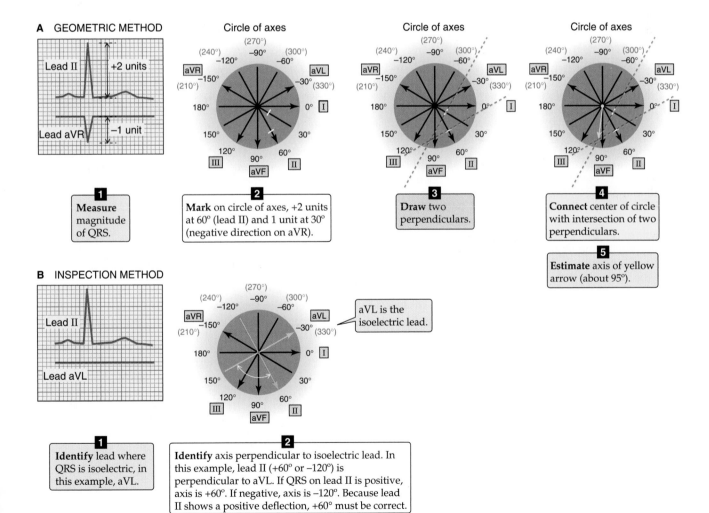

Figure 21-12 Estimation of the ECG axis in the frontal plane.

frightened or startled individuals or during normal exercise. Rarely, sinus tachycardia can be pathological, for example, in patients with acute hyperthyroidism (see Chapter 49).

Sinus arrhythmia is the name given to a normal phenomenon: a subtle change in heart rate that occurs with each respiratory cycle. Inspiration accelerates the heart rate (see Chapter 19); expiration slows it. Deepening of the respirations exaggerates these cyclic changes. The magnitude of the effect can vary significantly among individuals. The heart rate is still under the control of the SA node, but cyclic variations in sympathetic and parasympathetic tone modulate the SA node's pacemaker rate. The loss of sinus arrhythmia can be a sign of autonomic system dysfunction, as may be seen in patients with diabetes.

Although the list of pathological arrhythmias is long, two basic problems are responsible for nearly all arrhythmias: altered conduction and altered automaticity.

Conduction abnormalities are a major cause of arrhythmias

Disturbances of conduction make up the first major category of cardiac arrhythmias. Conduction disturbances can have multiple causes and can occur at any point in the conduction pathway. Conduction disturbances can be partial or complete. The two major causes of conduction disturbances are depolarization and abnormal anatomy.

If a tissue is injured (e.g., by stretch or anoxia), an altered balance of ionic currents can lead to a **depolarization**. The depolarization, in turn, partially inactivates I_{Na} and I_{Ca}, slowing the spread of current (i.e., slowing conduction). As a result, the tissue may become less excitable (partial conduction block) or completely inexcitable (complete conduction block).

Another type of conduction disturbance is the presence of an aberrant conduction pathway, reflecting **abnormal anatomy**. One such example is an accessory conduction pathway that rapidly transmits the action potential from the atria to the ventricles, bypassing the AV node, which normally imposes a conduction delay. Patients with the common Wolff-Parkinson-White syndrome have a bypass pathway called the bundle of Kent. The existence of a second pathway between the atria and ventricles predisposes affected individuals to supraventricular arrhythmias (see Accessory Conduction Pathways).

Myocardial Infarction

An acute myocardial infarction, or heart attack, begins with the occlusion of a coronary artery. The region of myocardium subserved by that coronary artery is deprived of oxygen and will die unless blood flow resumes shortly. During the initial stages, the myocardial cells are electrically active but their function is impaired, producing characteristic changes in the ECG. Complete but transient blockade of blood flow to the myocardium—even though it does not lead to cell death—may lead to a pattern of ECG changes similar to that seen during the acute phase of myocardial infarction. Because blood flow is regional, the areas of infarction are also regional. Thus, the physician can best observe the changes in electrical activity by examining the specific ECG leads that provide the best view of the involved region of myocardium.

The first electrical change associated with an acute myocardial infarction is **peaking of the T waves**, followed soon after by **T-wave inversion**. These T-wave changes are not specific for infarction and are reversible if blood flow is restored.

The next change, and one that is more characteristic of an acute myocardial infarction, is **elevation of the ST segment**. This change occurs because the myocytes closest to the epicardium become depolarized by the cellular anoxic injury, but they are still electrically coupled. Returning to the two-cell model (Fig. 21-13A), consider the cell on the left (cell A) to be normal and the cell on the right (cell B) to be damaged. Figure 21-13B shows the extracellular current, which is proportional to the differences in the action potentials of the two cells shown in Figure 21-13A. Because cell B has a more positive resting potential than cell A but the same plateau during the action potential, the difference in voltage between cell A and cell B is depressed everywhere but at the ST segment—making the ST segment appear elevated. This is also the ECG change that one views with an acute myocardial infarction.

Brief periods of **coronary artery spasm** can also produce ST elevation, presumably by the same mechanism. Rapid reperfusion of coronary arteries after acute blockage may lead to rapid and complete recovery of the myocardial cells, as indicated by the evanescent nature of the ECG changes.

Ischemia without cell death due to a "fixed" degree of occlusion (e.g., that caused by a thrombus or atherosclerosis) is often associated with changes in the ECG, typically ST-segment and T-wave changes. However, these changes are quite variable, presumably brought about by altered action potential duration in the affected regions. Patients experiencing exertional chest pain (angina) due to diminished coronary blood flow frequently have ECG changes during the anginal episode that include **ST-segment depression** and T-wave inversion.

With irreversible cell death, the ECG typically shows the evolution of **deep Q waves** (a large negative deflection at the beginning of the QRS complex). Q waves develop only in those leads overlying or near the region of the infarction. The Q waves indicate an area of myocardium that has become electrically silent. Because action potentials cannot propagate into the infarcted area, the net vector of the remaining areas of ventricular depolarization—by default—points *away* from this area. The result is a deep *negative* deflection on the ECG in the appropriate leads. Thus, an inferior wall infarction inscribes deep Q waves in leads II, III, and aVF. An infarction affecting the large, muscular anterior wall of the heart will inscribe deep Q waves in some of the precordial leads (V_1 through V_6).

Not all infarctions create deep Q waves; the only visible changes may be T-wave inversion and ST-segment depression. Clinically, these infarctions behave like incomplete infarctions, and patients are at risk of a second, "completing" event. Therefore, these patients are investigated and treated aggressively to prevent further infarction.

A ACTION POTENTIALS OF TWO SEPARATE CELLS

B SUBTRACTED ACTION POTENTIALS

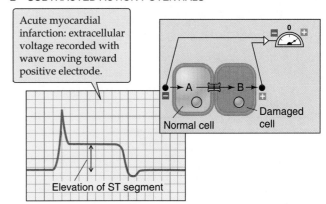

Figure 21-13 Two-cell model of a myocardial infarction. **A,** The damaged cell B *(blue record)* has a lower resting potential, but the plateau of its action potential is at the same level as the normal cell A *(green record)*. **B,** After the records in **A** are subtracted, the apparent elevation of ST segment is the same as the difference in resting potentials; the TP and PR regions are actually depressed.

Partial (or Incomplete) Conduction Block   Three major types of partial conduction block exist: slowed conduction, intermittent block, and unidirectional block. We defer the discussion of unidirectional block until we consider re-entry phenomena.

In **slowed conduction**, the tissue conducts all the impulses, but more slowly than normal. **First-degree AV block** reflects a *slowing* of conduction through the AV node. On an ECG, first-degree AV block appears as an unusually long PR interval (compare A and B of Fig. 21-14).

A second example of partial conduction block is **intermittent block**, in which the tissue conducts some impulses but not others. In the AV node, intermittent block leads to **second-degree AV block**, of which there are two types. Both reflect incomplete (i.e., intermittent) coupling of the atria to the ventricles. In a **Mobitz type I block** (or Wenckebach block), the PR interval gradually lengthens from one cycle to the next until the AV node fails completely, skipping a ventricular depolarization (Fig. 21-14C). With Mobitz type I block, it is most common to see every third or fourth atrial beat fail to conduct to the ventricles. In a **Mobitz type II block**, the PR interval is constant from beat to beat, but every nth ventricular depolarization is missing. In Figure 21-14D, the first cardiac cycle is normal. However, the second P wave is not followed by a QRS or T. Instead, the ECG record is flat until the third P wave arrives at the expected time, followed by a QRS and a T. Thus, we say that every second QRS is dropped (2:1 block).

Another form of intermittent conduction block, called **rate-dependent block**, reflects disease often seen in the large branches of the His-Purkinje fiber system (i.e., the bundle branches). When the heart rate exceeds a critical level, the ventricular conduction system fails, presumably because a part of the conducting system lacks sufficient time to repolarize. With intermittent failure of the His-Purkinje fiber system, the impulse is left to spread slowly and inefficiently through the ventricles by conducting from one myocyte to the next. Such a failure, whether intermittent or continuous, is known as a **bundle branch block** and appears on the

ECG as an intermittently wide QRS complex (Fig. 21-14E). Because this block impairs the coordinated spread of the action potential throughout the ventricles, the resulting contraction loses some efficiency.

Complete Conduction Block   In complete block, or **third-degree AV block**, no impulses conduct through the affected area, in either direction. For example, **complete block** at the AV node stops any supraventricular electrical impulse from triggering a ventricular contraction. Thus, AV nodal block electrically severs the atria and ventricles, each of which beats under control of its own pacemakers. This situation is called **AV dissociation**. The only ventricular pacemakers that are available to initiate cardiac contraction are the Purkinje fiber cells, which are notoriously unreliable and slow. Thus, cardiac output may fall, and blood pressure along with it. AV dissociation can therefore constitute a medical emergency, and placement of an artificial ventricular pacemaker can prove lifesaving. On an ECG, complete block appears as regularly spaced P waves (i.e., the SA node properly triggers the atria) and as irregularly spaced QRS and T waves that have a low frequency and no fixed relationship to the P waves (Fig. 21-14F).

Re-entry   An independent focus of pacemaker activity can develop as a consequence of a conduction disturbance. This class of conduction disturbance is called re-entry (or re-entrant excitation or circus movement). It is one of the major causes of clinical arrhythmias. It occurs when a wave of depolarization travels in an apparently endless circle. Re-entry has three requirements: (1) a closed conduction loop, (2) a region of unidirectional block (at least briefly), and (3) a sufficiently slow conduction of action potentials around the loop.

Before further considering re-entry, we need to discuss a conduction defect that is essential for re-entry—unidirectional block. **Unidirectional block** is a type of partial conduction block in which impulses travel in one direction but not in the opposite one. Unidirectional block may arise as a

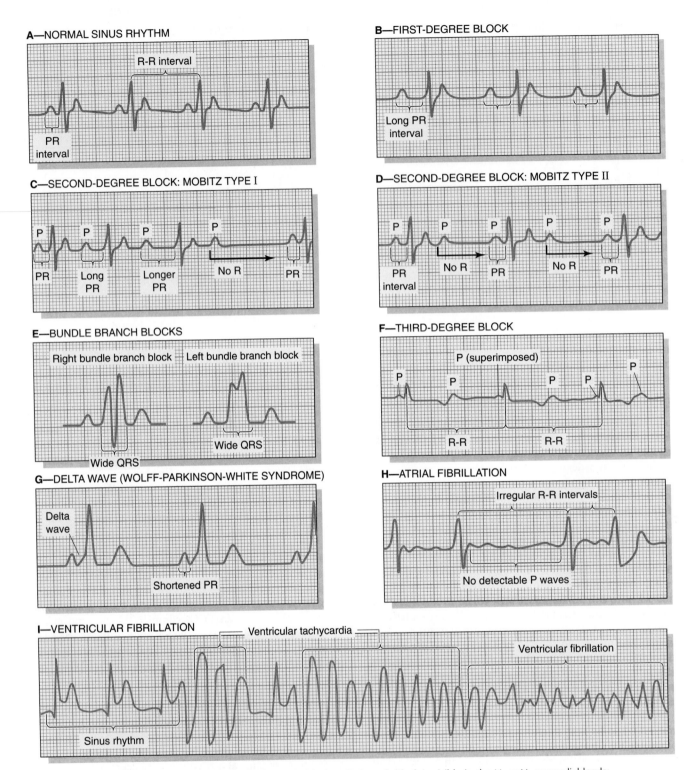

Figure 21-14 Pathological ECGs. In **E,** right bundle branch block is visible in the V₁ or V₂ precordial leads; left bundle branch block is visible in the V₅ or V₆ leads. *(Data from Chernoff HM: Workbook in Clinical Electrocardiography. New York, Medcom, 1972.)*

result of a local depolarization or may be due to pathological changes in functional anatomy. Normal cardiac tissue can conduct impulses in both directions (Fig. 21-15A). However, after an asymmetric anatomical lesion develops, many more healthy cells may remain on one side of the lesion than on

the other. When conduction proceeds in the direction from the many healthy cells to the few healthy cells, the current from the many may be sufficient to excite the few (right to left in Fig. 21-15B). On the other hand, when conduction proceeds in the opposite direction, the few healthy cells

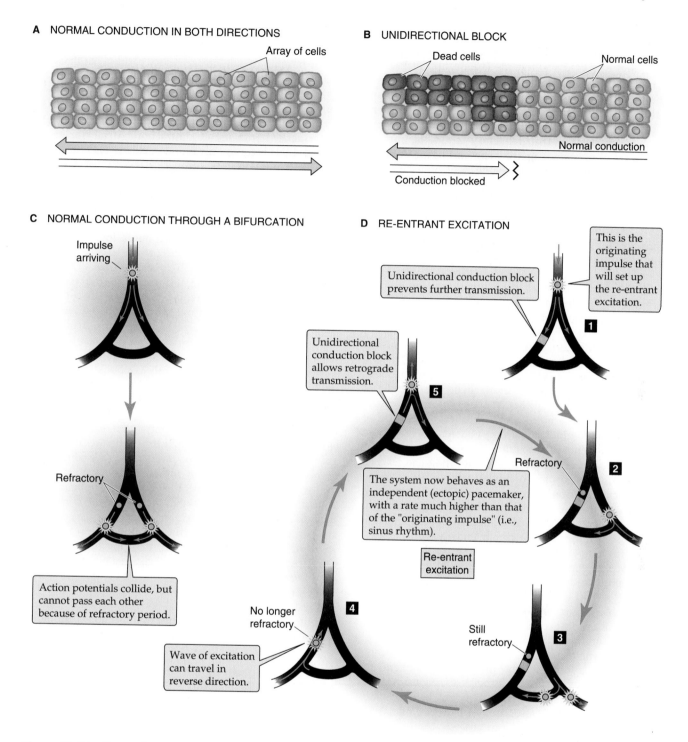

Figure 21-15 Abnormal conduction.

cannot generate enough current to excite the region of many healthy cells (left to right in Fig. 21-15B). The result is a unidirectional block.

We return now to the problem of re-entry. Imagine that an impulse is traveling down a bifurcating Purkinje fiber and is about to reach a group of ventricular myocytes—a *closed conduction loop* (Fig. 21-15C). However, the refractory zones prevent the re-entry of impulses from the right to the left, and vice versa. We now introduce a lesion that causes a

unidirectional conduction block in the left branch of the Purkinje fiber. When the impulse reaches the fork in the road, it spreads in both directions (Fig. 21-15D, step 1). However, the impulse cannot continue past the unidirectional block in the left branch. The impulse traveling down the right branch stimulates the distal conducting cells (Fig. 21-15D, step 2), leaving them in an effective refractory period. When the impulse reaches the ventricular muscle, it begins to travel back toward the damaged left branch (step 3). At this point, the cells in the normal right branch may still be refractory to excitation. The impulse finally reaches the damaged left branch and travels in a retrograde fashion up this branch, reaching and passing through the region of the unidirectional conduction block (step 4). Finally, the impulse again reaches the bifurcation (step 5). Because enough time has elapsed for the cells at the bifurcation as well as in the right branch to recover from their refractory period, the impulse can now travel retrograde up the main part of the Purkinje fiber as well as orthograde down the right branch—for a second time.

If this re-entrant movement (steps 2 → 5 → 2, and so on) continues, the frequency of re-entry will generally outpace the SA nodal pacemaker (frequency of step 1) and is often responsible for diverse tachyarrhythmias because the fastest pacemaker sets the heart rate. Re-entry excitation may be responsible for atrial and ventricular tachycardia, atrial and ventricular fibrillation, and many other arrhythmias. Re-entry can occur in big loops (Fig. 21-15D) or in small loops consisting entirely of myocardial cells.

Accessory Conduction Pathways The **Wolff-Parkinson-White (WPW) syndrome**, briefly mentioned earlier, is a common example of an accessory conduction pathway, which in this case provides a short circuit (i.e., bundle of Kent) around the delay in the AV node. The fast accessory pathway is composed not of Purkinje fibers but instead of muscle cells. It conducts the action potential directly from the atria to the ventricular septum, depolarizing some of the septal muscle earlier than if the depolarization had reached it by the slower, normal AV nodal pathway. As a result, ventricular depolarization is more spread out in time than is normal, giving rise to a broader than normal QRS complex. The general direction of ventricular depolarization is reversed, so that the events normally underlying the Q wave of the QRS complex have an axis opposite to that normally seen. This early depolarization, or **pre-excitation**, appears as a small, positive **delta wave** at the beginning of the QRS complex (Fig. 21-14G). In addition, because the time between atrial depolarization and ventricular depolarization (i.e., beginning of delta wave) is shortened, the interval between the P wave and the QRS complex is shortened.

The aberrant conduction pathway in WPW syndrome also establishes a loop that may meet the requirements for re-entry and may therefore be associated with a **supraventricular tachycardia**. Although in general a benign condition, WPW syndrome is associated with at least one attack of supraventricular tachycardia in at least 50% of affected individuals. The two most common supraventricular tachycardias seen in this population are paroxysmal supraventricular tachycardia and atrial fibrillation (described later). **Paroxysmal supraventricular tachycardia (PSVT)** is a regular tachycardia with a ventricular rate usually exceeding 150 beats per minute. Because ventricular depolarization still occurs through the normal conducting pathways, the QRS complex appears normal.

If, during an episode of PSVT, the conduction direction for re-entry is in the reverse direction (i.e., down the accessory pathway and back up through the AV node), the QRS shape may be unusual. This arrangement may produce a PSVT with wide and bizarre QRS complexes because ventricular depolarization does not occur along the normal bundle branches. A small number of people with WPW syndrome have more than one accessory pathway, so that multiple re-entry loops are possible.

Fibrillation In fibrillation, many regions of re-entrant electrical activity are present, creating electrical chaos that is not associated with useful contraction. **Atrial fibrillation** (Fig. 21-14H) is commonly found in elderly patients, sometimes with mitral valve or coronary artery disease, but often without any evidence of underlying cardiac disease. The re-entry loop within the atria moves wildly and rapidly, generating a rapid succession of action potentials—as many as 500 per minute. This wandering re-entry circuit easily becomes the fastest pacemaker in the heart, outpacing the SA node and bombarding the AV node. Fortunately, the AV node cannot repolarize fast enough to pass along all of these impulses. Only some make it through to the ventricles, resulting in the irregular appearance of QRS complexes without any detectable P waves. The baseline between QRS complexes may appear straight or may show small, rapid fluctuations. Although only some atrial impulses reach the ventricles, the ventricular rate can still be quite high.

Because the atria function mainly as a booster pump (see the box on atrial contraction in Chapter 22), many patients tolerate atrial fibrillation without harm and may even be unaware that they have it. Others may suffer greatly from the loss of a coordinated atrial contraction, particularly the elderly or those with coexisting cardiac disease. If possible, attempts should be made to convert most individuals back to normal sinus rhythm by either electrical or chemical means. If this is not possible, then attempts can be made to at least slow conduction through the AV node. For example, digitalis compounds increase parasympathetic and decrease sympathetic stimulation to the AV node, decreasing the speed of AV conduction and thus reducing the ventricular rate. β-Adrenergic blockers or Ca^{2+} channel blockers are also used to control ventricular rate.

Ventricular fibrillation (Fig. 21-14I) is a life-threatening medical emergency. The heart cannot generate cardiac output because the ventricles are not able to pump blood without a coordinated ventricular depolarization.

Altered automaticity can originate from the sinus node or from an ectopic locus

The automaticity of any cardiac tissue can change. Pacemaker cells can experience an alteration or even a complete absence of automaticity. Conversely, other cells that normally have no automaticity (e.g., ventricular muscle) can become "ectopic" pacemakers. These disturbances of automaticity make up the second major category of cardiac arrhythmias.

Depolarization-Dependent Triggered Activity A positive shift in the maximum diastolic potential brings V_m closer to the threshold for an action potential and can induce automaticity in cardiac tissue that otherwise has no pacemaker activity. The development of depolarization-induced triggered activity depends on the interaction of the Ca^{2+} current (I_{Ca}) and the repolarizing K^+ current (I_K). This mechanism

A PROLONGED ACTION POTENTIAL LEADS
TO EARLY AFTERDEPOLARIZATION

B PROLONGED ACTION POTENTIAL LEADS
TO A "RUN" OF SPONTANEOUS ACTIVITY

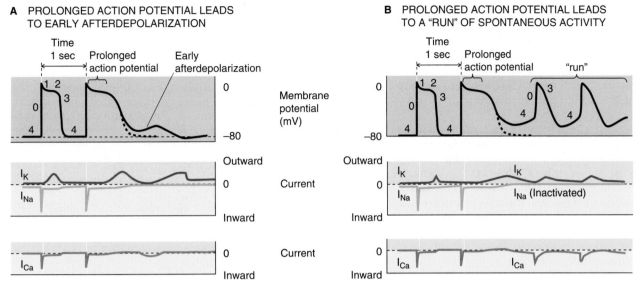

Figure 21-16   Abnormal automaticity in ventricular muscle. The records in this figure are idealized. **A,** The prolonged action potential keeps I_{Na} inactivated but permits I_{Ca} and I_K to interact and thereby produce a spontaneous depolarization—the early afterdepolarization. **B,** The afterdepolarization reaches threshold, triggering a sequence of several slow pacemaker-like action potentials that generate extrasystoles.

can produce a more rapid pacemaker depolarization in the SA or AV nodal cells, causing them to accelerate their pacemakers. It can also increase the intrinsic pacemaker rate in Purkinje fiber cells, which normally have a very slow pacemaker.

Depolarization-induced triggered activity is particularly dramatic in non-pacemaker tissues (e.g., ventricular muscle), which normally exhibit no diastolic depolarization. Factors that significantly prolong action potential duration can cause depolarization-dependent triggered activity. During the repolarization phase, I_{Na} remains inactivated because the cell is so depolarized (Fig. 21-16A). On the other hand, I_{Ca} has had enough time to recover from inactivation and—because the cell is still depolarized—triggers a slow, positive deflection in V_m known as an **early afterdepolarization**. Eventually, I_K increases and returns V_m toward the resting potential. Such early afterdepolarizations, if they are larger than the one shown in Figure 21-16A, may trigger an extrasystole. Isolated ventricular extrasystoles (known by many names, including premature ventricular contractions, or PVCs) may occur in normal individuals. Alterations in cellular Ca^{2+} metabolism (discussed in the next section) may increase the tendency of a prolonged action potential to produce an extrasystole. Ironically, a class of drugs used to treat arrhythmias can become *arrhythmogenic* by producing early afterdepolarizations. For example, quinidine can produce this dangerous adverse effect, presumably by inhibiting Na^+ channels and some K^+ channels and thus prolonging the ventricular muscle action potential.

More than one extrasystole—a **run of extrasystoles** (Fig. 21-16B)—is pathological. A run of three or more ventricular extrasystoles is the minimal requirement for diagnosis of **ventricular tachycardia**. This arrhythmia is life-threatening because it can degenerate into ventricular fibrillation (Fig. 21-14I), which is associated with no meaningful cardiac

output. The heart rate in ventricular tachycardia is much faster than normal, usually between 120 and 150 beats per minute (or faster), and the pacemaker driving the heartbeat is located in the ventricle itself. The heart rate in ventricular tachycardia may be so fast that the heart cannot pump blood effectively.

Long QT Syndrome (LQTS)   Patients with LQTS have a prolonged ventricular action potential and are prone to ventricular arrhythmias. In particular, these patients are susceptible to a form of ventricular tachycardia called **torsades de pointes**, or "twisting of the points," in which the QRS complexes appear to spiral around the baseline, constantly changing their axes and amplitude. LQTS can be congenital or acquired. The congenital form can involve mutations of cardiac Na^+ channels or K^+ channels (see the boxes on Na^+ channel and human heart defects in Chapter 7). The acquired form of LQTS, which is much more common, can result from various electrolyte disturbances (especially hypokalemia and hypocalcemia) or from prescribed or over-the-counter medications (e.g., several antiarrhythmic drugs, tricyclic antidepressants, and some nonsedating antihistamines when they are taken together with certain antibiotics, notably erythromycin).

Ca^{2+} overload and metabolic changes can also cause arrhythmias

Ca^{2+} Overload Ca^{2+} overload in the heart has many potential causes. One frequent factor is digitalis intoxication. Another is injury-related cellular depolarization. Ca^{2+} overload occurs when $[Ca^{2+}]_i$ increases, causing the SR to sequester too much Ca^{2+}. Thus overloaded, the SR begins to cyclically—and spontaneously—dump Ca^{2+} and then take it back up. The Ca^{2+} release may be large enough to stimulate a Ca^{2+}-activated nonselective cation channel and the Na-Ca exchanger (see Chapter 5). These current sources combine to produce I_{ti}, a **transient inward current** that produces a **delayed afterdepolarization**. When it is large enough, I_{ti} can depolarize the cell beyond threshold and produce a spontaneous action potential.

Metabolism-Dependent Conduction Changes   During ischemia and anoxia, many cellular events take place, including a fall in intracellular ATP levels. This fall in $[ATP]_i$ activates the ATP-sensitive K^+ channel (K_{ATP}), which is plentiful in cardiac myocytes. Thus, when $[ATP]_i$ falls sufficiently, K_{ATP} is less inhibited and the cells tend to become less excitable (i.e., K_{ATP} helps keep V_m close to E_K). The activation of this channel may explain, in part, the slowing or blocking of conduction that may occur during ischemia or in the peri-infarction period.

Electromechanical Dissociation   Rarely, patients being resuscitated from cardiac arrest exhibit a phenomenon called electromechanical dissociation, in which the heart's ECG activity is not accompanied by the pumping of blood. In many cases, the basis of electromechanical dissociation is not understood. However, in other cases, the cause is obvious. For example, the heart of a patient with a large pericardial effusion may manifest normal electrical activity, but the fluid between the heart and the pericardium may press in on the heart (cardiac tamponade) and prevent effective pumping.

REFERENCES

Books and Reviews

Antzelevitch C: Cellular basis and mechanism underlying normal and abnormal myocardial repolarization and arrhythmogenesis. Ann Med 2004; 36(Suppl 1):5-14.

Bers DM: Cardiac excitation-contraction coupling. Nature 2002; 415:198-205.

Chernoff HM: Workbook in Clinical Electrocardiography. New York: Medcom Press, 1972.

Einthoven W: The string galvanometer and the measurement of action currents of the heart. Nobel Lecture in Physiology or Medicine, vol 2. Amsterdam: Elsevier, 1964.

Keating MT, Sanguinetti MC: Molecular and cellular mechanisms of cardiac arrhythmias. Cell 2001; 104:569-580.

Kleber AG, Rudy Y: Basic mechanisms of cardiac impulse propagation and associated arrhythmias. Physiol Rev 2004; 84:431-488.

Noble D: Modeling the heart. Physiology 2004; 19:191-197.

Journal Articles

Cheng H, Lederer WJ, Cannell MB: Calcium sparks: Elementary events underlying excitation-contraction coupling in heart muscle. Science 1993; 262:740-744.

Pogwizd SM, Schlotthauer K, Li L, et al: Arrhythmogenesis and contractile dysfunction in heart failure: Roles of sodium-calcium exchange, inward rectifier potassium current, and residual beta-adrenergic responsiveness. Circ Res 2001; 88:1159-1167.

Weidmann S: Effect of current flow on the membrane potential of cardiac muscle. J Physiol 1951; 115:227-236.

CHAPTER 22

THE HEART AS A PUMP

Emile L. Boulpaep

THE CARDIAC CYCLE

The sequence of mechanical and electrical events that repeats with every heartbeat is called the **cardiac cycle**. The **duration** of the cardiac cycle is the reciprocal of heart rate:

$$\text{Duration (s/beat)} = \frac{60\,(\text{s/min})}{\text{Heart rate (beats/min)}} \quad (22\text{-}1)$$

For example, for a heart rate of 75 beats/min, the cardiac cycle lasts 0.8 s or 800 ms.

The closing and opening of the cardiac valves define four phases of the cardiac cycle

The cardiac pump is of the two-stroke variety. Like a pump with a reciprocating piston, the heart alternates between a filling phase and an emptying phase. Under normal circumstances, the electrical pacemaker in the sinoatrial node (see Chapter 21) determines the duration of the cardiac cycle, and the electrical properties of the cardiac conduction system and cardiac myocytes determine the relative duration of contraction and relaxation. As long as the heart rate remains unchanged, this pattern remains steady.

The cardiac **atria** are small chambers. The right atrium receives deoxygenated systemic venous return from the inferior and superior vena cava. The left atrium receives oxygenated blood from the lungs through the pulmonary circulation. Both atria operate as passive reservoirs more than as mechanical pumps. However, they do contract, and this contraction does enhance ventricular filling and cardiac output to a small degree (see the box on the importance of atrial contractions).

The inlet valves of the ventricles are called the **AV (atrioventricular) valves**. They permit blood to flow in one direction only, from the atria to the ventricles. The valve located between the *right* atrium and the right ventricle is the **tricuspid valve** because it has three flaps, or cusps. The valve located between the *left* atrium and the left ventricle is the **mitral valve** because it has only two cusps, which resemble a bishop's miter.

The outlet valves of the ventricles are called **semilunar valves**. They also allow blood to flow in just a single direction, from each ventricle into a large outflow tract vessel. Both the **pulmonary valve**, located between the right ventricle and pulmonary artery, and the **aortic valve**, located between the left ventricle and aorta, have three cusps.

Cardiac valves open passively when upstream pressure exceeds downstream pressure. They close passively when downstream pressure exceeds upstream pressure. The movement of the valve leaflets can be detected by echocardiography (see Chapter 17); their closure makes **heart sounds** that can be heard with a stethoscope. The stethoscope can also detect leaks in the valves that permit jets of blood to flow backward across the valvular orifice (i.e., regurgitation) as well as stenotic lesions that narrow the valve opening, forcing the blood to pass through a narrower space (i.e., stenosis). During certain parts of the cardiac cycle, blood passing through either **regurgitant** or **stenotic** lesions makes characteristic sounds that are called **murmurs** (see Chapter 17 for the box on this topic).

The cardiac cycle can be artificially divided into phases in any number of ways. However, from the point of view of the ventricles and the positions of their valves, we must consider a minimum of four distinct **phases**:

Inflow phase. The inlet valve is open and the outlet valve is closed.
Isovolumetric contraction. Both valves are closed, with no blood flow.
Outflow phase. The outlet valve is open and the inlet valve is closed.
Isovolumetric relaxation. Both valves are closed, with no blood flow.

Table 22-1 summarizes these four phases and the key events of the cardiac cycle. Note that the same events occur on the right side of the heart as on the left side.

It is common to separate these phases into two parts. **Systole** includes phases 2 and 3, when the ventricles are contracting; **diastole** includes phases 4 and 1, when the ventricles are relaxing. For a heart rate of 75 (cycle duration = 800 ms), systole occupies ~300 ms, and diastole ~500 ms.

Table 22-1   Events in the Cardiac Cycle

Valvular Events	Cardiac Chamber Events		Phase
Opening of AV valves (tricuspid and mitral)			
	Rapid ventricular filling	1	Diastole
	Decreased ventricular filling; diastasis	1	Diastole
	Atrial contraction (additional ventricular filling)	1	Diastole
Closing of AV valves (tricuspid and mitral)			
	Isovolumetric ventricular contraction (with all valves closed)	2	Systole
Opening of semilunar valves (pulmonary and aortic)			
	Rapid ventricular ejection (fast muscle shortening)	3	Systole
	Decreased ventricular ejection (slower muscle shortening)	3	Systole
Closing of semilunar valves (pulmonary and aortic)			
	Isovolumetric ventricular relaxation (with all valves closed)	4	Diastole
Opening of AV valves (tricuspid and mitral)			

With increasing heart rate—and thus decreasing cycle length—diastole shortens relatively more than systole does.

For convenience, the events in Table 22-1 start a short time after the beginning of diastole, with the opening of the AV valves and the start of ventricular filling (*phase 1*).

Changes in ventricular volume, pressure, and flow accompany the four phases of the cardiac cycle

Figure 22-1 illustrates the changes in pressure and volume that occur during the cardiac cycle. The four vertical lines indicate the timing of the four *valvular events*, which terminate each of the four phases defined previously:

AV valve closure terminates phase 1.
Semilunar valve opening terminates phase 2.
Semilunar valve closing terminates phase 3.
AV valve opening terminates phase 4.

The shapes of pressure tracings for the right side of the heart (Fig. 22-1A) and the left side of the heart (Fig. 22-1B) are similar except that the pressures on the right are a scaled-down version of those on the left. In both cases, the tracings begin in the *middle* of phase 1, that is, the period of decreased filling toward the end of diastole called **diastasis** (from the Greek *dia* [apart] + *histanai* [to stand]). Note that the volume changes in the left ventricle are exactly the same as those in the right ventricle because the cardiac outputs of the right and left sides of the heart are virtually identical (see Chapter 17). For purposes of illustration, we now focus on the records for the *left* side of the heart (Fig. 22-1B).

Diastasis Period (Middle of Phase 1)   During the diastasis, the mitral valve is open, but little blood flows from the left atrium to the left ventricle; ventricular volume slowly rises and approaches a plateau. The pressures in both the left atrium and the left ventricle rise slowly, driven by the pressure in the pulmonary veins, which is only slightly higher. The atrial pressure parallels—and is only slightly above—the ventricular pressure because the mitral valve is wide open, and the flow between the two chambers is minimal. The P wave of the electrocardiogram (ECG; see Chapter 21), which corresponds to atrial excitation, occurs at the end of this phase.

Atrial Contraction (End of Phase 1)   Immediately following the P wave is the atrial contraction, which causes a variable amount of blood to enter the left ventricle. In a person at rest, the atrial contraction transfers into the left ventricle a volume of blood that represents less than 20% of the subsequent stroke volume and often only a few percent. During heavy exercise, this figure can rise to 40% (see the box). Atrial contraction causes a slight rise in intra-atrial pressure and a comparable rise in ventricular pressure and volume. All during this period, the aortic pressure decreases as blood flows out to the periphery.

Isovolumetric Contraction (Phase 2)   When the ventricles begin to depolarize, as evidenced by the QRS complex on the ECG, systole commences. The ventricles contract, and very soon the pressure in the left ventricle exceeds that in the left atrium (first crossover of blue and orange pressure tracings in Fig. 22-1B, top panel). As a result, the *mitral valve closes*. The aortic valve has been closed this entire time. Thus, the left ventricle contracts with both mitral and aortic valves closed. Because the blood has no place to go, the result is an isovolumetric contraction that causes the pressure in the left ventricle to rise rapidly, eventually exceeding the pressure in the aorta (first crossover of blue and red tracings) and causing the aortic valve to open.

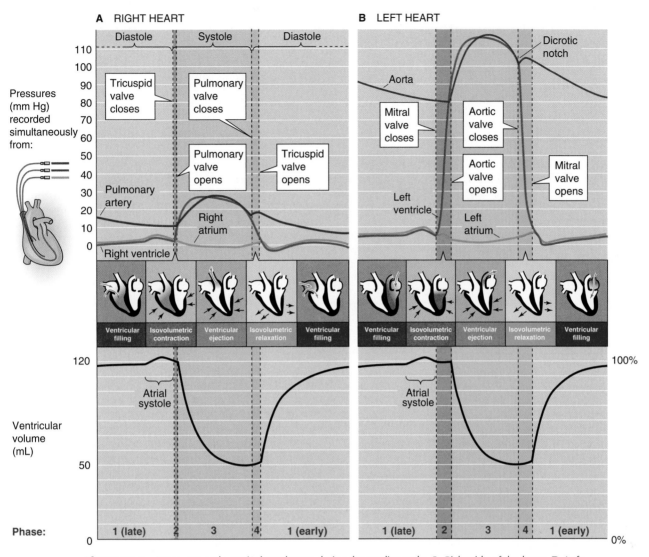

Figure 22-1 Pressures and ventricular volumes during the cardiac cycle. **A,** Right side of the heart. **B,** Left side of the heart. The *inset* shows the placement of catheters used for pressure measurements in the right side of the heart.

Ejection or Outflow (Phase 3) As the *aortic valve opens,* the ejection phase begins. During the first part of phase 3—**rapid ejection**—ventricular pressure (blue tracing in Fig. 22-1B, top) continues to rise, closely followed by a rapid elevation of aortic pressure, which at first is slightly less (red tracing). Accompanying these rapid pressure increases is a precipitous reduction in ventricular volume (Fig. 22-1B, bottom), as blood flows into the aorta. Aortic pressure continues to rise and eventually exceeds ventricular pressure (second crossover of blue and red tracings in Fig. 22-1B, top) just before both the aortic and ventricular pressures begin to fall. Despite the reversal of the pressure gradient across the aortic valve, the cusps of the aortic valve do not immediately snap shut because of the inertia of blood flow, which imparts considerable kinetic energy to the blood. During the latter part of phase 3—**decreased ejection**—the decrease in ventricular volume becomes less rapid, and both the ventricular and aortic pressures fall off. During the entire ejection phase, about 70 mL of blood flows into the aorta, leaving about 50 mL behind in the ventricle.

Isovolumetric Relaxation (Phase 4) Late in the ejection phase, blood flow across the aortic valve falls to extremely low values, until it actually reverses direction (i.e., retrograde or negative flow). At this point, the *aortic valve closes,* defining the onset of diastole. As blood flow in the aorta again becomes briefly positive (i.e., forward), there is a small upward deflection in the aortic pressure trace. The result is the **dicrotic notch** (from the Greek *dikrotos,* "double-beat"), or **incisura,** and the subsequent dicrotic wave, which interrupts the generally downward trend of aortic pressure. Because both the aortic and mitral valves are closed and no blood can enter the left ventricle, this is the period of isovolumetric relaxation. Pressure falls rapidly in the left ventricle.

Rapid Ventricular Filling Period (Beginning of Phase 1) When ventricular pressure falls below that in the left atrium (second crossover of blue and orange tracings in Fig. 22-1B), the *mitral valve opens.* Immediately following mitral valve opening, left ventricular volume begins to increase

Importance (and Unimportance) of Atrial Contraction

The relative importance of atrial contraction to overall cardiac function is evident in patients who develop atrial fibrillation (see Fig. 21-14H), an arrhythmia associated with loss of this atrial "kick." In atrial fibrillation, chaotic electrical activity, bombarding the atria with as many as 500 impulses per minute from all directions, prevents the concerted action of atrial cardiac muscle fibers that is necessary for coordinated atrial contraction. As a result, the atria fibrillate—they look like a wriggling bag of worms. In healthy persons with otherwise normal hearts, the loss of atrial contraction usually causes no symptoms at rest or perhaps only a sensation of an irregular or rapid heartbeat (i.e., the result of atrial fibrillation). However, if the patient already has a compromised myocardium (e.g., from ischemic heart disease, prolonged hypertension, or mitral stenosis), or if the patient is debilitated by dysfunction of other organs (e.g., chronic emphysema), the loss of the atrial contraction may further reduce cardiac output just enough to send the patient into florid congestive heart failure (see the box on cardiac hypertrophy) or even shock (i.e., arterial pressure so low that it compromises perfusion of peripheral tissues). The physician may treat a patient with an otherwise normal heart in a leisurely fashion or perhaps not at all—keeping in mind that patients with atrial fibrillation are at high risk for development of atrial thrombosis and thus possibly cerebral embolism and stroke. In patients with a compromised myocardium, emergency chemical or electrical cardioversion may be necessary.

rapidly (Fig. 22-1B, bottom). During this period of rapid ventricular filling, the left atrial and ventricular pressures evolve in parallel because the mitral valve is wide open. A period of relatively decreased filling follows, the period of diastasis with which we began our discussion. Thus, diastole includes both the rapid ventricular filling period and diastasis. As already noted, the length of diastole decreases with elevations in heart rate. This decrease comes first at the expense of the period of slower ventricular filling (i.e., diastasis).

During rapid ventricular filling, the aortic valve remains closed. Because blood continues to flow out to the periphery, owing to the recoil of the aorta's elastic wall (see the box on the effect of aortic compliance later in this chapter), the aortic pressure falls. This fall continues during diastasis.

The electrocardiogram, phonocardiogram, and echocardiogram follow the cyclic pattern of the cardiac cycle

Accompanying the basic cyclic pattern of cardiac pressure and volume changes are characteristic mechanical, electrical, acoustic, and echocardiographic changes. Figure 22-2 illustrates these events for the left side of the heart and the systemic circulation. Notice that the pressure records in the top panel of Figure 22-2 start with the atrial contraction, that is, slightly later than in Figure 22-1.

Aortic Blood Flow   Blood flow from the left ventricle to the ascending aorta rises most rapidly during the rapid ejection phase of the left ventricle. The peaking of aortic flow defines the beginning of the decreased ejection phase. See Figure 22-2, second panel.

Jugular Venous Pulse   The third panel of Figure 22-2 includes the jugular venous pulse, for comparison with the timing of other events. We discuss the jugular venous pulse later in the chapter.

Electrocardiogram   The ECG (discussed in Chapter 21) begins with the middle of the P wave (atrial depolarization). The QRS complex (ventricular depolarization) is the prelude to the upswing in ventricular pressure. The T wave (ventricular repolarization) occurs in the decreased ejection phase. See Figure 22-2, fourth panel.

Phonocardiogram and Heart Sounds   The opening and closing of the valves are accompanied by **heart sounds**, easily heard through a stethoscope or recorded with a digital stethoscope and stored as a phonocardiogram (Table 22-2). The dominant frequencies of heart sounds are lower (110 to 180 Hz) than those of heart murmurs (see Chapter 17), which result from turbulence (180 to 500 Hz). Each of the vertical dotted lines in Figure 22-2 indicates the movement of two valves, one on the right side of the heart and one on the left. Thus, two valves can contribute to a single heart sound, although the two components can often be separated by the ear. The phonocardiogram in Figure 22-2 shows the timing of the two major, or physiological, heart sounds (S_1 and S_2) as well as two other sounds (S_3 and S_4) that are occasionally heard. See Figure 22-2, fifth panel.

The physiological heart sounds S_1 and S_2 are heard following the closure of the cardiac valves: the mitral and tricuspid valves for S_1, and the aortic and pulmonary valves for S_2. However, the actual apposition of the valve leaflets (i.e., "slamming the door") does not produce the sound. Instead, vibrations resulting from sudden tension in the AV valves and the adjacent ventricular walls produce the **first heart sound**, S_1. Similarly, vibrations of the large vessel walls and columns of blood produce the **second heart sound**, S_2, following closure of the semilunar valves. These vibrations propagate through adjacent tissues to the chest wall, where one can normally hear the first and second heart sounds through a stethoscope. S_1 is usually stronger, longer, and of lower frequency than S_2.

Although the four vertical lines that define the four phases of the cardiac cycle are similar for the right and left sides of the heart, they do not line up perfectly with one another, as can be seen by comparing A and B of Figure 22-1. For example, the aortic valve usually closes just before the pulmonary valve. This timing difference produces the **physiological splitting** of the A_2 (i.e., aortic) and P_2 (i.e., pulmonary) components of the second heart sound. As we shall see later, inspiration accentuates the splitting of S_2. Pathological change that accentuates the asynchrony between the left and right sides of the heart (e.g., right bundle branch block) may also lead to splitting of the *first* heart sound.

With stiffening of the mitral valve, seen in mitral stenosis, the opening of the mitral valve may produce an additional

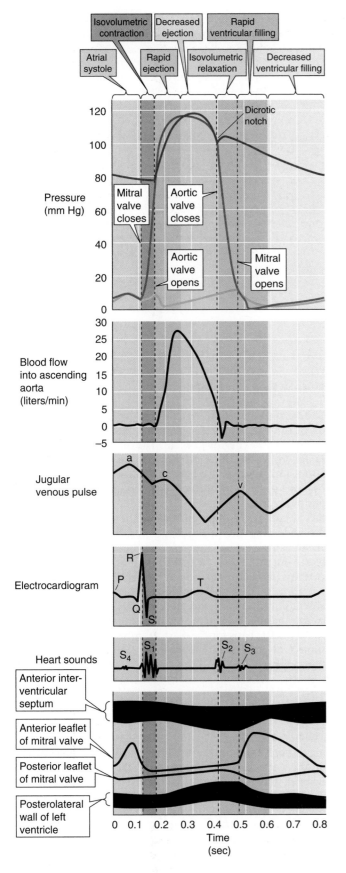

Figure 22-2 Mechanical, electrical, acoustic, and echocardiographic events in the cardiac cycle. *Top*, A repeat of Figure 22-1B, with three modifications: (1) the cardiac cycle begins with atrial contraction; (2) phase 1 of the cardiac cycle has three subparts: rapid ventricular filling, decreased ventricular filling, and atrial systole; (3) phase 3 has two subparts: rapid and decreased ventricular ejection.

sound, an **opening snap (OS)**, in early diastole just after S_2.

A physiological **third heart sound, S_3**, is present in some normal individuals, particularly children. S_3 occurs in early diastole when rapid filling of the ventricles results in recoil of ventricular walls that have a limited distensibility. An S_3 also can be heard in adults when the ventricle is so overfilled at the end of systole that the addition of 70 mL more blood during diastole brings the ventricle into a volume range in which ventricular compliance is very low. The result is an accentuated recoil, heard as an S_3. An S_3 can originate from the left or the right side of the heart. A gallop rhythm is a grouping of three heart sounds that together sound like hoofs of a galloping horse. Thus, the addition of an S_3 to the physiological S_1 and S_2 creates a three-sound sequence, S_1-S_2-S_3, that is termed a **protodiastolic gallop** or ventricular gallop.

When present, a **fourth heart sound, S_4**, coincides with atrial contraction. It is usually heard in pathological conditions in which an unusually strong atrial contraction occurs in combination with low compliance of the left ventricle. The addition of an S_4 produces another three-sound sequence, S_4-S_1-S_2, which is also a gallop rhythm, a **presystolic gallop** or atrial gallop.

Echocardiogram We discussed echocardiography in Chapter 17. The echocardiogram in the bottom panel of Figure 22-2 shows that the separation between the anterior and posterior leaflets of the mitral valve increases during atrial contraction. The leaflets meet at the beginning of phase 2 and remain together until rapid ventricular filling occurs in the beginning of phase 1, when the separation between leaflets becomes maximal. During the decreased phase of ventricular filling, the leaflets once again move closer together, until the next atrial contraction.

The cardiac cycle causes flow waves in the aorta and peripheral vessels

With the closing and opening of the heart's exit valves (i.e., pulmonary and aortic valves), blood flow and blood velocity across these valves oscillate from near zero, when the valves are closed, to high values, when the valves are open. *Blood flow* in the aortic arch actually oscillates between slightly negative and highly positive values (Fig. 22-3A, panel 1). *Pressure* in the aortic arch typically oscillates between about 80 and about 120 mm Hg (Fig. 22-3B, panel 1) but varies greatly among individuals. Phasic changes in pressure and flow also occur in the peripheral arteries. Arterial pressure is usually measured in a large artery, such as the brachial artery. Because very little pressure drop occurs between the aorta and such a large, proximate artery, the measured **systolic** and

Table 22-2 The Heart Sounds

Sound		Associated Events
S₁	First heart sound (sounds like *lub*)	Closure of mitral and tricuspid valves
	Two bursts, a mitral M₁ and a tricuspid T₁ component	
S₂	Second heart sound (sounds like *dub*)	Closure of aortic and pulmonary valves
	An aortic A₂ and a pulmonary P₂ component	
OS	Opening snap	Opening of a stenotic mitral valve
S₃	Third heart sound	Diastolic filling gallop or ventricular or protodiastolic gallop
S₄	Fourth heart sound	Atrial sound that creates an atrial or presystolic gallop

diastolic arterial pressures, as well as the pulse pressure and mean arterial pressure, closely approximate the corresponding aortic pressures. (See Chapter 17.)

If blood vessels were rigid tubes, so that the resistance (R) were constant, and if the driving pressure (ΔP) were also constant throughout the cardiac cycle, we could describe blood flow (F) by a simple Ohm's law–like relationship, as we did in Chapter 17 (see Equation 17-1). However, because blood vessels are compliant (so that R varies with pressure, as in Fig. 19-7B) and because both aortic pressure and flow vary during the cardiac cycle, we cannot describe real arteries in this way. In the field of hydraulics, oscillating flows and pressures have not only an **amplitude** but also a **phase**. As a result, the ratio $\Delta P/F$ is no longer resistance—a simple, time-*in*dependent quantity—but a *complex* quantity called the **mechanical impedance** that depends on the classical "resistance" as well as the compliance and inertial properties of the vessels and blood.

Because of these resistive, compliant, and inertial properties, the pressure and flow waves in vessels distal to the aorta are not quite the same as in the aorta. Instead, the farther the vessels are from the aorta, the more different the pressure and flow waves become.

Aortic Arch During the rapid ejection phase, peak *flow* through the aortic arch is remarkably high, ~30 L/min (dark beige band in Fig. 22-3A, panel 1). The peak linear velocity is ~100 cm/s, which makes it more likely that the blood will reach the critical Reynolds number value for turbulence (see Chapter 17). The rapid ejection of blood also causes a rapid rise of the *pressure* in the aorta to above that in the ventricle (Fig. 22-3B, panel 1). Even though the pressure gradient across the valve reverses, the valve does not close, as is evidenced by the continuous flow of blood from the ventricle into the aorta. The reason that flow continues in the forward direction is the *inertial* component of the blood flow, which represents considerable kinetic energy. Eventually, blood in the aortic arch decelerates sufficiently that the flow becomes

zero and eventually negative (producing reflux through the valve). As the aortic valve closes, it produces the dicrotic notch in the aortic pressure trace.

Thoracic-Abdominal Aorta and Large Arteries Just distal to the aortic arch, a transformation of the flow and pressure curves begins to occur. The records in panels 2 to 4 in Figure 22-3A show the flow curves for the abdominal aorta and some of its large branches. Peak systolic flow becomes smaller as one moves from the aorta toward the periphery (i.e., iliac and femoral arteries), as would be predicted because of the branching of the vessels. However, in the abdominal aorta, a new phenomenon is seen. As the elastic aorta—which stored blood during systole—releases blood during diastole, a second peak of flow appears. Note that this *diastolic component* of flow is larger in the abdominal aorta than in the more distal iliac artery and almost absent in the femoral artery. Of particular importance is the sizable diastolic flow in the carotid and renal arteries (panels 5 and 6). The basis for the diastolic component of flow is the subject of the box titled Effect of Aortic Compliance on Blood Flow.

The cardiac cycle also causes pressure waves in the aorta and peripheral vessels

The *pressure* curves in Figure 22-3B show that with increasing distance from the heart (panels 1 to 4), the rising portion of the wave becomes steeper and the peak is narrower. Because the peak gradually increases in height and the minimum pressure gradually decreases, the pulse pressure becomes greater. With increasing distance from the heart, an important secondary pressure oscillation appears during diastole (Fig. 22-3B, fourth panel). Thus, although the pressure waves are distorted, they are not damped. Although it might seem counterintuitive that the peak arterial pressure should increase as we get farther from the heart (i.e., Is the blood flowing against a pressure gradient?), it turns out that

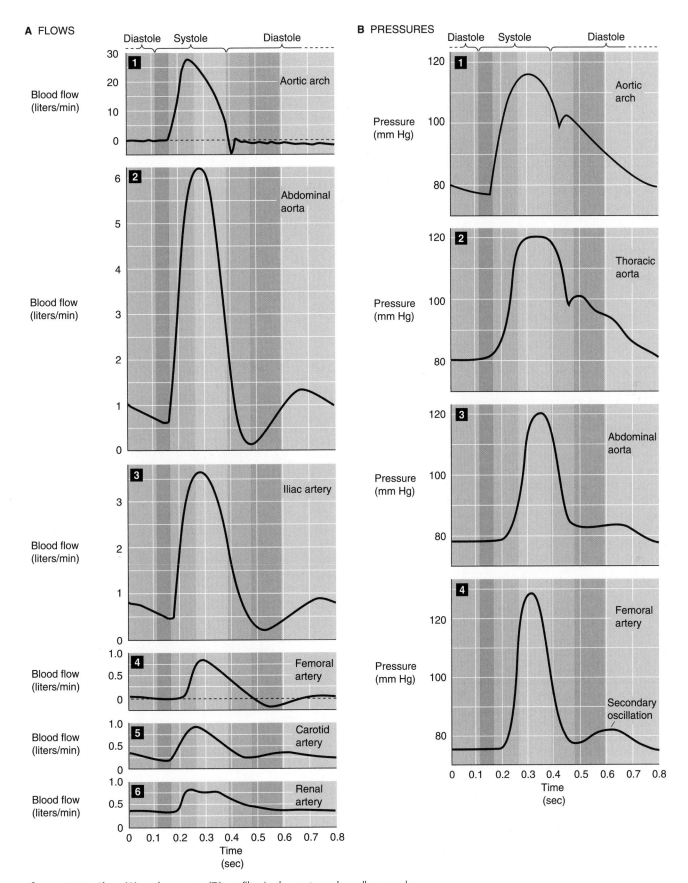

Figure 22-3 Flow (**A**) and pressure (**B**) profiles in the aorta and smaller vessels.

Effect of Aortic Compliance on Blood Flow

There is a large diastolic component to total blood flow in the large arteries that lie close to the aorta, such as the carotid and renal arteries (panels 5 and 6 in Fig. 22-3A). This sizeable diastolic component is largely the result of the high **compliance** of the vessel walls and the **radial expansion** of the vessels that occurs during ventricular ejection. We can reach at least an intuitive understanding of the radial contribution to flow in the aorta and large arteries by examining the ability of the aorta to store and to give up energy during the acceleration and deceleration of flow.

Figure 22-4 compares two branches of a hydraulic system that are identical in radius and length. One branch (branch 1) is rigid and made of glass, the other (branch 2) is elastic and made of rubber. Both branches terminate in a spout with an outflow resistance that is analogous to the resistance of arterioles. We assume that the resistance of the spout is much greater than that of the glass or rubber tube, so that we can ignore small changes in the diameter of the rubber tube on overall resistance. If we apply a *steady pressure* to both branches, the flows through the two branches are continuous and identical (Fig. 22-4A).

However, if we apply the *pressure in square pulses*, the flows in the two branches are quite different (Fig. 22-4B). The flow through the glass tubing instantly rises to a maximum value with the onset of the pressure wave and then instantly falls to zero when the driving pressure falls to zero. Thus, the plot of flow through the glass tube perfectly mirrors the plot of the applied square wave pressure. The flow through the rubber tube has a very different profile. During the interval of peak pressure, the rubber vessel gradually dilates, storing a volume of fluid. Therefore, the flow rises slowly to its maximum value. During the interval of the cycle when the driving pressure falls to zero, the expanded rubber vessel delivers its stored volume downstream, resulting in some forward flow despite the absence of any pressure head. The time-averaged outflow from the rubber tube exceeds that from the glass tube.

The aorta and large vessels behave like the rubber tube in Figure 22-4B. The oscillating pressure head in our model (i.e., between zero and a peak value) represents ventricular pressure. The maintenance of flow during interruption of the pressure head is equivalent to the continuing flow from the aorta during diastole.

Figure 22-4C shows an alternative mechanical model, that of a Windkessel (German for "wind chamber"), in which we replace the compliance of a distensible rubber tube with the compressible air within a chamber above the blood.

The two models illustrated in Figure 22-4B and C show how compliant blood vessels can convert discontinuous flow into a more continuous flow. The so-called Windkessel action of the arterial system considerably improves the efficiency of the pump (i.e., the heart) because the vessels are able to convert the phasic flow peaks of the pump into a more continuous flow.

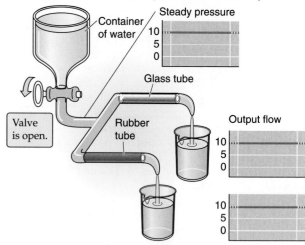

A STEADY INPUT PRESSURE (CONTINUOUS FLOW)

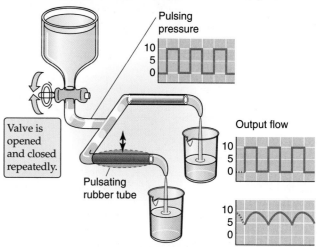

B SQUARE-PULSE PRESSURE (PULSATILE FLOW)

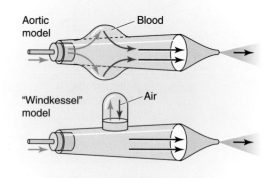

C "WINDKESSEL" MODEL OF AORTA

Figure 22-4 **A** and **B,** Effect of pulsatile pressure on flow through a compliant vessel. In **C,** the *gold arrows* indicate movements analogous to systole, and the *violet arrows*, diastole.

the *mean* arterial pressure does fall slightly with increasing distance from the heart.

Terminal Arteries and Arterioles

In the smallest arteries, the flows must be small. Here, the trend toward an increased peak pressure reverses. Instead, the pulse wave gets damped out for two reasons. First, because we are dealing with many parallel vessels with a large aggregate wall area, the aggregate compliance increases, damping the pressure wave. Second, because these smaller arteries have a smaller radius and thus a far greater resistance, the mean arterial pressure must fall in proportion to the much higher resistance. Thus, in contrast to the situation in the larger arteries, damping predominates over distortion.

Capillaries

By the time the blood reaches the capillaries, the damping is so severe that pulsations (i.e., pressure oscillations) do not normally occur—blood flow is continuous. The pulmonary capillaries are an exception; their upstream vessels are short, and they have low resistance and high compliance. The pulsation of systemic capillaries occurs only in cases of markedly increased pulse pressure, such as in patients with aortic regurgitation or hyperthyroidism, or in cases of generalized peripheral vasodilation.

Distortion of pressure waves is the result of their propagation along the arterial tree

Imagine that you are listening to a patient's heart with a stethoscope while simultaneously feeling the pulse of the radial artery near the wrist. For each heartbeat that you hear, you feel a radial pulse. You know that the peak pressure in the left ventricle occurs about midway between the first and second heart sounds, but the delay between the midpoint of the two heart sounds and the peak of the radial pulse is only ~0.1 s. Red blood cells take several seconds to flow from the heart to the wrist. Why, then, are you able to feel the pulse so soon after the heartbeat?

The answer is that the blood vessels conduct the palpable pulse as a **pressure wave**. The linear velocity of red blood cells—carried in the blood by convection—ranges from approximately 1 m/s in the aorta to vanishingly small values in the capillaries (see Chapter 19). However, the pressure wave travels at a velocity of 5 to 6 m/s in the aorta, increasing to 10 to 15 m/s in the small arteries.

The following example illustrates the difference between the velocity of a pressure wave and that of convection. Imagine that two people are submerged in a river, floating downstream (convection). Now the person upstream makes a sound under water. The sound waves (an example of a pressure wave) travel to the person downstream with a velocity that is far greater than the velocity of the river.

We could illustrate how pressure waves propagate along arteries by replotting the arterial pressure profiles from Figure 22-3B and stacking them one on top of the other. The four pressure waves in Figure 22-5 actually represent data obtained simultaneously in a dog with four catheters, the first placed in the aortic arch and the last three placed precisely 10 cm downstream from the previous one. The downstream propagation of the wave through the larger arteries is accompanied by a serious *distortion* of the

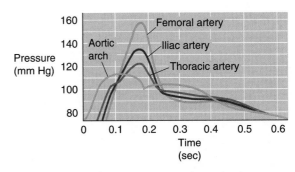

Figure 22-5 Arterial pressure waves. These simultaneous pressure records are from a dog, with catheters placed at 0, 10, 20, and 30 cm from the aortic arch. As the wave moves down the vessel, the upstroke is delayed, but the peak is higher.

pressure profile: it gets narrower and taller as we move downstream.

Effect of Frequency on Wave Velocity and Damping

The pressure wave moving from the aorta to the periphery is actually an ensemble of many individual waves, each with its own frequency. Higher frequency waves travel faster and undergo more damping than low-frequency waves (Fig. 22-6A). Recombination of these waves at a more peripheral site thus produces a new wave with a shape that is a distorted version of the original aortic wave.

Effect of Wall Stiffness on Wave Velocity

As the pressure wave reaches vessels that have a stiffer wall (e.g., greater ratio of wall thickness to vessel diameter), the velocity of the wave increases (Fig. 22-6B). Conversely, with a more compliant vessel, some of the energy of the pressure pulse goes into dilation of the vessel, so that the pressure wave spreads out and slows down. Because aging causes a decrease in vessel compliance (i.e., distensibility), the velocity of propagation actually increases.

Pressure waves in veins do not originate from arterial waves

We have seen earlier in this chapter that flow in *capillaries* is usually not pulsatile. Nevertheless, blood flow in systemic capillaries can exhibit slow oscillations, unrelated to the cardiac cycle. The action of upstream vasomotor control elements in arterioles and precapillary sphincters can cause fluctuations. In addition, changes in tissue pressure (e.g., caused by muscle contraction) can compress capillaries and cause further fluctuations in capillary flow. Pulmonary capillaries are especially susceptible to changes in the surrounding alveolar pressure (see Chapter 31).

Although systemic *veins* have pressure waves, these waves do not originate from arterial waves propagating through the capillary beds, which are nonpulsatile. Three mechanisms can contribute to the **venous pulse**: (1) retrograde action of the heartbeat during the cardiac cycle, (2) the respiratory cycle, and (3) the contraction of skeletal muscles.

Effect of the Cardiac Cycle

A large vein close to the heart, such as the **jugular vein**, has a complex pulse wave (Fig.

A   DISTORTION IN A VESSEL WITH UNIFORM DISTENSIBILITY

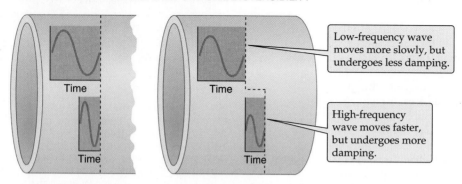

Low-frequency wave moves more slowly, but undergoes less damping.

High-frequency wave moves faster, but undergoes more damping.

B   DISTORTION IN A VESSEL WITH DECREASING DOWNSTREAM DISTENSIBILITY

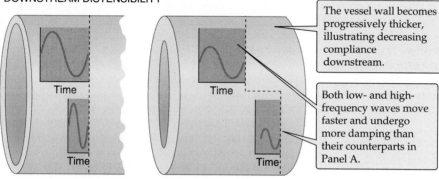

The vessel wall becomes progressively thicker, illustrating decreasing compliance downstream.

Both low- and high-frequency waves move faster and undergo more damping than their counterparts in Panel A.

Figure 22-6 Propagation of pressure waves. In **A** and **B,** the flow is from left to right. The left pair of pressure waves is at the same early time, whereas the right pair of pressure waves is at the same late time. If on the right (i.e., end of the vessel) we summate waves of different frequency at the same instant in time, then the composite wave is distorted (like the green femoral artery curve in Fig. 22-5).

22-7A) synchronized to the cardiac cycle. The three maxima, or peaks, in the jugular pulse wave are labeled *a*, *c*, and *v*. The three minima, or dips, are labeled *av*, *x*, and *y*. These pressure transients reflect events in the cardiac cycle:

The ***a* peak** is caused by the contraction of the right atrium.

The ***av* minimum** is due to relaxation of the right atrium and closure of the tricuspid valve.

The ***c* peak** reflects the pressure rise in the right ventricle early during systole and the resultant bulging of the tricuspid valve—which has just closed—into the right atrium.

The ***x* minimum** occurs as the ventricle contracts and shortens during the ejection phase, later in systole. The shortening heart—with tricuspid valve still closed—pulls on and therefore elongates the veins, lowering their pressure.

The ***v* peak** is related to filling of the right atrium against a closed tricuspid valve, which causes right atrial pressure to rise. As the tricuspid valve opens, the *v* peak begins to wane.

The ***y* minimum** reflects a fall in right atrial pressure during rapid ventricular filling, as blood leaves the right atrium through an open tricuspid valve and enters the right ventricle. The increase in venous pressure after the *y* minimum occurs as venous return continues in the face of reduced ventricular filling.

Effect of the Respiratory Cycle   Poiseuille was the first to observe that the pressure in the jugular vein becomes negative during inspiration (Fig. 22-7B). During inspiration, the diaphragm descends, causing intrathoracic pressure (and therefore the pressure inside the thoracic vessels) to decrease and intra-abdominal pressure to increase (see Chapter 27). Consequently, the venous return from the head and upper extremities transiently increases, as low-pressure vessels literally suck blood into the thoracic cavity. Simultaneously, the venous flow decreases from the lower extremities because of the relatively high pressure of the abdominal veins during inspiration. Therefore, during inspiration, pressure in the jugular vein falls while pressure in the femoral vein rises.

Effect of Skeletal Muscle Contraction ("Muscle Pump")
The contraction of skeletal muscle can also affect pressure and flow in veins. Large veins in the lower limbs are equipped with valves that prevent retrograde movement of blood (see Chapter 17). When a person is at rest and in the recumbent position, all venous valves are open and venous blood flow toward the heart is continuous. Standing causes the venous pressure in the foot to rise gradually to the hydrostatic pressure dictated by the vertical blood column from the foot to the heart (Fig. 22-7C). If the person begins to walk, the combination of the pumping action of the leg muscles on the leg veins and the action of the venous valves as hydrostatic relay stations causes the venous pressure in the foot to decrease. Each step causes both a small oscillation and a small net decrease in foot vein pressure. Once foot vein pressure has bottomed out, each step simply causes a small pressure oscillation. Walking causes a net decrease in pressure in both the superficial and deep foot veins as well as in the corresponding capillaries. When the exercise ceases, the venous pressure again rises.

A JUGULAR VENOUS PRESSURE CHANGES
CAUSED BY CARDIAC CYCLE

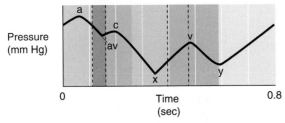

B JUGULAR VENOUS PRESSURE CHANGES
CAUSED BY RESPIRATORY CYCLE

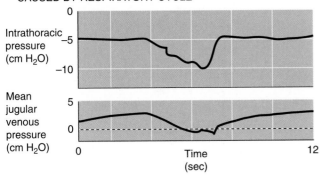

C VENOUS PRESSURE CHANGES IN FOOT
CAUSED BY MUSCLE CONTRACTION

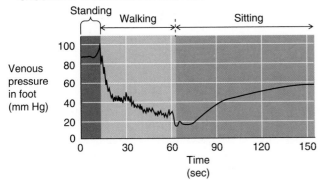

Figure 22-7 Venous pressure changes. In **A,** the time scale is a single cardiac cycle. The relative heights of the peaks and valleys are variable. In **B** and **C,** the time scale surrounds one protracted inspiration (i.e., several heartbeats); the y-axis shows the *mean* jugular venous pressure. (**B,** *Data from Brecher GA: Venous Return. New York, Grune & Stratton, 1956.* **C,** *Data from Pollack AA, Wood EH: Venous pressure in the saphenous vein at the ankle in man during exercise and changes in posture. J Appl Physiol 1949; 1:649-662.*)

CARDIAC DYNAMICS

The heart is a system of two pumps linked in series. The muscular wall of the left ventricle is thicker and more powerful than that of the right. The interventricular septum welding the two pumps together is even thicker. The thick muscular walls of the ventricles are responsible for exerting the heart's pumping action.

The heart does not depend on a rhythm generator in the brain, like the central pattern generators (see Chapter 16) that drive other rhythmic behaviors, such as respiration, locomotion, chewing, and shivering. Instead, pacemaker cells within the heart itself initiate cardiac excitation. When the heart is in a normal sinus rhythm, the pacemaker cells setting the rate are located in the sinoatrial (SA) node of the right atrium (see Chapter 21). The action potential then spreads through atrial myocytes and specialized tracts or bundles. The impulse cannot cross from the atria to the ventricles except through the atrioventricular (AV) node. The AV node inserts a time delay into the conduction that is essential to allow the ventricles to finish filling with blood before contraction and ejection occur. From the AV node, the impulse spreads through the bundle of His and then the right and left bundle branches; the left bundle branch divides in an anterior and posterior fascicle. Finally, the system of Purkinje fibers excites the ventricular myocytes, where the impulse propagates from cell to cell through gap junctions.

The right ventricle contracts like a bellows, whereas the left ventricle contracts like a hand squeezing a tube of toothpaste

The two ventricles share a common envelope of spiral and circular muscle layers. The arrangement of the spiral bundles ensures that ventricular contraction virtually wrings the blood out of the heart, although incompletely. The apex contracts before some of the basal portions of the ventricle, a sequence that propels blood upward to the aortic and pulmonary valves.

The mechanical action of the **right ventricle** resembles that of a bellows used to fan a fire (Fig. 22-8A). Although the distance between the free wall and the septum is small, the free wall has such a large surface area that a small movement of the free wall toward the septum ejects a large volume.

The mechanism of emptying of the right ventricle involves three motions. First, the longitudinal axis of the right ventricle shortens when spiral muscles pull the tricuspid valve ring toward the apex. Second, the free wall of the right ventricle moves toward the septum in a bellows-like motion. Third, the contraction of the deep circular fibers of the *left* ventricle forces the septum into a convex shape, so that the septum bulges into the right ventricle. This bulging of the septum stretches the free wall of the right ventricle over the septum. These three motions are well suited for ejection of a large volume but not for development of a high pressure. The right ventricle ejects the same blood volume as the left ventricle does, but it does so at much lower intraventricular pressures.

The mechanical action of the **left ventricle** occurs by a dual motion (Fig. 22-8B). First, constriction of the *circular muscle layers* reduces the diameter of the chamber, progressing from apex to base, akin to squeezing a tube of toothpaste. Second, contraction of the *spiral muscles* pulls the mitral valve ring toward the apex, thereby shortening the long axis. The first mechanism is the more powerful and is responsible for the high pressures developed by the left ventricle. The conical shape of the lumen gives the left ventricle a smaller surface-to-volume ratio than the right ventricle and contributes to the ability of the left ventricle to generate high pressures.

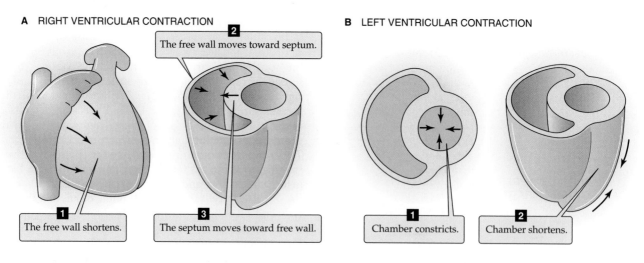

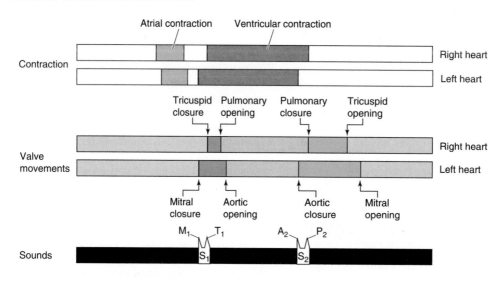

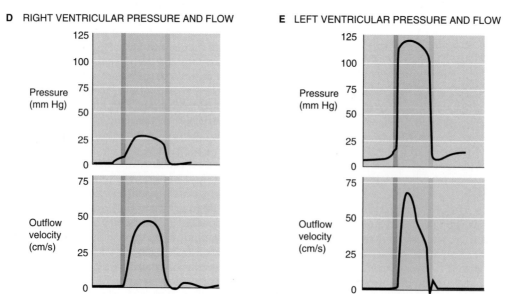

Figure 22-8 Comparison of the dynamics of the left and right ventricles.

The contraction of the **atria** normally makes only a minor contribution to the filling of the two ventricles when the subject is at rest (see the box on the importance of atrial contraction). However, the contraction of the atria is a useful safety factor in at least two circumstances. During tachycardia, when the diastolic interval—and thus the time for passive filling—is short, the atrial contraction can provide a much-needed boost. Atrial contraction is also useful in certain pathological conditions. For example, when a narrowed (i.e., stenotic) AV valve offers substantial resistance to the flow of blood from atrium to ventricle, the atrial pump can make an important contribution to ventricular filling.

The right atrium contracts before the left, but the left ventricle contracts before the right

When the cardiac cycle was introduced earlier in the chapter, we assumed that the events on the right and left sides of the heart happen simultaneously. However, as we have already noted in our discussion of the splitting of heart sounds, the timing of the two sides of the heart is slightly different (Fig. 22-8C).

Atrial Contraction Because the SA node is located in the right atrium, atrial contraction begins and ends earlier in the right atrium than in the left (Fig. 22-8C, Contraction).

Initiation of Ventricular Contraction Ventricular contraction starts slightly earlier on the *left* side, and the mitral valve closes before the tricuspid valve. However, this timing difference in the closure of the AV valves (Fig. 22-8C, Valve movements) is so small that it is unusual to hear a split S_1. On the other hand, the right ventricle has a briefer period of isovolumetric contraction because it does not need to build up as much pressure to open its semilunar (i.e., outflow) valve and to initiate ejection. Thus, the pulmonary valve opens slightly ahead of the aortic valve.

Ventricular Ejection Ejection from the right ventricle lasts longer than that from the left. The semilunar valves do not close simultaneously. The aortic valve, with its higher downstream pressure, closes before the pulmonary valve. Therefore, the pulmonary valve—with its lower downstream pressure—opens first and closes last. This timing difference in the closure of the semilunar valves explains the normal physiological splitting of S_2 (Fig. 22-8C, Sounds). During inspiration, the relatively negative intrathoracic pressure enhances filling of the right side of the heart, causing it to have a larger end-diastolic volume and therefore more blood to eject. The additional time required for right ventricular ejection postpones the closure of the pulmonary valve (P_2), broadening the physiological splitting of S_2.

Ventricular Relaxation Isovolumetric relaxation is briefer in the right side of the heart than in the left. The pulmonary valve closes *after* the aortic valve, and the tricuspid valve opens *before* the mitral valve. Therefore, the right ventricle begins filling before the left.

Measurements of ventricular volumes, pressures, and flows allow clinicians to judge cardiac performance

Definitions of Cardiac Volumes The cardiac output is the product of heart rate and stroke volume (see Chapter 17). The **stroke volume (SV)** is the difference between ventricular **end-diastolic volume (EDV)** and ventricular **end-systolic volume (ESV)**, that is, the difference between the maximal and minimal ventricular volumes. EDV is typically 120 mL, and the ESV is 50 mL, so that

$$
\begin{aligned}
SV &= EDV - ESV \\
&= 120\,mL - 50\,mL \qquad \text{(22-2)} \\
&= 70\,mL
\end{aligned}
$$

The **ejection fraction (EF)** is a dimensionless value, defined as the stroke volume normalized to the end-diastolic volume:

$$
EF = \frac{SV}{EDV} \qquad \text{(22-3)}
$$

In our example, the EF is (70 mL)/(120 mL) or ~0.6. The value should exceed 55% in a healthy person. Whereas the ejection fractions of the left and right ventricles are as a rule equal, clinicians normally measure left ventricular ejection fraction (LVEF).

Measurements of Cardiac Volumes Clinicians routinely measure the volume of the cardiac chambers by means of angiography or echocardiography (see Chapter 17). **One-dimensional (or M-mode) echocardiography** allows one to assess left ventricular performance in terms of linear dimensions and velocities by providing measurements of velocity of the posterior left ventricular wall, fractional shortening of the left ventricular circumference, and rate of fractional circumferential shortening. **Two-dimensional echocardiography** makes it possible to determine several ventricular volumes:

Left ventricular end-diastolic volume (LVEDV)
Left ventricular end-systolic volume (LVESV)
Stroke volume (SV = LVEDV – LVESV)
Left ventricular ejection fraction (LVEF = SV/LVEDV)

Measurement of Ventricular Pressures For right-sided heart catheterizations, clinicians use a Swan-Ganz catheter, which consists of three parallel tubes of different lengths. The longest is an end-hole catheter with a balloon flotation device that directs the tip in the direction of the blood flow. The other two tubes are side-hole catheters that terminate at two points proximal to the tip. The physician advances the catheter percutaneously through a large systemic vein, into the right side of the heart, and then into the pulmonary circulation where the tip of the longest tube literally *wedges* in a small pulmonary artery. Because a continuous and presumably closed column of blood connects the probe's end and the left atrium, the **wedge pressure** is taken as an index of left atrial pressure. For left-sided heart catheterizations,

Table 22-3 Comparison of Pressures in the Right and Left Circulations

PRESSURES (mm Hg)				
Right Atrium		**Left Atrium**		
Mean	2	Mean		8
		a wave		13
		c wave		12
		v wave		15
Right Ventricle		**Left Ventricle**		
Peak systolic	30	Peak systolic		130
End diastolic	6	End diastolic		10
Pulmonary Artery		**Aorta**		
Mean	15	Mean		95
Peak systolic	25	Peak systolic		130
End diastolic	8	End diastolic		80
Pulmonary Capillaries		**Systemic Capillaries**		
Mean	10	Mean		25

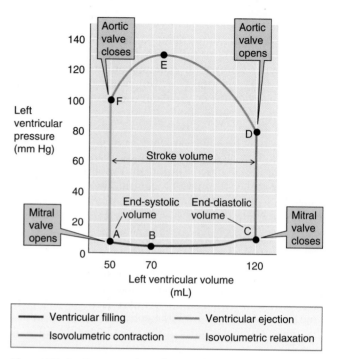

Legend:
— Ventricular filling — Ventricular ejection
— Isovolumetric contraction — Isovolumetric relaxation

Figure 22-9 Pressure-volume loop of the left ventricle.

clinicians insert a simple catheter percutaneously into an artery and then advance the catheter tip upstream to the left side of the heart. Table 22-3 lists some of the most important pressure values for the right and left sides of the heart.

Measurement of Flows The cardiologist can calculate flow from changes in ventricular volume, as measured by echocardiography and the Doppler ultrasound technique (see Chapter 17), both of which measure the flow of blood in the outflow tract (i.e., aorta). Figure 22-8D and E illustrates the profiles of outflow pressure and velocity for the two ventricles. Although the two ventricles expel on average the same *amount* of blood in a single cardiac cycle, the peak *velocity* is much higher in the left ventricle. In addition, the velocity rises far more rapidly in the left ventricle, indicating greater acceleration of the blood during ejection. The *pressure* wave is about five times larger in the left ventricle than in the right, and the rate at which the pressure rises ($\Delta P/\Delta t$) is more rapid in the left ventricle.

The pressure-volume loop of a ventricle illustrates the ejection work of the ventricle

In Figure 22-1, we saw separate plots of ventricular *pressure* against time and *volume* against time. If, at each point in time, we now plot pressure against volume, the result is a **pressure-volume loop**, as shown in Figure 22-9 for the left

ventricle. This loop is a "phase plot" that describes the relationship between left ventricular pressure and left ventricular volume during the cardiac cycle. Notice that although *time* does not explicitly appear in this plot, as we make one complete counterclockwise cycle around the loop, we sequentially plot pressure and volume at all time points of the cardiac cycle. However, the distance between two points on the loop is not proportional to elapsed time.

In examining this pressure-volume loop, we will arbitrarily start at point A in Figure 22-9 and then consider each of the segments of the loop (e.g., AB, BC, and so on) before again returning to point A. Although we use the left ventricle as an example, a similar analysis applies to the right ventricle.

Segment AB Point A represents the instant at which the *mitral valve opens*. At this point, left ventricular volume is at its minimal value of ~50 mL, and left ventricular pressure is at the fairly low value of ~7 mm Hg. As the mitral valve opens, the ventricle begins to fill passively because atrial pressure is higher than ventricular pressure. During interval AB, ventricular pressure falls slightly to ~5 mm Hg because the ventricular muscle is continuing to relax during diastole. Thus, despite the rapid entry of blood, ventricular pressure falls to its lowest value in the cardiac cycle.

Segment BC During a second phase of ventricular filling, volume rises markedly from ~70 to ~120 mL, accompanied by a rather modest increase in pressure from ~5 to ~10 mm Hg. The modest rise in pressure, despite a doubling of ventricular volume, reflects the high compliance ($C = \Delta V/\Delta P$) of the ventricular wall during late diastole. The relationship between pressure and volume during segment BC is similar to that in blood vessels (see Chapter 19).

Segment CD Point C represents the *closure of the mitral valve*. At this point, ventricular filling has ended and **isovolumetric contraction**—represented by the vertical line CD—is about to begin. Thus, by the definition of *isovolumetric*, ventricular volume remains at 120 mL while left ventricular pressure rises to ~80 mm Hg, about equal to the aortic end-diastolic pressure.

Segment DE Point D represents the *opening of the aortic valve*. With the outlet to the aorta now open, the ventricular muscle can begin to shorten and to eject blood. During this period of rapid ejection, ventricular volume decreases from ~120 to ~75 mL. Notice that as contraction continues during interval DE, the ventricular pressure rises even farther, reaching a peak systolic value of ~130 mm Hg at point E.

Segment EF Point E represents the instant at which the ventricular muscle starts to relax. During this period of decreased ejection, ventricular pressure falls from ~130 to ~100 mm Hg. Nevertheless, blood continues to leave the ventricle, and ventricular volume falls from ~75 mL at point E to ~50 mL at point F. Point F represents end-systolic volume and pressure. Notice that the ventricle does not shrink to zero volume at the end of systole. In total, 120 − 50 or 70 mL of blood has left the ventricle during systole (i.e., between points D and F). Therefore, the stroke volume is substantially less than the maximum ventricular volume (i.e., EDV). The ejection fraction in this example is ~60%, which is in the normal range. Ejection occurs against aortic pressures ranging between 80 and 130 mm Hg. Therefore, ejection is not "isotonic" (see Chapter 9).

Segment FA Point F represents the *closing of the aortic valve*. At this point, ejection has ended and **isovolumetric relaxation** is about to begin. The ventricular volume remains at 50 mL, while left ventricular pressure falls from ~100 mm Hg at point F to ~7 mm Hg at point A. At the end of isovolumetric relaxation, the mitral valve opens and the cardiac cycle starts all over again with ventricular filling.

The six segments of the pressure-volume loop correspond to different phases of the cardiac cycle:

Phase 1, the inflow phase, includes segments AB and BC.
Phase 2, isovolumetric contraction, includes segment CD.
Phase 3, the outflow phase, includes segments DE and EF.
Phase 4, isovolumetric relaxation, includes segment FA.

Segments CDEF represent systole, whereas segments FABC represent diastole.

The "pumping work" done by the heart is a small fraction of the total energy the heart consumes

The heart does its useful work as a pump by imparting momentum to the blood and propelling it against the resistance of the periphery.

Work, in its simplest definition, is the product of the force applied to an object and the distance the object moves ($W = $ force × distance). In considering **pressure-volume work**, we must revise this definition. Imagine that we have a volume of blood in a syringe. If we apply a *constant* force to the plunger, that is, if we apply a *constant* pressure to the blood, the plunger moves a certain distance as we eject the blood through a needle, thereby reducing blood volume by an amount ΔV. How much work have we done? For pressure moving a fluid, the external work is

$$W = P \cdot \Delta V \qquad (22\text{-}4)$$

If the aortic pressure were constant, the work done with each heartbeat would be simply the product of the aortic pressure (P) and the stroke volume ($\Delta V = SV = EDV - ESV$).

The pressure-volume relationships in Figure 22-10 illustrate the pressure-volume work of the **left ventricle**. The surface below the *segment* ABC (i.e., filling phase) is the work done *by the blood* (previously contained in the venous reservoirs and atria at a low pressure) on the ventricle (Fig. 22-10A). The surface below DEF (i.e., ejection phase) is the work done *by the heart* on the blood during the ejection (Fig. 22-10B). The difference between the areas in parts A and B of Figure 22-10—that is, the area within the single-cycle loop—is the *net* external work done by the heart (Fig. 22-10C).

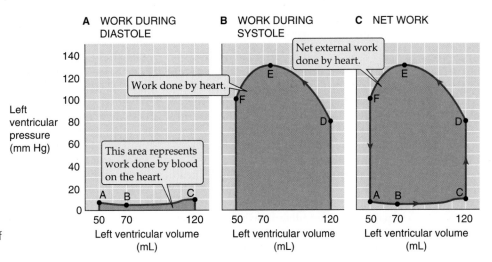

Figure 22-10 External work of the left ventricle.

The pressure-volume diagram for the **right ventricle** has the same general shape. However, the area (i.e., *net* external work) is only about one fifth as large because the pressures are so much lower.

The area of the loop in Figure 22-10C—that is, the pressure-volume work ($P \cdot V$)—ignores the speed at which the ventricle pumps the blood (i.e., acceleration that the heart imparts to the blood, or the time it takes to complete one cardiac cycle). Thus, the work per beat should also include the **kinetic energy** ($\frac{1}{2}mv^2$) that the heart imparts to the ejected blood:

$$\underbrace{W}_{\substack{\text{Total} \\ \text{external} \\ \text{work}}} = \underbrace{P \cdot V}_{\substack{\text{Pressure-} \\ \text{volume} \\ \text{work}}} + \underbrace{\tfrac{1}{2}mv^2}_{\substack{\text{Kinetic} \\ \text{energy}}} \qquad \text{(22-5)}$$

Of its total external work, the heart delivers only a relatively small fraction as kinetic energy. Moreover, the total external work is itself only a small portion of the total energy that the heart actually expends. Like other muscles, the heart not only shortens and performs *classical* work (e.g., isotonic contraction) but also maintains active tension without shortening (i.e., isometric contraction; see Chapter 9). During the isovolumetric contraction, the ventricle develops and maintains a high pressure without performing any total external work—just as we perform no useful work when we hold a weight without lifting it. However, in both isometric exercises, the muscle breaks down adenosine triphosphate (ATP) as long as it maintains isometric tension; the energy ends up as heat. This type of energy cost in heart muscle is called **tension heat**, which is proportional to the product of the tension of the ventricular wall (T) and the length of time (Δt) that the ventricle maintains this tension (i.e., tension-time integral). In the case of the heart, the pressure against which the ventricle must pump is a major determinant of the wall tension.

The total energy transformed in one cardiac cycle is the sum of the total external work done on the blood and the tension heat:

$$E = \underbrace{\underbrace{P \cdot V}_{\substack{\text{Pressure-} \\ \text{volume} \\ \text{work}}} + \underbrace{\tfrac{1}{2}mv^2}_{\substack{\text{Kinetic} \\ \text{energy}}}}_{\text{Total external work}} + \underbrace{k \cdot T \cdot \Delta t}_{\substack{\text{Tension} \\ \text{heat}}} \qquad \text{(22-6)}$$

k is a proportionality constant that converts $T \cdot \Delta t$ into units of energy. The tension heat is the *major* determinant of the total energy requirements of the heart. Total external work represents a relatively small fraction (3%) of the total energy needs of the heart at rest, rising to as much as 10% during exercise. The heat developed as part of the tension-time integral remains the major component of the total energy consumption, even during exercise.

The tension heat is not only far more costly for the heart than the pressure-volume work but also of considerable practical interest for the patient with coronary artery disease who wishes to step up cardiac output during increased physical activity. The major burden for such an individual may be not so much the total external work expended in driving additional blood through the circulation (i.e., increasing the cardiac output) but rather an increase in *tension heat* ($k \cdot T \cdot \Delta t$). Thus, it is advantageous to the patient to have a low wall tension (T)—that is, a low blood pressure. It is also advantageous for the patient not to spend too much time (Δt) in systole. The heart spends a greater fraction of its time in systole when the heart rate is high. Thus, the cardiac patient is better off to increase cardiac output at low pressure and low heart rate (i.e., a low $T \cdot \Delta t$ product). The only option left is to increase stroke volume.

The ratio of the ventricle's total external work ($P \cdot V + \frac{1}{2}mv^2$) to the total energy cost (i.e., W/E) is the heart's **mechanical efficiency**. Note that the mechanical efficiency has nothing to do with how effective the ventricle is at expelling blood (i.e., ejection fraction).

FROM CONTRACTILE FILAMENTS TO A REGULATED PUMP

In Chapter 9, we examined the general features of muscle contraction and compared the properties of skeletal, cardiac, and smooth muscle. In this chapter, we examine how some of the features of cardiac muscle underlie cardiac performance.

The entry of Ca²⁺ from the outside triggers Ca²⁺-induced Ca²⁺ release from the SR, initiating contraction of cardiac myocytes

Excitation-contraction (EC) coupling in cardiac ventricular myocytes is similar to EC coupling in skeletal muscle (see Chapter 9). One major difference is that in the case of skeletal muscle, the initiating event is the arrival of an action potential at the neuromuscular junction, the release of acetylcholine, and the initiation of an end-plate potential. In the ventricular myocyte, action potentials in adjacent myocytes depolarize the target cell through gap junctions (see Chapter 21) and thereby generate an action potential.

As in a skeletal muscle fiber (see Chapter 9), the depolarization of the plasma membrane in the ventricular myocyte invades T tubules that run radially to the long axis of the myocyte. Unlike skeletal muscle cells, cardiac myocytes also have *axial* T tubules that run parallel to the long axis of the cell and interconnect adjacent radial T tubules.

Another major difference in EC coupling between cardiac and skeletal muscle is in the way that the L-type Ca²⁺ channels (Cav1.2, dihydropyridine receptors) in the T-tubule membrane activate the Ca²⁺ release channels made up of four RYR2 molecules in the sarcoplasmic reticulum (SR) membrane. In skeletal muscle, the linkage is mechanical and does not require Ca²⁺ entry per se. If you place skeletal muscle in a Ca²⁺-free solution, the muscle can continue contracting until its intracellular Ca²⁺ stores become depleted. In contrast, cardiac muscle quickly stops beating. Why?

In cardiac muscle, Ca²⁺ entry through the L-type Ca²⁺ channel is essential for raising of [Ca²⁺]$_i$ in the vicinity of the RYR2 on the SR. A subset of Cav1.2 channels may be part of caveolae. This trigger Ca²⁺ activates an adjacent cluster of RYRs in concert, causing them to release Ca²⁺ locally into the cytoplasm (**Ca²⁺-induced Ca²⁺ release**). Such single events of Ca^{2+}-induced Ca^{2+} release can raise $[Ca^{2+}]_i$ as high as $10\,\mu M$ in microdomains of ~$1\,\mu m$ in diameter. These localized increases in $[Ca^{2+}]_i$ appear as **calcium sparks** when they are monitored with a Ca^{2+}-sensitive dye by confocal microscopy. If many L-type Ca^{2+} channels open simultaneously, the spatial and temporal summation of many elementary Ca^{2+} sparks leads to a global increase in $[Ca^{2+}]_i$.

The basic structure of the thin and thick filaments in cardiac muscle is the same as in skeletal muscle (see Fig. 9-5). After $[Ca^{2+}]_i$ increases, Ca^{2+} binds to the cardiac isoform of troponin C (TNNC1; see Table 9-1), and the Ca^{2+}-TNNC1 complex releases the inhibition of the cardiac isoform of troponin I (TNNI3) on actin. As a result, the tropomyosin (TPM1) filaments bound to cardiac troponin T (TNNT2) on the thin filament shift out of the way (see Fig. 9-6), allowing myosin to interact with active sites on the actin. ATP fuels the subsequent cross-bridge cycling (see Fig. 9-7). Because the heart can never rest, cardiac myocytes have a very high density of mitochondria and thus are capable of sustaining very high rates of oxidative phosphorylation (i.e., ATP synthesis).

The cross-bridge cycling causes thick filaments to slide past thin filaments, generating tension. When we discussed the mechanics of skeletal muscle in Chapter 9, we introduced the concept of a length-tension diagram (see Fig. 9-9), which is a plot of muscle tension as a function of muscle length. The length parameter in such a plot can be either the length of the whole skeletal muscle or the length of a single sarcomere. For heart muscle, which wraps around the ventricle, the length parameter can be either the ventricular volume, which is analogous to whole-muscle length, or the sarcomere length. The sarcomere, stretching from one Z line to another, is the functional unit in both skeletal and cardiac muscle.

Phosphorylation of phospholamban and of troponin I speeds cardiac muscle relaxation

With the waning of the phase 2 plateau of the cardiac action potential (see Fig. 21-4B), the influx of Ca^{2+} through L-type Ca^{2+} channels decreases, lessening the release of Ca^{2+} by the SR. By itself, halting of Ca^{2+} entry and release can only prevent a further increase in $[Ca^{2+}]_i$. The actual relaxation of the contractile proteins depends on three processes: (1) extrusion of Ca^{2+} into the extracellular fluid, (2) re-uptake of Ca^{2+} from the cytosol by the SR, and (3) dissociation of Ca^{2+} from troponin C. The last two of these processes are highly regulated.

Extrusion of Ca^{2+} into the Extracellular Fluid Even during the plateau of the action potential, the myocyte extrudes some Ca^{2+}. After the membrane potential returns to more negative values, the extrusion processes gain the upper hand and $[Ca^{2+}]_i$ falls. In the steady state (i.e., during the course of several action potentials), the cell must extrude all the Ca^{2+} that enters the cytosol from the extracellular fluid through L-type Ca^{2+} channels. As in most other cells (see Chapter 7), this extrusion of Ca^{2+} into the extracellular fluid occurs by two pathways: (1) a sarcolemmal Na-Ca exchanger (NCX1), which operates at relatively high levels of $[Ca^{2+}]_i$; and (2) a sarcolemmal Ca^{2+} pump (cardiac subtype 1, 2, and 4 of PMCA), which may function at even low levels of $[Ca^{2+}]_i$.

However, PMCA contributes only modestly to relaxation. Because PMCA is concentrated in caveolae, which contain receptors for various ligands, its role may be to modulate signal transduction.

Re-uptake of Ca^{2+} by the SR Even during the plateau of the action potential, some of the Ca^{2+} accumulating in the cytoplasm is sequestered into the SR by the cardiac subtype of the Ca^{2+} pump SERCA2a (see Chapter 5). **Phospholamban (PLN)**, an integral SR membrane protein with a single transmembrane segment, is an important regulator of SERCA2a. In SR membranes of cardiac, smooth, and slow-twitch skeletal muscle, unphosphorylated PLN can exist as a homopentamer that may function in the SR as an ion channel or as a regulator of Cl^- channels. The dissociation of the pentamer allows the hydrophilic cytoplasmic domain of PLN monomers to inhibit SERCA2a. However, phosphorylation of PLN by any of several kinases relieves phospholamban's inhibition of SERCA2a, allowing Ca^{2+} resequestration to accelerate. The net effect of phosphorylation is an increase in the rate of cardiac muscle relaxation. PLN knockout mice have uninhibited SERCA2a Ca^{2+} pumps and thus an increased velocity of muscle relaxation.

Phosphorylation of PLN by protein kinase A (PKA) explains why β_1-adrenergic agonists (e.g., epinephrine), which act through the PKA pathway (see Chapter 3), speed up the relaxation of cardiac muscle.

Dissociation of Ca^{2+} from Troponin C As $[Ca^{2+}]_i$ falls, Ca^{2+} dissociates from troponin C (see Chapter 9), blocking actin-myosin interactions and causing relaxation. β_1-Adrenergic agonists accelerate relaxation by promoting phosphorylation of troponin I, which in turn enhances the dissociation of Ca^{2+} from troponin C.

The overlap of thick and thin filaments cannot explain the unusual shape of the cardiac length-tension diagram

We discussed passive and active length-tension diagrams for skeletal muscle in Chapter 9 (see Fig. 9-9C and D). We obtain a *passive* length-tension diagram by holding a piece of resting skeletal or cardiac muscle at several predefined lengths and measuring the tension at each length (Fig. 22-11A, green and violet curves). We obtain the *active* length-tension diagram by stimulating the muscle at each predefined length (i.e., isometric conditions) and measuring the *increment* in tension from its resting or passive value (turquoise and brown curves).

The **passive length-tension diagrams** for skeletal and cardiac muscle are quite different. The passive tension of a skeletal muscle (Fig. 22-11A, green curve) is practically nil until the length of the sarcomere exceeds $2.6\,\mu m$. Beyond this length, passive tension rises slowly. On the other hand, the passive tension of cardiac muscle (violet curve) begins to rise at much lower sarcomere lengths and rises much more steeply. As a result, cardiac muscle will break if it is stretched beyond a sarcomere length of $2.6\,\mu m$, whereas it is possible to stretch skeletal muscle to a sarcomere length of $3.6\,\mu m$.

The reason for the higher passive tension is that the non-contractile (i.e., elastic) components of cardiac muscle are

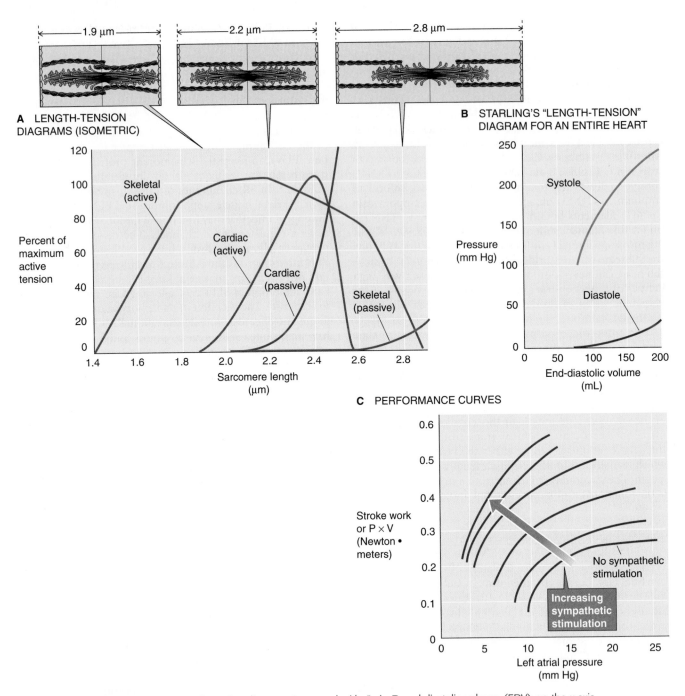

Figure 22-11 Length-tension diagram. Compared with **A,** in **B** end-diastolic volume (EDV) on the x-axis is used as an index of sarcomere length. (Because EDV was difficult to measure before the days of echocardiography, Starling actually used left atrial pressure as an index of the degree of filling.) Starling measured pressure on the y-axis as an index of tension. Thus, systolic pressure replaces active tension, and diastolic pressure replaces passive tension. In **C,** left atrial pressure on the x-axis is used as an index of sarcomere length, and stroke work (systolic pressure × ejected volume) on the y-axis is used instead of tension.

less distensible. The most important elastic component is the giant protein **titin**, which acts as a spring that provides the opposing force during stretch and the restoring force during shortening (see Fig. 9-4B).

The **active length-tension diagrams** also differ between skeletal and cardiac muscle. The active tension of skeletal muscle (turquoise curve) is high and varies only modestly between sarcomere lengths of 1.8 and 2.6 µm (Fig. 22-11A).

In Chapter 9, we accounted for the shape of this curve as caused by the degree of myofilament overlap. In cardiac muscle (brown curve), active tension has a relatively sharp peak when the muscle is prestretched to an initial sarcomere length of ~2.4 µm. As the prestretched sarcomere length increases from 1.8 to 2.4 µm, active tension rises steeply. We cannot account for this rise by an increase in the overlap of thick and thin filaments because the filament dimensions of cardiac and skeletal muscle are similar. Rather, the rise in tension at longer sarcomere lengths in cardiac muscle probably has two general causes. (1) Raising the sarcomere length above 1.8 μm increases the Ca^{2+} sensitivity of the myofilaments. One mechanism controlling the Ca^{2+} sensitivity may be interfilament spacing between thick and thin filaments because fiber diameter varies inversely with fiber length. As we stretch the muscle to greater sarcomere lengths, the lateral filament lattice spacing is less than in an unstretched fiber so that the probability of cross-bridge interaction increases. Increased cross-bridge formation in turn increases the Ca^{2+} affinity of TNNC1, thereby recruiting more cross-bridges and therefore producing greater force. Another mechanism could be that as the muscle elongates, increased strain on titin either alters lattice spacing or alters the packing of myosin molecules within the thick filament. (2) Raising the sarcomere length above 1.8 μm increases tension on stretch-activated Ca^{2+} channels, thereby increasing Ca^{2+} entry from the extracellular fluid and thus enhancing Ca^{2+}-induced Ca^{2+} release.

As cardiac sarcomere length increases above 2.4 μm, active tension declines precipitously, compared with the gradual fall in skeletal muscle. Once again, this fall-off does not reflect a problem in the overlap of thin and thick filaments. Instead, titin increases the passive *stiffness* of cardiac muscle and may also impede development of *active tension* at high sarcomere lengths.

Starling's law states that a greater fiber length (i.e., greater ventricular volume) causes the heart to deliver more mechanical energy

Long before the development of the sliding filament hypothesis and our understanding that active tension should depend on sarcomere length, Ernest Starling in 1914 anticipated the results of Figure 22-11A, using an isolated heart-lung preparation. **Starling's law** states that "the mechanical energy set free in the passage from the resting to the active state is a function of the length of the fiber." Therefore, the initial length of myocardial fibers determines the work done during the cardiac cycle. Figure 22-11B shows the results of experiments that Starling performed on the intact heart. Starling assumed that the initial *length* of the myocardial fibers is proportional to the end-diastolic volume (EDV). Further, he assumed that *tension* in the myocardial fibers is proportional to the systolic pressure. Therefore, starting from a volume-pressure diagram, Starling was able to reconstruct an equivalent length-tension diagram (Table 22-4).

His diagram for *diastole* (Fig. 22-11B, purple curve), which shows a rising pressure (tension) with increased EDV (fiber length), is very similar to the early part of the *passive* length-tension diagram for cardiac muscle (Fig. 22-11A, violet curve). His diagram for *systole* (Fig. 22-11B, red curve) is more or less equivalent to the ascending phase of the *active* length-tension diagram for cardiac muscle (Fig. 22-11A, brown curve). Therefore, Starling's systole curve shows that the heart is able to generate more pressure (i.e., deliver more blood) when more is presented to it.

A **ventricular performance curve** (Fig. 22-11C) is another representation of Starling's length-tension diagram, but it is one a clinician can obtain on a patient. A ventricular perfor-

Table 22-4 Equivalent Units for Converting Between a Three-Dimensional Heart and a Linear Muscle Fiber

ISOLATED MUSCLE = LINEAR		CARDIAC VENTRICLE = HOLLOW ORGAN	
Parameter	Units	Parameter	Units
Length	mm	Volume	mL
Extent of shortening	mm	Stroke volume	mL
Velocity of shortening	mm/s	Velocity of ejection	mL/s
Load	gram	Pressure	mm Hg
or force	dyne		
or tension	dyne/cm^2		

This table shows the equivalence between dimensions in converting from the contraction of a hollow organ, such as a cardiac ventricle, to a linear model of a single muscle contraction.

mance curve shows, on the y-axis, stroke work ($P \cdot \Delta V$, see Equation 22-4), which includes Starling's systolic pressure (itself an estimate of muscle tension), plotted against left atrial pressure, which corresponds to Starling's end-diastolic volume (itself an estimate of muscle length). What we learn from performance curves obtained on living subjects is that Starling's law *is not a fixed relationship*. For instance, the norepinephrine released during sympathetic stimulation—which increases myocardial contractility (as we will see later in this chapter)—steepens the performance curve and shifts it upward and to the left (Fig. 22-11C, brown arrow). Similar shifts occur with other **positive inotropic** agents (e.g., cardiac glycosides), that is, drugs that increase myocardial contractility. Note also that ventricular performance curves show no descending component because sarcomere length does not increase beyond 2.2 to 2.4 μm in healthy hearts.

The velocity of cardiac muscle shortening falls when the contraction occurs against a greater opposing force (or pressure) or at a shorter muscle length (or lower volume)

The functional properties of cardiac muscle—how much tension it can develop, how rapidly it can contract—depend on many factors but especially on two properties intrinsic to the cardiac myocyte.

1. *Initial sarcomere length.* For the beating heart, a convenient index of initial sarcomere length is *end-diastolic volume*. Both initial sarcomere length and EDV are measures of the **preload** imposed on the cardiac muscle *just before* it ejects blood from the ventricle during systole. *Starling's law*, in which the independent variable is EDV, focuses on preload.

2. *Force that the contracting myocytes must overcome.* In the beating heart, a convenient index of opposing force is the *arterial pressure* that opposes the outflow of blood from

the ventricle. Both opposing force and arterial pressure are measures of the **afterload** the ventricular muscle must overcome *as* it ejects blood during systole. Experiments on *isotonic contractions* focus on the afterload, factors that the ventricle can sense only *after* the contraction has begun.

Figure 22-12 shows how one might measure the *velocity of shortening* in a way that is relevant for a cardiac muscle facing both a preload and an afterload. In Figure 22-12A, the muscle starts off at rest, stretched between a fixed support (bottom of the muscle) and the left end of a lever (top of the muscle). A weight attached to the other end of the lever, but resting on a table, applies stretch to the muscle—to the extent allowed by the screw, which adjusts the "stop" of the lever's left end. Thus, the combination of the weight and the screw determines initial sarcomere length (i.e., preload). At this time, the muscle cannot sense the full extent of the weight. The more we stretch the muscle by retracting the screw, the greater the preload. When we begin to stimulate the muscle, it develops a gradually increasing tension (Fig. 22-12C, lower blue curve), but the length between the fixed point and the left end of the lever (Fig. 22-12A) remains constant. That is, the muscle cannot shorten. Therefore, in the first phase of the experiment, the muscle exerts increasing *isometric tension*.

When the muscle has built up enough tension, it can now begin lifting the weight off the table (Fig. 22-12B). This phase of the contraction is termed afterloaded shortening. The tension now remains at a fixed afterload value (flat portion of lower curve in Fig. 22-12C), but the muscle gradually shortens (rising portion of upper blue curve). Therefore, in the second phase of the experiment, the muscle exerts *isotonic contraction*. From the slope of the upper curve in Figure 22-12C, we can compute the velocity of shortening at a particular afterload.

This experiment roughly mimics the actions of ventricular muscle during systole. Initially, during its iso*metric* contraction, our hypothetical muscle increases its tension at constant length, as during the iso*volumetric* contraction of the cardiac cycle shown in segment CD of Figure 22-9. The initial length corresponds to EDV, the preload. Later, the muscle shortens while overcoming a constant force (i.e., generating a constant tension), as during the ejection phase of the cardiac cycle shown in segment DEF of Figure 22-9. The tension corresponds to arterial pressure, the afterload.

What happens if we vary the afterload (i.e., change the weight)? As we already observed in our discussion of skeletal muscle, it is easier to lift a feather than a barbell. Thus, with a heavier weight, the muscle develops a lot of tension but shortens slowly (Fig. 22-12D, red tracings). Conversely, with a lighter weight, the muscle develops only a little bit of tension but shortens rapidly (purple curves).

If we plot the velocities of shortening in Figure 22-12D as a function of the three different afterloads being lifted, we obtain the purple, blue, and red points on the load-velocity curve in Figure 22-12E. The velocity of muscle shortening corresponds to outflow velocity of the ventricle (Fig. 22-8D, E). Thus, at higher opposing arterial pressures, the outflow velocity should decrease. The black curve in Figure 22-12E applies to a muscle that we stretched only slightly in the preload phase (i.e., low preload in Fig. 22-12A). The red curve in Figure 22-12E shows a similar load-velocity relationship for a muscle that we stretched greatly in the preload phase (i.e., high preload). In both cases, the velocity of shortening increases as the tension (i.e., afterload) falls.

When the afterload is so large that no shortening ever occurs, that afterload is the **isometric tension**, shown as the point of zero velocity on the x-axis of Figure 22-12E. As expected from Starling's law, the greater the initial stretch (i.e., preload), the greater the isometric tension. In fact, at *any* velocity (Fig. 22-12E, dashed horizontal line), the tension is greater in the muscle that was stretched more in the preload phase (red curve)—a restatement of Starling's law.

In summary, at a given preload (i.e., walking up the black curve in Fig. 22-12E), the velocity of shortening for cardiac muscle becomes greater with lower afterloads (i.e., opposing pressure). Conversely, at a given afterload—that is, comparing the black and red curves for any common *x* value (Fig. 22-12E, dashed vertical line)—the velocity of shortening for cardiac muscle becomes greater with a greater preload (i.e., sarcomere length).

Finally, the curves in Figure 22-12E do not represent a fixed set of relationships. Positive inotropic agents shift all curves up and to the right. Thus, a positive inotropic agent allows the heart to achieve a given velocity against a greater load or to push a given load with a greater velocity.

Another way of representing how velocity of shortening depends on the initial muscle length (i.e., preload) is to monitor velocity of shortening during a single isotonic contraction. If we first apply a large preload to stretch a piece of muscle to an initial length of 9.0 mm (Fig. 22-12F) and then stimulate it, the velocity instantly rises to a peak value of ~8.5 mm/s; it then gradually falls to zero as the muscle shortens to 7.5 mm. If we start by applying a smaller preload, thereby stretching the muscle to an initial length of 8.5 or 8.0 mm, the peak velocity falls. Thus, initial length determines not only the tension that cardiac muscle can generate but also the speed with which the muscle can shorten.

Increases in heart rate enhance myocardial tension

Heart muscle tension has a special dependence on the frequency of contraction. If we stimulate isolated heart muscle only a few times per minute, the tension developed is much smaller than if we stimulate it at a physiological rate of 70/min. The progressive rise of tension after an increase in rate—the positive **staircase phenomenon**—was first observed by Henry Bowditch in 1871. Underlying the staircase phenomenon is an increase in SR Ca^{2+} content and release. The larger SR Ca^{2+} content has three causes. First, during each action potential plateau, more Ca^{2+} enters the cell through Cav1.2 L-type Ca^{2+} channels, and the larger number of action potentials per minute provides a longer aggregate period of Ca^{2+} entry through these channels. Second, the depolarization during the plateau of an action potential causes the Na-Ca exchanger NCX1 to operate in the reverse mode, allowing Ca^{2+} to enter the cell. At higher heart rates, these depolarizations occur more frequently and are accompanied by an increase in $[Na^+]_i$, which accentuates the reversal of NCX1, both of which enhance Ca^{2+} uptake.

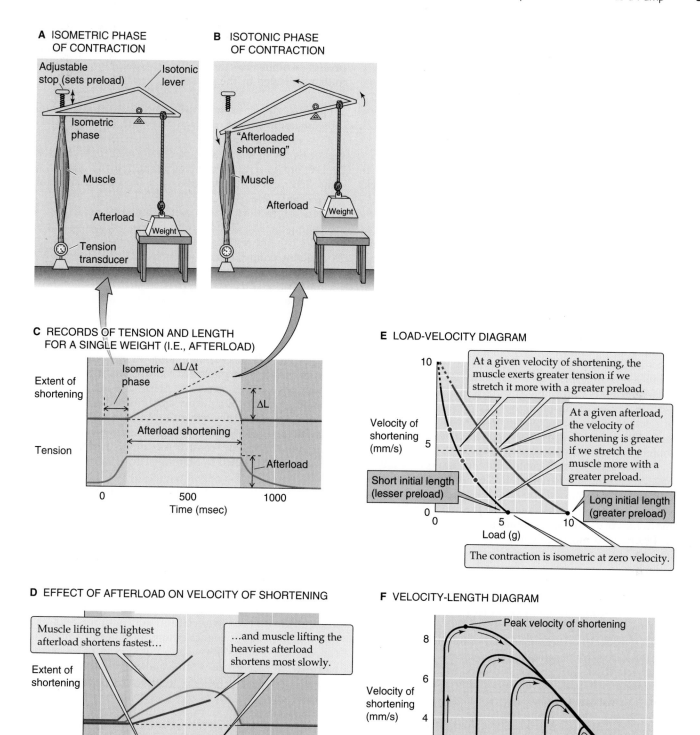

A ISOMETRIC PHASE OF CONTRACTION

Adjustable stop (sets preload)
Isotonic lever
Isometric phase
Muscle
Afterload
Weight
Tension transducer

B ISOTONIC PHASE OF CONTRACTION

"Afterloaded shortening"
Muscle
Afterload
Weight

C RECORDS OF TENSION AND LENGTH FOR A SINGLE WEIGHT (I.E., AFTERLOAD)

Extent of shortening
Isometric phase
ΔL/Δt
ΔL
Afterload shortening
Tension
Afterload
Time (msec)

E LOAD-VELOCITY DIAGRAM

Velocity of shortening (mm/s)

At a given velocity of shortening, the muscle exerts greater tension if we stretch it more with a greater preload.

At a given afterload, the velocity of shortening is greater if we stretch the muscle more with a greater preload.

Short initial length (lesser preload)
Long initial length (greater preload)
Load (g)
The contraction is isometric at zero velocity.

D EFFECT OF AFTERLOAD ON VELOCITY OF SHORTENING

Muscle lifting the lightest afterload shortens fastest…
…and muscle lifting the heaviest afterload shortens most slowly.

Extent of shortening
Tension
Time (msec)

F VELOCITY-LENGTH DIAGRAM

Peak velocity of shortening
Velocity of shortening (mm/s)
Muscle length (mm)
Long initial length (greater preload)
Short initial length (lesser preload)

Figure 22-12 Effect of preload and afterload on velocity of shortening. In **A,** the developed tension is not yet sufficient to lift the weight (i.e., afterload). In **B,** the muscle, which has now developed sufficient tension to lift the weight, shortens against a constant afterload. In **C,** the slope of the *blue curve* ($\Delta L/\Delta t$) is the velocity of shortening. The velocities of shortening for three different afterloads (tensions) in **D** are plotted as the three colored points of the lower curve in **E.** In **F,** the x-axis has the longest lengths on the left, so that "time" runs from left to right *(arrows)*. Note that the family of curves is enclosed by the envelope created by the curve for the greatest initial length.

Third, the increased heart rate stimulates SERCA2a, thereby sequestering in the SR the Ca^{2+} that entered the cell because of the first two mechanisms. The mechanism of this stimulation is that the rising $[Ca^{2+}]_i$, through calmodulin, activates CaM kinase II, leading to phosphorylation of PLN, enhancing SERCA2a.

Contractility is an intrinsic measure of cardiac performance

Now that we know that the performance of the heart depends on such factors as degree of filling (i.e., preload), arterial pressure (i.e., afterload), and heart rate, it would be useful to have a measure of the heart's *intrinsic* contractile performance, independent of these *extrinsic* factors. **Contractility** is such a measure.

Contractility is a somewhat vague but clinically useful term that distinguishes a better performing heart from a poorly performing one. In a patient, it is difficult to assess cardiac performance by use of the approaches in Figures 22-11 and 22-12. One clinically useful measurement of contractility is the ejection fraction (see earlier). However, according to Starling's law, ejection depends on end-diastolic volume (i.e., preload), which is *external* to the heart. Two somewhat better gauges of contractility are the **rate of pressure development** during ejection ($\Delta P/\Delta t$) and the **velocity of ejection**. Both correlate well with the velocity of shortening in Figure 22-12E and F, and they are very sensitive guides to the effect of inotropic interventions.

A third assessment of contractility focuses on the physiological relationship between pressure and volume during the cardiac cycle. In the era of echocardiography, these volume data are now reasonably easy to obtain. We return to the ventricular **pressure-volume loop** that we introduced in Figure 22-9 and redraw it as the purple loop in Figure 22-13A. In this example, the end-diastolic volume is 120 mL. Point D′ on the loop represents the relationship between pressure and volume at the end of the isovolumetric contraction, when the aortic valve opens. If we had prevented the aortic valve from opening, ventricular pressure would have continued to rise until the ventricle could generate no additional tension. In this case, the pressure would rise to point G′, the theoretical maximum isovolumetric pressure. We could repeat the measurement at very different EDVs by decreasing or increasing the venous return. Point G represents the maximum isovolumetric pressure for an EDV below 120 mL (orange loop), and point G″ for an EDV above 120 mL (green loop). The gold dashed line through points G, G′, and G″ in Figure 22-13A would describe the relationship between pressure and EDV under isometric (i.e., aortic valve closed) conditions—the equivalent of an isometric *Starling curve* (e.g., brown curve in Fig. 22-11A). The steeper this line, the greater the contractility.

It is impossible to measure maximum isovolumetric pressures in a patient because it is hardly advisable to prevent the aortic valve from opening. However, we can use the **end-systolic pressure** at point F′, on the normal pressure-volume loop with an EDV of 120 mL (purple loop). For an EDV below 120 mL (orange loop), the corner point would slide down and to the left (F). Conversely, for an EDV above 120 mL (green loop), the corner point would slide upward

and to the right (F″). The corner points of many such pressure-volume loops fall along a line—**the end-systolic pressure-volume relation (ESPVR)**—that is very similar to that generated by the points G, G′, and G″.

Effect of Changes in Contractility   The ESPVR is a clinically useful measure of contractility. Enhancing the contractility increases the slope of the ESPVR line, just as it increases the steepness of the ventricular performance curves (Fig. 22-11C, brown arrow). For example, imagine that—with the same EDV and aortic pressure as in the control situation (purple area and gold ESPVR line in Fig. 22-13B)—we increase contractility. We represent increased contractility by steepening the ESPVR line (from gold to red dashed line in Fig. 22-13B). The result is that ejection continues from point D′ to a new point F (red loop in Fig. 22-13B) until the left ventricular volume reaches a much lower value than normal. In other words, enhanced contractility increases *stroke volume*. Decreasing contractility would flatten the slope of the ESPVR and decrease stroke volume.

Effect of Changes in Preload (i.e., Initial Sarcomere Length)   A pressure-volume loop nicely illustrates the effect of an increased preload (i.e., increased filling or EDV) without changing contractility. Starting from the control situation (Fig. 22-13C, purple area), increase of the EDV shifts the isovolumetric segment to the right (CD on the red loop). Because the volume change along segment DEF is larger than for the control situation, stroke volume increases—as predicted by Starling's law.

Effect of Changes in Afterload   A pressure-volume loop also illustrates the effect of an increased afterload (i.e., increase in aortic pressure). Starting from the control situation (Fig. 22-13D, purple area), increase of the aortic pressure shifts the upper right corner of the loop from point D′ (purple loop) to D (red loop) because the ventricle cannot open the aortic valve until ventricular pressure reaches the higher aortic pressure. During the ejection phase—assuming that contractility (i.e., slope of the ESPVR) does not change—the ventricle necessarily ejects less blood until segment DEF intersects the ESPVR line. Therefore, an increase in afterload (at constant contractility) causes the loop to be taller and narrower, so that stroke volume and ejection fraction both decrease. However, if we were to increase contractility (i.e., increase the slope of the ESPVR), we could return the stroke volume to normal.

Positive inotropic agents increase myocardial contractility by raising $[Ca^{2+}]_i$

Modifiers of contractility can affect the dynamics of cardiac muscle contraction, independent of preload or afterload. These factors have in common their ability to change $[Ca^{2+}]_i$. When these factors increase myocardial contractility, they are called positive inotropic agents. When they decrease myocardial contractility, they are called negative inotropic agents.

Positive Inotropic Agents   Factors that increase myocardial contractility increase $[Ca^{2+}]_i$, either by opening Ca^{2+}

A STANDARD CONTRACTILITY CONDITIONS

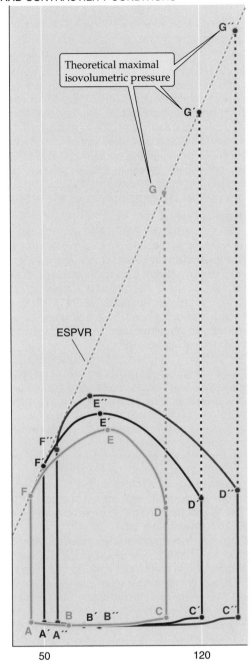

B INCREASED CONTRACTILITY

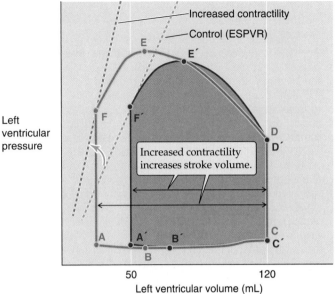

C INCREASED PRELOAD (FILLING)

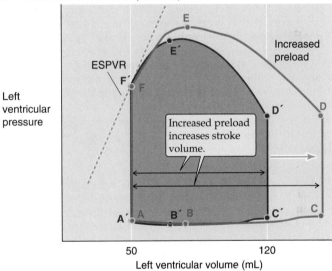

D INCREASED AFTERLOAD (AORTIC PRESSURE)

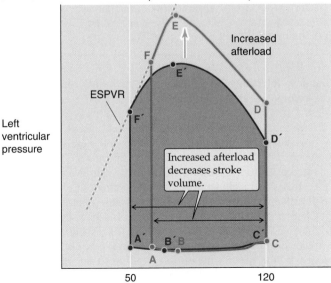

Figure 22-13 Assessment of contractility by use of a ventricular pressure-volume loop. The *purple pressure-volume loop* is the normal curve in Figure 22-9. In **A,** at the same normal state of cardiac contractility, the *red loop* is generated by decreasing EDV, and the *green loop* is generated by increasing EDV. The slope of the line through the points at the end of systole (F, F', and F") represents the end-systolic pressure-volume relation (ESPVR).

Cardiac Hypertrophy

Either volume overload or pressure overload can mechanically compromise the heart. A **volume overload** is an excessive EDV (i.e., preload). For example, a large arteriovenous shunt would volume overload both the left and right sides of the heart. The increased EDV leads to an increase in stroke volume (Fig. 22-13C), which elevates cardiac output. Systemic arterial pressure usually remains normal. A **pressure overload** is an excessive pressure in the ventricle's outflow tract (i.e., afterload). For the left side of the heart, the problem would be an increase in systemic arterial pressure (i.e., hypertension). The increased aortic pressure leads to a decrease in stroke volume (Fig. 22-13D). However, because of a compensatory increase in heart rate, cardiac output usually remains normal. When, over time, the adaptive process of hypertrophy becomes inadequate to cope with demand, the result is mechanical dysfunction and, ultimately, heart failure (see the box titled Cellular Basis of Heart Failure).

Because cells of the adult heart are terminally differentiated, stimuli that might be mitogenic in other cells cannot elicit cell division in the heart but rather cause the cardiac myocytes to hypertrophy and increase muscle mass. Elite athletes develop **physiological hypertrophy**, whereby the cardiac cells increase proportionally both in length and in width. Volume overload leads to **eccentric hypertrophy** characterized by increases of myocyte length out of proportion to width. Pressure overload causes **concentric hypertrophy** with a relatively greater increase in myocyte width.

A host of events may trigger hypertrophy, including various hypertrophic factors, increases in $[Ca^{2+}]_i$, and mechanical forces.

Hypertrophic Factors

Agents implicated in cardiac hypertrophy include the cardiac cytosolic protein **myotrophin (Myo/V1)** and the cytokine **cardiotrophin 1 (CT-1)** as well as catecholamines, angiotensin II, endothelin 1, insulin-like growth factor 2, transforming growth factor β, and interleukin 1. Catecholamines and angiotensin II both activate the MAP kinase cascade. Farther downstream the signal transduction pathway, the transcriptional response to hypertrophic stimuli includes the zinc finger transcription factor GATA4 and perhaps also the transcription factors SRF and Sp1 as well as the TEF-1 family. (See Chapter 4.)

Calcium

Elevated $[Ca^{2+}]_i$ may be both a trigger for hypertrophy and part of signal transduction pathways that lead to hypertrophy. $[Ca^{2+}]_i$ in heart cells is probably elevated initially during chronic volume or pressure overloads, just as $[Ca^{2+}]_i$ would be elevated in a normal heart that is working hard. Elevated $[Ca^{2+}]_i$ may activate calcineurin, a Ca^{2+}-dependent phosphatase (see Chapter 3). After being dephosphorylated by calcineurin, the transcription factor NF-AT3 can enter the nucleus and bind to GATA4 (see earlier), which transcriptionally activates genes responsible for hypertrophy. Mice that express constitutively activated forms of calcineurin develop cardiac hypertrophy and heart failure.

Mechanical Factors

Mechanical stretch induces the expression of specific genes. The mechanical sensor that triggers cardiac hypertrophy may be **MLP (muscle LIM protein)**, part of the myocardial cytoskeleton. Stretch activates a phosphorylation cascade of protein kinases: Raf-1 kinase, extracellular signal–regulated kinase (ERK), and a separate subfamily of the MAP kinases called SAPKs (for stretch-activated protein kinases). These various kinases regulate gene expression by activating the transcription factor AP-1 (see Chapter 4).

The pathways we have just discussed lead to several changes in gene expression within cardiac myocytes during hypertrophy. In addition to synthesizing many housekeeping proteins, hypertrophic cardiac myocytes undergo other changes that are more specific for contraction. Some of the most striking changes include *reduced* levels of the mRNA encoding three critical proteins in the membrane of the SR: (1) the Ca^{2+} release channel, (2) phospholamban, and (3) the SR Ca^{2+} pump (SERCA2). In addition, cardiac hypertrophy is associated with increased levels of mRNA for the skeletal α-actin, which is normally expressed in fetal but not in adult heart. Hypertrophic hearts also have increased expression of the angiogenic factor VEGF (see Chapter 20).

Although a hypertrophied myocardial cell may be able to do more work than a nonhypertrophied cell, it has a lower "contractility" when normalized to its cross-sectional area. Why should hypertrophied cardiac muscle not be as good as normal muscle? Possibilities include alterations in the transient increases in $[Ca^{2+}]_i$ during the cardiac action potential and alterations in the expression of the contractile filaments, particularly the myosin isoenzymes.

---

channels, inhibiting Na-Ca exchange, or by inhibiting the Ca^{2+} pump—all at the plasma membrane.

1. *Adrenergic agonists.* Catecholamines (e.g., epinephrine, norepinephrine) act on β_1 adrenoceptors to activate the α subunit of G_s-type heterotrimeric G proteins. The activated α_s subunits produce effects by two pathways. First, α_s raises intracellular levels of cyclic adenosine monophosphate (cAMP) and stimulates protein kinase A (see Chapter 3), which can then act by the mechanisms summarized in Table 22-2 to increase contractility and speed relaxation. Second, α_s can directly open L-type Ca^{2+} channels in the plasma membrane, leading to an increased Ca^{2+} influx during action potentials, increased $[Ca^{2+}]_i$, and enhanced contractility.

2. *Cardiac glycosides.* Digitalis derivatives inhibit the Na-K pump on the plasma membrane (see Chapter 5) and therefore raise $[Na^+]_i$. We would expect the increased $[Na^+]_i$ to slow down the Na-Ca exchanger NCX1, to raise steady-state $[Ca^{2+}]_i$, and to enhance contractility. Recent evidence suggests that cardiac glycosides may also increase $[Ca^{2+}]_i$ by a novel pathway—increasing the Ca^{2+} permeability of Na^+ channels in the plasma membrane.

3. *High extracellular $[Ca^{2+}]$.* Acting in two ways, elevated $[Ca^{2+}]_o$ increases $[Ca^{2+}]_i$ and thereby enhances contractility. First, it decreases the exchange of external Na^+ for internal Ca^{2+}. Second, more Ca^{2+} enters the myocardial cell through L-type Ca^{2+} channels during the action potential.

Cellular Basis of Heart Failure

Heart failure is among the most common causes of hospitalization in developed countries for people aged 65 years or older and is a leading cause of death. People whose hearts cannot sustain an adequate cardiac output become breathless (because blood backs up from the left side of the heart into the lungs) and have swollen feet and ankles (because blood backs up from the right side of the heart and promotes net filtration in systemic capillaries; see the box on edema in Chapter 20). On the cellular level, decreased contractility in heart failure could be a result of cardiac hypertrophy (see the box titled Cardiac Hypertrophy), reflecting alterations in the transient increases of $[Ca^{2+}]_i$, the expression of the contractile filaments, or both.

Changes in $[Ca^{2+}]_i$ physiology could reflect altered properties of the Cav1.2 L-type Ca^{2+} channel in the plasma membrane or the Ca^{2+} release channel RYR2 in the SR membrane. In an animal model of hypertension-induced cardiac hypertrophy that leads to heart failure, the Cav1.2 channels exhibit an impaired ability to activate RYR2 through Ca^{2+}-induced Ca^{2+} release. A distortion of the microarchitecture in hypertrophic cells, and thus a distortion of the spacing between Cav1.2 channels and RYR2, could be responsible for impaired coupling. Each of the four RYR2 molecules in the Ca^{2+} release channel associates with a molecule of **calstabin 2** (also known as the FK506-binding protein FKBP12.6) that, together with other proteins, forms a macromolecular complex regulating the Ca^{2+} release channel. Depletion of calstabin 2 in heart failure results in leaky RYR2 channels that continually release Ca^{2+} into the cytosol. High $[Ca^{2+}]_i$ makes the heart prone to delayed afterdepolarizations (see Chapter 21), ventricular arrhythmias, and sudden death.

Changes in the expression of contractile proteins can reduce contractility. Two isoforms of myosin heavy chain, αMHC and βMHC, are present in heart (see Table 9-1). The speed of muscle shortening increases with the relative expression of αMHC. In human heart failure, the amount of αMHC mRNA, relative to total MHC mRNA, falls from ~35% to ~2%.

An interesting animal model of heart failure is the knockout mouse that lacks the gene encoding MLP, the muscle LIM protein (see the box on cardiac hypertrophy). MLP-deficient mice have the same disrupted cytoskeletal architecture seen in failing hearts. In addition, these mice have a dilated cardiomyopathy. Although humans with failing hearts are generally not deficient in MLP, the evidence from these knockout mice suggests that the MLP system could play a role in certain forms of cardiomyopathy.

4. *Low extracellular $[Na^+]$.* Reducing the Na^+ gradient decreases Ca^{2+} extrusion through NCX1, raising $[Ca^{2+}]_i$ and enhancing contractility.
5. *Increased heart rate.* As we noted in introducing the staircase phenomenon, an increased heart rate increases SR stores of Ca^{2+} and also increases Ca^{2+} influx during the action potential.

Negative Inotropic Agents Factors that decrease myocardial contractility all decrease $[Ca^{2+}]_i$.

1. *Ca^{2+} channel blockers.* Inhibitors of L-type Ca^{2+} channels (see Chapter 7)—such as verapamil, diltiazem, and nifedipine—reduce Ca^{2+} entry during the plateau of the cardiac action potential. By reducing $[Ca^{2+}]_i$, they decrease contractility.
2. *Low extracellular $[Ca^{2+}]$.* Depressed $[Ca^{2+}]_o$ lowers $[Ca^{2+}]_i$, both by increasing Ca^{2+} extrusion through NCX1 and by reducing Ca^{2+} entry through L-type Ca^{2+} channels during the plateau of the cardiac action potential.
3. *High extracellular $[Na^+]$.* Elevated $[Na^+]_o$ increases Ca^{2+} extrusion through NCX1, thereby decreasing $[Ca^{2+}]_i$.

REFERENCES

Books and Reviews

Kobayashi T, Solaro RJ: Calcium, thin filaments, and the integrative biology of cardiac contractility. Annu Rev Physiol 2005; 67:39-46.

Moss RL, Fitzsimons DP: Frank-Starling relationship: Long on importance, short on mechanism. Circ Res 2002; 90:11-13.

Simmerman HKB, Jones LR: Phospholamban: Protein structure, mechanism of action, and role in cardiac function. Physiol Rev 1998; 78:921-947.

Wehrens XH, Marks AR: Molecular determinants of altered contractility in heart failure. Ann Med 2004; 36(Suppl 1):70-80.

Zimmer H-G: The isolated perfused heart and its pioneers. News Physiol Sci 1998; 13:203-210.

Journal Articles

Collins SP, Arand P, Lindsell CJ, et al: Prevalence of the third and fourth heart sound in asymptomatic adults. Congest Heart Fail 2005; 11:242-247.

Fukuda N, Wu Y, Nair P, Granzier HL: Phosphorylation of titin modulates passive stiffness of cardiac muscle in a titin isoform–dependent manner. J Gen Physiol 2005; 125:257-271.

Gómez AM, Valdivia HH, Cheng H, et al: Defective excitation-contraction coupling in experimental cardiac hypertrophy and heart failure. Science 1997; 276:800-806.

Sarnoff JS, Berglund E: Ventricular function. I. Starling's law of the heart studied by means of simultaneous right and left ventricular function curves in the dog. Circulation 1954; 9:706-718.

Wiggers CJ, Katz LN: The contours of ventricular volume curves under different conditions. Am J Physiol 1922; 58:439-475.

CHAPTER 23

REGULATION OF ARTERIAL PRESSURE AND CARDIAC OUTPUT

Emile L. Boulpaep

When faced with a patient who appears seriously ill, clinicians focus their immediate attention on the patient's vital signs: temperature, respiratory rate, pulse, and blood pressure. These parameters are aptly named vital because they reflect the most fundamental aspects of health and even survival; a significant abnormality in any of these components indicates that emergent care is required.

In this chapter, we focus on blood pressure, a critical hemodynamic factor and one that is easily measured. An adequate blood pressure is necessary for proper organ perfusion. Too low, and we say that the patient is in shock. Too high, and we say that the patient is hypertensive; an acute and profound elevation of the blood pressure can be just as dangerous as one that suddenly plummets. Here, we examine both the short- and long-term mechanisms that the body uses to regulate arterial blood pressure.

Because the arterial blood pressure depends to a large degree on the cardiac output, we also examine the regulation of this critical parameter. Finally, because cardiac output also depends on the venous return of blood to the heart, we discuss the matching between input (i.e., venous return) and cardiac output.

SHORT-TERM REGULATION OF ARTERIAL PRESSURE

Systemic mean arterial blood pressure is the principal variable that the cardiovascular system controls

Imagine that we must distribute city water to 1000 houses. We could decide in advance that each house uses 500 L/day and then pump this amount to each house at a constant rate. In other words, we would deliver ~20 L/hr, regardless of actual water usage. The cardiovascular equivalent of such a system would be a circulation in which the cardiac output and the delivery of blood to each tissue remain constant.

Alternatively, we could connect all the houses to a single, large water tower that provides a constant pressure head. Because the height of the water level in the tower is fairly stable, all faucets in all houses see the same pressure at all times. This system offers several advantages. First, each house can regulate its water usage by opening faucets according to need. Second, heavy water usage in one house with all faucets open does not affect the pressure head in the other houses with only one faucet open. Third, the pressure head in the water tower guarantees that each house will receive sufficiently high pressure to send water to houses with upper floors. This water tower system is analogous to our own circulatory system, which provides the same flexibility for distribution of blood flow by, first and foremost, *controlling the systemic mean arterial blood pressure.*

The priority given to arterial pressure control is necessary because of the anatomy of the circulatory system. A network of branched arteries delivers to each organ a mean arterial pressure that approximates the mean aortic pressure. Thus, all organs, whether close to or distant from the heart, receive the same mean arterial pressure. Each organ, in turn, controls local blood flow by increasing or decreasing local arteriolar resistance. In Chapter 20, we described these local control mechanisms in a general way, and in Chapter 24, we will discuss specific vascular beds.

The system that we just introduced works because a change in blood flow in one vascular bed does not affect blood flow in other beds—as long as the heart can maintain the mean arterial pressure. However, the circulatory system must keep mean arterial pressure not only *constant* but also *high enough* for glomerular filtration to occur in the kidneys or to overcome high tissue pressures in organs such as the eye.

Since Chapter 17, we have regarded the heart as the generator of a constant driving pressure. The principles of the feedback loops that the body uses to control the circulation are similar to those involved in the regulation of many other physiological systems. The short-term regulation of arterial pressure—on a time scale of seconds to minutes—occurs through neural pathways and targets the heart, vessels, and adrenal medulla. This short-term regulation is the topic of the present discussion. The long-term regulation of arterial pressure—on a time scale of hours or days—occurs through pathways that target the blood vessels, as well as the kidneys, in their control of extracellular fluid volume. This long-term regulation is the topic of the final portion of the chapter.

Neural reflexes mediate the short-term regulation of mean arterial blood pressure

The neural reflex systems that regulate mean arterial pressure operate as a series of **negative feedback loops**. All such loops are composed of the following elements:

1. **A detector.** A sensor or receptor quantitates the controlled variable and transduces it into an electrical signal that is a measure of the controlled variable.
2. **Afferent neural pathways.** These convey the message away from the detector, to the central nervous system (CNS).
3. **A coordinating center.** A control center in the CNS compares the signal detected in the periphery to a set-point, generates an error signal, processes the information, and generates a message that encodes the appropriate response.
4. **Efferent neural pathways.** These convey the message from the coordinating center to the periphery.
5. **Effectors.** These elements execute the appropriate response and alter the controlled variable, thereby correcting its deviation from the set-point.

A dual system of sensors and neural reflexes controls mean arterial pressure. The primary sensors are baroreceptors, which are actually stretch receptors or mechanoreceptors that detect distention of the vascular walls. The secondary sensors are chemoreceptors that detect changes in blood P_{O_2}, P_{CO_2}, and pH. The control centers are located within the CNS, mostly in the medulla, but sites within the cerebral cortex and hypothalamus also exert control. The effectors include the pacemaker and muscle cells in the heart, the vascular smooth muscle cells (VSMCs) in arteries and veins, and the adrenal medulla.

We all know from common experience that the CNS influences the circulation. Emotional stress can cause blushing of the skin or an increase in heart rate. Pain—or the stress of your first day in a gross anatomy laboratory—can elicit fainting because of a profound, generalized vasodilation and a decrease in heart rate (i.e., bradycardia).

Early physiologists, such as Claude Bernard, observed that stimulation of peripheral sympathetic nerves causes vasoconstriction and that interruption of the spinal cord in the lower cervical region drastically reduces blood pressure (i.e., produces hypotension). However, the first idea that a *reflex* might be involved in regulating the cardiovascular system came from experiments in which stimulation of a particular sensory (i.e., afferent) nerve caused a change in heart rate and blood pressure. In 1866, E. de Cyon and Carl Ludwig studied the depressor nerve, a branch of the vagus nerve. After they transected this nerve, they found that stimulation of the central (i.e., cranial) end of the cut nerve slows down the heart and produces hypotension. Hering showed that stimulation of the central end of another cut nerve—the sinus nerve (nerve of Hering), which innervates the carotid sinus—also causes bradycardia and hypotension. These two experiments strongly suggested that the depressor and sinus nerves carry sensory information to the brain and that the brain in some fashion uses this information to control cardiovascular function.

High-pressure baroreceptors at the carotid sinus and aortic arch are stretch receptors that sense changes in arterial pressure

Corneille Heymans was the first to demonstrate that pressure receptors—called **baroreceptors**—are located in arteries and are part of a neural feedback mechanism that regulates mean arterial pressure. He found that injection of epinephrine—also known as adrenaline—into a dog raises blood pressure and, later, lowers heart rate. Heymans hypothesized that increased blood pressure stimulates arterial sensors, which send a neural signal to the brain, and that the brain in turn transmits a neural signal to the heart, resulting in bradycardia.

To demonstrate that the posited feedback loop did not depend on the blood-borne traffic of chemicals between the periphery and the CNS, Heymans cross-perfused two dogs, so that only nerves connected the head of the dog to the rest of the animal's body. The dog's head received its blood flow from a second animal. (Today, one would use a heart-lung machine to perfuse the head of the first dog.) Heymans found that the vagus nerve carried both the upward and the downward traffic for the reflex arc and that agents carried in the blood played no role. He used a similar approach to demonstrate the role of the peripheral chemoreceptors in the control of respiration (see Chapter 32). For his work on the neural control of respiration, Heymans received the Nobel Prize in Physiology or Medicine for 1938.

The entire control process, known as the **baroreceptor control of arterial pressure** (Fig. 23-1), consists of baroreceptors (i.e., the detectors), afferent neuronal pathways, control centers in the medulla, efferent neuronal pathways, and the heart and blood vessels (i.e., the effectors). The negative feedback loop is designed so that *increased mean arterial pressure causes vasodilation and bradycardia*, whereas *decreased mean arterial pressure causes vasoconstriction and tachycardia* (i.e., increased heart rate).

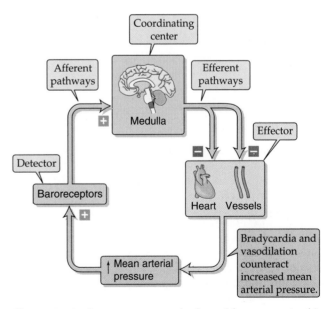

Figure 23-1 Baroreceptor control of arterial pressure. In this example, we assume that an increase in mean arterial pressure (*violet box*) is the primary insult.

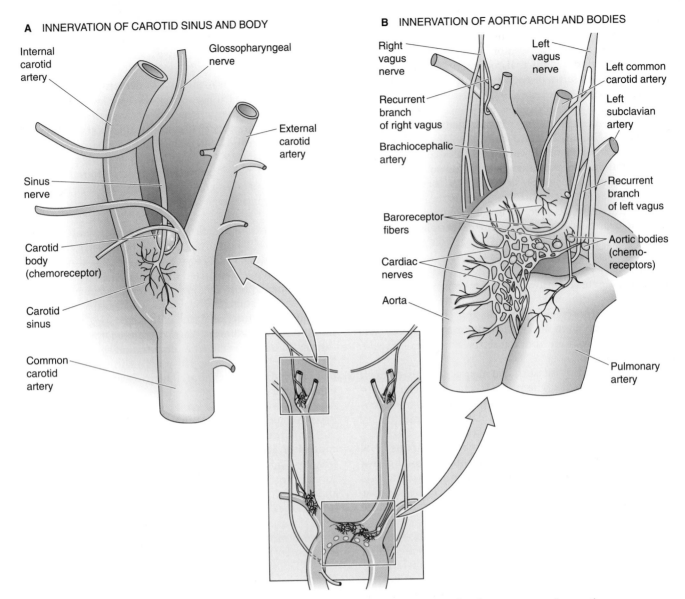

A INNERVATION OF CAROTID SINUS AND BODY

Internal carotid artery

Glossopharyngeal nerve

External carotid artery

Sinus nerve

Carotid body (chemoreceptor)

Carotid sinus

Common carotid artery

B INNERVATION OF AORTIC ARCH AND BODIES

Right vagus nerve

Left vagus nerve

Recurrent branch of right vagus

Left common carotid artery

Left subclavian artery

Brachiocephalic artery

Recurrent branch of left vagus

Baroreceptor fibers

Aortic bodies (chemoreceptors)

Cardiac nerves

Aorta

Pulmonary artery

Figure 23-2 Afferent pathways of the high-pressure baroreceptors. In **B,** the chemoreceptors (i.e., aortic bodies) are located on the underside of the aortic arch as well as at the bifurcation of the right brachiocephalic artery. On the left, aortic bodies, if present, are in a notch between the common carotid and the left subclavian arteries.

The sensor component consists of a set of mechanoreceptors located at strategic *high-pressure sites* within the cardiovascular system. As discussed later, the cardiovascular system also has *low-pressure* sensors that detect changes in venous pressure. The two most important high-pressure loci are the carotid sinus and the aortic arch. Stretching of the vessel walls at either of these sites causes vasodilation and bradycardia. The **carotid sinus** (Fig. 23-2A) is a very distensible portion of the wall of the internal carotid artery, located just above the branching of the common carotid artery into the external and internal carotid arteries. The arterial wall at the carotid sinus contains thin lamellae of elastic fibers but very little collagen or smooth muscle. The **aortic arch** (Fig. 23-2B) is also a highly compliant portion of the arterial tree that distends during each left ventricular ejection.

The baroreceptors in both the carotid sinus and the aortic arch are the branched and varicose (or coiled) terminals of myelinated and unmyelinated sensory nerve fibers, which are intermeshed within the elastic layers. The terminals express several nonselective cation channels in the TRP family: TRPC1, TRPC3, TRPC4, and TRPC5. TRPC channels may play a role both as primary electromechanical transducers and as modulators of transduction. An increase in the transmural pressure difference enlarges the vessel and thereby deforms the receptors. Baroreceptors are not really pressure sensitive but *stretch sensitive*. Indeed, TRPC1 is stretch sensitive. Direct stretching of the receptors results in increased firing of the baroreceptor's sensory nerve. The difference between stretch sensitivity and pressure sensitivity becomes apparent when one prevents the expansion of the vessel by surrounding the arterial wall with a plaster cast. When this is done, increase of the transmural pressure fails to increase the firing rate of the baroreceptor nerve. Removal of the cast restores the response. Other tissues surrounding the receptors act as a sort of mechanical filter, although much less so than the plaster cast.

As shown by the red records in the upper two panels of Figure 23-3A, a step increase in transmural pressure (i.e., stretch) produces an inward current that depolarizes the receptor, generating a **receptor potential** (see Chapter 15). The pressure increase actually causes a biphasic response in the receptor voltage. Following a large initial depolarization (the *dynamic* component) is a more modest but steady depolarization (the *static* component). This receptor potential, unlike a regenerative action potential, is a graded response whose amplitude is proportional to the degree of stretch (compare red and purple records).

These sensory neurons are *bipolar neurons* (see Chapter 10) whose cell bodies are located in ganglia near the brainstem. The central ends of these neurons project to the medulla. The cell bodies of the aortic baroreceptor neurons, which are located in the nodose ganglion (a sensory ganglion of the vagus nerve), express several TRPC channels. Although these nonselective cation channels are stretch sensitive and blocked by Gd^{3+}, they probably set only the *sensitivity* of the baroreceptor response.

Increased arterial pressure raises the firing rate of afferent baroreceptor nerves

If, in the absence of a pressure step, we depolarize the baroreceptor nerve ending, the result is an increase in the frequency of action potentials in the sensory nerve. Therefore, it is not surprising that graded increases in pressure produce graded depolarizations, resulting in graded increases in the spike frequency (Fig. 23-3A, lower two panels). Graded *decreases* in pressure gradually diminish receptor activity until the firing falls to vanishingly low frequencies at pressures around 40 to 60 mm Hg. Therefore, the baroreceptor encodes the mechanical response as a **frequency-modulated signal**.

A step increase in pressure generates a large initial depolarization, accompanied by a transient high-frequency discharge. The smaller, steady depolarization is accompanied by a steady but lower spike frequency. Because baroreceptors have both a dynamic and a static response, they are sensitive to both the *waveform* and the *amplitude* of a pressure oscillation. Therefore, bursts of action potentials occurring in phase with the cardiac cycle encode information on the pulse pressure (i.e., difference between the peak systolic and lowest diastolic pressures). The **static** pressure-activity curve in Figure 23-3B—obtained on single units of the sinus nerve—shows that the spike frequency rises sigmoidally with increases in *steady* blood pressure. The **pulsatile** pressure-activity curve in Figure 23-3B shows that when the pressure is *oscillating*, the mean discharge frequency at low mean pressures is higher than when pressure is steady.

Not all arterial receptors have the same properties. As we gradually increase intravascular pressure, different single units in the isolated carotid sinus begin to fire at different static pressures. Thus, the overall baroreceptor response to a pressure increase includes both an increased firing rate of

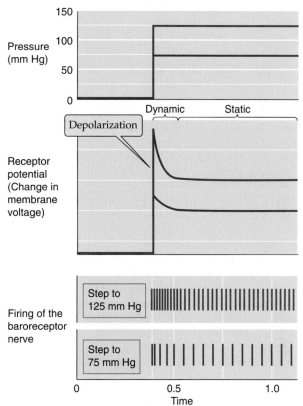

A RESPONSE TO INCREASED PRESSURE

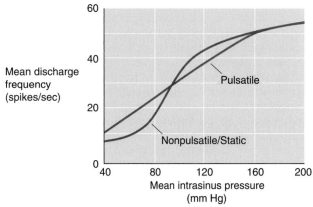

B PRESSURE-ACTIVITY RELATIONSHIPS

Figure 23-3 Afferent pathways of the high-pressure baroreceptors. In **A,** the records refer to hypothetical experiments on a baroreceptor in which one suddenly raises blood pressure to 75 mm Hg *(purple)* or to 125 mm Hg *(red)*. In **B,** the records refer to results from the carotid sinus nerve. *(Data from Chapleau MW, Abboud FM: Contrasting effects of static and pulsatile pressure on carotid baroreceptor activity in dogs. Circ Res 1987; 61:648-658.)*

active units and the **recruitment** of more units, until a saturation level is reached at ~200 mm Hg. The carotid sinus in some individuals is unusually sensitive. When wearing a tight collar, such a person may faint just from turning the head because compression or stretching of the carotid sinus orders the medulla to lower blood pressure.

The responses of the receptors in the carotid sinus and the aortic arch are different. In a given individual, a change in the carotid sinus pressure has a greater effect on the systemic arterial pressure than does a change in the aortic pressure. Compared with the carotid sinus receptor, the **aortic arch receptor**

has a higher threshold for activating the static response (~110 mm Hg vs. ~50 mm Hg);
has a higher threshold, likewise, for the dynamic response;
continues responding to pressure increases at pressures at which the carotid baroreceptor has already saturated;
is less sensitive to the rate of pressure change; and
responds less effectively to a decrease in pressure than to an increase in pressure (over the same pressure range).

Once a change in the arterial pressure has produced a change in the firing rate of the sensory nerve, the signal travels to the medulla. The afferent pathway for the carotid sinus reflex is the **sinus nerve**, which then joins the **glossopharyngeal** trunk (CN IX; Fig. 23-2A). The cell bodies of the carotid baroreceptors are located in the petrosal (or inferior) ganglion of the glossopharyngeal nerve (Fig. 23-4A). The afferent pathways for the aortic arch reflex are sensory fibers in the **depressor branch** of the **vagus nerve** (CN X; Fig. 23-2B). After joining the superior laryngeal nerves, the sensory fibers run cranially to their cell bodies in the nodose (or inferior) ganglion of the vagus (Fig. 23-4A).

The medulla coordinates afferent baroreceptor signals

The entire complex of medullary nuclei involved in cardiovascular regulation is called the **medullary cardiovascular center**. Within this center, broad subdivisions can be distinguished, such as a vasomotor area and a cardioinhibitory area. The medullary cardiovascular center receives all important information from the baroreceptors and is the major coordinating center for cardiovascular homeostasis.

Most afferent fibers from the two high-pressure baroreceptors project to the **nucleus tractus solitarii** (NTS, from the Latin *tractus solitarii* [of the solitary tract]; see Chapter 14), one of which is located on each side of the dorsal medulla (Fig. 23-4A, B). The neurotransmitter released by the baroreceptor afferents onto the NTS neurons is glutamate, which binds to the GluR2 subunits of AMPA receptors (see Chapter 13 and Fig. 15-15). Some neurons in the NTS (and also in the dorsal motor nucleus of the vagus, see later) have P_{2X} purinoceptors that are activated by extracellular ATP.

Inhibitory interneurons project from the NTS onto the **vasomotor area** in the ventrolateral medulla (Fig. 23-4B). This vasomotor area includes the A1 and C1 areas in the rostral ventrolateral medulla as well as the inferior olivary complex and other nuclei. Stimulation of the neurons in the **C1 area** produces a vasoconstrictor response. Unless inhibited by output from the NTS interneurons, neurons within the C1 area produce a tonic output that promotes vasoconstriction. Therefore, an increase in pressure stimulates baroreceptor firing, which in turn causes NTS interneurons to inhibit C1 neurons, resulting in vaso*dilation*. This C1 pathway largely accounts for the *vascular* component of the baroreceptor reflex. The bursting pattern of C1 neurons is locked to the cardiac cycle.

Excitatory interneurons project from the NTS onto a **cardioinhibitory area**, which includes the **nucleus ambiguus** and the **dorsal motor nucleus of the vagus** (see Chapter 14). Neurons in the dorsal motor nucleus of the vagus largely account for the *cardiac* component of the baroreceptor reflex (i.e., bradycardia). Some *inhibitory* interneurons probably project from the NTS onto a **cardioacceleratory** area, also located in the dorsal medulla. Stimulation of neurons in this area causes heart rate and cardiac contractility to increase.

The efferent pathways of the baroreceptor response include both sympathetic and parasympathetic divisions of the autonomic nervous system

After the medullary cardiovascular center has processed the information from the afferent baroreceptor pathways and integrated it with data coming from other pathways, this center must send signals back to the periphery through efferent (i.e., motor) pathways. The baroreceptor response has two major efferent pathways: the sympathetic and parasympathetic divisions of the autonomic nervous system.

Sympathetic Efferents   As discussed earlier, increased baroreceptor activity instructs the NTS to *inhibit* the C1 (i.e., vasomotor) and cardioacceleratory areas of the medulla. Functionally diverse bulbospinal neurons in both areas send axons down the spinal cord to synapse on and to stimulate preganglionic sympathetic neurons in the intermediolateral column of the spinal cord. Thus, we can think of these bulbospinal neurons as being presympathetic or prepreganglionic. The synapse can be adrenergic (in the case of the C1 neurons), peptidergic (e.g., neuropeptide Y), or glutamatergic. The glutamatergic synapses are the most important for the vasomotor response; the released glutamate acts on both NMDA and non-NMDA receptors on the preganglionic sympathetic neurons.

The cell bodies of the preganglionic sympathetic neurons are located in the intermediolateral gray matter of the spinal cord, between levels T1 and L3 (see Fig. 14-4). After considerable convergence and divergence, most of the axons from these preganglionic neurons synapse with postganglionic sympathetic neurons located within ganglia of the paravertebral sympathetic chain as well as within prevertebral ganglia (see Fig. 14-2). The neurotransmitter between the preganglionic and postganglionic sympathetic neurons is acetylcholine (ACh), which acts at N_2 nicotinic acetylcholine receptors (nAChR). Because of the convergence and divergence, sympathetic output does not distribute according to dermatomes (see Chapter 14). Postganglionic sympathetic fibers control a wide range of functions (see Fig. 14-4). Those that control blood pressure run with the large blood vessels and innervate both *muscular arteries and arterioles and veins.*

Increased sympathetic activity produces vasoconstriction. Indeed, the baroreceptor reflex produces *vasodilation* because it *inhibits* the tonic stimulatory output of the vasomotor C1 neurons. Because the bulbospinal neurons synapse with preganglionic sympathetic neurons between T1 and L3, severing of the spinal cord above T1 causes a severe fall in

A   LATERAL VIEW OF BRAINSTEM

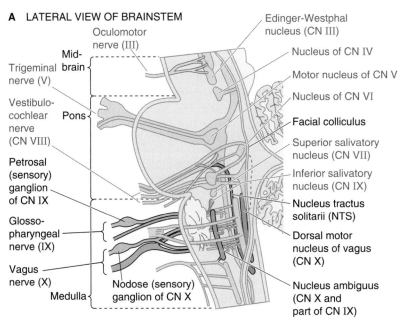

Figure 23-4 Medullary control centers for the cardiovascular system. In **A,** the relevant nuclei and cranial nerves are colorized and labeled in dark type. **B,** Hypothetical section through the medulla, showing projections of structures that do not necessarily coexist in a single cross section. ACh, acetylcholine; CN, cranial nerve; "Glu, etc.", glutamate and other neurotransmitters (i.e., norepinephrine and peptides); NE, norepinephrine; NTS, nucleus tractus solitarii.

B   AFFERENT AND EFFERENT PATHWAYS

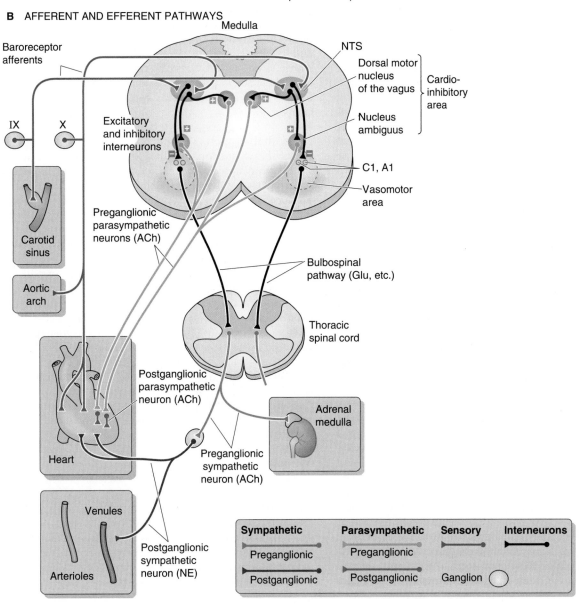

blood pressure. Sectioning of the cord below L3 produces no fall in blood pressure.

Another important target of postganglionic neurons with a cardiovascular mission is the heart. Output from the middle cervical and stellate ganglia, along with that from several upper thoracic ganglia (see Fig. 14-4), ramifies and after extensive convergence and divergence forms the cardiac nerves. Thus, severing of the spinal cord above T1 would block the input to the preganglionic sympathetic fibers to the heart. In addition, some preganglionic fibers do not synapse in sympathetic ganglia at all but directly innervate the chromaffin cells of the *adrenal medulla* through the splanchnic nerve. These cells release epinephrine, which acts on the heart and blood vessels (see later).

Parasympathetic Efferents   As noted earlier, increased baroreceptor activity instructs the NTS to stimulate neurons in the nucleus ambiguus and the dorsal motor nucleus of the vagus (cardioinhibitory area). The target neurons in these two nuclei are preganglionic parasympathetic fibers of the vagus nerve (CN X) that project to the heart. These efferent vagal fibers follow the common carotid arteries, ultimately synapsing in small ganglia in the walls of the atria. There, they release ACh onto the N_2-type nAChRs of the postganglionic parasympathetic neurons. The short postganglionic fibers then innervate the *sinoatrial (SA) node, the atria, and the ventricles*, where they act primarily to slow conduction through the heart (see later).

The principal effectors in the neural control of arterial pressure are the heart, the arteries, the veins, and the adrenal medulla

The cardiovascular system uses several effector organs to control systemic arterial pressure: the heart, arteries, veins, and adrenal medulla (Fig. 23-5).

Sympathetic Input to the Heart (Cardiac Nerves)   The sympathetic division of the autonomic nervous system influences the heart through the cardiac nerves, which form a plexus near the heart (Fig. 23-2). The postganglionic fibers, which release **norepinephrine**, innervate the SA node, atria, and ventricles. Their effect is to increase both heart rate and contractility (Table 23-1). Because it dominates the innervation of the SA node (which is in the right atrium), sympathetic input from the *right* cardiac nerve has more effect on the *heart rate* than does input from the left cardiac nerve. On the other hand, sympathetic input from the *left* cardiac nerve has more effect on *contractility*. In general, the cardiac nerves do not exert a strong tonic cardioacceleratory activity on the heart. At rest, their firing rate is less than that of the vagus nerve.

Parasympathetic Input to the Heart (Vagus Nerve)   The vagus normally exerts an intense tonic, parasympathetic activity on the heart through **ACh** released by the postganglionic fibers. Severing of the vagus nerve or administration of atropine (which blocks the action of ACh) increases heart rate. Indeed, experiments on the effects of the vagus on the heart led to the discovery of the first neurohumoral transmitter, ACh (see Chapter 8). Vagal stimulation decreases

heart rate by its effect on pacemaker activity (see Chapter 21). Just as the actions of the right and left cardiac nerves are somewhat different, the right vagus is a more effective inhibitor of the SA node than the left. The left vagus is a more effective inhibitor of conduction through the AV node. Vagal stimulation, to some extent, also reduces cardiac contractility.

Sympathetic Input to Blood Vessels (Vasoconstrictor Response)   The vasoconstrictor sympathetic fibers are disseminated widely throughout the blood vessels of the body. These fibers are most abundant in the kidney and the skin, relatively sparse in the coronary and cerebral vessels, and absent in the placenta. They release norepinephrine, which binds to adrenoceptors on the membrane of VSMCs. In most vascular beds, *vasodilation* is the result of a decrease in the tonic discharge of the vasoconstrictor sympathetic nerves.

Parasympathetic Input to Blood Vessels (Vasodilator Response)   Parasympathetic vaso*dilator* fibers are far less common than sympathetic vaso*constrictor* fibers. The parasympathetic vasodilator fibers supply the salivary and some gastrointestinal glands and are also crucial for vasodilation of erectile tissue in the external genitalia (see Chapters 54 and 55). Postganglionic parasympathetic fibers release ACh, which, as we shall see, *indirectly* causes vasodilation. In addition, these fibers produce vasodilation by releasing nitric oxide (NO) and vasoactive intestinal polypeptide (see Chapter 13).

Sympathetic Input to Blood Vessels in Skeletal Muscle (Vasodilator Response)   In addition to the more widespread sympathetic vasoconstrictor fibers, skeletal muscle in nonprimates has a special system of sympathetic fibers that produce *vasodilation* (see Chapter 14). These special fibers innervate the large precapillary vessels in skeletal muscle. The origin of the sympathetic vasodilator pathway is very different from that of the vasoconstrictor pathway, which receives its instructions—ultimately—from the vasomotor area of the medulla. Instead, the sympathetic vasodilator fibers receive their instructions—ultimately—from neurons in the cerebral cortex, which synapse on other neurons in the hypothalamus or in the mesencephalon. The fibers from these second neurons (analogous to the bulbospinal neurons discussed earlier) transit through the medulla without interruption and reach the spinal cord. There, these fibers synapse on preganglionic sympathetic neurons in the intermediolateral column, just as other descending neurons do. The vasodilatory preganglionic fibers synapse in the sympathetic ganglia on postganglionic neurons that terminate on VSMCs surrounding skeletal muscle blood vessels. These postganglionic vasodilatory fibers release ACh and perhaps other transmitters.

Therefore, blood vessels within skeletal muscle receive both sympathetic adrenergic and sympathetic cholinergic innervation. The cholinergic system, acting directly through muscarinic receptors, relaxes VSMCs and causes rapid vasodilation. This vasodilation in skeletal muscle occurs in the fight-or-flight response as well as perhaps during the anticipatory response in exercise (see Chapter 14). In both cases, mobilization of the sympathetic vasodilator system is accom-

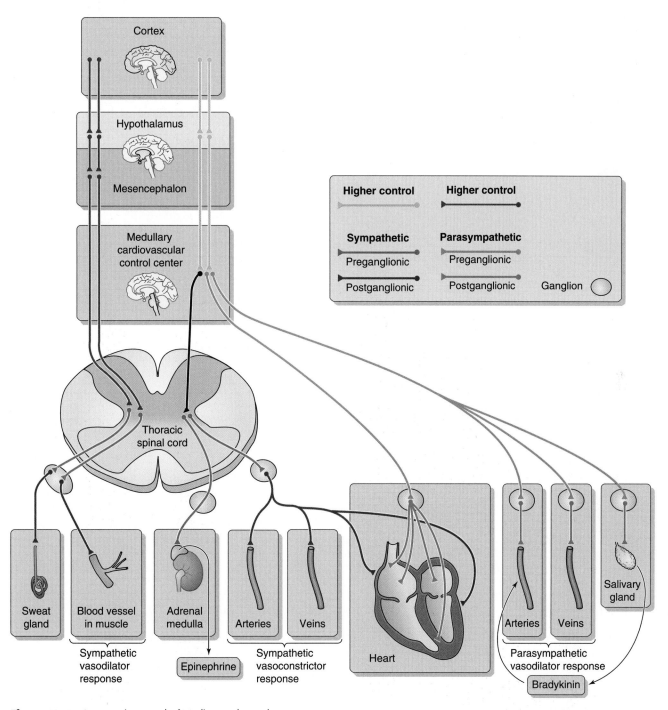

Figure 23-5 Autonomic control of cardiovascular end organs.

panied by extensive activation of the sympathetic division, including cardiac effects (i.e., increased heart rate and contractility) and generalized vasoconstriction of all vascular beds *except those in skeletal muscle.* (Little vasoconstriction occurs in cerebral and coronary beds, which have sparse sympathetic vasoconstrictor innervation.)

Adrenal Medulla   We have already mentioned that some preganglionic sympathetic fibers in the sympathetic splanchnic nerves also innervate the chromaffin cells in the adrenal medulla. Therefore, the adrenal medulla is the equivalent of

a sympathetic ganglion. The synaptic terminals of the preganglionic fibers release ACh, which acts on **nAChRs** of the **chromaffin cells** of the adrenal medulla (see Chapter 50). Chromaffin cells are thus modified postganglionic neurons that release their transmitters—**epinephrine** and, to a far lesser degree, norepinephrine—into the bloodstream rather than onto a specific end organ. Thus, the adrenal medulla participates as a global effector that through its release of epinephrine causes generalized effects on the circulation. As we will see in the next section, the epinephrine released by the adrenal medulla acts on both the heart and the blood

Table 23-1 Effects of Sympathetic and Parasympathetic Pathways on the Cardiovascular System

Effector Response	Anatomical Pathway	Neurotransmitter	Receptor	G Protein	Enzyme or Protein	Second Messenger
Tachycardia	Sympathetic	NE	β_1 on cardiac pacemaker	$G\alpha_s$	↑AC	↑$[cAMP]_i$
Bradycardia	Parasympathetic	ACh	M_2 on cardiac pacemaker	Direct action of dimeric $G_i\beta\gamma$	GIRK1 K⁺ channels	ΔV_m
Increase cardiac contractility	Sympathetic	NE	β_1 on cardiac myocyte	$G\alpha_s$ Direct action of $G\alpha_s$ on Cav1.2	↑AC	↑$[cAMP]_i$
Decrease cardiac contractility	Parasympathetic	ACh	M_2 on cardiac myocyte; Presynaptic M_2 receptor on noradrenergic neuron; M_3 receptor on cardiac myocyte	$G\alpha_i$ $G\alpha_i$ $G\alpha_q$	↓AC ↓AC ↑PLC → ↑$[Ca^{2+}]_i$ → ↑GC	↓$[cAMP]_i$ ↓$[cAMP]_i$ in neuron ↑$[cGMP]_i$ → ↑Cav1.2
Vasoconstriction in most blood vessels (e.g., skin)	Sympathetic	NE	α_1 on VSMC	$G\alpha_q$	↑PLC	↑$[Ca^{2+}]_i$
Vasoconstriction in some blood vessels	Sympathetic	NE	α_2 on VSMC	$G\alpha_{i/o}$	↓AC	↓$[cAMP]_i$
Vasodilation in most blood vessels (e.g., muscle)	Adrenal medulla	Epi	β_2 on VSMC	$G\alpha_s$	↑AC	↑$[cAMP]_i$
Vasodilation in erectile blood vessels	Parasympathetic	ACh	Presynaptic M_2 receptor on noradrenergic neurons	$G\alpha_i$	↓AC	↓$[cAMP]_i$ in neuron
	Parasympathetic	ACh	M_3 on endothelial cell	$G\alpha_q$	↑PLC → ↑$[Ca^{2+}]_i$ → ↑NOS	NO diffuses to VSMC
		NO	NO receptor (i.e., GC) inside VSMC	—	↑GC	↑$[cGMP]_i$
		VIP	VIP receptor on VSMC	$G\alpha_s$	↑AC	↑$[cAMP]_i$
Vasodilation in blood vessels of salivary gland	Parasympathetic	ACh	M_3 receptor on gland cell	$G\alpha_q$	↑Kallikrein	Kinins
Vasodilation in blood vessels of muscle in fight-or-flight response	Sympathetic	ACh NANC	Presynaptic M_2 receptor on noradrenergic neurons Receptor on VSMC	$G\alpha_i$	↓AC	↓$[cAMP]_i$ in neuron

AC, adenylyl cyclase; ACh, acetylcholine; cAMP, cyclic adenosine monophosphate; cGMP, cyclic guanosine monophosphate; Epi, Epinephrine; GC, guanylyl cyclase; GIRK1, G protein–activated/inwardly rectifying K⁺ channel (Kir3.1); NANC, nonadrenergic, noncholinergic; NE, norepinephrine; NO, nitric oxide; NOS, nitric oxide synthase; PLC, phospholipase C; VIP, vasoactive intestinal peptide; VSMC, vascular smooth muscle cell.

Table 23-2   Effects of Activating the β_1-Adrenergic Receptor in Ventricular Muscle*

β_1 Adrenoceptor
↓
Activated α_s
↓
↑ Adenylyl cyclase
↓
↑ cAMP
↓
↑ Protein kinase A
↓

Phosphorylation of L-type Ca^{2+} channels, Cav1.2	Phosphorylation of ryanodine receptor RYR2	Phosphorylation of phospholamban (PLN)	Phosphorylation of troponin I (TNNI3)	Interaction of α_s with Cav1.2
↑Open probability of Cav1.2	Dissociation of FKBP12.6 (calstabin 2) from RYR2-FKBP12.6 complex	↑SR Ca^{2+} pump (SERCA2a)	↑Off-rate of Ca^{2+} from Ca^{2+}-TNNC1 complex	↑Open probability of Cav1.2
↑Ca^{2+} influx	↑Open probability of RYR2	↑Ca^{2+} reuptake into SR ↑Ca^{2+} stores	↑Speed of relaxation (lusitropic)	↑Ca^{2+} influx
↑[Ca^{2+}]$_i$	↑Ca^{2+} release by SR	↑Speed of relaxation (lusitropic effect)	↓Duration of contraction	↑[Ca^{2+}]$_i$
↑Ca^{2+}-induced Ca^{2+} release from the SR (CICR)	↑[Ca^{2+}]$_i$	↓Duration of contraction		↑Ca^{2+}-induced Ca^{2+} release from the SR (CICR)
↑Contractility	↑Contractility			↑Contractility

*See Chapter 22 for a discussion of calstabin 2, Cav1.2, PLN, RYR2, SERCA2, TNNC1, and TNNI3.

vessels and thereby contributes to the control of the systemic arterial pressure.

The unique combination of agonists and receptors determines the end response in cardiac and vascular effector cells

Adrenergic Receptors in the Heart The *sympathetic* output to the heart affects both heart rate and contractility. Norepinephrine, released by the postganglionic sympathetic neurons, acts on postsynaptic β_1-adrenergic receptors of pacemaker cells in the SA node as well as on similar receptors of myocardial cells in the atria and ventricles. The β_1 adrenoceptor, through the G protein G$_s$, acts through the cAMP–protein kinase A pathway (see Chapter 3) to phosphorylate multiple effector molecules in both pacemaker cells and cardiac myocytes (Table 23-1).

In **pacemaker cells**, β_1 agonists stimulate (1) I_f, the diastolic Na$^+$ current, through HCN channels and (2) I_{Ca}, a Ca^{2+} current, through T- and L-type Ca^{2+} channels. The net effect of these two changes is an increased rate of diastolic depolarization (i.e., phase 4 of action potential; see Fig. 21-4A) and a negative shift in the threshold for the action potential (see Chapter 21). Because diastole shortens, the *heart rate* increases.

In **myocardial cells**, β_1 agonists exert several parallel **positive inotropic** effects through protein kinase A (Table 23-2). In addition, the activated α_s subunit of the G protein can directly activate L-type Ca^{2+} channels. The net effects of these pathways are contractions that are both stronger (see Chapter 21) and briefer (see Chapter 22).

Cholinergic Receptors in the Heart Parasympathetic output to the heart affects heart rate and, to a much lesser extent, contractility. ACh released by postsynaptic parasympathetic neurons binds to M$_2$ muscarinic (i.e., G protein–coupled) receptors on pacemaker cells of the SA node and on ventricular myocytes (Table 23-1).

In **pacemaker cells**, ACh acts by three mechanisms. (1) ACh triggers a membrane-delimited signaling pathway mediated not by the G protein α subunits but rather by the $\beta\gamma$ heterodimers (see Chapter 3). The newly released $\beta\gamma$ subunits directly open inward rectifier K$^+$ channels (GIRK1 or Kir3.1) in pacemaker cells (see Chapters 7 and 21). The resulting elevation of the K$^+$ conductance makes the maximum diastolic potential more negative during phase 4 of the action potential. (2) ACh also decreases I_f, thereby reducing the rate of diastolic depolarization. (3) ACh decreases I_{Ca}, thereby both reducing the rate of diastolic depolarization and making the threshold more positive (see Chapter 21). The net effect is a reduction in heart rate.

In **myocardial cells**, ACh has a *minor* **negative inotropic effect**, which could occur by two mechanisms. (1) Activation of the M$_2$ receptor, through Gα_i, inhibits adenylyl cyclase, reducing [cAMP]$_i$, thereby counteracting the effects of adrenergic stimulation. (2) Activation of the M_3 receptor, through $G\alpha_q$, stimulates phospholipase C, raising $[Ca^{2+}]_i$ and thus stimulating nitric oxide synthase (NOS; see Chapter 3). The newly formed NO stimulates guanylyl cyclase and increases $[cGMP]_i$, which somehow inhibits L-type Ca^{2+} channels and decreases Ca^{2+} influx.

Adrenergic Receptors in Blood Vessels The sympathetic division of the autonomic nervous system can modulate the tone of vascular smooth muscle in arteries, arterioles, and veins through two distinct routes—postganglionic sympathetic neurons and the adrenal medulla. Whether the net effect of sympathetic stimulation in a particular vessel is vasoconstriction (increased VSMC tone) or vasodilation (decreased VSMC tone) depends on four factors: (1) which agonist is released, (2) which adrenoceptors that agonist binds to, (3) whether receptor occupancy tends to cause vasoconstriction or vasodilation, and (4) which receptor subtypes happen to be present on a particular VSMC.

Which agonist is released is the most straightforward of the factors. Postganglionic sympathetic neurons release norepinephrine, and the adrenal medulla releases primarily epinephrine.

Which receptors the agonist binds to is more complex. Norepinephrine and epinephrine do not have exclusive affinity for a single type of adrenoceptor. The original α and β designations followed from the observation that norepinephrine appeared to have its greatest activity on α receptors, and epinephrine, on β receptors. However, although norepinephrine binds with a greater affinity to α receptors than to β receptors, it also can activate β receptors. Similarly, although epinephrine binds with a greater affinity to β receptors than to α receptors, it can also activate α receptors. Of course, synthetic agonists may be more specific and potent than either norepinephrine or epinephrine (e.g., the α agonist phenylephrine and β agonist isoproterenol). A finer pharmacological and molecular dissection reveals that both α and β receptors have subgroups (e.g., β_1 and β_2), and even the subgroups have subgroups (see Chapter 14). Each of these many adrenoceptor types has a unique pharmacology. Thus, the β_1 receptor has about the same affinity for epinephrine and norepinephrine, but the β_2 receptor has a higher affinity for epinephrine than for norepinephrine.

Whether receptor occupancy tends to cause vasoconstriction or vasodilation is straightforward (Table 23-1). The *vasoconstriction* elicited by catecholamines is an α effect, in particular, an α_1 effect. Thus, norepinephrine released from nerve terminals acts on the α_1 adrenoceptor, which is coupled to the G protein G_q. The resulting activation of phospholipase C (see Chapter 3) and formation of inositol 1,4,5-trisphosphate (IP_3) lead to a rise in $[Ca^{2+}]_i$ and smooth muscle contraction (see Table 20-7). In contrast, *vasodilation*, elicited by epinephrine released from the adrenal medulla, is a β_2 effect. Occupancy of the β_2 adrenoceptor triggers the cAMP–protein kinase A pathway, leading to phosphorylation of myosin light chain kinase (MLCK; see Chapter 9), which reduces the sensitivity of MLCK to the Ca^{2+}-calmodulin complex, resulting by default in smooth muscle relaxation (see Table 20-7).

Which receptor subtypes happen to be present on a particular VSMC is a complex issue. Many blood vessels are populated with a mixture of α-receptor or β-receptor subtypes, each stimulated to varying degrees by norepinephrine and epinephrine. Therefore, the response of the cell depends on the relative dominance of the subtype of receptor present on the cell surface. Fortunately, the only two subtypes in blood vessels that matter clinically are α_1 and β_2.

The ultimate outcome in the target tissue (vasoconstriction versus vasodilation) depends on both the heterogeneous mixture of agonists (norepinephrine versus epinephrine) applied and the heterogeneous mixture of VSMC receptors (α_1 and β_2) present in tissues. As an example, consider blood vessels in the skin and heart. Because cutaneous blood vessels have only α_1 receptors, they can only vasoconstrict, regardless of whether the agonist is norepinephrine or epinephrine. On the other hand, epinephrine causes coronary blood vessels to dilate because they have a greater number of β_2 receptors than α_1 receptors.

Cholinergic Receptors in or near Blood Vessels The addition of ACh to an isolated VSMC causes contraction (see Table 20-7). Thus, in an artificial situation in which the nerve terminals release only ACh and in which no other tissues are present, ACh would lead to vasoconstriction. In real life, however, ACh dilates blood vessels by binding to muscarinic receptors on neighboring cells and generating *other* messengers that indirectly cause vasodilation (Table 23-1). For example, in **skeletal muscle**, ACh may bind to M_2 receptors on the presynaptic membranes of postganglionic sympathetic neurons, decreasing $[cAMP]_i$ and inhibiting the release of norepinephrine. Thus, inhibition of vasoconstriction produces vasodilation.

In **erectile tissue**, ACh not only binds to presynaptic M_2 receptors as before but also binds to M_3 receptors on vascular *endothelial cells* and, through the phospholipase C pathway, releases IP_3 and raises $[Ca^{2+}]_i$ (see Fig. 14-11). The Ca^{2+} stimulates NOS to produce NO (see Chapter 3), which diffuses from the endothelial cell to the VSMC. Inside the VSMC, the NO activates soluble guanylyl cyclase, resulting in the production of cGMP and activation of protein kinase G. The subsequent phosphorylation of MLCK causes relaxation (see Chapter 20).

In **salivary glands**, postganglionic parasympathetic neurons release ACh, which may stimulate gland cells to secrete kallikrein, an enzyme that cleaves kininogens to vasodilating kinins (e.g., bradykinin). A similar paracrine sequence of events may occur in the **sweat glands** of nonapical skin, where postganglionic sympathetic fibers release ACh, indirectly leading to local vasodilation (see Chapter 24).

Nonadrenergic, Noncholinergic Receptors in Blood Vessels Postganglionic parasympathetic nerve terminals may cause vasodilation by co-releasing neurotransmitters other than ACh (Table 23-1), such as NO, neuropeptide Y, vasoactive intestinal peptide, and calcitonin gene–related peptide. NO of neuronal origin acts in the same way as endothelium-derived NO. Neuropeptide Y acts by lowering $[cAMP]_i$; vasoactive intestinal peptide and presumably calcitonin gene–related peptide act by raising [cAMP]$_i$ (see Table 20-7).

The medullary cardiovascular center tonically maintains blood pressure and is under the control of higher brain centers

The medullary cardiovascular center normally exerts its tonic activity on the sympathetic preganglionic neurons, whose cell bodies lie in the thoracolumbar segments of the spinal cord. However, a variety of somatic and visceral afferents also make connections with this efferent pathway in the spinal cord, and such afferents are responsible for several reflexes that occur at the spinal level. The sympathetic preganglionic neurons are normally so dependent on medullary input that they are not very sensitive to local afferents. Rather, these somatic and visceral afferents exert their major effect by ascending to the medulla and synapsing in the NTS. Nevertheless, some spinal (i.e., segmental) cardiovascular reflexes do exist. For example, the skin blanches in response to both pain and inflammation. These spinal reflexes become most powerful after a spinal transverse lesion.

Neurons of the C1 area of the medulla (Fig. 23-4) are responsible for maintaining a normal mean arterial pressure. In general, C1 neurons are tonically active and excite sympathetic preganglionic neurons to produce vasoconstriction (see Chapter 22). The presence of tonically active neurons in the C1 area raises the possibility that these neurons play a role in some forms of hypertension. Interestingly, clonidine, an antihypertensive agent, acts by binding to imidazole receptors on C1 area neurons.

Besides the afferents from the baroreceptors, the medullary cardiovascular center receives afferents from respiratory centers and from higher CNS centers, such as the hypothalamus and cerebral cortex (Fig. 23-5). The **hypothalamus** integrates many cardiovascular responses. Indeed, one can use a microelectrode to stimulate particular sites in the hypothalamus to reproduce a variety of physiological responses. The dorsomedial hypothalamic nucleus in the hypothalamus acts on the rostral ventrolateral medulla to mediate vasomotor and cardiac responses (e.g., during exercise and acute stress). The **cerebral cortex** influences the hypothalamic integration areas along both excitatory and inhibitory pathways. Thus, a strong emotion can lead to precipitous hypotension with syncope (i.e., fainting). Conditioned reflexes can also elicit cardiovascular responses. For example, it is possible, by reward conditioning, to train an animal to increase or to decrease its heart rate.

Secondary neural regulation of arterial blood pressure depends on chemoreceptors

Although baroreceptors are the primary sensors for blood pressure control, a second set of receptors, the peripheral chemoreceptors, also play a role. Whereas input from baroreceptors exerts a *negative* drive on the medullary *vasomotor center*, causing vasodilation, the peripheral chemoreceptors exert a *positive* drive on the vasomotor center, causing vasoconstriction (Fig. 23-6A). As far as the heart is concerned, input from *both* the baroreceptors and the peripheral

A INTRINSIC CARDIOVASCULAR RESPONSE

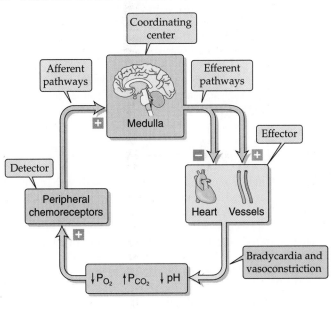

B INTEGRATED RESPONSE

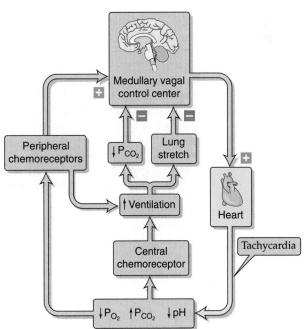

Figure 23-6 Chemoreceptor control of the cardiovascular system. In this example, we assume that a decrease in P_{O_2}, an increase in P_{CO_2}, or a decrease in pH is the primary insult *(violet box)*. In **A,** the bradycardia occurs only when ventilation is fixed or prevented (e.g., breath-holding). In **B,** the effects of breathing overcome the intrinsic cardiovascular response, producing tachycardia.

chemoreceptors exerts a positive drive on the *cardioinhibitory center;* that is, they both decrease heart rate (compare Figs. 23-1 and 23-6A).

The medullary *respiratory* centers—which include the areas that integrate the input from the peripheral chemoreceptors—strongly influence medullary *cardiovascular* centers. A fall in arterial P_{O_2}, a rise in P_{CO_2}, or a fall in pH stimulates the peripheral chemoreceptors to increase the firing frequency of the afferent nerves to the medulla. In the absence of conflicting input, which we discuss next, the intrinsic response of the medulla to this peripheral chemoreceptor input is to direct efferent pathways to cause *vasoconstriction* and *bradycardia* (Fig. 23-6A). Opposite changes in the P_{O_2}, P_{CO_2}, and pH have the opposite effects.

The **peripheral chemoreceptors**—whose primary role is to regulate ventilation (see Chapter 32)—lie close to the baroreceptors. Just as there are two types of high-pressure baroreceptors (i.e., carotid sinus and aortic arch), there are also two types of peripheral chemoreceptors: the carotid bodies and the aortic bodies (compare the location of the baroreceptor and chemoreceptor systems in Fig. 23-2A, B).

Carotid Bodies   The carotid body—or glomus caroticum—is located between the external and internal carotid artery. Although the human carotid body is small (i.e., ~1 mm³), it has an extraordinarily high blood flow per unit mass and a minuscule arteriovenous difference for P_{O_2}, P_{CO_2}, and pH—putting it in an excellent position to monitor the composition of the *arterial blood.* The chemosensitive cell in the carotid body is the **glomus cell**, which synapses with nerve fibers that join the glossopharyngeal nerve (CN IX). A fall in arterial P_{O_2}, a rise in arterial P_{CO_2}, or a fall in the pH increases the spike frequency in the sensory fibers of the afferent sinus nerve.

Aortic Bodies   The aortic bodies are situated immediately under the concavity of the aortic arch and in the angle between the *right* subclavian and carotid arteries. Aortic bodies may also be present at the angle between the *left* subclavian and common carotid arteries. The aortic glomus cells synapse with nerve fibers that are afferent pathways in the vagus nerve (CN X).

Afferent Fiber Input to the Medulla   The most important signal affecting the glomus cells is a low P_{O_2}, which triggers an increase in the firing rate of the sensory fibers. We will discuss ways in which this signal triggers neuronal firing in Chapter 32. Like the afferent fibers from the baroreceptors, the afferent fibers from both the carotid body (CN IX) and the aortic bodies (CN X) project to the NTS in the medulla. Indeed, the responses to input from the peripheral chemoreceptors overlap with those to input from the baroreceptors.

Physiological Role of the Peripheral Chemoreceptors in Cardiovascular Control   The fluctuations in P_{O_2} that normally occur in humans are not large enough to affect the blood pressure or heart rate. For the cardiovascular system, the peripheral chemoreceptors play a role only during severe hypoxia (e.g., hemorrhagic hypotension). As already noted, the *intrinsic* cardiovascular effects of hypoxia on the periph-

eral chemoreceptors include vasoconstriction and bradycardia (Fig. 23-6A). However, it is not easy to demonstrate this primary reflex bradycardia; indeed, it is observed only during forced apnea. Under real-life conditions, *hypoxia causes tachycardia.* Why? Hypoxia—through the peripheral chemoreceptors—normally stimulates the medullary respiratory centers, which in turn stimulate ventilation (Fig. 23-6B). As discussed later, the high P_{CO_2} that may accompany hypoxia stimulates the central chemoreceptors, which independently stimulates ventilation. This increased ventilation has two effects. First, it stretches the lungs, which in turn stimulates pulmonary stretch receptors. Afferent impulses from these pulmonary stretch receptors ultimately inhibit the cardioinhibitory center, causing reflex tachycardia. Second, as discussed in Chapter 31, increased alveolar ventilation caused by hypoxia lowers systemic P_{CO_2}, raising the pH of the brain extracellular fluid and inhibiting the cardioinhibitory center. Again, the net effect is tachycardia. Thus, the physiological response to hypoxia is tachycardia.

Central Chemoreceptors   In addition to peripheral chemoreceptors, *central* chemoreceptors are present in the medulla (see Chapter 32). However, in contrast to the peripheral chemoreceptors, which primarily sense a low P_{O_2}, the central chemoreceptors mainly sense a low brain pH, which generally reflects a high arterial P_{CO_2}.

As already noted (Fig. 23-4B), tonic baroreceptor input to the NTS in the medulla stimulates inhibitory interneurons that project onto the vasomotor area. This pathway exerts a considerable restraining influence on sympathetic output, which would otherwise cause vasoconstriction. Thus, cutting of these baroreceptor afferents causes vasoconstriction. The central chemoreceptor also influences the vasomotor area. Indeed, a high arterial P_{CO_2} (i.e., low brain pH), which stimulates the central chemoreceptor, disinhibits the vasomotor area—just as cutting of baroreceptor afferents disinhibits the vasomotor area. The result is also the same: an increase in the sympathetic output and vasoconstriction.

In summary, a low P_{O_2} acting on the peripheral chemoreceptor and a high P_{CO_2} acting on the central chemoreceptor act in concert to enhance vasoconstriction.

REGULATION OF CARDIAC OUTPUT

Other things being unchanged, an increased cardiac output raises mean arterial pressure. Therefore, it is not surprising that as we have just seen, the heart is an important effector organ in the feedback loops that regulate mean arterial pressure. Cardiac output is the product of the heart rate and stroke volume (see Equation 17-6), and both factors are under the dual control of (1) regulatory mechanisms intrinsic to the heart and (2) neural and hormonal pathways that are extrinsic to the heart.

Mechanisms intrinsic to the heart modulate both heart rate and stroke volume

Intrinsic Control of Heart Rate   As the length of diastole increases, the heart rate necessarily decreases. The diastolic interval is determined by the nature of the action potential fired off by the SA node. Such factors as the maximum diastolic potential, the slope of the diastolic depolarization (phase 4), and the threshold potential all influence the period between one SA node action potential and the next (see Fig. 21-6). Intrinsic modifiers of the SA node pacemaker, such as $[K^+]_o$ and $[Ca^{2+}]_o$, greatly influence the ionic currents responsible for SA node pacemaker activity but are not part of any cardiovascular feedback loops.

Intrinsic Control of Stroke Volume   Stroke volume is the difference between end-diastolic volume and end-systolic volume (see Equation 22-2). Various processes intrinsic to the heart affect both of these variables.

The **end-*diastolic* volume (EDV)** depends on the following:

1. **Filling pressure.** Ventricular filling pressure depends to a large degree on *atrial* filling pressure. When increased venous return causes atrial filling pressure to rise, EDV rises as well.
2. **Filling time.** The *longer* the filling time, the greater the EDV. As heart rate rises, diastole shortens to a greater extent than does systole, thereby decreasing EDV.
3. **Ventricular compliance** (reciprocal of the slope of the diastole curve in Fig. 22-11B). As ventricular compliance increases, a given filling pressure will produce a greater increase in ventricular volume, thus resulting in a greater EDV.

The **end-*systolic* volume (ESV)** depends on the following:

1. **Preload** (i.e., end-*diastolic* volume). According to Starling's law of the heart, increase of the EDV increases the stretch on the cardiac muscle and the force of the contraction (see the systole curve in Fig. 22-11B) and thus the stroke volume. Only at a very large EDV does contraction begin to weaken as the muscle fibers are too stretched to generate maximal power (see Fig. 22-11A).
2. **Afterload** (force against which the ventricle ejects its contents). The afterload of the left ventricle is the mean systemic arterial pressure; the afterload of the right ventricle is the mean pulmonary arterial pressure. Increased afterload impedes the heart's ability to empty and thereby increases ESV.
3. **Heart rate.** An increased heart rate leads to greater Ca^{2+} entry into myocardial cells, thereby increasing contractility and reducing ESV (see Chapter 22).
4. **Contractility.** Positive inotropic agents act by increasing $[Ca^{2+}]_i$ within the myocardial cells (see Chapter 22), thereby enhancing the force of contraction and decreasing ESV.

Note that a particular variable may affect both end-diastolic and end-systolic volumes. For example, an increased heart rate decreases EDV and decreases ESV. Therefore, its effect on stroke volume—the *difference* between these two volumes—may be difficult to predict.

Mechanisms extrinsic to the heart also modulate heart rate and stroke volume

We have already seen that the sympathetic and parasympathetic pathways are the efferent limbs of the feedback loops that control mean arterial pressure (Fig. 23-5). These efferent limbs also control cardiac output through heart rate and stroke volume. Because we have already described the anatomy, neurotransmitters, and transduction mechanisms involved in these pathways, we focus here on how these pathways specifically affect the heart rate and stroke volume.

Baroreceptor Regulation   Baroreceptor responses affect both heart rate and stroke volume, the *product* of which is *cardiac output*. However, baroreceptors do not monitor cardiac output per se but rather arterial pressure. Thus, the baroreceptor response does *not* correct spontaneous alterations in cardiac output unless they happen to change mean arterial pressure. For example, when an increase in the cardiac output matches a commensurate decrease in the peripheral resistance, leaving the mean arterial pressure unchanged, the baroreceptors do not respond. On the other hand, even if cardiac output is unchanged, it will be the target of the baroreceptor response if other factors (e.g., changes in peripheral resistance) alter arterial pressure.

Chemoreceptor Regulation   In Figure 23-6B, we saw that the integrated response to hypoxia and respiratory acidosis is *tachycardia*. This tachycardia response turns out to be a very helpful feedback mechanism for maintaining cardiac output. For example, a reduced cardiac output lowers arterial P_{O_2}, raises P_{CO_2}, and lowers pH. These changes stimulate the peripheral chemoreceptors, indirectly producing tachycardia and thereby increasing cardiac output. Thus, the chemoreceptor response corrects changes in blood chemistry that are likely to result from reduced cardiac output. Once again, the detector (i.e., the peripheral chemoreceptors) does not sense changes in the cardiac output per se but rather in the metabolic consequences of altered cardiac output. Changes in cardiac output go unnoticed by the chemoreceptors if they do not affect arterial P_{O_2}, P_{CO_2}, or pH.

It is fortunate that a high P_{CO_2} increases the heart rate (Fig. 23-6B) because a high P_{CO_2} has a direct effect on the heart, *decreasing* myocardial contractility. High P_{CO_2} leads to intracellular acidosis of the myocardial cells (see Chapter 28). The low pH_i shifts the $[Ca^{2+}]_i$–tension curve of cardiac muscle to higher $[Ca^{2+}]_i$ values, reflecting a lower sensitivity of TNNC1 to $[Ca^{2+}]_i$. Thus, in the absence of reflex tachycardia, high P_{CO_2} would decrease myocardial force and thereby lower cardiac output.

Low-pressure baroreceptors in the atria respond to increased "fullness" of the vascular system, triggering tachycardia, renal vasodilation, and diuresis

The baroreceptors located at *high*-pressure sites (i.e., the carotid sinus and aortic arch) are not the only stretch receptors involved in feedback regulation of the circulation. **Low-pressure baroreceptors**—bare ends of myelinated nerve fibers—are located at strategic *low*-pressure sites, including

A ANATOMICAL DISTRIBUTION

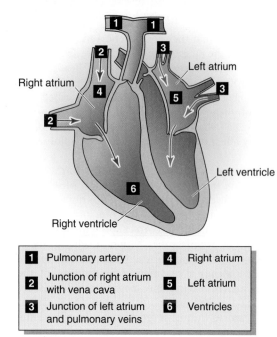

B RESPONSE OF ATRIAL A– AND B–TYPE RECEPTORS

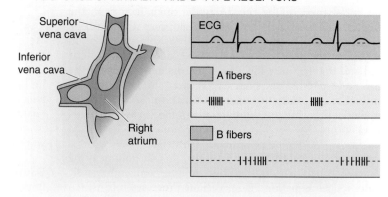

1	Pulmonary artery	4	Right atrium
2	Junction of right atrium with vena cava	5	Left atrium
3	Junction of left atrium and pulmonary veins	6	Ventricles

Figure 23-7 Low-pressure receptors. In **B,** A-type receptors *(orange)*, located mainly in the body of right atrium; B-type receptors *(green)*, located mainly in superior and inferior vena cava. ECG, electrocardiogram.

the pulmonary artery, the junction of the atria with their corresponding veins, the atria themselves, and the ventricles (Fig. 23-7A). Distention of these receptors depends largely on venous return to the heart. Therefore, these mechanoreceptors detect the "fullness" of the circulation and are part of a larger system of volume sensors that control the **effective circulating volume** of blood (see Chapter 40). These low-pressure receptors also help control cardiac output. By regulating both effective circulating volume and cardiac output, these receptors also *indirectly* regulate mean arterial blood pressure.

Atrial Receptors The most extensively studied low-pressure receptors are the atrial receptors. These are located at the ends of afferent axons—either A or B fibers—that join the vagus nerve (CN X). The A fibers fire in synchrony with atrial systole and therefore monitor heart rate (Fig. 23-7B). The B fibers fire in a burst during ventricular systole (Fig. 23-7B) and gradually increase their firing rate as the atria fill, reaching maximum firing frequency at the peak of the *v* wave of the atrial (i.e., jugular) pulse (Fig. 23-7A). Thus, the B fibers monitor the rising atrial volume. Because the **central venous pressure (CVP)**—the pressure inside large systemic veins leading to the right side of the heart—is the main determinant of right atrial filling, the B fibers also detect changes in CVP. By inference, the atrial B-type stretch receptors primarily monitor effective circulating volume and venous return.

The afferent pathways for the low-pressure receptors are similar to those for high-pressure baroreceptors and peripheral chemoreceptors traveling along the vagus nerve and projecting to the NTS and other nuclei of the medullary cardiovascular center. To some extent, the efferent pathways

and effector organs (i.e., heart and blood vessels) also are similar. However, whereas increased stretch of the high-pressure receptors *lowers* heart rate, increased stretch of the atrial B-type receptors *raises* heart rate (the **Bainbridge reflex**, which we discuss in the next section). Moreover, whereas increased stretch of the high-pressure receptors causes *generalized* vasodilation, increased stretch of the atrial B-type receptors decreases sympathetic vasoconstrictor output *only to the kidney*. The net effect of increased atrial stretch (i.e., tachycardia and renal vasodilation) is an increase in renal blood flow and—as seen in Chapter 35—an increase in urine output (i.e., diuresis). Decreased atrial stretch has little effect on heart rate but increases sympathetic output to the kidney. Therefore, as far as their direct cardiovascular effects are concerned, the high-pressure baroreceptors respond to stretch (i.e., increased blood pressure) by attempting to decrease blood pressure. The low-pressure baroreceptors respond to stretch (i.e., increased fullness) by attempting to eliminate fluid.

The afferent fibers of the atrial receptors that project to the NTS also synapse there with neurons that project to magnocellular neurons in the paraventricular nucleus of the hypothalamus (see Fig. 41-8). These hypothalamic neurons synthesize **arginine vasopressin (AVP)**—also known as antidiuretic hormone (see Chapter 38)—and then transport it down their axons to the posterior pituitary for release into the blood (see Chapter 47). Increased atrial stretch lowers AVP secretion, producing a water diuresis and thus decreasing total body water (see Chapter 40).

In addition to stimulating bare nerve endings, atrial stretch causes a *non*-neural response by stretching the atrial myocytes themselves. When stretched, atrial myocytes release **atrial natriuretic peptide (ANP)** or factor (ANF). ANP is a powerful vasodilator. It also causes diuresis (see Chapter 40) and thus enhances the renal excretion of Na^+ (i.e., it causes natriuresis). In these ways, it lowers effective circulating volume blood pressure.

Thus, enhanced atrial filling with consequent stretching of the atrial mechanoreceptors promotes diuresis by at least three efferent mechanisms, the first two of which are neurally mediated. (1) Tachycardia in combination with a reduced sympathetic vasoconstrictor output to the kidney increases renal blood flow. (2) Atrial baroreceptors cause decreased secretion of AVP. (3) The stretch of the atrial myocytes themselves enhances the release of ANP.

Ventricular Receptors Stretching of the ventricular *low*-pressure stretch receptors causes bradycardia and vasodilation, responses similar to those associated with stretching of the arterial *high*-pressure receptors. However, these ventricular receptors do not contribute appreciably to homeostasis of the cardiac output.

Cardiac output is roughly proportional to effective circulating blood volume

The **Bainbridge reflex** is the name given to the tachycardia caused by an increase in venous return. An increase in blood volume leads to increased firing of low-pressure B fibers (Fig. 23-7B) during atrial filling. The efferent limb of this Bainbridge reflex is limited to instructions carried by both parasympathetic and sympathetic pathways to the SA node, which determines heart rate. Effects on cardiac contractility and stroke volume are insignificant. Because the Bainbridge reflex saturates, the increase in heart rate is greatest at low baseline heart rates.

The Bainbridge reflex acts as a counterbalance to the baroreceptor reflex in the control of **heart rate**. The orange curve on the right upper quadrant of Figure 23-8 illustrates the Bainbridge reflex: increase of the effective circulating volume (i.e., increase of venous return and stimulation of *low-pressure* receptors) increases heart rate. On the other hand, we have already noted that decreased atrial stretch has little effect on heart rate by the Bainbridge reflex. The orange curve in the left upper quadrant of Figure 23-8 illustrates the intervention of the *high-pressure* baroreceptors. That is, a decrease in blood volume does not cause heart rate to fall but rather causes it to rise. Indeed, a significant reduction in blood volume leads to a fall in mean arterial pressure, reduced baroreceptor firing, and—through the cardioinhibitory and cardioaccelatory areas in the medulla (Fig. 23-4B)—stimulation of the SA node. Therefore, on examination of the full orange curve in Figure 23-8, we see that changes in blood volume or venous return have a biphasic effect on heart rate. By different mechanisms, volume loading and volume depletion *both* cause a graded increase in heart rate. In general, during volume loading, the Bainbridge reflex prevails, whereas during volume depletion, the high-pressure baroreceptor reflex dominates. *Heart rate is at its minimum when effective circulating volume is normal.*

Like heart rate (Fig. 23-8, orange curve), **stroke volume** also shows a peculiar, biphasic dependence on effective circulating volume (blue curve) that is the result of two competing effects. In the case of stroke volume, the competitors

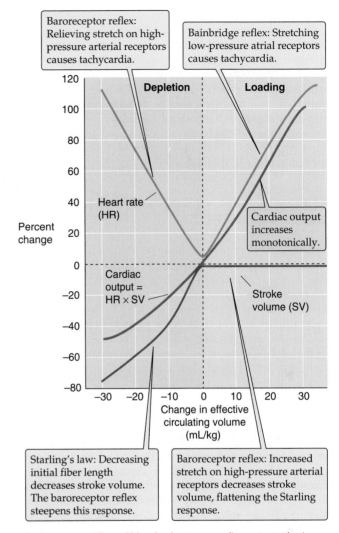

Figure 23-8 Effect of blood volume on cardiac output. The investigators changed effective circulating volume (x-axis) by altering blood volume.

are Starling's law and the baroreceptor reflex. According to Starling's law, as venous blood volume increases, enhanced ventricular filling increases EDV, thereby improving cardiac performance and thus stroke volume (see Chapter 22). The Starling relationship reflects the *intrinsic* properties of the heart muscle. However, in a real person, the baroreceptor reflex has a major influence on the dependence of stroke volume on blood volume. At low blood volumes, the baroreceptor reflex produces high sympathetic output, increasing contractility and steepening the Starling relationship (blue curve in the left lower quadrant of Fig. 23-8). At high blood volumes, the Starling relationship normally tends to be less steep. Moreover, the baroreceptor reflex reduces sympathetic output, thereby decreasing contractility and further flattening the blue curve in the right half of Figure 23-8.

In contrast to the biphasic response of heart rate and stroke volume to changes in effective circulating volume, **cardiac output** rises monotonically (Fig. 23-8, red curve). The reason for this smooth increase is that cardiac output is the product of heart rate *and* stroke volume. Starting from very low blood volumes (see the extreme left of Fig. 23-8), increase in the blood volume causes a gradual rise in stroke volume (blue curve), offset by a fall in heart rate (orange curve), resulting in an overall rise of cardiac output (red curve) until blood volume and stroke volume reach normal levels. Further increases in blood volume have no effect on stroke volume (blue curve) but increase heart rate (orange curve), further increasing cardiac output (red curve). Consequently, the dependence of cardiac output on effective circulating volume is the result of the complex interplay among three responses: (1) the Bainbridge reflex, (2) the baroreceptor reflex, and (3) Starling's law.

MATCHING OF VENOUS RETURN AND CARDIAC OUTPUT

Venous return is the blood flow returning to the heart. Most often, the term is used to mean the *systemic* venous return, that is, return of blood to the right side of the heart. Because the input of the right side of the heart must equal its output in the steady state, and because the cardiac outputs of the right and left sides of the heart are almost exactly the same, the input to the right side of the heart must equal the output of the left side of the heart. Thus, the systemic venous return must match the systemic cardiac output.

Increases in cardiac output cause right atrial pressure to fall

The right atrial pressure (RAP) determines the extent of ventricular filling and indeed was the first of the three determinants of end-diastolic volume discussed earlier in the chapter. In turn, RAP depends on the venous return of blood to the heart. Imagine that we replace the heart and lungs with a simple pump—with adjustable flow—that delivers blood into the aorta and simultaneously takes it back up from the right atrium (Fig. 23-9A). Using this simple pump, we can study the factors that govern venous return from the peripheral systemic circulation to the right side of the heart by varying flow (the *independent* variable) while recording RAP (the *dependent* variable).

We start our experiment with the pump generating a normal cardiac output of 5 L/min; the RAP is 2 mm Hg. This situation is represented by point A in Figure 23-9B, which is a plot of RAP versus venous return (i.e., our pump rate). When we reverse the axes, the plot is known as a **vascular function curve**. Note that we express venous return (i.e., cardiac *input*) in the same units as cardiac *output*. We now turn off the pump, a situation analogous to cardiac arrest. For several seconds, blood continues to flow from the arteries and capillaries into the veins because the arterial pressure continues to exceed the venous pressure. Remember that the aortic pressure does not fall to zero during diastole because of the potential energy stored in the elastic recoil of the arterial walls (see Chapter 22 for the box titled Effect of Aortic Compliance on Blood Flow). Similarly, after a cardiac arrest, this potential energy continues to push blood to the venous side until all pressures are equal throughout the vascular tree, and flow stops everywhere.

When blood flow finally ceases after a cardiac arrest, the pressures in the arteries, capillaries, veins, and right atrium

A MODEL OF SYSTEMIC CIRCULATION

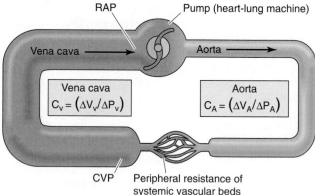

B VASCULAR FUNCTION CURVE WITH REVERSED AXES

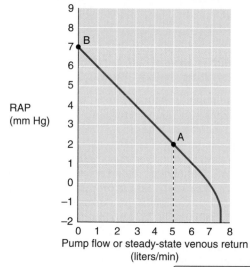

C VASCULAR FUNCTION CURVE

> When cardiac output, and thus venous return, is zero, RAP equals mean systemic filling pressure (MSFP).

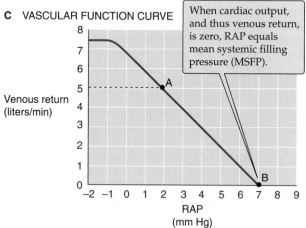

Figure 23-9 Vascular function. In **A,** a heart-lung machine replaces the right side of the heart, the pulmonary circulation, and the left side of the heart. We can set the pump flow to predetermined values and examine how cardiac output determines central venous pressure (CVP) and right atrial pressure (RAP). CV and CA are vascular compliances. **B** shows dependent variable (RAP) on the y-axis, whereas **C** shows RAP on the x-axis.

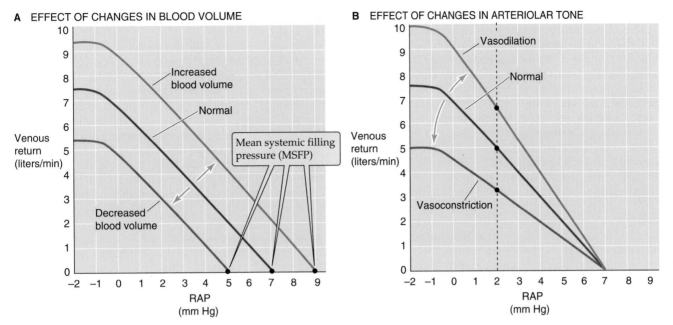

Figure 23-10   Effect of changes in blood volume and vasomotor tone on the vascular function curve. The *purple curves* are the same as the vascular function curve in Figure 23-9C. In **B,** dilation of the arterioles increases CVP and thus raises the driving force (CVP – RAP) for venous return. Constriction of arterioles has the opposite effects.

are uniform. This pressure is called the **mean systemic filling pressure (MSFP)** and is ~7 mm Hg (point B in Fig. 23-9B). Why is the MSFP not zero? When you fill an elastic container (e.g., a balloon) with fluid, the pressure inside depends on how much fluid you put in as well as the compliance of the container (see Equation 19-5). In the case of the cardiovascular system, MSFP depends on the blood volume and the overall compliance of the entire vascular system. Now that blood flow has ceased, there is obviously no longer any force (i.e., no ΔP) driving the blood from the veins into the pump. Therefore, RAP equals MSFP.

Now, starting with the system at a standstill (point B in Fig. 23-9B), we increase pump rate to some level, measure the steady-state RAP, and repeat this procedure several times at different pump rates. As the pump rate increases, RAP falls (Fig. 23-9B) because the inflow to the pump draws blood out of the right atrium, the site closest to the inlet of the pump. Because the upstream central venous pressure (CVP) exceeds RAP, blood flows from the large veins into the right atrium. At a pump rate of 5 L/min, the RAP falls to about +2 mm Hg, its original value. At even higher pump rates, RAP eventually falls to negative values.

Cardiovascular physiologists usually work with the vascular function curve with the axes reversed from those shown in Figure 23-9B, treating RAP as the independent variable and plotting it on the abscissa (Fig. 23-9C). As RAP becomes less positive, it provides a greater driving pressure (i.e., greater ΔP = CVP – RAP) for the return of blood from the periphery to the right atrium, as it must for cardiac output to increase. Thus, the cardiac output steadily rises as RAP falls. However, as RAP becomes increasingly negative, the transmural pressure of the large veins becomes negative, so that the large veins feeding blood to the right atrium col-

lapse. No further increment in venous return can occur, even though the driving pressure, ΔP, is increasing. Therefore, the vascular function curve plateaus at negative values of RAP, around –1 mm Hg (Fig. 23-9C).

Two different theories attempt to explain the shape of the vascular function curve in Figure 23-9C. One explanation for the curve's steepness emphasizes the high compliance of the venous capacitance vessels; the other focuses on their small viscous resistance. In reality, both compliance and resistance are responsible for the steepness of the vascular function curve.

Changes in blood volume shift the vascular function curve to different right atrial pressures, whereas changes in arteriolar tone alter the slope of the curve

Because the vascular function curve depends on how full the capacitance vessels are, *changing the blood volume* affects the vascular function curve. An increase in blood volume (e.g., a transfusion) shifts the curve to the right. In the example in Figure 23-10A, the intercept with the x-axis (i.e., MSFP) moves from 7 to 9 mm Hg, as would be expected if more blood were put into a distensible container, whether it is a balloon or the circulatory system. A decrease in blood volume (e.g., hemorrhage) shifts the curve and the x-intercept to the left. Thus, MSFP increases with transfusion and decreases with hemorrhage. However, changes in blood volume do *not* affect the *slope* of the linear portion of the vascular function curve as long as there is no change in either vessel compliance or resistance.

Change in the venomotor tone, by constriction or dilation of *only the veins,* is equivalent to change in the blood volume.

Returning to our balloon analogy, even if we hold the amount of blood constant, we can increase pressure inside the balloon by increasing the tension in the wall. Because most of the blood volume is in the veins, a pure increase in venomotor tone would be equivalent to a blood transfusion (Fig. 23-10A). Conversely, a pure decrease in venomotor tone would reduce the tension in the wall of the container, shifting the curve to the left, just as in a hemorrhage.

Change in the tone of the arterioles has a very different effect on the vascular function curve. Because the arterioles contain only a minor fraction of the blood volume, changes in the arteriolar tone have little effect on MSFP and thus on the x-intercept. However, changes in the arteriolar tone can have a marked effect on the CVP, which along with the RAP determines the driving force for the venous return. Arteriolar constriction flattens the vascular function curve; arteriolar dilation has the opposite effect (Fig. 23-10B). We can understand this effect by examining the vertical line through the three curves at an RAP of 2 mm Hg. For the middle or normal curve, the difference between a CVP of, say, 5 mm Hg and a RAP of 2 mm Hg ($\Delta P = \text{CVP} - \text{RAP} = 3 \text{ mm Hg}$) produces a venous return of 5 L/min. Arteriolar constriction might lower the CVP from 5 to 4 mm Hg, thereby reducing ΔP from 3 to 2 mm Hg. Because the driving pressure (ΔP) drops to $^2/_3$ of normal, venous return also falls to $^2/_3$ of normal. Thus, arteriolar constriction flattens the vascular function curve. Similarly, arteriolar dilation might raise CVP from 5 to 6 mm Hg, so that the ΔP increases from 3 to 4 mm Hg, producing a venous return that is $^4/_3$ of normal. Thus, arteriolar dilation steepens the vascular function curve.

In the preceding analysis, we assumed "pure" changes in blood volume or vessel tone. In real life, things can be more complicated. For example, hemorrhage is typically followed by arteriolar constriction for maintenance of the systemic arterial pressure. Thus, real situations may both shift the x-intercept and change the slope of the vascular function curve.

Because vascular function and cardiac function depend on each other, cardiac output and venous return match at exactly one value of right atrial pressure

Just as there is a vascular function curve, there is also a **cardiac function curve** that in effect is Starling's law. The classical Starling's law relationship (see the red curve in Fig. 22-11B), which is valid for both ventricles, is a plot of developed pressure versus EDV. However, we already expressed Starling's law as a cardiac performance curve in Figure 22-11C, plotting stroke work on the y-axis and atrial pressure on the x-axis. Because stroke work—at a fixed arterial pressure and heart rate—is proportional to cardiac output, we can replace stroke work with *cardiac output* on the y-axis of the cardiac performance curve. The result is the red cardiac function curve in Figure 23-11A. Note that the cardiac function curve is a plot of cardiac output versus RAP, and it has the same *units* as the vascular function curve. We can plot the two relationships on the same graph (Fig. 23-11A). However, the y-axis for the cardiac function curve is *cardiac output*, whereas the y-axis for the vascular function curve is *venous return*. Of course, cardiac output

and venous return (i.e., cardiac input) must be the same in the steady state.

We can now ask, Do the cardiac output and venous return depend on RAP? Does RAP depend on the cardiac output and venous return? The answer to both questions is an emphatic yes! They all depend on each other. There is no absolute dependent or independent variable in this closed circuit because, in the steady state, venous return and cardiac output must be equal. Venous return (from the vascular function curve) and cardiac output (from the cardiac function curve) can be equal only at the single point where the two curves intersect (point A in Fig. 23-11A). Only transient and small deviations in these two curves are possible unless either or both of the function curves change in shape.

Imagine what would happen if RAP transiently increased from 2 to 4 mm Hg (Fig. 23-11A). Starling's law states that the increased ventricular filling initially increases cardiac output from starting point A (5 L/min) to point B (7.3 L/min). Simultaneously, the increase in RAP causes a decrease in the driving pressure ΔP for venous return, that is, the difference CVP − RAP. Thus, the increase in RAP would initially reduce the venous return from point A (5 L/min) to point B′ (3 L/min). This imbalance between cardiac output and venous return cannot last very long. The transiently elevated cardiac output will have two effects. First, by sucking the right atrium dry, it will tend to lower RAP. Second, by pumping blood out of the heart and toward the veins, it will raise CVP. As a result, the difference CVP − RAP increases, and venous return moves from point B′ to C′. Because RAP at point C′ is lower than at B′, the cardiac output must also be less at point C than at point B. The imbalance between C and C′ (6.5 vs. 4 L/min) is now less than that between B and B′ (7.3 vs. 3 L/min). In this way, venous return gradually increases, cardiac output gradually decreases, and RAP gradually decreases until once again they all come into balance at point A. Thus, the cardiovascular system has an intrinsic mechanism for counteracting small, transient imbalances between cardiac input and output.

The only way to produce a *permanent change* in cardiac output, venous return, and RAP is to change at least one of the two function curves. The vascular function curve may be any one of a large family of such curves (Fig. 23-10A, B), depending on the precise blood volume, venomotor tone, and arteriolar tone. Thus, a transfusion of blood shifts the vascular function curve to the right, establishing a new steady-state operating point at a higher RAP (point A → point B in Fig. 23-11B). Similarly, vasodilation would rotate the vascular function curve to a steeper slope, also establishing a new steady-state operating point at a higher RAP.

The cardiac function curve also may be any one of a large family (see Fig. 22-11C), depending on afterload, heart rate, and, above all, the heart's contractile state. Therefore, increasing contractility by adding a cardiac glycoside such as digitalis shifts the cardiac function curve upward and to the left, establishing another steady-state operating point (point A → point B in Fig. 23-11C). Both physiological and pathological conditions can reset the vascular and cardiac function curves, resulting in a wide range of operating points for the match between venous return and cardiac output.

A MATCHING OF A SINGLE CARDIAC FUNCTION CURVE
WITH A SINGLE VASCULAR FUNCTION CURVE

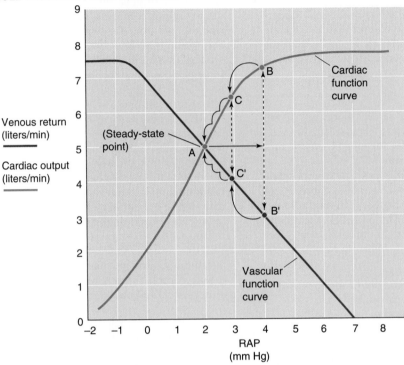

B SHIFT OF VASCULAR FUNCTION CURVE

C SHIFT OF CARDIAC FUNCTION CURVE

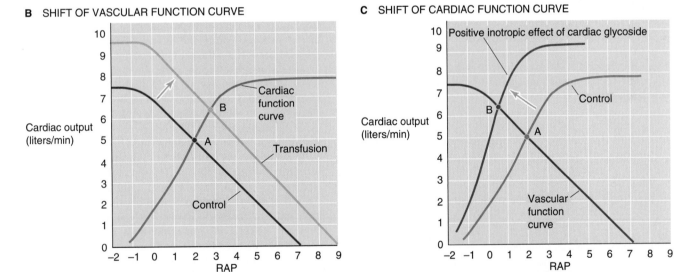

Figure 23-11 Matching of cardiac output with venous return. The *purple curves* are the same as the vascular curve in Figure 23-9C. The *red cardiac function curves* represent Starling's law. In **A,** point A is the single RAP at which venous return and cardiac output match. A transient increase in RAP from 2 to 4 mm Hg causes an initial mismatch between cardiac output (point B) and venous return (point B′), which eventually resolves (B′C′A and BCA). In **B,** permanently increasing blood volume (transfusion) shifts the vascular function curve to the right (as in Fig. 23-10A), so that a match between the cardiac output and venous return now occurs at a higher RAP (point B). In **C,** permanently increasing cardiac contractility shifts the cardiac function curve upward, so that a match between the cardiac output and the venous return now occurs at a lower RAP (point B).

INTERMEDIATE AND LONG-TERM CONTROL OF THE CIRCULATION

In addition to the rapidly acting neural mechanisms that control the total peripheral resistance and cardiac output, humoral controls contribute to the homeostasis of the circulation. In most instances, these control systems operate on a time scale of hours or days, far more slowly than the neurotransmitter-mediated reflex control by the CNS.

Two classes of humoral controls influence the circulation.

1. Vasoactive substances released in the blood, or in the proximity of vascular smooth muscle, modulate the vasomotor tone of arteries and veins, affecting blood pressure and the distribution of blood flow.
2. Nonvasoactive substances, which act on targets other than the cardiovascular system, control the effective circulating volume by modulating extracellular fluid volume. By determining the filling of the blood vessels, these nonvasoactive agents also modulate the mean arterial pressure and cardiac output.

Endocrine and paracrine vasoactive compounds control the circulatory system on an intermediate to long-term basis

Vasoactive substances, both endocrine and paracrine, cause blood vessels to contract or to relax (Table 23-3). In many instances, paracrine control dominates over endocrine control. The chemical messengers controlling the blood vessels can be amines, peptides, or proteins; derivatives of arachidonic acid; or gases such as NO.

Biogenic Amines Monoamines may be either vasoconstrictors (epinephrine and serotonin) or vasodilators (histamine).

1. **Epinephrine.** The source of this hormone is the adrenal medulla (see Chapter 50). Epinephrine binds to α_1 **receptors** on VSMCs, causing *vasoconstriction* (see Table 20-7), and to β_2 **receptors** on VSMCs, causing *vasodilation* (see Table 20-7). Because β_2 receptors are largely confined to the blood vessels of skeletal muscle, the heart, the liver,

and the adrenal medulla itself, epinephrine is not a systemic vasodilator. Epinephrine also binds to β_1 receptors in the heart, thereby *increasing the heart rate and contractility*. For the cardiovascular system, the effects of catecholamines originating from the adrenal medulla are usually minor compared with those of the norepinephrine released from the sympathetic nerve endings.

2. **Serotonin.** Also known as 5-hydroxytryptamine (5-HT; see Fig. 13-8B), this monoamine is synthesized by serotonergic nerves, enterochromaffin cells, and adrenal chromaffin cells. 5-HT is also present in platelets and mast cells. Serotonin binds to **5-HT$_{2A}$ or 5-HT$_{2B}$ receptors** on VSMCs, causing *vasoconstriction* (see Table 20-7). Circulating serotonin is generally not involved in normal systemic control of the circulation but rather in local control. Serotonin is particularly important with vessel damage, where it contributes to hemostasis (see Chapter 18).

3. **Histamine.** Like serotonin, histamine (see Fig. 13-8B) may also be present in nerve terminals. In addition, mast cells release histamine in response to tissue injury and inflammation. Histamine binds to **H$_2$ receptors** on VSMCs, causing *vasodilation* (see Table 20-7). Although histamine causes vascular smooth muscle to relax, it causes visceral smooth muscle (e.g., bronchial smooth muscle in asthma) to contract.

Peptides Vasoactive peptides may be either vasoconstrictors or vasodilators (Table 23-3).

1. **Angiotensin II (ANG II).** Part of the renin-angiotensin-aldosterone cascade (see Chapter 40), ANG II, as its name implies, is a powerful *vasoconstrictor*. The liver secretes angiotensinogen into the blood. The enzyme renin, released into the blood by the kidney, then converts angiotensinogen to the decapeptide ANG I. Finally, angiotensin-converting enzyme (ACE), which is present primarily on endothelial cells, particularly those of the lung, cleaves ANG I to the octapeptide ANG II. Aminopeptidases further cleave it to the heptapeptide ANG III, which is somewhat less vasoactive than ANG II.

In VSMCs, ANG II binds to G protein–coupled **AT$_{1A}$ receptors**, activating phospholipase C, raising $[Ca^{2+}]_i$, and leading to *vasoconstriction* (see Table 20-7). However, ANG II is *normally* not present in plasma concentrations high enough to produce systemic vasoconstriction. In contrast, ANG II plays a major role in cardiovascular control during blood loss (see Chapter 25), exercise, and similar circumstances that reduce renal blood flow. Reduced perfusion pressure in the kidney causes the release of renin (see Chapter 40). Plasma ANG II levels rise, leading to an intense vasoconstriction in the splanchnic and renal circulations. The resulting reduced renal blood flow leads to even more renin release and higher ANG II levels, a dangerous positive feedback system that can lead to acute renal failure. A widely studied model of hypertension that demonstrates the importance of this mechanism is the Goldblatt model for hypertension (see the box on hypertension).

ANG II has a range of other effects—besides direct vasoactive effects—that indirectly increase mean arterial pressure: (1) ANG II increases cardiac contractility; (2) it

Table 23-3 Vasoactive Compounds

Vasoconstrictors	Vasodilators
Epinephrine (through α_1 receptors)	Epinephrine (through β_2 receptors)
Serotonin	Histamine
ANG II	ANP
AVP	Bradykinins
Endothelin	PGE$_2$, PGI$_2$ NO

reduces renal plasma flow, thereby enhancing Na^+ reabsorption in the kidney; (3) as discussed in the next section, ANG II and ANG III also stimulate the adrenal cortex to release aldosterone; (4) in the CNS, ANG II stimulates thirst and leads to the release of another vasoconstrictor, AVP; (5) ANG II facilitates the release of norepinephrine by postganglionic sympathetic nerve terminals; and (6) finally, ANG II also acts as a cardiac growth factor (see the box in Chapter 22 on cardiac hypertrophy).

2. **Arginine vasopressin (AVP).** The posterior pituitary releases AVP, also known as antidiuretic hormone. AVP binds to V_{1a} **receptors** on VSMCs, causing *vasoconstriction* (see Table 20-7), but only at concentrations higher than those that are strongly antidiuretic (see Chapter 38). Hemorrhagic shock causes enhanced AVP release and a vasoconstriction that contributes to a transient restoration of arterial pressure (see Chapter 25).

3. **Endothelins (ETs).** Endothelial cells produce ETs (see Chapter 20) that bind to ET_A **receptors** on VSMCs, causing *vasoconstriction* (see Table 20-7). Although, on a molar basis, ETs are the most powerful vasoconstrictors, it is not clear whether these paracrine agents play a dominant role in overall blood pressure homeostasis.

4. **Atrial natriuretic peptide (ANP or ANF).** Released from atrial myocytes in response to stretch, this 28–amino acid peptide binds to **ANP receptor A (NPR1)** on VSMCs, which is membrane-bound guanylyl cyclase, causing *vasodilation* (see Table 20-7). Although ANP lowers blood pressure, its role in the overall regulation of mean arterial pressure is doubtful. Because ANP also has powerful diuretic and natriuretic actions, it ultimately reduces plasma volume and therefore blood pressure.

5. **Kinins.** At least three different kinins exist: (1) the nonapeptide **bradykinin**, which is formed in plasma; (2) the decapeptide **lysyl-bradykinin**, which is liberated from tissues; and (3) **methionyl-lysyl-bradykinin**, which is present in the urine. These kinins are breakdown products of **kininogens**, catalyzed by **kallikreins**—enzymes that are present in plasma and in tissues such as the salivary glands, pancreas, sweat glands, intestine, and kidney. Kallikreins form in the blood from the following cascade. Plasmin acts on clotting factor XII, releasing fragments with proteolytic activity. These factor XII fragments convert an inactive precursor, prekallikrein, to kallikreins. The kinins formed by the action of these kallikreins are eliminated by the **kininases** (kininase I and II). Kininase II is the same as angiotensin-converting enzyme. Thus, the same enzyme (ACE) that generates a vasoconstrictor (ANG II) also disposes of vasodilators (bradykinin). Bradykinin binds to **B2 receptors** on endothelial cells, causing release of NO and prostaglandins and thereby *vasodilation* (see Table 20-7). Like histamine, the kinins *relax* vascular smooth muscle but *contract* visceral smooth muscle.

Prostaglandins Many tissues synthesize these derivatives of arachidonic acid (see Chapter 3). Prostacyclin (PGI_2) binds to prostanoid **IP receptors** on VSMCs, causing strong *vasodilation* (see Table 20-7). Prostaglandin E_2 (PGE_2) binds to prostanoid **EP_2 and EP_4 receptors** on VSMCs, also causing *vasodilation* (see Table 20-7). It is doubtful that prostaglandins play a role in systemic vascular control. In veins and also in some arteries, arachidonic acid or Ca^{2+} ionophores cause endothelium-dependent contractions. Because cyclooxygenase inhibitors prevent this vasoconstrictor response, venous endothelial cells probably metabolize arachidonic acid into a vasoconstrictive cyclooxygenase product, presumably thromboxane A_2.

Nitric Oxide Nitric oxide synthase (NOS) produces NO from arginine in endothelial cells (see Chapter 20). NO activates the **soluble guanylyl cyclase** in VSMCs, causing *vasodilation* (see Table 20-7). Although NO is a powerful paracrine *vasodilator*, it is not clear that it plays an important role in overall blood pressure homeostasis.

Pathways for the renal control of extracellular fluid volume are the primary long-term regulators of mean arterial pressure

The *volume of the extracellular fluid* (ECF) includes both the blood plasma and the interstitial fluid. The small solutes in the plasma and interstitial fluid exchange freely across the capillary wall, so that the entire ECF constitutes a single osmotic compartment. Because the plasma volume is a more or less constant fraction (~20%) of the ECF volume, changes in the ECF volume produce proportional changes in plasma volume. Thus, assuming that the compliance of the vasculature is constant (see Equation 19-5), such an increase in plasma volume will lead to an increase in transmural blood pressure.

We saw in Chapter 20 that the *Starling forces* across a capillary (i.e., the hydrostatic and colloid osmotic pressure differences) determine the traffic of fluid between the plasma and the interstitial fluid (see Chapter 20 for the box on interstitial edema). Thus, alterations in the Starling forces acting across the capillary wall can affect the plasma volume and therefore blood pressure.

Because of the importance of the ECF volume and Starling forces in determining the plasma volume, one might expect that the body would have specific sensors for ECF volume, interstitial fluid volume, and blood volume. However, the parameter that the body controls in the intermediate and long-term regulation of the mean arterial pressure is none of these but rather a more vague parameter termed the **effective circulating volume**. The effective circulating volume is not an anatomical volume but the *functional* blood volume that reflects the extent of tissue perfusion, as sensed by the fullness or pressure in the vessels. The control mechanisms that defend effective circulating volume include the two classes of stretch receptors described in this chapter. First, the high-pressure receptors in the carotid sinus and aorta do double duty. In the short term, these baroreceptors regulate blood pressure by their direct cardiovascular effects, as was already discussed. In the longer term, they regulate effective circulating volume. Second, the low-pressure receptors—located in the pulmonary artery, the junction of the atria with their corresponding veins, the atria themselves, and the ventricles—regulate effective circulating volume by direct and indirect effects on the cardiovascular system. In addition to these already familiar receptors involved in neural control of the circulation, other sensors monitor effective circulating

Hypertension

Hypertension is found in ~20% of the adult population. It can damage endothelial cells, producing a number of proliferative responses, including arteriosclerosis. In the long term, hypertension can lead to coronary artery disease, myocardial infarction, heart failure, stroke, and renal failure. In the great majority of cases, hypertension is the result of dysfunction of the mechanisms used by the circulation for the long-term rather than short-term control of arterial pressure. In fact, chronically hypertensive patients may have diminished sensitivity of their arterial baroreceptors.

Most people with an elevated blood pressure have "primary hypertension," in which it is not possible to identify a single, specific cause. Renal artery stenosis, which compromises renal blood flow, is the most common cause of secondary hypertension. An experimental equivalent of renal artery stenosis is the "one-clip two-kidney" model of hypertension first described by Goldblatt (see the box on renal hypertension in Chapter 40). This model does not explain most cases of hypertension, but it does give us our best description of the pathophysiological mechanism involved in at least some patients with elevated blood pressure. The most common cause of renal artery stenosis is the narrowing of the renal artery by atherosclerotic plaque. Fibromuscular disease of the renal arterial wall can also be responsible, usually in young women, as can any space-occupying lesion (e.g., metastatic cancer or benign cysts). If the stenosis is removed by angioplasty or surgery, and if preliminary test results show that the stenosis is the likely cause of the elevation in blood pressure, then a significant percentage of patients will experience resolution of their hypertension.

The cumulative obstruction of smaller arteries and arterioles may also produce hypertension, as is often seen in diseases of the renal parenchyma or any end-stage renal disease. Conversely, constriction of larger vessels proximal to the kidneys can also cause hypertension, as is the case with coarctation of the aorta, a congenital malformation that constricts flow through the aorta to the lower parts of the body. Another cause of secondary hypertension is chronic volume overload. Volume overload can be acquired, such as in primary aldosteronism (caused by either a benign adenoma or bilateral hyperplasia) and pheochromocytoma (a tumor of the adrenal medulla that releases excessive amounts of catecholamines into the circulation). Volume overload can be genetic, as in rare mendelian forms of hypertension, such as Liddle disease, and pseudohypoaldosteronism type 2.

volume (see Table 40-2): the baroreceptors in the renal artery, the stretch receptors in the liver, and the atrial myocytes themselves as well as—to some extent—osmoreceptors in the CNS.

As we will see in Chapter 40, these sensors of effective circulating volume send signals to the dominant effector organ—the kidney—to change the rate of Na^+ excretion in the urine. These signals to the kidney follow four parallel effector pathways (see Chapter 40): (1) the renin–ANG II–aldosterone axis, (2) the autonomic nervous system, (3) the posterior pituitary that releases AVP, and (4) the atrial myocytes that release ANP. Among these four parallel pathways, the most important is the **renin-angiotensin-aldosterone** system. By regulating total body Na^+ content, the kidney determines ECF volume. Therefore, the kidney ultimately governs the blood volume and is thus the principal agent in the long-term control of mean arterial pressure.

REFERENCES

Books and Reviews

Andresen MC, Kunze DL: Nucleus tractus solitarius: Gateway to neural circulatory control. Annu Rev Physiol 1994; 56:93-116.

Cowley AW Jr: Long-term control of arterial blood pressure. Physiol Rev 1992; 72:231-300.

Navar LG, Zou L, Von Thun A, et al: Unraveling the mystery of Goldblatt hypertension. News Physiol Sci 1998; 13:170-176.

Pilowsky PM, Goodchild AK: Baroreceptor reflex pathways and neurotransmitters: 10 years on. J Hypertens 2002; 20:1675-1688.

Thrasher TN: Baroreceptors, baroreceptor unloading, and the long-term control of blood pressure. Am J Physiol Regul Integr Comp Physiol 2005; 288:R819-R827.

Journal Articles

Chapleau MW, Abboud FM: Contrasting effects of static and pulsatile pressure on carotid baroreceptor activity in dogs. Circ Res 1987; 61:648-658.

Hajdu MA, Cornish KG, Tan W, et al: The interaction of the Bainbridge and Bezold-Jarisch reflexes in the conscious dog. Basic Res Cardiol 1991; 86:175-185.

Mukkamala R, Cohen RJ, Mark RG: A computational model-based validation of Guyton's analysis of cardiac output and venous return curves. Comput Cardiol 2002; 29:561-564.

Potts JT: Inhibitory neurotransmission in the NTS in the nucleus tractus solitarii: Implications for baroreflex resetting during exercise. Exp Physiol 2006; 91:59-72.

Wang JJ, Flewitt JA, Shrive NG, et al: The systemic venous circulation—waves propagating on a windkessel: Relation of arterial and venous windkessels to the systemic vascular resistance. Am J Physiol Heart Circ Physiol 2006; 290:H154-H162.

CHAPTER 24

SPECIAL CIRCULATIONS

Steven S. Segal

In the preceding chapters, we considered blood flow to peripheral capillary beds as if the "periphery" were a single entity. In this chapter, we break that entity down into some of its component parts. Because each organ in the body has its own unique set of requirements, special circulations within each organ have evolved with their own particular features and regulatory mechanisms. Especially for times of great stress to the body, each organ possesses circulatory adaptations that allow it to make the changes appropriate for causing minimal harm to the overall organism. Here, we focus on the circulations of the brain, heart, skeletal muscle, abdominal viscera, and skin. We discuss other special circulations in the context of particular organs—the lungs in Chapter 31, the kidneys in Chapter 34, the placenta in Chapter 56, and the fetal circulation in Chapter 57.

The blood flow to individual organs must vary to meet the needs of the particular organ as well as of the whole body

The blood flow to each tissue must meet the nutritional needs of that tissue's parenchymal cells while at the same time allowing those cells to play their role in the homeostasis of the whole individual. The way in which the circulatory system distributes blood flow must be flexible so that changing demands can be met. In the process of meeting these demands, the body makes compromises. Consider the circulatory changes that accompany exercise. Blood flow to active skeletal muscle increases tremendously through both an increase and a redistribution of cardiac output. Blood flow to the coronary circulation must also rise to meet the demands of exercise. Furthermore, to dispose of the heat generated during exercise, the vessels in the skin dilate, thereby promoting heat transfer to the environment. As cardiac output is increasingly directed to active muscle and skin, circulation to the splanchnic and renal circulations decreases while blood flow to the brain is preserved.

This chapter focuses on the perfusion of select *systemic* vascular beds, but keep in mind that the lungs receive the entire cardiac output and therefore must also be able to accommodate any changes in total blood flow.

Neural, myogenic, metabolic, and endothelial mechanisms control regional blood flow

Several mechanisms govern vascular resistance and thus the distribution of blood circulating throughout the body. The extent to which a particular bed depends on a particular blood flow control mechanism varies from organ to organ. We have discussed these mechanisms in the preceding chapters and briefly review them here.

The interplay among these four mechanisms establishes a resting level of vasomotor tone. Vascular smooth muscle cells (VSMCs) and endothelial cells also use gap junctions for electrical and chemical signaling between themselves, thereby coordinating their activity during vasomotor control.

In addition to these mechanisms, which are part of a sophisticated feedback control system, other factors—which are *not* regulatory in nature—can affect the local circulation. These *other* factors are all mechanical forces that are external to the blood vessels and that tend either to collapse or to open them (see Chapter 22). For example, in the heart and skeletal muscle, muscle contraction transiently halts blood flow by compressing blood vessels within the tissue.

Neural Mechanisms The resistance vessels of nearly every organ are invested with fibers of the autonomic nervous system (ANS), particularly those of the sympathetic division (see Chapter 23). In addition to its critical role in controlling blood pressure and cardiac output, the ANS modulates local blood flow to meet the needs of particular tissues.

Myogenic Mechanisms Many vessels, particularly the muscular arteries and arterioles that govern vascular resistance, are inherently responsive to changes in transmural pressure. Increased pressure and the accompanying stretch of VSMCs elicit vasoconstriction, whereas decreased pressure elicits vasodilation. This myogenic response plays an important role in the autoregulation that occurs in the vessels of the brain, heart, skeletal muscle, and kidneys. (See Chapter 20.)

Metabolic Mechanisms Throughout the body, the vessels that govern blood flow are sensitive to the local metabolic needs of parenchymal cells. Table 20-8 lists several changes that act synergistically to increase local blood flow. For example, a decrease in P_{O_2} or pH promotes relaxation of VSMCs, thereby causing vasodilation. In response to activity, excitable cells raise extracellular K^+ concentration ($[K^+]_o$), which also causes vasodilation. Tissues with high energy demands—such as the brain, heart, and skeletal muscle during exercise—rely heavily on such local control mechanisms.

Endothelial Mechanisms Endothelial cells release a variety of vasoactive substances (see Table 20-9). For example, the shear stress exerted by the movement of blood through the vessel lumen stimulates the release of nitric oxide (NO), which relaxes VSMCs and prevents leukocyte adhesion.

THE BRAIN

Anastomoses at the circle of Willis and among the branches of distributing arteries protect the blood supply to the brain, which is approximately 15% of cardiac output

The brain accounts for only ~2% of the body's weight, yet it receives ~15% of the resting cardiac output. Of all the tissues in the body, the brain is the least tolerant of ischemia. It depends entirely on oxidative sources of energy production. Each day, the human brain oxidizes ~100 g of glucose, which is roughly equivalent to the amount stored as glycogen in the liver. Interruption of cerebral blood flow for just a few seconds causes unconsciousness. If ischemia persists for even a few minutes, irreversible cellular damage is likely.

Arteries Blood reaches the brain through four *source arteries*—the two internal carotid arteries and the two vertebral arteries (Fig. 24-1). The vertebral arteries join to form the basilar artery, which then splits to form the two posterior cerebral arteries, which in turn are part of the **circle of Willis** at the base of the brain. The internal carotid arteries are the major source of blood to the circle. Three bilateral pairs of *distributing arteries* (anterior, middle, and posterior cerebral arteries) arise from the circle of Willis to envelop the cerebral hemispheres. Smaller branches from the vertebral and basilar arteries distribute blood to the brainstem and cerebellum. The distributing arteries give rise to pial arteries that course over the surface of the brain, forming anastomoses, and then branch again into arterioles that penetrate the tissue at right angles to the brain surface. These penetrating arterioles branch centripetally to give rise to capillaries. The anastomoses on the cortical surface provide the collateral circulation that is so important should a distributing artery or one of its branches become occluded. Each of the four source arteries tends to supply the brain region closest to where the source artery joins the circle of Willis. If a stenosis develops in one source artery, other source arteries to the circle of Willis can provide alternative flow. Nevertheless, if flow through a carotid artery becomes severely restricted (e.g., with atherosclerotic plaque), ischemia may occur in the ipsilateral hemisphere, with impairment of function.

A MAJOR ARTERIAL SUPPLY AND CIRCLE OF WILLIS

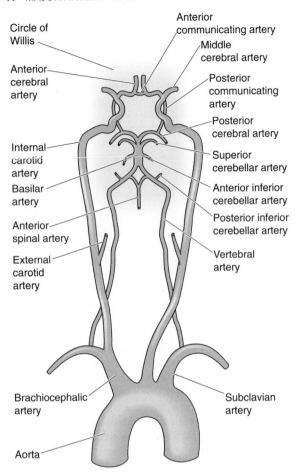

B DISTRIBUTING ARTERIES

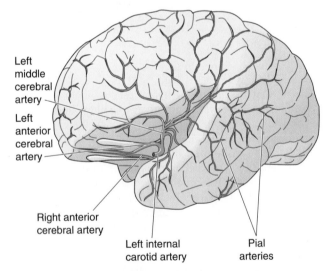

Figure 24-1 Vascular anatomy of the brain. The illustration in **B,** with the temporal lobe pulled away, depicts the major branches of the left middle cerebral artery, one of the distributing arteries. Pial arteries course over the surface of the brain and give rise to penetrating arterioles that supply the microcirculation within the brain.

Veins The veins of the brain are wide, thin-walled structures that are nearly devoid of smooth muscle and have no valves. In general, the veins drain the brain radially, in a centrifugal direction. The intracerebral veins converge into a superficial pial plexus lying under the arteries. The plexus drains into collecting veins, which course over the distributing arteries and empty into the **dural sinuses** (see Fig. 11-1B). The exception to this radial pattern is the deep white matter of the cerebral hemispheres and basal ganglia; these regions drain centrally into veins that course along the walls of the lateral ventricles to form a deep venous system, which also empties into the dural sinuses. Nearly all of the venous blood from the brain leaves the cranium by way of the **internal jugular vein**.

Capillaries One of the most characteristic features of the brain vasculature is the **blood-brain barrier** (see Chapter 11), which prevents the solutes in the lumen of the capillaries from having direct access to the brain extracellular fluid (BECF). For this reason, many drugs that act on other organs or vascular beds have no effect on the brain. Polar and water-soluble compounds cross the blood-brain barrier slowly, and the ability of proteins to cross the barrier is extremely limited. Only water, O_2, and CO_2 (or other gases) can readily diffuse across the cerebral capillaries. Glucose crosses more slowly by facilitated diffusion. No substance is *entirely* excluded from the brain; the critical variable is the rate of transfer. The blood-brain barrier protects the brain from abrupt changes in the composition of arterial blood. In a similar manner, a blood-testis barrier protects the germinal epithelia in males. The blood-brain barrier may become damaged in regions of the brain that are injured, infected, or occupied by tumors. Such damage can be helpful in identifying the location of tumors because tracers that are excluded from healthy central nervous system (CNS) tissue can enter the tumor. In specialized areas of the brain—the **circumventricular organs** (see Chapter 11)—the capillaries are fenestrated and have permeability characteristics similar to those of capillaries in the intestinal circulation.

Lymphatics The brain lacks lymphatic vessels.

Vascular Volume The skull encloses all of the cerebral vasculature, along with the brain and the cerebrospinal fluid compartments. Because the rigid cranium has a fixed total volume, vasodilation and an increase in vascular volume in one region of the brain must be met by reciprocal volume changes elsewhere within the cranium. Tight control of the cerebral blood volume is essential for preventing elevation of the intracranial pressure. With cerebral edema or hemorrhage, or with the growth of a brain tumor, neurological dysfunction can result from the restriction of blood flow due to vascular compression. An analogous situation can occur in the eyes of patients with glaucoma (see Chapter 15). Pressure buildup within the eye compresses the optic nerve and retinal artery, and blindness can result from the damage caused by diminished blood flow to the retinal cells.

Neural, metabolic, and myogenic mechanisms control blood flow to the brain

Cerebral blood flow averages 50 mL/min for each 100 g of brain tissue and, because of autoregulation, is relatively constant. Nevertheless, regional changes in blood distribution occur in response to changing patterns of neuronal activity (Fig. 24-2).

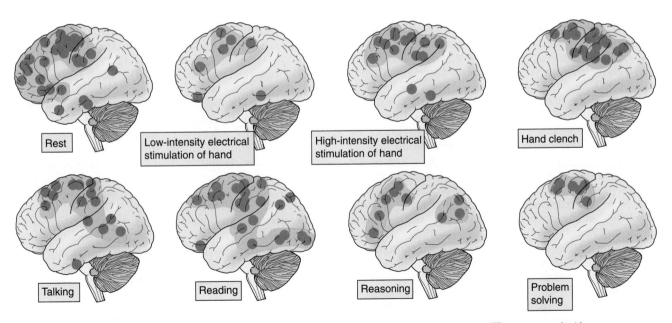

Figure 24-2 Changes in regional blood flow. The investigators used the washout of ^{133}Xe, measured with detectors placed over the side of the patient's head, as an index of regional blood flow in the dominant cerebral hemisphere. The turquoise "hot spots" represent regions where blood flow is more than 20% above mean blood flow for the entire brain. At rest, blood flow is greatest in the frontal and premotor regions. The patterns of blood flow change in characteristic ways with the other seven forms of cerebral activity. *(Data from Ingvar DH: Functional landscapes of the dominant hemisphere. Brain Res 1976; 107:181-197.)*

Neural Control *Sympathetic* nerve fibers supplying the brain vasculature originate from postganglionic neurons in the superior cervical ganglia and travel with the internal carotid and vertebral arteries into the skull, branching with the arterial supply. The sympathetic nerve terminals release norepinephrine, which causes contraction of VSMCs. *Parasympathetic* innervation of the cerebral vessels arises from branches of the facial nerve; they elicit a modest vasodilation when activated. The cerebral vessels are also supplied with sensory nerves, whose cell bodies are located in the trigeminal ganglia and whose sensory processes contain substance P and calcitonin gene–related peptide, both of which are vasodilatory neurotransmitters. Local perturbations (e.g., changes in pressure or chemistry) may stimulate the sensory nerve endings to release these vasodilators, an example of an axon reflex.

Despite this innervation, neural control of the cerebral vasculature is relatively weak. Instead, it is the local metabolic requirements of the brain cells that primarily govern vasomotor activity in the brain.

Metabolic Control Neural activity leads to ATP breakdown and to the local production and release of adenosine, a potent vasodilator. A local increase in brain metabolism also lowers P_{O_2} while raising P_{CO_2} and lowering pH in the nearby BECF. These changes trigger vasodilation and thus a compensatory increase in blood flow. Cerebral VSMCs relax mainly in response to low *extra*cellular pH; these cells are insensitive to increased P_{CO_2} per se, and decreased intracellular pH actually causes a weak vasoconstriction.

How does brain blood flow respond to systemic changes in pH? Lowering of *arterial* pH at a constant P_{CO_2} (metabolic acidosis; see Chapter 28) has little effect on cerebral blood flow because arterial H^+ cannot easily penetrate the blood-brain barrier and therefore does not readily reach cerebral VSMCs. On the other hand, lowering of arterial pH by increasing P_{CO_2} (respiratory acidosis; see Chapter 28) rapidly leads to a fall in the pH around VSMCs because CO_2 readily crosses the blood-brain barrier. This fall in pH of the BECF evokes pronounced dilation of the cerebral vasculature, with an increase in blood flow that occurs within seconds. The rise in arterial P_{CO_2} caused by inhalation of 7% CO_2 can cause cerebral blood flow to double. Conversely, the fall in arterial P_{CO_2} caused by hyperventilation raises the pH of the BECF, producing cerebral vasoconstriction, decreased blood flow, and dizziness. Clinically, hyperventilation is used to lower cerebral blood flow in the emergency treatment of acute cerebral edema and glaucoma.

A fall in the blood and tissue P_{O_2}—from hypoxemia or impaired cardiac output—may also contribute to cerebral vasodilation, although the effects are less dramatic than those produced by arterial hypercapnia. The vasodilatory effects of hypoxia may be direct or may be mediated by release of adenosine, K^+, or NO into the BECF.

Myogenic Control Cerebral resistance vessels are inherently responsive to changes in their transmural pressure. Increases in pressure lead to vasoconstriction, whereas decreases in pressure produce vasodilation.

The neurovascular unit matches blood flow to local brain activity

Neurons, glia, and cerebral blood vessels function as an integrated unit to distribute cerebral blood flow according to local activity within the brain (Fig. 24-2). This "neurovascular coupling" involves several signaling pathways that complement the metabolic control discussed before. Some neurotransmitters and neuromodulators are vasoactive (e.g., acetylcholine, catecholamines, and neuropeptides) and can control blood vessels in the region of synaptic activity. The endfeet of astrocytes (see Fig. 11-9) come into direct contact with the smooth muscle penetrating arterioles and the endothelial cells of capillaries. The release of neurotransmitters (e.g., glutamate and γ-aminobutyric acid) from neurons initiates $[Ca^{2+}]_i$ waves in astrocytes as well as in dendrites of adjacent neurons. These $[Ca^{2+}]_i$ waves stimulate the release of powerful vasodilators, including NO and metabolites of arachidonic acid. Thus, synaptic activity generates vasoactive mediators in neurons and astrocytes that can produce vasodilation. Concurrent activation of local interneurons with vascular projections helps focus the vasomotor response. The vasodilator signal conducts through gap junctions from cell to cell along the endothelium and smooth muscle cells of penetrating arterioles, retrograde to the pial arteries, which are a major part of vascular resistance. This reduction in proximal resistance directs increased blood flow to the region of increased neural activity.

Autoregulation maintains a fairly constant cerebral blood flow across a broad range of perfusion pressures

The perfusion pressure to the brain is the difference between the systemic arterial pressure (mean pressure, ~95 mm Hg) and intracranial venous pressure, which is nearly equal to the intracranial pressure (<10 mm Hg). A decrease in cerebral blood flow could thus result from a fall in arterial pressure or a rise in intracranial (or venous) pressure. However, the local control of cerebral blood flow maintains a nearly constant blood flow through perfusion pressures ranging from ~70 to 150 mm Hg. This constancy of blood flow—**autoregulation** (see Chapter 20)—maintains a continuous supply of O_2 and nutrients. In patients with hypertension, the cerebral blood flow remains normal because cerebral vascular resistance increases. Conversely, vascular resistance falls with hypotension. This autoregulation of blood flow has both myogenic and metabolic components.

Increases in intracranial pressure compress the brain vasculature and tend to reduce blood flow despite autoregulatory vasodilation. In such cases, the brain regulates its blood flow by inducing reflexive changes in *systemic arterial pressure*. This principle is exemplified by the **Cushing reflex**, an increase in arterial pressure that occurs in response to an increase in intracranial pressure. It appears that intracranial compression causes a local ischemia that stimulates vasomotor centers in the medulla. Increased sympathetic nerve activity in the systemic circulation then triggers a rise in total peripheral resistance. The Cushing reflex may occur acutely with the swelling that follows a head injury or more gradually with growth of a brain tumor. Over a considerable pressure range, the Cushing reflex ensures that the perfusion pressure can offset the effects of vascular compression and thereby maintain the constancy of cerebral blood flow.

THE HEART

The coronary circulation receives 5% of the resting cardiac output from the left side of the heart and mostly returns it to the right side of the heart

The heart receives ~5% of the resting cardiac output, although it represents less than 0.5% of total body weight. The heart normally uses oxidative phosphorylation to generate the ATP required to pump blood. However, of all the O_2 that the heart consumes, no more than 40% reflects the oxidation of carbohydrate. More than 60% of myocardial O_2 consumption in the fasting state is due to the oxidation of fatty acids. The myocardium readily oxidizes ketone bodies (see Chapter 51), which can provide considerable energy during starvation or during diabetic ketoacidosis. When the O_2 supply is adequate, the heart takes up and oxidizes both lactate and pyruvate, as do red (i.e., oxidative) skeletal muscle fibers, although the arterial concentration of pyruvate is usually low. When the energetic demand for ATP exceeds the supply of O_2, the heart can no longer take up lactate but instead releases lactate by breaking down its own glycogen stores. In this manner, the heart can continue to function for a short time when it is deprived of O_2. If hypoxia develops in the myocardium, nociceptive fibers trigger the sensation of referred pain, known as **angina pectoris**. More severe or prolonged insults damage the myocardial tissue, which eventually becomes necrotic (**myocardial infarction**).

The entire blood supply to the myocardium derives from the right and left coronary arteries, which originate at the root of the aorta behind the cusps of the aortic valves (Fig. 24-3). Although anatomy is subject to individual variation, the **right coronary artery** generally supplies the right ventricle and atrium, and the left coronary artery supplies the

left ventricle and atrium. The **left coronary artery** divides near its origin into two principal branches: the **left circumflex artery** sends branches to the left atrium and ventricle, and the **left anterior descending artery** descends to the apex of the heart and branches to supply the interventricular septum and a portion of the right as well as the left ventricle. These arteries course over the heart, branching into segments that penetrate into the tissue and dividing into capillary networks. Capillary density in histological sections of the human heart exceeds $3000/mm^2$ (skeletal muscle has only ~$400/mm^2$). The small diameter of cardiac muscle fibers ($<20\mu m$), less than half that of skeletal muscle (~$50\mu m$), facilitates O_2 diffusion into the cardiac cells, which have a high energetic demand.

Once blood passes through the capillaries, it collects in venules, which drain outward from the myocardium to converge into the epicardial veins. These veins empty into the right atrium through the **coronary sinus**. Other vascular channels drain directly into the cardiac chambers. These include the **thebesian veins**, which drain capillary beds within the ventricular wall. Because the deoxygenated blood carried by the thebesian veins exits predominantly into the ventricles, this blood flow bypasses the pulmonary circulation. Numerous *collateral* vessels among branches of the arterial vessels and throughout the venous system act as anastomoses; these provide alternative routes for blood flow should a primary vessel become occluded.

Extravascular compression impairs coronary blood flow during systole

In other systemic vascular beds, blood flow roughly parallels the pressure profile in the aorta, rising in systole and falling in diastole (see Fig. 22-3A). However, in the coronary circulation, flow is somewhat paradoxical. Although the heart is the source of its own perfusion pressure, myocardial contraction effectively compresses its own vascular supply. Therefore, the profile of blood flow through the coronary arteries depends on both the perfusion pressure in the aorta (Fig. 24-4, top panel) and the extravascular compression

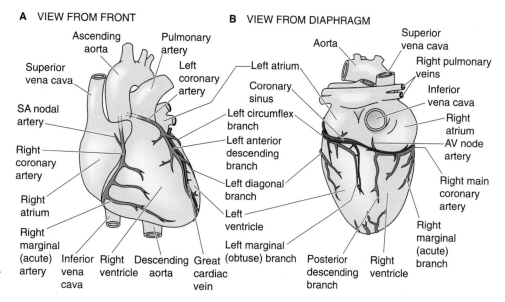

Figure 24-3 Heart and coronary circulation.

A VIEW FROM FRONT

Ascending aorta
Pulmonary artery
Superior vena cava
Left coronary artery
SA nodal artery
Right coronary artery
Right atrium
Right marginal (acute) artery
Inferior vena cava
Right ventricle
Descending aorta
Great cardiac vein

B VIEW FROM DIAPHRAGM

Aorta
Superior vena cava
Left atrium
Right pulmonary veins
Coronary sinus
Inferior vena cava
Left circumflex branch
Right atrium
Left anterior descending branch
AV node artery
Left diagonal branch
Right main coronary artery
Left ventricle
Left marginal (obtuse) branch
Right marginal (acute) branch
Posterior descending branch
Right ventricle

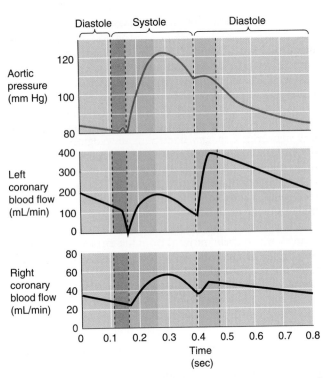

Figure 24-4 Coronary blood flow cycle. Bands at beginning of systole and diastole reflect isovolumetric contraction and relaxation, respectively.

resulting from the contracting ventricles, particularly the left ventricle.

Blood flow in the *left coronary artery* may actually reverse transiently in early systole (Fig. 24-4, middle panel), as the force of the left ventricle's isovolumetric contraction compresses the left coronary vessels, while the aortic pressure has not yet begun to rise (i.e., aortic valve is still closed). As aortic pressure increases later during systole, coronary blood flow increases but never reaches peak values. However, early during diastole, when the relaxed ventricles no longer compress the left coronary vessels and aortic pressure is still high, left coronary flow rises rapidly to extremely high levels. All told, ~80% of total left coronary blood flow occurs during diastole.

In contrast, the profile of flow through the *right coronary artery* (Fig. 24-4, lower panel) is very similar to the pressure profile of its feed vessel, the aorta. Here, systole contributes a greater proportion of the total flow, and systolic reversal does not occur. The reason for this difference is the lower wall tension developed by the right side of the heart, which pumps against the low resistance of the pulmonary circulation and does not occlude the right coronary vessels during contraction.

The impact of systolic contraction on the perfusion of the left coronary vessels is highlighted by the effect of ventricular fibrillation (see Fig. 21-14I). At the onset of this lethal arrhythmia, left coronary perfusion transiently *increases*, reflecting the loss of mechanical compression of the vasculature.

Changes in heart rate, because they affect the duration of diastole more than that of systole, also affect coronary flow. During tachycardia, the fraction of the cardiac cycle spent in diastole decreases, minimizing the time available for maximal left coronary perfusion. If the heart is healthy, the coronary vessels can adequately dilate in response to the metabolic signals generated by increased cardiac work, which offsets the negative effects of the shorter diastole. On the other hand, a high heart rate can be dangerous when severe coronary artery disease restricts blood flow.

Coronary blood flow not only varies in *time* during the cardiac cycle, it also varies with *depth* in the wall of the heart. Blood flows to cardiac myocytes through arteries that penetrate from the epicardium toward the endocardium. During systole, the intramuscular pressure is greatest near the endocardium and least near the epicardium. All things being equal, the perfusion of the endocardium would therefore be less than that of the epicardium. However, total blood flows to the endocardial and epicardial halves are approximately equal because the endocardium has a lower intrinsic vascular resistance and thus a greater blood flow during *diastole*. When the diastolic pressure at the root of the aorta is pathologically low (e.g., aortic regurgitation) or coronary arterial resistance is high (e.g., coronary artery occlusion), endocardial blood flow falls below the epicardial flow. Thus, the inner wall of the left ventricle often experiences the greatest damage with atherosclerotic heart disease.

Myocardial blood flow parallels myocardial metabolism

A striking feature of the coronary circulation is the nearly linear correspondence between myocardial O_2 consumption and myocardial blood flow. This relationship persists in isolated heart preparations, emphasizing that metabolic signals are the principal determinants of O_2 delivery to the myocardium. In a resting individual, each 100 g of heart tissue receives 60 to 70 mL/min of blood flow. Normally, the heart extracts 70% to 80% of the O_2 content of arterial blood (normally ~20 mL/dL blood), thereby producing an extremely low venous O_2 content (~5 mL/dL). Therefore, the myocardium cannot respond to increased metabolic demands by extracting much more O_2 than it already does when the individual is at rest. The heart can meet large increases in O_2 demand only by increasing coronary blood flow, which can exceed 250 mL/min per 100 g with exercise.

Because blood pressure normally varies within fairly narrow limits, the only way to substantially increase blood flow through the coronary circulation during exercise is by vasodilation. The heart relies primarily on metabolic mechanisms to increase the caliber of its coronary vessels. **Adenosine** has received particular emphasis in this regard. An increased metabolic activity of the heart, an insufficient coronary blood flow, or a fall in myocardial P_{O_2} results in adenosine release. Adenosine then diffuses to the VSMCs, activating purinoceptors to induce vasodilation by lowering $[Ca^{2+}]_i$ (see Table 20-7). Thus, inadequate perfusion to a region of tissue would elevate interstitial adenosine levels, causing vasodilation and restoration of flow to the affected region.

When cardiac demand outstrips the blood supply, a transient rise in $[K^+]_o$ may also contribute to the initial increase in coronary perfusion (see Table 20-8). However, it is unlikely that K^+ mediates sustained elevations in blood flow. When O_2 demand exceeds O_2 supply, a rise in the P_{CO_2} and a fall in P_{O_2} may also lower coronary vascular resistance.

Coronary blood flow is relatively stable between perfusion pressures of ~70 mm Hg and more than 150 mm Hg. Thus, like that of the brain, the blood flow to the heart exhibits autoregulation. In addition to the myogenic response, fluctuations in adenosine and P_{O_2} contribute to coronary autoregulation.

Although sympathetic stimulation directly constricts coronary vessels, accompanying metabolic effects predominate, producing an overall vasodilation

Sympathetic nerves course throughout the heart, following the arterial supply. Stimulation of these nerves causes the heart to beat more frequently and more forcefully. β_1 Adrenoceptors on the cardiac myocytes mediate these chronotropic and inotropic responses. As discussed in the preceding section, the increased metabolic work of the myocardium leads to coronary vasodilation through metabolic pathways. However, during pharmacological inhibition of the β_1 receptors on the cardiac myocytes, which prevents the increase in metabolism, sympathetic nerve stimulation causes a coronary *vasoconstriction*. This response is the direct effect of sympathetic nerve activity on α adrenoceptors on the VSMCs of the coronary resistance vessels. Thus, blocking of β_1 receptors "unmasks" adrenergic vasoconstriction. However, under normal circumstances (i.e., no β blockade), the tendency of the *metabolic* pathways to vasodilate far overwhelms the tendency of the *sympathetic* pathways to vasoconstrict.

Activation of the **vagus nerve** has only a mild vasodilatory effect on the coronary resistance vessels. This muted response is not due to insensitivity of the resistance vessels to acetylcholine, which elicits a pronounced vasodilation when it is administered directly. Rather, the release of acetylcholine from the vagus nerve is restricted to the vicinity of the sinoatrial node. Thus, the vagus nerve has a much greater effect on heart rate than on coronary resistance.

Collateral vessel growth can provide blood flow to ischemic regions

When a coronary artery or one of its primary branches becomes abruptly occluded, ischemia can produce necrosis (i.e., a myocardial infarct) in the region deprived of blood flow. However, if a coronary artery narrows *gradually* over time, collateral blood vessels may develop and at least partially ameliorate the reduced delivery of O_2 and nutrients to the compromised area, preventing or at least diminishing tissue damage. Collateral vessels originate from existing branches that undergo remodeling with the proliferation of endothelial and smooth muscle cells. Stimuli for collateral development include angiogenic molecules (see Chapter 20) released from the ischemic tissue and changes in mechanical stress in the walls of vessels supplying the affected region.

Vasodilator drugs may compromise myocardial flow through "coronary steal"

A variety of drugs can promote vasodilation of the coronary arteries. These are typically prescribed for patients suffering from angina pectoris, the chest pain associated with inadequate blood flow to the heart (see box titled Treating Coronary Artery Disease). If the buildup of atherosclerotic plaque—which underlies angina pectoris—occurs in the large epicardial arteries, the increased resistance lowers the pressure in the downstream microvessels. Under such conditions, the physician should be cautious in using pharmacological agents to dilate the coronary vessels. In an ischemic area of the myocardium downstream from a stenosis, metabolic stimuli may have already maximally dilated the arterioles. Administration of a vasodilator can then only increase the diameter of blood vessels in *nonischemic* vascular beds that are parallel to the ischemic ones. The result is **coronary steal**, a further reduction in the pressure downstream from the site of stenosis and further compromise of the blood flow to the ischemic region. When vasodilator therapy relieves angina, the favorable result is more likely to be attributable to the vasodilation of the *noncoronary* systemic vessels, which reduces peripheral resistance, thereby reducing the afterload during systole and thus the work of the heart.

THE SKELETAL MUSCLE

Perhaps the most impressive characteristic of the blood flow to skeletal muscle is its extreme range. Muscle blood flow at rest is 5 to 10 mL/min for each 100 g of tissue. With maximal aerobic exercise, it may increase 50-fold, reaching 250 mL/min or more for each 100 g of active muscle. The linear correspondence among work rate, O_2 consumption, and muscle blood flow implies a "coupling" between muscle fiber activity and O_2 delivery to capillaries. Muscle blood flow during exercise is the subject of Chapter 60. Here we discuss the key features of the organization of the skeletal muscle vasculature and the integration of its blood flow control mechanisms.

A microvascular unit is the capillary bed supplied by a single terminal arteriole

The vascular supply to skeletal muscle begins external to the tissue in the **feed arteries**. These muscular vessels are the last branches of the arterial supply, located just before entry into the tissue. As much as 30% to 50% of the total resistance to blood flow through skeletal muscle resides in these feed arteries. Therefore, an important site of blood flow control is located *proximal* to the microvessels that are in direct contact with skeletal muscle fibers.

The arteriolar network originates from the site at which a feed artery enters the muscle. Within the muscle, arterioles branch through several orders (Fig. 24-5A) until reaching the **terminal arterioles** (Fig. 24-5B), which are the last branches to contain smooth muscle and therefore the last branches still able to control blood flow. Thus, the terminal arteriole is the functional equivalent of the precapillary sphincter (see Chapter 20). The group of capillaries supplied by a terminal arteriole represents one **microvascular unit**, which is the smallest functional unit of blood flow control in skeletal muscle. Each unit consists of 15 to 20 capillaries that run parallel to the muscle fibers in each direction, for a distance of 1 mm or less, ending in a **collecting venule**.

A SKELETAL-MUSCLE CIRCULATION

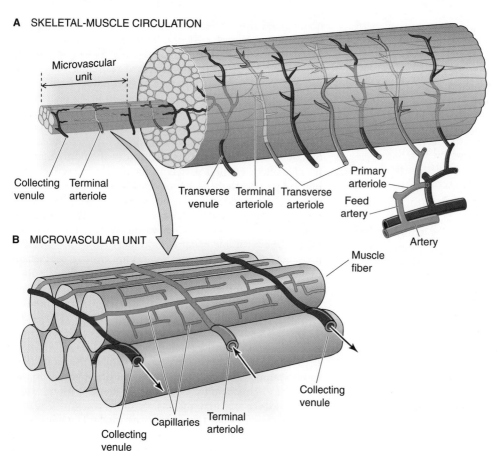

Figure 24-5 Microvascular units in skeletal muscle. **A,** A feed artery (FA) branches into primary arterioles, which after two more orders of branching gives rise to transverse arterioles (3A), which in turn gives rise to terminal arterioles (4A). **B,** The terminal arteriole supplies a microvascular unit (<1 mm in length).

Owing to the profound differences in length between capillaries (≤1 mm) and muscle fibers (centimeters), many microvascular units are required to span the distance of each muscle fiber. When a muscle fiber contracts, blood flow must increase throughout all of the microvascular units that supply that fiber to provide O_2 and to remove metabolites.

Metabolites released by active muscle trigger vasodilation and an increase in blood flow

When skeletal muscle is at rest, its vascular resistance is high, blood flow is low, and the venous O_2 content is only a few milliliters per deciliter lower than the arterial O_2 content. As exercise begins, the terminal arterioles (those closest to the capillaries) dilate first. This vasodilation increases blood flow through capillaries that are already conducting blood and also opens up quiescent capillaries, thus increasing the number of perfused capillaries and decreasing the effective intercapillary distance. If total blood flow has not yet increased very much, the increased muscle demand for O_2 produces a large increase in the O_2 extraction ratio (see Chapter 20). As metabolic demand later increases, additional O_2 delivery is required. The vasculature meets this demand by progressively dilating the terminal arterioles, then the more proximal arteriolar branches and feed arteries. Thus, vasodilation "ascends" the resistance network.

A coordinated vasodilation throughout the resistance network is essential when segments having substantial resistance are organized *in series* with each other. Dilation of the

downstream arterioles, without dilation of the proximal arterioles and feed arteries, would result in only a limited ability to increase muscle blood flow because of the high resistance of upstream vessels. Thus, when feed arteries dilate in concert with arterioles, the increase in muscle blood flow is profound.

The primary stimulus triggering vasodilation is the release of vasodilator substances (e.g., adenosine, CO_2, K^+) from active muscle fibers in proportion to the energy expenditure. These metabolites diffuse locally and—acting either directly on VSMCs or indirectly on adjacent endothelial cells—relax the VSMCs of resistance vessels, thereby increasing blood flow in proportion to local demand. Although a variety of substances released by muscle fibers can contribute to the hyperemia, no single stimulus yet explains the integrated response of blood-flow control to muscle contraction. Furthermore, the hyperemic response to increased muscle activity begins within a second or two of the onset of exercise. In contrast, it would take several seconds for these substances to be produced by the skeletal muscle fibers, to reach the interstitium, and to diffuse to the arteriolar VSMCs in sufficient concentration to elicit vasodilation.

The initiation of muscle fiber contraction leads to a release of K^+ that may hyperpolarize the nearby VSMCs (see Table 20-8). Once triggered, this hyperpolarization causes the small proximal arterioles to dilate, and the electrical signal spreads from cell to cell through gap junctions along the endothelium and into VSMCs, conducting upstream to the larger vessels and causing them to dilate in concert. This mechanism of conducted vasodilation, together with the

Treating Coronary Artery Disease

For many patients with gradual narrowing of their coronary arteries by atherosclerotic plaque, the first sign of disease may be the development of **angina pectoris**. Pain results when the metabolic demands of a region of myocardium exceed the ability of the compromised blood supply to satisfy those needs. Attacks of angina are often accompanied by characteristic changes on the electrocardiogram. If the diagnosis is in doubt—the chest pain of angina can sometimes be mimicked by gastroesophageal reflux, hyperventilation, costochondritis, and other clinical entities—an exercise test may stress the heart sufficiently to bring on the pain, to induce electrocardiographic changes, or to alter coronary blood flow as monitored by a thallium scan (see Chapter 17). Some patients with significant coronary artery narrowing never experience angina and are said to have silent *ischemia*. In these patients, only an astute clinician may detect the coronary disease.

Many patients with a stable anginal pattern respond well to medication. *Nitrates* induce vasodilation by releasing NO (see Chapter 3). The nitrates dilate peripheral veins, reducing venous return and thus the preload to the heart (see Chapter 22); they also dilate the arteries and arterioles, reducing blood pressure and therefore the afterload. Finally, nitrates may increase coronary collateral flow to the involved region of myocardium (see discussion of coronary steal). *Beta blockers* prevent the sympathetic nervous system from stimulating myocardial β_1 receptors, thereby reducing both heart rate and contractility and thus metabolic demand. *Calcium channel blockers* lessen the contractility of the heart muscle and the vascular smooth muscle. These interventions all reduce the metabolic demands of the heart.

In patients for whom medication cannot control the angina or who develop a pattern of unstable angina with an increasing frequency and severity of anginal attacks, mechanical revascularization may be required. For a long time, the only option was coronary artery bypass grafting, but **percutaneous transluminal coronary angioplasty** may now often be successful. A cardiologist can perform this procedure at the same time as a diagnostic coronary artery catheterization. The physician advances a balloon-tipped catheter through a peripheral artery into the left ventricle and then loops the catheter back out the left ventricle to have a favorable angle for entering the coronary vessels from the aorta. Inflation of the balloon at the site of the obstruction flattens the plaque into the wall of the vessel and restores blood flow. Recurrence of the obstruction may be due to proliferation of VSMCs. Refinements in the technique, placement of stents at the treated site, and use of aggressive anticoagulation have all contributed to the technique's growing success. Variants of this technique, in which lasers are used, are coming under study increasingly.

Given the continued prevalence of coronary artery disease, a great deal of research has been aimed at developing alternatives to medication and mechanical revascularization. Among the most promising of these is the use of angiogenesis promoters that promote the growth of new blood vessels (see Chapter 20).

action of the muscle pump, probably contributes to the rapid onset of hyperemia (discussed later). Increases in levels of other metabolites (e.g., adenosine and CO_2 levels) or decreases in P_{O_2} contribute to and sustain the hyperemic response.

Sympathetic innervation increases the intrinsic tone of resistance vessels

Sympathetic nerve fibers invest the entire resistance network, from feed arteries to terminal arterioles. The release of norepinephrine by these nerve terminals leads to vasoconstriction. Increased transmural pressure results in increased myogenic tone, also producing vasoconstriction. On the other hand, the shear stress of blood flowing past the endothelial cells produces vasodilators, such as NO. The interactions among these vasoconstrictor and vasodilatory mechanisms maintain the intrinsic basal tone of the VSMCs. Venules also constrict in response to sympathetic nerve stimulation but are not directly innervated and instead respond to norepinephrine that diffuses from the nearby arterioles.

With nearly one third of total body mass composed of muscle, the sympathetic control of vasomotor tone to skeletal muscle is an integral component of the regulation of both systemic arterial pressure (through total peripheral resistance) and cardiac filling (through venous capacitance and return). This principle is particularly true during maximal aerobic exercise, when more than 80% of the cardiac output flows to the active skeletal muscles.

The basal firing rate of the sympathetic nerves to skeletal muscle is 1 to 2 Hz, which contributes only modestly to the resting vasomotor tone. However, when high-pressure baroreceptors detect a fall in blood pressure (see Chapter 23), sympathetic firing to skeletal muscle may increase to 8 to 16 Hz. This degree of sympathetic nerve activity can close the lumens of arterioles in skeletal muscle.

During exercise, the proportion of cardiac output flowing through skeletal muscle increases. This redistribution of systemic blood flow occurs for two reasons. First, an increase in sympathetic tone constricts splanchnic circulation (see later), renal circulation (see Chapter 34), and the vessels of *inactive* skeletal muscle. Indeed, only the brain and heart are spared. Second, the metabolites released by *active* skeletal muscle overcome the vasoconstriction that sympathetic activity would otherwise produce. In addition, substances released during muscle fiber contraction (e.g., NO and adenosine) may inhibit norepinephrine release from sympathetic neurons.

The vasodilatory effects of the metabolites notwithstanding, sympathetic vasoconstrictor activity can be overwhelming, particularly when another large mass of muscle is active simultaneously and requires a substantial portion of cardiac output. Thus, during "whole-body" exercise, each muscle group may receive only a fraction of the blood flow it would otherwise get if it were the *only* active group in the body. It is at the level of the feed arteries—which are external to the muscle and thus physically removed from the direct influence of the vasoactive products of muscular activity—that sympathetic vasoconstriction puts an upper limit on blood

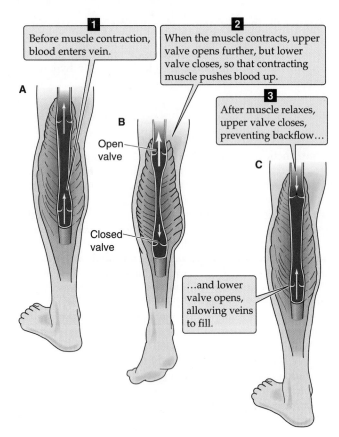

1 Before muscle contraction, blood enters vein.

2 When the muscle contracts, upper valve opens further, but lower valve closes, so that contracting muscle pushes blood up.

3 After muscle relaxes, upper valve closes, preventing backflow…

Open valve

Closed valve

…and lower valve opens, allowing veins to fill.

Figure 24-6 Muscle pump.

flow during intense aerobic exercise. At the same time, dilation of arterioles *within* the active muscle maximizes O_2 extraction by promoting capillary perfusion.

Rhythmic contraction promotes blood flow through the muscle pump

During exercise, skeletal muscle undergoes rhythmic changes in length and tension, giving rise to mechanical forces within the tissue analogous to those of the beating heart. The contraction of muscle forces venous blood out of the muscle and impedes arterial inflow (Fig. 24-6). Because valves in the veins prevent backflow of blood, each muscle contraction squeezes and empties the veins, driving blood toward the heart (see Chapter 22). During the subsequent relaxation, the reduction in venous pressure increases the driving force for capillary perfusion. In addition, peak arterial inflow occurs during relaxation between contractions. This pumping action of skeletal muscle on the vasculature imparts substantial kinetic energy to the blood, thereby reducing the work of the heart. Remarkably, the skeletal muscle pump may generate up to half of the energy required to circulate blood, an essential contribution for achieving the high blood flows experienced during maximal aerobic exercise. By contrast, use of drugs to dilate blood vessels of inactive muscle can increase blood flow to a lesser extent than is observed with rhythmic contractions.

THE SPLANCHNIC CIRCULATION

The splanchnic circulation includes the blood flow through the stomach, small intestine, large intestine, pancreas, spleen, and liver (Fig. 24-7A). The majority of flow to the liver occurs through the portal vein, which carries the venous blood draining from all of these organs except the liver itself.

The vascular supply to the gut is highly interconnected

The **celiac artery** is the primary blood supply to the stomach, pancreas, and spleen. The **superior and inferior mesenteric arteries** supply the large and small intestines as well as parts of the stomach and pancreas. The superior mesenteric artery is the largest of all the splanchnic branches from the aorta, carrying more than 10% of the cardiac output. The extensive interconnections between the arcading arterial branches (Fig. 24-7B) provide multiple collateral pathways through which blood can reach each portion of the intestines. This arrangement lessens the risk that the intestines may become ischemic should one of the arteries become occluded.

The microvascular network in the small intestine (Fig. 24-7C) is representative of that throughout the gastrointestinal tract. After penetrating the wall of the intestine, small arteries course through the various muscle layers and reach the submucosa, where they branch into arterioles. Some arterioles remain in the submucosa to form a submucosal vascular plexus. Others project toward the intestinal lumen and into the mucosa, including the villi. Still others project away from the mucosa and course along the smooth muscle bundles. Venules emerging from the villi and mucosal and muscularis layers converge into veins. These exit the intestinal wall, paralleling the arterial supply.

The arrangement of microvessels within a villus is like a fountain (Fig. 24-7D). The incoming arteriole courses up the center of the villus, branching into many capillaries along the way to the tip of the villus. Capillaries converge into venules and carry blood back to the base of the villus. Capillaries also interconnect the arteriole and the venule all along the villus. These microvessels are permeable to solutes of low molecular weight or high lipid solubility.

The arrangement just described can create a **countercurrent exchange** system that enables permeable solutes to move from the arteriole to the venule without having to traverse the entire length of the villus, particularly under conditions of *low flow*. With prolonged transit times, blood-borne O_2 can diffuse from the arteriole to the venule before reaching the tip of the villus, which makes it susceptible to anoxic damage. The situation is just the opposite for solutes (e.g., Na^+) that the villus epithelium absorbs during digestion. These solutes enter capillaries and then pass into venules. As the venous blood travels toward the base of the villus, the solute can diffuse out of the venules, into the interstitium, and then into the arterioles. In this way, the solute concentration in the arterial blood increases as the blood flows to the tip of the villus. This "trapping" process increases the interstitial osmolarity near the tip of the villus, in a manner analogous to the mechanism that maintains

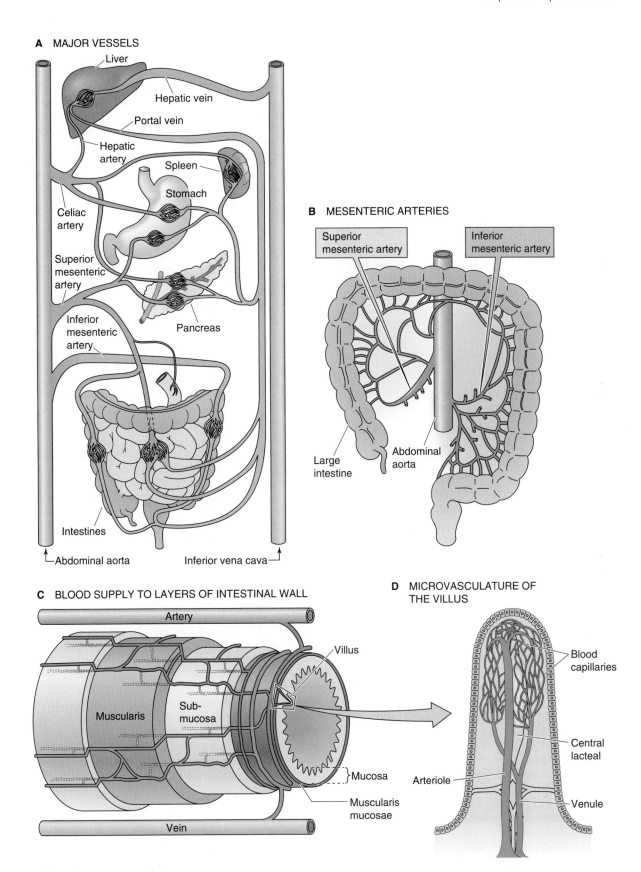

A MAJOR VESSELS

Liver
Hepatic vein
Portal vein
Hepatic artery
Spleen
Stomach
Celiac artery
Superior mesenteric artery
Inferior mesenteric artery
Pancreas
Intestines
Abdominal aorta
Inferior vena cava

B MESENTERIC ARTERIES

Superior mesenteric artery
Inferior mesenteric artery
Large intestine
Abdominal aorta

C BLOOD SUPPLY TO LAYERS OF INTESTINAL WALL

Artery
Villus
Muscularis
Sub-mucosa
Mucosa
Muscularis mucosae
Vein

D MICROVASCULATURE OF THE VILLUS

Blood capillaries
Central lacteal
Arteriole
Venule

Figure 24-7 Splanchnic circulation.

high osmolality at the tip of the renal medulla (see Chapter 38).

In contrast, when the intestinal mucosa is *adequately perfused* (e.g., at rest and particularly after a meal), the tips of the villi are well oxygenated (as in Fig. 24-7D), the effects of countercurrent exchange are reduced, and the osmolality within the villi falls.

Because the capillaries in the villi are fenestrated (i.e., they have large pores) and have a large surface area, they are well suited for absorbing nutrients from the intestinal lumen. The venous blood carries away the majority of **water-soluble nutrients** absorbed from the gut, eventually delivering them to the portal vein. **Lipophilic nutrients** absorbed from the intestinal lumen enter the central lacteal of the villus (Fig. 24-7D), which merges with the intestinal lymphatics. The lymph then delivers these substances into the bloodstream through the thoracic duct.

Blood flow to the gastrointestinal tract increases up to eight-fold after a meal (postprandial hyperemia)

Throughout the gastrointestinal tract, blood flow in each layer of the gut wall closely correlates with the local metabolism (which reflects digestive and absorptive activity). Intestinal blood flow at rest, in the fasting state, is typically 30 mL/min for each 100 g of tissue. However, flow can reach 250 mL/min for each 100 g during peak hyperemia after a meal. The increase in blood flow with the ingestion and digestion of a meal reflects a complex interplay of several factors.

First, the CNS initiates an "anticipatory" response that increases splanchnic blood flow with the mere thought of food—corresponding to the "cephalic phase" of gastric (see Chapter 42) and pancreatic (see Chapter 43) secretion.

Second, mucosal metabolic activity during digestion and absorption primarily depends on the rate of active transport of substances across the epithelium. These activities consume O_2 and produce **vasodilator metabolites** (e.g., adenosine and CO_2) that increase blood flow locally.

Third, the absorption of nutrients generates hyperosmolality in both the blood and the lymphatic vessels of the villus. Hyperosmolality itself stimulates an increase in blood flow.

Fourth, during digestion, the gastrointestinal tract releases several hormones, some of which are vasoactive. Of these, **cholecystokinin** and **neurotensin** (see Table 41-1) may reach high enough concentrations in the local circulation to promote intestinal blood flow. The intestinal epithelium also releases various kinins (e.g., bradykinin and kallidin), which are powerful vasodilators. The magnitude of the postprandial hyperemia further depends on the nature of the luminal content. Bile acids and partially digested fats are particularly effective in promoting hyperemia by acting on chemoreceptors in the intestinal mucosa.

The circulatory system does not distribute the increased splanchnic blood flow equally to all digestive organs, nor does it distribute the flow equally throughout the wall of even one segment of bowel. During and after a meal, blood flow increases sequentially along the gastrointestinal tract, first in the stomach and then in more distal segments of the

intestine as digestion proceeds. In all segments, blood flow through the muscularis layers primarily provides nutrition for the smooth muscle cells. However, flow through the villi and submucosal vessels supports the absorption of foodstuffs as well as the secretion of electrolytes, fluids, and enzymes. After a meal, splanchnic blood flow is elevated for 2 to 4 hours, primarily reflecting the vasodilation in the *mucosal* layer.

As in the heart and skeletal muscle, muscle contraction in the intestine (i.e., peristalsis) decreases blood flow, probably as a result of the compression applied by the muscularis in conjunction with the distending pressure of the luminal contents.

Sympathetic activity directly constricts splanchnic vessels, whereas parasympathetic activity indirectly dilates them

The gastrointestinal tract is endowed with its own division of the ANS, the **enteric nervous system** (ENS; see Chapters 14 and 41). At one level, the ENS is its own independent nervous system, with sensory neurons, the capacity to integrate and to process sensory data, and motor neurons. One of the components of the ENS, the myenteric (or Auerbach) plexus, releases vasoactive neurotransmitters. However, this plexus probably achieves its major influence on blood flow by controlling the peristaltic activity of the intestinal smooth muscle.

The enteric division sends sensory information upstream to the peripheral ganglia and to the CNS. The ENS also receives important input from the sympathetic and parasympathetic divisions of the ANS. Postganglionic **sympathetic neurons** originate in the celiac, superior mesenteric, and inferior mesenteric ganglia and send nerve fibers that travel along the corresponding major arteries to all splanchnic organs. Except for the capillaries, all splanchnic blood vessels receive sympathetic innervation. The predominant neural influence is *sympathetic vasoconstriction*, mediated by norepinephrine acting on α adrenoceptors on VSMCs. The vasoconstriction occurs to a similar extent in both the muscularis and mucosal layers, without redistribution of flow between the layers. Vasoconstriction elicited by sympathetic nerve activity can reduce blood flow to less than 10 mL/min per 100 g of tissue (i.e., ~25% of resting values).

Parasympathetic preganglionic fibers travel to the intestine through vagal or pelvic nerves, which contact postganglionic parasympathetic neurons in the intestinal wall. The effect of parasympathetic activity on blood flow is indirect. Parasympathetic activity stimulates intestinal motility and glandular secretion, which in turn increases intestinal metabolism, thereby enhancing blood flow to the gut.

Changes in the splanchnic circulation regulate total peripheral resistance and the distribution of blood volume

The splanchnic circulation serves both as a site of adjustable resistance and as a major reservoir of blood. During exercise, when blood flow increases to active skeletal muscle, sympathetic constriction of the splanchnic resistance vessels decreases the proportion of cardiac output directed to the viscera. Therefore, abdominal cramping can result from attempts to exercise too soon after eating, when the gastrointestinal tract still demands blood flow to support its digestive and absorptive activities.

The splanchnic circulation contains ~15% of the total blood volume, with the majority contained in the liver; sympathetic constriction of the capacitance vessels can rapidly mobilize about half of this blood volume. During increases in sympathetic tone, splanchnic arteriolar constriction reduces perfusion, resulting in the passive collapse of the splanchnic veins. Blood contained in these veins moves into the inferior vena cava, thus increasing the circulating blood volume. With a greater increase in sympathetic activity, as would occur with intense exercise or severe hemorrhage, active venoconstriction mobilizes even more venous blood, thereby helping to maintain arterial pressure.

Exercise and hemorrhage can substantially reduce splanchnic blood flow

A reduction in blood flow leads to the production of vasodilator metabolites (e.g., adenosine and CO_2), which stimulate arteriolar dilation and increase O_2 delivery. Nevertheless, during maximal exercise or severe hemorrhage, blood flow through the gut may fall to less than 25% of its resting value. Fortunately, temporary reductions in splanchnic flow can occur without serious O_2 deprivation; at rest, the viscera normally extract only ~20% of the O_2 carried in the blood, so that extraction can increase several-fold. However, extended periods of compromised splanchnic blood flow can irreversibly damage the intestinal parenchyma.

After a severe hemorrhage and sustained splanchnic vasoconstriction, the ischemic mucosal epithelia slough off, even after repletion of the blood volume and restoration of blood flow. Sloughing occurs particularly at the tips of the villi, where the epithelial cells are particularly susceptible to ischemia because of countercurrent flow. As these cells slough, it appears that pancreatic enzymes generate "activators" that enter the circulation and produce multiple organ failure. For example, such factors can lead to an irreversible decline in cardiovascular function. In an experimental setting, one can avoid damage to the heart by collecting the blood draining from the gut during the first several minutes of reperfusion, thereby preventing access of these blood-borne substances to the heart. Another major consequence of damage to the epithelium is **endotoxic shock**, which results from disruption of the barrier that normally prevents bacteria and toxins from escaping the intestinal lumen and entering the systemic circulation and peritoneal cavity.

The liver receives its blood flow from both the systemic and the portal circulations

The liver receives nearly one fourth of resting cardiac output. Of this blood flow, ~25% is arterial blood that arrives by the hepatic artery. The remaining 75% of the hepatic blood flow comes from the portal vein, which drains the stomach, intestines, pancreas, and spleen (Fig. 24-7A). Because the portal venous blood has already given up much of its O_2 to the gut, the hepatic artery is left to supply ~75% of the O_2 used by the liver.

We discuss the anatomy of the hepatic circulation in more detail in Chapter 46. Small branches of the portal vein give rise to terminal portal venules, and branches of the hepatic artery give rise to hepatic arterioles. These two independent sources of blood flow enter the liver lobule at its periphery. Blood flows from these terminal vessels into the sinusoids, which form the capillary network of the liver. The sinusoids converge at the center of the lobule to form terminal hepatic venules (i.e., central veins), which drain into progressively larger branches of the hepatic veins and finally into the inferior vena cava. Within the sinusoids, rapid exchange occurs between the blood and the hepatocytes because the vascular endothelial cells have large fenestrations and gaps and thus do not meet to form interendothelial junctions as in other capillaries. Thus, the liver sinusoids are more permeable to protein than are capillaries elsewhere in the body. The passage of blood from the gastrointestinal tract past the reticuloendothelial cells of the liver (see Chapter 46) also removes bacteria and particulate matter, thereby preventing the access of potentially harmful material to the general circulation.

The mean blood pressure in the portal vein is normally 10 to 12 mm Hg. In contrast, the pressure in the hepatic artery averages 90 mm Hg. These two systems, with very different pressures, feed into the sinusoids (8 to 9 mm Hg). The sinusoids drain into the hepatic veins (~5 mm Hg), and these in turn drain into the vena cava (2 to 5 mm Hg). These remarkable values lead us to three conclusions. First, there must be a very high "precapillary" resistance between the hepatic artery (90 mm Hg) and the sinusoids (8 to 9 mm Hg), causing the arterial pressure to step down to sinusoidal values. If the sinusoidal pressure were as high as in typical capillaries (e.g., 25 mm Hg), blood would flow from the hepatic artery to the sinusoids and then backward into the portal vein. Second, because the pressure in the portal vein (10 to 12 mm Hg) is only slightly higher than that in the sinusoids (8 to 9 mm Hg), the precapillary resistance of the portal inflow (75% of the total flow) must be very low. Third, because the pressure in the sinusoids is only slightly higher than that in the hepatic vein (~5 mm Hg), the resistance of the sinusoids must also be extremely low.

As a result of the unique hemodynamics of the liver, changes in pressure within the hepatic vein have profound effects on fluid exchange across the wall of sinusoids. For example, in right-sided congestive heart failure, an elevated vena cava pressure can result in transudation of fluid from the liver into the peritoneal cavity, a condition known as **ascites**.

A change in the blood flow through one of the inputs to the liver (e.g., portal vein) leads to a reciprocal change in flow through the other input (i.e., hepatic artery). However, these adjustments do not fully stabilize total hepatic blood flow. For example, if the inflow through the hepatic artery decreases, the pressure inside the sinusoids falls slightly, leading to an increase in flow from the portal vein into the sinusoids. When the inflow through the portal vein decreases, metabolic factors (e.g., decreases in metabolites carried by the portal blood) trigger an increase in flow from the hepatic arteriolar system. The hepatic arterial supply displays autoregulation (see Chapter 20), which is absent in the portal venous system. With changes in O_2 delivery, the liver

Portal Hypertension

The cirrhotic liver is hard, shrunken, scarred, and laced with thick bands of fibrotic tissue. The most common cause of this in the United States is chronic alcoholism, but worldwide, hepatitis B and hepatitis C are also leading causes. Less commonly, inherited diseases, such as hemochromatosis (iron overload) and Wilson disease (altered copper metabolism), can be responsible, as can diseases of unclear etiology, such as biliary cirrhosis and sclerosing cholangitis.

When damage to the liver becomes severe, the clinical consequences of cirrhosis can become life-threatening. The 5-year survival rate is the same as that for primary lung cancer—less than 10%. The three major complications of cirrhosis are metabolic abnormalities, portal hypertension, and hepatic encephalopathy.

Metabolic Abnormalities

The liver's inability to maintain its normal synthetic activities (see Chapter 46) results in a range of metabolic problems. Both albumin and cholesterol levels fall, and the prothrombin time rises, indicating failure of the liver to manufacture proteins in the coagulation cascade. Decreased plasma levels of K^+ and Na^+ often herald the onset of renal failure, a consequence of the *hepatorenal syndrome*.

Portal Hypertension

The scarring that accompanies cirrhosis causes increased resistance to blood flow through the liver. When the portal venous pressure rises, the signs and symptoms of portal hypertension can appear. The increased portal venous pressure leads to increased pressure in the splanchnic capillaries. The Starling forces (see Chapter 20) thus promote the filtration and extravasation of fluid. The result is abdominal edema (i.e., fluid accumulation in the interstitium), which can progress to frank **ascites** (i.e., fluid in the peritoneal cavity). As the portal pressure rises farther, a portion of the portal blood begins to flow through and dilate the portal anastomoses with systemic veins. These anastomoses are present in the lower esophagus, around the umbilicus, at the rectum, and in the retroperitoneum.

Dilation of the vessels in the lower esophagus can lead to the development of *esophageal varices*. These veins, and similar veins in the stomach, can burst and cause life-threatening hemorrhage. When varices are associated with persistent or recurrent bleeding, the physician can inject sclerosing agents directly into the varices, a procedure called sclerotherapy. However, even after sclerotherapy, recurrent bleeding is not uncommon, and complications include perforation, stricture formation, infection, and aspiration. It is possible to prevent rupture of the varices in some patients by placing an intrahepatic portosystemic shunt. One introduces a catheter through the jugular vein and into the liver and then places a stent between a branch of the hepatic vein and a branch of the portal vein, allowing portal blood to shunt directly into the vena cava.

In some cases of portal hypertension, surgical intervention is necessary. Portacaval shunts (i.e., those linking the portal vein and inferior vena cava) can stop rebleeding and reduce portal hypertension, but hepatic encephalopathy (see next) can occur and overall mortality is not improved. The distal splenorenal shunt is now the more popular choice of treatment. It is effective in preventing rebleeding, and because it diverts only a portion of the blood flow away from the liver (i.e., just the blood exiting the spleen; Fig. 24-7A), it is associated with a much lower incidence of encephalopathy.

Hepatic Encephalopathy

Even as hepatic scarring increases vascular resistance through the liver, hepatic perfusion continues for a while. However, as we have just seen, eventually some of the portal blood flow shunts around the damaged liver into systemic veins, through preexisting anastomoses. Because the liver is critical for removal and inactivation of naturally occurring toxic metabolites (see Chapter 46) as well as pharmacological agents, toxins that bypass the liver directly enter the systemic veins and can build up in the plasma. If these toxins (e.g., NH_3; see Fig. 39-6) cross the blood-brain barrier, they can cause acute delirium.

---

compensates with corresponding changes in O_2 extraction ratio. Hence, the liver tends to maintain constant O_2 consumption.

THE SKIN

The skin is the largest organ of the body

The skin is the major barrier between the internal milieu of the body and the unregulated environment of the outside world. The skin is normally overperfused in relation to its nutritional requirements. Thus, local metabolic control of skin blood flow is of little functional importance. However, changes in blood flow to the skin also play a central role in the body's temperature regulation (see Chapter 59).

In terms of blood flow, we can divide the skin into apical skin (Fig. 24-8A), which is present on the nose, lips, ears, hands, and feet, and nonapical skin (Fig. 24-8B). As in other

vascular beds, arterioles break up into capillaries, which reunite to form venules. The capillaries reach only as superficially as the dermis; the epidermis does not have a blood supply. The venules that are part of a plexus of vessels near the dermal-epidermal border (i.e., the most superficial vessels) may contain an appreciable volume of blood, thereby imparting a pinkish hue to individuals with light-colored skin. When cutaneous blood flow decreases, this volume of blood also decreases, lessening the reddish component of skin color (i.e., pallor). Local nutritional flow through the precapillary sphincters and capillaries is under the control of local vasodilator metabolites and sensory stimuli (e.g., temperature, touch, pain). For example, the vascular beds can respond to local thermal changes, largely independent of sympathetic nerve activity: the blood vessels dilate when the skin is directly heated and constrict when it is cooled.

In addition to the effects of local metabolites and local warming and cooling, the blood flow to the skin is under sympathetic neural control. Increases in body core tempera-

A   APICAL SKIN

B   NONAPICAL SKIN

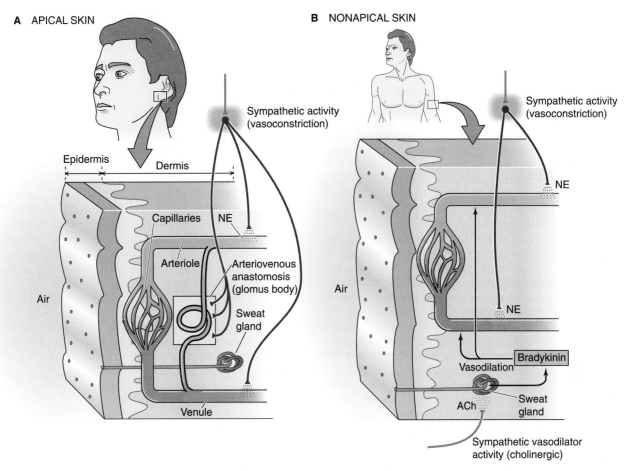

Figure 24-8   Blood flow to the skin. **A,** In apical skin, glomus bodies (arteriovenous anastomoses) can reach a density of ~500 per cm² in the nail beds. **B,** The nonapical skin lacks glomus bodies. Postganglionic sympathetic fibers release norepinephrine (NE), causing the usual vasoconstriction. Preganglionic sympathetic fibers release acetylcholine (ACh) and cause vasodilation, perhaps mediated by formation of bradykinin.

ture increase blood flow to the skin, leading to a loss of heat. Decreases in core temperature result in the opposite effect of conserving heat. In contrast to other vascular beds, this neural control is far more important than local metabolic control in the overall regulation of skin blood flow.

Specialized arteriovenous anastomoses in apical skin help control heat loss

Apical Skin   The apical skin at the extremities of the body has a very high surface-to-volume ratio that favors heat loss. Circulation to these apical regions has an unusual feature— *arteriovenous (a-v) anastomoses* called **glomus bodies**. (These glomus bodies are unrelated to the glomus cells of the peripheral chemoreceptors.) Glomus bodies are tiny nodules found in many parts of the body, including the ears, the pads of the fingers and toes, and the nail beds. As the afferent arteriole enters the connective tissue capsule of the glomus body, it becomes a vessel with a small lumen and a thick, muscular wall comprising multiple layers of myoepithelioid cells. These vessels—which have a rich sympathetic innervation—connect with short, thin-walled veins that eventually drain into larger skin veins. The a-v anastomoses, which are

involved in heat exchange, are in parallel with the capillaries of the skin, which are involved in nutrient exchange (Fig. 24-8A).

The anastomotic vessels are under neural control, rather than the control of local metabolites, and play a critical role in temperature regulation. In these apical regions, blood flow is under the control of sympathetic fibers that release norepinephrine and thereby constrict the arterioles, anastomotic vessels, and venules. Therefore, the increase in sympathetic tone that occurs in response to decreases in core temperature elicits vasoconstriction in the a-v anastomoses, a fall in blood flow, and a reduction in heat loss. Maximal sympathetic stimulation can completely obliterate the lumen of an anastomotic vessel, thus greatly reducing total blood flow to the skin. On the other hand, when the core temperature rises, the withdrawal of sympathetic tone leads to passive vasodilation; there is no active vasodilation. Indeed, blocking of the sympathetic input to a hand in a neutral thermal environment can increase blood flow 4-fold above basal levels—as much as heat stress can produce. Thus, sympathetic tone to the vasculature of apical skin is substantial at rest.

Nonapical Skin   The body uses a very different approach for regulating blood flow in nonapical skin. One important difference is that the vasculature of this skin almost completely lacks a-v anastomoses. A second important difference is that there are two types of sympathetic neurons innervating the vessels of the skin. Some release *norepinephrine* and some release *acetylcholine*.

Vasoconstriction occurs in response to the release of norepinephrine. In contrast to the situation in *apical* skin, blockade of sympathetic innervation to *nonapical* skin in a thermoneutral environment produces little change in skin blood flow, demonstrating little vasoconstrictor activity at rest.

Vasodilation in nonapical skin occurs in response to sympathetic neurons that release acetylcholine (see Chapter 14). Indeed, blockade of sympathetic innervation to the nonapical skin in a warm environment produces vasoconstriction and a decrease in skin blood flow, demonstrating neurally directed vasodilation before the blockade. The precise mechanism of this vasodilation is obscure. One proposal is that the acetylcholine stimulates eccrine sweat glands, causing the secretion of sweat as well as enzymes that lead to the local formation of vasoactive molecules. For instance, gland cells release kallikrein, a protease that converts kininogens to kinins, one of which is bradykinin (see Chapter 23). These kinins may act in a paracrine fashion on nearby blood vessels to relax VSMCs and thereby increase local perfusion. Cholinergic sympathetic neurons may cause vasodilation by means of a second pathway involving the co-release of vasodilatory neurotransmitters (e.g., calcitonin gene–related peptide, vasoactive intestinal polypeptide) that act directly on VSMCs, independent of sweat gland activity. Evidence for the second pathway is that the vasodilation cannot be blocked by atropine.

Mechanical stimuli elicit local vascular responses in the skin

The White Reaction
If the skin is stroked mildly with a sharp instrument, a blanched line appears in the trailing path of the instrument. The immediate response is attributable to passive expulsion of the blood by the external mechanical force. During the next 15 to 60 seconds, the **white reaction** that ensues is caused by contraction of microvascular VSMCs and pericytes in response to mechanical stimulation. This active response has the effect of emptying the capillary loops, the collecting venules, and the subpapillary venous plexus of blood in a sharply delineated manner.

The Triple Response
If a pointed instrument is drawn across the skin more forcefully, a series of reactions ensues that is collectively known as the **triple response**. Within several seconds, a band of increased redness due to a local dilation and increased perfusion of capillaries and venules appears within the perturbed area. This **red reaction** is independent of innervation and may persist for one to several minutes. The presumed cause is the local release of a vaso-

dilator substance (e.g., histamine) from cells that were disturbed by the mechanical response.

If the stimulus is sufficiently strong or repeated, the reddening of the skin is no longer restricted to the line that was stroked but spreads to the surrounding region. This **flare reaction** appears several seconds after the localized redness and is due to dilation of arterioles. The flare reaction depends on a local nervous mechanism, known as the **axon reflex**, that depends on the branching of a single nerve fiber (see Fig. 15-29). A stimulus applied to one branch (containing the sensory receptor) gives rise to an action potential that travels centrally to the point of fiber branching. From this branch point, the afferent signal travels both orthodromically to the spinal cord and antidromically along the collateral branch. As a result, this collateral branch releases the vasodilating neurotransmitters. Sectioning of the nerve fiber central to the site of the collateral branch eliminates the awareness of the stimulus but does not eliminate the flare reaction until the nerve fiber degenerates.

When the stimulus is even more intense, as by the lash of a whip, the skin along the line of injury develops localized swelling known as the **wheal**. This local edema results from an increase in capillary permeability (e.g., in response to histamine) as filtration exceeds absorption. The wheal is preceded by and ultimately replaces the red reaction, appearing within a few minutes from the time of injury, and it is often surrounded by the flare reaction.

REFERENCES

Books and Reviews

Faraci FM, Heistad DD: Regulation of the cerebral circulation: Role of endothelium and potassium channels. Physiol Rev 1998; 78:53-97.

Hoffman JIE, Spaan JAE: Pressure-flow relations in coronary circulation. Physiol Rev 1990; 70:331-390.

Iadecola C: Neurovascular regulation in the normal brain and in Alzheimer's disease. Nat Rev Neurosci 2004; 5:347-360.

Lauritzen M: Reading vascular changes in brain imaging: Is dendritic calcium the key? Nat Rev Neurosci 2005; 6:77-85.

Segal SS: Regulation of blood flow in the microcirculation. Microcirculation 2005; 12:33-45.

Journal Articles

Apkon M, Boron WF: Extracellular but not intracellular alkalinization constricts rat cerebral arterioles. J Physiol 1995; 484: 743-753.

Berne RM: Role of adenosine in the regulation of coronary blood flow. Circ Res 1980; 47:807-813.

Bohlen HG, Lash JM: Resting oxygenation of rat and rabbit intestine: Arteriolar and capillary contributions. Am J Physiol 1995; 269:H1342-H1348.

Duza T, Sarelius IH: Increase in endothelial cell Ca²⁺ in response to mouse cremaster muscle contraction. J Physiol 2004; 555:459-469.

VanTeeffelen JW, Segal SS: Interaction between sympathetic nerve activation and muscle fibre contraction in resistance vessels of hamster retractor muscle. J Physiol 2003; 550:563-574.

CHAPTER 25

INTEGRATED CONTROL OF
THE CARDIOVASCULAR SYSTEM

Emile L. Boulpaep

In the preceding chapters, we examined cardiovascular regulation at several different levels. Powerful *systemic* mechanisms operate over both the short term and the long term to control mean arterial pressure and cardiac output. Operating independently of these are *local* mechanisms of control that regulate blood flow at the microcirculatory level. In addition, individual organs have their own unique tools for managing specific circulatory requirements. In this chapter, we put it all together and learn how the cardiovascular system integrates the complex systemic, local, and individualized regulatory mechanisms in response to the demands of everyday life.

INTERACTION AMONG THE DIFFERENT CARDIOVASCULAR CONTROL SYSTEMS

The control of the cardiovascular system involves linear, branched, and connected interactions

In the previous chapters, we often presented physiological responses in a linear sequence or on a **linear chart**. For instance, we might represent the carotid-baroreceptor feedback loop (see Chapter 23) as a linear sequence of events (Fig. 25-1A). However, cardiovascular parameters and associated physiological responses are often related by multiple factors, requiring a more complex diagram called a **branching tree** (or an algorithmic tree). For example, in our discussion of the control of cardiac output (see Chapter 23), we started with the knowledge that cardiac output depends on *two* parameters—stroke volume and heart rate. Therefore, with our very first step, we come to a fork in the road—an example of a branching tree (Fig. 25-1B). At the next level, we encounter a pair of forks because stroke volume and heart rate both depend on two parameters. Finally, at the third level, we see that each of the determinants of stroke volume and heart rate depends on multiple factors (i.e., multiple forks).

The control of some cardiovascular parameters is even more complex, requiring that we graft branches from smaller trees. For example, we know from Ohm's law that *mean arterial pressure* depends on both *cardiac output* (and all the elements in its branching tree in Fig. 25-1B) and *total peripheral resistance*, which requires a branching tree of its own (Fig. 25-1C). Moreover, sometimes an element in one part of the "forest" interacts with another element that is far away. A physiological system with such complex interactions is best represented by a **connected diagram**, which may include feedback loops (Fig. 25-1C, red arrows), parameters that appear more than once in the tree (connected by a red dashed line), or factors that modulate parameters in two different branches of the tree (connected by brown arrows). Although not shown in Figure 25-1C, several feedback loops may impinge on a single element, and some loops are more dominant than others. The complex interactions among parameters make it difficult to distinguish factors of overriding importance from those of lesser weight. Moreover, when one disturbs a single parameter in a complex physiological system, the initial state of other parameters determines the end-state of the system. In previous chapters, we have chosen situations that artificially isolate one portion of the cardiovascular system (e.g., heart, microcirculation) to explain in a simple way the homeostatic control mechanisms that govern that subsystem. However, conditions isolating subsystems rarely apply to a real person.

How can we evaluate which parameters are crucial? As an example, consider one subsystem, the heart. Let us assume that we can rigorously analyze all determinants of cardiac function—such as Starling's law, force-velocity relationships, effect of heart rate on contractility, and so forth. These analyses take the form of mathematical expressions, which we can combine by **systems analysis** to create a model that describes the behavior of the entire heart—at least theoretically. How can we test whether our model is reasonable? We can compare the physiological response of the heart in vivo with the response predicted by a computer simulation of the model. Using this approach, we may be able to establish whether we have used the correct feedback loops, whether we have assigned proper values to various elements, and whether we have assigned the proper weight to each interaction. In this way, we can use any agreement between the experimental data and the performance of the model as evidence—but not proof—that the concepts contained in the model are reasonable.

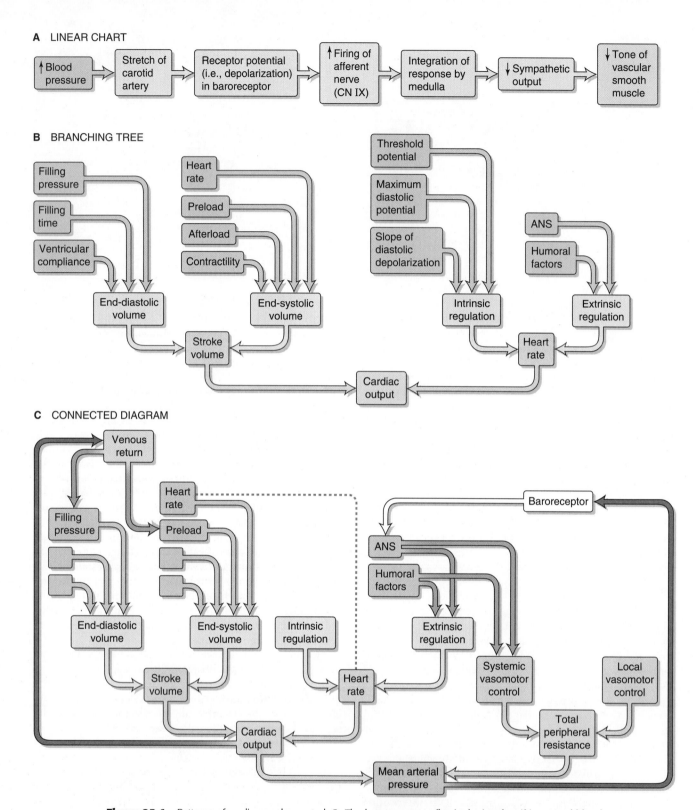

Figure 25-1 Patterns of cardiovascular control. **A,** The baroreceptor reflex is depicted as if increased blood pressure affected a single stretch receptor, which ultimately would influence a single effector (i.e., vascular smooth muscle). **B,** Cardiac output depends on multiple parameters, which in turn depend on multiple parameters, and so on. However, we ignore potential interactions among parameters. **C,** A branching tree represents the control of mean arterial pressure. The left limb repeats **B**. Superimposed on this simple tree are three more complex interactions: (1) feedback loops *(red arrows)*, (2) two occurrences of the same parameter *(connected by the red dashed line)*, and (3) examples of parameters exerting effects on two different branches of the tree *(brown arrows)*. ANS, autonomic nervous system.

Regulation of the entire cardiovascular system depends on the integrated action of multiple subsystem controls as well as noncardiovascular controls

In performing a systems analysis of the entire cardiovascular system, we must consider the interrelationships among the various "subsystems" summarized in the central yellow block of Figure 25-2. Not surprisingly, we cannot fully understand how a particular disturbance affects the overall circulation unless we consider all subsystems in an integrated fashion. For instance, consider the effects of administering norepinephrine, which has a high affinity for α_1 adrenoceptors, less for β_1 adrenoreceptors, and far less for β_2 adrenoceptors. These receptors are present, in varying degrees, in both the blood vessels and the heart. A *branching tree* would predict the following. Because α_1 adrenoceptors (high affinity) are present in most vascular beds, we expect widespread vasoconstriction. Because β_2 adrenoceptors (low affinity) are present in only a few vascular beds, we predict little vasodilation. Because β_1 adrenoceptors (intermediate affinity) are present in pacemaker and myocardial cells of the heart, we would anticipate an increase in both heart rate and contractility and therefore an increase in cardiac output.

Although our analysis predicts that the *heart rate* should increase, in most cases, the dominant effect of intravenous norepinephrine injection is to slow down the heart. The explanation, which relies on a *connected diagram*, is that increased peripheral resistance (caused by stimulation of α_1 receptors) and increased cardiac output (caused by stimulation of β_1 receptors) combine to cause a substantial rise in mean arterial pressure. The baroreceptor reflex (see red arrow on right in Fig. 25-1C) then intervenes to instruct the heart to slow down (see Chapter 23). However, bradycardia may not occur if many vascular beds were dilated before the administration of norepinephrine; in this case, the rise in blood pressure would be modest. Bradycardia might also not occur if the baroreceptor reflex were less sensitive, as would be the case in a chronically hypertensive patient (see Chapter 23 for the box on this topic). Thus, the effect of intravenous administration of norepinephrine on heart rate depends on the preexisting state of various subsystems.

In trying to understand the integrated response of the cardiovascular system to an insult, we must include in our analysis not only all the subsystems of the cardiovascular system but also the pertinent control systems outside the circulation (see blue boxes in Fig. 25-2):

1. **Autonomic nervous system.** Part of the autonomic nervous system (ANS) is intimately involved in cardiovascular control (e.g., high-pressure baroreceptor response). On the other hand, a generalized activation of the ANS, such as occurs with the fight-or-flight response (see Chapter 14), also affects the circulation.
2. **Respiratory system.** We have already seen that ventilatory activity converts the intrinsic bradycardia response to tachycardia during stimulation of the peripheral chemoreceptors (see Chapter 23). In addition, the action of the respiratory muscles during inspiration causes intrathoracic pressure to become more negative, thereby increasing venous return. A third example is that the

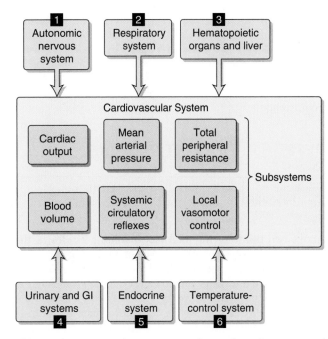

Figure 25-2 Interaction among cardiovascular subsystems and noncirculatory systems. GI, gastrointestinal.

evaporative loss of water during breathing reduces total body water and, ultimately, blood volume.

3. **Hematopoietic organs and liver.** These systems control blood composition in terms of cell constituents and plasma proteins. The hematocrit and large proteins (e.g., fibrinogen) are major determinants of blood viscosity (see Chapter 17) and therefore of blood flow. Because the plasma proteins also determine colloid osmotic pressure, they are a major component of the Starling forces, which determine the distribution of extracellular fluid between the interstitium and the blood plasma. (See Chapter 20.)
4. **Gastrointestinal and urinary systems.** Because the gastrointestinal tract and kidneys are the principal organs determining input and output of electrolytes and water, they are mainly responsible for controlling the volume and electrolyte composition of extracellular fluid. Extracellular fluid volume plays a central role in the long-term control of blood pressure (see Chapter 40).
5. **Endocrine system.** Part of the endocrine system is intimately involved in cardiovascular control (e.g., epinephrine release by the adrenal medulla). Other hormones influence the cardiovascular system either because they are vasoactive agents (see Chapter 23) or because they regulate fluid volume and electrolyte composition by acting on the kidney and gastrointestinal system.
6. **Temperature control system.** The cardiovascular system is a major effector organ for thermoregulation, carrying blood from the body core to the skin, where heat loss then occurs (see Chapter 59). In part, this heat loss occurs as sweat glands secrete fluid that then evaporates. However, the loss of extracellular fluid volume reduces the effective circulating volume (see Chapter 23).

Inclusion of control elements outside the circulation (Fig. 25-2) in our connected diagram of the cardiovascular system

(Fig. 25-1C) would expand the computer model to include hundreds of independent and dependent variables. Rather than trying to grasp such an exhaustive model, we work here through the integrated cardiovascular responses to four important circulatory "stresses": (1) orthostasis (i.e., standing up), (2) emotional stress, (3) exercise, and (4) hemorrhage.

RESPONSE TO ERECT POSTURE

Because of gravity, standing up (orthostasis) tends to shift blood from the head and heart to veins in the legs

About two thirds of the total blood volume resides in the systemic veins (see Chapter 19). When a recumbent subject assumes an upright position, the blood shifts from the central blood volume reservoirs and other veins to large veins in the dependent limbs. In discussing Figure 17-8B, we assumed that the cardiovascular system somehow made the adjustments necessary to keep right atrial pressure (RAP) constant at about +2 mm Hg. Indeed, unless compensatory mechanisms intervene, blood redistribution will lower not only arterial blood pressure but also venous return and thus cardiac output.

To illustrate the effect of blood redistribution on venous return, we will represent the entire circulatory system by a horizontal, distensible cylinder 180 cm in length (the height of our person) and 3 cm in radius (Fig. 25-3A). This cylinder holds ~5000 mL of blood (the normal blood volume). We know that immediately after a cardiac arrest, the entire vascular system will have a mean systemic filling pressure (MSFP) of ~7 mm Hg (see Chapter 23). The MSFP is the pressure in the circulation that would remain in the absence of any pumping or any gravity effects. Thus, if a subject is recumbent and has no heartbeat, and if the cardiovascular system is filled with a normal blood volume of 5000 mL, the overall compliance of the system will produce a uniform pressure of ~7 mm Hg. If we were to transfuse an additional 100 mL of blood into our cylinder, the MSFP would rise by ~1 mm Hg. We can conclude that the compliance, expressed as a normalized distensibility (see Chapter 19), is

$$\text{Relative distensibility} = \frac{(\Delta V / V_o)}{\Delta P}$$
$$= \frac{(100\,\text{mL}/5000\,\text{mL})}{1\,\text{mm}\,\text{Hg}}$$
$$= 0.02\,\frac{\text{mL}}{\text{mL} \times \text{mm}\,\text{Hg}}$$
$$= 0.02/(\text{mm}\,\text{Hg}) \qquad (25\text{-}1)$$

Thus, for every 2% increase in blood volume, the MSFP of the cylinder increases by 1 mm Hg.

What will happen to our cylinder if we now turn it upright? This position is called orthostasis (from the Greek *orthos* [upright] + *histanai* [to stand]). Because we have a vertical column of blood 180 cm tall, we must now consider gravity (Fig. 25-3B). The highest pressures will be at the

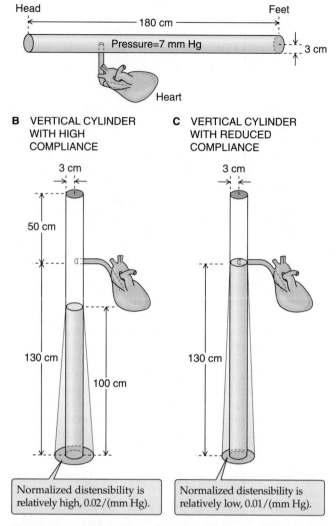

A HORIZONTAL CYLINDER

B VERTICAL CYLINDER WITH HIGH COMPLIANCE

C VERTICAL CYLINDER WITH REDUCED COMPLIANCE

Normalized distensibility is relatively high, 0.02/(mm Hg).

Normalized distensibility is relatively low, 0.01/(mm Hg).

Figure 25-3 Model of the orthostatic redistribution of blood. **A,** A horizontal tube (3-cm radius, 180 cm long) contains the entire blood volume (5 L). With no blood flow, pressure inside the tube is uniform and corresponds to a mean systemic filling pressure of 7 mm Hg. **B,** With the cylinder upright (orthostasis), pressure gradually increases toward the bottom, causing increasingly greater distention of this compliant tube. Because blood volume has shifted to the bottom, the upper level of the blood column is 30 cm below the level of the heart, preventing venous return. **C,** Reducing compliance of the tube by half also causes distention to fall by half. With the reduced shift of blood volume, the upper level of the blood column now just reaches the heart.

bottom of the cylinder. (Figure 17-8B shows that orthostasis causes venous pressure at the ankle to rise from 5 to 100 mm Hg.) Therefore, our cylinder will distend maximally at the bottom, and this distention represents a shift in blood volume. The bottom of the cylinder (corresponding to the "dependent areas" of a person) gains volume, whereas the top (i.e., corresponding to the cranial portion of a person) loses blood volume. In fact, there would be no blood at all at the top of the cylinder.

By just how much would the column of blood fall in our upright, 180-cm-tall cylinder? If the overall vascular volume distensibility were 0.02/(mm Hg), then the actual height of the blood column inside the cylinder would be only about 100 cm. If the heart were 50 cm below the top of the cylinder, then the top of the column would now be ~30 cm below the level of the heart. Therefore, there would be no blood to return to the heart. Moreover, the RAP would be negative (−30 cm H_2O, or about −22 mm Hg). Because the heart cannot create a vacuum this large at its input by "sucking" blood—in fact, the heart must be filled by a positive RAP—cardiac output would fall to zero.

The autonomic nervous system mediates an "orthostatic response" that raises heart rate and peripheral vascular resistance and thus tends to restore mean arterial pressure

If our model predicts that orthostasis should cause RAP to fall to −22 mm Hg, how is it that the body manages to maintain RAP at about +2 mm Hg in the upright position? The answer is that pooling of blood in the dependent vessels is much less pronounced during orthostasis than would be predicted by Figure 25-3B, where ~2.2 L disappeared from the top of the cylinder. The actual amount of pooling in both legs of a real person is only ~500 mL. Four major factors help reduce pooling and maintain RAP.

Nonuniform Initial Distribution of Blood   In our cylinder example, the blood was initially distributed evenly throughout the length of the cylinder. In a recumbent human, however, most of the blood in large veins is located in the central blood volume (see Chapter 19), that is, the vessels near the heart. If a large fraction of the blood had started off in the head, the orthostatic shift of blood would have been more dramatic, as in Figure 25-3B. The majority of the 500 mL of blood that pools in the legs during orthostasis comes from the intrathoracic vascular compartments. What is the sequence of events by which blood volume redistributes during orthostasis? As one stands, the output from the heart for a number of beats exceeds the venous return into the thoracic pool. This excess blood ends up filling the vessels in the dependent regions of the body. The result is a net transfer of blood—by way of the heart—from the intrathoracic vascular compartments to the dependent vessels.

Nonuniform Distensibility of the Vessels   In Figure 25-3B, we assumed a relative distensibility of 0.02/(mm Hg). If we had instead used a value of 0.01/(mm Hg)—that is, if the vessels were *less* distensible—standing would cause a less dramatic shift of blood to the dependent vessels, ~1.4 L (Fig. 25-3C) instead of ~2.2 L (Fig. 25-3B). As a result, the height of the blood column would fall from 180 to only 130 cm (Fig. 25-3C) in the upright position, rather than to 100 cm (Fig. 25-3B). Assuming a lower distensibility for the leg veins is reasonable because small vessels are far stiffer than larger ones, such as the aorta and vena cava. With the lower relative distensibility of 0.01/(mm Hg), the column of blood would just reach the heart. Indeed, when a subject stands quietly, the zero effective pressure level—the height in the body where vascular pressure equals atmospheric pressure—is about at the level of the right atrium. Obviously, if the circulatory system reduces its distensibility even further through the regulated contraction of vascular smooth muscle (dis-

cussed later), the height of the column of blood will increase and improve venous return.

Muscle Pumps   An important compensation for blood pooling during orthostasis comes from skeletal muscle contraction. When a person stands, the muscles of the legs and abdomen tighten. The presence of valves in the veins, as well as intermittent muscular movement, contributes to the flow of blood upward along the veins (see Figs. 22-7C and 24-6). Vessels of the abdominal region remain nearly unaffected by orthostasis because the abdominal viscera are contained in a water-filled jacket that is maintained by the tone of the abdominal muscles.

Autonomic Reflexes   Because of decreased venous return, cardiac output tends to fall by ~20% soon after one assumes an erect position. However, the fall in cardiac output would be even greater in the absence of autonomic reflexes. The decreased venous return leads to a fall in RAP, which in turn leads to a decrease in stroke volume and thus arterial pressure. High-pressure baroreceptors (see Chapter 23) sense this decrease in arterial pressure, which leads to an increased sympathetic output that raises vascular tone throughout the body and increases heart rate and contractility. Together, the constriction of arterioles (which raises total peripheral resistance) and the increased heart rate restore the systemic mean arterial pressure, despite a small decrease in stroke volume. In the dependent regions of the body, the sympathetic response also increases the tone of the veins, thereby decreasing their diameter and their capacity (compare B and C in Fig. 25-3).

In summary, of the four factors that contribute to the stability of RAP during orthostasis, two are anatomical (i.e., nonuniformities of initial blood volume distribution and distensibility) and two are physiological (i.e., muscle pumps and autonomic reflexes). The two physiological mechanisms are both important. Indeed, after a lumbar sympathectomy, patients tend to faint when standing. However, after some months, they are able to compensate, perhaps by using the muscle pumps more effectively or by enhancing the sympathetic response of the heart.

The extent of the **orthostatic response**—how much the heart rate or peripheral vascular resistance increases under the control of the ANS—depends on a variety of factors (Table 25-1), which involve nearly the entire cardiovascular system. Because these factors may differ from person to person or within any one individual according to the circumstances, the orthostatic response is highly variable. We now discuss two examples of this variability.

Postural Hypotension   In very sensitive subjects lying on a tilt table, a sudden orthostatic tilt can cause such a large fall in arterial pressure that the individual becomes dizzy or even faints. **Fainting** is caused by a transient fall in arterial pressure that causes cerebral perfusion to become inadequate.

Temperature Effects   In a *cool environment*, where the arterioles in the lower extremities are constricted, the initial dip in arterial pressure can be small, despite the decrease in stroke volume. The explanation is that the high arteriolar

Table 25-1 Factors Influencing the Degree of Orthostatic Response*

Total blood volume
Distribution of blood volume
Size of vessels in dependent regions of the body
Vascular distensibility
Mean systemic filling pressure (pressure in the absence of cardiac output)
Level at which zero effective pressure is normally located in a particular individual
Degree of tilt
Skeletal muscle tone; strength and rate of intermittent contraction of skeletal muscles
Vascular sufficiency
Abdominal muscle tone
Temperature
Response of low-pressure receptors
Response of high-pressure baroreceptors
Activity of the sympathetic system
Initial heart rate
Initial myocardial contractility
Sensitivity of vascular smooth muscle to sympathetic stimulation

*That is, by how much does standing up increase heart rate and peripheral vascular resistance?

resistance delays the transfer of blood from the thoracic pool to the legs. As a result, the sympathetic response to the small drop in mean arterial pressure may already be in effect before further pooling can occur. In a *warm environment*, where the arterioles in the skin are more dilated, orthostasis leads to faster transfer of blood from the thoracic pool to the legs so that—before the sympathetic response can develop—the initial decreases in stroke volume, mean arterial pressure, and pulse pressure can be large. Thus, soldiers standing quietly at attention in hot weather are more likely to faint than are soldiers marching in a cold environment because of differences in muscle pump activity and vasoconstriction.

RESPONSES TO ACUTE EMOTIONAL STRESS

The fight-or-flight reaction is a sympathetic response that is centrally controlled in the cortex and hypothalamus

Emotional responses vary greatly among people. A severe emotional reaction can resemble the **fight-or-flight response** in animals (see Chapter 14). This defense reaction causes a generalized increase in skeletal muscle tone and increased sensory attention.

Fight-or-flight behavior is an extreme example of an integrated acute stress response that originates entirely within the central nervous system (CNS), without involvement of peripheral sensors or reflexes. The response is due to the activation of sensory centers in the **cortex** (Fig. 25-4), which activate a part of the limbic system called the **amygdalae**. The amygdalae in turn activate the **locus coeruleus** (see

Chapter 13), which is in the pons, as well as hypothalamic nuclei. Noradrenergic neurons in the locus coeruleus project to nearly every part of the CNS (see Fig. 13-7), including the **hypothalamic paraventricular nucleus (PVN)**, which produces both an endocrine and an ANS response. The *endocrine response* of the PVN involves (1) release of arginine vasopressin (AVP) by magnocellular neurons in the PVN (see Fig. 40-8), thereby reducing urine output (see Chapter 38); and (2) release of corticotropin-releasing hormone (see Chapter 50) by parvocellular neurons in the PVN, activating the hypothalamic-pituitary-adrenal axis and thereby releasing cortisol, which is important for the metabolic response to stress. The *ANS response* of the PVN involves projections to (1) autonomic nuclei in the brainstem (dorsal motor nucleus of the vagus, rostral ventrolateral medulla, and NTS) that are part of the **medullary cardiovascular center** (see Chapter 23) and (2) direct projections to the **spinal intermediolateral column** (Fig. 25-4).

The overall fight-or-flight response involves the following:

1. **Skeletal muscle blood flow.** In animals—but perhaps not in humans—activation of postganglionic sympathetic cholinergic neurons (see Chapter 14) *directly* causes a rapid increase in blood flow to skeletal muscle (see Chapter 23). In humans as well as in other mammals, flow also increases *secondarily* more slowly and less dramatically because the adrenal medulla releases epinephrine, which acts on β_2 adrenoceptors on skeletal muscle blood vessels. The result is dilation and an increase in blood flow. In a full-blown fight-or-flight reaction, muscle exercise generates metabolites that further increase skeletal muscle blood flow (see Chapter 24). Of course, humans may not exercise skeletal muscle in responding to internal stress (e.g., anxiety or panic).

2. **Cutaneous blood flow.** The **sympathetic** response causes little change in blood flow to skin unless it stimulates sweating. The neural pathway involves sympathetic cholinergic neurons (see Chapter 14), which release acetylcholine and perhaps vasodilatory neurotransmitters (e.g., calcitonin gene–related peptide, vasoactive intestinal peptide). The acetylcholine causes the secretion of sweat and possibly also the local formation of kinins (see Chapter 23). These kinins increase capillary permeability and presumably also dilate arterioles but constrict venules (i.e., increasing the midcapillary pressure). The result would be an increased filtration of fluid from the skin capillaries into the interstitium, causing dermal swelling.

3. **Adrenal medulla.** Preganglionic sympathetic neurons stimulate the chromaffin cells to release epinephrine, which causes vasodilation in muscle (through β_2 adrenoceptors) and vasoconstriction in the kidney and splanchnic beds (through α_1 adrenoceptors).

4. **Renal and splanchnic blood flow.** In virtually all vascular beds, increased sympathetic output causes vasoconstriction and thereby decreases blood flow. The systemic release of epinephrine also vasoconstricts these vascular beds rich in α_1 adrenoceptors.

5. **Veins.** Most veins constrict in response to sympathetic output.

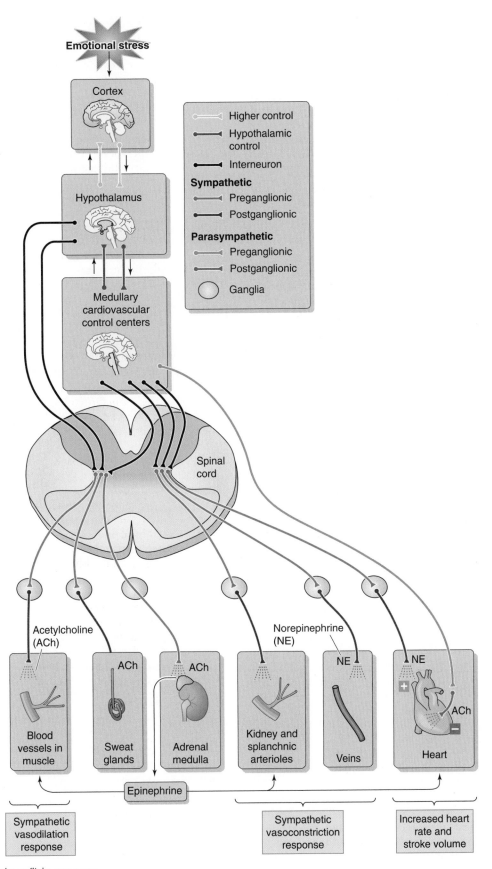

Figure 25-4 Fight-or-flight response.

6. **The heart.** Increased sympathetic output and decreased vagal output cause a rise in heart rate and contractility, so that cardiac output increases.
7. **Blood volume.** High plasma levels of AVP reduce urine output and maintain blood volume.
8. **Mean arterial pressure.** Depending on the balance of vasodilation and vasoconstriction, the overall result of vascular resistance changes may be either a decrease or an increase in total peripheral resistance. Nevertheless, because cardiac output increases, the net result of an increased cardiac output and a resistance change is an increase in arterial pressure.

The common faint reflects mainly a parasympathetic response caused by sudden emotional stress

About one fifth of humans experience one or more episodes of fainting during adolescence. This type of fainting is known as vasodepressor syncope or **vasovagal syncope** (**VVS**). About 40% of syncope cases seen in outpatient settings are vasovagal in nature. VVS can occur in response to a sudden emotional stress, phlebotomy, the sight of blood, or acute pain. Fainting usually starts when the individual is standing or sitting, rarely when the individual is recumbent. The loss of consciousness is due to a transient fall in perfusion pressure to the brain. The "playing dead" reaction in animals is the equivalent of VVS in humans.

VVS originates with activation of specific areas in the cerebral cortex. Indeed, stimulation of areas in the anterior cingulate gyrus can trigger a faint. Although the exact trigger is not known, VVS has been attributed to activation of the **Bezold-Jarisch reflex**. This reflex—originally described as the cardiorespiratory response to the intravenous injection of veratrum alkaloids—causes bradycardia, hypotension, and apnea. In experimental animals, stimulation of arterial baroreceptors or ventricular baroreceptors (see Chapter 23) by any of a host of chemicals—veratrum alkaloids, nicotine, capsaicin, histamine, serotonin, snake and insect venoms—can also trigger the Bezold-Jarisch reflex. In patients, coronary injection of contrast material or of thrombolytic agents can cause VVS, presumably by stimulating ventricular receptors. It is possible that these chemical stimuli activate the same stretch-sensitive TRPC channels of arterial baroreceptors (see Chapter 23) that are usually activated by high blood pressure. In humans, triggers clearly distinct from those known to initiate a Bezold-Jarisch reflex can also elicit VVS. Whatever the actual trigger, vagal afferents carry signals to higher CNS centers, which act through autonomic nuclei in the medulla to cause a massive stimulation of the parasympathetic system and abolition of sympathetic tone.

VVS involves changes in several parameters (Fig. 25-5):

1. **Total peripheral resistance.** A massive vasodilation results from the removal of sympathetic tone from the resistance vessels of the skeletal muscle, splanchnic, renal, and cerebral circulations. The resulting fall in blood pressure fails to activate a normal baroreceptor response.

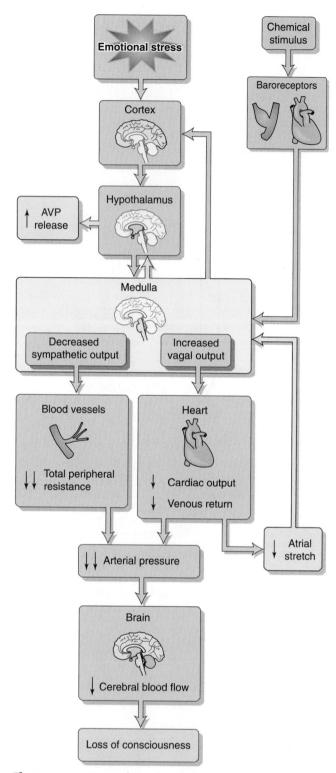

Figure 25-5 Vasovagal syncope. AVP, arginine vasopressin.

2. **Cardiac output.** Intense vagal output to the heart causes bradycardia and decreased stroke volume, resulting in a marked decrease in cardiac output. Because atropine, a muscarinic receptor blocker, does not reliably prevent syncope, decreased sympathetic tone to the heart may also play a role in causing bradycardia.

3. **Arterial pressure.** The combination of a sudden decrease in both total peripheral resistance and cardiac output causes a profound fall in mean arterial pressure.

4. **Cerebral blood flow.** The fall in mean arterial pressure causes global cerebral ischemia. If the decreased cerebral blood flow persists for only a few seconds, the result is dizziness or faintness. If it lasts for ~10 seconds, the subject loses consciousness. The stress underlying the common faint also may provoke hyperventilation, which lowers arterial P_{CO_2} (see Chapter 31). The resulting constriction of cerebral blood vessels (see Chapter 24) further impairs cerebral blood flow, which increases the likelihood of a faint.

5. **Other manifestations of altered ANS activity.** Pallor of the skin and sweating (beads of perspiration) are signs that often appear before the loss of consciousness. Intense vagal stimulation of the gastrointestinal tract may cause epigastric pain that is interpreted as nausea. Mydriasis (pupillary dilation) as well as visual blurring can also result from parasympathetic stimulation.

Fainting is more likely to occur in a warm room, after a volume loss (e.g., dehydration or hemorrhage), or after standing up or other maneuvers that tend to lower mean arterial pressure. You might think that these stresses would trigger baroreceptor responses that increase cardiac output and vascular resistance, thereby making fainting less likely. However, the same integrated pattern of brain activity that orchestrates VVS also appears to suppress the expected baroreceptor reflexes that would otherwise counteract the syncope.

After regaining consciousness, the patient often notices oliguria (reduced urine output), caused by high plasma levels of AVP (also known as antidiuretic hormone; see Chapter 38). Elevated levels of AVP can result in part from the reduced atrial stretch that occurs during periods of decreased venous return (see Chapter 23). The pallor and nausea that persist after fainting may also result from the high levels of circulating AVP.

RESPONSE TO EXERCISE

Adaptation to exercise probably places the greatest demands on circulatory function. The main feature of the cardiovascular response to exercise is an increased cardiac output, up to 4 or 5 times the resting cardiac output. The increase in cardiac output during exercise is the result of increased heart rate (~3 times control) more than of increased stroke volume (~1.5 times control). The cardiovascular response to exercise has both early and late components and originates from higher centers in the CNS (early), from mechanical and chemical changes triggered by contracting skeletal muscle (delayed), and from various reflexes (delayed).

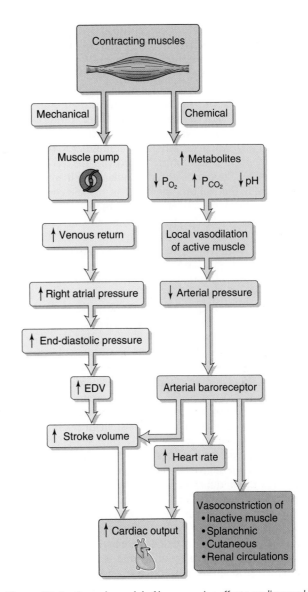

Figure 25-6 An early model of how exercise affects cardiovascular function. EDV, end-diastolic volume.

Early physiologists suggested that muscle contraction leads to mechanical and chemical changes that trigger an increase in cardiac output

Contracting skeletal muscle produces cardiovascular changes that mimic many of those that occur during exercise. In fact, early physiologists believed that these skeletal muscle effects triggered *all* of the cardiovascular changes associated with exercise. We now know that these skeletal muscle effects are important only for the *delayed* cardiovascular responses in exercise. Muscle contraction directly affects the cardiovascular system in two ways (Fig. 25-6)—a mechanical response that increases venous return and a chemical response that dilates blood vessels in active muscle.

Mechanical Response: Increased Venous Return The pumping action of contracting skeletal muscle improves venous return (see Chapters 22 and 24). As a result, RAP, ventricular end-diastolic pressure, and end-diastolic volume should all increase. According to the Starling mechanism (see Chapter 22), the result should be an increase in stroke volume.

Chemical Response: Local Vasodilation in Active Muscle

Enhanced skeletal muscle metabolism produces multiple changes in the chemistry of the interstitial fluid. The P_{O_2} and pH fall, whereas other metabolites (CO_2, lactic acid, K^+, and adenosine) accumulate. Moreover, the accumulation of metabolites causes interstitial osmolarity to increase. After a small delay that follows the onset of muscle contraction, the developing chemical changes cause the arterioles to dilate (see Chapters 20 and 24), which may lead to an initial fall in arterial pressure. However, this fall is transient because of the intervening baroreceptor response (see Chapter 23), which increases heart rate and stroke volume, both of which enhance cardiac output. At the same time, the baroreceptor reflex vasoconstricts inactive muscle regions as well as the splanchnic, renal, and cutaneous circulations.

Cardiovascular physiologists believed for a long time that the mechanical and chemical limbs in Figure 25-6, both of which originate in active muscle, are responsible for the increased cardiac output during exercise. However, not only is Figure 25-6 incomplete, some of its predictions are incorrect or do not occur in the predicted order. As far as the *mechanical effect* on venous return is concerned, the model predicts a rise in ventricular end-diastolic pressure and thus end-diastolic volume. As far as the *chemical effect* is concerned, the model predicts that it should take time for chemical changes in active skeletal muscle to produce local vasodilation. Therefore, there ought to be a time lag between the initiation of exercise and the fall in mean arterial pressure that triggers the baroreceptor response (e.g., increased heart rate).

In the 1950s, Rushmer tested these predictions on trained unanesthetized dogs. Recording the *mechanical limb* of Figure 25-6, he found that at the onset of exercise, left ventricular end-diastolic pressure does *not* rise and that left ventricular end-diastolic volume diminishes rather than increases. These findings cast doubt on the primary role of the Starling mechanism in raising stroke volume during exercise. Recording the *chemical limb* of Figure 25-6, Rushmer found *no* transient fall in mean arterial pressure, thus casting doubt on the importance of the baroreceptor reflex. Furthermore, he saw *no* delay between the onset of exercise and the increase of heart rate, thus calling into question the idea that the chemically induced vasodilation is at the root of the tachycardia.

The explanation for the discrepancies between the predicted and actual findings is the presence of a central command that rapidly activates the sympathetic division of the ANS.

Central command organizes an integrated cardiovascular response to exercise

During exercise, a **central command** controls the parallel activation of both the motor cortex (see Chapter 16) and cardiovascular centers. The central command involves such brain areas as the **medial prefrontal cortex** (involved in the mental state of thinking and planning exercise) as well as the insula and anterior cingulate gyrus, which are **cortical parts of the limbic system** (see Chapter 14). Indeed, the medial prefrontal cortex receives multiple limbic inputs. Moreover, both cortical centers modulate stress-related sympathetic outflow, including the sympathetic outflow related to exercise. Rushmer and his colleagues explored various sites in the diencephalon (see Chapter 10) of dogs to determine if stimulation of any of them might mimic the integrated sympathetic response to exercise. In the 1950s, Rushmer found that stimulation of the H_2 fields of Forel in the ventral thalamus or neurons in the periventricular gray matter of the hypothalamus reproduced all the details of the cardiac response to exercise, even though the muscles of the dog were completely quiescent. The central command centers project to the lateral hypothalamus, rostral ventrolateral medulla, and NTS to make autonomic adaptations appropriate for exercise (Fig. 25-7):

1. **Increased cardiac output.** Increased sympathetic output to the heart causes early tachycardia and increased contractility, resulting in a rapid upsurge of cardiac output.
2. **Vasoconstriction.** Sympathetic output from the medulla causes vasoconstriction in inactive muscle regions as well as in the renal, splanchnic, and cutaneous circulations. The net effect is to make more blood available for diversion to the contracting muscles. Except during maximal exercise, the increase in splanchnic and renal resistance does not result in a fall in local blood flow to the abdominal viscera and kidneys. Rather, because the arterial pressure increases along with the renal and splanchnic vascular resistance, the *absolute* blood flow remains close to resting levels in these tissues, even as the flow to the skeletal muscle increases markedly. However, *fractional* blood flow (i.e., local blood flow normalized to cardiac output) does fall in these regions. In the early phase of exercise, skin blood flow also decreases. However, cutaneous blood flow eventually rises, reflecting the attempt of the temperature regulatory system to prevent body temperature from rising too much (see Chapter 59).
3. **Early vasodilation in active muscle.** In dogs—although not in humans or other primates—at the initiation of exercise, central command stimulates hypothalamic neurons whose axons bypass the medullary cardiovascular centers and synapse on preganglionic sympathetic neurons in the spinal cord (see Chapter 23). The postganglionic neurons synapse on cholinergic sympathetic vasodilator fibers that innervate the vascular smooth muscle of skeletal muscle and trigger early peripheral vasodilation in active skeletal muscle. As discussed in the next section, the delayed local "chemical" response later reinforces this vasodilation.

The increased alertness that accompanies the anticipation of exercise can elicit all the components of the early response to exercise. The early response resembles the fight-or-flight reaction. In humans, the anticipatory cardiovascular adjustments prepare the body for the increased metabolism of the exercising skeletal muscle. For sprinters at the start of a 100-m dash, the anticipatory response prepares them to deliver an increased cardiac output and simultaneously to

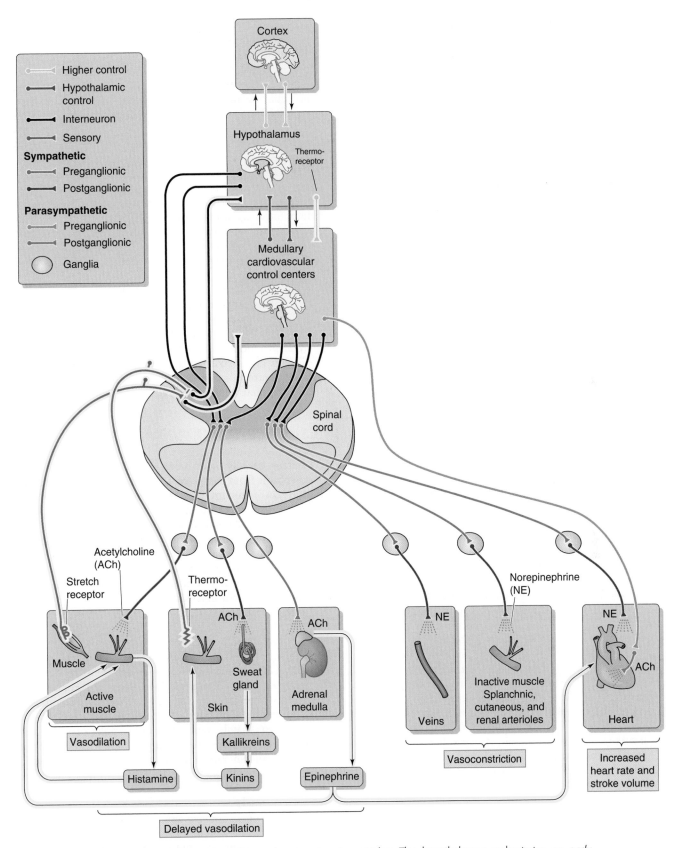

Figure 25-7 Integrated cardiovascular response to exercise. The hypothalamus orchestrates an *early* response, which includes vasodilation of active muscle (the mechanism of which is controversial in humans), vasoconstriction of certain inactive tissues, and increased cardiac output. In addition to those responses shown in Figure 25-6, the *delayed* responses (highlighted in *yellow*) include release of histamine, kallikreins, and epinephrine, leading to delayed vasodilation. Delayed local chemical responses from contracting muscles sustain early cardiovascular responses. Cutaneous thermoreceptors trigger delayed vasodilation in the skin.

divert the increased blood flow away from tissues that do not require increased blood flow.

Muscle and baroreceptor reflexes, metabolites, venous return, histamine, epinephrine, and increased temperature reinforce the response to exercise

In addition to the events orchestrated by the command center, the integrated cardiovascular response to exercise includes the following.

1. **Exercise pressor reflex.** A neural drive called the exercise pressure reflex originates within the exercising muscle itself. Contraction activates stretch receptors that sense muscle tension and may also activate chemoreceptors that sense metabolites. Signals from these receptors travel through small thinly myelinated (Aδ or group III in Table 12-1) and unmyelinated (C or group IV) sensory fibers from skeletal muscle to the spinal cord and then on to the medullary cardiovascular control centers. This sensory input reinforces the central input to the cardiovascular control center and thus sustains the sympathetic outflow.

2. **Arterial baroreflexes.** Elevated mean arterial pressure resulting from high cardiac output and vasoconstriction outside active muscle would normally slow the heart. However, during exercise, central command resets the sensitivity of the **arterial baroreflex** so that the heart slows only at much higher arterial pressures. Conversely, if massive vasodilation in exercising skeletal muscle would reduce total peripheral resistance, the baroreceptor reflex maintains mean arterial pressure.

3. **Vasodilation triggered by metabolites in skeletal muscle.** *Metabolites* released locally (Fig. 25-7) dilate the resistance vessels and recruit capillaries that had received no blood flow at rest (see Chapter 24). As a result of this decrease in resistance, in concert with the increase in cardiac output, blood flow to active skeletal muscle can be as much as 20 times that to resting skeletal muscle. This vasodilator effect of metabolites thus more than overcomes any vasoconstrictive tendency produced by norepinephrine.

4. **Increased venous return.** The central command discussed in the preceding section explains the early increase in cardiac output during exercise. The mechanical and the chemical limbs described in Figure 25-6 further sustain the high cardiac output. Mechanically, the **muscle pump** increases venous return, and stroke volume rises by the **Starling mechanism.** Chemical mediators cause a vasodilation of active muscle beds that results in the rapid mobilization of blood from the central blood volume to exercising muscle.

5. **Histamine release.** Cells near the arterioles may release their intracellular stores of histamine, a potent vasodilator (see Table 20-7). Although these histamine-containing cells are quiescent when sympathetic nerves release *norepinephrine*, they release histamine when sympathetic tone wanes. Because of relaxation of the arterioles and precapillary sphincters, the pressure in the muscle capil-

laries rises, leading to increased extravasation of fluid and enhanced lymph flow.

6. **Epinephrine release.** During severe exercise, preganglionic sympathetic fibers to the adrenal medulla stimulate epinephrine release. The systemic effects of circulating epinephrine on cardiac β₁ adrenoceptors enhance the neural effects on the heart, thus increasing cardiac output. Circulating epinephrine also acts on vascular β₂ adrenoceptors, augmenting vasodilation mainly in skeletal muscle and heart.

7. **Regulation of body core temperature.** As exercise continues, increased metabolism causes body core temperature to rise, activating **temperature-sensitive cells** in the hypothalamus. This activation has two effects, both of which promote heat loss through the skin as part of a temperature regulatory response. (See Chapter 59.) First, the hypothalamus signals the medulla to inhibit its sympathetic vasoconstrictor outflow to the skin, thereby increasing cutaneous blood flow. Recall that vasoconstriction is part of the early response to exercise (see earlier). Second, the hypothalamus activates sympathetic cholinergic fibers to sweat glands, causing an increase in sweat production as well as an indirect cutaneous vasodilation that may involve kinin formation. In addition, these neurons may co-release neurotransmitters that directly dilate cutaneous vessels (see Chapter 24).

RESPONSE TO HEMORRHAGE

If a person rapidly loses more than 10% or 20% of total blood volume from a large *vein*, the inadequate intravascular volume causes sequential decreases in central blood volume, venous return, ventricular filling, stroke volume, cardiac output, and thus mean arterial pressure. However, if the blood loss comes from a large peripheral *artery*, the mean arterial pressure in central arteries does not fall until cardiac output falls secondary to decreased venous return. Of course, if the blood loss occurs from a blown aortic aneurysm, mean arterial pressure falls immediately.

Large hemorrhages, in which one loses 30% or more of total blood volume, produce **hypovolemic shock**. Shock is a state of peripheral circulatory failure that is characterized by inadequate perfusion of the peripheral tissues. During shock, the *systolic* arterial pressure is usually below 90 mm Hg, and the *mean* arterial pressure is below 70 mm Hg. For reasons that will become clear, by the time one records a significant fall in mean arterial pressure, other signs of shock are evident. The first signs may be narrowing of the pulse pressure and a sensation of faintness when sitting or standing. The subject in hypovolemic shock has cold and moist (i.e., "clammy") skin as well as a rapid and weak pulse. Moreover, urine output drops to less than 25 mL/hr, even though fluid intake had been normal.

After its abrupt initial fall, arterial pressure tends to return to normal (Fig. 25-8, red curve), although blood pressure falls irreversibly (blue dashed curve) in some cases. Under favorable circumstances, the body restores blood pressure toward normal values by mobilizing two lines of defense. First, circulatory control mechanisms act on the heart and blood vessels to restore cardiac output and to increase

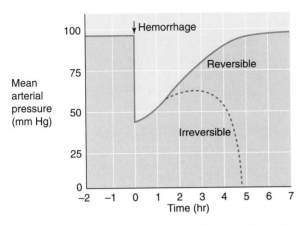

Figure 25-8 Changes in blood pressure with hemorrhage. At time zero, the investigator removes enough blood from the experimental animal to lower mean arterial pressure to 45 mm Hg.

peripheral resistance. Second, mechanisms of capillary exchange and fluid conservation restore the intravascular volume.

After hemorrhage, cardiovascular reflexes restore mean arterial pressure

Several cardiovascular reflexes cooperate to compensate for the fall in mean arterial pressure. These reflexes originate from four major groups of receptors (numbered 1 to 4 in Fig. 25-9).

1. **High-pressure baroreceptors.** The fall in arterial pressure leads to a decrease in the firing rate of afferents from the carotid and aortic baroreceptors (see Chapter 23). The resulting enhanced sympathetic output and diminished vagal output increase heart rate and cardiac contractility and also produce venoconstriction and selective arteriolar constriction. These responses cooperate to re-establish the arterial pressure.

2. **Low-pressure baroreceptors.** Reduced blood volume directly decreases effective circulating volume, which in turn lessens the activity of low-pressure stretch receptors (see Chapter 23). The resulting increased sympathetic outflow causes vasoconstriction in a number of vascular beds, particularly the kidney, reducing glomerular filtration rate and urine output. In response to decreased stretch, low-pressure receptors at various sites in the circulation ultimately have divergent effects on heart rate. The atrial stretch receptors also instruct the hypothalamus to enhance release of AVP, which reduces renal water excretion (see Chapter 38). During shock, the vasoconstrictor effects of AVP appear to be important for maintaining peripheral vascular resistance. Reduced atrial stretch also lowers the level of circulating atrial natriuretic peptide (see Chapter 23), thereby reducing salt and water loss by the kidneys (see Chapter 40).

3. **Peripheral chemoreceptors.** As blood pressure drops, perfusion of the carotid and aortic bodies declines, causing local hypoxia near the glomus cells and an increase in the firing rate of the chemoreceptor afferents,

a response enhanced by increased sympathetic tone to the peripheral chemoreceptor vessels (see Chapter 32). Increased *chemoreceptor* discharge leads to increased firing of the sympathetic vasoconstrictor fibers and ventilatory changes that indirectly increase heart rate (see Chapter 23).

4. **Central chemoreceptors.** Severe hypotension results in brain ischemia, which leads to a fall in the P_{O_2} of brain extracellular fluid as well as a rise in P_{CO_2} and a fall in pH. The acidosis has a profound effect on the central chemoreceptors in the medulla, leading to a sympathetic output several-fold more powerful than that caused by baroreceptor reflexes (see Chapter 23).

These four reflex pathways have in common the activation of a massive sympathetic response that results in the release of norepinephrine from postganglionic sympathetic neurons. In addition, the sympathetic response triggers the **adrenal medulla** to release epinephrine and norepinephrine roughly in proportion to the severity of the hemorrhage. Lowering of the mean arterial pressure to 40 mm Hg causes circulating levels of epinephrine to rise 50-fold, and norepinephrine, 10-fold. The consequences of the four combined reflex actions are the following responses (Fig. 25-9).

Tachycardia and Increased Contractility Increased sympathetic activity increases heart rate roughly in proportion to the volume of shed blood. Thus, the degree of tachycardia is an index of the severity of the hemorrhage. Increased sympathetic tone increases myocardial contractility but can increase stroke volume only after venous return also improves.

Arteriolar Constriction Sympathetic constriction of the resistance vessels is most pronounced in the blood vessels of the *extremities, skin, skeletal muscle, and abdominal viscera.* Although both precapillary and postcapillary resistance vessels constrict, the *precapillary* response initially dominates. As a result, capillary pressure falls precipitously, leading to the transcapillary refill discussed in the next section. *Renal blood flow falls rapidly after hemorrhage as a result of the fall in blood pressure but recovers after a few minutes because of autoregulation (see Chapter 34). The responses of both high- and low-pressure stretch receptors lead to enhanced sympathetic vasoconstrictor traffic to the kidney. Although renal blood flow has a high threshold for this sympathetic traffic, the sympathetic vasoconstriction eventually overrides renal autoregulation if arterial pressure remains low or continues to fall. In hypovolemic shock, renal blood flow falls to a proportionately greater extent than does cardiac output, which explains why severe hemorrhage often results in acute renal failure. Blood flow in the medulla of the kidney is less compromised than in the cortex, leading to "medullary washout" of the hypertonic interstitial fluid in the renal medulla (see Chapter 38) and an inability to produce a concentrated urine. Both coronary blood flow and cerebral blood flow initially fall after hemorrhage, but autoregulation can largely restore blood flow to normal.

Venous Constriction The fall in blood volume with hemorrhage occurs primarily in the large capacitance vessels, espe-

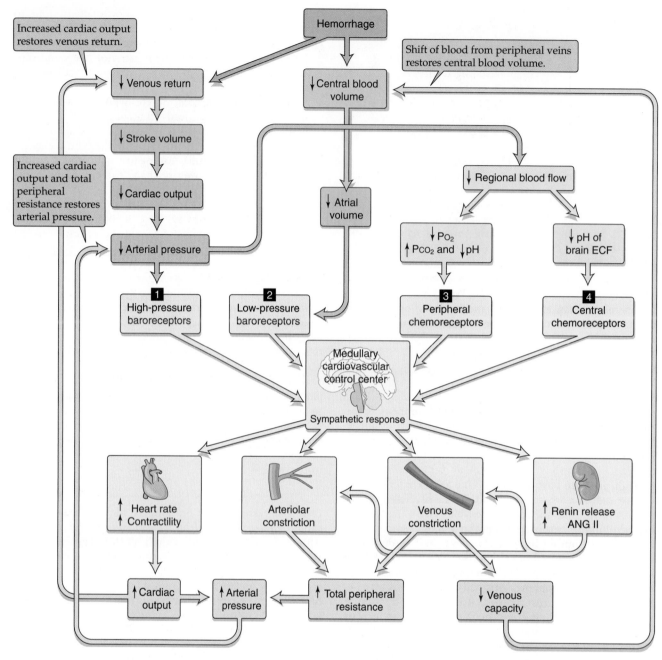

Figure 25-9 Integrated response to hemorrhage. Blood loss triggers four kinds of receptors (numbered 1 to 4) to produce an integrated response orchestrated by the medulla. ANG, angiotensin; ECF, extracellular fluid.

cially those that contain the central blood volume. These vessels are very sensitive to sympathetic stimulation (which causes constriction) and less so to local metabolites (which causes dilation). The sympathetic venous constriction decreases both the *capacity* and the compliance of the large veins, thereby tending to restore central venous pressure. In addition, sympathetic venous constriction increases **postcapillary resistance**, which is important for transcapillary refill (see later).

Circulating Vasoactive Agonists As already discussed, sympathetic stimulation of the adrenal medulla causes circulating epinephrine levels to rise. In addition, sympathetic

stimulation of the granular cells in the juxtaglomerular apparatus of the kidney leads to an increased release of renin and, ultimately, increased plasma levels of angiotensin II (ANG II; see Chapter 23). In hemorrhagic shock, ANG II rises to concentrations that are vasoconstrictive. Activation of the sympathetic system also triggers sympathetic cholinergic stimulation of the sweat glands (see Chapter 24), causing the patient's extremities to become clammy.

With moderate blood losses (10% to 20%), these four responses can increase total peripheral resistance sufficiently to keep arterial pressure at about normal levels. However, cardiac output remains depressed.

After hemorrhage, transcapillary refill, fluid conservation, and thirst restore the blood volume

The reflexes discussed in the preceding section compensate for the principal *consequences* of blood loss—decreased blood pressure and reduced cardiac output. The responses discussed here compensate for the *primary disturbance*, the loss of blood volume.

Transcapillary Refill   The movement of fluid from the interstitium to the blood plasma is the major defense against reduced blood volume. Starling forces (see Chapter 20) are critically important during hemorrhage and hypovolemic shock. Immediately after hemorrhage, a phase of **hemodilution** develops, as was first observed during World War I, when medics noted that injured soldiers arrived at the first-aid station with diluted blood (i.e., low hematocrit). Within an hour, interstitial fluid replaces ~75% of the shed blood volume. Studies performed around World War II showed that the dilution of **hemoglobin** is more pronounced than the dilution of **plasma proteins** after hemorrhage. Therefore, not only do fluid and electrolytes move from the interstitium to the blood, but proteins also enter the vascular compartment.

Transcapillary refill involves two steps. The first is **fluid movement** from the interstitium to the vasculature. Capillary hydrostatic pressure (P_c) (Fig. 25-10A) depends on arteriolar and venular pressures as well as on the relation of the precapillary to the postcapillary resistance (see Chapter 19). Immediately after the hemorrhage, the upstream arteriolar pressure and the downstream venular pressure both fall, causing P_c to fall (Fig. 25-10B). The Starling forces thus produce a large net movement of fluid and small electrolytes from the interstitium into the capillaries. As compensation occurs, total peripheral resistance increases, in part restoring arteriolar pressure (Fig. 25-10C). However, because precapillary resistance increases more than does postcapillary resistance, P_c remains relatively low, sustaining the net movement of fluid into the capillaries. Normally, little protein would enter with the fluid because nonfenestrated capillary walls reflect proteins very effectively (see Chapter 20). The entry of protein-free fluid into the capillary gradually modifies the three other Starling forces. First, the interstitial fluid volume decreases, lowering interstitial hydrostatic pressure (P_{if}). Second, the plasma proteins become diluted, so that capillary colloid osmotic pressure (π_c) falls. Finally, the removal of a protein-free solution from the interstitium raises colloid osmotic pressure in the bulk interstitium (π_{if}) and in the subglycocalyx fluid (π_{sg}; see Chapter 20). The result of these dissipating Starling forces is that transcapillary refill gradually wanes and eventually ceases.

The second step in transcapillary refill is the appearance of **plasma proteins** in the blood. These proteins probably enter the blood across fenestrae of the mesenteric and hepatic capillaries, two regions in which the interstitium has a very high interstitial colloid osmotic pressure. In addition, hemorrhage rapidly stimulates albumin synthesis by the liver. Plasmapheresis, the artificial removal of plasma proteins from the blood, has the same effect on albumin synthesis, suggesting that a reduction in the concentration

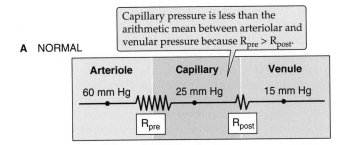

A NORMAL

> Capillary pressure is less than the arithmetic mean between arteriolar and venular pressure because $R_{pre} > R_{post}$.

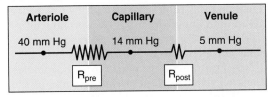

B UNCOMPENSATED HEMORRHAGE

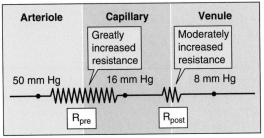

C COMPENSATED HEMORRHAGE

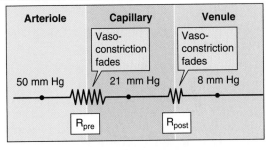

D DECOMPENSATED HEMORRHAGE

Figure 25-10   Effect of hemorrhage on capillary hydrostatic pressure. **A,** In this figure (which is similar to Fig. 19-4A), R_{pre} and R_{post} are the precapillary and postcapillary resistances, respectively. Here, the ratio $R_{post}/R_{pre} = 0.35$. **B,** The fall in capillary hydrostatic pressure reverses the Starling forces, causing net movement of fluid from the interstitium to the capillary lumen. **C,** Sympathetic stimulation increases total peripheral resistance ($R_{post}/R_{pre} = 0.25$ in this example). **D,** Capillary pressure rises ($R_{post}/R_{pre} = 0.45$ in this example).

of plasma proteins per se stimulates the liver to make albumin.

Water from the **intracellular** compartments ultimately replaces the lost **interstitial** fluid. What the driving force is for water to leave the cells and to enter the interstitium is somewhat controversial. The blood osmolality often rises after hemorrhage, presumably reflecting interstitial hyperosmolality. The additional interstitial osmoles come from ischemic tissues that release the products of proteolysis, glycolysis, and lipolysis. Therefore, interstitial hyperosmolality may provide the **osmotic** drive for the movement of water from the intracellular to the interstitial compartment.

Renal Conservation of Salt and Water   Arterial hypotension and lowered renal blood flow reduce the glomerular filtration rate (see Chapter 34) and therefore diminish the urinary excretion of salt and water. In addition to the direct hemodynamic effects, the reduced effective circulating volume promotes the renal retention of Na^+ by four mechanisms, which are discussed more fully in Chapter 40. First, reduced effective circulating volume activates the renin-angiotensin cascade, increasing aldosterone release and thus enhancing salt and water reabsorption by the distal nephron. Second, increased sympathetic nerve activity promotes Na^+ retention by altering renal hemodynamics, enhancing renin release and stimulating Na^+ reabsorption by renal tubule cells. Third, the release of AVP reduces water excretion. Finally, reduced effective circulating volume inhibits release of atrial natriuretic peptide and thus promotes renal Na^+ retention. Therefore, the overall response of the kidney to blood loss is to reduce the excretion of water and salt, thereby contributing to the conservation of extracellular fluid. However, the renal response only *conserves* fluid; by itself, it does not *add* any water to the extracellular fluid. (See Chapter 40.)

Thirst   The blood hyperosmolality caused by hemorrhage (discussed two paragraphs before) stimulates thirst osmoreceptors. A far more potent stimulus for thirst—as well as salt appetite—is the reduced effective circulating volume and blood pressure caused by severe hemorrhage. (See Chapter 40.) These urges, if fulfilled, actually provide some of the raw materials for replacement of the blood lost in hemorrhage.

Positive feedback mechanisms cause irreversible hemorrhagic shock

In some cases, hemorrhagic shock can be irreversible. After an initial fall in arterial pressure and perhaps some recovery, arterial pressure and the perfusion of peripheral tissues may inexorably deteriorate (Fig. 25-8, blue dashed curve). Moreover, in these cases, the fall in arterial pressure does not reverse even if the physician intervenes at this time and replaces the volume of blood lost as the result of hemorrhage.

The best experimental model for irreversible hemorrhagic shock is **prolonged hypotension**. Typically, the researcher acutely removes blood from an experimental animal—thereby reducing blood pressure to some low target value—and then *clamps* the mean arterial pressure at this low target by either removing or infusing blood as the normal physiological responses evolve. Studies of this kind reveal that hemorrhagic shock can become irreversible as a result of the failure of multiple response components: (1) the vasoconstrictor response, (2) the capillary refill response, (3) the cardiac response, and (4) the CNS response.

Failure of the Vasoconstrictor Response   With prolonged hemorrhagic hypotension, the total peripheral resistance—which first increases in response to sympathetic stimulation—tends to return to prehemorrhage levels. This failure to maintain vasoconstriction has several origins. First, desensitization of the vascular adrenoceptors or depletion of neurotransmitters in the nerve terminals close to the blood

vessels may cause "sympathetic escape." Second, the ischemic tissues release metabolites and other vasodilator compounds that act on local blood vessels, thereby counteracting the vasoconstricting stimuli. In the late phases of irreversible shock, humans may become completely unresponsive to a range of vasoconstrictor drugs. Third, plasma AVP levels may have fallen substantially from the peak value during the early phase of hemorrhage—perhaps reflecting a decreased ability of the low-pressure baroreceptor reflex to trigger hypothalamic neurons to release AVP or a depletion of AVP stores. Under these conditions, restoration of AVP levels to their initial peak can markedly increase blood pressure.

Failure of the Capillary Refill   Some blood vessels are able to sustain the initial increase in resistance better than others are. Over time, precapillary sphincters fail first, followed by the precapillary resistance vessels (i.e., arterioles), the postcapillary resistance vessels, and the capacitance vessels. Figure 25-10D shows an example in which, after prolonged hypotension, the precapillary constrictor response has fully faded, whereas the postcapillary response is partially maintained. Because the ratio R_{post}/R_{pre} has risen, the midcapillary pressure (see Chapter 19) increases from 16 mm Hg (Fig. 25-10C) to 21 mm Hg (Fig. 25-10D). You will recall that early during hemorrhage, the net Starling forces reverse, favoring the movement of fluid from the interstitium to the blood. The gradual increase of R_{post}/R_{pre} (Fig. 25-10D) reverses this reversal, so that fluid once again leaves the capillary, even though the blood volume has not yet been restored. Thus, after the initial large influx of water and electrolytes into the capillary lumen, not only does transcapillary refill decline, but a net loss occurs. This phenomenon contributes to the hemoconcentration that occasionally occurs in prolonged hemorrhagic states.

Failure of the Heart   Several factors may contribute to the weakening of the heart. Acidosis reduces $[Ca^{2+}]_i$ in the myocardium and thus reduces contractility. In severe cases, subendocardial hemorrhage and necrosis of the heart muscle render the myocardium nonfunctional. Various organs may also release cardiotoxic shock factors, which exert a negative inotropic effect on the heart (see Chapter 22). Ultimately, hypovolemic shock converts to cardiogenic shock.

Central Nervous System Depression   Moderate ischemia, by its effects on the central chemoreceptors, stimulates the cardiovascular control centers in the brain. However, prolonged cerebral ischemia depresses neural activity throughout the brain, thereby weakening the sympathetic output and in turn causing a decay in both vascular and cardiac responses. A progressive fall in the circulating levels of catecholamines of adrenal origin further worsens the outcome.

REFERENCES

Books and Reviews
Butler PJ, Jones DR: Physiology of diving of birds and mammals. Physiol Rev 1997; 77:837-899.
Gutierrez G, Reines HD, Wulf-Gutierrez ME: Clinical review: Hemorrhagic shock. Crit Care 2004; 8:373-380.

Kunze DL: Role of baroreceptor resetting in cardiovascular regulation: Acute resetting. Fed Proc 1995; 44:2408-2411.

Persson PB: Modulation of cardiovascular control mechanisms and their interaction. Physiol Rev 1996; 76:193-244.

Williamson JW, Fadel PJ, Mitchell JH: New insights into central cardiovascular control during exercise in humans: A central command update. Exp Physiol 2006; 91:51-58.

Journal Articles

Gulli G, Cooper VL, Claydon VE, Hainsworth R: Prolonged latency in the baroreflex mediated vascular resistance response in subjects with postural related syncope. Clin Auton Res 2005; 15:207-212.

Guyton AC, Coleman TG, Cowley AW Jr, et al: A systems analysis approach to understanding long-range arterial blood pressure control and hypertension. Circ Res 1974; 35:159-176.

Jacobsen TN, Morgan BJ, Scherrer U, et al: Relative contributions of cardiopulmonary and sinoaortic baroreflexes in causing sympathetic stimulation in the human skeletal muscle circulation during orthostatic stress. Circ Res 1993; 73:367-378.

Mellander S: Comparative studies on the adrenergic neurohormonal control of resistance and capacitance blood vessels in the cat. Acta Physiol Scand Suppl 1960; 50:1-86.

Smith OA Jr, Rushmer RF, Lasher EP: Similarity of cardiovascular responses to exercise and to diencephalic stimulation. Am J Physiol 1960; 198:1139-1142.

THE RESPIRATORY SYSTEM

CHAPTER 26

ORGANIZATION OF THE RESPIRATORY SYSTEM

Walter F. Boron

COMPARATIVE PHYSIOLOGY OF RESPIRATION

External respiration is the exchange of O_2 and CO_2 between the atmosphere and the mitochondria

For millennia, people have regarded breathing as being synonymous with life. Life begins and ends with breathing. The Bible states that God "breathed into [Adam's] nostrils the breath of life" and then later used part of Adam's ventilatory apparatus—a rib—to give life to Eve.

In the fourth and fifth centuries BC, writings attributed to Hippocrates suggested that the primary purpose of breathing is to cool the heart. It was not until the 18th century that the true role of breathing began to emerge as several investigators studied the chemistry of gases. Chemists had recognized similarities between combustion and breathing but thought that both involved the release of a "fire-essence" called phlogiston. According to their theory, neither combustion nor life could be supported once air became saturated with phlogiston.

In the 1750s, Joseph Black found that heating calcium carbonate produces a gas he called fixed air, now known to be **carbon dioxide (CO_2)**. This work revolutionized chemistry by showing that other gases exist besides ordinary "air" and that a chemical reaction can involve a gas. Shortly thereafter, Henry Cavendish found that fermentation and putrefaction also produce "fixed air." Joseph Priestley discovered several new gases between the late 1760s and mid-1770s, including "dephlogistonated air," co-discovered by Carl Scheele. Priestley found that combustion, putrefaction, and breathing all *consume* dephlogistonated air and all reduce the volume of room air by ~20%. Conversely, he found that green plants *produce* dephlogistonated air, which he quantitated by reacting it with nitric oxide (a colorless gas) to produce nitrogen dioxide (a red gas).

In the mid-1770s, Priestley presented his findings to Antoine Lavoisier—often regarded as the father of modern chemistry. Lavoisier quickly put Priestley's empirical observations into a theoretical framework that he used to demolish the phlogiston theory, which Priestley held to his death.

Lavoisier recognized that dephlogistonated air, which he named **oxygen (O_2)**, represents the ~20% of room air consumed by combustion in Priestley's experiments, leaving behind "nonvital" air, or **nitrogen**. Furthermore, he proposed that O_2 is consumed because it reacts with one substance to produce another. The mathematician Joseph-Louis Lagrange suggested that O_2 consumption and CO_2 production occur not in the lungs but in isolated tissues, as Lazzaro Spallanzani later rigorously demonstrated in the late 18th century.

Thus, by the end of the 18th century, chemists and physiologists appreciated that combustion, putrefaction, and respiration all involve chemical reactions that consume O_2 and produce CO_2. Subsequent advances in the chemistry of gases by Boyle, Henry, Avogadro, and others laid the theoretical foundation for the physiology of O_2 and CO_2. Thus, respiration was a unifying theme in the early histories of physiology, chemistry, and biochemistry.

Later work showed that mitochondrial respiration (i.e., the oxidation of carbon-containing compounds to form CO_2) is responsible for the O_2 consumption and CO_2 production observed by Spallanzani. This aspect of respiration is often called **internal respiration** or oxidative phosphorylation (see Chapter 58).

In the chapters on respiratory physiology, we focus on **external respiration**, the dual processes of (1) transporting O_2 from the atmosphere to the mitochondria and (2) transporting CO_2 from the mitochondria to the atmosphere. We will also see that CO_2 transport is intimately related to acid-base homeostasis.

Diffusion is the major mechanism of external respiration for small aquatic organisms

The most fundamental mechanism of O_2 and CO_2 transport is **diffusion** (see Chapter 5). Random movements of molecules such as O_2 and CO_2, whether in a gaseous phase or dissolved in water, result in a net movement of the substance from regions of high concentration to regions of low concentration (Fig. 26-1A, inset). No expenditure of energy is involved. The driving force for diffusion is the concentration gradient.

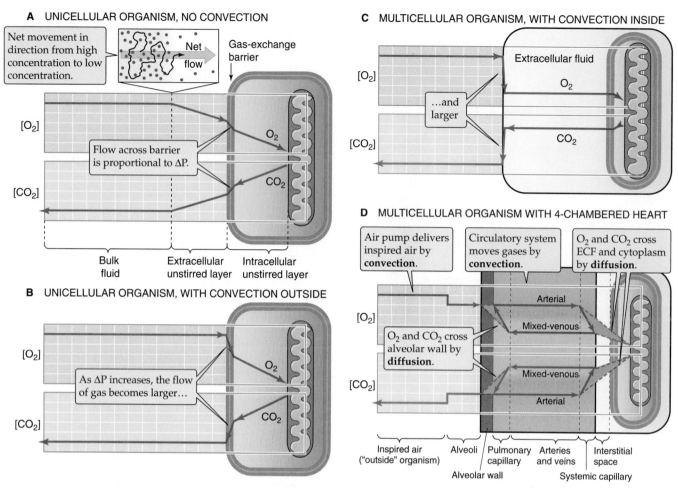

Figure 26-1 Diffusion of O_2 and CO_2 for a single-celled organism. In **A** to **D**, the y-axis of grids shows the dissolved concentration (or partial pressure) of O_2 and CO_2. The x-axis represents distance (not to scale). In **D**, the *broken red* and *blue lines* and the enclosed *violet triangles* represent the magnitude of the gradients driving O_2 and CO_2 diffusion. The *red* (O_2) and *blue* (CO_2) pathways represent the circuit of blood from the pulmonary capillaries to the systemic capillaries and back again.

Imagine a unicellular organism suspended in a beaker of pond water at 37°C. The water is in equilibrium with an atmosphere that has the usual composition of O_2 and CO_2 (Table 26-1). The partial pressures of O_2 (P_{O_2}) and of CO_2 (P_{CO_2}) in the *dry* air are slightly higher than their corresponding values in the *wet* air immediately above the surface of the water (see the box on wet gases). It is these partial pressures in wet air that determine the concentrations of dissolved O_2 ($[O_2]_{Dis}$) and dissolved CO_2 ($[CO_2]_{Dis}$) in the water (see the box on partial pressures and Henry's law). Thus, the P_{O_2} in the wet air—as well as the water beneath it—will be ~149 mm Hg (or torr), and the P_{CO_2} will be an almost negligible 0.2 mm Hg. These numbers describe the composition of the **bulk phase** of the pond water (Fig. 26-1A, left side), at some distance from the organism. However, because the mitochondria within the organism continuously consume O_2 and produce CO_2, the P_{O_2} at the surface of the mitochondria will be lower than the bulk-phase P_{O_2}, whereas the P_{CO_2} at the mitochondrial surface will be higher than the bulk-phase P_{CO_2} (Fig. 26-1A, right side). These differences in partial pressure cause O_2 to diffuse from the bulk pond water toward

Table 26-1 Composition of Air

Gas	DRY AIR, ATMOSPHERE		WET AIR, TRACHEA	
	Fraction in Air (%)	Partial Pressure at Sea Level (mm Hg)	Fraction in Air (%)	Partial Pressure at Sea Level (mm Hg)
N_2	78.09	593.48	73.26	556.78
O_2	20.95	159.22	19.65	149.37
CO_2	0.03	0.23	0.03	0.21
Ar	0.93	7.07	0.87	6.63
H_2O	0	0	6.18	47
Total	100	760	100	760

N_2, nitrogen; Ar, argon.

Wet Gases: Partial Pressures of O_2 and CO_2 in Solutions That Are Equilibrated with Wet Air

Imagine that a beaker of water is equilibrated with a normal atmosphere and that both water and atmosphere have a temperature of 37°C. For dry air (i.e., air containing no water vapor), O_2 makes up ~21% of the total gas by volume (Table 26-1). Thus, if the ambient pressure—or **barometric pressure (P_B)**—is 760 mm Hg, the partial pressure of O_2 (P_{O_2}) is 21% of 760 mm Hg, or 159 mm Hg (Fig. 26-2). However, if the air-water interface is reasonably stationary, water vapor will saturate the air immediately adjacent to the liquid. What is the P_{O_2} in this wet air? At 37°C, the partial pressure of water (P_{H_2O}) is 47 mm Hg. Of the total pressure of the wet air, P_{H_2O} makes up 47 mm Hg, and the components of the dry air make up the remaining 760 − 47, or 713 mm Hg. Thus, the partial pressure of O_2 in this wet air is

$$P_{O_2} = \overbrace{F_{O_2}}^{\text{Fraction of dry air that is } O_2} \cdot (P_B - P_{H_2O})$$
$$= (21\%) \cdot (760 \text{ mm Hg} - 47 \text{ mm Hg})$$
$$= 149 \text{ mm Hg}$$

The CO_2 composition of dry air is ~0.03% (Table 26-1). Thus, the partial pressure of CO_2 in wet air is

$$P_{CO_2} = F_{CO_2} \cdot (P_B - P_{H_2O})$$
$$= (0.03\%) \cdot (760 \text{ mm Hg} - 47 \text{ mm Hg})$$
$$= 0.21 \text{ mm Hg}$$

These examples are realistic for respiratory physiology. As we inhale relatively cool and dry air, the nose and other upper respiratory passages rapidly warm and moisturize the passing air so that it assumes the composition of wet air given in Table 26-1.

Partial Pressures and Henry's Law

Respiratory physiologists generally express the concentration of a gas, whether it is mixed with another gas (e.g., O_2 mixed with N_2, as is the case for air) or dissolved in an aqueous solution (e.g., O_2 dissolved in water), in terms of partial pressure. **Dalton's law** states that the total pressure (P_{total}) of a mixture of gases is the sum of their individual **partial pressures**. Imagine that we are dealing with an ideal gas (Z) mixed with other gases. Because the ratio of the partial pressure of Z (P_Z) to the total pressure (P_{total}) is its mole fraction (X_Z),

$$P_Z = X_Z \cdot P_{total}$$

Thus, if P_Z in one sample of gas were twice as high as in another, X_Z (i.e., concentration of Z) would also be twice as high.

It may not be immediately obvious why—when Z is dissolved in aqueous solutions—it is still reasonable to express the concentration of Z in terms of P_Z. According to **Henry's law**, the concentration of O_2 dissolved in water ($[O_2]_{Dis}$) is proportional to P_{O_2} in the gas phase:

$$[O_2]_{Dis} = s \cdot P_{O_2}$$

The proportionality constant s is the **solubility**; for O_2, s is ~0.0013 mM/mm Hg at 37°C for a solution mimicking blood plasma. The solubility of CO_2 is ~23-fold higher. Consider a beaker of water at 37°C equilibrated with an atmosphere having a P_{O_2} of 100 mm Hg, the partial pressure in mammalian *arterial* blood plasma (Fig. 26-3A, solution 1):

$$[O_2]_{Dis} = \left(0.0013 \frac{\text{mM}}{\text{mm Hg}}\right) \cdot (100 \text{ mm Hg})$$
$$= 0.13 \text{ mM}$$

Now consider a second beaker equilibrated with an atmosphere having a P_{O_2} of 40 mm Hg, the partial pressure of O_2 in *mixed-venous* blood (Fig. 26-3A, solution 2):

$$[O_2]_{Dis} = \left(0.0013 \frac{\text{mM}}{\text{mm Hg}}\right) \cdot (40 \text{ mm Hg})$$
$$= 0.05 \text{ mM}$$

If we now place samples of these two solutions on opposite sides of a semipermeable barrier in a closed container (Fig. 26-3B), the O_2 gradient across this barrier expressed in terms of concentrations ($\Delta[O_2]$) is 0.13 − 0.05 or 0.08 mM. Expressed in terms of partial pressures (ΔP_{O_2}), this same gradient is 100 − 40 = 60 mm Hg.

Imagine now that we take a 5-mL sample of each of the solutions in the beakers in Figure 26-3A, drawing the fluid up into syringes, sealing the syringes, putting them on ice, and sending them to a clinical laboratory for analysis—as is routinely done with samples of arterial blood. Even though there is no gas phase in equilibrium with either of the solutions in the syringes, the laboratory will report the O_2 levels in millimeters of mercury (mm Hg). These are the partial pressures of O_2 with which the solutions were or would have to be equilibrated to achieve the $[O_2]_{Dis}$ in the liquid samples.

the mitochondria and the CO_2 to diffuse in the opposite direction.

The diffusion of O_2 follows a gradient of decreasing P_{O_2} (Fig. 26-1A). The region over which P_{O_2} falls gradually from the bulk pond water toward the outer surface of the plasma membrane is the **extracellular unstirred layer**, so named because no convective mixing occurs in this zone. A similar gradual decline in P_{O_2} drives O_2 diffusion through the **intracellular unstirred layer**, from the inner surface of the plasma membrane to the mitochondria. The abrupt fall in P_{O_2} across the plasma membrane reflects some resistance to gas flow. The profile for P_{CO_2} is similar, although with the opposite orientation.

The rate at which O_2 or CO_2 moves across the surface of the organism is the **flow** (units: moles/s). According to a simplified version of **Fick's law** (see Chapter 5), flow is proportional to the concentration difference across this barrier. Because we know from Henry's law that the concentration of a dissolved gas is proportional to its partial pressure in the

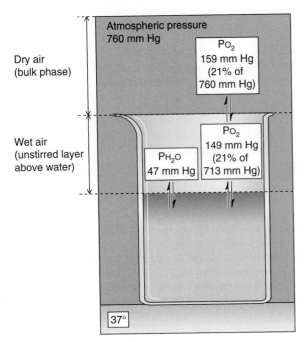

Figure 26-2 Wet versus dry gases.

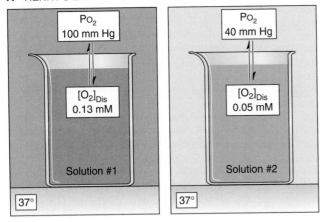

A HENRY'S LAW

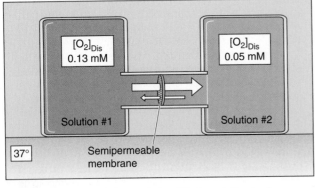

B DIFFUSION OF DISSOLVED GAS

Figure 26-3 Henry's law and the diffusion of dissolved gases.

gas phase, flow is also proportional to the partial pressure difference (ΔP):

$$\text{Flow} \propto \Delta P \qquad (26\text{-}1)$$

Simple diffusion is the mechanism by which O_2 and CO_2 move *short* distances in the respiratory system: between the air and blood in the alveoli, and between the mitochondria and blood of the peripheral circulation.

Convection enhances diffusion by producing steeper gradients across the diffusion barrier

A purely diffusive system can establish only a relatively small ΔP across the gas-exchange barrier of the organism (Fig. 26-1A). Yet, for small organisms, even this relatively small ΔP is adequate to meet the demands for O_2 uptake and CO_2 removal. However, when the organism's diameter exceeds ~1 mm, simple diffusion becomes inadequate for gas exchange. One way of ameliorating this problem is to introduce a mechanism for **convection** on the outside surface of the organism. For a paramecium, the beating cilia bring bulk-phase water—having a P_{O_2} of ~154 mm Hg at 25°C and a P_{CO_2} of ~0.2 mm Hg—very near to the cell's surface. This mixing reduces the size of the extracellular unstirred layer, thereby increasing the P_{O_2} and decreasing the P_{CO_2} on the outer surface of the organism. The net effect is that the partial pressure gradients for both O_2 and CO_2 increase across the gas exchange barrier (Fig. 26-1B), leading to a proportionate increase in the flow of both substances.

A filter feeder, such as an oyster or a clam, pumps bulk-phase water past its organ of gas exchange. Because of the relatively low solubility of O_2 in water, such an organism may need to pump 16,000 mL of water to extract a mere 1 mL of O_2 gas. In fish, which are far more efficient, the ratio may be considerably lower, ~400 : 1.

In mammals, the bulk phase is the atmosphere and the external convective system is an air pump that includes the chest wall, the respiratory muscles, and the passages through which the air flows (i.e., from the nose up to the alveoli). **Ventilation** is the process of moving air into and out of the lungs. Amphibians move air into their lungs by swallowing it. Reptiles, birds, and mammals expand their lungs by developing a negative pressure inside the thorax. Because of the much higher O_2 content of air (about 210 mL O_2/L of air at standard temperature and pressure/dry or STPD; see the box on page 617) as opposed to water (~35 mL O_2/L of water), humans need to move far less air than oysters need to move water. For example, a human may ventilate the alveoli with 4000 mL of fresh air every minute and extract from this air 250 mL of O_2 gas, a ratio of 16 : 1.

Although we are 1000-fold more efficient than oysters, the principle of external convective systems is the same: ensure that the external surface of the gas exchange barrier is in close contact with a fluid whose composition matches—as closely as is practical—that of the bulk phase. How "closely" is "practical"? The composition of alveolar air approaches that of wet inspired air as alveolar ventilation approaches infinity (see Chapter 31). Because high ventilatory rates have a significant metabolic cost, the body must

Conventions for Measurement of Volumes of Gases

BTPS

Gases within the lung are saturated with water vapor at 37°C (310 K). At this temperature, P_{H_2O} is 47 mm Hg (see the box on wet gases). If the glottis is open and no air is flowing, then the total pressure of the air in the lungs is P_B, which we will assume to be 760 mm Hg. In this case, the partial pressure of *dry* gases in the lungs is (760 − 47) = 713 mm Hg. The convention is to report the volume of gases in the lungs—and changes in the volume of these gases—at body temperature and pressure, saturated with water or **BTPS**. Such volumes include both wet and dry gases.

ATPS

If we exhale a volume of air from the lungs (ΔV_{BTPS}) into a spirometer, the "floor" of which is formed by water (Fig. 26-8), the exhaled air will now be at ambient temperature and pressure, saturated with water or **ATPS**. Thus, we must correct the volume change (ΔV_{ATPS}) registered by the spirometer (at ATPS) to know the volume that this same gas had occupied in the lungs (at BTPS). Two factors are at work as warm alveolar air moves into a cooler spirometer: (1) P_{H_2O} decreases and some gaseous H_2O condenses into liquid H_2O, according to the temperature dependence of P_{H_2O}; and (2) the pressure exerted by the dry gas molecules decreases, according to Charles' law. Starting from the Boyle-Charles law:

$$\frac{P_{BTPS} \cdot \Delta V_{BTPS}}{T_{BTPS}} = \frac{P_{ATPS} \cdot \Delta V_{ATPS}}{T_{ATPS}}$$

it is possible to show that

$$\Delta V_{BTPS} = \frac{(P_B - P_{H_2O \text{ at } T_{ambient}})}{(P_B - P_{H_2O \text{ at } T_{body}})} \cdot \frac{T_{body}}{T_{ambient}} \cdot \Delta V_{ATPS}$$

Here, T_{body} and $T_{ambient}$ are absolute temperatures.

If T_{body} is 37°C (310 K), then the corresponding P_{H_2O} is 47 mm Hg. If $T_{ambient}$ is 25°C (or 298 K), then the corresponding P_{H_2O} is 24 mm Hg. For these conditions, the conversion from an ATPS volume to a BTPS volume becomes

$$\Delta V_{BTPS} = \frac{(760 - 24)}{(760 - 47)} \cdot \frac{310 \text{ K}}{298 \text{ K}} \cdot \Delta V_{ATPS} = 1.074 \cdot \Delta V_{ATPS}$$

Thus, the same wet gas that occupies 1000 mL in the spirometer at ATPS occupies 1074 mL in the lungs at BTPS.

STPD

The convention is to report the volume of gases in the blood (e.g., dissolved CO_2 or O_2 bound to hemoglobin) in the same way that chemists would—at standard temperature and pressure/dry or **STPD**. The standard temperature is 0°C (273 K), and the standard pressure is 760 mm Hg. You may recall from introductory chemistry that a mole of an ideal gas occupies 22.4 L at STPD. If you wish to convert a ΔV_{STPD} to a ΔV_{BTPS}, it is possible to show that

$$\Delta V_{BTPS} = \frac{P_B}{P_B - P_{H2O \text{ at } T_{body}}} \cdot \frac{T_{body}}{T_{standard}} \cdot \Delta V_{STPD}$$

For a body temperature of 37°C, the conversion from a BTPS volume to an STPD volume becomes

$$\Delta V_{BTPS} = \frac{760}{760 - 47} \cdot \frac{310}{273} \cdot \Delta V_{STPD} = 1.21 \cdot \Delta V_{STPD}$$

Thus, the same dry gas that occupies 1000 mL under standard chemical conditions occupies 1210 mL in the body at BTPS.

---

trade off optimizing alveolar P_{O_2} and P_{CO_2} on the one hand against minimizing the work of ventilation on the other. In the average adult human, the compromise that has evolved is an alveolar ventilation of ~4000 mL/min, an alveolar P_{O_2} of ~100 mm Hg (versus 149 mm Hg in a wet atmosphere at 37°C), and an alveolar P_{CO_2} of ~40 mm Hg (versus 0.2 mm Hg).

A clinical example in which the external convective system fails is barbiturate poisoning. Here, drug intoxication inhibits the respiratory control centers in the medulla (see Chapter 32), so that ventilation slows or even stops. The consequence is that the unstirred layer between the bulk-phase atmosphere and the alveolar blood-gas barrier becomes extremely large (i.e., the distance between the nose and the alveoli). As a result, alveolar P_{O_2} falls to such low levels that the ΔP_{O_2} across the alveolar wall cannot support an O_2 flow and an arterial $[O_2]$ that is compatible with life. Cessation of ventilation also causes the alveolar P_{CO_2} to rise to such high levels that the CO_2 flow from blood to alveolar air is unacceptably low.

An *external* convective system maximizes gas exchange by continuously supplying bulk-phase water or air to the exter-

nal surface of the gas exchange barrier, thereby maintaining a high external P_{O_2} and a low external P_{CO_2}. A **circulatory system** is an *internal* convective system that maximizes flow of O_2 and CO_2 across the gas exchange barrier by delivering, to the inner surface of this barrier, blood that has as low a P_{O_2} and as high a P_{CO_2} as is practical. **Perfusion** is the process of delivering blood to the lungs. Figure 26-1C shows a primitive—and hypothetical—internal convective system, one that essentially stirs the entire internal contents of the organism, so that the P_{O_2} of the bulk internal fluids is uniform, right up to the surface of the mitochondria. The result is that the ΔP_{O_2} across the gas exchange barrier is rather large, but the ΔP_{O_2} between the bulk internal fluid and the mitochondria is rather small.

Figure 26-1D summarizes the P_{O_2} and P_{CO_2} profiles for a sophisticated circulatory system built around a four-chambered heart and separate pulmonary and systemic circulations. The circulatory system carries (by convection) low-P_{O_2} blood from a systemic capillary near the mitochondria to the alveolar wall. At the beginning of a pulmonary capillary, a high alveolar-to-blood P_{O_2} gradient ensures a high O_2 inflow (by diffusion), and blood P_{O_2} rises to match the alveolar (i.e., external) P_{O_2} by the time the blood leaves the pulmonary capillary. Finally, the systemic arterial blood carries (by convection) this high-P_{O_2} blood to the systemic capillaries, where a high blood-to-mitochondria P_{O_2} gradient maximizes the O_2 flux into the mitochondria (by diffusion). The opposite happens with CO_2. Thus, separate pulmonary and systemic circulations ensure maximal gradients for gas diffusion in both the pulmonary and systemic capillaries.

The scenario outlined in Figure 26-1D requires the four-chambered heart characteristic of mammals as well as of advanced reptiles and birds. The right ventricle pumps low-P_{O_2}/high-P_{CO_2} blood received from the peripheral veins to the lungs, whereas the left ventricle pumps high-P_{O_2}/low-P_{CO_2} blood received from pulmonary veins to the periphery (i.e., mitochondria). Maintenance of maximal gradients for O_2 and CO_2 diffusion in both the pulmonary and systemic capillaries at the mitochondria requires that right and left ventricular blood not mix. However, this sort of mixing is exactly what occurs in fish and amphibians, whose hearts have a common ventricle. In these animals, the aortic blood has P_{O_2} and P_{CO_2} values that are intermediate between the extreme values of venous blood returning from the systemic circulation and the blood returning from the gas-exchange barrier. The result is less than optimal P_{O_2} and P_{CO_2} gradients at both the gas exchange barrier and the mitochondria.

In humans, the internal convective system may fail when diseased heart valves cause a decrease in cardiac output. Another example is the shunting of blood between the pulmonary and the systemic circulations, as may occur in newborns with congenital anomalies (e.g., atrial or ventricular septal defects). The result is the same sort of mixing of systemic venous and gas exchange barrier blood that occurs in amphibians and fish. Thus, patients with shunts cannot establish normal P_{O_2} and P_{CO_2} gradients in the pulmonary and peripheral capillaries and thus cannot generate normal flows of O_2 and CO_2.

Surface area amplification enhances diffusion

the passive flow of O_2 or CO_2 across a barrier is proportional not only to the concentration gradient but also to the area of the barrier:

$$\text{Flow} \propto \Delta P \times \text{Area} \qquad (26\text{-}2)$$

Indeed, higher animals have increased their ability to exchange O_2 and CO_2 with their environment by increasing the **surface area** across which gas exchange takes place. For example, mollusks (e.g., squid) and fish have gills, which they form by evaginating the gas exchange barrier, thus greatly amplifying its surface area. Higher land animals amplify their gas exchange barriers by invaginating them, forming lungs. In an amphibian such as the adult frog, the lungs are simple air sacs with a relatively small surface area. Not surprisingly, a large portion of their gas exchange must occur across the skin. The gas exchange barrier is considerably more sophisticated in reptiles, which line their lungs with alveoli or even subdivide them with alveoli-lined barriers. The net effect is to increase the surface-to-volume ratio of the lungs. Mammals increase the area available for diffu-

sion even more, by developing highly complex lungs with bronchi and a large number of alveoli.

In humans, the lung surface is so large and so thin that O_2 and CO_2 transport across the alveolar wall is ~3-fold faster than necessary—at least when the person is resting at sea level. Nevertheless, this redundancy is extremely important during exercise (when cardiac output can increase markedly), for life at high altitude (where the P_{O_2} is low), and in old age (when lung function diminishes). A substantial decrease in surface area, or thickening of the barrier, can be deleterious. Examples are the surgical removal of a lung (which reduces the total surface for gas exchange by about half) and pulmonary edema (which increases the effective thickness of the barrier). Thus, if an individual with a thickened barrier loses a lung, the remaining surface area may not be large enough to sustain adequate rates of gas exchange.

Respiratory pigments such as hemoglobin increase the carrying capacity of the blood for both O_2 and CO_2

In mammals, the external convective system (i.e., ventilatory apparatus), the internal convective system (i.e., circulatory system), and the barrier itself (i.e., alveolar wall) are so efficient that the diffusion of O_2 and CO_2 is not what limits the exchange of gases, at least not in healthy subjects at sea level.

Imagine what would happen if the mixed-venous blood flowing down a pulmonary capillary contained only water and salts. The diffusion of O_2 from the alveolar air space into the "blood" is so fast—and the solubility of O_2 in saline is so low (see the box on Henry's law)—that before the blood could move ~1% of the way down the capillary, the P_{O_2} of the blood would match the P_{O_2} of the alveolar air (i.e., all of the O_2 that *could* move *would* have moved). For the remaining ~99% of the capillary, the P_{O_2} gradient across the barrier would be nil, and no more O_2 would flow into the blood. As a result, at a normal cardiac output, the "blood" could never carry away enough O_2 from the lungs to the tissues to sustain life. The same is true in reverse for the elimination of CO_2.

Animals solve this problem with respiratory pigments, specialized metalloproteins that—via the metal—reversibly bind O_2, greatly increasing the carrying capacity of blood for O_2. In some arthropods and mollusks, the pigment is **hemocyanin**, which coordinates two copper atoms. Polychaete worms and brachiopods use **hemerythrins**, which coordinate two iron atoms. However, the most common—and most efficient—respiratory pigments are the **hemoglobins**, which coordinate a porphyrin ring that contains iron. All vertebrates as well as numerous unrelated groups of animals use hemoglobin, which is the chief component of erythrocytes or red blood cells.

The presence of hemoglobin markedly improves the dynamics of O_2 uptake by blood passing through the lungs. Under normal conditions, hemoglobin reversibly binds ~96% of the O_2 that diffuses from the alveolar air spaces to the pulmonary capillary blood, greatly increasing the carrying capacity of blood for O_2. Hemoglobin also plays a key role in the transport or **carriage** of CO_2 by reversibly binding CO_2 and by acting as a powerful pH buffer. In **anemia**, the hemoglobin content of blood is reduced, thus lowering the carrying capacity of blood for O_2 and CO_2. An individual with anemia can compensate only if the systemic tissues extract more O_2 from each liter of blood or if cardiac output increases. However, there are limits to the amount of O_2 that tissues can extract or to the level to which the heart can increase its output.

Pathophysiology recapitulates phylogeny—in reverse

It should be clear from the pathophysiological examples discussed that when a key component of the respiratory system fails in a higher organism, external respiration becomes more like that of an organism lower on the evolutionary ladder. For example, a failure of a mammal's air pump makes this individual behave more like a unicellular aquatic organism without cilia. A reduction in the surface area of the alveoli in a mammal creates the same problems faced by an amphibian with simple sack-like lungs. A major shunt in the circulatory system makes a mammal behave more like a fish. In severe anemia, a mammal faces the same problems as a lower life form with a less efficient respiratory pigment.

ORGANIZATION OF THE RESPIRATORY SYSTEM IN HUMANS

Humans optimize each aspect of external respiration—ventilation, circulation, area amplification, gas carriage, local control, and central control

The human respiratory system (Fig. 26-4) has two important characteristics. First, it uses highly efficient convective systems (i.e., ventilatory and circulatory systems) for long-distance transport of O_2 and CO_2. Second, it reserves diffusion exclusively for short-distance movements of O_2 and CO_2. The key components of this respiratory system are the following:

1. **An air pump.** The external convective system consists of the upper respiratory tract and large pulmonary airways, the thoracic cavity and associated skeletal elements, and the muscles of respiration. These components deliver air to and remove air from the alveolar air spaces—**alveolar ventilation.** Inspiration occurs when muscle contractions increase the volume of the thoracic cavity, thereby lowering intrathoracic pressure, which causes the alveoli to expand passively, which in turn lowers alveolar pressure. Air then flows from the environment to the alveoli, down a pressure gradient. A quiet expiration occurs when the muscles relax. We discuss the mechanics of ventilation in Chapter 27.

2. **Mechanisms for carrying O_2 and CO_2 in the blood.** Red blood cells are highly specialized for transporting O_2 from the lungs to the peripheral tissues and for transporting CO_2 in the opposite direction. They have extremely high levels of hemoglobin and other components that help to rapidly load and unload huge amounts of O_2 and CO_2. In the pulmonary capillaries, hemoglobin binds O_2, thereby

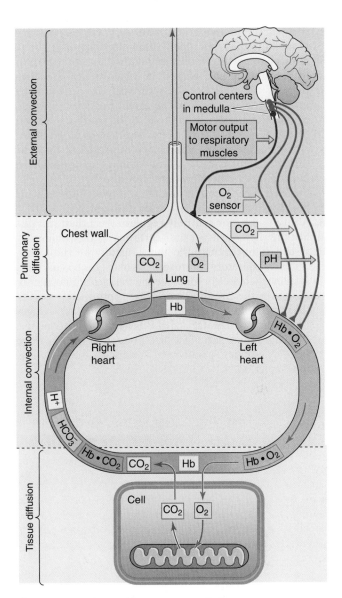

Figure 26-4 The respiratory apparatus in humans.

enabling the blood to carry ~65-fold more O_2 than saline. In the systemic capillaries, hemoglobin plays a key role in the carriage of CO_2—produced by the mitochondria—to the lungs. Hemoglobin accomplishes this task by chemically reacting with some of the CO_2 and by buffering the H^+ formed as carbonic anhydrase converts CO_2 to HCO_3^- and H^+. Thus, hemoglobin plays a central role in acid-base chemistry, as discussed in Chapter 28, as well as for the carriage of O_2 and CO_2, treated in Chapter 29.

3. **A surface for gas exchange.** The gas exchange barrier in humans consists of the alveoli, which provide a huge but extremely thin surface area for passive diffusion of gases between the alveolar air spaces and the pulmonary capillaries. We discuss the anatomy of the alveoli later in this chapter and explore pulmonary gas exchange in Chapter 30. A similar process of gas exchange occurs between the systemic capillaries and mitochondria.

4. **A circulatory system.** The internal convective system in humans consists of a four-chambered heart and separate

systemic and pulmonary circulations. We discuss the flow of blood to the lungs—**perfusion**—in Chapter 31.

5. **A mechanism for locally regulating the distribution of ventilation and perfusion.** Efficient gas exchange requires that the ratio of ventilation to perfusion be uniform for all alveoli to the extent possible. However, neither the delivery of fresh air to the entire population of alveoli nor the delivery of mixed-venous blood to the entire population of pulmonary capillaries is uniform throughout the lungs. The lungs attempt to maximize the uniformity of ventilation-perfusion ratios by using sophisticated feedback control mechanisms to regulate local air flow and blood flow, as discussed in Chapter 31.

6. **A mechanism for centrally regulating ventilation.** Unlike the rhythmicity of the heart, that of the respiratory system is not intrinsic to the lungs or the chest wall. Instead, respiratory control centers in the **central nervous system** rhythmically stimulate the muscles of inspiration. Moreover, these respiratory centers appropriately modify the pattern of ventilation during exercise or other changes in physical or mental activity. Sensors for arterial P_{O_2}, P_{CO_2}, and pH are part of feedback loops that stabilize these three "blood gas" parameters. We discuss these subjects in Chapter 32.

Respiratory physiologists have agreed on a set of symbols to describe parameters that are important for pulmonary physiology and pulmonary function tests (Table 26-2).

Conducting airways deliver fresh air to the alveolar spaces

We will discuss lung development in Chapter 57. In the embryo, each lung invaginates into a separate pleural sac, which reflects over the surface of the lung.

The **parietal pleura**, the wall of the sac that is farthest from the lung, contains blood vessels that are believed to produce an ultrafiltrate of the plasma called **pleural fluid**. About 10 mL of this fluid normally occupies the virtual space between the parietal and the **visceral pleura**. The visceral pleura lies directly on the lung and contains lymphatics that drain the fluid from the pleural space. When the production of pleural fluid exceeds its removal, the volume of pleural fluid increases (**pleural effusion**), limiting the expansion of the lung. Under normal circumstances, the pleural fluid probably lubricates the pleural space, facilitating physiological changes in lung size and shape.

The lungs themselves are divided into **lobes**, three in the right lung (i.e., upper, middle, and lower lobes) and two in

Table 26-2 Symbol Conventions in Respiratory Physiology

RESPIRATORY MECHANICS		GAS EXCHANGE	
Main Symbols		**Main Symbols**	
C	Compliance	C	Concentration (or content) in a liquid
f	Respiratory frequency	D	Diffusion capacity
P	Pressure	f	Respiratory frequency
R	Resistance	F	Fraction
V	Volume of gas	P	Pressure
$\dot{V}$	Flow of gas	$\dot{Q}$	Flow of blood (perfusion)
		R	Gas exchange ratio
		S	Saturation of hemoglobin
		V	Volume of gas
		$\dot{V}$	Ventilation
Modifiers		**Modifiers**	
A	Alveolar	a	Systemic arterial
AW	Airway	A	Alveolar
B	Barometric	B	Barometric
		c	Pulmonary capillary
		E	Expired
		I	Inspired
		v	Systemic venous (in any vascular bed)
		$\bar{v}$	Mixed systemic venous

Data from Macklem PT: Symbols and abbreviations. In Handbook of Physiology, Section 3: The Respiratory System, vol 1. Bethesda, MD: American Physiological Society, 1985.

the left (i.e., upper and lower lobes). The right lung, which is less encumbered than the left by the presence of the heart, makes up ~55% of total lung mass and function.

We refer to the progressively bifurcating pulmonary airways by their **generation number** (Fig. 26-5). The zeroth generation is the trachea, the first-generation airways are the right and left mainstem bronchi, and so on. Inasmuch as the right mainstem bronchus has a greater diameter than the left and is more nearly parallel with the trachea, inhaled foreign bodies more commonly lodge in the right lung than in the left. Humans have ~23 generations of airways. As generation number increases (i.e., as airways become smaller), the amount of cilia, the number of mucus-secreting cells, the presence of submucosal glands, and the amount of cartilage in the airway walls all gradually decrease. The mucus is important for trapping small foreign particles. The cilia sweep the carpet of mucus—kept moist by secretions from the submucosal glands—up toward the pharynx, where

swallowing eventually disposes of the mucus. The cartilage is important for preventing airway collapse, which is especially a problem during expiration (see Chapter 27). Airways maintain some cartilage to about the 10th generation, up to which point they are referred to as **bronchi**.

Beginning at about the 11th generation, the now cartilage-free airways are called **bronchioles**. Because they lack cartilage, bronchioles can maintain a patent lumen only because the pressure surrounding them may be more negative than the pressure inside and because of the outward pull (radial traction or tethering) of surrounding tissues. Thus, bronchioles are especially susceptible to collapse during expiration. Up until generation ~16, no alveoli are present, and the air cannot exchange with the pulmonary capillary blood. The airways from the nose and lips down to the alveoli-free bronchioles are the **conducting airways**, which serve only to move air by convection (i.e., like water moving through a pipe) to those regions of the lung that participate

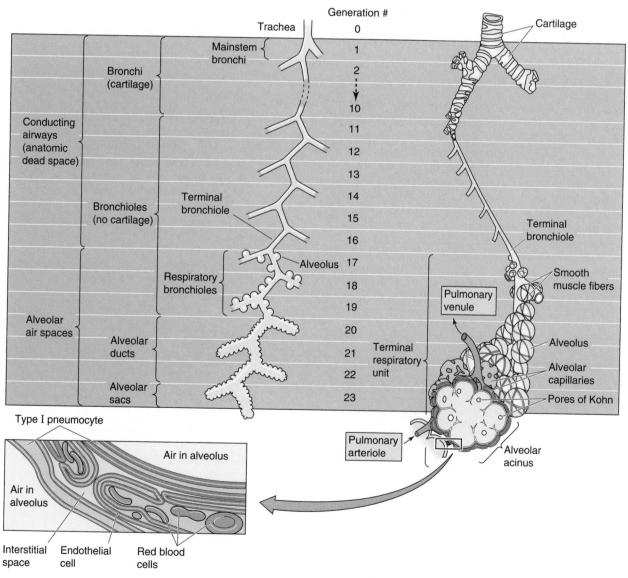

Figure 26-5 Generations of airways.

in gas exchange. The most distal conducting airways are the **terminal bronchioles** (generation ~16). The aggregate volume of conducting airways, the **anatomical dead space**, amounts to ~150 mL in healthy young males and somewhat more than 100 mL in females. The anatomical dead space is only a small fraction of the total lung capacity, which averages 5 to 6 L in adults, depending on the size and health of the individual.

Alveolar air spaces are the site of gas exchange

Alveoli first appear budding off bronchioles at generation ~17. These **respiratory bronchioles** participate in gas exchange over at least part of their surface. Respiratory bronchioles extend from generation ~17 to generation ~19, the density of alveoli gradually increasing with generation number (Fig. 26-5). Eventually, alveoli completely line the airways. These **alveolar ducts** (generations 20 to 22) finally terminate blindly as **alveolar sacs** (generation 23). The aggregation of all airways arising from a single terminal bronchiole (i.e., the respiratory bronchioles, alveolar ducts, and alveolar sacs), along with their associated blood and lymphatic vessels, is a **terminal respiratory unit** or **primary lobule**.

The cross-sectional area of the trachea is ~2.5 cm². Unlike the situation in systemic arteries (see Chapter 19), wherein the aggregate cross-sectional area of the branches always exceeds the cross-sectional area of the parent vessel, the aggregate cross-sectional area falls from the trachea through the first four generations of airways (Fig. 26-6). Because all of the air that passes through the trachea also passes through the two mainstem bronchi and so on, the product of aggregate cross-sectional area and linear velocity is the same for each generation of conducting airways. Thus, the linear velocity of air in the first four generations is higher than that in the trachea, which may be important during coughing (see Chapter 32). In succeeding generations, the aggregate cross-sectional area rises, at first slowly and then very steeply. As a result, the linear velocity falls to very low values. For example, the terminal bronchioles (generation 16) have an

aggregate cross-sectional area of ~180 cm², so that the average linear velocity of the air is only (2.5 cm²)/(180 cm²) = 1.4% of the value in the trachea.

As air moves into the respiratory bronchioles and further into the terminal respiratory unit, where linear velocity is minuscule, convection becomes less and less important for the movement of gas molecules, and diffusion dominates. Notice that the long-distance movement of gases from the nose and lips to the end of the generation-16 airways occurs by *convection*. However, the short-distance movement of gases from generation-17 airways to the farthest reaches of the alveolar ducts occurs by *diffusion*, as does the movement of gases across the gas-exchange barrier (~0.6 µm).

The **alveolus** is the fundamental unit of gas exchange. Alveoli are hemispheric structures with diameters that range from 75 to 300 µm. The ~300 million alveoli have a combined surface area of 50 to 100 m² and an aggregate maximal volume of 5 to 6 L in the two lungs. Both the diameter and the surface area depend on the degree of lung inflation. The lungs have a relatively modest total volume (i.e., ~5.5 L), very little of which is invested in conducting airways (i.e., ~0.15 L). However, the alveolar area is tremendously amplified. For example, a sphere with a volume of 5.5 L would have a surface area of only 0.16 m², which is far less than 1% of the alveolar surface area.

The alveolar lining consists of two types of epithelial cells, type I and type II alveolar pneumocytes. The cuboidal type II cells exist in clusters and are responsible for elaborating **pulmonary surfactant**, which substantially eases the expansion of the lungs (see Chapter 27). The type I cells are much thinner than the type II cells. Thus, even though the two cell types are present in about equal numbers, the type I cells cover 90% to 95% of the alveolar surface and represent the shortest route for gas diffusion. After an injury, type I cells slough and degenerate, whereas type II cells proliferate and line the alveolar space, re-establishing a continuous epithelial layer. Thus, the type II cells appear to serve as repair cells.

The pulmonary capillaries are usually sandwiched between two alveolar air spaces. In fact, the blood forms an almost

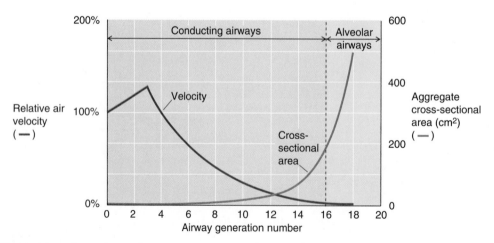

Figure 26-6 Dependence of aggregate cross-sectional area and of linear velocity on generation number. At generation 3, the aggregate cross-sectional area has a minimum (not visible) where velocity has its maximum. (*Data from Bouhuys A, The Physiology of Breathing. New York: Grune & Stratton, 1977.*)

uninterrupted sheet that flows like a twisted ribbon between abutting alveoli. At the type I cells, the alveolar wall (i.e., pneumocyte plus endothelial cell) is typically 0.15 to 0.30 μm thick. Small holes (**pores of Kohn**) perforate the septum separating two abutting alveoli. The function of these pores, which are surrounded by capillaries, is unknown.

The lung receives two blood supplies: the pulmonary arteries and the bronchial arteries (Fig. 26-7). The **pulmonary arteries**, by far the major blood supply to the lung, carry the relatively deoxygenated mixed-venous blood. After arising from the right ventricle, they bifurcate as they follow the bronchial tree, and their divisions ultimately form a dense, richly anastomosing, hexagonal array of capillary segments that supply the alveoli of the terminal respiratory unit. The pulmonary capillaries have an average internal diameter of ~8 μm, and each segment of the capillary network is ~10 μm in length. The average erythrocyte spends ~0.75 second in the pulmonary capillaries as it traverses up to three alveoli. After gas exchange in the alveoli, the blood eventually collects in the pulmonary veins.

The **bronchial arteries** are branches of the aorta and thus carry freshly oxygenated blood. They supply the conducting airways. At the level of the respiratory bronchioles, capillaries derived from bronchial arteries anastomose with those derived from pulmonary arteries. Because capillaries of the bronchial circulation drain partially into pulmonary veins, there is some **venous admixture** of the partially deoxygenated blood from the bronchial circulation and the newly oxygenated blood (see Chapter 31). This mixing represents part of a small physiological **shunt**. A small amount of the bronchial blood drains into the azygos and accessory hemiazygos veins.

The lungs play important nonrespiratory roles, including filtering the blood, serving as a reservoir for the left ventricle, and performing several biochemical conversions

Although their main function is to exchange O_2 and CO_2 between the atmosphere and the blood, the lungs also play important roles that are not directly related to external respiration.

Olfaction   Ventilation is essential for delivery of odorants to the olfactory epithelium (see Chapter 15). Sniffing behavior, especially important for some animals, allows one to sample the chemicals in the air without the risk of bringing potentially noxious agents deep into the lungs.

Processing of Inhaled Air Before It Reaches the Alveoli
Strictly speaking, the warming, moisturizing, and filtering of inhaled air in the conducting airways *is* a respiratory function. It is part of the cost of doing the business of ventilation. **Warming** of cool, inhaled air is important so that gas exchange in the alveoli takes place at body temperature. If the alveoli and the associated blood were substantially cooler than body temperature, the solubility of these alveolar gases in the cool pulmonary capillary blood would be relatively high. As the blood later warmed, the solubility of these gases would decrease, resulting in air bubbles (i.e., emboli) that could lodge in small systemic vessels and cause infarction. **Moisturizing** is important to prevent the alveoli from becoming desiccated. Finally, **filtering** of large particles is important to prevent small airways from being clogged with debris that may also be toxic.

Warming, moisturizing, and filtering are all more efficient with nose breathing rather than with mouth breathing. The nose, including the nasal turbinates, has a huge surface area and a rich blood supply. Nasal hairs tend to filter out large particles (greater than ~15 μm in diameter). The turbulence set up by these hairs—as well as the highly irregular surface topography of the nasal passages—increases the likelihood that particles larger than ~10 μm in diameter will **impact** and embed themselves in the mucus that coats the nasal mucosa. Moreover, air inspired through the nose makes a right-angle turn as it heads toward the trachea. The inertia of larger particles causes them to strike the posterior wall of the nasopharynx, which coincidentally is endowed with large amounts of lymphatic tissue that can mount an immunological attack on inspired microbes. Of the larger particles that manage to escape filtration in the upper

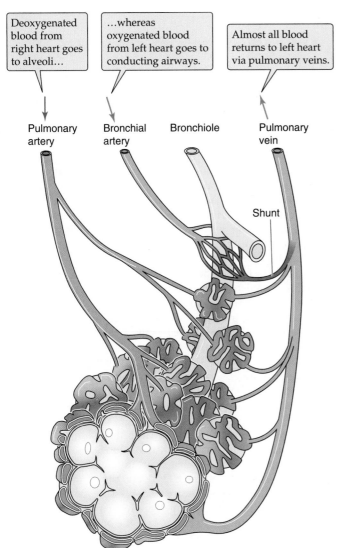

Figure 26-7   The blood supply to the airways.

Deoxygenated blood from right heart goes to alveoli...

...whereas oxygenated blood from left heart goes to conducting airways.

Almost all blood returns to left heart via pulmonary veins.

Pulmonary artery

Bronchial artery

Bronchiole

Pulmonary vein

Shunt

airways, almost all will impact on the mucus of the trachea and the bronchi.

Smaller particles (2 to 10 µm in diameter) also may impact a mucus layer. In addition, gravity may cause them to **sediment** from the slowly moving air in small airways and to become embedded in mucus. Particles with diameters below ~0.5 µm tend to reach the alveoli suspended in the air as **aerosols**. The airways do not trap most (~80%) of these aerosols but expel them in the exhaled air.

The lung has a variety of strategies for dealing with particles that remain on the surface of the alveoli or penetrate into the interstitial space. Alveolar macrophages (on the surface) or interstitial macrophages may phagocytose these particles, enzymes may degrade them, or lymphatics may carry them away. In addition, particles suspended in the fluid covering the alveolar surface may flow with this fluid up to terminal bronchioles, where they meet a layer of mucus that the cilia propel up to progressively larger airways. There, they join larger particles—which entered the mucus by impaction or sedimentation—on their journey to the oropharynx. Coughing and sneezing (see Chapter 32 for the box on sighs, yawns, coughs, and sneezes), reflexes triggered by airway irritation, accelerate the movement of particulates up the conducting airways.

Left Ventricular Reservoir   The highly compliant pulmonary vessels of the prototypic 70-kg human contain ~500 mL of blood (see Table 19-2), which is an important buffer for filling of the left ventricle. For example, if one clamps the pulmonary artery of an experimental animal so that no blood may enter the lungs, the left side of the heart can suck enough blood from the pulmonary circulation to sustain cardiac output for about two beats.

Filtering Small Emboli from the Blood   The mixed-venous blood contains microscopic emboli, small particles (e.g., blood clots, fat, air bubbles) capable of occluding blood vessels. If these emboli were to reach the systemic circulation and lodge in small vessels that feed tissues with no collateral circulation, the consequences—over time—could be catastrophic. Fortunately, the pulmonary vasculature can trap these emboli before they have a chance to reach the left side of the heart. If the emboli are sufficiently few and small, the affected alveoli can recover their function. Keep in mind that alveolar cells do not need the circulation to provide them with O_2 or to remove their CO_2. In addition, after a small **pulmonary embolism**, alveolar cells may obtain nutrients from anastomoses with the bronchial circulation. However, if pulmonary emboli are sufficiently large or frequent, they can cause serious symptoms or even death. A liability of the blood filtration function is that emboli made up of cancer cells may find the perfect breeding ground for support of metastatic disease.

Biochemical Reactions   The entire cardiac output passes through the lungs, exposing the blood to the tremendous surface area of the pulmonary capillary endothelium. It is apparently these cells that are responsible for executing biochemical reactions that selectively remove many agents from the circulation while leaving others unaffected (Table 26-3). Thus, the lung can be instrumental in determining which

Table 26-3   Handling of Agents by the Pulmonary Circulation

Unaffected	Largely Removed
PGA_1, PGA_2, PGI_2	PGE_1, PGE_2, $PGF_{2\alpha}$, leukotrienes
Histamine, epinephrine, dopamine	Serotonin, bradykinin
Angiotensin II, arginine vasopressin, gastrin, oxytocin	Angiotensin I (converted to angiotensin II)

Data from Levitzky MG: Pulmonary Physiology, 4th ed. New York: McGraw-Hill, 1999.

signaling molecules in the mixed-venous blood reach the systemic arterial blood. The pulmonary endothelium also plays an important role in converting angiotensin I (a decapeptide) to angiotensin II (an octapeptide), a reaction that is catalyzed by angiotensin-converting enzyme (see Chapter 40).

LUNG VOLUMES AND CAPACITIES

The spirometer measures changes in lung volume

The maximal volume of all the airways in an adult—the nasopharynx, the trachea, and all airways down to the alveolar sacs—is typically 5 to 6 L. Respiratory physiologists have defined a series of lung "volumes" and "capacities" that, although not corresponding to a particular anatomical locus, are easy to measure with simple laboratory instruments and that convey useful information for clinical assessment.

A **spirometer** measures the volume of air inspired and expired and therefore the change in lung volume. Spirometers today are complex computers, many so small that they can easily be held in the palm of one hand. The subject blows against a predetermined resistance, and the device performs all the calculations and interpretations. Nevertheless, the principles of spirometric analysis are very much the same as those for the "old-fashioned" spirometer shown in Figure 26-8A, which is far easier to conceptualize. This simple spirometer has a movable, inverted bell that is partially submerged in water. An air tube extends from the subject's mouth, through the water, and emerges in the bell, just above water level. Thus, when the subject exhales, air enters the bell and lifts it. The change in bell elevation, which we can record on moving paper, is proportional to the volume of air that the subject exhales. Because air in the lungs is saturated with water vapor at 37°C (body temperature and pressure, saturated with water vapor or **BTPS**), and the air in the spirometer is ambient temperature and pressure, saturated with water vapor or **ATPS**, we must apply a temperature correction to the spirometer reading (see the box on page 617).

The amount of air entering and leaving the lungs with each breath is the **tidal volume** (V_T). During quiet respirations, the V_T is ~500 mL. The initial portion of the spiro-

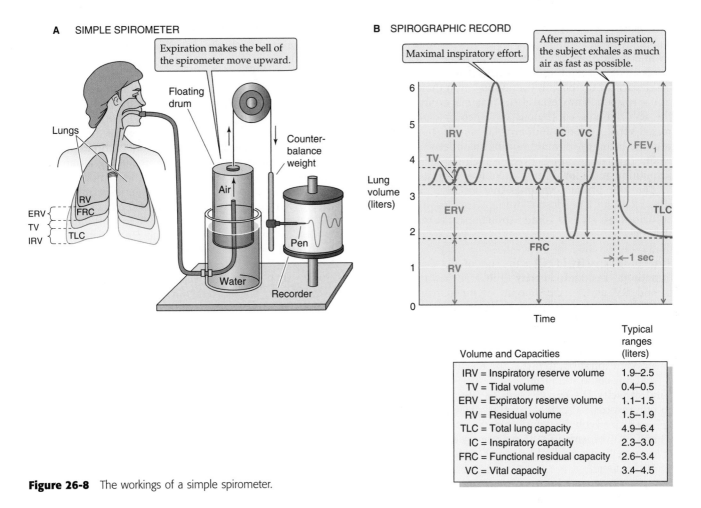

A SIMPLE SPIROMETER

Expiration makes the bell of the spirometer move upward.

Floating drum

Lungs

Counter-balance weight

Air

Pen

Water

Recorder

RV
ERV
TV
FRC
IRV
TLC

B SPIROGRAPHIC RECORD

Maximal inspiratory effort.

After maximal inspiration, the subject exhales as much air as fast as possible.

Lung volume (liters)

IRV
TV
ERV
RV
IC VC
FRC
FEV$_1$
TLC
1 sec

Time

Volume and Capacities	Typical ranges (liters)
IRV = Inspiratory reserve volume	1.9–2.5
TV = Tidal volume	0.4–0.5
ERV = Expiratory reserve volume	1.1–1.5
RV = Residual volume	1.5–1.9
TLC = Total lung capacity	4.9–6.4
IC = Inspiratory capacity	2.3–3.0
FRC = Functional residual capacity	2.6–3.4
VC = Vital capacity	3.4–4.5

Figure 26-8 The workings of a simple spirometer.

graph of Figure 26-8B illustrates changes in lung volume during quiet breathing. The product of tidal volume and the frequency of breaths is **total ventilation**, given in liters (BTPS) per minute.

Because, with a typical Western diet, metabolism consumes more O_2 (~250 mL/min) than it produces CO_2 (~200 mL/min; see Chapter 28), the volume of air entering the body with each breath is slightly greater (~1%) than the volume leaving. In reporting changes in lung volume, respiratory physiologists have chosen to measure the volume leaving—the **expired lung volume (V_E)**.

At the end of a quiet inspiration, the additional volume of air that the subject *could* inhale with a maximal effort is known as the **inspiratory reserve volume (IRV)**. The magnitude of IRV depends on several factors, including the following:

1. **Current lung volume.** The greater the lung volume after inspiration, the smaller the IRV.
2. **Lung compliance.** A decrease in compliance, a measure of how easy it is to inflate the lungs, will cause IRV to fall as well.
3. **Muscle strength.** If the respiratory muscles are weak, or if their innervation is compromised, IRV will decrease.

4. **Comfort.** Pain associated with injury or disease limits the desire or ability to make a maximal inspiratory effort.
5. **Flexibility of skeleton.** Joint stiffness, caused by diseases such as arthritis and kyphoscoliosis (i.e., curvature of the spine), reduces the maximal volume to which one can inflate the lungs.
6. **Posture.** IRV falls when a subject is in a recumbent position because it is more difficult for the diaphragm to move the abdominal contents.

After a quiet expiration, the additional volume of air that one can expire with a maximal effort is the **expiratory reserve volume (ERV)**. The magnitude of the ERV depends on the same factors listed before and on the strength of abdominal and other muscles needed to produce a maximal expiratory effort.

Even after a maximal expiratory effort, a considerable amount of air remains inside the lungs—the **residual volume (RV)**. Because a spirometer can measure only the air entering or leaving the lungs, it obviously is of no use in ascertaining the RV. However, we will see that other methods are available to measure RV. Is it a design flaw for the lungs to contain air that they cannot exhale? Would it not be better for the lungs to exhale all their air and to collapse completely during a maximal expiration? Total collapse would be detrimental for at least two reasons. (1) After an airway collapses, an unusually high pressure is required to re-inflate it. By minimizing airway collapse, the presence of an RV optimizes energy expenditure. (2) Blood flow to the lungs and other parts of the body is continuous, even though ventilation is episodic. Thus, even after a maximal expiratory effort, the RV allows a continuous exchange of gases between mixed-venous blood and alveolar air. If the RV were extremely low, the composition of blood leaving the lungs would oscillate widely between a high P_{O_2} at the peak of inspiration and a low P_{O_2} at the nadir of expiration.

The four primary **volumes** that we have defined—V_T, IRV, ERV, and RV—do not overlap (Fig. 26-8B). The lung capacities are various combinations of these four primary volumes:

Total lung capacity (TLC) is the sum of all four volumes.
Functional residual capacity (FRC) is the sum of ERV and RV and is the amount of air remaining inside the respiratory system after a quiet expiration. Because FRC includes RV, we cannot measure it using only a spirometer.
Inspiratory capacity (IC) is the sum of IRV and TV. After a quiet expiration, the IC is the maximal amount of air that one could still inspire.
Vital capacity (VC) is the sum of IRV, TV, and ERV. In other words, VC is the maximal achievable tidal volume and depends on the same factors discussed earlier for IRV and ERV. In patients with pulmonary disease, the physician may periodically monitor VC to follow the progress of the disease.

At the end of the spirographic record in Figure 26-8B, the subject made a maximal inspiratory effort and then exhaled as rapidly and completely as possible. The volume of air exhaled in 1 second under these conditions is the **forced expiratory volume in 1 second (FEV$_1$)**. In healthy young adults, FEV$_1$ is ~80% of VC. FEV$_1$ depends on all the factors that affect VC as well as on airway resistance. Thus, FEV$_1$ is a valuable measurement for monitoring a variety of pulmonary disorders and the effectiveness of treatment.

The volume of distribution of helium or nitrogen in the lung is an estimate of the residual volume

Although we cannot use a spirometer to measure residual volume or any capacity containing RV (i.e., FRC or TLC), we can use two general approaches to measure RV, both based on the **law of conservation of mass**. In the first approach, we compute RV from the volume of distribution of either helium (He) or nitrogen (N_2). However, any nontoxic gas would do, as long as it does not rapidly cross the blood-gas barrier. In the second approach, discussed in the next section, we compute RV by use of Boyle's law.

The principle underlying the **volume of distribution** approach is that the concentration of a substance is the ratio of mass (moles) to volume (liters). If the mass is constant, and if we can measure the mass and concentration, then we can calculate the volume of the physiological compartment in which the mass is distributed. In our case, we ask the

subject to breathe a gas that cannot escape from the airways. From the experimentally determined mass and concentration of that gas, we calculate lung volume.

Helium-Dilution Technique We begin with a spirometer containing air with 10% He—this is the *initial* helium concentration, $[He]_{initial} = 10\%$ (Fig. 26-9A). We use He because it is poorly soluble in water and therefore diffuses slowly across the alveolar wall (see Chapter 30). In this example, the initial spirometer volume, $V_{S(initial)}$, including all air up to the valve at the subject's mouth, is 2 L. The amount of He in the spirometer system at the outset of our experiment is thus $[He]_{initial} \times V_{S(initial)}$, or $(10\%) \times (2\ L) = 0.2\ L$.

We now open the valve at the mouth and allow the subject to breathe spirometer air until the He distributes evenly throughout the spirometer and airways. After equilibration, the *final* He concentration ($[He]_{final}$) is the same in the airways as it is in the spirometer. The volume of the "system"—the spirometer volume (V_S) plus lung volume (V_L)—is fixed from the instant that we open the valve between the spirometer and the mouth. When the subject inhales, V_L increases and V_S decreases by equal amounts. When the subject exhales, V_L decreases and V_S increases, but ($V_L + V_S$) remains unchanged. Because the system does not lose He, the total He content after equilibration must be the same as it was at the outset. In our example, we assume that $[He]_{final}$ is 5%.

If the spirometer and lung volumes at the end of the experiment are the same as those at the beginning,

$$[He]_{initial} \cdot V_S = [He]_{final} \cdot (V_S + V_L) \tag{26-3}$$

Solving for lung volume,

$$V_L = V_S \cdot \left(\frac{[He]_{initial}}{[He]_{final}} - 1 \right) \tag{26-4}$$

If we now insert the values from our experiment:

$$V_L = 2\,L \cdot \left(\frac{10\%}{5\%} - 1 \right) = 2\,L$$

V_L corresponds to the lung volume at the instant we open the valve and allow He to begin equilibrating. If we wish to measure FRC, we open the valve just after the completion of a *quiet* expiration. If we open the valve after a *maximal* expiration, then the computed V_L is RV. Because the subject rebreathes the air mixture in the spirometer until [He] stabilizes, the He-dilution approach is a **closed-circuit** method.

Nitrogen-Washout Method Imagine that you have a paper cup that contains a red soft drink. You plan to "empty" the cup but wish to know the "residual volume" of soft drink that will remain stuck to the inside of the cup (V_{cup}) after it is emptied. First, before emptying the cup, you determine the concentration of red dye in the soft drink; this is [red dye]$_{cup}$. Now empty the cup. Although you do not yet know V_{cup}, the product [red dye]$_{cup} \times V_{cup}$ is the *mass* of residual red dye that remains in the cup. Next, add hot water to the

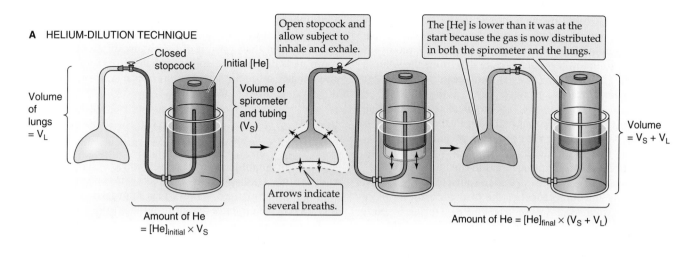

A HELIUM-DILUTION TECHNIQUE

Closed stopcock

Initial [He]

Volume of lungs = V_L

Volume of spirometer and tubing (V_S)

Open stopcock and allow subject to inhale and exhale.

Arrows indicate several breaths.

The [He] is lower than it was at the start because the gas is now distributed in both the spirometer and the lungs.

Volume = $V_S + V_L$

Amount of He = [He]$_{initial}$ × V_S

Amount of He = [He]$_{final}$ × ($V_S + V_L$)

B NITROGEN-WASHOUT TECHNIQUE

Special valve: Inspired air is 100% O_2. Expired air goes to an expandable sack.

Tank of 100% O_2

Initial [N_2]

Volume of lungs = V_L

100% O_2 dilutes N_2 in alveoli.

All expired gases go to sack.

All the N_2 is now in sack.

Amount of N_2 in lungs = [N_2]$_{initial}$ × V_L

Amount of N_2 = [N_2]$_{sack}$ × V_{sack}

After 7 minutes, almost no N_2 is left in the lungs.

Alveolar [N_2]

Time (min): −1 0 1 2 3 4 5 6 7

C PLETHYSMOGRAPHIC APPROACH

Electronically controlled shutter that can obstruct airflow.

Pressure gauge

Airtight booth

Outside air source

ΔV_L

Spirometer

The Mead plethysmograph is an airtight box. Every time the subject inspires, air moves into the spirometer, which registers the change in lung volume (ΔV_L).

Volume (L): 3.16, 3.15, 3.14, 3.13, 3.12, 3.11, V_L, 3.09

← $V_L + \Delta V$

ΔV

Pressure (mm Hg): 762, P, 758, 756, 754, 752, 750, 748, 746

ΔP

← P − ΔP

Time (seconds): 0 0.2 0.4 0.6 0.8 1

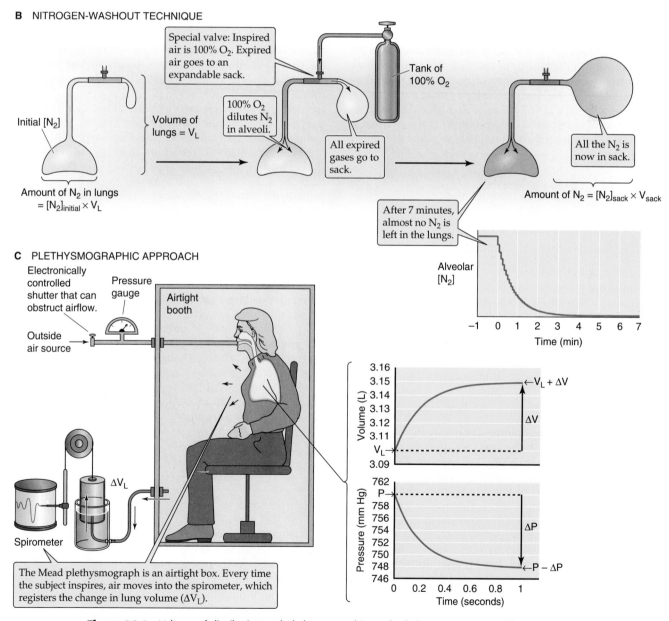

Figure 26-9 Volume of distribution and plethysmographic methods for measurement of lung volume. In **C,** the spirometer is usually replaced in modern plethysmographs by an electronic pressure gauge. In such instruments, the change in lung volume is computed from the change in pressure inside the plethysmograph (see Fig. 27-10).

cup, swish it around inside the glass, and dump the now reddish water into a graduated cylinder. After repeating this exercise several times, you see that virtually all the red dye is now in the graduated cylinder. Finally, determine the volume of fluid in the cylinder ($V_{cylinder}$) and measure its red dye concentration. Because [red dye]$_{cup}$ × V_{cup} is the same as [red dye]$_{cylinder}$ × $V_{cylinder}$, you can easily calculate the residual volume of the soft drink that had been in the glass. This is the principle behind the nitrogen-washout method.

Assume that the initial lung volume is V_L and that the initial concentration of nitrogen gas in the lungs is $[N_2]_{initial}$. Thus, the *mass* of N_2 in the lungs at the outset is $[N_2]_{initial} \times V_L$. We now ask the subject to breathe through a mouthpiece equipped with a special valve (Fig. 26-9B). During inspiration, the air comes from a reservoir of 100% O_2; the key point is that this inspired air contains no N_2. During expiration, the exhaled air goes to a sack with an initial volume of zero. Each inspiration of 100% O_2 dilutes the N_2 in the lungs. Each expiration sends a fraction of the remaining N_2 into the sack. Thus, the $[N_2]$ in the lungs falls stepwise with each breath until eventually the subject has washed out into the sack virtually all the N_2 that had initially been in the lungs. Also entering the sack are some of the inspired O_2 and all expired CO_2. The standard period for washing out of the N_2 with normal breathing is 7 minutes, after which the sack has a volume of V_{sack} and an N_2 concentration of $[N_2]_{sack}$. Because the mass of N_2 now in the sack is the same as that previously in the lungs:

$$[N_2]_{initial} \cdot V_L = [N_2]_{sack} \cdot V_{sack} \tag{26-5}$$

Thus, the lung volume is

$$V_L = V_{sack} \cdot \frac{[N_2]_{sack}}{[N_2]_{initial}} \tag{26-6}$$

To illustrate, consider an instance in which $[N_2]_{initial}$ is 75%. If the volume of gas washed into the sack is 40 L, roughly a total ventilation of 6 L/min for 7 minutes, and $[N_2]_{sack}$ is 3.75%, then:

$$V_L = 40\,L \cdot \frac{3.75\%}{75\%} = 2\,L \tag{26-7}$$

What particular lung volume or capacity does V_L represent? The computed V_L is the lung volume at the instant the subject begins to inhale the 100% O_2. Therefore, if the subject had just finished a quiet expiration before beginning to inhale the O_2, V_L would be FRC; if the subject had just finished a maximal expiratory effort, V_L would represent RV.

The key element in the nitrogen-washout method is the requirement that during the period of O_2 breathing, all N_2 previously in the lungs—and no more—ends up in the sack. In other words, we assume that N_2 does not significantly diffuse between blood and alveolar air during our 7-minute experiment. Because N_2 has a low water solubility, and therefore the amount dissolved in body fluids is very low at normal barometric pressure, the rate of N_2 diffusion across the alveolar wall is very low (see Chapter 30). Therefore, our

assumption is very nearly correct. In principle, we could preload the lung with any nontoxic, water-insoluble gas (e.g., He) and then wash it out with any different gas (e.g., room air). Because the subject inhales from one reservoir and exhales into another in the nitrogen-washout method, it is an **open-system** technique.

The plethysmograph, together with Boyle's law, is a tool for estimation of residual volume

We also can compute V_L from small *changes* in lung pressure and volume that occur as a subject attempts to inspire through an obstructed airway. This approach is based on **Boyle's law**, which states that if the temperature and number of gas molecules are constant, the product of pressure and volume is a constant:

$$P \cdot V_L = Constant \tag{26-8}$$

To take advantage of this relationship, we have the subject step inside an airtight box called a **plethysmograph** (from the Greek *plethein* [to be full]), which is similar to a telephone booth. The subject breathes through a tube that is connected to the outside world (Fig. 26-9C). Attached to this tube is a gauge that registers pressure at the mouth and an electronically controlled shutter that can, on command, completely obstruct the tube. The Mead-type plethysmograph in Figure 26-9C has an attached spirometer. As the subject inhales, lung volume and the volume of the subject's body increase by the same amount, displacing an equal volume of air from the plethysmograph into the spirometer, which registers the increase in lung volume (ΔV_L).

As the experiment starts, the shutter is open, and the subject quietly exhales, so that V_L is FRC. Because no air is flowing at the end of the expiration, the mouth and alveoli are both at barometric pressure, which is registered by the pressure gauge (P). We now close the shutter, and the subject makes a small inspiratory effort, typically only ~50 mL, against the closed inlet tube. The subject's inspiratory effort will cause lung volume to increase to a new value, $V_L + \Delta V_L$ (see graph in Fig. 26-9C). However, the number of gas molecules in the airways is unchanged, so this *increase* in volume must be accompanied by a *decrease* in airway pressure (ΔP) to a new value, $P - \Delta P$. Because no air is flowing at the peak of this inspiratory effort, the pressure measured by the gauge at the mouth is once again the same as the alveolar pressure. According to Boyle's law:

$$\underbrace{P \cdot V_L}_{\substack{\text{Initial} \\ \text{PV} \\ \text{product}}} = \underbrace{(P - \Delta P) \cdot (V_L + \Delta V_L)}_{\substack{\text{PV product} \\ \text{at peak of} \\ \text{inspiratory effort}}} \tag{26-9}$$

Rearranging Equation 26-9 yields the initial lung volume:

$$V_L = \Delta V_L \cdot \frac{P - \Delta P}{\Delta P} \tag{26-10}$$

As an example, assume that ΔV_L at the peak of the inspiratory effort is 50 mL and that the corresponding pressure decrease in the airways is 12 mm Hg. If the initial pressure (P) was 760 mm Hg,

$$V_L = 0.050\,L \cdot \frac{(760-12)\,\text{mm Hg}}{12\,\text{mm Hg}} = 3.1\,L \quad \textbf{(26-11)}$$

What lung volume or capacity does 3.1 L represent? Because, in our example, the inspiratory effort against the closed shutter began after a quiet expiratory effort, the computed V_L is FRC. If it had begun after a maximal expiration, the measured V_L would be RV.

REFERENCES

Books and Reviews

Macklem PT: Symbols and abbreviations. In Handbook of Physiology, Section 3: The Respiratory System, vol I, p. ix. Bethesda, MD: American Physiological Society, 1985.

Mortola JP, Frappell PB: On the barometric method for measurements of ventilation, and its use in small animals. Can J Physiol Pharmacol 1998; 76:937-944.

Satir P, Sleigh MA: The physiology of cilia and mucociliary interactions. Annu Rev Physiol 1990; 52:137-155.

Journal Articles

Fowler WS: Lung function studies. II. The respiratory dead space. Am J Physiol 1948; 154:405-416.

MECHANICS OF VENTILATION

Walter F. Boron

The field of **pulmonary mechanics**—the physics of the lungs, airways, and chest wall—deals with how the body moves air in and out of the lungs, producing a *change* in lung volume (V_L). When we examine these mechanical properties while no air is flowing, we are studying **static** properties. The situation becomes more complicated under **dynamic** conditions, when the lungs are changing volume and air is flowing either in or out.

STATIC PROPERTIES OF THE LUNG

The balance between the outward elastic recoil of the chest wall and the inward elastic recoil of the lungs generates a subatmospheric intrapleural pressure

The interaction between the lungs and the thoracic cage determines V_L. The lungs have a tendency to collapse because of their **elastic recoil**, a *static property* represented by the inwardly directed arrows in Figure 27-1A. The chest wall also has an elastic recoil. However, this elastic recoil tends to pull the thoracic cage outward (Fig. 27-1B). The stage is thus set for an interaction between the lungs and the chest wall: at equilibrium, the inward elastic recoil of the lungs exactly balances the outward elastic recoil of the chest wall (Fig. 27-1C). This interaction between lungs and chest wall does not occur by direct attachment but through the **intrapleural space** between the visceral and parietal pleurae (see Chapter 26). This space is filled with a small amount of pleural fluid and is extremely thin (5 to 35 μm). Because the lungs and chest wall pull away from each other on opposite sides of the intrapleural space, the **intrapleural pressure** (P_{IP}) is less than barometric pressure (P_B); that is, the intrapleural space is a *relative vacuum*. Although the designation P_{IP} implies that we are referring exclusively to the intrapleural space, this description is not entirely accurate. Indeed, in addition to the intrapleural space, P_{IP} is probably similar to the pressure in several other regions of the chest cavity:

1. the virtual space between the chest wall or diaphragm and the parietal pleura;

2. the virtual space between the lung and the visceral pleura;
3. the interstitial space that surrounds all pulmonary airways;
4. around the heart and vessels;
5. around and—to the extent that smooth muscle tone can be neglected—inside the esophagus.

It is helpful to think of P_{IP} as the intrathoracic pressure—the pressure everywhere in the thorax except in the lumens of blood vessels, lymphatics, or airways.

The vacuum is not uniform throughout the intrapleural space. When the subject is upright, the vacuum is greatest (i.e., P_{IP} is least) near the apex of the lungs and progressively falls along the longitudinal axis to its lowest value near the bases of the lungs (Fig. 27-2). If a subject whose lungs are ~30 cm tall has finished a quiet expiration, and if P_B is 760 mm Hg, P_{IP} is ~753 mm Hg near the apices of the lungs and ~758 mm Hg near the bases. The P_{IP} gradient is about what one would expect, given the density of the lungs. Note that P_{IP} is subatmospheric throughout the chest cavity. Because respiratory physiologists historically measured these small pressures with water manometers rather than with less sensitive mercury manometers, it has become customary to express P_{IP} in *cm H_2O* relative to a P_B of 0 cm H_2O. Thus, P_{IP} is about −10 cm H_2O at the apex and −2.5 cm H_2O at the base of the lungs.

The reasons for the apex-to-base P_{IP} gradient are **gravity** and **posture**. When an individual stands vertically on the surface of the earth, gravity pulls the lungs downward and away from the apex of the thoracic cage. This force creates a greater vacuum (i.e., a lower P_{IP}) at the apex. Gravity also pushes the bases of the lungs into the thoracic cavity, reducing the vacuum there. Standing on one's head would invert these relationships. Lying on one's side would create a P_{IP} gradient along a frontal-horizontal axis (i.e., from side to side), although the P_{IP} gradient would be much smaller because the side-to-side dimension of the thorax (and therefore the gradient created by the weight of the lungs) is less than the longitudinal dimension. In outer space, the P_{IP} gradient would vanish. Thus, the local P_{IP} depends on the position within the gravitational field.

A ELASTIC RECOIL OF LUNGS

B ELASTIC RECOIL OF CHEST WALL

C ELASTIC RECOILS OF LUNGS AND CHEST WALL IN BALANCE

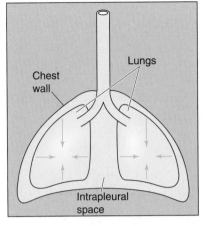
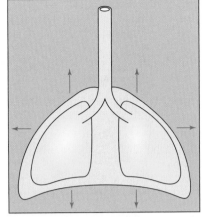
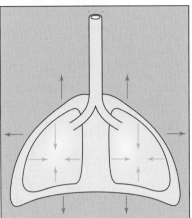

Figure 27-1 Opposing elastic recoils of the lungs and chest wall.

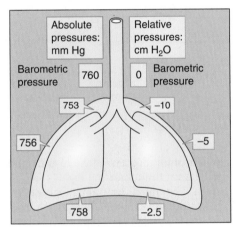

Figure 27-2 Intrapleural pressures. The values are those after a quiet expiration (i.e., functional residual capacity [FRC]).

For most of the remainder of this book, we ignore the P_{IP} gradient and refer to an average P_{IP} of about −5 cm H_2O after a quiet expiration (Fig. 27-2).

Contraction of the diaphragm and selected intercostal muscles increases the volume of the thorax, producing an inspiration

We have seen that the opposing elastic recoils of the lungs and chest wall create a negative P_{IP} that keeps the lungs expanded. Any change in the balance between these elastic recoils will cause V_L to change as well. For example, imagine a healthy person with a functional residual capacity (FRC) of 3 L and a P_{IP} of −5 cm H_2O. If that person now develops **pulmonary fibrosis**, which increases the elastic recoil of the lungs, FRC would decrease because a P_{IP} of −5 cm H_2O would no longer be adequate to keep the resting V_L at 3 L. Moreover, as the lungs shrink, P_{IP} would become more negative, causing chest volume to decrease as well. Under normal circumstances, the key elastic recoil is the one *we* control: the elastic recoil of the chest wall, which we change moment

to moment by modulating the tension of the muscles of respiration.

The **muscles of inspiration** expand the chest, increasing the elastic recoil of the chest wall and making P_{IP} more negative. Despite the P_{IP} gradient from the apex to the base of the lungs when no air is flowing at FRC (Fig. 27-2), the ΔP_{IP} during inspiration is similar throughout the thoracic cavity. Responding to this enhanced intrathoracic vacuum, the lungs expand passively. The increase in V_L is virtually the same as the increase in thoracic volume. The muscles that produce a quiet inspiration are called the **primary muscles of inspiration** and include the diaphragm and many intercostal muscles.

The most important component of the increase in chest volume is the rise in the chest cavity's rostral-caudal diameter, a result of the action of the **diaphragm**. Stimulated by the phrenic nerves (derived from cervical roots C3 to C5), the diaphragm contracts and moves downward into the abdomen ~1 cm during quiet ventilation.

The **external and internal intercostal muscles**, innervated by segmental spinal nerves, span the space between adjacent ribs. The action of each such muscle depends partly on its orientation but especially—because of the shape of the rib cage—on its position along the rostral-caudal axis and around the dorsal-ventral circumference of the rib cage. Thus, not all external intercostals are inspiratory, and not all internal intercostals are expiratory. Inspiratory neurons preferentially stimulate the most rostral and dorsal *external* intercostals and the parasternal *internal* intercostals, both of which have inspiratory mechanical advantages. The contraction of these muscles has two consequences (Fig. 27-3A). First, the rib cage and the tissues between the ribs stiffen and are therefore better able to withstand the increasingly negative P_{IP}. Second, thoracic volume increases as ribs 2 through 10 rotate upward and outward, increasing the transverse diameter (bucket-handle effect, Fig. 27-3B), and the upper ribs rotate the sternum upward and outward, increasing the anterior-posterior diameter (water pump–handle effect).

During a **forced** inspiration, the **accessory** (or **secondary**) **muscles** of inspiration also come into play:

A INSPIRATION

The most rostral and dorsal subsets of the **external** intercostal muscles (gold)—as well as the parasternal subset of the **internal** intercostal muscles (blue)—have an *inspiratory* mechanical advantage.

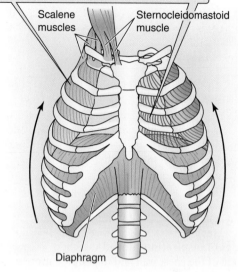

Scalene muscles

Sternocleidomastoid muscle

Diaphragm

B BUCKET-HANDLE AND WATER-PUMP– HANDLE EFFECTS

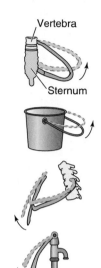

Vertebra

Sternum

C EXPIRATION

The most caudal subset of the **internal** intercostal muscles (blue)—as well as the caudal-ventral subset of the **external** intercostal muscles (gold) and the triangularis sterni muscle (transversus thoracis)—have an *expiratory* mechanical advantage.

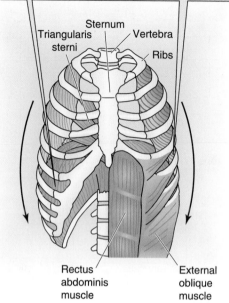

Triangularis sterni

Sternum

Vertebra

Ribs

Rectus abdominis muscle

External oblique muscle

Figure 27-3 Actions of major respiratory muscles. External intercostal muscles slope obliquely between ribs, mostly forward and downward. Internal intercostal muscles also slope obliquely between ribs, but mostly backward and downward.

1. **Scalenes.** These muscles lift the first two ribs.
2. **Sternocleidomastoids.** These muscles lift the sternum outward, contributing to the water pump–handle effect.
3. **Neck and back muscles.** These elevate the pectoral girdle (increasing the cross-sectional area of the thorax) and extend the back (increasing the rostral-caudal length).
4. **Upper respiratory tract muscles.** The actions of these muscles decrease airway resistance.

Relaxation of the muscles of inspiration produces a quiet expiration

During a *quiet* inspiration, *normal* lungs store enough energy in their elastic recoil to fuel a quiet expiration, just as stretching of a rubber band stores enough energy to fuel the return to initial length. Thus, a quiet expiration is normally passive, accomplished simply by relaxation of the muscles of inspiration. Thus, *there are no primary muscles of expiration.*

Expiration is not *always* entirely passive. One example is a forced expiration in an individual with normal airway resistance. Another is even a quiet expiration of a person with a disease that increases airway resistance (e.g., asthma, chronic bronchitis, emphysema). In either case, the **accessory muscles of expiration** help make P_{IP} more positive:

1. **Abdominal muscles** (internal and external oblique, rectoabdominal and transverse abdominal muscles). Contraction of these muscles (Fig. 27-3C) increases intra-abdominal pressure and forces the diaphragm upward

into the chest cavity, decreasing the rostral-caudal diameter of the thorax and increasing P_{IP}.
2. **Intercostals.** The most ventral-caudal *external* intercostals, the most caudal *internal* intercostals, and an intercostal-like muscle called the triangularis sterni all have an expiratory mechanical advantage. Expiratory neurons selectively stimulate these muscles, reducing both the anterior-posterior and the transverse diameters of the thorax. These actions are particularly important for coughing.
3. **Neck and back muscles.** Lowering of the pectoral girdle reduces the cross-sectional area of the thorax, whereas flexion of the trunk reduces the rostral-caudal diameter.

During a forced *inspiration*, the accessory muscles of inspiration use their energy mainly to increase V_L (rather than to overcome resistance to airflow); the lungs store this extra energy in their elastic recoil. During a forced *expiration*, the accessory muscles of expiration use their energy mainly to overcome the resistance to airflow, as discussed later.

Increase of the static compliance makes it easier to inflate the lungs

Imagine that a person suffers a puncture wound to the chest cavity, so that air enters the thorax from the atmosphere, raising P_{IP} to the same level as P_B. This condition is called a **pneumothorax** (from the Greek *pneuma* [air]). With no vacuum to counter their elastic recoil, alveoli will collapse—a condition known as **atelectasis**. The upper part of Figure 27-4A illustrates an extreme hypothetical case in which pres-

A PNEUMOTHORAX AND LUNG RE-INFLATION

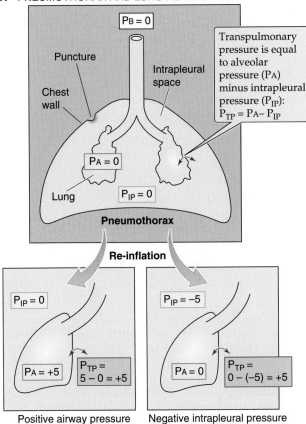

Re-inflation

Positive airway pressure   Negative intrapleural pressure

B STATIC PRESSURE-VOLUME DIAGRAM

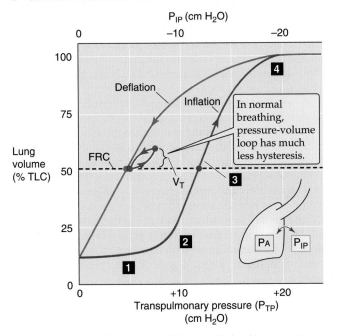

Figure 27-4 Collapse and re-inflation of the lungs. In **A,** we assume that intrapleural pressure (P_{IP}) rises to barometric pressure (P_B), so that transpulmonary pressure (P_{TP}) falls to 0, collapsing the lungs.

sure is atmospheric throughout the thorax. Even though the lungs are collapsed, V_L is not 0 because proximal airways collapse before smaller ones farther downstream, trapping air. The resulting **minimal air volume** is ~10% of total lung capacity (TLC), ~500 mL.

We now wish to re-expand the collapsed lungs to their original volume (i.e., FRC). What are the forces at work during such a re-expansion? The force responsible for distending an airway is the **transmural pressure** (P_{TM})—the *radial* pressure difference across an airway wall at any point along the tracheobronchial tree:

$$P_{TM} = P_{AW} - P_{IP} \qquad (27\text{-}1)$$

P_{AW} is the pressure inside the airway, and P_{IP} is the pressure in the interstitial space surrounding the airway. A special case of P_{TM} is the transmural pressure across the *alveolar* wall—**trans*pulmonary* pressure** (P_{TP}):

$$P_{TP} = P_A - P_{IP} \qquad (27\text{-}2)$$

P_A is **alveolar pressure**. When the glottis is open and no air is flowing, the lungs are under **static conditions**, and P_A must be 0 cm H_2O:

$$\text{Static conditions:} \quad P_{TP} = 0 - P_{IP} = -P_{IP} \qquad (27\text{-}3)$$
(glottis open)

Thus, with the glottis open under static conditions, the pressure that inflates the alveoli (i.e., P_{TP}) is simply the negative of P_{IP}. We can re-expand the lungs to FRC by any combination of an increase in P_A and a decrease in P_{IP}, as long as P_{TP} ends up at 5 cm H_2O (Fig. 27-4A, lower panels). Thus, it makes no difference whether we increase P_A from 0 to +5 cm H_2O with P_{IP} fixed at 0 (the principle behind positive-pressure ventilation in an intensive care unit) or whether we decrease P_{IP} from 0 to −5 cm H_2O with P_A fixed at 0 (the principle behind physiological ventilation). In both cases, V_L increases by the same amount.

A clinician would treat the pneumothorax by inserting a chest tube through the wound into the thoracic cavity and gradually pumping out the intrathoracic air. The clinician might also insert a tube through the mouth and into the upper trachea (to ensure a patent airway), use a mechanical ventilator (to ensure gas exchange), and sedate the patient (to prevent the patient from fighting the ventilator). Between the inspiratory cycles of the ventilator, the *lungs are under static conditions* and V_L depends only on P_{TP}— that is, the difference between P_A (which is set by the ventilator) and P_{IP}. As we remove air from the thorax, P_{IP} becomes more negative and the alveoli re-expand. We can characterize the elastic (or static) properties of the lungs by plotting V_L versus P_{TP} as V_L increases (Fig. 27-4B, purple curve). How do we obtain the necessary data? In principle, we could determine V_L by using one of the methods discussed in Equation 26-4. We could read off P_A (needed to compute P_{TP}) directly from the ventilator. Finally, we could in principle measure P_{IP} by using a pressure transducer at the tip of the chest tube. Most important, we must take our readings between inspiratory cycles of the ventilator—under *static conditions*.

During the re-inflation, measured under static conditions, we can divide the effect on V_L into four stages, starting at the left end of the purple curve in Figure 27-4B:

Stage 1: **Stable V_L.** In the lowest range of P_{IP} values, making P_{IP} more negative has little or no effect on V_L. For example, decreasing P_{IP} from 0 to -1 cm H_2O (i.e., increase P_{TP} from 0 to $+1$ cm H_2O), we record no change in V_L. Why? As discussed later, it is very difficult—because of the surface tension created by the air-water interface—to pop open an airway that is completely collapsed. Until P_{TP} is large enough to overcome the collapsing effects of surface tension, a decrease in P_{IP} has no effect on V_L.

Stage 2: **Opening of airways.** Decreasing P_{IP} beyond about -8 cm H_2O produces V_L increases that are at first small, reflecting the popping open of proximal airways with the greatest compliance. Further decreasing P_{IP} produces larger increases in V_L, reflecting the expansion of already open airways as well as recruitment of others.

Stage 3: **Linear expansion of open airways.** After all the airways are already open, making P_{IP} increasingly more negative inflates all airways further, causing V_L to increase in a roughly linear fashion.

Stage 4: **Limit of airway inflation.** As V_L approaches TLC, decreases in P_{IP} produce ever smaller increases in V_L, reflecting decreased airway and chest wall compliance and the limits of muscle strength.

What would happen if, having inflated the lungs to TLC, we allowed P_{IP} to increase to 0 cm H_2O once again? Obviously, the V_L would decrease. However, the lungs follow a different path during deflation (Fig. 27-4B, red curve), creating a **P_{IP}-V_L loop.** The difference between the inflation and the deflation paths—**hysteresis**—exists because a greater P_{TP} is required *to open* a previously closed airway, owing to a deficit of surfactant at the air-water interface, than *to keep* an open airway from closing, reflecting abundant surfactant. We will discuss surfactant in the next section. The horizontal dashed line in Figure 27-4B shows that *inflating* collapsed lungs to FRC requires a P_{IP} of -12 cm H_2O (purple point), whereas *maintaining* previously inflated lungs at FRC requires a P_{IP} slightly less negative than -5 cm H_2O (red point). During normal ventilation, the lungs exhibit much less hysteresis, and the green P_{IP}-V_L loop in Figure 27-4B lies close to the red deflation limb of our original loop. The changes in V_L in Figure 27-4B reflect mainly changes in the volume of *alveoli*, with a small contribution from conducting airways.

We will now focus on just the red curve in Figure 27-4B, a portion of which is the middle curve in Figure 27-5. Here, P_{TP} is $+5$ cm H_2O when V_L is at FRC. As the subject makes a normal inspiration with a tidal volume (V_T) of 500 mL, P_{TP} increases (i.e., P_{IP} decreases) by 2.5 cm H_2O. The ratio of ΔV_L to ΔP_{TP} (i.e., the slope of the P_{TP}-V_L curve) is the compliance and a measure of the distensibility of the lungs. In our example,

$$C = \frac{\Delta V_T}{\Delta P_{TP}} = \frac{0.5\,\text{L}}{(7.5 - 5.0)\,\text{cm}\;H_2O} = 0.2\,\frac{\text{L}}{\text{cm}\;H_2O} \quad (27\text{-}4)$$

Because we made this measurement under conditions of zero airflow, C is the **static compliance.** Static compliance,

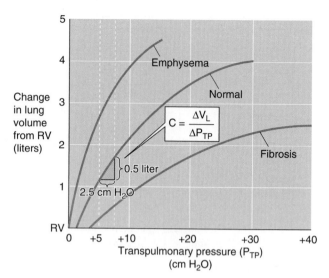

Figure 27-5   Static pressure-volume curves for lungs in health and disease.

like V_L, is mainly a property of the alveoli. The elastance of the lungs, which is a measure of their *elastic recoil*, is the reciprocal of the compliance ($E = 1/C$). Lungs with a high compliance have a low elastic recoil, and vice versa.

Figure 27-5 also shows representative P_{TP}-V_L relationships for lungs of patients with pulmonary fibrosis (bottom curve) and emphysema (top curve). In **pulmonary fibrosis**, the disease process causes deposition of fibrous tissue, so that the lung is stiff and difficult to inflate. Patients with **restrictive lung disease**, by definition, have a decreased C (i.e., a decreased slope of the V_L versus P_{TP} relationship in Fig. 27-5) at a given V_L. The same ΔP_{TP} that produces a 500-mL V_L increase in normal lungs produces a substantially *smaller* V_L increase in fibrotic lungs. In other words, static compliance ($\Delta V_L/\Delta P_{TP}$) is much less, or elastic recoil is much greater.

In **emphysema**, the situation is reversed. The disease process, a common consequence of cigarette smoking, destroys pulmonary tissue and makes the lungs floppy. An important part of the disease process is the destruction of the extracellular matrix, including elastin, by elastase released from macrophages. Normal mice that are exposed to cigarette smoke develop emphysema rapidly, whereas the disease does not develop in "smoker" mice lacking the macrophage elastase gene. The same increase in P_{TP} that produces a 500-mL V_L increase in normal lungs produces a substantially *larger* V_L increase in lungs with emphysema. In other words, static compliance is much greater (i.e., much less elastic recoil).

Because it requires work to inflate the lungs against their elastic recoil, one might think that a little emphysema might be a good thing. Although it is true that patients with emphysema exert less effort to inflate their lungs, the cigarette smoker pays a terrible price for this small advantage. The destruction of pulmonary architecture also makes emphysematous airways more prone to collapse during expiration, drastically increasing airway resistance.

Two additional points are worth noting. First, compliance (i.e., slope of P_{TP}-V_L curve) decreases as V_L increases

Restrictive Pulmonary Disease

Two major categories of pulmonary disease—restrictive and obstructive—can severely reduce total ventilation, that is, the amount of air entering and leaving the lungs per unit of time. Pulmonologists use the term **restrictive lung disease** in an inclusive sense to refer to any disorder that reduces functional residual capacity, vital capacity, or total lung capacity (see Fig. 26-8), thereby making the lungs difficult to inflate. Pure restrictive disease does not affect airway resistance. Restrictive disease can affect the *lung parenchyma* or three *extrapulmonary* structures.

Lung Parenchyma

Restrictive diseases of the lung parenchyma decrease the static compliance of the lung—mainly a property of the alveoli. To overcome increased elastic recoil, the patient must make extra effort to inhale. The patient compensates by making rapid but shallow inspirations. In newborns, an example is **infant respiratory distress syndrome**, caused by a deficiency in surfactant. **Pulmonary edema** is a buildup of fluid in the interstitial space between the alveolar and capillary walls and, eventually, the alveolar space. Interstitial inflammation of a variety of causes (e.g., infection, drugs, environmental exposure) can lead to the deposition of fibrous tissue and a group of diseases called **diffuse interstitial pulmonary fibrosis**.

Pleura

A buildup in the intrapleural space of either air (pneumothorax) or fluid (pleural effusion) can restrict the expansion of a vast number of alveoli.

Chest Wall

Rigidity of the chest wall makes it difficult to increase thoracic volume even if the neuromuscular system (see next) can generate normal forces. **Ankylosing spondylitis** is an inflammatory disorder of the axial skeleton that may reduce the bucket-handle rotation of the ribs during quiet inspirations and the flexion and extension of the trunk during forced inspirations and expirations. In **kyphoscoliosis** (angulation and rotation of the spine), deformation of the vertebrae and ribs may reduce ventilation. In both conditions, impairment of coughing predisposes to lung infections.

Neuromuscular System

The central nervous system may fail to stimulate the respiratory muscles adequately, or the muscles may fail to respond appropriately to stimulation. In **polio**, the virus occasionally attacks respiratory control centers in the brainstem. **Amyotrophic lateral sclerosis** (ALS or Lou Gehrig's disease) leads to the destruction of premotor and motor neurons, including those to the muscles of respiration. (See Chapter 32.) Indeed, dyspnea on exertion is a common early symptom of ALS. Certain **drug overdoses** (e.g., barbiturate poisoning) may temporarily inhibit respiratory control centers in the brainstem. In the absence of supportive therapy (i.e., mechanical ventilation), the respiratory failure can be fatal. The pain that accompanies surgery or other injuries to the chest can also severely limit the ability to ventilate. **Local paralysis** of intercostal muscles allows the enhanced intrathoracic vacuum to suck in intercostal tissues during inspiration. This paradoxical movement reduces the efficiency of inspiration. Paradoxical movement may also occur with broken ribs, a condition known as **flail chest**.

---

from FRC to TLC (Fig. 27-5). Second, the P_{TP}-V_L curve is the amalgam of pressure-volume relationships of all alveoli. Different alveoli have different P_{TP}-V_L curves and may experience different intrapleural pressures, depending on their position within a gravitational field (Fig. 27-2). This inhomogeneity of static parameters contributes to regional differences in ventilation (see Chapter 31).

Surface tension at the air-water interface of the airways accounts for most of the elastic recoil of the lungs

What is the basis of the elastic recoil that determines the static compliance of the lungs? The elasticity of pulmonary cells and the extracellular matrix (e.g., elastin and collagen), what we might think of as the "anatomical" component of elastic recoil, generally accounts for a small part. The basis of most of the recoil was suggested in 1929 by von Neergaard, who excised lungs from cats and inflated them by applying positive pressure to the trachea under two conditions. When he filled the lungs with air, the P_{TP}-V_L curve looked similar to the one we have seen before (Fig. 27-6A, blue curve). However, when he degassed the airways and re-inflated them with saline, he found that (1) the P_{TP}-V_L relationship (Fig. 27-6A, orange curve) exhibited far less

hysteresis and (2) the static compliance was substantially greater (i.e., much less pressure was required to inflate the lungs). These changes occurred because the saline-filled lungs lacked the air-water interface that generated surface tension in the air-filled lungs. It is this surface tension that is responsible for a large fraction of the lung's elastic recoil.

Surface tension is a measure of the force acting to pull a liquid's surface molecules together at an air-liquid interface (Fig. 27-6B). Water molecules in the bulk liquid phase are equally attracted to surrounding water molecules in all directions, so that the net force acting on these "deep" water molecules is zero. However, water molecules at the surface are equally attracted to others in all directions but "up," where no molecules are available to pull surface water molecules toward the air phase. Thus, a net force pulls surface molecules away from the air-water interface toward the bulk water phase.

We can think of the surface water molecules as beads connected by an elastic band. The force that pulls a water molecule down into the bulk also creates a *tension* between the molecules that remain at the surface, in a direction that is *parallel* to the surface. If we try to overcome this tension and stretch the air-water interface (Fig. 27-6C), thus increasing its area, we must apply force (F) to bring water molecules

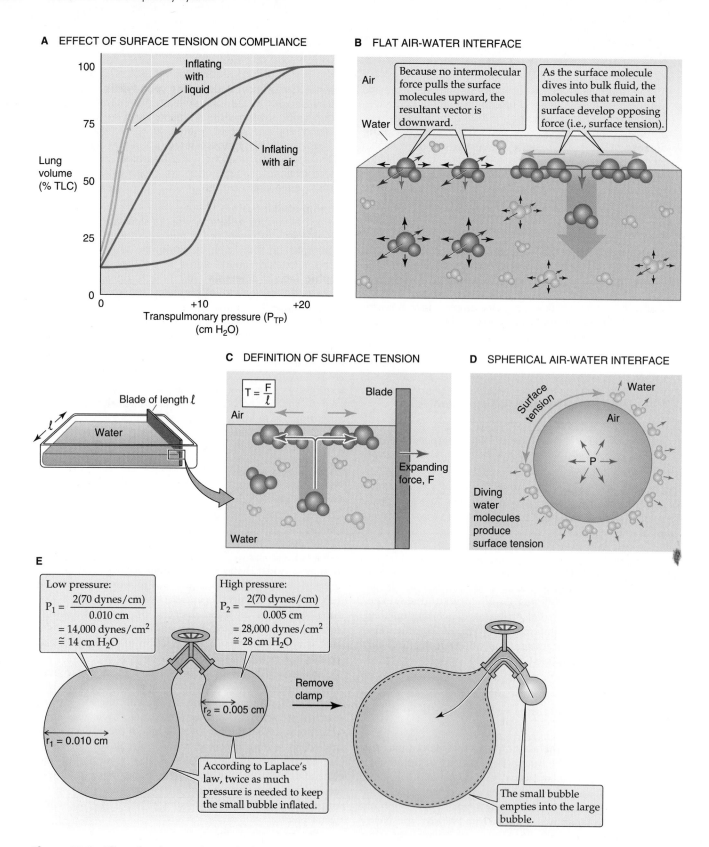

A EFFECT OF SURFACE TENSION ON COMPLIANCE

Inflating with liquid

Inflating with air

Lung volume (% TLC)

Transpulmonary pressure (P_{TP}) (cm H_2O)

B FLAT AIR-WATER INTERFACE

Air

Water

Because no intermolecular force pulls the surface molecules upward, the resultant vector is downward.

As the surface molecule dives into bulk fluid, the molecules that remain at surface develop opposing force (i.e., surface tension).

C DEFINITION OF SURFACE TENSION

Blade of length ℓ

Water

$T = \dfrac{F}{\ell}$

Blade

Air

Water

Expanding force, F

D SPHERICAL AIR-WATER INTERFACE

Surface tension

Water

Air

P

Diving water molecules produce surface tension

E

Low pressure:
$$P_1 = \frac{2(70 \text{ dynes/cm})}{0.010 \text{ cm}}$$
$$= 14{,}000 \text{ dynes/cm}^2$$
$$\cong 14 \text{ cm } H_2O$$

High pressure:
$$P_2 = \frac{2(70 \text{ dynes/cm})}{0.005 \text{ cm}}$$
$$= 28{,}000 \text{ dynes/cm}^2$$
$$\cong 28 \text{ cm } H_2O$$

$r_2 = 0.005$ cm

$r_1 = 0.010$ cm

Remove clamp

According to Laplace's law, twice as much pressure is needed to keep the small bubble inflated.

The small bubble empties into the large bubble.

Figure 27-6 Effect of surface tension on the lung.

from the bulk liquid (a low-energy state) to the surface (a high-energy state). If the body of water on which we tug has a length of l, then the surface tension (T) is

$$T = \frac{F}{l} \qquad (27\text{-}5)$$

For a simple air-water interface at 37°C, the surface tension is ~70 dynes/cm.

A drop of water falling through the air tends to form into a sphere because this shape has the smallest surface area and thus the lowest energy. Put differently, when the drop is spherical, it is impossible for any additional water molecules to leave the surface.

In the reverse scenario, a spherical air bubble surrounded by water (Fig. 27-6D), unbalanced forces acting on surface water molecules cause them to dive into the bulk, decreasing the surface area and creating tension in the plane of the air-water interface. This surface tension acts like a belt tightening around one's waist. It tends to decrease the volume of compressible gas inside the bubble and increases its pressure. At equilibrium, the tendency of increased pressure to expand the gas bubble balances the tendency of surface tension to collapse it. Laplace's equation describes this equilibrium:

$$P = \frac{2T}{r} \qquad (27\text{-}6)$$

P is the *dependent* variable; the surface tension T is a *constant* for a particular interface, and the bubble radius r is the *independent* variable. Therefore, the smaller the bubble's radius, the greater the pressure needed to keep the bubble inflated. See Chapter 19 for a description of how Laplace's treatment applies to blood vessels.

Our bubble-in-water analysis is important for the lung because a thin layer of water covers the inner surface of the alveolus. Just as surface tension at the air-water interface of our gas bubble causes the bubble to constrict, it also causes alveoli and other airways to constrict, contributing greatly to elastic recoil.

The analogy between air bubbles and alveoli breaks down somewhat because an alveolus only approximates a part of a sphere. A second complicating factor is that not all alveoli are the same size; some may have a diameter that is three or four times larger than that of others. Third, alveoli are interconnected.

Figure 27-6E shows what would happen if two imaginary air bubbles in water were connected by a tube with a valve that allows us to make or break the connection between the bubbles. For both, assume that the surface tension T is 70 dynes/cm. The valve is initially closed. The first bubble has a radius of 0.010 cm. The second is only half as wide. At equilibrium, the pressure required to keep the smaller bubble inflated is twice that necessary to keep the larger bubble inflated (see calculations in Fig. 27-6E). If we now open the valve between the two bubbles, air will flow from the smaller bubble to the larger bubble. To make matters worse for the smaller bubble, the smaller it becomes, the greater is the pressure needed to stabilize its shrinking radius. Because its pressure is less than required, air continues to flow out of the smaller bubble until it implodes completely.

In principle, the lung faces a similar problem. Smaller alveoli tend to collapse into larger ones. As we shall see, pulmonary surfactant minimizes this collapsing tendency by lowering surface tension. However, even without surfactant, the collapse of small alveoli could proceed only so far because each alveolus is tethered to adjacent alveoli, which help hold it open—the **principle of interdependence**.

Why would it matter if many smaller alveoli collapsed into a few larger alveoli? Such a collapse would reduce the total alveolar surface area available for diffusion of O_2 and CO_2 (see Chapter 29). Thus, from a teleological point of view, it is important for the lung to keep the alveoli as uniformly inflated as possible.

Pulmonary surfactant is a mixture of lipids—mainly dipalmitoylphosphatidylcholine—and apoproteins

As noted earlier, surface tension accounts for most of the elastic recoil in normal lungs. However, if it were not for pulmonary surfactant, total elastic recoil would be even higher, and the lungs would be far more difficult to inflate. During quiet breathing, surfactant reduces surface tension to ~25 dynes/cm or less, far below the value of 70 dynes/cm that exists at a pure air-water interface.

The term **surfactant** means a surface-active agent. Because surfactants have both a hydro*philic* region (strongly attracted to water) and a hydro*phobic* region (strongly repelled by water), they localize to the surface of an air-water interface. An example of a synthetic surfactant is dishwashing detergent. As a younger student, you may have done a simple experiment in which you filled a small-diameter cup with water and carefully floated a thin sewing needle—lengthwise—on the surface. The needle, like an insect that walks on water, is supported by surface tension, which pulls in the plane of the air-water interface. When you add a drop of liquid detergent to the surface of the water, the needle instantly sinks. Why? The detergent greatly reduces the surface tension.

Detergent molecules orient themselves so that their hydrophilic heads point toward (and interact with) the most superficial water molecules, whereas the hydrophobic tails point toward the air (Fig. 27-7A). The hydrophilic surfactant *heads* pull strongly upward on the most superficial water molecules, greatly reducing the net force on these surface water molecules and minimizing their tendency to dive into the bulk water. What prevents surfactant at the air-surfactant interface from diving into the bulk water? The hydrophobic *tails* exert a counterforce, pulling the surfactant upward toward the air. The situation is not unlike that of a fishing line with a bobber at one end and a sinker at the other: as long as the bobber is sufficiently buoyant, it remains at the water's surface. Thus, unlike surface water molecules, which are subjected to a large net force pulling them into the bulk, surfactant experiences a much smaller net force. The greater the surface density of surfactant molecules at the air-water interface (i.e., the smaller the surface occupied by water molecules), the smaller the surface tension.

Pulmonary surfactant is a complex mixture of lipids and proteins. Type II alveolar cells (see Chapter 26), cuboidal epithelial cells that coexist with the much thinner type I cells,

A EFFECT OF SURFACTANT ON SURFACE TENSION

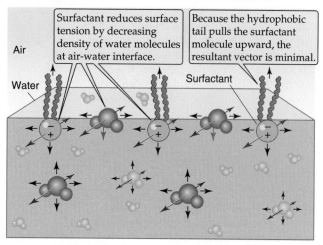

Surfactant reduces surface tension by decreasing density of water molecules at air-water interface.

Because the hydrophobic tail pulls the surfactant molecule upward, the resultant vector is minimal.

Table 27-1 Surfactant Apoproteins

Apoprotein	Solubility	Role
SP-A	Water	Innate immunity Formation of tubular myelin
SP-B	Lipid	Speeds formation of monolayer Formation of tubular myelin
SP-C	Lipid	Speeds formation of monolayer
SP-D	Water	Innate immunity Metabolism of surfactant?

B DIPALMITOYL PHOSPHATIDYL-CHOLINE (DPPC)

C THE SURFACTANT APOPROTEIN SP-A

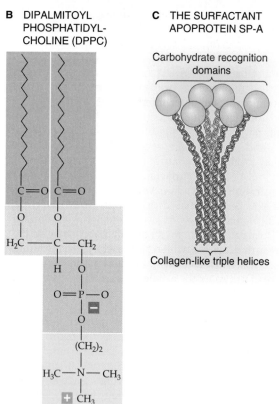

Carbohydrate recognition domains

Collagen-like triple helices

Figure 27-7 Effect of a surface-active agent on surface tension.

Proteins account for the remaining ~10% of pulmonary surfactant. Plasma proteins (mainly albumin) and secretory IgA make up about half of the protein, and four **apoproteins** (SP-A, SP-B, SP-C, and SP-D) make up the rest. **SP-A** and **SP-D** are water soluble and have collagen-like domains (Table 27-1). Both contribute to "innate immunity" by acting as opsonins to coat bacteria and viruses, thereby promoting phagocytosis by macrophages resident in the alveoli. In addition, SP-A (Fig. 27-7C) may be important for exertion of feedback control that limits surfactant secretion. The two hydrophobic apoproteins, **SP-B** and **SP-C**, are intrinsic membrane proteins that greatly increase the rate at which surfactant enters the air-water interface and then spreads as a surface film. The hereditary absence of SP-B leads to respiratory distress that is fatal unless the newborn receives a lung transplant.

The lipid components of pulmonary surfactant enter type II cells from the bloodstream (Fig. 27-8A). Type II cells use the secretory pathway (see Chapter 2) to synthesize the four apoproteins, all of which undergo substantial post-translational modification. The final assembly of surfactant occurs in **lamellar bodies**, which are ~1 μm in diameter and consist of concentric layers of lipid and protein (Fig. 27-8B). Some of the material in these lamellar bodies represents newly synthesized components, and some of it represents recycled surfactant components retrieved from the alveolar surface. Each hour, the normal lung secretes into the alveolar space ~10% of the material present in the lamellar bodies.

The secretion of pulmonary surfactant occurs by constitutive exocytosis (see Chapter 2). Both synthesis and secretion are quite low until immediately before birth, when a surge in maternal glucocorticoid levels triggers these processes (see Chapter 57). Infants born prematurely may thus lack sufficient levels of surfactant and may develop **infant respiratory distress syndrome** (IRDS; see Chapter 57 for the box on this topic). In postnatal life, several stimuli enhance the surfactant secretion, including hyperinflation of the lungs (e.g., sighing and yawning), exercise, and pharmacological agents (e.g., β-adrenergic agonists, Ca^{2+} ionophores).

After its secretion into the thin layer of water that covers the alveolar epithelium, freed from the physical constraints of confinement to a lamellar body, pulmonary surfactant undergoes major structural changes. In this aqueous layer, surfactant takes on the form of a meshwork known as

synthesize and secrete pulmonary surfactant. Clara cells in the respiratory bronchioles manufacture at least some components of pulmonary surfactant. Lipids make up ~90% of surfactant and are responsible for the surface-active properties. About half of the lipid is **dipalmitoylphosphatidylcholine** (DPPC; Fig. 27-7B), also known as dipalmitoyllecithin, which contains two fully saturated 16-carbon fatty acid chains (i.e., palmitates). The second most common lipids in pulmonary surfactant are phosphatidylcholine molecules with *unsaturated* fatty acid chains. Compared with cell membranes, phosphatidylglycerol (~11% of lipid) is overrepresented in surfactant.

A SURFACTANT METABOLISM

B

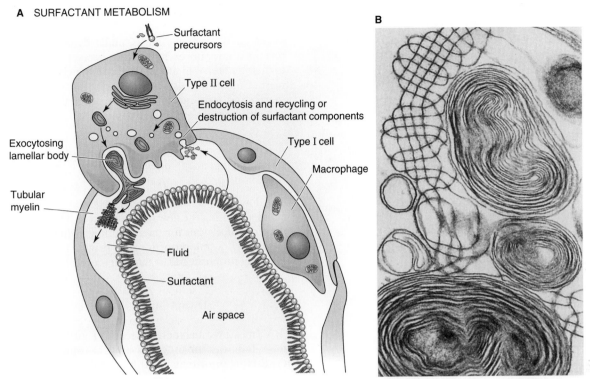

Figure 27-8 Generation of pulmonary surfactant. In **B,** the structures with concentric layers are lamellar bodies, which are continuous with tubular myelin (grid-like structures). (**B** courtesy of Dr. M. C. Williams, University of California, San Diego.)

tubular myelin (Fig. 27-8B), which is rich in surfactant apoproteins. It is not clear whether surfactant normally passes through the tubular myelin state before forming a surface film at the air-water interface. However, tubular myelin is not *required;* SP-A knockout mice lack tubular myelin but have a normal surface film.

Two mechanisms remove components of pulmonary surfactant from the surface of alveoli. Alveolar macrophages degrade some of the surfactant. Type II cells take up the rest and either recycle or destroy it.

Pulmonary surfactant reduces surface tension and increases compliance

The pulmonary surfactant present at the alveolar air-water interface has three major effects.

First, because surfactant reduces surface tension, it increases compliance, making it far easier to inflate the lungs. If surfactant suddenly disappeared from the lungs, mimicking the situation in IRDS, total elastic recoil would increase (i.e., compliance would *decrease*) twofold or more, causing small airways to collapse partially. The situation would be similar to that described by the fibrosis curve in Figure 27-5. Because the compliance of the lungs is far lower than normal, an infant with IRDS—compared with a normal infant—must produce far larger changes in P_{TP} (or P_{IP}) to achieve the same increase in V_L. Therefore, infants with low surfactant levels must expend tremendous effort to contract their inspiratory muscles and expand the lungs.

Second, by reducing surface tension, surfactant minimizes fluid accumulation in the alveolus. In the absence of surfactant, the large surface tension of the liquid layer between the air and the alveolar type I cells would cause the "air bubble" to collapse, drawing fluid into the alveolar space from the interstitium. The net effect would be to increase the thickness of the liquid layer, thereby impairing gas diffusion. With normal levels of surfactant, the surface tension of the water layer is low, and the tendency to draw fluid from the interstitium to the alveolar space is balanced by the negative interstitial hydrostatic pressure (i.e., P_{IP}), which favors fluid movement from the alveolar space into the interstitium.

Third, surfactant helps keep alveolar size relatively uniform during the respiratory cycle. Imagine that we start—after a quiet expiration—with two alveoli having the same radius (e.g., 100 μm) and the same surface density of surfactant (to yield a surface tension of 20 dynes/cm), as indicated by the inner dashed circles of the two alveoli in Figure 27-9. However, either the conducting airway leading to the lower alveolus has a higher resistance or the lower alveolus itself has more fibrous tissue. Either way, the lower alveolus inflates more slowly during inspiration and—at any time—has a smaller volume than the upper one. This size difference has two negative consequences. (1) The total surface area of the two alveoli is less than if they had inflated equally, impairing gas diffusion. (2) Because the final volume increase of the upper alveolus may be greater than that of the lower one, its ventilation may be greater. Such unevenness of ventilation impairs effective gas exchange (see Chapter 31).

Fortunately, surfactant helps alveoli dynamically adjust their rates of inflation and deflation, making ventilation more uniform among alveoli. During rapid inflation, the

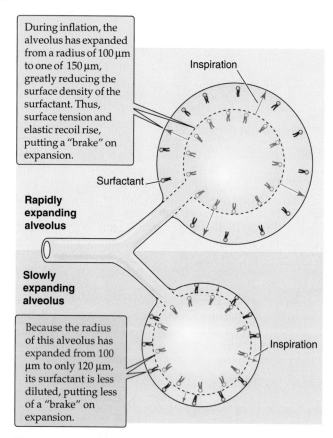

During inflation, the alveolus has expanded from a radius of 100 μm to one of 150 μm, greatly reducing the surface density of the surfactant. Thus, surface tension and elastic recoil rise, putting a "brake" on expansion.

Inspiration

Surfactant

Rapidly expanding alveolus

Slowly expanding alveolus

Because the radius of this alveolus has expanded from 100 μm to only 120 μm, its surfactant is less diluted, putting less of a "brake" on expansion.

Inspiration

Figure 27-9   Braking action of surfactant on inflation.

alveolar surface expands more rapidly than additional surfactant can reach the surface from a surfactant pool beneath the surface. Thus, surfactant on the surface is thought to break up like a flow of ice on the sea, with open areas of pure water between clusters of surfactant. With more exposed water at the surface, surface tension increases. Surface tension may double during inspiration, compared with the resting value at FRC. This effect would be exaggerated in rapidly expanding alveoli, which would develop a higher surface tension more quickly than slowly expanding alveoli. This higher surface tension produces a greater elastic recoil that opposes further expansion. Thus, the dilution of surfactant tends to put more of a brake on rapidly expanding airways, slowing their expansion to more nearly match that of alveoli that tend to inflate more slowly.

The opposite appears to happen during expiration, when the surface area of rapidly contracting alveoli falls more rapidly than surfactant can dive back down into the subsurface pool. The compression of surfactant causes surface tension to fall precipitously. Surface tension during expiration may fall to half the resting value at FRC. The more rapidly an alveolus shrinks, the more quickly its surface tension falls, the lower is its elastic recoil, and the greater is its tendency to re-expand. This action puts a brake on rapidly contracting alveoli, slowing their rate of shrinkage to more closely match that of slowly contracting alveoli. These changes in surfactant contribute to the small amount of hysteresis in a P_{IP}-V_L loop during quiet breathing (green loop in Fig. 27-4B).

DYNAMIC PROPERTIES OF THE LUNG

When air is flowing—that is, under dynamic conditions—one must not only exert the force necessary to maintain the lung and chest wall at a certain volume (i.e., static component of force) but also exert an extra force to overcome the inertia and resistance of the tissues and air molecules (i.e., dynamic component of force).

Airflow is proportional to the difference between alveolar and atmospheric pressure but inversely proportional to airway resistance

The flow of air through tubes is governed by the same principles governing the flow of blood through blood vessels and the flow of electrical current through wires (see Equation 17-1). Airflow is proportional to driving pressure (ΔP) but inversely proportional to **total airway resistance (R_{AW})**:

$$\dot{V} = \frac{\Delta P}{R_{AW}} = \frac{P_A - P_B}{R_{AW}} \qquad (27\text{-}7)$$

$\dot{V}$ (measured in liters per second) is airflow; the dot above the V indicates the time derivative of volume. For the lung, the driving pressure is the difference between alveolar pressure (P_A) and barometric pressure (P_B). Thus, for a fixed resistance, more *airflow* requires a greater ΔP (i.e., more effort). Viewed differently, to achieve a desired airflow, a greater *resistance* requires a greater ΔP.

When airflow is laminar—that is, when air molecules move smoothly in the same direction—we can apply Poiseuille's law, which states that the resistance (R) of a tube is proportional to the viscosity of the gas (η) and length of the tube (l) but inversely proportional to the fourth power of radius:

$$R = \frac{8}{\pi} \cdot \frac{\eta l}{r^4} \qquad (27\text{-}8)$$

This equation is the same as Equation 17-11 for laminar blood flow. In general, changes in viscosity and length are not very important for the lung, although the resistance while breathing helium is greater than that for nitrogen, the major component of air, because helium has a greater viscosity. However, the key aspect of Equation 27-8 is that airflow is extraordinarily sensitive to changes in airway **radius**. The fourth-power dependence of R on radius means that a 10% decrease in radius causes a 52% increase in R—that is, a 34% *decrease* in airflow. Although Poiseuille's law strictly applies only to laminar flow conditions, as discussed later, airflow is even more sensitive to changes in radius when airflow is *not* laminar.

In principle, it is possible to compute the total airway resistance of the tracheobronchial tree from anatomical measurements, applying Poiseuille's law when the flow is laminar and analogous expressions for airways in which the flow is not laminar. In 1915, Rohrer used this approach, along with painstaking measurements of the lengths and diameters of the airways of an autopsy specimen, to calculate the R_{AW} of the tracheobronchial tree. However, it is not practical to *compute* R_{AW} values, especially if we are interested in physiological or pathological changes in R_{AW}. Therefore, for both physiologists and physicians, it is important to *measure* R_{AW} directly. Rearrangement of Equation 27-7 yields an expression for R_{AW} that we can compute after measurement of the driving pressure and the airflow that it produces:

$$R_{AW} = \frac{\Delta P}{\dot{V}} = \frac{P_A - P_B}{\dot{V}} \left(\text{units: } \frac{\text{cm H}_2\text{O}}{\text{L/s}} \right) \quad (27\text{-}9)$$

We can measure airflow directly with a **flowmeter** (pneumotachometer) built into a tube through which the subject breathes. The driving pressure is more of a problem because of the difficulty in measuring P_A during breathing. In 1956, DuBois and colleagues met this challenge by cleverly using Boyle's law and a **plethysmograph** to measure the P_A (Fig. 27-10). For example, if the peak $\dot{V}$ during a quiet inspiration is −0.5 L/s (by convention, a negative value denotes inflow) and P_A at the same instant is −1 cm H_2O (from the plethysmograph), then

$$R_{AW} = \frac{\Delta P}{\dot{V}} = \frac{P_A - P_B}{\dot{V}} = \frac{-1 \text{cm H}_2\text{O}}{-0.5 \text{L/s}} = 2 \frac{\text{cm H}_2\text{O}}{\text{L/s}} \quad (27\text{-}10)$$

In normal individuals, R_{AW} is ~1.5 cm H_2O/(L/s) but can range from 0.6 to 2.3. Resistance values are higher in patients with respiratory disease and can exceed 10 cm H_2O/(L/s) in extreme cases.

The resistance that we measure in this way is the *airway resistance*, which represents ~80% of total pulmonary resistance. The remaining 20% represents **tissue resistance**—that is, the friction of pulmonary and thoracic tissues as they slide past one another as the lungs expand or contract.

In the lung, airflow is transitional in most of the tracheobronchial tree

We have seen that laminar airflow is governed by a relationship that is similar to Ohm's law. What happens when the airflow is not laminar? How can we predict whether the airflow is likely to be laminar? The flow of a fluid down a tube is **laminar** when particles passing any particular point always have the same speed and direction. Because of their viscosity, real fluids move fastest down the midline of the tube, and velocity falls to 0 as we approach the wall of the tube (Fig. 27-11A), as discussed for blood in Chapter 17. If the average velocity of the fluid flowing down the tube passes a critical value, flow becomes **turbulent**; local irregular currents, called vortices, develop randomly, and they greatly increase resistance to flow. Under ideal laboratory conditions, airflow generally is laminar when the dimensionless **Reynolds number** (*Re*) is less than 2000 (see Chapter 17):

$$Re = \frac{2r\bar{v}\rho}{\eta} \quad (27\text{-}11)$$

r is the radius of the tube, $\bar{v}$ is the velocity of the gas averaged over the cross section of the tube, ρ is the density of the gas, and η is its viscosity. When *Re* exceeds ~3000, flow tends to be turbulent. Between *Re* values of 2000 and 3000, flow is unstable and may switch between laminar and turbulent.

Reynolds developed Equation 27-11 to predict turbulence when fluids flow through tubes that are long, straight, smooth, and unbranched. Pulmonary airways, however, are short, curved, bumpy, and bifurcated. The branches are especially a problem because they set up small eddies (Fig. 27-11B). Although these eddies resolve farther along the airways, the air soon encounters yet other bifurcations, which establish new eddies. This sort of airflow is termed **transitional**. Because of the complex geometry of pulmonary airways, the critical *Re* in the lungs is far lower than the ideal value of 2000. In fact, *Re* must be less than ~1 for lung airflow to be laminar. Such low *Re* values and thus laminar flow are present only in the small airways that are distal to terminal bronchioles (see Chapter 26).

Airflow is transitional throughout most of the tracheobronchial tree. Only in the trachea, where the airway radius is large and linear air velocities may be extremely high (e.g., exercise, coughing), is airflow truly turbulent (Fig. 27-11C).

The distinction among laminar, transitional, and turbulent airflow is important because these patterns influence how much energy one must invest to produce airflow. When flow is *laminar* (see Equation 27-7), airflow is proportional to ΔP and requires relatively little energy. When flow is *transitional*, one must apply more ΔP to produce the same airflow because producing vortices requires extra energy. Thus, the "effective resistance" increases. When flow is *turbulent*, airflow is proportional not to ΔP but to $\sqrt{\Delta P}$. Thus, we must apply an even greater ΔP to achieve a given flow (i.e., effective resistance is even greater).

The smallest airways contribute only slightly to total airway resistance in healthy lungs

As discussed earlier, airway resistance for healthy individuals is ~1.5 cm H_2O/(L/s). Because effective resistance can increase markedly with increases in airflow—owing to transitional and turbulent airflow—it is customary to measure resistances at a fixed, relatively low flow of ~0.5 L/s. The second column of Table 27-2 shows how R_{AW} normally varies with location as air moves from lips to alveoli during a quiet inspiration. A striking feature is that the greatest aggregate resistance is in the pharynx-larynx and large airways (diameter > 2 mm, or before about generation 8). Of the R_{AW} of 1.5 cm H_2O/(L/s) in this normal subject, 0.6 is in the upper air passages, 0.6 is in the large airways, and only 0.3 is in the small airways.

Because R increases with the fourth power of airway radius (see Equation 27-8), it might seem counterintuitive that the small airways have the lowest aggregate resistance. However, although each small airway has a high individual resistance, so many are aligned in parallel that their aggregate resistance is very low. We see this same pattern of resistance in the vascular system, where capillaries make a smaller contribution than arterioles to aggregate resistance (see Chapter 19).

Table 27-2 also shows an example of a patient with moderately severe **chronic obstructive pulmonary disease (COPD)**, a condition in which emphysema or chronic bronchitis increases R_{AW} (see the box on obstructive pulmonary diseases). COPD is a common and debilitating consequence

A SUBJECT AT REST

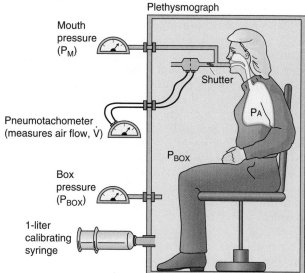

Plethysmograph

Mouth pressure (P_M)

Shutter

P_A

P_{BOX}

Pneumotachometer (measures air flow, $\dot{V}$)

Box pressure (P_{BOX})

1-liter calibrating syringe

B SUBJECT BREATHING AGAINST A CLOSED SHUTTER   **C** SUBJECT BREATHING THROUGH AN OPEN SHUTTER

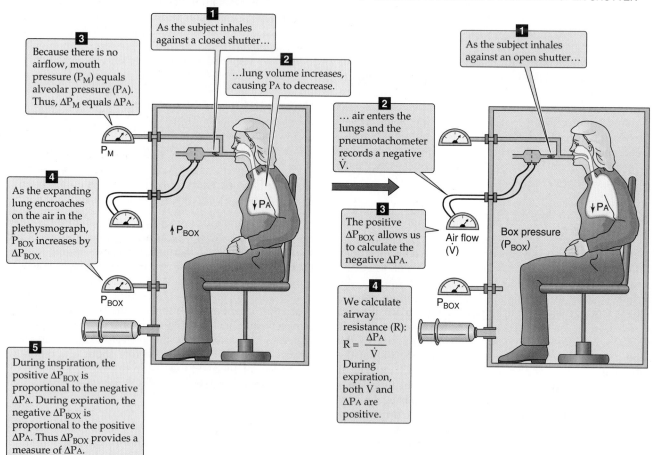

1 As the subject inhales against a closed shutter…

2 …lung volume increases, causing P_A to decrease.

3 Because there is no airflow, mouth pressure (P_M) equals alveolar pressure (P_A). Thus, ΔP_M equals ΔP_A.

P_M

4 As the expanding lung encroaches on the air in the plethysmograph, P_{BOX} increases by ΔP_{BOX}.

$\uparrow P_{BOX}$

$\downarrow P_A$

P_{BOX}

5 During inspiration, the positive ΔP_{BOX} is proportional to the negative ΔP_A. During expiration, the negative ΔP_{BOX} is proportional to the positive ΔP_A. Thus ΔP_{BOX} provides a measure of ΔP_A.

1 As the subject inhales against an open shutter…

2 … air enters the lungs and the pneumotachometer records a negative $\dot{V}$.

3 The positive ΔP_{BOX} allows us to calculate the negative ΔP_A.

Air flow ($\dot{V}$)

4 We calculate airway resistance (R):
$$R = \frac{\Delta P_A}{\dot{V}}$$
During expiration, both $\dot{V}$ and ΔP_A are positive.

$\downarrow P_A$

Box pressure (P_{BOX})

P_{BOX}

Figure 27-10 Measurement of alveolar pressure (P_A) during airflow. This plethysmograph is similar to the one in Figure 26-9C, except that the spirometer is replaced by a sensitive device for measurement of the pressure inside the plethysmograph (P_{BOX}). The subject breathes plethysmograph air through a tube that has an electronically controlled shutter as well as meters for measurement of airflow and pressure at the mouth. In **B**, with the subject making an inspiratory effort against a closed shutter, pressure at the mouth equals P_A. We obtain the calibration ratio $\Delta P_A/\Delta P_{BOX}$, which allows us to convert future changes in the P_{BOX} to changes in P_A. In **C**, the subject inspires through an open shutter. During the first moments of inspiration, the thorax expands before much air enters the lungs. Because alveoli expand without much of an increase in the number of gas molecules, P_A must fall. Conversely, because the thorax encroaches on the plethysmograph air, which has hardly lost any gas molecules to the lungs, P_{BOX} must rise. From the calibration ratio $\Delta P_A/\Delta P_{BOX}$, we calculate ΔP_A from ΔP_{BOX} *during* inspiration. P_A at any point during the respiratory cycle is the sum of the known P_B and the measured ΔP_A.

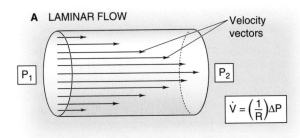

A LAMINAR FLOW

Velocity vectors

P_1 P_2

$$\dot{V} = \left(\frac{1}{R}\right)\Delta P$$

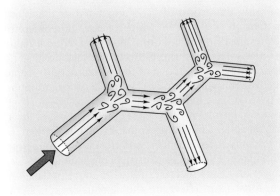

B TRANSITIONAL FLOW

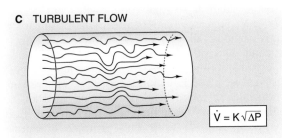

C TURBULENT FLOW

$$\dot{V} = K\sqrt{\Delta P}$$

Figure 27-11 Laminar, transitional, and turbulent flow. In **A,** laminar airflow ($\dot{V}$) is proportional to the driving pressure ($\Delta P = P_1 - P_2$). In **C,** where turbulent airflow is proportional to the square root of the driving pressure, a greater ΔP (i.e., effort) is needed to produce the same $\dot{V}$ as in panel **A.**

Table 27-2 Airway Resistance*

Locus	Normal	COPD
Pharynx-larynx	0.6	0.6
Airways > 2 mm diameter	0.6	0.9
Airways < 2 mm diameter	0.3	3.5
Total airway resistance	1.5	5.0

*Units of resistance, cm H_2O/(L/s).

Obstructive Pulmonary Disease

Two major categories of pulmonary disease can markedly reduce total ventilation: the *restrictive* pulmonary diseases (discussed in the box on diseases affecting ventilation); and the **obstructive pulmonary diseases**, in which the pathological process causes a decrease in airway resistance—primarily a property of the **conducting airways** (see Chapter 26).

The condition can be acute, as with the aspiration of a **foreign body**, the buildup of **mucus** in an airway lumen, or the constriction of the airway lumen due to the contraction of smooth muscle in **asthma** (see the box on that topic).

Chronic obstructive pulmonary disease (COPD) is defined as an increase in airway resistance caused by **chronic bronchitis** (long-standing inflammation of the bronchi or bronchioles), **emphysema** (destruction of alveolar walls, producing a smaller number of large alveoli), or a combination of the two. In the United States, COPD is the fourth leading cause of death. The major risk factor is cigarette smoking, although the inherited absence of α_1-antitrypsin (see Table 18-1) also predisposes to COPD. Inflammation leads to the infiltration of the walls of conducting airways by macrophages, activated T lymphocytes, and neutrophils and the infiltration of alveolar walls by activated lymphocytes. The release of neutrophil elastase and other proteases overwhelms natural antiproteases, such as α_1-antitrypsin. Bronchitis increases airway resistance by narrowing the lumen. With its destruction of alveolar walls, emphysema increases the static compliance, which, by itself, would make it easier to inhale. However, the destruction of parenchyma also reduces the mechanical tethering of conducting airways, leading to an exaggerated collapse of these airways during expiration and thus an increase in airway resistance.

of cigarette smoking, far more common than the lung cancer that receives so much attention in the lay press. Notice *where* the disease strikes. Even though COPD increases total airway resistance to 5.0 cm H_2O/(L/s)—3.3-fold greater than in our normal subject—pharynx-larynx resistance does not change at all, and large-airway resistance increases only modestly. Almost all of the increment in R_{AW} is due to a nearly 12-fold increase in the resistance of the smallest airways! According to Equation 27-8, we could produce a 12-fold increase in R_{AW} by decreasing radius by about half.

Although small airways normally have a very low aggregate resistance, it is within these small airways that COPD has its greatest and earliest effects. Even a doubling of small-airway resistance from 0.3 to 0.6 cm H_2O/(L/s) in the early stages of COPD would produce such a small incre-

ment in R_{AW} that it would be impossible to identify the COPD patient in a screening test based on resistance measurements. As discussed in Chapter 31, approaches that detect the nonuniformity of ventilation are more sensitive for detection of early airway disease. In addition to COPD, the other common cause of increased R_{AW} is **asthma** (see the box on asthma).

Asthma

Asthma, a common condition, occurs in 5% to 10% of the American population. Asthma is primarily an *inflammatory* disorder; the familiar bronchospasm is secondary to the underlying inflammation. One hypothesis is that asthma represents the inappropriate activation of immune responses designed to combat parasites in the airways. When a susceptible person inhales a trigger (e.g., pollen), inflammatory cells rush into the airways, releasing a multitude of cytokines, leukotrienes, and other humoral substances (e.g., histamine) that induce bronchospasm.

The patient suffering an acute asthma attack is usually easy to recognize. The classic presentation includes shortness of breath, wheezing, and coughing. Triggers include allergens, heat or cold, a host of occupational irritants, and exercise. The patient can often identify the specific trigger. Spirometry can confirm the diagnosis; the most characteristic feature is a decreased FEV_1. Many asthmatics use peak flowmeters at home because the severity of symptoms does not always correlate with objective measurements of the disease's severity.

The type of treatment depends on the frequency and severity of the attacks. Patients with infrequent attacks that are not particularly severe can often be treated with an inhaled β_2-adrenergic agonist, only when needed. These medications, easily delivered by a metered-dose inhaler that can be carried around in one's pocket or purse, act on β_2-adrenergic receptors to oppose bronchoconstriction. A patient who requires such an agent more than one or two times a week should receive an inhaled corticosteroid on a regular basis to suppress inflammation. Inhaled corticosteroids generally lack the side effects of oral corticosteroids, but oral corticosteroids may be required in a patient with sustained and severe asthma. Many patients rely on regular dosing of long-acting β-agonist inhalers and inhaled corticosteroids to keep their asthma under control. Theophylline (a phosphodiesterase inhibitor that raises $[cAMP]_i$; see Chapter 3), once a mainstay of asthma therapy, is now used far less commonly. Inhaled anticholinergic agents are more useful with COPD patients than with asthmatics but can be beneficial in some patients who cannot tolerate the side effects of β-adrenergic agonists (notably tachycardia). Smooth muscle relaxants (e.g., cromakalim-related drugs; see Chapter 7) and other anti-inflammatory agents (e.g., leukotriene inhibitors) also play a role in asthma therapy.

Vagal tone, histamine, and reduced lung volume all increase airway resistance

Several factors can modulate R_{AW}, including the autonomic nervous system (ANS), humoral factors, and changes in the volume of the lungs themselves. The vagus nerve, part of the **parasympathetic** division of the ANS, releases acetylcholine, which acts on an M_3 muscarinic receptor on bronchial smooth muscle (see Chapter 14). The result is bronchoconstriction and therefore an increase in R_{AW}. The muscarinic antagonist atropine blocks this action. Irritants such as cigarette smoke cause a reflex bronchoconstriction (see Chapter 32) in which the vagus nerve is the efferent limb.

Opposing the action of the vagus nerve is the **sympathetic** division of the ANS, which releases norepinephrine and dilates the bronchi and bronchioles but reduces glandular secretions. However, these effects are weak because norepinephrine is a poor agonist of the β_2-adrenergic receptors that mediate this effect through cyclic adenosine monophosphate (cAMP; see Chapter 14).

Humoral factors include **epinephrine**, released by the adrenal medulla. Circulating epinephrine is a far better β_2 agonist than is norepinephrine and therefore a more potent bronchodilator. **Histamine** constricts bronchioles and alveolar ducts and thus increases R_{AW}. Far more potent is the bronchoconstrictor effect of the leukotrienes LTC_4 and LTD_4.

One of the most powerful determinants of R_{AW} is V_L. R_{AW} is extremely high at residual volume (RV) but decreases steeply as V_L increases (Fig. 27-12A). One reason for this effect is obvious: all pulmonary airways—including the conducting airways, which account for virtually all of R_{AW}—expand at high V_L, and resistance falls steeply as radius increases (see Equation 27-8). A second reason is the principle of interdependence—alveoli tend to hold open their neighbors by exerting radial traction or **mechanical tethering** (Fig. 27-12B). This principle is especially important for conducting airways, which have thicker walls than alveoli and thus a lower compliance. At high V_L, alveoli dilate more than the adjacent bronchioles, pulling the bronchioles farther open by mechanical tethering. Patients with **obstructive lung disease**, by definition, have an increased R_{AW} at a given V_L (Fig. 27-12A). However, because these patients tend to have a higher than normal FRC, they breathe at a higher V_L, where airway resistance is—for them—relatively low.

Intrapleural pressure has a static component ($-P_{TP}$) that determines lung volume and a dynamic component (PA) that determines airflow

In Equation 27-2, we defined transpulmonary pressure as the difference between alveolar and intrapleural pressure ($P_{TP} = P_A - P_{IP}$). What is the physiological significance of these three pressures, and how do we control them?

P_{IP} is the parameter that the brain—through the muscles of respiration—directly controls. Rearranging the definition of P_{TP} in Equation 27-2:

$$P_{IP} = (-P_{TP}) + P_A \qquad (27\text{-}12)$$

Regardless of its cause, increased R_{AW} greatly increases the energy required to move air into and out of the lungs. If the increase in R_{AW} is severe enough, it can markedly limit exercise. In extreme cases, even walking may be more exercise than the patient can manage. The reason is obvious from the pulmonary version of Ohm's law (see Equation 27-7). The maximal ΔP (ΔP_{max}) that we can generate between atmosphere and alveoli during inspiration, for example, depends on how low we can drive *alveolar pressure* using our muscles of inspiration. For a given ΔP_{max}, a 3.3-fold increase in R_{AW} (COPD patient in Table 27-2) translates to a 3.3-fold reduction in maximal airflow ($\dot{V}_{max}$).

A DEPENDENCE OF TOTAL AIRWAY RESISTANCE ON LUNG VOLUME

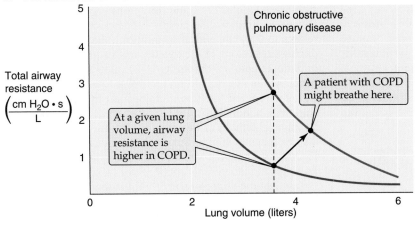

B MECHANICAL TETHERING

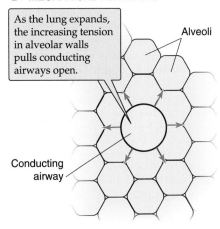

Figure 27-12 Airway resistance.

Table 27-3 Static Versus Dynamic Properties of the Lungs

Property	Static	Dynamic
Anatomical correlate	Alveoli	Conducting airways
Key "constant"	Static compliance, C	Airway resistance, R_{AW}
Key pressure	P_{TP} ($P_{TP} = P_A - P_{IP}$)	P_A
Key parameter	V_L ($C = \Delta V_L / \Delta P_{TP}$)	$\dot{V}$ ($\dot{V} = P_A / R_{AW}$)
Pathological change	Restrictive disease (e.g., fibrosis), caused by $\downarrow C$	Obstructive disease (e.g., COPD), caused by $\uparrow R_{AW}$

Thus, P_{IP} has two components, $-P_{TP}$ and P_A, as summarized in Figure 27-13 and Table 27-3. As we will see in the next section, P_{TP} and P_A literally flow from P_{IP}.

Transpulmonary Pressure P_{TP} is a *static* parameter. It does not cause airflow. Rather, along with static compliance, P_{TP} determines V_L. The curve in the lower left part of Figure 27-13—like the middle plot of Figure 27-5—describes how V_L depends on P_{TP}. That is, this curve describes the P_{TP} required to overcome the elastic (i.e., static) forces that oppose lung expansion but makes no statement about $\dot{V}$. We have already seen that the slope of this curve is static compliance, a property mainly of the alveoli, and that a decrease in C can produce *restrictive* lung disease. Note that P_{TP} not only determines V_L under static conditions, when there is no airflow, but also under dynamic conditions (i.e., during inspiration and expiration). However, the brain does not directly control P_{TP}.

Alveolar Pressure P_A is a dynamic parameter. It does not determine V_L directly. Instead, along with airway resistance, P_A determines *airflow*. The curve in the lower right part of Figure 27-13 describes how $\dot{V}$ depends on P_A. That is, this curve describes the P_A required to overcome inertial and

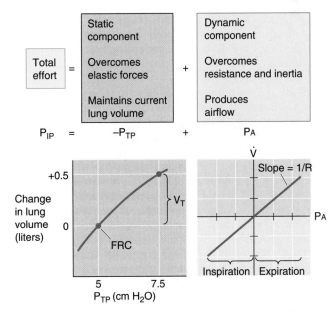

Figure 27-13 The static and dynamic components of intrapleural pressure.

resistive (i.e., dynamic) forces that oppose airflow but makes no statement about V_L. The slope of this plot is airway **conductance**, the reciprocal of R_{AW}, which is mainly a property of the conducting airways. A decrease in R_{AW} can produce *obstructive* lung disease. When PA is 0, $\dot{V}$ must be 0, regardless of whether V_L is at RV or TLC or anywhere in between. If the PA is positive and the glottis is open, air flows from alveoli to atmosphere, regardless of V_L. If PA is negative, air flows in the opposite direction. As is the case with P_{TP}, the brain does not directly control PA.

During inspiration, a sustained negative shift in P_{IP} causes PA to become transiently more negative

During a quiet respiratory cycle—an inspiration of 500 mL, followed by an expiration—the body first generates negative and then positive values of PA. The four large gray panels of Figure 27-14 show an idealized time course of five key parameters. The uppermost panel is a record of V_L. The next panel is a pair of plots, $-P_{TP}$ and P_{IP}. The third shows the record of PA. The bottom panel shows a simultaneous record of $\dot{V}$.

On the right side of Figure 27-14 are the static P_{TP}-V_L curve and the dynamic PA-$\dot{V}$relationship (both copied from Fig. 27-13). On the left side is a series of four cartoons that represent snapshots of the key pressures (i.e., P_{IP}, P_{TP}, and PA) at four points during the respiratory cycle:

a. Before inspiration begins. The lungs are under static conditions at a volume of FRC.
b. Halfway through inspiration. The lungs are under dynamic conditions at a volume of FRC + 250 mL.
c. At the completion of inspiration. The lungs are once again under static conditions but at a volume of FRC + 500 mL.
d. Halfway through expiration. The lungs are under dynamic conditions at a volume of FRC + 250 mL.
a. At the end of expiration/ready for the next inspiration. The lungs are once again under static conditions at a volume of FRC.

The V_L record in the top gray panel of Figure 27-14 shows that V_L rises more or less exponentially during inspiration and similarly falls during expiration.

Knowing the time course of V_L, we obtained the P_{TP} values in the second gray panel by reading them off the static P_{TP}-V_L diagram to the right and plotted them as $-P_{TP}$ (for consistency with Equation 27-12). As V_L increases during inspiration, P_{TP} increases (i.e., $-P_{TP}$ becomes more negative). The opposite is true during expiration. Remember that P_{TP} (along with static compliance) determines V_L at any time.

The P_{IP} record in the second gray panel shows that P_{IP} is the same as $-P_{TP}$ whenever the lungs are under static conditions (points *a*, *c*, and *a*). During inspiration, P_{IP} rapidly becomes more negative than $-P_{TP}$ but then merges with $-P_{TP}$ by the end of inspiration. The difference between P_{IP} and $-P_{TP}$ is PA, which must be negative to produce airflow into the lungs. During expiration, P_{IP} is more positive than $-P_{TP}$.

The PA record in the third gray panel shows that alveolar pressure is zero under static conditions (points *a*, *c*, and *a*). During inspiration, PA rapidly becomes negative but then relaxes to 0 by the end of inspiration. The opposite is true during expiration. The PA values in this plot represent the differences between the P_{IP} and $-P_{TP}$ plots in the preceding panel.

We computed $\dot{V}$ (bottom gray panel) from the relationship in Equation 27-7: $\dot{V} = (PA - P_B)/R_{AW}$. Remember that PA (along with R_{AW}) determines $\dot{V}$ at any time. Here, we assume that R_{AW} is fixed during the respiratory cycle at 1 cm $H_2O/(L/s)$. Thus, the $\dot{V}$ record has the same time course as PA.

The key message in Figure 27-14 is that during inspiration, the negative shift in P_{IP} has two effects. The body invests some of the energy represented by ΔP_{IP} into transiently making PA more negative (dynamic component). The result is that air *flows* into the lungs and V_L increases; but this investment in PA is only transient. Throughout inspiration, the body invests an increasingly greater fraction of its energy in making P_{TP} more positive (static component). The result is that the body *maintains* the new, higher V_L. By the end of inspiration, the body invests all of the energy represented by ΔP_{IP} in maintaining V_L and none in further expansion. The situation is not unlike that faced by Julius Caesar as he, with finite resources, conquered Gaul. At first, he invested all of his resources in expanding his territory at the expense of the feisty Belgians; but as the conquered territory grew, he was forced to invest an increasingly greater fraction of his resources in maintaining the newly conquered territory. In the end, he necessarily invested all of his resources in maintaining his territory and was unable to expand further.

Dynamic compliance falls as respiratory frequency rises

In the preceding section, we examined pressure, volume, and flow changes during an idealized respiratory cycle of 5 seconds, which corresponds to a respiratory frequency of 12/minute. The top curve in Figure 27-15A shows a normal V_L time course during an inspiration. As for any exponential process, the **time constant** (τ) is the interval required for ΔV_L to be ~63% complete. For healthy lungs, τ is ~0.2 second. Thus, for inspiration, the increase in V_L is 63% complete after 0.2 second, 86% complete after 0.4 second, 95% complete after 0.6 second, and so on. We will make the simplifying assumption that the time available for inspiration is half this time or 2.5 seconds, which represents more than 12 time constants! Thus, if the V_T after infinite time were 500 mL, the ΔV_L measured 2.5 seconds after initiation of inspiration would also be ~500 mL (Fig. 27-15A, green point). In Figure 27-15B, we replot this value as the green point at a frequency of 12/minute on the top curve (i.e., normal lungs).

For a respiratory frequency of 24/minute, 1.25 seconds is available for inspiration. At the end of this time, the ΔV_L is ~499 mL (Fig. 27-15B, blue point on the top curve).

If we further increase the respiratory frequency to 48/minute, only 0.625 second is available for inspiration. At the end of this period, only slightly more than 3 time constants, the ΔV_L is ~478 mL (Fig. 27-15B, red point on top curve).

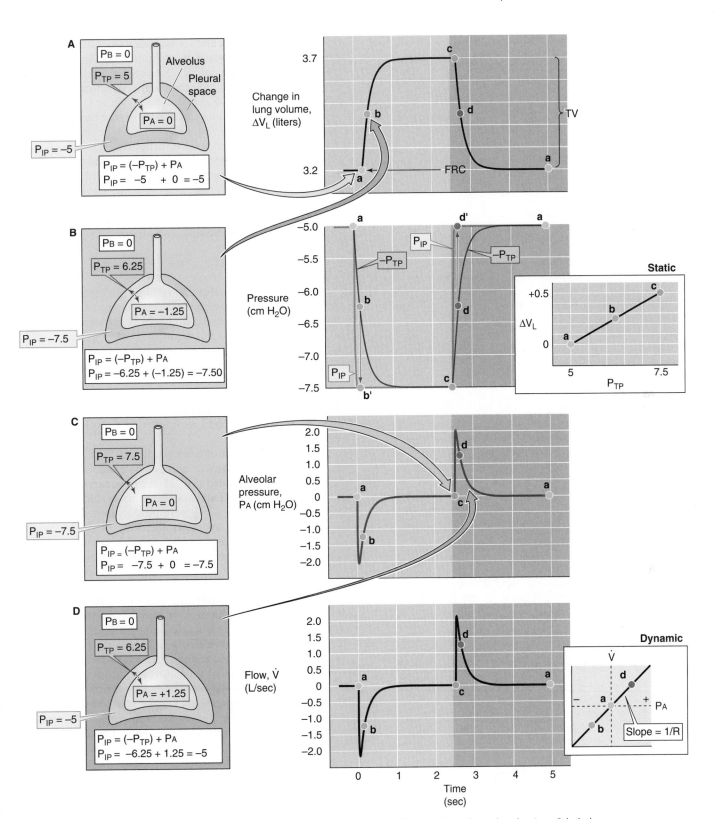

Figure 27-14 The respiratory cycle. P_B, P_{IP}, P_{TP}, and P_A are all in cm H_2O. The colored points (labeled *a*, *b*, *c*, and *d*) in each of the central panels correspond to the illustrations (on the *left*) with the same colored background. The two panels on the *right* are taken from Figure 27-13. V_L, lung volume; $\dot{V}$, airflow.

A EFFECT OF AIRWAY RESISTANCE ON RATE OF INFLATION

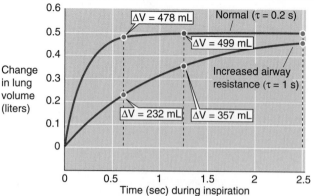

B EFFECT OF AIRWAY RESISTANCE ON TIDAL VOLUME

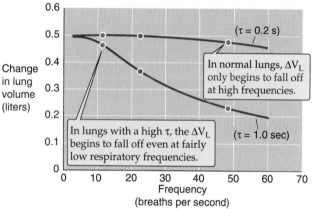

C EFFECT OF RESPIRATORY FREQUENCY ON TIDAL VOLUME

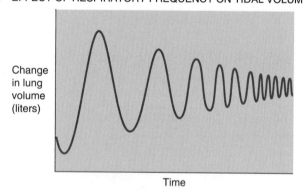

Figure 27-15 Dynamic compliance. In **A** and **B,** the colored points represent changes in volume at respiratory frequencies of 12, 24, and 48 breaths per minute.

Thus, over a wide range of frequencies, ΔV_L is largely unchanged. Only when respiratory frequency approaches extremely high values does ΔV_L begin to fall off.

 The situation is very different for a subject with substantially increased airway resistance. If R_{AW} increased 5-fold, τ would also increase 5-fold to 1 second. As a result, the trajectory of V_L also would slow by a factor of 5 (Fig. 27-15A, bottom curve). If we could wait long enough during an inspiration, these unhealthy lungs would eventually achieve a ΔV_L of 500 mL. The problem is that we cannot wait that long. Therefore, if the frequency is 12/minute and inspira-

tion terminates after only 2.5 seconds (i.e., only 2.5 time constants), the ΔV_L would be only 459 mL (Fig. 27-15B, green point on bottom curve). Thus, even at a relatively low frequency, the patient with increased R_{AW} achieves a ΔV_L that is well below normal.

For a respiratory frequency of 24/minute, when only 1.25 seconds is available for inspiration, the ΔV_L is only 357 mL (Fig. 27-15B, blue point on bottom curve). At a respiratory frequency of 48/minute, when only 0.625 second is available for inspiration, the ΔV_L is only 232 mL (Fig. 27-15B, red point on the bottom curve). Thus, the ΔV_L for the subject with increased R_{AW} falls rapidly as frequency increases.

We can represent the *change* in V_L during cyclic breathing by a parameter called **dynamic compliance**:

$$C_{dynamic} = \frac{\Delta V_L}{-\Delta P_{IP}} \qquad (27\text{-}13)$$

Note that $C_{dynamic}$ is proportional to ΔV_L in Figure 27-15B. Under truly static conditions (i.e., frequency of 0), $-\Delta P_{IP}$ equals ΔP_{TP}, and *dynamic* compliance is the same as *static* compliance (C or C_{static}) that we introduced in Equation 27-4. As frequency increases, $C_{dynamic}$ falls below C_{static}. The degree of divergence increases with resistance. For the normal lung in Figure 27-15B, ΔV_L and thus $C_{dynamic}$ fall by only ~5% as frequency rises from 0 to 48/minute. However, for the lung with a 5-fold increased airway resistance, $C_{dynamic}$ falls by more than 50% as frequency rises from 0 to 48/minute.

This pathological pattern is typical of asthma; R_{AW} is elevated, but C_{static} is relatively normal. In emphysema, both R_{AW} and C_{static} are elevated (Fig. 27-5, upper curve). Thus, a plot of $C_{dynamic}$ versus frequency would show that $C_{dynamic}$ is initially greater than C_{static} at low respiratory frequencies, but it falls below C_{static} as frequency increases. What do these frequency-dependent decreases in $C_{dynamic}$ mean for a patient? The greater the respiratory frequency, the less time is available for inspiration or expiration, and the smaller the V_T (Fig. 27-15C).

This analysis greatly oversimplifies what happens in the lungs of real people. Although we have treated the lungs as if there were one value for R_{AW} and one for C_{static}, each conducting airway has its own airway resistance and each alveolar unit has its own static compliance, and these values vary with parameters such as V_L, posture, and hormonal status. As a result, some alveolar units have greater time constants than others. Airway disease may make some of these time constants substantially higher. As respiratory frequency increases, alveoli with relatively high time constants will have less time to undergo volume changes. As a result, these "slow" airways—compared with the "faster" airways—will make progressively smaller contributions to the overall ventilation of the lungs. At sufficiently high frequencies, very slow airways may drop out of the picture entirely.

Transmural pressure differences cause airways to dilate during inspiration and to compress during expiration

We have noted three factors that modulate airway caliber: (1) the ANS, (2) humoral substances, and (3) V_L (Fig. 27-12). A fourth factor that modulates R_{AW} is flow of air through the conducting airway itself. Airflow alters the pressure difference across the walls of an airway, and this change in **transmural pressure (P_{TM})** can cause the airway to dilate or to collapse. Figure 27-16A-C depicts the pressures along a single hypothetical airway, extending from the level of the alveolus to the lips, under three conditions: during inspiration (Fig. 27-16A), at rest (Fig. 27-16B), and during expiration (Fig. 27-16C). In all three cases, the lung is at the same volume, FRC; the only difference is whether air is flowing into the lung, not flowing at all, or flowing out of the lung. Because V_L is at FRC, P_{TP} (the P_{TM} for the alveoli) is 5 cm H_2O in all three cases.

Static Conditions First consider what happens under static conditions (Fig. 27-16B). In the absence of airflow, the pressures inside all airways must be 0. Considering first the alveoli, P_{TP} is 5 cm H_2O and the P_A is 0, and thus P_{IP} is −5 cm H_2O. We will ignore the effects of gravity on P_{IP} and thus assume that P_{IP} is uniform throughout the chest cavity. The P_{IP} of −5 cm H_2O acts not only on alveoli but on *all* conducting airways within the thoracic cavity. For these, P_{TM} at any point is the difference between the pressure inside the airway (P_{AW}) and P_{IP} (see Equation 27-1):

$$P_{TM} = P_{AW} - P_{IP} = 0 - (-5\,cm\,H_2O) = +5\,cm\,H_2O \quad (27\text{-}14)$$

In other words, a transmural pressure of +5 cm H_2O acts on *all* thoracic airways (but *not* the trachea in the neck, for example), tending to expand them to the extent that their compliance permits.

Inspiration Now consider what happens during a vigorous inspiration (Fig. 27-16A). We first exhale to a V_L below FRC and then vigorously inhale, so that the P_A is −15 cm H_2O at the instant that V_L passes through FRC. Because the lung is at FRC, P_{TP} is +5 cm H_2O. The P_{IP} needed to produce a P_A of −15 cm H_2O is

$$\begin{aligned} P_{IP} &= (-P_{TP}) + P_A \\ &= -5\,cm\,H_2O + (-15\,cm\,H_2O) \quad (27\text{-}15) \\ &= -20\,cm\,H_2O \end{aligned}$$

This "inspiring" P_{IP} of −20 cm H_2O is just enough to produce the desired airflow and also to maintain the alveoli at precisely the same volume that they had under static conditions. But how does this exceptionally negative P_{IP} affect airways upstream from the alveoli? P_{AW} gradually decays from −15 cm H_2O in the alveoli to 0 at the lips. The farther we move from the alveoli, the less negative is P_{AW}, and thus the greater is P_{TM}.

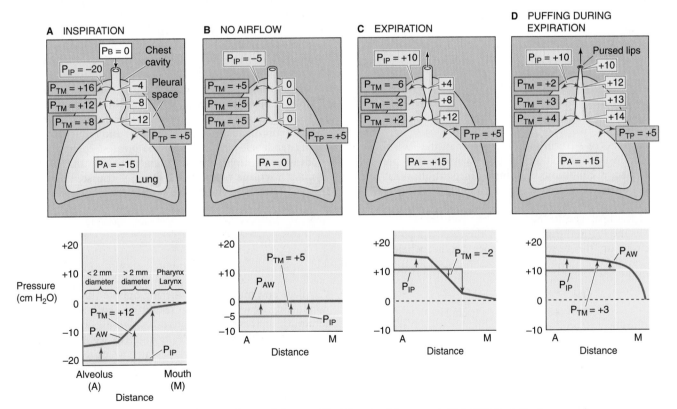

Figure 27-16 Dilation and collapse of airways with airflow. In all four panels, V_L is FRC. P_{TM} is the transmural pressure across conducting airways. Airway pressure (P_{AW}) and values in *pale blue balloons* represent pressures inside conducting airways (all in cm H_2O). Graphs at bottom show P_{AW} profiles along airways *(blue curve)* from alveolus to mouth. P_{IP} is constant throughout the thorax *(green curve)*. The *upward arrows* tend to expand the airways, whereas the *downward arrows* tend to squeeze them.

As an illustration, consider a point about halfway up the airway's resistance profile, where P_{AW} is −8 cm H_2O:

$$P_{TM} = P_{AW} - P_{IP}$$
$$= -8 \text{cm } H_2O - (-20 \text{cm } H_2O) \quad \textbf{(27-16)}$$
$$= +12 \text{cm } H_2O$$

Thus, the transmural pressure opposing the elastic recoil at this point has increased from +5 cm H_2O at rest (Fig. 27-16B) to +12 cm H_2O during this vigorous inspiration (Fig. 27-16A). Because P_{TM} has increased, the airway will dilate. The tendency to dilate increases as we move from the alveoli to larger airways. As shown in the graph in the lower part of Figure 27-16A, P_{AW} (and thus P_{TM}, as indicated by the upward arrows) gradually increases. Note that the very positive P_{TM} values that develop in the larger airways determine only the *tendency* to dilate. The extent to which an airway *actually* dilates also depends on its compliance. The amount of cartilage supporting the airways gradually increases from none for 11th-generation airways to a substantial amount for the mainstem bronchi. Because the increasing amount of cartilage in the larger airways decreases their compliance, they have an increasing ability to resist changes in caliber produced by a given change in P_{TM}.

Expiration   As might be expected, conducting airways tend to collapse during expiration (Fig. 27-16C). We first inhale to a V_L above FRC and then exhale vigorously, so that P_A is +15 cm H_2O at the instant that V_L passes through FRC. Because the lung is at FRC, P_{TP} is +5 cm H_2O. The P_{IP} needed to produce a P_A of +15 cm H_2O is

$$P_{IP} = (-P_{TP}) + P_A$$
$$= -5 \text{cm } H_2O + (+15 \text{cm } H_2O) \quad \textbf{(27-17)}$$
$$= +10 \text{cm } H_2O$$

This P_{IP} of +10 cm H_2O is 5 less than the P_A and thus maintains the alveoli at the same volume that prevailed under static conditions and during inspiration. What is the effect of this very positive P_{IP} on the upstream airways? P_{AW} must decrease gradually from +15 cm H_2O in the alveoli to 0 at the lips. The farther we move from the alveolus, the lower the P_{AW} and thus the lower the P_{TM}. At a point about halfway up the airway's resistance profile, where P_{AW} is +8 cm H_2O:

$$P_{TM} = P_{AW} - P_{IP}$$
$$= +8 \text{cm } H_2O - (+10 \text{cm } H_2O) \quad \textbf{(27-18)}$$
$$= -2 \text{cm } H_2O$$

Thus, at this point during a vigorous expiration, the transmural pressure opposing elastic recoil has fallen sharply from +5 cm H_2O at rest (which tends to mildly inflate the airway) to −2 cm H_2O during expiration (which actually tends to squeeze the airway). As we move from the alveoli to larger airways, P_{AW} gradually decreases. That is, P_{TM} gradually shifts from an ever-decreasing inflating force (positive values) to an ever-increasing squeezing force (negative

values), as indicated by the change in the orientation of the arrows in the lower panel of Figure 27-16C. Fortunately, these larger airways—with the greatest collapsing tendency—have the most cartilage and thus some resistance to the natural collapsing tendency that develops during expiration. In addition, mechanical tethering helps all conducting airways surrounded by alveoli to resist collapse. Nevertheless, R_{AW} is greater during expiration than it is during inspiration.

The problem of airway compression during expiration is exaggerated in patients with **emphysema**, a condition in which the alveolar walls break down. This process results in fewer and larger air spaces with fewer points of attachment and less mutual buttressing of air spaces. Although the affected alveoli have an increased compliance and thus a larger diameter at the end of an inspiration, they are flimsy and exert less mechanical tethering on the conducting airways they surround. Thus, patients with emphysema have great difficulty exhaling because their conducting airways are less able to resist the tendency to collapse. However, these patients make their expirations easier in three ways. We could predict them all from our knowledge of dynamic respiratory mechanics:

1. **They exhale slowly.** A low $\dot{V}$ during expiration translates to a less positive P_A and thus a less positive P_{IP}, minimizing the tendency to collapse.
2. **They breathe at higher V_L.** A high V_L maximizes the mechanical tethering that opposes airway collapse during expiration and thus minimizes R_{AW} (Fig. 27-12A).
3. **They exhale through pursed lips.** This maneuver—known as puffing—creates an artificial, high resistance at the lips. Because the greatest pressure drop occurs at the location of the greatest resistance, puffing causes a greater share of the P_{AW} drop to occur across the lips rather than along collapsible, cartilage-free airways. Thus, puffing maintains relatively high P_{AW} values farther along the tracheobronchial tree (Fig. 27-16D) and reduces collapsing tendencies throughout. The greatest collapsing tendencies are reserved for the largest airways that have the most cartilage (see Chapter 26). Of course, the patient pays a price for puffing: $\dot{V}$ and thus the ventilation of the alveoli is low.

Because of airway collapse, expiratory flow rates become independent of effort at low lung volumes

Cartilage and mechanical tethering oppose the tendency of conducting airways to collapse during expiration. Because tethering increases as V_L increases, we expect airways to better resist collapse when V_L is high. To see if this is true, we will examine how expiratory airflow varies with effort (i.e., alveolar pressure) at different V_L.

Imagine that we make a maximal inspiration and then hold our breath with glottis open (Fig. 27-17A). Thus, P_A is 0. In addition, P_{TP} is +30 cm H_2O to maintain TLC. From Equation 27-12, $P_{IP} = (-P_{TP}) + P_A = -30$ cm H_2O. Now, starting from TLC, we make a maximal expiratory effort. Figure 27-17B summarizes the pressures in the alveoli and thorax at the instant we begin exhaling but before V_L has had

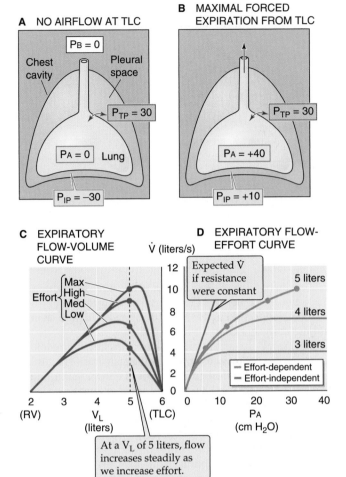

A NO AIRFLOW AT TLC

P$_B$ = 0

Chest cavity

Pleural space

P$_{TP}$ = 30

P$_A$ = 0   Lung

P$_{IP}$ = −30

B MAXIMAL FORCED EXPIRATION FROM TLC

P$_{TP}$ = 30

P$_A$ = +40

P$_{IP}$ = +10

C EXPIRATORY FLOW-VOLUME CURVE

$\dot{V}$ (liters/s)

Effort { Max, High, Med, Low }

12
10
8
6
4
2
0

2 (RV)   3   4   5   6 (TLC)

V$_L$ (liters)

At a V$_L$ of 5 liters, flow increases steadily as we increase effort.

D EXPIRATORY FLOW-EFFORT CURVE

Expected $\dot{V}$ if resistance were constant

5 liters
4 liters
3 liters

— Effort-dependent
— Effort-independent

0   10   20   30   40

P$_A$ (cm H$_2$O)

Figure 27-17 Dependence of airflow on effort. In **D,** note that if airway resistance were fixed, increased effort (i.e., increased P$_A$) would yield a proportionate increase in $\dot{V}$, as indicated by the *red line*. However, increased effort tends to narrow airways, raising resistance and tending to flatten the curves. As V$_L$ decreases (e.g., 4 or 3 L), airflow becomes independent of effort with increasingly low effort. P$_B$, P$_{IP}$, P$_{TP}$, and P$_A$ are all in cm H$_2$O.

time to change. P$_{TP}$ is still +30 cm H$_2$O, but P$_A$ is now +40 cm H$_2$O (to produce a maximal expiration) and P$_{IP}$ is therefore +10 cm H$_2$O. As V$_L$ decreases during the course of the expiration, we will monitor $\dot{V}$, V$_L$, and P$_A$.

The top curve in Figure 27-17C shows how $\dot{V}$ changes as a function of V$_L$ when, starting from TLC, we make a maximal expiratory effort. Notice that $\dot{V}$ rises to its maximal value at a V$_L$ that is somewhat less than TLC and then gradually falls to 0 as V$_L$ approaches RV. The data in this top curve, obtained with maximal expiratory effort (i.e., at maximal P$_A$), will help us determine how expiratory flow varies with effort. To get the rest of the necessary data, we repeat our experiment by again inhaling to TLC and again exhaling to RV. However, with each trial, we exhale with less effort (i.e., at smaller P$_A$)—efforts labeled as high, medium, and low in Figure 27-17C.

If we draw a vertical line upward from a V$_L$ of 5 L in Figure 27-17C, we see that at this very high V$_L$, $\dot{V}$ gets larger and larger as the effort increases from low to medium to high

to maximal. Because these efforts correspond to increasing P$_A$ values, we can plot these four $\dot{V}$ data points (all obtained at a V$_L$ of 5 L) versus P$_A$ in the top curve of Figure 27-17D. Because $\dot{V}$ increases continuously with the P$_A$, flow is **effort dependent** at a V$_L$ of 5 L. If the airways were made of steel, this plot of $\dot{V}$ versus P$_A$ would be a straight line. Because the actual plot bends downward at higher values of P$_A$ (i.e., greater efforts), R$_{AW}$ must have increased with effort (i.e., the airways collapsed somewhat).

Returning to Figure 27-17C, we see that an important characteristic of these data is that the $\dot{V}$ versus V$_L$ curve for maximal expiratory effort defines an envelope that none of the other three curves could penetrate. Thus, at a V$_L$ of 4 L, $\dot{V}$ is ~7 L/s, regardless of whether the expiratory effort is high or maximal (i.e., the two points overlie one another on the graph). At a V$_L$ of 3 L, the four curves have practically merged, so that $\dot{V}$ is ~3.5 L/s regardless of effort. Thus, at lung volumes that are below 3 L, it does not matter how much effort we make; the expiratory flow can never exceed a certain value defined by the envelope.

Shifting back to Figure 27-17D, we see that for the lower two $\dot{V}$ versus P$_A$ plots, $\dot{V}$ increases with P$_A$—up to a point. Further increases in effort (i.e., P$_A$) are to no avail because they produce a proportional increase in R$_{AW}$—expiration-induced airway collapse. Thus, the more positive values of P$_{IP}$ not only produce more positive values of P$_A$ but also increase R$_{AW}$, so that P$_A$/R$_{AW}$ and thus $\dot{V}$ remain constant.

At low lung volumes, flow becomes **effort independent** because the reduced mechanical tethering cannot oppose the tendency toward airway collapse that always exists during expiration. Moreover, at progressively lower V$_L$, flow becomes effort independent earlier. In other words, particularly at low lung volumes, it simply does not pay to try any harder.

REFERENCES

Books and Reviews

De Troyer A, Kirkwood PA, Wilson TA: Respiratory action of the intercostal muscles. Physiol Rev 2005; 85:717-756.

Dietl P, Haller T: Exocytosis of lung surfactant: From the secretory vesicle to the air-liquid interface. Annu Rev Physiol 2005; 67:595-621.

Floros J, Kala P: Surfactant proteins: Molecular genetics of neonatal pulmonary diseases. Annu Rev Physiol 1998; 60:365-384.

Fryer AD, Jacoby DB: Muscarinic receptors and control of airway smooth muscle. Am J Respir Crit Care Med 1998; 158: S154-S160.

Lai-Fook S: Pleural mechanics and fluid exchange. Physiol Rev 2005; 84:385-410.

Wright JR: Immunomodulatory functions of surfactant. Physiol Rev 1997; 77:931-962.

Journal Articles

Avery ME, Mead J: Surface properties in relation to atelectasis and hyaline membrane disease. Am J Dis Child 1959; 97:517-523.

Clements JA: Surface tension of lung extracts. Proc Soc Exp Biol Med 1957; 95:170-172.

Mead J, Whittenberger JL, Radford EP Jr: Surface tension as a factor in pulmonary volume-pressure hysteresis. J Appl Physiol 1957; 10:191-196.

Perkins WR, Dause RB, Parente RA: Role of lipid polymorphism in pulmonary surfactant. Science 1996; 273:330-332.

CHAPTER 28

ACID-BASE PHYSIOLOGY

Walter F. Boron

Acid-base physiology is really the study of the proton, or hydrogen ion (H^+). Although they are present in exceedingly low concentrations in most intracellular and extracellular fluids, protons nevertheless have a major impact on biochemical reactions and on a variety of physiological processes that are critical for the homeostasis of the entire body and individual cells. Not surprisingly, the body has evolved sophisticated systems to maintain $[H^+]$ values within narrow and precise ranges in the blood plasma, intracellular fluid, and other compartments.

This chapter provides the introduction to acid-base physiology, including the chemistry of buffers, the CO_2/HCO_3^- buffer system, the competition between the CO_2/HCO_3^- buffer system and other buffers, and the regulation of intracellular pH. In other chapters, we will discuss how blood pH—and, by extension, the pH of extracellular fluid—is under the dual control of the respiratory system, which regulates plasma $[CO_2]$ (see Chapter 31), and the kidneys, which regulate plasma $[HCO_3^-]$ (see Chapter 39). In addition, we discuss the control of cerebrospinal fluid pH in Chapter 32.

pH AND BUFFERS

pH values vary enormously among different intracellular and extracellular compartments

According to Brønsted's definition, an **acid** is any chemical substance (e.g., CH_3COOH, NH_4^+) that can donate an H^+. A **base** is any chemical substance (e.g., CH_3COO^-, NH_3) that can accept an H^+. The term **alkali** can be used interchangeably with **base**.

$[H^+]$ varies over a large range in biological solutions, from more than 100 mM in gastric secretions to less than 10 nM in pancreatic secretions. In 1909, the chemist Sørensen introduced the **pH scale** in an effort to simplify the notation in experiments in which he was examining the influence of $[H^+]$ on enzymatic reactions. He based the pH scale on powers of 10:

$$pH \equiv -\log_{10}[H^+] \qquad (28\text{-}1)$$

Thus, when $[H^+]$ is 10^{-7} M, the pH is 7.0. The higher the $[H^+]$, the lower the pH (Table 28-1). A 10-fold change in $[H^+]$ corresponds to a pH shift of 1, whereas a 2-fold change in $[H^+]$ corresponds to a pH shift of ~0.3.

Even small changes in pH can have substantial physiological consequences because most biologically important molecules contain chemical groups that can either donate an H^+ (e.g., $R\text{—}COOH \rightarrow R\text{—}COO^- + H^+$) and thereby act as a weak acid or accept an H^+ (e.g., $R\text{—}NH_2 + H^+ \rightarrow R\text{—}NH_3^+$) and thus behave as a weak base. To the extent that these groups donate or accept protons, a pH shift causes a change in their net electrical charge (or valence) that can, in turn, alter a molecule's conformation and thus its biological activity.

pH-sensitive molecules include a variety of enzymes, receptors and their ligands, ion channels, transporters, and structural proteins. For most proteins, pH sensitivity is modest. The activity of the Na-K pump (see Chapter 5), for example, falls by about half when the pH shifts by ~1 pH unit from the optimum pH, which is near the resting pH of the typical cell. However, the activity of phosphofructokinase, a key glycolytic enzyme (see Chapter 58), falls by ~90% when pH falls by only 0.1. The overall impact of pH changes on cellular processes can be impressive. Therefore, cell proliferation in response to mitogenic activation is maximal at the normal, resting intracellular pH but may fall as much as 85% when intracellular pH falls by only 0.4.

Table 28-2 summarizes the pH values in several body fluids. Because the pH of neutral water at 37°C is 6.81, most major body compartments are alkaline.

Buffers minimize the size of the pH changes produced by the addition of acid or alkali to a solution

A **buffer** is any substance that reversibly consumes or releases H^+. In this way, buffers help stabilize pH. Buffers do not *prevent* pH changes; they only help to *minimize* them.

Consider a hypothetical buffer B for which the protonated form $HB^{(n+1)}$, with a valence of $n+1$, is in equilibrium with its deprotonated form $B^{(n)}$, which has the valence of n:

Table 28-1 Relationship Between [H⁺] and pH Values

	[H⁺] (M)	pH	
× 10	1×10^{-6} 1×10^{-7} 1×10^{-8}	6.0 7.0 8.0	1 pH unit
× 2	8×10^{-8} 4×10^{-8} 2×10^{-8} 1×10^{-8}	7.1 7.4 7.7 8.0	0.3 pH unit

Table 28-2 Approximate pH Values of Various Body Fluids

Compartment	pH
Gastric secretions (under conditions of maximal acidity)	0.7
Lysosome	5.5
Chromaffin granule	5.5
Neutral H_2O at 37°C	6.81
Cytosol of a typical cell	7.2
Cerebrospinal fluid	7.3
Arterial blood plasma	7.4
Mitochondrial inner matrix	7.5
Secreted pancreatic fluid	8.1

$$HB^{(n+1)} \rightleftarrows B^{(n)} + H^+ \tag{28-2}$$

Here, $HB^{(n+1)}$ is a **weak acid** because it does not fully dissociate; $B^{(n)}$ is its **conjugate weak base**. Conversely, $B^{(n)}$ is a **weak base** and $HB^{(n+1)}$ is its conjugate weak acid. The **total buffer concentration**, [TB], is the sum of the concentrations of the protonated and unprotonated forms:

$$[TB] = [HB^{(n+1)}] + [B^{(n)}] \tag{28-3}$$

The valence of the acidic (i.e., protonated) form can be positive, zero, or negative:

Weak acid $(HB^{(n+1)})$ Conjugate weak base $(B^{(n)})$

$$
\begin{aligned}
NH_4^+ &\rightleftarrows NH_3 &&+ H^+ \\
H_2CO_3 &\rightleftarrows HCO_3^- &&+ H^+ \\
H_2PO_4^- &\rightleftarrows HPO_4^{2-} &&+ H^+
\end{aligned}
\tag{28-4}
$$

In these examples, NH_4^+ (ammonium), H_2CO_3 (carbonic acid), and $H_2PO_4^-$ ("monobasic" inorganic phosphate) are all

weak acids; NH_3 (ammonia), HCO_3^- (bicarbonate), and HPO_4^{2-} ("dibasic" inorganic phosphate) are the respective conjugate weak bases. Each buffer reaction is governed by a **dissociation constant**, K:

$$K = \frac{[B^{(n)}][H^+]}{[HB^{(n+1)}]} \tag{28-5}$$

If we add to a physiological solution a small amount of HCl—which is a strong acid because it fully dissociates—the buffers in the solution consume almost all added H^+:

$$H^+ + Cl^- + B^{(n)} \rightarrow HB^{(n+1)} + Cl^- \tag{28-6}$$

For each H^+ buffered, one $B^{(n)}$ is *consumed*. The tiny amount of H^+ that is *not buffered* remains free in solution and is responsible for the decrease in pH.

If we instead titrate this same solution with a strong base such as NaOH, H^+ derived from $HB^{(n+1)}$ neutralizes almost all the added OH^-:

$$Na^+ + OH^- + HB^{(n+1)} \rightarrow Na^+ + B^{(n)} + H_2O \tag{28-7}$$

For each OH^- buffered, one $B^{(n)}$ is *formed*. The tiny amount of added OH^- that is not neutralized by the buffer equilibrates with H^+ and H_2O and is responsible for an increase in pH.

A useful measure of the strength of a buffer is its **buffering power (β)**, which is the number of moles of strong base (e.g., NaOH) that one must add to a liter of solution to increase pH by one pH unit. This value is equivalent to the amount of strong acid (e.g., HCl) that one must add to decrease the pH by one pH unit. Thus, buffering power is

$$\beta \equiv \frac{\overbrace{\Delta[\text{Strong base}]}^{\text{moles/liter}}}{\Delta pH} = -\frac{\overbrace{\Delta[\text{Strong acid}]}^{\text{moles/liter}}}{\Delta pH} \tag{28-8}$$

In the absence of CO_2/HCO_3^-, the buffering power of whole blood (which contains erythrocytes, leukocytes, and platelets) is ~25 mM/pH unit. This value is known as the **non-HCO_3^- buffering power** ($\beta_{\text{non-}HCO_3^-}$). In other words, we would have to add 25 mmol of NaOH to a liter of whole blood to increase the pH by one unit, assuming that β is constant over this wide pH range. For blood plasma, which lacks the cellular elements of whole blood, the non-HCO_3^- buffering power is only ~5 mM/pH unit, which means that only about one fifth as much strong base would be needed to produce the same pH increase.

According to the Henderson-Hasselbalch equation, pH depends on the ratio [CO₂]/[HCO₃⁻]

The most important physiological buffer pair is CO_2 and HCO_3^-. The impressive strength of this buffer pair is due to the volatility of CO_2, which allows the lungs to maintain stable CO_2 concentrations in the blood plasma despite ongoing metabolic and buffer reactions that produce or consume CO_2. Imagine that a beaker contains an aqueous solution of 145 mM NaCl (pH = 6.81) but no buffers. We now expose this solution to an atmosphere containing CO_2 (Fig. 28-1). The concentration of dissolved CO_2 ($[CO_2]_{Dis}$) is governed by **Henry's law** (see Chapter 26 for the box on that topic):

$$[CO_2]_{Dis} = s \cdot P_{CO_2} \qquad (28\text{-}9)$$

At the temperature (37°C) and ionic strength of mammalian blood plasma, the **solubility coefficient**, s, is ~0.03 mM/mm Hg. Because the alveolar air with which arterial blood equilibrates has a P_{CO_2} of ~40 mm Hg, or torr, $[CO_2]_{Dis}$ in arterial blood is

$$[CO_2]_a = (0.03 \text{ mM/mm Hg}) \cdot 40 \text{ mm Hg} = 1.2 \text{ mM} \qquad (28\text{-}10)$$

So far, the entry of CO_2 from the atmosphere into the aqueous solution has had *no effect* on pH. The reason is that we have neither generated nor consumed H^+. CO_2 itself is neither an acid nor a base. If we were considering dissolved N_2 or O_2, our analysis would end here because these gases do not further interact with simple aqueous solutions. The aqueous chemistry of CO_2, however, is more complicated because CO_2 reacts with the solvent (i.e., H_2O) to form carbonic acid:

$$CO_2 + H_2O \xrightarrow{\text{slow}} H_2CO_3 \qquad (28\text{-}11)$$

This **CO_2 hydration reaction** is very slow. In fact, it is far too slow to meet certain physiological needs. The enzyme **carbonic anhydrase**, present in erythrocytes and elsewhere, catalyzes a reaction that effectively bypasses this slow hydration reaction. Carbonic acid is a weak acid that rapidly dissociates into H^+ and HCO_3^-:

$$H_2CO_3 \xrightarrow{\text{fast}} H^+ + HCO_3^- \qquad (28\text{-}12)$$

This **dissociation reaction** is the first point at which pH falls. Note that the formation of HCO_3^- (the conjugate weak base of H_2CO_3) necessarily accompanies the formation of H^+ in a stoichiometry of 1:1. The observation that pH decreases, even though this reaction produces the weak base HCO_3^-, is sometimes confusing. A safe way to reason through such an apparent paradox is to focus always on the fate of the proton. If the reaction forms H^+, pH falls. Thus, even though the dissociation of H_2CO_3 leads to generation of a weak base, pH falls because H^+ forms along with the weak base.

Unlike the hydration of CO_2, the dissociation of H_2CO_3 is extremely fast. Thus, in the absence of carbonic anhydrase, the slow CO_2 hydration reaction limits the speed at which increased $[CO_2]_{Dis}$ leads to the production of H^+. HCO_3^- can accept a proton to form its conjugate weak acid (i.e., H_2CO_3) or release a second proton to form its conjugate weak base (i.e., CO_3^{2-}). Because this reaction generally is of only minor physiological significance for buffering in mammals, we will not discuss it further.

We may treat the hydration and dissociation reactions that occur when we expose water to CO_2 as if only one reaction were involved:

$$CO_2 + H_2O \rightleftarrows H_2CO_3 \rightleftarrows H^+ + HCO_3^-$$
$$CO_2 + H_2O \rightleftarrows H^+ + HCO_3^- \qquad (28\text{-}13)$$

Moreover, we may define a dissociation constant for this pseudoequilibrium:

$$K = \frac{[H^+][HCO_3^-]}{[CO_2]} \qquad (28\text{-}14)$$

In logarithmic form, this equation becomes

$$pH = pK + \log\frac{[HCO_3^-]}{[CO_2]} \qquad (28\text{-}15)$$

Finally, we may express $[CO_2]$ in terms of P_{CO_2}, recalling from Henry's law that $[CO_2] = s \cdot P_{CO_2}$:

$$pH = pK + \log\frac{[HCO_3^-]}{s \cdot P_{CO_2}} \qquad (28\text{-}16)$$

This is the **Henderson-Hasselbalch** equation, a logarithmic restatement of the CO_2/HCO_3^- equilibrium in Equation 28-14. Its central message is that pH depends not on $[HCO_3^-]$ or P_{CO_2} but on their ratio. Human arterial blood has a P_{CO_2} of ~40 mm Hg and a $[HCO_3^-]$ of ~24 mM. If we assume that the pK governing the CO_2/HCO_3^- equilibrium is 6.1 at 37°C, then

$$pH = 6.1 + \log\frac{24 \text{ mM}}{(0.03 \text{ mM/mm Hg}) \times 40 \text{ mm Hg}} = 7.40 \qquad (28\text{-}17)$$

Thus, the Henderson-Hasselbalch equation correctly predicts the normal pH of arterial blood.

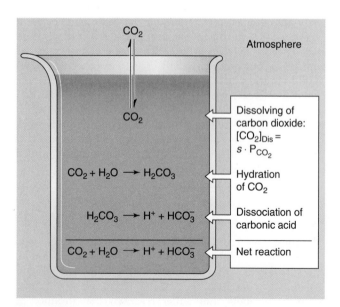

Figure 28-1 Interaction of CO_2 with water.

CO₂/HCO₃⁻ has a far higher buffering power in an open than in a closed system

The buffering power of a buffer pair such as CO_2/HCO_3^- depends on three factors:

1. **Total concentration of the buffer pair, [TB].** Other things being equal, β is proportional to [TB].
2. **The pH of the solution.** The precise dependence on pH will become clear later.
3. **Whether the system is open or closed.** That is, can one member of the buffer pair equilibrate between the "system" (the solution in which the buffer is dissolved) and the "environment" (everything else)?

If neither member of the buffer pair can enter or leave the system, then $HB^{(n+1)}$ can become $B^{(n)}$, and vice versa, but [TB] is fixed. This is a **closed system**. An example of a closed-system buffer is inorganic phosphate in a beaker of water or a titratable group on a protein in blood plasma. In a closed system, the buffering power of a buffer pair is

$$\beta_{closed} = 2.3[TB]\frac{[H^+]\cdot K}{([H^+ + K])^2} \quad (28\text{-}18)$$

Two aspects of Equation 28-18 are of interest. First, at a given $[H^+]$, β_{closed} is proportional to [TB]. Second, at a given [TB], β_{closed} has a bell-shaped dependence on pH (green curve in Fig. 28-2A). β_{closed} is maximal when $[H^+] = K$ (i.e., when pH = pK). Most non-HCO_3^- buffers in biological fluids behave as if they are in a closed system. Although many fluids are actually *mixtures* of several non-HCO_3^- buffers, the total $\beta_{non\text{-}HCO_3^-}$ in such a mixture is the sum of their β_{closed} values, each described by Equation 28-18. The red curve in Figure 28-2B shows how total $\beta_{non\text{-}HCO_3^-}$ varies with pH for a solution containing a mixture of nine buffers (including the one described by the green curve), each present at a [TB] of 12.6 mM, with pK values evenly spaced at intervals of 0.5 pH unit. In this example, total $\beta_{non\text{-}HCO_3^-}$ is remarkably stable over a broad pH range and has a peak value that is the same as that of whole blood: 25 mM/pH unit. Indeed, whole blood

is a complex mixture of many non-HCO_3^- buffers. The most important of these are titratable groups on hemoglobin and, to a far lesser extent, other proteins. Even less important than the "other proteins" are small molecules such as inorganic phosphate. The [TB] values for these many buffers are not identical, and the pK values are not evenly spaced. Nevertheless, the buffering power of whole blood is nearly constant near the physiological pH.

The second physiologically important condition under which a buffer can function is in an **open system**. Here, one buffer species (e.g., CO_2) equilibrates between the system and the environment. A laboratory example is a solution containing CO_2 and HCO_3^-, in which dissolved CO_2 equilibrates with gaseous CO_2 in the atmosphere (Fig. 28-1). A physiological example is blood plasma, in which dissolved CO_2 equilibrates with gaseous CO_2 in the alveoli. In either case, $[CO_2]_{Dis}$ is fixed during buffering reactions. However, the **total CO_2**—$[CO_2] + [HCO_3^-]$—can vary widely. Because total CO_2 can rise to very high values, CO_2/HCO_3^- in an open system can be an extremely powerful buffer. Consider, for example, a liter of a solution having a pH of 7.4, a P_{CO_2} of 40 mm Hg (1.2 mM CO_2), and 24 mM $[HCO_3^-]$—*but no other buffers* (Fig. 28-3, stage 1). What happens when we add 10 mmol of HCl? Available $[HCO_3^-]$ neutralizes almost all of the added H^+, forming nearly 10 mmol H_2CO_3 and then nearly 10 mmol CO_2 plus nearly 10 mmol H_2O (Fig. 28-3, stage 2A). The CO_2 that forms does not accumulate but evolves to the atmosphere so that $[CO_2]_{Dis}$ is constant. What is the final pH? If $[CO_2]_{Dis}$ remains at 1.2 mM in our open system, and if $[HCO_3^-]$ decreases by almost exactly 10 mM (i.e., the amount of added H^+) from 24 to 14 mM, the Henderson-Hasselbalch equation predicts a fall in pH from 7.40 to 7.17, corresponding to an increase in free $[H^+]$ of

$$\Delta[H^+] = (10^{-7.17} - 10^{-7.40})\,M$$
$$= 0.000,068\,mM - 0.000,040\,mM \quad (28\text{-}19)$$
$$= 0.000,028\,mM$$

Even though we have added 10 *milli*moles HCl to 1 L, $[H^+]$ increased by only 28 *nano*molar (Fig. 28-3, stage 3A). Therefore, the open-system buffer has neutralized

A   SINGLE BUFFER

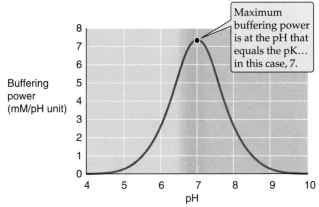

Maximum buffering power is at the pH that equals the pK... in this case, 7.

Buffering power (mM/pH unit)

B   MULTIPLE BUFFERS

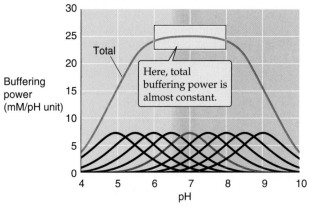

Total

Here, total buffering power is almost constant.

Buffering power (mM/pH unit)

Figure 28-2   Buffering power in a closed system. In **B,** the solution contains nine buffers, each at a concentration of 12.6 mM and with pK values evenly spaced 0.5 pH unit apart.

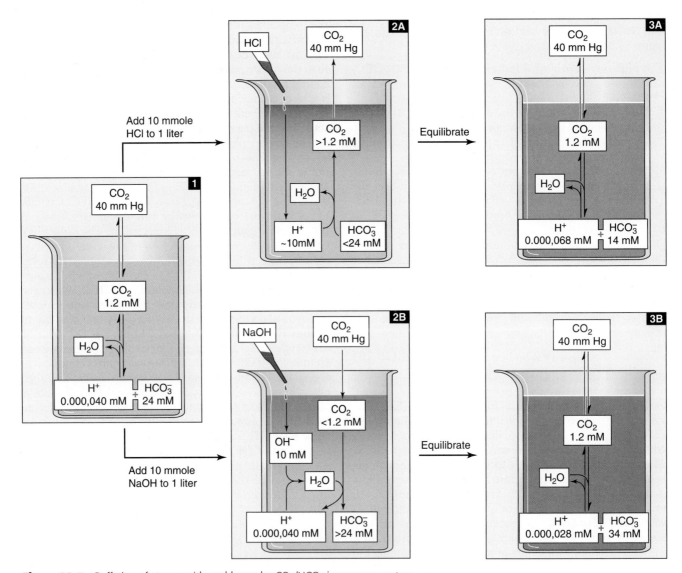

Figure 28-3 Buffering of strong acids and bases by CO_2/HCO_3^- in an open system.

9.999,972 mmol of the added 10 mmol H^+. The buffering provided by CO_2/HCO_3^- in an open system (β_{open}) is so powerful because only depletion of HCO_3^- limits neutralization of H^+. The buildup of CO_2 is not a limiting factor because the atmosphere is an infinite sink for newly produced CO_2.

The opposite acid-base disturbance occurs when we add a strong base such as NaOH. Here, the buffering reactions are just the reverse of those in the preceding example. If we add 10 mmol of NaOH to 1 L of solution, almost all added OH^- combines with H^+ derived from CO_2 that enters from the atmosphere (Fig. 28-3, stage 2B). One HCO_3^- ion forms for each OH^- neutralized. Buffering power in this *open system* is far higher than that in a closed system because CO_2 availability does not limit neutralization of added OH^-. Only the buildup of HCO_3^- limits neutralization of more OH^-. In this example, even though we added 10 mmol NaOH, free $[H^+]$ decreased by only 12 nM (Fig. 28-3, stage 3B) as pH rose from 7.40 to 7.55.

Whether CO_2/HCO_3^- neutralizes an acid or a base, the open-system buffering power is

$$\beta_{open} = 2.3 \cdot [HCO_3^-] \qquad (28\text{-}20)$$

Notice that β_{open} does not have a maximum. Because β_{open} is proportional to $[HCO_3^-]$, β_{open} rises exponentially with pH when P_{CO_2} is fixed (Fig. 28-4, blue curve). In normal arterial blood (i.e., $[HCO_3^-]$ = 24 mM), β_{open} is ~55 mM/pH unit. As we have already noted, the buffering power of all non-HCO_3^- buffers ($\beta_{non\text{-}HCO_3^-}$) in whole blood is ~25 mM/pH unit. Thus, in whole blood, β_{open} represents more than two thirds of the total buffering power. The relative contribution of β_{open} is far more striking in interstitial fluid, which lacks the cellular elements of blood and also has a lower protein concentration.

CO_2/HCO_3^- does not *necessarily* behave as an open-system buffer. In the preceding example, we could have added NaOH to a CO_2/HCO_3^- solution in a capped syringe. In such a closed system, not only does accumulation of HCO_3^- limit neutralization of OH^-, but the availability of CO_2 is limiting as well. Indeed, for fluid having the composition of normal

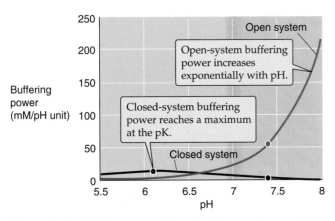

Figure 28-4 Buffering power of the CO_2/HCO_3^- system. At pH 7.4 on the *blue curve*, the solution has the same composition as does arterial blood plasma: a P_{CO_2} of 40 mm Hg and an $[HCO_3^-]$ of 24 mM. If the system is open (i.e., CO_2 equilibrates with atmosphere), β_{open} is ~55 mM/pH unit at pH 7.40 and rises exponentially with pH (see Equation 28-20). If the system is closed, β_{closed} is only ~2.6 mM/pH unit at pH 7.4 and is maximal at the pK of the buffer (see Equation 28-18).

arterial blood, the *closed-system* CO_2/HCO_3^- buffering power is only 2.6 mM/pH unit (Fig. 28-4, black curve), less than 5% of the β_{open} value of 55 mM/pH unit. You might think that the only reason the closed-system buffering power is so low in this example is that the pH of 7.4 is 1.3 pH units above the pK. However, even if pH were equal to the pK of 6.1, the closed-system CO_2/HCO_3^- buffering power in our example would be only ~14 mM/pH unit, about one quarter of the open-system value at pH 7.4. A physiological example in which the CO_2/HCO_3^- system is "poorly open" is **ischemia**, wherein a lack of blood flow minimizes the equilibration of tissue CO_2 with blood CO_2. Thus, ischemic tissues are especially susceptible to large pH shifts.

ACID-BASE CHEMISTRY WHEN CO_2/HCO_3^- IS THE ONLY BUFFER

In this section, we consider buffering by CO_2 and HCO_3^- when these are the *only* buffers present in the solution. We defer to the following section the more complex example, in which *both* CO_2/HCO_3^- and non-HCO_3^- buffers are present in the same solution.

In the absence of other buffers, doubling of P_{CO_2} causes pH to fall by 0.3 but causes almost no change in $[HCO_3^-]$

Figure 28-5 represents 1 L of a solution with the same CO_2/HCO_3^- composition as arterial blood plasma but no buffers other than CO_2/HCO_3^-. What are the consequences of increasing P_{CO_2} in the gas phase? The resulting increase in $[CO_2]_{Dis}$ causes the CO_2/HCO_3^- equilibrium to shift toward formation of H^+ and HCO_3^-. This disturbance is an example of a **CO_2 titration** because we initiated it by altering P_{CO_2}. More specifically, it is a **respiratory acidosis**—"acidosis" because pH falls, and "respiratory" because pulmonary problems (Table

28-3) are the most common causes of an increase in the P_{CO_2} of arterial blood (see Chapter 31).

In the absence of non-HCO_3^- buffers, how far pH falls during respiratory acidosis depends on the initial pH and P_{CO_2} as well as on the final P_{CO_2}. For example, doubling of P_{CO_2} from 40 mm Hg (Fig. 28-5, stage 1) to 80 mm Hg causes $[CO_2]_{Dis}$ to double to 2.4 mM (Fig. 28-5, stage 2A). At this point, the 1-L system is far *out* of equilibrium and can return to equilibrium only if some CO_2 (x mmol) combines with x H_2O to form x H^+ and x HCO_3^-. Thus, according to Equation 28-14, the following must be true at equilibrium:

$$\underbrace{\begin{matrix}10^{-6.1}\,\text{M}\\ \text{or}\\ 10^{-3.1}\,\text{mM}\end{matrix}}_{K} = \frac{\overbrace{(0.000,040\,\text{mM}+x)}^{[H^+]}\overbrace{(24\,\text{mM}+x)}^{[HCO_3^-]}}{\underbrace{2.4\,\text{mM}}_{[CO_2]}} \quad (28\text{-}21)$$

Solving this equation for x yields an extremely small value, nearly 40 nmol, or 0.000,040 mmol. x represents the **flux** of CO_2 that passes through the reaction sequence $CO_2 + H_2O \rightarrow H_2CO_3 \rightarrow H^+ + HCO_3^-$ to re-establish the equilibrium. CO_2 from the atmosphere replenishes the CO_2 consumed in this reaction, so that $[CO_2]_{Dis}$ remains at 2.4 mM after the new equilibrium is achieved (Fig. 28-5, stage 3A). The reason that the flux x is so small is that with no other buffers present, every H^+ formed remains free in solution. Thus, only a minuscule amount of H^+ needs to be formed before $[H^+]$ nearly doubles from 40 to ~80 nM. However, $[HCO_3^-]$ undergoes only a tiny fractional increase, from 24 to 24.000,040 mM. The doubling of the denominator in Equation 28-21 is matched by a doubling of the numerator, nearly all of which is due to the near-doubling of $[H^+]$. The final pH in this example of respiratory acidosis is

$$pH = -\log(80\,\text{nM}) = 7.10 \quad (28\text{-}22)$$

Another way of arriving at the same answer is to insert the final values for $[HCO_3^-]$ and P_{CO_2} into the Henderson-Hasselbalch equation:

$$pH = 6.1 + \log\frac{24.000,040\,\text{mM}}{(0.03\,\text{nM/mm Hg})\cdot(80\,\text{mm Hg})} = 7.10 \quad (28\text{-}23)$$

The opposite acid-base disturbance, in which P_{CO_2} falls, is **respiratory alkalosis**. In a solution containing no buffers other than CO_2/HCO_3^- reducing P_{CO_2} by half, from 40 to 20 mm Hg, would cause all of the aforementioned reactions to shift in the opposite direction, so that pH would rise by 0.3, from 7.4 to 7.7. We could produce respiratory alkalosis in a beaker by lowering the P_{CO_2} in the gas phase. In humans, hyperventilation (Table 28-3) lowers alveolar and thus arterial P_{CO_2} (see Chapter 31).

Thus, in the absence of non-HCO_3^- buffers, doubling of $[CO_2]$ causes pH to fall by 0.3, whereas halving of $[CO_2]$ causes pH to rise by 0.3 (Table 28-1). Remember, the log of 2 is 0.3.

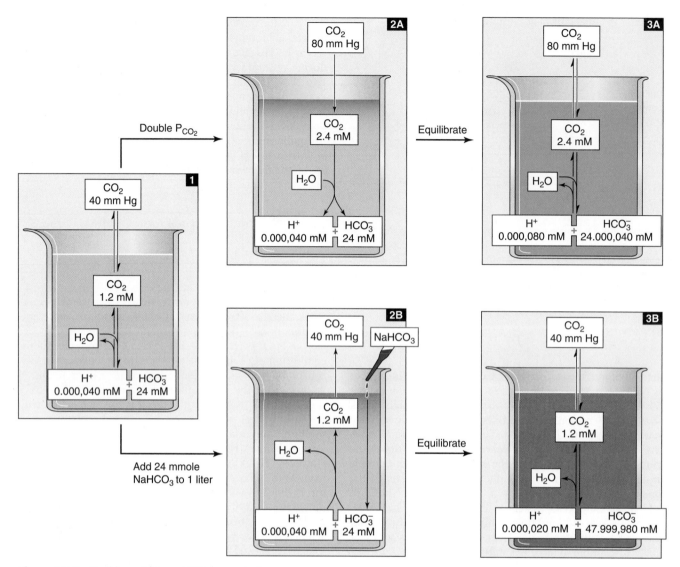

Figure 28-5 Doubling of CO_2 or HCO_3^- concentrations.

In the absence of other buffers, doubling of [HCO_3^-] causes pH to rise by 0.3

What would happen if we doubled [HCO_3^-] rather than P_{CO_2}? Starting with 1 L of solution that has the ionic composition of arterial blood (Fig. 28-5, stage 1), adding 24 mmol of HCO_3^- (e.g., $NaHCO_3$) drives the CO_2/HCO_3^- equilibrium toward CO_2 (Fig. 28-5, stage 2B). The new equilibrium is achieved when x mmol of HCO_3^- combines with x H^+ to produce x CO_2 and x H_2O. Because the system is *open to CO_2*, the generation of x mmol CO_2 causes no change in [CO_2]$_{Dis}$; the newly formed CO_2 simply evolves into the atmosphere. Thus, according to Equation 28-14, the following must be true at equilibrium:

$$\underbrace{\substack{10^{-6.1}\,M \\ \text{or} \\ 10^{-3.1}\,\text{mM}}}_{K} = \frac{\overbrace{(0.000,040\,\text{mM} - x)}^{[H^+]}\overbrace{(48\,\text{mM} - x)}^{[HCO_3^-]}}{\underbrace{1.2\,\text{mM}}_{\text{fixed}\,[CO_2]}} \quad \text{(28-24)}$$

Solving this equation yields an x of nearly 0.000,020 mM. Thus, in the absence of other buffers, an initial doubling of [HCO_3^-] from 24 to 48 mM causes [H^+] to fall by nearly half, from 40 to 20 nM. Although [HCO_3^-] also decreases by 20 nM, its fractional change from 48 to 47.999,980 mM is insignificant. The final pH is

$$pH = -\log(20\,nM) = 7.70 \quad \text{(28-25)}$$

The Henderson-Hasselbalch equation yields the same result:

$$pH = 6.1 + \log \frac{47.999,980\,\text{mM}}{(0.03\,\text{mM/mm Hg}) \cdot (40\,\text{mm Hg})} = 7.70 \quad \text{(28-26)}$$

Thus, in the absence of non-HCO_3^- buffers, doubling of [HCO_3^-] causes pH to increase by ~0.3. Rather than adding HCO_3^-, we could produce an identical effect by adding the same amount of strong base (e.g., NaOH), as we did in

Table 28-3 The Four Major Acid-Base Disorders

Disorder	Proximate Causes	Clinical Causes	Changes in Arterial Acid-Base Parameters
Respiratory acidosis	Increased P_{CO_2}	Decreased alveolar ventilation (e.g., drug overdose) ↓ Lung diffusing capacity (e.g., pulmonary edema) Ventilation-perfusion mismatch	pH ↓ [HCO_3^-] ↑ P_{CO_2} ↑
Respiratory alkalosis	Decreased P_{CO_2}	Increased alveolar ventilation caused by: Hypoxia (e.g., acclimatization to high altitude) Anxiety Aspirin intoxication	pH ↑ [HCO_3^-] ↓ P_{CO_2} ↓
Metabolic acidosis	Addition of acids other than CO_2 or H_2CO_3 Removal of alkali (fixed P_{CO_2})	↓Urinary secretion of H^+ (e.g., renal failure) Ketoacidosis (e.g., diabetes mellitus) Lactic acidosis (e.g., shock) HCO_3^- loss (e.g., severe diarrhea)	pH ↓ [HCO_3^-] ↓ P_{CO_2}: no change
Metabolic alkalosis	Addition of alkali Removal of acids other than CO_2 or H_2CO_3 (fixed P_{CO_2})	HCO_3^- load (e.g., $NaHCO_3$ therapy) Loss of H^+ (e.g., severe vomiting)	pH ↑ [HCO_3^-] ↑ P_{CO_2}: no change

Figure 28-3 (stages 2B and 3B), or by *removing* the same amount of strong acid (e.g., HCl). Although the removal of HCl from a solution in a beaker may seem artificial, the removal of gastric HCl from the body occurs during vomiting (Table 28-3). We also could add a *weak* base (e.g., NH_3) or remove any *weak* acid (e.g., lactic acid) other than CO_2 or H_2CO_3. However, to produce the same alkali load, we would have to add or remove more of a *weak* base or acid than for a *strong* base or acid. All of these maneuvers, carried out at a fixed P_{CO_2}, are examples of **metabolic alkalosis**—"alkalosis" because the pH increases, and "metabolic" because derangements in metabolism are common clinical causes.

The opposite acid-base disturbance—in which we remove HCO_3^- or another alkali or add an acid other than CO_2 or H_2CO_3—is **metabolic acidosis**. Starting with a solution having the ionic composition of arterial blood, removing half of the initial HCO_3^- or removing 12 mM NaOH or adding 12 mM HCl would cause all of the aforementioned reactions to shift in the opposite direction, so that pH would fall by 0.3, from 7.4 to 7.1. Common causes of metabolic acidosis in humans are renal failure and metabolic problems (Table 28-3).

We saw in Equation 28-26 that the pH of a CO_2/HCO_3^- solution does not depend on [HCO_3^-] or P_{CO_2} but on their ratio. Because it is the kidney that controls [HCO_3^-] in the blood plasma (see Chapter 39), and because it is the lung that controls P_{CO_2} (see Chapter 31), the pH of blood plasma is under the dual control of both organ systems, a concept embodied by a whimsical variant of the Henderson-Hasselbalch equation:

$$pH = Constant + \frac{Kidney}{Lungs} \qquad (28\text{-}27)$$

ACID-BASE CHEMISTRY IN THE PRESENCE OF CO_2/HCO_3^- AND NON-HCO_3^- BUFFERS—THE DAVENPORT DIAGRAM

So far, our discussion has focused on simple systems in which the only pH buffers are either (1) one or more non-HCO_3^- buffers or (2) CO_2/HCO_3^-. Under these circumstances, it is relatively easy to predict the effects of acid-base disturbances. Real biological systems, however, are mixtures of CO_2/HCO_3^- and many non-HCO_3^- buffers. Thus, to understand the effects of respiratory and metabolic acid-base disturbances in a biological system, we must consider multiple competing equilibria—one for CO_2/HCO_3^- (described by Equation 28-16) and one for each of the non-HCO_3^- buffers (each described by its version of Equation 28-5). Obtaining a precise solution to such clinically relevant problems is impossible. One approach is to use a computer to make increasingly more precise approximations of the correct answer. Another, more intuitive approach is to use a graphical method to estimate the final pH. The Davenport diagram is the best such tool.

The Davenport diagram is a graphical tool for interpretation of acid-base disturbances in blood

What happens to the pH of blood—a complex mixture that includes many non-HCO_3^- buffers—when P_{CO_2} doubles? We simplify matters by lumping together the actions of all non-HCO_3^- buffers, so that $H^+ + B^{(n)} \rightleftarrows HB^{(n+1)}$ represents the reactions of *all* non-HCO_3^- buffers. When we raise P_{CO_2}, almost all of the newly formed H^+ reacts with $B^{(n)}$ to form $HB^{(n+1)}$ so that the free [H^+] rises only slightly.

$$CO_2 + H_2O \rightarrow HCO_3^- + H^+$$

Non-HCO$_3^-$ buffers consume almost all the H$^+$ produced by CO$_2$.

$$B^{(n)}$$
$$HB^{(n+1)}$$

$$(28\text{-}28)$$

In this simplified approach, the final pH depends on two competing buffer reactions—one involving CO_2/HCO_3^-, and the other involving $HB^{(n+1)}/B^{(n)}$. Computation of the final pH requires solving of two simultaneous equations, one for each buffer reaction.

The CO$_2$/HCO$_3^-$ Buffer The first of the two equations that we must solve simultaneously is a rearrangement of the Henderson-Hasselbalch equation (Equation 28-16):

$$[HCO_3^-] = s \cdot P_{CO_2} \cdot 10^{(pH - pK_{CO_2})} \qquad (28\text{-}29)$$

For a P_{CO_2} of 40 mm Hg, the equation requires that $[HCO_3^-]$ be 24 mM when pH is 7.40—as in normal arterial blood plasma. If pH decreases by 0.3 at this same P_{CO_2}, Equation 28-29 states that $[HCO_3^-]$ must fall by half to 12 mM. Conversely, if pH increases by 0.3, $[HCO_3^-]$ must double to 48 mM. The blue column of Table 28-4 lists the $[HCO_3^-]$ values that Equation 28-29 predicts for various pH values when P_{CO_2} is 40 mm Hg. Plotting these $[HCO_3^-]$ values against pH yields the blue curve labeled P_{CO_2} = 40 mm Hg in Figure 28-6A. This curve, which is known as a CO$_2$ isobar or **isopleth** (from the Greek *isos* [equal] + *plethein* [to be full]), represents all possible combinations of $[HCO_3^-]$ and pH at a P_{CO_2} of 40 mm Hg. Table 28-4 also summarizes $[HCO_3^-]$ values prevailing at P_{CO_2} values of 20 mm Hg and 80 mm Hg. Note that at a P_{CO_2} of 20 mm Hg (orange column), representing respiratory alkalosis, $[HCO_3^-]$ values are half those for a P_{CO_2} of 40 mm Hg at the same pH. At a P_{CO_2} of 80 mm Hg (green column), representing respiratory acidosis, $[HCO_3^-]$ values are twice those at a P_{CO_2} of 40 mm Hg. Each of the isopleths in Figure 28-6A rises exponentially with pH. The slope of each isopleth also rises exponentially with pH and

Table 28-4 Relationship Between [HCO$_3^-$] and pH at Three Fixed Levels of PCO$_2$

pH	[HCO$_3^-$] (mM)		
	P$_{CO_2}$ = 20 mm Hg	P$_{CO_2}$ = 40 mm Hg	P$_{CO_2}$ = 80 mm Hg
7.1	6 mM	12 mM	24 mM
7.2	8	15	30
7.3	10	19	38
7.4	12	**24**	48
7.5	15	30	60
7.6	19	38	76
7.7	24	48	96

represents β_{open} for CO_2/HCO_3^-. At a particular pH, an isopleth representing a higher P_{CO_2} (i.e., a higher $[HCO_3^-]$) has a steeper slope, as Equation 28-20 predicts.

Non-HCO$_3^-$ Buffers The second of the two equations that we must solve simultaneously describes the lumped reaction of all non-HCO$_3^-$ buffers. To understand the origin of this equation, we begin with the green curve in Figure 28-6B, the **titration curve** of a single non-HCO$_3^-$ buffer with a pK of 7 and total buffer concentration of 12.6 mM (as for the green curve in Fig. 28-2B). At a pH of 10, $[HB^{(n+1)}]$ for this single buffer is extremely low because almost all of the "B" is in the form $B^{(n)}$. As we lower pH by successively adding small amounts of HCl, $[HB^{(n+1)}]$ gradually rises—most steeply when pH equals pK. Indeed, at any pH, the slope of this curve is the negative of β for this single buffer. The black curves in Figure 28-6B are the titration curves for eight other buffers, each present at a [TB] of 12.6 mM, with pK values evenly spaced at intervals of 0.5 pH unit on either side of 7. The red curve in Figure 28-6B is the sum of the titration curves for all nine buffers. Its slope—the negative of the total buffering power of all nine buffers—is remarkably constant over a broad pH range. (The red curve in Figure 28-2B shows how β, the slope of the red curve here in Figure 28-6B, varies with pH.) The red curve in Figure 28-6B represents the second of the two equations that we must solve simultaneously.

Solving the Problem Figure 28-6C is a Davenport diagram, a combination of the three CO$_2$ isopleths in Figure 28-6A and the linear part of the red non-HCO$_3^-$ titration curve in Figure 28-6B. The red non-HCO$_3^-$ titration line (representing $\beta_{non-HCO_3^-}$ for whole blood, 25 mM/pH unit) intersects with the CO$_2$ isopleth for a P_{CO_2} of 40 mm Hg at the point labeled Start, which represents the initial conditions for arterial blood. At this intersection, both CO_2/HCO_3^- and non-HCO$_3^-$ buffers are simultaneously in equilibrium.

We are now in a position to answer the question raised at the beginning of this section: What will be the final pH when we increase the P_{CO_2} of whole blood from 40 to 80 mm Hg? The final equilibrium conditions for this case of *respiratory acidosis* must be described by a point that lies simultaneously on the red non-HCO$_3^-$ titration line and the green isopleth for 80 mm Hg. Obtaining the answer by use of the Davenport diagram requires a three-step process:

Step 1: Identify the point at the intersection of the initial P_{CO_2} isopleth and the initial non-HCO$_3^-$ titration line (Fig. 28-6C, Start).

Step 2: Identify the isopleth describing the *final* P_{CO_2} (80 mm Hg in this case).

Step 3: Follow the non-HCO$_3^-$ titration line to its intersection with the final P_{CO_2} isopleth. In Figure 28-6C, this intersection occurs at point A, which corresponds to a pH of 7.19 and an $[HCO_3^-]$ of 29.25 mM.

As discussed earlier, in the *absence* of non-HCO$_3^-$ buffers, this same doubling of P_{CO_2} causes a larger pH decrease, from 7.4 to 7.1.

By following three similar steps, we can use the Davenport diagram to predict the final pH and $[HCO_3^-]$ under condi-

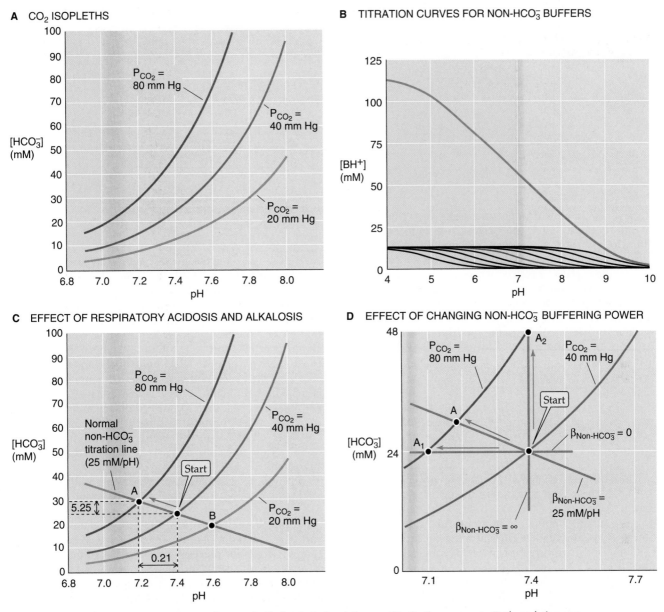

A CO$_2$ ISOPLETHS

B TITRATION CURVES FOR NON-HCO$_3^-$ BUFFERS

C EFFECT OF RESPIRATORY ACIDOSIS AND ALKALOSIS

D EFFECT OF CHANGING NON-HCO$_3^-$ BUFFERING POWER

Figure 28-6 Davenport diagram. In **A,** the three *isopleths* are CO$_2$ titration curves. In **B,** the solution contains nine buffers, each at a concentration of 12.6 mM and with pK values evenly spaced 0.5 pH unit apart, as in Figure 28-2B. In **C,** the *red arrow* represents the transition from a normal acid-base status (Start) for blood to respiratory acidosis (point A) produced by raising P$_{CO_2}$ to 80 mm Hg. Point B represents respiratory alkalosis produced by lowering P$_{CO_2}$ to 20 mm Hg. In **D,** the labeled points represent the results of respiratory acidosis when the non-HCO$_3^-$ buffering power β$_{non-HCO_3^-}$ is zero (point A$_1$), 25 mM/pH (point A), and infinity (point A$_2$).

tions of a *respiratory alkalosis*. For example, what would be the effect of decreasing P$_{CO_2}$ by half, from 40 to 20 mm Hg? Follow the red non-HCO$_3^-$ titration line from Start to its intersection with the orange isopleth for a P$_{CO_2}$ of 20 mm Hg (point B), which corresponds to a pH of 7.60 and an [HCO$_3^-$] of 19 mM. If the solution had *not* contained non-HCO$_3^-$ buffers, halving of the P$_{CO_2}$ would have caused a larger pH increase, from 7.4 to 7.7.

The amount of HCO$_3^-$ formed or consumed during respiratory acid-base disturbances increases with the non-HCO$_3^-$ buffering power

Although it is reasonable to focus on CO$_2$ during respiratory acid-base disturbances, it would be wrong to assume that [HCO$_3^-$] is constant. For example, in Figure 28-6C, where

Table 28-5 Relationship Between HCO_3^- Buffering Power and the Amount of HCO_3^- Formed in Response to a Doubling of P_{CO_2}

Non-HCO_3^- Buffering Power	ΔpH	HCO_3^- Formed (mM)	Fractional $\Delta[H^+]$	Fractional $\Delta[HCO_3^-]$	Fractional $\Delta[HCO_3^-] \times \Delta[H^+]$
0	−0.30	0.000,040	1.999,997	1.000,002	2.00
25	−0.21	5.25	1.71	1.17	2.00
∞	0	24.0	1.00	2.00	2.00

$\beta_{non-HCO_3^-}$ is 25 mM/pH unit, increasing P_{CO_2} from 40 to 80 mm Hg causes $[HCO_3^-]$ to increase from 24 to 29.25 mM. Thus, in each liter of solution, 5.25 mmol CO_2 combines with 5.25 mmol H_2O to form 5.25 mmol HCO_3^- (which we see as the $\Delta[HCO_3^-]$ value between Start and A) and 5.25 mmol H^+. Nearly all of this H^+ disappears as nearly 5.25 mmol of the deprotonated non-HCO_3^- buffers ($B^{(n)}$) consumes H^+ to form nearly 5.25 mmol of their conjugate weak acids ($HB^{(n+1)}$). Thus, the flux through the reaction sequence in Equation 28-28 is nearly 5.25 mmol for each liter of solution.

$$CO_2 + H_2O \xrightarrow{5.25mM} HCO_3^- + H^+$$
$$\sim 5.25mM \left. \right| \begin{matrix} B^{(n)} \\ \\ HB^{(n+1)} \end{matrix} \quad (28\text{-}30)$$

Thus, the non-HCO_3^- buffers drive the conversion of CO_2 to HCO_3^-. These buffers minimize the increase in free $[H^+]$ that a given flux of CO_2 can produce. Thus, with a high $\beta_{non-HCO_3^-}$, a large amount of CO_2 must "flux" through Equation 28-30 before the free concentrations of HCO_3^- and H^+ rise sufficiently to satisfy the CO_2/HCO_3^- equilibrium (Equation 28-14).

$\beta_{non-HCO_3^-}$ varies with the hemoglobin content of blood. Thus, patients with anemia have a low $\beta_{non-HCO_3^-}$, whereas patients with polycythemia have a high $\beta_{non-HCO_3^-}$.

Figure 28-6D illustrates the importance of $\beta_{non-HCO_3^-}$. If $\beta_{non-HCO_3^-}$ is zero, the non-HCO_3^- titration line is horizontal, and doubling of P_{CO_2} from 40 to 80 mm Hg does not change $[HCO_3^-]$ significantly (Fig. 28-6D, point A_1), verifying our earlier conclusion (Fig. 28-5, stage 3A). Simultaneously, pH falls by 0.3, which corresponds to a near-doubling of $[H^+]$. Thus, doubling of $[CO_2]$ leads to a doubling of the product $[HCO_3^-][H^+]$, so that the ratio $[HCO_3^-][H^+]/[CO_2]$—the equilibrium constant, K—is unchanged (Table 28-5, top row). Figure 28-6D also shows what happens if $\beta_{non-HCO_3^-}$ has the normal value of 25 mM/pH unit. Here, point A is the same as point A in Figure 28-6C, and it shows that $[HCO_3^-]$ increases by 5.25 mM, or 17% (Table 28-5, middle row). Finally, if $\beta_{non-HCO_3^-}$ were ∞, the non-HCO_3^- titration line would be vertical, and doubling of P_{CO_2} would not change pH at all (point A_2 in Fig. 28-6D). In this case, $[HCO_3^-]$ would double, so that the doubling of the product $[HCO_3^-]\cdot[H^+]$ would match the doubling of P_{CO_2} (Table 28-5, bottom row).

Adding or removing an acid or base—at a constant P_{CO_2}—produces a metabolic acid-base disturbance

Earlier, we examined the effect of adding HCl in the *absence* of other buffers (Fig. 28-3). Predicting the pH change for such an acid-base disturbance was straightforward because the titration of HCO_3^- to CO_2 consumed all buffered H^+. The situation is more complex when the solution also contains non-HCO_3^- buffers (Fig. 28-7, stage 1). When we add 10 mmol of HCl to 1 L of solution, the open-system CO_2/HCO_3^- buffer pair neutralizes most of the added H^+, non-HCO_3^- buffers handle some, and a minute amount of added H^+ remains free and lowers pH (Fig. 28-7, stage 2A). Because the system is open, the CO_2 formed during buffering of the added H^+ escapes to the atmosphere. If this buffering reaction were occurring in the blood, the newly formed CO_2 would escape first into the alveolar air and then into the atmosphere.

How much of the added H^+ ($\Delta[Strong\ acid] = 10$ mM) follows each of the three pathways in this example of *metabolic acidosis*? Answering this question requires dealing with two competing equilibria, the CO_2/HCO_3^- and the non-HCO_3^- buffering reactions. As for respiratory acid-base disturbances, we cannot precisely solve the equations governing metabolic acid-base disturbances. However, we can use the Davenport diagram on the left of Figure 28-7 to obtain a graphical estimate of the final pH and $[HCO_3^-]$ through a four-step process:

Step 1: Identify the point describing the initial conditions (Fig. 28-7, Start, graph on left).

Step 2: Following the arrow labeled #2, move downward (in the direction of decreased $[HCO_3^-]$) by 10 mM—the concentration of added H^+—to the point labeled *. In this maneuver, we assume that the reaction $HCO_3^- + H^+ \rightarrow CO_2 + H_2O$ has initially consumed *all* of the added H^+. Of course, if this were true, the CO_2/HCO_3^- reaction would be far out of equilibrium and the pH would not have changed at all. Also, the non-HCO_3^- buffers would not have had a chance to participate in the buffering of H^+.

Step 3: Through *, draw a line (Fig. 28-7, black line on left) that is parallel to the non-HCO_3^- titration line.

Step 4: Following the arrow labeled #4, move to the intersection of the new black line and the original P_{CO_2} isopleth. In Figure 28-7, left, this intersection occurs at point C, which corresponds to a pH of 7.26 and an $[HCO_3^-]$ of 17.4 mM. This maneuver tracks the reaction

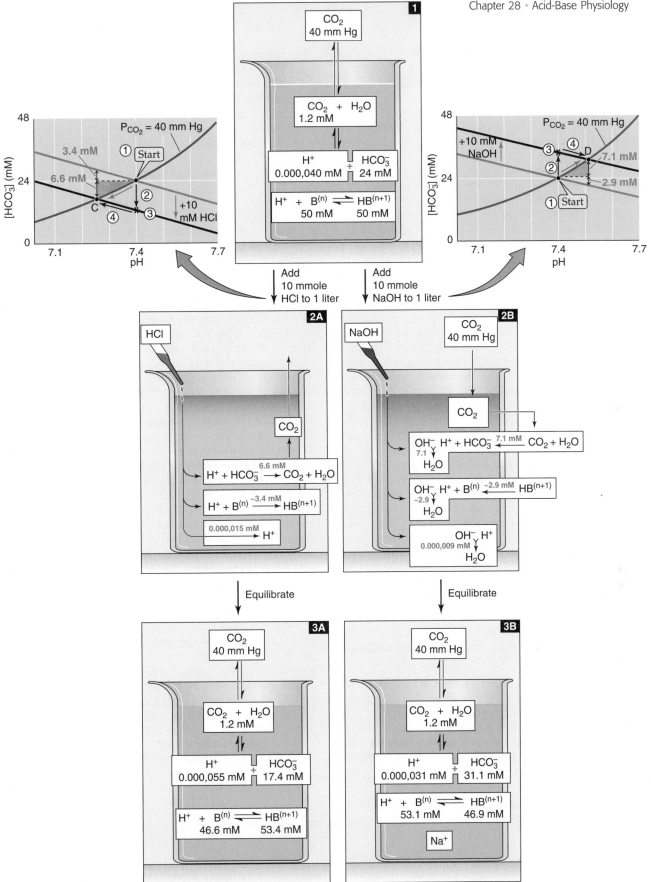

Figure 28-7 Metabolic acidosis and alkalosis in the presence of non-HCO_3^- buffers. The *red arrows* in the Davenport diagrams represent the transition to metabolic acidosis (point C) and metabolic alkalosis (point D). This example differs from Figure 28-3, in which the solution contained no buffers other than CO_2/HCO_3.

$CO_2 + H_2O \rightarrow HCO_3^- + H^+$. Non-$HCO_3^-$ buffers consume nearly all of this H^+ in the reaction $H^+ + B^{(n)} \rightarrow HB^{(n+1)}$. As a result, $[HCO_3^-]$, $[H^+]$, and $[HB^{(n+1)}]$ all rise and the system equilibrates.

As a shortcut, we could bypass the two black arrows and simply follow the red arrow along the CO_2 isopleth from Start to point C.

We now can return to the question of how much of the added H^+ follows each of the three pathways in Figure 28-7, stage 2A. Because $[HCO_3^-]$ decreased by $24 - 17.4 = 6.6$ mM, the amount of H^+ buffered by CO_2/HCO_3^- must have been 6.6 mmol in each liter. Almost all of the remaining H^+ that we added, nearly 3.6 mmol, must have been buffered by non-HCO_3^- buffers. A tiny amount of the added H^+, ~0.000,015 mmol, must have remained unbuffered and was responsible for decreasing pH from 7.40 to 7.26 (Fig. 28-7, stage 3A).

Figure 28-7 also shows what would happen if we added 10 mmol of a strong base such as NaOH to our 1-L solution. The open-system CO_2/HCO_3^- buffer pair neutralizes most of the added OH^-, non-HCO_3^- buffers handle some, and a minute amount of added OH^- remains unbuffered, thus raising pH (Fig. 28-7, stage 2B). The Davenport diagram on the right of Figure 28-7 shows how much of the added OH^- follows each of the three pathways in this example of *metabolic alkalosis*. The approach is similar to the one we used earlier for metabolic acidosis, except that in this case, we generate a new black line that is displaced 10 mM *above* the non-HCO_3^- titration line. We follow the P_{CO_2} isopleth to its intersection with this black line at point D, which corresponds to a final pH of 7.51 and an $[HCO_3^-]$ of 31.1 mM. Thus, $[HCO_3^-]$ rose by $31.1 - 24.0 = 7.1$ mM. This is the amount of added OH^- that CO_2/HCO_3^- buffered. Non-HCO_3^- buffers must have buffered almost all of the remaining OH^- that we added, ~2.9 mmol in each liter. The unbuffered OH^-, which was responsible for the pH increase, must have been in the nanomolar range (Fig. 28-7, stage 3B).

During metabolic disturbances, CO_2/HCO_3^- makes a greater contribution to total buffering when pH and P_{CO_2} are high and when $\beta_{non-HCO_3^-}$ is low

In Figure 28-7, CO_2/HCO_3^- neutralized 7.1 mmol of the 10 mmol of OH^- added to 1 L ($\Delta pH = +0.11$) but only 6.6 mmol of the added 10 mmol H^+ ($\Delta pH = -0.14$). The reason for this difference is that the buffering power of CO_2/HCO_3^- in an open system increases exponentially with pH (Fig. 28-4, blue curve). In the Davenport diagram, this pH

dependence of β_{open} appears as the slope of the CO_2 isopleth, which increases exponentially with pH. *Thus, adding alkali will always cause a smaller pH change than adding an equivalent amount of acid.* In our example of metabolic alkalosis (Fig. 28-7, right), the mean β_{open} is $(7.1 \text{ mM})/(0.11 \text{ pH unit})$ = 65 mM/pH unit in the pH range 7.40 to 7.51 (Table 28-6). On the other hand, in our example of metabolic acidosis (Fig. 28-7, left), the mean β_{open} is $(6.6 \text{ mM})/(0.14 \text{ pH unit})$ = 47 mM/pH unit in the pH range 7.26 to 7.40, substantially less than in the more alkaline range. Because $\beta_{non-HCO_3^-}$ is 25 mM/pH unit over the entire pH range, β_{total} is greater in the alkaline pH range.

We have already seen that β_{open} is proportional to $[HCO_3^-]$ (see Equation 28-20) and that—at a fixed pH—$[HCO_3^-]$ is proportional to P_{CO_2} (see Equation 28-29). Thus, other things being equal, the contribution of β_{open} to total buffering increases with P_{CO_2}. Patients with a high P_{CO_2} due to respiratory failure will therefore have a higher buffering power than normal individuals at the same pH.

Because CO_2/HCO_3^- and non-HCO_3^- buffers compete for added OH^- or H^+, the contribution of CO_2/HCO_3^- to total buffering also depends on $\beta_{non-HCO_3^-}$. Figure 28-8 illustrates the effects of adding 10 mmol NaOH to our standard 1-L CO_2/HCO_3^- solution at $\beta_{non-HCO_3^-}$ values of 0, 25 mM/pH unit, and ∞. We saw in Figure 28-3 (stage 3B) that adding 10 mmol NaOH to a 1-L solution containing CO_2/HCO_3^- but no other buffers causes $[HCO_3^-]$ to increase from 24 to 34 mM and pH to increase from 7.40 to 7.55. To use a Davenport diagram to solve the same problem (Fig. 28-8A), we generate a non-HCO_3^- titration line, with slope of zero (because $\beta_{non-HCO_3^-}$ = 0), through the Start point. We also draw a black line with the same slope but displaced 10 mM higher. Following the blue $P_{CO_2} = 40$ mm Hg isopleth from Start to the point where the isopleth intersects with the black line at point D_1, we see that—as expected—the final pH is 7.55 and the final $[HCO_3^-]$ is 34 mM. Thus, CO_2/HCO_3^- must buffer virtually all 10 mmol of OH^- added to 1 L. Because the total buffering power is simply β_{open}, the pH increase must be rather large, 0.15.

When $\beta_{non-HCO_3^-}$ is 25 mM/pH unit, as in the Davenport diagram on the upper right panel of Figure 28-7 (replotted in Fig. 28-8B), CO_2/HCO_3^- can buffer only 7.1 mmol because the non-HCO_3^- buffers neutralize 2.9 mmol. With the increased total buffering power, the pH increase is only 0.11.

Finally, when $\beta_{non-HCO_3^-}$ is ∞, the black line lies right on top of the vertical non-HCO_3^- titration line (Fig. 28-8C). Thus, neither $[HCO_3^-]$ nor pH changes at all. However, $[HB^{(n+1)}]$ increases by 10 mM because the infinitely powerful non-HCO_3^- buffers do all of the buffering.

Table 28-6 Buffering Produced by CO_2/HCO_3^- and Non-HCO_3^- Buffers*

Addition	ΔpH	$\Delta[HCO_3^-]$	$\beta_{open} = \dfrac{\Delta[HCO_3^-]}{\Delta pH}$	$\Delta[B^{(n)}]$	$\beta_{non-HCO_3^-} = \dfrac{\Delta[B^{(n)}]}{\Delta pH}$	β_{total}
+10 mmol H^+	~ −0.14	~6.6 mM	47 mM/pH unit	~3.4 mM	25 mM/pH unit	72 mM/pH
+10 mmol OH^-	~ +0.11	~7.1 mM	65 mM/pH unit	~2.9 mM	25 mM/pH unit	89 mM/pH

*The "additions" are made to 1 L of solution. Initial pH = 7.40, P_{CO_2} = 40 mm Hg, $[HCO_3^-]$ = 24 mM. $\beta_{non-HCO_3^-}$ is assumed to be 25 mM/pH unit.

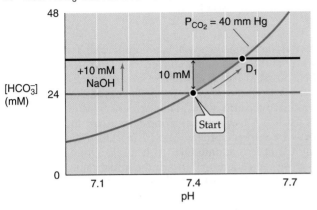

A NON-HCO$_3^-$ BUFFERING POWER OF ZERO

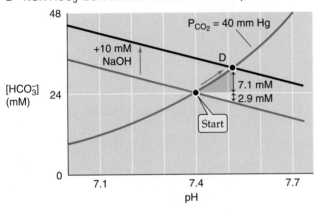

B NON-HCO$_3^-$ BUFFERING POWER OF 25 mM/pH UNIT

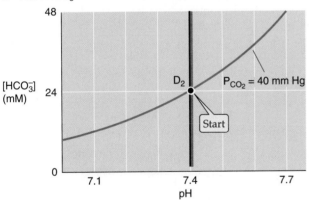

C NON-HCO$_3^-$ BUFFERING POWER OF INFINITY

Figure 28-8 The effect of non-HCO$_3^-$ buffering power on the pH increase caused by metabolic alkalosis.

A metabolic change can compensate for a respiratory disturbance

Thus far, we have considered what happens during *primary* respiratory and metabolic acid-base disturbances. When it is

challenged by such acid or alkaline loads in the blood plasma, the body **compensates** by altering [HCO$_3^-$] or P$_{CO_2}$, returning pH toward its initial value and minimizing the magnitude of the overall pH change.

In Figure 28-9A we revisit an example, originally introduced in Figure 28-6C, in which we produced a primary respiratory acidosis by increasing P$_{CO_2}$ from 40 to 80 mm Hg (red arrow in Figure 28-9A between Start and point A at pH 7.19). If the high P$_{CO_2}$ persists, the only way we can restore pH toward its initial value of 7.40 is to add an alkali (e.g., HCO$_3^-$ or OH$^-$) or to remove an acid (e.g., H$^+$), which are equivalent. Adding 10 mmol of OH$^-$ to 1 L, for example, superimposes a metabolic *alkalosis* on the primary respiratory *acidosis*—a **metabolic compensation to respiratory acidosis.**

The Davenport diagram predicts the consequences of adding 10 mmol of OH$^-$ to 1 L. We start by generating a black line that is parallel to the red non-HCO$_3^-$ titration line but displaced upward by 10 mM. Point A$_1$, the intersection of the black line and the P$_{CO_2}$ isopleth for 80 mm Hg, represents a final pH of 7.29, still lower than the normal 7.40 but much higher than the 7.19 prevailing before compensation.

If we add an additional 14 mmol OH$^-$, for a total addition of 24 mmol OH$^-$ to 1 L, pH returns to exactly its initial value of 7.40 (point A$_2$ in Fig. 28-9A). In other words, we can perfectly compensate for doubling of P$_{CO_2}$ from 40 mm Hg (Start) to 80 mm Hg (point A) by adding an amount of OH$^-$ equivalent to the amount of HCO$_3^-$ that was present (i.e., 24 mM) at Start. *Perfect* compensation of respiratory acidosis is an example of **isohydric hypercapnia** (i.e., the *same* pH at a *higher* P$_{CO_2}$):

$$pH = 6.1 + \log \frac{\overbrace{48 \text{ mM}}^{\text{Doubled[HCO}_3^-]}}{(0.03 \text{ mM/mm Hg}) \times \underbrace{80 \text{ mm Hg}}_{\text{Doubled P}_{CO_2}}} \quad (28\text{-}31)$$

$$= 7.4$$

The kidneys are responsible for the metabolic compensation to a primary respiratory acidosis. They acutely sense high P$_{CO_2}$ and may also chronically sense low blood pH. The response is to increase both the secretion of acid into the urine and the transport of HCO$_3^-$ into the blood (see Chapter 39), thereby raising plasma pH—a compensatory metabolic alkalosis. The renal compensation to a substantial respiratory acidosis is not perfect, so that pH remains below the normal value of 7.40.

The kidneys can also perform a **metabolic compensation to a respiratory alkalosis.** In Figure 28-9B we revisit a second example, originally introduced in Figure 28-6C, in which we produced a primary respiratory alkalosis by decreasing P$_{CO_2}$ from 40 to 20 mm Hg (red arrow in Figure 28-9B between Start and point B at pH 7.60). We can compensate for most of this respiratory alkalosis by adding 10 mmol of H$^+$ to each liter of solution or by removing 10 mmol NaHCO$_3$ or NaOH, which produces the same effect. A black line is generated parallel to the red non-HCO$_3^-$ titration line but displaced downward by 10 mM. Point B$_1$ (pH 7.44), at the intersection of the black line and the P_{CO_2} isopleth for 20 mm Hg, represents a partial compensation.

If we add an additional 2 mmol H^+, for a total addition of 12 mmol of H^+ to each liter, pH returns to exactly its initial value of 7.40 (point B_2 in Fig. 28-9B). Why is this amount so much less than the 24 mmol of OH^- that we added to each liter to compensate perfectly for a *doubling* of P_{CO_2}? When we halve P_{CO_2}, we need only add an amount of H^+ equivalent to half the amount of HCO_3^- that was present (24/2 = 12 mM) at Start.

In response to a primary respiratory alkalosis, the kidneys secrete less acid into the urine and transport less HCO_3^- into the blood (see Chapter 39), thereby lowering plasma pH—a compensatory metabolic acidosis.

A respiratory change can compensate for a metabolic disturbance

Just as metabolic changes can compensate for respiratory disturbances, respiratory changes can compensate for metabolic ones. In Figure 28-10A we return to an example originally introduced on the left of Figure 28-7, in which we produced a primary metabolic acidosis by adding 10 mmol of HCl to 1 L of arterial blood (red arrow in Fig. 28-10A between Start and point C at pH 7.26). Other than by removing the H^+ (or adding OH^- to neutralize the H^+), the only way we can restore pH toward the initial value of 7.40 is to lower P_{CO_2}. That is, we can superimpose a respiratory *alka-*

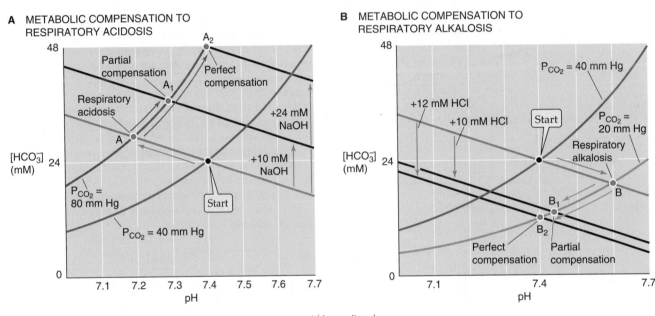

Figure 28-9   Metabolic compensation to primary respiratory acid-base disturbances.

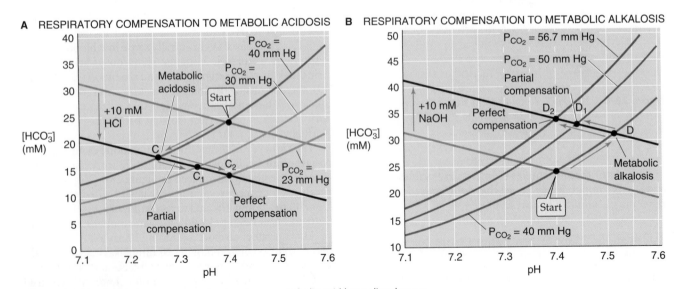

Figure 28-10   Respiratory compensation to primary metabolic acid-base disturbances.

losis on the primary metabolic *acidosis*—a **respiratory compensation to a metabolic acidosis**. For example, we can compensate for most of the metabolic acidosis by reducing P_{CO_2} from 40 to 30 mm Hg. Starting at C, follow the black line from the P_{CO_2} isopleth for 40 mm Hg to the new isopleth for 30 mm Hg at point C_1 (pH 7.34). This maneuver represents a *partial* compensation.

If we reduce P_{CO_2} by an additional 6.6 mm Hg to 23.4 mm Hg, we produce a perfect compensation, which we represent in Figure 28-10A by following the black line from C until we reach pH 7.40 at point C_2, which is on the P_{CO_2} isopleth for 23.4 mm Hg. Perfect compensation requires that we reduce P_{CO_2} by a fraction (i.e., $[40 - 23.4]/40 \cong 0.42$) that is identical to the ratio of added HCl to the original $[HCO_3^-]$ (i.e., 10/24 $\cong 0.42$).

Not surprisingly, the respiratory system is responsible for the respiratory compensation to a primary metabolic acidosis. The low plasma pH or $[HCO_3^-]$ stimulates the peripheral chemoreceptors and, if sufficiently long-standing, also the central chemoreceptors. (See Chapter 32.) The result is an increase in alveolar ventilation, which lowers P_{CO_2} (see Chapter 31) and thus provides the respiratory compensation.

The body achieves a **respiratory compensation to a primary metabolic alkalosis** in just the opposite manner. In Figure 28-10B we revisit an example originally presented in the right of Figure 28-7, in which we produced a primary metabolic alkalosis by adding 10 mmol of NaOH to 1 L (red arrow in Fig. 28-10B between Start and point D at pH 7.51). If we now increase P_{CO_2} from 40 to 50 mm Hg, we partially compensate for the metabolic alkalosis by moving from D to D_1 (pH 7.44). If we raise P_{CO_2} by an additional 6.7 mm Hg to ~56.7 mm Hg, the compensation is perfect, and pH returns to 7.40 (D_2).

In response to a primary metabolic alkalosis, the respiratory system decreases alveolar ventilation and thereby raises P_{CO_2}. The compensatory respiratory acidosis is the least "perfect" of the four types of compensation we have discussed. The reason is that one can decrease alveolar ventilation—and thus oxygenation—only so far before compromising one's very existence.

In a real person, each of the four primary acid-base disturbances—points A, B, C, and D in Figures 28-9 and 28-10—occurs in the extracellular fluid. In each case, the body's first and almost instantaneous response is to use extracellular buffers to neutralize part of the acid or alkaline load. In addition, cells rapidly take up some of the acid or alkaline load and thus participate in the buffering, as discussed later. Furthermore, renal tubule cells may respond to a *metabolic* acidosis of extrarenal origin (e.g., diabetic ketoacidosis) by increasing acid secretion into the urine or to a metabolic alkalosis (e.g., $NaHCO_3$ therapy) by decreasing acid secretion—examples of *metabolic* compensation to a *metabolic* disturbance. Points C and D in Figure 28-10 include the effects of the actual acid or alkaline load, extracellular and intracellular buffering, and any renal (i.e., metabolic) response.

Position on a Davenport diagram defines the nature of an acid-base disturbance

The only tools needed to characterize acid-base status (i.e., pH, $[HCO_3^-]$, and P_{CO_2}) are a Davenport diagram and elec-

trodes for measurement of pH and P_{CO_2}. From these last two parameters, we can compute $[HCO_3^-]$ by use of the Henderson-Hasselbalch equation. The acid-base status of blood plasma—or of any aqueous solution—must fall into one of five major categories:

1. **Normal.** For arterial blood, pH is 7.40, $[HCO_3^-]$ is 24 mM, and P_{CO_2} is 40 mm Hg. This point was Start in the previous figures and is the central point in Figure 28-11A-D.

2. **One of the four primary (or uncompensated) acid-base disturbances.** The coordinates for pH and $[HCO_3^-]$ fall on either of the following: the non-HCO_3^- titration line but off the 40 mm Hg isopleth for uncompensated respiratory acidosis (point A, Fig. 28-11A) or alkalosis (point B); or the 40 mm Hg isopleth but off the non-HCO_3^- titration line for an uncompensated metabolic acidosis (point C) or alkalosis (point D).

3. **A partially compensated disturbance.** The coordinates for pH and $[HCO_3^-]$ fall in any of the four colored regions of Figure 28-11B. For example, point A_1 in the blue region represents a partially compensated respiratory acidosis. In a subject for whom a respiratory acidosis has existed for longer than a few hours, increased renal H^+ excretion has probably already begun producing a metabolic compensation. Depending on the extent of the original acidosis and the degree of compensation, point A_1 could lie anywhere in the blue region. We can reach similar conclusions for the other three disturbances and compensations.

4. **A perfectly compensated disturbance.** The point falls on the vertical line through pH 7.4. As indicated by point A_2D_2 in Figure 28-11C, a perfect compensation following respiratory acidosis is indistinguishable from that following metabolic alkalosis. In either case, the final outcome is isohydric hypercapnia. Similarly, point B_2C_2 represents a perfect compensation from either metabolic acidosis or respiratory alkalosis (isohydric hypocapnia).

5. **A compound respiratory-metabolic disturbance.** The point falls in one of the two colored regions in Figure 28-11D. For example, points A_3 and C_3 represent a respiratory acidosis complicated by metabolic acidosis, or vice versa. The second disturbance causes the pH to move even farther away from "normal," as might occur in an individual with both respiratory and renal failure (Table 28-3). Of course, it is impossible to determine if one of the two compounding disturbances developed before the other.

pH REGULATION OF INTRACELLULAR FLUID

Clinicians focus on the acid-base status of blood plasma, the fluid compartment whose acid-base status is easiest to assess. However, the number of biochemical reactions and other processes that occur *outside* a cell pales in comparison to the number of those that occur *inside*. It stands to reason that the most important biological fluid for pH regulation is the cytosol. It is possible to monitor intracellular pH (pH_i) continuously in isolated cells and tissues by use of pH-sensitive dyes or microelectrodes. Moreover, with magnetic resonance

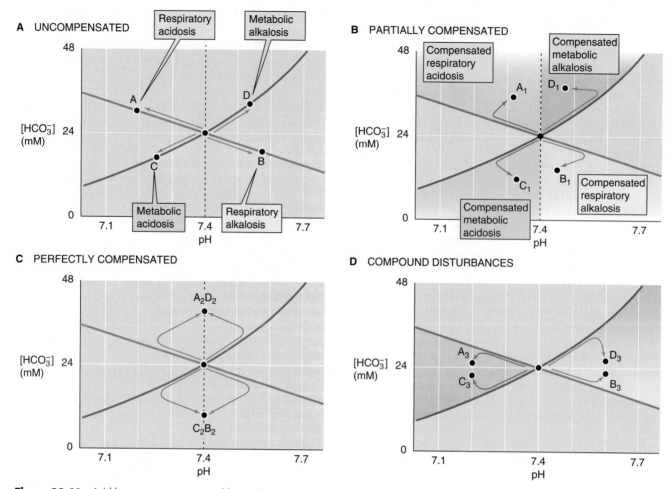

Figure 28-11 Acid-base states represented by position on a Davenport diagram.

techniques, one can monitor pH_i in living humans (e.g., skeletal muscle). The pH of cells both influences and is influenced by extracellular pH.

Ion transporters at the plasma membrane closely regulate the pH inside of cells

Figure 28-12A shows a hypothetical cell with two acid-base transporters, a Na-H exchanger, and a Cl-HCO_3 exchanger. We will use the Na-H exchanger as a prototypic **acid extruder**, a transporter that tends to raise intracellular pH (pH_i). The Na-H exchanger uses the energy of the Na^+ gradient to move H^+ out of the cell. We will take the Cl-HCO_3 exchanger as a prototypic **acid loader**. This exchanger, driven by the steep out-to-in Cl^- gradient, moves HCO_3^- out of the cell. The intracellular acid loading produced by Cl-HCO_3 exchange is a **chronic acid load** because it tends to acidify the cell as long as the transporter is active. In our example, the chronic acid extrusion through Na-H exchange balances the chronic acid loading through Cl-HCO_3 exchange, producing a steady state. In real cells, several other acid extruders and acid loaders may contribute to pH_i regulation. (See Chapter 5.)

Imagine that we use a micropipette to inject HCl into the cell in Figure 28-12A. This injection of an **acute acid load**—a one time–only introduction of a fixed quantity of acid—

causes an immediate fall in pH_i (Fig. 28-12B, black curve), an example of **intracellular metabolic acidosis**. If we add HCl to a beaker, the pH remains low indefinitely. However, when we acutely acid load a cell, pH_i spontaneously recovers to the initial value. This pH_i recovery cannot be due to passive H^+ efflux out of the cell, inasmuch as the electrochemical gradient for H^+ (see Chapter 5) usually favors H^+ influx. Hence, the pH_i recovery reflects the active transport of acid from the cell—*a metabolic compensation to a metabolic acid load.*

During the recovery of pH_i from the acid load in Figure 28-12B, the Na-H exchanger not only must extrude the quantity of H^+ previously injected into the cell (the *acute* acid load), it also must counteract whatever acid loading the Cl-HCO_3 exchanger continues to impose on the cell (the *chronic* acid load).

Acid extrusion rates tend to be greatest at low pH_i values and fall off as pH_i approaches its resting value (Fig. 28-12C, black curve). As discussed later, low pH_i also *inhibits* Cl-HCO_3 exchange and thus acid loading. The response to low pH_i therefore involves two feedback loops operating in push-pull fashion, stimulating acid extrusion and inhibiting acid loading.

In addition to pH_i, hormones, growth factors, oncogenes, cell volume, and extracellular pH (pH_o) all can modulate these transporters. The pH_o effect is especially important.

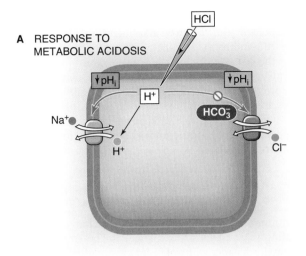

A RESPONSE TO METABOLIC ACIDOSIS

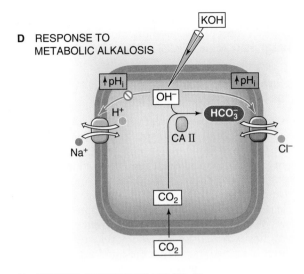

D RESPONSE TO METABOLIC ALKALOSIS

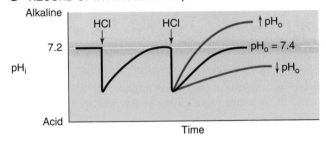

B RECORD OF INTRACELLULAR pH

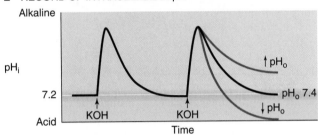

E RECORD OF INTRACELLULAR pH

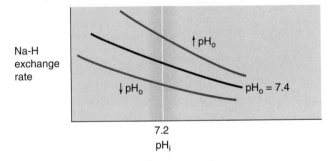

C pH_i DEPENDENCE OF ACID EXTRUDERS

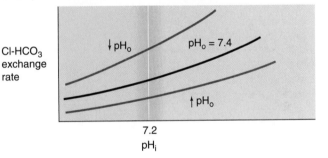

F pH_i DEPENDENCE OF ACID LOADERS

Figure 28-12 Recovery of a cell from intracellular acid and alkali loads.

In general, a low pH_o slows the rate of pH_i recovery from acute acid loads and reduces the final steady-state pH_i (Fig. 28-12B, red curve), whereas a high pH_o does the opposite (blue curve). The underlying cause of these pH_o effects is a shift of the pH_i dependence of acid extrusion (Fig. 28-12C, red and blue curves) and, as we shall see, changes in acid loading.

Cells also spontaneously recover from acute alkaline loads. If we inject a cell with potassium hydroxide (KOH; Fig. 28-12D), pH_i rapidly increases but then slowly recovers to its initial value (Fig. 28-12E, black curve), reflecting stimulation of acid loading and inhibition of acid extrusion. The injection of OH^- represents a metabolic alkalosis, whereas increased $Cl-HCO_3$ exchange represents a metabolic compensation. The $Cl-HCO_3$ exchanger is most active at high pH_i values (Fig. 28-12F). As discussed previously, increases

in pH_i generally inhibit acid extruders. Thus, the response to alkaline loads—like the response to acid loads—includes dual feedback loops operating in push-pull fashion, stimulating acid loading and inhibiting acid extrusion. During the pH_i recovery from an acute alkaline load, $Cl-HCO_3$ exchange must not only neutralize the alkali previously injected into the cell (the acute alkali load) but also counteract the alkalinizing effect of acid extruders such as the Na-H exchanger.

Like the Na-H exchanger, the $Cl-HCO_3$ exchanger is under the control of hormones and growth factors. It also probably has a pH_o sensitivity that is opposite to that of the acid extruders, with low pH_o enhancing $Cl-HCO_3$ exchange. In general, an extracellular metabolic acidosis, with its simultaneous fall in *both* pH_o and $[HCO_3]$ (Table 28-3), should stimulate $Cl-HCO_3$ exchange (Fig. 28-12F, red curve).

During the recovery from acute alkali loads, metabolic acidosis therefore causes pH_i to fall more rapidly and to reach a lower steady-state value (Fig. 28-12E, red curve).

Indirect interactions between K^+ and H^+ make it appear as if cells have a K-H exchanger

Clinicians have long known that extracellular acidosis leads to a release of K^+ from cells and thus hyperkalemia. Conversely, hyperkalemia leads to the exit of H^+ from cells, resulting in extracellular acidosis. These observations, which one can duplicate at the level of single cells, led to the suggestion that cells generally have a K-H exchanger. It is true that specialized cells in the stomach (see Chapter 42) and kidney (see Chapter 39) do have an ATP-driven pump that extrudes H^+ in exchange for K^+. Moreover, the K/HCO_3 cotransporter described in certain cells could mimic a K-H exchanger. Nevertheless, the effects that long ago led to the K-H exchange hypothesis probably reflect *indirect* interactions of H^+ and K^+.

One example of apparent K-H exchange is that hyperkalemia causes an intracellular alkalosis. Not only is this effect *not* due to a 1:1 exchange of K^+ for H^+, it is not even due to the increase in $[K^+]_o$ per se. Instead, the high $[K^+]_o$ depolarizes the cell, and this positive shift in membrane voltage can promote the net uptake of HCO_3^- through the electrogenic

Na/HCO_3 cotransporter (see Chapter 5) and thus a rise in pH_i—a **depolarization-induced alkalinization**. Depolarization also can indirectly stimulate other transporters that alkalinize the cell. We discuss the converse example of acidemia causing hyperkalemia in Chapter 37: extracellular acidosis lowers pH_i and inhibits transporters responsible for K^+ uptake, leading to net K^+ release from cells. Although we have no evidence that a K-H exchanger exists in humans, imagining that it exists is sometimes a helpful tool for quickly predicting interactions of H^+ and K^+ in a clinical setting.

Changes in intracellular pH are often a sign of changes in extracellular pH and vice versa

By definition, acid extrusion (e.g., Na-H exchange) equals acid loading (e.g., Cl-HCO_3 exchange) in the steady state. Disturbing this balance shifts pH_i. For example, extracellular *metabolic* acidosis inhibits acid extrusion and stimulates acid loading, thus lowering steady-state pH_i. This intracellular acidosis is not instantaneous but develops during a few minutes. Conversely, extracellular metabolic alkalosis leads to a slow increase in steady-state pH_i. In general, a change in pH_o shifts pH_i in the same direction, but ΔpH_i is usually only 20% to 60% of ΔpH_o. In other words, an extracellular metabolic acidosis causes a net transfer of acid from the extracellular to the intracellular space, and an extracellular

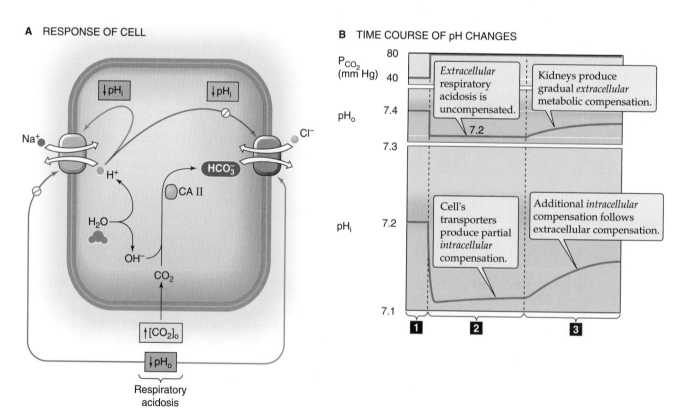

Figure 28-13 Response of cell to extracellular respiratory acidosis. In **A,** respiratory acidosis sends conflicting messages to the acid-base transporters. The rise in $[CO_2]$ leads to a fall in intracellular pH (pH_i), which stimulates the Na-H exchanger but inhibits the Cl-HCO_3 exchanger—tending to cause pH_i to recover. However, the low extracellular pH (pH_o) directly inhibits the Na-H exchanger but stimulates the Cl-HCO_3 exchanger. In **B,** the influx of CO_2 produces a rapid intracellular metabolic acidosis (1). The low pH_o initially hampers the ability of the cell to recover from the acid load (2). The delayed recovery of pH_o, through its effects on the transporters, leads to an additional recovery of pH_i as well (3).

metabolic alkalosis has the opposite effect. Thus, cells participate in buffering of extracellular acid and alkali loads.

Extracellular *respiratory* acidosis generally affects pH_i in three phases. First, the increase in extracellular $[CO_2]_{Dis}$ creates an inwardly directed gradient for CO_2. This dissolved gas rapidly enters the cell (Fig. 28-13A) and produces HCO_3^- and H^+. This **intracellular respiratory acidosis** manifests itself as a rapid fall in pH_i (Fig. 28-13B, phase 1 in lower panel). Carbonic anhydrase greatly accelerates the formation of HCO_3^- and H^+ from CO_2, so that pH_i can complete its decline in just a few seconds.

In the second phase, the cell recovers from this acid load, but only feebly (Fig. 28-13B, phase 2 in lower panel) because the decrease in pH_o inhibits acid extrusion and stimulates acid loading. During a period of minutes, pH_i may recover only partially if at all.

In the third phase, the extracellular respiratory acidosis stimulates the kidneys to upregulate acid-base transporters and thus stimulate urinary acid secretion (see Chapter 39). The net effect, during a period of hours or days, is an extracellular metabolic compensation that causes pH_o to increase gradually (Fig. 28-13B, phase 3 in upper panel). As pH_o rises, it gradually relieves the inhibition of Na-H exchange and other acid extruders and cancels the stimulation of Cl-HCO_3 exchange and other acid loaders. Thus, *intra*cellular pH recovers in parallel with *extra*cellular pH, albeit by only 20% to 60% as much as pH_o (Fig. 28-13B, phase 3 in lower panel). The pH_i recovery represents an **intracellular metabolic compensation** to the intracellular respiratory acidosis.

Not all cell types have the same resting pH_i. Moreover, different cell types often have very different complements of acid-base transporters and very different ways of regulating these transporters. Nevertheless, the example in Figure 28-13 illustrates that the fate of pH_i is closely intertwined with that of interstitial fluid and thus blood plasma. During respiratory acid-base disturbances, the lungs generate the insult, and virtually every other cell in the body must defend itself against it. In the case of metabolic acid-base disturbances, however, some cells may generate the insult, whereas the others attempt to defend themselves against it. From a teleological point of view, one can imagine that the primary reason that the body regulates the pH of the blood plasma and extracellular fluids is to allow the cells to properly regulate their pH_i. The primary reason that the clinical assessment of blood acid-base parameters can be useful is that these parameters tend to parallel cellular acid-base status.

REFERENCES

Books and Reviews

Bevensee MO, Alper S, Aronson PS, Boron WF: Control of intracellular pH. In Seldin DW, Giebisch G (eds): The Kidney: Physiology and Pathophysiology, 3rd ed, pp 391-442. Philadelphia: JB Lippincott, 2000.

Davenport HW: The ABC of Acid Base Chemistry, 6th ed. Chicago: University of Chicago Press, 1974.

Mount DB, Romero MF: The SLC26 gene family of multifunctional anion exchangers. Pflügers Arch 2004; 447:710-721.

Orlowski J, Grinstein S: Diversity of the mammalian sodium/proton exchanger SLC9 gene family. Pflügers Arch 2004; 447:549-565.

Romero MF, Fulton CM, Boron WF: The SLC4 family of HCO_3^- transporters. Pflügers Arch 2004; 447:495-509.

Roos A, Boron WF: Intracellular pH. Physiol Rev 1981; 61:296-434.

Journal Articles

Boron WF, De Weer P: Intracellular pH transients in squid giant axons caused by CO_2, NH_3, and metabolic inhibitors. J Gen Physiol 1976; 67:91-112.

Thomas RC: The effect of carbon dioxide on the intracellular pH and buffering power of snail neurones. J Physiol 1976; 255:715-735.

Zhao J, Hogan EM, Bevensee MO, Boron WF: Out-of-equilibrium CO_2/HCO_3^- solutions and their use in characterizing a novel K/HCO_3 cotransporter. Nature 1995; 374:636-639.

CHAPTER 29

TRANSPORT OF OXYGEN AND CARBON DIOXIDE IN THE BLOOD

Walter F. Boron

CARRIAGE OF OXYGEN

The amount of O_2 dissolved in blood is far too small to meet the metabolic demands of the body

Blood carries O_2 in two forms. More than 98% of the O_2 normally binds to hemoglobin within the **erythrocytes**, also known as red blood cells (RBCs). A tiny fraction physically dissolves in the aqueous phases of both blood plasma and the cytoplasm of blood cells (predominantly RBCs). What is the significance of the O_2 that is bound to hemoglobin?

Imagine that we expose a liter of blood plasma, initially free of O_2, to an atmosphere having the same P_{O_2} as alveolar air—100 mm Hg. Oxygen will move from the atmosphere to the plasma until an equilibrium is established, at which time the concentration of **dissolved O_2** ($[O_2]_{Dis}$) in the blood obeys **Henry's law** (see Chapter 26 for the box on this topic):

$$[O_2]_{Dis} = k_{O_2} \cdot P_{O_2} \qquad (29\text{-}1)$$

If we express P_{O_2} in millimeters of mercury (mm Hg) and $[O_2]_{Dis}$ in milliliters of O_2 gas (measured at standard temperature and pressure or STP) per 100 mL (or dL) of blood, then the solubility k_{O_2} is ~0.003 mL O_2 for each deciliter of blood and each millimeter of mercury of O_2 partial pressure at 37°C. For arterial blood:

$$[O_2]_{Dis} = \frac{0.3 \text{ mL } O_2}{100 \text{ mL blood} \cdot \text{mm Hg}} \cdot 100 \text{ mm Hg} \qquad (29\text{-}2)$$
$$= 0.3 \text{ mL } O_2/100 \text{ mL blood}$$

Is such an O_2-carrying capacity adequate to supply O_2 to the systemic tissues? If these tissues could extract all the O_2 dissolved in arterial blood so that no O_2 remained in venous blood, and if cardiac output were 5000 mL/min, then—according to the Fick principle (see Chapter 17)—the delivery of dissolved O_2 to the tissues would be

$$\dot{V}_{O_2} = \overbrace{\frac{5000 \text{ mL blood}}{\text{min}}}^{\text{Blood flow}} \cdot \overbrace{\frac{0.3 \text{ mL } O_2}{100 \text{ mL blood}}}^{\substack{O_2 \text{ concentration} \\ \text{in plasma}}} \qquad (29\text{-}3)$$

where $\dot{V}_{O_2}$ is labeled "O_2 delivery."

$$= 15 \text{ mL } O_2/\text{min}$$

However, the average 70-kg human at rest consumes O_2 at the rate of ~250 mL/min. Dissolved O_2 could supply the body's metabolic demands only if cardiac output increased by a factor of 250/15 or nearly 17-fold! Thus, the body cannot rely on dissolved O_2 as a mechanism for O_2 carriage.

Hemoglobin consists of two α and two β subunits, each of which has an iron-containing heme and a polypeptide globin

Normal adult **hemoglobin (Hb)** is a tetramer having a molecular mass of ~68 kDa, each monomer consisting of a heme and a globin (Fig. 29-1A). The heme is a porphyrin compound coordinated to a single iron atom. The **globin** is a polypeptide, either an α chain (141 amino acids) or a β chain (146 amino acids). The homology between the α and β chains is sufficient that they have similar conformations, a series of seven helices enveloping a single heme. Thus, the complete Hb molecule has the stoichiometry [α (heme)]₂ [β (heme)]₂ and can bind as many as four O_2 molecules, one for each iron atom. The erythroblasts that synthesize Hb closely coordinate the production of α chains, β chains, and heme.

Heme is a general term for a metal ion chelated to a porphyrin ring. In the case of Hb, the metal is iron in the Fe^{2+} or ferrous state (Fig. 29-1B). The porphyrin consists of four linked pyrrole rings that through their nitrogen atoms coordinate a single, centrally located Fe^{2+}. Because the iron-porphyrin complex is rich in conjugated double bonds, it absorbs photons of relatively low energy (i.e., light in the visible range). The interaction among O_2, Fe^{2+}, and porphyrin causes the complex to have a red color when it is fully saturated with O_2 (e.g., arterial blood) and a purple color when it is devoid of O_2 (e.g., venous blood).

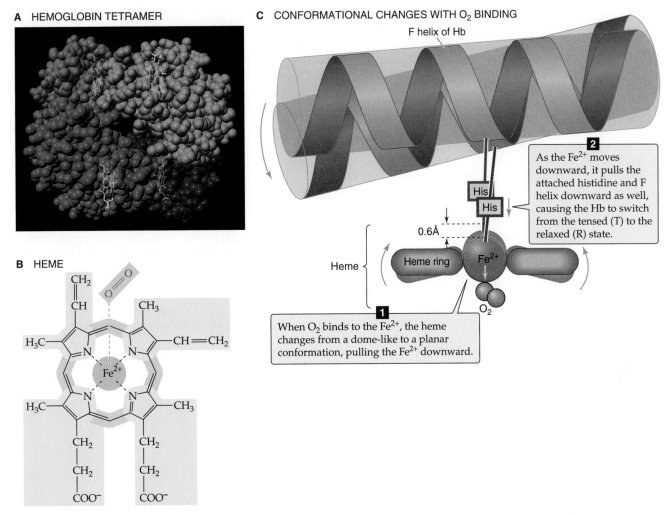

A HEMOGLOBIN TETRAMER

B HEME

C CONFORMATIONAL CHANGES WITH O_2 BINDING

F helix of Hb

His
His

0.6Å

Heme { Heme ring Fe^{2+}

O_2

2 As the Fe^{2+} moves downward, it pulls the attached histidine and F helix downward as well, causing the Hb to switch from the tensed (T) to the relaxed (R) state.

1 When O_2 binds to the Fe^{2+}, the heme changes from a dome-like to a planar conformation, pulling the Fe^{2+} downward.

CH_2
CH
CH_3
H_3C
$CH=CH_2$
Fe^{2+}
N N
N N
H_3C
CH_3
CH_2
CH_2
CH_2
CH_2
COO^-
COO^-

Figure 29-1 The structure of hemoglobin (Hb).

Hb can bind O_2 only when the iron is in the Fe^{2+} state. The Fe^{2+} in Hb can become oxidized to ferric iron (Fe^{3+}), either spontaneously or under the influence of compounds such as nitrites and sulfonamides. The result of such an oxidation is **methemoglobin** (metHb), which is incapable of binding O_2. Inside the RBC, the heme-containing enzyme **methemoglobin reductase** uses the reduced form of nicotinamide adenine dinucleotide (NADH) to reduce metHb back to Hb, so that only about 1.5% of total Hb is in the metHb state. In the rare case in which a genetic defect results in a deficiency of this enzyme, metHb may represent 25% or more of the total Hb. Such a deficiency results in a decreased O_2-carrying capacity, leading to tissue hypoxia.

The environment provided by the globin portion of Hb is crucial for the O_2-heme interaction. To be useful, this interaction must be fully reversible under physiological conditions, allowing repetitive capture and release of O_2. The interaction of O_2 with free Fe^{2+} normally produces Fe^{3+}, the simplest example of which is rust. Even with isolated heme, O_2 *irreversibly* oxidizes Fe^{2+} to Fe^{3+}. However, when heme is part of Hb, interactions with ~20 amino acids cradle the heme in the globin, so that O_2 loosely and *reversibly* binds to Fe^{2+}. The crucial residue is a histidine that bonds to the Fe^{2+}

and donates negative charge that stabilizes the Fe^{2+}-O_2 complex. This histidine is also crucial for transmitting, to the rest of the Hb tetramer, the information that an O_2 molecule is or is not bound to the Fe^{2+}. When all four hemes are devoid of O_2, each of the four histidines pulls its Fe^{2+} above the *plane of its porphyrin ring* by ~0.06 nm (the blue conformation in Fig. 29-1C), distorting the porphyrin ring. Thus, the Fe^{2+}-histidine bond is under strain in deoxyhemoglobin, a strain that it transmits to the rest of the α or β subunit and thence to the rest of the Hb molecule. The various components of the Hb tetramer are so tightly interlinked, as if by a snugly fitting system of levers and joints, that no one subunit can leave this **tensed (T) state** unless they all leave it together. Because the shape of the heme in the T state sterically inhibits the approach of O_2, empty Hb has a very low affinity for O_2.

When one O_2 binds to one of the Fe^{2+} atoms, the Fe^{2+} tends to move down into the plane of the porphyrin ring. If the Fe^{2+} actually *could* move, it would flatten the ring and relieve the strain on the Fe^{2+}-histidine bond. When enough O_2 molecules bind, enough energy builds up and all four subunits of the Hb simultaneously snap into the **relaxed (R) state**, whether or not they are bound to O_2. In this R state, with its flattened heme, the Hb molecule has an O_2 affinity that is ~150-fold greater than that in the T state. Thus, when P_{O_2} is zero, all Hb molecules are in the T state and have a low O_2 affinity. When P_{O_2} is very high, all Hb molecules are in the R state and have a high O_2 affinity. At intermediate P_{O_2} values, an equilibrium exists between Hb molecules in the T and R states.

Myoglobin (Mb) is another heme-containing, O_2-binding protein that is specific for muscle (see Chapter 9). The globin portion of Mb arose in a gene duplication event from a primordial globin. Additional duplications along the nonmyoglobin branch of the globin family led first to the α and β chains of Hb and then to other α-like and β-like chains (see the box on forms of hemoglobin). Mb functions as a *monomer*, homologous to either an α or a β chain of Hb. Although it is capable of binding only a single O_2, Mb has a much higher O_2 affinity than Hb does. In the capillaries, Hb can thus hand off O_2 to an Mb inside a muscle cell; this Mb then transfers its O_2 to the next Mb, and so on, speeding diffusion of O_2 through the muscle cell. Because of the low solubility of O_2, this action is essential. There is insufficient dissolved O_2, by itself, to establish an intracellular O_2 gradient large enough to deliver adequate O_2 to mitochondria.

The Hb-O_2 dissociation curve has a sigmoidal shape because of cooperativity among the four subunits of the hemoglobin molecule

Imagine that we expose whole blood to a gas phase with a P_{O_2} that we can set at any one of several values (Fig. 29-2). For example, we could incubate the blood with a P_{O_2} of 40 mm Hg, typical of mixed-venous blood, and centrifuge a sample to separate plasma from erythrocytes, as one would for determination of the hematocrit (see Chapter 5). Next, we individually determine the O_2 content of the plasma (i.e, dissolved O_2) and packed RBCs. If we know how much water is inside the RBCs, we can subtract the amount of O_2 dissolved in this water from the total O_2, arriving at the amount of O_2 bound to Hb.

Repeating this exercise over a range of P_{O_2} values, we obtain the red curve in Figure 29-3. The right-hand ordinate gives the O_2 bound to Hb (in the units of mL O_2/dL blood). The left-hand ordinate gives the same data in terms of **% O_2 saturation** of Hb (S_{O_2} or "Sat"). To compute S_{O_2}, we need to know the maximal amount of O_2 that can bind to Hb at extremely high P_{O_2} values. Expressed in terms of grams of Hb protein, this **O_2 capacity** is ~1.39 mL O_2/g Hb—assuming that no metHb is present. In real life, the O_2 capacity may be closer to 1.35 mL O_2/g Hb because O_2 cannot bind to Hb that is either in the Fe^{3+} state (e.g., metHb) or, as discussed later, bound to carbon monoxide. We can translate this O_2 capacity to a value for the maximal amount of O_2 that can bind to Hb in 100 mL of blood. If the Hb content is 15 g Hb/dL blood (i.e., normal for an adult man), then

Maximal O_2 bound to Hb

$$= (O_2 \text{ capacity of Hb}) \times (\text{Hb content of blood})$$

$$= \frac{1.35 \text{ mL } O_2}{\text{g Hb}} \cdot \frac{15 \text{ g Hb}}{\text{dL blood}} \qquad (29\text{-}4)$$

$$= \sim 20.3 \, (\text{mL } O_2)/\text{dL blood}$$

The percent saturation of Hb is

$$\% \text{ Saturation of Hb} = \frac{O_2 \text{ actually bound to Hb}}{O_2 \text{ capacity of Hb}} \cdot 100$$

$$(29\text{-}5)$$

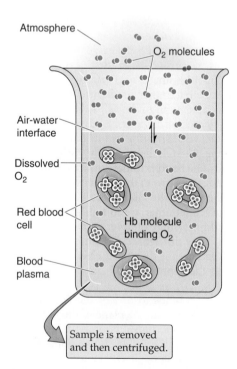

Figure 29-2 Determination of O_2 content in blood plasma and erythrocytes. RBCs, red blood cells; WBCs, white blood cells.

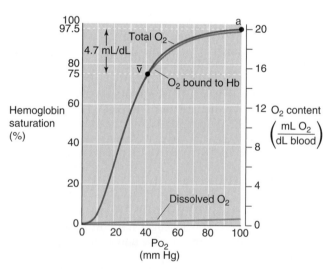

Figure 29-3 A normal Hb-O_2 dissociation curve. The y-axis on the right shows O_2 content. For the *red curve* (O_2 content of Hb), we assume 15 g Hb/dL of blood and an O_2 capacity of 1.35 mL O_2/g Hb. The *brown curve* is the sum of the red and *purple curves*. The y-axis on the left, which pertains only to the red curve, gives the percentage of Hb saturation or S_{O_2}.

Notice that the curve in Figure 29-3 is sigmoidal or S shaped because of the cooperativity among the four O_2 binding sites on the Hb molecule. At low P_{O_2} values, increases in P_{O_2} produce relatively small increases in O_2 binding, reflecting the relatively low O_2 affinity of Hb in the T state. At moderate P_{O_2} values, the amount of bound O_2 increases more steeply with increases in P_{O_2}, reflecting the increased O_2 affinity as more Hb molecules shift to the R state. The P_{O_2} at which the Hb is half saturated is known as the **P_{50}**. Finally, the Hb-O_2 versus P_{O_2} curve flattens at high P_{O_2} values as the Hb saturates. The difference in Hb saturation at low versus high P_{O_2} values is the basis for an important clinical tool, the pulse oximeter (see the box on measuring O_2 saturation).

At the P_{O_2} prevailing in normal arterial blood (Pa_{O_2}), ~100 mm Hg, the Hb saturation (Sa_{O_2}) is ~97.5% or 19.7 mL O_2/dL bound to Hb (Table 29-1). The dissolved O_2 (purple curve in Fig. 29-3) would add an additional 0.3 mL O_2/dL for a **total O_2 content** of 20.0 mL O_2/dL (point *a* on the brown curve in Fig. 29-3). In mixed-venous blood, in which P_{O_2} ($P\bar{v}_{O_2}$) is ~40 mm Hg, the Hb saturation ($S\bar{v}_{O_2}$) is ~75% or 15.2 mL O_2/dL bound to Hb (Table 29-1). The dissolved O_2 would add 0.1 mL O_2/dL for a total of 15.3 mL O_2/dL (point $\bar{v}$ in Fig. 29-3). The difference in total O_2 content between points *a* and $\bar{v}$, the a-$\bar{v}$ difference, is the amount of O_2 that the lungs add to the blood in the pulmonary capillaries, which is the same amount that all the tissues extract from the blood in the systemic capillaries:

$$\underbrace{\Delta C(a-\bar{v})_{O_2}}_{\substack{\text{a-}\bar{v} \\ \text{difference for total} \\ O_2 \text{ content}}} = \underbrace{\frac{20.0\,\text{mL}\,O_2}{\text{dL blood}}}_{\substack{O_2 \text{ content of} \\ \text{arterial} \\ \text{blood}}} - \underbrace{\frac{15.3\,\text{mL}\,O_2}{\text{dL blood}}}_{\substack{O_2 \text{ content of} \\ \text{mixed-venous} \\ \text{blood}}} \quad (29\text{-}6)$$

$$= \frac{4.7\,\text{mL}\,O_2}{\text{dL blood}}$$

Of the total a-$\bar{v}$ difference of 4.7 mL O_2/dL, Hb provides 4.5 mL O_2/dL or nearly 96% of the O_2 that the lungs add and the systemic tissues extract from blood (Table 29-1). Is this a-$\bar{v}$ difference in O_2 content enough to satisfy the metabolic demands of the body (i.e., ~250 mL O_2/min)? Using the Fick principle, as we did in Equation 29-3, we see that the combination of a cardiac output of 5 L/min and an a-$\bar{v}$ difference of 4.7 mL/dL would be nearly adequate:

$$\underbrace{\dot{V}_{O_2}}_{\substack{O_2 \\ \text{consumption} \\ \text{by tissues}}} = \underbrace{\frac{5000\,\text{mL blood}}{\text{min}}}_{\text{Blood flow}} \cdot \underbrace{\frac{4.7\,\text{mL}\,O_2}{100\,\text{mL blood}}}_{\substack{\text{a-}\bar{v} \\ \text{difference} \\ \text{for total} \\ O_2 \text{ content}}} \quad (29\text{-}7)$$

$$= \sim 235\,\text{mL}\,O_2/\text{min}$$

By either increasing cardiac output by ~6% or decreasing the P_{O_2} of mixed-venous blood, the body could meet a demand of 250 mL O_2/min. We spend our lives moving endlessly from point *a* in Figure 29-3 to point $\bar{v}$ (as we deliver O_2 to the tissues) and then back to point *a* (as we take up more O_2 from alveolar air).

Because the plot of $[O_2]_{Dis}$ versus P_{O_2} is linear (Fig. 29-3, purple curve), the amount of O_2 that can dissolve in blood plasma has no theoretical maximum. Thus, breathing of 100% O_2 would raise arterial P_{O_2} by ~6-fold, so that ~1.8 mL of O_2 would be dissolved in each deciliter of arterial blood. Although dissolved O_2 would make a correspondingly greater contribution to overall O_2 carriage under such unphysiological conditions, Hb would still carry the vast majority of O_2. Hence, a decrease in Hb content of the blood—known as **anemia**—can markedly reduce O_2 carriage. The body can compensate for decreased Hb content in the same two ways that, in the earlier example, we increased the $\dot{V}_{O_2}$ from 235 to 250 mL O_2/min. First, it can increase cardiac output. Second, it can increase O_2 extraction, thereby reducing mixed-venous O_2 content. Anemia leads to pallor of the mucous membranes and skin, reflecting the decrease in the red Hb pigment. Impaired O_2 delivery may cause lethargy and fatigue. The accompanying increase in cardiac output may be manifested as palpitations and a systolic murmur. Shortness of breath may also be a part of the syndrome.

If decreased Hb levels are detrimental, then increasing Hb content should increase the maximal O_2 content, thus providing a competitive advantage for athletes. Even in normal individuals, [Hb] in RBC cytoplasm is already extremely high. Hypoxia (e.g., adaptation to high altitude) leads to the increased production of erythropoietin, a hormone that somewhat increases the amount of Hb per erythrocyte but especially increases RBC number. Indeed, a few instances have been highly publicized in the international press in which elite athletes have infused themselves with erythrocytes or injected themselves with recombinant erythropoietin. However, an excessive increase

Table 29-1 Summary of a-$\bar{v}$ Difference in O_2 Composition of Blood

	P_{O_2} (mm Hg)	Hb Saturation (S_{O_2})	O_2 Bound to Hb (mL/dL)*	O_2 Dissolved (mL/dL)	Total O_2 Content (mL/dL)
a	100	97.5%	19.7	0.3	20.0
$\bar{v}$	40	75%	15.2	~0.1	15.3
a-$\bar{v}$ difference	60	22.5%	4.5	~0.2	4.7

*Assuming a hemoglobin content of 15 g Hb/dL blood and an O_2 capacity of 1.35 mL O_2/g Hb. Here, fully saturated hemoglobin would carry 20.3 mL O_2/dL blood.

in hematocrit—**polycythemia**—has the adverse effect of increasing blood viscosity and thus vascular resistance (see Chapter 17). The consequences include increased blood pressure in both the systemic and pulmonary circulations and a mismatch of ventilation to perfusion within the lung. Such a ventilation-perfusion mismatch leads to hypoxia (see Chapter 31) and thus *desaturation* of arterial Hb. Thus, the optimal hematocrit—presumably ~45%—is one that achieves a high maximal O_2 content but at a reasonable blood viscosity.

The purplish color of desaturated Hb produces the physical sign known as **cyanosis**, a purplish coloration of the skin and mucous membranes. Cyanosis results not from the *absence* of saturated or oxygenated Hb but from the *presence* of desaturated Hb. Thus, an anemic patient with poorly saturated Hb might have too little unsaturated Hb for it to be manifested as cyanosis. The physician's ability to detect cyanosis also depends on other factors, such as the subject's skin pigmentation and the lighting conditions for the physical examination.

Increases in temperature, [CO₂], and [H⁺], all of which are characteristic of metabolically active tissues, cause hemoglobin to dump O₂

Metabolically active tissues not only have a high demand for O_2, they also are warm, produce large amounts of CO_2, and are acidic. Indeed, high temperature, high P_{CO_2}, and low pH of metabolically active tissues all decrease the O_2 affinity of Hb by acting at nonheme sites to shift the equilibrium between the T and R states of Hb more toward the low-affinity T state. The net effect is that metabolically active tissues can signal Hb in the *systemic* capillaries to release more O_2 than usual, whereas less active tissues can signal Hb to release less. In the *pulmonary* capillaries—where temperature is lower than in active tissues, P_{CO_2} is relatively low, and pH is high—these same properties promote O_2 uptake by Hb.

Temperature Increasing the temperature causes the Hb-O_2 dissociation curve to *shift to the right*, whereas decreasing the temperature has the opposite effect (Fig. 29-4). Compar-

---

Forms of Hemoglobin

The normal **adult form of hemoglobin** ($\alpha_2\beta_2$), known as HbA, is only one of several normal forms that are present in prenatal or postnatal life. Some of these other hemoglobins contain naturally occurring α-like chains (e.g., α and ζ) or β-like chains (e.g., β, γ, δ, and ϵ); others reflect post-translational modifications. Three genes for α-**like chains** (all encoding 141 amino acids) cluster on chromosome 16; at the 5' end of the cluster is one gene for a ζ chain, followed by two for the α chain. Pseudogenes for ζ and α are also present. Five genes for β-**like chains** (all encoding 146 amino acids) are clustered on chromosome 11; starting at the 5' end is one for ϵ, followed by two for γ (γ_G coding for glycine at position 136, γ_A for alanine), and one each for δ and β. A pseudogene for β is also present. A locus control region regulates the expression of these β-like chains during development (see Chapter 4).

The four **prenatal hemoglobins** (Table 29-2) consist of various combinations of two α-like chains (e.g., α and ζ) and two β-like chains (e.g., ϵ and γ). Very early in life, when erythropoiesis occurs in the yolk sac, the Hb products are the three **embryonic hemoglobins**. When erythropoiesis shifts to the liver and spleen at ~10 weeks of gestation, the Hb product is **fetal hemoglobin**, or HbF ($\alpha_2\gamma_2$). Erythrocytes containing HbF have a higher O_2 affinity than do those containing HbA owing to special properties of γ chains. The newborn's blood contains both HbA and HbF; the HbF gradually falls by 1 year of age to the minute levels that are characteristic of the adult (rarely more than 1% to 2% of total Hb). With severe stress to the erythroid system—such as marked hemolysis, bone marrow failure, or recovery from bone marrow transplantation—immature erythroid precursors may be forced to mature before they have differentiated sufficiently to produce HbA. In these conditions, circulating levels of HbF may increase considerably. In some hereditary cases, normal HbF persists in the adult, with no clinically significant consequences.

Even adult blood contains several normal **minor-component hemoglobins** (Table 29-3), which account for 5% to 10% of the total blood Hb. In HbA₂ (~2.5% of total Hb), δ chains replace the β chains of HbA. Although the physiological significance of HbA₂ is unknown, the δ chains reduce the sickling of sickle hemoglobin (see later). Three other minor-component hemoglobins are the result of the nonenzymatic glycosylation of HbA. HbA₁ₐ, HbA₁ᵦ, and HbA₁ᵤ form when intracellular glucose 6-phosphate (G6P) reacts with the terminal amino groups of the β chains of HbA. In poorly controlled diabetes mellitus, a disease characterized by decreased insulin or insulin sensitivity (see Chapter 51), blood glucose concentrations rise and, with them, intracellular concentrations of G6P. As a result, glycosylated hemoglobins may represent 10% or more of the total Hb. Because Hb glycosylation is irreversible, and because the RBC has a mean lifetime of 120 days, levels of these glycosylated hemoglobins are clinically useful for assessing the long-term control of blood glucose levels in diabetics.

Numerous abnormal hemoglobins exist, most of which are caused by single amino acid substitutions on one of the polypeptide chains. One of the most clinically important is HbS, or **sickle hemoglobin**, in which a valine replaces the glutamate normally present at position 6 of the β chain. Although oxygenated HbS has a normal solubility, deoxygenated HbS is only about half as soluble as deoxygenated HbA. As a result, in low-O_2 environments, HbS can crystallize into long fibers, giving the cells a sickle-like appearance. The sickled erythrocytes may disrupt blood flow in small vessels, causing many of the acute symptoms of sickle cell crisis, including pain, renal dysfunction, retinal bleeding, and aseptic necrosis of bone. In addition, sickle cells are prone to hemolysis (mean lifetime, <20 days), leading to a chronic **hemolytic anemia**.

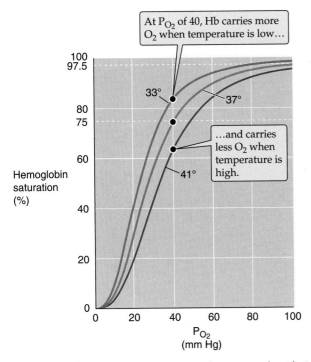

At P_{O_2} of 40, Hb carries more O_2 when temperature is low...

...and carries less O_2 when temperature is high.

33°   37°

41°

Figure 29-4 The effect of temperature changes on the Hb-O_2 dissociation curve.

Table 29-2 Subunit Structures of Prenatal and Minor-Component Hemoglobins

Hemoglobin	α-Like Subunit	β-Like Subunit	Time of Expression
Gower 1	ζ	ε	Embryonic
Gower 2	α	ε	Embryonic
Portland	ζ	γ	Embryonic
HbF (fetal)	α	γ	Fetal
HbA$_2$	α	δ	Postnatal
HbA (adult)	α	β	Postnatal

Table 29-3 Makeup of Total Hemoglobin in Adult Human Blood

Hemoglobin Type	Fraction of Total Hemoglobin
HbA	~92%
HbA$_{1a}$	0.75%
HbA$_{1b}$	1.5%
HbA$_{1c}$	3%-6%
HbA$_2$	2.5%
Total	100%

ing the three Hb-O_2 dissociation curves in Figure 29-4 at the P_{O_2} of mixed-venous blood (40 mm Hg), we see that the amount of O_2 bound to Hb becomes progressively less at higher temperatures. In other words, high temperature decreases the O_2 affinity of Hb, releasing O_2. One mechanism of this temperature effect may be small shifts in the pK values of various amino acid side chains, which cause shifts in net charge and thus a conformational change.

The maximal temperatures achieved in active muscle are ~40°C. Of course, very low temperatures can prevail in the skin of extremities exposed to extreme cold.

Acid In 1904, Christian Bohr, a physiologist and father of atomic physicist Niels Bohr, observed that respiratory acidosis shifts the Hb-O_2 dissociation curve to the right (Fig. 29-5A). This decrease in O_2 affinity has come to be known as the **Bohr effect**. A mild respiratory acidosis occurs physiologically as erythrocytes enter the systemic capillaries. There, the increase in extracellular P_{CO_2} causes CO_2 to enter erythrocytes, leading to a fall in intracellular pH (see Chapter 28). Other acidic metabolites may also lower extracellular and therefore intracellular pH. Thus, this intracellular respiratory acidosis has two components—a decrease in pH and an increase in P_{CO_2}. We now appreciate that *both* contribute to the rightward shift of the Hb-O_2 dissociation curve observed by Bohr.

The effect of acidosis on the Hb-O_2 dissociation curve (Fig. 29-5B)—**pH-Bohr effect**—accounts for most of the overall Bohr effect. One can readily demonstrate the pH-Bohr effect in a solution of Hb by imposing a metabolic acidosis (e.g., decreasing pH at a fixed P_{CO_2}). It should not be surprising that Hb is sensitive to changes in pH because Hb is an outstanding H$^+$ buffer (see Chapter 28):

$$Hb + H^+ \rightleftarrows Hb\text{—}H^+ \quad \text{(29-8)}$$

Although Hb has many titratable groups, the ones important here are those with pK values in the physiological pH range. As we acidify the solution, raising the ratio [Hb-H$^+$]/[Hb] for susceptible groups, we change the conformation of the Hb molecule, thus lowering its O_2 affinity:

$$Hb(O_2)_4 + 2H^+ \rightleftarrows Hb(H^+)_2 + 4O_2 \quad \text{(29-9)}$$

This is an extreme example in which we added enough H$^+$ to cause Hb to dump *all* of its O_2. Under more physiological conditions, the binding of ~0.7 mol of H$^+$ causes Hb to release 1 mole of O_2. This property is important in the systemic tissues, where [H$^+$] is high. The converse is also true: O_2 binding causes a conformational change in the Hb molecule, which lowers the affinity of Hb for H$^+$.

Carbon Dioxide The isolated effect of hypercapnia on the Hb-O_2 dissociation curve (Fig. 29-5C) represents a small portion of the overall Bohr effect. Demonstration of such a **CO_2-Bohr effect** requires that we study the O_2 affinity of Hb at a fixed pH, increasing P_{CO_2} and HCO$_3^-$ proportionally—an example of **isohydric hypercapnia**. As P_{CO_2} increases, CO_2 combines with unprotonated amino groups on Hb (Hb—NH$_2$) to form **carbamino groups** (Hb—NH—COO$^-$).

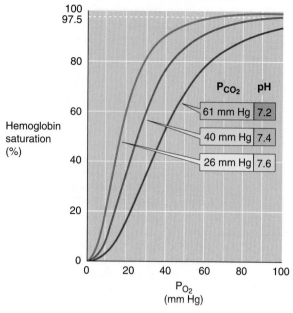

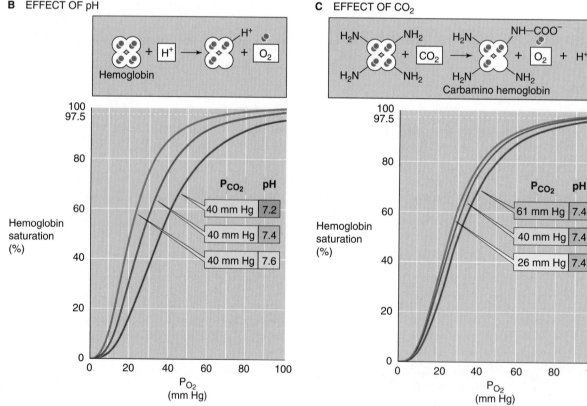

Figure 29-5 The effect of acidosis and hypercapnia on the Hb-O_2 dissociation curve (Bohr effect).

Although Hb has other amino groups, only the four amino termini of the globin chains are susceptible to appreciable carbamino formation, the β chains more so than the α chains. Because amino groups exist in a protonated form (Hb-NH_3^+) in equilibrium with an unprotonated form, the reaction of CO_2 with Hb-NH_2 tends to shift Hb away from the Hb-NH_3^+ form and toward the Hb-NH-COO^- form:

$$\text{Hb-NH}_3^+ \xrightarrow[]{\text{H}^+} \text{Hb-NH}_2 \xrightarrow[]{\text{CO}_2 \quad \text{H}^+} \text{Hb-NH-COO}^-$$

(29-10)

The overall effect of carbamino formation is therefore a negative shift in the charge on one amino acid side chain, causing a shift in the conformation of Hb and reducing its O_2 affinity:

$$(O_2)_4 \text{Hb-NH}_3^+ + CO_2 \rightleftharpoons (O_2)_3 \text{Hb-NH-COO}^- + O_2 + 2H^+$$

$$(29\text{-}11)$$

Thus, an increased P_{CO_2} causes Hb to unload O_2, which is important in the systemic tissues. Conversely, an increased P_{O_2} causes Hb to unload CO_2, which is important in the lungs.

In conclusion, the Hb-O_2 dissociation curve shifts to the right under conditions prevailing in the capillaries of metabolically active systemic tissues—increased temperature (Fig. 29-4), decreased pH (Fig. 29-5B), and increased P_{CO_2} (Fig. 29-5C). These right shifts are synonymous with decreased O_2 affinity. Thus, high metabolic rates promote the unloading of O_2 from Hb. Clearly, blood cannot unload O_2 unless the blood gets to the tissues. Indeed, in most systemic arterioles, local hypercapnia and acidosis also are powerful stimuli for vasodilation (see Chapter 24), enhancing O_2 *delivery* to metabolically active tissues.

2,3-Diphosphoglycerate reduces the affinity of adult but not of fetal hemoglobin

The affinity of Hb for O_2 is very sensitive to the presence of the glycolytic metabolite 2,3-diphosphoglycerate (2,3-DPG) and, to a lesser extent, organic phosphates such as adenosine triphosphate (ATP). The concentration of **2,3-DPG** is about the same as that of Hb. Indeed, 2,3-DPG binds to Hb in a 1:1 stoichiometry, interacting with a central cavity formed by the two β chains. At physiological pH, 2,3-DPG has an average of ~3.5 negative charges, which interact with 8 positively charged amino acid residues in this central cavity. O_2 binding, however, changes the shape of the central cavity, destabilizing DPG-bound Hb. As a result, deoxygenated Hb has a 100-fold higher affinity for 2,3-DPG than does oxygenated Hb. Conversely, binding of 2,3-DPG to Hb destabilizes the interaction of Hb with O_2, promoting the release of O_2:

$$\text{Hb}(O_2)_4 + 2,3\text{-DPG} \rightleftharpoons \text{Hb}(2,3\text{-DPG}) + 4O_2 \quad (29\text{-}12)$$

The result is a right shift in the Hb-O_2 dissociation curve (Fig. 29-6). This effect of 2,3-DPG on the O_2 affinity of Hb is important both in hypoxia and in understanding the physiology of fetal Hb.

Decrease of the P_{O_2} of RBCs stimulates glycolysis, leading to increased levels of 2,3-DPG. Indeed, chronic hypoxia, anemia, and acclimation to high altitude are all associated with an increase in 2,3-DPG levels, thus lowering the O_2 affinity of Hb. Reducing the affinity is a two-edged sword. At the relatively high P_{O_2} in alveoli, where the Hb-O_2 dissociation curve is fairly flat, this decrease in O_2 affinity reduces O_2 *uptake*—but only slightly. At the low P_{O_2} in systemic tissues, where the Hb-O_2 dissociation curve is steep, this decrease in O_2 affinity markedly increases the O_2 *release*. The net effect is enhanced O_2 unloading to metabolizing tissues, which is more important than P_{O_2} per se.

In Figure 29-7, the blue Hb-O_2 dissociation curve represents pure or "stripped" Hb (i.e., in the absence of CO_2, 2,3-DPG, and other organic phosphates). The O_2 affinity of pure Hb is quite high, as evidenced by the left shift of the curve.

Measuring the Oxygen Saturation of Hemoglobin Clinically: The Pulse Oximeter

The different colors of venous and arterial blood reflect the difference in light absorbance between oxygenated Hb and deoxygenated Hb. Clinicians now routinely exploit these differences to obtain simple, noninvasive measurements of the arterial O_2 saturation (Sa_{O_2}) of Hb in patients. The **pulse oximeter** has a probe that one attaches to the ear, finger, or any part of the body at which pulsating blood vessels are accessible externally. On one side of the pulsating vascular bed, the pulse oximeter shines red and infrared light; on the other side, it detects the light transmitted through the bed and calculates absorbances. These total absorbances have two components: (1) a nonpulsatile component that arises from stationary tissues, including blood inside capillaries and veins; and (2) a pulsatile component that arises from blood inside arterioles and arteries. The difference between the total and nonpulsatile absorbance is thus the pulsatile component, which represents only arterial or oxygenated blood. Because oxygenated Hb and deoxygenated Hb absorb red and infrared light differently, the pulse oximeter can calculate Sa_{O_2} from the ratio of pulsatile light absorbed at the two wavelengths. The pulse oximeter accomplishes this magic by using a sophisticated microprocessor and software to produce results that strongly agree with those provided by blood gas analysis of a sample of arterial blood.

The pulse oximeter measures Sa_{O_2} in arterial blood. Because systemic capillaries and veins do not pulsate, they do not contribute to the measurement. Thus, a patient with peripheral cyanosis (e.g., purple fingertips caused by cold-induced vasoconstriction) may have a perfectly normal "central" (i.e., arterial) Sa_{O_2}. Pulse oximetry cannot detect carbon monoxide poisoning because the absorbance spectra of Hb-CO and Hb-O_2 are similar.

Health professionals widely employ pulse oximetry in hospitalized patients, particularly those in intensive care units, where continuous monitoring of Sa_{O_2} is critical. These patients include those on mechanical ventilators and others, less severely ill, who suffer some degree of respiratory compromise. Pulse oximetry has also become popular as an outpatient tool for assessment of the presence of hypoxemia during sleep and thus for screening of **sleep apnea** (see Chapter 32 for the box on sleep apnea). Because of the insidious nature of hypoxia, pilots of light aircraft have begun to use pulse oximeters to detect developing hypoxia at high altitudes.

Adding only CO_2 (orange curve) or only 2,3-DPG (green curve) to the solution shifts the curve somewhat to the right, and adding both yields the brown curve that is indistinguishable from the red curve for intact RBCs under physiological conditions.

The fetal Hb (HbF) in fetal erythrocytes (see the box on forms of hemoglobin) has a higher O_2 affinity than the Hb inside adult RBCs (HbA). This difference is crucial for the fetus, whose blood must abstract O_2 from maternal blood in the placenta (see Chapter 56). The difference in

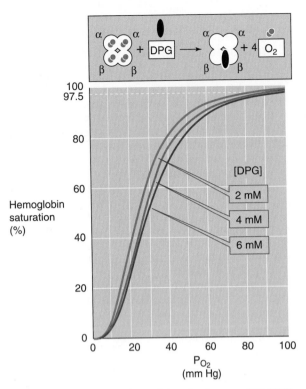

Figure 29-6 The effect of 2,3-diphosphoglycerate (2,3-DPG) on O_2 affinity of hemoglobin. After lowlanders spent about 2 days at an altitude of ~4500 m, their cytosolic [2,3-DPG] increased by ~50%, shifting the Hb-O_2 dissociation curve to the right.

O_2 affinities does not, however, reflect differences in O_2 affinities of *stripped* HbA and HbF, which are nearly identical. The crucial difference is that the γ chains of HbF bind 2,3-DPG less avidly than do the β chains of HbA. With less 2,3-DPG bound, the dissociation curve of HbF is left shifted, similar to the HbA curve labeled Hb + CO_2 in Figure 29-7.

O_2 is not the only gas that can bind to the Fe^{2+} of Hb; carbon monoxide (CO), nitric oxide (NO), and H_2S can also bind to Hb and snap it into the R state. In **carbon monoxide poisoning**, CO binds to Hb with an affinity that is ~200-fold greater than that of O_2. Thus, the maximal O_2 capacity falls to the extent that CO binds to Hb. However, the major reason that CO is toxic is that as it snaps Hb into the R state, CO increases the O_2 affinity of Hb and shifts the Hb-O_2 dissociation curve far to the left. Thus, when Hb reaches the systemic capillaries in CO poisoning, its tenacity for O_2 is so high that the bright red blood cannot release enough O_2 to the tissues.

CARRIAGE OF CARBON DIOXIDE

Blood carries total CO_2 mainly as HCO_3^-

The blood carries CO_2 and related compounds in five forms:

1. **Dissolved CO_2.** $[CO_2]_{Dis}$ follows Henry's law (see Chapter 26 for the box on that topic), and it is in the millimolar range in both blood plasma and blood cells. It makes up only ~5% of the total CO_2 of arterial blood (gold portion of leftmost bar in Fig. 29-8).

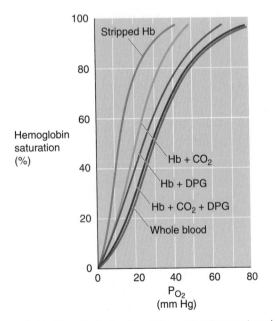

Figure 29-7 The effect of adding CO_2 or 2,3-DPG to stripped Hb. The four brown curves are Hb-O_2 dissociation curves for pure Hb (2 mM) in artificial solutions. Stripped Hb is devoid of both CO_2 and 2,3-DPG. When CO_2 or 2,3-DPG was present, P_{CO_2} was 40 mm Hg and [2,3-DPG] was 2.4 mM. The cytosol of erythrocytes in blood *(red curve)* had the same composition as the artificial solutions.

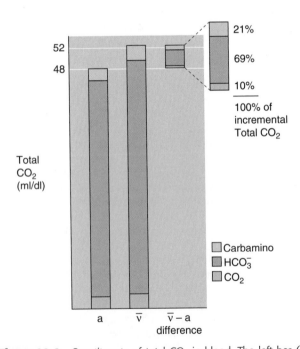

Figure 29-8 Constituents of total CO_2 in blood. The left bar (*a*) represents arterial blood; the *middle bar* ($\bar{v}$), mixed-venous blood; and the *right bar*, the incremental CO_2 that the blood picks up in the systemic capillaries.

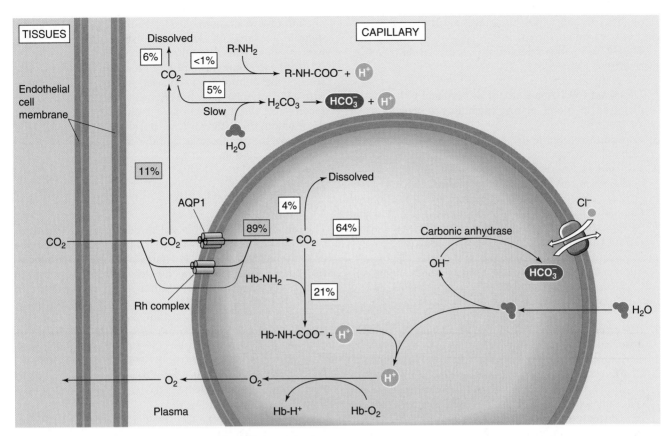

Figure 29-9 Carriage of CO_2 from systemic capillaries to the lungs.

2. **Carbonic acid.** H_2CO_3 can form either from CO_2 and H_2O or from H^+ and HCO_3^- (see Chapter 28). Because the equilibrium constant governing the reaction $CO_2 + H_2O \rightleftharpoons H_2CO_3$ is ~0.0025, $[H_2CO_3]$ is only $^1/_{400}$ as large as $[CO_2]$. Thus, H_2CO_3 is not quantitatively important for CO_2 carriage.

3. **Bicarbonate.** HCO_3^- can form in three ways. First, H_2CO_3 can dissociate into HCO_3^- and H^+. Second, CO_2 can combine directly with OH^- to form HCO_3^-, the reaction catalyzed by carbonic anhydrase. Third, HCO_3^- forms when carbonate combines with H^+. In arterial blood, HCO_3^- is ~24 mM, so that HCO_3^- represents ~90% of total CO_2 (purple portion of leftmost bar in Fig. 29-8).

4. **Carbonate.** CO_3^{2-} forms from the dissociation of bicarbonate: $HCO_3^- \rightarrow CO_3^{2-} + H^+$. Because the p$K$ of this reaction is so high (~10.3), $[CO_3^{2-}]$ is only ~$^1/_{1000}$ as high as HCO_3^- at pH 7.4. Thus, like H_2CO_3, CO_3^{2-} is not quantitatively important for CO_2 carriage.

5. **Carbamino compounds.** By far the most important carbamino compound is carbamino hemoglobin (Hb-NH-COO$^-$), which forms rapidly and reversibly as CO_2 reacts with free amino groups on Hb. In arterial blood, carbamino compounds account for ~5% of total CO_2 (blue portion of leftmost bar in Fig. 29-8).

The reason we group together these five CO_2-related compounds under the term **total CO_2** is that the method Van Slyke introduced in the 1920s—which remains the basis

for assay of blood HCO_3^- in modern clinical laboratories—cannot distinguish among the five.

CO_2 transport depends critically on carbonic anhydrase, the Cl-HCO$_3$ exchanger, and hemoglobin

The total CO_2 concentration of arterial blood is ~26 mM, or ~48 mL of CO_2 gas per deciliter (measured at STP). HCO_3^- constitutes ~90% of this 48 mL/dL, with CO_2 and carbamino compounds contributing ~5% each (*a* bar in Fig. 29-8). As blood courses through the systemic capillary beds, it picks up ~4 mL/dL of CO_2, so that the total CO_2 of mixed-venous blood is ~52 mL/dL ($\bar{v}$ bar in Fig. 29-8). In what forms does blood carry this *incremental* 4 mL/dL of CO_2 to the lungs? About 10% of the incremental CO_2 moves as dissolved CO_2, ~69% as HCO_3^-, and ~21% as carbamino compounds (rightmost two bars in Fig. 29-8). Therefore, dissolved CO_2 and carbamino CO_2 are far more important for carrying *incremental* CO_2 to the lungs than we might have surmised, given their contribution to *total* CO_2 in arterial blood.

Figure 29-9 summarizes the events that occur as incremental CO_2 enters systemic capillaries. As fast as biological oxidations in the mitochondria produce CO_2, this gas diffuses out of cells, through the extracellular space, across the capillary endothelium, and into the blood plasma. Some of the incremental CO_2 (~11%) remains in blood plasma throughout its journey to the lungs, but most (~89%), at least initially, enters the RBCs.

The ~11% of the incremental CO_2 in plasma travels in three forms:

1. **Dissolved CO_2.** About 6% of incremental CO_2 remains dissolved in blood plasma (assuming a hematocrit of 40%).
2. **Carbamino compounds.** An insignificant amount forms carbamino compounds with plasma proteins.
3. **Bicarbonate.** About 5% of incremental CO_2 forms HCO_3^- in the plasma and remains in the plasma: $CO_2 + H_2O \rightarrow H_2CO_3 \rightarrow H^+ + HCO_3^-$. The amount of HCO_3^- that follows this path depends critically on non-HCO_3^- buffering power (see Chapter 28), which is very low in plasma (~5 mM/pH unit).

The remaining ~89% of incremental CO_2 enters the RBCs, predominantly through two "gas channels," **AQP1** and the Rh complex. This CO_2 also has three fates:

1. **Dissolved CO_2.** About 4% of incremental CO_2 remains dissolved inside the RBC.
2. **Carbamino compounds.** About 21% of incremental CO_2 forms carbamino compounds with Hb. Why does so much CO_2 travel as carbamino compounds inside the red cell, whereas so little does in the blood plasma? First, the Hb concentration inside RBCs (~33 g/dL) is far higher than that of albumin and globulins in plasma (~7 g/dL). Second, Hb forms carbamino compounds far more easily than do major plasma proteins. Moreover, Hb forms carbamino compounds even more easily as it loses O_2 in the systemic capillaries (reverse of the CO_2-Bohr effect). Finally, Hb is a far better buffer than the plasma proteins for the H^+ formed as a byproduct in carbamino formation and becomes an even better buffer as it loses O_2 in the systemic capillaries (reverse of the pH-Bohr effect).
3. **Bicarbonate.** About 64% of the incremental CO_2 forms HCO_3^-. Why does so much more CO_2 form HCO_3^- in the erythrocyte than in plasma? First, erythrocytes contain a high level of **carbonic anhydrases**, greatly accelerating the conversion of CO_2 to HCO_3^-. In the absence of enzyme, hardly any HCO_3^- would form inside erythrocytes during the brief time the cells spend in their passage through a typical systemic capillary. Second, the **Cl-HCO_3 exchanger AE1** (see Chapter 5) transports some of the newly formed HCO_3^- out of the cell, promoting formation of more HCO_3^-. This uptake of Cl^- in exchange for HCO_3^- is known as the chloride or Hamburger shift. Third, the buffering of H^+ by Hb (see point 2) also pulls the reaction to the right.

The combined effects of the described intracellular and extracellular events is that ~10% of incremental CO_2 formed in systemic tissues moves to the lungs as dissolved CO_2, 6% in plasma and 4% inside erythrocytes (gold portion of rightmost bar in Fig. 29-8). About 21% moves as carbamino compounds, almost exclusively inside erythrocytes as carbamino Hb (blue portion of rightmost bar in Fig. 29-8). Finally, ~69% of incremental CO_2 moves as HCO_3^-, 5% that forms in plasma and 64% that forms inside the RBC (purple portion of rightmost bar in Fig. 29-8). Because H_2O enters the cell during HCO_3^- formation, erythrocytes swell as they pass through systemic capillaries.

When mixed-venous blood (with a P_{CO_2} of ~46 mm Hg) reaches the pulmonary capillaries (surrounded by alveoli with a P_{CO_2} of only ~40 mm Hg), CO_2 moves from the erythrocytes and blood plasma into the alveolar air space. All of the reactions discussed earlier reverse. In the process, Cl^- and H_2O leave the erythrocytes, and the cells shrink.

The high P_{O_2} in the lungs causes the blood to dump CO_2

The carriage of total CO_2 in the blood depends on the three blood gas parameters—P_{CO_2}, plasma pH, and P_{O_2}. The three plots in the main portion of Figure 29-10 are **CO_2 dissociation curves**. Each plot shows how changes in P_{CO_2} affect the total CO_2 content of blood. Although pH per se does not appear in this diagram, pH decreases as P_{CO_2} increases along the x-axis (i.e., respiratory acidosis; see Chapter 28). The blue plot is the CO_2 dissociation curve when P_{O_2} is zero ($S_{O_2} \cong 0\%$ Hb). The next two plots are CO_2 dissociation curves for P_{O_2} values of 40 mm Hg ($S_{O_2} \cong 75\%$; purple) and 100 mm Hg ($S_{O_2} \cong 97.5\%$; red). The green line at the bottom of Figure 29-10 shows that the *dissolved* component of total CO_2 rises only slightly with increases in P_{CO_2}.

Three features of the CO_2 dissociation curves in Figure 29-10 are noteworthy:

1. **Near-linear relationship in the physiological range of P_{CO_2} and P_{O_2} values** (Fig. 29-10, inset). In contrast, the O_2 dissociation curve is highly nonlinear in its physiological range (i.e., 40 to 100 mm Hg).
2. **Up-shift of curve with decreasing P_{O_2}.** At any P_{CO_2}, total CO_2 content rises as P_{O_2} (or Hb saturation) falls—the **Haldane effect**. Thus, as blood enters systemic capillaries and releases O_2, the CO_2-carrying capacity rises so that blood picks up extra CO_2. Conversely, as blood enters the pulmonary capillaries and binds O_2, the CO_2-carrying capacity falls so that blood dumps extra CO_2 (Table 29-4). The Haldane effect is the flip side of the coin from the pH-Bohr and CO_2-Bohr effects. First, just as H^+ binding lowers the O_2 affinity of Hb (Equation 29-9), O_2 binding destabilizes protonated hemoglobin (Hb-H^+), promoting H^+ release. By mass action, this H^+ reduces CO_2-carrying capacity by favoring the formation of CO_2 from both carbamino Hb and HCO_3^- (Fig. 29-9). Second, just as carbamino formation lowers the O_2 affinity of Hb (Equation 29-11), O_2 binding destabilizes carbamino Hb (Hb-NH-COO$^-$), promoting CO_2 release.
3. **Steepness.** Because CO_2 dissociation curves (Fig. 29-10) are much steeper than O_2 dissociation curves (Fig. 29-3), P_{CO_2} must increase from 40 mm Hg in arterial blood to only 46 mm Hg in mixed-venous blood to increase the CO_2 content by the ~4 mL/dL of CO_2 required to remove CO_2 as fast as the mitochondria produce it. In contrast, P_{O_2} must decrease from 100 to 40 mm Hg to dump enough O_2 to meet metabolic demands.

In the inset to Figure 29-10, point *a* on the red curve represents arterial blood, with a P_{CO_2} of 40 mm Hg and a P_{O_2}

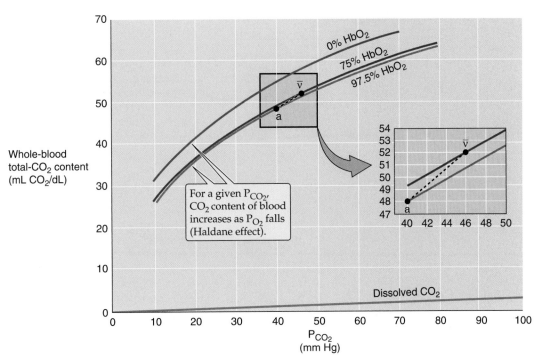

Figure 29-10 CO_2 dissociation curves (Haldane effect).

Table 29-4 Factors Affecting the Amount of Total CO_2 Carried by Blood

Parameter	Effects of Increasing the Parameter
P_{CO_2}	Increased $[CO_2]_{Dis}$ (Henry's law) Increased formation of HCO_3^- ($CO_2 + H_2O \rightarrow HCO_3^- + H^+$) Increased formation of carbamino ($CO_2 + Hb\text{-}NH_3^+ + \rightarrow Hb\text{-}NH\text{-}COO^- + 2H^+$)
[Plasma protein]	Increased plasma buffering power. The increased capacity for consuming H^+ indirectly promotes formation of HCO_3^-.
Plasma pH	Increased formation of HCO_3^- in plasma (Henderson-Hasselbalch equation) Increased pH inside red cell, promoting formation of HCO_3^- and carbamino hemoglobin
[Hemoglobin]	Increased formation of carbamino hemoglobin *(direct)* Increased buffering power inside erythrocyte. The increased capacity for consuming H^+ *indirectly* promotes formation of HCO_3^- and carbamino hemoglobin.
P_{O_2}	Decreased buffering power of hemoglobin (inverse of pH-Bohr effect). The decreased capacity for consuming H^+ indirectly restrains formation of HCO_3^- and carbamino hemoglobin. Decreased formation of carbamino hemoglobin (inverse of CO_2-Bohr effect)

of 100 mm Hg ($S_{O_2} \cong 97.5\%$). Point $\bar{v}$ on the purple curve represents mixed-venous blood, with a P_{CO_2} of 46 mm Hg but a P_{O_2} of only 40 mm Hg ($S_{O_2} \cong 75\%$). The difference between the total CO_2 contents represented by the two points (i.e., 52 versus 48 mL/dL) represents the 4 mL/dL of CO_2 the blood takes up as it passes through systemic capillaries. If it were not for the Haldane effect, the blood would remain on the red curve, and the P_{CO_2} increase would cause the CO_2 content to increase by only ~2.7 mL/dL. Thus, at a P_{CO_2} of 46 mm Hg, the fall in P_{O_2} that occurs as blood flows through systemic capillaries allows the blood to pick up ~50% more CO_2 (i.e., 4 versus 2.7 mL/dL). Viewed differently, if it were not for the Haldane effect, mixed-venous P_{CO_2} would have to increase to ~49 mm Hg for blood to carry 4 mL/dL of CO_2. Table 29-4 summarizes how changes in blood parameters can influence the amount of total CO_2 that the blood is able to carry.

The O_2-CO_2 diagram describes the interaction of P_{O_2} and P_{CO_2} in the blood

We have seen that Hb plays a key role in transporting O_2 from the lungs to peripheral tissues, transporting CO_2 in the opposite direction, and buffering H^+. These functions are intimately interrelated: P_{CO_2} and pH influence the O_2-Hb dissociation curve (Bohr effects; Fig. 29-5), and P_{O_2} influences the CO_2 dissociation curve (Haldane effect; Fig. 29-10). A useful way of illustrating this mutual dependence is the **O_2-CO_2 diagram**, which we will revisit in Chapter 31 to understand regional differences between alveolar P_{O_2} and P_{CO_2}.

On a coordinate system with P_{CO_2} on the ordinate and P_{O_2} on the abscissa, each blue curve in Figure 29-11 represents an **isopleth of identical O_2 content** in whole blood (from the Greek *isos* [equal] + *plethein* [to be full]). For example,

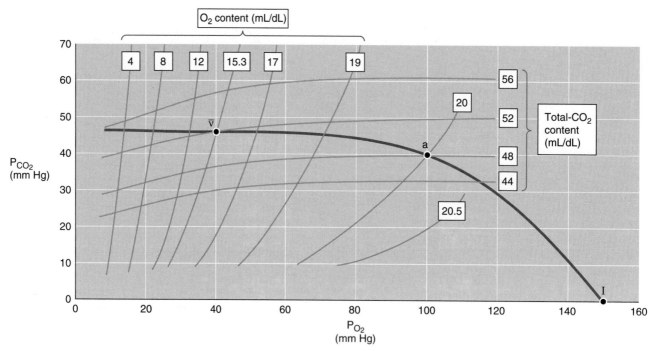

Figure 29-11   The O_2-CO_2 diagram.

arterial blood (point *a*) lies on the isopleth for an O_2 content of 20.0 mL/dL, with coordinates of P_{O_2} = 100 mm Hg and P_{CO_2} = 40 mm Hg. Following this isopleth from a P_{CO_2} of 40 mm Hg (point *a*) to, say, 46 mm Hg, we see that the blood could carry the same 20.0 mL/dL of O_2 only if we increase P_{O_2} from 100 to nearly 105 mm Hg. *Thus, as P_{CO_2} increases, the O_2 content of blood decreases (Bohr effect).* If it were not for the Bohr effect, all blue curves would be vertical lines. Mixed-venous blood (point $\bar{v}$) is on the O_2 content isopleth for 15.3 mL/dL, at a P_{O_2} of 40 mm Hg and a P_{CO_2} of 46 mm Hg. If blood were equilibrated with inspired air (point *I*), it would have a P_{O_2} of 150 mm Hg and a P_{CO_2} of 0.

Each red curve is an **isopleth of identical CO_2 content**. Arterial blood (point *a*) lies on the isopleth for 48 mL/dL. Similarly, mixed-venous blood (point $\bar{v}$) lies on the isopleth for 52 mL/dL. Following this 52 mL/dL isopleth from a P_{O_2} of 40 mm Hg (point $\bar{v}$) to, say, 100 mm Hg, we see that the blood could carry the same 52 mL/dL of CO_2 only if we increase P_{CO_2} from 46 to nearly 50 mm Hg. *Thus, as the P_{O_2} increases, the CO_2 content of blood decreases (Haldane effect).* If it were not for the Haldane effect, all red curves would be horizontal lines. Blood equilibrated with inspired air (point *I*) would have a CO_2 content of 0.

In Figure 29-11, the green curve connecting the points $\bar{v}$, *a*, and *I* represents all possible combinations of P_{O_2} and P_{CO_2} in normal lungs.

REFERENCES

Books and Reviews

Bauer C: Structural biology of hemoglobin. In Crystal RG, West JB (eds): The Lung, pp 1215-1223. New York: Lippincott-Raven, 1991.

Jelkmann W: Erythropoietin: Structure, control of production, and function. Physiol Rev 1992; 72:449-487.

Kilmartin JV, Rossi-Bernardi L: Interactions of hemoglobin with hydrogen ion, carbon dioxide and organic phosphates. Physiol Rev 1973; 53:836-890.

Klocke RA: Carbon dioxide. In Crystal RG, West JB (eds): The Lung, pp 1233-1239. New York: Lippincott-Raven, 1991.

Percy MJ, McFerran NV, Lappin TR: Disorders of oxidised haemoglobin. Blood Rev 2005; 19:61-68.

Journal Articles

Arnone A: X-ray studies of the interaction of CO_2 with human deoxyhaemoglobin. Nature 1974; 247:143-145.

Benesch R, Benesch RE: Intracellular organic phosphates as regulators of oxygen release by haemoglobin. Nature 1969; 221:618-622.

Endeward V, Musa-Aziz R, Boron WF, et al: Evidence that aquaporin 1 is a major pathway for CO_2 transport across the human erythrocyte membrane. FASEB J 2006; 20:1974-1981.

Perutz MF, Kilmartin JV, Nishidura K, et al: Identification of residues contributing to the Bohr effect of human haemoglobin. J Mol Biol 1980; 138:649-670.

Perutz MF, Lehmann H: Molecular pathology of human haemoglobin. Nature 1968; 219:902-909.

CHAPTER 30

GAS EXCHANGE IN THE LUNGS

Walter F. Boron

The complex anatomy of the pulmonary tree, the mechanics of the respiratory system, and the sophisticated carriage mechanisms for O_2 and CO_2 combine to serve two essential purposes: the ready diffusion of O_2 from the alveoli to the pulmonary capillary blood and the movement of CO_2 in the opposite direction. In this chapter, we consider principles that govern these diffusive events and factors that in certain diseases can limit gas exchange.

DIFFUSION OF GASES

Gas flow across a barrier is proportional to diffusing capacity (D_L) and concentration gradient (Fick's law)

Although, early on, physiologists thought that the lung actively secretes O_2 into the blood, we now know that the movements of both O_2 and CO_2 across the alveolar blood-gas barrier occur by simple **diffusion** (see Chapter 5). Random motion alone causes a net movement of molecules from areas of high concentration to areas of low concentration. Although diffusion per se involves no expenditure of energy, the body must do work—in the form of ventilation and circulation—to create the concentration gradients down which O_2 and CO_2 diffuse. Over short distances, diffusion can be highly effective.

Suppose that a barrier that is permeable to O_2 separates two air-filled compartments (Fig. 30-1A). The partial pressures (see Chapter 26 for the box on partial pressures and Henry's law) of O_2 on the two sides are P_1 and P_2. The probability that an O_2 molecule on side 1 will collide with the barrier and move to the opposite side is proportional to P_1:

$$Flow_{1 \to 2} \propto P_1 \qquad (30\text{-}1)$$

The **unidirectional movement** of O_2 in the opposite direction, from side 2 to side 1, is proportional to the partial pressure of O_2 on side 2:

$$Flow_{2 \to 1} \propto P_2 \qquad (30\text{-}2)$$

The **net movement** of O_2 from side 1 to side 2 is the difference between the two unidirectional flows:

$$Flow_{net} \propto (P_1 - P_2) \qquad (30\text{-}3)$$

Note that net flow is proportional to the difference in partial pressures, not the ratio. Thus, when P_1 is 100 mm Hg (or torr) and P_2 is 95 mm Hg (ratio of 1.05), the net flow is 5-fold greater than when P_1 is 2 mm Hg and P_2 is 1 mm Hg (ratio of 2).

The term **flow** describes the number of O_2 molecules moving across the entire area of the barrier per unit time (units: moles/s). If we normalize flow for the area of the barrier, the result is a **flux** [units: moles/($cm^2 \cdot s$)]. Respiratory physiologists usually measure the flow of a gas such as O_2 as the volume of gas (measured at standard temperature and pressure/dry; see Chapter 26) moving per unit time. V refers to the volume and $\dot{V}$ is its time derivative (volume of gas moving per unit time), or flow.

The proportionality constant in Equation 30-3 is the **diffusing capacity** for the lung, D_L [units: mL/(min · mm Hg)]. Thus, the flow of gas becomes

$$\dot{V}_{net} = D_L \cdot (P_1 - P_2) \qquad (30\text{-}4)$$

This equation is a simplified version of **Fick's law** (see Chapter 5), which states that net flow is proportional to the concentration gradient, expressed here as the partial pressure gradient.

Applying Fick's law to the diffusion of gas across the alveolar wall requires that we extend our model somewhat. Rather than a simple barrier separating two compartments filled with dry gas, a wet barrier covered with a film of water on one side will separate a volume filled with moist air from a volume of blood plasma at 37°C (Fig. 30-1B). Now we can examine how the physical characteristics of the gas and the barrier contribute to D_L.

Two *properties of the gas* contribute to D_L—molecular weight and solubility in water. First, the mobility of the gas should decrease as its molecular weight (MW) increases. Indeed, **Graham's law** states that diffusion is inversely proportional to the square root of MW. Second, Fick's law states

A DRY, HOMOGENEOUS BARRIER

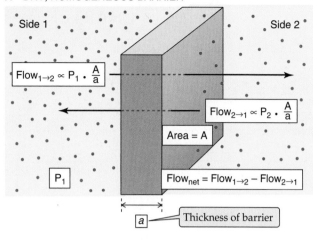

B ALVEOLAR WALL

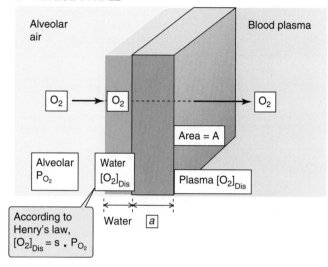

Figure 30-1 Diffusion of a gas across a barrier.

that the flow of the gas across the wet barrier is proportional to the *concentration* gradient of the gas dissolved in water. According to **Henry's law** (see Chapter 26 for the box on that topic), these concentrations are proportional to the respective partial pressures, and the proportionality constant is the solubility of the gas (s). Therefore, poorly soluble gases (e.g., N_2, He) diffuse poorly across the alveolar wall.

Two *properties of the barrier* contribute to D_L—area and thickness. First, the net flow of O_2 is proportional to the **area** (**A**) of the barrier, describing the odds that an O_2 molecule will collide with the barrier. Second, the net flow is inversely proportional to the **thickness** (**a**) of the barrier, including the water layer. The thicker the barrier, the smaller the O_2 partial pressure gradient ($\Delta P_{O_2}/a$) through the barrier (Fig. 30-2). An analogy is the slope of the trail that a skier takes from a mountain peak to the base. Whether the skier takes a steep expert trail or a shallow beginner's trail, the endpoints of the journey are the same. However, the trip is much faster along the steeper trail!

Finally, a combined property of both the barrier and the gas also contributes to D_L, a proportionality constant k that describes the interaction of the gas with the barrier.

Replacing D_L in Equation 30-4 with an area, solubility, thickness, molecular weight, and the proportionality constant (k):

$$\dot{V}_{net} = \underbrace{\left[k \frac{A \cdot s}{a \sqrt{MW}} \right]}_{D_L} (P_1 - P_2) \qquad (30\text{-}5)$$

Equations 30-4 and 30-5 are analogous to **Ohm's law** for electricity:

$$I = \left(\frac{1}{R} \right) \cdot \Delta V \qquad (30\text{-}6)$$

Electrical current (I) in Ohm's law corresponds to the net flow of gas ($\dot{V}_{net}$); the reciprocal of resistance (i.e., conductance) corresponds to diffusing capacity (D_L); and the voltage

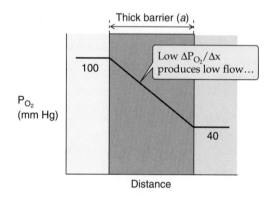

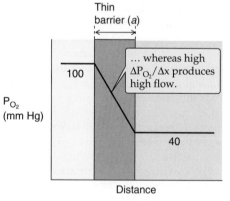

Figure 30-2 Effect of barrier thickness.

difference (ΔV) that drives electrical current corresponds to the pressure difference ($P_1 - P_2$ or ΔP).

The total flux of a gas between alveolar air and blood is the summation of multiple diffusion events along each pulmonary capillary during the respiratory cycle

Equation 30-5 describes O_2 diffusion between two compartments whose properties are uniform both spatially and temporally. Does this equation work for the lungs? If we assume that the alveolar air, blood-gas barrier, and pulmonary capillary blood are uniform in space and time, then the net diffusion of O_2 ($\dot{V}_{O_2}$) from alveolar air to pulmonary capillary blood is

$$\dot{V}_{O_2} = \underbrace{\left[k \frac{A \cdot s}{a\sqrt{MW}} \right]}_{D_{L_{O_2}}} (P_{A_{O_2}} - P_{c_{O_2}}) \qquad (30\text{-}7)$$

$D_{L_{O_2}}$ is the diffusing capacity for O_2, $P_{A_{O_2}}$ is the O_2 partial pressure in the alveolar air, and $P_{c_{O_2}}$ is the comparable parameter in pulmonary capillary blood. Although Equation 30-7 may seem sophisticated, a closer examination reveals that $D_{L_{O_2}}$, $P_{A_{O_2}}$, and $P_{c_{O_2}}$ are more complicated than they at first appear.

$D_{L_{O_2}}$ Among the five terms that make up $D_{L_{O_2}}$, two vary both temporally (during the respiratory cycle) and spatially (from one piece of alveolar wall to another). During inspiration, lung expansion causes the surface area (A) available for diffusion to increase and the thickness of the barrier (a) to decrease (Fig. 30-3A). Because of these *temporal* differences, $D_{L_{O_2}}$ should be maximal at the end of inspiration. However, even at one instant in time, barrier thickness—and the surface area of alveolar wall with this thickness—differs among pieces of alveolar wall. These *spatial* differences exist both at rest and during the respiratory cycle.

$P_{A_{O_2}}$ Like area and thickness, alveolar P_{O_2} varies both temporally and spatially (Fig. 30-3B). In any given alveolus, $P_{A_{O_2}}$ is greatest during inspiration (when O_2-rich air enters the lungs) and least just before the initiation of the next inspiration (after perfusion has maximally drained O_2 from the alveoli), as discussed in Chapter 31. These are *temporal* differences. We will see that when an individual is standing, $P_{A_{O_2}}$ is greatest near the lung apex and least near the base (see Chapter 31). Moreover, mechanical variations in the resistance of conducting airways and the compliance of alveoli cause ventilation—and thus P_{O_2}—to vary among alveoli. These are *spatial* differences.

$P_{c_{O_2}}$ As discussed later, as the blood flows down the capillary, capillary P_{O_2} rises to match $P_{A_{O_2}}$ (Fig. 30-3C). Therefore, O_2 diffusion is maximal at the beginning of the pulmonary capillary and gradually falls to zero farther along the capillary. Moreover, this profile varies during the respiratory cycle.

The complications that we have raised for O_2 diffusion apply as well to CO_2 diffusion. Of these complications, by far the most serious is the change in $P_{c_{O_2}}$ with distance along the pulmonary capillary. How, then, can we use Fick's law to understand the diffusion of O_2 and CO_2? Clearly, we cannot insert a single set of fixed values for $D_{L_{O_2}}$, $P_{A_{O_2}}$, and $P_{c_{O_2}}$ into Equation 30-7 and hope to describe the overall flow of O_2 between all alveoli and their pulmonary capillaries throughout the entire respiratory cycle. However, Fick's law does describe gas flow between air and blood for a *single piece of alveolar wall* (and its apposed capillary wall) at a *single time* during the respiratory cycle. For O_2:

$$\begin{array}{c} \dot{V}_{O_2}\text{ for one piece} \\ \text{of alveolar wall,} \\ \text{at one time} \end{array} = \underbrace{\left[k \frac{A \cdot s}{a\sqrt{MW}} \right]}_{D_{L_{O_2}}} (P_{A_{O_2}} - P_{c_{O_2}}) \qquad (30\text{-}8)$$

For one piece of alveolar wall and at one instant in time, A and a (and thus $D_{L_{O_2}}$) have well-defined values, as do $P_{A_{O_2}}$ and $P_{c_{O_2}}$. The total amount of O_2 flowing from all alveoli to all pulmonary capillaries throughout the entire respiratory cycle is simply the sum of all individual diffusion events, added up over all pieces of alveolar wall (and their apposed pieces of capillary wall) and over all times in the respiratory cycle:

$$\text{Overall } \dot{V}_{O_2} = \overset{\substack{\text{All pieces} \\ \text{of alveolar} \\ \text{wall}}}{\sum} \overset{\substack{\text{All times} \\ \text{in respiratory} \\ \text{cycle}}}{\sum} \left(D_{L_{O_2}}(P_{A_{O_2}} - P_{c_{O_2}}) \right)$$

$$(30\text{-}9)$$

Here, $D_{L_{O_2}}$, $P_{A_{O_2}}$, and $P_{c_{O_2}}$ are the "microscopic" values for one piece of alveolar wall, at one instant in time.

Even though the version of Fick's law in Equation 30-9 does indeed describe O_2 diffusion from alveolar air to pulmonary capillary blood—and a comparable equation would do the same for CO_2 diffusion in the opposite direction—it is not of much practical value for *predicting* O_2 uptake. However, we can easily compute the uptake of O_2 *that has already taken place* by use of the **Fick principle** (see Chapter 17). The rate of O_2 uptake by the lungs is the difference between the rate at which O_2 leaves the lungs through the pulmonary veins and the rate at which O_2 enters the lungs through the pulmonary arteries. The rate of O_2 *departure from* the lungs is the product of blood flow (i.e., cardiac output, $\dot{Q}$) and the O_2 content of pulmonary venous blood, which is virtually the same as that of systemic arterial blood (Ca_{O_2}). Remember that "content" (see Chapter 29) is the sum of dissolved O_2 and O_2 bound to hemoglobin (Hb). Similarly, the rate of O_2 *delivery to* the lungs is the product of $\dot{Q}$ and the O_2 content of pulmonary arterial blood, which is the same as that of the mixed-venous blood ($C\bar{v}_{O_2}$). Thus, the difference between the rates of O_2 departure and O_2 delivery is

$$\overset{\substack{\text{Rate of} \\ O_2\text{ uptake} \\ \text{by lungs}}}{\overbrace{\text{Overall }\dot{V}_{O_2}}} = \overset{\substack{\text{Rate of} \\ O_2\text{ departure} \\ \text{from lungs}}}{\overbrace{\dot{Q} \cdot Ca_{O_2}}} - \overset{\substack{\text{Rate of} \\ O_2\text{ delivery} \\ \text{to lungs}}}{\overbrace{\dot{Q} \cdot C\bar{v}_{O_2}}} \qquad (30\text{-}10)$$

$$= \dot{Q} \cdot (Ca_{O_2} - C\bar{v}_{O_2})$$

For a cardiac output of 5 L/min, a Ca_{O_2} of 20 mL O_2/dL blood, and a $C\bar{v}_{O_2}$ of 15 mL O_2/dL blood, the rate of O_2 uptake by the pulmonary capillary blood is

$$\overset{\substack{\text{Rate of} \\ O_2\text{ uptake} \\ \text{by lungs}}}{\overbrace{\text{Overall }\dot{V}_{O_2}}} = \overset{\text{Cardiac output}}{\overbrace{\frac{5000 \text{ mL of blood}}{\text{min}}}} \times (20-15)\overset{\substack{a-\bar{v}\text{ difference of} \\ O_2\text{ content}}}{\overbrace{\frac{\text{mL } O_2}{100 \text{ mL blood}}}}$$

$$= 250 \text{ mL } O_2 / \text{min}$$

$$(30\text{-}11)$$

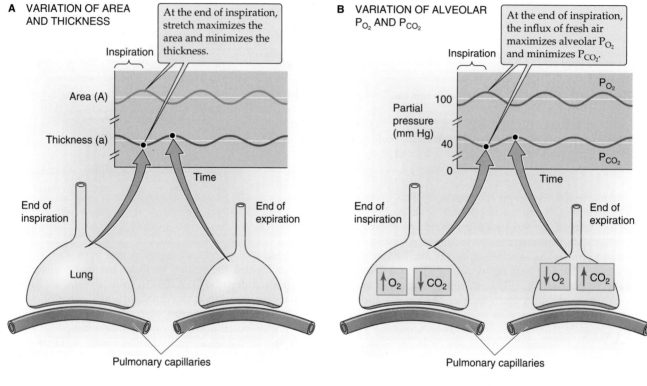

A VARIATION OF AREA AND THICKNESS

At the end of inspiration, stretch maximizes the area and minimizes the thickness.

Area (A)

Thickness (a)

Time

Inspiration

End of inspiration

Lung

End of expiration

Pulmonary capillaries

B VARIATION OF ALVEOLAR P_{O_2} AND P_{CO_2}

At the end of inspiration, the influx of fresh air maximizes alveolar P_{O_2} and minimizes P_{CO_2}.

Partial pressure (mm Hg)

100

40

0

P_{O_2}

P_{CO_2}

Time

Inspiration

End of inspiration

↑O_2 ↓CO_2

End of expiration

↓O_2 ↑CO_2

Pulmonary capillaries

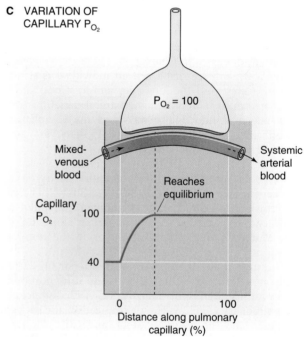

C VARIATION OF CAPILLARY P_{O_2}

$P_{O_2} = 100$

Mixed-venous blood

Systemic arterial blood

Reaches equilibrium

Capillary P_{O_2}

100

40

0   100

Distance along pulmonary capillary (%)

Figure 30-3 Complications of using Fick's law.

Figure 30-4 Transport of O_2 from alveolar air to hemoglobin (Hb). The 12 diffusion constants (D_1-D_{12}) govern 12 diffusive steps across a series of 12 barriers: (1) the interface between the alveolar air and water layer; (2) the water layer itself; (3-5) the two membranes and cytoplasm of the type I alveolar pneumocyte (i.e., epithelial cell); (6) the interstitial space containing the extracellular matrix; (7-9) the two membranes and cytoplasm of the capillary endothelial cell; (10) a thin layer of blood plasma (<0.2 μm in mammals); and (11-12) the membrane and cytoplasm of the erythrocyte. $\theta \cdot V_c$ describes how fast O_2 binds to Hb.

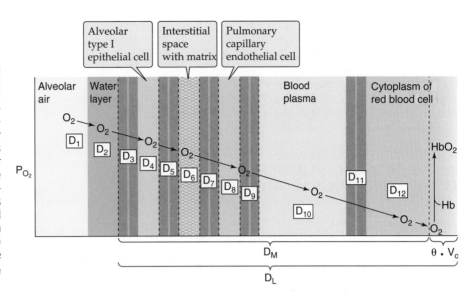

Obviously, the amount of O_2 that the lungs take up must be the same regardless of whether we *predict* it by repeated application of Fick's law of diffusion (Equation 30-9) or *measure* it by use of the Fick principle (Equation 30-10):

$$\underbrace{\overbrace{\sum_{\substack{\text{All pieces} \\ \text{of alveolar} \\ \text{wall}}} \overbrace{\sum_{\substack{\text{All times} \\ \text{in respiratory} \\ \text{cycle}}}}^{\text{Fick's law}} (D_{L_{O_2}}(P_{A_{O_2}} - P_{c_{O_2}}))}_{} = \overbrace{\dot{Q} \cdot (C_{a_{O_2}} - C_{\bar{v}_{O_2}})}^{\text{Fick principle}}$$

$$(30\text{-}12)$$

The flow of O_2, CO, and CO_2 between alveolar air and blood depends on the interaction of these gases with red blood cells

We have been treating O_2 transport as if it involved only the diffusion of the gas across a homogeneous barrier. In fact, the barrier is a three-ply structure comprising an alveolar epithelial cell, a capillary endothelial cell, and the intervening interstitial space containing extracellular matrix. The barrier is remarkable not only for its impressive surface area (50 to 100 m^2) and thinness (~0.6 μm) but also for its strength, which derives mainly from type IV collagen in the lamina densa of the basement membrane (often <50 nm) within the extracellular matrix.

One could imagine that as O_2 diffuses from the alveolar air to the Hb inside an erythrocyte (red blood cell), the O_2 must cross 12 discrete mini-barriers (Fig. 30-4). A mini-diffusing capacity (D_1-D_{12}) governs each of the 12 steps and contributes to a so-called **membrane diffusing capacity** (**D_M**) because it primarily describes how O_2 diffuses through various membranes. How do these mini-diffusing capacities contribute to D_M? Returning to our electrical model (Equation 30-6), we recognize that D is analogous to the reciprocal of resistance. Therefore, we can represent the 12 diffusive steps by 12 resistors in series. Because the total resistance is the sum of the individual resistances, the reciprocal of D_M is the sum of the reciprocals of the mini-diffusing capacities:

$$\frac{1}{D_M} = \frac{1}{D_1} + \frac{1}{D_2} + \frac{1}{D_3} + \cdots + \frac{1}{D_{10}} + \frac{1}{D_{11}} + \frac{1}{D_{12}} \quad (30\text{-}13)$$

Of course, these parameters vary with location in the lung and position in the respiratory cycle.

For most of the O_2 entering the blood, the final step is binding to Hb (see Chapter 29), which occurs at a finite rate:

$$\text{Rate of } O_2 \text{ uptake by hemoglobin} = (\theta \cdot V_c)P_{O_2} \quad (30\text{-}14)$$

θ is a rate constant that describes how many milliliters of O_2 gas bind to the Hb in 1 mL of blood each minute and for each millimeter of mercury (mm Hg) of partial pressure. V_c is the volume of blood in the pulmonary *capillaries*. The product $\theta \cdot V_c$ has the same dimensions as D_M [units: mL/(min · mm Hg)], and both contribute to the overall diffusing capacity:

$$\frac{1}{D_L} = \frac{1}{D_M} + \frac{1}{\theta \cdot V_c} \quad (30\text{-}15)$$

Because O_2 binds to Hb so rapidly, its "Hb" term $1/(\theta \cdot V_c)$ is probably only ~5% as large as its "membrane" term $1/D_M$.

For CO, which binds to Hb even more tightly than does O_2 (see Chapter 29)—but far more slowly—$\theta \cdot V_c$ is quantitatively far more important. The overall uptake of CO, which pulmonary specialists use to compute D_L, seems to depend about equally on the D_M and $\theta \cdot V_c$ terms.

As far as the movement of CO_2 is concerned, one might expect the D_L for CO_2 to be substantially higher than that for O_2, inasmuch as the solubility of CO_2 in water is ~23-fold higher than that of O_2 (see Chapter 26). However, measurements show that $D_{L_{CO_2}}$ is only 3- to 5-fold greater than $D_{L_{O_2}}$. The likely explanation is that the interaction of CO_2 with the red blood cell is more complicated than that for O_2, involving interactions with Hb, carbonic anhydrase, and the Cl-HCO_3 exchanger (see Chapter 29).

In summary, the movement of O_2, CO, and CO_2 between the alveolus and the pulmonary capillary involves not only diffusion but also interactions with Hb. Although these interactions have only a minor effect on the diffusing capacity for O_2, they are extremely important for CO and CO_2. Although we will generally refer to "diffusing capacity" as if it represented only the diffusion across a homogeneous barrier, one must keep in mind its more complex nature.

DIFFUSION AND PERFUSION LIMITATIONS ON GAS TRANSPORT

The diffusing capacity normally limits the uptake of carbon monoxide from alveolar air to blood

Imagine that a subject breathes air containing a very low level of CO, say 0.1%, for a brief time. Breathing of higher levels of CO for longer periods could be fatal because CO,

which binds to Hb with an affinity that is 200 to 300 times higher than that of O_2, prevents Hb from releasing O_2 to the tissues (see Chapter 29). If we assume that barometric pressure (P_B) is 760 mm Hg and that P_{H_2O} is 47 mm Hg at 37°C, then we can compute the P_{CO} of the wet inspired air entering the alveoli (see Chapter 26 for the box on wet gases):

$$
P_{CO} = \overbrace{F_{I_{CO}}}^{\substack{\text{Fraction of inspired} \\ \text{dry air that is CO}}} \cdot (P_B - P_{H_2O}) \tag{30-16}
$$
$$
= 0.1\% \cdot (760 - 47)\,\text{mm Hg}
$$
$$
= {\sim}0.7\,\text{mm Hg}
$$

If the subject smokes cigarettes or lives in a polluted environment, CO will be present in the mixed-venous blood—and therefore the alveolar air—even before our test begins. If not, the initial P_{CO} of the mixed-venous blood entering the pulmonary capillaries will be ~0 mm Hg. Thus, a small gradient (~0.7 mm Hg) drives CO diffusion from alveolar air into blood plasma (Fig. 30-5A). As CO enters the blood plasma, it diffuses into the cytoplasm of red blood cells,

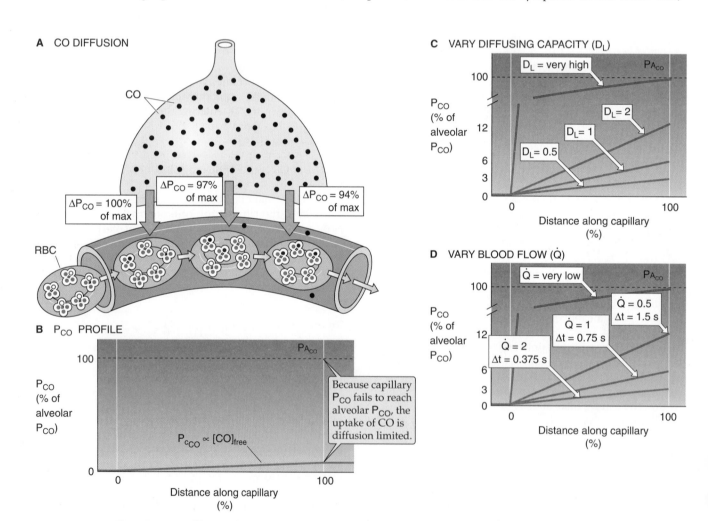

Figure 30-5 Diffusion of CO. In **A,** ΔP_{CO} is CO partial pressure gradient from alveolar air to pulmonary capillary blood. As the red blood cell (RBC) enters the capillary, O_2 occupies three of the four sites on hemoglobin. In **B,** PA_{CO} is alveolar P_{CO}. In **C,** the blood flow Q̇ has a relative value of 1. In **D,** the diffusing capacity D_L has a relative value of 1. Because P_{CO} is very low in **B-D,** we are on the linear portion of the Hb-CO dissociation curve. Thus, the CO content at the end of the capillary is approximately proportional to the capillary P_{CO}.

where Hb binds it avidly. The flow of CO from alveolus to red blood cell is so slow, and the affinity and capacity of Hb to bind CO is so great, that Hb binds almost all incoming CO. Because only a small fraction of the total CO in the pulmonary capillary blood remains free in solution, the aqueous phase of the blood remains nearly a perfect sink for CO. That is, P_{CO} in the capillary (Pc_{CO}), which is proportional to *free* [CO] in the capillary, rises only slightly above 0 mm Hg as the blood courses down the capillary (Fig. 30-5B). Thus, by the time the blood reaches the end of the capillary (~0.75 second later), Pc_{CO} is still far below alveolar P_{CO} (PA_{CO}). In other words, CO fails to reach **diffusion equilibrium** between the alveolus and the blood.

There are two reasons that Pc_{CO} rises so slowly as blood flows down the pulmonary capillary:

1. **The CO flux ($\dot{V}_{CO}$) is low.** According to Fick's law, $\dot{V}_{CO} = D_{L_{CO}} (PA_{CO} - Pc_{CO})$. Because we chose to use an extremely low inspired P_{CO}, the alveolar P_{CO} driving CO diffusion was likewise extremely low, causing Pc_{CO} to rise slowly. In addition, the physiological $D_{L_{CO}}$ is moderate.
2. **Hb continuously traps incoming CO.** Hb has a high affinity and high capacity for CO. Thus, for a low $\dot{V}_{CO}$, Pc_{CO}—proportional to the free [CO]—rises very slowly.

We will now explore factors that influence how much CO the blood takes up as it flows down the capillary. The principles that we develop here apply equally well to O_2 and CO_2. First, we use the Fick principle (Equation 30-10) to quantitate, after the fact, how much CO has entered the blood:

$$\text{Overall } \dot{V}_{CO} = \dot{Q} \cdot (Cc'_{CO} - C\bar{v}_{CO}) \quad (30\text{-}17)$$

Overall $\dot{V}_{CO}$ is the total flow of CO along the entire length of all capillaries throughout the lungs, $\dot{Q}$ is cardiac output, Cc'_{CO} is the CO content of blood at the end of the pulmonary capillary (dissolved and bound to Hb), and $C\bar{v}_{CO}$ is the CO content of mixed-venous blood at the *beginning* of the capillary. If we assume that $C\bar{v}_{CO}$ is 0, then Equation 30-17 simplifies to

$$\text{Overall } \dot{V}_{CO} = \dot{Q} \cdot Cc'_{CO} \quad (30\text{-}18)$$

Of course, this overall $\dot{V}_{CO}$, computed from the Fick principle, must be the same as the sum of the individual diffusion events, computed from Fick's law (analogous to Equation 30-12):

$$\underbrace{\dot{Q} \cdot Cc'_{CO}}_{\text{Fick principle}} = \overbrace{\underbrace{\sum}_{\substack{\text{All pieces} \\ \text{of alveolar} \\ \text{wall}}} \underbrace{\sum}_{\substack{\text{All times} \\ \text{in respiratory} \\ \text{cycle}}} (D_{L_{CO}} \cdot (PA_{CO} - Pc_{CO}))}^{\text{Fick's law}}$$
$$(30\text{-}19)$$

How does CO uptake depend on $D_{L_{CO}}$ and $\dot{Q}$? For basal conditions, we assume that $D_{L_{CO}}$ and $\dot{Q}$ both have relative values of 1 and that the curve labeled $D_L = 1$ in Figure 30-5C describes the trajectory of Pc_{CO}. As a result, Cc'_{CO} also has a relative value of 1. According to the Fick principle, the total amount of CO moving into the blood along the capillary is

$$\begin{aligned} \text{Overall } \dot{V}_{CO} &= \dot{Q} \cdot Cc'_{CO} \\ &= 1 \cdot 1 \quad\quad\quad\quad (30\text{-}20) \\ &= 1 \end{aligned}$$

What would happen if we keep $\dot{Q}$ constant but double $D_{L_{CO}}$? Fick's law (Equation 30-19) predicts that the flow of CO into the blood for each diffusion event along the capillary would double. Thus, along the entire capillary, Pc_{CO} would rise twice as steeply (Fig. 30-5C, curve labeled $D_L = 2$) as before. As a result, Cc'_{CO} and thus $\dot{V}_{CO}$ would also double.

Halving of $D_{L_{CO}}$ would have the opposite effect: Cc'_{CO} and thus $\dot{V}_{CO}$ would also halve (Fig. 30-5C, bottom curve). Therefore, CO uptake is proportional to $D_{L_{CO}}$ over a wide range of $D_{L_{CO}}$ values (Table 30-1, upper half). Of course, if it were possible to make $D_{L_{CO}}$ extremely high, then capillary Pc_{CO} would rise so fast that CO would equilibrate with the Hb before the end of the capillary, and capillary Pc_{CO} would reach alveolar P_{CO} (Fig. 30-5C, top curve). However, for realistic values of $D_{L_{CO}}$—as well as low alveolar P_{CO} levels and normal Hb concentrations—CO would fail to reach equilibrium by the end of the capillary.

How would alteration of blood flow affect $\dot{V}_{CO}$? If $\dot{Q}$ were halved and the dimensions of the capillary remained constant, then the contact time of the blood with the alveolar capillary would double. Thus, at any distance down the capillary, twice as much cumulative time would be available for CO diffusion. The trajectory of capillary Pc_{CO} versus distance would be twice as steep (Fig. 30-5D, curve labeled $\dot{Q} = 0.5$) as in the basal state (curve labeled $\dot{Q} = 1$), and Cc'_{CO} would also be twice as great. However, because we achieved this increase in Cc'_{CO} by cutting $\dot{Q}$ in half, the product $\dot{Q} \cdot Cc'_{CO} = \dot{V}_{CO}$ would be the same as that in the basal state (Table 30-1, lower half).

Doubling of blood flow would cause capillary Pc_{CO} to rise only half as steeply (Fig. 30-5D, bottom curve) as in the basal state but still have no effect on $\dot{V}_{CO}$. Thus, for the range of D_L and $\dot{Q}$ values in this example, *CO uptake is unaffected by changes in blood flow.* Of course, if we were to reduce $\dot{Q}$ to

Table 30-1 Alveolar Transport of CO

	$D_{L_{CO}}$	$\dot{Q}$	×	Cc'_{CO}	=	$\dot{V}_{CO}$
Vary D_L ($\dot{Q}$ constant)	2	1		2		2
	1	1		1		1
	½	1		½		½
Vary $\dot{Q}$ (D_L constant)	1	½		2		1
	1	1		1		1
	1	2		½		1

$D_{L_{CO}}$ is the diffusing capacity of the lungs for CO. $\dot{Q}$ is the cardiac output. Cc'_{CO} is the CO content of the blood at the end of the capillary. $\dot{V}_{CO}$ is the overall rate of CO uptake by the pulmonary capillary blood. The values in the table are all relative to "control" values of unity.

extremely low values, then capillary P_{CO} would reach alveolar P_{CO} by the end of the capillary (Fig. 30-5D, top curve).

In our example, we have assumed that the Pc_{CO} profile along the capillary is linear and that changes in $\dot{Q}$ do not affect capillary dimensions. In fact, these assumptions are not entirely valid. Nevertheless, the uptake of CO is more or less proportional to the D_L for CO and rather insensitive to perfusion. Therefore, we say that the uptake of CO is **diffusion limited** because it is the diffusing capacity that predominantly limits CO transport. We can judge whether the transport of a gas is predominantly diffusion limited by comparing the partial pressure of the gas at the end of the pulmonary capillary with the alveolar partial pressure. *If the gas does not reach diffusion equilibrium (i.e., if the end-capillary partial pressure fails to reach the alveolar partial pressure), then transport is predominantly diffusion limited.* However, if the gas does reach diffusion equilibrium, then its transport is perfusion limited, as discussed next.

Perfusion normally limits the uptake of nitrous oxide from alveolar air to blood

Unlike CO, nitrous oxide ("laughing gas," N_2O) does not bind to Hb. Therefore, when a subject inhales N_2O, the gas enters the blood plasma and the red blood cell cytoplasm but has nowhere else to go (Fig. 30-6A). Consequently, as blood courses down the pulmonary capillary, the concentration of free N_2O—and thus capillary P_{N_2O} (Pc_{N_2O})—rises very rapidly (Fig. 30-6B). By the time the blood is ~10% of the way along the capillary, Pc_{N_2O} has reached alveolar P_{N_2O} (PA_{N_2O}), and N_2O is thus in diffusion equilibrium between alveolus and blood. The reason N_2O reaches diffusion equilibrium—whereas CO does not—is not that its $D_{L_{N_2O}}$ is particularly high or that we chose a high inspired P_{N_2O}. The key difference is that Hb does not bind to N_2O.

How does N_2O uptake by the lungs depend on $D_{L_{N_2O}}$ and $\dot{Q}$? If we assume that the N_2O content of the mixed-venous blood entering the pulmonary capillary ($C\bar{v}_{N_2O}$) is 0:

$$\text{Overall } \dot{V}_{N_2O} = \dot{Q} \cdot Cc'_{N_2O} \qquad (30\text{-}21)$$

Cc'_{N_2O} is the N_2O content of the blood at the end of the pulmonary capillary and represents entirely N_2O physically dissolved in blood, which according to Henry's law (see Chapter 26 for the box on that topic) is proportional to Pc_{N_2O}. The overall $\dot{V}_{N_2O}$ computed from the Fick principle in Equation 30-21 is the sum of individual diffusion events along the capillary:

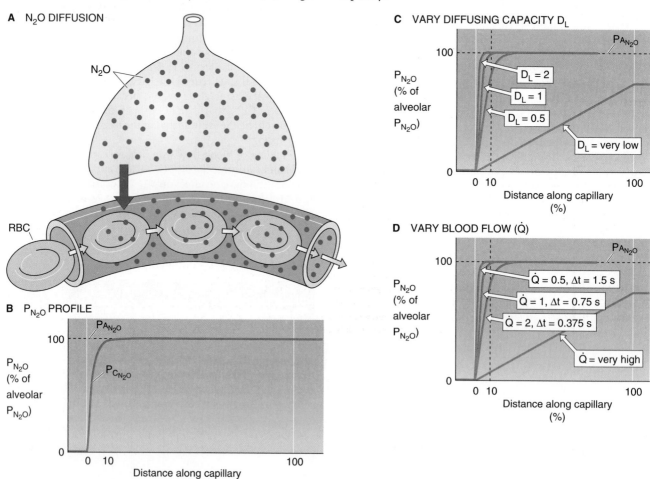

Figure 30-6 Diffusion of N_2O. In **B,** PA_{N_2O} is alveolar P_{N_2O} and Pc_{N_2O} is capillary P_{N_2O}. In **C,** the blood flow $\dot{Q}$ has a relative value of 1. In **D,** the diffusing capacity D_L has a relative value of 1. The N_2O content at the end of the capillary is proportional to P_{N_2O}.

$$\underbrace{\dot{Q} \cdot Cc'_{N_2O}}_{\text{Fick principle}} = \underbrace{\overbrace{\sum_{\substack{\text{All pieces} \\ \text{of alveolar} \\ \text{wall}}}^{\text{Fick's law}} \sum_{\substack{\text{All times} \\ \text{in respiratory} \\ \text{cycle}}} \left(D_{L_{N_2O}} \cdot (P_{A_{N_2O}} - P_{C_{N_2O}}) \right)}$$

(30-22)

Because N_2O reached diffusion equilibrium at ~10% of the way down the capillary (i.e., $P_{C_{N_2O}} = P_{A_{N_2O}}$), the individual diffusion terms in Equation 30-22 equate to 0 for the distal 90% of the capillary!

We can approach the uptake of N_2O in the same way we did the uptake of CO. We begin, under basal conditions, with relative values of 1 for $D_{L_{N_2O}}$, $\dot{Q}$, and end-capillary N_2O content. Thus, the initial $\dot{V}_{N_2O}$ is $\dot{Q} \times Cc'_{N_2O} = 1$.

Figure 30-6C shows that doubling of $D_{L_{N_2O}}$ doubles the flow of N_2O into the blood for each diffusion event, causing $P_{C_{N_2O}}$ to rise twice as steeply as before along the capillary. However, even though this doubling of $D_{L_{N_2O}}$ causes N_2O to come into diffusion equilibrium twice as fast as before, it has no effect on either the N_2O content of end-capillary blood or $\dot{V}_{N_2O}$, both of which remain at 1. Cutting $D_{L_{N_2O}}$ in half also would have no effect on $\dot{V}_{N_2O}$. Thus, N_2O uptake is insensitive to changes in $D_{L_{N_2O}}$ at least over the range of values that we examined (Table 30-2, upper half). In other words, the *uptake* of N_2O is not *diffusion* limited.

What would be the effect of reducing $\dot{Q}$ by half while holding $D_{L_{N_2O}}$ constant? If we assume that capillary dimensions remain constant, then halving of $\dot{Q}$ would double the contact time of blood with the alveolus and make the $P_{C_{N_2O}}$ trajectory along the capillary twice as steep as before (Fig. 30-6D). Nevertheless Cc'_{N_2O} remains unchanged at 1. However, because we reduced $\dot{Q}$ by half, $\dot{V}_{N_2O}$ also falls by half. Conversely, doubling of $\dot{Q}$ causes $\dot{V}_{N_2O}$ to double. Thus, N_2O uptake is more or less proportional to blood flow (i.e., perfusion) over a wide range of $\dot{Q}$ values (Table 30-2, lower half). For this reason, we say that N_2O transport is predominantly **perfusion limited**. *The transport of a gas is predominantly perfusion limited if the gas in the capillary comes into equilibrium with the gas in the alveolar air by the end of the capillary.*

In principle, CO transport could become perfusion limited and N_2O could become diffusion limited under special conditions

Although normally CO transport is diffusion limited and N_2O transport is perfusion limited, changes in certain parameters could, at least in theory, make CO uptake perfusion limited or make N_2O uptake diffusion limited. To illustrate, we introduce an analogy (Fig. 30-7): workers at a railroad siding trying to load boxes (transport gas at a rate $\dot{V}$) onto the cars of a passing train. Each worker (the diffusive event) has a limited rate for putting boxes on the train, and the total rate is the sum for all the workers (D_L). Each railway car (the red blood cell) has a limited capacity for holding boxes, and the total capacity is the sum for all cars (Hb concentration). Finally, because the train is moving (the perfusion rate, $\dot{Q}$), a limited time is available to load each railway car.

First imagine that the speed of the train perfectly matches the number of workers (Fig. 30-7A). Thus, all workers are always fully occupied, and the railway cars depart the siding fully loaded; the last box is put on each car just as the car leaves the siding. Any decrease in worker number, any increase in the carrying capacity of each car, or any increase in train speed causes the railway cars to leave the siding at least partially empty. Thus, if we fix train speed at "normal," *a decrease in the number of workers* below "normal" (Fig. 30-7B) would cause a proportional decrease in the shipping rate—the number of boxes the train carries away per hour. In other words, when the number of workers is between 0 and normal, the shipping rate is worker (diffusion) limited.

Now return to the original "perfect-match" condition in which both worker number and train speed are normal. An increase in the worker number at constant train speed has no effect on either the number of boxes loaded onto each railway car (which remain filled to capacity) or the shipping rate (Fig. 30-7C). In this higher range of worker number, the shipping rate is no longer limited by the workers but by the speed of the train or by the carrying capacity of the railway cars. Thus, we could say that the shipping rate is speed (perfusion) limited, although it would be equally true to say that it is carrying capacity (Hb) limited.

Let us return again to the original condition in which worker number perfectly matches train speed. An increase in the train speed while the worker number is fixed at the normal value causes railway cars to leave the siding partially empty (Fig. 30-7D). However, shipping rate is unaffected because the normal number of boxes is simply distributed over a greater number of cars. Under these conditions, shipping rate is again worker (diffusion) limited because the increase in the number of workers would proportionally increase shipping rate. In fact, whenever you see cars leaving the siding only partially filled, you can conclude that shipping rate is worker (diffusion) limited, regardless of whether this situation arose because of a decrease in worker number, an increase in train speed, or an increase in car carrying capacity.

Finally, let us again return to the perfectly matched initial condition and now decrease train speed while holding worker number fixed at the normal value. As velocity

Table 30-2 Alveolar Transport of N_2O

	$D_{L_{N_2O}}$	$\dot{Q}$	$\times$	Cc'_{N_2O}	$=$	$\dot{V}_{N_2O}$
Vary D_L ($\dot{Q}$ constant)	2	1		1		1
	1	1		1		1
	½	1		1		1
Vary $\dot{Q}$ (D_L constant)	1	½		1		½
	1	1		1		1
	1	2		1		2

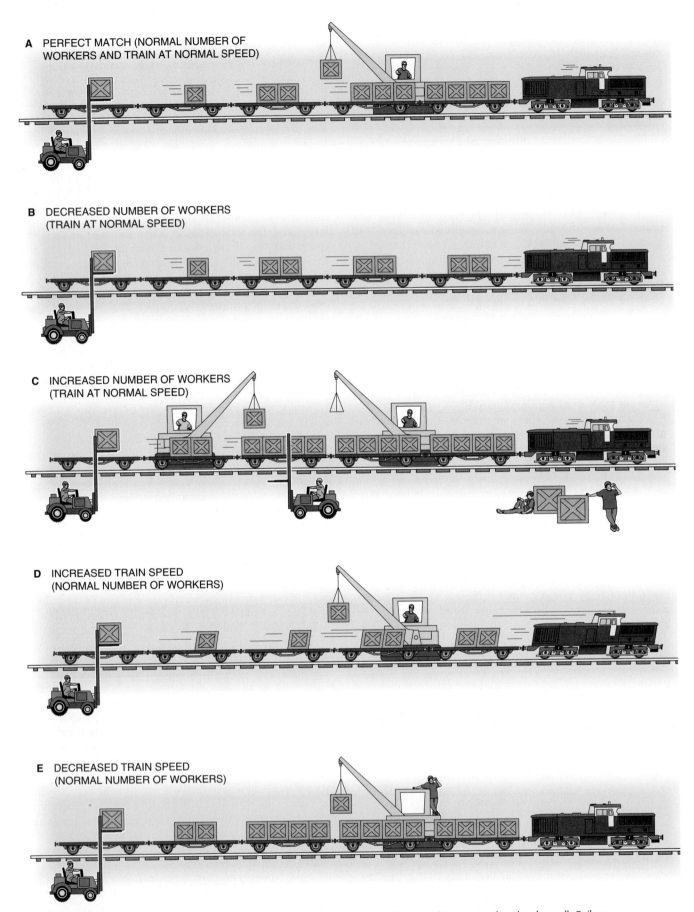

Figure 30-7 Railway car analogy. Workers represent the diffusion of O_2 across the alveolar wall. Railway cars represent capacity of blood to carry O_2. The speed of the train represents blood flow.

decreases below normal, shipping rate decreases proportionally (Fig. 30-7E), even though the railway cars leave the siding fully loaded. Thus, shipping rate is speed (perfusion) limited. It would be equally true to characterize the system as being limited by carrying capacity (Hb). In fact, whenever you see cars leaving the siding fully filled, you can conclude that shipping rate is speed (perfusion) limited, regardless of whether this situation arose because of an increase in worker number, a decrease in train speed, or a decrease in car carrying capacity.

The reader is now in a position to consider factors that could render CO transport predominantly *perfusion* limited or N_2O transport *diffusion* limited. Several changes to the system would cause CO transport to be no longer limited by $D_{L_{CO}}$. Conversely, several other changes would cause the transport of N_2O to be no longer limited by $\dot{Q}$.

The uptake of carbon monoxide provides an estimate of D_L

Because the **pulmonary diffusing capacity** plays such an important role in determining the partial pressure profile of a gas along the pulmonary capillary, being able to measure D_L would be valuable. Moreover, an approach that is easily applicable to patients could be useful both as a diagnostic tool and to follow the progression of diseases affecting D_L.

We have already seen (Equation 30-9) that we can use Fick's law to compute the overall uptake of a gas if we summate many individual diffusion events for all pieces of alveolar wall and all times in the respiratory cycle:

$$\text{Overall } \dot{V}_{gas} = \overset{\substack{\text{All pieces}\\ \text{of alveolar}\\ \text{wall}}}{\sum} \overset{\substack{\text{All times}\\ \text{in respiratory}\\ \text{cycle}}}{\sum} (D_{L_{gas}} \cdot (P_{A_{gas}} - P_{c_{gas}}))$$

$$(30\text{-}23)$$

If we could ignore spatial and temporal nonuniformities, then we could eliminate the two troublesome Σ symbols and compute an *overall* $D_{L_{gas}}$ from the *overall* $\dot{V}_{gas}$. We could accommodate modest spatial and temporal variations in $P_{A_{gas}}$ by computing an *average* alveolar partial pressure $(\bar{P}_{A_{gas}})$. Furthermore, if the partial pressure profile of the gas along the capillary were linear, we could use an *average* capillary partial pressure $(\bar{P}_{c_{gas}})$ as well. If we could identify a gas for which these assumptions are reasonable, we could simplify Equation 30-23 to an expression that is similar to the version of Fick's law with which we started this chapter (Equation 30-7):

$$\text{Overall } \dot{V}_{gas} = D_{L_{gas}} \cdot (\bar{P}_{A_{gas}} - \bar{P}_{c_{gas}}) \quad (30\text{-}24)$$

Which gas could we use to estimate D_L? We certainly do *not* want to use N_2O, whose uptake is *perfusion* limited. After all, $\dot{V}_{N_2O}$ is more or less proportional to changes in $\dot{Q}$ but virtually insensitive to changes in D_L (Table 30-2). Viewed differently, the driving pressure between alveolus and capillary $(P_{A_{N_2O}} - P_{c_{N_2O}})$ is high at the beginning of the capillary but soon falls to zero (Fig. 30-6B). Thus, it would be very difficult to pick a reasonable value for the *average* capillary

P_{N_2O} to insert into Equation 30-24. However, CO is an excellent choice because its uptake is diffusion limited, so that changes in the parameter of interest (i.e., D_L) have nearly a proportionate effect on $\dot{V}_{CO}$. Viewed differently, the driving pressure between alveolus and capillary $(P_{A_{CO}} - P_{c_{CO}})$ is nearly ideal because it falls more or less linearly as blood courses down the pulmonary capillary (Fig. 30-5B). Thus, we might solve Equation 30-24 for $D_{L_{CO}}$:

$$D_{L_{CO}} = \frac{\dot{V}_{CO}}{(\bar{P}_{A_{CO}} - \bar{P}_{c_{CO}})} \quad (30\text{-}25)$$

Note that $D_{L_{CO}}$ and $\dot{V}_{CO}$ are *average* values that reflect properties of all alveoli throughout both lungs at all times in the respiratory cycle. $\bar{P}_{A_{CO}}$ reflects minor changes during the respiratory cycle as well as more substantial variations in $P_{A_{CO}}$ from alveolus to alveolus due to local differences in ventilation and perfusion (see Chapter 31). Finally, $\bar{P}_{c_{CO}}$ reflects not only the small increase in $P_{c_{CO}}$ as blood flows down the capillary but also any CO that may be present in the mixed-venous blood that enters the pulmonary capillary. For nonsmokers who live in a nonpolluted environment, $P\bar{v}_{CO}$ is nearly zero and thus we often can ignore $\bar{P}_{c_{CO}}$.

We will discuss two general methods for estimation of $D_{L_{CO}}$, the steady-state technique and the single-breath test. These tests, both using CO, are useful for estimation of pulmonary diffusing capacity in a clinical setting, even among very ill patients in the intensive care unit.

In the **steady-state technique** (Fig. 30-8), the subject breathes a low CO/air mixture (e.g., 0.1% to 0.2%) for

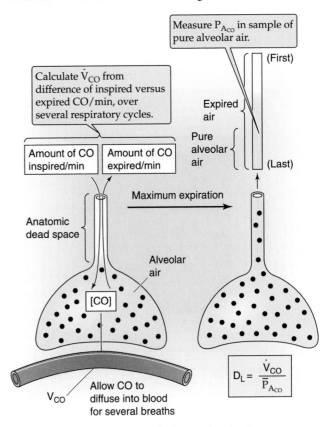

Figure 30-8 Steady-state method for estimating $D_{L_{CO}}$.

approximately a dozen breaths to allow $P_{A_{CO}}$ to stabilize. Calculation of $D_{L_{CO}}$ requires at least two measurements: $\dot{V}_{CO}$ and $\bar{P}_{A_{CO}}$. We compute the rate of CO uptake from the difference between the amounts of CO in inspired air versus expired air over time. We can directly measure $\bar{P}_{A_{CO}}$ in an alveolar air sample (see Chapter 31). D_L is then $\dot{V}_{CO}/\bar{P}_{A_{CO}}$. If the subject happens to be a smoker or to live in a polluted environment, an accurate measurement of D_L requires a venous blood sample to estimate the mixed-venous P_{CO}. In this case, we calculate D_L from the more complete expression in Equation 30-25.

In the **single-breath technique** (Fig. 30-9), the subject makes a maximal expiratory effort to residual volume (see Chapter 27) and then makes a maximal inspiration of air containing CO and holds the breath for 10 seconds. The inhaled air is a mixture of dilute CO (e.g., 0.3%) plus a gas such as helium, which has a low water solubility and thus a negligible transport across the blood-gas barrier (see Equation 30-5). We can use helium to compute the extent to which the inhaled CO/He mixture becomes diluted as it first enters the alveoli and also to calculate the alveolar volume into which the CO/He mixture distributes (see Chapter 27). This information allows us to calculate two crucial parameters at the *beginning* of the breath-holding period: (1) $P_{A_{CO}}$ and (2) the amount of CO in the alveoli. During the 10 seconds of breath-holding, some of the inhaled CO diffuses into the blood. The greater the $D_{L_{CO}}$, the greater the diffusion of CO, and the more $P_{A_{CO}}$ falls. As the subject exhales, we obtain a sample of alveolar air and use it to determine two crucial parameters at the *end* of the breath-holding period: (1) $P_{A_{CO}}$ and (2) the amount of CO in the alveoli.

The initial and final $P_{A_{CO}}$ values allow us to compute $\bar{P}_{A_{CO}}$. The initial and final alveolar CO amounts allow us to compute $\dot{V}_{CO}$ during the 10-second breath-holding period.

Bear in mind that the value of $D_{L_{CO}}$ determined by use of either of these methods is an *average* pulmonary diffusing capacity. As discussed in Chapter 31, pulmonary disease can cause ventilation to become nonuniform, making it difficult to obtain alveolar air samples that are representative of the entire lung. A normal value for $D_{L_{CO}}$ is ~25 mL CO taken up per minute for each millimeter of mercury of partial pressure driving CO diffusion and for each milliliter of blood having a normal Hb content. This value of $D_{L_{CO}}$ depends not only on D_M (i.e., the "membrane" or truly diffusive component of D_L) in Equation 30-15 but also on $\theta \cdot V_c$. For CO transport, D_M and $\theta \cdot V_c$ are each ~50 mL CO/(min·mL blood):

$$\frac{1}{D_L} = \frac{1}{50} + \frac{1}{50} = \frac{1}{25} \qquad (30\text{-}26)$$

Thus, $1/(\theta \cdot V_c)$ makes a major contribution to the final $D_{L_{CO}}$. Because V_c is proportional to the Hb content of the blood, and because Hb content is decreased in **anemia**, a subject can have a reduced $D_{L_{CO}}$ even though the diffusion pathways in the lung (i.e., D_M) are perfectly normal. Recall that $1/(\theta \cdot V_c)$ makes an insignificant contribution to the D_L for O_2. Nevertheless, it is the D_L for CO—and not that for O_2—that one uses for a clinical index of diffusing capacity. Table 30-3 summarizes several factors that can affect the calculated $D_{L_{CO}}$.

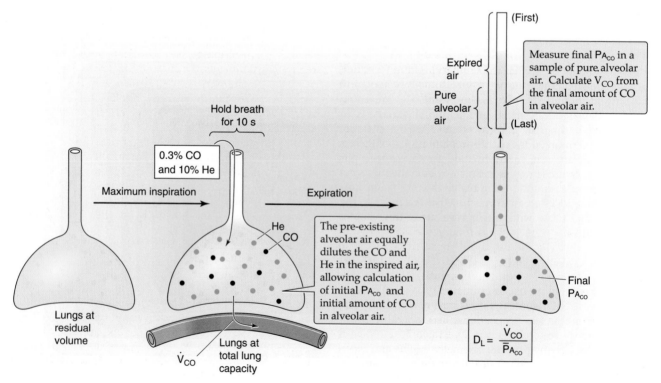

Figure 30-9 • Single-breath method for estimating $D_{L_{CO}}$.

Table 30-3 Factors That Affect the Diffusing Capacity for CO

Factor	Effect	Explanation
Body size	↑Size → ↑DL_{CO}	With ↑ in lung size, diffusion area (A) and volume of pulmonary capillary blood (V_c) both ↑.
Age	↑Age → ↓DL_{CO}	DL_{CO} decreases by ~2% per year after the age of 20 years.
Sex	Male → ↑DL_{CO}	Corrected for age and body size, DL_{CO} is about 10% greater in men than in women.
Lung volume	↑Volume → ↑DL_{CO}	In an individual, ↑ in lung volume causes an ↑ in volume of pulmonary capillary blood (V_c), an ↑ in diffusion area (A), and a ↓ in diffusion distance (a).
Exercise	Exercise → ↑DL_{CO}	An ↑ in $\dot{Q}$ causes dilation of pulmonary capillaries, which in turn causes an ↑ in area for diffusion (A) and volume of pulmonary capillary blood (V_c).
Body position	DL_{CO}: supine > sitting > standing	Changes in posture presumably ↑ volume of pulmonary capillary blood (V_c).
PA_{O_2}	↑PA_{O_2} → ↓DL_{CO}	O_2 lowers the rate at which CO combines with hemoglobin.
PA_{CO_2}	↑PA_{CO_2} → ↑DL_{CO}	CO_2 causes an ↑ in volume of pulmonary capillary blood (V_c).

DL_{CO}, diffusion capacity of CO; PA_{O_2}, partial pressure of O_2 in alveolar blood; PA_{CO_2}, partial pressure CO_2 in alveolar air.

For both O₂ and CO₂, transport is normally perfusion limited

Uptake of O₂ Blood enters the pulmonary capillaries (Fig. 30-10A) with the P_{O_2} of mixed-venous blood, typically 40 mm Hg. Capillary P_{O_2} reaches the alveolar P_{O_2} of ~100 mm Hg about one third of the way along the capillary (Fig. 30-10B, black curve). This P_{O_2} profile along the pulmonary capillary is intermediate between that of CO in Figure 30-5B (where CO fails to reach diffusion equilibrium) and N₂O in Figure 30-6B (where N₂O reaches diffusion equilibrium ~10% of the way along the capillary). The transport of O₂ is similar to that of CO in that both molecules bind to Hb. Why, then, does O₂ reach **diffusion equilibrium**, whereas CO does not?

The uptake of O₂ differs from that of CO in three important respects. First, Hb that enters the pulmonary capillary is already heavily preloaded with O₂. Because Hb in the mixed-venous blood is ~75% saturated with O₂ (see Chapter 29)—versus ~0% for CO—the available O₂-binding capacity of Hb is relatively low. Second, because the alveolar P_{O_2} is rather high (i.e., ~100 mm Hg)—versus <1 mm Hg for CO—the alveolar blood P_{O_2} gradient is large (i.e., ~60 mm Hg) and the initial rate of O₂ diffusion from the alveolus into pulmonary capillary blood is immense. Third, D_L for O₂ is higher than that for CO owing to a greater $\theta \cdot V_c$. As a result of these three factors, Hb in pulmonary capillary blood rapidly approaches its equilibrium carrying capacity for O₂ along the first third of the capillary. Because capillary P_{O_2} reaches alveolar P_{O_2}, O₂ transport is **perfusion limited**, as is the case for N₂O. Because O₂ normally reaches diffusion equilibrium so soon along the capillary, the lung has a tremendous **D_L reserve** for O₂ uptake. Even if we reduce DL_{O_2} by half, O₂ still reaches diffusion equilibrium about two

thirds of the way along the capillary (Fig. 30-10B, blue curve). If we could double DL_{O_2}, O₂ would reach diffusion equilibrium much earlier than usual (Fig. 30-10B, red curve). However, neither change in DL_{O_2} would affect O₂ uptake, which is *not* diffusion limited.

The D_L reserve for O₂ uptake is extremely important during **exercise**, when cardiac output can increase by up to a factor of 5 (see Chapter 17), substantially decreasing the contact time of the blood with the pulmonary capillaries. The contact time appears not to decrease by more than a factor of ~3, probably because the slightly increased pressure recruits and distends the pulmonary vessels (see Chapter 31). As a result, even with vigorous exercise, P_{CO_2} reaches virtual equilibrium with the alveolar air by the end of the capillary (Fig. 30-10C, green curve)—except in some elite athletes. Thus, the increase in $\dot{Q}$ during exercise leads to a corresponding increase in $\dot{V}_{O_2}$, which carries obvious survival benefits. In patients with pulmonary disease, thickening of the alveolar blood-gas barrier can reduce DL_{O_2} sufficiently that equilibration of P_{O_2} fails to occur by capillary's end during exercise (Fig. 30-10C, brown curve). In this case, O₂ transport becomes diffusion limited.

Like exercise, **high altitude** stretches out the P_{O_2} profile along the capillary (Fig. 30-10D, red curve). At altitude, barometric pressure and ambient P_{O_2} decrease proportionally (see Chapter 61), leading to a fall in alveolar P_{O_2}. Because of O₂ extraction by the systemic tissues, P_{O_2} also is lower in the mixed-venous blood entering the pulmonary capillaries. This lower $P\bar{v}_{O_2}$ has two consequences. First, the alveolar capillary P_{O_2} gradient at the beginning of the capillary is low, reducing the absolute O₂ transport rate. Second, because at altitude the mixed-venous P_{O_2} is lower, we now operate on a steeper part of the Hb-O₂ dissociation curve (see Fig. 29-3).

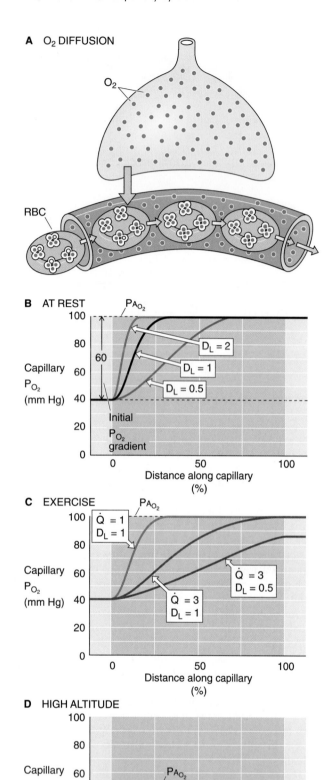

Figure 30-10   Diffusion of O_2. In **A,** as the red blood cell (RBC) enters the capillary, O_2 occupies three of the four sites on hemoglobin. In **B-D,** $P_{A_{O_2}}$ is alveolar P_{O_2}. In **B** and **D,** $\dot{Q}$ is constant.

Thus, a given increment in the O_2 content of the pulmonary capillary blood causes a smaller increase in P_{O_2}.

The combination of exercise and high altitude can cause O_2 transport to become diffusion limited even in healthy individuals (Fig. 30-10D, green curve). If the subject also has a pathological condition that lowers $D_{L_{O_2}}$, then transport may become diffusion limited even more readily at altitude. Obviously, any combination of exercise, high altitude, and reduced $D_{L_{O_2}}$ compounds the problems for O_2 transport.

Escape of CO_2   Mixed-venous blood entering the pulmonary capillary has a P_{CO_2} of ~46 mm Hg, whereas the alveolar P_{CO_2} is ~40 mm Hg (Fig. 30-11A). Thus, CO_2 diffuses in the opposite direction of O_2—from blood to alveolus—and P_{CO_2} falls along the pulmonary capillary (Fig. 30-11B, black curve), reaching **diffusion equilibrium**. Compared with O_2, one factor that tends to speed CO_2 equilibration is that the D_L for CO_2 is 3-fold to 5-fold greater than that for O_2. However, two factors tend to slow the equilibration of CO_2. First, the initial P_{CO_2} gradient across the blood-gas barrier is only ~6 mm Hg at the beginning of the capillary, ~10% as large as the initial P_{O_2} gradient. Second, in their physiological ranges, the CO_2 dissociation curve (see Fig. 29-10) is far steeper than the Hb-O_2 dissociation curve (see Fig. 29-3). Thus, a decrement in the CO_2 content of the pulmonary capillary blood causes a relatively small decrease in P_{CO_2}. Thus, a smaller gradient and a steeper dissociation curve counteract the larger D_L. Many authors believe that as indicated by the black curve in Figure 30-11B, capillary P_{CO_2} reaches alveolar P_{CO_2} about one third of the way along the pulmonary capillary (as is the case for O_2). Others have suggested that CO_2 equilibration is slower, occurring just before the end of the pulmonary capillary. In either case, a decrease in D_L in certain lung diseases (see next section) or heavy exercise (Fig. 30-11B, red and blue curves) may cause the transport of CO_2 to become diffusion limited.

Pathological changes that reduce D_L do not necessarily produce hypoxia

The measured pulmonary diffusing capacity for CO falls in disease states accompanied by a thickening of the alveolar blood-gas barrier, a reduction in the surface area (i.e., capillaries) available for diffusion, or a decrease in the amount of Hb in the pulmonary capillaries. Examples of pathological processes accompanied by a decrease in D_L include the following:

Diffuse interstitial pulmonary fibrosis, which is a fibrotic process causing a thickening of the interstitium, thickening of alveolar walls, and destruction of capillaries—sometimes with marked decreases in D_L. In some cases, the cause is unknown (i.e., idiopathic); in others, it is secondary to such disorders as sarcoidosis, scleroderma, and exposure to occupational agents (e.g., asbestos).
Chronic obstructive pulmonary disease (COPD), which not only increases the resistance of conducting airways but can lead to a destruction of pulmonary capillaries and thus a reduction in both (1) surface area available for diffusion and (2) total pulmonary capillary Hb content (see Chapter 27).

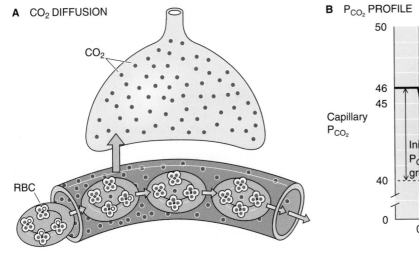

Figure 30-11 Diffusion of CO_2. In **B,** $P_{A_{CO_2}}$ is alveolar P_{CO_2}.

Loss of functional lung tissue, as caused by either a tumor or surgery. Surgical removal of lung tissue reduces D_L because of a decrease in both (1) surface area and (2) total pulmonary capillary Hb content.

Anemia, in which the fall in total Hb content decreases the $\theta \cdot V_c$ component of $D_{L_{CO}}$.

Although pulmonary diseases can cause both a decrease in D_L and hypoxemia (i.e., a decrease in arterial P_{O_2}), it is not necessarily true that the decrease in D_L is the sole or even the major cause of the hypoxemia. The same diseases that lower D_L also upset the distribution of ventilation and perfusion throughout the lung. As discussed in Chapter 31, mismatching of ventilation to perfusion among various regions of the lungs can be a powerful influence leading to hypoxemia. Furthermore, because the lung has a sizeable D_L reserve for O_2 (and perhaps for CO_2 as well), D_L would have to decrease to about one third of its normal value for O_2 transport to become diffusion limited. Thus, in a disease causing both a decrease in D_L and disturbances in the distribution of ventilation and perfusion, it is difficult to determine the extent to which an accompanying reduction of D_L is responsible for the resulting hypoxemia.

REFERENCES

Books and Reviews

Cerretelli P, Di Prampero PE: Gas exchange in exercise. In Handbook of Physiology, Section 3: The Respiratory System, vol 1, pp 297-339. Bethesda, MD: American Physiological Society, 1985.

Forster RE: Exchange of gases between alveolar air and pulmonary capillary blood: Pulmonary diffusion capacity. Physiol Rev 1957; 37:391-452.

Hlastala MP: Diffusing-capacity heterogeneity. In Handbook of Physiology, Section 3: The Respiratory System, vol 1, pp 217-232. Bethesda, MD: American Physiological Society, 1985.

Maina JN, West JB: Thin and strong! The bioengineering dilemma in the structural and functional design of the blood-gas barrier. Physiol Rev 2005; 85:811-844.

Weibel ER: Morphological basis of alveolar-capillary gas exchange. Physiol Rev 1973; 53:419-495.

Journal Articles

Crapo JD, Crapo RO: Comparison of total lung diffusion capacity and the membrane component of diffusion capacity as determined by physiologic and morphometric techniques. Respir Physiol 1983; 51:181-194.

Krogh M: The diffusion of gases through the lungs of man. J Physiol 1914-1915; 49:271-300.

Roughton FJW, Forster RE: Relative importance of diffusion and chemical reaction rates in determining rate of exchange of gases in the human lung, with special reference to true diffusing capacity of pulmonary membrane and volume of blood in the lung capillaries. J Appl Physiol 1957; 11:290-302.

Torre-Bueno JR, Wagner PD, Saltzman HA, et al: Diffusion limitation in normal humans during exercise at sea level and simulated altitude. J Appl Physiol 1985; 58:989-995.

Wagner PD, West JB: Effects of diffusion impairment on O_2 and CO_2 time courses in pulmonary capillaries. J Appl Physiol 1972; 33:62-71.

CHAPTER 31

VENTILATION AND PERFUSION OF THE LUNGS

Walter F. Boron

Although diffusion is at the very heart of the gas exchange, as we discussed in Chapter 30, two other parameters are also extremely important. Ventilation and perfusion—both of which require energy—are critical because they set up the partial pressure gradients along which O_2 and CO_2 diffuse. **Ventilation** is the convective movement of air that exchanges gases between the atmosphere and the alveoli. In Chapter 27, we discussed the mechanics of ventilation. In the first part of this chapter, we consider the importance of ventilation for determination of alveolar P_{O_2} and P_{CO_2} and also see that ventilation varies from one group of alveoli to the next. **Perfusion** is the convective movement of blood that carries the dissolved gases to and from the lung. In Chapters 17 to 25, we discussed the cardiovascular system. In the second part of this chapter, we examine the special properties of the pulmonary circulation and see that, like ventilation, perfusion varies in different regions of the lung. Finally, in the third part of this chapter, we see that the ratio of ventilation to perfusion—and the distribution of ventilation-perfusion ratio among alveolar units—is critically important for gas exchange and thus for the composition of the *arterial blood gases*: P_{O_2}, P_{CO_2}, and pH.

VENTILATION

About 30% of total ventilation in a respiratory cycle is wasted ventilating anatomical dead space (i.e., conducting airways)

Total ventilation (V_T) is the volume of air moved out of the lungs per unit of time:

$$\dot{V}_T = \frac{V}{t} \qquad (31\text{-}1)$$

Here, V is the volume of air exiting the lungs during a *series of breaths*. Note that we are using $\dot{V}$ differently than in Chapter 27, where $\dot{V}$ represented flow through an airway at a particular *instant* in time. A practical definition is that $\dot{V}_T$ is the product of tidal volume (TV or V_T) and the respiratory frequency (f). Thus, for someone with a tidal volume of 0.5 L, breathing 12 breaths/min:

$$\begin{aligned} \dot{V}_T &= V_T \cdot f \\ &= (0.5\,\text{L}) \cdot (12/\text{min}) \qquad (31\text{-}2) \\ &= 6\,\text{L/min} \end{aligned}$$

Because total ventilation is usually reported as liters per minute, it is sometimes called **minute ventilation**.

Before an inspiration, the conducting airways are filled with "stale" air having the same composition as alveolar air (Fig. 31-1, step 1); we will see why shortly. During inspiration, ~500 mL of "fresh" atmospheric air (high P_{O_2}/low P_{CO_2}) enters the body (step 2). However, only the first 350 mL reaches the alveoli; the final 150 mL remains in the conducting airways (nose, pharynx, larynx, trachea, and other airways without alveoli)—that is, the **anatomical dead space**. These figures are typical for a 70-kg person; V_T and V_d are roughly proportional to body size. During inspiration, ~500 mL of air also enters the alveoli. However, the first 150 mL is stale air previously in the conducting airways; only the final 350 mL is fresh air. By the end of inspiration, the 500 mL of air that entered the alveoli (150 mL of stale air plus 350 mL of fresh air) has mixed by diffusion with the preexisting alveolar air (step 3). During expiration (step 4), the first 150 mL of air emerging from the body is the fresh air left in the conducting airways from the previous inspiration. As the expiration continues, 350 mL of stale alveolar air sequentially moves into the conducting airways and then exits the body—for a total of 500 mL of air leaving the body. Simultaneously, 500 mL of air leaves the alveoli. The first 350 mL is the same 350 mL that exited the body. The final 150 mL of stale air to exit the alveoli remains in the conducting airways, as we are ready to begin the next inspiration.

Thus, with each 500-mL inspiration, only the *initial* 350 mL of fresh air entering the body reaches the alveoli. With each 500-mL expiration, only the *final* 350 mL of air exiting the body comes from the alveoli. One 150-mL bolus of *fresh air* shuttles back and forth between the atmosphere and conducting airways. Another 150-mL bolus of *stale air* shuttles back and forth between the conducting airways and

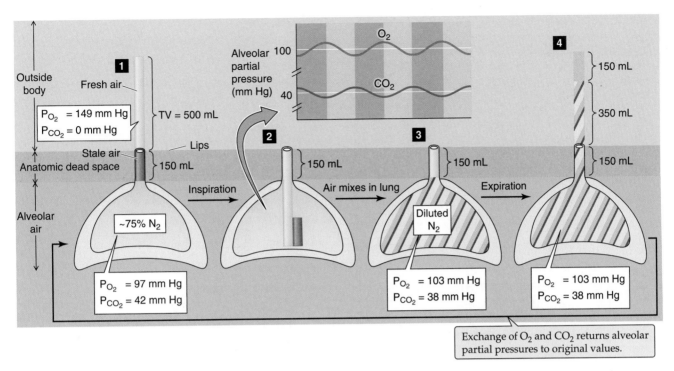

Figure 31-1 Ventilation of dead space and alveolar space during a respiratory cycle.

alveoli. **Dead-space ventilation** ($\dot{V}_D$) is the volume of the stale air so shuttled per minute. **Alveolar ventilation** ($\dot{V}_A$) is the volume of fresh air per minute that actually reaches the alveoli, or the volume of stale alveolar air that reaches the atmosphere. Thus, total ventilation—a reflection of the work invested in breathing—is the sum of the wasted dead-space ventilation and the useful alveolar ventilation. In our example,

$$
\begin{array}{llll}
 & \dfrac{\text{liters}}{\text{breath}} & \dfrac{\text{breaths}}{\text{minute}} & \dfrac{\text{liters}}{\text{minute}} \\[2ex]
\dot{V}_D = \quad V_D \cdot f & = 0\ 150 \ \cdot & 12 & = 1\ 8 \\
\dot{V}_A = (V_T - V_D) \cdot f & = 0\ 350 \ \cdot & 12 & = 4\ 2 \\
\hline
\dot{V}_T = \quad V_T \cdot f & = 0\ 500 \ \cdot & 12 & = 6\ 0
\end{array}
\qquad (31\text{-}3)
$$

so that the dead-space ventilation is 30% of the total ventilation.

The inset of Figure 31-1 illustrates how inspiration and expiration lead to small fluctuations in the alveolar partial pressures for O_2 and CO_2, noted earlier in Figure 30-3B. Throughout the respiratory cycle, blood flowing through the pulmonary capillaries continuously draws O_2 out of the alveolar air and adds CO_2. Just before an inspiration, alveolar P_{O_2} has fallen to its lowest point, and alveolar P_{CO_2} has risen to its highest. During inspiration, a new bolus of inspired fresh air mixes with preexisting alveolar air, causing alveolar P_{O_2} to rise and alveolar P_{CO_2} to fall. During expiration and until the next inspiration, alveolar P_{O_2} and P_{CO_2} gradually drift to the values that we saw at the start of the respiratory cycle. Assuming that functional residual capacity (FRC) is 3 L and that each breath adds 350 mL of fresh air, one can calculate that alveolar P_{O_2} oscillates with an amplitude of

~6 mm Hg, whereas alveolar P_{CO_2} oscillates with an amplitude of ~4 mm Hg.

Fowler's single-breath N_2 washout estimates anatomical dead space

In 1948, Ward Fowler introduced an approach for estimation of the anatomical dead space based on the washout from the lungs of N_2. The key concept is that N_2 is physiologically inert. After the subject has been breathing room air, the alveolar air is ~75% N_2. After a quiet expiration, when lung volume is FRC (Fig. 31-2A, step 1), the subject takes a single, normal-sized breath (~500 mL). The inspired air is 100% O_2, although in principle we could use any nontoxic gas mixture lacking N_2. The *first portion* of inspired O_2 enters the alveolar spaces (step 2), where it rapidly mixes by diffusion and dilutes the N_2 and other gases remaining after the previous breaths of room air (step 3). The *last portion* of the inspired O_2 (~150 mL) remains in the conducting airways, which have a P_{N_2} of zero.

The subject now exhales ~500 mL of air (step 4). If no mixing occurred between the N_2-free air in the most distal conducting airways and the N_2-containing air in the most proximal alveolar spaces, then the first ~150 mL of air emerging from the body would have an $[N_2]$ of zero (Fig. 31-2B, red lines). After this would come a sharp transition to a much higher $[N_2]$ for the final ~350 mL of expired air. Thus, the expired volume with an $[N_2]$ of zero would represent air from the conducting airways (anatomical dead space), whereas the remainder would represent air from the alveoli.

In reality, some mixing occurs between the air in the conducting airways and alveoli, so that the transition is S

A DILUTION OF INSPIRED 100% O₂

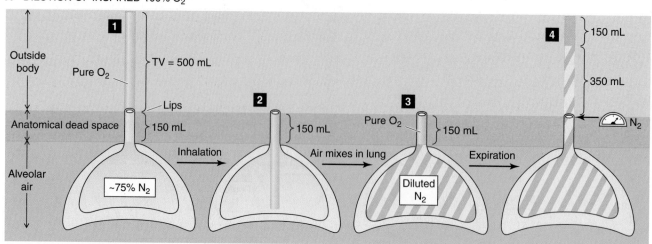

B [N₂] PROFILE OF EXPIRED AIR WITH NO MIXING

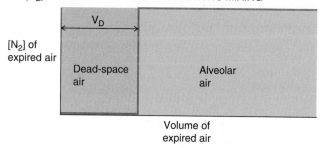

C MEASURED [N₂] PROFILE

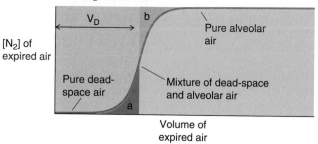

Figure 31-2 Fowler's technique for measurement of anatomical dead space.

shaped (Fig. 31-2C, red curve). A vertical line drawn through the S-shaped curve, so that *area a* is the same as *area b*, marks the idealized transition between air from conducting and alveolar airways—as in Figure 31-2B. The expired lung volume at the point of this vertical line is thus the anatomical dead space. In Figure 31-2C, the part of the S-shaped curve with an expired [N₂] of zero represents pure dead-space air, the part where [N₂] gradually rises represents a mixture of dead-space and alveolar air, and the part where [N₂] is high and flat represents pure alveolar air. This plateau is important because it is during this plateau that one obtains an **alveolar gas sample.**

Bohr's expired [CO₂] approach estimates physiological dead space

In principle, we could compute the dead space using *any* gas whose expiration profile looks like that of N₂. Nitrogen is useful because we can easily create an artificial situation in which the subject makes a single inhalation of N₂-free air (e.g., a single breath of 100% O₂). Another possibility is CO₂. Its profile during expiration is similar to that of N₂. Moreover, we do not need to use any special tricks to get it to work because room air has practically no CO₂. Yet plenty of CO₂ is in the alveoli, where it evolves from the incoming mixed-venous blood. After a quiet expiration (Fig. 31-3A, step 1), the P₍CO₂₎ of the alveolar air is virtually the same as the P₍CO₂₎ of

the arterial blood (see Chapter 30), ~40 mm Hg. The subject now inhales a normal tidal volume (~500 mL) of room air, although any CO₂-free gas mixture would do. The first portion enters the alveoli (step 2), where it rapidly dilutes the CO₂ and other gases remaining after the previous breath (step 3). The rest (~150 mL) remains in the conducting airways, which now have a P₍CO₂₎ of ~0. When the subject now expires (step 4), the first air that exits the body is the CO₂-free gas that had filled the conducting airways, followed by the CO₂-containing alveolar air. Thus, the idealized profile of expired [CO₂] (Fig. 31-3B, red lines) is similar to the idealized [N₂] profile (Fig. 31-2B). In particular, the volume of expired air at the vertical line in Figure 31-3B is the estimated *anatomical* dead space.

One could use a CO₂ probe to record the expired [CO₂] profile during a single-breath CO₂ washout rather than the [N₂] profile that Fowler used to measure anatomical dead space. However, because CO₂ probes did not exist in his day, Christian Bohr used a single-breath CO₂ washout but analyzed the *average* P₍CO₂₎ in the *mixed*-expired air (i.e., averaged over the dead space plus expired alveolar air).

The principle of Bohr's approach is that the amount of CO₂ present in the volume of mixed-expired air (V₍E₎) is the sum of the CO₂ contributed by the volume of air from the dead space (V₍D₎) plus the CO₂ contributed by the volume of air coming from the *alveoli* (V₍E₎ − V₍D₎). As summarized in Figure 31-3B:

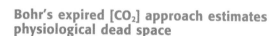

A DILUTION OF INSPIRED ROOM AIR

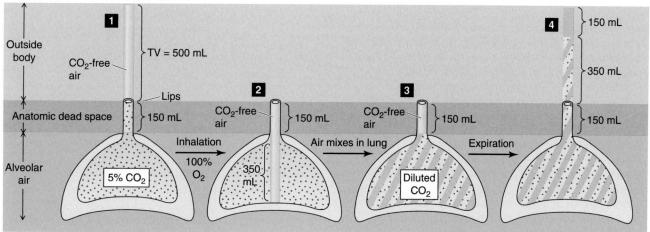

B [CO₂] PROFILE OF EXPIRED AIR

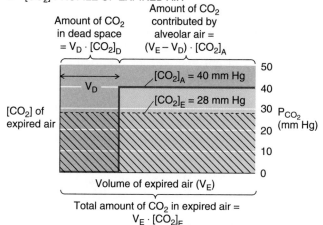

C EFFECT OF ALVEOLAR DEAD-SPACE VENTILATION ON EXPIRED-CO₂ PROFILE

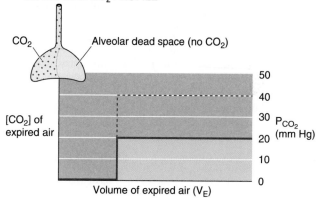

Figure 31-3 Bohr's method for measurement of physiological dead space.

1. The amount of CO_2 coming from the **dead space** is the product of V_D and $[CO_2]$ in this dead-space air. Because $[CO_2]_d$ is zero, the area beneath V_D is also zero.
2. The amount of CO_2 coming from **alveolar air** is the product of $(V_E - V_D)$ and alveolar $[CO_2]$ and is represented by the rose area in Figure 31-3B.
3. The total amount of CO_2 in the **mixed-expired air** is the product of V_E and the average $[CO_2]$ in this air and is represented by the hatched area in Figure 31-3B.

Because the rose and hatched areas in Figure 31-3B must be equal, and because the alveolar and expired $[CO_2]$ values are proportional to their respective P_{CO_2} values, it is possible to show that

$$\frac{V_D}{V_E} = \frac{P_{A_{CO_2}} - P_{E_{CO_2}}}{P_{A_{CO_2}}} \qquad (31\text{-}4)$$

This is the **Bohr equation**. Typically, V_D/V_E ranges between 0.20 and 0.35. For a V_D of 150 mL and a V_E of 500 mL, V_D/V_E would be 0.30. For example, if the alveolar P_{CO_2} is 40 mm Hg and the mixed-expired P_{CO_2} is 28 mm Hg, then

$$\frac{V_D}{V_E} = \frac{40 - 28}{40} = 30\% \qquad (31\text{-}5)$$

Equation 31-4 makes good intuitive sense. In an imaginary case in which we reduced V_D to zero, the expired air would be entirely from the alveoli, so that

$$\frac{V_D}{V_E} = \frac{40 - 40}{40} = 0\% \qquad (31\text{-}6)$$

On the other hand, if we reduced the tidal volume to a value at or below the dead-space volume, then *all* of the expired air would be dead-space air. In this case, $P_{E_{CO_2}}$ would be zero and

$$\frac{V_D}{V_E} = \frac{40 - 0}{40} = 100\% \qquad (31\text{-}7)$$

Two examples of this principle are of practical importance. During **panting**, the respiratory frequency is very high, but the tidal volume is only slightly greater than the anatomical dead space. Thus, most of the total ventilation is wasted as dead-space ventilation. If we reduced tidal volume below V_D, then in principle there would be no alveolar ventilation at all! During **snorkeling**, a swimmer breathes through a tube that increases V_D. If the snorkeling tube had a volume of 350 mL and the dead space within the body of the swimmer were 150 mL, then a tidal volume of 500 mL would in principle produce no alveolar ventilation. Consequently, the swimmer would suffocate, even though total ventilation was normal! Thus, the fractional dead space (V_D/V_E) depends critically on tidal volume.

Although Fowler's and Bohr's methods yield about the same estimate for V_D in healthy individuals, the two techniques actually measure somewhat different things. Fowler's approach measures **anatomical dead space**—the volume of the conducting airways from the mouth and nose up to the point where N_2 in the alveolar gas rapidly dilutes inspired 100% O_2. Bohr's approach, on the other hand, measures the **physiological dead space**—the volume of airways *not* receiving CO_2 from the pulmonary circulation and therefore *not* engaging in gas exchange. In a healthy person, the anatomical and physiological dead spaces are identical—the volume of the conducting airways. However, if some alveoli are ventilated but not perfused by pulmonary capillary blood, these unperfused alveoli, like conducting airways, do not contain CO_2. The air in such unperfused alveoli, known as **alveolar dead space**, contributes to the physiological dead space:

$$\underbrace{\text{Physiological dead space}}_{\text{Bohr's method}} = \underbrace{\text{Anatomical dead space}}_{\text{Fowler's method}} + \text{Alveolar dead space} \quad (31\text{-}8)$$

Fowler's and Bohr's methods could yield very different results in a patient with a **pulmonary embolism**, a condition in which a mass such as a blood clot wedges into and obstructs part or all of the pulmonary circulation. Alveoli downstream from the embolus are ventilated but not perfused; that is, they are alveolar dead space (Fig. 31-3C). Thus, Bohr's method—but not Fowler's method—could detect an increase in the physiological dead space caused by a pulmonary embolism.

Alveolar ventilation is the ratio of CO₂ production rate to CO₂ mole fraction in alveolar air

One way of computing alveolar ventilation is to subtract the dead space from the tidal volume and multiply the difference by the respiratory frequency (see Equation 31-3). We can also calculate $\dot{V}_A$ from alveolar P_{CO_2}. The body produces CO_2 by oxidative metabolism at a rate of ~200 mL/min. In the steady state, this rate of CO_2 production ($\dot{V}_{CO_2}$) must equal the rate at which the CO_2 enters the alveoli and the rate at which we exhale the CO_2. Of course, this 200 mL/min of exhaled CO_2 is part of the ~4200 mL of total alveolar air that we exhale each minute. Therefore, the exhaled 200 mL of CO_2 is ~5% of the exhaled 4200 mL of alveolar air:

$$\frac{\text{Volume of CO}_2 \text{ leaving alveoli in 1 min}}{\text{Volume of air leaving alveoli in 1 min}} = \left(\begin{array}{c} \text{Volume} \\ \text{fraction} \\ \text{of CO}_2 \text{ in} \\ \text{alveolar air} \end{array} \right) = (\text{CO}_2 \text{ mole fraction})_A$$

$$\frac{\dot{V}_{CO_2}}{\dot{V}_A} = \frac{200 \text{ mL}}{4200 \text{ mL}} = 5\%$$

$$(31\text{-}9)$$

Rearrangement of this equation and solving for $\dot{V}_A$ yields

$$\dot{V}_A = \underbrace{\frac{\dot{V}_{CO_2}}{(\text{CO}_2 \text{ mole fraction})_A}}_{} = k \frac{\dot{V}_{CO_2}}{P_{A_{CO_2}}} \quad (31\text{-}10)$$

The equation above the brace is true only when we *measure all parameters under the same conditions*. This obvious point would hardly be worth noting if respiratory physiologists had not managed, by historical accident, to measure the two volume terms under different conditions:

1. Body temperature and pressure, saturated with water vapor (BTPS; see Chapter 26) for $\dot{V}_A$.
2. Standard temperature and pressure, dry (STPD; see Chapter 26) for $\dot{V}_{CO_2}$.

Thus, in Equation 31-10, we introduce a constant k that not only indicates that $P_{A_{CO_2}}$ (alveolar P_{CO_2}—measured at 37°C) is proportional to the mole fraction of CO_2 in alveolar air but also accounts for the different conditions for measuring the parameters.

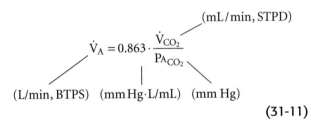

$$\dot{V}_A = 0.863 \cdot \frac{\dot{V}_{CO_2}}{P_{A_{CO_2}}}$$

(mL/min, STPD)

(L/min, BTPS)   (mm Hg·L/mL)   (mm Hg)

$$(31\text{-}11)$$

This is the **alveolar ventilation equation**, which we can use to compute $\dot{V}_A$. We determine $\dot{V}_{CO_2}$ by collecting a known volume of expired air during a fixed time period and analyzing its CO_2. For a 70-kg human, $\dot{V}_{CO_2}$ is ~200 mL/min. We can determine $P_{A_{CO_2}}$ by sampling the expired air at the end of an expiration—an alveolar gas sample. This **end-tidal** P_{CO_2} (Fig. 31-2C) is ~40 mm Hg. In practice, clinicians generally measure *arterial* P_{CO_2} (Pa_{CO_2}) and assume that alveolar and arterial P_{CO_2} are identical (see Chapter 30). Inserting these values into the alveolar ventilation equation, we have

$$\dot{V}_A = 0.863 \cdot \frac{\dot{V}_{CO_2}}{P_{A_{CO_2}}} = 0.863 \cdot \frac{200 \text{ mL/min}}{40 \text{ mm Hg}} \quad (31\text{-}12)$$

$$= 4.315 \text{ L/min}$$

For the sake of simplicity—and consistency with our example in Equation 31-3—we round this figure to 4.2 L/min.

Although it is usually safe to regard $\dot{V}_{CO_2}$ as being constant for a person at rest, a clinical example in which $\dot{V}_{CO_2}$ can increase markedly is **malignant hyperthermia** (see Chapter 9 for the box on this topic), which is associated with increased oxidative metabolism. One hallmark of this clinical catastrophe is that the increase in $\dot{V}_{CO_2}$ leads to an increase in $P_{A_{CO_2}}$ even though $\dot{V}_{CO_2}$ is normal.

Alveolar and arterial P_{CO_2} are inversely proportional to alveolar ventilation

Viewed from a different perspective, Equation 31-11 illustrates one of the most important concepts in respiratory physiology: other things being equal, alveolar P_{CO_2} is inversely proportional to alveolar ventilation. This conclusion makes intuitive sense because the greater the $\dot{V}_A$, the more that the fresh, inspired air dilutes the alveolar CO_2. Rearrangement of Equation 31-11 yields

$$P_{A_{CO_2}} = 0.863 \cdot \frac{\dot{V}_{CO_2}}{\dot{V}_A} \qquad (31\text{-}13)$$

In other words, if CO_2 production is fixed, then doubling of $\dot{V}_A$ causes $P_{A_{CO_2}}$ to fall to half of its initial value. Conversely, halving of $\dot{V}_A$ causes $P_{A_{CO_2}}$ to double. Because *arterial* P_{CO_2} is virtually the same as *alveolar* P_{CO_2} (see Chapter 30), changes in $\dot{V}_A$ affect $P_{A_{CO_2}}$ and $P_{a_{CO_2}}$.

The blue curve in Figure 31-4 helps illustrate the principle. Imagine that your tissues are producing 200 mL/min of CO_2. In a steady state, your lungs must blow off 200 mL of CO_2 each minute. Also, imagine that your lungs are exhaling 4200 mL/min of alveolar air. Because the 200 mL of expired

CO_2 must dissolve in the 4200 mL of exhaled alveolar air (center point in Fig. 31-4), Equation 31-13 tells us that your alveolar P_{CO_2} (and thus $P_{A_{CO_2}}$) must be ~40 mm Hg.

What would happen if the excitement of reading about respiratory physiology caused your alveolar ventilation to double, to 8400 mL/min? This is an example of **hyperventilation**. You could double $\dot{V}_A$ either by doubling respiratory frequency or by doubling the difference between tidal volume and dead space, or a combination of the two (see Equation 31-3). Immediately on doubling of $\dot{V}_A$, you would be blowing off at twice the previous rate not only alveolar air (i.e., 8400 mL/min) but also CO_2 (i.e., 400 mL/min). Because your body would continue to produce only 200 mL/min of CO_2— assuming that doubling of $\dot{V}_A$ does not increase $\dot{V}_{CO_2}$—you would initially blow off CO_2 faster than you made it, causing CO_2 levels throughout your body to fall. However, the falling P_{CO_2} of mixed-venous blood would cause alveolar P_{CO_2} to fall as well, and thus the rate at which you blow off CO_2 would gradually fall. Eventually, you would reach a new steady state in which the rate at which you blow off CO_2 would exactly match the rate at which you produce CO_2 (i.e., 200 mL/min).

On reaching a new steady state, the P_{CO_2} values in your mixed-venous blood, arterial blood, and alveolar air would be stable. But what would be the $P_{A_{CO_2}}$? Because each minute you now are blowing off 8400 mL of alveolar air (i.e., twice normal) but still only 200 mL of CO_2 (right point in Fig. 31-4), your alveolar P_{CO_2} must be half normal, or ~20 mm Hg. Not only does the hyperventilation cause *alveolar* P_{CO_2} to fall by half, it also causes *arterial* P_{CO_2} to fall by half. Thus, hyperventilation leads to **respiratory alkalosis** (see Chapter 28). This respiratory alkalosis causes the arterioles in the brain to constrict (see Chapter 24), reducing blood flow to the brain, which causes dizziness.

What would happen if instead of doubling alveolar ventilation, you halved it from 4200 to 2100 mL/min? This is an example of **hypoventilation**. At the instant you began hypoventilating, the volume of CO_2 expired per unit time would fall by half, to 100 mL/min, even though CO_2 production by the tissues would remain at 200 mL/min. Thus, CO_2 would build up throughout the body, causing $P_{A_{CO_2}}$ to rise. To what value would $P_{A_{CO_2}}$ have to increase before you would reach a new steady state? Because each minute you must exhale 200 mL of CO_2, but this can be diluted in only 2100 mL or half the usual amount of alveolar air (left point in Fig. 31-4), the alveolar $[CO_2]$ must double from ~40 to 80 mm Hg. Of course, this doubling of *alveolar* P_{CO_2} is paralleled by a doubling of *arterial* P_{CO_2}, leading to a **respiratory acidosis** (see Chapter 28).

Therefore, the steady-state alveolar P_{CO_2} is inversely proportional to alveolar ventilation. The higher the $\dot{V}_A$, the lower the $P_{A_{CO_2}}$. If $\dot{V}_A$ were infinitely high, then $P_{A_{CO_2}}$ would theoretically fall to zero, the P_{CO_2} of inspired air.

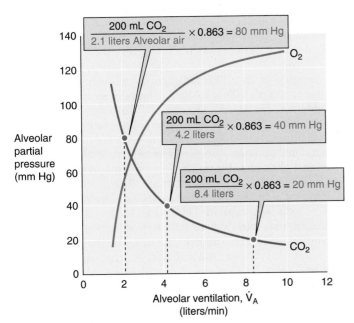

Figure 31-4 Dependence of alveolar CO_2 and O_2 on alveolar ventilation. As alveolar ventilation increases, alveolar P_{O_2} and P_{CO_2} approach their values in inspired air. At extremely low or high $\dot{V}_A$, where O_2 consumption and CO_2 production do not remain constant, these idealized curves are no longer valid.

Alveolar and arterial P_{O_2} rise with increased alveolar ventilation

As illustrated by the orange curve in Figure 31-4, increases in alveolar ventilation cause alveolar P_{O_2} to rise and—at an infinite $\dot{V}_A$—to approach the inspired P_{O_2} of ~149 mm Hg.

Although alveolar P_{O_2} obviously depends critically on $\dot{V}_A$, it is also influenced to a lesser extent by alveolar gases other than O_2—namely, H_2O, N_2, and CO_2. The partial pressure of H_2O at 37°C is 47 mm Hg, and P_{H_2O} will not change unless body temperature changes. The partial pressures of all of the other gases "fit" into what remains of barometric pressure (P_B) after P_{H_2O} has claimed its mandatory 47 mm Hg. We can think of N_2 as a "spectator molecule" because it is not metabolized; P_{N_2} is whatever it has to be to keep the total pressure of the dry alveolar air at $760 - 47 = 713$ mm Hg. That leaves us to deal with CO_2.

Because inspired air contains virtually no CO_2, we can think of the alveolar CO_2 as coming exclusively from metabolism. However, $\dot{V}_{CO_2}$ depends not only on how fast the tissues burn O_2 but also on the *kind of fuel* they burn. If the fuel is carbohydrate, then the tissues produce one molecule of CO_2 for each O_2 consumed (see Chapter 58). This ratio is termed the **respiratory quotient (RQ)**:

$$RQ = \frac{\dot{V}_{CO_2}}{\dot{V}_{O_2}} \qquad \text{(31-14)}$$

In this example, the RQ is 1, which is a good place to start when considering how alveolar P_{CO_2} affects alveolar P_{O_2}. If we consider only the *dry* part of the inspired air that enters the alveoli (see Table 26-1), then $P_{I_{N_2}}$ is $713 \times 0.78 = 557$, $P_{I_{O_2}}$ is $713 \times 0.2095 = 149$ mm Hg, and $P_{I_{CO_2}}$ is ~0. As pulmonary capillary blood takes up incoming O_2, it replaces the O_2 with an equal number of CO_2 molecules in the steady state (RQ = 1). Because the exchange of O_2 for CO_2 is precisely 1 for 1, alveolar P_{O_2} is what is left of the inspired P_{O_2} after metabolism replaces some alveolar O_2 with CO_2 (P_{ACO_2}= 40 mm Hg):

$$\begin{aligned} P_{A_{O_2}} &= P_{I_{O_2}} - P_{A_{CO_2}} \\ &= 149 - 40 \\ &= 109 \text{ mm Hg} \end{aligned} \qquad \text{(31-15)}$$

A typical fat-containing diet in industrialized nations produces an RQ of ~0.8 (see Chapter 58), so that 8 molecules of CO_2 replace 10 molecules of O_2 in the alveolar air. This 8-for-10 replacement has two consequences. First, the volume of alveolar air falls slightly during gas exchange. Because the non-H_2O pressure remains at 713 mm Hg, this volume contraction concentrates the N_2 and dilutes the O_2. Second, the volume of *expired* alveolar air is slightly less than the volume of *inspired* air.

The **alveolar gas equation** describes how alveolar P_{O_2} depends on RQ:

$$\textbf{RQ = 1: } P_{A_{O_2}} = P_{I_{O_2}} - P_{A_{CO_2}} \qquad \text{(31-16)}$$

General case: $P_{A_{O_2}} = P_{I_{O_2}} - P_{A_{CO_2}} \cdot \left(F_{I_{O_2}} + \dfrac{1-F_{I_{O_2}}}{RQ} \right)$ (31-17)

$F_{I_{O_2}}$ is the fraction of inspired *dry* air that is O_2, which is 0.21 for room air (see Table 26-1). Note that when RQ is 1, the term in parentheses becomes unity, and Equation 31-17 reduces to Equation 31-16. The term in parentheses also becomes unity, regardless of RQ, if $F_{I_{O_2}}$ is 100% (i.e., the subject breathes pure O_2)—in this case, no N_2 is present to dilute the O_2.

A simplified version of Equation 31-17 is nearly as accurate:

$$P_{A_{O_2}} = P_{I_{O_2}} - \frac{P_{A_{CO_2}}}{RQ} \qquad \text{(31-18)}$$

The concepts developed in the last two sections allow us to compute both alveolar P_{CO_2} and P_{O_2}. The approach is to first use Equation 31-13 to calculate $P_{A_{CO_2}}$ from $\dot{V}_{CO_2}$ and $\dot{V}_A$ and then use Equation 31-17 to calculate $P_{A_{O_2}}$ from $P_{A_{CO_2}}$ and RQ. Imagine that we first found that $P_{A_{CO_2}}$ is 40 mm Hg, and that we know that RQ is 0.8. What is $P_{A_{O_2}}$?

$$P_{A_{O_2}} = P_{I_{O_2}} - P_{A_{CO_2}} \cdot \left(F_{I_{O_2}} + \frac{1-F_{I_{O_2}}}{RQ} \right)$$

$$P_{A_{O_2}} = 149 - 40 \cdot \underbrace{\left(0.21 + \frac{1-0.21}{0.8} \right)}_{1.2} \qquad \text{(31-19)}$$

$$= 149 - 48$$

$$= 101 \text{ mm Hg}$$

By default, the partial pressure of N_2 and other gases (e.g., argon) is $P_B - P_{A_{CO_2}} - P_{A_{O_2}}$, or $713 - 40 - 101 = 572$ mm Hg. For simplicity, we round down this $P_{A_{O_2}}$ to 100 mm Hg in our examples.

Because of the action of gravity on the lung, regional ventilation in an upright subject is normally greater at the base than at the apex

Until now, we have assumed that all alveoli are ventilated to the same extent. We could test this hypothesis by use of an imaging technique to assess the uniformity of ventilation. Imagine that a subject who is standing up breathes air containing ^{133}Xe. Because Xe has very low water solubility, it (like He and N_2) has a very low diffusing capacity (see Chapter 30); during a short period, it remains almost entirely within the alveoli.

Imaging of the ^{133}Xe radioactivity immediately after a single breath of [^{133}Xe] provides an index of *absolute regional ventilation* (Fig. 31-5A). However, [^{133}Xe] might be low in a particular region either because the alveoli truly receive little ventilation or because the region has relatively little tissue. Therefore, we normalize the *absolute* data to the maximal regional alveolar volume. The subject continues to breathe the ^{133}Xe until [^{133}Xe] values stabilize throughout the lungs. When the subject now makes a maximal inspiratory effort (V_L = total lung capacity [TLC]), the level of radioactivity detected over any region reflects that region's maximal volume. Dividing the single-breath image by the steady-state image at TLC yields a ratio that describes *regional ventilation per unit volume*.

This sort of analysis shows that alveolar ventilation in a standing person gradually falls from the base to the apex of the lung (Fig. 31-5B). Why? The answers are **posture** and **gravity**. In Chapter 27 we saw that because of the lung's weight, intrapleural pressure (P_{IP}) is more negative at the apex than at the base when the subject is upright (Fig. 31-5C). The practical consequences of this P_{IP} gradient become clear when we examine a static pressure-volume

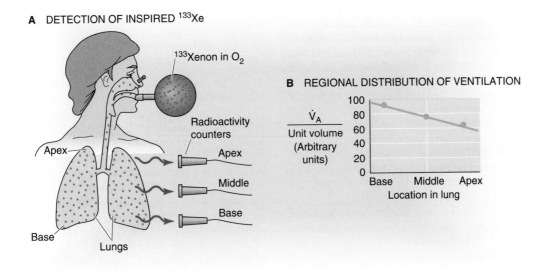

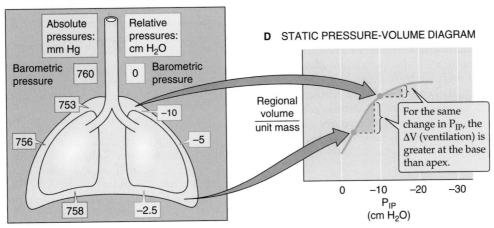

Figure 31-5 Distribution of ventilation. *(Data from West JB: Respiratory Physiology—The Essentials, 4th ed. Baltimore, Williams & Wilkins, 1990.)*

diagram not for the lungs as a whole (as we did in Fig. 27-5) but rather for a small piece of lung (Fig. 31-5D). We assume that the intrinsic mechanical properties of the airways are the same, regardless of whether the tissue is at the base or at the apex. At the base, where P_{IP} might be only −2.5 cm H_2O at FRC, the alveoli are relatively underinflated compared with tissues at the apex, where P_{IP} might be −10 cm H_2O and the alveoli are relatively overinflated. However, because the base of the lung is underinflated at FRC, it is on a steeper part of the pressure-volume curve (i.e., it has a greater **static compliance**) than the overinflated apex. Thus, during an inspiration, the same ΔP_{IP} (e.g., 2.5 cm H_2O) produces a larger ΔV_L near the base than near the apex. Keep in mind that it is the *change* in volume per unit time, not the initial volume, that defines ventilation.

The relationship between ventilation and basal versus apical location in the lung would be reversed if the subject hung by the knees from a trapeze. A person reclining on the right side would ventilate the dependent lung tissue on the right side better than the elevated lung tissue on the left. Of course, the right-to-left P_{IP} gradient in the reclining subject would be smaller than the apex-to-base P_{IP} gradient in the standing subject, reflecting the smaller distance (i.e., smaller hydrostatic pressure difference). Subjects under microgravity conditions (see Chapter 58), such as astronauts aboard the International Space Station, experience no P_{IP} gradients and thus no gravity-dependent regional differences in ventilation.

Restrictive and obstructive pulmonary diseases can exacerbate the nonuniformity of ventilation

Even in microgravity, where we would expect no regional differences in ventilation, ventilation would still be nonuniform at the *microscopic* or *local* level because of seemingly random differences in local static compliance (C) and airway resistance (R). In fact, such local differences in the ventilation of alveolar units are probably more impressive than gravity-dependent regional differences. Moreover, pathological changes in compliance and resistance can substantially increase the local differences and thus the nonuniformity of ventilation.

Restrictive Pulmonary Disease As discussed in the box on diseases affecting ventilation in Chapter 27, restrictive pulmonary diseases include disorders that decrease the static compliance of alveoli (e.g., fibrosis) as well as disorders that limit the expansion of the lung (e.g., pulmonary effusion). Figure 31-6A shows a hypothetical example in which R is normal and disease has halved the static compliance of one lung but left the other unaffected. Thus, for the usual change in P_{IP}, the final volume change (ΔV) of the diseased lung is only half normal, so that its ventilation is also halved. Because the ventilation of the other unit is normal, decreased local compliance has increased the nonuniformity of ventilation.

Obstructive Pulmonary Disease As discussed in the box on asthma in Chapter 27, obstructive pulmonary diseases include disorders (e.g., asthma, COPD) that increase the resistance of conducting airways. Scar tissue or a local mass, such as a neoplasm, can also occlude a conducting airway or compress it from the outside. Even if the effect is not sufficiently severe to increase overall airway resistance, a local increase in R causes an increase in the time constant τ for filling or emptying of the affected alveoli (Fig. 31-6B, lower curve). An isolated increase in R would not affect ΔV if sufficient time were available for the inspiration. However, if sufficient time is not available, then alveoli with an elevated τ will not completely fill or empty, and their ventilation will decrease. Of course, the mismatching of ventilation between the two units worsens as respiratory frequency increases, as we saw in our discussion of dynamic compliance (see Chapter 27).

PERFUSION OF THE LUNG

The pulmonary circulation has low pressure and resistance but high compliance

The pulmonary circulatory system handles the same cardiac output as the systemic circulation but in a very different way. The systemic circulation is a *high-pressure* system. This high pressure is necessary to pump blood to the top of the brain while standing or even to a maximally elevated fingertip. The systemic circulation also needs to be a high-pressure system because it is a high-*resistance* system. It uses this high resistance to control the distribution of blood flow. Thus, at rest, a substantial fraction of the systemic capillaries are closed, giving the system the flexibility to redistribute large amounts of blood (e.g., to muscle during exercise). The mean pressure of the aorta is ~95 mm Hg (Table 31-1). At the opposite end of the circuit is the right atrium, which has a mean pressure of ~2 mm Hg. Thus, the driving pressure for blood flow through the systemic circulation is ~93 mm Hg. Given a cardiac output ($\dot{Q}$) of 5 L/min or 83 mL/s, we can compute the resistance of the systemic system by use of an equation like Ohm's law (see Equation 17-10):

$$R_{systemic} = \frac{\Delta P}{\dot{Q}} = \frac{93 \, \text{mm Hg}}{83 \, \text{mL blood/s}} \qquad (31\text{-}20)$$
$$= 1.1 \, \text{PRU}$$

PRU is a peripheral resistance unit (see Chapter 17), which has the dimensions mm Hg/(mL/s).

A REDUCE COMPLIANCE OF ONE LUNG TO HALF NORMAL

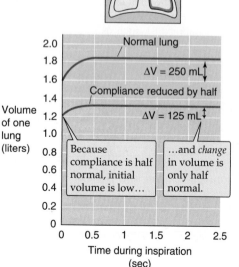

B INCREASE AIRWAY RESISTANCE OF ONE LUNG 5-FOLD

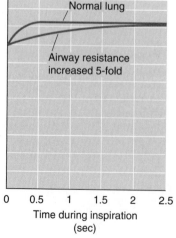

Figure 31-6 Pathologic nonuniformity of ventilation.

Table 31-1 Comparison of Pressures in the Pulmonary and Systemic Circulatory System*

PULMONARY CIRCULATION		SYSTEMIC CIRCULATION	
	Mean Pressure (mm Hg)		Mean Pressure (mm Hg)
Pulmonary artery	15	Aorta	95
Beginning of capillary	12	Beginning of capillary	35
End of capillary	9	End of capillary	15
Left atrium	8	Right atrium	2
Net driving pressure	15 − 8 = 7	Net driving pressure	95 − 2 = 93

*The reference point for all pressures is the pressure outside the heart at the level of the left atrium.

In contrast, the pulmonary circulation is a low-pressure system. It can afford to be a low-pressure system because it needs to pump blood only to the top of the lung. Moreover, it *must* be a low-pressure system to avoid the consequences of Starling forces (see Chapter 20), which would otherwise flood the lung with edema fluid. The mean pressure in the pulmonary artery is only ~15 mm Hg. Because the mean pressure of the left atrium, at the other end of the circuit, is ~8 mm Hg, and because the cardiac output of the right side of the heart is the same as for the left side, we have

$$R_{pulmonary} = \frac{\Delta P}{\dot{Q}} = \frac{7\,mm\,Hg}{83\,mL\,blood/s} \quad (31\text{-}21)$$
$$= 0.08\,PRU$$

Thus, the total resistance of the pulmonary circulation is less than one tenth that of the systemic system, which explains how the pulmonary circulation accomplishes its mission at such low pressures. Unlike in the systemic circulation, where most of the pressure drop occurs in the arterioles (i.e., between the terminal arteries and beginning of the capillaries), in the pulmonary circulation almost the entire pressure drop occurs rather uniformly between the pulmonary artery and the end of the capillaries. In particular, the arterioles make a much smaller contribution to resistance in the pulmonary circulation than in the systemic circulation.

What are the properties of the pulmonary vasculature that give it such a low resistance? First, let us examine the complete circuit. The **pulmonary artery** arises from the right ventricle, bifurcates, and carries relatively deoxygenated blood to each lung. The two main branches of the pulmonary artery follow the two mainstem bronchi into the lungs and bifurcate along with the bronchi and bronchioles. A single pulmonary arteriole supplies all of the capillaries of a terminal respiratory unit (see Chapter 26). Together, the two lungs have ~300 *million* alveoli. However, they may have as many as 280 *billion* highly anastomosing capillary seg-

ments (each looking like the edge of a hexagon in a piece of chicken wire), or nearly 1000 such capillary segments per alveolus—creating a surface for gas exchange of ~100 m². It is easy to imagine why some have described the pulmonary capillary bed as a nearly continuous flowing sheet of blood surrounding the alveoli. At rest, the erythrocytes spend ~0.75 second navigating this capillary bed, which contains ~75 mL of blood. During exercise, capillary blood volume may increase to ~200 mL. Pulmonary venules collect the oxygenated blood from the capillary network, converge, course between the lobules, converge some more, and eventually enter the left atrium through the pulmonary veins. The total circulation time through the pulmonary system is 4 to 5 seconds.

Pulmonary blood vessels are generally shorter and wider than their counterparts on the systemic side. Arterioles are also present in much higher numbers in the pulmonary circulation. Although the pulmonary arterioles contain smooth muscle and can constrict, these vessels are far less muscular than their systemic counterparts, and their resting tone is low. These properties combine to produce a system with an unusually **low resistance**.

The walls of pulmonary vessels have another key property: thinness, like the walls of veins elsewhere in the body. The thin walls and paucity of smooth muscle give the pulmonary vessels a **high compliance**, which has three consequences. First, pulmonary vessels can accept relatively large amounts of blood that shift from the legs to the lungs when a person changes from a standing to a recumbent position. Second, as we discuss later, the high compliance also allows the vessels to dilate in response to modest increases in pulmonary arterial pressure. Third, the pulse pressure in the pulmonary system is rather low (on an absolute scale). The systolic and diastolic pressures in the pulmonary artery are typically 25 and 8 mm Hg, yielding a **pulse pressure** of ~17 mm Hg. In contrast, the systolic and diastolic pressures in the aorta are ~120 and 80 mm Hg, for a pulse pressure of ~40 mm Hg. Nonetheless, relative to the *mean* pulmonary artery pressure of 15 mm Hg, the pulmonary pulse pressure of 17 mm Hg is quite high.

Overall pulmonary vascular resistance is minimal at functional residual capacity

Because pulmonary blood vessels are so compliant, they are especially susceptible to deformation by external forces. These forces are very different for vessels that are surrounded by alveoli (i.e., alveolar vessels) compared with those that are not (i.e., extra-alveolar vessels). In both types, the key consideration is whether these external forces pull vessels open or crush them.

Alveolar Vessels Alveolar vessels include the capillaries as well as slightly larger vessels that are also surrounded on all sides by alveoli (Fig. 31-7A). The resistance of these alveolar vessels depends on both the transmural pressure gradient and lung volume.

We have already introduced the **transmural pressure gradient** (P_{TM}) in our discussions of systemic blood vessels (see Chapter 17) and conducting airways (see Chapter 27). For

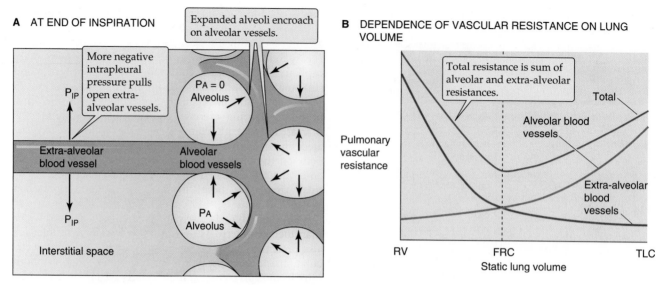

Figure 31-7   **A** and **B,** Pulmonary vascular resistance. FRC, functional residual capacity; RV, respiratory volume; TLC, total lung capacity. (**B,** Data from Murray JF: The Normal Lung, 2nd ed. Philadelphia, WB Saunders, 1986.)

alveolar vessels, P_{TM} is the difference between the pressures in the vessel *lumen* and in the surrounding *alveoli* (P_A). For simplicity, we consider the factors affecting P_{TM} at a fixed lung volume.

The pressure inside these vessels varies with the *cardiac cycle*; indeed, the pulmonary capillary bed is one of the few in which flow is pulsatile (see Chapter 22). The pressure inside the alveolar vessels also depends greatly on their vertical position relative to the left atrium: the higher the vessel, the lower the pressure.

The pressure in the alveoli varies with the *respiratory cycle*. With no airflow and the glottis open, P_A is the same as P_B (i.e., 0 cm H_2O). On the other hand, P_B is negative during inspiration and positive during expiration. A combination of a high intravascular pressure and a negative P_A tends to dilate the compliant alveolar vessels, lowering their resistance. But a combination of a low intravascular pressure and a positive P_A crushes these vessels, raising their resistance.

Changes in *lung volume* (V_L) have characteristic effects on alveolar vessels. For simplicity, here we assume that each time we examine a new V_L, airflow has stopped, so that P_A is zero. As V_L increases, the alveolar walls become more stretched out. Consequently, the alveolar vessels become stretched along their longitudinal axis but crushed when viewed in cross section. Both of these effects tend to raise vessel resistance. Thus, as V_L increases, the resistance of the alveolar vessels also increases (Fig. 31-7B, red curve).

Extra-alveolar Vessels   Because they are not surrounded by alveoli, the extra-alveolar vessels are sensitive to intrapleural pressure (Fig. 31-7A). Again for simplicity, we examine the effect of changing V_L after airflow has already stopped. The increasingly negative values of P_{IP} needed to achieve increasingly higher lung volumes also increase the P_{TM} of the extra-alveolar vessels and tend to dilate them. Thus, as V_L increases, the resistance of the extra-alveolar vessels decreases (Fig. 31-7B, blue curve).

In summary, increases in V_L tend to crush alveolar vessels and thus increase their resistance but to expand extra-alveolar vessels and thus decrease their resistance. The net effect on overall pulmonary vascular resistance of increasing V_L from residual volume (RV) to TLC is biphasic (Fig. 31-7B, violet curve). Starting at RV, an increase in V_L first causes pulmonary vascular resistance to fall, as the dilation of extra-alveolar vessels dominates. Pulmonary vascular resistance reaches its minimum value at about FRC. Further increases in V_L (as during a normal inspiration) increase overall resistance, as the crushing of alveolar vessels dominates.

Increases in pulmonary arterial pressure reduce pulmonary vascular resistance by recruiting and distending pulmonary capillaries

Although the pulmonary circulation is normally a low-resistance system under resting conditions, it has a remarkable ability to lower its resistance even further. During exercise, 2-fold to 3-fold increases in cardiac output may elicit only a minor increase in mean pulmonary arterial pressure. In other words, a slight increase in pulmonary arterial pressure is somehow able to markedly *decrease* resistance (Fig. 31-8A) and thus markedly *increase* flow (Fig. 31-8B). This behavior is a general property of a passive/elastic vascular bed (see Fig. 19-7A, red curve). Two "passive" mechanisms—that is, mechanisms not related to "active" changes in the tone of vascular smooth muscle—are at work here: the recruitment and distention of pulmonary capillaries. However, before we can understand either change, we must more completely describe the pulmonary capillaries at "rest."

Under "resting" conditions (i.e., at relatively low values of pulmonary arterial pressure), some pulmonary capillaries are open and conducting blood, others are open but not conducting substantial amounts of blood, and still others are closed (Fig. 31-8C). Why should some capillaries be **open** but have no flow? In a highly anastomosing capillary network,

A EFFECT OF PULMONARY ARTERIAL PRESSURE ON VASCULAR RESISTANCE

B EFFECT OF PULMONARY ARTERIAL PRESSURE ON BLOOD FLOW

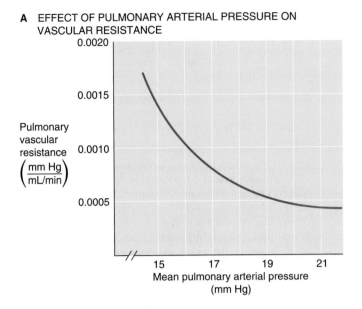

C RECRUITMENT AND DISTENTION OF ALVEOLAR VESSELS

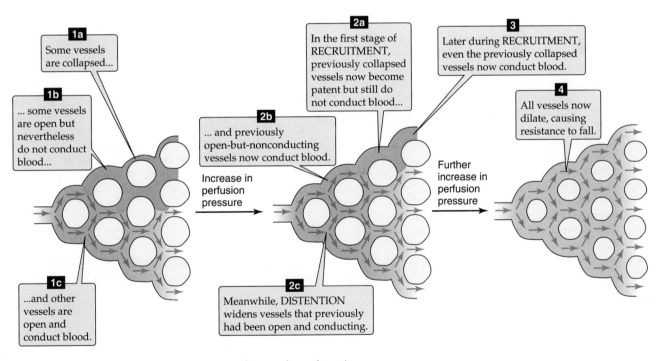

Figure 31-8 Effects of perfusion pressure on pulmonary hemodynamics.

tiny differences in driving pressure might exist. In addition, seemingly random differences in the dimensions of parallel capillaries may lead to differences in resistance. In low-pressure systems, such slight differences in absolute resistance allow pathways with relatively low resistances to steal flow from neighbors with slightly higher resistances, leaving some "open" pathways heavily underused. A familiar example is a type of garden hose used to drizzle water on a flower bed; this hose is closed at its distal end but perforated with hundreds of tiny holes. If water pressure is low, only some of the holes conduct water.

Why should some parallel vessels be **closed**? Popping open a previously closed vessel requires that the perfusion pressure overcome the tone of the vascular smooth muscle and reach that vessel's **critical closing pressure** (see Chapter 19), which varies from vessel to vessel. As we discuss later, alveolar vessels also may be closed because the alveolar pressure exceeds intravascular pressure, thereby crushing the vessel.

Recruitment Imagine that the pressure inside a pulmonary arteriole starts out at a fairly low level. As pressure increases, some vessels that were completely *closed* may now open (Fig. 31-8C). Similarly, capillaries that previously had been *open but not conducting* now begin to conduct blood. The greater the increase in perfusion pressure, the greater the number of open and conducting vessels. This recruitment of additional parallel capillary pathways reduces overall vascular resistance.

Distention   Once a vessel is open and conducting, further pressure increases will increase P_{TM} and thus cause the vessel to dilate (Fig. 31-8C). The net effect is a reduction in overall pulmonary resistance. Although a pressure increase can simultaneously recruit and distend various vessels, distention probably tends to occur later; that is, distention is the primary mechanism for lowering resistance under conditions in which the initial pressure was already relatively high.

Hypoxia is a strong vasoconstrictor, opposite to its effect in the systemic circulation

In addition to lung volume and perfusion pressure, several other factors can modulate pulmonary vascular resistance.

Oxygen   The effects of changes in P_{O_2}, P_{CO_2}, and pH on pulmonary vascular resistance are opposite to those observed in the systemic circulation. Thus, hypoxia causes pulmonary vasoconstriction. What appears to be critical is not so much the P_{O_2} in the lumen of the arterioles and venules but rather the P_{O_2} in the *alveolar air* adjacent to the vessel. Indeed, perfusion of the pulmonary vasculature with a hypoxic solution is far less effective than ventilation of the airways with a low-P_{O_2} air mixture.

Hypoxic vasoconstriction occurs in isolated lung tissue and thus does not rely on either the nervous system or systemic hormones. Rather, the low P_{O_2} is generally believed to act directly on the pulmonary vascular smooth muscle cells. How this occurs is unknown, but hypothesized mechanisms include all those proposed for the sensing of hypoxia by the peripheral chemoreceptor, which we discuss in Chapter 32. Somehow, the hypoxia inhibits one or more K^+ channels, causing the membrane potential of vascular smooth muscle cells to move away from E_K. This depolarization opens voltage-gated Ca^{2+} channels, leading to an influx of Ca^{2+} and smooth muscle contraction (see Chapter 9).

CO₂ and Low pH   High P_{CO_2} and low interstitial pH promote vasoconstriction, although with far less potency than hypoxia. Elevated P_{CO_2} may produce its effect by decreasing the pH of either the extracellular or intracellular fluid. Following a general pattern that is repeated in the control of Ventilation, hypoxia makes the vascular smooth muscle cells more sensitive to respiratory acidosis.

Autonomic Nervous System   The sympathetic and parasympathetic innervation of the pulmonary vasculature is far less impressive than that of the systemic circulation. Increased sympathetic tone seems to reduce the compliance of (i.e., stiffen) the pulmonary artery walls without increasing resistance per se. Increased parasympathetic tone causes a mild vasodilation, the relevance of which is unknown.

Hormones and Other Humoral Agents   The pulmonary blood vessels are relatively *unresponsive* to hormones and other signaling molecules. Table 31-2 summarizes the actions of some factors that modify pulmonary vascular resistance.

Because of gravity, regional perfusion in an upright subject is far greater near the base than the apex of the lung

When it comes to perfusion—like ventilation—not all alveoli are created equal. First of all, *microscopic* or *local* differences in pulmonary vascular resistance lead to corresponding local differences in perfusion. Of course, disease can exacerbate these differences. In addition, gravity causes large *regional* differences in perfusion that we can assess by use of a ^{133}Xe imaging technique. In Figure 31-5A, we used the inhalation of ^{133}Xe gas to measure the uniformity of *ventilation*. In Figure 31-9A, we equilibrate a saline solution with ^{133}Xe and then inject the solution intravenously as the patient holds his or her breath. When the ^{133}Xe reaches the lungs, it rapidly enters the alveolar air, inasmuch as Xe is poorly soluble in water. A lung scan reveals the distribution of radioactivity, which now reflects the regional uniformity of *perfusion*. If we normalize the ^{133}Xe to account for differences in regional lung volume—as we did for the ventilation scan—then we can obtain a graph showing how blood flow varies from the bottom to the top of the lung of an upright subject.

The results of such a ^{133}Xe perfusion study show that when the patient is upright, perfusion ($\dot{Q}$) is greatest near the base of the lungs and falls toward low levels near the apex (Fig. 31-9B). Note that although regional $\dot{Q}$ is highest *near* the base of the lung, $\dot{Q}$ falls off somewhat from this peak as we approach the extreme base. With exercise, perfusion increases in all regions of the lung but more so near the apex, so that the nonuniformity of perfusion is less.

Table 31-2   Changes or Agents That Affect Pulmonary Vascular Resistance

Dilators	Constrictors
↑ $P_{A_{O_2}}$	↓ $P_{A_{O_2}}$
↓ $P_{A_{CO_2}}$	↑ $P_{A_{CO_2}}$
↑ pH	↓ pH
Histamine H_2 agonists	Histamine H_1 agonists
PGI₂ (prostacyclin), PGE₁	Thromboxane A₂, PGF₂α, PGE₂
β-Adrenergic agonists (e.g., isoproterenol)	α-Adrenergic agonists
Bradykinin	Serotonin
Theophylline	Angiotensin II
Acetylcholine	
NO	

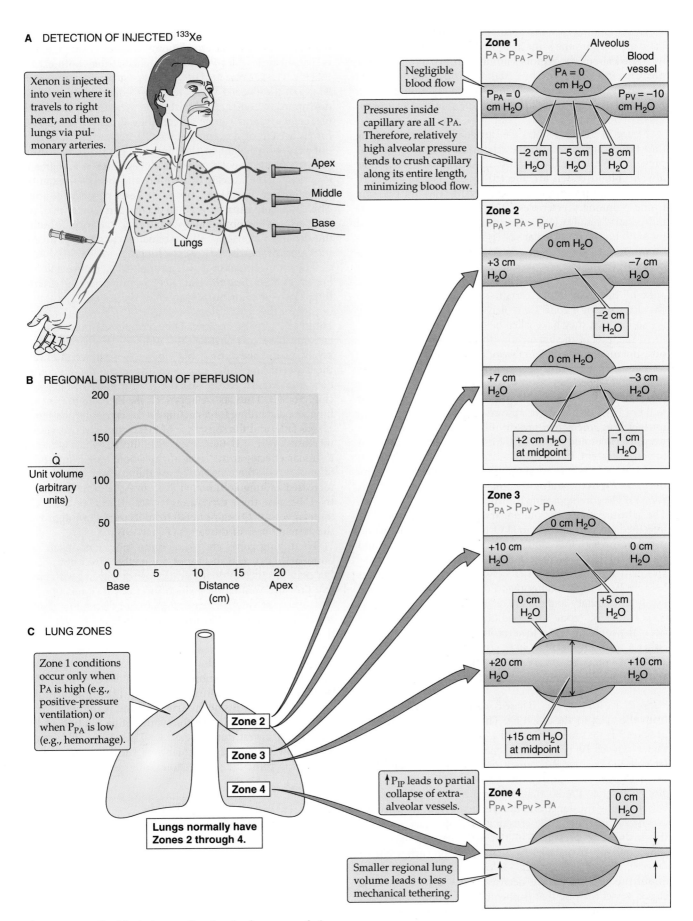

A DETECTION OF INJECTED ^{133}Xe

Xenon is injected into vein where it travels to right heart, and then to lungs via pulmonary arteries.

Apex
Middle
Base
Lungs

B REGIONAL DISTRIBUTION OF PERFUSION

$\dfrac{\dot{Q}}{\text{Unit volume (arbitrary units)}}$

200
150
100
50
0

0 5 10 15 20
Base   Distance   Apex
(cm)

C LUNG ZONES

Zone 1 conditions occur only when P_A is high (e.g., positive-pressure ventilation) or when P_{PA} is low (e.g., hemorrhage).

Zone 2
Zone 3
Zone 4

Lungs normally have Zones 2 through 4.

Zone 1
$P_A > P_{PA} > P_{PV}$

Negligible blood flow

Alveolus
Blood vessel

$P_A = 0$ cm H_2O
$P_{PA} = 0$ cm H_2O
$P_{PV} = -10$ cm H_2O

Pressures inside capillary are all < P_A. Therefore, relatively high alveolar pressure tends to crush capillary along its entire length, minimizing blood flow.

-2 cm H_2O -5 cm H_2O -8 cm H_2O

Zone 2
$P_{PA} > P_A > P_{PV}$

0 cm H_2O
$+3$ cm H_2O
-7 cm H_2O
-2 cm H_2O

0 cm H_2O
$+7$ cm H_2O
-3 cm H_2O
$+2$ cm H_2O at midpoint
-1 cm H_2O

Zone 3
$P_{PA} > P_{PV} > P_A$

0 cm H_2O
$+10$ cm H_2O
0 cm H_2O

0 cm H_2O
$+5$ cm H_2O

$+20$ cm H_2O
$+10$ cm H_2O

$+15$ cm H_2O at midpoint

↑P_{IP} leads to partial collapse of extraalveolar vessels.

Zone 4
$P_{PA} > P_{PV} > P_A$

0 cm H_2O

Smaller regional lung volume leads to less mechanical tethering.

Figure 31-9 Physiological nonuniformity of pulmonary perfusion.

Why should $\dot{Q}$ have this peculiar height dependence? The basic answers are the same as those for the similar question we raised about the regional nonuniformity of *ventilation*: **posture** and **gravity**. Thus, standing on your head will reverse the flow-height relationship, and we would expect height-related differences in flow to be minimal in microgravity conditions.

Figure 31-9C shows how we can divide the upright lung into four zones based on the relationships among various pressures. We define the first three zones on the basis of how *alveolar* blood vessels are affected by the relative values of three different pressures: alveolar pressure (P_A), the pressure inside pulmonary arterioles (P_{PA}), and the pressure inside pulmonary venules (P_{PV}). In the fourth zone, we instead focus on how extra-alveolar vessels are affected by intrapleural pressure (P_{IP}).

Zone 1: $P_A > P_{PA} > P_{PV}$ These conditions prevail at the apex of the lung under certain conditions. The defining characteristic of a zone 1 alveolar vessel is that P_{PA} and P_{PV} are so low that they have fallen below P_A.

At the level of the left atrium (the reference point for the pressure measurements), the *mean* P_{PA} is ~15 mm Hg (Table 31-1), which—because mercury is 13.6-fold more dense than water—corresponds to ~20 cm H_2O (Fig. 31-9C, lower panel of zone 3). Similarly, mean P_{PV} is ~8 mm Hg, or ~10 cm H_2O. As we move upward closer to the apex of an upright lung, the actual pressures in the lumens of pulmonary arterioles and venules fall by 1 cm H_2O for each 1 cm of vertical ascent. In the hypothetical case in which alveoli at the lung apex are 20 cm above the level of the left atrium, the mean P_{PA} of these alveoli would be 0 cm H_2O (Fig. 31-9C, zone 1). The corresponding P_{PV} would be about −10 cm H_2O. The pressure inside the pulmonary capillary (Pc) would be intermediate, perhaps −5 cm H_2O. In principle, blood would still flow through this capillary—the driving pressure would be ~10 cm H_2O—were it not for the pressure inside the alveoli, which is 0 cm H_2O between breaths. Therefore, because P_A is much higher than Pc, the negative P_{TM} would crush the capillary and greatly reduce blood flow.

Fortunately, zone 1 conditions do not exist for normal people at rest. However, they can arise if there is either a sufficient decrease in P_{PA} (e.g., in hemorrhage) or a sufficient increase in P_A (e.g., in **positive-pressure ventilation**).

Zone 2: $P_{PA} > P_A > P_{PV}$ These conditions normally prevail from the apex to the midlung. The defining characteristic of zone 2 is that mean P_{PA} and P_{PV} are high enough so that they sandwich P_A (Fig. 31-9C, zone 2). Thus, at the arteriolar end, the positive P_{TM} causes the alveolar vessel to dilate. Farther down the capillary, though, luminal pressure gradually falls below P_A, so that the negative P_{TM} squeezes the vessel, raising resistance and thus reducing flow. As we move downward in zone 2, the crushing force decreases because the hydrostatic pressures in the arteriole, capillary, and venule all rise in parallel by 1 cm H_2O for each 1 cm of descent (Fig. 31-9C, upper → lower panels of zone 2). Simultaneously, resistance decreases. The conversion of a closed vessel (or one that is open but not conducting) to a conducting one by increased P_{PA} and P_{PV} is an example of **recruitment.**

Zone 3: $P_{PA} > P_{PV} > P_A$ These conditions prevail in the middle to lower lung. The defining characteristic of zone 3 is that mean P_{PA} and P_{PV} are so high that they both exceed P_A (Fig. 31-9C, zone 3). Thus, P_{TM} is positive along the entire length of the alveolar vessel, tending to dilate it. As we move downward in zone 3, the hydrostatic pressures in the arteriole, capillary, and venule all continue to rise by 1 cm H_2O for each 1 cm of descent. Because P_A between breaths does not vary with height in the lung, the gradually increasing pressure of the alveolar vessel produces a greater and greater P_{TM}, causing the vessel to dilate more and more—an example of **distention** (Fig. 31-9C, upper → lower panels of zone 3). This distention causes a gradual decrease in resistance of the capillaries as we move downward in zone 3. Hence, although the driving force ($P_{PA} - P_{PV}$) remains constant, perfusion increases toward the base of the lung.

The arrangement in which a variable P_{TM} controls flow is known as a **Starling resistor**. Keep in mind that the driving force ($P_{PA} - P_{PV}$) is constant in all of the zones.

Zone 4: $P_{PA} > P_{PV} > P_A$ These conditions prevail at the extreme base of the lungs. In zone 4, the *alveolar vessels* behave as in zone 3; they dilate more as we descend toward the base of the lung. However, the *extra-alveolar vessels* behave differently. At the base of the lung, P_{IP} is least negative (Fig. 31-5C). Thus, as we approach the extreme base of the lung, the distending forces acting on the extra-alveolar blood vessels fade, and the resistance of these extra-alveolar vessels increases (Fig. 31-9C, zone 4). Recall that we saw a similar effect—at the level of the whole lung (Fig. 31-7B, blue curve)—where resistance of the extra-alveolar vessels increased as lung volume fell (i.e., as P_{IP} became less negative). Because these extra-alveolar vessels feed or drain the alveolar vessels, $\dot{Q}$ begins to fall from its peak as we approach the extreme base of the lungs (Fig. 31-9B).

These lung zones are *physiological*, not anatomical. The boundaries between the zones are neither fixed nor sharp. For example, the boundaries can move downward with positive-pressure ventilation (which increases P_A) and upward with exercise (which increases P_{PA}). In our discussion of lung zones, we have tacitly assumed that P_A is always zero and that the values of P_{PA} and P_{PV} are stable and depend only on height in the lung. In real life, of course, things are more complicated. During the respiratory cycle, P_A becomes negative during inspiration (promoting dilation of alveolar vessels) but positive during expiration. During the cardiac cycle, the pressure inside the arterioles and pulmonary capillaries is greatest during systole (promoting dilation of the vessel) and lowest during diastole. Thus, we would expect blood flow through an alveolar vessel to be greatest when inspiration coincides with systole.

MATCHING VENTILATION AND PERFUSION

The greater the ventilation-perfusion ratio, the higher the P_{O_2} and the lower the P_{CO_2} in the alveolar air

In Figure 31-4, we saw that all other factors being equal, alveolar ventilation determines alveolar P_{O_2} and P_{CO_2}. The greater the ventilation, the more closely $P_{A_{O_2}}$ and $P_{A_{CO_2}}$ approach their respective values in inspired air. However, in Figure 31-4, we were really focusing on *total* alveolar ventilation and how this influences the *average*, or idealized, alveolar P_{O_2} and P_{CO_2}. In fact, we have already learned that both ventilation and perfusion vary among alveoli. In any group of alveoli, the greater the local ventilation, the more closely the composition of local alveolar air approaches that of the inspired air. Similarly, because blood flow removes O_2 from the alveolar air and adds CO_2, the greater the perfusion, the more closely the composition of local alveolar air approaches that of mixed-venous blood. Thus, the local **ventilation-perfusion ratio** ($\dot{V}_A/\dot{Q}$) determines the local $P_{A_{O_2}}$ and $P_{A_{CO_2}}$.

You might view the alveoli as a sports venue where ventilation and perfusion are engaged in a continuous struggle over control of the composition of alveolar air. To the extent that ventilation gains the upper hand, $P_{A_{O_2}}$ rises and $P_{A_{CO_2}}$ falls. To the extent that perfusion holds sway, these parameters change in the opposite direction.

As a physical analogue of this struggle over control of alveolar P_{O_2}, consider water flowing (analogous to $\dot{V}_A$) from a faucet into a sink (alveoli); the water exits ($\dot{Q}$) through a drain with an adjustable opening. If the drain opening is in midposition and we begin flowing water moderately fast, then the water level ($P_{A_{O_2}}$) will gradually increase and reach a steady state. Increasing the inflow of water ($\dot{V}_A$) will cause the water level ($P_{A_{O_2}}$) to rise until the product of pressure head and drain conductance is high enough to drive water down the drain as fast as the water flows in. If we increase the drain opening and thus the outflow of water ($\dot{Q}$), then the water level ($P_{A_{O_2}}$) will fall until the decrease in the pressure head matches the increase in drain conductance, so that once again water inflow and outflow are balanced. Just as a high faucet/drain ratio will raise the water level, a high $\dot{V}_A/\dot{Q}$ ratio will increase alveolar P_{O_2}.

Because of the action of gravity, the regional ventilation-perfusion ratio ($\dot{V}_A/\dot{Q}$) in an upright subject is greater at the apex of the lung than at the base

We have already seen that when a subject is upright in a gravitational field, ventilation falls from the base to the apex

of the lung (Fig. 31-5B), and perfusion also falls, but more steeply (Fig. 31-9B). Thus, it is not surprising that the ratio $\dot{V}_A/\dot{Q}$ itself varies with height in the lung (Fig. 31-10A). $\dot{V}_A/\dot{Q}$ is lowest near the base, where $\dot{Q}$ exceeds $\dot{V}_A$. The ratio gradually increases to 1 at about the level of the third rib and further increases toward the apex, where $\dot{Q}$ falls more precipitously than $\dot{V}_A$.

Table 31-3 shows how differences in $\dot{V}_A/\dot{Q}$ at the apex and base of the lungs influence the regional composition of alveolar air. At the apex (the most rostral 7% of lung volume in this example), where $\dot{V}_A/\dot{Q}$ is highest, alveolar P_{O_2} and P_{CO_2} most closely approach their values in inspired air. Because both O_2 and CO_2 transport across the blood-gas barrier are **perfusion limited** (see Chapter 30), O_2 and CO_2 have completely equilibrated between the alveolar air and the blood by the end of the pulmonary capillaries. Thus, blood leaving the apex has the same high P_{O_2} and low P_{CO_2} as the alveolar air. Of course, the relatively low P_{CO_2} produces a *respiratory alkalosis* (see Chapter 28) in the blood leaving the apex.

The situation is just the opposite near the base of the lung (the most caudal 13% of lung volume in this example). Because $\dot{V}_A/\dot{Q}$ here is lowest, alveolar P_{O_2} and P_{CO_2} tend more

Table 31-3 Effect of Regional Differences in $\dot{V}_A/\dot{Q}$ on the Composition of Alveolar Air and Pulmonary Capillary Blood

Location	Fraction of Total Lung Volume	$\dot{V}_A/\dot{Q}$	P_{O_2} (mm Hg)	P_{CO_2} (mm Hg)	pH	$\dot{Q}$ (L/min)
Apex	7%	3.3	132	28	7.55	0.07
Base	13%	0.6	89	42	7.38	1.3
Overall	100%	0.84*	100	40	7.40	5.0

*Because the transport of both O_2 and CO_2 is perfusion limited, we assume that end-capillary values of P_{O_2} and P_{CO_2} are the same as their respective alveolar values. If the overall alveolar ventilation for the two lungs is 4.2 L/min, and if the cardiac output (i.e., perfusion) is 5 L/min, then the overall $\dot{V}_A/\dot{Q}$ ratio for the two lungs is (4.2 L/min)/(5 L/min) = 0.84.

Data from West JB: Ventilation/Blood Flow and Gas Exchange. Oxford, UK: Blackwell, 1989.

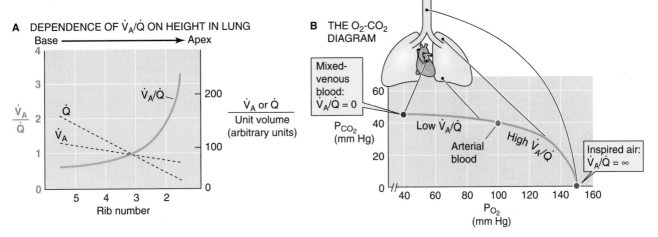

Figure 31-10 Regional differences in $\dot{V}_A/\dot{Q}$ ratio and alveolar gas composition. (*Data from West JB: Ventilation/Blood Flow and Gas Exchange. Oxford, UK, Blackwell, 1985.*)

toward their values in mixed-venous blood. What impact do these different regions of the lung, each with its own $\dot{V}_A/\dot{Q}$ ratio, have on the composition of systemic arterial blood? Each region makes a contribution that is proportional to its blood flow (see the rightmost column in Table 31-3). Because the apex is poorly perfused, it makes only a small contribution to the overall composition of arterial blood. On the other hand, pulmonary tissue at the base of the lungs, which receives ~26% of total cardiac output, makes a major contribution. As a result, the average composition of blood exiting the lung more closely reflects the composition of the blood that had equilibrated with the air in the base of the lung.

The **O₂-CO₂ diagram** introduced as Figure 29-11 is a helpful tool to depict how different $\dot{V}_A/\dot{Q}$ ratios throughout the lung produce different blood gas compositions. The curve in Figure 31-10B represents all possible combinations of P_{O_2} and P_{CO_2} in the alveolar air or end–pulmonary capillary blood. The H₂O-saturated **inspired air** (P_{O_2} = 149 mm Hg, P_{CO_2} = ~0 mm Hg) represents the rightmost extreme of the diagram. By definition, the $\dot{V}_A/\dot{Q}$ ratio of inspired air is ∞ because it does not come into contact with pulmonary capillary blood. The **mixed-venous blood** (P_{O_2} = 40 mm Hg, P_{CO_2} = 46 mm Hg) represents the other extreme. By definition, the $\dot{V}_A/\dot{Q}$ ratio of mixed-venous blood is 0 because it has not yet come into contact with alveolar air. With the endpoints of the diagram established, we can now predict—with the help of the alveolar gas equation (Equation 31-17) and the Bohr effect and the Haldane effect (see Chapter 29)—all possible combinations of P_{O_2} and P_{CO_2} throughout the lung. As shown in Figure 31-10B, the base, midportion, and apex of the lungs correspond to points along the O₂-CO₂ diagram between mixed-venous blood at one extreme and inspired air at the other.

The ventilation of unperfused alveoli (local $\dot{V}_A/\dot{Q}$ = ∞) triggers compensatory bronchoconstriction and a fall in surfactant production

The effects of gravity on ventilation and perfusion cause regional $\dot{V}_A/\dot{Q}$ to vary widely, even in idealized lungs (Fig. 31-10A). However, microscopic or local physiological and pathological variations in ventilation and perfusion can cause even greater mismatches of $\dot{V}_A/\dot{Q}$, the extremes of which are alveolar dead-space ventilation (this section) and shunt (next section).

Alveolar Dead-Space Ventilation   At one end of the spectrum of $\dot{V}_A/\dot{Q}$ mismatches is the elimination of blood flow to a group of alveoli. For example, if we ligated the pulmonary artery feeding one lung, the affected alveoli would receive no perfusion even though ventilation would initially continue normally (Fig. 31-11A). Earlier, we saw that such alveolar dead space together with the anatomical dead space constitutes the physiological dead space (Equation 31-8). The ventilation of the unperfused alveoli is called *alveolar dead-space ventilation* because it does not contribute to gas exchange. Thus, these alveoli behave like conducting airways.

A natural cause of alveolar dead-space ventilation is a pulmonary embolism, which obstructs blood flow to a group of alveoli. Because one task of the lung is to filter small emboli from the blood (see Chapter 26), the lung must deal with small regions of alveolar dead-space ventilation on a recurring basis. At the instant the blood flow ceases, the alveoli supplied by the affected vessels contain normal alveolar air. However, each cycle of inspiration and expiration replaces some stale alveolar air with fresh, inspired air. Because no exchange of O₂ and CO₂ occurs between these

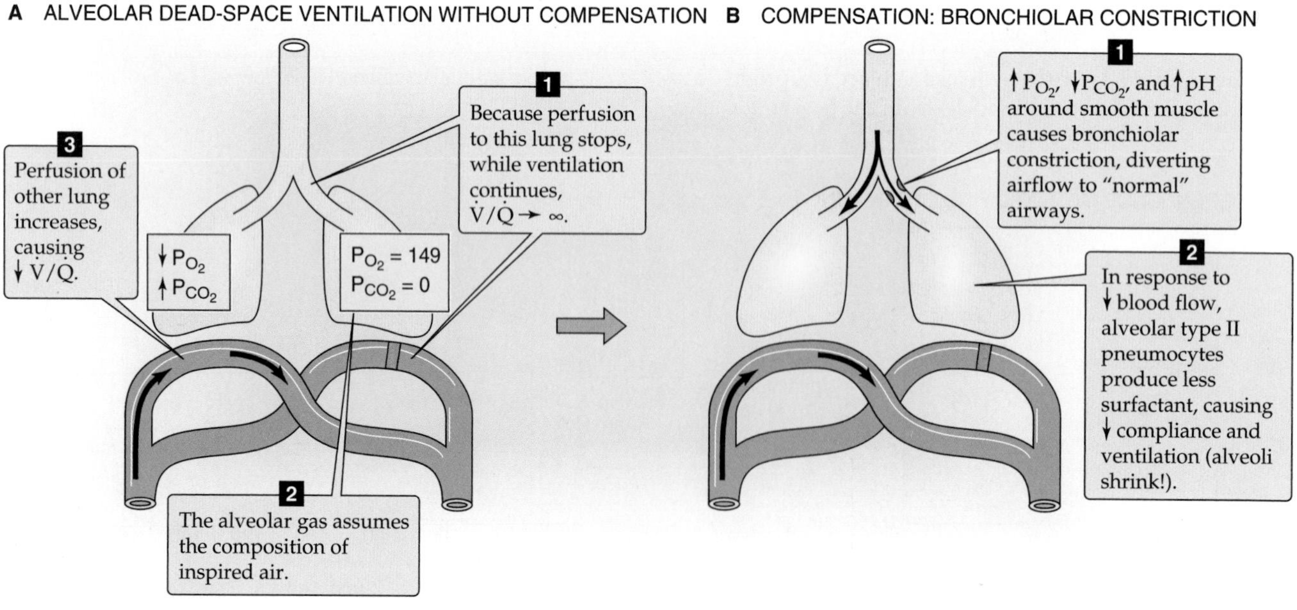

Figure 31-11 Extreme $\dot{V}_A/\dot{Q}$ mismatch and compensatory response—alveolar dead-space ventilation.

unperfused alveoli and pulmonary capillary blood, the alveolar gas gradually achieves the composition of moist inspired air, with alveolar P_{O_2} rising to ~149 mm Hg and P_{CO_2} falling to ~0 mm Hg (Fig. 31-11A, step 2). By definition, alveolar dead space has a $\dot{V}_A/\dot{Q}$ ratio of ∞, as described by the "inspired air" point on the x-axis of an O_2-CO_2 diagram (Fig. 31-10B).

Redirection of Blood Flow   Blocking of blood flow to one group of alveoli diverts blood to other "normal" alveoli, which then become somewhat hyperperfused. Thus, the blockage not only increases $\dot{V}_A/\dot{Q}$ in alveoli downstream from the blockage but also decreases $\dot{V}_A/\dot{Q}$ in other regions. Redirection of blood flow thus accentuates the nonuniformity of ventilation.

Regulation of Local Ventilation   Because alveolar dead-space ventilation causes alveolar P_{CO_2} to fall to ~0 mm Hg in downstream alveoli, it leads to a respiratory alkalosis (see Chapter 28) in the surrounding interstitial fluid. These local changes trigger a compensatory **bronchiolar constriction** in the adjacent tissues (Fig. 31-11B), so that during a period of seconds to minutes, airflow partially diverts away from the unperfused alveoli and toward normal alveoli, to which blood flow is also being diverted. This compensation makes teleological sense because it tends to correct the $\dot{V}_A/\dot{Q}$ shift in both the unperfused and normal alveoli. The precise mechanism of bronchiolar constriction is unknown, although bronchiolar smooth muscle may contract—at least in part—in response to a high extracellular pH.

In addition to a local respiratory alkalosis, the elimination of perfusion has a second consequence. Downstream from the blockage, alveolar type II pneumocytes become starved for various nutrients, including the lipids they need to make surfactant. (These cells never become starved for O_2!) As a result of the decreased blood flow, **surfactant production** *falls* during a period of hours to days. The result is a local decrease in compliance, further reducing local ventilation.

These compensatory responses—bronchiolar constriction (i.e., increased resistance, a property of conducting airways) and reduced surfactant production (i.e., decreased compliance, a property of alveoli)—work well only if the alveolar dead space is relatively small, so that an ample volume of healthy tissue remains into which the airflow can be diverted.

The perfusion of unventilated alveoli (local $\dot{V}_A/\dot{Q}$ = 0) triggers a compensatory hypoxic vasoconstriction

Shunt   Alveolar dead-space ventilation is at one end of the spectrum of $\dot{V}_A/\dot{Q}$ mismatches. At the opposite end is shunt—the flow of blood past unventilated alveoli. For example, if we ligate a mainstem bronchus, then inspired air cannot refresh alveoli distal to the obstruction (Fig. 31-12A). As a result, mixed-venous blood perfusing the unventilated alveoli "shunts" from the right side to the left side of the heart, without benefit of ventilation. When the low-O_2 shunted blood mixes with high-O_2 unshunted blood (which *is* ventilated), the result is that the mixture has a lower than normal P_{O_2}, causing hypoxia in the systemic arteries. It is possible to calculate the extent of the shunt from the degree of hypoxia.

Natural causes of airway obstruction include the aspiration of a **foreign body** or the presence of a **tumor** in the lumen of a conducting airway. The collapse of alveoli (**atel-**

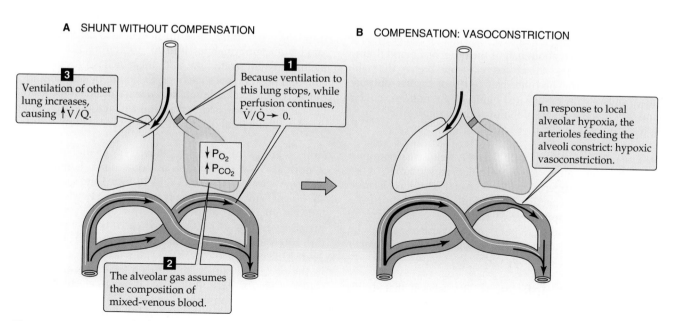

A   SHUNT WITHOUT COMPENSATION

3 Ventilation of other lung increases, causing ↑$\dot{V}/\dot{Q}$.

1 Because ventilation to this lung stops, while perfusion continues, $\dot{V}/\dot{Q}$ → 0.

↓P_{O_2}
↑P_{CO_2}

2 The alveolar gas assumes the composition of mixed-venous blood.

B   COMPENSATION: VASOCONSTRICTION

In response to local alveolar hypoxia, the arterioles feeding the alveoli constrict: hypoxic vasoconstriction.

Figure 31-12   Extreme $\dot{V}_A/\dot{Q}$ mismatch and compensatory response—shunt.

ectasis) also produces a right-to-left shunt, a pathological example of which is pneumothorax (see Chapter 27). Atelectasis also occurs naturally in dependent regions of the lungs, where P_{IP} is not so negative (Fig. 31-5C) and surfactant levels gradually decline. Sighing or yawning stimulates surfactant release (see Chapter 27) and can reverse physiological atelectasis.

Imagine that an infant aspirates a peanut. Initially, the air trapped distal to the obstruction has the composition of normal alveolar air. However, pulmonary capillary blood gradually extracts O_2 from the trapped air and adds CO_2. Eventually, the P_{O_2} and P_{CO_2} of the trapped air drift to their values in **mixed-venous blood**. If the shunt is small, so that it does not materially affect the P_{O_2} or P_{CO_2} of the systemic arterial blood, then the alveoli will have a P_{O_2} of 40 mm Hg and a P_{CO_2} of 46 mm Hg. By definition, shunted alveoli have a $\dot{V}_A/\dot{Q}$ of 0 and are represented by the "mixed-venous blood" point on an O_2-CO_2 diagram (Fig. 31-10B).

Redirection of Airflow Blocking of airflow to one group of alveoli simultaneously diverts air to normal parts of the lung, which then become somewhat hyperventilated. Thus, shunt not only decreases $\dot{V}_A/\dot{Q}$ in unventilated alveoli but also increases $\dot{V}_A/\dot{Q}$ in other regions. The net effect is a widening of the nonuniformity of $\dot{V}_A/\dot{Q}$ ratios.

Asthma Although it is less dramatic than complete airway obstruction, an incomplete occlusion also decreases $\dot{V}_A/\dot{Q}$. An example is asthma, in which hyperreactivity of airway smooth muscle increases local airway resistance and decreases ventilation of alveoli distal to the pathological process.

Normal Anatomical Shunts The **thebesian veins** drain some of the venous blood from the heart muscle, particularly the left ventricle, directly into the corresponding cardiac chamber. Thus, delivery of deoxygenated blood from thebesian veins into the left ventricle (<1% of cardiac output) represents a right-to-left shunt. The **bronchial arteries**, branches of the aorta that carry ~2% of the cardiac output, supply the *conducting* airways (see Chapter 26). After passing through capillaries, about half of the bronchial blood drains into a systemic vein—the azygos vein—and then to the right side of the heart. The other half (~1% of cardiac output) anastomoses with oxygenated blood in pulmonary venules and thus represents part of the anatomical right-to-left shunt (see Chapter 17).

Pathological Shunts In Chapter 57, we discuss examples of right-to-left shunts. Respiratory distress syndrome of the newborn (see Chapter 57 for the box on this topic) can cause airway collapse. Generalized hypoxemia in the newborn can constrict the pulmonary vasculature, as we will see in the next paragraph, leading to pulmonary hypertension and the shunting of blood through the foramen ovale or a patent ductus arteriosus (see Chapter 57).

Regulation of Local Perfusion The alveoli that derive from a single terminal bronchiole surround the pulmonary arteriole that supplies these alveoli. Thus, the vascular smooth muscle cells (VSMCs) of this pulmonary arteriole

are bathed in an interstitial fluid whose composition reflects that of the local alveolar gas. In the case of shunt, VSMCs sense a decrease in P_{O_2}, an increase in P_{CO_2}, and a fall in pH. The decrease in local alveolar P_{O_2} triggers a compensatory **hypoxic pulmonary vasoconstriction**, which the accompanying respiratory acidosis augments (Fig. 31-12B). Note that this response is just the opposite of that of *systemic* arterioles, which *dilate* in response to hypoxia (see Chapter 20). Hypoxic pulmonary vasoconstriction makes teleological sense because it diverts blood flow away from unventilated alveoli toward normal alveoli, to which airflow is also being diverted. This compensation tends to correct the $\dot{V}_A/\dot{Q}$ shift in both the unventilated and normal alveoli.

If the amount of pulmonary tissue involved is sufficiently small (<20%), then hypoxic vasoconstriction has a minimal effect on overall pulmonary vascular resistance. The vasoconstriction causes a slight increase in pulmonary arterial pressure, which recruits and distends pulmonary vessels outside of the shunt zone. In contrast, *global* alveolar hypoxia—caused, for example, by ascending to high altitude—produces a generalized hypoxic vasoconstriction that may cause the resistance of the pulmonary vasculature to more than double. In susceptible individuals, the result can be acute mountain sickness (see Chapter 61).

Even if whole-lung $\dot{V}_A$ and $\dot{Q}$ are normal, exaggerated local $\dot{V}_A/\dot{Q}$ mismatches produce hypoxia and respiratory acidosis

As we saw in Table 31-3, even a normal person has lung regions with $\dot{V}_A/\dot{Q}$ values ranging from ~0.6 to 3.3. In addition, even a normal person has local variations in $\dot{V}_A/\dot{Q}$ due to alveolar dead-space ventilation as well as physiological and anatomical shunts. These physiological $\dot{V}_A/\dot{Q}$ mismatches produce an arterial P_{CO_2} (i.e., ~40 mm Hg) that we regard as normal and an arterial P_{O_2} (i.e., ~100 mm Hg) that we also regard as normal. If pathological processes exaggerate this $\dot{V}_A/\dot{Q}$ mismatch, the result is respiratory acidosis and hypoxia. The sophisticated compensatory responses—discussed before—to alveolar dead-space ventilation and shunt help minimize these mismatches. Thus, uncompensated $\dot{V}_A/\dot{Q}$ abnormalities lead to respiratory acidosis and hypoxia. To illustrate how $\dot{V}_A/\dot{Q}$ mismatches produce these consequences, here we examine CO_2 and O_2 handling in a normal individual and then in two extreme, idealized examples: alveolar dead-space ventilation and shunt—each in the absence of any local or system-wide compensation.

Normal Lungs Figure 31-13 shows how an individual with a normal $\dot{V}_A/\dot{Q}$ distribution in each lung handles CO_2 and O_2. We assume that total $\dot{V}_A$ (4.2 L/min) and $\dot{Q}$ (5 L/min) are normal and divided equally between the two lungs. Each lung eliminates half of the 200 mL/min of CO_2 produced by metabolism (Fig. 31-13A), and each takes up half of the 250 mL/min of O_2 consumed by metabolism (Fig. 31-13B). The physiological $\dot{V}_A/\dot{Q}$ distribution, as discussed in the preceding paragraph, yields a mean alveolar P_{CO_2} of ~40 mm Hg in each lung and a mean alveolar P_{O_2} of ~100 mm Hg. Because the fluxes of CO_2 and O_2 across the alveolar blood-gas barrier are each perfusion limited (see Chapter 30), the CO_2 and O_2 partial pressures in the systemic

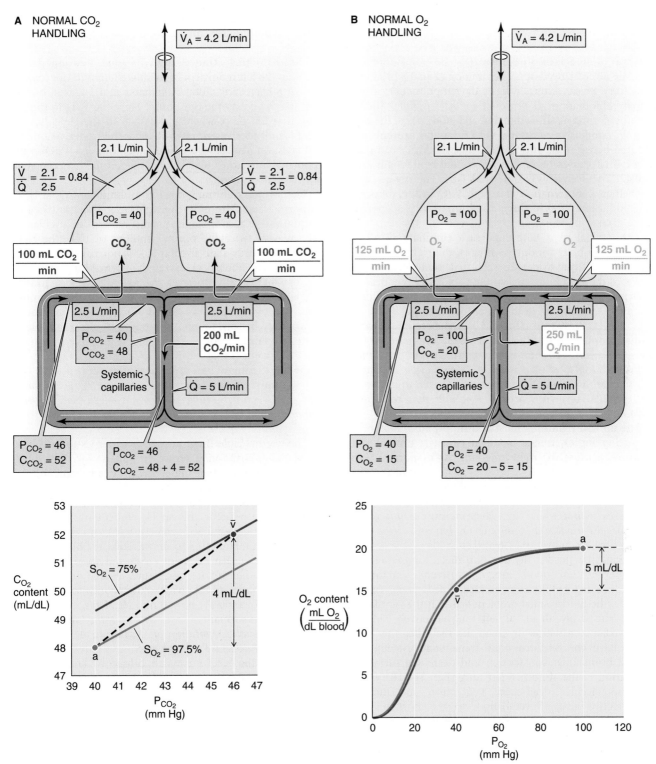

Figure 31-13 Normal distribution of $\dot{V}_A$ and $\dot{Q}$. This is an idealized example. In the upper panels of **A** and **B,** the light beige boxes give the alveolar ventilation to each lung as well as the total alveolar ventilation ($\dot{V}_A$). The pink boxes give the blood flow to each lung as well as the total cardiac output ($\dot{Q}$). The white boxes give the rates of CO_2 or O_2 transport (mL/min) at either the pulmonary or systemic capillaries. The blue boxes give the CO_2 and O_2 partial pressures (mm Hg) in alveolar air. The lavender boxes give the CO_2 partial pressure (mm Hg) and CO_2 content (mL/dL) in the mixed-venous blood, in the blood leaving each of the lungs, and in the mixed-arterial blood. The dark beige boxes give the same information for O_2. The lower panel of **A** shows hypothetical plots of how total CO_2 content varies with P_{CO_2} at the Hb-O_2 saturations typical of arterial blood (*red line*) and mixed-venous blood (*violet line*). The *vertical arrow* indicates the decrease in total CO_2 content between the mixed-venous and arterial blood (4 mL/dL). The lower panel of **B** shows comparable plots for how total O_2 content varies with P_{O_2} at the pH and P_{CO_2} values typical of mixed-venous blood (*violet curve*) and arterial blood (*red curve*). The *vertical arrow* indicates the increase in total O_2 content between the mixed-venous and arterial blood (5 mL/dL).

arterial blood are the same as in the alveoli, and arterial pH is normal.

Alveolar Dead-Space Ventilation Affecting One Lung

To simulate alveolar dead-space ventilation (Fig. 31-14) in the laboratory, we can surgically ligate the left pulmonary artery, thereby eliminating all *perfusion to the left lung*. Total $\dot{Q}$ remains at its normal 5 L/min, but all blood goes to the right lung. $\dot{V}_A$ remains at its normal 4.2 L/min and is evenly distributed between the two lungs. Thus, the $\dot{V}_A/\dot{Q}$ to the left lung is 2.1/0 or ∞, whereas the $\dot{V}_A/\dot{Q}$ to the right lung is 2.1/5 or 0.42. The overall $\dot{V}_A/\dot{Q}$ is normal, 0.84. The key question is whether a combination of a high $\dot{V}_A/\dot{Q}$ in the abnormal lung and a low $\dot{V}_A/\dot{Q}$ in the normal lung can yield normal blood gases.

The normal right lung must now eliminate all of the CO_2 that the body produces—that is, the right lung must eliminate CO_2 at twice the rate that it normally does. However, the right lung has its usual $\dot{V}_A$ of 2.1 L/min. Because a normal amount of alveolar air must carry away twice as much CO_2 in the new steady state, the right lung's alveolar P_{CO_2} doubles to ~80 mm Hg (Fig. 31-14A). Because the entire cardiac output perfuses the normal right lung, arterial P_{CO_2} is also ~80 mm Hg. *Thus, even with the severe $\dot{V}_A/\dot{Q}$ abnormality produced by alveolar dead-space ventilation, the lung is able to expel the usual 200 mL/min of CO_2, but at a tremendous price: a very high arterial P_{CO_2} and thus respiratory acidosis.*

The normal right lung must also supply all of the body's O_2—delivering O_2 to the blood at twice its normal rate. However, because the right lung still has its normal $\dot{V}_A$ of 2.1 L/min, its alveolar P_{O_2} falls to ~51 mm Hg in the new steady state. The blood leaving the right lung, which is identical to systemic arterial blood, also has a P_{O_2} of ~51 mm Hg. *Thus, even with a severe $\dot{V}_A/\dot{Q}$ abnormality, the lung is able to import the usual 250 mL/min of O_2, but at a tremendous price: a very low arterial P_{O_2} (hypoxia).*

We can now answer the question that we posed earlier: the hyperperfused "good" lung cannot make up for the deficit incurred by the hypoperfused "bad" lung. In our example, the fundamental problem was that the ventilation of unperfused alveoli in the left lung effectively reduced the alveolar ventilation by half. In real life, the body would have compensated both locally and systemically. Locally, bronchiolar constriction and decreased surfactant production in the abnormal left lung (Fig. 31-11B) would diminish alveolar dead-space ventilation and increase the effective alveolar ventilation to the normal right lung. Systemically, as we discuss in the next chapter, the respiratory acidosis and hypoxia would stimulate chemoreceptors to increase ventilation. If the body could double $\dot{V}_A$ to the right lung—and if this right lung has a normal diffusing capacity—then it would be matching the doubled perfusion of the right lung with a doubled ventilation, and all resting blood gas parameters would return to normal.

A massive pulmonary embolism that obstructs the left pulmonary artery is superficially similar to the example that we have just discussed. However, other associated problems (e.g., right-sided heart failure secondary to an increase in pulmonary vascular resistance, release of vasoactive agents) make the pulmonary embolism potentially fatal.

Shunt Affecting One Lung

Imagine that an object occludes the left mainstem bronchus, *eliminating all ventilation to the left lung*. Total $\dot{V}_A$ remains at 4.2 L/min, but all ventilation goes to the right lung. Thus, the $\dot{V}_A/\dot{Q}$ to the left lung is 0/2.5, or 0, whereas the $\dot{V}_A/\dot{Q}$ to the right lung is 4.2/2.5, or 1.68. The overall $\dot{V}_A/\dot{Q}$ is normal, 0.84. Again, the key question is whether a combination of a low $\dot{V}_A/\dot{Q}$ in the abnormal lung and a high $\dot{V}_A/\dot{Q}$ in the normal lung can yield normal blood gases.

The normal right lung must now eliminate CO_2 at twice its normal rate. However, the right lung also has twice its normal $\dot{V}_A$. Because twice the normal amount of alveolar air carries away twice the normal amount of CO_2, the right lung's new steady-state alveolar P_{CO_2} is normal, ~40 mm Hg (Fig. 31-15A). The blood leaving the normal lung also has a P_{CO_2} of ~40 mm Hg. However, the unventilated lung has the P_{CO_2} of *mixed-venous blood*, ~51 mm Hg in this example. After the two streams of blood mix—known as **venous admixture**, because venous blood combines with blood from ventilated alveoli—arterial blood in the left ventricle has a *CO_2 content* that is midway between the CO_2 contents of the two streams of blood, corresponding to an arterial P_{CO_2} of ~46 mm Hg. *Thus, even with the severe $\dot{V}_A/\dot{Q}$ abnormality produced by shunt, the lung is once again able to expel the usual 200 mL/min of CO_2, but once again at a price: a high arterial P_{CO_2} (respiratory acidosis).*

The normal right lung must also deliver O_2 to the blood at twice the normal rate. However, because the right lung's $\dot{V}_A$ is also twice its usual value, its new steady-state alveolar P_{O_2} is normal, ~100 mm Hg. The blood leaving the right lung also has a P_{O_2} of ~100 mm Hg, a hemoglobin (Hb) saturation (S_{O_2}) of ~97.5%, and an O_2 content of ~20 mL/dL. However, the unventilated lung has a P_{O_2} of mixed-venous blood, ~29 mm Hg in this example. Thus, the blood leaving the shunted lung has an S_{O_2} of ~49% and an O_2 content of ~10 mL/dL. After venous admixture, arterial O_2 content is $(20 + 10)/2$ or 15 mL/dL, which corresponds to an arterial S_{O_2} (Sa_{O_2}) of 73 and a P_{O_2} of ~40 mm Hg. *Thus, even with the severe $\dot{V}_A/\dot{Q}$ abnormality caused by shunt, the lung is able to import the usual 250 mL/min of O_2, but at the price of an extremely low arterial P_{O_2} (hypoxia).*

Why did the $\dot{V}_A/\dot{Q}$ mismatch caused by shunt lead to only a mild respiratory acidosis but a severe hypoxia? The fundamental problem is that the Hb-O_2 dissociation curve (see Fig. 29-3) is nearly saturated at the normal arterial P_{O_2}. If O_2 content were proportional to P_{O_2}, then mixing of unshunted blood (P_{O_2} = 100 mm Hg) with shunted blood (P_{O_2} = 29 mm Hg) would have yielded arterial blood with a P_{O_2} of $(100 + 29)/2 = ~65$ mm Hg, which is far higher than the arterial P_{O_2} of ~40 mm Hg in our example.

In our example, shunt would trigger compensation at two levels. Locally, hypoxic vasoconstriction would divert blood to well-ventilated alveoli. Systemically, an increase in $\dot{V}_A$ would lower P_{CO_2} and raise P_{O_2} in the normal right lung. In fact, even a modest increase in $\dot{V}_A$ would be sufficient to lower arterial P_{CO_2} to 40 mm Hg. However, even if $\dot{V}_A$ approached

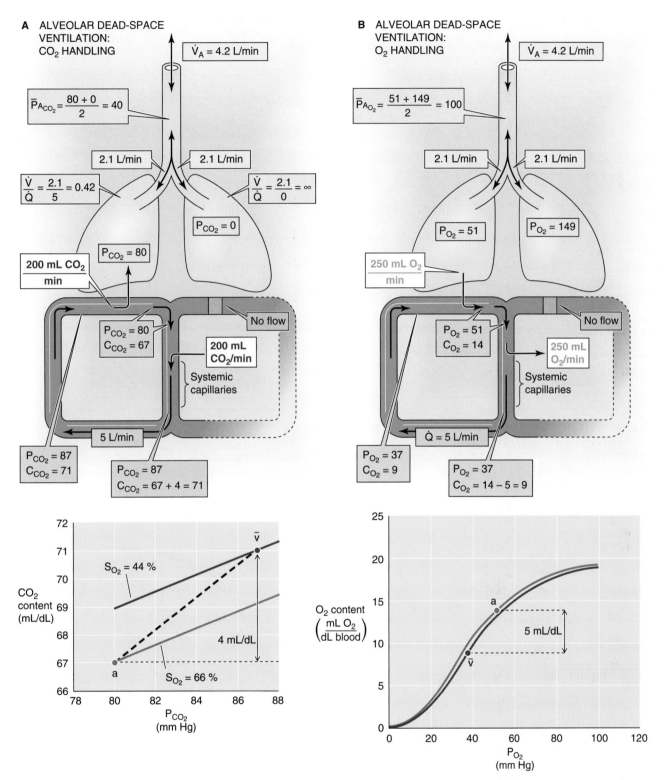

Figure 31-14 Alveolar dead-space ventilation. The numbers in this idealized example refer to a time after the individual has achieved a new steady state. In the upper panels of **A** and **B,** the light beige boxes give the alveolar ventilation to each lung as well as the total alveolar ventilation ($\dot{V}_A$). The green boxes give the blood flow to each lung as well as the total cardiac output ($\dot{Q}$). The white boxes give the rates of CO_2 or O_2 transport (mL/min) at either the pulmonary or systemic capillaries. The blue boxes give the CO_2 and O_2 partial pressures (mm Hg) in alveolar air. The lavender boxes give the CO_2 partial pressure (mm Hg) and CO_2 content (mL/dL) in the mixed-venous blood, in the blood leaving each of the lungs, and in the mixed-arterial blood. The dark beige boxes give the same information for O_2. The lower panel of **A** shows plots of how total CO_2 content in this example varies with P_{CO_2} at the Hb-O_2 saturations of arterial blood *(red line)* and mixed-venous blood *(violet line)*. Despite the severe respiratory acidosis, the decrease in total CO_2 content between the mixed-venous and arterial blood is normal (4 mL/dL). The lower panel of **B** shows comparable plots for how total O_2 content varies with P_{O_2} at the pH and P_{CO_2} values of mixed-venous blood *(violet curve)* and arterial blood *(red curve)*. Despite the severe hypoxia, the increase in total O_2 content between the mixed-venous and arterial blood is normal (5 mL/dL).

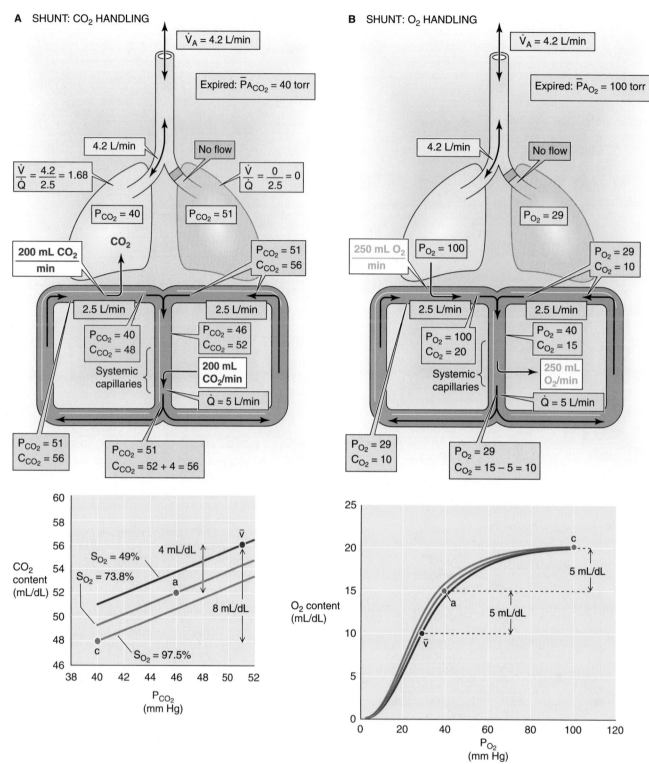

Figure 31-15 Shunt. The numbers in this idealized example refer to a time after the individual has achieved a new steady state. In the upper panels of **A** and **B,** the light beige boxes give the alveolar ventilation to each lung as well as the total alveolar ventilation ($\dot{V}_A$). The green boxes give the blood flow to each lung as well as the total cardiac output ($\dot{Q}$). The white boxes give the rates of CO_2 or O_2 transport (mL/min) at either the pulmonary or systemic capillaries. The blue boxes give the CO_2 and O_2 partial pressures (mm Hg) in alveolar air. The lavender boxes give the CO_2 partial pressure (mm Hg) and CO_2 content (mL/dL) in the mixed-venous blood, in the blood leaving each of the lungs, and in the mixed-arterial blood. The dark beige boxes give the same information for O_2. The lower panel of **A** shows plots of how total CO_2 content in this example varies with P_{CO_2} at the Hb-O_2 saturations for unshunted blood at the end of the pulmonary capillary *(red line)*, for shunted/mixed-venous blood *(violet line)*, and for mixed-arterial blood *(green line)*. Because of the 50% shunt, the decrease in total CO_2 content between mixed-venous blood (point $\bar{v}$) and unshunted blood (point c) must be twice normal (8 mL/dL) to produce a normal decrease (4 mL/dL) between mixed-venous blood (point $\bar{v}$) and mixed-arterial blood (point a). The lower panel of **B** shows comparable plots for how total O_2 content varies with P_{O_2} at the pH and P_{CO_2} values of mixed-venous blood *(violet curve)* and arterial blood *(red curve)*. Because of the 50% shunt, the increase in total O_2 content between mixed-venous blood (point $\bar{v}$) and unshunted blood (point c) must be twice normal (10 mL/dL) to produce a normal increase (5 mL/dL) between mixed-venous blood (point $\bar{v}$) and mixed-arterial blood (point a).

infinity (raising the right lung's alveolar P_{O_2} to the inspired P_{O_2} of ~149 mm Hg), arterial P_{O_2} would still be well under 100 mm Hg. In fact, even if the inspired air were 100% O_2, the arterial P_{O_2} would still fail to reach 100 mm Hg; because of the shape of the Hb-O_2 dissociation curve, an increased alveolar P_{O_2} can increase the O_2 content of arterial blood only marginally (see the box titled Clinical Approaches for Diagnosis of a $\dot{V}_A/\dot{Q}$ Mismatch).

Mixed $\dot{V}_A/\dot{Q}$ Mismatches Pathological $\dot{V}_A/\dot{Q}$ mismatches cause the range of $\dot{V}_A/\dot{Q}$ ratios to broaden beyond the physiological range. Some alveoli may be true alveolar dead space (i.e., perfusion absent, $\dot{V}_A/\dot{Q} = \infty$), but others are more modestly underperfused. Some alveoli may be totally shunted (i.e., ventilation absent, $\dot{V}_A/\dot{Q} = 0$), but others are more modestly underventilated. Thus, the left ventricle receives a mixture of blood from alveoli with $\dot{V}_A/\dot{Q}$ ratios from ∞ to 0, corresponding to all of the points along the O_2-CO_2 diagram in Figure 31-10B. What is the composition of this mixed blood? The principles that we developed in our simplified examples of alveolar dead-space ventilation and shunt still hold. Even if total $\dot{V}_A$ and total $\dot{Q}$

Clinical Approaches for Diagnosis of a $\dot{V}_A/\dot{Q}$ Mismatch

Simple diagnostic methods are available to detect the presence of a $\dot{V}_A/\dot{Q}$ mismatch, to assess its severity, and to identify a shunt.

Diagnosis of Exclusion
The physician can often diagnose a pathological nonuniformity of $\dot{V}_A/\dot{Q}$ by excluding other possibilities. In general, low arterial P_{O_2}—under basal metabolic conditions—could be due to reduced inspired P_{O_2} (e.g., high altitude), reduced alveolar ventilation, decreased diffusing capacity (D_L), or $\dot{V}_A/\dot{Q}$ mismatch. Let us assume that arterial P_{O_2} is appropriate for the altitude (see Equations 31-16 and 31-17) and that simple spirometry test results indicate that respiratory mechanics are normal. Because D_L is normally about 3-fold greater than necessary for achieving diffusion equilibrium for O_2 and CO_2, a problem with D_L is unlikely in the absence of a positive history. By default, the most likely cause is a $\dot{V}_A/\dot{Q}$ defect.

Alveolar-Arterial Gradient for O_2
The difference between the *mean* alveolar P_{O_2} and the systemic arterial P_{O_2} is known as the **alveolar-arterial (A-a) gradient for P_{O_2}**. In our "normal" example in Figure 31-13B, both mean alveolar P_{O_2} and arterial P_{O_2} were 100 mm Hg. In real life, however, physiological $\dot{V}_A/\dot{Q}$ mismatches cause arterial P_{O_2} to be 5 to 15 mm Hg below the mean alveolar value.

A defining characteristic of $\dot{V}_A/\dot{Q}$ mismatches is that they widen the A-a P_{O_2} gradient. In our example of alveolar dead space in Figure 31-14B, the mean alveolar P_{O_2} was (51 + 149)/2 = 100 mm Hg, whereas the systemic arterial P_{O_2} was 51 mm Hg, for an A-a gradient of 49 mm Hg. In our example of shunt in Figure 31-15B, the mean alveolar P_{O_2} was 100 mm Hg, whereas the arterial P_{O_2} was only 40 mm Hg—an A-a gradient of 60 mm Hg.

Because the A-a gradient for P_{O_2} is an index of the severity of the $\dot{V}_A/\dot{Q}$ mismatch, physicians routinely estimate the A-a gradient in the intensive care unit. The approach is (1) to obtain the arterial blood gas values, which include Pa_{O_2} and Pa_{CO_2}; (2) to assume that the mean PA_{CO_2} is the same as the measured Pa_{CO_2}; (3) to use the alveolar gas equation (see Equation 31-17) to compute the mean PA_{O_2} from mean PA_{CO_2}; and (4) to compute the difference $PA_{O_2} - Pa_{O_2}$. However, the assumption in point 2 is not entirely true because $\dot{V}_A/\dot{Q}$ mismatches cause an A-a gradient for CO_2 just as they do for O_2.

Effect of Breathing 100% O_2
Once a $\dot{V}_A/\dot{Q}$ mismatch has been identified, it is important to distinguish between a shunt, which might be corrected surgically, and other causes. Imagine two patients with similar degrees of hypoxia. In the first patient, one lung is relatively hypoventilated (low $\dot{V}_A/\dot{Q}$) and the other lung is relatively hyperventilated (high $\dot{V}_A/\dot{Q}$). However, no alveoli are shunted. In the second patient, a complete shunting of blood makes one lung totally unventilated (a $\dot{V}_A/\dot{Q}$ of 0, as in Fig 31-15). The normal lung has a high $\dot{V}_A/\dot{Q}$. We can distinguish between the two cases by having both subjects inspire 100% O_2.

When the patient without predominant shunt breathes 100% O_2, the P_{O_2} of the blood leaving both lungs will be far higher than normal (Fig. 31-16A). Blood leaving the hypoventilated lung has a P_{O_2} somewhat lower than that of the blood leaving the hyperventilated lung. However, because the P_{O_2} is on the flat part of the Hb-O_2 dissociation curve in both cases, the S_{O_2} values are virtually identical. The miniscule difference in O_2 contents between the two streams of blood is due to a difference in dissolved O_2. Thus, the mixed systemic arterial blood will have slightly elevated O_2 content, Sa_{O_2} of ~100%, and markedly elevated P_{O_2}.

The situation is very different in the patient with a severe shunt (Fig. 31-16B). Because blood leaving the shunted lung does not equilibrate with the alveoli ventilated with 100% O_2, it has the low P_{O_2}, S_{O_2}, and O_2 content characteristic of mixed-venous blood. Although blood leaving the normal lung will have an extremely high P_{O_2}, both the S_{O_2} and O_2 content will be only slightly above normal—like the hyperventilated lung in Figure 31-16. Thus, when one stream of blood with a slightly increased O_2 content ("normal" lung) mixes with another stream with a markedly decreased O_2 content ("shunted" lung), the mixed systemic arterial blood has a lower than normal O_2 content. This low O_2 content translates to a low Sa_{O_2} and thus to a low systemic arterial P_{O_2}. Thus, unlike subjects with other kinds of $\dot{V}_A/\dot{Q}$ mismatches that do not include substantial shunt (e.g., alveolar dead-space ventilation in Fig. 31-14), those with substantial shunt have low arterial P_{O_2} values, even while breathing 100% O_2. Because breathing of 100% O_2 greatly increases mean alveolar P_{O_2} without substantially increasing arterial P_{O_2}, this maneuver greatly exaggerates the A-a difference for P_{O_2}.

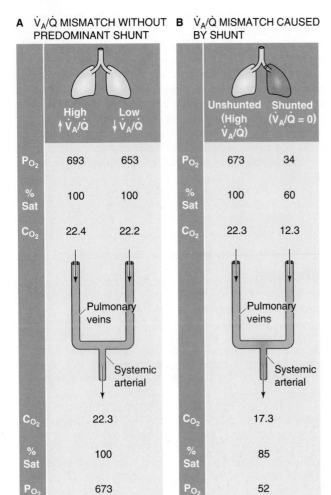

Figure 31-16 Analysis of $\dot{V}_A/\dot{Q}$ mismatch by administration of 100% O_2.

remain normal, pathologically high $\dot{V}_A/\dot{Q}$ ratios in some alveoli cannot make up for pathologically low ratios in others, and vice versa. The result of uncompensated pathological $\dot{V}_A/\dot{Q}$ mismatching is always respiratory acidosis and hypoxia.

REFERENCES

Books and Reviews

Canning BJ: Reflex regulation of airway smooth muscle tone. J Appl Physiol 2006; 101:971-985.

Forster RE, DuBois AB, Briscoe WA, Fisher AB: The Lung: Physiological Basis of Pulmonary Function Tests, 3rd ed. Chicago: Year Book, 1986.

Milic-Emili J: Topographical inequality of ventilation. In Crystal RG, West JB: The Lung, pp 1043-1052. New York: Raven Press, 1991.

Moudgil R, Michelakis ED, Archer SL: The role of K^+ channels in determining pulmonary vascular tone, oxygen sensing, cell proliferation, and apoptosis: Implications in hypoxic pulmonary vasoconstriction and pulmonary arterial hypertension. Microcirculation 2006; 13:615-632.

Journal Articles

Fowler W: Lung function studies II. The respiratory dead space. Am J Physiol 1948; 154:405-416.

Lenfant C: Measurement of ventilation/perfusion distribution with alveolar arterial differences. J Appl Physiol 1963; 18:1090-1094.

Riley RL, Cournand A: Analysis of factors affecting partial pressures of O_2 and CO_2 in gas and blood of lungs: Theory. J Appl Physiol 1951; 4:77-101.

Riley RL, Cournand A, Donald KW: Analysis of factors affecting partial pressures of O_2 and CO_2 in gas and blood of lungs: Methods. J Appl Physiol 1951; 4:102-120.

West JB, Dollery CT, Naimark A: Distribution of blood flow in isolated lung: Relation to vascular and alveolar pressures. J Appl Physiol 1964; 19:713-724.

CHAPTER 32

CONTROL OF VENTILATION

George B. Richerson and Walter F. Boron

OVERVIEW OF THE RESPIRATORY CONTROL SYSTEM

Breathing is one of those things in life that you almost never think about until something goes wrong with it. However, those with pulmonary disease become intensely aware of breathing, as do people who overexert themselves, especially at high altitude. The feeling of dyspnea that they experience (see the box on this topic) is one of the most unpleasant sensations in life. Swimmers and SCUBA divers, professional singers, practitioners of the Lamaze technique, and anyone with a bed partner who snores also focus intensely on breathing. It is common for respiratory output to be the last brain function to be lost in comatose patients, in which case its cessation marks the onset of brain death. Thus, despite our common tendency to ignore it, control of ventilation is one of the most important of all brain functions.

The ventilatory control mechanism must accomplish two tasks. First, it must establish the *automatic rhythm* for contraction of the respiratory muscles. Second, it must adjust this rhythm to accommodate changing *metabolic* demands (as reflected by changes in blood P_{O_2}, P_{CO_2}, and pH), varying *mechanical* conditions (e.g., changing posture), and a range of episodic, *nonventilatory* behaviors (e.g., speaking, sniffing, eating).

Automatic centers in the brainstem activate the respiratory muscles rhythmically and subconsciously

The rhythmic output of the central nervous system (CNS) to muscles of ventilation normally occurs automatically, without any conscious effort. Neurons within the medulla generate signals that are distributed appropriately to various pools of cranial and spinal motor neurons (see Chapter 9), which directly innervate the respiratory muscles (Fig. 32-1). The specific site containing the neurons that generate the respiratory rhythm—the **central pattern generator** (CPG; see Chapter 16)—under normal conditions is still unknown. A vast array of neurons—located primarily in the medulla but also in the pons and other brainstem regions—fire more action potentials during specific parts of the respiratory cycle.

For example, some neurons have peak activity during inspiration, and others, during expiration. These neurons are called **respiratory-related neurons** (RRNs) because their activity patterns correlate with breathing. Some RRNs are **interneurons** (i.e., making local connections), others are **premotor neurons** (i.e., innervating motor neurons), and still others are **motor neurons** (i.e., innervating muscles of respiration).

The most important respiratory motor neurons are those that send axons through the phrenic nerve to innervate the diaphragm (Table 32-1), one of the *primary muscles of inspiration*. When respiratory output increases (e.g., during exercise), activity also appears in motor neurons that innervate a wide variety of *accessory* muscles of inspiration and expiration. (See Chapter 26.)

Each of these muscles is active at different times within the respiratory cycle, and the brain can alter this timing, depending on prevailing conditions. It is the job of the premotor neurons to orchestrate the appropriate patterns of activity among the different pools of motor neurons. The pattern of alternating inspiratory and expiratory activity that occurs under normal conditions during non-rapid eye movement (NREM) sleep, at rest, and during mild exercise is called **eupnea**. During eupnea, neural output to respiratory muscles is highly regular, with rhythmic bursts of activity during inspiration only to the diaphragm and certain intercostal muscles. Expiration occurs purely as a result of cessation of inspiration and passive, elastic recoil of the chest wall and lungs. During more intense exercise, the amplitude and frequency of phrenic nerve activity increase, and additional activity appears in nerves that supply accessory muscles of inspiration. With this increased effort, the accessory muscles of expiration also become active (see Chapter 26), thereby producing more rapid exhalation and permitting the next inspiration to begin sooner (i.e., increasing respiratory frequency).

Peripheral and central chemoreceptors—which sense P_{O_2}, P_{CO_2}, and pH—drive the central pattern generator

The CPG for breathing is the clock that times the automatic cycling of inspiration and expiration. In some cases, the CPG

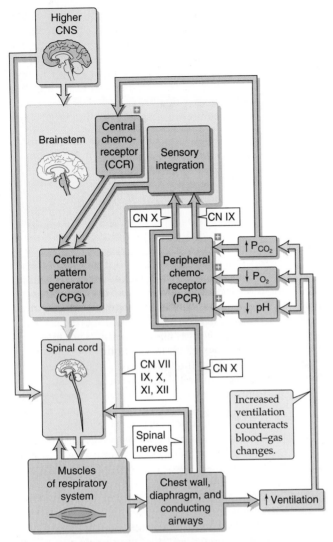

Figure 32-1   Control of ventilation.

stops "ticking" in the absence of **tonic drive** inputs, resulting in the absence of ventilation, or **apnea**. Although this tonic drive comes from many sources, the most important are the central and peripheral chemoreceptors, which monitor the **arterial blood gases**—O_2, CO_2, and pH. Unlike a clock, the frequency of the respiratory CPG changes with the strength of the drive from the chemoreceptors, resulting in changes in both depth and frequency of ventilation.

The **peripheral chemoreceptors**, located in the carotid bodies in the neck and aortic bodies in the thorax, are primarily sensitive to decreases in arterial P_{O_2}, although high P_{CO_2} and low pH also stimulate them and enhance their sensitivity to hypoxia. They convey their sensory information to the medulla through the glossopharyngeal nerve (CN IX) and vagus nerve (CN X). The **central chemoreceptors**, located on the "brain" side of the blood-brain barrier (see Chapter 11), sense increases in arterial P_{CO_2} and—much

Dyspnea

Dyspnea is the feeling of being short of breath, or the unpleasant conscious awareness of difficulty in breathing. In some cases, dyspnea is an adaptive response. For example, when arterial P_{O_2} falls or P_{CO_2} rises from breath-holding, asphyxia, or pulmonary disease, dyspnea leads to efforts to increase ventilation and thus to restore blood gases to normal. However, dyspnea can occur even with a normal arterial P_{O_2} and P_{CO_2}. For example, increased airway resistance can cause dyspnea, even if blood gases do not change. Intense exercise also causes dyspnea, even though P_{CO_2} usually falls. Other causes of dyspnea seem maladaptive. For example, claustrophobia and panic attacks can induce the feeling of suffocation—that is, dyspnea—despite normal ventilatory parameters. The central neural mechanisms and pathways responsible for dyspnea are unknown.

Table 32-1   Innervation of the Primary and Some Secondary Muscles of Respiration

Muscles	Nerve	Location of Cell Body of Motor Neuron
Primary Muscles of Inspiration		
Diaphragm	Phrenic nerve	Phrenic motor nuclei in ventral horn of spinal cord, C3-C5
Intercostal muscles	Intercostal nerves	Ventral horn of thoracic spinal cord
Secondary Muscles of Inspiration		
Larynx and pharynx	Vagus (CN X) and glossopharyngeal (CN IX) nerves	Primarily within the nucleus ambiguus
Tongue	Hypoglossal nerve (CN XII)	Hypoglossal motor nucleus
Sternocleidomastoid and trapezius muscles	Accessory nerve (CN XI)	Spinal accessory nucleus, C1-C5
Nares	Facial nerve (CN VII)	Facial motor nucleus
Secondary Muscles of Expiration		
Intercostal muscles	Intercostal nerves	Ventral horn of thoracic spinal cord
Abdominal muscles	Spinal nerves	Ventral horn of lumbar spinal cord

more slowly—decreases in arterial pH but not in arterial P_{O_2}. All three signals trigger an increase in alveolar ventilation that tends to return these arterial blood gas parameters to normal. Thus, the peripheral and central chemoreceptors, in addition to supplying tonic drive to the CPG, form the critical sensory end of a **negative feedback system** that uses respiratory output to stabilize arterial P_{O_2}, P_{CO_2}, and pH (Fig. 32-1).

Other receptors and higher brain centers also modulate ventilation

Left alone, the respiratory CPG would tick regularly for an indefinite period. However, many inputs to the CPG reset the clock. For example, respiratory output is often highly irregular during many behaviors that use the respiratory muscles (e.g., eating, talking, and yawning). During NREM sleep or quiet wakefulness and with anesthesia, the CPG is unperturbed and *does* run regularly; it is under these conditions that neuroscientists usually study mechanisms of respiratory control.

A variety of receptors in the lungs and airways provide sensory feedback that the medulla integrates and uses to alter respiratory output. Stretch receptors monitor pulmonary mechanics (e.g., lung volume, muscle length) and may help optimize breathing parameters during changes in posture or activity. Activation of pulmonary stretch receptors also can terminate inspiratory efforts, thereby preventing overinflation. Other sensors that detect the presence of foreign bodies or chemicals in the airways are important for protecting the lungs by triggering a cough or a sneeze. Still others detect the movement of joints, which may be important for raising ventilation with exercise. The mechanoreceptors and chemoreceptors from the lungs and lower (i.e., distal conducting) airways send their sensory information to the respiratory neurons of the medulla through CN X, and those from the upper airways send information through CN IX.

Nonrespiratory brainstem nuclei and higher centers in the CNS also interact with respiratory control centers, allowing the ventilatory system to accommodate such activities as speaking, playing a musical instrument, swallowing, and vomiting. These interconnections also allow respiratory control to be highly integrated with the autonomic nervous system, the sleep-wake cycle, emotions, and other aspects of brain function.

In the remainder of this chapter, we examine (1) respiratory neurons, (2) how these neurons generate the automatic rhythm of ventilation, (3) the control of ventilation by arterial blood gases, and (4) how afferent feedback and higher CNS centers modulate ventilation.

NEURONS THAT CONTROL VENTILATION

The neurons that generate the respiratory rhythm are located in the medulla

A classic method for determining which parts of the CNS are responsible for controlling respiratory output is to transect the neuraxis at different levels and to observe changes

in breathing. Using this approach in the 2nd century, Galen performed the first experiments to determine the location of the respiratory controller. As a physician for gladiators in the Greek city of Pergamon, he observed that breathing stopped after a sword blow to the high cervical spine. A similar blow to the lower cervical spine paralyzed the arms and legs but allowed respiration to continue. He reproduced these lesions in live animals and correctly concluded that the brain sends information through the midcervical spinal cord to the diaphragm.

Eighteen centuries later, Lumsden used a similar approach in cats. He found that transection of the CNS between the medulla and spinal cord (Fig. 32-2; spinomedullary transection) causes ventilation to cease as a result of loss of the descending input to phrenic and intercostal motor neurons in the spinal cord. However, even after a spinomedullary transection, respiratory activity continues in muscles innervated by motor neurons whose cell bodies reside in the brainstem. During the period that would have been an inspiration, the nostrils continue to flare, and the muscles of the tongue, pharynx, and larynx continue to maximize airway caliber—although this respiratory activity cannot sustain life. Thus, spinomedullary transection blocks ventilation by interrupting output to the diaphragm, not by eliminating the respiratory rhythm. In other words, the neural machinery driving ventilation lies above the spinal cord.

When Lumsden, in the 1940s, made a transection between the pons and the medulla (Fig. 32-2; pontomedullary transection), he noticed that breathing continued, but with an abnormal "gasping" pattern. Others have since observed relatively normal breathing after a transection at this level and concluded that the gasping seen by Lumsden is due to surgical damage to the respiratory CPG in the rostral medulla. Today, some respiratory neurophysiologists believe, like Lumsden, that the medulla can generate only gasping and that eupnea requires the pons as well as the medulla. However, the consensus is that the respiratory CPG is located in the medulla but that other sites, including the pons, *shape* the respiratory output to produce the normal pattern.

The pons modulates—but is not essential for—respiratory output

Although the medulla alone can generate a basic respiratory rhythm, both higher CNS centers and sensory inputs finetune this rhythm. For example, the pons contains neurons that affect respiratory output.

Lumsden found that a *midpons transection* has only a modest effect—an increase in tidal volume and a slight decrease in respiratory rate. A *bilateral vagotomy*—interrupting the two vagus nerves, which carry sensory information from pulmonary stretch receptors—has a similar but smaller effect. However, combining a *midpons transection with a bilateral vagotomy* causes the animal to make prolonged inspiratory efforts (**inspiratory apneuses**) that are interrupted by only brief expirations. A brainstem *transection above the pons* did not alter the basic respiratory pattern of eupnea. These observations led Lumsden to propose that (1) the caudal pons contains an **apneustic center** (i.e., it can

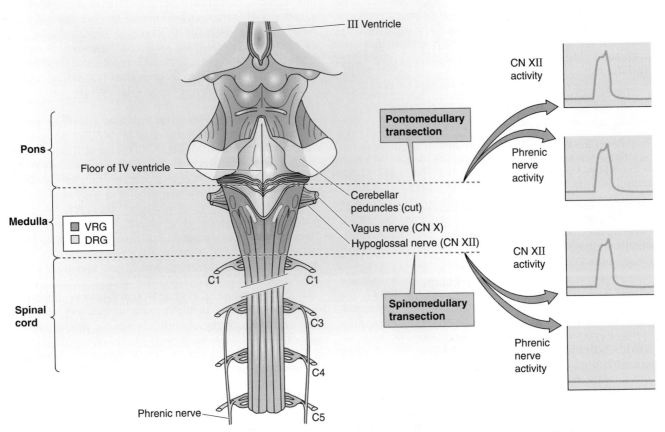

Figure 32-2 Effect of brainstem transections. A dorsal view of the brainstem and spinal cord, with the cerebellum removed, and records of integrated nerve activity during one respiratory cycle, following the indicated transection. During inspiration, *integrated nerve activity* (a moving average of the amplitude of action potentials) increases in the nerves to the tongue (e.g., CN XII) and the diaphragm (phrenic nerve). CN, cranial nerve; DRG, dorsal respiratory group; VRG, ventral respiratory group.

cause apneuses) and (2) the rostral pons contains a **pneumotaxic center** that prevents apneuses (i.e., it promotes coordinated respirations). He believed that these regions and the medulla are required for normal breathing.

What is the modern view? We now appreciate that the apneustic center is not a specific nucleus but is distributed diffusely throughout the caudal pons. The pneumotaxic center is located in the **nucleus parabrachialis medialis** and adjacent **Kölliker-Fuse nucleus** in the rostral pons. However, the pneumotaxic center is not unique in preventing apneuses because simply increasing the temperature of the animal can reverse apneuses induced by lesions in the pneumotaxic center. Moreover, by making lesions in many locations *outside* the pneumotaxic center, apneuses can also be induced. Today, we still do not understand the role of the apneustic center, and the consensus is that the pneumotaxic center plays a general role in a variety of brainstem functions—including breathing—but is not required for eupnea. Thus, the terms *apneustic center* and *pneumotaxic center* are used primarily because of their historical significance.

The dorsal and ventral respiratory groups contain many neurons that fire in phase with respiratory motor output

In the 1930s, Gesell and colleagues used extracellular microelectrode recordings to monitor single neurons, finding that many neurons within the medulla increase their firing rate during one of the phases of the respiratory cycle. Some of these neurons fire more frequently during inspiration (**inspiratory neurons**), whereas others fire more often during expiration (**expiratory neurons**).

Not all neurons that fire in phase with the respiratory cycle are involved in respiration. For example, because they are located within the chest cavity, aortic baroreceptors (see Chapter 23) produce an output that varies with lung inflation, but they are primarily involved in the control of cardiovascular—not respiratory—function. Conversely, some neurons whose firing does not correlate with the respiratory cycle may be essential for respiratory control. For example, central chemoreceptors may fire tonically (i.e., they do not burst during inspiration) and yet are critical for

Normal and Abnormal Respiratory Patterns

Respiratory output can change for a variety of reasons. Many patterns, both normal and abnormal, have recognizable characteristics summarized here. Figure 32-3 illustrates some of these.

Eupnea   Normal breathing.

Sighs   Larger than normal breaths that occur automatically at regular intervals in normal subjects, possibly to counteract collapse of alveoli (atelectasis).

Yawn   An exaggerated sigh.

Tachypnea   An increase in respiratory rate.

Hyperventilation   An increase in alveolar ventilation—caused by an increase in respiratory frequency or an increase in tidal volume—that decreases arterial P_{CO_2}. Seen in pregnancy and liver cirrhosis (due to increased progesterone), in panic attacks, and as a compensation to metabolic acidosis.

Kussmaul breathing   Refers to extremely deep, rapid breathing seen with metabolic acidosis, such as in diabetic ketoacidosis (see Chapter 51 for the box on diabetes mellitus).

Central neurogenic hyperventilation   Rapid, deep breathing causing a decrease in arterial P_{CO_2}. Although described in some patients with focal brain lesions, this pattern may actually reflect coexisting lung disease or other systemic illness.

Cheyne-Stokes respiration   A benign respiratory pattern. Cycles of a gradual increase in tidal volume, followed by a gradual decrease in tidal volume, and then a period of apnea. Seen with bilateral cortical disease or congestive heart failure or in healthy people during sleep at high altitude.

Gasping   Maximal, brief inspiratory efforts separated by long periods of expiration. Seen in severe anoxia, as well as a terminal, agonal breathing pattern in patients with brainstem lesions.

Apneusis (inspiratory)   Prolonged inspirations separated by brief expirations. Rarely seen in humans.

Apnea   Cessation of respiration.

Vagal breathing   Slow, deep inspirations caused by interruption of vagus nerve input to the brainstem. Rarely seen in humans.

Cluster breathing   Similar to ataxic breathing, with groups of breaths, often of differing amplitude, separated by long periods of apnea. Seen with medullary or pontine lesions.

Ataxic breathing   Highly irregular inspirations, often separated by long periods of apnea. Seen mainly with medullary lesions.

Biot breathing   First described in patients with meningitis by Biot (in 1876) as a variant of cluster breathing (see above), with breaths of nearly equal volume separated by periods of apnea. Biot breathing is also considered to be a variant of ataxic breathing.

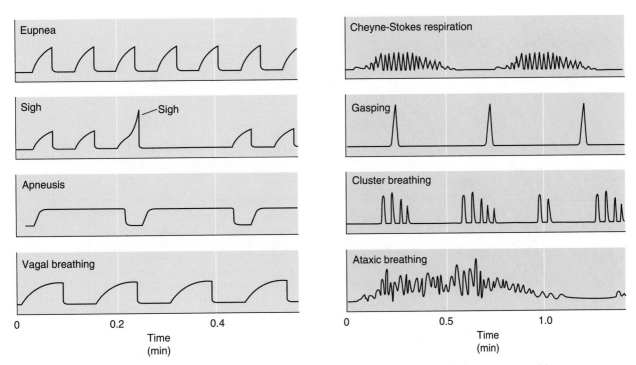

Figure 32-3   Respiratory patterns. These records are typical of either integrated phrenic nerve activity or lung volume. Those on the left come from experimental animals, and those on the right, from humans. All of the patterns, theoretically, could occur in experimental animals or humans, and many occur in clinical settings.

maintaining respiratory output by providing tonic drive. Thus, not all RRNs (e.g., those stimulated by the aortic baroreceptor) play a *direct* role in respiration, and respiratory control involves more than just RRNs (e.g., chemoreceptor neurons).

Although electrical recordings from RRNs cannot identify *all* neurons necessary for producing respiratory output, this mapping has proved very useful in defining neurons that are candidates for *controlling* ventilation. On each side of the medulla, two large concentrations of RRNs—the dorsal and ventral respiratory groups—are grossly organized into sausage-shaped columns, oriented along the long axis of the medulla (Fig. 32-4). Many neurons of these two regions tend to fire exclusively during either inspiration or expiration.

The pons also contains RRNs. Although, as discussed before, pontine neurons may not be needed to *produce* a normal respiratory rhythm, they can influence respiratory output.

The dorsal respiratory group processes sensory input and contains primarily inspiratory neurons

The **dorsal respiratory group (DRG)** primarily contains inspiratory neurons (Table 32-2). It extends for about one third of the length of the medulla and is located bilaterally in and around the **nucleus tractus solitarii (NTS)**, which receives *sensory* input from all viscera of the thorax and abdomen and plays an important role in control of the autonomic nervous system (see Chapter 14). The NTS is viscerotopically organized, with the respiratory portion of the NTS ventrolateral to the **tractus solitarius**, just beneath the floor of the caudal end of the fourth ventricle (Fig. 32-4). These NTS neurons, as well as some immediately adjacent neurons in the dorsal medulla, make up the DRG.

As might be surmised from the sensory role of the NTS, one of the major functions of the DRG is the *integration* of sensory information from the respiratory system. Indeed, some of the DRG neurons receive sensory input—through the glossopharyngeal (CN IX) and vagus (CN X) nerves—from peripheral chemoreceptors as well as from receptors in the lungs and airways (see earlier). Some of the RRNs in the DRG are local *interneurons*. Others are *premotor neurons*, projecting directly to various pools of motor neurons—primarily inspiratory—in the spinal cord and ventral respiratory group (Fig. 32-4).

The ventral respiratory group is primarily motor and contains both inspiratory and expiratory neurons

The **ventral respiratory group (VRG)** contains both inspiratory and expiratory neurons (Table 32-2). It is ventral to the DRG, about midway between the dorsal and ventral surfaces

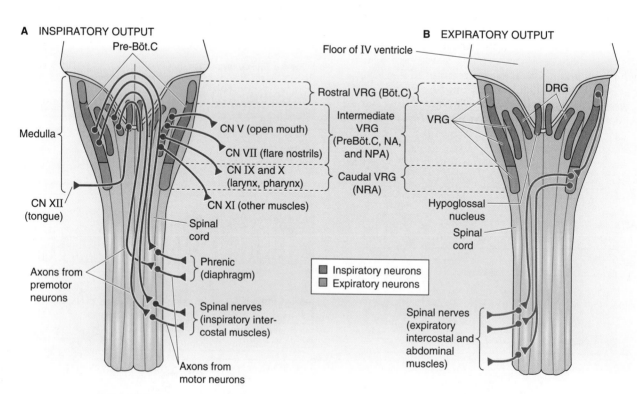

Figure 32-4 Dorsal and ventral respiratory groups and their motor output. **A,** Inspiratory output. **B,** Expiratory output. These are dorsal views of the brainstem and spinal cord, with the cerebellum removed. The dorsal respiratory group (DRG) includes the nucleus tractus solitarii (NTS). The ventral respiratory group (VRG) includes the Bötzinger complex (BötC), pre-Bötzinger complex (preBötC), nucleus ambiguus (NA), nucleus para-ambigualis (NPA), and nucleus retroambigualis (NRA). The color coding indicates whether the neurons are primarily inspiratory (*red*) or primarily expiratory (*green*).

Table 32-2 Properties of the DRG and VRG

Property	DRG	VRG		
		Rostral	Intermediate	Caudal
Location	Dorsal medulla	Midway between dorsal and ventral surfaces of medulla		
Major component	Nucleus tractus solitarii (NTS)	Nucleus retrofacialis (NRF) or Bötzinger complex	Pre-Bötzinger complex, nucleus ambiguus (NA), and nucleus para-ambigualis (NPA)	Nucleus retroambigualis (NRA)
Dominant activity	Inspiratory	Expiratory	Inspiratory	Expiratory

DRG, dorsal respiratory group; VRG, ventral respiratory group.

of the medulla. The VRG lies within and around a series of nuclei that form a column of neurons extending from the pons nearly to the spinal cord and is thus considerably longer than the DRG (Fig. 32-4). Like the DRG, the VRG contains local *interneurons* and *premotor* neurons. In contrast to the DRG, the VRG also contains *motor* neurons that innervate muscles of the pharynx and larynx as well as viscera of the thorax and abdomen. Sensory information related to pulmonary function comes indirectly through the DRG. Thus, the VRG plays more of an efferent role, whereas the DRG primarily plays an afferent role.

The VRG consists of three regions that perform specific functions. (1) The **rostral VRG** (or **Bötzinger complex, BötC**) contains *interneurons* that drive the expiratory activity of the caudal region. (2) The **intermediate VRG** contains somatic *motor* neurons whose axons leave the medulla through CN IX and CN X. These fibers supply the pharynx, larynx, and other structures, thus maximizing the caliber of the upper airways during inspiration. The intermediate VRG also contains *premotor* neurons that project to inspiratory motor neurons in the spinal cord and medulla. Within the rostral pole of the intermediate VRG is a group of inspiratory neurons defined as the **pre-Bötzinger complex (preBötC)**, which, as we will see later, is involved in generating the respiratory rhythm. (3) The **caudal VRG** contains *premotor* neurons that travel down the spinal cord to synapse on motor neurons that innervate accessory muscles of expiration, such as abdominal and certain intercostal muscles (see Chapter 27).

GENERATION OF THE RESPIRATORY RHYTHM

Different RRNs fire at different times during inspiration and expiration

Eupneic breathing is highly stereotyped and consists of two phases—inspiration and expiration (Fig. 32-5A, B). During the **inspiratory phase**, phrenic nerve output to the diaphragm gradually increases in activity during 0.5 to 2 seconds and then declines precipitously at the onset of expiration (Fig. 32-5C). The ramp increase in activity helps ensure a smooth increase in lung volume. During the **expiratory**

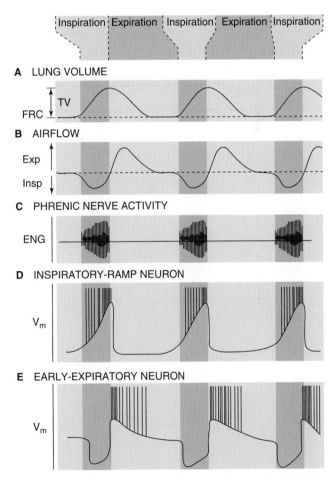

Figure 32-5 Neural activity during the respiratory cycle. The activity of respiratory-related neurons in the medulla (examples of which are shown in **D** and **E**) leads to the phasic activity of the phrenic nerve (**C**) and other respiratory nerves, which produces airflow (**B**), causing lung volume to change (**A**). ENG, electroneurogram; Exp, expiration; FRC, functional residual capacity; Insp, inspiration; TV, tidal volume; V_m, membrane potential.

phase, the phrenic nerve is inactive, except—in some cases—for a brief burst at the onset.

Underlying the activity of the phrenic nerve—and the other motor nerves supplying the muscles of inspiration and expiration—is a spectrum of firing patterns of different

RRNs located within the DRG and VRG (see earlier). RRNs can be broadly classified as inspiratory or expiratory, but each class includes many subtypes, based on how their firing patterns correlate with the respiratory cycle. Figure 32-5D, E shows two such patterns. Each subtype presumably plays a unique role in generating and shaping respiratory output—that is, the activity of the nerves to each respiratory muscle. RRNs may be further subclassified on the basis of their responses to afferent inputs, such as lung inflation and changes in arterial P_{CO_2}.

The firing patterns of RRNs depend on the ion channels in their membranes and the synaptic inputs they receive

What are the mechanisms for generating so many types of activity in RRNs? For example, if the RRN is a premotor neuron, its firing pattern must be appropriate for driving a motor neuron, such as one in the phrenic nerve nucleus. Two complementary mechanisms appear to contribute to the firing patterns necessary for the neuron to do its job. (1) The intrinsic membrane properties of RRNs—the complement and distribution of ion channels present in a neuron—influence the firing pattern of that neuron. (2) The synaptic input—excitatory postsynaptic potentials (EPSPs) and inhibitory postsynaptic potentials (IPSPs)—changes with an appropriate pattern during the respiratory cycle and thereby generates a specific firing pattern.

Intrinsic Membrane Properties   Many neurons in respiratory nuclei have intrinsic membrane properties that influence the types of firing patterns they are able to produce. For example, many DRG neurons have a K^+ current called a **transient A-type current** (see Chapter 7). If we first hyperpolarize and then depolarize such a neuron, it begins firing action potentials, but only after a delay. The hyperpolarization removes the inactivation of the A-type current, and the subsequent depolarization transiently activates the A-type K^+ current and transiently slows depolarization of the membrane and inhibits generation of action potentials (see Fig. 7-18C). If the A-type current is large, the neuron cannot begin to fire until after the A-type current sufficiently inactivates (see Fig. 7-18D). The delay in firing of a neuron with A-type current can explain why some RRNs fire only late during inspiration, even though they receive EPSPs continuously during inspiration. As we will see, other neurons have pacemaker properties due to their complement of ion channels, allowing them to fire action potentials spontaneously without synaptic input.

Synaptic Input   The most obvious explanation for a neuron's having a specific firing pattern is that it receives excitatory synaptic input when it is supposed to fire action potentials and receives inhibitory synaptic input when it is quiet. Indeed, some RRNs fire only during early inspiration, when they receive strong excitatory synaptic input. These early inspiratory neurons also inhibit late-onset inspiratory neurons, and vice versa (Fig. 32-6). As a result of this reciprocal inhibition, only one of the two subtypes of inspiratory neurons can be maximally active at a time.

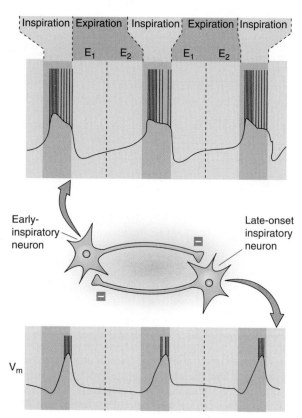

Figure 32-6 Patterned synaptic input: reciprocal inhibition. Because of reciprocal inhibition between the early-burst neuron and the late-onset inspiratory neuron, only one can be maximally active at a time.

In addition to synaptic input from RRNs that occurs rhythmically, in phase with breathing, respiratory neurons also receive input from other neuronal systems. This input can either interrupt regular breathing or control the level of ventilation, allowing the respiratory system to respond appropriately to challenges and to be integrated with many different brain functions.

Pacemaker properties and synaptic interactions may both contribute to the generation of the respiratory rhythm

Perhaps the most important questions that still need to be answered about the neural control of breathing revolve around the mechanism and identity (or location) of the respiratory CPG. We address the mechanism in this section and which cells are involved in the next.

Two general theories have evolved for the mechanism of the respiratory CPG. The first posits that subsets of neurons have pacemaker activity; the second, that synaptic interactions create the rhythm.

Pacemaker Activity   Some cells have ion channels that endow them with pacemaker properties (see Chapter 16). For example, isolated cardiac myocytes produce rhythmic activity by "pacemaker currents" (see Chapter 21). Some neurons have similar pacemaker activity and repeatedly fire one spike at a time (i.e., beating pacemakers). Other pacemaker neurons repeatedly generate bursts of spikes (i.e., bursting pacemakers).

The first evidence for pacemaker activity in a mammalian respiratory nucleus came from the laboratory of Peter Getting. In brain slices from the guinea pig, putative premotor respiratory neurons in the NTS fire erratically at a low rate, with no apparent respiratory rhythm. However, adding thyrotropin-releasing hormone (TRH; see Chapter 49) to the bathing medium causes these neurons to generate bursts of action potentials (Fig. 32-7A), similar to inspiratory bursts in RRNs of the DRG during eupnea in an intact animal (Fig. 32-7B). Indeed, axons that come from the medullary raphe nuclei (see Chapter 13) project to the NTS, where they release TRH and thereby could induce bursting pacemaker activity in NTS neurons. This pacemaker activity might either contribute to generation of the respiratory rhythm or augment respiratory output generated within another site. Pacemaker activity is also present in neurons within another respiratory nucleus—the pre-Bötzinger complex (see later).

Synaptic Interactions Even neural circuits without pacemaker neurons can generate rhythmic output (see Chapter 16). Indeed, synaptic connections within and between the DRG and VRG establish neural circuits and generate EPSPs and IPSPs with a timing that could explain the neurons' oscillatory behavior during the respiratory cycle (Fig. 32-5). Computational neurobiologists have proposed a variety of pure **network models** of respiratory rhythm generation. According to these models, the CPG that produces the respi-

ratory rhythm depends solely on synaptic connections between subtypes of RRNs and not at all on the pacemaker activity of individual neurons. Thus, the rhythm would be an emergent property of the network.

One of the difficulties with network models of breathing is that not all of the neurons within the respiratory network are known. Network models also must take into account the presence of the rich complement of intrinsic membrane properties that exist in the component neurons, but also not all of these are fully characterized. As a result, *pure* network models must be very complex to explain all aspects of the normal respiratory rhythm. Supplementing network models with intrinsic membrane properties (e.g., pacemaker activity) allows the models to be simpler. Moreover, from an evolutionary perspective, it is reasonable to infer that pacemaker cells may have driven primitive respiratory systems (e.g., gills). In higher organisms, both pacemaker activity and synaptic interactions are probably important for generating the normal respiratory rhythm.

The respiratory CPG for eupnea could reside in a single site or in multiple sites or could emerge from a complex network

Where is the respiratory CPG for eupnea? In 1851, Flourens proposed a *noeud vital* ("vital node") in the medulla, a small region that is the sole site producing respiratory output. In 1909, the neuroanatomist Santiago Ramón y Cajal reported that neurons in the NTS receive afferents from pulmonary

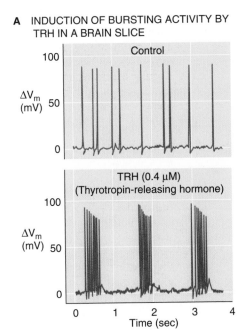

A INDUCTION OF BURSTING ACTIVITY BY TRH IN A BRAIN SLICE

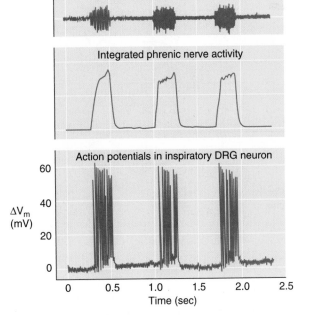

B BURSTING ACTIVITY IN INTACT BRAIN

Figure 32-7 Pacemaker activity in respiratory-related neurons. (**A,** *Data from Dekin MS, Richerson GB, Getting PA: Thyrotropin-releasing hormone induces rhythmic bursting in neurons of the nucleus tractus solitarii. Science 1985; 229:67.* **B,** *Data from Richerson GB, Getting PA: Maintenance of complex neural function during perfusion of the mammalian brain. Brain Res 1987; 409:128.*)

stretch receptors and that NTS neurons project directly to the phrenic motor nucleus. He concluded that the NTS is the site of respiratory rhythm generation. However, today—in spite of considerable progress—the question of where in the medulla the CPG is located remains unanswered. Here we discuss three major proposals for the location of the respiratory CPG.

Restricted-Site Model

Toshihiko Suzue first introduced the in vitro brainstem/spinal cord preparation from the neonatal rat, and Jeffrey Smith and Jack Feldman further developed this preparation to study the generation of respiratory output. In this preparation, a small region in the rostral VRG—the pre-Bötzinger complex (Fig. 32-4)—generates rhythmic motor output in the phrenic nerve and hypoglossal nerve (CN XII, which innervates the tongue, an accessory muscle of inspiration). Destroying the pre-Bötzinger complex in the isolated brainstem causes respiratory output to cease. In a slice preparation, the pre-Bötzinger complex generates rhythmic bursts of activity that one can record from the hypoglossal nerve rootlets (Fig. 32-8). These experiments have led to the hypothesis that the pre-Bötzinger complex is the site of the respiratory CPG.

Distributed Oscillator Models

Another possibility is that there is more than one CPG, any one of which could take over the job of generating the respiratory rhythm, depending on the conditions. As already noted, TRH can induce bursting pacemaker activity in DRG neurons. Moreover, a group of neurons in the parafacial respiratory group near the ventral surface of the medulla can also produce rhythmic activity. One interpretation is that various groups of respiratory neurons are latent CPGs and that the location of the dominant CPG can shift during different behaviors. A second interpretation is that the presence of rhythmicity in multiple areas represents a redundancy, ensuring that respiratory output does not fail. This design would be analogous to initiation of the heartbeat, in which many cells within the sinoatrial node can be the first to fire, and cells in other parts of the heart can take over if the sinoatrial node fails (see Chapter 21). In this model, some respiratory neurons with intrinsic oscillatory behavior would contribute to rhythm generation only under unusual conditions (e.g., hypoxia, anesthesia, early in development); under these conditions, the neurons might generate abnormal or pathological respiratory output (e.g., gasping). A third interpretation is that only one CPG exists for eupnea and that other regions augment the rhythm (and make it more robust) but are unable to generate a rhythm on their own.

Emergent Property Model

The most common early explanation for generation of the respiratory rhythm (e.g., that proposed by Lumsden) is that no individual region of the DRG or VRG is *sufficient* to generate the rhythm but that many of them are *necessary*. A normal rhythm would require the component neurons in multiple brainstem regions to be "wired up" in a specific way. Some still believe that this view is essentially correct, arguing that none of the individual regions proposed to contain *the* CPG can produce a pattern of activity with all of the features described during eupnea.

None of the models we have discussed is universally accepted, and some of their elements are not mutually exclusive. The challenges in testing these hypotheses include the complexity of the CNS even at the level of the medulla, the

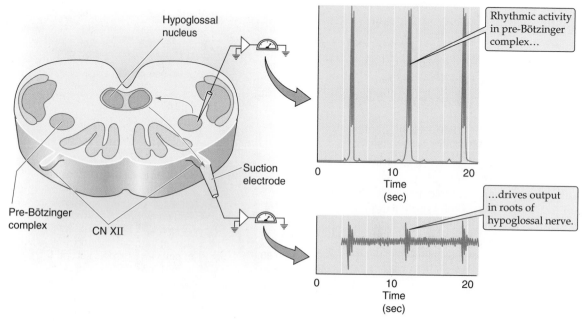

Figure 32-8 Possible role of pre-Bötzinger complex as the respiratory central pattern generator. The recordings were made in a brain slice containing the pre-Bötzinger complex, a piece of the hypoglossal nucleus, and some rootlets of the hypoglossal nerve. (*Data from Smith JC, Ellenberger HH, Ballanyi K, et al: Pre-Bötzinger complex: A brainstem region that may generate respiratory rhythm in mammals. Science 1991; 254:726.*)

technical difficulty in studying neurons of the mammalian brainstem, and the large number of nonrespiratory neurons in the medulla. Yet, because it is primitive both ontogenetically and phylogenetically, the respiratory CPG will probably prove to be far easier to define than most other mammalian neural networks, such as those responsible for consciousness or memory.

CHEMICAL CONTROL OF VENTILATION

In fulfilling its mission to exchange O_2 and CO_2 between the atmosphere and the capillaries of the systemic circulation, the respiratory system attempts to regulate the blood gas parameters, that is, the arterial levels of O_2, CO_2, and pH. These are overwhelmingly the most important influences on breathing. The body senses these parameters through two sets of chemoreceptors—the peripheral chemoreceptors and the central chemoreceptors. Hypoxia, hypercapnia, and acidosis all cause an increase in ventilation, which tends to raise P_{O_2}, to lower P_{CO_2}, and to raise pH, thereby correcting deviations in the three blood-gas parameters. Although small variations in arterial P_{CO_2} and P_{O_2} occur with activities such as sleep, exercise, talking, and panting, the control of blood gases is so tight in normal individuals that it is rare for arterial P_{CO_2} to change from the normal 40 mm Hg by more than a few millimeters of mercury. Thus, the peripheral and central chemoreceptors form the vital sensory arm of a negative feedback mechanism that stabilizes arterial P_{O_2}, P_{CO_2}, and pH.

PERIPHERAL CHEMORECEPTORS

Peripheral chemoreceptors (carotid and aortic bodies) respond to hypoxia, hypercapnia, and acidosis

A decrease in arterial P_{O_2} is the primary stimulus for the peripheral chemoreceptors. Increases in P_{CO_2} and decreases in pH also stimulate these receptors and make them more responsive to hypoxia.

Sensitivity to Decreased Arterial P_{O_2} Perfusion of the carotid body with blood having a low P_{O_2}—but a normal P_{CO_2} and pH—causes a prompt and reversible increase in the firing rate of axons in the carotid sinus nerve. Figure 32-9A shows a comparable experiment on an isolated chemoreceptor cell of the carotid body. Under normal acid-base conditions, increase of P_{O_2} above the normal value of ~100 mm Hg has only trivial effects on the firing rate of the nerve. However, at normal values of P_{CO_2} and pH (Fig. 32-9B, blue curve), decrease of P_{O_2} to values below 100 mm Hg causes a progressive increase in the firing rate.

Sensitivity to Increased Arterial P_{CO_2} The carotid body can sense hypercapnia in the absence of hypoxia or acidosis. It is possible to maintain a constant extracellular pH (pH_o) while increasing P_{CO_2} by keeping the ratio $[HCO_3^-]/P_{CO_2}$ constant (see Chapter 28). The maroon curve in Figure 32-9C shows the results of experiments in which graded increases

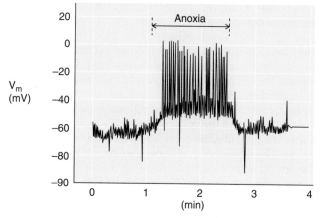

A EFFECT OF ANOXIA ON SINGLE, ISOLATED GLOMUS CELL

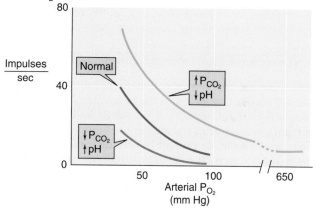

B EFFECT OF RESPIRATORY ACID-BASE DISTURBANCES ON O_2 SENSITIVITY

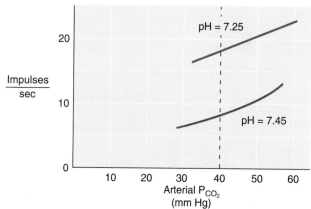

C EFFECT OF pH CHANGES ON CO_2 SENSITIVITY

Figure 32-9 Chemosensitivity of the carotid body. **A,** Effect of anoxia on a single, isolated glomus cell. Anoxia elicits a depolarization and small action potentials, as measured with a patch pipette. **B,** Effect of respiratory acid-base disturbances on O_2 sensitivity. **C,** Effect of pH changes on CO_2 sensitivity. In **B** and **C**, the y-axis represents the frequency of action potentials in single sensory fibers from the carotid body. (**A,** Data from Buckler KJ, Vaughan-Jones RD: Effects of hypoxia on membrane potential and intracellular calcium in rat neonatal carotid body type I cells. J Physiol 1994; 476:423-428. **B,** Data from Cunningham DJC, Robbins PA, Wolff CB: Integration of respiratory responses to changes in alveolar partial pressures of CO_2 and O_2 and in arterial pH. In Cherniack NS, Widdicombe J: Handbook of Physiology, Section 3: The Respiratory System, vol II, pp 475-528. Bethesda, MD: American Physiological Society, 1986. **C,** Data from Biscoe TJ, Purves MJ, Sampson SR: The frequency of nerve impulse in single carotid body chemoreceptor afferent fibers recorded in vivo with intact circulation. J Physiol 1970; 208:121-131.)

in P_{CO_2}—at a fixed blood pH of 7.45 and a fixed P_{O_2} of 80 mm Hg—produced graded increases in the firing rate of the carotid sinus nerve.

Sensitivity to Decreased Arterial pH The carotid body also can sense acidosis in the absence of hypoxia or hypercapnia. The green curve in Figure 32-9C shows the results of experiments that are the same as those represented by the maroon curve, except that blood pH was fixed at 7.25 rather than at 7.45. Over the entire range of P_{CO_2} values, the firing rate of the carotid sinus nerve is greater at a pH of 7.25 than at 7.45. Thus, metabolic acidosis (see Chapter 28) stimulates the carotid body.

In summary, besides being sensitive to hypoxia, the carotid body is sensitive to *both* components of respiratory acidosis (see Chapter 28)—high P_{CO_2} and low pH. In fact, respiratory acidosis makes the carotid body more sensitive to hypoxia (Fig. 32-9B, orange curve), whereas respiratory alkalosis has the opposite effect (Fig. 32-9B, red curve).

The glomus cell is the chemosensor in the carotid and aortic bodies

The body has two sets of peripheral chemoreceptors: the **carotid bodies**, one located at the bifurcation of each of the common carotid arteries; and the **aortic bodies**, scattered along the underside of the arch of the aorta (Fig. 32-10A). The carotid *bodies* should not be confused with the carotid *sinus* (see Chapter 23), which is the bulbous initial portion of the internal carotid artery that serves as a *baroreceptor*. Similarly, the aortic *bodies* should not be confused with baroreceptors of the aortic arch.

The major function of the carotid and aortic bodies is to sense hypoxia in the arterial blood and signal cells in the medulla to increase ventilation. This signaling occurs through afferents of the glossopharyngeal nerve (CN IX) for the carotid bodies and of the vagus nerve (CN X) for the aortic bodies. The carotid bodies have been more extensively studied than the aortic bodies, which are smaller and less accessible. The first description of their function as chemoreceptors was provided by Corneille Heymans, for which he was awarded the 1938 Nobel Prize for Physiology or Medicine.

Aside from their chemosensitivity, three features characterize the carotid bodies. First, they are extremely small: each weighs only ~2 mg. Second, for their size, they receive an extraordinarily high blood flow—the largest of any tissue in the body. Their blood flow, normalized for weight, is ~40-fold higher than that of the brain. Third, they have a very high metabolic rate, 2- to 3-fold greater than that of the brain. Thus, even though the metabolic rate is high, the blood flow is so much higher that the composition of the blood (e.g., P_{O_2}, P_{CO_2}, and pH) in the carotid body capillaries is virtually the same as in the systemic arteries.

The chemosensitive cells of the carotid body are the type I or **glomus cells**. They are ~10 μm in diameter, are roughly spherical, and occur in clusters (Fig. 32-10B). Adjacent glomus cells may communicate with each other through gap

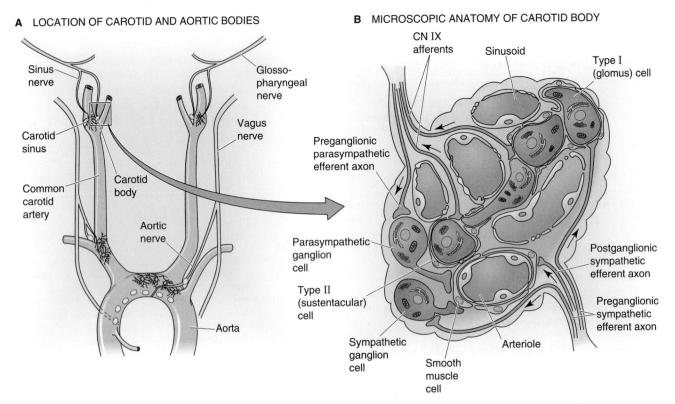

A LOCATION OF CAROTID AND AORTIC BODIES

B MICROSCOPIC ANATOMY OF CAROTID BODY

Figure 32-10 Anatomy of the peripheral chemoreceptors. (**B,** *Data from Williams PL, Warwick R [eds]: Splanchnology. In Gray's Anatomy. Philadelphia: WB Saunders, 1980.*)

junctions. Embryologically, the glomus cell is neuroectodermal in origin and shares many characteristics with neurons of the peripheral nervous system as well as with adrenal chromaffin cells (see Chapter 49). Indeed, glomus cells have four neuron-like characteristics. (1) Some are innervated by *preganglionic* sympathetic neurons. (2) Glomus cells have a variety of voltage-gated ion channels. (3) Depolarization triggers action potentials. (4) Glomus cells have numerous intracellular vesicles containing a variety of neurotransmitters—acetylcholine, dopamine, norepinephrine, substance P, and met-enkephalin. Stimulation causes the release of these neurotransmitters and controls the firing of the sensory nerve endings.

Sensory endings of the carotid sinus nerve (a branch of CN IX) impinge on carotid body glomus cells. Neurotransmitter release from the glomus cells triggers action potentials in the carotid sinus nerve, which makes its first synapse on neurons of the NTS (part of the DRG), thereby signaling the medulla that the systemic arterial blood has a low P_{O_2}, a high P_{CO_2}, or a low pH.

Surrounding individual clusters of glomus cells are the type II or **sustentacular cells** (Fig. 32-10B), which are supporting cells similar to glia. Also close to the glomus cells is a dense network of **fenestrated capillaries**. This vascular anatomy as well as the exceptionally high blood flow puts the glomus cells in an ideal position to monitor the arterial blood gases with fidelity.

Both the sympathetic and parasympathetic divisions of the autonomic nervous system innervate the carotid body. As already noted, preganglionic sympathetic neurons synapse on glomus cells and presumably can alter their function. Autonomic fibers also contact blood vessels; increased sympathetic tone decreases local blood flow. Because the metabolic rate of the carotid body is high, a large decrease in blood flow produces a local fall in P_{O_2} near the glomus cells, even when systemic arterial P_{O_2} remains constant. Increased sympathetic tone thus "fools" the carotid body into behaving as if a hypoxic state existed. Hence, by modulating blood flow to the carotid body, the autonomic nervous system can fine-tune the response of the peripheral chemoreceptors.

The aortic bodies also include scattered glomus cells that presumably have a function similar to that of glomus cells in the carotid bodies. However, there are distinct differences between their responses to stimuli and the effects they have on ventilation. For the purposes of this section, we focus our discussion here on the carotid bodies, about which more is known.

Hypoxia, hypercapnia, and acidosis inhibit K+ channels, raise glomus cell [Ca2+]i, and release neurotransmitters

The sensitivity of the glomus cell to hypoxia, hypercapnia, and acidosis is a special case of chemoreception that we discussed in connection with sensory transduction (see Chapter 15). It is interesting that one cell type—the glomus cell—is able to sense all three blood-gas modalities. The final common pathway for the response to all three stimuli (Fig. 32-11) is an inhibition of BK K+ channels, depolarization of the glomus cell, possible firing of action potentials, opening of voltage-gated Ca^{2+} channels, increase in $[Ca^{2+}]_i$, secretion

of neurotransmitters, and stimulation of the afferent nerve fiber. What differs among the three pathways is how the stimulus inhibits K+ channels.

Hypoxia Investigators have proposed three mechanisms by which low P_{O_2} might inhibit K+ channels. First, some evidence suggests that a heme-containing protein responds to a decrease in P_{O_2} by lowering the open probability of closely associated K+ channels. Second, in rabbit glomus cells, hypoxia raises $[cAMP]_i$, which inhibits a cAMP-sensitive K+ current. Third, small decreases in P_{O_2} inhibit NADPH oxidase in mitochondria, thus increasing the ratio of reduced glutathione versus oxidized glutathione, which directly inhibits certain K+ channels. The relative roles of the three pathways may depend on the species. Regardless of how hypoxia inhibits which K+ channels, the resulting depolarization activates voltage-gated Ca^{2+} channels.

Hypercapnia An increase in P_{CO_2} causes CO_2 to move into the glomus cell, thereby generating H+ (see Chapter 28) and leading to a virtually instantaneous fall of intracellular pH (pH_i). As pH_i decreases, the protons appear to inhibit high-conductance BK K+ channels by displacing Ca^{2+} from their binding sites. The result is a depolarization, a rise in $[Ca^{2+}]_i$, and the release of neurotransmitter.

Extracellular Acidosis A decrease in pH_o inhibits acid-base transporters (e.g., Na-H exchangers) that elevate pH_i and stimulates acid-base transporters (e.g., Cl-HCO3 exchangers) that lower pH_i, thereby leading to a slow fall in pH_i (see Chapter 28). Thus, even at a constant P_{CO_2}, extracellular acidosis (i.e., metabolic acidosis) triggers the same cascade of events outlined for hypercapnia, albeit more slowly.

CENTRAL CHEMORECEPTORS

When the blood-gas parameters are nearly normal, the central chemoreceptors are the primary source of feedback for assessing the effectiveness of ventilation and also the major source of tonic drive for breathing. Just as the peripheral chemoreceptors are primarily sensitive to arterial hypoxia, the neurons that act as central chemoreceptors are primarily sensitive to arterial *hypercapnia*, which generally presents itself as respiratory acidosis (i.e., a decrease in pH_o brought about by a rise in P_{CO_2}; see Chapter 28). However, the actual parameter sensed appears to be a low pH in or around the chemoreceptor neurons.

The blood-brain barrier separates the central chemoreceptors in the medulla from arterial blood

In the 1950s, Isidore Leusen—working on dogs with denervated peripheral chemoreceptors—found that ventilation increased when he perfused the cerebral ventricles with an acidic solution having a high P_{CO_2}. Because the resultant hyperventilation caused a respiratory *alkalosis* in the blood, it must have been the *local acidosis* in the brain that raised ventilation. From this and later experiments, we now believe

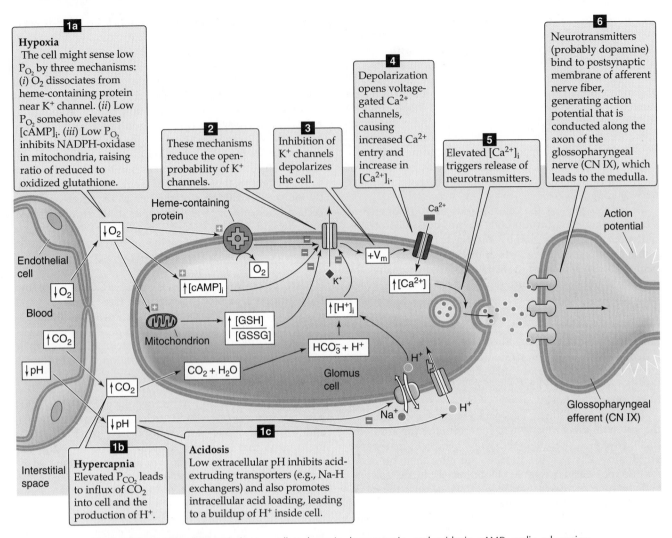

Figure 32-11 Response of glomus cell to hypoxia, hypercapnia, and acidosis. cAMP, cyclic adenosine monophosphate; GSH, reduced glutathione; GSSG, oxidized glutathione.

that the primary stimulus driving respiration during respiratory acidosis is not actually an increase in arterial P_{CO_2} but probably the ensuing pH decrease within brain tissue. Most evidence indicates that the central chemoreceptors are at a site within the brain parenchyma that responds to changes both in arterial P_{CO_2} and in cerebrospinal fluid (CSF) pH.

Starting from normal blood gas parameters, an increase in the arterial P_{CO_2} from 40 to ~45 mm Hg (an increase of only ~12.5%) doubles ventilation. By contrast, hypoxia doubles ventilation only if P_{O_2} falls by ~50%. If P_{CO_2} increases suddenly, the increase in ventilation begins rapidly, augmenting first the *depth* and later the *frequency* of inspirations. However, the response may take as long as 10 minutes to develop fully (Fig. 32-12A). If, instead, the acid-base disturbance in arterial blood is a *metabolic* acidosis (i.e., a decrease in pH_o and $[HCO_3^-]_o$ at a fixed P_{CO_2}; see Chapter 28) of comparable magnitude, ventilation increases much more slowly and the steady-state increase is substantially less.

The reason for these observations is that the central chemoreceptors are located within the brain parenchyma (Fig. 32-12B) and are bathed in **brain extracellular fluid (BECF)**, which is separated from arterial blood by the **blood-brain barrier (BBB)**. The BBB has a high permeability to small, neutral molecules such as O_2 and CO_2 but a low permeability to ions such as Na^+, Cl^-, H^+, and $[HCO_3^-]_o$ (see Chapter 11). An increase in arterial P_{CO_2} rapidly leads to a P_{CO_2} increase of similar magnitude in the BECF, in the CSF, and inside brain cells. The result is an acidosis in each of these compartments. In fact, because the protein concentration of CSF or BECF is lower than that of blood plasma (see Table 11-1), the non-HCO_3^- buffering power (see Chapter 28) of CSF and BECF is also substantially less. Thus, at least initially, raising P_{CO_2} produces a larger signal (i.e., pH decrease) in the CSF and BECF than in the blood.

Although raising arterial P_{CO_2} causes the pH of the BECF and CSF to fall rapidly, the choroid plexus (see Chapter 11) and perhaps the BBB partially restore the pH of these compartments by actively transporting HCO_3^- from the blood into the CSF. Thus, after many hours of respiratory acidosis in the arterial blood, the low-pH signal in the BECF and CSF gradually wanes. Even so, respiratory acid-base disturbances

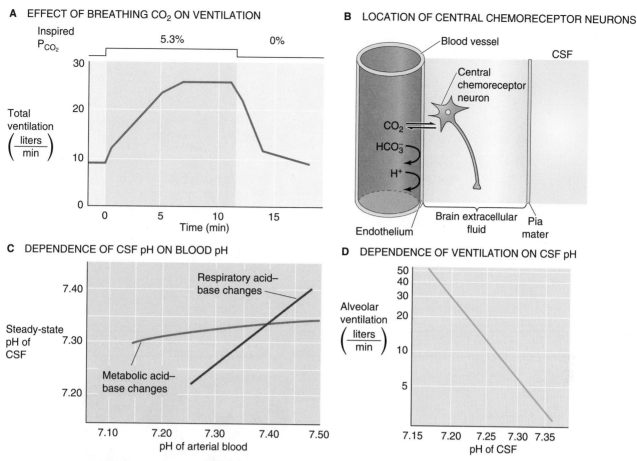

Figure 32-12 Effect of arterial hypercapnia on brain pH and ventilation. (*A, Data from Padget P: The respiratory response to carbon dioxide. Am J Physiol 1928; 83:384-389. **B**, Data from Fencl V: Acid-base balance in cerebral fluids. In Cherniack NS, Widdicombe J: Handbook of Physiology, Section 3: The Respiratory System, vol II, part 1, pp 115-140. Bethesda, MD: American Physiological Society, 1986. **C**, Data from Fencl V, Miller TB, Pappenheimer JR: Studies on the respiratory response to disturbances of acid-base balance, with deductions concerning the ionic composition of cerebral interstitial fluid. Am J Physiol 1966; 210:459-472.*)

lead to substantial changes in the steady-state pH of the BECF and CSF (Fig. 32-12C, purple curve).

In contrast to its high CO_2 permeability, the BBB's permeability to ions such as H^+ and HCO_3^- is low. For this reason, and because the BBB actively regulates the pH of the BECF and CSF, *metabolic* acid-base disturbances alter steady-state brain pH only 10% to 35% as much as identical blood pH changes during *respiratory* acid-base disturbances (Fig. 32-12C, red curve). Therefore, ventilation is much less sensitive to changes in arterial pH and $[HCO_3^-]$ at constant arterial P_{CO_2}. Ventilation correlates uniquely with the pH of the BECF (Fig. 32-12D), regardless of whether respiratory or metabolic acid-base disturbances produce the pH changes in the BECF.

Central chemoreceptors are located in the ventrolateral medulla and other brainstem nuclei or areas

Early work on the central chemoreceptor by Hans Loeschcke, Marianne Schläfke, and Robert Mitchell identified candidate regions near the surface of the ventrolateral medulla (VLM; Fig. 32-13A). The application of acidic solutions to the rostral or caudal VLM leads to a prompt increase in ventilation. Moreover, focal cooling of these areas to 20°C to reversibly inhibit neurons—or placement of lesions to permanently destroy the neurons—blunts the ventilatory response to respiratory acidosis. This and other work led to the conclusion that the central chemoreceptors are located near the surface of the VLM.

More recent work indicates that the VLM is not the only location of central chemoreceptors. For example, studies on brain slices and cultured cells show that acidosis stimulates neurons in many brainstem nuclei. Besides the VLM, these include the medullary raphe (Fig. 32-13A, inset), the nucleus ambiguus, and the NTS—all in the medulla—as well as the locus coeruleus and hypothalamus. Experiments in the laboratory of Eugene Nattie show that focal acidosis within many of these areas stimulates breathing in intact animals. It is not clear whether all of these chemosensitive areas play a role in the control of ventilation. If they do, multiple sensors may be another example of redundancy in a critical system. Some

A CHEMOSENSITIVE REGIONS

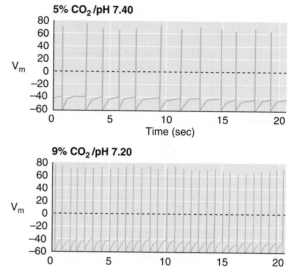

B NEURON STIMULATED BY ACIDOSIS

C RECIPROCAL CONTROL OF RESPIRATORY NEURONS

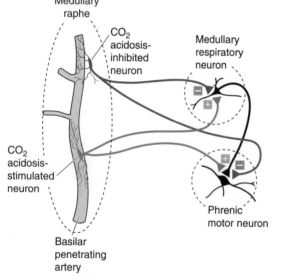

D ASSOCIATION OF SEROTONERGIC NEURONS WITH ARTERIES

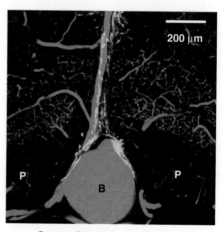

Green - Serotonin neurons
Red - Blood
Yellow - Overlap of red and green

Figure 32-13 Chemosensitive neurons in the ventrolateral medulla and raphe. Illustrated in **A** is a ventral view of a cat medulla showing chemosensitive areas named after the three physiologists who first described them. The slice to the right shows the location of serotonergic neurons in the ventrolateral medulla and medullary raphe nuclei. **B,** Patch pipette recordings of neurons cultured from the medullary raphe of rats. Those that are stimulated by acidosis are serotonergic. **D,** Transverse section of rostral medulla, near the ventral surface, with blood vessels colored *red* and serotonergic neurons colored *green. Yellow* shows the overlap of red and green. B, basilar artery; P, pyramidal tracts. (**A,** *Data from Dermietzel R: Central chemosensitivity, morphological studies. In Loeschcke HH [ed]: Acid-Base Homeostasis of the Brain Extracellular Fluid and the Respiratory Control System, pp 52-66. Stuttgart: Thieme, 1976.* **B,** *Data from Wang W, Pizzonia JH, Richerson GB: Chemosensitivity of rat medullary raphe neurones in primary tissues culture. J Physiol 1998; 511:433-450).* **D,** *Data from Risso-Bradley A, Pieribone VA, Wang W, et al: Chemosensitive serotonergic neurons are closely associated with large medullary arteries. Nat Neurosci 2002; 5:401-402.)*

may come into play only under special circumstances, such as during severe acid-base disturbances; others may be responsible for arousal from sleep only when airways are obstructed.

Some neurons of the medullary raphe and ventrolateral medulla are unusually pH sensitive

Certain medullary raphe neurons are unusually pH sensitive. In brain slices and in tissue culture, small decreases in extracellular pH raise the firing rate of one subset of medullary raphe neurons (Fig. 32-13B) and lower the firing rate of another. In both types of chemosensitive neurons, metabolic and respiratory disturbances have similar effects on firing, indicating that the primary stimulus is a decrease in either extracellular or intracellular pH, rather than an increase in P_{CO_2}.

The two types of chemosensitive neurons have other distinguishing properties, including different shapes, basal firing patterns, and neurotransmitter content. For example, the neurons stimulated by acidosis contain the *stimulatory* neurotransmitter **serotonin**, whereas those that are inhibited by acidosis may contain the *inhibitory* neurotransmitter **GABA**. Serotonergic neurons are also present in the VLM. When arterial P_{CO_2} rises, acidosis-stimulated neurons may stimulate breathing like an accelerator on a car, whereas acidosis-inhibited neurons may decrease the inhibition of breathing, as when one is letting off on the brake (Fig. 32-13C).

The serotonergic neurons in the medullary raphe are in close apposition to branches of the basilar artery (Fig. 32-13D), which puts them—like the glomus cells of the peripheral chemoreceptors—in a position to sense arterial P_{CO_2} with fidelity. Thus, serotonergic neurons of the raphe and VLM have many properties that would be expected of central respiratory chemoreceptors. Many infants who have died of **sudden infant death syndrome (SIDS)** have a deficit of serotonergic neurons, which is consistent with a prevailing theory that a subset of SIDS infants have a defect in central respiratory chemoreception.

INTEGRATED RESPONSES TO HYPOXIA, HYPERCAPNIA, AND ACIDOSIS

In real life, it is rare for arterial P_{O_2} to fall without accompanying changes in P_{CO_2} and pH. In addition, changes in individual blood-gas parameters may independently affect both the peripheral and the central chemoreceptors. How does the respiratory system as a whole respond to changes in multiple blood-gas parameters?

Hypoxia accentuates the acute response to respiratory acidosis

Respiratory Acidosis When the blood gas parameters are nearly normal, respiratory acidosis (increased P_{CO_2}/decreased pH) stimulates ventilation more than does hypoxia. If an animal breathes an air mixture containing CO_2, the resultant respiratory acidosis causes ventilation to increase rapidly. Because both peripheral and central chemoreceptors respond to respiratory acidosis, both could contribute to the response. It is possible to isolate the function of the two sets of chemoreceptors by (1) denervating the peripheral chemoreceptors to study the response of the central chemoreceptors alone or (2) perfusing the carotid bodies to study the response of the peripheral chemoreceptors alone. On the basis of approaches such as these, it appears that the central chemoreceptors account for 65% to 80% of the integrated response to respiratory acidosis under normoxic conditions. However, the response of the peripheral chemoreceptors is considerably more rapid than that of the central chemoreceptors, which require several minutes to develop a full-blown response.

At an alveolar P_{O_2} that is somewhat higher than normal, raising the alveolar P_{CO_2} causes a linear increase in steady-state ventilation (Fig. 32-14A, red curve). Lowering the alveolar P_{O_2} has two effects (Fig. 32-14A, other two curves). First, at a given P_{CO_2}, hypoxia increases ventilation, reflecting the response of the peripheral chemoreceptors to hypoxia. Second, hypoxia increases the *sensitivity* of the integrated response to respiratory acidosis. That is, the slopes of the curves increase. At least part of the explanation for this increase in slopes is that the peripheral chemoreceptor itself—as judged by the activity of the carotid sinus nerve—becomes more sensitive to respiratory acidosis with coexisting hypoxia.

Metabolic Acidosis Severe metabolic acidosis (e.g., diabetic ketoacidosis) leads to profound hyperventilation, known as **Kussmaul breathing**. This hyperventilation can drive arterial P_{CO_2} down to low levels, in an attempt to compensate for the metabolic acidosis. Acutely, the main stimulus for hyperventilation comes from peripheral chemoreceptors. Because a severe decrease in arterial pH does produce a small fall in CSF pH, central chemoreceptors also participate in this response. If the insult persists for many hours, CSF pH falls even farther, and central chemoreceptor drive becomes more prominent.

Respiratory acidosis accentuates the acute response to hypoxia

If an animal breathes an O_2-free air mixture, the resulting hypoxia causes ventilation to increase rapidly. As already discussed, the peripheral chemoreceptors respond primarily to hypoxia. To what extent do central mechanisms contribute to the integrated response to acute hypoxia? In an animal with denervated peripheral chemoreceptors, hypoxia actually *depresses* respiratory output. Thus, the integrated response actually underestimates the stimulatory contribution of the peripheral chemoreceptors.

At an arterial P_{CO_2} that is slightly lower than normal, lowering of alveolar P_{O_2} has very little effect on ventilation until P_{O_2} falls below 50 mm Hg (Fig. 32-14B, red curve). The eventual response at very low P_{O_2} values indicates that the peripheral chemoreceptors play a vital, fail-safe role in responding to extreme hypoxia, as at high altitudes (see Chapter 61). Raising the arterial P_{CO_2} (i.e., respiratory acidosis) has two effects (Fig. 32-14B, other two curves). First, at

A DEPENDENCE ON P_{CO_2}

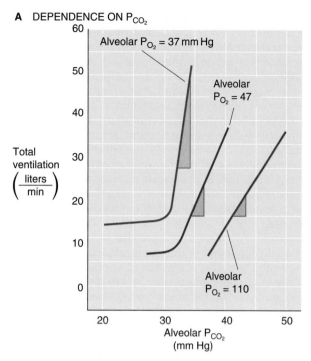

B DEPENDENCE ON P_{O_2}

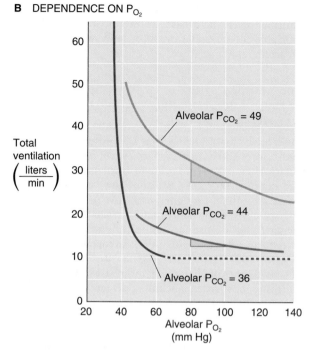

Figure 32-14 Integrated ventilatory response to changes in P_{CO_2} (**A**) and P_{O_2} (**B**). The *shaded triangles* indicate the slopes. (**A,** *Data from Nielsen M, Smith H: Studies on the regulation of respiration in acute hypoxia. Acta Physiol Scand 1952; 24:293-313.* **B,** *Data from Loeschcke HH, Gertz KH: Einfluss des O_2-Druckes in der Einatmungsluft auf die Atemtätigkeit der Menschen, gepruüft unter Konstanthaltung des alveolaren CO_2-Druckes. Pflugers Arch Gesamte Physiol 1958; 267:460-477.*)

Chronic Hypercapnia in Pulmonary Disease

Chronic hypercapnia occurs in many people with lung disease (e.g., emphysema—destruction of alveoli and loss of proper gas exchange) or with muscle weakness (e.g., amyotrophic lateral sclerosis, neuropathies, and myopathies). An increase in P_{CO_2} leads to an immediate respiratory acidosis in the arterial blood and brain. If CO_2 remains elevated, the pH of the CSF/BECF slowly recovers (i.e., increases) during the following 8 to 24 hours. The mechanism of this pH_{CSF} increase is probably an increase in HCO_3^- flux into the CSF/BECF across the choroid plexus and BBB, representing a metabolic compensation to the respiratory acidosis (see Chapter 28). The increased CSF pH shifts the CO_2 response curves in Figure 32-14A to the right because, compared with reference conditions, a higher P_{CO_2} is needed to produce a given degree of CSF acidity (i.e., ventilatory drive). Such a resetting of the central chemoreceptors may be important clinically for patients who chronically retain CO_2. Even though P_{CO_2} may be quite high, adaptation of the CSF/BECF restores pH_{CSF} toward normal. With central chemoreceptor drive for ventilation now decreased, the main drive for ventilation may become hypoxia through peripheral chemoreceptors. Administration of supplemental O_2 to such a patient may remove the hypoxic drive as well, causing ventilation to decrease and P_{CO_2} to rise to very high levels (e.g., $P_{CO_2} > 100$ mm Hg). At such high levels, CO_2 acts as a narcotic, depressing respiration. This "CO_2 narcosis" then directly inhibits ventilation and can cause death from hypoventilation—a classic example of "too much of a good thing."

a given P_{O_2}, respiratory acidosis increases ventilation, reflecting the dual contributions of the peripheral and central chemoreceptors to hypercapnia and acidosis. Second, respiratory acidosis increases the *sensitivity* of the integrated response to hypoxia. That is, the curves become steeper. These effects on the integrated response (Fig. 32-14B) are similar to—although more exaggerated than—the effects of respiratory acidosis on the response of the peripheral chemoreceptor to hypoxia (Fig. 32-9B).

MODULATION OF VENTILATORY CONTROL

The major parameters that feed back on the respiratory control system are the blood gases—P_{O_2}, P_{CO_2}, and pH. In addition, the respiratory system receives input from two other major sources: (1) a variety of stretch and chemical/irritant receptors that monitor the size of the airways and the presence of noxious agents and (2) higher CNS centers that modulate respiratory activity for the sake of nonrespiratory activities.

Stretch and chemical/irritant receptors in the airways and lung parenchyma provide feedback about lung volume and the presence of irritants

Sensors within the lungs and upper airways detect foreign bodies, chemical irritants, or immunological challenges and help protect the lungs—one of the few organs that have direct access to the outside world. Sensors also detect changes in lung volume to help control output to the respiratory muscles. These sensors are part of respiratory afferent fibers from the thorax that travel with CN X, and those from the upper airways travel with CN IX. Both synapse within the DRG in the medulla.

Slowly Adapting Pulmonary Stretch Receptors (PSRs)

Within the tracheobronchial tree are mechanoreceptors that detect changes in lung volume by sensing stretch of the airway walls. One type of PSR—the slowly adapting PSR—responds to stretch with an increase in firing that then decays very slowly over time. One of their functions may be to inform the brain about lung volume to optimize respiratory output.

A reflex that involves slowly adapting PSRs is the **Hering-Breuer reflex**, one of the first examples in physiology of *negative feedback*. In 1868, Hering and Breuer found that lung inflation inhibits the output of phrenic motor neurons (Fig. 32-15), thereby protecting the lungs from overinflation. Because the reflex also increases respiratory frequency, it maintains a constant alveolar ventilation. This reflex may be important in controlling tidal volume during eupnea in human infants. In adults, this reflex does not occur until lung volume is greater than during a normal inspiration. However, the sensor may provide feedback that the medulla uses to choose a combination of tidal volume and respiratory frequency that minimizes the work of breathing.

Rapidly Adapting Pulmonary Stretch (Irritant) Receptors

This PSR responds to a sudden, maintained inflation with a rapid increase in firing rate, which then decreases by 80% or more within 1 second. Unlike slowly adapting PSRs, rapidly adapting PSRs are very sensitive to a variety of chemical stimuli, hence the term *irritant receptors*. These agents include serotonin, prostaglandins, bradykinin, ammonia, cigarette smoke, and ether. An important function of these receptors may be to detect pathophysiological processes in the airway, such as chemical irritation, congestion, and inflammation. These receptors also detect histamine, which produces bronchoconstriction in asthma.

C-Fiber Receptors

A rich network of small, *unmyelinated* axons (C fibers) have nerve endings in the alveoli (**juxtacapillary** or **J receptors**) and conducting airways. Like slowly adapting PSRs, which are extensions of myelinated axons, C-fiber receptors respond to both chemical and mechanical stimuli. Stimulation of C-fiber receptors elicits a triad of rapid and shallow breathing, bronchoconstriction, and increased secretion of mucus into airways—all of which may be defense mechanisms. Bronchoconstriction and rapid, shallow breathing enhance turbulence (see Chapter 27), favoring the deposition of foreign substances in mucus higher up in the bronchial tree, where mucus-secreting cells are located.

Higher brain centers coordinate ventilation with other behaviors and can override the brainstem's control of breathing

The role of the CNS in controlling ventilation is far more complex than generating a regular pattern of inspirations and expirations and then modifying this pattern in response to input from mechanical and chemical sensors. The CNS also must balance the need to control P_{O_2}, P_{CO_2}, and pH with the need to control ventilation for nonrespiratory purposes, such as speaking, sniffing, and regulating temperature (e.g., panting in dogs). In addition, the CNS must coordinate breathing with behaviors that require the *absence* of airflow, such as chewing, swallowing, and vomiting.

Many nonrespiratory regions of the CNS tonically stimulate or inhibit respiration. For example, the **reticular activating system** (see Chapter 10) in the brainstem is one of the sources of tonic drive to the respiratory CPG. An increase in this drive occurs during arousal from sleep, when a *general alerting reaction* increases ventilation and heart rate and activates the brain as evidenced on an electroencephalogram.

Coordination with Voluntary Behaviors That Use Respiratory Muscles

Numerous voluntary actions initiated in the cerebral cortex involve a change in airflow—voluntarily hyperventilating, breath-holding, speaking, singing, whistling, and playing musical wind instruments. Although voluntary control over muscles of respiration can be exquisitely precise, this control is not absolute. For example, voluntary breath-holding can last only so long before being

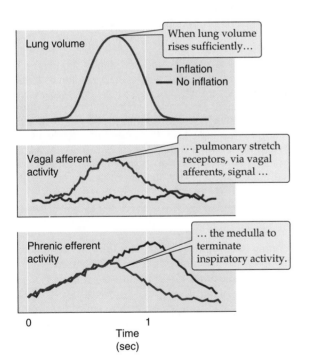

Figure 32-15 The Hering-Breuer reflex. In a paralyzed and artificially ventilated animal, prevention of lung inflation during inspiratory activity (*blue curves*) leads to prolonged phrenic nerve output (i.e., if the animal were not paralyzed, then tidal volume would be large). Inflation of the lungs during inspiratory activity (*red curves*) produces feedback that shortens the duration of inspiratory activity (i.e., if the animal were not paralyzed, then the tidal volume would be smaller) and also causes the next breath to occur earlier (respiratory frequency would increase). *(Data from von Euler C: Brainstem mechanisms for generation and control of breathing pattern. In Cherniack NS, Widdicombe J: Handbook of Physiology, Section 3: The Respiratory System, vol II, part 1, pp 1-67. Bethesda, MD: American Physiological Society, 1986.)*

Sighs, Yawns, Coughs, and Sneezes

The respiratory apparatus engages in a variety of motor behaviors that help maintain normal lung function and gas exchange by protecting the alveoli from collapse or preventing obstruction of the upper airways.

Sigh or "Augmented Breath"

A sigh is a slow and deep inspiration, held for just a moment, followed by a longer than normal expiratory period (Fig. 32-3A). A normal person sighs ~6 times per hour. Local collapse of alveoli (atelectasis) may initiate a sigh, which is an important mechanism for stimulating release of surfactant (see Chapter 27) and thus reopening these alveoli. Hypoxia and respiratory acidosis increase sigh frequency, consistent with the idea that sighs counteract decreased alveolar ventilation.

Yawn

An exaggerated sigh, a yawn takes lung volume to total lung capacity for several seconds. The mouth is fully open. In the extreme case, the arms are stretched upward, the neck is extended to elevate the pectoral girdle, and the back is extended—maneuvers that maximize lung volume (see Chapter 27). Yawning is even more effective than sighing in opening up the most resistant atelectatic alveoli. Everyone "knows" that yawns are contagious, and some evidence suggests that this is actually true. Yawns may (1) minimize atelectasis as one prepares for a long period of sleep or anticipates sleep (as during a boring cell biology lecture) and (2) reverse—on arousal—the atelectasis that has accumulated during sleep.

Cough Reflex

Coughing is important for ridding the tracheobronchial tree of inhaled foreign substances. There is probably no single class of "cough receptors." The tickling sensation that is relieved by a cough is analogous to the cutaneous itch and is probably mediated by C-fiber receptors. *Thus, a cough is a respiratory scratch.*

When *lower airway* receptors trigger a cough, it begins with a small inspiration that increases the coughing force. Mecha-nosensitive and irritant receptors in the *larynx* can trigger either coughing or apnea. When they trigger a cough, the inspiration is absent, minimizing the chances that the offending foreign body will be pulled deeper into the lungs. In either case, a forced expiratory effort against a closed glottis raises intrathoracic and intra-abdominal pressures to very high levels. The glottis then opens suddenly, and the pressure inside the larynx falls almost instantaneously to near-atmospheric levels. This sudden drop in luminal pressure produces dramatic increases in the *axial* (alveolus to trachea) pressure gradient that drives airflow. In the trachea, this pressure drop also decreases the *radial* transmural pressure difference across the tracheal wall, thereby collapsing the trachea, especially the membranous (i.e., noncartilaginous) part of the trachea. (See Chapter 27.) As a result, tracheal cross-sectional area may fall to as little as one-sixth its original value. The net effect is a brief but violent rush of air out of the trachea at velocities near 800 km/hr (~65% of the speed of sound) that loosens mucus or foreign bodies and moves them upward. Protracted bouts of severe coughing can lead to syncope (lightheadedness) because the high intrathoracic pressure decreases venous return and reduces cardiac output (see Chapter 23).

Sneeze

Sensors in the nose detect irritants and can evoke a sneeze. Curiously, these same receptors are probably also responsible for apnea in response to water applied to the face or nose, which is part of the diving reflex that evolved in diving mammals such as the seal to prevent aspiration during submersion. A sneeze differs from a cough in that a sneeze is almost always preceded by a deep inspiration. Like a cough, a sneeze involves an initial buildup of intrathoracic pressure behind a closed glottis. Unlike a cough, a sneeze involves pharyngeal constriction during the buildup phase and an explosive forced expiration through the nose as well as the mouth. This expiration is accompanied by contraction of facial and nasal muscles, so that the effect is to dislodge foreign bodies from the nasal mucosa.

---

overwhelmed by ventilatory drive from chemoreceptors. The cerebral cortex controls the respiratory system by at least two major mechanisms. First, some cortical neurons send axons to respiratory centers in the medulla. Second, some cortical premotor neurons send axons to motor neurons that control muscles of respiration. One consequence of this dual control mechanism is that lesions in specific areas of the cerebral cortex can abolish voluntary breath-holding, a condition known as **respiratory apraxia.** Another consequence is that small CNS lesions may specifically knock out one set of connections. For example, patients with intractable pain are sometimes treated with partial transection of the upper cervical ventrolateral spinal cord to cut axons carrying pain sensation to the thalamus (spinothalamic tract). When this procedure inadvertently damages respiratory projections within the reticulospinal tract, patients breathe properly while awake but experience respiratory failure while asleep (**Ondine's curse;** see the box on this topic). The lesion may cut automatic premotor neurons descending to the spinal cord from respiratory centers in the medulla, but not voluntary ones from the cortex.

Coordination with Complex Nonventilatory Behaviors   One of the jobs of the brain is to coordinate complex behaviors such as yawning, chewing, swallowing, sucking, defecating, grunting, and vomiting. During yawning and vomiting, for example, groups of neurons orchestrate an array of simultaneous actions, only some involving the respiratory system. The premotor neurons that project from medullary respiratory centers to respiratory motor neurons are probably distinct from descending pathways involved in these complex nonventilatory behaviors.

Modification by Affective States   Fear, horror, rage, and passion can be associated with major and highly characteristic changes in the respiratory pattern. For example, if a child runs in front of a car you are driving, the sudden application of the brakes is almost always accompanied by

the limbic system (see Chapter 14) of the forebrain may mediate these emotional effects on breathing.

Balancing Conflicting Demands of Gas Exchange and Other Behaviors Ventilation, or lack thereof, is involved in a wide variety of behaviors, many of which have nothing to do with alveolar gas exchange per se. How is it that the brain is able to weigh the need for alveolar gas exchange against these competing demands on the respiratory system? Playing of a musical wind instrument is an example in which respiratory and nonrespiratory needs are reconciled. Musicians must make rapid and deep inspirations, followed by slow and prolonged expirations that can lead to considerable breath-to-breath variations in alveolar P_{CO_2}. Nevertheless, these variations balance out, so that professionals can follow a musical score for prolonged periods without significant changes in average alveolar ventilation.

In other cases, conflicting demands are not so easily resolved. In infants, suckling relegates alveolar ventilation to a lower priority, and P_{CO_2} rises. Subjects reading aloud tend to increase their alveolar ventilation by ~25%, and P_{CO_2} falls. Thus, during speech, chemical drive is overwhelmed by voluntary behavior. On the other hand, when strenuous exercise increases the need for alveolar ventilation, the CNS permits only brief gasps for speech—the ability of voluntary behavior to subvert body homeostasis can go only so far.

Ondine's Curse, Sleep, and Sleep Apnea

Ondine's Curse

Ondine, a water nymph in a German legend, was immortalized in the 1811 fairy tale by Friedrich Heinrich Karl, Baron de la Motte-Fouqué. In the play *Ondine* by Jean Giraudoux in 1939, Ondine married a mortal man, Hans, with the understanding that Hans would never marry a mortal woman. However, when Ondine later returned to the sea, her husband did remarry. Ondine's father punished Hans by requiring him to make a continuous conscious effort to maintain lung ventilation (and all other automatic body functions). If he fell asleep, he would stop breathing and die. Hans explained to Ondine how hard it is to live with his curse: "One moment of inattention and I shall forget to hear, to breathe. They will say he died because breathing bored him." Rare patients have been identified who have the same disorder—minus the relationship with a water nymph. These patients can be treated with a ventilator when they sleep and can maintain normal ventilation on their own while awake.

Sleep

Sleep, or even closing one's eyes, has powerful effects on the breathing pattern and CO_2 responsiveness. During non–rapid eye movement (NREM) sleep, the regularity of eupneic breathing increases; also, the sensitivity of the respiratory system to CO_2 decreases compared with wakefulness, and the outflow to the muscles of the pharynx decreases. During rapid eye movement (REM) sleep, the pattern of breathing becomes markedly irregular, sometimes with no discernible rhythm, and the sensitivity of the respiratory system to CO_2 decreases further. Thus, P_{CO_2} often increases during NREM sleep and usually even more so during REM sleep. Barbiturates at low doses depress drive to the respiratory system and, if superimposed on normal sleep, can halt ventilation altogether.

Sleep Apnea

The collection of disorders in which ventilation ceases during deeper stages of sleep, particularly during REM sleep, is known as sleep apnea. Some cases of sleep apnea are related to Ondine's curse and are due to a lack of central drive (central sleep apnea). However, most cases are due to collapse of the airway with sleep (obstructive sleep apnea), usually in obese people. The airway collapse is due to an exaggeration of the normal decrease in airway tone during sleep, superimposed on the structural problem of reduced airway diameter due to obesity. This is a common disorder associated with severe and excessive snoring, poor and interrupted sleep, daytime somnolence, and behavioral changes, possibly leading ultimately to hypertension and cardiac arrhythmias.

---

an equally sudden and rapid inspiration, with mouth open wide, increasing lung volume to nearly total lung capacity. The tendency of prevarications to be associated with changes in the breathing pattern is the basis for one part of the polygraph test used as a **lie detector**. Descending pathways from

REFERENCES

Books and Reviews
Coleridge JCG: Pulmonary reflexes: Neural mechanisms of pulmonary defense. Annu Rev Physiol 1994; 56:69-91.
Feldman JL: Neurophysiology of breathing in mammals. In Bloom FE: Handbook of Physiology, Section 1: The Nervous System, vol IV, pp 463-525. Bethesda, MD: American Physiological Society, 1986.
Loeschcke HH: Central chemosensitivity and the reaction theory. J Physiol 1982; 332:1-24.
Peers C, Buckler KJ: Transduction of chemostimuli by the type I carotid body cell. J Membrane Biol 1995; 144:1-9.
Richerson GB: Serotonergic neurons as carbon dioxide sensors that maintain pH homeostasis. Nat Rev Neurosci 2004; 5:449-461.

Journal Articles
Gray PA, Janczewski WA, Mellen N, et al: Normal breathing requires pre-Bötzinger complex neurokinin-1 receptor–expressing neurons. Nat Neurosci 2001; 4:1-4.
Pappenheimer, JR, Fencl V, Heisey SR, Held D: Role of cerebral fluids in control of respiration as studied in unanesthetized goats. Am J Physiol 1965; 208:436-450.
Schläfke ME, See WR, Loeschcke HH: Ventilatory response to alterations of H⁺ ion concentration in small areas of the ventral medullary surface. Resp Physiol 1970; 10:198-212.
Wang W, Zaykin AV, Tiwari JK, et al: Acidosis-stimulated neurons of the medullary raphe are serotonergic. J Neurophysiol 2001; 85:2224-2235.
Williams SEJ, Wootton P, Mason HS, et al: Hemoxygenase-2 is an oxygen sensor for a calcium-sensitive potassium channel. Science 2004; 206: 2093-2097.

THE URINARY SYSTEM

CHAPTER 33

ORGANIZATION OF
THE URINARY SYSTEM

Gerhard Giebisch and Erich Windhager

The kidneys serve three essential functions. First, they function as filters, removing metabolic products and toxins from the blood and excreting them through the urine. Second, they regulate the body's fluid status, electrolyte balance, and acid-base balance. Third, the kidneys produce or activate hormones that are involved in erythrogenesis, Ca^{2+} metabolism, and the regulation of blood pressure and blood flow.

FUNCTIONAL ANATOMY OF THE KIDNEY

We begin this discussion with a macroscopic view and progress to the microscopic level as we describe the **nephron**, the functional unit of the kidney that is repeated approximately 1 million times within each kidney.

The kidneys are paired, retroperitoneal organs that comprise a complex mixture of vascular and epithelial elements

The human kidneys are paired, bean-shaped structures that lie behind the peritoneum on each side of the vertebral column (Fig. 33-1A). They extend from the 12th thoracic vertebra to the third lumbar vertebra. The two kidneys together comprise somewhat less than 0.5% of the total body weight; in men, each kidney weighs 125 to 170 g, whereas in women, each kidney weighs 115 to 155 g.

A fibrous, almost nondistensible capsule covers each kidney (Fig. 33-1B). In the middle of the concave surface, a slit in the capsule—the **hilus**—serves as the port of entry for the renal artery and nerves and as the site of exit for the renal vein, the lymphatics, and the ureter. The hilus opens into a shallow space called the **renal sinus**, which is completely surrounded by renal parenchyma except where it connects with the upper end of the ureter. The renal sinus includes the urine-filled spaces: the **renal pelvis** proper and its extensions, the **major** and the **minor calyces**. Blood vessels and nerves also pass through the sinus. The renal capsule reflects into the sinus at the hilus so that its inner layers line the sinus and the outer layers anchor to the blood vessels and renal pelvis.

A section of the kidney (Fig. 33-1B) reveals two basic layers, the cortex (granular outer region) and the medulla (darker inner region). The granularity of the **cortex** results from the presence of glomeruli, microscopic tufts of capillaries, and a large number of highly convoluted epithelial structures in the form of tubules. The **medulla** lacks glomeruli and consists of a parallel arrangement of tubules and small blood vessels.

The medulla is subdivided into 8 to 18 conical **renal pyramids**, whose bases face the cortical-medullary border; the tip of each pyramid terminates in the renal pelvis. At the tip of each pyramid are perforations, almost invisible to the naked eye, through which urine flows into the minor calyces of the renal sinus.

The kidneys are unique in having a very high blood flow and glomerular capillaries that are bounded by upstream and downstream arterioles

Although the kidneys comprise less than 0.5% of total body weight, they receive ~20% of the cardiac output. This high blood flow provides the blood plasma necessary for forming an ultrafiltrate in the glomeruli. The renal circulation has a unique sequence of vascular elements: a high-resistance arteriole (the afferent arteriole), followed by a high-pressure glomerular capillary network for filtration, followed by a second high-resistance arteriole (the efferent arteriole), which is followed by a low-pressure capillary network that surrounds the renal tubules (peritubular capillaries) and takes up the fluid absorbed by these tubules.

The main features of the renal vascular system are illustrated in Figure 33-1B and C. A single **renal artery** enters the hilus and divides into anterior and posterior branches, which give rise to interlobar and then arcuate arteries. The latter arteries skirt the corticomedullary junction, where they branch into ascending interlobular arteries that enter the cortex and give rise to numerous **afferent arterioles**. These give rise to glomerular capillaries that rejoin to form **efferent arterioles**. For nephrons in the *superficial* portion of the cortex, the efferent arterioles are the origin of a dense peritubular capillary network that supplies oxygen and

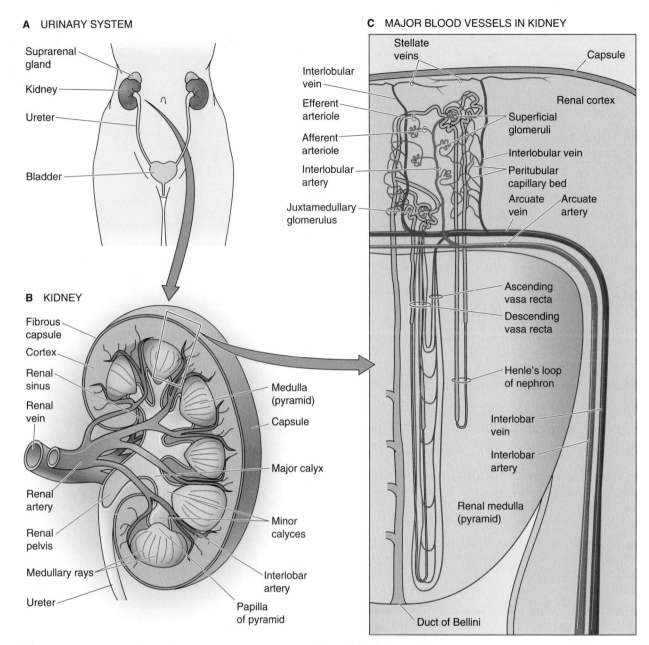

Figure 33-1   Structure of the urinary system. **B,** Posterior view of the right kidney.

nutrients to the tubules in the cortex. The afferent and efferent arterioles determine the hydrostatic pressure in the interposed glomerular capillaries. The tone of both arterioles is under the control of a rich sympathetic innervation, as well as a wide variety of chemical mediators.

Very small branches of the arcuate artery, or the proximal portion of the interlobular artery, supply a subpopulation of juxtamedullary glomeruli that are located at or near the junction of cortex and medulla. The efferent arterioles of these nephrons descend into the renal papillae to form hairpin-shaped vessels called the **vasa recta**, which provide capillary networks for tubules in the medulla. Some 90% of the blood entering the kidney perfuses superficial glomeruli and cortex; only ~10% perfuses juxtamedullary glomeruli and medulla.

Lymph vessels, which drain the interstitial fluid of the cortex and may contain high concentrations of renal hormones such as erythropoietin (EPO), leave the kidney by following arteries toward the hilus. Lymphatics are absent from the renal medulla, where they would otherwise tend to drain the high-osmolality interstitial fluid, which is necessary for producing concentrated urine (see Chapter 38).

The functional unit of the kidney is the nephron

Each kidney consists of 800,000 to 1,200,000 nephrons. Each nephron is an independent entity until the point at which its collecting duct merges with the collecting duct or ducts from one or more other nephrons.

A nephron consists of a glomerulus and a tubule. The **glomerulus** is a cluster of blood vessels from which the plasma filtrate originates. The **tubule** is an epithelial structure consisting of many subdivisions, designed to convert the filtrate into urine. These two entities—vascular and epithelial—meet at the blind end of the tubule epithelium, which is called **Bowman's capsule** or the **glomerular capsule**. This capsule surrounds the glomerulus and contains **Bowman's space**, which is contiguous with the lumen of the tubule. It is here that filtrate passes from the vascular system into the tubule system.

The remainder of the nephron consists of subdivisions of the tubule (Fig. 33-2). The epithelial elements of the nephron include Bowman's capsule, the proximal tubule, the thin descending and thin ascending limbs of the loop of Henle, the thick ascending limb of the loop of Henle, the distal convoluted tubule, and the connecting tubule. The connecting tubule leads further into the initial collecting tubule, the cortical collecting tubule, and the medullary collecting ducts.

Within the renal cortex, as noted earlier, one can distinguish two populations of nephrons (Fig. 33-2). **Superficial nephrons** have short loops extending to the boundary between outer and inner medulla. **Juxtamedullary nephrons**, which play a special role in the production of concentrated urine, have long loops that extend as far as the tip of the medulla.

The renal corpuscle has three components: vascular elements, the mesangium, and Bowman's capsule and space

The **renal corpuscle**, the site of formation of the glomerular filtrate, comprises the glomerulus, Bowman's space, and Bowman's capsule. During the development of the kidney, the interaction between the ureteric bud—which gives rise to the urinary system from the collecting duct to the ureters—and the surrounding loose mesenchyme (Fig. 33-3A) leads to the branching of the ureteric bud and condensation of the mesenchyme (Fig. 33-3B). These condensed

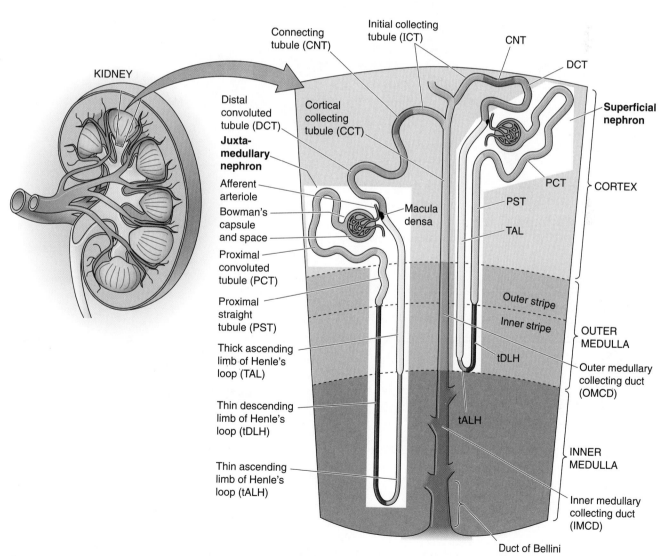

Figure 33-2 Structure of the nephron.

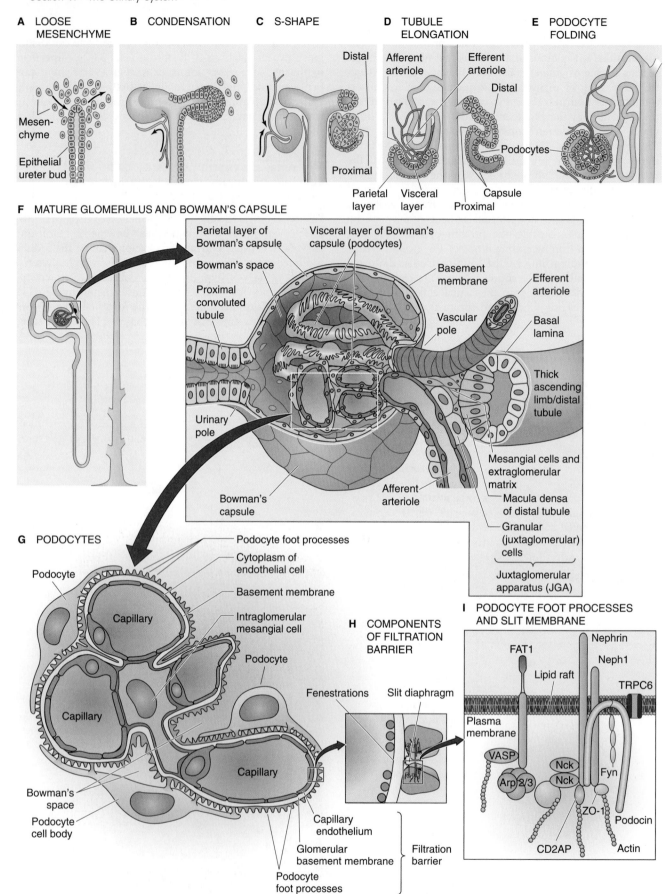

A LOOSE MESENCHYME

Mesenchyme

Epithelial ureter bud

B CONDENSATION

C S-SHAPE

Distal

Proximal

D TUBULE ELONGATION

Afferent arteriole

Efferent arteriole

Distal

Podocytes

Parietal layer

Visceral layer

Capsule

Proximal

E PODOCYTE FOLDING

F MATURE GLOMERULUS AND BOWMAN'S CAPSULE

Parietal layer of Bowman's capsule

Visceral layer of Bowman's capsule (podocytes)

Bowman's space

Basement membrane

Proximal convoluted tubule

Efferent arteriole

Vascular pole

Basal lamina

Thick ascending limb/distal tubule

Urinary pole

Mesangial cells and extraglomerular matrix

Bowman's capsule

Afferent arteriole

Macula densa of distal tubule

Granular (juxtaglomerular) cells

Juxtaglomerular apparatus (JGA)

G PODOCYTES

Podocyte

Capillary

Capillary

Bowman's space

Podocyte cell body

Podocyte foot processes

Cytoplasm of endothelial cell

Basement membrane

Intraglomerular mesangial cell

Podocyte

Capillary

Capillary endothelium

Glomerular basement membrane

Podocyte foot processes

Filtration barrier

H COMPONENTS OF FILTRATION BARRIER

Fenestrations

Slit diaphragm

I PODOCYTE FOOT PROCESSES AND SLIT MEMBRANE

FAT1

Nephrin

Neph1

Lipid raft

TRPC6

Plasma membrane

VASP

Nck

Nck

Fyn

Arp 2/3

ZO-1

Podocin

CD2AP

Actin

Figure 33-3 **A-G**, Development of glomerulus and Bowman's capsule. **H**, The capillary lumen. The four major layers of the glomerular filtration barrier. **I**, Model of podocyte foot processes and slit membrane. The diagram shows nephrin and other proteins of the slit diaphragm. (**A-E** modified from Ekblom P: In Seldin DW, Giebisch G: The Kidney, 2nd ed, pp 475-501. New York: Raven Press, 1992; **H** modified from Kriz W, Kaissling B: In Seldin DW, Giebisch G [eds]: The Kidney: Physiology and Pathophysiology, 3rd ed, pp 587-854. New York: Raven Press, 2000.)

cells differentiate into epithelium that forms a hollow, S-shaped tubular structure (Fig. 33-3C) that gives rise to the nephron's tubular elements between Bowman's capsule and the connecting segment. The distal portion of the S-shaped tubular structure elongates and connects with branches of the developing ureteric bud (Fig. 33-3D). At the same time, the blind proximal end of this S-shaped tubule closely attaches to the arterial vascular bundle that develops into the glomerular capillary tuft. Thinning of the epithelium on one circumference of the blind end of the S-shaped tubule leads to the emergence of the future parietal layer of Bowman's capsule. In contrast, the opposite visceral layer thickens and attaches to the glomerular capillaries (Fig. 33-3D). These visceral epithelial cells later fold and develop into podocytes (Fig. 33-3E).

In the mature kidney (Fig. 33-3F), foot processes of the podocytes cover the glomerular capillaries. These podocytes, modified epithelial cells, thus represent the *visceral* layer of Bowman's capsule. Beginning at the vascular pole, the podocytes are continuous with the *parietal* layer of Bowman's capsule. Glomerular filtrate drains into the space between these two layers (Bowman's space) and flows into the proximal tubule at the urinary pole of the renal corpuscle.

The glomerular filtration barrier between the glomerular capillary lumen and Bowman's space comprises four elements with different functional properties (Fig. 33-3G): (1) a glycocalyx covering the luminal surface of endothelial cells, (2) the endothelial cells, (3) the glomerular basement membrane, and (4) epithelial podocytes.

The **glycocalyx** consists of negatively charged glycosaminoglycans (see Chapter 2) that may play a role in preventing leakage of large negatively charged macromolecules. **Endothelial cells** of the glomerular capillaries are almost completely surrounded by the glomerular basement membrane and a layer of podocyte foot processes (Fig. 33-4). The exception is a small region toward the center of the glomerulus, where the endothelial cells have neither basement membrane nor podocytes and come into direct contact with mesangial cells resembling smooth muscle. Filtration occurs away from the mesangial cells, at the peripheral portion of the capillary wall, which is covered with basement membrane and podocytes. The endothelial cells contain large **fenestrations**, 70-nm holes that provide no restriction to the movement of water and small solutes—including proteins or other large molecules—out of the lumen of the capillary (Fig. 33-5). Thus, the endothelial cells probably serve only to limit the filtration of cellular elements (e.g., erythrocytes).

The **basement membrane**, located between endothelial cells and podocyte foot processes (Fig. 33-3G), separates the endothelial layer from the epithelial layer in all parts of the glomerular tuft. The basement membrane itself has three layers (Fig. 33-3H): (1) an inner thin layer (*lamina rara interna*); (2) a thick layer (*lamina densa*), and (3) an outer thin layer (*lamina rara externa*). The basement membrane makes an important contribution to the permeability characteristics of the filtration barrier by restricting intermediate-sized to large solutes (molecular weight >1 kDa). Because the basement membrane contains heparan sulfate proteoglycans, it is especially restricts large, negatively charged solutes (see Fig. 34-4).

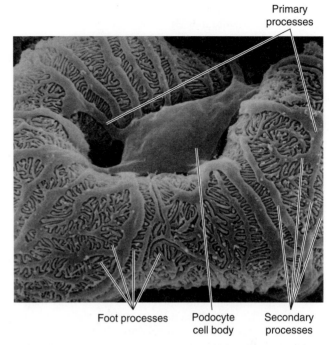

Figure 33-4 Glomerular capillaries covered by the foot processes of podocytes. This scanning electron micrograph shows a view of glomerular capillaries from the vantage point of Bowman's space. The outer surfaces of the capillary endothelial cells are covered by a layer of interdigitating foot processes of the podocytes. The podocyte cell body links to the foot processes by leg-like connections. *(Courtesy of Don W. Fawcett.)*

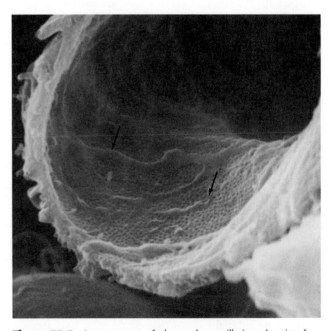

Figure 33-5 Inner aspect of glomerular capillaries, showing fenestrations of endothelial cells (*arrows*). This scanning electron micrograph shows a view of the glomerular capillary wall from the vantage point of the capillary lumen. Multiple fenestrations, each ~70 nm in diameter, perforate the endothelial cells. *(From Brenner BM: Brenner and Rector's The Kidney, 7th ed, vol 1, p 10. Philadelphia: Saunders, 2004.)*

Podocytes have foot interdigitating processes that cover the basement membrane (Fig. 33-4). Between the interdigitations are **filtration slits** (Fig. 33-3H), which are connected by a thin diaphragmatic structure—the **slit diaphragm**—with pores ranging in size from 4 to 14 nm. Glycoproteins with negative charges cover the podocytes, filtration slits, and slit diaphragms. These negative charges contribute to the restriction of filtration of large anions (Fig. 33-4). **Nephrin, neph1, podocin,** and other membranes organized on lipid rafts of podocytes form the slit diaphragm (Fig. 33-3I). Phosphotyrosine motifs on the intracellular domains of some of these proteins may recruit other molecules involved in signaling events that control slit permeability. The extracellular domains of nephrin, neph1, and FAT1 from adjacent podocytes may zip together to help form the filtration slit. In Finnish-type nephrosis, the genetic absence of nephrin leads to severe proteinuria.

Supporting the glomerular capillary loops is a network of contractile **mesangial cells**, which secrete the extracellular matrix. This network is continuous with the smooth muscle cells of the afferent and efferent arterioles. The matrix extends to the extraglomerular mesangial cells (Fig. 33-3F). The **juxtaglomerular apparatus (JGA)** includes the extraglomerular mesangial cells, the macula densa, and the granular cells. The **macula densa** (Latin [dense spot]) is a region of specialized epithelial cells of the thick ascending limb, where it contacts its glomerulus (Fig. 33-3F). These cells have strikingly large nuclei and are closely packed, and thus they have a plaque-like appearance. The **granular cells**, also called juxtaglomerular or epithelioid cells, in the wall of afferent arterioles are specialized smooth muscle cells that produce, store, and release renin (see Chapter 40). The JGA is part of a complex feedback mechanism that regulates renal blood flow and filtration rate (see Chapter 34), and it also indirectly modulates Na$^+$ balance (see Chapter 40) and systemic blood pressure (see Chapter 23).

The tubule components of the nephron include the proximal tubule, loop of Henle, distal tubule, and collecting duct

Figure 33-6 illustrates the ultrastructure of the cells of the different tubule segments. Table 33-1 lists these segments and their abbreviations. Based on its appearance at low magnification, the **proximal tubule** can be divided into the proximal convoluted tubule (Fig. 33-6A), and the proximal straight tubule (Fig. 33-6B). However, based on ultrastructure, the proximal tubule can alternatively be subdivided into three segments: S1, S2, and S3. The S1 segment starts at the glomerulus and includes the first portion of the proximal convoluted tubule. The S2 segment starts in the second half of the proximal convoluted tubule and continues into the first half of the proximal straight tubule. Finally, the S3 segment includes the distal half of the proximal straight tubule that extends into the medulla.

Both the apical (luminal) and basolateral (peritubular) membranes of proximal tubule cells are extensively amplified (Fig. 33-6A, B). The apical membrane has infoldings in the form of a well-developed *brush border*. This enlargement of the apical surface area correlates with the main function

of this nephron segment, namely, to reabsorb the bulk of the filtered fluid back into the circulation. A central cilium, which may play a role in sensing fluid flow, protrudes from the apical pole of proximal tubule cells and nearly all tubule cells.

The *basolateral membranes* of adjacent proximal tubule cells form numerous interdigitations, bringing abundant mitochondria in close contact with the plasma membrane. The interdigitations of the lateral membranes also form an extensive extracellular compartment bounded by the tight junctions at one end and by the basement membrane of the epithelium at the other end. Proximal tubule cells contain lysosomes, endocytic vacuoles, and a well-developed endoplasmic reticulum. Proximal tubule cells are also characterized by a prominent Golgi apparatus (see Chapter 2), which is important for synthesizing many membrane components, sorting them, and targeting them to specific surface sites. From the S1 to the S3 segments, cell complexity progressively declines, correlating with a gradual decrease of reabsorptive rates along the tubule. Thus, the cells exhibit a progressively less developed brush border, diminished complexity of lateral cell interdigitations, a lower basolateral cell membrane area, and a decrease in the number of mitochondria.

In comparison with the S3 segment of the proximal tubule, the cells lining the **descending** and **ascending thin limbs** of the loop of Henle are far less complex (Fig. 33-6C, D), with few mitochondria and little cell membrane amplification. In superficial nephrons, the *thin ascending* limbs are extremely abbreviated (Fig. 33-2). However, they form a major part of the long loops of the juxtamedullary nephrons.

Epithelial cells lining the **thick ascending limb** of the loop of Henle, which terminates at the macula densa, are characterized by tall interdigitations and numerous mitochondria within extensively invaginated basolateral membranes (Fig. 33-6E). This complex cell machinery correlates with the key role these cells play in making the medullary interstitium hyperosmotic.

Until the latter part of the 20th century, morphologists defined the **classic distal tubule**—on the basis of light microscopic studies—as the nephron segment stretching from the macula densa to the first confluence of two nephrons in the collecting duct system. Today, we subdivide the classic distal tubule into three segments, based on ultrastructural studies: the distal convoluted tubule (starting at the macula densa), the connecting tubule, and the initial collecting tubule. What was classically termed the early distal tubule is mainly the distal convoluted tubule, whereas the classically termed late distal tubule is mainly the initial collecting tubule.

The **distal convoluted tubule** begins at the macula densa and ends at the transition to the connecting tubule (Fig. 33-6F). The cells of the distal convoluted tubule are similar in structure to those of the thick ascending limb. However, significant cell heterogeneity characterizes the tubule segments that follow.

The **connecting tubule**, which ends at the transition to the initial collecting tubule, consists of two cell types: connecting tubule cells and intercalated cells. Connecting tubule cells (Fig. 33-6G) are unique in that they produce and release

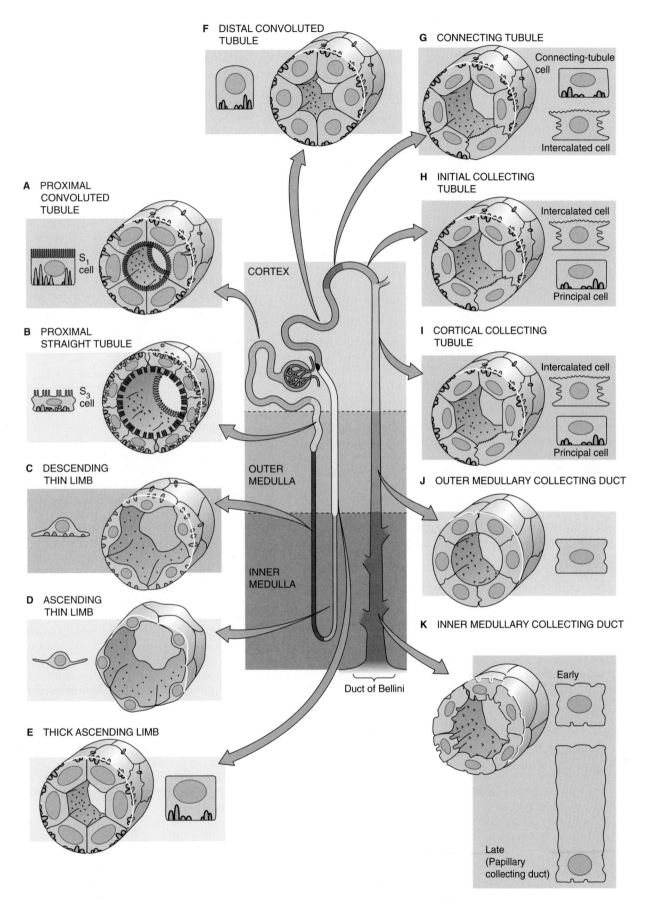

Figure 33-6   Structure of tubule cells along the nephron. Because of the variability among tubule segments, the cross sections of the tubule are not to scale.

Table 33-1 Tubule Segments of the Nephron

Tubule Segment	Abbreviation
Proximal convoluted tubule	PCT
Proximal straight tubule	PST
Thin descending limb of loop of Henle	tDLH
Thin ascending limb of loop of Henle	tALH
Thick ascending limb of loop of Henle	TAL
Distal convoluted tubule	DCT
Connecting tubule	CNT
Initial collecting tubule	ICT
Cortical collecting tubule	CCT
Outer medullary collecting duct	OMCD
Inner medullary collecting duct	IMCD

renal **kallikrein**, a local hormone whose precise function is still uncertain. We discuss intercalated cells later.

The two segments following the connecting tubule, the **initial collecting tubule** (up to the first confluence) and the **cortical collecting tubule** (after the confluence), are identical. They are composed of intercalated and principal cells, which exhibit striking morphological and functional differences. **Intercalated cells**, similar in structure to the intercalated cells of the connecting tubule, make up about one third of the lining of these collecting tubule segments (Fig. 33-6H, I). They are unusual among tubule cells in that they lack a central cilium. One subpopulation of these cells (A- or α-intercalated cells) secretes H^+ and reabsorbs K^+, whereas another (B- or ß-intercalated cells) secretes HCO_3^-. **Principal cells** make up about two thirds of the cells of the initial collecting tubule and cortical collecting tubule (Fig. 33-6H, I). Compared with intercalated cells, principal cells have fewer mitochondria, only modestly developed invaginations of the basolateral membrane, and a central *cilium* on the apical membrane. Principal cells reabsorb Na^+ and Cl^- and secrete K^+.

The **medullary collecting duct** is lined mostly by one cell type that increases in cell height toward the papilla (Fig. 33-6J, K). The number of intercalated cells diminishes, beginning at the outer medullary collecting duct. Cells in this segment continue the transport of electrolytes and participate in the hormonally regulated transport of water and of urea. At the extreme end of the medullary collecting duct (i.e., the "papillary" collecting duct or duct of Bellini), the cells are extremely tall.

The tightness of tubule epithelia increases from the proximal to the medullary collecting tubule

Epithelia may be either "tight" or "leaky," depending on the permeability of their **tight junctions** (see Chapter 5). In general, the tightness of the tubule epithelium increases from the proximal tubule to the collecting duct. In the leaky *proximal tubule*, junctional complexes are shallow and, in freeze-fracture studies, show only a few strands of membrane proteins (see Chapter 2). In contrast, in the relatively tight *collecting tubule*, tight junctions extend deep into the intercellular space and consist of multiple strands of membrane proteins. Tubule segments with tight junctions consisting of only one strand have low electrical resistance and high solute permeability, whereas tubules with several strands tend to have high electrical resistance and low permeability.

Gap junctions (see Chapter 6) provide low-resistance pathways between some, but not all, neighboring tubule cells. These gap junctions are located at various sites along the lateral cell membranes. Electrical coupling exists among proximal tubule cells, but not among heterogenous cell types, such as those found in the connecting and collecting tubules.

MAIN ELEMENTS OF RENAL FUNCTION

The nephron forms an ultrafiltrate of the blood plasma and then selectively reabsorbs the tubule fluid or secretes solutes into it

As they do for capillaries elsewhere in the body, Starling forces (see Chapter 20) govern the flow of fluid across the capillary walls in the **glomerulus** and result in net filtration. However, in the case of the glomerular capillaries, the filtrate flows not into the interstitium, but into Bowman's space, which is contiguous with the lumen of the proximal tubule.

The main function of renal tubules is to recover most of the fluid and solutes filtered at the glomerulus. If the fluid were not recovered, the kidney would excrete the volume of the entire blood plasma in less than half an hour. The retrieval of the largest fraction of glomerular filtrate occurs in the **proximal tubule**, which *reabsorbs* NaCl, $NaHCO_3$, filtered nutrients (e.g., glucose and amino acids), divalent ions (e.g., Ca^{2+}, HPO_4^{2-}, and SO_4^{2-}), and water. Finally, the proximal tubule *secretes* NH_4^+ and a variety of endogenous and exogenous solutes into the lumen.

The main function of the **loop of Henle** (i.e., thin descending limb of loop of Henle [tDLH], thin ascending limb of loop of Henle [tALH], thick ascending limb of loop of Henle [TAL]) is to participate in forming concentrated or dilute urine. The loop does this by pumping NaCl into the interstitium of the medulla without appreciable water flow, thus making the interstitium hypertonic. Downstream, the medullary collecting duct exploits this hypertonicity by either permitting or not permitting water to flow by osmosis into the hypertonic interstitium. In humans, only ~15% of the nephrons, the juxtamedullary nephrons, have long loops that descend to the tip of the papilla. Nevertheless, this *subpopulation* of nephrons (Fig. 33-2) is extremely important for creating the osmotic gradients within the papilla that allow water movement out of the lumen of the *entire population* of medullary collecting ducts. As a result of this water movement, urine osmolality in the collecting ducts can far exceed that in the plasma.

TAL cells secrete the Tamm-Horsfall glycoprotein (THP). Normal subjects excrete 30 to 50 mg/day into the urine, thus accounting—along with albumin (<20 mg/day)—for most of the protein normally present in urine. THP adheres to certain strains of *Escherichia coli* and may be part of the innate defense against urinary tract infections. THP also constitutes the matrix of all urinary casts, defined as cylindrical debris in the urine that takes the shape of the tubule lumens in which it is formed.

The classic **distal tubule** and the **collecting duct system** perform the fine control of NaCl and water excretion. Although only small fractions of the glomerular filtrate reach these most distally located nephron sites, these tubule segments are where several hormones (e.g., aldosterone, arginine vasopressin) exert their main effects on electrolyte and water excretion.

The juxtaglomerular apparatus is a region where each thick ascending limb contacts its glomerulus

Elements of the JGA play two important regulatory roles. First, if the amount of fluid and NaCl reaching a nephron's **macula densa** (Fig. 33-3F) increases, the glomerular filtration rate (GFR) of *that nephron* falls. We discuss this phenomenon of **tubuloglomerular feedback** in Chapter 34.

The second regulatory mechanism comes into play during a decrease in the pressure of the renal artery feeding the various afferent arterioles. When the afferent arteriole senses decreased stretch in its wall, this baroreceptor (see Chapter 23) directs neighboring granular cells to increase their release of **renin** into the general circulation. We discuss the renin-angiotensin-aldosterone axis, which is important in the long-term control of **systemic arterial blood pressure**, in Chapter 40.

Sympathetic nerve fibers to the kidney regulate renal blood flow, glomerular filtration, and tubule reabsorption

The autonomic innervation to the kidneys is entirely **sympathetic**; the kidneys lack parasympathetic nerve fibers. The sympathetic supply to the kidneys originates from the celiac plexus (see Fig. 14-3), and it generally follows the arterial vessels into the kidney. The varicosities of the sympathetic fibers release norepinephrine and dopamine into the loose connective tissue near the smooth muscle cells of the vasculature (i.e., renal artery as well as afferent and efferent arterioles) and near the proximal tubules. Sympathetic stimulation to the kidneys has three major effects. First, the catecholamines cause vasoconstriction. Second, the catecholamines strongly enhance Na^+ reabsorption by proximal tubule cells. Third, as a result of the dense accumulation of sympathetic fibers near the granular cells of the JGA, increased sympathetic nerve activity dramatically stimulates renin secretion.

Renal nerves also include afferent (i.e., sensory) fibers. A few myelinated nerve fibers conduct baroreceptor and chemoreceptor impulses that originate in the kidney. Increased perfusion pressure stimulates renal **baroreceptors** in the interlobular arteries and afferent arterioles. Renal ischemia

and abnormal ion composition of the interstitial fluid stimulate **chemoreceptors** located in the renal pelvis. These pelvic chemoreceptors probably respond to high extracellular levels of K^+ and H^+ and may elicit changes in capillary blood flow.

The kidneys are also endocrine organs: they produce renin, the biologically active form of vitamin D, erythropoietin, prostaglandins, and bradykinin

Besides **renin** production by the JGA granular cells (see Chapter 40), the kidneys play several other endocrine roles. Proximal tubule cells convert circulating 25-hydroxyvitamin D to the active metabolite, **1,25-dihydroxyvitamin D**. This hormone controls Ca^{2+} and phosphorus metabolism by acting on the intestines, kidneys, and bone (see Chapter 52), and is important for developing and maintaining bone structure.

Fibroblast-like cells in the interstitium of the cortex and outer medulla secrete **EPO** in response to a fall in the local tissue P_{O_2} (see p. 453). EPO stimulates the development of red blood cells by action on hematopoietic stem cells in bone marrow. In chronic renal failure, the deficiency of EPO leads to severe anemia that can be treated with recombinant EPO.

The kidney releases **prostaglandins** and several **kinins**, paracrine agents that control circulation within the kidney. These substances are generally vasodilators and may play a protective role when renal blood flow is compromised. Tubule cells also secrete angiotensin, bradykinin, cAMP, and ATP into the lumen, but the precise function of such local secretion is poorly understood.

MEASURING RENAL CLEARANCE AND TRANSPORT

Numerous tests can assess renal function. Some are applicable only in animal experiments. Others are useful in clinical settings and fall into two general categories:

1. Modern imaging techniques provide outstanding macroscopic views of renal blood flow, filtration, and excretory function.
2. Measurements of so-called renal clearance of various substances evaluate the ability of the kidneys to handle solutes and water.

This section focuses on clearance measurements, which compare the rate at which the glomeruli filter a substance (water or a solute) with the rate at which the kidneys excrete it into the urine. By measuring the difference between the amounts filtered and excreted for a particular substance, we can estimate the net amount reabsorbed or secreted by the renal tubules and can thus gain insight into the three basic functions of the kidney: glomerular **filtration**, tubule **reabsorption**, and tubule **secretion**. Although widely used, clearance methods have the inherent limitation that they measure *overall* nephron function. This function is overall in two different senses. First, clearance sums many individual transport operations occurring sequentially along a nephron.

Second, clearance sums the output of all 2 million nephrons in parallel. Hence, clearance cannot provide information on precise sites and mechanisms of transport. Such information can, however, come from studies of individual nephrons, tubule cells, or cell membranes. One can also apply the clearance concept to other problems, such as clearance of bile by the liver (see Chapter 46) or clearance of hormones from the blood.

The clearance of a solute is the virtual volume of plasma that would be totally cleared of a solute in a given time

All solutes excreted into the urine ultimately come from the blood plasma perfusing the kidneys. Thus, the rate at which the kidney excretes a solute into the urine equals the rate at which the solute disappears from the plasma, provided the kidney does not produce, consume, or store the solute. Imagine that, in 1 minute, 700 mL of plasma will flow through the kidneys. This plasma contains 0.7 L × 142 mM or ~100 mmol of Na^+. Of this Na^+, the kidneys remove and excrete into the urine only a tiny amount, ~0.14 mmol. In principle, these 0.14 mmol of Na^+ could have come from only 1 mL of plasma, had all Na^+ ions been removed (i.e., cleared) from this volume. The **clearance** of a solute is defined as the virtual volume of blood plasma (per unit time) needed to supply the amount of solute that appears in the urine. Thus, in our example, Na^+ clearance was 1 mL/min, even though 700 mL of plasma flowed through the kidneys.

Renal clearance methods are based on the principle of mass balance and the special anatomy of the kidney (Fig. 33-7). For any solute (X) that the kidney does not synthesize, degrade, or accumulate, the only route of entry to the kidney is the renal artery, and the only two routes of exit are the renal vein and the ureter. Because the input of X equals the output of X,

$$\underbrace{\underbrace{P_{X,a}}_{\frac{mmole}{mL}} \cdot \underbrace{RPF_a}_{\frac{mL}{min}}}_{\text{Arterial input of X}} = \underbrace{\left(\underbrace{P_{X,v}}_{\frac{mmole}{mL}} \cdot \underbrace{RPF_v}_{\frac{mL}{min}}\right)}_{\text{Venous output of X}} + \underbrace{\left(\underbrace{U_X}_{\frac{mmole}{mL}} \cdot \underbrace{\dot{V}}_{\frac{mL}{min}}\right)}_{\text{Urine output of X}} \quad (33\text{-}1)$$

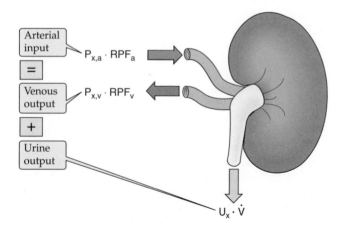

Figure 33-7 Solute mass balance in the kidney. See text for details.

$P_{X,a}$ and $P_{X,v}$ are the plasma concentrations of X in the renal artery and renal vein, respectively. RPF_a and RPF_v are the rates of renal plasma flow (RPF) in the renal artery and vein, respectively. U_X is the concentration of X in urine. $\dot{V}$ is urine flow (the overdot represents the time derivative of volume). The product $U_X \cdot \dot{V}$ is the **urinary excretion rate**, the amount of X excreted in urine per unit time.

In developing the concept of renal clearance, we transform Equation 33-1 in two ways, both based on the assumption that the kidneys clear all X from an incoming volume of arterial plasma. First, we replace RPF_a with the inflow of the virtual volume—the clearance of X (C_X)—that provides just that amount of X that appears in the urine. Second, we assign the virtual venous output a value of zero. Thus, Equation 33-1 becomes the following:

$$\underbrace{P_{X,a} \cdot C_X}_{\substack{\text{Virtual} \\ \text{arterial input}}} = \underbrace{0}_{\substack{\text{Virtual} \\ \text{venous output}}} + \underbrace{(U_X \cdot \dot{V})}_{\substack{\text{Actual} \\ \text{urine output}}} \quad (33\text{-}2)$$

Solving for clearance,

$$C_X = \frac{U_X \cdot \dot{V}}{P_X} \quad (33\text{-}3)$$

This is the classic **clearance equation** that describes the virtual volume of plasma that would be *totally cleared* of a solute in a given time (Table 33-2A). We need to know only three parameters to compute the clearance of a solute X:

1. the concentration of X in the urine (U_X);
2. the volume of urine formed in a given time ($\dot{V}$); and
3. the concentration of X in systemic blood plasma (P_X), which is the same as $P_{X,a}$ in Equation 33-1.

Table 33-2 Renal Clearance

A. Clearance of Any Substance X

$$C_X = \frac{U_X \cdot \dot{V}}{P_X} = \frac{(mg \text{ or } mol/mL) \cdot (mL/min)}{mg \text{ or } mol/mL} = \frac{mL}{min}$$

C_X may vary between zero, for a substance that does not appear in the urine (e.g., glucose), and ~700 mL/min (i.e., total RPF) for a substance (e.g., PAH) that is totally removed from the blood in a single pass through the kidney.

B. Clearance of PAH Approximates RPF (at Low Plasma PAH Concentration)

$$C_{PAH} = RPF = \frac{U_{PAH} \cdot \dot{V}}{P_{PAH}}$$

C. Clearance of Inulin equals GFR

$$C_{In} = GFR = \frac{U_{In} \cdot \dot{V}}{P_{In}}$$

C, clearance; GFR, glomerular filtration rate; In, inulin; P, plasma; PAH, p-aminohippurate; RPF, renal plasma flow; U, urine; $\dot{V}$, volume per unit of time.

Together, the three basic functions of the kidney—glomerular filtration, tubule reabsorption, and tubule secretion—determine the renal clearance of a solute. In the special case in which the kidneys completely clear X from plasma during a *single passage* through the kidneys ($P_{X,v} = 0$ in Equation 33-1), the renal clearance of X equals RPF_a in Equation 33-1. Because *p-aminohippurate (PAH)* is just such a special solute, its clearance is a good estimate of RPF_a, which we simplify to **RPF** (Table 33-2B). We discuss RPF in Chapter 34.

For all solutes that *do not* behave like PAH, the renal venous plasma still contains some X. Thus, the virtual volume cleared of X in a given time is less than the total RPF. For most solutes, then, clearance describes a virtual volume of plasma that would be *totally cleared* of a solute, whereas in reality a much larger volume of plasma is *partially cleared* of the solute.

We can use a clearance approach to estimate another important renal parameter: **GFR**, which is the volume of fluid filtered into Bowman's capsule per unit time. Imagine a solute X that fulfills two criteria. First, X is freely filtered (i.e., concentration of X in Bowman's space is the same as that in blood plasma). Second, the tubules do not absorb, secrete, synthesize, degrade, or accumulate X. Thus, the amount of X that appears in the urine per unit time ($U_X \cdot \dot{V}$) is the same as the amount of X that the glomerulus filters per unit time ($P_X \cdot GFR$):

$$\overbrace{P_X \cdot GFR}^{\substack{\text{Input to} \\ \text{Bowman's space}}} = \overbrace{U_X \cdot \dot{V}}^{\substack{\text{Output into} \\ \text{urine}}} \quad (33\text{-}4)$$

The input to Bowman's space is also known as the **filtered solute load** and is generally given in millimoles (or milligrams) per minute. Rearranging Equation 33-4.

$$GFR = \frac{U_X \cdot \dot{V}}{P_X} \quad (33\text{-}5)$$

Equation 33-5 is in exactly the same form as the classic clearance equation (Equation 33-3). In other words, GFR is C_X if X has the required properties. As discussed in Chapter 34, **inulin** is just such a solute (Table 33-2C).

A solute's urinary excretion is the algebraic sum of its filtered load, reabsorption by tubules, and secretion by tubules

The homeostasis of body fluids critically depends on the ability of the kidneys to determine the amount of a given solute that they excrete into the urine. Renal excretion rate (E_X) depends on three factors (Fig. 33-8):

1. the rate of filtration of X (F_X): the **filtered load** ($F_X = GFR \cdot P_X$);
2. the rate of reabsorption of X (R_X) by the tubules; and
3. the rate of secretion of X (S_X) by the tubules.

This interrelationship is expressed quantitatively as follows:

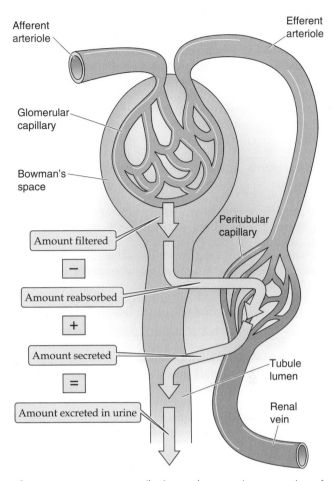

Figure 33-8 Factors contributing to the net urinary excretion of a substance.

$$\overbrace{E_X}^{\substack{\text{Amount} \\ \textit{excreted} \\ \text{per unit} \\ \text{time}}} = \overbrace{F_X}^{\substack{\text{Amount} \\ \textit{filtered} \\ \text{per unit} \\ \text{time}}} - \overbrace{R_X}^{\substack{\text{Amount} \\ \textit{reabsorbed} \\ \text{per unit} \\ \text{time}}} + \overbrace{S_X}^{\substack{\text{Amount} \\ \textit{secreted} \\ \text{per unit} \\ \text{time}}} \quad (33\text{-}6)$$

For some substances (e.g., inulin), no reabsorption or secretion occurs. For most substances, *either* reabsorption *or* secretion determines the amount present in the final urine. However, for some substances, *both* reabsorption *and* secretion determine excretion.

If a solute is only reabsorbed, *but not secreted*, we can rearrange Equation 33-6 to obtain the rate of **reabsorption** Equation 33-6:

$$\overbrace{R_X}^{\substack{\text{Reabsorption rate} \\ \text{(mg/min)}}} = \overbrace{GFR \cdot P_X}^{\substack{\text{Filtered load} \\ \text{(mg/min)}}} - \overbrace{U_X \cdot \dot{V}}^{\substack{\text{Excretion rate} \\ \text{(mg/min)}}} \quad (33\text{-}7)$$

Conversely, if a solute is only secreted, *but not reabsorbed*, the rate of **secretion** is as follows:

$$\overbrace{S_X}^{\substack{\text{Secretion rate} \\ \text{(mg/min)}}} = \overbrace{U_X \cdot \dot{V}}^{\substack{\text{Excretion rate} \\ \text{(mg/min)}}} - \overbrace{GFR \cdot P_X}^{\substack{\text{Filtered rate} \\ \text{(mg/min)}}} \quad (33\text{-}8)$$

In applying Equations 33-7 and 33-8, we must keep in mind two important limitations. First, to estimate the rate at which a substance appears in the filtrate—the filtered load—from the product $GFR \cdot P_X$, we assume that P_X is the *freely filterable* concentration of X. Indeed, many substances, particularly univalent electrolytes, urea, glucose, and amino acids, are freely filterable. However, if the solute binds to protein, for example, then it will not be freely filterable. For these solutes, including Ca^{2+}, phosphate, Mg^{2+}, and PAH, it is necessary to measure plasma binding and correct for the nonfilterable fraction of the solute. Second, for us to apply the mass balance equation (Equation 33-6), the kidney must not synthesize, degrade, or accumulate the solute. An example of a solute that is synthesized by the kidney is ammonium. Examples of solutes degraded by the kidney include glutamine and glutamate (which are deaminated to yield ammonium) as well as several other amino acids and monocarboxylic and dicarboxylic acids.

When the kidney both *reabsorbs* and *secretes* a substance, clearance data are inadequate to describe renal handling. For example, if the proximal tubule completely reabsorbed a solute that a later segment then secreted, clearance data alone would imply that only filtration and some reabsorption occurred. We would have no reason to implicate secretion. Complex combinations of reabsorption and secretion occur with K^+, uric acid, and urea.

Another useful parameter for gauging how the kidney handles a freely filtered solute is the **fractional excretion** (FE), which is the ratio of the amount excreted in the urine $(U_X \cdot \dot{V})$ to the filtered load $(P_X \cdot GFR)$:

$$FE_X = \frac{U_X \cdot \dot{V}}{P_X \cdot GFR} \qquad (33\text{-}9)$$

According to Equation 33-3, however, the term $(U_X \cdot \dot{V}/P_X)$ is simply the clearance of X (C_X):

$$FE_X = \frac{C_X}{GFR} \qquad (33\text{-}10)$$

As discussed in Chapter 34, one estimates GFR by measuring the clearance of inulin (C_{In}). Thus, the fractional excretion of a freely filterable solute is the same as the **clearance ratio**:

$$FE_X = \frac{C_X}{C_{In}} \qquad (33\text{-}11)$$

Microscopic techniques make it possible to measure single-nephron rates of filtration, absorption, and secretion

Because clearance methods treat the kidney as a "black box," reflecting the activity of many single nephrons and nephron segments, it is very difficult to determine which nephron segments are responsible for which transport processes. It is also impossible to determine which nephrons

are responsible for overall urinary excretion. To learn how single nephrons function, and to understand how individual nephron segments contribute to overall nephron function, physiologists developed a series of invasive techniques for studying renal cells in the research laboratory (Fig. 33-9).

To apply the concept of clearance to a single nephron site, one uses the free-flow micropuncture approach (Fig. 33-9A) and measures the concentration of the solute in the tubule fluid at that site (TF_X), volume flow at that site (i.e., the collection rate), and plasma concentration (P_X). By analogy with the *macroscopic* clearance equation, we can write a clearance equation for a single nephron:

$$C_X = \frac{TF_X \times \text{Volume collection rate}}{P_X} \qquad (33\text{-}12)$$

Compared with Equation 33-3, here TF_X replaces U_X and "Volume collection rate" replaces $\dot{V}$. We can use this basic equation to compute the amount of fluid that a single nephron filters, as well as the amounts of fluid and solutes that a single tubule segment handles.

Single-Nephron Glomerular Filtration Rate If X in Equation 33-12 is a marker for GFR (e.g., inulin or In), one can calculate single-nephron GFR (SNGFR) using an equation that is similar to that in Table 33-2C to calculate total GFR:

$$SNGFR = \frac{TF_{In} \times \text{Volume collection rate}}{P_{In}} \qquad (33\text{-}13)$$

Using the numeric values for rat kidney shown in Figure 33-10, we can use Equation 33-13 to compute the SNGFR:

$$SNGFR = \frac{(3\,mg/mL) \times (10\,nL/min)}{(1\,mg/mL)} = 30\,nL/min \qquad (33\text{-}14)$$

Handling of Water by Tubule Segments In a Single Nephron We also can use the same information that we used to compute SNGFR to calculate the rate of water reabsorption between the glomerulus and the micropuncture site. The fraction of filtered water remaining at the micropuncture site is as follows:

$$\frac{\text{Fraction of filtered}}{\text{water remaining}} = \frac{\text{Volume collection rate}}{SNGFR} \qquad (33\text{-}15)$$

Substituting the expression for SNGFR (Equation 33-13) into Equation 33-15, we have the following:

$$\frac{\text{Fraction of filtered}}{\text{water remaining}} = \frac{\text{Volume collection rate}}{(TF_{In} \times \text{Volume collection rate})/P_{In}}$$

$$= \frac{P_{In}}{TF_{In}}$$

$$(33\text{-}16)$$

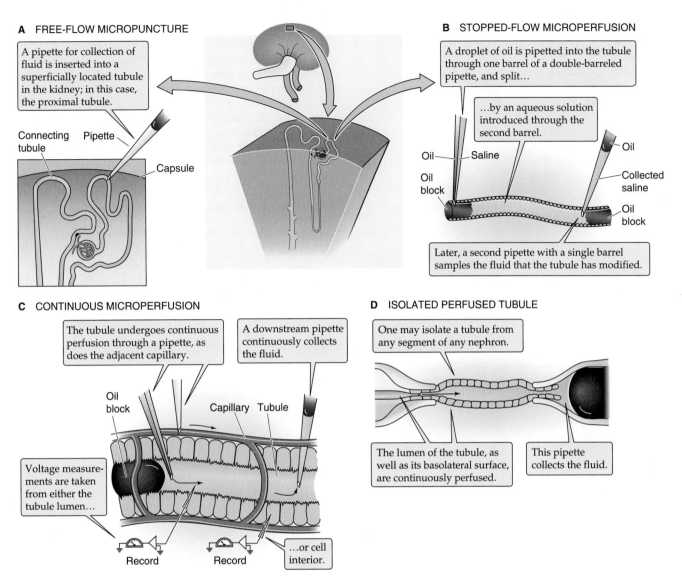

Figure 33-9 Methods for studying renal function in the research laboratory.

Thus, to know the *fraction* of filtered water remaining at the collection site, we do not need to know the collection rate, only the concentrations of inulin in blood plasma and at the collection site. In the example of Figure 33-10, in which the tubule reabsorbed two thirds of the fluid, the fraction of filtered water remaining at the sampling site is (1 mg/mL)/(3 mg/mL) or ~0.33.

The **fraction of filtered water reabsorbed** is 1 minus the fraction of filtered water remaining:

$$\text{Fraction of filtered water reabsorbed} = 1 - \frac{P_{In}}{TF_{In}} \quad (33\text{-}17)$$

In our example, the fraction of filtered water reabsorbed is 1 − 0.33 or ~0.67.

Handling of Solutes by Tubule Segments in a Single Nephron We can use the same concepts of single-nephron clearance to quantitate the reabsorption or secretion of any

solute along the tubule. The first step is to estimate the fraction of the filtered solute remaining at the puncture site. This parameter—the **fractional solute delivery**—is the ratio of the amount of solute appearing at the micropuncture site to the amount of solute filtered at the glomerulus (i.e., **single-nephron filtered load**):

$$\text{Fractional solute delivery} = \frac{\begin{array}{c}\text{Rate of solute delivery to}\\\text{micropuncture site}\end{array}}{\text{Single-nephron filtered load}}$$

$$(33\text{-}18)$$

The numerator is the product of volume collection rate and tubule solute concentration (TF_X), and the denominator is the product of SNGFR and the plasma solute concentration (P_X):

$$\begin{array}{c}\text{Fractional solute}\\\text{delivery}\end{array} = \frac{\text{Volume collection rate} \times TF_X}{\text{SNGFR} \times P_X} \quad (33\text{-}19)$$

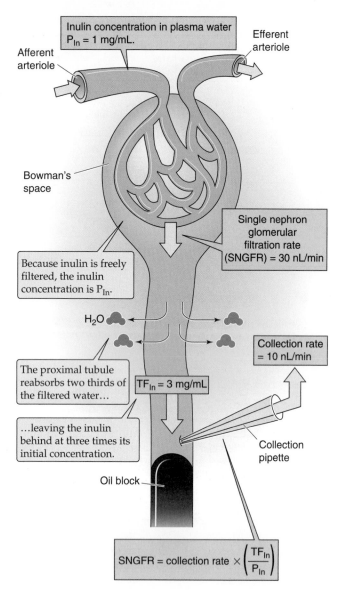

Figure 33-10 Measurement of single-nephron glomerular filtration rate. Data are for the rat.

In Equations 33-15 and 33-16, we saw that the ratio (Volume collection rate/SNGFR) is (P_{In}/TF_{In}). Making this substitution in Equation 33-19, we obtain an alternative expression for fractional solute excretion:

$$\text{Fractional solute delivery} = \frac{TF_X/P_X}{TF_{In}/P_{In}} \qquad (33\text{-}20)$$

The advantage of Equation 33-20 over Equation 33-19 is that no measurements of collection rates are required.

Equation 33-20 is important for understanding the transport of a solute along the nephron. If $(TF_X/P_X)/(TF_{In}/P_{In})$ is greater than 1, **secretion** has occurred. Merely observing that the solute *concentration* in tubule fluid increases along the length of the nephron does not necessarily mean that the tubule secreted the solute; the concentration would also

increase if water were reabsorbed. We can conclude that secretion has occurred only if the solute concentration in tubule fluid, relative to its concentration in filtrate, exceeds the concentration ratio of inulin. If $(TF_X/P_X)/(TF_{In}/P_{In})$ is less than 1, **reabsorption** has occurred.

Rather than referring to the fraction of the solute excreted (i.e., remaining) up to the point of the micropuncture site, we can also refer to the **fractional solute reabsorption** at the puncture site. By analogy to Equation 33-17 for water, this parameter for a solute is merely 1 minus the fractional solute excretion:

$$\text{Fractional solute reabsorption} = 1 - \frac{TF_X/P_X}{TF_{In}/P_{In}} \qquad (33\text{-}21)$$

Thus, applying the principles of clearance and mass balance to a single nephron, we can calculate SNGFR as well as the fractional reabsorption of water and solutes at the micropuncture site.

THE URETERS AND BLADDER

As discussed in Chapters 44 and 45, the epithelium of the gastrointestinal system continues to modify the contents of the gastrointestinal tract up until the point where the contents finally exit the body. The situation is very different in the mammalian urinary system. By the time the fluid leaves the most distal portion of the collecting duct, the fluid has the composition of final urine. Thus, the renal pelvis, ureters, bladder, and urethra do not substantially modify the urine volume or composition.

The ureters propel urine from the renal pelvis to the bladder by peristaltic waves conducted along a syncytium of smooth muscle cells

The **ureters** serve as conduits for the passage of urine from the renal pelvis into the urinary bladder (Fig. 33-1A). Located in the retroperitoneum, each ureter loops over the top of the common iliac artery and vein on the same side of the body and courses through the pelvis. The ureters enter the lower, posterior portion of the bladder (**ureterovesical junction**), pass obliquely through its muscular wall, and open into the bladder lumen 1 to 2 cm above, and lateral to, the orifice of the urethra (Fig. 33-11A). The two ureteral orifices, connected by a ridge of tissue, and the urethral orifice form the corners of a triangle (**bladder trigone**). A flap-like valve of mucous membrane covers each ureteral orifice. This anatomical valve, in conjunction with the physiological valve-like effect created by the ureter's oblique pathway through the bladder wall, prevents reflux of urine back into the ureters during contraction of the bladder.

The lumen of each ureter is lined by **transitional epithelium**, which is above a submucosal layer of connective tissue, as well as an inner longitudinal and an outer circular layer of smooth muscle. Ureteral **smooth muscle** functions as a syncytium and is thus an example of unitary smooth muscle (see Chapter 9). Gap junctions (see Chapter 6) conduct electrical activity from cell to cell at a velocity of 2 to

A URETERS AND BLADDER

B SMOOTH-MUSCLE
ACTION POTENTIAL

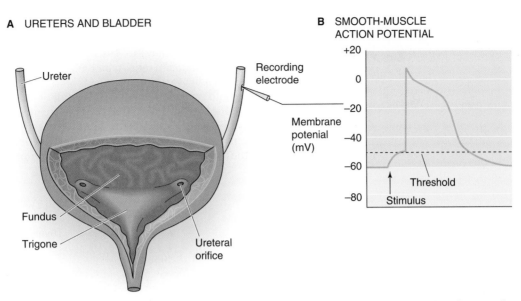

Figure 33-11 **A** and **B,** Anatomy of the ureters and bladder. In **B,** ureteral smooth muscle cells generally have a resting membrane potential of ~−60 mV, mainly determined by a high K⁺ membrane permeability. Na⁺ channels speed the upstroke of the action potential, although Ca²⁺ channels are mainly responsible for the action potential.

6 cm/s. Chemical or mechanical stimuli (e.g., stretch) or a suprathreshold membrane depolarization may trigger an **action potential** (Fig. 33-11B) of the plateau type (see Chapter 9).

Contraction of ureteral smooth muscle is similar to that of other smooth muscle (see Chapter 9), in which Ca²⁺-calmodulin activates myosin light chain kinase (MLCK). cAMP-dependent protein kinase (PKA) can phosphorylate MLCK, thereby lowering the affinity of MLCK for Ca²⁺-calmodulin and impairing phosphorylation of myosin light chains. This mechanism may, at least in part, account for the relaxing effect of cAMP on smooth muscle.

Ureteral **peristaltic waves** originate from electrical **pacemakers** in the proximal portion of the renal pelvis. These waves propel urine along the ureters and into the bladder in a series of spurts, at frequencies of two to six per minute. The intraureteral hydrostatic pressure is 0 to 5 cm H₂O at baseline, but it increases to 20 to 80 cm H₂O during peristaltic waves. Blockade of ureteral outflow to the bladder, as by a kidney stone, causes the ureter to dilate and increases the baseline hydrostatic pressure to 70 to 80 cm H₂O over a period of 1 to 3 hours. This pressure is transmitted in retrograde fashion to the nephrons and thus creates a stopped-flow condition in which glomerular filtration nearly comes to a halt. **Hydronephrosis**, dilation of the pelvis and calyces of the kidney, can evolve over hours to days. Patients complain of severe pain (renal colic) resulting from distention of involved structures. If not cleared, the obstruction can cause marked renal dysfunction and even acute renal failure. With persistent obstruction, the pressure inside the ureter declines to a level that is only slightly higher than the normal baseline. Even though the patient produces no urine (anuria), glomerular filtration continues, albeit at a markedly reduced rate, a condition reflecting a balance between filtration and fluid reabsorption by the tubules.

Although ureteral peristalsis can occur without innervation, the autonomic nervous system can modulate peristalsis. As in other syncytial smooth muscle, autonomic control of the ureters occurs by diffuse transmitter release from multiple varicosities formed as the postganglionic axon courses over the smooth muscle cell. *Sympathetic* input (through aortic, hypogastric, and ovarian or spermatic plexuses) modulates ureteral contractility as norepinephrine acts by excitatory α-adrenergic receptors and inhibitory ß-adrenergic receptors. *Parasympathetic* input enhances ureteral contractility through acetylcholine, either by directly stimulating muscarinic cholinergic receptors (see Chapter 3) or by causing postganglionic sympathetic fibers to release norepinephrine, which then can stimulate α-adrenoceptors. Some autonomic fibers innervating the ureters are afferent **pain fibers**. In fact, the pain of renal colic associated with violent peristaltic contractions proximal to an obstruction is one of the most severe encountered in clinical practice.

Sympathetic, parasympathetic, and somatic fibers innervate the urinary bladder and its sphincters

The urinary bladder consists of a main portion (body) that collects urine and a funnel-shaped extension (neck) that connects with the urethra (Fig. 33-11A). Transitional epithelium lines the bladder lumen. Three poorly defined layers of smooth muscle make up the bulk of the bladder wall, the so-called **detrusor muscle**. At the lower tip of the trigone, the bladder lumen opens into the posterior urethra (i.e., distal part of bladder neck), which extends over 2 to 3 cm. The wall of the posterior urethra contains *smooth* muscle fibers of the detrusor muscle interspersed with elastic tissue, together forming the **internal sphincter** (Table 33-3). Immediately adjacent is the **external sphincter**, made up of voluntary, mainly slow-twitch *striated*-muscle fibers.

Table 33-3   Overview of the Urethral Sphincters

Characteristic	Internal Sphincter	External Sphincter
Type of muscle	Smooth	Skeletal
Nerve reaching the structure	Hypogastric	Pudendal
Nature of innervation	Autonomic	Somatic

In humans, bladder smooth muscle appears to lack gap junctions, a finding suggesting the absence of electrotonic coupling between cells. Thus, bladder smooth muscle is probably "multiunit" (see Chapter 9), with a 1:1 ratio between nerve endings and smooth muscle cells. Contraction of bladder smooth muscle is typical of other smooth muscle cells.

The bladder and sphincters receive sympathetic and parasympathetic (autonomic) as well as somatic (voluntary) innervation (Fig. 33-12). The **sympathetic innervation** to the bladder and internal sphincter arises from neurons in the

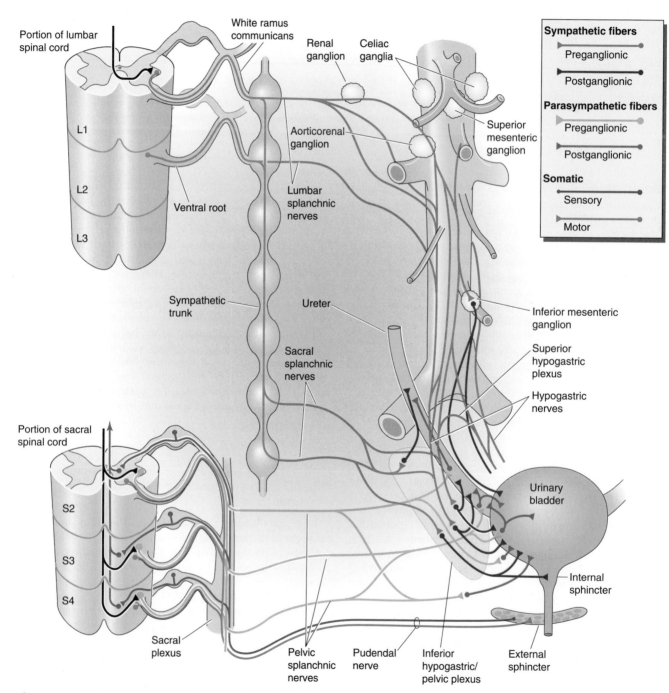

Figure 33-12 • Autonomic and somatic innervation of the bladder.

intermediolateral cell column of the tenth thoracic to the second lumbar spinal cord segment (see Chapter 14). The preganglionic fibers then pass through lumbar splanchnic nerves to the superior hypogastric plexus, where they give rise to the left and right hypogastric nerves. These nerves lead to the inferior hypogastric/pelvic plexus, where preganglionic sympathetic fibers synapse with postganglionic fibers. The postganglionic fibers continue to the bladder wall through the distal portion of the hypogastric nerve. This distal portion also contains the preganglionic *parasympathetic* axons discussed in the next paragraph.

The **parasympathetic innervation** of the bladder originates from the intermediolateral cell column in segments S2 through S4 of the sacral spinal cord. The *parasympathetic* fibers approaching the bladder via the pelvic splanchnic nerve are still preganglionic. They synapse with postganglionic neurons in the body and neck of the urinary bladder.

The **somatic innervation** originates from motor neurons arising from segments S2 to S4. Through the pudendal nerve, these motor neurons innervate and control the voluntary skeletal muscle of the external sphincter (Fig. 33-12).

Filling the bladder activates stretch receptors that initiate the micturition reflex, a spinal reflex arc also under the control of higher central nervous system centers

Bladder **tone** is defined by the relationship between bladder volume and internal (intravesical) pressure. One can measure the volume-pressure relationship by first inserting a catheter through the urethra and emptying the bladder and then recording the pressure while filling the bladder with 50-mL increments of water. The record of the relationship between volume and pressure is a **cystometrogram** (Fig. 33-13, blue curve). Increasing bladder volume from 0 to ~50 mL produces a moderately steep increase in pressure. Additional volume increases up to ~300 mL produce almost no pressure increase; this high compliance reflects relaxation of

bladder smooth muscle. At volumes higher than 400 mL, additional increases in volume produce steep rises in "passive" pressure. Bladder tone, up to the point of triggering the micturition reflex, is independent of extrinsic bladder innervation.

Cortical and suprapontine centers in the brain normally inhibit the micturition reflex, which the **pontine micturition center** coordinates. The pontine micturition center controls both the bladder detrusor muscle and the urinary sphincters. During the **storage phase**, stretch receptors in the bladder send afferent signals to the brain through the pelvic splanchnic nerves. One first senses the urge for voluntary bladder emptying at a volume of ~150 mL and senses fullness at 400 to 500 mL. Nevertheless, until a socially acceptable opportunity to void presents itself, efferent impulses from the brain, in a learned reflex, inhibit presynaptic parasympathetic neurons in the sacral spinal cord that

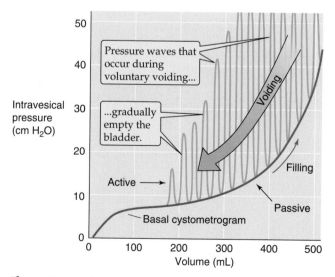

Figure 33-13 A cystometrogram.

Pathophysiology of Micturition

Lesions in the nervous system can lead to bladder dysfunction, the characteristics of which will depend on the site of the neural lesion. Three major classes of lesions can be distinguished.

1. **Combined afferent and efferent lesions.** Severing both afferent and efferent nerves initially causes the bladder to become distended and flaccid. In the chronic state of the so-called "decentralized bladder," many small contractions of the progressively hypertrophied bladder muscles replace the coordinated micturition events. Although small amounts of urine can be expelled, a residual volume of urine remains in the bladder after urination.

2. **Afferent lesions.** When only the sacral dorsal roots (sensory fibers) are interrupted, reflex contractions of the bladder, in response to stimulation of the stretch receptors, are totally abolished. The bladder frequently becomes distended, the wall thins, and bladder tone decreases. However, some residual contractions remain because of the intrinsic contractile response of smooth muscle to stretch. As a rule, a residual urine volume is present after urination.

3. **Spinal cord lesions.** The effects of spinal cord transection (e.g., in paraplegic patients) include the initial state of **spinal shock** in which the bladder becomes overfilled and exhibits sporadic voiding ("overflow incontinence"). With time, the voiding reflex is re-established, but with no voluntary control. Bladder capacity is often reduced and reflex hyperactivity may lead to a state called "spastic neurogenic bladder." Again, the bladder cannot empty completely, resulting in the presence of significant residual urine. Urinary tract infections are frequent because the residual urine volume in the bladder serves as an incubator for bacteria. In addition, during the period of "overflow incontinence," before the voiding reflex is re-established, these patients have to be catheterized frequently, further predisposing to urinary tract infections.

would otherwise stimulate the detrusor muscle. Voluntary contraction of the external urinary sphincter probably also contributes to storage.

The **voiding phase** begins with a voluntary relaxation of the external urinary sphincter, followed by the internal sphincter. When a small amount of urine reaches the proximal (posterior) urethra, afferents signal the cortex that voiding is imminent. The micturition reflex now continues as pontine centers no longer inhibit the parasympathetic preganglionic neurons that innervate the detrusor muscle. As a result, the bladder contracts, expelling urine. Once this micturition reflex has started, the initial bladder contractions lead to further trains of sensory impulses from stretch receptors, thus establishing a self-regenerating process (Fig. 33-13, red spikes moving to the left). At the same time, the cortical centers inhibit the external sphincter muscles. Voluntary urination also involves the voluntary contraction of abdominal muscles, which further raises bladder pressure and thus contributes to voiding and complete bladder emptying.

The basic bladder reflex that we have just discussed, although inherently an autonomic spinal cord reflex, may be either facilitated or inhibited by higher centers in the central nervous system that set the level at which the threshold for voiding occurs. Because of the continuous flow of urine from the kidneys to the bladder, the function of the various sphincters, and the nearly complete emptying of the bladder during micturition, the entire urinary system is normally sterile.

REFERENCES

Books and Reviews

Benzing T: Signaling at the slit diaphragm. J Am Soc Nephrol 2004; 15:1382-1391.

Kriz W, Bankir L: A standard nomenclature for structures of the kidney. Kidney Int 1988; 33:1-7.

Seldin DW, Giebisch G (eds): The Kidney: Physiology and Pathophysiology, 3rd ed. Philadelphia: Lippincott Williams & Wilkins, 2000.

Smith H: The Kidney: Structure and Function in Health and Disease. New York: Oxford University Press, 1951.

Weiss RW: Physiology and pharmacology of the renal pelvis and ureter. In Walsh PC, Rettig AB, Vaughan E, Wein AJ (eds): Campbell's Urology, 7th ed, pp 839-870. Philadelphia: WB Saunders, 1998.

Journal Articles

Maxwell PH, Osmond MK, Pugh CW, et al: Identification of the renal erythropoietin-producing cells using transgenic mice. Kidney Int 1993; 44:1149-1162.

Shannon JA: The excretion of inulin by the dog. Am J Physiol 1935; 112:405-413.

Smith HW, Finklestein N, Aliminosa L, et al: The renal clearances of substituted hippuric acid derivatives and other aromatic acids in dog and man. J Clin Invest 1945; 24:388-404.

Tamm I, Horsfall FL Jr: A mucoprotein derived from human urine which reacts with influenza, mumps, and Newcastle disease viruses. J Exp Med 1952; 95:71-97.

Walker AM, Bott PA, Oliver J, MacDowell MC: The collection and analysis of fluid from single nephrons of the mammalian kidney. Am J Physiol 1941; 134:580-595.

CHAPTER 34

GLOMERULAR FILTRATION AND RENAL BLOOD FLOW

Gerhard Giebisch and Erich Windhager

GLOMERULAR FILTRATION

A high glomerular filtration rate is essential for maintaining stable and optimal extracellular levels of solutes and water

Qualitatively, the filtration of blood plasma by the renal glomeruli is the same as the filtration of blood plasma across capillaries in other vascular beds (see Chapter 20). Glomerular ultrafiltration results in the formation of a fluid—the **glomerular filtrate**—with solute concentrations that are similar to those in plasma water. However, proteins, other high-molecular-weight compounds, and protein-bound solutes are present at reduced concentration. The glomerular filtrate, like filtrates formed across other body capillaries, is free of formed blood elements, such as red and white blood cells.

Quantitatively, the rate of filtration that occurs in the glomeruli greatly exceeds that in all the other capillaries of the circulation combined because of greater Starling forces (see Chapter 20) and higher capillary permeability. Compared with other organs, the kidneys receive an extraordinarily large amount of blood flow—normalized to the mass of the organ—and filter an unusually high fraction of this blood flow. Under normal conditions, the **glomerular filtration rate** (GFR; see Chapter 33) of the two kidneys is 125 mL/min or 180 L/day. Such a large rate of filtrate formation is required to expose the entire extracellular fluid frequently (>10 times/day) to the scrutiny of the renal tubule epithelium. If it were not for such a high turnover of the extracellular fluid, only small volumes of blood would be "cleared" per unit time (see Chapter 33) of certain solutes and water. Such a low clearance would have two harmful consequences for the renal excretion of solutes that renal tubules *cannot adequately secrete*.

First, in the presence of a sudden increase in the plasma level of a toxic material—originating either from metabolism or from food or fluid intake—the excretion of the material would be delayed. High blood flow and a high GFR allow the kidneys to eliminate harmful materials rapidly by filtration.

A second consequence of low clearance would be that steady-state plasma levels would be very high for waste materials that depend on filtration for excretion. The following example by Robert Pitts, a major contributor to renal physiology, illustrates the importance of this concept. Consider two individuals on a diet that contains 70 g/day of protein, one person with normal renal function (e.g., GFR of 180 L/day) and the other a renal patient with sharply reduced glomerular filtration (e.g., GFR of 18 L/day). Each individual produces 12 g/day of nitrogen in the form of urea (urea nitrogen) derived from dietary protein and must excrete this into the urine. However, these two individuals achieve urea balance at very different blood urea levels. We make the simplifying assumption that the tubules neither absorb nor secrete urea, so that *only* filtered urea can be excreted, and *all* filtered urea is excreted. The physiologically normal individual can excrete 12 g/day of urea nitrogen from 180 L of blood plasma having a blood urea nitrogen value of 12 g/180 L, or 6.7 mg/dL. In the patient whose GFR is reduced to 10% of normal, excreting 12 g/day of urea nitrogen requires that each of the 18 L of filtered blood plasma has a blood urea nitrogen that is 10 times higher, or 67 mg/dL. Thus, excreting the same amount of urea nitrogen—to maintain a steady state—requires a much higher plasma blood urea nitrogen in the renal patient than in the normal individual.

The clearance of inulin is a measure of glomerular filtration rate

The ideal **glomerular marker** for measuring GFR would be a substance X that has the same concentration in the glomerular filtrate as in plasma and that also is not reabsorbed, secreted, synthesized, broken down, or accumulated by the tubules (Table 34-1). In Equation 33-4, we saw the following:

$$\underset{\substack{\text{Input into}\\\text{Bowman's space}}}{\underbrace{\underset{\frac{mg}{mL}}{P_X} \cdot \underset{\frac{mL}{min}}{GFR}}} = \underset{\substack{\text{Output into}\\\text{urine}}}{\underbrace{\underset{\frac{mg}{mL}}{U_X} \cdot \underset{\frac{mL}{min}}{\dot{V}}}} \qquad (34\text{-}1)$$

P_X is the concentration of the solute in plasma, GFR is the sum of volume flow from the plasma into all Bowman's spaces, U_X is the urine concentration of the solute, and $\dot{V}$ is the urine flow. Rearranging this equation,

$$GFR = \frac{U_X \times \dot{V}}{P_X}$$

$$\frac{mL}{min} = \frac{(mg/mL) \times (mL/min)}{(mg/mL)} \quad \text{(34-2)}$$

Note that Equation 34-2 has the same form as the clearance equation (see Equation 33-3) and is identical to Equation 33-5. Thus, the plasma clearance of a glomerular marker is the *GFR*.

Inulin is an exogenous starch-like fructose polymer that is extracted from the Jerusalem artichoke and has a molecular weight of 5000 Da. Inulin is freely filtered at the glomerulus but is neither reabsorbed nor secreted by the renal tubules (Fig. 34-1A). Inulin also fulfills the additional requirements listed in Table 34-1 for an ideal glomerular marker.

Assuming that GFR does not change, three tests prove that inulin clearance is an accurate marker of GFR. First,

as shown in Figure 34-1B, the rate of inulin excretion ($U_{In} \cdot \dot{V}$) is directly proportional to the plasma inulin concentration (P_{In}), as implied by Equation 34-2. The slope in Figure 34-1B is the inulin clearance. Second, inulin clearance is independent of the plasma inulin concentration (Fig. 34-1C). This conclusion was already implicit in Figure 34-1B, in which the slope (i.e., inulin clearance) does not vary with P_{In}. Third, inulin clearance is independent of urine flow (Fig. 34-1D). Given a particular P_{In}, after the renal corpuscles filter the

Table 34-1 Criteria for Use of a Substance to Measure Glomerular Filtration Rate

1.	Substance must be freely filterable in the glomeruli.
2.	Substance must be neither reabsorbed nor secreted by the renal tubules.
3.	Substance must not be synthesized, broken down, or accumulated by the kidney.
4.	Substance must be physiologically inert (not toxic and without effect on renal function).

A HANDLING OF INULIN

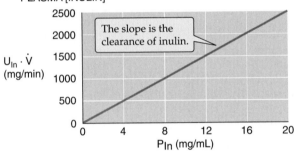

B DEPENDENCE OF INULIN EXCRETION ON PLASMA [INULIN]

The slope is the clearance of inulin.

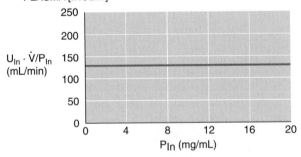

C DEPENDENCE OF INULIN CLEARANCE ON PLASMA [INULIN]

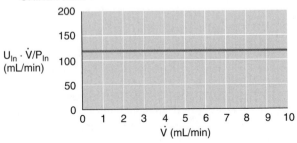

D DEPENDENCE OF INULIN CLEARANCE ON URINE FLOW

Figure 34-1 Clearance of inulin.

inulin, the total amount of inulin in the urine does not change. Thus, diluting this glomerular marker in a large amount of urine or concentrating it in a small volume, does not affect the total amount of inulin excreted ($U_{In} \cdot \dot{V}$). If the urine flow is high, the urine inulin concentration will be proportionally low, and vice versa. Because ($U_{In} \cdot \dot{V}$) is fixed, ($U_{In} \cdot \dot{V}$)/P_{In} is also fixed.

Two lines of evidence provide direct proof that inulin clearance represents GFR. First, by collecting filtrate from single glomeruli, Richards and coworkers showed in 1941 that the concentration of inulin in Bowman's space of the mammalian kidney is the same as in plasma. Thus, inulin is freely filtered. Second, by perfusing single tubules with known amounts of labeled inulin, Marsh and Frasier showed that the renal tubules neither secrete nor reabsorb inulin.

Although the inulin clearance is the most reliable method for measuring GFR, it is not practical for clinical use. One must administer inulin intravenously to achieve reasonably constant plasma inulin levels. Another deterrent is that the chemical analysis for determining inulin levels in plasma and urine is sufficiently demanding to render inulin unsuitable for routine use in a clinical laboratory.

The normal value for GFR in a 70-kg man is ~125 mL/min. Population studies show that GFR is proportional to body surface area. Because the surface area of an average 70-kg man is 1.73 m², the normal GFR in men is often reported as 125 mL/min/1.73 m² of body surface area. In women, this figure is 110 mL/min/1.73 m². Age is a second variable. GFR is very low in the newborn, owing to incomplete development of functioning glomerular units. Beginning at ~2 years of age, GFR normalizes for body surface area and gradually falls off with age as a consequence of progressive loss of functioning nephrons.

The clearance of creatinine is a useful clinical index of glomerular filtration rate

Because inulin is not a convenient marker for routine clinical testing, nephrologists use other compounds that can be labeled with radioisotopes and that have clearances similar to those of inulin. The most commonly used compounds in human studies are ^{125}I-iothalamate, radioactive vitamin B_{12} ([57]Co- or [58]Co-cyanocobalamin) and ^{51}Cr-ethylenediaminetetraacetic acid (EDTA). However, these compounds are of limited reliability in GFR measurements because of variable binding to proteins and the loss of labeled iodine from the iothalamate.

The problems of intravenous infusion of a GFR marker can be completely avoided by using an *endogenous* substance with inulin-like properties. **Creatinine** is such a substance, and its clearance is a reasonable estimate of GFR in humans, but not all species. Tubules, to variable degree, secrete creatinine, which, by itself, would lead to an ~20% overestimate of GFR in humans. However, because commonly used colorimetric methods overestimate plasma creatinine concentrations, the calculated creatinine clearance turns out to be close to the inulin clearance. Thus, the effects of these two errors (i.e., tubule secretion and overestimated plasma levels) tend to cancel out each other. In clinical practice, determining the creatinine clearance is an easy and reliable means of assessing the GFR, and such determination avoids the need

to inject anything into the patient. One merely obtains samples of venous blood and urine, analyzes them for creatinine concentration, and makes a simple calculation.

The source of plasma creatinine is the normal metabolism of **creatine phosphate** in muscle. In men, this metabolism generates creatinine at the rate of 20 to 25 mg/kg body weight/day (i.e., ~1.5 g/day in a 70-kg man). In women, the value is 15 to 20 mg/kg body weight/day (i.e., ~1.2 g/day in a 70-kg woman), owing to lower muscle mass. In the steady state, the rate of urinary creatinine excretion equals this rate of metabolic production. Therefore, to avoid errors in estimating the GFR from the creatinine clearance, one must take care to exclude non–steady-state pathologic conditions of creatinine release, such as hyperthermia or other conditions of muscle wasting or damage. Ingestion of meat, which has a high creatinine content, also produces non–steady-state conditions. To minimize the effects of such an ingestion, the patient collects urine over an entire 24-hour period, and the plasma sample is obtained by venipuncture in the morning before breakfast.

Frequently, clinicians use the **endogenous plasma concentration of creatinine**, normally 1 mg/dL, as an instant index of GFR. This use rests on the inverse relationship between the plasma creatinine concentration (P_{Cr}) and the creatinine clearance (C_{Cr}):

$$C_{Cr} = \frac{U_{Cr} \cdot \dot{V}}{P_{Cr}} \qquad (34\text{-}3)$$

In the steady state, when metabolic production in muscle equals the urinary excretion rate ($U_{Cr} \cdot \dot{V}$) of creatinine, and both remain fairly constant, this equation predicts that a plot of P_{Cr} versus C_{Cr} (i.e., P_{Cr} versus GFR) is a rectangular hyperbola (Fig. 34-2). For example, in a healthy person whose GFR is 100 mL/min, plasma creatinine is ~1 mg/dL. The product of GFR (100 mL/min) and P_{Cr} (1 mg/dL) is thus 1 mg/min, which is the rate of both creatinine production

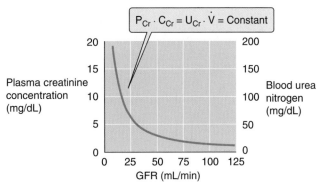

Figure 34-2 Dependence of plasma creatinine and blood urea nitrogen on the GFR. In the steady state, the amount of creatinine appearing in the urine per day ($U_{Cr} \cdot \dot{V}$) equals the production rate. Because all filtered creatinine ($P_{Cr} \cdot C_{Cr}$) appears in the urine, ($P_{Cr} \cdot C_{Cr}$) equals ($U_{Cr} \cdot \dot{V}$), which is constant. Thus, P_{Cr} must increase as C_{Cr} (i.e., GFR) decreases, and vice versa. If we assume that the kidney handles urea in the same way that it handles inulin, then a plot of blood urea nitrogen versus GFR will have the same shape as that of creatinine concentration versus GFR.

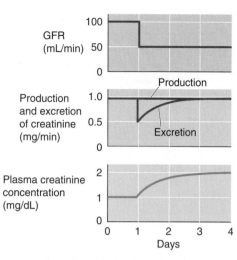

Figure 34-3 Effect of suddenly decreasing the GFR on plasma creatinine concentration.

Table 34-2 Permselectivity of the Glomerular Barrier

Substance	Molecular Weight (Da)	Effective Molecular Radius* (nm)	Filtrate (UF_X/P_X)
Na^+	23	0.10	1.0
K^+	39	0.14	1.0
Cl^-	35	0.18	1.0
H_2O	18	0.15	1.0
Urea	60	0.16	1.0
Glucose	180	0.33	1.0
Sucrose	342	0.44	1.0
Polyethylene glycol	1,000	0.70	1.0
Inulin	5,200	1.48	0.98
Lysozyme	14,600	1.90	0.8
Myoglobin	16,900	1.88	0.75
Lactoglobulin	36,000	2.16	0.4
Egg albumin	43,500	2.80	0.22
Bence Jones protein	44,000	2.77	0.09
Hemoglobin	68,000	3.25	0.03
Serum albumin	69,000	3.55	<0.01

*The effective molecular radius is the Einstein-Stokes radius, which is the radius of a sphere that diffuses at the same rate as the substance under study.

Data from Pitts RF: Physiology of the Kidney and Body Fluids, 3rd ed. Chicago: Year Book, 1974.

and of creatinine excretion. If GFR suddenly drops to 50 mL/min (Fig. 34-3, top), the kidneys will initially filter and excrete less creatinine (Fig. 34-3, middle), although the production rate is unchanged. As a result, the plasma creatinine level will rise to a new steady state, which is reached at a P_{Cr} of 2 mg/dL (Fig. 34-3, bottom). At this point, the product of the reduced GFR (50 mL/min) and the elevated P_{Cr} (2 mg/dL) will again equal 1 mg/min, the rate of endogenous production of creatinine. Similarly, if GFR were to fall to one fourth of normal, P_{Cr} would rise to 4 mg/dL. This concept is reflected in the right-rectangular hyperbola of Figure 34-2.

Molecular size, electrical charge, and shape determine the filterability of solutes across the glomerular filtration barrier

The glomerular filtration barrier consists of three elements (see Chapter 33): (1) endothelial cells, (2) the glomerular basement membrane, and (3) epithelial podocytes. The latter two layers are covered with negative charges. Table 34-2 summarizes the permselectivity of the glomerular barrier for different solutes, as estimated by the ratio of solute concentration in the ultrafiltrate versus the plasma (UF_X/P_X). The ratio UF_X/P_X, also known as the **sieving coefficient** for the solute X, depends on molecular weight and effective molecular radius. Investigators have used two approaches to estimate UF_X/P_X. The first, which is valid for all solutes, is the **micropuncture** technique (see Fig. 33-9A). Sampling fluid from Bowman's space yields a direct measurement of UF_X, from which we can compute UF_X/P_X. The second approach, which is only valid for solutes that the kidney neither absorbs nor secretes, is to compute the **clearance ratio** (see Chapter 33), the ratio of the clearances of X (C_X) and inulin (C_{In}).

Inspection of Table 34-2 shows that substances of low **molecular weight** (<5500 Da) and small **effective molecular radius** (e.g., water, urea, glucose, and inulin) appear in the filtrate in the same concentration as in plasma $(UF_X/P_X = 1)$. In these instances, no sieving of the contents of the fluid moving through the glomerular "pores" occurs, so that the water moving through the filtration slits by convection carries the solutes with it. As a result, the concentration of the solute in the filtrate is the same as in bulk plasma. The situation is different for substances with a molecular weight that is greater than ~14 kDa, such as lysozyme. Larger and larger macromolecules are increasingly restricted from passage, so that only traces of plasma albumin (69 kDa) are normally present in the glomerular filtrate.

In addition to molecular weight and radius, **electrical charge** also makes a major contribution to the permselectivity of the glomerular barrier. Figure 34-4A is a plot of the clearance ratio for uncharged, positively charged, and negatively charged dextran molecules of varying molecular size. Two conclusions can be drawn from these data. First, *neutral* dextrans with an effective molecular radius smaller than 2 nm pass readily across the glomerular barrier. For dextrans with a larger radius, the clearance ratio decreases with an increase in molecular size, so that passage ceases when the radius exceeds 4.2 nm. Second, *anionic* dextrans (e.g.,

A DEPENDENCE OF FILTERABILITY ON CHARGE AND SIZE

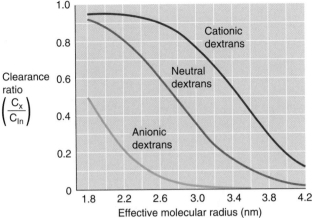

B DEPENDENCE OF FILTERABILITY OF ANIONIC DEXTRANS ON CHARGE OF GLOMERULAR BARRIER

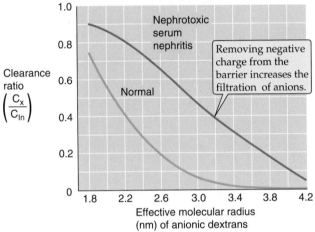

Figure 34-4 Clearance ratios of dextrans. *(Data from Brenner BM, Hostetter TH, Humes HD: N Engl J Med 1978; 298:826-833.)*

dextran sulfates) are restricted from filtration, whereas *cationic* dextrans (e.g., diethylaminoethyl dextrans) pass more readily into the filtrate. For negatively charged dextrans, the relationship between charge and filterability is characterized by a left shift of the curve relating molecular size to clearance ratio, whereas the opposite is true for positively charged dextrans.

The previously discussed results suggest that the glomerular filtration barrier carries a net negative charge that restricts the movement of anions but enhances the movement of cations. In some experimental models of glomerulonephritis, in which the glomerular barrier loses its negative charge, the permeability of the barrier to negatively charged macromolecules is enhanced. Figure 34-4B compares clearance ratios of dextran sulfate in normal rats and in rats with nephrotoxic serum nephritis. Clearance ratios of dextran sulfate are uniformly greater in the animals with nephritis. Thus, the disease process destroys negative charges in the filtration barrier and accelerates the passage of negatively charged dextrans. Because albumin is also negatively charged at physiological pH, loss of negative charge in the glomerular barrier probably contributes in an important way to the

development of albuminuria in the early stages of renal diseases such as glomerulonephritis.

Finally, the **shape** of macromolecules also affects the permselectivity of the glomerular barrier. Rigid or globular molecules have lower clearance ratios (i.e., sieving coefficients) than molecules of a similar size (e.g., dextrans), which are highly deformable.

The hydrostatic pressure in the glomerular capillary favors glomerular ultrafiltration, whereas the oncotic pressures in the capillary and the hydrostatic pressure in Bowman's space oppose it

As is the case for filtration in other capillary beds (see Chapter 20), glomerular ultrafiltration depends on the product of the ultrafiltration coefficient (K_f) and net Starling forces.

$$GFR = K_f \cdot \underbrace{[(P_{GC} - P_{BS}) - (\pi_{GC} - \pi_{BS})]}_{P_{UF}} \quad (34\text{-}4)$$

Figure 34-5A provides a schematic overview of the driving forces affecting ultrafiltration. P_{GC} is the **hydrostatic pressure in the glomerular capillary**, which favors ultrafiltration. P_{BS} is the **hydrostatic pressure in Bowman's space**, which opposes ultrafiltration. π_{GC} is the **oncotic pressure in the glomerular capillary**, which opposes ultrafiltration. Finally, π_{BS} is the **oncotic pressure of the filtrate in Bowman's space**, which favors ultrafiltration. Thus, two forces favor filtration (P_{GC} and π_{BS}), and two oppose it (P_{BS} and π_{GC}).

The **net driving force favoring ultrafiltration (P_{UF})** at any point along the glomerular capillaries is the difference between the hydrostatic pressure difference and the oncotic pressure difference between the capillary and Bowman's space. Thus, the GFR is proportional to the net **hydrostatic force** ($P_{GC} - P_{BS}$) minus the net **oncotic force** ($\pi_{GC} - \pi_{BS}$). The first term of the hydrostatic pressure difference is the P_{GC}. As discussed later, the unique arrangement in which afferent and efferent arterioles flank the glomerular capillary keeps P_{GC} at ~50 mm Hg (Fig. 34-5B), a value that is twice as high as in most other capillaries. Moreover, direct measurements of pressure in rodents show that P_{GC} decays little between the afferent and efferent ends of glomerular capillaries. The second term of the hydrostatic pressure difference is the P_{BS}. This pressure is ~10 mm Hg and does not vary along the capillary.

As far as the oncotic driving forces are concerned, the first term is the π_{BS}, which is very small (Fig. 34-5B). The π_{GC} starts off at 25 mm Hg at the beginning of the capillary. As a consequence of the continuous production of a protein-free glomerular filtrate, the oncotic pressure of the fluid left behind in the glomerular capillary progressively rises along the capillary.

Figure 34-5C compares the two forces *favoring* ultrafiltration ($P_{GC} + \pi_{BS}$) with the two forces *opposing* ultrafiltration ($P_{BS} + \pi_{GC}$) and shows how they vary along the glomerular capillary. The rapid increase in the oncotic pressure of capillary blood (π_{GC}) is the major reason why the forces favoring and opposing filtration may balance

A FORCES AFFECTING ULTRAFILTRATION

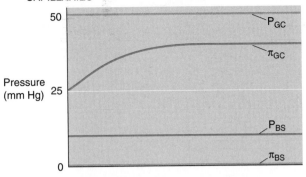

P_GC = Glomerular capillary hydrostatic pressure
π_BS = Bowman's space oncotic pressure
P_BS = Bowman's space hydrostatic pressure
π_GC = Glomerular capillary oncotic pressure

B STARLING FORCES ALONG THE GLOMERULAR
CAPILLARIES

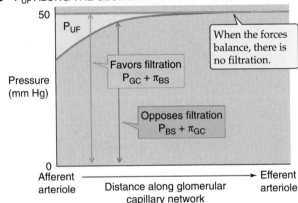

C P_UF ALONG THE GLOMERULAR CAPILLARIES

Figure 34-5   **A–C,** Glomerular ultrafiltration. In **B,** the oncotic pressure of the glomerular capillary (π_{GC}), which starts off at the value of normal arterial blood, rises as ultrafiltration removes fluid from the capillary. In **C,** P_{UF} is the net driving force favoring ultrafiltration.

each other at a point some distance before the end of the glomerular capillary. Beyond this point, P_{UF} is zero, and the system is said to be in **filtration equilibrium** (i.e., no further filtration).

Note that K_f in Equation 34-4 is the product of the hydraulic conductivity of the capillary (L_p) and the effective surface area available for filtration (S_f), as defined earlier (see Chapter 20). We use K_f because it is experimentally difficult to assign values to either L_p or S_f. Whereas P_{UF} is of similar order of magnitude in glomerular and systemic capillaries, the value of K_f of the glomerular filtration barrier exceeds—by more than an order of magnitude—the K_f of all other systemic capillary beds combined. This difference in K_f values underlies the tremendous difference in filtration, ~180 L/day in the kidneys (which receive ~20% of the cardiac output) compared with ~20 L/day (see Chapter 20) in the combined *arteriolar* ends of capillary beds in the rest of the body (which receive the other ~80%).

Alterations in the glomerular capillary surface area—owing to changes in mesangial cell contractility (see Chapter 33)—can produce substantial changes in the S_f component of K_f. These cells respond to extrarenal hormones such as systemically circulating angiotensin II (ANG II), arginine vasopressin (AVP), and parathyroid hormone. Mesangial cells also produce several vasoactive agents, such as prostaglandins and ANG II.

RENAL BLOOD FLOW

Renal blood flow (RBF) is ~1 L/min out of the total cardiac output of 5 L/min. Normalized for weight, this blood flow amounts to ~350 mL/min for each 100 g of tissue, which is 7-fold higher than the normalized blood flow to the brain (see Chapter 24). Renal *plasma* flow (RPF) is

$$RPF = (1 - Hct) \cdot RBF \qquad (34\text{-}5)$$

Given a hematocrit (Hct) of 0.40 (see Chapter 5), the "normal" RPF is ~600 mL/min.

Increased glomerular plasma flow leads to an increase in glomerular filtration rate

At low glomerular plasma flow (Fig. 34-6A), **filtration equilibrium** occurs halfway down the capillary. At higher plasma flow (i.e., normal for humans), the profile of net ultrafiltration forces (P_{UF}) along the glomerular capillary stretches out considerably to the right (Fig. 34-6B), so that the point of equilibrium would be reached at a site actually beyond the end of the capillary. Failure to reach equilibrium (**filtration *disequilibrium***) occurs because the increased delivery of plasma to the capillary outstrips the ability of the filtration

A LOW GLOMERULAR PLASMA FLOW

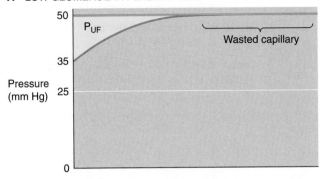

B NORMAL GLOMERULAR PLASMA FLOW

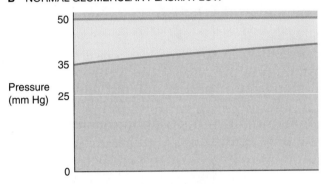

C HIGH GLOMERULAR PLASMA FLOW

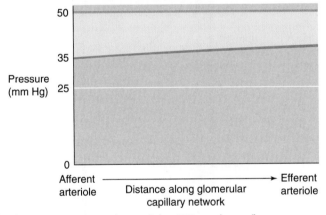

D GFR vs. PLASMA FLOW

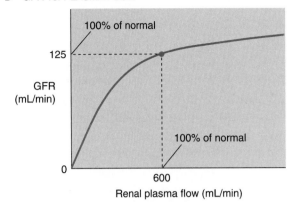

E FF vs. PLASMA FLOW

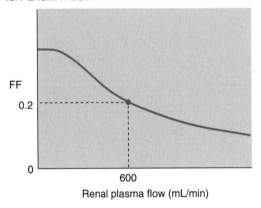

Figure 34-6 Dependence of the GFR on plasma flow.

apparatus to remove fluid and simultaneously increase capillary oncotic pressure. As a result, π_{GC} rises more slowly along the length of the capillary.

The shift of filtration equilibrium toward the efferent arteriole has two important consequences. First, as one progresses along the capillary, P_{UF} (and hence filtration) remains greater. Second, filtration occurs along a greater stretch of the glomerular capillary, thereby increasing the useful surface area for filtration. Thus, the end of the capillary that is "wasted" at low plasma flow rates really is "in reserve" to contribute at higher rates.

A further increase in plasma flow stretches out the π_{GC} profile even more, so that P_{UF} is even higher at each point along the capillary (Fig. 34-6C). Single-nephron GFR (SNGFR) is the sum of individual filtration events along the capillary. Thus, SNGFR is proportional to the *yellow area* that represents the product of P_{UF} and effective (i.e., non-wasted) length along the capillary. Because the yellow areas progressively increase in Figure 34-6A to C, SNGFR increases with glomerular plasma flow. However, this increase is not linear. Compared with the normal situation, the GFR summed for both kidneys increases only moderately with *increasing* RPF, but it decreases greatly with *decreasing* RPF (Fig. 34-6D).

The relationship between GFR and RPF also defines a parameter known as the **filtration fraction** (FF), which is the volume of filtrate that forms from a given volume of plasma entering the glomeruli:

$$FF = \frac{GFR}{RPF} \qquad (34\text{-}6)$$

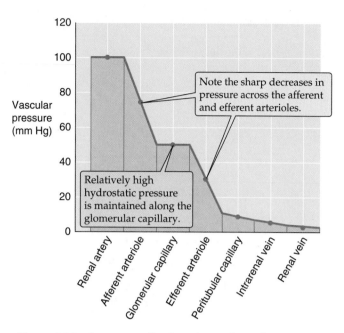

Figure 34-7 Pressure profile along the renal vasculature.

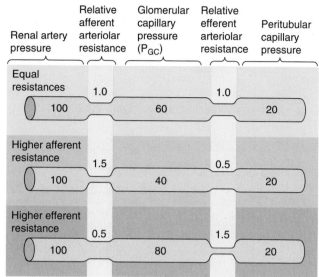

Because the normal GFR is ~125 mL/min and the normal RPF is ~600 mL/min, the normal FF is ~0.2. Because GFR saturates at high values of RPF, FF is greater at low plasma flows than it is at high plasma flows. The dependence of GFR on plasma flow through the glomerular capillaries is similar to the dependence of alveolar O_2 and CO_2 transport on pulmonary blood flow (see Chapter 30).

Afferent and efferent arteriolar resistances control both glomerular plasma flow and glomerular filtration rate

The renal microvasculature has two unique features. First, this vascular bed has two major sites of resistance control, the afferent and the efferent arterioles. Second, it has two capillary beds in series, the glomerular and the peritubular capillaries. As a consequence of this unique architecture, significant pressure drops occur in both arterioles (Fig. 34-7), glomerular capillary pressure is relatively high throughout, and peritubular capillary pressure is relatively low. Selective constriction or relaxation of the afferent and efferent arterioles allows for highly sensitive control of the hydrostatic pressure in the intervening glomerular capillary and thus of glomerular filtration.

Figure 34-8A illustrates an idealized example in which we reciprocally change afferent and efferent arteriolar resistance while keeping total arteriolar resistance—and thus glomerular plasma flow—constant. Compared with an initial condition in which the afferent and efferent arteriolar resistances are the same (Fig. 34-8A, top panel), constricting the *afferent* arteriole—while relaxing the efferent arteriole—lowers P_{GC} (Fig. 34-8A, middle panel). Conversely, constricting the *effer-*

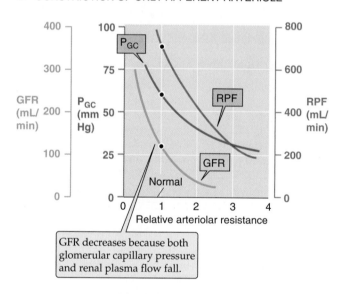

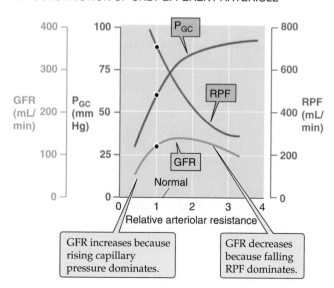

Figure 34-8 Role of afferent and efferent arteriolar resistance on pressure and flows. In **A**, the sum of afferent and efferent arteriolar resistance is always 2, whereas in **B** and **C**, the total resistance changes.

ent arteriole—while relaxing the afferent arteriole—raises P_{GC} (Fig. 34-8A, lower panel). From these idealized P_{GC} responses, one could predict that an increase in afferent arteriolar resistance would decrease the GFR and that an increase in efferent arteriolar resistance should have the opposite effect. However, physiological changes in the afferent and efferent arteriolar resistance usually do not keep overall arteriolar resistance constant. Thus, changes in arteriolar resistance generally lead to changes in glomerular plasma flow, which, as discussed earlier, can influence GFR independent of glomerular capillary pressure.

Figure 34-8B and C show somewhat more realistic effects on RPF and GFR as we change the resistance of a *single* arteriole. With a selective increase of *afferent* arteriolar resistance (Fig. 34-8B), both capillary pressure and RPF decrease, leading to a monotonic decline in the GFR. In contrast, a selective increase of *efferent* arteriolar resistance (Fig. 34-8C) causes a steep increase in glomerular capillary pressure as well as a decrease in RPF. As a result, over the lower range of resistances, GFR increases with efferent resistance as an increasing P_{GC} dominates. Conversely, at higher resistances, GFR begins to fall as the effect of a declining RPF dominates. These opposing effects on glomerular capillary pressure and RPF account for the biphasic dependence of GFR on efferent resistance.

The examples in Figure 34-8B and C, in which only afferent or efferent resistance increased, are still somewhat artificial. During sympathetic stimulation, or in response to ANG II, both afferent *and* efferent resistances increase. Thus, RPF decreases. The generally opposing effects on GFR of increasing both afferent resistance (Fig. 34-8B) and efferent resistance (Fig. 34-8C) explain why the combination of both keeps GFR fairly constant despite a decline in RPF.

In certain realistic examples, changes in either the afferent or the efferent arteriolar resistance dominate. A striking case in which a decrease in *afferent arteriolar* resistance dominates is the large increase in RPF that occurs with the loss of renal tissue, as after nephrectomy in a kidney donor. GFR in the **remnant kidney** nearly doubles, owing primarily to a dramatic *decrease* in the resistance of the afferent arteriole (Fig. 34-8B).

An example of a predominantly *efferent arteriolar* effect is seen after administration of ANG II inhibitors (e.g., captopril) to patients with hypertension resulting from increased endogenous angiotensin levels. Administering such agents not only decreases blood pressure, but also often leads to a significant fall in GFR. If we imagine that the peak of the GFR curve in Figure 34-8C represents the patient before treatment, then reducing the resistance of the efferent arteriole would indeed cause GFR to decrease.

The peritubular capillaries provide nutrients for tubules and retrieve the fluid the tubules reabsorb

Peritubular capillaries originate from the efferent arterioles of the superficial and juxtamedullary glomeruli (see Fig. 33-1C). The capillaries from the superficial glomeruli form a dense network in the cortex, and those from the juxtamedullary glomeruli follow the tubules down into the medulla, where the capillaries are known as the **vasa recta** (see Chapter 33). The peritubular capillaries have two main functions.

First, these vessels deliver oxygen and nutrients to the epithelial cells. Second, they are responsible for taking up from the interstitial space the fluid that the renal tubules reabsorb.

The Starling forces that govern filtration in other capillary beds apply here as well (Fig. 34-9A). However, in peritubular capillaries, the pattern is unique. In "standard" systemic capillaries, Starling forces favor filtration at the arteriolar end and absorption at the venular end (see Chapter 20). Glomerular capillaries resemble the early part of these standard capillaries: the Starling forces always favor filtration (Fig. 34-9B, yellow area). The peritubular capillaries are like the late part of standard capillaries: the Starling forces always favor absorption (Fig. 34-9C, brown area).

What makes peritubular capillaries unique is that glomerular capillaries and the efferent arteriole precede them. Glomerular filtration elevates the oncotic pressure of blood entering the peritubular capillary network (π_{PC}) to ~35 mm Hg. In addition, the resistance of the efferent arteriole decreases the intravascular hydrostatic pressure (P_{PC}) to ~20 mm Hg (Fig. 34-9A). Interstitial oncotic pressure (π_O) is 4 to 8 mm Hg, and interstitial hydrostatic pressure (P_O) is probably 6 to 10 mm Hg. The net effect is a large net absorptive pressure at the beginning of the peritubular capillary. Along the peritubular capillary, π_{PC} falls modestly because of the reabsorption of protein-poor fluid from the interstitium into the capillary, and hydrostatic pressure probably falls modestly as well. Even so, the Starling forces remain solidly in favor of absorption along the entire length of the peritubular capillary, falling from ~17 mm Hg at the arteriolar end to ~12 mm Hg at the venular end (Fig. 34-9C).

The net absorptive force at the beginning of the peritubular capillaries is subject to the vagaries of glomerular fluid dynamics. For instance, expansion of the extracellular fluid volume (Fig. 34-10) inhibits the renin-angiotensin system (see Chapter 40), thus leading to a relatively larger decrease in efferent than in afferent arteriolar resistance and therefore a rise in P_{PC}. The fall in total arteriolar resistance causes a rise in RPF that is larger than the increase in GFR, thereby resulting in a fall in filtration fraction. Thus, more fluid remains inside the glomerular capillary, and the blood entering the peritubular capillaries has an oncotic pressure that is not as high as it otherwise would be (e.g., π_{PC} of <35 mm Hg). The fall in efferent arteriolar resistance also raises the P_{PC} (e.g., P_{PC} of >20 mm Hg). As a consequence of the low π_{PC} and high P_{PC}, the peritubular capillaries take up less interstitial fluid (see Chapter 35). The reverse sequence of events takes place during volume contraction and in chronic heart failure.

Lymphatic capillaries are mainly found in the cortex. They provide an important route for removing protein from the interstitial fluid. Proteins leak continuously from the peritubular capillaries into the interstitial fluid. Total renal lymph flow is small and amounts to less than 1% of RPF.

Blood flow in the renal cortex exceeds that in the renal medulla

Measurements of regional blood flow in the kidney show that ~90% of the blood leaving the glomeruli in efferent

A GLOMERULAR AND PERITUBULAR CAPILLARIES

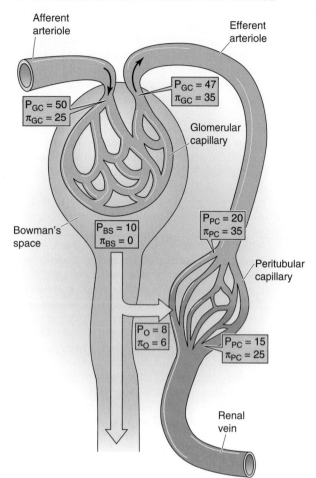

B NORMAL GLOMERULAR PLASMA FLOW

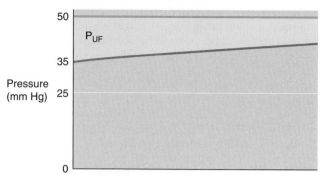

C NET ABSORPTIVE PRESSURE ALONG PERITUBULAR CAPILLARIES

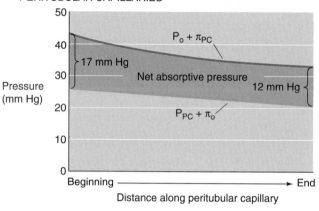

Figure 34-9 Starling forces along the *peritubular* capillaries. See text for discussion.

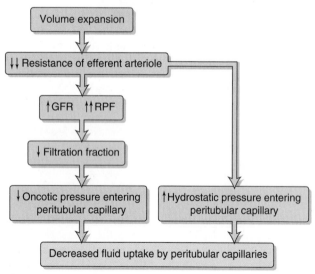

Figure 34-10 Effect of volume expansion on fluid uptake by the peritubular capillaries.

arterioles perfuses cortical tissue. The remaining 10% perfuses the renal medulla, with only 1% to 2% reaching the papilla. The relatively low blood flow through the medulla, a consequence of the high resistance of the long vasa recta, is important for minimizing washout of the hypertonic medullary interstitium and thus for producing a concentrated urine (see Chapter 38).

The clearance of *p*-aminohippurate is a measure of renal plasma flow

As discussed in Chapter 32, for any solute (X) that the kidney neither metabolizes nor produces, the only route of entry to the kidney is the renal artery, and the only two routes of exit are the renal vein and the ureter (see Chapter 33):

$$\underbrace{\underbrace{P_{X,a}}_{\frac{mmol}{mL}} \cdot \underbrace{RPF_a}_{\frac{mL}{min}}}_{\substack{\text{Arterial input} \\ \text{of X}}} = \underbrace{\left(\underbrace{P_{X,v}}_{\frac{mmol}{mL}} \cdot \underbrace{RPF_v}_{\frac{mL}{min}}\right)}_{\substack{\text{Venous output} \\ \text{of X}}} + \underbrace{\left(\underbrace{U_X}_{\frac{mmol}{mL}} \cdot \underbrace{\dot{V}}_{\frac{mL}{min}}\right)}_{\substack{\text{Urine output} \\ \text{of X}}} \quad (34\text{-}7)$$

The foregoing equation (a restatement of Equation 33-1) is an application of the Fick principle used for measurements of regional blood flow (see Chapter 17). To estimate arterial RPF (RPF_a)—or, more simply, RPF—we could in principle use the clearance of *any substance* that the kidney measurably excretes into the urine, as long as it is practical to obtain samples of systemic arterial plasma, renal venous plasma, and urine. The problem, of course, is sampling blood from the renal vein.

However, we can avoid the need for sampling the renal vein if we choose a substance that the kidneys clear so efficiently that they leave almost *none* in the renal vein. **p-Aminohippuric acid** (PAH) is just such a substance (see Chapter 33). Because PAH is an organic acid that is not normally present in the body, PAH must be administered by continuous intravenous infusion. Some PAH binds to plasma proteins, but a significant amount remains freely dissolved in the plasma and therefore filters into Bowman's space. However, the kidney filters only ~20% of the renal plasma flow (i.e., FF = ~0.2), and a major portion of the PAH remains in the plasma that flows out of the efferent arterioles. PAH diffuses out of the peritubular capillary network and reaches the basolateral surface of the proximal tubule cells. These cells have a high capacity to secrete PAH from blood into the tubule lumen against large concentration gradients. This PAH secretory system (see Chapter 36) is so efficient that—as long as we do not overwhelm it by infusing too much PAH—almost no PAH (~10%) remains in the renal venous blood. We assume that all the PAH presented to the kidney appears in the urine:

$$\text{PAH excreted} = \text{PAH filtered} + \text{PAH secreted in urine} \\ \text{in glomerulus by tubules}$$

(34-8)

In the example of Figure 34-11, the concentration of filterable PAH in the arterial blood plasma (P_{PAH}) is 10 mg/dL or 0.1 mg/mL. If RPF is 600 mL/min, then the arterial load of PAH to the kidney is 60 mg/min. Of this amount, 10 mg/min appears in the glomerular filtrate. If the tubules secrete the remaining 50 mg/min, then the entire 60 mg/min of PAH presented to the kidney appears in the urine (i.e., the kidneys clear the entire quantity of PAH that is presented to them during a single passage of blood). In practice, the kidneys excrete ~90% of the arterial load of PAH when P_{PAH} does not exceed 12 mg/dL.

As long as we do not infuse too much PAH (i.e., as long as virtually no PAH remains in the renal venous blood), Equation 34-7 reduces to the equation for the clearance of PAH, as introduced in Table 33-2B:

$$C_{PAH} = RPF = \frac{U_{PAH} \cdot \dot{V}}{P_{PAH}}$$

(34-9)

If we apply this equation to the example in Figure 34-11:

$$C_{PAH} = RPF = \frac{60\,\text{mg/min}}{10\,\text{mg/dL}} = \frac{60\,\text{mg/min}}{0.1\,\text{mg/mL}} = 600\,\text{mL/min}$$

(34-10)

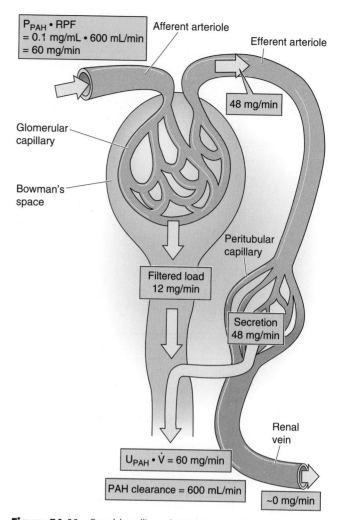

Figure 34-11 Renal handling of PAH. P_{PAH} and U_{PAH} are plasma and urine concentrations of PAH.

To compute RPF, we need to collect a urine sample to obtain ($U_{PAH} \cdot \dot{V}$) and a blood sample to obtain P_{PAH}. However, the blood sample need not be arterial. For example, one can obtain venous blood from the arm, inasmuch as skeletal muscle extracts negligible amounts of PAH.

CONTROL OF RENAL BLOOD FLOW AND GLOMERULAR FILTRATION

Autoregulation, which involves both a renal myogenic and a tubuloglomerular feedback mechanism, keeps renal blood flow and glomerular filtration rate relatively constant

An important feature of the renal circulation is its remarkable ability to maintain RBF and GFR within narrow limits, although mean arterial pressure may vary between ~80 and 170 mm Hg (Fig. 34-12, middle and bottom panels). Stability of blood flow—**autoregulation** (see Chapter 20)—is also a property of the vascular beds serving two other vital organs, the brain and the heart. Perfusion to all three of these organs must be preserved in emergency situations, such as hypoten-

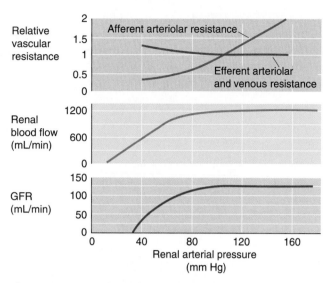

Figure 34-12 Autoregulation of renal blood flow and GFR. *(Data from Arendshorst WJ, Finn WF, Gottschalk CW: Am J Physiol 1975; 228:127-133.)*

sive shock. Autoregulation of the renal blood supply is independent of the influence of renal nerves and circulating hormones, and it persists even when one perfuses isolated kidneys with erythrocyte-free solutions. Autoregulation of RBF and, consequently, autoregulation of GFR, which depends on RBF (Fig. 34-6D), stabilize the filtered load of solutes that reach the tubules over a wide range of arterial pressures. Autoregulation of RBF also protects the fragile glomerular capillaries against increases in perfusion pressure that could lead to structural damage.

The kidney autoregulates RBF by responding to a rise in renal arterial pressure with a proportional increase in the resistance of the afferent arterioles. Autoregulation comes into play during alterations in arterial pressure that occur, for example, during changes in posture, light to moderate exercise, and sleep. It is the *afferent arteriole* where the autoregulatory response occurs, and where the resistance to flow rises with increasing perfusion pressure (Fig. 34-12, top panel). In contrast, *efferent* arteriolar resistance, capillary resistance, and venous resistance all change very little over a wide range of renal arterial pressures.

Two basic mechanisms—equally important—underlie renal autoregulation: a myogenic response of the smooth muscle of the afferent arterioles and a tubuloglomerular feedback (TGF) mechanism.

Myogenic Response The afferent arterioles have the inherent ability to respond to changes in vessel circumference by contracting or relaxing—a myogenic response (see Chapter 20). The mechanism of contraction is the opening of stretch-activated, nonselective cation channels in vascular smooth muscle. The resultant depolarizing leads to an influx of Ca^{2+} that stimulates contraction (see Table 20-7).

Tubuloglomerular Feedback The juxtaglomerular apparatus (see Chapter 33) mediates the TGF mechanism. The **macula densa** cells in the thick ascending limb sense an

increase in GFR and, in classic feedback fashion, translate this to a contraction of the afferent arteriole, a fall in P_{GC} and RPF, and hence a decrease in GFR.

Experimental evidence for the existence of a TGF mechanism rests on measurements of SNGFR. One introduces a wax block into the lumen of the proximal tubule to block luminal flow (Fig. 34-13A). Upstream from the wax block, a pipette collects the fluid needed to compute SNGFR (see Equation 33-13). Downstream to this oil block, another pipette perfuses the loop of Henle with known solutions and at selected flows. The key observation is that an inverse relationship exists between the late proximal perfusion rate (i.e., fluid delivery to macula densa) and SNGFR (Fig. 34-13B).

The mechanism of this TGF is thought to be the following. An increase in arterial pressure leads to increases in glomerular capillary pressure, RPF, and GFR. The increase in GFR leads to an increased delivery of Na^+, Cl^-, and fluid into the proximal tubule and, ultimately, to the macula densa cells of the juxtaglomerular apparatus. The macula densa does not sense flow per se, but the higher luminal $[Na^+]$ or $[Cl^-]$ resulting from high flow. Because of high Na/K/Cl cotransporter activity at the apical membrane of the macula densa cell, increases in luminal $[Na^+]$ and $[Cl^-]$ translate to parallel increases in intracellular concentrations of these two ions. Indeed, blocking the Na/K/Cl cotransporter with furosemide (see Chapter 5) not only blocks the uptake of Na^+ and Cl^- into the macula densa cells, but also interrupts TGF. The rise in $[Cl^-]_i$, in conjunction with a Cl^- channel at the basolateral membrane, apparently leads to a depolarization, which activates a nonselective cation channel, which, in turn, allows Ca^{2+} to enter the macula densa cell. The result is an increase in $[Ca^{2+}]_i$ that causes the macula densa cell to release paracrine agents (ATP, adenosine, thromboxane, or other substances) that may trigger contraction of nearby vascular smooth muscle cells. A1 adenosine receptors on the smooth muscle cells may be particularly important in this response. The net effect is an increase in afferent arteriolar resistance and a decrease in GFR, thereby counteracting the initial increase in GFR.

Several factors increase or decrease the sensitivity of the TGF mechanism (Fig. 34-13B). Indeed, investigators have suggested that several of these factors may be physiological signals from the macula densa cells or modulators of these signals (Table 34-3).

Volume expansion and a high-protein diet increase glomerular filtration rate by reducing tubuloglomerular feedback

The **sensitivity** of TGF is defined as the change in SNGFR for a given change in the perfusion rate of the loop of Henle. Thus, sensitivity is the absolute value of the slope of the curves in Figure 34-13B. The **set point** of the feedback system is defined as the loop perfusion rate at which SNGFR falls by 50%.

Both the intrinsic sensitivity of the macula densa mechanism and the initial set point for changes in flow are sensitive to changes in the extracellular fluid volume. Expansion of the extracellular fluid decreases the sensitivity (i.e., steepness) of the overall feedback

A EXPERIMENTAL PREPARATION

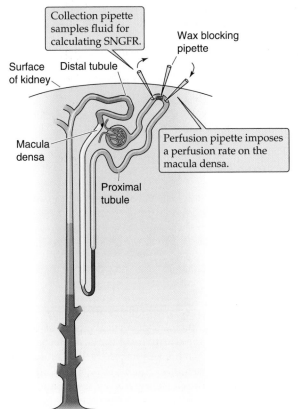

B DEPENDENCE OF SNGFR ON DISTAL TUBULE FLOW

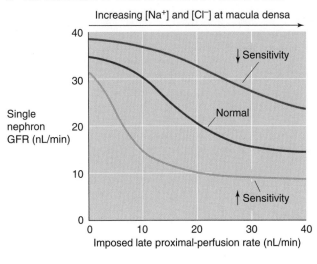

Figure 34-13 Tubuloglomerular feedback. *(Data from **B** modified from Navar LG: Adv Physiol Educ 1998; 20:S221-S235.)*

Table 34-3 Modulation of Tubuloglomerular Feedback

Factors That Increase Sensitivity of TGF Volume Contraction
Adenosine
Prostaglandin E_2
Thromboxane
Hydroxyeicosatetraenoic acid
Angiotensin II

Factors That Decrease Sensitivity of TGF Volume Expansion
ANP
NO
cAMP
Prostaglandin I_2
High-protein diet

loop. Conversely, volume contraction increases the sensitivity of TGF, thus helping preserve fluid by reducing GFR.

Of clinical importance may be the observation that a **high-protein diet** increases the GFR and RPF by indirectly lowering the sensitivity of the TGF mechanism. A high-protein diet somehow enhances NaCl reabsorption proximal to the macula densa, so that luminal [NaCl] at the macula densa falls. As a consequence, the flow in the loop of Henle (and thus GFR) must be higher to raise [NaCl] to a particular level at the macula densa. A high-protein diet may decrease TGF and may thereby increase glomerular capillary pressure. This sequence of events may lead, particularly in the presence of intrinsic renal disease, to permanent glomerular damage.

Four factors that modulate renal blood flow and glomerular filtration rate play key roles in regulating effective circulating volume

Changes in effective circulating volume (see Chapter 23) trigger responses in four parallel effector pathways that ultimately modulate either renal hemodynamics or renal Na^+ reabsorption. The four effector pathways are (1) the renin-angiotensin-aldosterone axis, (2) the sympathetic nervous system, (3) AVP, and (4) atrial natriuretic peptide (ANP). In Chapter 39, we discuss the integrated control of effective circulating volume. Here, we focus on the direct actions of the four effector pathways on renal hemodynamics.

Renin-Angiotensin-Aldosterone Axis In terms of renal hemodynamic effects, the most important part of this axis is its middle member, the peptide hormone ANG II (see Chapter 40). ANG II has multiple actions on renal hemodynamics (Table 34-4), the overall effect of which is to reduce blood flow and GFR.

Sympathetic Nerves Sympathetic tone to the kidney may increase either as part of a general response—as occurs with pain, stress, trauma, hemorrhage, or exercise—or as part of

Table 34-4 Hemodynamic Actions of Angiotensin II on the Kidney

Site	Action	Properties
Renal artery and afferent arteriole	Constriction	Ca^{2+} influx through voltage-gated channels Inhibited by prostaglandins
Efferent arteriole	Constriction	May depend on Ca^{2+} mobilization from internal stores Insensitive to Ca^{2+} channel blockers Prostaglandins may counteract the constriction during volume contraction or low effective circulating volume
Mesangial cells	Contraction with reduction in K_f	Ca^{2+} influx Ca^{2+} mobilization from internal stores
Tubuloglomerular feedback mechanism	Increased sensitivity	Increased responsiveness of afferent arteriole to signal from macula densa
Medullary blood flow	Reduction	May be independent of changes in cortical blood flow

Modified from Arendshorst WJ, Navar LG. In Schrier RW, Gottschalk CW: Diseases of the Kidney, vol 1, 5th ed, pp 65-117. Boston: Little, Brown, 1993.

a more selective renal response to a decrease in effective circulating volume (see Chapter 40). In either case, sympathetic nerve terminals release **norepinephrine** into the interstitial space. At relatively high levels of nerve stimulation, both afferent and efferent arteriolar resistances rise, thus generally decreasing RBF and GFR. The observation that the RBF may fall more than the GFR is consistent with a preferential *efferent* arteriolar constriction. With maximal nerve stimulation, however, afferent vasoconstriction predominates and leads to drastic reductions in both RBF and GFR.

In addition, sympathetic stimulation triggers granular cells to increase their release of renin, raising levels of ANG II (see Chapter 40), which acts as described earlier. Finally, sympathetic tone signals tubule cells to increase their reabsorption of Na^+ (see Chapter 35).

Arginine Vasopressin In response to increases in the osmotic pressure of the extracellular fluid, the posterior pituitary releases AVP, also known as antidiuretic hormone (see Chapter 38). Although the principal effect of this small polypeptide is to increase water absorption in the collecting duct, AVP also increases vascular resistance. Despite physiological fluctuations of circulating AVP levels, total RBF and GFR remain nearly constant. Nevertheless, AVP may decrease blood flow to the renal *medulla*, thereby minimizing the washout of the hypertonic medulla; this hypertonicity is essential for forming a concentrated urine.

In amphibians, reptiles, and birds, the generalized vascular effects of AVP are more pronounced than they are in mammals. In humans, severe decreases in effective circulating volume (e.g., shock) cause a massive release of AVP through nonosmotic stimuli (see Chapter 25). Only under these conditions does AVP produce systemic vasoconstriction and thus contribute to maintaining systemic blood pressure (see Chapter 23).

Atrial Natriuretic Peptide Atrial myocytes release ANP in response to increased atrial pressure and thus effective circulating volume (see Chapter 40). The major effect of ANP is hemodynamic: it markedly vasodilates afferent and efferent arterioles, thereby increasing cortical and medullary blood flow, and lowers the sensitivity of the TGF mechanism (Table 34-3). The net effect is an increase in RPF and GFR. ANP also affects renal hemodynamics indirectly, by inhibiting secretion of renin (thus lowering ANG II levels) and AVP. At higher levels, ANP decreases systemic arterial pressure and increases capillary permeability. ANP plays a role in the diuretic response to the redistribution of extracellular fluid and plasma volume into the thorax that occurs during space flight and water immersion (see Chapter 61).

Other vasoactive agents modulate renal blood flow and glomerular filtration rate

Many vasoactive agents—in addition to the ones discussed in the previous section—modulate RBF and GFR when these agents are infused systemically or are applied locally to the renal vasculature. Despite considerable research on such hemodynamic actions, the precise role of individual vasoactive agents in the response to physiological and pathophysiological stimuli remains uncertain. At least three kinds of observations have complicated our understanding: (1) several agents with opposing actions are often released simultaneously; (2) blocking a specific vasoactive messenger may have relatively little effect on renal hemodynamics; and (3) a single vasoactive agent may have different, or even opposing, actions at low and high concentrations. Nevertheless, renal and extrarenal agents may cooperate to provide a full and physiologically adequate response to a wide spectrum of challenges.

Epinephrine Released by the chromaffin cells of the adrenal medulla (see Chapter 50), epinephrine exerts dose-dependent effects on the kidney that are similar to those of norepinephrine (see earlier).

Dopamine Dopaminergic nerve fibers terminate in the kidney, and dopamine receptors are present in renal blood vessels. The renal effect of dopamine is to vasodilate, which is opposite to the effects of epinephrine and norepinephrine.

Endothelins The endothelins are peptides with strong vasoconstrictor action (see Chapter 20) but a very short half-life. The hemodynamic actions of endothelins are limited to local effects because little of this hormone escapes into the general circulation. In the kidney, several agents—ANG II, epinephrine, higher doses of AVP, thrombins, and shear stress—trigger release of endothelins from the endothelium of renal cortical vessels and mesangial cells. The endothelins act locally to constrict smooth muscles of renal vessels and thus most likely are a link in the complex network of local messengers between endothelium and smooth muscle. When administered systemically, endothelins constrict the afferent and efferent arterioles and reduce the ultrafiltration coefficient (K_f). The result is a sharp reduction in both RBF and GFR.

Prostaglandins In the kidney, vascular smooth muscle cells, endothelial cells, mesangial cells, and tubule and interstitial cells of the renal medulla are particularly important for synthesizing the locally acting prostaglandins from arachidonic acid, through the cyclooxygenase pathway (see Chapter 3). The effects of prostaglandins are complex and depend on the baseline vasoconstriction exerted by ANG II. Indeed, prostaglandins appear mainly to be protective and are important under conditions in which the integrity of the renal circulation is threatened. In particular, local intrarenal effects of prostaglandins prevent excessive vasoconstriction, especially during increased sympathetic simulation or activation of the renin-angiotensin system. Accelerated prostaglandin synthesis and release are responsible for maintaining fairly constant blood flow and GFR in conditions of high ANG II levels (e.g., during surgery, following blood loss, or in the course of salt depletion).

Leukotrienes Probably in response to inflammation, the renal vascular smooth muscle cells and glomeruli—as well as leukocytes and blood platelets—synthesize several leukotrienes from arachidonic acid, through the lipoxygenase pathway (see Chapter 3). These locally acting vasoactive agents are strong vasoconstrictors; their infusion reduces RBF and GFR.

Nitric Oxide The endothelial cells of the kidney use nitrous oxide synthase (NOS) to generate NO from L-arginine (see Chapter 3). NO has a strong smooth muscle relaxing effect and—under physiological, unstressed conditions—produces significant renal vasodilation. NO probably defends against excess vasoconstrictor effects of agents such as ANG II and epinephrine. Injecting NOS inhibitors into the systemic circulation constricts afferent and efferent arterioles, thus increasing renal vascular resistance and producing a sustained fall of RBF and GFR. Moreover, NOS inhibitors blunt the vasodilatation that is triggered by low rates of fluid delivery to the macula densa part of the TGF mechanism.

REFERENCES

Books and Reviews

Komlosi P, Fintha A, Bell PD: Renal cell-to-cell communication via extracellular ATP. Physiology 2005; 20:86-90.

Maddox DA, Brenner BM: Glomerular ultrafiltration. In Brenner BM (ed): The Kidney, 6th ed, pp 319-374. Philadelphia: WB Saunders, 2000.

Navar LG, Inscho WE, Majid DSA, et al: Paracrine regulation of the renal microcirculation. Physiol Rev 1996; 76:425-537.

Pallone TL, Zhang Z, Rhinehart K: Physiology of the renal medullary microcirculation. Am J Physiol 2003; 284:F253-F266.

Schnermann J: The juxtaglomerular apparatus: From anatomical peculiarity to physiological relevance. J Am Soc Nephrol 2003; 14:1681-1694.

Stockand JD, Sansom SC: Glomerular mesangial cells: Electrophysiology and regulation of contraction. Physiol Rev 1998; 78:723-744.

Journal Articles

Arendshorst WJ, Finn WF, Gottschalk CW: Autoregulation of renal blood flow in the rat kidney. Am J Physiol 1975; 228:127-133.

Brenner BM, Troy JL, Daugharty TM, et al: Dynamics of glomerular ultrafiltration in the rat. II. Plasma flow dependence of GFR. Am J Physiol 1972; 223:1184-1190.

Lapointe JY, Laamarti A, Bell PD: Ionic transport in macula densa cells. Kidney Int 1998; 54:S58-S64.

Robertson CR, Deen WM, Troy JL, Brenner BM: Dynamics of glomerular ultrafiltration in the rat. III. Hemodynamics and autoregulation. Am J Physiol 1972; 223:1191-1200.

Tucker BJ, Blantz RC: An analysis of the determinants of nephron filtration rate. Am J Physiol 1977; 232:F477-F483.

Wilcox CS, Welch WJ, Murad F, et al: Nitric oxide synthase in macula densa regulates glomerular capillary pressure. Proc Natl Acad Sci U S A 1992; 89:11993-11997.

CHAPTER 35

TRANSPORT OF SODIUM AND CHLORIDE

Gerhard Giebisch and Erich Windhager

The kidneys help to maintain the body's extracellular fluid (ECF) volume by regulating the amount of Na^+ in the urine. Na^+ is the most important contributor to the osmolality of the ECF; hence, where Na^+ goes, water follows. This chapter focuses on how the kidneys maintain the ECF volume by regulating Na^+ and its most prevalent anion, Cl^-.

The normal daily urinary excretion of Na^+ is only a tiny fraction of the total Na^+ filtered by the kidneys (Fig. 35-1). The filtered load of Na^+ is the product of the glomerular filtration rate (GFR, ~180 L/day) and the plasma Na^+ concentration (~142 mM; see Table 5-2), or ~25,500 mmol/day. This amount is equivalent to the Na^+ in ~1.5 kg of table salt, more than nine times the total quantity of Na^+ present in the body fluids. With a typical Western diet containing ~120 mmol of Na^+, the kidneys reabsorb ~99.6% of the filtered Na^+ by the time the tubule fluid (TF) reaches the renal pelvis. Therefore, even minute variations in the fractional reabsorptive rate could lead to changes in total body Na^+ that markedly alter ECF volume and, hence, body weight. Thus, it is not surprising that each nephron segment makes its own unique contribution to Na^+ homeostasis.

Na+ AND Cl− TRANSPORT BY DIFFERENT SEGMENTS OF THE NEPHRON

Na+ and Cl− reabsorption is largest in the proximal tubule, followed by Henle's loop, the classic distal tubule, and the collecting tubules and ducts

Figure 35-2 summarizes the segmental distribution of Na^+ reabsorption along the nephron. The **proximal tubule** reabsorbs the largest fraction of filtered Na^+ (~67%). Because [Na^+] in *TF* (or TF_{Na}) remains the same as that in *plasma* (i.e., $TF_{Na}/P_{Na} = 1.0$; see Chapter 33) throughout the length of the proximal tubule, it follows that the [Na^+] in the *reabsorbate* is the same as that in plasma. Because Na^+ salts are the dominant osmotically active solutes in the filtrate, reabsorption must be a nearly isosmotic process.

The **loop of Henle** reabsorbs a smaller but significant fraction of filtered Na^+ (~25%). Because of the low water

permeability of the thick ascending limb (TAL), this nephron segment reabsorbs Na^+ faster than it reabsorbs water, so that [Na^+] in the TF entering the distal convoluted tubule (DCT) has decreased substantially ($TF_{Na}/P_{Na} \cong 0.45$).

The **classic distal tubule** (see Chapter 33) and **collecting ducts** reabsorb smaller fractions of filtered Na^+ and water than do more proximal segments. The segments between the DCT and the cortical collecting tubule (CCT), inclusive, reabsorb ~5% of the filtered Na^+ load. Finally, the medullary collecting duct reabsorbs ~3% of the filtered Na^+ load. Although the distal nephron reabsorbs only small amounts of Na^+, it can establish a steep transepithelial concentration gradient and can respond to several hormones, including mineralocorticoids and arginine vasopressin (AVP).

The tubule reabsorbs Na+ through both the transcellular and the paracellular pathways

The tubule can reabsorb Na^+ and Cl^- through both transcellular and paracellular pathways (Fig. 35-3A). In the **transcellular pathway**, Na^+ and Cl^- sequentially traverse the apical and basolateral membranes before entering the blood. In the **paracellular pathway**, these ions move entirely by an extracellular route, through the tight junctions between cells. In the transcellular pathway, transport rates depend on the electrochemical gradients, ion channels, and transporters at the apical and basolateral membranes. However, in the paracellular pathway, transepithelial electrochemical driving forces and permeability properties of the tight junctions govern ion movements.

Transcellular Na+ Reabsorption The basic mechanism of transcellular Na^+ reabsorption is similar in all nephron segments and is a variation on the classic two-membrane model of epithelial transport (see Chapter 5). The *first step* is the passive entry of Na^+ into the cell across the **apical membrane**. Because the intracellular Na^+ concentration ([Na^+]$_i$) is low and the cell voltage is negative with respect to the lumen, the electrochemical gradient is favorable for passive Na^+ entry across the apical membrane (Fig. 35-3B). However, different tubule segments use different mechanisms of passive Na^+ entry across the apical membrane. The proximal

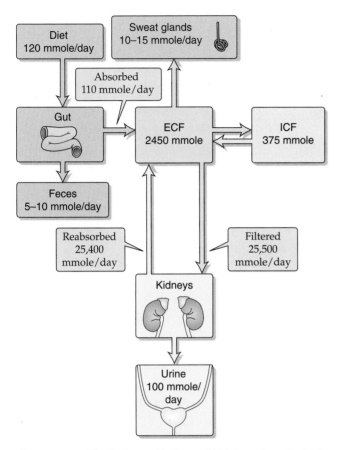

Figure 35-1 Distribution and balance of Na$^+$ throughout the body. The values in the boxes are approximations. ICF, intracellular fluid.

tubule, the TAL, and the DCT all use a combination of Na$^+$-coupled cotransporters and exchangers to move Na$^+$ across the apical membrane; however, in the cortical and medullary collecting ducts, Na$^+$ enters the cell through epithelial Na$^+$ channels (ENaC).

The *second step* of transcellular Na$^+$ reabsorption is the active extrusion of Na$^+$ out of the cell across the **basolateral membrane** (Fig. 35-3B). This Na$^+$ extrusion is mediated by the Na-K pump (see Chapter 5), which keeps [Na$^+$]$_i$ low (~15 mM) and [K$^+$]$_i$ high (~120 mM). Because the basolateral membrane is primarily permeable to K$^+$, it develops a voltage of ~70 mV, with the cell interior negative with respect to the interstitial space. Across the apical membrane, the cell is negative with respect to the lumen. The magnitude of the apical membrane voltage may be either lower or higher than that of the basolateral membrane, depending on the nephron segment and its transport activity.

Paracellular Na$^+$ Reabsorption The basic mechanism of paracellular Na$^+$ transport is similar among nephron segments: the transepithelial electrochemical gradient for Na$^+$ drives transport. However, both the transepithelial voltage and the luminal [Na$^+$] vary along the nephron (Table 35-1). As a result, the net driving force for Na$^+$ is positive—favoring passive Na$^+$ reabsorption—only in the S2 and S3 segment of the proximal tubule and in the TAL. In the other segments, the net driving force is negative—favoring passive Na$^+$ dif-

fusion from blood to lumen ("backleak"). In addition to the purely passive, paracellular reabsorption of Na$^+$ in the S2 and S3 segments and TAL, Na$^+$ can also move uphill from lumen to blood through **solvent drag** across the tight junctions. In this case, the movement of H$_2$O—energized by the active transport of Na$^+$ into the lateral intercellular space—from the lumen to the lateral intercellular space also sweeps Na$^+$ and Cl$^-$ in the same direction.

Nephron segments also vary in their **leakiness** to Na$^+$ ions. This leakiness is largely a function of the varying ionic conductance of the paracellular pathway between cells across the tight junction. In general, the leakiness of the paracellular pathway decreases along the nephron from the proximal tubule (the most leaky) to the papillary collecting ducts. However, even the tightest renal epithelia have only what may be regarded as a moderate degree of tightness compared with truly "tight" epithelia, such as the skin, the gastric mucosa, and the urinary bladder (see Chapter 5).

The leakiness of an epithelium has serious repercussions for the steepness of the ion gradients that the epithelium can develop and maintain. For both Na$^+$ and Cl$^-$, the ability of specific nephron segments to establish large concentration gradients correlates with the degree of tightness, which limits the backflux of ions between cells. Thus, the luminal fluid in the distal nephron attains much lower concentrations of Na$^+$ and Cl$^-$ than it does in the proximal tubule.

An important consequence of a highly leaky paracellular pathway is that it provides a mechanism by which the basolateral membrane voltage can generate a current that flows through the tight junctions and charges up the apical membrane, and vice versa (Fig. 35-3B). For example, hyperpolarization of the basolateral membrane leads to hyperpolarization of the apical membrane. A consequence of this **paracellular electrical coupling** is that the apical membrane of a leaky epithelium, such as the proximal tubule, has a membrane voltage that is negative (−67 mV in Fig. 35-3B) and close to that of the basolateral membrane (−70 mV in Fig. 35-3B), whereas one would expect that, based on the complement of channels and ion gradients at the apical membrane, the apical membrane would have a far less negative voltage. A practical benefit of this crosstalk is that it helps couple the activity of the basolateral electrogenic Na-K pump to the passive entry of Na$^+$ across the apical membrane. If the Na-K pump rate increases, not only does [Na$^+$]$_i$ decrease, enhancing the *chemical* Na$^+$ gradient across the apical membrane, but also the basolateral membrane hyperpolarizes (i.e., the cell becomes more negative with respect to the blood). Electrical coupling translates this basolateral hyperpolarization to a concomitant apical hyperpolarization, thus also enhancing the electrical gradient favoring apical Na$^+$ entry.

Na$^+$, Cl$^-$, AND WATER TRANSPORT AT THE CELLULAR AND MOLECULAR LEVEL

Na$^+$ reabsorption involves apical transporters or ENaC and a basolateral Na-K pump

Proximal Tubule Along the first half of the tubule (Fig. 35-4A), a variety of cotransporters in the *apical membrane*

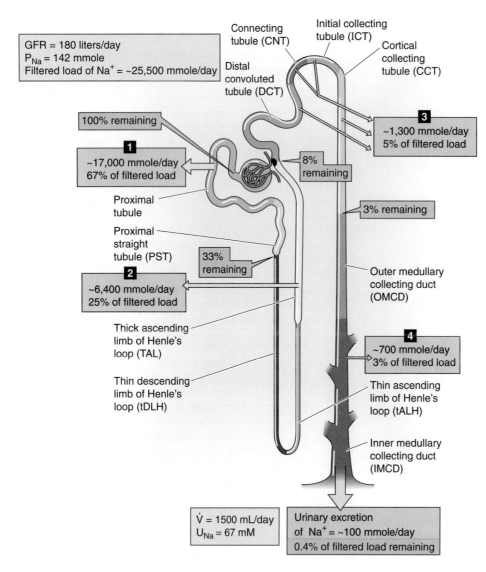

GFR = 180 liters/day
P_{Na} = 142 mmole
Filtered load of Na^+ = ~25,500 mmole/day

Connecting tubule (CNT)

Initial collecting tubule (ICT)

Cortical collecting tubule (CCT)

Distal convoluted tubule (DCT)

1 100% remaining

~17,000 mmole/day
67% of filtered load

3 ~1,300 mmole/day
5% of filtered load

8% remaining

3% remaining

Proximal tubule

Proximal straight tubule (PST)

33% remaining

2 ~6,400 mmole/day
25% of filtered load

Outer medullary collecting duct (OMCD)

Thick ascending limb of Henle's loop (TAL)

4 ~700 mmole/day
3% of filtered load

Thin descending limb of Henle's loop (tDLH)

Thin ascending limb of Henle's loop (tALH)

Inner medullary collecting duct (IMCD)

$\dot{V}$ = 1500 mL/day
U_{Na} = 67 mM

Urinary excretion of Na^+ = ~100 mmole/day
0.4% of filtered load remaining

Figure 35-2 Estimates of renal handling of Na^+ along the nephron. The numbered *yellow boxes* indicate the absolute amount of Na^+—as well as the fraction of the filtered load—that various nephron segments reabsorb. The *green boxes* indicate the fraction of the filtered load that remains in the lumen at these sites. The values in the boxes are approximations. P_{Na}, plasma Na^+ concentration; U_{Na}, urine Na^+ concentration.

couples the downhill uptake of Na^+ to the uphill uptake of solutes such as glucose, amino acids, phosphate, sulfate, lactate, and other monocarboxylic and dicarboxylic acids. Many of these Na^+-driven cotransporters are electrogenic, carrying net positive charge into the cell. Thus, both the low $[Na^+]_i$ and the negative apical membrane voltage fuel the secondary active uptake of these other solutes, which we discuss in Chapter 35. In addition to the cotransporters, Na^+ entry is also coupled to the extrusion of H^+ through the electroneutral **Na-H exchanger** (NHE3). The role of NHE3 in renal acid secretion is discussed in Chapter 39.

Both cotransporters and exchangers exploit the downhill Na^+ gradient across the apical cell membrane that is established by the **Na-K pump** in the *basolateral membrane*. The Na-K pump and, to a lesser extent, the electrogenic **Na/HCO₃ cotransporter** (NBC) are also responsible for the second step in Na^+ reabsorption, moving Na^+ from cell to blood. The presence of K^+ channels in the basolateral membrane is important for two reasons. First, these channels establish the negative voltage across the basolateral membrane and establish a similar negative voltage across the

apical membrane through paracellular electrical coupling. Second, these channels permit the recycling of K^+ that had been transported into the cell by the Na-K pump.

Because of a lumen-negative transepithelial voltage in the early proximal tubule, as well as a paracellular pathway that is permeable to Na^+, approximately one third of the Na^+ that is transported from lumen to blood by the transcellular pathway diffuses back to the lumen by the *paracellular pathway* ("backleak").

Thin Limbs of Henle's Loop Na^+ transport by the thin descending and thin ascending limbs of Henle's loop is almost entirely passive and paracellular (see Chapter 38).

Thick Ascending Limb Two major pathways contribute to Na^+ reabsorption in the TAL: transcellular and paracellular (Fig. 35-4B). The *transcellular pathway* includes two major mechanisms for taking up Na^+ across the apical membrane. The **Na/K/Cl cotransporter** (NKCC2) couples the inward movement of 1 Na^+, 1 K^+, and 2 Cl^- ions in an electroneutral process driven by the downhill concentration

A PARACELLULAR AND TRANSCELLULAR ROUTES

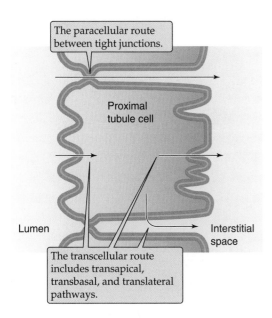

The paracellular route between tight junctions.

Proximal tubule cell

Lumen

Interstitial space

The transcellular route includes transapical, transbasal, and translateral pathways.

B DRIVING FORCES FOR Na⁺ TRANSPORT

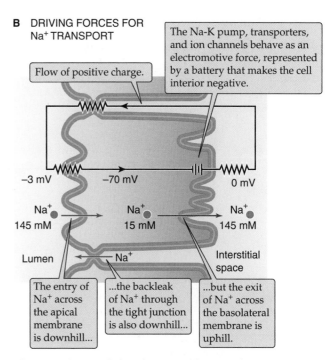

The Na-K pump, transporters, and ion channels behave as an electromotive force, represented by a battery that makes the cell interior negative.

Flow of positive charge.

−3 mV   −70 mV   0 mV

Na^+ 145 mM Na^+ 15 mM Na^+ 145 mM

Lumen Na^+ Interstitial space

The entry of Na^+ across the apical membrane is downhill...

...the backleak of Na^+ through the tight junction is also downhill...

...but the exit of Na^+ across the basolateral membrane is uphill.

Figure 35-3 **A** and **B**, Transcellular and paracellular mechanisms of Na⁺ and Cl⁻ reabsorption. The example in **B** illustrates the electrochemical driving forces for Na⁺ in the early proximal tubule. The equivalent circuit demonstrates that the flow of positive charge across the apical membrane makes the apical membrane voltage more negative.

Table 35-1 Transepithelial Driving Forces for Sodium

	Luminal [Na⁺]	Transepithelial Chemical Driving Force*†	Transepithelial Voltage (i.e., Electrical Driving Force)†‡	Transepithelial Electrochemical Driving Force†
Proximal tubule, S1	142 mM	0 mV	−3 mV	−3 mV
Proximal tubule, S3	142 mM	0 mV	+3 mV	+3 mV
TAL	100 mM	−9 mV	+15 mV	+6 mV
DCT	70 mM	−19 mV	−5 to +5 mV	−24 to −14 mV
CCT	40 mM	−34 mV	−40 mV	−74 mV

*The chemical driving force is calculated assuming a plasma [Na⁺] of 142 mM and is given in mV.
†A negative value promotes passive Na⁺ movement from blood to lumen (i.e., backleak or secretion), whereas a positive value promotes passive Na⁺ movement from lumen to blood (i.e., reabsorption).
‡A negative value indicates that the lumen is negative with respect to the blood.

gradients of Na⁺ and Cl⁻ (see Chapter 5). The second entry pathway for Na⁺ is an **NHE3**. As in the proximal tubule, the basolateral Na-K pump keeps [Na⁺]ᵢ low and moves Na⁺ to the blood.

Two features of the apical step of Na⁺ reabsorption in the TAL are noteworthy. First, the **loop diuretics** (e.g., furosemide and bumetanide) inhibit Na/K/Cl cotransport. Second, a large fraction of the K⁺ that the NKCC2 brings into the cell recycles to the lumen through apical K⁺ channels. These channels are essential for replenishing luminal K⁺ and thus for maintaining adequate Na/K/Cl cotransport.

A key aspect of the *paracellular pathway* for Na⁺ reabsorption in the TAL is lumen-positive voltage (Fig. 35-4B). Nearly all other epithelia have lumen-negative voltage because the apical membrane voltage is less negative than the basolateral membrane voltage (see Fig. 5-18D). The TAL is just the opposite. Because K⁺ channels dominate the apical membrane conductance, the voltage of the TAL apical membrane is more negative than that of the basolateral membrane, thereby resulting in lumen-positive transepithelial voltage. This lumen-positive voltage provides the driving force for the diffusion of Na⁺ across the tight junctions, thus

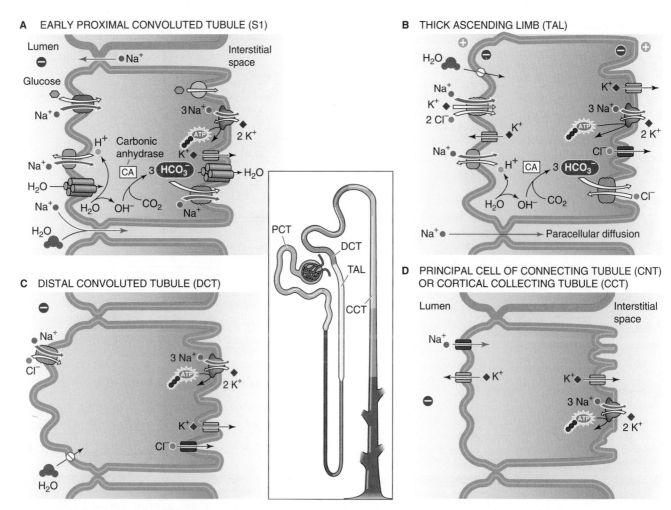

Figure 35-4   **A** to **D**, Cell models of Na⁺ reabsorption. PCT, proximal convoluted tube.

accounting for approximately half of the Na⁺ reabsorption by the TAL. The lumen-positive voltage also drives the passive reabsorption of K⁺ (see Chapter 37) and of Ca^{2+} and Mg^{2+} (see Chapter 36) through the paracellular pathway. Because the TAL has low water permeability, removing luminal NaCl leaves the remaining TF *hypo-osmotic*. Hence, the TAL is sometimes referred to as the diluting segment.

Distal Convoluted Tubule   Na⁺ reabsorption in the DCT occurs almost exclusively by the transcellular route (Fig. 35-4C). The *apical step* of Na⁺ uptake is mediated by an electroneutral **Na/Cl cotransporter** (**NCC**; see Chapter 5) that belongs to the same family as the NKCC2 in the TAL. However, the NCC differs from the NKCC2 in being independent of K⁺ and highly sensitive to thiazide diuretics. Although the thiazides produce less diuresis than do the loop diuretics, the thiazides are nevertheless effective in removing excess Na⁺ from the body. The *basolateral step* of Na⁺ reabsorption, as in other cells, is mediated by the Na-K pump.

Initial and Cortical Collecting Tubules   Na⁺ reabsorption in these nephron segments and in the connecting tubule is transcellular and is mediated by the majority cell type, the **principal cell** (Fig. 35-4D). The neighboring ß-intercalated cells are important for reabsorbing Cl⁻, as discussed later. Na⁺ crosses the *apical membrane* of the principal cell through the **ENaCs**, which are distinct from the voltage-gated Na⁺ channels expressed by excitable tissues (see Chapter 7). ENaC is a heteromer comprising homologous α, ß, and γ subunits, each of which has two membrane-spanning segments. These ENaCs are unique in that low levels of the diuretic drug **amiloride** block them in a specific way. This compound is a relatively mild diuretic because Na⁺ reabsorption along the collecting duct is modest. The *basolateral step* of Na⁺ reabsorption is mediated by the Na-K pump, which also provides the electrochemical driving force for the apical entry of Na⁺.

The unique transport properties of the apical and basolateral membranes of the principal cells are also the basis for the lumen-negative transepithelial potential difference of approximately −40 mV in the CCT (Table 35-1). In addition to ENaCs, the CCT has both apical and basolateral K⁺ channels, which play a key role in K⁺ transport (see Chapter 37). The apical entry of Na⁺ (which tends to make the lumen negative) and the basolateral exit of K⁺ (which tends to make the cell negative) are, in effect, two batteries of identical sign, arranged in series. In principle, these two batteries could add up to a transepithelial voltage of ~100 mV (lumen negative).

However, under most conditions, K^+ *exit* from cell to lumen partially opposes the lumen-negative potential generated by Na^+ entry. The net effect of these three batteries is a transepithelial voltage of ~−40 mV (lumen negative).

The transepithelial voltage of the CCT can fluctuate considerably, particularly because of changes in the apical Na^+ battery owing to, for example, changes in luminal $[Na^+]$. In addition, changing levels of aldosterone or AVP may modulate the *number* of ENaCs that are open in the apical membrane and may thus affect the relative contribution of this Na^+ battery to apical membrane voltage.

Medullary Collecting Duct The inner and outer medullary collecting ducts reabsorb only a minute amount of Na^+, ~3% of the filtered load (Fig. 35-2). It is likely that ENaCs mediate the apical entry of Na^+ in these segments and that the Na-K pump extrudes Na^+ from the cell across the basolateral membrane (Fig. 35-4D).

Cl⁻ reabsorption involves both paracellular and transcellular pathways

Most of the filtered Na^+ is reabsorbed with Cl^-. However, the segmental handling of Cl^- differs somewhat from that of Na^+. Both transcellular and paracellular pathways participate in Cl^- reabsorption.

Proximal Tubule The proximal tubule reabsorbs Cl^- by both the transcellular and the paracellular routes, with the *paracellular* believed to be the dominant route in the early proximal tubule (Fig. 35-5A). The transcellular pathway is dominant in the late proximal tubule (Fig. 35-5B), where the energetically uphill influx of Cl^- across the apical membrane occurs through an exchange of luminal Cl^- for cellular anions (e.g., formate, oxalate, HCO_3^-, and OH^-), mediated by CFEX (SLC26A6). Cl-base exchange is an example of *tertiary* active transport: the apical NHE3, itself a *secondary* active transporter (see Chapter 5), provides the H^+ that neutralizes base in the lumen, thereby sustaining the gradient for Cl-anion exchange. The basolateral exit step for transcellular Cl^- movement may occur in part through a Cl^- **channel** that is analogous in function to the cystic fibrosis transmembrane conductance regulator (CFTR; see Chapter 43). In addition, the basolateral membrane of the proximal tubule may also have a **K/Cl cotransporter** (**KCC**), which is in the same family as NKCC2 and NCC.

Passive Cl^- reabsorption through the *paracellular pathway* is driven by different electrochemical Cl^- gradients in the early versus the late proximal tubule. The S1 segment initially has no Cl^- concentration gradient between lumen and blood. However, the lumen-negative voltage (Table 35-1)—generated by electrogenic Na/glucose and Na/amino acid cotransport—establishes a favorable *electrical* gradient for passive Cl^- reabsorption. Solvent drag also makes a contribution in the S1 segment. In the S2 and S3 segments, the lumen-positive voltage opposes paracellular Cl^- absorption (Table 35-1). However, preferential HCO_3^- reabsorption in the earlier portions of the proximal tubule leaves Cl^- behind (see Chapter 39), so that $[Cl^-]$ in the lumen becomes higher than that in the blood. This favorable lumen-to-blood *chemical* gradient for Cl^- overcomes the electrical gradient so that

paracellular movement of Cl^- in the late proximal tubule proceeds in the reabsorptive direction.

The upper part of Figure 35-6 shows the profile of the ratio of concentrations in TF versus plasma (TF/P) (see Chapter 33) for the major solutes in TF along the proximal tubule. Only minor changes occur in the TF/P for osmolality or Na^+. Because the tubule does not reabsorb inulin, the substantial increase in TF_{In}/P_{In} indicates net fluid reabsorption. The fall in $TF_{HCO_3^-}/P_{HCO_3^-}$ mirrors an increase in TF_{Cl}/P_{Cl} because the tubule reabsorbs HCO_3^- more rapidly than it does Cl^-. The early proximal tubule avidly reabsorbs glucose and amino acids, leading to sharp decreases in the concentrations of these substances in the TF.

An important characteristic of the proximal tubule is that the transepithelial voltage reverses polarity between the S1 and the S2 segments (Fig. 35-6, lower panel). The early proximal tubule is lumen negative because it reabsorbs Na^+ electrogenically, both through electrogenic apical Na^+ transporters (e.g., Na/glucose cotransporter) and the basolateral Na-K pump. The late proximal tubule reabsorbs Na^+ at a lower rate. Moreover, because TF_{Cl} is greater than P_{Cl}, the paracellular diffusion of Cl^- from lumen to bath generates a lumen-positive potential that facilitates passive Na^+ reabsorption by the same paracellular route.

Thick Ascending Limb Cl^- reabsorption in the TAL takes place largely by Na/K/Cl cotransport across the apical membrane (Fig. 35-5C), as we already noted in our discussion of Na^+ reabsorption (Fig. 35-4B). The exit of Cl^- across the basolateral cell membrane through Cl^- channels of the ClC family (see Table 6-2, number 15) overwhelms any entry of Cl^- through the Cl-HCO_3 exchanger. You may recall that only *half* of the Na^+ reabsorption by the TAL is transcellular, whereas *all* Cl^- reabsorption is transcellular. Overall, Na^+ reabsorption and Cl^- reabsorption are identical because the apical NKCC2 moves two Cl^- for each Na^+.

Distal Convoluted Tubule Cl^- reabsorption by the DCT (Fig. 35-5D) occurs by a mechanism that is somewhat similar to that in the TAL, except the apical step occurs through the NCC, as discussed earlier in connection with Na^+ reabsorption by the DCT (Fig. 35-4C). Cl^- channels that are probably similar to those in the TAL mediate the basolateral Cl^- exit step.

Collecting Ducts The initial cortical tubule and the CCT reabsorb Cl^- by two mechanisms. First, the principal cell generates a transepithelial voltage (~40 mV, lumen negative) that is favorable for *paracellular* diffusion of Cl^- (Fig. 35-5E). Second, the ß-type intercalated cells reabsorb Cl^- using a *transcellular* process that involves Cl-HCO_3 exchange across the apical membranes and Cl^- channels in the basolateral membrane (Fig. 35-5F). Neither the α-type intercalated cells nor the principal cells are involved in transcellular Cl^- reabsorption.

Water reabsorption is passive and secondary to solute transport

Proximal Tubule If water reabsorption by the proximal tubule were to follow solute reabsorption *passively*, then one

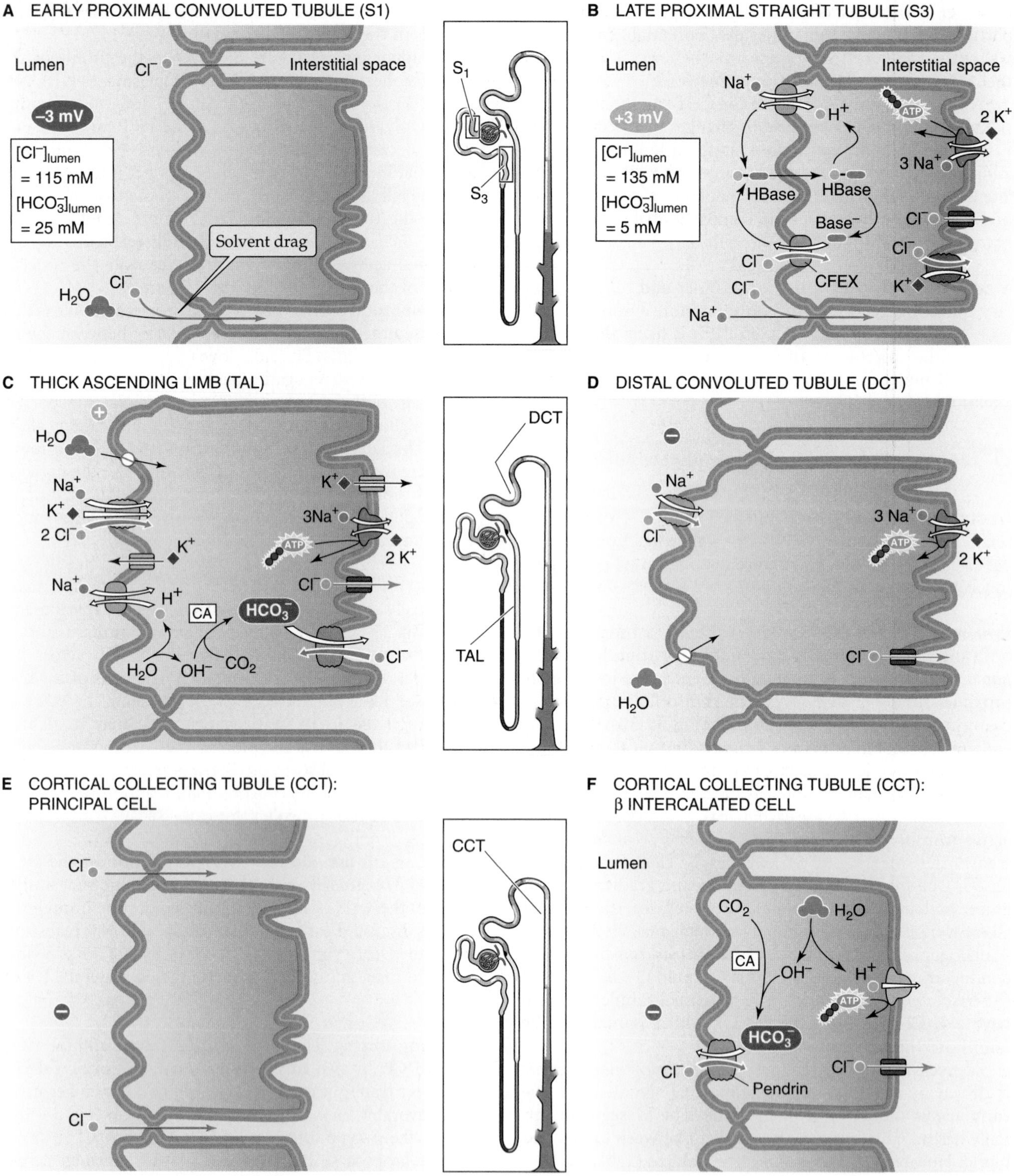

A EARLY PROXIMAL CONVOLUTED TUBULE (S1)

Lumen

Interstitial space

−3 mV

$[Cl^-]_{lumen}$ = 115 mM

$[HCO_3^-]_{lumen}$ = 25 mM

Solvent drag

H_2O Cl^-

B LATE PROXIMAL STRAIGHT TUBULE (S3)

Lumen

Interstitial space

+3 mV

$[Cl^-]_{lumen}$ = 135 mM

$[HCO_3^-]_{lumen}$ = 5 mM

Na^+ H^+ $2 K^+$ $3 Na^+$

HBase   HBase

Base$^-$ Cl^- Cl^-

Cl^- CFEX K^+

Cl^-

Na^+

ATP

C THICK ASCENDING LIMB (TAL)

H_2O

Na^+

K^+

$2 Cl^-$

Na^+

H^+

H_2O OH^- CO_2

CA

HCO_3^-

K^+

$3 Na^+$

$2 K^+$

Cl^-

Cl^-

ATP

DCT

TAL

D DISTAL CONVOLUTED TUBULE (DCT)

Na^+

Cl^-

H_2O

$3 Na^+$

$2 K^+$

Cl^-

ATP

E CORTICAL COLLECTING TUBULE (CCT): PRINCIPAL CELL

Cl^-

Cl^-

CCT

F CORTICAL COLLECTING TUBULE (CCT): β INTERCALATED CELL

Lumen

CO_2 H_2O

CA

OH^- H^+

HCO_3^-

Cl^- Pendrin Cl^-

ATP

Figure 35-5 **A** to **F**, Cell models of Cl$^-$ transport. In **B**, base may include formate, oxalate, HCO$_3^-$, and OH$^-$. HBase represents the conjugate weak acid (e.g., formic acid).

would expect the osmolality inside the peritubular capillaries to be greater than that in the luminal fluid. Indeed, investigators have found that the lumen is slightly hypo-osmolar.

If, conversely, proximal tubule water reabsorption were active, one would expect it to be independent of Na$^+$ reab-

sorption. Actually, the opposite was found by Windhager and colleagues in 1959. Using the stationary microperfusion technique, these investigators introduced solutions having various [Na$^+$] values into the proximal tubule lumen, and they kept luminal osmolality constant by adding mannitol

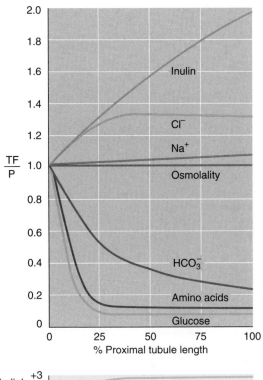

Figure 35-6 Changes in solute composition along the proximal tubule. In the *upper panel*, TF/P is the ratio of concentration or osmolality in TF versus blood plasma (P). Because we assume that the proximal tubule reabsorbs half of the filtered water, TF_{In}/P_{In} rises from 1 to 2. The *lower panel* shows the transition of transepithelial voltage from a negative to a positive value. In, inulin.

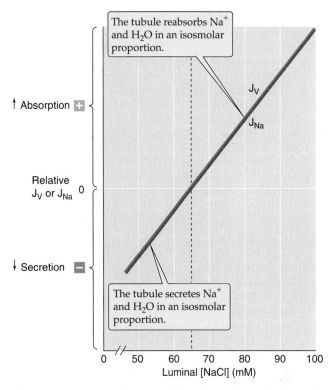

Figure 35-7 Isosmotic water reabsorption in the proximal tubule. J_V and J_{Na} are the rates of fluid (or *volume*) and Na^+ reabsorption, respectively, in stationary microperfusion experiments.

(which is poorly reabsorbed). Because these experiments were performed on amphibian proximal tubules, the maximal $[Na^+]$ was only 100 mM, the same as that in blood plasma. After a known time interval, these investigators measured the volume of fluid remaining in the tubule lumen and calculated the rate of fluid reabsorption (J_V). They also measured $[Na^+]$ of the luminal fluid and calculated the rate of Na^+ reabsorption (J_{Na}). These experiments showed that both J_V and J_{Na} are directly proportional to the initial luminal $[Na^+]$ (Fig. 35-7). Moreover, the ratio J_{Na}/J_V is constant and is equal to the osmolality of the lumen, findings indicating that Na^+ reabsorption and secretion are approximately **isosmotic**.

Windhager and colleagues also found that at a luminal $[Na^+]$ of 100 mM, the J_{Na} and J_V were large and in the reabsorptive direction. When luminal $[Na^+]$ was only 65 mM, both J_{Na} and J_V were zero. At lower luminal $[Na^+]$ values, both J_{Na} and J_V reversed (i.e., the tubule secreted both Na^+ and water). At these low luminal $[Na^+]$ values, active transcellular movement of Na^+ from lumen to blood cannot overcome the increasing paracellular backleak of Na^+, and the result is net secretion of an isosmotic NaCl solution. This experiment shows that Na^+ can move uphill from lumen to blood, as long as the opposing Na^+ gradient is not too steep,

and it also suggests that the movement of water is not active, but passively follows the reabsorption of Na^+.

If water movement is passive, why is the difference in osmolality so small between the proximal tubule lumen and blood? The answer is that, because the water permeability of the proximal tubule epithelium to water is so high, the osmolality gradient needed to generate the observed passive reabsorption of water is only 2 to 3 mOsm. A somewhat greater osmolality gradient probably exists between the lumen and an inaccessible basolateral compartment comprising the lateral intercellular space and the microscopic unstirred layer that surrounds the highly folded basolateral membrane of the proximal tubule cell.

The pathway for water movement across the proximal tubule epithelium appears to be a combination of transcellular and paracellular transit, with the transcellular route dominating. The reason for the high rate of water movement through the proximal tubule cell is the presence of a high density of aquaporin 1 (AQP1) **water channels** in both the apical and basolateral membranes. Indeed, in the AQP1-null mouse, the fluid that the proximal tubule reabsorbs can be hyperosmotic to the luminal fluid.

Loop of Henle and Distal Nephron Two features distinguish water and Na^+ transport in the distal nephron. First, the TAL and all downstream segments have relatively low water permeability in the absence of AVP (or antidiuretic hormone). The upregulation of this water permeability by AVP is discussed in Chapter 37. Second, the combination of NaCl reabsorption and low water permeability allows these

Osmotic Diuresis

Normally, luminal [Na⁺] does not change along the proximal tubule. The only exception is **osmotic diuresis**, a state in which poorly permeable substances are present in the plasma and, therefore, in the glomerular filtrate. Examples are the infusion of sucrose and mannitol. Another is untreated diabetes mellitus (see Chapter 51 for the box on that topic), when the blood glucose level may become too high for the capacity of renal tubules to reabsorb the highly elevated glucose load. Glucose then acts as a poorly reabsorbed substance and as an osmotic diuretic. Because the proximal tubule must reabsorb isosmotic Na⁺ salts from a luminal mixture of Na⁺ salts and poorly reabsorbable solutes (e.g., mannitol), luminal [Na⁺] progressively falls and luminal [mannitol] rises, but luminal osmolality does not change (Fig. 35-8).

Because, as we have seen, the rate of Na⁺ and fluid reabsorption falls as the luminal [Na⁺] falls (Fig. 35-7), the proximal tubule reabsorbs progressively less Na⁺ and fluid as the fluid travels along the tubule. This decrease in Na⁺ and water reabsorption leaves a larger volume of TF, thereby producing osmotic diuresis. Clinicians use osmotic diuretics in several settings. For example, mannitol osmotically draws water out of brain tissue into the vascular system, for ultimate excretion by the kidneys. For this reason, osmotic diuresis has proven useful in treating patients with acutely increased intracranial pressure from an expanding tumor or abscess, hematoma or hemorrhage, or edema. Mannitol also reduces the risk of radiocontrast-induced acute renal failure in susceptible patients (e.g., those with underlying renal disease, volume depletion, diabetes mellitus, or congestive heart failure) who must undergo radiological procedures that require a substantial dye load.

It is common to distinguish between two types of diuresis: solute and water diuresis. The foregoing example of **solute or osmotic diuresis** is characterized by excretion of a larger than normal volume of urine that is rich in solutes. In contrast, **water diuresis** leads to excretion of larger than normal volumes of urine that is dilute (i.e., poor in solutes).

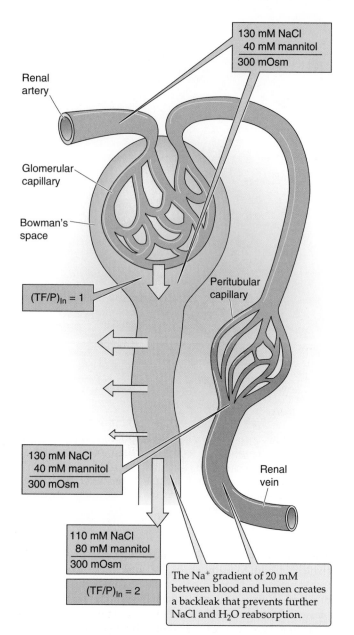

Figure 35-8 Osmotic diuresis and luminal [Na⁺] along the proximal tubule. In this example, blood and glomerular filtrate both contain 40 mM mannitol and have an osmolality of 300 mOsm. The isosmotic reabsorption of NaCl (but *not* mannitol) from proximal tubule lumen to blood causes luminal [mannitol] to rise and [NaCl] to fall, but causes no change in luminal osmolality. Once luminal [Na⁺] falls sufficiently, the Na⁺ backleak from peritubular capillaries balances active Na⁺ reabsorption, and net reabsorption of NaCl and water is zero. The absence of fluid absorption after this point causes osmotic diuresis. Viewed another way, the rising luminal [mannitol], with the osmotically obligated water the mannitol holds in the lumen, produces the diuresis. (TF/P)$_{In}$, the ratio of inulin concentrations in TF/P.

nephron segments to generate a low luminal [Na⁺] and osmolality with respect to the surrounding interstitial fluid. Given this large osmotic gradient across the epithelium, the distal nephron is poised to reabsorb water passively from a hypo-osmotic luminal fluid into the isosmotic blood when AVP increases the water permeability.

The kidney's high O₂ consumption reflects a high level of active Na⁺ transport

Because virtually all Na⁺ transport ultimately depends on the activity of the ATP-driven Na-K pump and, therefore, on the generation of ATP by oxidative metabolism, it is not surprising that renal O₂ consumption is large and parallels Na⁺ reabsorption. Despite their low weight (<0.5% of body weight), the kidneys are responsible for 7% to 10% of total O₂ consumption. Although it would seem that the high O₂ consumption would necessitate a large arteriovenous difference in P$_{O_2}$, actually the renal blood flow is so large that the

artery-vein P$_{O_2}$ difference is actually much smaller than that in cardiac muscle or brain.

If one varies Na⁺ reabsorption experimentally and measures renal O₂ consumption, the result is a straight-line relationship (Fig. 35-9). However, the kidneys continue to

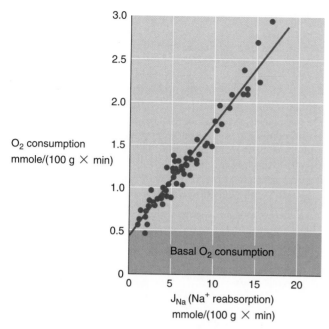

Figure 35-9 Dependence of O_2 consumption on Na^+ transport. Na^+ reabsorption (J_{Na}) was varied by changing GFR, administering diuretics, or imposing hypoxia. O_2 consumption was computed from the arteriovenous P_{O_2} difference.

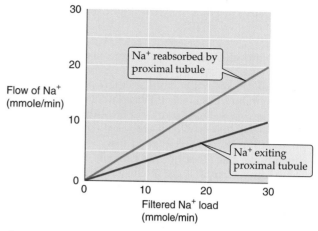

Figure 35-10 Constancy of fractional Na^+ reabsorption by the proximal tubule.

consume a modest but significant amount of O_2 even in the complete absence of net Na^+ reabsorption. This transport-independent component reflects the basic metabolic needs for the maintenance of cell viability.

REGULATION OF Na^+ AND Cl^- TRANSPORT

The body regulates Na^+ excretion through the following three major mechanisms:

1. Changes in renal hemodynamics alter the Na^+ load presented to the kidney and modulate the rate of NaCl reabsorption in the proximal tubule by a process known as glomerulotubular (GT) balance. We discuss these hemodynamic effects in the next three sections.
2. Three factors that regulate "effective circulating volume" (see Chapter 23) do so in part by increasing Na^+ reabsorption (i.e., producing **natriuresis**). A fourth does so in part by decreasing Na^+ reabsorption. We briefly introduce these four factors in the fourth section of this subchapter, and we discuss them more fully in Chapter 39.
3. In addition to the natriuretic factor alluded to in item 2, four other natriuretic humoral factors can decrease Na^+ reabsorption, as we see in the final section of this chapter.

GT balance stabilizes fractional Na^+ reabsorption by the proximal tubule in the presence of changes in the filtered Na^+ load

When hemodynamic changes (e.g., caused by changes in intake of Na^+ or protein or by extreme exercise, severe pain,

or anesthesia) alter GFR and thus the Na^+ load presented to the nephron, *proximal* tubules respond by reabsorbing a *constant fraction* of the Na^+ load. This constancy of fractional Na^+ reabsorption along the proximal tubule—**GT balance**—is independent of external neural and hormonal control and thus safeguards Na^+ balance.

Figure 35-10 shows how the *absolute reabsorption* of Na^+ increases proportionally with increases in the filtered Na^+ load, achieved by varying GFRs at constant plasma [Na^+]. The amount of luminal Na^+ remaining at the end of the proximal tubule also increases linearly with the filtered Na^+ load. Later, we discuss the impact of such altered Na^+ delivery to more distally located nephron segments.

When excessive Na^+ loss (e.g., sweating or diarrhea) contracts the ECF volume, the reduced renal perfusion pressure causes GFR to fall. In response, the proximal tubule excretes a constant fraction of Na^+ and water, corresponding to a smaller absolute amount. Thus, GT balance helps to prevent additional Na^+ and water loss. Conversely, when Na^+ retention expands ECF (causing GFR to rise), the proximal tubule excretes a constant fraction of filtered Na^+, corresponding to an increased absolute amount. This response tends to correct the volume expansion. At the level of the whole kidney, GT balance is not perfect, mainly because distal nephron Na^+ absorption is under neural and hormonal control.

The proximal tubule achieves GT balance by both peritubular and luminal mechanisms

How do the proximal tubule cells sense that the GFR has changed? Both peritubular and luminal control mechanisms contribute, although no agreement exists concerning their relative roles.

Peritubular Factors in the Proximal Tubule As discussed in the previous chapter, Starling forces across the peritubular capillary walls determine the uptake of interstitial fluid and thus the net reabsorption of NaCl and fluid from the tubule lumen into the peritubular capillaries (see Chapter 34). These peritubular **physical factors** also play a role in GT balance. We can distinguish a sequence of three transport steps as reabsorbed fluid moves from the tubule lumen into the blood (Fig. 35-11A):

Step 1: Solutes and water enter a tubule cell across the apical membrane.

Step 2: Solutes and water from step 1 (i.e., "reabsorbate") exit the tubule cell across the basolateral membrane and enter an *inter*cellular compartment—the **lateral interspace**—that is bounded by the apical tight junction, the basolateral tubule cell membranes, and a basement membrane that does not discriminate between solutes and solvent. Steps 1 and 2 constitute the *transcellular pathway*.

Step 3: The reabsorbate can either backleak into the lumen (step 3a) or move sequentially into the interstitial space and then into the blood (step 3b).

At normal GFR (Fig. 35-11A), reabsorptive Starling forces—the low hydrostatic and high oncotic pressure in the capillaries—cause an extensive uptake of reabsorbate into the capillaries. Because of GT balance, alterations in GFR lead to changes in peritubular pressures (both hydrostatic and oncotic) that, in turn, modulate the forces that govern step 3 in the foregoing list. Peritubular mechanisms of GT balance come into play only when the changes in GFR are associated with alterations in **filtration fraction** (FF = GFR/

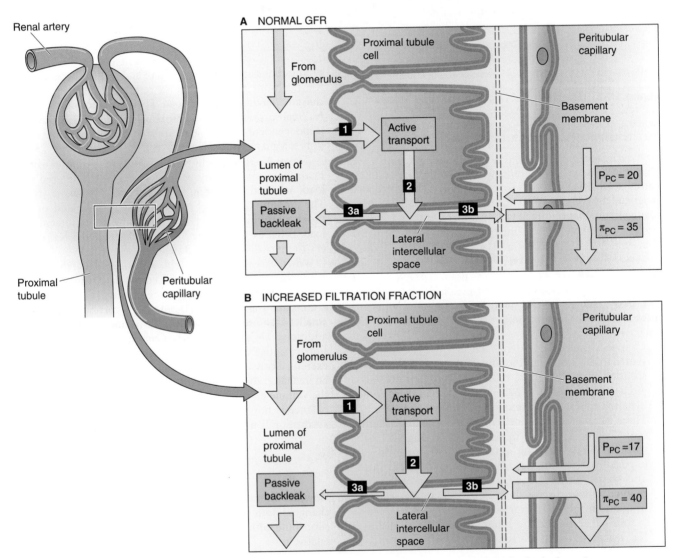

Figure 35-11   Peritubular mechanisms of GT balance. In **A**, P_{PC} and π_{PC} are, respectively, the hydrostatic and the oncotic pressures in the peritubular capillaries. At the level of the tubule, the net Na^+ reabsorption is the difference between active transcellular transport and passive backleak through the paracellular pathway. At the level of the peritubular capillary, net fluid absorption is the difference between fluid absorption (driven by π_{PC}) and fluid filtration (driven by P_{PC}). In **B**, increasing the filtered fraction has effects on both the tubule and the peritubular capillaries. At the level of the tubule, the increased concentrations of Na^+-coupled solutes (e.g., glucose) increase active transport. At the level of the capillaries, the lower P_{PC} and higher protein concentration (π_{PC}) pull more fluid from the interstitium. The net effect is reduced passive backleak.

RPF; see Chapter 34). Consider an example in which we increase GFR at constant glomerular plasma flow, thereby increasing FF (Fig. 35-11B). We can produce this effect by increasing efferent arteriolar resistance while concomitantly decreasing afferent arteriolar resistance (see Fig. 33-8A, lower panel). The result is an increase in glomerular capillary pressure (i.e., net filtration pressure) without a change in overall arteriolar resistance. These changes have two important consequences for peritubular capillaries. First, the increased GFR translates to less fluid remaining in the efferent arteriole, so that peritubular *oncotic pressure* (π_{PC}) rises. Second, the increased GFR also translates to less blood flowing into the efferent arteriole, thereby decreasing *hydrostatic pressure* in the peritubular capillaries (P_{PC}). As a consequence, the net driving force increases for the transport of fluid from the lateral interspace into the capillaries, thus leading to a more effective absorption of fluid and NaCl. The opposite sequence of events occurs during extracellular volume expansion.

Luminal Factors in the Proximal Tubule   Luminal factors also contribute to GT balance, as evidenced by the observation that increased flow along the proximal tubule—without any peritubular effects—leads to an increase in fluid and NaCl reabsorption. The luminal concentrations of solutes such as glucose, amino acids, and HCO_3^- fall along the length of the proximal tubule, as the tubule reabsorbs these solutes (Fig. 35-6). Increasing luminal flow would, for instance, cause luminal [glucose] to fall less steeply along the tubule length, and more glucose would be available for reabsorption at distal sites. The net effect is that, integrated over the entire proximal tubule, higher luminal flows increase the reabsorption of Na^+, glucose, and other Na^+-coupled solutes.

A second luminal mechanism may revolve around a flow sensor. It appears that increased flow causes increased bending of the **central cilium** on the apical membrane, an effect that may signal increased fluid reabsorption. Third, a hypothetical humoral factor may also contribute to GT balance. If one harvests TF and injects it into a single proximal tubule, Na^+ reabsorption increases. Angiotensin II (ANG II)—a small peptide hormone that is both filtered in the glomeruli and secreted by proximal tubule cells—increases Na^+ reabsorption in the proximal tubule.

The distal nephron also increases Na^+ reabsorption in response to an increased Na^+ load

The tubules of the distal nephron, like their proximal counterparts, also increase their absolute magnitude of Na^+ reabsorption in response to increased flow. The principle is the same as that for glucose transport in the proximal tubule, except here it is luminal $[Na^+]$ that falls less steeply when flow increases (Fig. 35-12A). Because the transport mechanisms responsible for Na^+ reabsorption by the distal nephron work faster at higher luminal $[Na^+]$ values, reabsorption at any site increases with flow (Fig. 35-12B). In contrast to GT balance in the proximal tubule, increasing flow by a factor of 4 in the distal nephron may cause cumulative Na^+ reabsorption to rise by only a factor of 2 (Fig. 35-12C).

The opposite changes in Na^+ and fluid transport occur when GFR—and thus distal flow—acutely *falls*, as in **circulatory shock**. Because of GT balance, the proximal nephron reabsorbs a constant fraction of Na^+, thereby delivering a lower absolute amount of Na^+ to the DCT. The distal nephron—under the influence of neural and humoral factors discussed later—lowers luminal $[Na^+]$ even further so that the final urine may contain only traces of Na^+.

Four parallel pathways that regulate effective circulating volume all modulate Na^+ reabsorption

GT balance is only one element in a larger, complex system for controlling Na^+ balance. As we see in Chapter 39, the control of effective circulating volume (i.e., Na^+ content) is under the powerful control of four parallel effectors (see Chapter 40): the renin-angiotensin-aldosterone axis, the

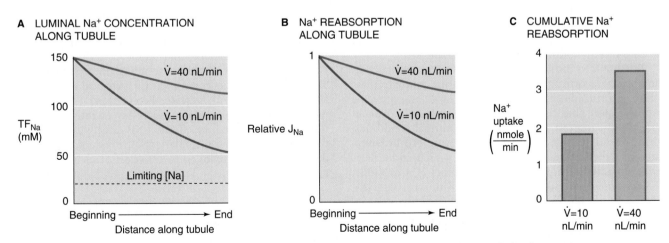

Figure 35-12   Flow dependence of Na^+ transport in the distal nephron. **A** and **B** are idealized representations of the effect of increased flow ($\dot{V}$) on luminal $[Na^+]$ and Na^+ reabsorption rate (J_{Na}) along the TAL. Limiting [Na] is the theoretical minimal value that the tubule could achieve at zero flow. **C** summarizes the effect of flow on cumulative Na^+ reabsorption.

sympathetic nervous system, AVP, and atrial natriuretic peptide (ANP). In the previous chapter, we saw how these factors modulate renal blood flow and GFR (see Chapter 34). Here, we briefly discuss how these four effectors modulate Na$^+$ reabsorption, a subject that we treat more comprehensively beginning in Chapter 40.

Renin-Angiotensin-Aldosterone Axis ANG II—the second element in the renin-angiotensin-aldosterone axis (see Chapter 40)—binds to AT$_1$ receptors at the apical and basolateral membranes of proximal tubule cells and, predominantly through protein kinase C, stimulates apical NHE3s. ANG II also stimulates Na-H exchange in the TAL and stimulates apical Na$^+$ channels in the initial collecting tubule. These effects promote Na$^+$ reabsorption.

Aldosterone—the final element in the renin-angiotensin-aldosterone axis—stimulates Na$^+$ reabsorption by the initial tubule and the CCT, and by medullary collecting ducts. Normally, only 2% to 3% of the filtered Na$^+$ load is under humoral control by aldosterone. Nevertheless, the sustained loss of even such a small fraction would exceed the daily Na$^+$ intake significantly. Accordingly, the lack of aldosterone that occurs in adrenal insufficiency (Addison disease) can lead to severe Na$^+$ depletion, contraction of the ECF volume, and circulatory insufficiency.

Aldosterone acts on the **principal cells** of the collecting ducts (Fig. 35-13A) by binding to cytoplasmic mineralocorticoid receptors (MRs) that then translocate to the nucleus and upregulate transcription (see Chapters 3 and 4). Thus, the effects of aldosterone require a few hours to manifest themselves because they depend on the increased production of aldosterone-induced proteins. One of these is **SGK** (serum- and glucocorticoid-regulated kinase), a key player in the early phase of aldosterone action. Early cellular actions of aldosterone action include upregulation of apical ENaCs, apical K$^+$ channels, the basolateral Na-K pump, and mitochondrial metabolism. The effects on ENaC involve an increase in the product of channel number and open probability (NP$_o$), and thus apical Na$^+$ permeability. The simultaneous activation of apical Na$^+$ entry and basolateral Na$^+$ extrusion ensures that, even with very high levels of Na$^+$ reabsorption, [Na$^+$]$_i$ and cell volume are stable. Long-term exposure to aldosterone leads to the targeting of newly synthesized Na-K pumps to the basolateral membrane and to amplification of the basolateral membrane area.

Because MRs distinguish poorly between glucocorticoids and mineralocorticoids, and because plasma concentrations of glucocorticoids greatly exceed those of aldosterone, one would expect glucocorticoids to exert a mineralocorticoid effect and cause Na$^+$ retention. Under normal conditions, this does not happen because of the enzyme **11β-hydroxysteroid dehydrogenase 2** (11β-HSD2), which co-localizes with intracellular adrenal steroid receptors (Fig. 35-13B). This enzyme irreversibly converts cortisol into cortisone (see Fig. 50-2), an inactive metabolite with low affinity for MRs. In sharp contrast, the enzyme does *not* metabolize aldosterone. Thus, 11β-HSD2 enhances the apparent specificity of MRs by protecting them from illicit occupancy by cortisol. As may be expected, an 11β-HSD2 deficiency may mimic a mineralocorticoid excess. Carbenoxolone, a specific inhibitor of 11β-HSD2, prevents metabolism of cortisol in target

cells, thus permitting abnormal activation of MRs by this glucocorticoid (Fig. 35-13C). Another inhibitor of 11β-HSD2 is glycyrrhetinic acid, a component of natural **licorice**. Thus, natural licorice can cause abnormal Na$^+$ retention and hypertension, a condition known as **mineralocorticoid excess syndrome** (MES).

Sympathetic Division of the Autonomic Nervous System Sympathetic nerve terminals in the kidney release norepinephrine, which has two major *direct* effects on Na$^+$ reabsorption. First, high levels of sympathetic stimulation markedly reduce renal blood flow and therefore GFR (see Chapter 34). Both proximal GT balance (Fig. 35-10) and the flow response of the distal nephron (Fig. 35-12) cause Na$^+$ excretion to fall. Second, even low levels of sympathetic stimulation activate α-adrenergic receptors in proximal tubules. This activation stimulates both the apical NHE3 and basolateral Na-K pump (Fig. 35-4A), thereby increasing Na$^+$ reabsorption, independent of any hemodynamic effects.

Arginine Vasopressin or Antidiuretic Hormone Released by the posterior pituitary, AVP binds to a V$_2$ receptor at the basolateral membrane of target cells. Acting through G$_s$, the AVP increases [cAMP]$_i$ (see Chapter 3). As discussed in Chapter 39, the overall renal effect of AVP in humans is to produce urine with a high osmolality and thereby retain water (see Chapter 38). However, AVP also stimulates Na$^+$ reabsorption. In the TAL, AVP stimulates the apical NKCC2 and K$^+$ channels (Fig. 35-4B). In principal cells of the initial collecting tubule and the CCT, AVP stimulates Na$^+$ transport by increasing the number of open Na$^+$ channels (NP$_o$) in the apical membrane.

Atrial Natriuretic Peptide Of the four parallel effectors (see Chapter 40) that control effective circulating volume, ANP is the only one that promotes natriuresis. A polypeptide released by atrial cardiomyocytes (see Chapter 19), ANP stimulates a receptor guanylyl cyclase to generate cGMP (see Chapter 3). The major effects of ANP are hemodynamic. It causes renal vasodilation, by massively increasing blood flow to both the cortex and the medulla. Increased blood flow to the *cortex* raises GFR and increases the Na$^+$ load to the proximal tubule and to TAL (see Chapter 34). Increased blood flow to the *medulla* washes out the medullary interstitium, thus decreasing osmolality and ultimately reducing passive Na$^+$ reabsorption in the thin ascending limb (see Chapter 38). The combined effect of increasing cortical and medullary blood flow is to increase the Na$^+$ load to the distal nephron and thus to increase urinary Na$^+$ excretion. In addition to its hemodynamic effects, ANP directly inhibits Na$^+$ transport in the inner medullary collecting duct, perhaps by decreasing the activity of nonselective cation channels in the apical membrane.

An endogenous steroid, prostaglandins, bradykinin, and dopamine all decrease Na$^+$ reabsorption

Aside from ANP (see previous section), three humoral agents have significant natriuretic action, in part due to inhibition of Na$^+$ reabsorption at the level of the tubule cell.

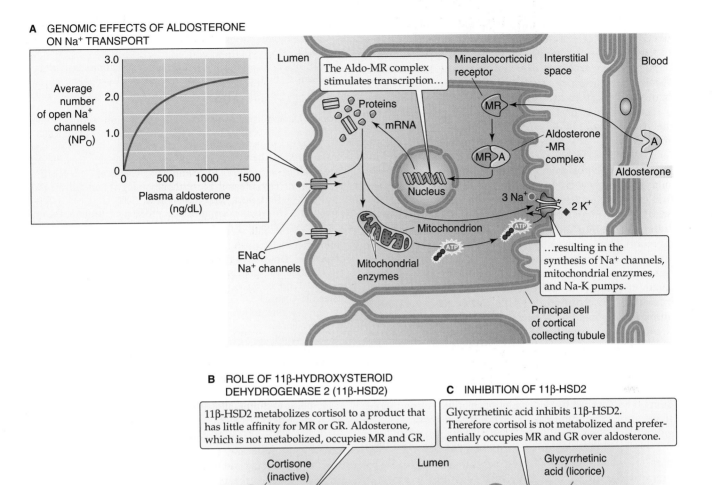

A GENOMIC EFFECTS OF ALDOSTERONE ON Na⁺ TRANSPORT

Average number of open Na⁺ channels (NP_O)

Plasma aldosterone (ng/dL)

The Aldo-MR complex stimulates transcription…

Proteins

mRNA

Mineralocorticoid receptor

Interstitial space

Blood

MR

Aldosterone-MR complex

A

Aldosterone

MR A

Nucleus

ENaC Na⁺ channels

3 Na⁺

2 K⁺

Mitochondrion

Mitochondrial enzymes

ATP

ATP

…resulting in the synthesis of Na⁺ channels, mitochondrial enzymes, and Na-K pumps.

Principal cell of cortical collecting tubule

B ROLE OF 11β-HYDROXYSTEROID DEHYDROGENASE 2 (11β-HSD2)

11β-HSD2 metabolizes cortisol to a product that has little affinity for MR or GR. Aldosterone, which is not metabolized, occupies MR and GR.

Cortisone (inactive)

Lumen

Cortisol

11β-HSD2

C

C

Glucocorticoid receptor

GR A

MR A

A

A

Principal cell

Aldosterone

Mineralocorticoid receptor

Interstitium

C INHIBITION OF 11β-HSD2

Glycyrrhetinic acid inhibits 11β-HSD2. Therefore cortisol is not metabolized and preferentially occupies MR and GR over aldosterone.

Glycyrrhetinic acid (licorice)

11β-HSD2

C

C

GR C

MR C

A

A

Principal cell

Figure 35-13 Cellular actions of aldosterone. The inset in **A** shows the upregulation of ENaCs, based on patch-clamp data from the rat CCT. *N* is the number of channels in the patch, and P_O is the open probability. In **B**, 11β-HSD2 prevents cortisol (a glucocorticoid), which is present at high plasma concentrations, from having mineralocorticoid effects in the target cell. In **C**, with the enzyme blocked, cortisol acts as a mineralocorticoid. GR, glucocorticoid receptor.

Endogenous Na-K Pump Inhibitor Human plasma contains an endogenous, ouabain-like steroid (see Chapter 5) that inhibits Na-K pumps in a wide variety of cells. This natural Na-K pump inhibitor increases with salt loading and is present in high levels in patients with hypertension. In response to Na⁺ loading, the body may increase levels of this inhibitor, which presumably would bind preferentially to Na-K pumps of collecting duct cells, thereby elevating $[Na^+]_i$ and enhancing Na⁺ excretion.

Prostaglandins and Bradykinin Produced locally in the kidney, these agents act through protein kinase C (see Chapter 3) to inhibit Na⁺ reabsorption, probably by phosphorylating K⁺ or Na⁺ channels. In the TAL, prostaglandin

E_2 (PGE_2) inhibits the apical *K⁺ channel*, depolarizing the apical and basolateral membranes, and diminishing passive Cl^- efflux across the basolateral membrane. $[Cl^-]_i$ therefore rises, impeding the turnover of the apical NKCC2 (Fig. 35-4B). In addition, the transepithelial voltage becomes less lumen positive, thus decreasing the driving force for passive paracellular reabsorption of Na^+ and other cations. In the CCT, both PGE_2 and bradykinin inhibit ENaCs (Fig. 35-4D).

Dopamine The kidney forms dopamine locally from circulating L-dopa. Na^+ loading increases the synthesis and urinary excretion rate of dopamine, whereas a low-Na^+ diet has the opposite effect. As noted earlier, dopamine causes renal vasodilation (see Chapter 34), which increases Na^+ excretion. Dopamine also directly inhibits Na^+ reabsorption at the level of tubule cells. Indeed, D_1 and D_2 dopamine receptors are present in the renal cortex, where they both apparently lead to an increase in $[cAMP]_i$. The result is an inhibition of both the apical NHE3 and the basolateral Na-K pump in proximal tubule and TAL cells. In humans, administering low doses of dopamine leads to natriuresis.

REFERENCES

Books and Reviews

Aronson PS, Giebisch G: Mechanisms of chloride transport in the proximal tubule. Am J Physiol 1997; 273:F179-F192.

Garcia NH, Ramsey CR, Knox FG: Understanding the role of paracellular transport in the proximal tubule. News Physiol Sci 1998; 13:38-243.

Reilly RF, Ellison DH: The mammalian distal tubule: Physiology, pathophysiology, and molecular anatomy. Physiol Rev 2000; 80:277-313.

Rossier BC, Pradervand S, Schild L, Hummler E: Epithelial sodium channel and the control of sodium balance: Interaction between genetic and environmental factors. Annu Rev Physiol 2002; 64:877-897.

Schafer JA: Abnormal regulation of ENaC: Syndromes of salt retention and salt wasting by the collecting duct. Am J Physiol 2002; 283:F221-F235.

Wilcox CS, Baylis C, Wingo C: Glomerulo-tubular balance and proximal regulation. In Seldin DW, Giebisch G (eds): The Kidney: Physiology and Pathophysiology, 2nd ed, vol 2, pp 1805-1841. New York: Raven Press, 1992.

Wright FS: Flow-dependent transport processes: Filtration, absorption, secretion. Am J Physiol 1982; 243:F1-F11.

Journal Articles

Alpern RJ, Howlin KJ, Preisig P: Active and passive components of chloride transport in the rat proximal convoluted tubule. J Clin Invest 1985; 76:1360-1366.

Green R, Giebisch G: Osmotic forces driving water reabsorption in the proximal tubule of the rat kidney. Am J Physiol 1989; 257: F669-F675.

Lewy J, Windhager EE: Peritubular control of proximal tubular fluid reabsorption in the rat kidney. Am J Physiol 1968; 214:943-954.

Quentin F, Chambrey R, Trinh-Trang-Tan MM, et al: The Cl^-/HCO_3^- exchanger pendrin in the rat kidney is regulated in response to chronic alterations in chloride balance. Am J Physiol 2004; 287:F1179-F1188.

CHAPTER 36

TRANSPORT OF UREA, GLUCOSE, PHOSPHATE, CALCIUM, MAGNESIUM, AND ORGANIC SOLUTES

Gerhard Giebisch and Erich Windhager

The kidney plays a central role in controlling the plasma levels of a wide range of solutes that are present at low concentrations in the body. The renal excretion of a solute depends on three processes—filtration, reabsorption, and secretion (see Chapter 33). The kidney filters and then totally reabsorbs some of the substances we discuss in this chapter (e.g., glucose). Others, it filters and also secretes (e.g., the organic anion *p*-aminohippurate [PAH]). Still others, the kidney filters, reabsorbs, and secretes (e.g., urea).

UREA

The kidney filters, reabsorbs, and secretes urea

The liver generates urea from NH_4^+, the primary nitrogenous end product of amino acid catabolism (see Chapter 46). The primary route for urea excretion is the urine, although some urea exits the body through the stool and sweat. The normal plasma concentration of urea is 2.5 to 6 mM. Clinical laboratories report plasma urea levels as **blood urea nitrogen** (**BUN**) in the units "mg of elemental nitrogen per dL plasma"; normal values are 7 to 18 mg/dL. For a 70-kg person ingesting a typical Western diet, and producing 1.5 to 2 L/day of urine, the urinary excretion of urea is ~450 mmol/day.

The kidney freely filters urea at the glomerulus, and then it both reabsorbs and secretes it. Because the tubules reabsorb more urea than they secrete, the amount of urea excreted in the urine is less than the quantity filtered. In the example shown in Figure 36-1A (i.e., average urine flow), the kidneys excrete ~40% of the filtered urea. The primary sites for urea reabsorption are the proximal tubule and the medullary collecting duct, whereas the primary sites for secretion are the thin limbs of the loop of Henle.

In the very early **proximal tubule** (Fig. 36-1B), [urea] in the lumen is the same as in blood plasma. However, paracellular fluid reabsorption along the proximal tubule sweeps some urea along with it through **solvent drag** (see Chapter 20). In addition, water reabsorption tends to increase [urea]

in the lumen, thereby generating a favorable transepithelial gradient that drives urea reabsorption by **diffusion** through the transcellular or paracellular pathway. The greater the fluid reabsorption along the proximal tubule, the greater is the reabsorption of urea through both solvent drag and diffusion.

In *juxtamedullary* nephrons, as the tubule fluid in the **thin descending limb** (tDLH) approaches the tip of the loop of Henle, [urea] is higher in the medullary interstitium than in the lumen (see Chapter 38). Thus, the deepest portion of the tDLH *secretes* urea through facilitated diffusion (Fig. 36-1C) mediated by the urea transporter **UT-A2**, which is encoded by the *SLC14A2* gene. As the fluid turns the corner to flow up the **thin ascending limb** (tALH), the tubule cells continue to secrete urea into the lumen, probably also by facilitated diffusion (Fig. 36-1D).

The tDLH of *superficial* nephrons is located in the inner stripe of the outer medulla. Here, the interstitial [urea] is higher than the luminal [urea] because the vasa recta carry urea from the inner medulla. Because the tDLH cells of these superficial nephrons appear to have **UT-A2** along their entire length, these cells *secrete* urea. Thus, both superficial and probably also juxtamedullary nephrons contribute to urea secretion, raising urea delivery to ~110% of the filtered load at the level of the cortical collecting ducts.

Finally, the **inner medullary collecting duct** (IMCD) *reabsorbs* urea by a transcellular route that is unusual in that both the apical and basolateral steps occur by facilitated diffusion (Fig. 36-1E). The **UT-A1** urea transporter moves urea across the apical membrane of the IMCD cell, whereas **UT-A3** probably mediates urea movement across the basolateral membrane. Arginine vasopressin (AVP)—also known as antidiuretic hormone (ADH)—stimulates UT-A1 but not UT-A3. In Chapter 38, we discuss the role of urea transport in the urinary concentrating mechanism.

UT-A2, the prototypical member of the UT family, is a glycosylated 55-kDa integral membrane protein with 10 putative membrane-spanning segments. UT-A2 is unusual among membrane proteins in that it is extremely hydrophobic; except for a large extracellular loop, almost the entire

A HANDLING OF UREA ALONG NEPHRON

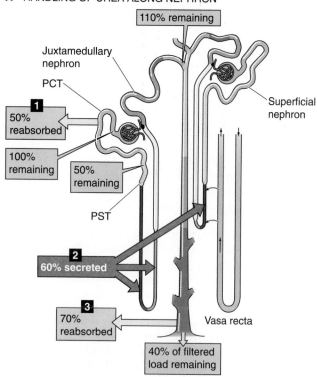

Figure 36-1 **A** to **E**, Urea handling by the kidney. In **A**, we assume a normal urine flow and thus a urea excretion of 40% of the filtered load. The numbered *yellow boxes* indicate the fraction of the filtered load that various nephron segments reabsorb. The tALH and the tip of the tDLH in juxtamedullary nephrons secrete urea. In superficial nephrons, the entire tDLH may secrete urea. The *red box* indicates the fraction of the filtered load jointly secreted by both nephron types. The *green boxes* indicate the fraction of the filtered load that remains in the lumen. The values in the boxes are approximations. UT-A1, UT-A2, and UT-A3 are urea transporters.

B PROXIMAL TUBULE

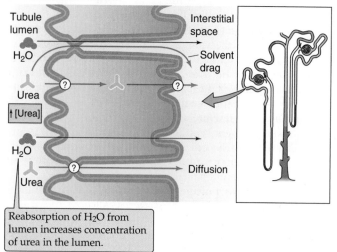

C THIN DESCENDING LIMB (tDLH)

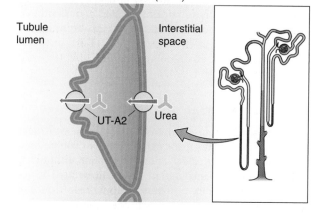

D THIN ASCENDING LIMB (tALH)

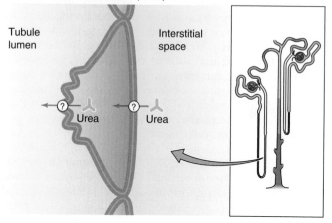

E INNER MEDULLARY COLLECTING DUCT (IMCD)

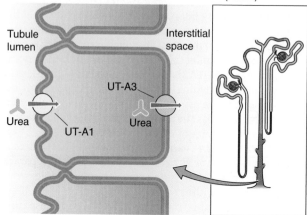

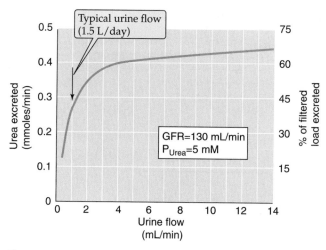

Figure 36-2 Urea excretion versus urine flow. *(Data from Austin JH, Stillman E, Van Slyke DD: J Biol Chem 1921; 46:91-112.)*

central portion of the protein may be embedded within the membrane. UT-A1, a splice variant of the same gene, is a 97-kDa protein with 20 membrane-spanning segments. UT-A1 is basically UT-A3 linked to UT-A2 by an intracellular loop. This loop has several putative phosphorylation sites for protein kinase A (PKA), a feature that explains why AVP—which acts through cAMP (see Chapter 3)—stimulates only UT-A1. As discussed in Chapter 38, **UT-B1** and **UT-B2**, which are encoded by a different gene *(SLC14A1)*, are present in the descending limb of the vasa recta.

Urea excretion rises with increasing urinary flow

Because urea transport depends primarily on urea concentration differences across the tubule epithelium, changes in urine flow unavoidably affect renal urea handling (Fig. 36-2). At low urine flow, when the tubule reabsorbs considerable water and therefore much urea, the kidneys excrete only ~15% of filtered urea (see Fig. 38-6). However, the kidneys may excrete as much as 70% of filtered urea at high urine flow, when the tubules reabsorb relatively less water and urea. During the progression of renal disease, the decline of the glomerular filtration rate (GFR) leads to a low urine flow and urea retention, and thus an increase in BUN.

In clinical conditions such as *volume depletion*, in which the urine flow declines sharply (see Chapter 40), urea excretion decreases out of proportion to the fall in GFR. The resulting high BUN can thus serve as laboratory confirmation of dehydration. The flow dependence of urea clearance contrasts with the behavior of creatinine clearance, which, like inulin clearance (see Chapter 34), is largely independent of urine flow. Consequently, in patients with reduced effective circulating volume (see Chapter 23), and hence low urine flow, the plasma [BUN]/[creatinine] ratio increases from its normal value of ~10 (both concentrations in mg/dL).

GLUCOSE

The proximal tubule reabsorbs glucose through an apical, electrogenic Na/glucose cotransporter and a basolateral facilitated diffusion mechanism (GLUT)

The fasting plasma glucose concentration (see Chapter 51) is normally 4 to 5 mM (70 to 100 mg/dL) and is regulated by insulin and other hormones. The kidneys freely filter glucose at the glomerulus and then reabsorb it, so that only trace amounts normally appear in the urine (Fig. 36-3A). The *proximal tubule* reabsorbs nearly all the filtered load of glucose, mostly along the first third of this segment. More distal segments reabsorb almost all the remainder. In the proximal tubule, luminal [glucose] is initially equal to plasma [glucose]. As the early proximal tubule reabsorbs glucose, luminal [glucose] drops sharply, falling to levels far lower than those in the interstitium. Accordingly, glucose reabsorption occurs against a concentration gradient and must therefore be active.

Glucose reabsorption is transcellular; glucose moves from the lumen to the proximal tubule cell through Na/glucose cotransport and from cytoplasm to blood by facilitated diffusion (Fig. 36-3B, C). At the apical membrane, a member of the **Na/glucose cotransporter** (SGLT) family (see Chapter 5) couples the movements of the electrically neutral D-glucose (but not L-glucose) and Na⁺. Phloridzin, extracted from the root bark of certain fruit trees (e.g., cherry, apple), inhibits the SGLTs. The basolateral Na-K pump maintains the intracellular Na⁺ concentration ($[Na^+]_i$) lower than that of the tubule fluid. Moreover, the electrically negative cell interior establishes a steep electrical gradient that favors the flux of Na⁺ from lumen to cell. Thus, the electrochemical gradient of Na⁺ drives the uphill transport of glucose into the cell (i.e., secondary active transport), thereby concentrating glucose in the cytoplasm (see Chapter 5).

In the early part of the proximal tubule (S1 segment), a high-capacity/low-affinity transporter called **SGLT2** mediates apical glucose uptake (Fig. 36-3B). This cotransporter has Na⁺/glucose stoichiometry of 1:1. In the later part of the proximal tubule (S3 segment), a high-affinity/low-capacity cotransporter called **SGLT1** is responsible for apical glucose uptake (Fig. 36-3C). Because this cotransporter has Na⁺/glucose stoichiometry of 2:1 (i.e., far more electrochemical energy per glucose), it can generate a far larger glucose gradient across the apical membrane (see Chapter 5). Paracellular glucose permeability progressively diminishes along the proximal tubule, further contributing to the tubule's ability to maintain high transepithelial glucose gradients and to generate near-zero glucose concentrations in the fluid emerging from the proximal tubule.

Once inside the cell, glucose exits across the basolateral membrane by a member of the **GLUT** family of glucose transporters (see Chapter 5). These transporters are Na⁺ *independent* and move glucose by facilitated diffusion. Thus, the GLUTs are quite distinct from the SGLTs. Like the apical

A HANDLING OF GLUCOSE ALONG NEPHRON

B EARLY PROXIMAL TUBULE (S1)

C LATE PROXIMAL TUBULE (S3)

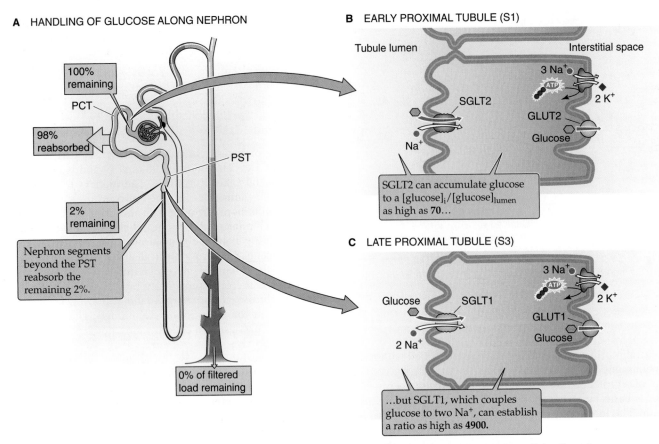

Figure 36-3 **A** to **C**, Glucose handling by the kidney. The *yellow box* indicates the fraction of the filtered load that the proximal tubule reabsorbs. The *green boxes* indicate the fraction of the filtered load that remains in the lumen at various sites. The values in the boxes are approximations. PCT, proximal convoluted tubule; PST, proximal straight tubule.

SGLTs, the basolateral GLUTs differ between early and late proximal tubule segments, with GLUT2 in the early proximal tubule (Fig. 36-3B) and GLUT1 in the late proximal tubule (Fig. 36-3C). In contrast to the apical SGLTs, the basolateral GLUTs have a much lower sensitivity to phloridzin.

Glucose excretion in the urine occurs only when the plasma concentration exceeds a threshold

The relationship between plasma [glucose] and the rate of glucose reabsorption is the **glucose titration curve**. Figure 36-4A shows how rates of glucose filtration (orange curve), excretion (green), and reabsorption (red) vary when one increases plasma [glucose] by infusing intravenous glucose. As plasma [glucose] rises—at a constant GFR—from control levels to ~200 mg/dL, glucose excretion remains zero. It is only above a **threshold** of ~200 mg/dL (~11 mM) that glucose appears in the urine. Glucose excretion rises linearly as plasma [glucose] increases further. Because the threshold is considerably higher than the normal plasma [glucose] of ~100 mg/dL (~5.5 mM), and because the body effectively regulates plasma [glucose] (see Chapter 51), healthy people do not excrete any glucose in the urine, even after a meal.

Likewise, patients with *diabetes mellitus*, who have chronically elevated plasma glucose concentrations, do not experience glucosuria until the blood sugar level exceeds this threshold value.

The glucose titration curve shows a second property—**saturation**. The rate of glucose reabsorption reaches a plateau (T_m) at ~400 mg/min. The reason for the T_m value is that the low-capacity SGLT (i.e., SGLT1) in the late proximal tubule—and perhaps even the high-capacity cotransporter (i.e., SGLT2) in the early proximal tubule—now become fully saturated. Therefore, these transporters cannot respond to further increases in filtered glucose.

Figure 36-4A also shows that the rate of glucose reabsorption reaches the T_m gradually, not abruptly. This **splay** in the titration curve probably reflects both anatomical and kinetic differences among nephrons. Therefore, a particular nephron's filtered load of glucose may be mismatched to its capacity to reabsorb glucose. For example, a nephron with a larger glomerulus has a larger load of glucose to reabsorb. Different nephrons may have different distributions and densities of SGLT2 and SGLT1 along the proximal tubule. Accordingly, saturation in different nephrons may occur at different plasma levels.

At low filtered glucose loads, when no glucose appears in the urine (Fig. 36-4A), the *clearance* (see Chapter 33) of

A GLUCOSE TITRATION CURVE

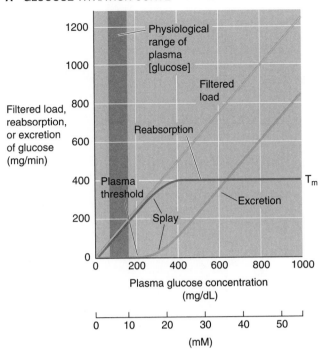

B GLUCOSE CLEARANCE

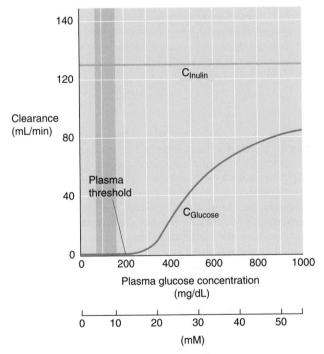

Figure 36-4 The effect of increasing plasma glucose concentrations on glucose excretion and clearance. In **A**, T_m is the transport maximum for reabsorption. In **A** and **B**, the *darker vertical bands* represent the physiological range of plasma [glucose], which spans from a fasting [glucose] to the peak value after a meal.

glucose is zero. As the filtered load increases beyond the threshold, and glucose excretion increases linearly with plasma [glucose], the clearance of glucose progressively increases. At extremely high glucose loads, when the amount of glucose reabsorbed becomes small compared with the filtered load, glucose behaves more like inulin (i.e., it remains in the tubule lumen). Thus, if we replot the glucose excretion data in Figure 36-4A as *clearance* (i.e., excretion divided by plasma [glucose]), we see that, as the filtered glucose load rises, glucose clearance (Fig. 36-4B, red curve) approaches inulin clearance (orange).

The four key characteristics of glucose transport—(1) threshold, (2) saturation (T_m), (3) splay, and (4) clearance approaching GFR at infinite plasma concentrations—apply to several other solutes as well, including amino acids, Krebs cycle intermediates (e.g., acetate, citrate, and α-ketoglutarate [α-KG]), PAH, and phosphate.

OTHER ORGANIC SOLUTES

The proximal tubule reabsorbs amino acids using a wide variety of apical and basolateral transporters

The total concentration of amino acids in the blood is ~2.4 mM. These L-amino acids are largely those absorbed by the gastrointestinal tract (see Chapter 45), although they also may be the products of protein catabolism or of the de novo synthesis of nonessential amino acids.

The glomeruli freely filter amino acids (Fig. 36-5A). Because amino acids are important nutrients, it is advantageous to retrieve them from the filtrate. The proximal tubule reabsorbs more than 98% of these amino acids by a transcellular route, using a wide variety of amino acid transporters, some of which have overlapping substrate specificity (Table 36-1). At the *apical* membrane, amino acids enter the cell by Na⁺-driven or H⁺-driven transporters as well as amino acid exchangers (Fig. 36-5B). At the *basolateral* membrane, amino acids exit the cell by amino acid exchangers—some of which are Na⁺ dependent—and also by facilitated diffusion (see Chapter 5). Particularly in the late proximal tubule and "postproximal" nephron segments, where the availability of luminal amino acids is low, SLC38A3 mediates the Na⁺-dependent uptake of amino acids across the basolateral membrane. This process is important for cellular nutrition or for metabolism. For example, in proximal tubule cells, SLC38A3 takes up glutamine—the precursor for NH_4^+ synthesis and gluconeogenesis (see Chapter 58 and Fig. 39-5A).

For an amino acid to cross the proximal tubule epithelium, it must move through both an apical and a basolateral transporter. For example, **glutamate** enters the cell across the apical membrane through SLC1A1. This transporter simultaneously takes up Na⁺ and H⁺ in exchange for K⁺ (Fig. 36-5B). Inside the cell, glutamate can be metabolized to α-KG in the synthesis of NH_4^+ and gluconeogenesis, or it can exit across the basolateral membrane, perhaps by SLC1A4 or SLC1A5. The positively charged **lysine** and **arginine** cross the apical membrane in exchange for neutral amino acids, mediated by the heterodimeric transporter SLC7A9/SLC3A1.

A HANDLING OF AMINO ACIDS ALONG NEPHRON

B AMINO-ACID REABSORPTION BY PROXIMAL TUBULE

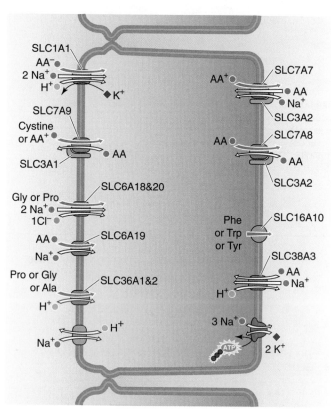

Figure 36-5 **A** and **B**, Amino acid handling by the kidney. In **A**, the *yellow box* indicates the fraction of the filtered load that the proximal tubule reabsorbs. The *green boxes* indicate the fraction of the filtered load that remains in the lumen at various sites. The values in the boxes are approximations. PCT, proximal convoluted tubule; PST, proximal straight tubule.

This process is driven by the cell-negative voltage and by relatively high intracellular concentrations of the neutral amino acids. Lysine and arginine exit across the basolateral membrane through the electroneutral, heterodimeric transporter SLC7A7/SLC3A2, which simultaneously takes up Na^+ and a neutral amino acid. **Neutral amino acids** other than proline can cross the apical membrane through SLC6A19, driven by Na^+, and exit across the basolateral membrane through the heterodimeric SLC7A8/SLC3A2, which exchanges neutral amino acids. Neutral aromatic amino acids such as tyrosine, can exit by facilitated diffusion, mediated by SLC16A10. **Proline** enters across the apical membrane together with H^+ through SLC36A1 and exits across the basolateral membrane through the neutral amino acid exchanger SLC7A8/SLC3A2.

Because the same carrier can reabsorb structurally similar amino acids, *competitive inhibition* may occur in the presence of two related amino acids. This effect may explain why the tubules do not fully reabsorb some amino acids (e.g., glycine, histidine, and some nonproteogenic amino acids, such as L-methylhistidine and taurine), even though the transporter itself is normal. Competition can also occur in patients with hyperargininemia (Table 36-2; see also the box titled Hyperaminoacidurias).

Apparent competition between transported solutes occurs when they compete for the same energy source. Because the apical uptake of many organic and some inorganic solutes

(e.g., phosphate, sulfate) depends on the electrochemical Na^+ gradient, increasing the activity of one such transporter can slow others. For example, glucose uptake by electrogenic Na^+/glucose cotransport may compromise the reabsorption of some amino acids for two reasons: (1) raising $[Na^+]$ diminishes the chemical Na^+ gradient for other Na^+-driven transporters; and (2) carrying net positive charge into the cell depolarizes the apical membrane, thus decreasing the electrical gradient.

With a few exceptions, the kinetics of amino acid reabsorption resembles that of glucose: The titration curves show saturation and transport maxima (T_m). In contrast to the case of glucose, in which the T_m is relatively high, the T_m values for amino acids are generally low. As a consequence, when plasma levels of amino acids increase, the kidneys excrete the amino acids in the urine, thus limiting the maximal plasma levels.

An H^+-driven cotransporter takes up oligopeptides across the apical membrane, whereas endocytosis takes up proteins and other large organic molecules

Oligopeptide The proximal tubules reabsorb ~99% of filtered oligopeptides (Fig. 36-6). Segments beyond the proximal tubule contribute little to peptide transport.

Table 36-1 Amino Acid Transporters*

Apical Uptake				
Human Gene Symbols	**Protein Names**	**Luminal Substrates**	**Other Transported Species**	**Location**
SLC1A1	(System X$_{AG}^-$) EAAT3, EAAC1	Anionic (or acidic) amino acids (Glu and Asp)	Cotransports 2 Na$^+$ and 1 H$^+$ inward, exchanges 1 K$^+$ outward (Electrogenic uptake of net + charge)	Kidney, small intestine, brain
Heterodimer: SLC7A9 SLC3A1	(System b^{0+}) b$^{0,+}$AT rBAT	Cationic (i.e., basic) amino acids (Lys$^+$ or Arg$^+$) or cystine (Cys-S-S-Cys)	Exchanges for neutral amino acid (Electrogenic uptake of + charge when substrate is Lys$^+$ or Arg$^+$)	Kidney—cystinuria
SLC6A14	(System B^{0+}) ATB^{0+}	Neutral and cationic amino acids	Cotransports 2 Na$^+$ and 1 Cl$^-$	Small intestine
SLC6A18	(System Gly) XT2	Gly	Cotransports with Na$^+$ and Cl$^-$	Kidney
SLC6A19 SLC6A15	(System B^0) B^{0}AT1 B^{0}AT2	Neutral amino acids (not Pro), including aromatic amino acids (Phe, Trp, Tyr)	Cotransports with Na$^+$ (No Cl$^-$)	Kidney—Hartnup Kidney, brain
SLC6A20	(System IMINO) SIT, XT3	Proline, imino acids	Cotransports 2 Na$^+$ and 1 Cl$^-$	Kidney, small intestine, brain
SLC36A1	PAT1, LYAAT1	Pro, Ala, Gly, and imino acids	Cotransports with H$^+$	Small intestine, colon, kidney, brain
SLC36A2	PAT2	Pro, Ala, Gly, and amino acids	Cotransports with H$^+$	Kidney, heart, lung

Basolateral Exit				
Human Gene Symbols	**Protein Names**	**Cytoplasmic Substrates**	**Other Transported Species**	**Location**
SLC6A5 SLC6A9	(System GLY) GLYT2 GLYT1	Glycine (also *N*-methylglycine, i.e., sarcosine)	Cotransports Na$^+$ and Cl$^-$	Small intestine
Heterodimer: SLC7A7 SLC3A2	(System y$^+$L) y$^+$LAT1 4F2hc	Cationic (i.e., basic) amino acids (Arg$^+$, Lys$^+$, ornithine$^+$)	Exchanges for extracellular neutral amino acid plus Na$^+$	Kidney, small intestine
Heterodimer: SLC7A8 SLC3A2	(System L) LAT2 4F2hc	Neutral amino acids	Exchanges for neutral extracellular amino acid	Kidney
SLC16A10	TAT1	Aromatic amino acids (Phe, Trp, Tyr)	None (facilitated diffusion)	Kidney
SLC38A1,2,4	(System A) SNAT1,2,4	Gln, Ala, Asn, Cys, His, Ser	Cotransports Na$^+$	Small intestine

Basolateral Nutritional Uptake				
Human Gene Symbols	**Protein Names**	**Basolateral Substrates**	**Other Transported Species**	**Location**
SLC38A3	(System N) SNAT3	Gln, Asn, His	Cotransports Na$^+$ inward, exchanges H$^+$ outward	Kidney
SLC1A4 SLC1A5	(System ASC) ASCT1 ASCT2	Ala, Ser, Cys, Thr	Exchanges for extracellular neutral amino acids. Na$^+$ dependent	Kidney, small intestine

Continued

Table 36-1 Amino Acid Transporters—cont'd

Uptake by Other Tissues				
Human Gene Symbols	**Protein Names**	**Extracellular Substrates**	**Other Transported Species**	**Location**
SLC1A2	EAAT2, GLT-1	Anionic (or acidic) amino acids (Glu and Asp)	Cotransports 2 Na^+ and 1 H^+ inward, exchanges 1 K^+ outward (Electrogenic uptake of net + charge)	Brain (astrocytes), liver
SLC1A3	EAAT1, GLAST			Brain (astrocytes), heart, skeletal muscle
SLC1A6	EAAT4			Brain (cerebellum)
SLC1A7	EAAT5			Retina
SLC6A1	GAT1	GABA (also betaine, β-alanine, taurine)	Cotransports Na^+ and Cl^-	Brain (GABAergic neurons)
SLC6A11	GAT3			Brain (GABAergic neurons), kidney
SLC6A12	BGT1			Kidney, brain
SLC6A13	GAT2			Brain (choroid plexus), retina, liver, kidney

*The "System" designation is a historical classification is based on functional characteristics in intact epithelia, intact cells, or membrane vesicles.

Table 36-2 Patterns of Hyperaminoacidurias

	Disease	**Amino Acids**	**Mechanism**
A. Prerenal Hyperaminoaciduria ("Overflow")	Hyperargininemia	Arg	Elevated plasma concentration and thus elevated filtered load overwhelms T_m
B. Competition	Side effect of hyperargininemia	Lys Ornithine	High filtered load of one amino acid (e.g., Arg) inhibits the reabsorption of another, both carried SLC7A9(b^{0+}AT1)/ SLC3A1 (rBAT)
C. Renal Aminoaciduria	Anionic aminoaciduria	Glu Asp	Defective SLC1A1 (EAAT3); autosomal recessive disease
	Hartnup disease (neutral aminoaciduria)	Neutral and ring-structure amino acids (e.g., phenylalanine)	Defective SLC6A19 (B^0AT1); autosomal recessive disease
	Cystinuria (cationic aminoaciduria)	Cystine (Cys-S-S-Cys) and cationic amino acids	Defective SLC7A9 (b^{0+}AT1) or SLC3A1 (rBAT); autosomal recessive disease
	Lysinuric protein intolerance (cationic aminoaciduria)	Lys Arg	Defective SLC7A7 (y^+LAT1) or SLC3A2 (4F2hc) Autosomal recessive disease
D. Generalized Proximal Tubule Dysfunction	Fanconi syndrome	All amino acids	Metabolic, immune, or toxic conditions (inherited or acquired) that impair function of the proximal tubule cell

Several peptidases are present at the outer surface of the brush border membrane of proximal tubule cells (Fig. 36-6B), just as they are in the small intestine (see Chapter 45). These brush border enzymes (e.g., γ-glutamyltransferase, aminopeptidases, endopeptidases, and dipeptidases) hydrolyze many peptides, including angiotensin II (see Chapter 40), thereby releasing into the tubule lumen the free constituent amino acids and oligopeptides. Tubule cells reabsorb the resulting free amino acids as described in the previous section. The cell also absorbs the resulting oligopeptides (2 to 5 residues)—as well as other peptides (e.g., carnosine) that are resistant to brush border enzymes—using the apical H/oligopeptide cotransporters **PepT1** and **PepT2** (see Chapter 5). PepT1 is a low-affinity/high-capacity system in the early proximal tubule, whereas PepT2 is a high-affinity/low-capacity transporter in the late proximal segments, analogous to the properties of SGLT2 and SGLT1.

Hyperaminoacidurias

In general, an increase in the renal excretion of an amino acid (**hyperaminoaciduria**) may occur when the plasma concentration increases owing to any of several metabolic derangements, or when the carrier-mediated reabsorption of the amino acid decreases abnormally.

Prerenal (i.e., the Defect Is *Before* the Kidney) Hyperaminoacidurias

Hyperargininemia (Table 36-2A) is an inherited condition in which a metabolic defect leads to an increase in plasma arginine (Arg) levels that, in turn, increases the filtered load of Arg. Although the reabsorption of Arg increases, the filtered load exceeds the T_m, and the renal excretion increases.

Competition

Because the same transporter (the heterodimeric SLC7A9/SLC3A1 in Table 45-3) that carries Arg across the apical membrane also transports lysine (Lys) and ornithine, competition from Arg decreases the reabsorption of the other two (Table 36-2B). As a result, the urinary excretion of Lys and ornithine also increases. Because the metabolic production of Lys and ornithine does not change, plasma concentrations of these two amino acids, in contrast to that of Arg, usually fall.

Renal Aminoacidurias

This category of diseases results from an autosomal recessive defect in an amino acid transporter (Table 36-2C), and thus also affects absorption in the gastrointestinal tract (see Chapter 45 for the box on Defects in Apical Amino Acid Transport:

Hartnup Disease and Cystinuria). In **Hartnup disease**, the defective apical transporter (SLC6A19) normally handles neutral amino acids (e.g., Ala, Ser), including those with rings (i.e., Phe, Trp, Tyr). In **cystinuria,** the affected apical transporter is the heterodimeric SLC7A9/SLC3A1 that carries cystine (Cys-S-S-Cys) and cationic amino acids (i.e., Arg, Lys, ornithine). An increased filtered load of one of these amino acids leads to increased excretion of all of them. Nephrolithiasis (i.e., kidney stones) may be a consequence of the increased excretion of the poorly soluble cystine.

Probably the most severe renal hyperaminoaciduria is **lysinuric protein intolerance** (LPI), resulting from the reduced reabsorption of Lys and Arg. The resulting low blood [Arg] impairs the urea cycle and detoxification of ammonium (hyperammonemia). Other features include alveolar proteinosis (the leading cause of death), hepatosplenomegaly, and—in severe cases—mental deterioration. The defective proximal tubule basolateral transporter (the heterodimeric SLC7A7/SLC3A2) normally mediates the efflux of Arg and Lys into blood in exchange for the uptake of Na^+ and neutral amino acids.

Generalized Proximal Tubule Dysfunction

The Fanconi syndrome (Table 36-2D), which can be inherited or acquired, is characterized by a generalized loss of proximal tubule function. The kidney fails to reabsorb appropriately not only amino acids, but also Na^+, Cl^-, HCO_3^-, glucose, and water.

A HANDLING OF OLIGOPEPTIDES ALONG NEPHRON

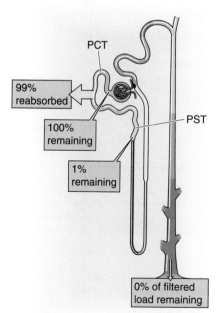

B PROXIMAL TUBULE: OLIGOPEPTIDES

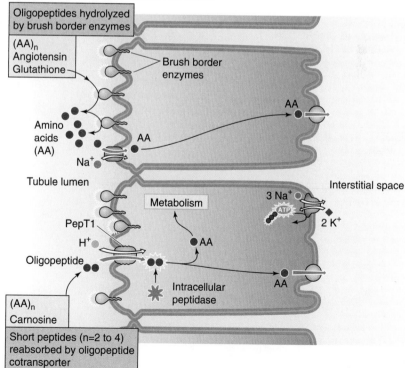

Figure 36-6 **A** and **B**, Oligopeptide handling by the kidney. In **A**, the *yellow box* indicates the fraction of the filtered load that the proximal tubule reabsorbs. The *green boxes* indicate the fraction of the filtered load that remains in the lumen at various sites. The values in the boxes are approximations. PCT, proximal convoluted tubule; PST, proximal straight tubule.

Once inside the cell, the oligopeptides undergo hydrolysis by cytosolic peptidases; this pathway is involved in the degradation of neurotensin and bradykinin. The distinction between which oligopeptides the cells fully digest in the lumen and which they take up through a PepT is not clearcut. Oligopeptides that are more resistant to hydrolysis by peptidases are probably more likely to enter through a PepT.

Proteins Although the glomerular filtration barrier (see Chapter 33) generally prevents the filtration of large amounts of protein, this restriction is incomplete (see Chapter 34). For example, the albumin concentration in the filtrate is very low (4 to 20 mg/L), only 0.01% to 0.05% of the plasma albumin concentration. Nevertheless, given a GFR of 180 L/day, the filtered albumin amounts to 0.7 to 3.6 g/day. In contrast, albumin excretion in the urine normally is only ~30 mg/day. Thus, the tubules reabsorb some 96% to 99% of filtered albumin (Fig. 36-7A). In addition to albumin, the tubules extensively reabsorb other proteins (e.g., lysozyme, light chains of immunoglobulins, and β_2-microglobulin), SH-containing peptides (e.g., insulin), and other polypeptide hormones (e.g., parathyroid hormone [PTH], atrial natriuretic peptide [ANP], and glucagon). It is not surprising that tubule injury can give rise to proteinuria even in the absence of glomerular injury.

Proximal tubule cells use **receptor-mediated endocytosis** (see Chapter 5) to reabsorb proteins and polypeptides (Fig. 36-7B). The first step is binding to receptors at the apical membrane (e.g., megalin, cubilin), followed by internalization into clathrin-coated endocytic vesicles. Factors that interfere with vesicle formation or internalization, such as metabolic inhibitors and cytochalasin B, inhibit this selective absorption. The vesicles fuse with endosomes; this fusion recycles the vesicle membrane to the apical surface and targets their content for delivery to lysosomes. At the lysosomes, acid-dependent proteases largely digest the contents over a period that is on the order of minutes for peptide hormones and many hours or even days for other proteins. The cells ultimately release the low-molecular-weight end products of digestion, largely amino acids, across the basolateral membrane into the peritubular circulation. Although the proximal tubule hardly reabsorbs any protein in an intact state, a small subset of proteins avoids the lysosomes and moves by transcytosis for release at the basolateral membrane.

In addition to the apical absorption and degradation pathway, the kidney has two other pathways for protein degradation. The first may be important for several bioactive proteins, particularly those for which receptors are present on the basolateral membrane (e.g., insulin, ANP, AVP, and PTH). After transcytosis, the proximal tubule cell partially hydrolyzes peptide hormones at the basolateral cell membrane. The resulting peptide fragments re-enter the circulation, where they are available for glomerular filtration and ultimate handling by the apical absorption/degradation pathway. The second alternative pathway for protein degradation involves receptor-mediated endocytosis by endothelial cells of the renal vascular and glomerular structures. This pathway participates in the catabolism of small peptides, such as ANP.

In conclusion, the kidney plays a major role in the metabolism of small proteins and peptide hormones. Renal extraction rates may be large, and they account for as much as 80%

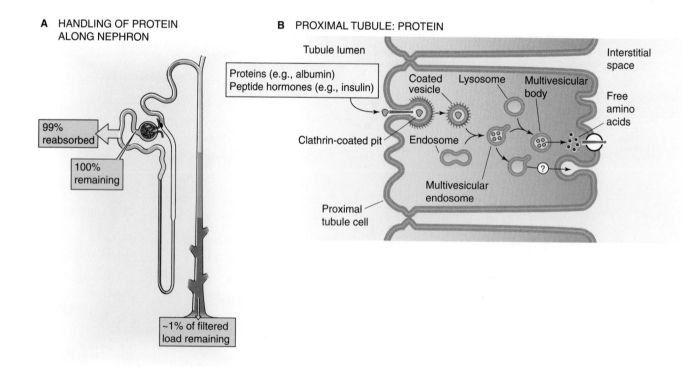

A HANDLING OF PROTEIN ALONG NEPHRON

99% reabsorbed

100% remaining

~1% of filtered load remaining

B PROXIMAL TUBULE: PROTEIN

Tubule lumen

Proteins (e.g., albumin)
Peptide hormones (e.g., insulin)

Coated vesicle

Lysosome

Multivesicular body

Interstitial space

Free amino acids

Clathrin-coated pit

Endosome

Proximal tubule cell

Multivesicular endosome

Figure 36-7 **A** and **B**, Protein handling by the kidney. In **A**, the *yellow box* indicates the fraction of the filtered load that the proximal tubule reabsorbs. The *green boxes* indicate the fraction of the filtered load that remains in the lumen at various sites. The values in the boxes are approximations.

of the total metabolic clearance. Thus, it is not surprising that end-stage renal disease can lead to elevated levels of glucagon, PTH, gastrin, and ANP. Under physiological conditions, glomerular filtration represents the rate-limiting step for the removal of low-molecular-weight proteins from the circulation—apical absorption by the tubules, intracellular hydrolysis, and peritubular hydrolysis do not saturate over a wide range of filtered loads.

Two separate apical Na⁺-driven cotransporters reabsorb monocarboxylates and dicarboxylates/tricarboxylates

The combined concentration of carboxylates in the blood plasma is a few millimolars, of which lactate represents the largest fraction. The monocarboxylates pyruvate and lactate are products of anaerobic glucose metabolism (see Chapter 58). The dicarboxylates and tricarboxylates include intermediates of the **citric acid cycle**. Because these carboxylates are important for energy metabolism, their loss in the urine would be wasteful. Normally, the proximal tubule reabsorbs virtually all these substances (Fig. 36-8A).

At least two distinct Na⁺-dependent cotransporters carry carboxylates across the apical membranes (Fig. 36-8B). One system is specific for monocarboxylates, including lactate, pyruvate, acetoacetate, and β-hydroxybutyrate. A second cotransporter (NaDC1 or SLC13A2) carries dicarboxylates and tricarboxylates, such as α-KG, malate, succinate, and citrate. Once inside the cell, the monocarboxylates exit across

the basolateral membrane through an H⁺/monocarboxylate cotransporter 2 (MCT2, SLC16A7). Because monocarboxylates enter across the apical membrane coupled to Na⁺, and then exit across the basolateral membrane coupled to H⁺, monocarboxylate reabsorption leads to an accumulation of Na⁺ by the cell and a rise in intracellular pH.

Dicarboxylates exit the cell across the basolateral membrane through multiple organic anion-carboxylate exchangers (e.g., the renal organic anion transporter OAT1 and OAT3; see Chapter 5) that may overlap in substrate specificity or may even carry anions of different valence. Because the molecular identities and stoichiometries of some of these transporters are unknown, we present organic anion exchangers in a generic sense in this and the next three sections.

Although the proximal tubule normally reabsorbs carboxylates fully, carboxylates may appear in the urine when their plasma levels are elevated. Urinary excretion may occur when the filtered load of acetoacetate and β-hydroxybutyrate—ketone bodies (see Chapter 51) produced during starvation or during low-insulin states (diabetes mellitus)—exceeds the T_m in the proximal tubule.

Proximal tubule transport of PAH is an example of a T_m-limited secretory mechanism

The kidneys handle PAH (a monovalent anion), as well as many organic anions (e.g., many metabolites of endogenous compounds and administered drugs), by both filtration and

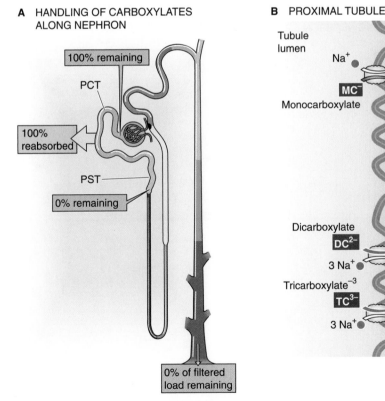

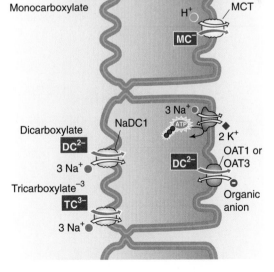

A HANDLING OF CARBOXYLATES ALONG NEPHRON

B PROXIMAL TUBULE

Figure 36-8 **A** and **B**, Monocarboxylate, dicarboxylate, and tricarboxylate handling by the kidney. In **A**, the *yellow box* indicates the fraction of the filtered load that the proximal tubule reabsorbs. The *green boxes* indicate the fraction of the filtered load that remains in the lumen at various sites. The values in the boxes are approximations. MCT, H⁺/monocarboxylate cotransporter; PCT, proximal convoluted tubule; PST, proximal straight tubule.

secretion (Fig. 36-9A). The synthetic anion PAH is somewhat unusual in that ~20% of it binds to plasma proteins, largely albumin. Thus, only ~80% of PAH is available for filtration. Assuming a filtration fraction (see Chapter 34) of 20%, only 80% × 20%, or 16%, of the arterial load of PAH appears in Bowman's space. Nevertheless, at low plasma [PAH], the kidneys excrete into the urine nearly all (~90%) of the PAH entering the renal arteries, so that very little PAH remains in the renal veins. Because the kidneys almost completely clear it from the blood in a single passage, PAH is useful for measuring renal plasma flow (see Chapter 34).

The nephron secretes PAH mainly in the late proximal tubule (S3 segment), and it does so by the transcellular route, against a sizable electrochemical gradient. PAH uptake across the *basolateral* membrane occurs through the high-affinity OAT1 and the lower-affinity OAT3 transporters, driven by the outward gradient of the α-KG, which is a dicarboxylate (Fig. 36-9B). This uptake of PAH is an example of *tertiary active transport* because the basolateral Na/dicarboxylate cotransporter NaDC3—in a process of *secondary active transport*—elevates α-KG in the cell, thereby creating the outward α-KG gradient. NaDC3 carries three Na^+ ions and one dicarboxylate into the cell. Finally, the basolateral Na-K pump—in a process of *primary active transport*—establishes the Na^+ gradient used to drive the accumulation of α-KG.

The apical step of PAH secretion probably occurs through exchange for luminal anions or through electrogenic facilitated diffusion, driving by the inside-negative membrane potential. Several anionic drugs (e.g., probenecid) that compete at the basolateral PAH-anion exchanger or the apical PAH-anion exchanger inhibit PAH secretion from blood to lumen.

Just as glucose reabsorption saturates at its T_m as one increases plasma [glucose], PAH secretion (Fig. 36-10A, red curve) saturates at a sufficiently high plasma [PAH]. Starting from an initially low value, increasing plasma [PAH] causes excretion (green) to rise much faster than filtration (orange). Subtracting the amount filtered from the amount excreted, we see that the rate of PAH secretion at first rises rapidly with plasma [PAH]. However, as plasma [PAH] approaches ~20 mg/dL, the amount of secreted PAH reaches a plateau (T_m), typically 60 to 80 mg/min, indicating saturation of secretory mechanisms.

After plasma [PAH] has increased enough to reach the T_m, further increases in plasma [PAH] increase urinary excretion, but only as a consequence of the increase in the filtered load, not because of increased tubule secretion. At these high plasma PAH levels, the kidneys can no longer fully remove PAH from the blood in a single pass, and therefore it would no longer be appropriate to use PAH secretion to estimate renal plasma flow. At low plasma [PAH] values (<12 mg/dL), PAH extraction from plasma flowing through the kidney is nearly complete (~90%), forming the basis for using PAH clearance as a measure of renal plasma flow.

Recall that as plasma [glucose] increases, glucose clearance *rises* to approach inulin clearance (Fig. 36-4B). In contrast, PAH clearance (Fig. 36-10B, red curve) *decreases* with

A HANDLING OF PAH ALONG NEPHRON

B LATE PROXIMAL TUBULE (S3)

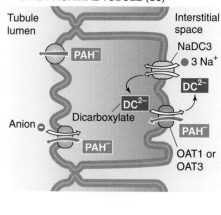

Figure 36-9 **A** and **B**, PAH handling by the kidney. In **A**, the *red box* indicates the fraction of the filtered load secreted by the proximal tubule. The *green boxes* indicate the fraction of the filtered load that remains in the lumen at various sites when plasma [PAH] is low (<12 mg/dL). The values in the boxes are approximations. PCT, proximal convoluted tubule; PST, proximal straight tubule.

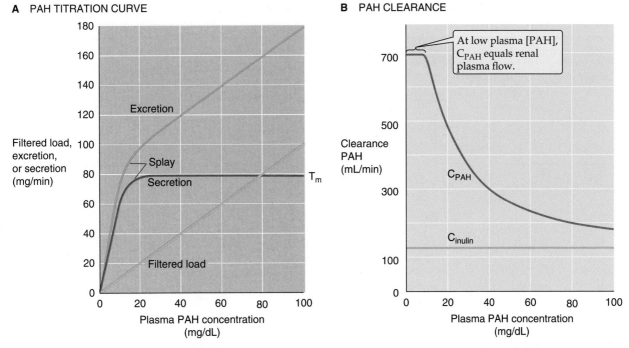

Figure 36-10 **A** and **B**, Effect of increasing plasma PAH concentrations on PAH excretion and clearance. In **A**, T_m represents the transport maximum for reabsorption.

increasing plasma [PAH] and falls to approach inulin clearance (orange). The reason is that, as plasma [PAH] increases, secreted PAH forms a progressively smaller fraction of the PAH appearing in the urine.

Transporters similar to those that secrete PAH also secrete a variety of organic anions

In addition to PAH, the late proximal tubule secretes a wide variety of organic anions. These anions include the following (Table 36-3): (1) endogenous anions, such as oxalate and bile salts; (2) exogenous anions, such as the drugs penicillin and furosemide; and (3) uncharged molecules *conjugated* to anionic groups, such as sulfate or glucuronate (see Chapter 46). The proximal tubule secretes these anions into the lumen by using basolateral and apical anion exchangers that are similar to those involved in PAH secretion (Fig. 36-9B). At the apical membrane, the secreted anion appears to exchange for luminal Cl⁻, urate, or OH⁻.

Although the proximal tubule both reabsorbs and secretes urate, reabsorption usually dominates

Urate, a monovalent anion, is the end product of purine catabolism (Fig. 36-11A). Plasma [urate] is typically 3 to 7 mg/dL (0.2 to 0.4 mM) and is elevated in gout. The glomeruli filter urate, and then the proximal tubule successively reabsorbs (S1 segment), secretes (S2 segment), and again reabsorbs (S3 segment) urate (Fig. 36-11B). Reabsorption is the more important transport pathway, so that the kidneys excrete only ~10% of filtered urate.

Reabsorption Reabsorption of urate occurs by both a paracellular route involving passive diffusion and a transcellular route involving active transport (Fig. 36-11C). The contribution of the paracellular pathway can become apparent during extracellular volume depletion, which can lead to a compensatory enhancement of proximal-tubule fluid reabsorption. Solvent drag (p. 488) can then enhance paracellular urate reabsorption, thereby decreasing urate excretion and raising plasma levels of urate. The transcellular mechanism predominates in the early proximal tubule. The active apical step does not involve Na⁺ cotransport, but rather the exchange of luminal urate for any of a host of intracellular anions. URAT1 exchanges luminal urate for monocarboxylates (e.g., lactate), whereas OAT4 exchanges luminal urate for dicarboxylates. Once inside the cell, urate exits across the basolateral membrane either by facilitated diffusion via OAT2, or by exchange with an organic anion via OAT1 or OAT3.

Uricosuric agents such as probenecid, salicylate, and other non-steroidal anti-inflammatory drugs inhibit URAT1. Indeed, probenecid is useful in the treatment of gout.

Secretion The basolateral step of urate *secretion* (Fig. 36-11D) is mediated by organic anion exchange via reversal of OAT1 and OAT3 (which also mediates basolateral PAH uptake, see Fig. 36-9B), as well as by facilitated diffusion via OAT2. Urate exits the cell across the apical membrane by reversal of OAT4 (Fig. 36-11D), as well as by facilitated diffusion via UAT. Under certain conditions, renal urate excretion can exceed the quantity filtered, indicating net secretion.

Table 36-3 Organic Anions and Cations Secreted by the Late Proximal Tubule

	Anions	Cations
Endogenous	cAMP and cGMP Bile salts Hippurate Oxalate α-Ketoglutarate Short-chain fatty acids Prostaglandins (e.g., PGE$_2$) Urate Creatinine (zwitterion) Uremic organic anions*	Epinephrine Acetylcholine Choline Dopamine Histamine Serotonin Thiamine Guanidine Creatinine (zwitterion)
Exogenous	Acetazolamide Chlorothiazide Furosemide PAH Penicillin G Probenecid Saccharin Salicylate Indomethacin	Atropine Quinine Amiloride Cimetidine NMN Morphine Paraquat Procainamide Tetraethylammonium Chlorpromazine
Conjugated (Endogenous and Exogenous)	Glucuronate conjugates† Glutathione conjugates† Sulfate conjugates†	

*Hippurate-like aryl organic anions that interfere with PAH transport.
†See Chapter 46.
NMN, *N*-methylnicotinamide; PGE$_2$, prostaglandin E$_2$.

The late proximal tubule secretes several organic cations

The late proximal tubule (Fig. 36-12A) is also responsible for secreting a wide range of both endogenous and exogenous organic *cations* (Table 36-3). Some of the most important endogenous organic cations are the monoamine neurotransmitters such as dopamine, epinephrine, norepinephrine, and histamine (see Chapter 13). Exogenous secreted organic cations include morphine, quinine, and the diuretic amiloride (see Chapter 35).

The polyspecific organic cation transporter OCT2 (see SLC22 family in Table 5-4 on p. 118) is responsible for the *basolateral* uptake of these organic cations (Fig. 36-12B). OCT2 mediates facilitated diffusion and is electrogenic.

At the *apical* membrane, an organic cation-H$^+$ exchanger OCTN1 (Fig. 36-12B) moves these cations from the cell to the lumen. The energy for the extrusion of the organic cation is the H$^+$ electrochemical gradient across the apical mem-

brane, from lumen to cell. Because the apical Na-H exchanger *(a secondary active transporter)* is largely responsible for establishing this H$^+$ gradient, the cation-H exchange is an example of tertiary active transport.

An organic cation secreting mechanism is also responsible for secreting creatinine, the breakdown product of phosphocreatine. Despite this modest secretion, creatinine is a useful index of GFR (see Chapter 34).

The nonionic diffusion of neutral weak acids and bases promotes their transport across tubules and explains why their excretion is pH dependent

Many cations or anions are, in fact, weak acids or bases in equilibrium with a neutral species (see Chapter 28), which generally diffuses across a membrane much faster than the corresponding cation or anion. This rapid diffusion usually occurs because the neutral species is far more soluble in the lipid bilayer of cell membranes than is the charged species.

Changing the luminal pH can substantially affect the overall transport of a buffer pair. For example, acidifying the tubule lumen promotes the reabsorption of a neutral weak acid and the secretion of a neutral weak base. In the case of a neutral weak acid such as salicylic acid (Fig. 36-13A), the glomerular filtrate contains both the neutral weak acid (HA) and its conjugate weak base, which is an anion (A$^-$). The secretion of H$^+$ into the lumen (see Chapter 39) titrates the A$^-$ to HA, thus raising luminal [HA] above intracellular [HA], so that HA rapidly diffuses across the apical membrane—by the process of **nonionic diffusion**—into the tubule cell and across the basolateral membrane into the blood. The more acidic the luminal fluid, the greater is the titration of A$^-$ to HA, and the greater is the nonionic diffusion of HA from lumen to blood.

In the case of a weak base such as ammonia (Fig. 36-13B), the glomerular filtrate contains both the neutral weak base (B) and the cationic species (BH$^+$). The secretion of H$^+$ into the lumen titrates B to BH$^+$, thus lowering luminal [B] below intracellular [B], so that B rapidly diffuses from cell to lumen. The resulting fall in intracellular [B] sets up a gradient for B to diffuse from blood to cell. The more acidic the luminal fluid, the greater is the titration of B to BH$^+$, and the greater is the nonionic diffusion of B from blood to lumen.

A striking example of how luminal pH affects the clearance of a weak acid is the renal handling of salicylic acid and its anion species, salicylate. At a urinary pH of ~7.5, the amount of total salicylate (salicylic acid + salicylate anion) excreted is the same as the filtered load (Fig. 36-13C); that is, the clearance of total salicylate (C$_{Salicylate}$) equals GFR. Lower urinary pH values favor the titration of luminal salicylate anion to salicylic acid, which the tubule readily reabsorbs. Hence, lowering pH causes the fractional excretion of total salicylate (FE$_{Salicylate}$ = C$_{Salicylate}$/GFR; see Chapter 33) to fall to less than unity. At very low urinary pH values, the kidney reabsorbs virtually all salicylate, and FE$_{Salicylate}$ approaches zero. However, at urinary pH values higher than ~7.5, FE$_{Salicylate}$ increases markedly because the alkalinity keeps luminal levels of the salicylate anion high and levels of salicylic acid low, so that the neutral weak acid now diffuses from blood to lumen.

A URIC ACID AND URATE

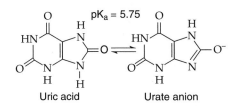

$pK_a = 5.75$

Uric acid ⇌ Urate anion

C PROXIMAL TUBULE: URATE REABSORPTION (S1,S3)

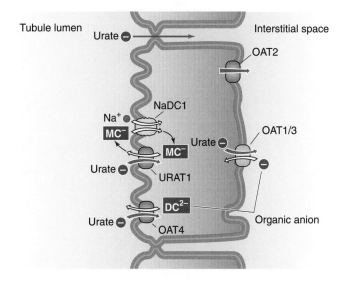

B HANDLING OF URATE ALONG NEPHRON

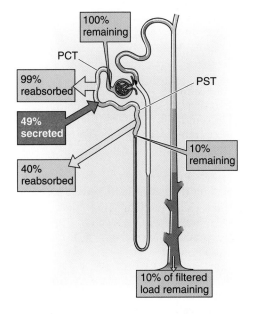

D PROXIMAL TUBULE: URATE SECRETION (S2)

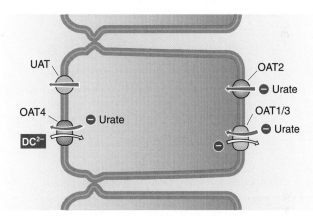

Figure 36-11 **A** and **B**, Urate handling by the kidney. In **A**, the *yellow arrows* indicate reabsorption, whereas the *red arrow* indicates secretion. The *green boxes* indicate the fraction of the filtered load remaining at various sites. The values in the boxes are approximations. In **B**, the molecular identities of the apical and basolateral urate transporters are unknown. PCT, proximal convoluted tubule; PST, proximal straight tubule.

It is possible to treat overdoses of salicylate or acetylsalicylate (i.e., aspirin) by alkalinizing the urine with HCO_3^- or by increasing urine flow with diuretics. The reason is that both high pH and high urine flow keep luminal levels of salicylic acid low, thereby maintaining a sink for salicylic acid in the lumen. Both treatments enhance the urinary excretion of the drug and lower plasma concentrations. The converse example of urinary pH dependence is seen in the excretion of a neutral weak base, such as ammonia or quinine (Fig. 36-13D).

PHOSPHATE

As discussed in Chapter 52, the metabolism of inorganic phosphate (P_i) depends on bone, the gastrointestinal tract,

and kidneys. About half of total plasma phosphate (Table 36-4) is in an ionized form, and the rest is either complexed to small solutes (~40%) or bound to protein (10% to 15%). The plasma concentration of total P_i varies rather widely, between 0.8 and 1.5 mM (2.5 to 4.5 mg/dL of elemental phosphorus). Thus, the filterable phosphate (i.e., both the ionized and complexed) varies between ~0.7 and 1.3 mM. At a normal blood pH of 7.4, 80% of the ionized plasma phosphate is HPO_4^{2-}, and the rest is $H_2PO_4^-$. Assuming that the total plasma phosphate concentration is 4.2 mg/dL, that only the free and complexed phosphate is filterable, and that the GFR is 180 L/day, each day the kidneys filter ~7000 mg of phosphate. Because this amount is more than an order of magnitude greater than the total extracellular pool of phosphate (see Chapter 52), it is clear that the kidney must reabsorb most of the phosphate filtered in the glomerulus.

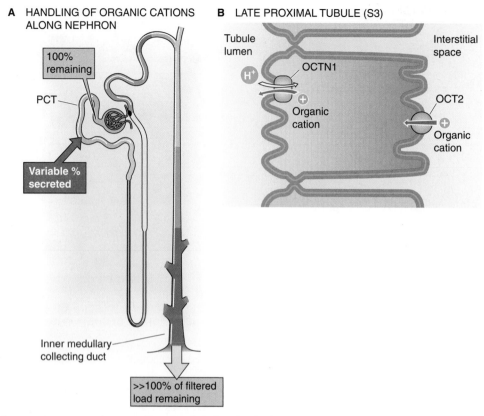

A HANDLING OF ORGANIC CATIONS ALONG NEPHRON

100% remaining

PCT

Variable % secreted

Inner medullary collecting duct

>>100% of filtered load remaining

B LATE PROXIMAL TUBULE (S3)

Tubule lumen

Interstitial space

H⁺

OCTN1

Organic cation

OCT2

Organic cation

Figure 36-12 **A** and **B**, Organic cation handling by the kidney. In **A**, the *red arrow* indicates secretion. The *green boxes* indicate the fraction of the filtered load remaining at various sites. The values in the boxes are approximations. OCT, organic cation transporter; PCT, proximal convoluted tubule.

Table 36-4 Components of Total Plasma Phosphate

	mg/dL	mM	% of Total
Ionized $H_2PO_4^-$ and HPO_4^{2-}	2.1	0.7	50
Diffusible phosphate complexes	1.5	0.5	40
Nondiffusible (protein-bound) phosphate	0.6	0.2	10
Total phosphate	4.2	1.4	100

The proximal tubule reabsorbs phosphate through an apical Na/phosphate cotransporter (NaP$_i$)

The proximal tubule reabsorbs ~80% of the filtered phosphate (Fig. 36-14A). The loop of Henle and the collecting ducts reabsorb only negligible amounts of phosphate, but the classic distal tubule (see Chapter 33) reabsorbs ~10% of the filtered load. The kidneys excrete the remaining ~10% in the urine.

The proximal tubule reabsorbs most of the filtered phosphate by the transcellular route (Fig. 36-14B). Phosphate ions enter the cell across the *apical* membrane by secondary active transport, energized by the apical electrochemical Na⁺ gradient. The apical Na/phosphate cotransporter NaP$_i$-IIa (SLC34A1) translocates three Na⁺ ions and one divalent phosphate ion (HPO_4^{2-}). Thus, the process is electrogenic (net positive charge into the cell). In contrast, NaP$_i$-IIc (SLC34A3)—which is in low abundance in adults—is electroneutral. As pH along the proximal tubule falls, the relative concentration of $H_2PO_4^-$ increases, and overall phosphate uptake becomes even more electrogenic.

Apical phosphate uptake is under the control of intracellular pH as well as luminal pH and [Na⁺]. Intracellular H⁺ appears to stimulate NaP$_i$ allosterically. However, *luminal* H⁺ is a competitive inhibitor of Na⁺ binding to the extracellular face of NaP$_i$, so that when luminal pH falls, it is more difficult for Na⁺ to bind. In addition, even when luminal [Na⁺] is saturating, an acidic luminal pH inhibits phosphate uptake, possibly by shifting the phosphate equilibrium toward $H_2PO_4^-$, which NaP$_i$ may not transport as well as HPO_4^{2-}.

The passive exit of phosphate across the *basolateral* membrane occurs by a mechanism that is not well understood. The basolateral membrane also has a *type III* Na/P$_i$ cotransporter that carries three Na⁺ with each phosphate. It thus mediates electrogenic *uptake* of phosphate—presumably for nutrition of the tubule cells—rather than exit across the basolateral membrane.

Although it is clear that the proximal tubule reabsorbs almost all filtered phosphate at low filtered loads, the role of

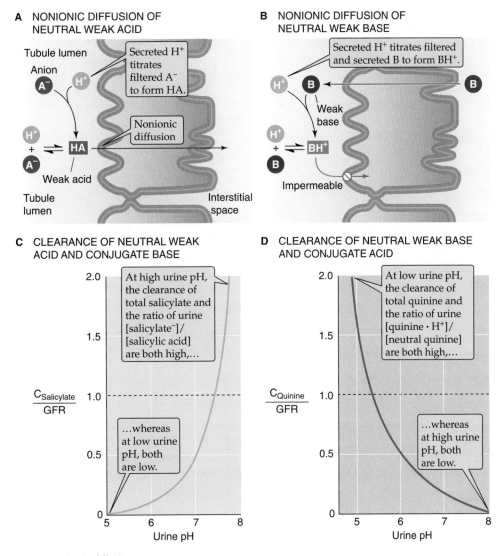

A NONIONIC DIFFUSION OF NEUTRAL WEAK ACID

Tubule lumen

Anion

A⁻

H⁺

Secreted H⁺ titrates filtered A⁻ to form HA.

Nonionic diffusion

H⁺
+
A⁻

HA

Weak acid

Tubule lumen

Interstitial space

B NONIONIC DIFFUSION OF NEUTRAL WEAK BASE

Secreted H⁺ titrates filtered and secreted B to form BH⁺.

H⁺   B   B

Weak base

H⁺
+
B

BH⁺

Impermeable

C CLEARANCE OF NEUTRAL WEAK ACID AND CONJUGATE BASE

$\dfrac{C_{Salicylate}}{GFR}$

At high urine pH, the clearance of total salicylate and the ratio of urine [salicylate⁻]/[salicylic acid] are both high,…

…whereas at low urine pH, both are low.

Urine pH

D CLEARANCE OF NEUTRAL WEAK BASE AND CONJUGATE ACID

$\dfrac{C_{Quinine}}{GFR}$

At low urine pH, the clearance of total quinine and the ratio of urine [quinine · H⁺]/[neutral quinine] are both high,…

…whereas at high urine pH, both are low.

Urine pH

Figure 36-13 **A** to **D**, Nonionic diffusion.

the distal nephron in phosphate handling is controversial. When experimental animals are maintained on a low-phosphate diet, the classic distal tubule absorbs a significant fraction of the filtered load of phosphate, thus minimizing phosphate loss in the urine.

Phosphate excretion in the urine already occurs at physiological plasma concentrations

Phosphate handling by the kidney shares some of the properties of renal glucose handling, including threshold, saturation with T_m kinetics, and splay (Fig. 36-15). However, important differences exist. First, some phosphate excretion (green curve) occurs even at normal levels of plasma [phosphate]. Thus, a small increment in the plasma [phosphate] results in significant acceleration of phosphate excretion (i.e., to higher values along the green curve), whereas plasma [glucose] must double before glucose excretion even commences. Accordingly, the kidney plays an important role in the regulation of plasma [phosphate], but it does not normally modulate plasma [glucose]. Second, the kidney reaches

the T_m for phosphate (red curve) at the high end of normal plasma [phosphate] values, whereas the kidney reaches the T_m for glucose at levels that are far higher than physiological plasma [glucose] levels. Third, the renal phosphate T_m is sensitive to a variety of stimuli, including hormones and acid-base balance, whereas the glucose T_m is insensitive to regulators of glucose metabolism, such as insulin.

Parathyroid hormone, the key regulator of phosphate excretion, inhibits apical sodium/phosphate uptake

Table 36-5 summarizes the major hormones and other factors that regulate phosphate transport by the proximal tubule. Although these factors affect phosphate transport through many different signaling pathways, they fall into two major categories. Some act rapidly and independently of protein synthesis. Others act more slowly, through mechanisms requiring protein synthesis.

The most important hormonal regulator is **PTH**, which inhibits phosphate reabsorption and thus promotes phos-

A HANDLING OF PHOSPHATE ALONG NEPHRON

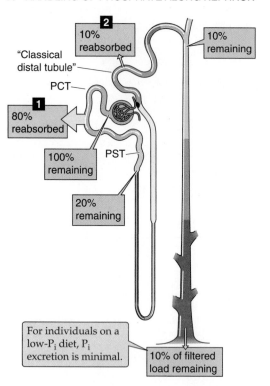

For individuals on a low-P$_i$ diet, P$_i$ excretion is minimal.

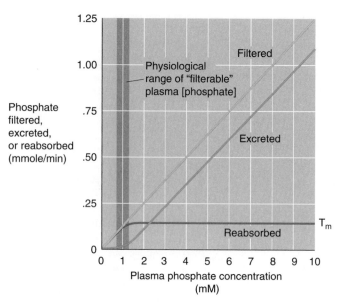

Figure 36-15 Phosphate titration curves. The plasma phosphate concentration is the filterable phosphate (i.e., ionized plus complexed to small solutes). The *dark vertical* band is the approximate range of normal filterable values.

B PROXIMAL TUBULE

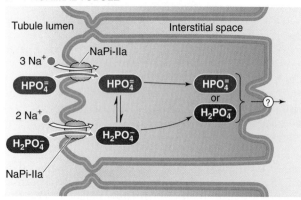

Figure 36-14 **A** and **B**, Phosphate handling by the kidney. In **A**, the numbered *yellow boxes* indicate the fraction of the filtered load that various nephron segments reabsorb. The *green boxes* indicate the fraction of the filtered load that remains in the lumen after these segments. The values in the boxes are approximations. In **B**, the top path illustrates reabsorption of divalent phosphate (HPO$_4^{2-}$), and the bottom path illustrates the reabsorption of monovalent phosphate (H$_2$PO$_4^-$). PCT, proximal convoluted tubule; PST, proximal straight tubule.

Table 36-5 Factors That Modulate Phosphate Excretion

↓ Reabsorption ↑ Excretion	↑ Reabsorption ↓ Excretion
PTH	1,25-dihydroxy-vitamin D
Extracellular volume expansion	High Ca^{2+} intake
High dietary phosphate intake	Phosphate deprivation
High plasma [phosphate]	
Glucocorticoids	Insulin
Acidosis	Alkalosis
Calcitonin	Thyroid hormone
ANP	Growth hormone
Dopamine	
Diuretics	
PTHrP	
Fasting	
Acute renal denervation	
Autosomal and X-linked hypophosphatemia	

PTHrP, PTH-related protein.

phate excretion. PTH is a classic example of a rapid regulator that does *not* require protein synthesis. PTH binds to PTH 1R receptors, which appear to couple to *two* heterotrimeric G proteins (see Chapter 52). The first (Gα$_s$) activates adenylyl cyclase and, through cAMP, stimulates PKA. The second (Gα$_q$), particularly at low PTH levels, activates phospholipase C (PLC), and then protein kinase C (PKC) (see Chapter 3). Once activated, PKA and PKC promote endocytotic removal of NaP$_i$ from the apical membrane, thus reducing phosphate reabsorption. Conversely, when PTH levels decrease, a net insertion of membrane vesicles containing NaP_i occurs, thereby leading to an increase in phosphate reabsorption.

Another inhibitor of phosphate reabsorption, ANP (see Chapter 40), may also activate protein kinase, but it does so through cGMP rather than through cAMP. An additional example of a rapid effect on phosphate reabsorption is extracellular fluid expansion, which accelerates proximal phosphate excretion along with Na^+ excretion (see Chapter 35).

Several modulators of phosphate transport are slow, acting by controlling protein synthesis and thus Na/P_i cotransporter mRNA levels. High dietary phosphate intake decreases phosphate reabsorption, even without changes in PTH levels. Changes in plasma [phosphate], such as those that occur in phosphate depletion or loading, also modulate the balance between retrieval and insertion of Na/P_i cotransporters. Both phosphate depletion and 1,25-dihydroxyvitamin D (see Chapter 52) upregulate the cotransporter. Glucocorticoid excess and metabolic acidosis downregulate the cotransporter; the latter effect is synergistic with the direct effects of H^+ on the NaP_i protein (see earlier). Because phosphate is the primary pH buffer in normal urine, factors that increase urinary [phosphate] (e.g., acidosis) increase the titratable acidity component of renal acid excretion (see Chapter 39).

CALCIUM

Binding to plasma proteins and formation of Ca^{2+}-anion complexes influence the filtration and reabsorption of Ca^{2+}

Whole-body Ca^{2+} balance—as well as the hormonal control of free, ionized plasma calcium (Ca^{2+}) levels—is the subject of Chapter 52. Here we discuss the role of the kidney in Ca^{2+} balance. The *total* concentration of Ca^{2+} in plasma is normally 2.2 to 2.6 mM (8.8 to 10.6 mg/dL). Table 36-6 summarizes the forms of total Ca^{2+} in the plasma. Some 40% binds to plasma proteins, mainly albumin, and constitutes the nonfilterable fraction. The **filterable** portion, ~60% of total plasma Ca^{2+}, consists of two moieties. The first, ~15% of the total, complexes with small anions such as carbonate, citrate, phosphate, and sulfate. The second, ~45% of total Ca^{2+}, is the ionized Ca^{2+} that one may measure with Ca^{2+}-sensitive electrodes or dyes. It is the concentration of this free, ionized Ca^{2+} that the body tightly regulates; plasma $[Ca^{2+}]$ normally is 1.0 to 1.3 mM (4.0 to 5.2 mg/dL).

Table 36-6 Components of Total Plasma Ca^{2+}

	mg/dL	mM	% of Total
Ionized Ca^{2+}	4.7	1.2	~45%
Diffusible Ca^{2+} complexes	1.4	0.3	~15%
Nondiffusible (protein-bound) Ca^{2+}	3.9	1.0	~40%
Total Ca^{2+}	10.0	2.5	100%

The distribution among the various forms of total Ca^{2+} is not fixed. Because H^+ competes with Ca^{2+} for binding to anionic sites on proteins or small molecules, acidosis generally increases plasma $[Ca^{2+}]$. Thus, the decrease in luminal pH that occurs along the nephron (see Chapter 39) makes additional Ca^{2+} available for recovery. In addition, Ca^{2+} binding to proteins in the plasma depends on the concentration of proteins, particularly albumin. A change in the level of the anions with which Ca^{2+} can form complexes also affects the distribution of different Ca^{2+} entities. Tubule cells probably reabsorb Ca^{2+}-anion complexes poorly. However, because the concentration of these anions declines along the nephron owing to anion reabsorption, free Ca^{2+} becomes available for transport.

The proximal tubule reabsorbs a large fraction of filtered Ca^{2+}, with the thick ascending limb and distal convoluted tubule reabsorbing smaller amounts

The kidney reabsorbs ~99% of the filtered load of Ca^{2+}, principally at the proximal tubule, the thick ascending limb (TAL), and the distal convoluted tubule (DCT) (Fig. 36-16A).

Proximal Tubule The proximal tubule reabsorbs ~65% of the filtered Ca^{2+}, a process that is *not* subject to hormonal control. A small part of the Ca^{2+} reabsorbed by the proximal tubule (~20% of the 65%) moves by the *transcellular* route that we discuss in the next section. However, most proximal tubule Ca^{2+} reabsorption (~80% of the ~65%) occurs by the paracellular route (Fig. 36-16B). The evidence for a large component of *paracellular Ca^{2+} transport* is the high Ca^{2+} permeability of the tubule, as well as the sensitivity of net Ca^{2+} transport to changes in the transepithelial electrochemical gradient for Ca^{2+}. For example, imposing a lumen-negative transepithelial voltage induces Ca^{2+} secretion, whereas a lumen-positive voltage induces reabsorption. Because the S2 and S3 segments of the proximal tubule normally have a small lumen-positive voltage, it is not surprising that they are responsible for reabsorbing a large fraction of filtered Ca^{2+} by the paracellular route. In addition to Ca^{2+} *diffusion* through tight junctions, proximal Ca^{2+} reabsorption parallels that of Na^+ and water, a finding suggesting participation of *solvent drag* (see Chapter 20).

Thick Ascending Limb The TAL reabsorbs ~25% of the filtered Ca^{2+} (Fig. 36-16C). Under normal conditions, about half of the Ca^{2+} reabsorption in the TAL occurs passively by a paracellular route, driven by the lumen-positive voltage. Thus, it is not surprising that hormones such as AVP, which make the transepithelial voltage more positive, indirectly increase Ca^{2+} reabsorption. The other half of Ca^{2+} reabsorption by the TAL occurs by the transcellular pathway (see next section), which PTH stimulates.

Distal Convoluted Tubule This segment reabsorbs ~8% of the filtered Ca^{2+} load (Fig. 36-16D). Despite the relatively small amount of Ca^{2+} delivered, the DCT is a major regulatory site for Ca^{2+} excretion. In contrast to the proximal tubule and TAL, the DCT reabsorbs Ca^{2+} predominantly by an active, transcellular route (see next section). Evidence against

A HANDLING OF Ca²⁺ ALONG NEPHRON

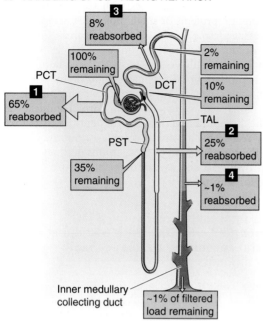

B PROXIMAL TUBULE

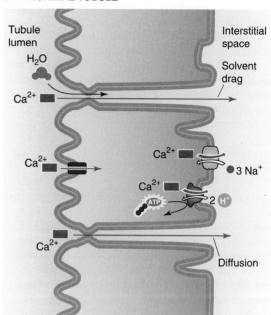

C THICK ASCENDING LIMB (TAL)

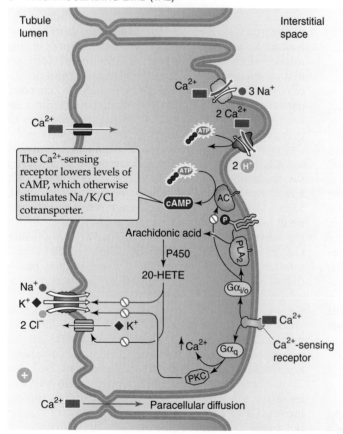

D DISTAL CONVOLUTED TUBULE (DCT)

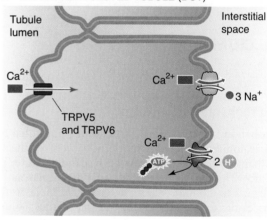

Figure 36-16 **A** to **D**, Calcium handling by the kidney. In **A**, the numbered *yellow boxes* indicate the approximate fraction of the filtered load that various nephron segments reabsorb. The *green boxes* indicate the fraction of the filtered load that remains in the lumen after these segments. The values in the boxes are approximations. AC, adenylyl cyclase; PCT, proximal convoluted tubule; PST, proximal straight tubule.

a substantial component of paracellular Ca^{2+} reabsorption is that—under a variety of experimental maneuvers (see Chapter 36)—it is easy to dissociate Ca^{2+} transport in the DCT from Na^+ and water reabsorption. The quantitative contribution of the collecting ducts and tubules to Ca^{2+} reabsorption is quite small (~1% of the filtered load), and their role in regulating renal Ca^{2+} excretion is not well defined.

Transcellular Ca^{2+} movement is a two-step process, involving passive Ca^{2+} entry through apical channels and basolateral extrusion by electrogenic Na/Ca exchange and a Ca^{2+} pump

We have seen that the contribution of the transcellular route to Ca^{2+} reabsorption increases steadily from the proximal tubule to the TAL and to the DCT. Regardless of the nephron segment, tubule cells apparently use the same general mechanism to move Ca^{2+} through the cell from lumen to blood (Fig. 36-16B-D).

Because $[Ca^{2+}]_i$ is only ~100 nM (~10,000-fold less than in extracellular fluid), and because the membrane voltage across the apical membrane is ~−70 mV, a steep electrochemical gradient favors Ca^{2+} entry across *the apical membrane*. Work on the DCT shows that apical Ca^{2+} entry is passive and is mediated by epithelial Ca^{2+} channels TRP5 and TRP6 (ECaC1 and ECaC2), which are not gated by voltage. This Ca^{2+} channel has consensus phosphorylation sites for PKA, PKC, and cGMP-stimulated protein kinase (PKG), as well as interaction sites for ankyrin (see Chapter 2), a component of the cytoskeleton. Mg^{2+} competes with Ca^{2+} for entry into the cytoplasm, and extracellular H^+ blocks channel activity. Whether similar Ca^{2+} channels play a role in transcellular Ca^{2+} reabsorption in the proximal tubule and TAL is unknown.

As Ca^{2+} enters the tubule cell across the apical membrane, Ca^{2+}-binding proteins buffer the Ca^{2+}, helping to keep $[Ca^{2+}]_i$ low, and maintaining a favorable gradient for Ca^{2+} influx. In addition, Ca^{2+} may temporarily enter certain organelles, particularly the endoplasmic reticulum and mitochondria. In the steady state, however, the cell must extrude across the basolateral membrane all the Ca^{2+} that enters across the apical membrane. Both primary and secondary active transporters participate in this Ca^{2+} extrusion against a steep electrochemical gradient. The primary active transporter is an ATP-driven plasma-membrane Ca^{2+} ATPase or pump (PMCA; see Chapter 5). PMCA is present in several nephron segments, with its highest density in the basolateral membrane of the DCT. Increases in $[Ca^{2+}]_i$—such as those triggered by PTH through PLC and inositol triphosphate (IP_3)—activate calmodulin and thus stimulate PMCA (see Chapter 3).

In addition to the Ca^{2+} pump, an Na-Ca exchanger (NCX; see Chapter 5) also extrudes Ca^{2+} across the basolateral membrane of tubule cells. At physiologically low $[Ca^{2+}]_i$ levels, when the NCX is not very active, the major pathway for Ca^{2+} extrusion is the Ca^{2+} pump. Only when $[Ca^{2+}]_i$ increases does the NCX begin to make a significant contribution. Conversely, if the $[Ca^{2+}]_i$ is normal and the inward Na^+ electrochemical gradient falls (e.g., $[Na^+]_i$ rises), the NCX can reverse direction and load the cell with Ca^{2+}.

Table 36-7 Factors Affecting Ca^{2+} Reabsorption Along the Nephron

Site	Increase Reabsorption	Decrease Reabsorption
Proximal tubule	Volume contraction	Volume expansion
Thick ascending limb	PTH Calcitonin	Furosemide and related diuretics
Distal convoluted tubule	PTH Vitamin D AVP Alkalosis Thiazide diuretics	Phosphate depletion
Collecting duct	Amiloride	—

PTH and vitamin D stimulate—whereas high plasma Ca^{2+} inhibits—Ca^{2+} reabsorption

Table 36-7 summarizes factors that modulate Ca^{2+} handling by various segments of the nephron.

Parathyroid Hormone The most important regulator of renal Ca^{2+} reabsorption is **PTH**, which stimulates Ca^{2+} reabsorption in the TAL, the DCT, and the connecting tubule. PTH appears to increase the open probability of apical Ca^{2+} channels (Fig. 36-16C, D). Such an increase in Ca^{2+} permeability would increase $[Ca^{2+}]_i$, which, in turn, would stimulate basolateral Ca^{2+} extrusion mechanisms, increase Ca^{2+} reabsorption, and raise plasma $[Ca^{2+}]$.

As we saw in our discussion of phosphate handling, PTH acts by binding to the PTH 1R receptor, which apparently couples to *two* heterotrimeric G proteins and activates two kinases (see Chapter 52). Activation of $G\alpha_s$ raises $[cAMP]_i$ and stimulates PKA. Activation of $G\alpha_q$ ultimately stimulates a PKC that is unusual in being *in*sensitive to phorbol esters (see Chapter 3). Both pathways are essential for the action of PTH on apical Ca^{2+} entry. Like PTH, **calcitonin** at low concentrations also increases Ca^{2+} reabsorption through cAMP in both the TAL and the DCT.

Vitamin D Acting on gene transcription, vitamin D (see Chapter 52) increases Ca^{2+} reabsorption in the distal nephron, thus complementing the major Ca^{2+}-retaining action of vitamin D, Ca^{2+} absorption in the gastrointestinal tract (see Chapter 45). In renal tubule cells, vitamin D upregulates the Ca^{2+}-binding protein, which contributes to enhanced Ca^{2+} reabsorption by keeping $[Ca^{2+}]_i$ low during increased Ca^{2+} traffic through the cell.

Plasma Ca^{2+} Levels The kidney, similar to the parathyroid gland (see Chapter 52), responds directly to changes in extracellular $[Ca^{2+}]$. In the cortical TAL, an increase in basolateral $[Ca^{2+}]$ inhibits both the Na/K/Cl cotransporter and K^+ channels on the apical membrane (Fig. 36-16C), thereby decreasing the lumen-positive transepithelial potential and reducing paracellular Ca^{2+} reabsorption. The mechanism appears to be the following: Extracellular Ca^{2+} binds to a basolateral **Ca^{2+}-sensing receptor** (CaSR), which couples to at least two G proteins. First, activation of $G\alpha_i$ decreases $[cAMP]_i$, thus reducing stimulation of Na/K/Cl cotransport by cAMP (see Chapter 35). Second, activation of a member of the G_i/G_o family stimulates phospholipase 2 (PLA_2; see Chapter 3), thereby increasing levels of arachidonic acid and one of its cytochrome P450 metabolites, probably 20-hydroxyeicosatetraenoic acid (HETE). The latter inhibits apical Na/K/Cl cotransporters and K^+ channels. Third, CaSR activates $G\alpha_q$, elevating $[Ca^{2+}]_i$ and stimulating PKC (see Chapter 3), which also inhibits Na/K/Cl cotransport. Regardless of the mechanism, inhibition of apical Na/K/Cl cotransport (1) lowers $[Cl^-]_i$ and thus hyperpolarizes the basolateral membrane and (2) lowers $[K^+]_i$ and thus depolarizes the apical membrane. Together, these two effects reduce the lumen-positive transepithelial voltage, thereby inhibiting the paracellular reabsorption of Ca^{2+} and Mg^{2+} (see later). The Ca^{2+}-sensing receptor is also present in the proximal tubule, the medullary TAL, the DCT, and the collecting ducts.

An interesting consequence of reduced Na^+ reabsorption induced by high plasma $[Ca^{2+}]$ is an inhibition of the kidney's ability to generate concentrated urine (see Chapter 38). Indeed, chronic hypercalcemia results in dilute urine, a form of nephrogenic diabetes insipidus (see Chapter 38 for the box on this topic). By keeping urine $[Ca^{2+}]$ relatively low, this effect may help to avoid Ca^{2+} stones under conditions of high Ca^{2+} excretion.

Diuretics Among diuretics, those acting on the TAL, such as furosemide, decrease Ca^{2+} reabsorption, whereas those acting on the distal nephron, such as thiazides and amiloride, increase Ca^{2+} reabsorption. Thus, of these drugs, only the powerful loop diuretic furosemide is appropriate for treating hypercalcemic states. In the TAL, **furosemide** (see Chapter 35) reduces the lumen-positive voltage and thus the driving force for passive, paracellular Ca^{2+} reabsorption. Accordingly, urinary Ca^{2+} excretion increases in parallel with Na^+ excretion.

In contrast, the effects of thiazides and amiloride are exceptions to the general rule that Ca^{2+} and Na^+ excretion parallel each other. **Thiazide diuretics** inhibit Na/Cl cotransport and stimulate Ca^{2+} reabsorption in the DCT. Inhibiting apical Na/Cl cotransport lowers $[Cl^-]_i$ in the DCT cell, thus hyperpolarizing the cell. The steeper electrical gradient increases apical Ca^{2+} entry, secondarily stimulating basolateral Ca^{2+} extrusion. **Amiloride** inhibits apical Na^+ channels in the initial and cortical collecting tubules and hyperpolarizes the apical membrane. Thus, like the thiazides, amiloride augments Ca^{2+} reabsorption by enhancing the gradient for apical Ca^{2+} entry. The stimulatory effects of thiazides and of amiloride on apical Ca^{2+} uptake require physiological PTH levels to keep the apical Ca^{2+} channels open (see Chapter 35).

MAGNESIUM

Most Mg^{2+} reabsorption takes place along the thick ascending limb

Approximately 99% of the total body stores of magnesium reside either within bone (~54%) or within the intracellular

Table 36-8 Patterns of Hyperaminoacidurias

	mg/dL	mM	% of Total
Ionized Mg^{2+}	1.3	0.56	62
Diffusible Mg^{2+} complexes	0.1	0.06	7
Nondiffusible (protein-bound) Mg^{2+}	0.6	0.28	31
Total Mg^{2+}	2.0	0.90	100

compartment (~45%), mostly muscle. Renal magnesium excretion plays an important role in maintaining physiological plasma magnesium levels. The body maintains the total magnesium concentration in blood plasma within narrow limits, 0.8 to 1.0 mM (1.8 to 2.2 mg/dL). Of this total, ~30% is protein-bound (Table 36-8). The remaining ~70% of total magnesium, which is filterable, is made up of two components. Less than 10% is complexed to anions such as phosphate, citrate, and oxalate, thus leaving ~60% of the total as free, ionized magnesium (Mg^{2+}).

Disturbances of Mg^{2+} metabolism usually involve abnormal *losses*, and these occur most frequently during gastrointestinal malabsorption (see Chapter 45) and diarrhea, in the course of renal disease, and following the administration of diuretics. Clinical manifestations of Mg^{2+} depletion include neurologic disturbances such as tetany (especially when associated with hypocalcemia), cardiac arrhythmias, and increased peripheral vascular resistance. Conversely, increased Mg^{2+} intake may lower blood pressure and may reduce the incidence of hypertension. Severe hypermagnesemia, which may occur following excessive intake or renal failure, results in a toxic syndrome involving nausea, hyporeflexia, respiratory insufficiency, and cardiac arrest.

Normally, 5% or less of the filtered magnesium load appears in the urine (Fig. 36-17A). In contrast to the predominantly "proximal" reabsorption pattern of the major components of the glomerular filtrate, Mg^{2+} reabsorption occurs mainly along the TAL. In all segments, Mg^{2+} reabsorption is mainly paracellular.

Normally, the **proximal tubule** reabsorbs only ~15% of the filtered magnesium load (Fig. 36-17B). Water reabsorption along the proximal tubule causes luminal $[Mg^{2+}]$ to double compared with the value in Bowman's space, thereby establishing a favorable Mg^{2+} electrochemical gradient for passive, paracellular Mg^{2+} reabsorption. Solvent drag may also contribute to the paracellular reabsorption of Mg^{2+}.

The **TAL** absorbs ~70% of the filtered magnesium load and is also the main site of *control* of Mg^{2+} transport (Fig. 36-17C). The driving force for paracellular Mg^{2+} reabsorption is the lumen-positive voltage of the TAL. In states of Mg^{2+} depletion (see later), the TAL may reabsorb some Mg^{2+} by a *transcellular* route.

In the TAL, a specific tight junction protein called **claudin 16** or paracellin-1 (see Chapter 5) is necessary for paracellular Mg^{2+} reabsorption. A mutation of the paracellin-1 gene leads to an autosomal recessive disorder characterized by severe renal Mg^{2+} wasting. Mg^{2+} reabsorption along the **DCT**

A HANDLING OF Mg²⁺ ALONG NEPHRON

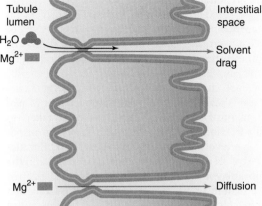

B PROXIMAL TUBULE

C THICK ASCENDING TUBULE (TAL)

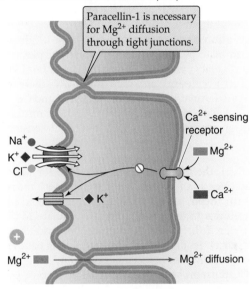

Figure 36-17 **A** to **C**, Magnesium handling by the kidney. In **A**, the numbered yellow boxes indicate the fraction of the filtered load that various nephron segments reabsorb. The DCT, initial collecting tubule (ICT), cortical collecting tubule (CCT), outer medullary collecting duct (OMCD), and IMCD together reabsorb 10% of the filtered load. The green boxes indicate the fraction of the filtered load that remains in the lumen after these segments. The values in the boxes are approximations. PCT, proximal convoluted tubule; PST, proximal straight tubule.

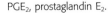

Table 36-9 Factors Affecting Mg²⁺ Reabsorption Along the Nephron

Site	Increase Reabsorption	Decrease Reabsorption
Proximal tubule	Volume contraction	Volume expansion
Thick ascending limb	PTH, calcitonin, glucagon, AVP Low plasma [Mg²⁺] Metabolic alkalosis	Furosemide and related loop diuretics Mannitol High plasma [Mg²⁺] or [Ca²⁺]
Distal convoluted tubule and collecting tubules/ducts	PTH, calcitonin, glucagon, AVP, aldosterone, PGE₂ Low plasma [Mg²⁺] Amiloride	High plasma [Mg²⁺] or [Ca²⁺] Metabolic acidosis K⁺ or phosphate depletion

PGE₂, prostaglandin E₂.

and the **collecting tubules** and **ducts** accounts for only ~10% of the filtered load.

Mg²⁺ Reabsorption Increases with Depletion of Mg²⁺ or Ca²⁺ or with Elevated PTH Levels

Table 36-9 shows the site of action of factors modulating renal Mg^{2+} excretion.

Mg^{2+} Depletion In response to low plasma $[Mg^{2+}]$, the TAL increases its reabsorption of Mg^{2+}, independent of Na^+ and Ca^{2+} transport. This observation has been taken to suggest that a fraction of Mg^{2+} reabsorption may be *transcellular* and may involve an active transport step. Because $[Mg^{2+}]_i$ in TAL cells is relatively low (0.5 to 0.6 mM) and the apical membrane voltage is cell negative, the apical electrochemical gradient favors passive Mg^{2+} uptake. It is likely that cation-selective channels, perhaps TRPV5/6, mediate apical Mg^{2+} uptake. The basolateral step for transcellular Mg^{2+} reabsorption is also uncertain, but it may include a unique ATP-dependent Mg^{2+} pump or an Na-Mg exchanger.

Hypermagnesemia and Hypercalcemia The kidney seems to discriminate poorly between increases in plasma $[Mg^{2+}]$ and $[Ca^{2+}]$. Thus, *each* of these disturbances inhibits the reabsorption of both Mg^{2+} and Ca^{2+} in the TAL, thereby leading to increased urinary excretion of both Mg^{2+} and Ca^{2+}. It is thought that high plasma $[Mg^{2+}]$ and $[Ca^{2+}]$ diminish Mg^{2+} reabsorption because each can bind to the Ca^{2+}-sensing receptor.

Hormones PTH, the most important hormone for Mg^{2+} regulation, increases both proximal and distal Mg^{2+} reabsorption. When tested separately in hormone-depleted animals, AVP, glucagons, and calcitonin all stimulate Mg^{2+} reabsorption in the TAL, by acting through cAMP and PKA. Many of these hormones probably act by modulating passive Mg^{2+} movement through the paracellular pathway, either by changing NaCl transport and transepithelial voltage or by increasing paracellular permeability.

Diuretics In general, diuretics decrease Mg^{2+} reabsorption and thus enhance Mg^{2+} excretion. This statement is particularly true for diuretics targeting the TAL. Similar to their effects on Ca^{2+}, loop diuretics act by depressing the lumen-positive voltage and thus the gradient for the passive, paracellular Mg^{2+} reabsorption. Osmotic diuretics, such as mannitol, also reduce Mg^{2+} reabsorption along the loop of Henle.

REFERENCES

Books and Reviews

Chattopadhyay N, Brown EM (eds): Calcium-Sensing Receptor, pp 69-102. Boston: Kluwer Academic, 2002.

Chillarón J, Roca R, Valencia A, et al: Heteromeric amino acid transporters: Biochemistry, genetics and physiology. Am J Physiol 2001; 281:F995-F1018.

Ciarimboli G, Schlatter E: Regulation of organic cation transport. Pflugers Arch Eur J Physiol 2005; 449:423-441.

Hoenderop JGJ, Bindels RJM: Epithelial Ca^{2+} and Mg^{2+} channels in health and disease. J Am Soc Nephrol 2005; 16:15-26.

Murer H, Hernando N, Forster I, Biber J: Proximal tubular phosphate reabsorption: Molecular mechanisms. Physiol Rev 2000; 80:1373-1409.

Sands JM: Mammalian urea transporters. Annu Rev Physiol 2003; 65:543-566.

Shayakul C, Hediger MA: The SLC14 gene family of urea transporters. Pflügers Arch 2004; 447:603-609.

Journal Articles

Austin JH, Stillman E, Van Slyke DD: Factors governing the excretion rate of urea. J Biol Chem 1921; 46:91-112.

Fei YJ, Kanai Y, Nussberger S, et al: Expression cloning of a mammalian proton-coupled oligopeptide transporter. Nature 1994; 368:563-566.

Forster IC, Wagner CA, Busch AE, et al: Electrophysiological characterization of the flounder type II Na/Pi cotransporter (NaPi-5) expressed in *Xenopus laevis* oocytes. J Membr Biol 1997; 160:9-25.

Hediger MA, Coady MJ, Ikeda IS, Wright EM: Expression cloning and cDNA sequencing of the Na^+/glucose transporter. Nature 1987; 330:379-381.

Simon DB, Lu Y, Choate KA, et al: Paracellin-1, a renal tight junction protein required for paracellular Mg^{2+} resorption. Science 1999; 285:103-106.

You G, Smith CP, Kanai Y, et al: Expression cloning and characterization of the vasopressin-regulated urea transporter. Nature 1993; 365:844-847.

Zhao H, Shiue H, Palkon S, et al: Ezrin regulates NHE3 translocation and activation after Na^+-glucose cotransport. Proc Natl Acad Sci U S A 2004; 101:9485-9490.

CHAPTER 37

TRANSPORT OF POTASSIUM

Gerhard Giebisch and Erich Windhager

POTASSIUM BALANCE AND THE OVERALL RENAL HANDLING OF POTASSIUM

Changes in K⁺ concentrations can have major effects on cell and organ function

The distribution of K^+ in the body differs strikingly from that of Na^+. Whereas Na^+ is largely extracellular, K^+ is the most abundant intracellular cation. Some 98% of the total body K^+ content (~50 mmol/kg body weight) is inside cells; only 2% is in the extracellular fluid (ECF). The body tightly maintains the plasma $[K^+]$ at 3.5 to 5.0 mM.

Table 37-1 summarizes the most important physiological functions of K^+ ions. A *high* $[K^+]$ inside cells and mitochondria is essential for maintaining cell volume, for regulating intracellular pH and controlling cell-enzyme function, for DNA and protein synthesis, and for cell growth. The relatively *low* extracellular $[K^+]$ is necessary for maintaining the steep K^+ gradient across cell membranes that is largely responsible for the membrane potential of excitable and nonexcitable cells. Therefore, changes in extracellular $[K^+]$ can cause severe disturbances in excitation and contraction. As a general rule, either doubling the normal plasma $[K^+]$ or reducing it by half results in severe disturbances in skeletal and cardiac muscle function. The potentially life-threatening disturbances of cardiac rhythmicity that result from a rise of plasma $[K^+]$ are particularly important (see the box titled Hyperkalemia and the Heart).

Chronic K^+ depletion leads to several metabolic disturbances. These include the following: (1) inability of the kidney to form concentrated urine; (2) a tendency to develop metabolic alkalosis; and, closely related to this acid-base disturbance, (3) a striking enhancement of renal ammonium excretion (see Chapters 38 and 39).

K⁺ homeostasis involves external K⁺ balance between environment and body and internal K⁺ balance between intracellular and extracellular compartments

Figure 37-1 illustrates processes that govern K^+ balance and the distribution of K^+ in the body: (1) gastrointestinal (GI) intake, (2) renal and extrarenal excretion, and (3) the internal distribution of K^+ between the intracellular and extracellular fluid compartments. The first two processes accomplish external K^+ balance (i.e., body versus environment), whereas the last achieves internal K^+ balance (i.e., intracellular versus extracellular fluids).

External K⁺ Balance **The relationship between dietary K^+ intake and K^+ excretion** determines external K^+ balance. The *dietary intake* of K^+ is approximately equal to that of Na^+, 80 to 120 mmol/day. This K^+ intake is more than the entire K^+ content of the ECF, which is only ~70 mmol. For the plasma K^+ content to remain constant, the body must excrete K^+ through renal and extrarenal mechanisms at the same rate as K^+ ingestion. Moreover, because dietary K^+ intake can vary over a wide range, it is important that these K^+ excretory mechanisms be able to adjust appropriately to variable K^+ intake. The kidney is largely responsible for K^+ excretion, although the GI tract plays a minor role. The kidneys excrete 90% to 95% of the daily K^+ intake; the colon excretes 5% to 10%. Although the colon can adjust its K^+ excretion in response to some stimuli (e.g., adrenal hormones, changes in dietary K^+, decreased capacity of the kidneys to excrete K^+), the colon—by itself—is incapable of increasing K^+ secretion sufficiently to maintain external K^+ balance.

Internal K⁺ Balance Maintaining normal intracellular and extracellular $[K^+]$ requires not only the *external* K^+ balance just described, but also the appropriate distribution of K^+ within the body. Most of the K^+ is inside cells—particularly muscle cells, which represent a high faction of body mass—with smaller quantities in liver, bone, and red blood cells. The markedly unequal distribution between the intracellular and extracellular K^+ content has important quantitative implications. Of the total intracellular K^+ content of ~3 mol, shuttling as little as 1% to or from the ECF would cause a 50% change in extracellular $[K^+]$, with severe consequences for neuromuscular function (Table 37-1).

Ingested K⁺ moves transiently into cells for storage before excretion by the kidney

What happens when the body is presented with a K^+ load? By far, the most common source of a K^+ load is dietary K^+. When one ingests K^+ salts, both the small intestine and the

Table 37-1 Physiological Role of K⁺ Ions

A. Roles of Intracellular K⁺	
Cell-volume maintenance	Net loss of K⁺ → cell shrinkage Net gain of K⁺ → cell swelling
Intracellular pH regulation	Net loss of K⁺ → cell acidosis Net gain of K⁺ → cell alkalosis
Cell enzyme functions	K⁺ dependence of enzymes (e.g., some ATPases, succinic dehydrogenase)
DNA/protein synthesis, growth	Lack of K⁺ → reduction of protein synthesis, stunted growth
B. Roles of Transmembrane [K⁺] Ratio	
Resting cell membrane potential	Reduced $[K^+]_i/[K^+]_o$ → membrane depolarization Increased $[K^+]_i/[K^+]_o$ → membrane hyperpolarization
Neuromuscular activity	Low plasma K⁺: muscle weakness, muscle paralysis, intestinal distention, respiratory failure High plasma K⁺: increased muscle excitability; later, muscle weakness (paralysis)
Cardiac activity	Low plasma K⁺: slowed conduction of pacemaker activity, arrhythmias High plasma K⁺: conduction disturbances, ventricular arrhythmias, and ventricular fibrillation
Vascular resistance	Low plasma K⁺: vasoconstriction High plasma K⁺: vasodilation

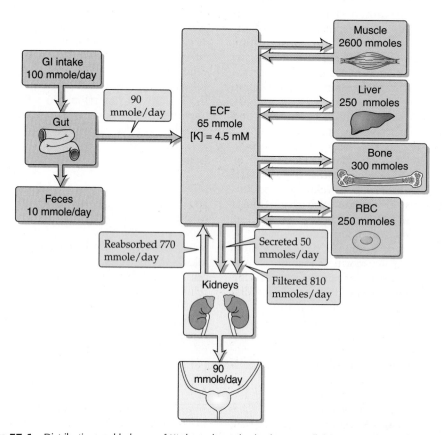

Figure 37-1 Distribution and balance of K⁺ throughout the body. Intracellular K⁺ concentrations are similar in all tissues in the four purple boxes. The values in the boxes are approximations. RBC, red blood cell.

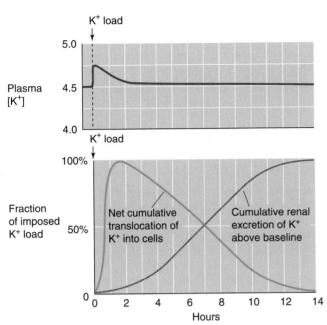

Figure 37-2 K⁺ handling following an acute K⁺ load. *(Data from Cogan MG: Fluid and Electrolytes: Physiology and Pathophysiology. Norwalk, CT: Appleton & Lange, 1991.)*

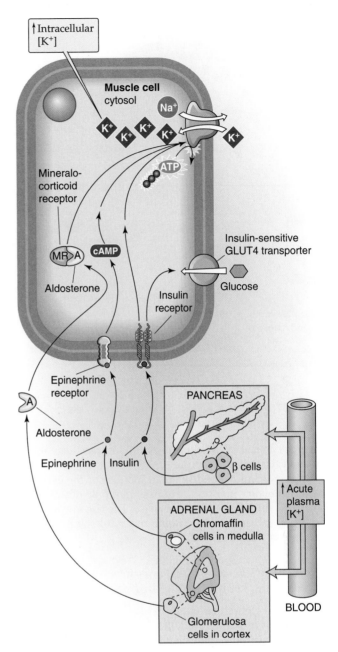

Figure 37-3 K⁺ uptake into cells in response to high plasma [K⁺].

colon (see Chapter 44) absorb the K⁺. In addition to external sources of K⁺, substantial amounts of K⁺ may enter the ECF from damaged tissues (see the box titled Clinical Implications: Evaluating Hypokalemia and Hyperkalemia in the Patient). Such K⁺ release from intracellular to extracellular fluid can lead to a severe, even lethal, increase in plasma [K⁺] (i.e., **hyperkalemia**). However, even a large meal presents the body with a K⁺ load that could produce hyperkalemia if it were not for mechanisms that buffer and ultimately excrete this K⁺.

Some four fifths of an ingested K⁺ load temporarily moves into cells, so that plasma [K⁺] rises only modestly, as shown in the upper panel of Figure 37-2. Were it not for this translocation, plasma [K⁺] could reach dangerous levels. The transfer of excess K⁺ into cells is rapid and almost complete after an hour (lower panel of Fig. 37-2, gold curve). With a delay, the kidneys begin to excrete the surfeit of K⁺ (lower panel of Fig. 37-2, brown curve), leaching from the cells the excess K⁺ that they had temporarily stored.

What processes mediate the temporary uptake of K⁺ into cells during K⁺ loading? As shown in Figure 37-3, the hormones insulin, epinephrine (a β-adrenergic agonist), and aldosterone all promote the transfer of K⁺ from extracellular to intracellular fluid through the ubiquitous **Na-K pump**. Indeed, the lack of **insulin** or a deficient renin-angiotensin-**aldosterone** system can significantly compromise tolerance to K⁺ loading and can predispose to hyperkalemia. Similarly, administering β-**adrenergic blockers** (in treatment of hypertension) impairs sequestration of an acute K⁺ load.

Acid-base disturbances also affect internal K⁺ distribution. As a rule, acidemia leads to hyperkalemia as tissues release K⁺. One can think of this K⁺ release as an "exchange" of intracellular K⁺ for extracellular H⁺, although a single transport protein generally does not mediate this "exchange"

(see Chapter 28). Extracellular acidosis probably leads to loss of cellular K⁺ because the resulting decrease in intracellular pH lessens the binding of K⁺ to nondiffusible intracellular anions (Fig. 37-4). Moreover, intracellular acidosis compromises both the Na-K pump and the Na/K/Cl cotransporter (NKCC2), both of which move K⁺ into cells. Interestingly, for the same degree of acidemia, mineral acids produce a greater degree of hyperkalemia than do organic acids.

Alkalemia causes cells to take up K⁺, thus leading to **hypokalemia**. Although the mechanism is not known, high HCO₃⁻ levels—even in the absence of extracellular pH changes—induce hypokalemia by stimulating K⁺ transfer into cells. Another example of this apparent exchange of K⁺ for H⁺ is the effect of K⁺ on acid-base homeostasis. As discussed in

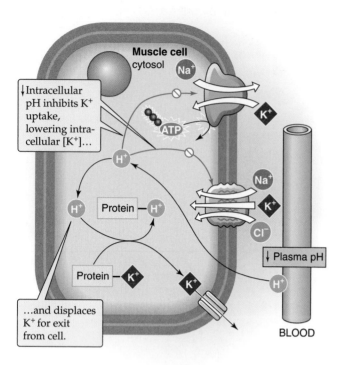

↓ Intracellular pH inhibits K⁺ uptake, lowering intracellular [K⁺]...

...and displaces K⁺ for exit from cell.

↓ Plasma pH

BLOOD

Figure 37-4   Effect of acidosis on K⁺ uptake into cells.

Chapters 28 and 39, K⁺ depletion causes intracellular acidosis and extracellular alkalosis.

In some clinical conditions, an increase of the **extracellular osmolality** induces the transfer, not only of water, but also of K⁺ into the extracellular space. The rise in plasma K⁺ following infusion of hypertonic mannitol solutions is an example of this phenomenon.

The kidney excretes K⁺ by a combination of filtration, reabsorption, and secretion

At a normal glomerular filtration rate (GFR) and at physiological levels of plasma [K⁺], the kidney filters ~800 mmol/day of K⁺, far more than the usual dietary intake of 80 to 120 mmol/day. Therefore, to achieve K⁺ balance, the kidneys normally need to excrete 10% to 15% of the filtered K⁺. Under conditions of low dietary K⁺ intake, the kidneys excrete 1% to 3% of filtered K⁺, so that—with a normal- or low-K⁺ diet—the kidneys could achieve K⁺ balance by *filtration* and *reabsorption* alone. Considering only the filtered K⁺ load and external K⁺ balance, we would have no reason to suspect that the kidneys would be capable of K⁺ secretion. However, with a chronically high dietary K⁺, when the kidneys must rid the body of excess K⁺, urinary K⁺ excretion may exceed 150% of the total amount of filtered K⁺. Therefore, even if the tubules reabsorbed none of the filtered K⁺, they must be capable of secreting an amount equivalent to at least 50% of the filtered K⁺ load.

As discussed later, even in the absence of a large dietary K⁺ load, K⁺ *secretion* by the tubules is an important component of urinary K⁺ excretion. Therefore, K⁺ handling is a complex combination of K⁺ filtration at the glomerulus

as well as both K⁺ reabsorption and secretion by the renal tubules.

POTASSIUM TRANSPORT BY DIFFERENT SEGMENTS OF THE NEPHRON

The proximal tubule consistently reabsorbs the bulk of the filtered K⁺, whereas the distal nephron may reabsorb or secrete K⁺, depending on dietary K⁺

Figure 37-5 summarizes the pattern of K⁺ transport along the nephron under conditions of low or normal/high K⁺ intake. In either case, the kidney filters K⁺ in the glomerulus and then extensively reabsorbs it along the proximal tubule (~80%) and the loop of Henle (~10%), so that only ~10% of the filtered K⁺ enters the distal convoluted tubule (DCT). Moreover, in either case, the medullary collecting duct (MCD) reabsorbs K⁺. The K⁺ handling depends critically on dietary K⁺ in five nephron segments: the DCT, the connecting tubule (CNT), the initial collecting tubule (ICT), the cortical collecting tubule (CCT), and the MCD.

Low Dietary K⁺   When the body is trying to conserve K⁺, the classic distal tubule (i.e., DCT, CNT, and ICT) and CCT all reabsorb K⁺, so that only a small fraction of the filtered load (1% to 3%) appears in the urine (Fig. 37-5A). In states of K⁺ depletion, this additional K⁺ reabsorption can be life-saving, by retrieving from the tubule lumen precious K⁺ that escaped reabsorption along the proximal tubule and loop of Henle. Despite the degree to which the kidneys can enhance K⁺ reabsorption, they cannot restrict K⁺ loss in the urine as effectively as they can restrict Na⁺ loss. Therefore, a negative K⁺ balance and hypokalemia may develop when K⁺ intake has been abnormally low for prolonged periods of time.

Normal or High Dietary K⁺   When external K⁺ balance demands that the kidneys excrete K⁺, the ICT, CCT, and the more proximal portion of the MCD *secrete* K⁺ into the tubule lumen (Fig. 37-5B). Together, these segments, known as the **distal K⁺ secretory system**, account for most of the urinary excretion of K⁺. It is also this distal K⁺ secretory system that responds to many stimuli that modulate K⁺ excretion. Even at normal rates of K⁺ excretion (10% to 15% of the filtered load), the proximal tubules and loop of Henle first absorb very large amounts of K⁺ (~90% of the filtered load), so that the K⁺ appearing in the urine may largely represent K⁺ secreted by more distal segments of the nephron.

Medullary trapping of K⁺ helps to maximize K⁺ excretion when K⁺ intake is high

The kidney traps K⁺ in the medullary interstitium, with the interstitial [K⁺] being highest at the tip of the papilla and falling toward the cortex. This **medullary K⁺ trapping** is the result of three steps along the nephron. First, because interstitial [K⁺] rises toward the tip of the papilla, **juxtamedullary nephrons**, whose long loops of Henle dip into the inner medulla (see Chapter 33), secrete K⁺ *passively* into the thin descending limb of the loop of Henle (tDLH). Indeed, analy-

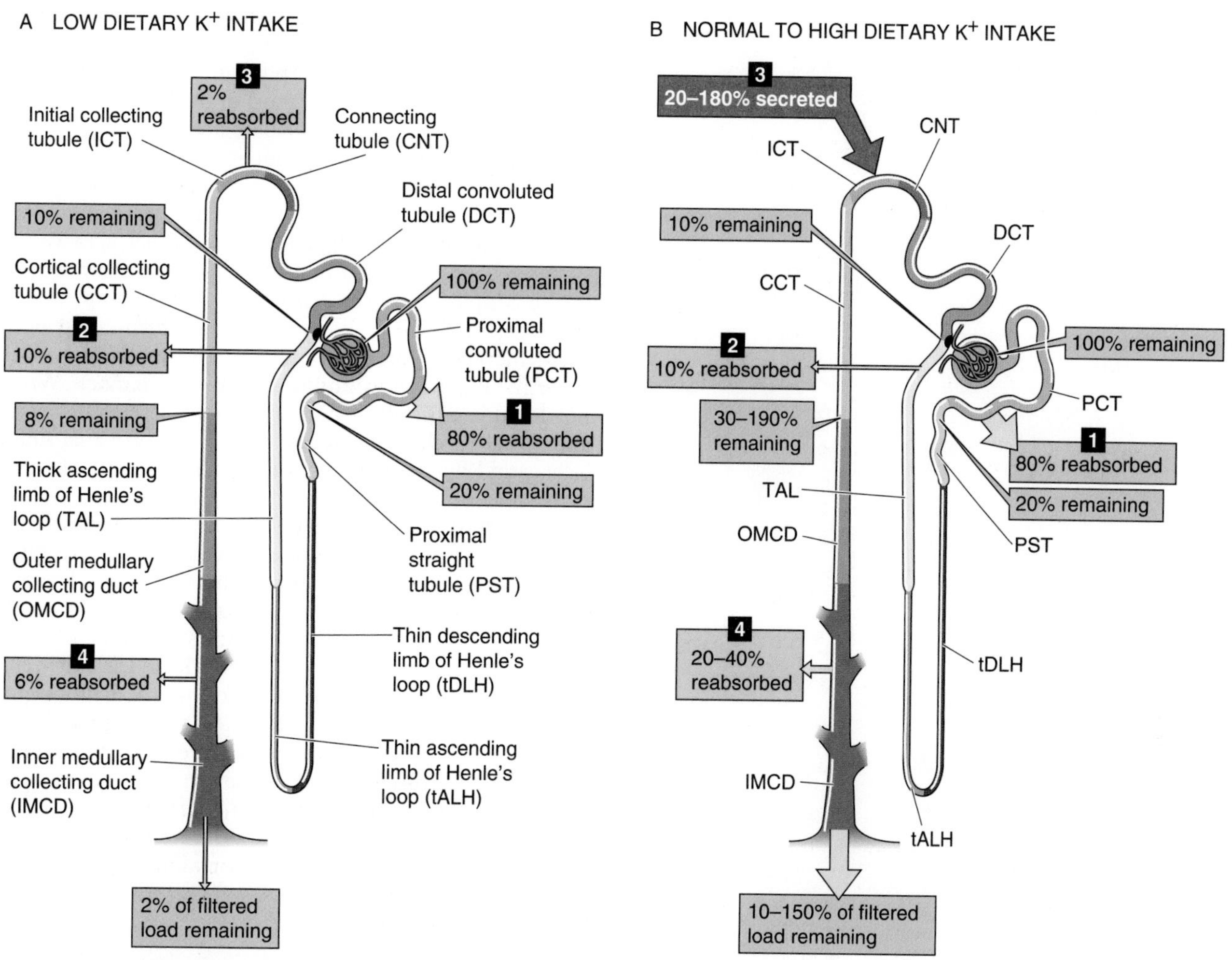

A LOW DIETARY K⁺ INTAKE

B NORMAL TO HIGH DIETARY K⁺ INTAKE

Figure 37-5 K⁺ handling along the nephron. In **A** and **B**, the numbered yellow boxes indicate the fraction of the filtered load that various nephron segments reabsorb, whereas the red box in **B** indicates the fraction of the filtered load secreted by the ICT and CCT. The green boxes indicate the fraction of the filtered load that remains in the lumen after these segments.

sis of fluid collected from the hairpin bend of the long loops of Henle of juxtamedullary nephrons shows that the amount of K⁺ delivered to the collection site at the hairpin bend can exceed not only the amount of K⁺ present at the end of the proximal tubule, but also the amount of K⁺ filtered. This K⁺ secretion by the tDLH is the *first step* of a process known as **medullary K⁺ recycling** (Fig. 37-6).

The second step of medullary K⁺ recycling is K⁺ reabsorption by the thin (tALH) and thick (TAL) ascending limbs, which deposit K⁺ in the medullary interstitium. This newly deposited interstitial K⁺ contributes to the high interstitial [K⁺]. Together, the tALH and TAL of a juxtamedullary loop reabsorb more K⁺ than the *descending* limb secretes, so that net K⁺ reabsorption occurs along the loop, thereby contributing to medullary K⁺ trapping.

The third step of medullary K⁺ recycling is the reabsorption of K⁺ by the MCDs. Regardless of whether the distal K⁺ secretory system (ICT, CCT, early MCD) reabsorbs K⁺ (Fig. 37-5A) or secretes K⁺ (Fig. 37-5B), the MCDs reabsorb some K⁺, thereby contributing to medullary K⁺ trapping.

One would think that—with respect to K⁺ excretion—medullary K⁺ recycling is inefficient because K⁺ exits the

ascending limb and MCD only to re-enter the nephron upstream, in the tDLH. However, medullary recycling and concomitant K⁺ trapping may be important in maximizing the excretion of K⁺ when K⁺ intake is high. Under these conditions, K⁺ secretion by the distal K⁺ secretory system is intense, so that luminal [K⁺] in the MCD may rise to 200 mM or higher. Thus, enhanced K⁺ trapping in the medullary interstitium minimizes the [K⁺] difference between the MCD lumen and its peritubular environment, thus reducing the passive loss of K⁺ from the MCD.

POTASSIUM TRANSPORT AT THE CELLULAR AND MOLECULAR LEVEL

K⁺ reabsorption along the proximal tubule is largely passive and follows the movement of Na⁺ and fluid

The proximal tubule reabsorbs most of the filtered K⁺ through two paracellular mechanisms (Fig. 37-7A): solvent drag and electrodiffusion. **Solvent drag** (see Chapter 20)

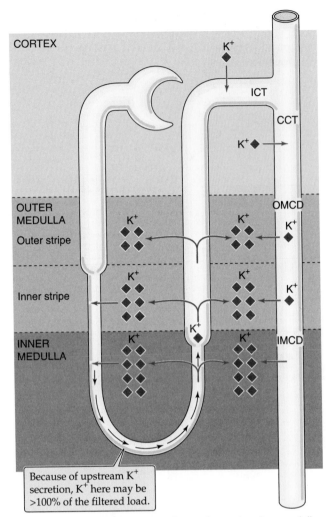

CORTEX

K⁺

ICT

CCT

K⁺◆

OUTER
MEDULLA

Outer stripe

K⁺

OMCD

K⁺

K⁺

Inner stripe

K⁺

K⁺

K⁺

INNER
MEDULLA

K⁺

K⁺

IMCD

Because of upstream K⁺
secretion, K⁺ here may be
>100% of the filtered load.

Figure 37-6 Medullary recycling of K⁺ by juxtamedullary nephrons.

occurs along the entire length of the proximal tubule. Active Na⁺ transport (see Chapter 35) drives net fluid reabsorption across the proximal tubule epithelium through the paracellular shunt pathway, thereby entraining K⁺ along with the fluid. Indeed, one of the distinguishing features of proximal tubule K⁺ reabsorption is its strong dependence on net fluid reabsorption. Thus, interventions that depress fluid reabsorption almost always inhibit K⁺ reabsorption.

As fluid flows down the proximal tubule, the luminal voltage shifts from negative to positive (see Chapter 35). By the late proximal tubule, the transepithelial voltage is sufficiently positive to provide a favorable gradient for K⁺ **electrodiffusion** (see Chapter 6) through the low-resistance paracellular pathway, from lumen to blood.

Although the proximal tubule reabsorbs K⁺ by paracellular pathways, the proximal tubule has several cellular pathways for K⁺ movement that do not directly participate in K⁺ reabsorption (Fig. 37-7A): (1) a basolateral Na-K pump, a feature common to all tubule cells; (2) apical and basolateral K⁺ channels; and (3) a basolateral K/Cl cotransporter (KCC).

The K⁺ conductance of the basolateral membrane greatly exceeds that of the apical membrane, and it appears that

different channels are responsible for the K⁺ conductances in these two membranes. The open probability of the *basolateral* K⁺ channel increases sharply with the turnover rate of the Na-K pump. Accordingly, most of the K⁺ taken up by the Na-K pump recycles across the basolateral membrane by K⁺ channels and a KCC and does not appear in the lumen. This basolateral K⁺ channel belongs to the class of inwardly rectifying K⁺ channels (**ROMK**) characterized by ATP sensitivity: a decrease in [ATP]ᵢ enhances channel activity (see Chapter 7). This regulation by [ATP]ᵢ is most likely involved in the coupling between basolateral Na-K pumps and K⁺ channels. An increase in pump rate—which could occur when increased apical Na⁺ entry increases [Na⁺]ᵢ—would lower [ATP]ᵢ, relieving inhibition of the K⁺ channels. Were it not for this crosstalk between the basolateral Na-K pump and apical K⁺ channels, the K⁺ content of proximal tubule cells would fluctuate dramatically during alterations in net Na⁺ transport.

In contrast to the high state of activity of the basolateral K⁺ channels, *apical* K⁺ channels are largely quiescent under normal conditions. They appear to become active, however, when tubule cells swell, possibly when entry of Na⁺ from the lumen increases rapidly. These channels, which may be activated by membrane stretch, then allow K⁺ to leave the cell, a process that causes cells to shrink toward their original volume (a volume-regulatory decrease; see Chapter 5).

Even if the apical K⁺ channels were open more often, uptake of K⁺ across the apical membrane would not occur, because the electrochemical K⁺ gradient favors K⁺ movement from cell to lumen. Because K⁺ cannot enter across the apical membrane, no transcellular reabsorption of K⁺ can take place. Thus, proximal tubule K⁺ reabsorption must occur exclusively by the paracellular pathway.

K⁺ reabsorption along the TAL occurs through both a passive paracellular route and a transcellular route that exploits secondary active Na/K/Cl cotransport

As discussed earlier, the **tDLHs** of the loop of Henle, particularly those originating from juxtamedullary nephrons, *secrete* K⁺ (Fig. 37-6). This secretion of K⁺ from the medullary interstitium into the tDLH lumen is passive, driven by the high [K⁺] of the medullary interstitium and made possible by a substantial K⁺ permeability. Both the tDLH lumen and the interstitium become increasingly K⁺ rich toward the tip of the papilla.

In the **tALH**, K⁺ moves from lumen to interstitium passively, by the paracellular pathway. The major driving force for this passive reabsorption of K⁺ is the lumen-to-interstitium K⁺ gradient, which becomes progressively larger as the fluid moves toward the cortex because interstitial [K⁺] becomes progressively lower toward the cortex.

The **TAL** of the loop of Henle reabsorbs K⁺ by both paracellular and transcellular mechanisms (Fig. 37-7B). The lumen-positive voltage, together with the relatively high paracellular K⁺ permeability, allows passive K⁺ reabsorption to occur by the *paracellular* pathway. The lumen-positive voltage develops because of a substantial difference in the ion permeabilities of the apical and basolateral membranes. The *apical* membrane is K⁺ selective, so that the apical mem-

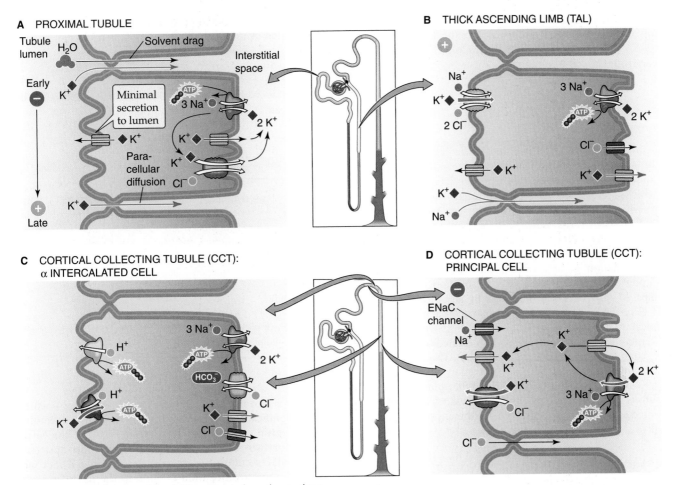

A PROXIMAL TUBULE

Tubule lumen

H_2O

Solvent drag

Interstitial space

Early

K^+

Minimal secretion to lumen

ATP

$3 Na^+$

$2 K^+$

K^+

Para-cellular diffusion

K^+

K^+

Cl^-

K^+

Late

B THICK ASCENDING LIMB (TAL)

Na^+

K^+

$2 Cl^-$

$3 Na^+$

ATP

$2 K^+$

Cl^-

K^+

K^+

Na^+

C CORTICAL COLLECTING TUBULE (CCT):
α INTERCALATED CELL

H^+

ATP

H^+

ATP

K^+

$3 Na^+$

ATP

$2 K^+$

HCO_3^-

K^+

Cl^-

Cl^-

D CORTICAL COLLECTING TUBULE (CCT):
PRINCIPAL CELL

ENaC channel

Na^+

K^+

K^+

K^+

Cl^-

$3 Na^+$

ATP

$2 K^+$

Cl^-

Figure 37-7 Cellular models of K^+ transport along the nephron.

brane potential depends mainly on the cell-to-lumen $[K^+]$ gradient. In contrast, the TAL *basolateral* membrane is permeable to both K^+ and Cl^-. Hence, the basolateral membrane potential lies between the equilibrium potentials of Cl^- (~–50 mV) and K^+ (~–90 mV), so that it is less negative than if the basolateral membrane were permeable only to K^+. Because the apical membrane potential is more negative than the basolateral membrane potential, the transepithelial voltage is lumen positive. This potential provides a substantial driving force for the passive, paracellular reabsorption of cations such as K^+ and Na^+. Half of the K^+ reabsorbed by the TAL exits by this paracellular pathway, with the lumen-positive potential being the main driving force.

The other half of K^+ reabsorption by the TAL occurs by a *transcellular* pathway, using the apical NKCC2 (see Chapter 5). The major evidence for such a mechanism is the mutual interdependence of Na^+, Cl^-, and K^+ transport. Removing any of the three cotransported ions from the lumen abolishes transcellular K^+ reabsorption. However, because inhibiting the NKCC2 also abolishes the lumen-positive potential (see Chapter 35), this inhibition also blocks passive, paracellular K^+ reabsorption.

The apical NKCC2 is a typical example of a "secondary" active transporter (see Chapter 5). Expressed in electrical terms, the apical membrane potential is some 10 to 12 mV

more positive than the K^+ equilibrium potential, so that K^+ would tend to diffuse passively from cell to lumen. Because the combined inward gradients of Na^+ and Cl^- across the apical membrane greatly exceed that of K^+, the energy is adequate for the coupled uptake of all three ion species. Ultimately, a primary active transporter (i.e., Na-K pump) at the basolateral membrane drives the secondary active transport of K^+ in the apical membrane. Inhibiting the basolateral Na-K pump leads to an increase in $[Na^+]_i$ and $[Cl^-]_i$, so that apical Na/K/Cl transport ceases. A characteristic feature of the NKCC2 is its sensitivity to a class of diuretics that have their main site of action in the TAL. Therefore, administering so-called **loop diuretics** such as furosemide or bumetanide blocks net reabsorption of Na^+, Cl^-, and K^+.

The apical K^+ conductance mentioned earlier—which mainly represents a K^+ channel called ROMK—is also important for the function of the NKCC2 (Fig. 37-7B). The major function of the apical K^+ channel is to provide a mechanism for recycling much of the K^+ from cell to lumen, so that luminal $[K^+]$ does not fall so low as to jeopardize Na/K/Cl cotransport (see Chapter 35). Nevertheless, some of the K^+ entering the cell by the NKCC2 exits across the basolateral membrane, thereby accounting for transcellular K^+ reabsorption. The presence of apical K^+ channels also explains why inhibiting Na/K/Cl cotransport—either with loop diuretics (e.g., furosemide) or by deleting from the lumen of any of the cotransported ions—causes the TAL to engage in net K⁺ *secretion*. Active K⁺ uptake no longer opposes the K⁺ leak from the cell to lumen.

K⁺ reabsorption by intercalated cells occurs through apical K⁺ uptake mediated by an H-K pump, followed by passive efflux of K⁺ across the basolateral membrane

Ultrastructurally, the ICT and CCT are nearly identical (see Chapter 33); they are made up of ~70% principal cells (which secrete K⁺) and ~30% intercalated cells (some of which reabsorb K⁺). As discussed earlier, the ICT, CCT, and MCD reabsorb K⁺ in response to K⁺ depletion (Fig. 37-5A). This K⁺ reabsorption is a transcellular process (Fig. 37-7C), mediated by α **intercalated cells**, a subpopulation of intercalated cells that are interspersed among the principal cells. K⁺ reabsorption occurs in two steps: (1) an *active step* mediated by an apical ATP-driven H-K pump (see Chapter 5), similar to that present at the apical membrane of parietal cells in gastric glands (see Chapter 42); and (2) a *passive step* mediated by a basolateral K⁺ channel, which allows K⁺ to leak out. The α intercalated cells are also responsible for H⁺ secretion (see Chapter 39). In K⁺ depletion, a condition in which the abundance of H-K pumps increases dramatically, is often associated with accelerated secretion of H⁺ and the development of hypokalemic alkalosis.

K⁺ secretion by principal cells of the ICT and CCT occurs by active K⁺ uptake across the basolateral membrane, followed by passive diffusion through apical K⁺ channels

The *early* portion of the classic distal tubule (i.e., DCT) secretes K⁺ but at a relatively low rate. However, a high rate of K⁺ secretion into the tubule fluid is one of the distinguishing features of *late* portions of the classic distal tubule (i.e., CNT and ICT) and of the CCT. Of the two cell types in the ICT and CCT, the **principal cell** secretes K⁺, by a transcellular process (Fig. 37-7D). The three key elements of the principal cell are (1) an Na-K pump for active K⁺ uptake at the basolateral membrane, (2) a relatively high (and variable) apical K⁺ permeability, and (3) a favorable electrochemical driving force for K⁺ exit across the apical membrane. In addition, K⁺ may move from cell to lumen through the apical KCC (see Chapter 5). The net effects are the active movement of K⁺ from blood to cell and the passive movement of K⁺ from cell to lumen. Changes in any of the three elements can affect the secretion of K⁺.

K⁺ reabsorption along the MCD is both passive and active

The capacity for K⁺ *secretion* diminishes from the cortical to the MCD. Indeed, the **MCD** is responsible for K⁺ *reabsorption*, which contributes to medullary K⁺ recycling (Fig. 37-6). This K⁺ loss from the MCD lumen can occur

Table 37-2 Luminal and Peritubular Factors That Modulate K⁺ Secretion by the Distal K⁺-Secretory System*

LUMINAL FACTORS	
Stimulators	**Inhibitors**
↑ Flow rate	↑ [K⁺]
↑ [Na⁺]	↑ [Cl⁻]
↓ [Cl⁻]	↑ [Ca²⁺]
↑ [HCO₃⁻]	Ba²⁺
Negative luminal voltage	Amiloride
Diuretics acting upstream of ICT/CCT	
PERITUBULAR FACTORS	
Stimulators	**Inhibitors**
↑ K⁺ intake	↓ pH
↑ [K⁺]	Epinephrine
↑ pH	
Aldosterone	
AVP	

*ICT, CCT, and proximal portion of MCD.

by *passive* movement by the paracellular pathway—which has a significant K⁺ permeability—driven by a favorable K⁺ concentration gradient. The luminal [K⁺] of the MCD is high for two reasons. First, the segments just upstream (i.e., distal K⁺ secretory system) may have secreted K⁺. Second, the continuing reabsorption of fluid in the medullary collecting tubules, particularly in the presence of high arginine vasopressin (AVP) levels, further increases luminal [K⁺]. In addition to passive K⁺ reabsorption, apical H-K pumps (similar to those in α intercalated cells in Fig. 37-7C) may mediate *active* K⁺ reabsorption, especially during low K⁺ intake.

REGULATION OF RENAL POTASSIUM EXCRETION

Table 37-2 summarizes factors that modulate K⁺ secretion. These may be grouped into luminal and peritubular (i.e., bathing basolateral membrane) factors.

Increased luminal flow increases K⁺ secretion

One of the most potent stimuli of K⁺ secretion is the rate of fluid flow along the distal K⁺ secretory system (i.e., ICT and CCT). Under almost all circumstances, an increase in luminal flow increases K⁺ secretion (Fig. 37-8), and a similar relationship holds between final urine flow and K⁺ excretion. Accordingly, the increased urine flow that occurs with extracellular volume expansion, osmotic diuresis, or administration of several diuretic agents (e.g., acetazolamide, furosemide, thiazides) leads to enhanced K⁺ excretion (**kaliuresis**). Almost uniformly, increased urinary flow is also associated with increased Na⁺ excretion

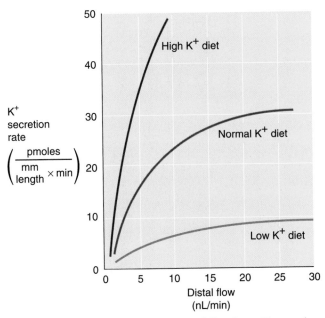

Figure 37-8 Effect of flow (i.e., Na⁺ delivery) on K⁺ excretion. *(Data from Stanton BA, Giebisch G: Renal potassium transport. In Windhager E [ed]: Handbook of Physiology: Renal Physiology, pp 813-874. New York: Oxford University Press, 1992.)*

(natriuresis), so that both solutes appear in increased amounts in the urine.

The strong flow dependence of distal K⁺ secretion is a consequence of the high apical K⁺ permeability of principal cells (Fig. 37-7D). When luminal flow is low, then as K⁺ moves from the principal cell to the lumen, luminal [K⁺] rises rapidly to a steady-state level, thereby inhibiting further K⁺ diffusion from the cell. Thus, total K⁺ secretion is relatively low. When luminal flow is high, it sweeps newly secreted K⁺ downstream. The resulting fall in luminal [K⁺] steepens the K⁺ gradient across the apical membrane and consequently increases passive K⁺ flux from cell to lumen.

Increased luminal flow also increases the Na⁺ delivery to tubule cells, thus raising luminal [Na⁺] and enhancing Na⁺ uptake. This incremental supply of Na⁺ to the principal cell stimulates its Na-K pump, increases basolateral K⁺ uptake, and further increases K⁺ secretion. The Na⁺ sensitivity of K⁺ secretion is most pronounced when luminal [Na⁺] is lower than 35 mM, as is often the case in the CCT.

An increased lumen-negative transepithelial potential increases K⁺ secretion

The apical step of K⁺ secretion in the ICT and CCT occurs by diffusion of K⁺ from the principal cell to the lumen, a process that depends on the apical electrochemical K⁺ gradient (Fig. 37-7D). Increases in luminal [Na⁺]—enhancing apical Na⁺ entry through epithelial Na⁺ channels (ENaCs) (see Chapter 35)—depolarize the apical membrane, favoring the exit of K⁺ from cell to lumen (i.e., K⁺ secretion). Conversely, a fall in luminal [Na⁺] hyperpolarizes the apical membrane, thereby inhibiting K⁺ secretion.

The diuretic **amiloride** (see Chapter 35) has the same effect on K⁺ secretion as decreasing luminal [Na⁺]. By blocking apical ENaCs, amiloride hyperpolarizes the apical membrane and reduces the electrochemical gradient for K⁺ secretion. Thus, amiloride is a K⁺-sparing diuretic.

Low luminal [Cl⁻] enhances K⁺ secretion

Lowering luminal Cl⁻—replacing it with an anion (e.g., SO_4^{2-} or HCO_3^-) that the tubule reabsorbs poorly—promotes K⁺ loss into the urine, independent of changes in the lumen-negative voltage. Underlying this effect may be the KCC in the apical membrane of the principal cell (Fig. 37-7D). Lowering luminal [Cl⁻] increases the cell-to-lumen Cl⁻ gradient, which presumably stimulates K/Cl cotransport and thus K⁺ secretion.

When luminal [Cl⁻] in the DCT is low, thiazide diuretics may indirectly *inhibit* K⁺ secretion. These drugs inhibit Cl⁻ uptake by a luminal Na/Cl cotransporter in the DCT (see Chapter 35), thus presenting a *higher* luminal [Cl⁻] to the downstream K⁺ secretory sites in the ICT and CCT. This elevation in luminal [Cl⁻] secondarily inhibits K⁺ efflux from the principal cell through the KCC (Fig. 37-7D) and thus reduces K⁺ secretion.

Aldosterone increases K⁺ secretion

Both mineralocorticoids and glucocorticoids cause kaliuresis (see Chapter 50). Primary hyperaldosteronism leads to K⁺ wasting and hypokalemia, whereas adrenocortical insufficiency (i.e., deficiency of both mineralocorticoids and glucocorticoids) leads to K⁺ retention and hyperkalemia.

Mineralocorticoids Aldosterone, the main native mineralocorticoid, induces K⁺ secretion in the ICT and CCT, particularly when its effects are prolonged. Aldosterone and desoxycorticosterone acetate (DOCA), a powerful synthetic mineralocorticoid, increase the transcription of genes that enhance Na⁺ reabsorption and, secondarily, K⁺ secretion in the *principal cells* of the ICT and CCT (see Chapter 35). Three factors act in concert to promote K⁺ secretion. First, over a period of a few hours, aldosterone increases the basolateral K⁺ uptake by stimulating the Na-K pump. Over a few days, elevated aldosterone also leads to a marked amplification of the area of the basolateral membrane of principal cells, as well as to a corresponding increase in the number of Na-K pump molecules. Conversely, adrenalectomy causes a significant reduction in basolateral surface area and Na-K pumps in principal cells. Second, mineralocorticoids stimulate apical ENaCs, thus depolarizing the apical membrane and increasing the driving force for K⁺ diffusion from cell to lumen. Third, aldosterone increases the K⁺ conductance of the apical membrane.

Considering its mechanisms of action, we could expect aldosterone to stimulate both K⁺ secretion and Na⁺ reabsorption. Therefore, one would think that the renal excretion of K⁺ and Na⁺ should always be inversely related. However, the extent to which aldosterone increases K⁺ excretion depends strongly on Na$^+$ excretion. For example, when Na$^+$ intake and excretion are low, the Na$^+$ retention induced by aldosterone reduces luminal flow, and Na$^+$ delivery to such low levels that K$^+$ excretion fails to increase. In contrast, under high-flow conditions (e.g., with a high Na$^+$ load or following administration of diuretics that act on the TAL or the DCT), aldosterone increases K$^+$ excretion.

Long-term administration of mineralocorticoids leads to a sequence of events known as **aldosterone escape**. Aldosterone leads to Na$^+$ retention and hence volume expansion. Eventually, the volume expansion causes proximal Na$^+$ reabsorption to fall (see Fig. 34-11), thereby increasing Na$^+$ delivery to the ICT and CCT and ultimately raising Na$^+$ excretion toward pre-aldosterone levels. Thus, the kidney can escape the Na$^+$-retaining effect of aldosterone, albeit at the price of expanding the extracellular volume. The situation is different with respect to K$^+$, because the increased Na$^+$ delivery to the distal K$^+$ secretory system continues to stimulate K$^+$ secretion. Once the body has become depleted of K$^+$, the aldosterone-stimulated K$^+$ secretion eventually wanes, and the distal nephron may return to net K$^+$ reabsorption.

Glucocorticoids   Under physiological conditions, glucocorticoids enhance K$^+$ excretion (Fig. 37-9). Corticosterone and dexamethasone, a synthetic glucocorticoid, produce this effect largely by increasing flow along the distal K$^+$ secretory system (i.e., ICT and CCT). Because glucocorticoids increase the GFR and probably lower the water permeability of the distal K$^+$ secretory system, they increase the amounts of fluid and Na$^+$ remaining in these segments. These two flow effects, by themselves, increase K$^+$ secretion. Indeed, when one per-

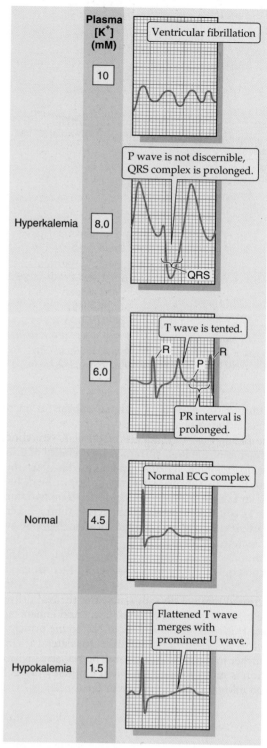

Figure 37-9   Effect of changes in plasma [K$^+$] on the ECG. These five traces show recordings from the precordial V$_4$ lead.

Hyperkalemia and the Heart

An electrocardiogram (ECG)—a measure of the electrical activity of the myocardial cells (see Chapter 21)—can be clinically useful for detecting rising plasma [K$^+$].

As plasma [K$^+$] begins to rise (Fig. 37-9, 6 mM), the T wave becomes tall and peaked, assuming a symmetric, "tented" shape. The PR interval becomes prolonged, and the P wave gradually flattens. Eventually, the P wave disappears (Fig. 37-9, 8 mM). Moreover, the QRS complex, which represents depolarization of the ventricles, widens and merges with the T wave, forming a sine-wave pattern. At higher concentrations, ventricular fibrillation, a lethal arrhythmia, may develop (Fig. 37-9, 10 mM). These changes on the ECG do not always occur in this precise order, and some patients with hyperkalemia may progress very rapidly to ventricular fibrillation. Any change in the ECG resulting from hyperkalemia requires immediate clinical attention.

Decreases in plasma [K$^+$] also affect the ECG. For example, moderate decreases in [K$^+$] to ~3 mM cause the QT interval to lengthen and the T wave to flatten. Lower values of [K$^+$] lead to the appearance of a U wave (Fig. 37-9, 1.5 mM), which represents the delayed repolarization of the ventricles.

---

fuses the distal K$^+$ secretory system at a *constant rate*, glucocorticoids have no effect on K$^+$ transport. In addition, administering unphysiologically high doses of glucocorticoids may stimulate K$^+$ transport directly as glucocorticoids bind to *mineralocorticoid* receptors; despite the presence of

11β-hydroxysteroid dehydrogenase in aldosterone target cells (see Chapter 35).

High K⁺ intake promotes renal K⁺ secretion

Dietary K⁺ Loading An increase in dietary K⁺ intake causes, after some delay, an increase in urinary K⁺ excretion (Fig. 37-5B). If the period of high-K⁺ intake is prolonged, a condition of tolerance (K⁺ adaptation) develops in which the kidneys become able to excrete large doses of K⁺—even previously lethal doses—efficiently, with only a small rise in plasma [K⁺].

The kaliuresis following an acute or chronic K⁺ load is the result of increased K⁺ secretion in the ICT and CCT (compare the three curves in Fig. 37-8 at a single flow), a process that occurs by three mechanisms. First, a transient rise in plasma [K⁺], even if maintained for only short periods, is an effective stimulus for K⁺ excretion. The mechanism is increased K⁺ uptake across the basolateral membrane of principal cells by the Na-K pump, a response shared by most of the cells of the body. As is the case with mineralocorticoid stimulation, the ultrastructure of the ICT and CCT correlates with changes in the rate of K⁺ transport induced by high dietary K⁺. Therefore, a high-K⁺ diet—independent of the effects of aldosterone—causes surface amplification of the basolateral membrane of principal cells. Second, the increased plasma [K⁺] stimulates glomerulosa cells in the adrenal cortex to synthesize and release aldosterone (see Chapter 55). This mineralocorticoid is a potent stimulus for K⁺ secretion both in the kidney by principal cells (see earlier) and in the colon (see Chapter 44). Third, acute K⁺ loading inhibits proximal Na⁺ and fluid reabsorption and increases the flow and Na⁺ delivery to the distal K⁺ secretory system, processes that stimulate K⁺ secretion.

Dietary K⁺ Deprivation In response to K⁺ restriction, the kidneys retain K⁺ (Fig. 37-5A). The rate of urinary K⁺ excretion may fall to 1% to 3% of the filtered load, a finding reflecting the action of two mechanisms at the level of the ICT and CCT. First, the low plasma [K⁺] suppresses K⁺ secretion by the principal cells (Fig. 37-8, lower curve) both by reducing basolateral K⁺ uptake by principal cells and by reducing aldosterone secretion. Second, the low plasma [K⁺] stimulates K⁺ reabsorption by intercalated cells through H-K pumps (Fig. 37-7C), thus causing the [K⁺] of the final urine to fall sharply, sometimes to levels lower than that of the plasma. In addition, the MCD responds to K⁺ depletion by increasing its reabsorption of K⁺, by enhancing both the activity of its apical K-H pump and its paracellular K⁺ permeability.

Whereas states of high K⁺ secretion (i.e., aldosterone or high-K⁺ diet) amplify the basolateral membrane area of principal cells, K⁺ deprivation amplifies the *apical* membrane of α *intercalated* cells. Moreover, K⁺ depletion causes an increased incorporation of rod-shaped particles in the apical membrane of α intercalated cells, and the density of these particles correlates well with enhanced K⁺ reabsorption. These morphological changes probably underlie the increased

active K⁺ reabsorption and H⁺ secretion mediated by H-K pumps.

Acidosis decreases K⁺ secretion

Acid-base disturbances have marked effects on renal K⁺ transport. In general, either metabolic alkalosis or respiratory alkalosis leads to increased K⁺ excretion (see Chapter 27). Conversely, acidosis reduces K⁺ excretion, although this response is more variable than that to alkalosis. Changes in systemic acid-base parameters affect K⁺ transport mainly by acting on the distal K⁺ secretory system.

As discussed, alkalosis leads to hypokalemia, owing to K⁺ uptake by cells throughout the body. Despite this fall in plasma [K⁺], alkalosis *stimulates* K⁺ secretion in the distal K⁺ secretory system, thereby worsening the hypokalemia. Conversely, K⁺ secretion falls in acidosis despite the shift of K⁺ from cells to ECF and the concomitant rise in plasma [K⁺].

The cellular events underlying the renal response to acid-base disturbances most likely involve effects of pH_i on both the basolateral Na-K pump and the apical K⁺ channels of the principal cells in the ICT and CCT. Tubule perfusion studies with ⁴²K indicate that decreasing the extracellular pH—which also decreases pH_i—inhibits the Na-K pump and thus K⁺ secretion. Even more important is that the decrease in pH_i also reduces the permeability of the apical K⁺ channels, which are exquisitely sensitive to acidification (Fig. 37-10). The reverse changes occur in alkalosis.

The changes in tubule flow (i.e., fluid delivery to the distal K⁺ secretory system) that occur in acid-base disturbances may modulate the effects of pH changes per se. For example, metabolic alkalosis increases the flow by delivering an HCO₃⁻-rich solution to the ICT and CCT. By itself, this increased flow enhances K⁺ secretion, and thus *potentiates* the effect of alkalosis per se. In contrast, acidosis also increases distal flow, in this case by inhibiting proximal fluid reabsorption, with the consequence that the tendency of increased flow to increase K⁺ secretion *opposes* the effect of acidosis per se to decrease it. Therefore, the net effect of acidosis on K⁺ excretion is variable.

Epinephrine reduces and AVP enhances K⁺ excretion

By both extrarenal and renal mechanisms, **epinephrine** lowers K⁺ excretion. First, epinephrine enhances K⁺ uptake by extrarenal tissues (see Chapter 27), thereby lowering plasma [K⁺] and reducing the filtered K⁺ load. Second, catecholamines directly inhibit K⁺ secretion in nephron segments downstream of the ICT.

Although it is not a major regulator of K⁺ excretion, **AVP**, also known as antidiuretic hormone [ADH], can stimulate the distal K⁺ secretory system by two mechanisms (Fig. 37-7D): (1) AVP increases the apical Na⁺ conductance, thus depolarizing the apical membrane and providing a larger driving force for K⁺ efflux from cell to lumen; and (2) AVP increases apical K⁺ permeability. However, AVP also reduces urine flow and thus inhibits K⁺ secretion. Therefore, the two opposing effects—a direct stimulation of K⁺ secretion and a

A SINGLE-CHANNEL CURRENTS

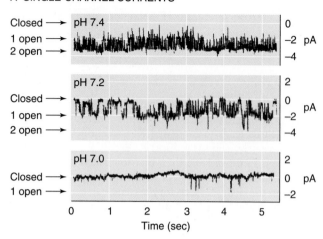

B OPEN PROBABILITY

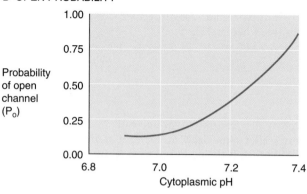

Figure 37-10 Effect of intracellular acidosis on K$^+$-channel activity in the apical membrane of a principal cell. In **A**, the recordings show single-channel K$^+$ currents from inside-out patches, with different pH values on the "cytoplasmic" side. As shown in **B**, channels are almost never open at pH values at 7.0 or lower. *(Data from Wang W, Geibel J, Giebisch G: Am J Physiol 1990; 259:F494-F502.)*

Clinical Implications: Evaluating Hypokalemia and Hyperkalemia in the Patient

We can directly apply the physiological principles discussed in this chapter to understanding the common causes and treatment of hypokalemia and hyperkalemia.

Hypokalemia

The body can lose K$^+$ from three sites: the kidneys, the GI tract, and the skin. Renal losses occur most commonly in patients taking diuretics (e.g., furosemide and thiazides) that act at sites upstream to the distal K$^+$ secretory system (i.e., ICT, CCT, and proximal portion of MCD). K$^+$ losses can also occur in individuals with renal tubule disorders or alterations in the renin-angiotensin-aldosterone system (e.g., hyperaldosteronism). Because gastric and intestinal secretions have a high [K$^+$], vomiting and severe diarrhea are common causes of hypokalemia. Significant K$^+$ depletion through the skin can occur in two situations: (1) strenuous exercise on a hot, humid day can cause dehydration and hypokalemia from the loss of many liters of perspiration; and (2) severe and extensive burns can result in the transudation of vast amounts of K$^+$-containing fluid through the skin. In both cases, the lost fluid is K$^+$ rich compared with plasma.

Low plasma [K$^+$] can also develop as the result of altered K$^+$ distribution within the body, without any net loss of whole-body K$^+$. Common causes include alkalosis, a catecholamine surge (e.g., as during any acute stress to the body, such as an acute myocardial infarction), and excessive insulin administration during the treatment of diabetic ketoacidosis.

Patients may develop hypokalemia because of inadequate dietary K$^+$ intake. Patients receiving large amounts of intravenous saline (which lacks K$^+$) may also waste K$^+$. Some persons in rural areas ingest clay (a behavior called pica), which binds K$^+$ in the GI tract and prevents K$^+$ absorption.

Hyperkalemia

Probably the most common cause of a high laboratory value for plasma [K$^+$] is **pseudohyperkalemia**, a falsely elevated value that results from traumatic hemolysis of red blood cells during blood drawing. Red blood cells release their intracellular stores of K$^+$ in the blood sample, and the laboratory reports a falsely elevated plasma [K$^+$]. Patients with myeloproliferative disorders associated with greatly increased numbers of platelets or white blood cells can also show a falsely elevated [K$^+$] because of K$^+$ released during clot formation within the blood sample tube.

Excessive intake of K$^+$ rarely causes hyperkalemia in persons with healthy kidneys. However, even in these individuals, a large K$^+$ bolus can cause transient hyperkalemia (Fig. 37-2, top), often from an ill-advised intravenous line. Altered distribution of K$^+$ can lead to elevated plasma levels in patients with acidosis and, rarely, as a result of β-adrenergic blockade. Digitalis, a cardiac glycoside that inhibits the Na-K pump (see Chapter 5), is another rare cause of hyperkalemia resulting from K$^+$ redistribution. Massive breakdown of cells can release large amounts of K$^+$ into the extracellular space. This release can occur in patients with intravascular hemolysis (e.g., from a mismatched blood transfusion), burns, crush injuries, rhabdomyolysis (massive muscle destruction such as can be seen with trauma or sepsis), GI bleeding with subsequent intestinal absorption of K$^+$-rich fluid, or destruction of tumor tissue or leukemic blood cells by chemotherapy.

Impaired renal excretion of K$^+$ is the primary cause of a sustained increase in plasma [K$^+$]. Hypoaldosteronism, high doses of amiloride, and distal renal tubular acidosis can be responsible, but advanced renal failure itself from any of a myriad number of disorders is the most common cause.

The treatment of hyperkalemia depends on the severity of the problem. For severe hyperkalemia (i.e., [K$^+$] > 8 mM) with accompanying ECG changes, the physician immediately infuses calcium gluconate intravenously to counter the electrophysiological effects of the hyperkalemia. (Ca^{2+} raises the threshold for action potentials and lessens membrane excitability). One may also simultaneously administer NaHCO$_3$, glucose, and often insulin to move some of the K$^+$ from the extracellular to the intracellular space. These are all temporizing measures. To remove the excess K$^+$ from the body, the physician administers a nonabsorbable Na-K cation exchange resin (e.g., sodium polystyrene sulfonamide) either orally or as an enema. The resin binds the K$^+$ and carries it out of the body through the GI tract. However, the resin takes several hours to work. Thus, for patients with hyperkalemia and ECG changes, the temporizing measures buy time for the resin to act. For patients with end-stage renal failure, dialysis is often necessary to return the plasma [K$^+$] to normal.

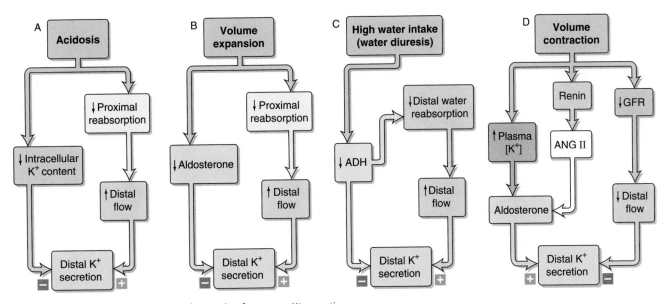

Figure 37-11 **A** to **D**, Interaction of opposing factors on K⁺ secretion.

flow-related reduction of K⁺ secretion—may cancel each other.

Increased distal flow enhances K⁺ secretion and adds to the direct effects of "regulatory factors"

It should be apparent from the foregoing discussion that the net effect of a specific disturbance on K⁺ excretion in the final urine often represents a result of two or more interacting factors. Changes in flow often indirectly amplify or attenuate the direct response of the distal K⁺ secretory system to a given stimulus. Figure 37-11 shows four examples of **attenuating effects**. The first three (acidosis, volume expansion, and high water intake) are characterized by the competition between a direct inhibitory effect on K⁺ secretion and an indirect stimulatory effect of increased flow (Fig. 37-11A through C).

Extracellular volume contraction (Fig. 37-11D) has three effects. First, it decreases distal flow and thus inhibits the distal K⁺ secretory system. Second, volume contraction increases angiotensin II (ANG II) levels, a process that, in turn, *increases* aldosterone release and hence K⁺ secretion. Third, volume contraction also produces a small rise in plasma [K⁺], the magnitude of which may normally not evoke much of an increase in aldosterone release. However, in the presence of elevated ANG II, even such a small increase in plasma [K⁺] is a potent stimulus for aldosterone release (see Chapter 50). Thus, the potentiation between K⁺ and ANG II ensures continued K⁺ excretion, even when low fluid delivery to the distal K⁺ secretory system would have the opposite effect.

In some instances, the direct actions of an agent and flow-related effects may have **additive effects**. Three examples follow.

First, metabolic alkalosis—as discussed—directly stimulates the distal K⁺ secretory system. In addition, the delivery of the poorly reabsorbable HCO₃⁻ in metabolic alkalosis increases distal flow, thereby potentiating K⁺ excretion.

Second, hyperkalemia directly stimulates the distal K⁺ secretory system. In addition, because increased plasma [K⁺] inhibits Na⁺ and fluid reabsorption in the proximal tubule, distal flow increases, again potentiating K⁺ excretion.

Third, administration of diuretics that act on a site upstream of the ICT and CCT increases Na⁺ delivery to the distal K⁺ secretory system and thereby stimulates K⁺ secretion. In addition, the volume contraction induced by the diuretic raises aldosterone levels, again potentiating K⁺ excretion. Hypokalemia is thus a possible harmful side effect of diuretic treatment.

REFERENCES

Books and Reviews
Giebisch G: Challenges to potassium metabolism: Internal distribution and external balance. Wien Klin Wochenschr 2004; 116:353-366.
Hebert SC, Desir G, Giebisch G, Wang W: Molecular diversity and regulation of renal potassium channels. Physiol Rev 2005; 85:319-371.
Jamison RL: Potassium recycling. Kidney Int 1987; 31:695-703.
Wingo CS, Cain BD: The renal H-K-ATPase: Physiological significance and role in potassium homeostasis. Annu Rev Physiol 1993; 55:323-347.

Journal Articles
Greger R, Schlatter E: Presence of luminal K⁺, a prerequisite for active NaCl transport in the cortical thick ascending limb of Henle's loop of rabbit kidney. Pflugers Arch 1981; 392:92-94.
Gu RM, Wei Y, Falck JR, et al: Effects of protein tyrosine kinase and protein tyrosine phosphatase on apical K⁺ channels in the TAL. Am J Physiol 2001; 281:C1188-C1195.
Ho K, Nichols CG, Lederer WJ, et al: Cloning and expression of an inwardly rectifying ATP-regulated potassium channel. Nature 1993; 362:31-38.

Liu W, Xu S, Woda C, et al: Effect of flow and stretch on the $[Ca^{2+}]_i$ response of principal and intercalated cells in cortical collecting duct. Am J Physiol 2003; 285:F998-F1012.

Malnic G, Klose R, Giebisch G: Micropuncture study of renal potassium excretion in the rat. Am J Physiol 1964; 206: 674-686.

Stokes J: Consequences of potassium recycling in the renal medulla: Effects on ion transport by the medullary thick ascending limb of Henle's loop. J Clin Invest 1982; 70:219-229.

Wade JB, O'Neil RG, Pryor JL, Boulpaep EL: Modulation of cell membrane area in renal cortical collecting tubules by corticosteroid hormones. J Cell Biol 1979; 81:439-445.

Wang W, Geibel J, Giebisch G: Regulation of small conductance K channel in the apical membrane of rat cortical collecting tubule. Am J Physiol 1990; 259:F494-F502.

CHAPTER 38

URINE CONCENTRATION AND DILUTION

Gerhard Giebisch and Erich Windhager

WATER BALANCE AND THE OVERALL RENAL HANDLING OF WATER

The kidney can generate a urine as dilute as 30 mOsm (1/10 of plasma osmolality) or as concentrated as 1200 mOsm (4× plasma osmolality)

In the steady state, water intake and output must be equal (Table 38-1). The body's three major sources of water are (1) water ingested, (2) water contained within foods that we eat, and (3) water produced by aerobic metabolism as mitochondria convert foodstuffs and O_2 to CO_2 and H_2O (see Chapter 58).

The major route of water loss is usually through the kidneys, the organs that play the central role in regulating water balance. The feces are usually a minor route of water output (see Chapter 44). Although the production of sweat can increase markedly during exercise or at high temperatures, sweat production is geared to help regulate body core temperature (see Chapter 59), not body water balance. Water also evaporates from the skin and is lost in the humidified air exhaled from the lungs and air passages. The figures summarized in Table 38-1 obviously vary, depending on diet, physical activity, and the environment (e.g., temperature and humidity).

The kidney adjusts its water output to compensate for either abnormally high or abnormally low water intake or for abnormally high water losses through other routes. The kidney excretes a variable amount of solute, depending especially on salt intake. However, for a normal diet, the excreted solute is ~600 mOsmol/day. For average conditions of water and solute intake and output, this 600 mOsmol is dissolved in a daily urine output of 1500 mL. A key principle is that, regardless of the volume of water they excrete, the kidneys must excrete ~600 mOsmol/day. Stated somewhat differently, the product of urine osmolality and urine output is approximately constant:

$$\text{Osmoles excreted/day} = \underbrace{U_{Osm}}_{\substack{\text{Urine} \\ \text{osmolality}}} \times \underbrace{\dot{V}}_{\substack{\text{Urine} \\ \text{output/day}}} \quad (38\text{-}1)$$

Therefore, to excrete a wide range of water volumes, the human kidney must produce urine having a wide range of osmolalities. For example, when the kidney excretes the 600 mOsmol dissolved in 1500 mL of urine each day, urine osmolality must be 400 mOsm:

$$U_{Osm} = \frac{\text{Osmol excreted/day}}{\dot{V}} = \frac{600 \text{ mOsmol/day}}{1.5 \text{ L/day}} \quad (38\text{-}2)$$
$$= 400 \; mOsm$$

When the intake of water is especially high, the human kidney can generate urine having an osmolality as low as ~30 mOsm. Because the kidneys may still need to excrete 600 mOsmol of solutes, the urine volume in an extreme **water diuresis** would be as high as 20 L/day.

$$\dot{V} = \frac{\text{Osmol excreted/day}}{U_{Osm}} = \frac{600 \text{ mOsmol/day}}{30 \text{ mOsm}} \quad (38\text{-}3)$$
$$= 20 \text{ L/day}$$

However, when it is necessary to conserve water (e.g., with restricted water intake; excessive loss by sweat or stool), the kidney is capable of generating urine with an osmolality as high as ~1200 mOsm. Therefore, with an average solute load, the minimal urine volume can be as low as ~0.5 L/day:

$$\dot{V} = \frac{\text{Osmol excreted/day}}{U_{Osm}} = \frac{600 \text{ mOsmol/day}}{1200 \text{ mOsm}} \quad (38\text{-}4)$$
$$= 0.5 \text{ L/day}$$

Therefore, the kidney is capable of diluting the urine ~10-fold with respect to blood plasma, but it is capable of concentrating the urine only ~4-fold. Renal failure reduces both the concentrating and diluting ability.

Table 38-1 Input and Output of Water

INPUT	
Source	**Amount (mL)**
Ingested fluids	1200
Ingested food	1000
Metabolism	300
Total	2500
OUTPUT	
Route	**Amount (mL)**
Urine	1500
Feces	100
Skin/sweat	550
Exhaled air	350
Total	2500

(Data from Valtin H: Renal Dysfunction: Mechanisms Involved in Fluid and Solute Imbalance, p 21. Boston: Little, Brown, 1979.)

Free water clearance is positive if the kidney produces urine that is less concentrated than plasma and negative if the kidney produces urine that is more concentrated than plasma

A urine sample can be thought of as consisting of two moieties: (1) the volume that would be necessary to dissolve all the excreted solutes at a concentration that is isosmotic with blood plasma; and (2) the volume of pure or solute-free water—or, simply, **free water**—that one must add (or subtract) to the previous volume to account for the entire urine volume. As discussed later, the kidney generates free water in the tubule lumen by reabsorbing solutes, mainly NaCl, in excess of water along nephron segments with low water permeability. When the kidney generates free water, the urine becomes dilute (hypo-osmotic). Conversely, when the kidney removes water from an isosmotic fluid, the urine becomes concentrated (hyperosmotic). When the kidney neither adds nor subtracts free water from the isosmotic moiety, the urine is isosmotic with blood plasma.

The urine output is the sum of the rate at which kidney excretes the isosmotic moiety of urine (**osmolal clearance**, C_{Osm}) and the rate at which it excretes free water (**free water clearance** [C_{H_2O}]):

$$\dot{V} = C_{Osm} + C_{H_2O} \qquad (38\text{-}5)$$

Of course, C_{H_2O} is negative (i.e., excretion of negative free water) if the kidney removes free water and produces concentrated urine. We compute C_{Osm} in the same way we would

compute the clearance of any substance from the blood (see Chapter 33):

$$C_{Osm} = \frac{U_{Osm} \cdot \dot{V}}{P_{Osm}} \qquad (38\text{-}6)$$

P_{Osm} is the osmolality of blood plasma. The osmolal clearance is the hypothetical volume of blood (in milliliters) that the kidneys fully clear of solutes (or osmoles) per unit time. For example, if the daily solute excretion ($U_{Osm} \cdot \dot{V}$) is fixed at 600 mOsmol/day, and P_{Osm} is 300 mOsmol/L, then Equation 38-6 tells us that C_{Osm} has a fixed value of 2 L/day.

We can obtain C_{H_2O} only by subtraction:

$$C_{H_2O} = \dot{V} - C_{Osm} \qquad (38\text{-}7)$$

Indeed, C_{H_2O} does not conform to the usual definition of clearance because C_{H_2O} is not $(U_{H_2O} \cdot \dot{V})/P_{H_2O}$. Nevertheless, this apparent misnomer has been accepted by renal physiologists and nephrologists.

The range of C_{H_2O} values for the human kidney is related to the extremes in urine osmolality, as shown for the following three examples:

Isosmotic Urine If the osmolalities of the urine and plasma are the *same* ($U_{Osm} = P_{Osm}$), then osmolal clearance equals urine flow:

$$C_{Osm} = \frac{U_{Osm} \cdot \dot{V}}{P_{Osm}} = \frac{300\,\text{mOsmol/L} \times 2\,\text{L/day}}{300\,\text{mOsmol/L}} \qquad (38\text{-}8)$$
$$= 2\,\text{L/day} = \dot{V}$$

Therefore, Equation 38-7 tells us that C_{H_2O} must be zero.

Dilute Urine If the urine is more dilute than plasma ($\dot{V} > C_{Osm}$), then the difference between $\dot{V}$ and C_{Osm} is the **positive C_{H_2O}**. When the kidney *maximally dilutes* the urine to 30 mOsm, the total urine flow ($\dot{V}$) must be 20 L/day (see Equation 38-3):

$$C_{H_2O} = \dot{V} - C_{Osm}$$
$$\text{Maximal dilution:} \quad C_{H_2O} = 20\,\text{L/day} - 2\,\text{L/day} \qquad (38\text{-}9)$$
$$= +18\,\text{L/day}$$

Concentrated Urine If the urine is more concentrated than plasma ($\dot{V} < C_{Osm}$), then the difference between $\dot{V}$ and C_{Osm} is a negative number, the **negative C_{H_2O}**. When the kidney *maximally concentrates* the urine to 1200 mOsm, the total urine flow must be 0.5 L/day (see Equation 38-4):

$$C_{H_2O} = \dot{V} - C_{Osm}$$
$$\text{Maximal concentration:} \quad C_{H_2O} = 0.5\,\text{L/day} - 2\,\text{L/day}$$
$$= -1.5\,\text{L/day}$$
$$(38\text{-}10)$$

Thus, the kidneys can generate C_{H_2O} of as much as +18 L/day under maximally diluting conditions, or as little as −1.5 L/day under maximally concentrating conditions. This wide range of C_{H_2O} represents the kidneys' attempt to stabilize the osmolality of extracellular fluid in the face of changing loads of solutes or water. From the extreme C_{H_2O} that the kidneys can achieve, we can conclude that the organism withstands the challenge of water load better than a water deficit.

WATER TRANSPORT BY DIFFERENT SEGMENTS OF THE NEPHRON

The kidney generates concentrated urine by using osmosis to drive water from the tubule lumen, across a water-permeable epithelium, into a hypertonic interstitium

The kidney generates *dilute* urine by pumping salts out of the lumen of tubule segments that are impermeable to water. What is left behind is tubule fluid that is hypo-osmotic (dilute) with respect to the blood.

How does the kidney generate *concentrated* urine? One approach could be to pump water actively out of the tubule lumen. However, water pumps do not exist (see Chapter 5). Instead, the kidney uses osmosis as the driving force to concentrate the contents of the tubule lumen. The kidney generates the osmotic gradient by creating a hypertonic interstitial fluid in a confined compartment, the renal medulla. The final step for making a hyperosmotic urine is to thread a water-permeable tube—the medullary collecting duct (MCD)—through this hyperosmolar compartment. The result is that the fluid in the tubule lumen can equilibrate with the hypertonic interstitium, thus generating concentrated urine.

Although net absorption of H_2O occurs all along the nephron, not all segments alter the osmolality of the tubule fluid. The proximal tubule, *regardless of the final osmolality of the urine*, reabsorbs two thirds of the filtered fluid isosmotically (i.e., the fluid reabsorbed has the same osmolality as plasma). The loop of Henle reabsorbs salt in excess of water, so that the fluid entering the distal convoluted tubule (DCT) is hypo-osmotic. *Whether the final urine is dilute or concentrated* depends on whether water reabsorption occurs in more distal segments: the initial and cortical collecting tubules (ICT and CCT) and the outer and inner MCDs (OMCD and IMCD). **Arginine vasopressin (AVP)**—also called **antidiuretic hormone** (ADH)—regulates the variable fraction of water reabsorption in these four nephron segments. Figure 13-9 shows the structure of AVP.

Tubule fluid is isosmotic in the proximal tubule, becomes dilute in the loop of Henle, and then either remains dilute or becomes concentrated by the end of the collecting duct

Figure 38-1 shows two examples of how tubule fluid osmolality (expressed as the ratio TF_{Osm}/P_{Osm}) changes along the nephron. The first is a case of water restriction, in which the kidneys maximally concentrate the urine and excrete a

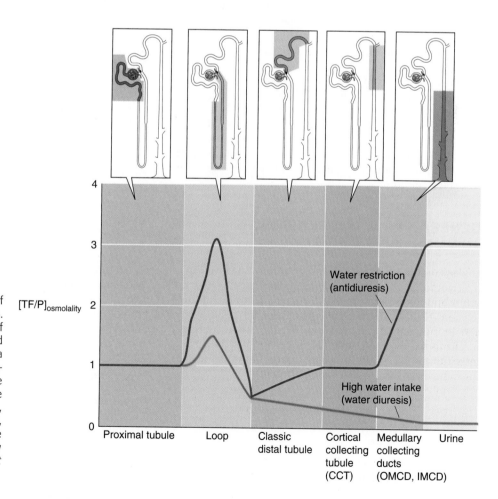

Figure 38-1 Relative osmolality of the tubule fluid along the nephron. Plotted on the y-axis is the ratio of the osmolality of the tubule fluid (TF) to the osmolality of the plasma (P); plotted on the x-axis is a representation of distance along the nephron. The *red record* is the profile of relative osmolality (i.e., $TF/P_{osmolality}$) for water restriction, whereas the *blue record* is the profile for high water intake. *(Data from Gottschalk CW: Physiologist 1961; 4:33-55.)*

minimal volume of water (**antidiuresis**). The second is a case of ingestion of excess water, in which the kidneys produce a large volume of dilute urine (**water diuresis**). In both cases, the tubule fluid does not change in osmolality along the proximal tubule, and it becomes hypotonic to plasma by the end of the thick ascending limb of the loop of Henle (TAL), also known as the diluting segment (see Chapter 35). Therefore, the fluid entering the DCT is hypo-osmotic with respect to plasma, regardless of the final urine osmolality.

Under conditions of restricted water intake or **hydropenia**, elevated levels of AVP increase the water permeability of the nephron from the ICT to the end of the IMCD. As a result, the osmolality of the tubule fluid increases along the ICT (Fig. 38-1, red curve), achieving the osmolality of the cortical interstitium—which is the same as the osmolality of plasma (~290 mOsm)—by the end of this nephron segment. No additional increase in osmolality occurs along the CCT, because the tubule fluid is already in osmotic equilibrium with the surrounding cortical interstitium. However, in the MCDs, the luminal osmolality rises sharply as the tubule fluid equilibrates with the surrounding medullary interstitium, which becomes increasingly more hyperosmotic from the corticomedullary junction to the papillary tip. Eventually the tubule fluid reaches osmolalities that are as much as four times higher than the plasma. Thus, the MCDs are responsible for concentrating the final urine.

In summary, the two key elements in producing a concentrated urine are the hyperosmotic medullary interstitium that provides the osmotic gradient and the AVP that raises the water permeability of the distal nephron. How the kidney generates this interstitial hyperosmolality is discussed in the next subchapter, and the role of AVP is discussed in the last subchapter.

Under conditions of **water loading**, depressed AVP levels cause the water permeability of the distal nephron to remain low. However, the continued reabsorption of NaCl along the distal nephron effectively separates salt from water and leaves a relatively hypotonic fluid behind in the tubule lumen. Thus, the tubule fluid becomes increasingly hypotonic from the DCT throughout the remainder of the nephron (Fig. 38-1, blue curve).

GENERATING A HYPEROSMOTIC MEDULLA AND URINE

Understanding the mechanisms involved in forming a hypertonic or hypotonic urine requires knowing (1) the solute and water permeability characteristics of each tubule segment, (2) the osmotic gradient between the tubule lumen and its surrounding interstitium, (3) the active transport mechanisms that generate the hyperosmotic medullary interstitium, and (4) the "exchange" mechanisms that sustain the hyperosmotic medullary compartment.

The renal medulla is hyperosmotic to blood plasma during both antidiuresis (low urine flow) and water diuresis

The loop of Henle plays a key role in both the dilution and the concentration of the urine. The main functions of the loop are to remove NaCl—more so than water—from the lumen and to deposit this NaCl in the interstitium of the renal medulla. By separating tubule NaCl from tubule water, the loop of Henle participates *directly* in forming dilute urine. Conversely, because the TAL deposits this NaCl into the medullary interstitium, thus making it hyperosmotic, the loop of Henle is *indirectly* responsible for elaborating concentrated urine. As discussed later, urea also contributes to the hypertonicity of the medulla.

Figure 38-2A shows approximate values of osmolality in the tubule fluid and interstitium during an *antidiuresis* produced, for example, by water restriction. Figure 38-2B, however, illustrates the comparable information during a *water diuresis* produced, for example, by high water intake. In *both* conditions, interstitial osmolality progressively rises from the cortex to the tip of the medulla (corticomedullary osmolality gradient). The difference between the two conditions is that the maximal interstitial osmolality during antidiuresis, ~1200 mOsm (Fig. 38-2A), is more than twice that achieved during water diuresis, ~500 mOsm (Fig. 38-2B).

Because of the NaCl pumped out of the rather water-impermeable TAL, the tubule fluid at the end of this segment is hypo-osmotic to the cortical interstitium during both antidiuresis and water diuresis. However, beyond the TAL, luminal osmolalities differ considerably between antidiuresis and diuresis. In *antidiuresis*, the fluid becomes progressively more concentrated from the ICT to the end of the nephron (Fig. 38-2A). In contrast, during *water diuresis*, the hypotonicity of the tubule fluid is further accentuated as the fluid passes along segments from the DCT to the end of the nephron segments that are relatively water impermeable and continue to pump NaCl out of the lumen (Fig. 38-2B). During *antidiuresis*, the tubule fluid in the ICT, CCT, OMCD, and IMCD more or less equilibrates with the interstitium, but it fails to do so during *water diuresis*. This marked difference in osmotic equilibration reflects the action of AVP, which increases water permeability in each of the previously mentioned four segments.

Although NaCl transport generates a gradient of only ~200 mOsm across any portion of the ascending limb, the countercurrent system can multiply this single effect to produce a 900-mOsm gradient between the cortex and the papilla

Developing and maintaining the hyperosmolality of the medullary interstitium depends on the net transport of NaCl across the rather water-impermeable wall of the ascending limb of the loop of Henle, from lumen to interstitium. This salt reabsorption increases the osmolality of the interstitium and decreases the osmolality of the fluid within the lumen. The limiting NaCl concentration gradient that the tubule can develop at any point along its length is only ~200 mOsm, and this concentration alone could not explain the ability of the kidney to raise the osmolality of the papilla to 1200 mOsm. The kidney can achieve such high solute levels only because the hairpin loops of Henle create a countercurrent flow mechanism that multiplies the single *transverse* gradient of 200 mOsm. The result is an osmotic gradient of 900 mOsm along both the axis of the lumen of the ascending limb and

A   WATER RESTRICTION (ANTIDIURESIS)

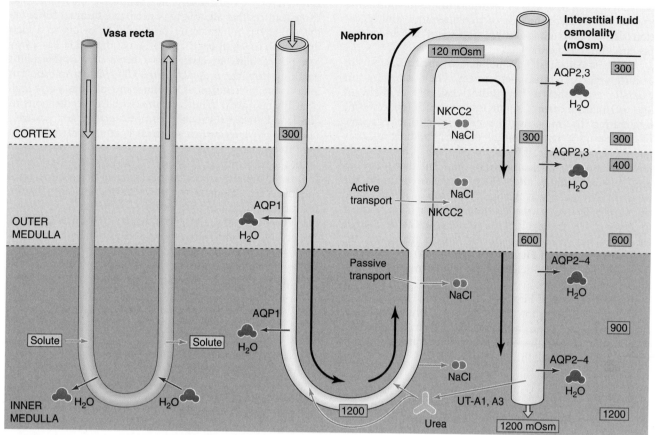

B   HIGH WATER INTAKE (WATER DIURESIS)

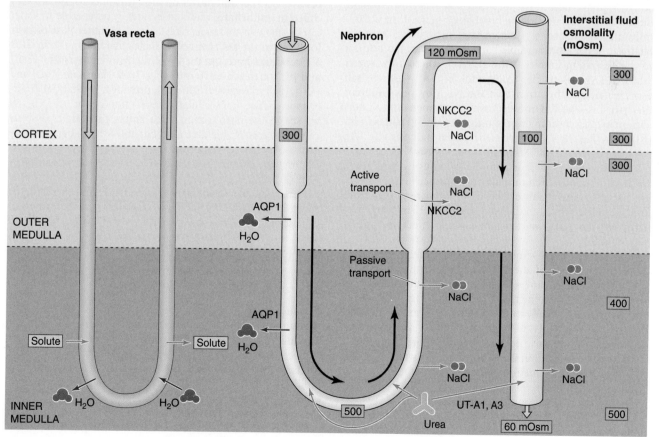

Figure 38-2   Nephron and interstitial osmolalities. **A**, Water restriction (antidiuresis). **B**, High water intake (water diuresis). The numbers in boxes are osmolalities (mOsm) along the lumen of the nephron and along the corticomedullary axis of the interstitium. The outflow of blood from the vasa recta is greater than the inflow, a finding reflecting the uptake of water reabsorbed from the collecting ducts.

the corticomedullary axis of the interstitium. In addition to the hairpin shape of the loop of Henle, osmotic multiplication also depends on a distinct pattern of salt and water permeabilities along the loop of Henle.

Figure 38-3 illustrates a simplified, schematized model of a **countercurrent-multiplier** system. The kidney in this example establishes a longitudinal osmotic gradient of 300 mOsm from cortex (300 mOsm) to papilla (600 mOsm) by iterating (i.e., multiplying) a single effect that is capable of generating a transepithelial osmotic gradient of only 200 mOsm. Of course, if we had used more cycles, we could have generated a corticomedullary gradient that was even greater. For example, after 39 cycles in our example, the interstitial osmolality at the tip of the loop of Henle would be ~1200. Therefore, the countercurrent arrangement of the loop of Henle magnifies the osmotic work that a single ascending limb cell can perform. Among mammals, the length of the loop of Henle—compared with the thickness of the renal cortex—determines the maximal osmolality of the medulla.

In the *last panel* of Figure 38-3, we include the collecting duct in the model to show the final event of urine concentration: allowing the fluid in the collecting duct to equilibrate osmotically with the hyperosmotic interstitium produces a concentrated urine.

The single effect is the result of passive NaCl reabsorption in the thin ascending limb and active NaCl reabsorption in the thick ascending limb

So far, we have treated the ascending limb as a functionally uniform epithelium that is capable of generating a 200-mOsm gradient between lumen and interstitium, across a relatively water-impermeable barrier. However, the bottom of the ascending limb is "thin" (tALH), whereas the top is "thick" (TAL). Both the tALH and the TAL separate salt from water, but they transport the NaCl by very different mechanisms. The **TAL** moves NaCl from lumen out to interstitium using a combination of transcellular and paracellular pathways (Fig. 38-4). For the transcellular pathway, the TAL cell takes up Na+ and Cl− through an apical Na/K/Cl cotransporter and exports these ions to the blood using basolateral Na-K pumps and Cl− channels. For the paracellular pathway, the lumen-positive transepithelial voltage drives Na+ from lumen to blood through the tight junctions. Using these two pathways, the TAL can generate a single effect as large as 200 mOsm.

In contrast, the movement of Na+ and Cl− from the lumen to the interstitium of the **tALH** appears to be an entirely passive process. During the debate on the mechanism of NaCl reabsorption in the tALH, several investigators pointed out that it was difficult to imagine how the extraordinarily thin cells of the tALH, with their paucity of mitochondria, could perform intensive active solute transport. Because the concentration of NaCl in the lumen exceeds that of the interstitium of the inner medulla, NaCl is reabsorbed passively. The key question for this model is: How did the luminal [NaCl] in the tALH become so high?

The work of concentrating the NaCl in the lumen was performed earlier, when the fluid was in the **thin descending limb** (tDLH) of juxtamedullary nephrons. This tDLH has three features that allow it to concentrate luminal NaCl: (1) the tDLH has a high water permeability, owing to a high expression of aquaporin 1 (AQP1); (2) the tDLH has a very low permeability to NaCl and a finite urea permeability, resulting from the presence of the UT-A2 urea transporter; and (3) the interstitium of the inner medulla has a very high [NaCl] and [urea]. The high interstitial concentrations of NaCl and urea provide the osmotic energy for passively reabsorbing water, which secondarily concentrates NaCl in the lumen of the tDLH.

In the interstitium, [Na+], [Cl−], and [urea] all rise along the axis from the cortex to the papillary tip of the renal medulla (Fig. 38-4). In the *outer* medulla, a steep rise in interstitial [Na+] and [Cl−] occurs—owing to the pumping of NaCl out of the TAL (see Chapter 35)—that is largely responsible for producing the hypertonicity. Although urea makes only a minor contribution in the outermost portion of the outer medulla, [urea] rises steeply from the middle of the outer medulla to the papilla. At the tip of the papilla, urea and NaCl each contribute half of the interstitial osmolality. As discussed in the next section, this steep interstitial [urea] profile in the inner medulla (Fig. 38-4) is the result of the unique water and urea permeabilities of the collecting tubules and ducts (Fig. 38-2A).

Knowing that NaCl and urea contribute to the high osmolality of the inner medullary interstitium, we can understand how the tDLH passively elevates [NaCl] in the lumen to levels higher than that in the interstitium. NaCl is the main solute in the lumen at the tip of the papilla but urea contributes to the luminal osmolality. As the luminal fluid turns the corner and moves up the tALH, it encounters a very different epithelium, one that is now impermeable to water but permeable to NaCl. The ClC-K1 channel is selectively localized to the tALH (overt diabetes insipidus [DI] in *ClC-K1* knockout mice). At the tip of the papilla interstitial [Na+] and [Cl−] are each ~300 mM (Fig. 38-4). Luminal [Na+] and [Cl−], each in excess of 300 mM, provide a substantial gradient for passive transcellular reabsorption of Na+ and Cl−. As we see in the next section, urea enters the tALH passively caused by a favorable urea gradient and by urea permeability of the tALH larger than that of the tDLH. The entry of urea opposes the osmotic work achieved by the passive reabsorption of NaCl. Even though the mechanism and magnitude of the single effect is different in the tALH and the TAL, the result is the same. At any level, osmolality in the lumen of the ascending limb is lower than it is in the interstitium.

The inner medullary collecting duct reabsorbs urea and produces high levels of urea in the interstitium of the inner medulla

Because urea comes from protein breakdown, urea delivery to the kidney, and therefore the contribution of urea to the medullary hyperosmolality, is larger with protein-rich diets. Indeed, investigators have long known that the higher the dietary protein content, the greater is the concentrating ability.

Urea Handling   The renal handling of urea is complex (see Chapter 36). The kidney filters urea in the glomerulus and

Figure 38-3 Stepwise generation of a high interstitial osmolality by a countercurrent multiplier. This example illustrates in a stepwise fashion how a countercurrent-multiplier system in the loop of Henle increases the osmolality of the medullary interstitium. Heavy boundaries of ascending limb and early DCT indicate that these nephron segments are rather impermeable to water, even in the presence of AVP. The numbers refer to the osmolality (mOsm) of tubule fluid and interstitium. The *top panel* shows the starting condition (step 0), with isosmotic fluid (~300 mOsm) throughout the ascending and descending limbs and in the interstitium. Each cycle comprises two steps. Step 1 is the "single effect": NaCl transport from the lumen of the ascending limb to the interstitium, which instantaneously equilibrates with the lumen of the descending limb (steps 1, 3, 5, and 7). Step 2 is an "axial shift" of tubule fluid along the loop of Henle (steps 2, 4, and 6), with an instantaneous equilibration between the lumen of the descending limb and the interstitium. Beginning with the conditions in step 0, the first single effect is NaCl absorption across the rather water-impermeable *ascending* limb. At each level, we assume that this single effect creates a 200-mOsm *difference* between the ascending limb (which is water *impermeable*) and a second compartment: the combination of the interstitium and descending limb (which is water *permeable*). Thus, the osmolality of the ascending limb falls to 200 mOsm, whereas the osmolality of the interstitium and descending limb rise to 400 mOsm (step 1). The shift of new isosmotic fluid (~300 mOsm) from the proximal tubule in the cortex into the descending limb pushes the column of tubule fluid along the loop of Henle, thus *decreasing* osmolality at the top of the descending limb and *increasing* osmolality at the bottom of the ascending limb. Through instantaneous equilibration, the interstitium—with an assumed negligible volume—acquires the osmolality of the descending limb, thereby diluting the top of the interstitium (step 2). A second cycle starts with net NaCl transport out of the ascending limb (step 3), again generating an osmotic gradient of 200 mOsm—at each transverse level—between the ascending limb on the one hand and the interstitium and descending limb on the other. After the axial shift of tubule fluid and instantaneous equilibration of the descending limb with the interstitium (step 4), osmolality at the bottom of the ascending limb exceeds that of the preceding cycle. With successive cycles, interstitial osmolality at tip of the loop of Henle rises progressively from 300 (step 0) to 400 (step 1) to 500 (step 3) to 550 (step 5) and then to 600 (step 7). Thus, in this example, the kidney establishes a longitudinal osmotic gradient of 300 mOsm from the cortex (300 mOsm) to the papilla (600 mOsm) by iterating (i.e., multiplying) a single effect that is capable of generating a transepithelial osmotic gradient of only 200 mOsm. Step 7A adds the collecting duct and shows the final event of urine concentration: allowing the fluid in the collecting duct to equilibrate osmotically with the hyperosmotic interstitium, producing a concentrated urine. *(Based on a model by Pitts RF: Physiology of the Kidney and Body Fluids. Chicago, Year Book, 1974.)*

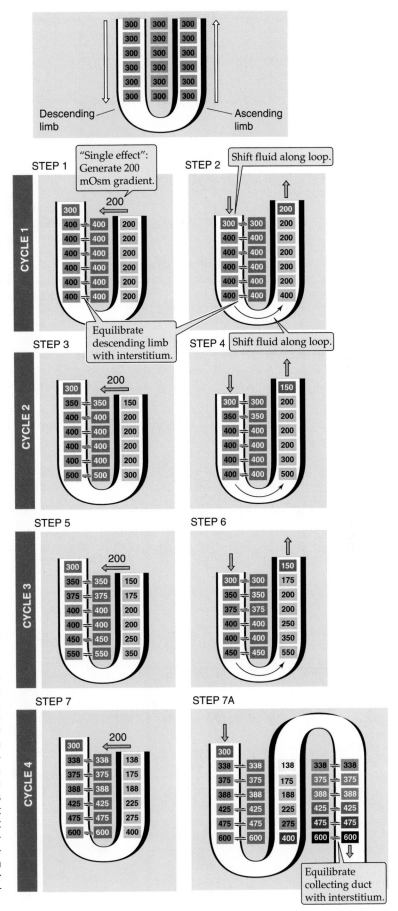

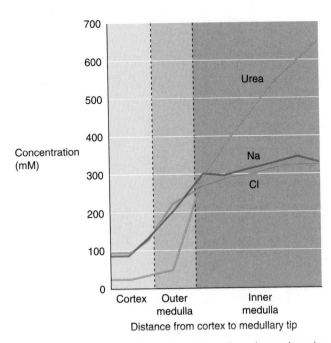

Figure 38-4 Concentration profiles of Na+, Cl−, and urea along the corticomedullary axis. The data are from hydropenic dogs. *(Data from Ullrich KJ, Kramer K, Boylan JW: Prog Cardiovasc Dis 1961; 3:395-431.)*

reabsorbs about half in the proximal tubule. In juxtamedullary nephrons, the tDLH and the tALH secrete urea into the tubule lumen. Finally, the IMCD reabsorbs urea. The net effect is that the kidney excretes less urea into the urine than it filters. Depending on urine flow (see Fig. 36-2), the fractional excretion may be as low as 15% (minimal urine flow) or as high as 60% or more (maximal urine flow). Because we are interested in understanding the role of urea in establishing a hypertonic medullary interstitium, in Figure 38-5 we consider an example in which maximal AVP produces minimal urine flow (i.e., antidiuresis), a condition already illustrated in Figure 38-2A.

As the tubule fluid enters the TAL, the [urea] is several-fold higher than it is in the plasma because ~100% of the filtered load of urea remains, even though earlier nephron segments have reabsorbed water. All nephron segments from TAL to the OMCD, inclusive, have low permeabilities to urea. In the presence of AVP, however, all segments from the ICT to the end of the nephron have high water permeabilities and continuously reabsorb fluid. As a result, luminal [urea] gradually rises, beginning at the ICT and reaching a concentration as much as 8-fold to 10-fold higher than that in blood plasma by the time the tubule fluid reaches the end of the OMCD.

The **IMCD** differs in an important way from the three upstream segments: Although AVP increases *only water per-*

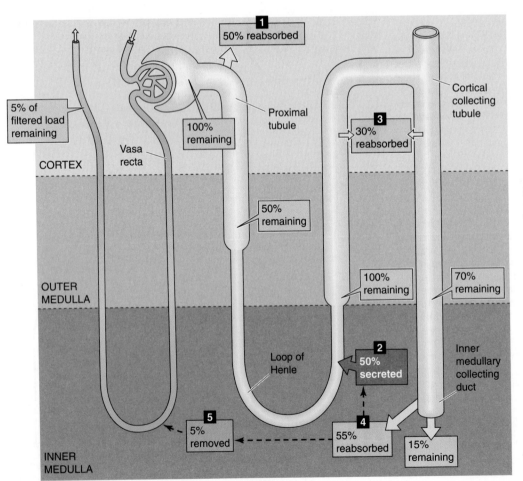

Figure 38-5 Urea recycling. Under conditions of water restriction (antidiuresis), the kidneys excrete ~15% of the filtered urea. The numbered *yellow boxes* indicate the fraction of the filtered load that various nephron segments *reabsorb*. The single *red box* indicates the fraction of the filtered load secreted by the tALH, and the single *brown box* indicates the fraction of the filtered load *carried away* by the vasa recta. The *green boxes* indicate the fraction of the filtered load that remains in the lumen after these segments. The values in the boxes are approximations.

meability in the ICT, CCT, and OMCD, AVP increases water *and urea permeability* in the IMCD. In the IMCD, the high luminal [urea] and the high urea permeabilities of the apical membrane (through the urea transporter **UT-A1**; see Chapter 36) and basolateral membrane (through **UT-A3**) promote the outward facilitated diffusion of urea from the IMCD lumen, through the IMCD cells, and into the medullary interstitium. As a result, urea accumulates in the interstitium and contributes about half of the total osmolality in the deepest portion of the inner medulla. In addition, in the outer portion of the inner medulla, active urea reabsorption occurs through a Na-urea cotransporter in the apical membrane of the early IMCD.

Because of the accumulation of urea in the inner medullary interstitium, [urea] is higher in the interstitium than it is in the lumen of the **tDHL** and **tALH** of juxtamedullary (i.e., long-loop) nephrons. This concentration gradient drives urea into the tDLH through UTA-2 and into the tALH through an as-yet unidentified transporter. The secretion of urea into the tDLH and tALH accounts for two important observations: First, more urea (i.e., a greater fraction of the filtered load) emerges from the tALH than entered the tDLH. Second, as noted earlier, [urea] in the TAL is considerably higher than that in blood plasma.

Urea Recycling   The processes that we have just described—(1) absorption of urea from IMCD into the interstitium, (2) secretion of urea from interstitium into the thin limbs, and (3) delivery of urea up into the cortex and back down through nephron segments from the TAL to the IMCD—are the three elements of a loop. This **urea recycling** is responsible for the buildup of a high [urea] in the inner medulla. A small fraction of the urea that the IMCD deposits in the interstitium moves into the vasa recta, which removes it from the medulla and returns it either to superficial nephrons or to the general circulation.

The preceding discussion focused on the situation in *antidiuresis*, in which AVP levels are high and the kidney concentrates urea in the inner medulla. The converse situation pertains in *water diuresis*, when circulating levels of AVP are low. The kidney reabsorbs *less* water along the ICT, CCT, OMCD, and IMCD. Furthermore, with low AVP levels, the IMCD has *lower* permeability to both urea and water. In addition, urea may be actively secreted by an apical Na-urea exchanger located in the apical membrane of the most distal portions of the IMCD. Therefore, during water diuresis, the interstitial [urea] is lower, and more urea appears in the urine.

The vasa recta's countercurrent exchange mechanism and relatively low blood flow minimize the washout of the medullary hypertonicity

The simplified scheme for the countercurrent multiplier presented in Figure 38-3 did not include blood vessels. If we were simply to introduce a straight, permeable blood vessel running from papilla to cortex, or vice versa, the blood flow would soon wash away the papillary hypertonicity that is critical for concentrating urine. Figure 38-6A shows a hypothetical, poorly designed kidney with only *descending* vasa

recta. Here, blood would flow from cortex to papilla and then exit the kidney. Because the blood vessel wall is permeable to small solutes and water, the osmolality of the blood would gradually increase from 300 to 1200 mOsm during transit from cortex to papilla, thus reflecting a loss of water or a gain of solutes. Because these movements occur at the expense of the medullary interstitium, the interstitium's hyperosmolality would be washed out into the blood. The greater the blood flow through this straight/unlooped blood vessel, the greater the medullary washout would be.

The kidney solves the medullary washout problem in two ways. First, compared with the blood flow in the renal cortex, which is one of the highest (per gram of tissue) of any tissue in the body, the blood flow through the medulla is relatively low, corresponding to no more than 5% to 10% of total renal plasma flow. This low flow represents a compromise between the need to deliver nutrients to the medulla and the need to avoid washout of medullary hypertonicity.

Second, and far more significant, the kidney uses a hairpin configuration, with the descending and ascending vasa recta both entering and leaving through the same region, thus creating an efficient **countercurrent exchange mechanism** (Fig. 38-6B) in the blood vessels. The vasa recta have a hairpin configuration, but no capacity for active transport. We start with the osmotic stratification in the medullary interstitium that the countercurrent multiplier generated in the presence of high AVP levels. This osmotic stratification results in part from a gradient of $[Na^+] + [Cl^-]$, but also from a similarly directed cortex-to-papilla gradient of [urea] (Fig. 38-4A). As isosmotic blood enters the hyperosmotic milieu of the medulla, which has high concentrations of NaCl and urea, NaCl and urea diffuse into the lumen of the descending vasa recta, whereas water moves in the opposite direction. This entry of urea into the descending vasa recta occurs through facilitated diffusion, mediated by the **UT-B1** and **UT-B2** urea transporter (see Chapter 36). The result is that the osmolality of the blood increases as the blood approaches the tip of the hairpin loop. As the blood rounds the curve and heads up toward the cortex inside the ascending vasa recta, that blood eventually develops a higher solute concentration than the surrounding interstitium. As a consequence, NaCl and urea now diffuse from the lumen of the vasa recta into the interstitium, whereas water moves into the ascending vasa recta.

Viewed as a whole, these passive exchange processes cause the descending vasa recta to gain solute and lose water, but they cause the ascending vessels to lose solute and gain water. Thus, at any level, the descending and ascending vessels exchange solutes and water through—and at the expense of—the medullary interstitium. Solute recirculates from the ascending vessel, through the interstitium, to the descending vessel. Conversely, the countercurrent exchange mechanism also "short circuits" the water, but in the opposite direction, from the descending vessel, through the interstitium, to the ascending vessel. The net effect is that the countercurrent exchanger tends to trap solutes in and exclude water from the medulla, thereby minimizing dissipation of the corticomedullary osmolality gradient.

The total mass of solute and water leaving the medulla each minute through the *ascending* vasa recta must exceed the total inflow of solute and water into the medulla through

A HYPOTHETICAL STRAIGHT-TUBE EXCHANGER

B HYPOTHETICAL COUNTERCURRENT EXCHANGER

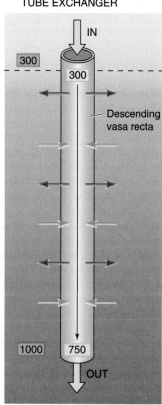

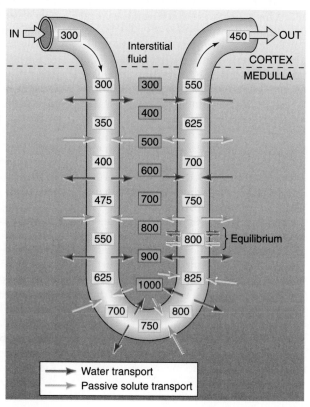

Figure 38-6 Model of countercurrent exchange. **A**, If blood simply flows from the cortex to the medulla through a straight tube, then the blood exiting the medulla will have a high osmolality (750 mOsm), thus washing out the osmolality gradient of the medullary interstitium. The numbers in the *yellow boxes indicate* the osmolality (in mOsm) inside the vasa recta, and the numbers in the *green boxes* indicate the osmolality of the interstitial fluid. **B**, If blood flows into and out of the medulla through a hairpin loop, then the water will leave the vessel, and solute will enter along the entire descending vessel and part of the ascending vessel. Along the rest of the ascending vessel, the fluxes of water and solute are reversed. The net effect is that the blood exiting the medulla is less hypertonic than that in **A** (450 versus 750 mOsm), so that the kidney better preserves the osmotic gradient in the medulla. The values in the boxes are approximations. *(Data from a model by Pitts RF: Physiology of the Kidney and Body Fluids. Chicago: Year Book, 1974.)*

the *descending* vasa recta. With regard to *solute balance*, the renal tubules continuously deposit NaCl and urea in the medullary interstitium. Thus, in the steady state, the vasa recta must remove these solutes lest they form crystals of NaCl and urea in the medullary interstitium. Almost all the urea in the interstitium of the inner medulla comes from the IMCD, and in the steady state most of this leaves the interstitium by way of the tALH (Fig. 38-5, red box). The blood of the vasa recta carries away the balance or excess urea (Fig. 38-5, brown box). The blood also carries off the excess NaCl that enters the interstitium from the ascending limb of the loop of Henle and, to some extent, from the MCDs.

With regard to *water balance* within the medulla, the descending limb of the loop of Henle and—in the presence of AVP—the MCD continuously gives up water to the medullary interstitium as the tubule fluid becomes more concentrated. Therefore, in the steady state, the ascending vasa recta must also remove excess water from the medulla.

The net effect of managing both solute and water balance in the medulla is that the ascending vasa recta carry out more

salt and more water than the descending vasa recta carry in. Although no precise measurements have been made, it is likely that the osmolality of blood leaving the ascending vasa recta exceeds that of the blood entering the descending vessels by a fairly small amount, perhaps 10 to 30 mOsm.

The medullary collecting duct produces concentrated urine by osmosis, driven by the osmotic gradient between the medullary interstitium and the lumen

In contrast to the loop of Henle, which acts as a *counter*current multiplier, and the loop-shaped vasa recta, which act as a *counter*current exchanger, the MCD is an unlooped or straight-tube exchanger. The wall of the MCD has three important permeability properties: (1) in the absence of AVP, it is relatively impermeable to water, urea, and NaCl along its entire length; (2) AVP increases its water permeability along its entire length; and (3) AVP increases its urea permeability along just the terminal portion of the tube

(IMCD). The collecting duct traverses a medullary interstitium that has a stratified, ever-increasing osmolality from the cortex to the tip of the papilla. Thus, along the entire length of the tubule, the osmotic gradient across the collecting duct epithelium favors the reabsorption of water from lumen to interstitium.

A complicating factor is that two solutes—NaCl and urea—contribute to the osmotic gradient across the tubule wall. As fluid in the collecting duct lumen moves from the corticomedullary junction to the papillary tip, the [NaCl] gradient across the tubule wall always favors the osmotic reabsorption of water (Fig. 38-7). For urea, the situation is just the opposite. However, because the ICT, CCT, and OMCD are all relatively impermeable to urea, water reabsorption predominates in the presence of AVP and gradually causes luminal [urea] to increase in these segments. Because the interstitial [urea] is low in the cortex, a rising luminal [urea] in the ICT and CCT *opposes* water reabsorption in these segments. Even when the tubule crosses the corticomedullary junction, courses toward the papilla, and is surrounded by interstitial fluid with an ever-increasing [urea], the transepithelial urea gradient still favors water movement into the lumen.

Thus, the presence of urea per se in the lumen of the collecting tubules and ducts is actually a handicap for the osmotic concentration of the urine, because the luminal urea tends to pull water back into the tubule lumen. Fortunately, the IMCD partially compensates for this problem by having a relatively low reflection coefficient for urea (Σ_{urea}), thus converting any transepithelial difference in urea concentration into a smaller difference in effective osmotic pressure (see Chapter 20). The Σ for urea is 0.74, whereas that for NaCl is 1.0. Thus, water reabsorption continues in the IMCD even though [urea] in tubule fluid exceeds that in the interstitium. The combination of a high interstitial [NaCl] and high Σ_{NaCl} promotes NaCl-driven water *absorption*. A low Σ_{urea} minimizes urea-driven water *secretion*.

The kidney also compensates for having a high [urea] in the lumen of the MCDs by having a high interstitial [urea], which—to some extent—osmotically balances the urea in the lumen of the papillary collecting ducts. Were it not for urea accumulation in the medullary interstitium, interstitial [NaCl] would have to be much higher, and this, in turn, would require increased NaCl transport in the TAL.

If luminal urea opposes the formation of a concentrated urine, why did the mammalian kidney evolve to have high levels of urea in the lumen of the collecting tubules and ducts? At least two reasons are known. First, because urea is the body's major excretable nitrogenous waste, the kidney's ability to achieve high urinary [urea] reduces the necessity to excrete large volumes of water for excreting nitrogenous waste. Second, as we have already seen, the kidney actually takes advantage of urea to generate maximally concentrated urine. Thus, in the presence of AVP, the permeability of the IMCD to urea is high, so that large amounts of urea can enter the medullary interstitium. The high interstitial [urea] energizes the increase in luminal [NaCl] in the tDLH, which, in turn, fuels the single effect in the tALH, thus creating the high inner medullary [NaCl] that is *directly* responsible for concentrating the urine.

As discussed, the composition of the inner medullary interstitium determines the composition of the final urine. However, to some extent, the composition of the final urine, as well as the rate of urine flow, also influences the composition of the interstitium. Figure 38-2 shows that the medullary interstitial osmolality is much lower, and the stratification of osmolality from cortex to papillary tip is much less, during water diuresis than during antidiuresis. Two factors contribute to the lesser degree of osmotic stratification under conditions of water diuresis, when levels of AVP are low. First, less urea moves from the IMCD lumen to the interstitium, both because of the low urea permeability of the IMCD and because of the low water permeability of the upstream segments that would otherwise concentrate urea. Second, the MCDs reabsorb some water despite the low AVP levels, and this water dilutes the medullary interstitium. The reasons for this apparent paradox are as follows: (1) even when AVP is low, the water permeability is not zero; (2) the ICT and CCT present a much larger fluid volume to the MCD, because they reabsorb less water when AVP levels are low; and (3) the tubule fluid is more hypotonic, so that a larger osmotic gradient exists for transepithelial water movement. With low AVP levels, this larger osmotic gradient overrides the effect of the lower water permeability. Table 38-2 summarizes factors that modulate urinary concentration ability.

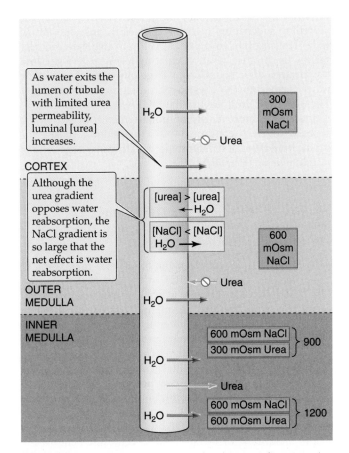

Figure 38-7 Opposing effects of NaCl and urea gradients on urine concentrating ability during antidiuresis. The numbers in the *green boxes* indicate the osmolalities (in mOsm) of the interstitial fluid.

Table 38-2 Factors That Modulate Urinary Concentration and Dilution

1. **Osmotic gradient of medullary interstitium from corticomedullary junction to papilla:**
   a. **Length of loops of Henle:** Species with long loops (e.g., desert rodents) concentrate more than those with short loops (e.g., beaver).
   b. **Rate of active NaCl reabsorption in the TAL:** Increased luminal Na^+ delivery to TAL (high GFR or filtration fraction, and low proximal tubule Na^+ reabsorption) enhances NaCl reabsorption, whereas low Na^+ delivery (low GFR, increased proximal Na^+ and fluid reabsorption) reduces concentrating ability. High Na-K pump turnover enhances NaCl reabsorption, whereas inhibiting transport (e.g., loop diuretics) reduces concentrating ability.

2. **Protein content of diet:** High-protein diet, up to a point, promotes urea accumulation in the inner medullary interstitium and increased concentrating ability.

3. **Medullary blood flow:** Low blood flow promotes high interstitial osmolality. High blood flow washes out medullary solutes.

4. **Osmotic permeability of the collecting tubules and ducts to water:** AVP enhances water permeability and thus water reabsorption.

5. **Luminal flow in the loop of Henle and the collecting duct:** High flow (osmotic diuresis) diminishes the efficiency of the countercurrent multiplier and thus reduces the osmolality of the medullary interstitium. In the MCD, high flow reduces the time available for equilibration of water and urea.

6. **Pathophysiology:** Central DI reduces plasma AVP levels, whereas nephrogenic DI reduces renal responsiveness to AVP (see the box titled Diabetes Insipidus).

REGULATION BY ARGININE VASOPRESSIN

Large-bodied neurons in the paraventricular and supraoptic nuclei of the hypothalamus synthesize AVP, a nonapeptide also known as ADH. These neurons package the AVP and transport it along their axons to the posterior pituitary, where they release AVP through a breech in the blood-brain barrier into the systemic circulation (see p. 875). In Chapter 40, we discuss how increased plasma osmolality and decreased effective circulating volume increase AVP release. AVP has synergistic effects on two target organs. First, at rather high circulating levels, such as those seen in hypovolemic shock, AVP acts on vascular smooth muscle to cause *vasoconstriction* (see Chapter 23) and thus to increase blood pressure. Second, and more importantly, AVP acts on the kidney, where it is the major regulator of water excretion. AVP increases water reabsorption by enhancing the water permeabilities of the collecting tubules and ducts and also by stimulating urea transport across the cells of the IMCD.

AVP increases water permeability in all nephron segments beyond the distal convoluted tubule

Of the water remaining in the DCT, the kidney reabsorbs a variable fraction in the segments from the ICT to the end of the nephron. Absorption of this final fraction of water is under the control of circulating AVP. In the kidney, AVP (1) increases water permeability in all the segments beyond the DCT, (2) increases urea permeability in the IMCD, and (3) increases active NaCl reabsorption in the TAL.

Figure 38-8 summarizes the water permeability of various nephron segments. The water permeability is highest in the proximal tubule and tDHL. The high water permeability in these segments reflects the abundant presence of **AQP1** water channels (see Chapter 3) in the apical and basolateral cell membranes.

In marked contrast to the proximal tubule and tDLH, the following few segments—from the tALH to the connecting tubule—have very low water permeabilities. In the absence of AVP, the next tubule segments, the ICT and CCT, have rather low water permeabilities, whereas the MCDs are virtually impermeable to water. However, AVP dramatically increases the water permeabilities of the collecting tubules (ICT and CCT) and ducts (OMCD and IMCD) by causing **AQP2** water channels to insert into the apical membrane (see later). A third type of water channel, **AQP3**, is present in the basolateral cell membranes of MCDs. Like AQP1, AQP3 is *insensitive* to AVP.

Given the favorable osmotic gradients discussed in the preceding subchapter, high levels of AVP cause substantial water reabsorption to occur in AVP-sensitive nephron segments. In contrast, when circulating levels of AVP are low, for instance after ingestion of large amounts of water, the water permeability of these nephron segments remains low. Therefore, the fluid leaving the DCT remains hypotonic as it flows down more distal nephron segments. In fact, in the absence of AVP, continued NaCl absorption makes the tubule fluid even more hypotonic, resulting in a large volume of dilute urine (Fig. 38-1).

AVP, acting through cAMP, causes vesicles containing aquaporin 2 water channels to fuse with the apical membrane of principal cells of the collecting tubules and ducts

AVP binds to V_2 receptors in the basolateral membrane of the principal cells from the ICT to the end of the nephron (Fig. 38-9). Receptor binding activates the G_s heterotrimeric G protein, thus stimulating adenylyl cyclase to generate cAMP (see Chapter 3). The latter activates protein kinase A, which phosphorylates unknown proteins that play a role in the trafficking of intracellular vesicles containing AQP2 and the fusion of these vesicles with the apical membrane. These water channels are AVP sensitive, not in the sense that AVP modulates their single-channel water conductance, but rather in the context of their *density* in the apical membrane. In conditions of low AVP, AQP2 water channels are mainly in the membrane of intracellular vesicles just beneath the apical membrane. In the membrane of these vesicles, the AQP2 water channels are present as **aggregophores**—aggregates of AQP2 proteins. Under the influence of AVP, the

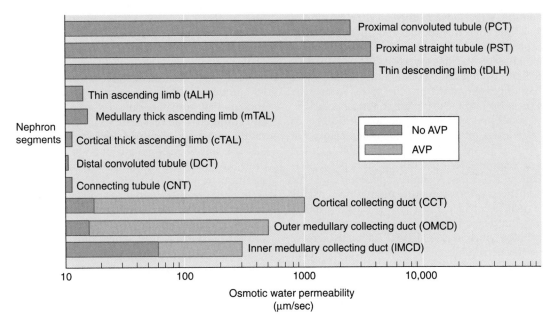

Figure 38-8 Water permeability in different nephron segments. Note that the x-axis scale is logarithmic. *(From Knepper MA, Rector FC: In Brenner BM [ed]: The Kidney, pp 532-570. Philadelphia: WB Saunders, 1996.)*

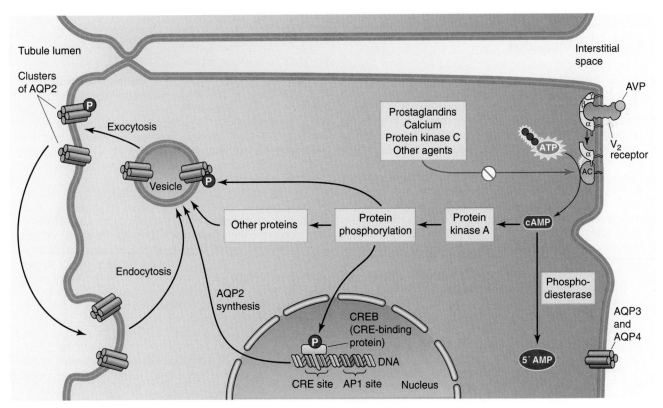

Figure 38-9 Cellular mechanism of AVP action in the collecting tubules and ducts.

vesicles containing AQP2 move to the apical membrane of principal cells of the collecting tubules and ducts. By exocytosis (see Chapter 2), these vesicles fuse with the apical membrane, thus increasing the density of AQP2. When AVP levels in the blood decline, endocytosis retrieves the water channel–containing aggregates from the apical membrane and shuttles them back to the cytoplasmic vesicle pool.

The apical water permeability of principal cells depends not only on AVP levels, but also on certain other factors. For example, high $[Ca^{2+}]_i$ and high $[Li^+]$ both inhibit adenylyl cyclase, thus decreasing $[cAMP]_i$, reducing water permeability, and producing a diuresis. A similar inhibition of AQP2 insertion, and hence a decrease in water permeability, occurs when agents such as colchicine disrupt the integrity of the cytoskeleton. Conversely, inhibitors of phosphodiesterase (e.g., theophylline), which increase $[cAMP]_i$, tend to increase the osmotic water permeability.

AVP enhances the urinary-concentrating mechanism by stimulating the urea transporter UT-A1 in the inner medullary collecting ducts, thus increasing urea reabsorption

AVP promotes water reabsorption not only by increasing the water permeability of the collecting tubules and ducts, but also by enhancing the osmotic gradients across the walls of the inner and perhaps the OMCD. In the *outer* medulla, AVP acts through the cAMP pathway to increase NaCl reabsorption by the TAL. AVP acts by stimulating apical Na/K/Cl cotransport and K^+ recycling across the apical membrane (see Chapter 35). The net effect is to increase the osmolality of the outer medullary interstitium and thus enhance the osmotic gradient favoring water reabsorption by the OMCD. In addition, AVP stimulates the growth of TAL cells in animals that are genetically devoid of AVP. This hormone also stimulates Na^+ reabsorption in the CCT, largely by activating apical Na^+ channels (ENaC). These observations on the TAL and CCT were all made on rodents. In humans, these TAL and CCT mechanisms may have only minor significance.

In the *inner* medulla, AVP enhances the urea permeability of the terminal two thirds of the IMCD. The AVP-dependent increase in $[cAMP]_i$ that triggers the apical insertion of AQP2-containing vesicles also leads to a phosphorylation of apical UT-A1 urea transporters (see Chapter 36), increasing their activity. The results are a substantial increase in urea reabsorption and thus the high interstitial [urea] that is indirectly responsible for generating the osmotic gradient that drives water reabsorption in the inner medulla.

Segments of the nephron other than the IMCD have varying degrees of urea permeability. However, AVP increases urea permeability only in the apical membrane of the IMCD. In particular, AVP has no effect on other urea transporters: UT-A2 (in tDLH), UT-B1/B2 (in vasa recta), or UT-A3 (basolateral membrane of the IMCD).

Diabetes Insipidus

DI is a fairly rare disorder that occurs in two varieties. The first, neurogenic or **central DI**, is caused by failure of AVP secretion. The lesion can be either at the level of the hypothalamus (where neurons synthesize AVP) or in the pituitary gland (where neurons release AVP). Central DI can be idiopathic, familial, or caused by any disorder of the hypothalamus or pituitary, such as injury, a tumor, infection, or autoimmune processes. In the second variety, **nephrogenic DI**, the kidneys respond inadequately to normal or even elevated levels of circulating AVP. Nephrogenic DI can also be idiopathic or familial and may be associated with electrolyte abnormalities (e.g., states of K^+ depletion or high plasma $[Ca^{2+}]$), the renal disease associated with sickle cell anemia, and various drugs (notably Li^+ and colchicine).

In both central and nephrogenic DI, patients present with polyuria and polydipsia. If allowed to progress unchecked, the disorder can result in marked hypernatremia, hypotension, and shock. Often the physician first suspects the diagnosis when the patient is deprived of access to water or other fluids. The patient may then quickly become dehydrated, and a random determination of plasma $[Na^+]$ may yield a very high value.

The physician can confirm the diagnosis of DI most easily by a fluid deprivation test. The patient will continue to produce a large output of dilute urine, despite the need to conserve fluids. If the patient has *central* DI, administering a subcutaneous dose of AVP will rapidly increase urine osmolality by more than 50%. In patients with *nephrogenic* DI, conversely, the increase in urine osmolality will be less. Simultaneous measurements of plasma AVP levels may confirm the diagnosis.

The treatment for central DI is **desmopressin acetate** (DDAVP) (see Fig. 56-10), a synthetic AVP analogue that patients can take intranasally. Nephrogenic DI, in which the kidneys are resistant to the effects of the hormone, does not respond to DDAVP. In these patients, it is best to treat the underlying disease and also to reduce the elevated plasma $[Na^+]$ by administering a diuretic (to produce natriuresis) and by restricting dietary Na^+.

The high urine flow in DI is associated with low rates of solute excretion. Therefore, the physician must distinguish DI from states of **polyuria** accompanied by high rates of solute excretion in the urine (**osmotic diuresis**). The most frequent cause is **chronic renal failure**, when a decreasing population of nephrons is charged with excreting the daily load of solutes or other renal diseases associated with compromised proximal fluid and solute transport. Polyuria with excretion of solute-rich urine also occurs in untreated **diabetes mellitus**. In that case, the polyuria occurs because the high plasma [glucose] leads to the filtration of an amount of glucose that exceeds the capacity of the proximal tubule to retrieve it from the lumen (see Chapter 36). A third cause of osmotic diuresis is the administration of poorly reabsorbable solutes, such as mannitol or HCO_3^-.

In an entirely distinct class of polyurias is **primary polydipsia**, a psychoneurotic disorder in which patients drink large amounts of fluid. Whereas simple water deprivation benefits a patient with primary polydipsia, it aggravates the condition of a patient with DI.

Role of Aquaporins in Renal Water Transport

Whereas AQP1 is the water channel responsible for a large amount of transcellular fluid movement in the proximal tubule and the tDLH, three related isoforms of the water channel protein—AQP2, AQP3, and AQP4—are present in the principal cells of the collecting ducts. These channels regulate water transport in collecting tubules and ducts. Apical AQP2 is the basis for AVP-regulated water permeability. AQP3 and AQP4 are present in the basolateral membrane of principal cells, where they provide an exit pathway for water movement into the peritubular fluid.

Short-term and long-term regulation of water permeability depends on an intact AQP2 system. In short-term regulation, AVP—through cAMP—causes water channel–containing vesicles from a subapical pool to fuse with the apical membrane (Fig. 38-9). As a result, the number of channels and the water permeability sharply increase. In long-term regulation, AVP—by enhancing transcription of the *AQP2* gene—increases the abundance of AQP2 protein in principal cells.

Mutations of several AQP genes lead to loss of function and marked abnormalities of water balance. Examples include sharply decreased fluid absorption along the proximal tubule in AQP1 knockout animals and nephrogenic DI (see the box on this topic) in patients with mutations of the gene for AQP2. An interesting situation may develop during the third trimester of pregnancy, when elevated plasma levels of vasopressinase—a placental aminopeptidase that degrades AVP—may lead to a clinical picture of central DI.

An acquired increase of AQP2 expression often accompanies states of abnormal fluid retention, such as congestive heart failure, hepatic cirrhosis, the nephrotic syndrome, and pregnancy. Some conditions—including acute and chronic renal failure, primary polydipsia, a low-protein diet, and SIADH (see the box titled Syndrome of Inappropriate Antidiuretic Hormone Secretion)—are associated with increased AQP2 levels in the apical membrane.

Syndrome of Inappropriate Antidiuretic Hormone Secretion

The syndrome of inappropriate ADH secretion (SIADH) is the opposite of DI. Patients with SIADH secrete levels of ADH (i.e., AVP) or AVP-like substances that are inappropriately *high*, given the plasma osmolality. Thus, the urine osmolality is inappropriately high as the kidneys salvage inappropriately large volumes of water from the urine. As a result, total body water increases, the blood becomes hypo-osmolar, plasma [Na⁺] drops (**hyponatremia**), and cells swell. If plasma [Na⁺] falls substantially, cell swelling can cause headaches, nausea, vomiting, and behavioral changes. Eventually, stupor, coma, and seizures may ensue.

Before making the diagnosis of SIADH, the physician must rule out other causes of hyponatremia in which AVP levels may be appropriate. In Chapter 40, we discuss how plasma osmolality and effective circulating volume *appropriately* regulate AVP secretion. SIADH has four major causes:

1. Certain **malignant tumors** (e.g., bronchogenic carcinoma, sarcomas, lymphomas, and leukemias) release AVP or AVP-like substances.

2. **Cranial disorders** (e.g., head trauma, meningitis, and brain abscesses) can increase AVP release.

3. **Nonmalignant pulmonary disorders** (e.g., tuberculosis, pneumonia, and abscesses) and positive-pressure ventilation also can cause SIADH.

4. Several **drugs** can either stimulate AVP release (e.g., clofibrate, phenothiazines), increase the sensitivity of renal tubules to AVP (e.g., chlorpropamide), or both (e.g., carbamazepine).

Treatment is best directed at the underlying disorder, combined, if necessary and clinically appropriate, with fluid restriction. Patients with a plasma [Na⁺] <110 mM must receive urgent attention. Infusing hypertonic Na⁺ is usually effective, but the correction must be gradual or severe neurologic damage can result owing to rapid changes in the volume of neurons, especially in the pontine area of the brainstem.

REFERENCES

Books and Reviews

Agre P, Preston GM, Smyth BL, et al: Aquaporin CHIP: The archetypal molecular water channel. Am J Physiol 1993; 265: F463-F476.

Greger R: Transport mechanisms in thick ascending limb of Henle's loop of mammalian nephron. Physiol Rev 1985; 65:760-797.

Knepper MA, Saidel GM, Hascall VC, Dwyer T. Concentration of solutes in the renal inner medulla: Interstitial hyaluronan as a mechano-osmotic transducer. Am J Physiol 2003; 284: F433-F446.

Sands JM: Mammalian urea transporters: Annu Rev Physiol 2003; 65:543-566.

Sasaki W, Ishibashi K, Marumo F: Aquaporin-2 and -3: Representatives of two subgroups of the aquaporin family colocalized in the kidney collecting duct. Annu Rev Physiol 1998; 60:199-220.

Shayakul C, Hediger MA: The SLC14 gene family of urea transporters. Pflügers Arch 2004; 447: 603-609.

Tsukaguchi H, Shayakul C, Berger UV, Hediger MA: Urea transporters in kidney: Molecular analysis and contribution to the urinary concentrating process. Am J Physiol 1998; 275: F319-F324.

Journal Articles

Deen PMT, Verdijk MAJ, Knoers NVAM, et al: Requirement of human renal water channel AQP-2 for vasopressin-dependent concentration of urine. Science 1994; 264:92-95.

Gottschalk CW: Micropuncture studies of tubular function in the mammalian kidney. Physiologist 1961; 4:33-55.

Gottschalk CW, Mylle M: Micropuncture study of composition of loop of Henle fluid in desert rodents. Am J Physiol 1959; 204:532-535.

Lassiter WE, Gottschalk CW, Mylle M: Micropuncture study of net transtubular movement of water and urea in nondiuretic kidney. Am J Physiol 1964; 200:1139-1146.

Pallone TL, Edwards A, Ma T, et al: The intrarenal distribution of blood flow. Adv Organ Biol 2000; 9:75-92.

Sanjana VM, Robertson CR, Jamison RL: Water extraction from the inner medullary collecting tubule system: A role for urea. Kidney Int 1976; 10:139-146.

Ullrich KJ, Kramer K, Boylan JW: Present knowledge of the counter-current system in the mammalian kidney. Prog Cardiovasc Dis 1961; 3:395-431.

CHAPTER 39

TRANSPORT OF ACIDS AND BASES

Gerhard Giebisch and Erich Windhager

The lungs and the kidneys are largely responsible for regulating the acid-base balance of the blood (see Chapter 28). They do so by independently controlling the two major components of the body's major buffering system: CO_2 and HCO_3^- (Fig. 39-1). Chapter 31 focuses on how the lungs control plasma $[CO_2]$. In this chapter, we see how the kidneys control plasma $[HCO_3^-]$.

ACID-BASE BALANCE AND THE OVERALL RENAL HANDLING OF ACID

Although the lungs excrete a large amount of CO_2, a potential acid formed by metabolism, the kidneys are crucial for excreting nonvolatile acids

The kidneys play a critical role in helping the body rid itself of excess acid that accompanies the intake of food or that forms in certain metabolic reactions. By far, the largest potential source of acid is **CO_2** production (Table 39-1A), which arises during oxidation of carbohydrates, fats, and most amino acids (see Chapter 58). An adult ingesting a typical Western diet produces ~15,000 mmol/day of CO_2. This CO_2 would act as an acid if it went on to form H^+ and HCO_3^- (see Chapter 28). Fortunately, the lungs excrete this prodigious amount of CO_2 by diffusion across the alveolar-capillary barrier (see Chapter 30), thus preventing the CO_2 from forming H^+.

However, metabolism also generates **nonvolatile acids**—such as sulfuric acid, phosphoric acid, and various organic acids—that the lungs cannot handle (Table 39-1B). In addition, metabolism generates **nonvolatile bases**, which end up as HCO_3^- (Table 39-1C). Subtracting the metabolically generated base from the metabolically generated acid leaves a net endogenous H^+ production of ~40 mmol/day for a person weighing 70 kg. The strong acids contained in a typical Western acid-ash diet (20 mmol/day of H^+ gained) and the obligatory loss of bases in stool (10 mmol/day of OH^- lost) represent an additional acid load to the body of 30 mmol/day. Thus, the body is faced with a total load of nonvolatile acids (i.e., not CO_2) of ~70 mmol/day—

or ~1 mmol/kg body weight—derived from metabolism, diet, and intestinal losses. The kidneys handle this acid load by "dividing" 70 mmol/day of carbonic acid (H_2CO_3): excreting ~70 mmol/day of H^+ into the urine and simultaneously transporting 70 mmol/day of new HCO_3^- into the blood. Once in the blood, this new HCO_3^- neutralizes the daily load of 70 mmol of nonvolatile acid.

Were it not for the tightly controlled excretion of H^+ by the kidney, the daily load of ~70 mmol of nonvolatile acids would progressively lower plasma pH and, in the process, exhaust the body's stores of bases, especially HCO_3^-. The result would be death by relentless acidification. Indeed, one of the characteristic symptoms of renal failure is severe acidosis caused by acid retention. The kidneys continuously monitor the acid-base parameters of the extracellular fluid and adjust their rate of acid secretion to maintain the pH of extracellular fluid within narrow limits.

In summary, although the lungs excrete an extremely large amount of a *potential* acid in the form of CO_2, the kidneys play an equally essential role in the defense of the normal acid-base equilibrium, because they are the sole effective route for neutralizing *nonvolatile* acids.

To maintain acid-base balance, the kidney must not only reabsorb virtually all filtered HCO_3^-, but must also secrete into the urine the daily production of nonvolatile acids

As discussed, the major functions of the kidney, in terms of acid-base balance, are to secrete acid into the urine and thus to neutralize the nonvolatile acids that metabolism produces. However, before the kidney can begin to accomplish these tasks, it has to deal with a related and even more serious problem: retrieving from the tubule fluid virtually all HCO_3^- filtered by the glomeruli.

Each day, the glomeruli filter 180 L of blood plasma, each liter containing 24 mmol of HCO_3^-, so that the daily filtered load of HCO_3^- is 180 L × 24 mM = 4320 mmol. If this filtered HCO_3^- were all left behind in the urine, the result would be equivalent to an acid load in the blood of 4320 mmol, or catastrophic metabolic acidosis (see Chapter 28). The kidneys

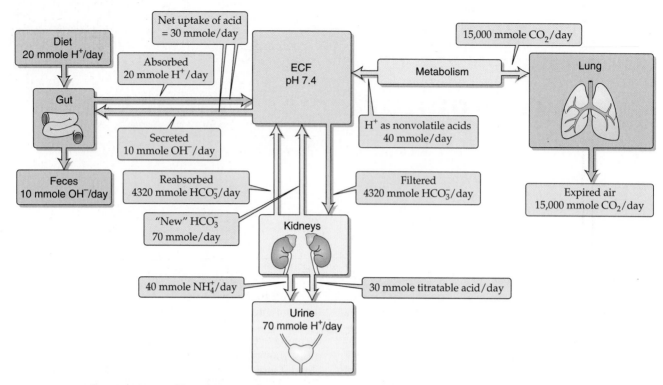

Figure 39-1 Acid-base balance. All values are for a 70-kg person ingesting a typical "Western" acid-ash diet. The values in the boxes are approximations. ECF, extracellular fluid.

Table 39-1 Metabolic Sources of Nonvolatile Acids and Bases

A. Reactions Producing CO_2 (Merely a Potential Acid)

1. Complete oxidation of neutral carbohydrate and fat → $CO_2 + H_2O$
2. Oxidation of *most* neutral amino acids → Urea + CO_2 + H_2O

B. Reactions Producing Nonvolatile Acids

1. Oxidation of sulfur-containing amino acids → Urea + $CO_2 + H_2O + H_2SO_4$ → $2 H^+ + SO_4^{2-}$ (examples: methionine, cysteine)
2. Metabolism of phosphorus-containing compounds → H_3PO_4 → $H^+ + H_2PO_4^-$
3. Oxidation of *cationic* amino acids → Urea + $CO_2 + H_2O$ + H^+ (examples: lysine+, arginine+)
4. Production of nonmetabolizable organic acids → HA → $H^+ + A^-$ (examples: uric acid, oxalic acid)
5. Incomplete oxidation of carbohydrate and fat → HA → $H^+ + A^-$ (examples: lactic acid, ketoacids)

C. Reactions Producing Nonvolatile Bases

1. Oxidation of *anionic* amino acids → Urea + $CO_2 + H_2O$ + HCO_3^- (e.g., glutamate⁻, aspartate⁻)
2. Oxidation of organic anions → $CO_2 + H_2O + HCO_3^-$ (e.g., lactate⁻, acetate⁻)

handle this problem by reclaiming virtually all the filtered HCO_3^-. As discussed in the next section, the kidney accomplishes this task by secreting H^+ into the tubule lumen and titrating the 4320 mmol/day of filtered HCO_3^- to CO_2 and H_2O.

After the kidney reclaims virtually all the filtered HCO_3^- (i.e., 4320 mmol/day), how does it deal with the acid load of 70 mmol/day produced by metabolism, diet, and intestinal losses? If we simply poured 70 mmol of nonvolatile acid into the ~1.5 L of "unbuffered" urine produced each day, urinary $[H^+]$ would be 0.070 mol/1.5 L = 0.047 M, which would correspond to a pH of ~1.3. The lowest urine pH that the kidney can achieve is ~4.4, which corresponds to an $[H^+]$ that is three orders of magnitude lower than required to excrete the 70 mmol/day of nonvolatile acids. The kidneys solve this problem by binding the H^+ to buffers that the kidney can excrete within the physiological range of urinary pH values. Some of these buffers the kidney *filters*—for example, phosphate, creatinine, and urate. Because of its favorable pK of 6.8 and its relatively high rate of excretion, phosphate is the most important nonvolatile filtered buffer. The other major urinary buffer is NH_3/NH_4^+, which the kidney *synthesizes*. After diffusing into the tubule lumen, the NH_3 reacts with secreted H^+ to form NH_4^+. Through adaptive increases in the synthesis of NH_3 and excretion of NH_4^+, the kidneys can respond to the body's need to excrete increased loads of H^+.

Does the kidney eliminate the 70 mmol/day of nonvolatile acids by simply filtering and then excreting them in the urine? After the 70 mmol/day nonvolatile **acid challenge** presents itself to the extracellular fluid, the body deals with this challenge in three steps:

Step 1: Extracellular HCO_3^- neutralizes *most* of the H^+ load:

$$HCO_3^- + \underbrace{H^+}_{\text{Acid load}} \rightarrow CO_2 + H_2O \qquad (39\text{-}1)$$

Thus, HCO_3^- decreases by an amount that is equal to the H^+ it consumes, thereby producing an equal amount of CO_2 in the process. Non-HCO_3^- buffers ($B^- + H^+ \rightleftharpoons BH^+$; see Chapter 28) in the blood neutralize most of the remaining H^+ load:

$$B^- + \underset{\text{Acid load}}{\underbrace{H^+}} \rightarrow BH \qquad (39\text{-}2)$$

Thus, B^-, too, decreases by an amount that is equal to the H^+ it consumes. A very tiny fraction of the H^+ load (<0.001%; see Chapter 28) escapes buffering by either HCO_3^- or B^-. This remnant H^+ is responsible for a small drop in the extracellular pH.

Step 2: The lungs excrete the CO_2 formed in Equation 39-1. The body does not excrete the HB generated in Equation 39-2, but rather converts it back into B^-, as discussed later.

Step 3: The kidneys regenerate the HCO_3^- and B^- in the extracellular fluid by creating new HCO_3^- at a rate that is equal to the rate of H^+ production (i.e., ~70 mmol/day). Thus, over the course of a day, 70 mmol more HCO_3^- exits the kidneys through the renal veins than entered through the renal arteries. Most of this new HCO_3^- replenishes the HCO_3^- consumed by the neutralization of nonvolatile acids, thereby maintaining extracellular $[HCO_3^-]$ at ~24 mM. The remainder of this new HCO_3^- regenerates B^-:

$$HCO_3^- + BH \rightarrow \underset{\substack{\text{Regenerated} \\ \text{base}}}{\underbrace{B^-}} + CO_2 + H_2O \qquad (39\text{-}3)$$

Again, the lungs excrete the CO_2 formed in Equation 39-3, just as they excrete the CO_2 formed in Equation 39-1. Thus, by generating new HCO_3^-, the kidneys maintain constant levels of both HCO_3^- and the deprotonated forms of non-HCO_3^- buffers (B^-) in the extracellular fluid.

Table 39-2 summarizes the three components of net urinary acid excretion. Historically, component 1 is referred to as **titratable acid**, the amount of base one must add to a sample of urine to bring its pH back up to the pH of blood plasma. The titratable acid does not include the H^+ the kidneys excrete as NH_4^+, which is component 2. Because the pK of the NH_3/NH_4^+ equilibrium is greater than 9, almost all the NH_4^+ buffer in the urine is in the form of NH_4^+, and titrating urine from an acid pH to a pH of 7.4 will not appreciably convert NH_4^+ to NH_3. If no filtered HCO_3^- were lost in component 3, the generation of new HCO_3^- by the kidneys would be the sum of components 1 and 2. To the extent that filtered

HCO_3^- is lost in the urine, the new HCO_3^- must exceed the sum of components 1 and 2.

The kidneys also can control HCO_3^- and B^- following an **alkaline challenge**, produced, for example, by ingesting alkali or by vomiting (which leads to a loss of HCl, equivalent to a gain in $NaHCO_3$). The kidney responds by decreasing net acid excretion—that is, by sharply reducing the excretion rates of titratable acid and NH_4^+. The result is a decrease in the production of new HCO_3^-. With an extreme alkali challenge, the excretion of urinary HCO_3^- also increases and may exceed the combined rates of titratable acid and NH_4^+ excretion. In other words, component 3 in Table 39-2 exceeds the sum of components 1 and 2, so that net acid excretion becomes negative, and the kidney becomes a net excretor of alkali. In this case, the kidneys return less HCO_3^- to the extracellular fluid through the renal veins than entered the kidneys through the renal arteries.

Secreted H^+ titrates HCO_3^- to CO_2 (HCO_3^- reabsorption) and also titrates filtered non-HCO_3^- buffers and endogenously produced NH_3 (nonvolatile acid excretion)

As we have seen, the kidney can reabsorb nearly all of the filtered HCO_3^- and excrete additional acid into the urine as both titratable acid and NH_4^+. The common theme of these three processes is **H^+ secretion** from the blood into the lumen. Thus, the secreted H^+ can have three fates. It can titrate (1) filtered HCO_3^-, (2) filtered phosphate (or other filtered buffers that contribute to the "titratable acid"), and (3) NH_3, both secreted and, to a lesser extent, filtered.

Titration of Filtered HCO_3^- (HCO_3^- Reabsorption) Extensive reabsorption reclaims almost all the filtered HCO_3^- (>99.9%). As discussed in the next major section, the kidney reabsorbs HCO_3^- at specialized sites along the nephron. However, regardless of the site, the basic mechanism of HCO_3^- reabsorption is the same (Fig. 39-2A): H^+ transported into the lumen by the tubule cell titrates filtered HCO_3^- to CO_2 plus H_2O. One way that this titration can occur is by H^+ interacting with HCO_3^- to form H_2CO_3, which, in turn, dissociates to yield H_2O and CO_2. However, the reaction $H_2CO_3 \rightarrow H_2O + CO_2$ is far too slow to convert the entire filtered load of HCO_3^- to CO_2 plus H_2O. The enzyme carbonic anhydrase (CA)—which is present in many tubule segments—bypasses this slow reaction by splitting HCO_3^- into CO_2 and OH^- (Table 39-1). The secreted H^+ neutralizes this OH^- so that the net effect is to accelerate the production of H_2O and CO_2.

The apical membranes of these H^+-secreting tubules are highly permeable to CO_2, so that CO_2 produced in the lumen,

Table 39-2 Components of Net Urinary Acid Excretion

		1		2		3
Net urinary acid excretion	=	Excreted H^+ bound to phosphate (as $H_2PO_4^-$), creatinine, and uric acid	+	Excreted H^+ bound to NH_3 (as NH_4^+)	−	Excretion of filtered HCO_3^-

A HCO₃⁻ REABSORPTION

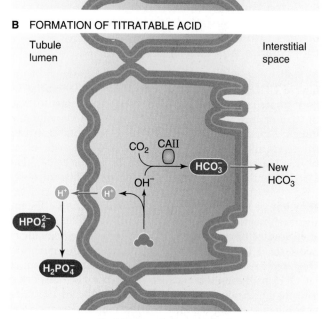

B FORMATION OF TITRATABLE ACID

C AMMONIUM EXCRETION

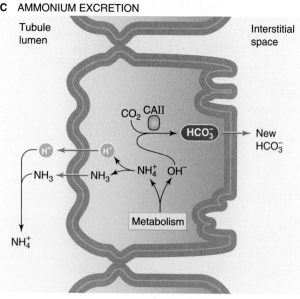

Figure 39-2 Titration of luminal buffers by secreted H^+. **A** and **B**, Generic models of H^+ secretion at various sites along the nephron. The *red arrows* represent diverse transport mechanisms. **C**, Ammonium handling by the proximal tubule.

as well as the H_2O, diffuses into the tubule cell. Inside the tubule cell, the CO_2 and H_2O regenerate intracellular H^+ and HCO_3^- with the aid of CA. Finally, the cell exports these two products, thereby moving the H^+ out across the apical membrane into the tubule lumen and the HCO_3^- out across the basolateral membrane into the blood. Thus, for each H^+ secreted into the lumen, one HCO_3^- disappears from the lumen, and one HCO_3^- appears in the blood. However, the HCO_3^- that disappears from the lumen and the HCO_3^- that appears in the blood are *not* the same molecule. To secrete H^+ and yet keep intracellular pH within narrow physiological limits (see Chapter 28), the cell closely coordinates the apical secretion of H^+ and the basolateral exit of HCO_3^-.

Two points are worth re-emphasizing. First, HCO_3^- reabsorption does not represent net H^+ excretion into the urine. It merely prevents the loss of the filtered alkali. Second, even though HCO_3^- reabsorption is simply a reclamation effort, this process consumes by far the largest fraction of the H^+ secreted into the tubule lumen. For example, reclaiming the 4320 mmol of HCO_3^- filtered each day requires 4320 mmol of H^+ secretion, far more than the additional 70 mmol/day of H^+ secretion necessary for neutralizing nonvolatile acids.

Titration of Filtered Non-HCO₃⁻ Buffers (Titratable Acid Formation) The H^+ secreted into the tubules can interact with buffers other than HCO_3^- and NH_3. The titration of the non-NH_3, non-HCO_3^- buffers (B^-)—mainly HPO_4^{2-}, creatinine, and urate—to their conjugate weak acids (BH) constitutes the titratable acid discussed earlier.

$$H^+ + B^- \rightarrow BH \qquad (39\text{-}4)$$

The major proton acceptor in this category of buffers excreted in the urine is HPO_4^{2-}, although creatinine also makes an important contribution; urate and other buffers contribute to a lesser extent. Figure 39-2B shows the fate of H^+ as it protonates phosphate from its divalent form (HPO_4^{2-}) to its monovalent form ($H_2PO_4^-$). Because low luminal pH inhibits the apical Na/phosphate cotransporter (NaP_i) in the proximal tubule, and NaP_i carries $H_2PO_4^-$ less effectively than HPO_4^{2-} (see Chapter 36), the kidneys tend to excrete H^+-bound phosphate in the urine. For each H^+ it transfers to the lumen to titrate HPO_4^{2-}, the tubule cell generates one new HCO_3^- and transfers it to the blood (Fig. 39-2B).

How much does the titratable acid contribute to net acid excretion? The following three factors determine the rate at which these buffers act as vehicles for excreting acid:

1. **The amount of the buffer in the glomerular filtrate and final urine**. The filtered load of HPO_4^{2-}, for example, is the product of plasma $[HPO_4^{2-}]$ and glomerular filtration rate (GFR) (see Chapter 33). Plasma phosphate levels may range from 0.8 to 1.5 mM (see Chapter 52). Therefore, increasing plasma $[HPO_4^{2-}]$ allows the kidneys to

excrete more H⁺ in the urine as $H_2PO_4^-$. Conversely, decreasing the GFR (as in chronic renal failure) reduces the amount of HPO_4^{2-} available for buffering, lowers the excretion of titratable acid, and thus contributes to metabolic acidosis. Ultimately, the key parameter is the amount of buffer excreted in the urine. In the case of phosphate, the fraction of the filtered load that the kidney excretes increases markedly as plasma [phosphate] exceeds the maximum saturation (T_m; see Chapter 36). For a plasma [phosphate] of 1.3 mM, the kidneys reabsorb ~90%, and ~30 mmol/day appear in the urine.

2. **The pK of the buffer.** To be most effective at accepting H⁺, the buffer (e.g., phosphate, creatinine, urate) should have a pK value that is between the pH of the glomerular filtrate and the pH of the final urine. For example, if blood plasma has a pH of 7.4, then only ~20% of its phosphate (pK = 6.8) will be in the form of $H_2PO_4^-$ (Table 39-3). Even if the final urine were only mildly acidic, with a pH of 6.2, ~80% of the phosphate in the urine would be in the form of $H_2PO_4^-$. In other words, the kidney would have titrated ~60% of the filtered phosphate from HPO_4^{2-} to $H_2PO_4^-$. Because creatinine has a pK of 5.0, lowering the pH of the tubule fluid from 7.4 to 6.2 increases the fractional protonation of creatinine from ~0.4% to only ~6%. However, urate has a pK of 5.8, so lowering pH from 7.4 to 6.2 would increase its fractional protonation from 2.5% to 28.5%.

3. **The pH of the urine.** Regardless of the pK of the buffer, the lower the urinary pH, the more protonated is the buffer, and the greater is the amount of acid excreted with this buffer. As discussed, lowering the pH of the tubule fluid from 7.4 to 6.2 increases the protonation of creatinine from 0.4% to only ~6%. However, if the final urine pH is 4.4, the fractional protonation of creatinine increases to ~80% (Table 39-3). Thus, creatinine becomes a much more effective buffer during acidosis, when the kidney maximally acidifies the urine.

Titration of Filtered and Secreted NH₃ (Ammonium Excretion) The third class of acceptors of luminal H⁺ is NH_3. However, unlike either HCO_3^- or the bases that give rise to titratable acid (e.g., HPO_4^{2-}), most of the luminal NH_3 is not filtered in the glomerulus. Instead, most NH_3 diffuses into the lumen from the tubule cell (Fig. 39-2C), and some NH_4^+ may enter the lumen directly through the apical Na-H exchanger NHE3. In the case of the proximal tubule, the conversion of glutamine to α-ketoglutarate (α-KG) generates two NH_4^+ ions, which form two NH_3 and two H⁺ ions.

Table 39-3 Titration of Buffers

	% PROTONATED BUFFER		
pH	Phosphate (pK = 6.8)	Urate (pK = 5.8)	Creatinine (pK = 5.0)
7.4	20.1	2.5	0.4
6.2	79.9	28.5	5.9
4.4	99.6	96.2	79.9

In addition, the metabolism of α-KG generates two OH⁻ ions, which CA converts to HCO_3^- ions. This new HCO_3^- then enters the blood.

In summary, when renal tubule cells secrete H⁺ into the lumen, this H⁺ simultaneously titrates three kinds of buffers: (1) HCO_3^-, (2) HPO_4^{2-} and other buffers that become the titratable acid, and (3) NH_3. Each of these three buffers competes with the other two for available H⁺. In our example, the kidneys secrete 4390 mmol/day of H⁺ into the tubule lumen. The kidneys use most of this secreted acid—4320 mmol/day or ~98% of the total—to reclaim filtered HCO_3^-. The balance of the total secreted H⁺ (70 mmol/day) the kidneys use to generate new HCO_3^-.

ACID-BASE TRANSPORT BY DIFFERENT SEGMENTS OF THE NEPHRON

Most nephron segments secrete H⁺ to varying degrees.

The nephron reclaims virtually all the filtered HCO_3^- in the proximal tubule (~80%), thick ascending limb (~10%), and distal nephron (~10%)

The kidney reabsorbs the largest fraction of filtered HCO_3^- (~80%) along the proximal tubule (Fig. 39-3A). By the end of the proximal tubule, luminal pH falls to ~6.8, which represents only a modest transepithelial H⁺ gradient, compared with the plasma pH of 7.4. Thus, the proximal tubule is a high-capacity, low-gradient system for H⁺ secretion. The thick ascending limb of the loop of Henle (TAL) reabsorbs an additional 10% of filtered HCO_3^-, so that by the time the tubule fluid reaches the distal convoluted tubule (DCT), the kidney has reclaimed ~90% of the filtered HCO_3^-. The rest of the distal nephron—from the DCT to the inner medullary collecting duct (IMCD)—reabsorbs almost all the remaining ~10% of the filtered HCO_3^-. Although the latter portion of the nephron reabsorbs only a small fraction of the filtered HCO_3^-, it can lower luminal pH to ~4.4. Thus, the collecting tubules and ducts are a low-capacity, high-gradient system for H⁺ transport.

The amount of HCO_3^- lost in the urine depends on urine pH. If the $[CO_2]$ in the urine were the same as that in the blood, and if urine pH were 5.4, the $[HCO_3^-]$ in the urine would be 0.24 mM, which is 1% of the 24 mM in blood (see Chapter 28). For a urine production of 1.5 L/day, the kidneys would excrete 0.36 mmol/day of HCO_3^-. For a filtered HCO_3^- load of 4320 mmol/day, this loss represents a fractional excretion of ~0.01%. In other words, the kidneys reclaim ~99.99% of the filtered HCO_3^-. Similarly, at a nearly maximally acidic urine pH of 4.4, urine $[HCO_3^-]$ would be only 0.024 mM. Therefore, the kidneys would excrete only 36 μmol/day of filtered HCO_3^- and would reabsorb ~99.999%.

The nephron generates new HCO_3^-, mostly in the proximal tubule

The kidney generates new HCO_3^- in two ways (Fig. 39-3B). It titrates filtered buffers such as HPO_4^{2-} to produce titratable

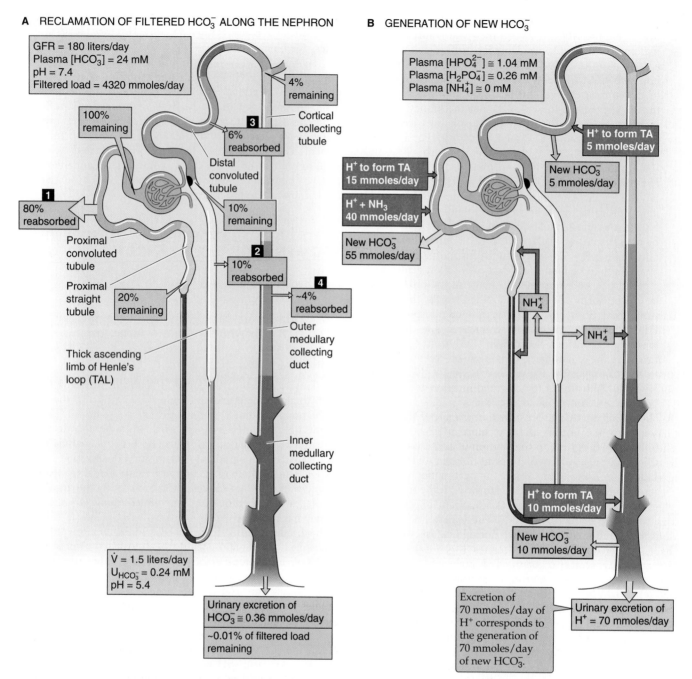

Figure 39-3 Acid-base handling along the nephron. **A,** The *numbered yellow boxes* indicate the fraction of the filtered load absorbed by various nephron segments. The *green boxes* indicate the fraction of the filtered load that remains in the lumen after these segments. **B,** The *red boxes* indicate the moieties of acid secretion associated with either the formation of titratable acid or the secretion of NH_4^+. The *yellow boxes* indicate the formation of new HCO_3^- or NH_4^+ reabsorption by the thick ascending limb. The values in the boxes are approximations.

acid, and it titrates secreted NH_3 to NH_4^+. In healthy people, NH_4^+ excretion is the more important of the two and contributes ~60% of *net* acid excretion or new HCO_3^-.

Formation of Titratable Acid   The extent to which a particular buffer contributes to titratable acid (Fig. 39-2B) depends on the amount of buffer in the lumen and luminal pH. The titratable acid resulting from *phosphate* is already

substantial at the end of the proximal tubule (Table 39-4), even though the proximal tubule reabsorbs ~80% of the filtered phosphate. The reason is that the luminal pH equals the pK of the buffer at the end of the proximal tubule. The titratable acid resulting from phosphate rises only slightly along the classical distal tubule (i.e., DCT, connecting tubule [CNT], and initial collecting tubule [ICT]), because acid secretion slightly exceeds phosphate reabsorption. The titrat-

Table 39-4 Titratable Acidity of Creatinine and Phosphate Along the Nephron*

| | pH | PHOSPHATE | | CREATININE | | Sum of Titratable Acid Resulting from Phosphate and Creatinine (mmol/day) |
		Filtered Load Remaining (%)	Titratable Acid Resulting from P_i (mmol/day)	Filtered Load Remaining (%)	Titratable Acid Resulting from Creatinine (mmol/day)	
Bowman's space	7.4	100	0	100	0	0
End of proximal tubule	6.8	20	14.0	120†	0.2	14.2
End of ICT	6.0	10	15.5	120	1.7	17.2
Final urine	5.4	10	17.8	120	5.5	23.3

*Note that other buffers in the urine contribute to the *total* titratable acid, which increases with the excreted amount of each buffer and with decreases in urine pH. In this example, we assume a plasma [phosphate] of 1.3 mM, a plasma [creatinine] of 0.09 mM, and a GFR of 180 L/day.
†We assume that the proximal tubule secretes an amount of creatinine that is equivalent to 20% of the filtered load.

able acid resulting from phosphate rises further as luminal pH falls to 4.4 along the collecting ducts in the absence of significant phosphate reabsorption.

Although the late proximal tubule secretes creatinine, the titratable acid resulting from *creatinine* (Table 39-4) is minuscule at the end of the proximal tubule, because luminal pH is so much higher than creatinine's pK. However, the titratable acidity resulting from creatinine increases substantially along the collecting ducts as luminal pH plummets. The urine contains other small organic acids (e.g., uric, lactic, pyruvic, and citric acids) that also contribute to titratable acid.

NH_4^+ Excretion   Of the new HCO_3^- that the nephron generates, ~60% (~40 mmol/day) is the product of net NH_4^+ excretion (Fig. 39-3B), which is the result of five processes: (1) the proximal tubule actually secretes slightly more than ~40 mmol/day of NH_4^+; (2) the TAL reabsorbs some NH_4^+ and deposits it in the interstitium; (3) some of this interstitial NH_4^+ recycles back to the proximal tubule and thin descending limb (tDLH); (4) some of the interstitial NH_4^+ enters the lumen of the collecting duct; and finally, (5) some of the interstitial NH_4^+ enters the vasa recta and leaves the kidney. As we shall see, the liver may use some of this NH_4^+ to generate urea. Thus, the net amount of new HCO_3^- attributable to NH_4^+ excretion is (1) − (2) + (3) + (4) − (5).

ACID-BASE TRANSPORT AT THE CELLULAR AND MOLECULAR LEVEL

The secretion of acid from the blood to the lumen (whether for reabsorption of filtered HCO_3^-, formation of titratable acid, or NH_4^+ excretion) requires at least three components: (1) transport of H^+ (derived from H_2O) from tubule cell to lumen, leaving behind intracellular OH^-; (2) conversion of intracellular OH^- to HCO_3^-, catalyzed by CA; and (3) transport of newly formed HCO_3^- from tubule cell to blood.

In addition, because the buffering power of filtered non-HCO_3^- buffers is not high enough for these buffers to accept

sufficient luminal H^+, the formation of new HCO_3^- requires that the kidney generate buffer de novo. This buffer is NH_3.

H^+ moves across the apical membrane from tubule cell to lumen by three mechanisms: Na-H exchange, electrogenic H^+ pumping, and K-H pumping

Although the kidney could, in principle, acidify the tubule fluid either by secreting H^+ or by reabsorbing OH^- or HCO_3^-, the secretion of H^+ appears to be solely responsible for acidifying tubule fluid. At least three mechanisms can extrude H^+ across the apical membrane; not all of these are present in any one cell.

Na-H Exchanger   NHE (see Chapter 5) is responsible for the largest fraction of net H^+ secretion. This exchanger is present not only throughout the proximal tubule (Fig. 39-4A, B) but also in the TAL (Fig. 39-4C) and DCT.

Of the known isoforms of NHE, NHE3 is particularly relevant for the kidney because it moves more H^+ from tubule cell to lumen than any other transporter. The apical **NHE3** secretes H^+ in exchange for luminal Na^+. Because a steep lumen-to-cell Na^+ gradient drives this exchange process (see Chapter 5), apical H^+ secretion ultimately depends on the activity of the basolateral Na-K pump.

The carboxy termini of the NHEs have phosphorylation sites for various protein kinases. Protein kinase C (PKC) phosphorylates all isoforms, whereas protein kinase A (PKA) phosphorylates only the apical NHE3. In the proximal tubule, PKC activates the apical NHE, but PKA inhibits it. For example, parathyroid hormone inhibits NHE3 through PKA.

Electrogenic H^+ Pump   A second mechanism for apical H^+ secretion by tubule cells is the electrogenic H^+ pump, which appears to be a vacuolar-type ATPase (see Chapter 5). The ATP-driven H^+ pump can establish steep transepithelial H^+ concentration gradients, thus lowering the urine pH to ~4.0 to 5.0. In contrast, NHE, which depends on the 10-fold Na^+

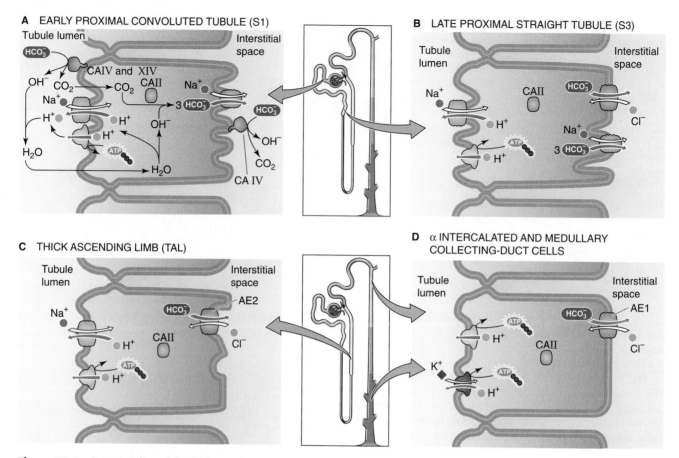

Figure 39-4 **A** to **D**, Cell models of H⁺ secretion.

gradient across the apical membrane, cannot generate an H⁺ gradient in excess of ~1 pH unit.

The apical electrogenic H⁺ pumps are located mainly in a subpopulation of intercalated cells (α cells) of the cortical collecting tubule (CCT) and in cells of the IMCD and outer medullary collecting duct (OMCD; Fig. 39-4D). However, H⁺ pumps are also present in the apical membrane of the proximal tubule (Fig. 39-4A, B), the TAL (Fig. 39-4C), and the DCT. In addition, an electrogenic H⁺ pump is also present in the basolateral membrane of β intercalated cells. Mutations in the gene encoding one of the subunits of this H⁺ pump cause metabolic acidosis (see Chapter 28) in the blood—**distal renal tubule acidosis.**

The regulation of the apical H⁺ pump probably involves several mechanisms. First, the transepithelial electrical potential appears to modulate the H⁺ pump rate. For instance, aldosterone induces increased apical Na⁺ uptake by the principal cells in the CCT (see Chapter 35), thus causing an increase in the lumen-negative potential, which, in turn, stimulates the H⁺ pump. Second, aldosterone stimulates the H⁺ pump independently of changes in voltage. Third, acidosis increases the recruitment and targeting of pump molecules to the apical membranes of α intercalated cells in the ICT and CCT, whereas alkalosis has the opposite effect.

H-K Exchange Pump A third type of H⁺-secretory mechanism is present in the ICT, the CCT, and the OMCD (Fig.

39-4D): an electroneutral H-K pump (see Chapter 5) that is related to the Na-K pump. Several isoforms of the H-K pump are present in the kidney, and exhibit differential sensitivities to inhibition by drugs such as omeprazole, SCH-28080, and ouabain. The H-K pump retrieves luminal K⁺ in animals on a low-K⁺ diet (see Chapter 37) and, as a side effect, produces enhanced H⁺ secretion that contributes to the generation of hypokalemic metabolic alkalosis.

Carbonic anhydrases in the lumen and cytosol stimulate H⁺ secretion by accelerating the interconversion of CO_2 and HCO_3^-

The CAs (see Fig. 28-3) play an important role in renal acidification by catalyzing the interconversion of CO_2 to HCO_3^-. Inhibition of CA by sulfonamides, such as acetazolamide, profoundly slows acid secretion. CA may act at three distinct sites of acid-secreting tubule cells (Fig. 39-4): the extracellular face of the apical membrane, the cytoplasm, and the extracellular face of the basolateral membrane. Two CA isoforms are especially important for tubule cells. The soluble CA II is present in the cytoplasm, whereas a GPI linkage (see Chapter 2) anchors CA IV to the outside of the apical membrane, predominantly in proximal cells.

Apical Action of Carbonic Anhydrase (CA IV) In the absence of apical CA, the H⁺ secreted accumulates in the lumen, thus inhibiting Na-H exchange and H^+ secretion. By promoting the conversion of luminal HCO_3^- to CO_2 plus OH^-, apical CA prevents the lumen from becoming overly acidic and thus substantially relieves this inhibition. Thus, CA promotes high rates of HCO_3^- reabsorption along the early proximal tubule (Fig. 39-4A).

In the distal nephron (Fig. 39-4D), H^+ secretion is less dependent on luminal CA than it is in the early proximal tubule, for two reasons. First, the H^+ secretion rate is lower than that in the proximal tubule. Thus, the uncatalyzed conversion of luminal H^+ and HCO_3^- to CO_2 and H_2O can more easily keep up with the lower H^+ secretion rate. Second, in the collecting tubules and ducts the electrogenic H^+ pump can extrude H^+ against a very high gradient. Therefore, even in the absence of CA, the collecting ducts can raise luminal $[H^+]$ substantially and consequently can accelerate the uncatalyzed reaction by mass action.

Cytoplasmic Action of Carbonic Anhydrase (CA II) Cytoplasmic CA accelerates the conversion of intracellular CO_2 and OH^- to HCO_3^- (Fig. 39-4). As a result, CA II increases the supply of H^+ for apical H^+ extrusion and the supply of HCO_3^- for the basolateral HCO_3^- exit step. In the ICT and CCT, the intercalated cells (which engage in acid-base transport) contain CA II, whereas the principal cells do not.

Basolateral Action of Carbonic Anhydrase The role played by basolateral CA IV and CA XIV (an integral membrane protein with an extracellular catalytic domain) is not yet understood.

Inhibition of Carbonic Anhydrase The administration of drugs that block CA, such as acetazolamide, strongly inhibits HCO_3^- reabsorption along the nephron and leads to the excretion of an alkaline urine. Because acetazolamide reduces the reabsorption of Na^+, HCO_3^-, and water, this drug is also a **diuretic** (i.e., it promotes urine output). However, a small amount of H^+ secretion and of HCO_3^- reabsorption remains despite the complete inhibition of CA. This remaining transport is related in part to the slow uncatalyzed hydration-dehydration reactions and in part to a buildup of luminal H_2CO_3, which may diffuse into the cell across the apical membrane (i.e., mimicking the uptake of CO_2 and H_2O).

HCO_3^- efflux across the basolateral membrane takes place by electrogenic Na/HCO_3 cotransport and Cl-HCO_3 exchange

The regulation of the intracellular pH of acid-secreting tubule cells requires that H^+ secretion across the apical membrane be tightly linked to, and matched by, the extrusion of HCO_3^- across the basolateral membrane. Two mechanisms are responsible for HCO_3^- transport from the cell into the peritubular fluid: electrogenic Na/HCO_3 cotransport and Cl-HCO_3 exchange.

Electrogenic Na/HCO_3 Cotransport (NBCe1) In proximal tubule cells, the electrogenic Na/HCO_3 cotransporter NBCe1 (see Chapter 5) is responsible for much of the HCO_3^- transport across the basolateral membrane. NBCe1 is expressed at highest levels in the S1 portion of the proximal

tubule (Fig. 39-4A) and gradually becomes less abundant in the more distal proximal tubule segments (Fig. 39-4B). NBCe1 (SLC4A4) is a 1035 amino acid protein with a molecular weight of ~130 kDa. 4,4′-Diisothiocyanostilbene-2,2′-disulfonate (DIDS), an inhibitor of most HCO_3^- transporters, also inhibits NBCe1. Because, in proximal tubule cells, this transporter usually transports three HCO_3^- ions for each Na^+, the electrochemical driving forces cause it to carry these ions from cell to blood. Renal NBCe1 carries two *net* negative charges and is thus electrogenic. Human mutations that reduce either NBCe1 activity or NBCe1 targeting to the basolateral membrane cause severe metabolic acidosis—**proximal renal tubule acidosis**.

Chronic metabolic and respiratory acidosis, hypokalemia, and hyperfiltration all increase NBCe1 activity. As would be expected, several factors cause parallel changes in the activities of the apical NHE and basolateral Na/HCO_3 cotransporter and minimize changes in cell pH and $[Na^+]$. Thus, angiotensin II (ANG II) and PKC stimulate both transporters, whereas parathyroid hormone and PKA markedly inhibit both.

Cl-HCO_3 Exchange In the S3 segment of the proximal tubule, as well as in the TAL and collecting tubules and ducts, Cl-HCO_3 exchangers participate in transepithelial acid-base transport. The AE1 anion exchanger (see Chapter 5) is found in the basolateral membranes of α intercalated cells of the CNT, the ICT, and the CCT (Fig. 39-4D). Basolateral AE2 is present in the TAL (Fig. 39-4C) and the DCT.

NH_4^+ is synthesized from glutamine by proximal tubules, partly reabsorbed in the loop of Henle, and secreted passively into papillary collecting ducts

As we saw in our discussion of the segmental handling of NH_4^+ (Fig. 39-3B), the **proximal tubule** is the main site of renal NH_4^+ synthesis, although almost all other tubule segments have the capacity to form NH_4^+. The proximal tubule forms NH_4^+ largely from glutamine (Fig. 39-5A), which enters tubule cells both from luminal and peritubular fluid through Na^+-coupled cotransporters. Inside the mitochondria, glutaminase splits glutamine into NH_4^+ and glutamate, and then glutamate dehydrogenase splits the glutamate into α-KG and a second NH_4^+. Ammonium is a weak acid that can dissociate to form H^+ and NH_3. Because the pK of the NH_3/NH_4^+ equilibrium is ~9.2, the NH_3/NH_4^+ ratio is 1:100 at a pH of 7.2. Whereas the cationic NH_4^+ is only poorly soluble in lipid membranes and therefore cannot readily diffuse across cell membranes, NH_3 readily crosses most, but not all, cell membranes. When NH_3 diffuses from a relatively alkaline proximal tubule or collecting duct cell into the more acidic lumen, the NH_3 becomes trapped in the lumen after buffering the newly secreted H^+ to form the relatively impermeant NH_4^+ (Fig. 39-5A). In addition to the diffusion of NH_3 across the apical membrane, the apical NHE may directly secrete some NH_4^+ into the proximal tubule lumen (with NH_4^+ taking the place of H^+).

A second consequence of NH_4^+ synthesis is that the byproduct α-KG participates in gluconeogenesis, which

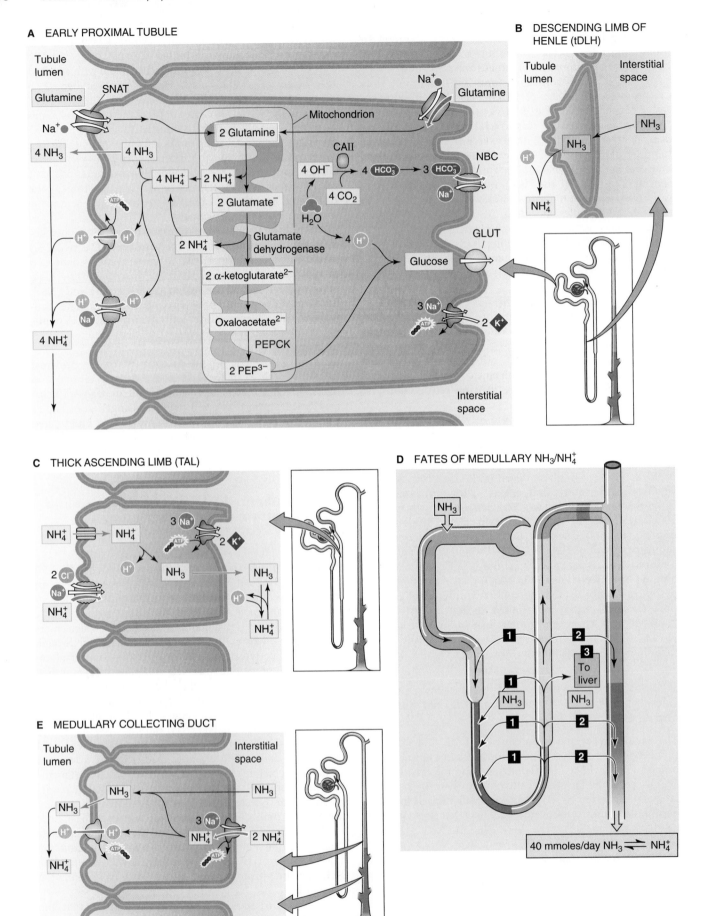

Figure 39-5 **A** to **E**, Ammonium handling. **B**, In juxtamedullary nephrons, the secretion of NH_4^+ into the tubule lumen of the tDLH occurs mainly in the outer portion of the medulla. In **D**, the *numbered boxes* indicate the three fates of the NH_4^+ reabsorbed by TAL. PEP, phosphoenolpyruvate.

indirectly generates HCO_3^- ions. As shown in Figure 39-5A, the metabolism of two glutamines generates four NH_3 and two α-KG. Gluconeogenesis of these two α-KG, along with four H^+, forms one glucose and four HCO_3^- ions. Accordingly, for each NH_4^+ secreted into the tubule lumen, the cell secretes one new HCO_3^- into the peritubular fluid.

In juxtamedullary nephrons, which have long loops of Henle, the **tDLH** may both secrete and reabsorb NH_3. Tubule fluid may become alkaline along the tDLH, titrating NH_4^+ to NH_3 and promoting NH_3 efflux from the tubule lumen (i.e., reabsorption). Conversely, reabsorption of NH_4^+ by the TAL (see following paragraph) creates a gradient favoring NH_3 diffusion into the lumen of the tDLH. Modeling of these processes predicts net secretion of NH_3 into the tDLH in the outer medulla (Fig. 39-5D) and net absorption in the inner medulla (not shown). In the **thin ascending limb,** NH_4^+ reabsorption may occur by diffusion of NH_4^+ into the interstitium.

In contrast to the earlier segments, the **TAL** *reabsorbs* NH_4^+ (Fig. 39-5C). Thus, much of the NH_4^+ secreted by the proximal tubule and tDLH does not reach the DCT. Because the apical membrane of the TAL is unusual in having very low NH_3 permeability, the TAL takes up NH_4^+ across the apical membrane by using two transport mechanisms, the Na/K/Cl cotransporter and the K^+ channels. Indeed, inhibiting the Na/K/Cl cotransporter blocks a significant fraction of NH_4^+ reabsorption, a finding suggesting that NH_4^+ can replace K^+ on the cotransporter. Ammonium leaves the cell across the basolateral membrane as NH_3, thus leading to accumulation of NH_4^+ in the renal medulla.

The NH_4^+ that has accumulated in the interstitium of the medulla has three possible fates (Fig. 39-5D). First, some dissociates into H^+ and NH_3. The late proximal tubule and the early tDLH take up this NH_3 by nonionic diffusion and trap it as NH_4^+ (Fig. 39-5B). Thus, NH_4^+ **recycles** between the proximal tubule/tDLH and the TAL.

Second, some of the interstitial NH_4^+ dissociates into H^+ and NH_3, which enters the lumen of the cortical and medullary collecting ducts by nonionic diffusion. There, H^+ actively secreted into the lumen titrates the NH_3 to NH_4^+ (Fig. 39-5E). In addition, the Na-K pump may carry NH_4^+ into cells of the medullary collecting ducts, and NH_4^+ may be substituted for K^+. To the extent that NH_4^+ moves directly from the TAL to the medullary collecting duct, it represents a **bypass** of the cortical portions of the distal nephron. This bypass prevents cortical portions of the distal nephron from losing NH_3 by diffusion from the lumen into the cortical interstitium and thus keeps the toxic NH_3 from entering the circulation.

The third fate of medullary NH_4^+ is **washout**, the return of a small fraction of the NH_4^+ to the systemic circulation for eventual detoxification by the liver. In the steady state, the buildup of NH_4^+ in the medulla leads to a sharp increase of $[NH_4^+]$ along the corticomedullary axis.

Because the liver synthesizes glutamine (see Chapter 46), the main starting material for NH_4^+ production in the kidney, hepatorenal interactions are important in the overall process of NH_4^+ excretion (Fig. 39-6). The liver disposes of ~1000 mmol/day of amino groups during the catabolism of amino acids. Some of these amino groups become NH_4^+ through deamination reactions, and some end up as amino

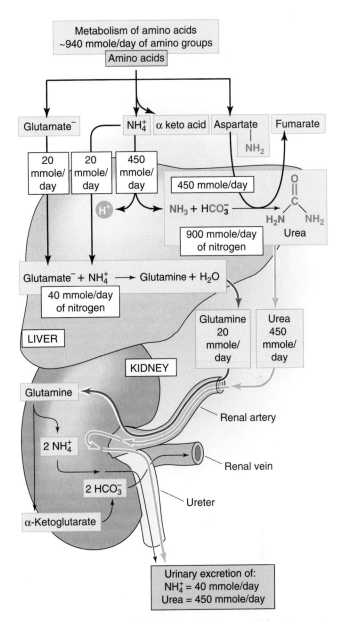

Figure 39-6 Cooperation between the liver and kidney in excreting nitrogen derived from amino acid breakdown. In this example, we assume a release of 940 mmol/day of amino groups, resulting in the urinary excretion of 450 mmol/day of urea (900 mmol/day of amino nitrogen) and 40 mmol/day of NH_4^+. The values in the boxes are approximations.

groups on either glutamate or aspartate through transamination reactions.

Of the ~1000 mmol/day of catabolized amino groups, the liver detoxifies ~95% by producing urea (see Chapter 46), which the kidneys excrete (see Chapter 36). One $-NH_2$ in urea comes from an NH_4^+ that had dissociated to form NH_3 and H^+, the other $-NH_2$ comes from aspartate, and the C=O comes from HCO_3^-. The net result is the generation of urea and two acid equivalents.

The liver detoxifies the remaining ~5% of catabolized amino groups by converting NH_4^+ and glutamate to glutamine. This reaction does not generate acid-base equivalents. The proximal tubule cells take up this hepatic glutamine and use it as the source of the NH_4^+ that they secrete into the tubule lumen as they generate one new HCO_3^- (Fig. 39-5A).

Thus, the two hepatorenal mechanisms for disposing of catabolized amino groups have opposite effects on HCO_3^-. For each catabolized amino group excreted as urea, the liver *consumes* the equivalent of one HCO_3^-. For each catabolized amino group excreted as NH_4^+ by the glutamine pathway, the proximal tubule *produces* one new HCO_3^- (Fig. 39-6). To the extent that the kidney excretes NH_4^+, the liver consumes less HCO_3^- as it synthesizes urea.

REGULATION OF RENAL ACID SECRETION

A variety of physiological and pathophysiological stimuli can modulate renal H^+ secretion as well as NH_3 synthesis. Most of these factors produce coordinated changes in apical and basolateral acid-base transport, as well as in NH_3 production.

Respiratory acidosis stimulates renal H^+ secretion

The four fundamental pH disturbances are respiratory acidosis and alkalosis and metabolic acidosis and alkalosis (see Fig. 28-11). In each case, the initial and almost instantaneous line of defense is the action of buffers—both in the extracellular and intracellular compartments—to *minimize* the magnitude of the pH changes (see Chapter 28). However, *restoring* the pH to a value as close to normal as possible requires slower, compensatory responses from the lungs or kidneys.

In respiratory acidosis, in which the primary disturbance is an increase in arterial P_{CO_2}, the compensatory response is an increase in renal H^+ secretion, which translates to increased production of new HCO_3^- through NH_4^+ excretion. The opposite occurs in respiratory alkalosis. These changes in H^+ secretion tend to correct the distorted $[HCO_3^-]/[CO_2]$ ratios that occur in primary respiratory acid-base derangements.

Respiratory acidosis stimulates H^+ secretion in at least two ways. First, an *acute* elevated P_{CO_2} directly stimulates proximal tubule cells to secrete H^+, as shown by applying solutions in which it is possible to change P_{CO_2} without altering basolateral pH or $[HCO_3^-]$. However, isolated changes in basolateral pH (i.e., without an accompanying change in $[HCO_3^-]$ or P_{CO_2})—which also produce large changes in pH_i—have a negligible effect in the short term. Thus, proximal tubule cells directly sense basolateral CO_2. Second, *chronic* respiratory acidosis leads to adaptive responses that upregulate acid-base transporters. For example, activities of the apical NHE and the basolateral Na/HCO_3 cotransporter are elevated in membrane vesicles that have been isolated from animals that were previously exposed to high

P_{CO_2} levels. These adaptive changes persist for some time, even after P_{CO_2} levels have returned to normal. Such a sustained increase in transporter activity may help to explain why, once H^+ secretion has adapted, reversing the original respiratory acidosis may produce rebound metabolic alkalosis.

Metabolic acidosis stimulates both proximal H^+ secretion and NH_3 production

The first compensatory response to metabolic acidosis is increased alveolar ventilation, which blows off CO_2 (see Chapter 32) and thus corrects the distorted $[HCO_3^-]/[CO_2]$ ratio in primary metabolic acidosis. The kidneys can also participate in the compensatory response, assuming, of course, that the acidosis is not the consequence of renal disease. An *acute* fall in basolateral $[HCO_3^-]$ stimulates proximal H^+ secretion, probably by enhancing HCO_3^- efflux from the proximal tubule cell through the Na/HCO_3 cotransporter and also by reducing HCO_3^- backleak through tight junctions from interstitial fluid to tubule lumen. Proximal tubule cells also directly sense basolateral HCO_3^- and respond to decreases in $[HCO_3^-]$ by increasing H^+-secretory rates.

In *chronic* metabolic acidosis, the adaptive responses of the proximal tubule are probably similar to those outlined earlier for chronic respiratory acidosis. These include upregulation of apical Na-H exchange and electrogenic H^+ pumping, as well as basolateral Na/HCO_3 cotransport (Fig. 39-7). For example, when one isolates brush border membranes from the renal cortex of animals made chronically acidotic, NHE3 activity is significantly increased. Therefore, the proximal tubule cell adapts to chronic acidosis, possibly by increasing the number of transporters. The upregulation appears to involve activation of PKC, a serine/threonine kinase (see Chapter 3). In proximal tubule cells, chronic

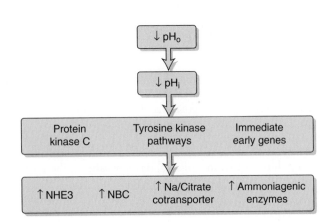

Figure 39-7 The effects of chronic acidosis on proximal tubule function. *Enhanced Na citrate reabsorption is a defense against acidosis by conversion of citrate to HCO_3^-. The price paid is enhanced stone formation because luminal citrate reduces stone formation by complexing with Ca^{2+}. Indeed, acidotic patients tend to develop Ca^{2+}-containing kidney stones. NBC, electrogenic Na/HCO_3 contransporter; NHE3, Na-H exchanger 3.

intracellular acidosis also stimulates a member of the Src family of receptor-associated tyrosine kinases (see Chapter 3). Indeed, herbimycin, a tyrosine-kinase inhibitor, blocks upregulation of NHE3 in chronic acidosis. Endothelin appears to be essential for the upregulation of NHE3 in chronic metabolic acidosis.

The parallel activation of apical and basolateral transporters minimizes changes in pH_i, whereas it increases transepithelial HCO_3^- reabsorption. An important and still unresolved question concerns the continued response of tubule cells to chronic acidosis even after the coordinated stimulation of apical and basolateral acid-base transporters has returned pH_i to normal.

In addition to the increased H^+ secretion, the other ingredient needed to produce new HCO_3^- is enhanced NH_3 production. Together, the two increase NH_4^+ excretion. Indeed, the excretion of NH_4^+ into the urine increases markedly as a result of the adaptive response to chronic metabolic acidosis (Fig. 39-8A). Thus, the ability to increase NH_3 synthesis is an important element in the kidney's defense against acidotic challenges. Indeed, as chronic metabolic acidosis develops, the kidneys progressively excrete a larger fraction of urinary H^+ as NH_4^+. As a consequence, the excretion of titratable acid becomes a progressively smaller fraction of total acid excretion.

The adaptive stimulation of NH_3 synthesis, which occurs in response to a fall in pH_i, involves stimulation of both glutaminase and phosphoenolpyruvate carboxykinase (PEPCK). The stimulation of mitochondrial glutaminase increases the conversion of glutamine to NH_4^+ and glutamate (Fig. 39-5A). The stimulation of PEPCK enhances gluconeogenesis and thus the conversion of α-KG (the product of glutamate deamination) to glucose.

Metabolic alkalosis reduces proximal H⁺ secretion and, in the cortical collecting tubule, may even provoke HCO₃⁻ secretion

Figure 39-8B illustrates the response of the proximal tubule to metabolic alkalosis. As shown in the *upper curve*, when the peritubular capillaries have a physiological $[HCO_3^-]$, increasing the *luminal* $[HCO_3^-]$ causes H^+ secretion to increase steeply up to a luminal $[HCO_3^-]$ of ~45 mM. The reason is that the incremental luminal HCO_3^- is an additional buffer that minimizes the luminal acidification in the vicinity of the apical H^+ transporters.

As shown in the *lower curve* in Figure 39-8B, when the peritubular blood has a higher than physiological $[HCO_3^-]$ —that is, metabolic alkalosis—H^+ secretion is lower for any luminal $[HCO_3^-]$. The likely explanation is that the increase in blood $[HCO_3^-]$ (1) depresses the rate at which the Na/HCO_3 cotransporter moves HCO_3^- from cell to blood and (2) increases paracellular HCO_3^- backleak from interstitium to lumen.

So far, we have discussed the effect of metabolic alkalosis on H^+ secretion by the proximal tubule. In the ICT and CCT, metabolic alkalosis can cause the tubule to switch from secreting H^+ to secreting HCO_3^- into the lumen. The α **intercalated cells** in the ICT and CCT secrete H^+, by using an apical H^+ pump and a basolateral Cl-HCO_3 exchanger, which is AE1 (SLC4A1; Fig. 39-4D). Metabolic alkalosis, over a period of days, shifts the intercalated cell population, thus increasing the proportion of β **intercalated cells** at the expense of α cells. Because β cells have the opposite apical versus basolateral distribution of H^+ pumps and Cl-HCO_3 exchangers, they *secrete* HCO_3^- into the lumen and tend to correct the metabolic alkalosis. The apical

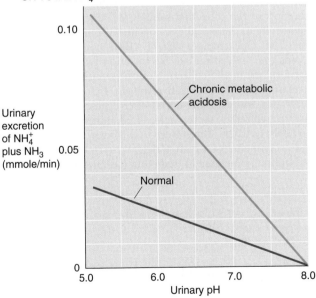

A EFFECT OF CHRONIC METABOLIC ACIDOSIS ON TOTAL NH₄⁺ EXCRETION INTO FINAL URINE

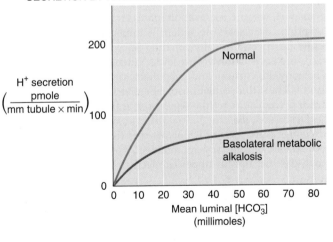

B EFFECT OF BASOLATERAL ALKALOSIS ON H⁺ SECRETION BY PROXIMAL TUBULES

Figure 39-8 Effect of acid-base disturbances on renal acid-base transport. (**A**, *Data from Pitts RF: Fed Proc 1948; 7:418-426;* **B**, *data from Alpern RJ, Cogan MG, Rector FC: J Clin Invest 1983; 71:736-746.*)

Cl-HCO$_3$ exchanger in β cells is **pendrin** (SLC26A4; see Fig. 35-5F).

By increasing HCO$_3^-$ delivery to the tubules, an increased glomerular filtration rate enhances HCO$_3^-$ reabsorption (glomerulotubular balance for HCO$_3^-$)

Increasing either luminal flow or luminal [HCO$_3^-$] significantly enhances HCO$_3^-$ reabsorption, probably by raising effective [HCO$_3^-$] (and thus pH) in the microenvironment of H$^+$ transporters in the brush border microvilli. Because a high luminal pH stimulates the NHEs and H$^+$ pumps located in the microvilli of the proximal tubule, increased flow translates to enhanced H$^+$ secretion. This flow dependence, an example of glomerulotubular (GT) balance (see Chapter 35), is important because it minimizes HCO$_3^-$ loss, and thus the development of a metabolic acidosis, when GFR increases. Conversely, this GT balance of HCO$_3^-$ reabsorption also prevents metabolic *alkalosis* when GFR decreases. The flow dependence of HCO$_3^-$ reabsorption also accounts for the stimulation of H$^+$ transport that occurs after uninephrectomy (i.e., surgical removal of one kidney), when GFR in the remnant kidney rises in response to the loss of renal tissue.

Extracellular volume contraction stimulates renal H$^+$ secretion by increasing levels of angiotensin II, aldosterone, and sympathetic activity

As discussed in Chapter 40, a decrease in *effective circulating volume* stimulates Na$^+$ reabsorption by four parallel pathways (see Chapter 40), including activation of the renin-angiotensin-aldosterone axis (and thus an increase in ANG II levels) and stimulation of renal sympathetic nerves (and thus the release of norepinephrine). Both ANG II and norepinephrine stimulate Na-H exchange in the proximal tubule. Because the proximal tubule couples Na$^+$ and H$^+$ transport, volume contraction increases not only Na$^+$ reabsorption but also H$^+$ secretion. Volume expansion has the opposite effect. On a longer time scale, volume depletion also increases aldosterone levels, thereby enhancing H$^+$ secretion in cortical and medullary collecting ducts (see later). Thus, the regulation of effective circulating volume takes precedence over the regulation of plasma pH.

Decreased *dietary Na$^+$ intake* increases apical Na-H exchange activity, even if one assesses the activity in brush border membrane vesicles removed from the animal. A high-Na$^+$ diet has the opposite effect.

Hypokalemia increases renal H$^+$ secretion

As discussed in Chapter 36, acid-base disturbances can cause changes in K$^+$ homeostasis. The opposite is also true. Because a side effect of K$^+$ depletion is increased renal H$^+$ secretion, K$^+$ depletion is frequently associated with metabolic alkalosis. Several lines of evidence indicate that, in the proximal tubule, hypokalemia leads to a marked increase in apical Na-H exchange and basolateral Na/HCO$_3$ cotransport. As in other cells, the pH of tubule cells falls during K$^+$ depletion (see Chapter 28). The resulting chronic cell acidification may

lead to adaptive responses that activate Na-H exchange and electrogenic Na/HCO$_3$ cotransport, presumably by the same mechanisms that stimulate H$^+$ secretion in chronic acidosis (Fig. 39-7). In the proximal tubule, K$^+$ depletion also markedly increases NH$_3$ synthesis and NH$_4^+$ excretion, thus increasing urinary H$^+$ excretion as NH$_4^+$. Finally, K$^+$ depletion stimulates apical K-H exchange in α intercalated cells of the ICT and CCT (see Chapter 37) and enhances H$^+$ secretion as a side effect of K$^+$ retention.

Just as hypokalemia can cause metabolic alkalosis, hyperkalemia is often associated with metabolic *acidosis*. A contributory factor may be reduced NH$_4^+$ excretion, perhaps because of lower synthesis in proximal tubule cells. In addition, with high luminal [K$^+$] in the TAL, K$^+$ competes with NH$_4^+$ for uptake by apical Na/K/Cl cotransporters and K$^+$ channels, thereby reducing NH$_4^+$ reabsorption. As a result, the reduced NH$_4^+$ levels in the medullary interstitium provide less NH$_3$ for diffusion into the medullary collecting duct. Finally, with high [K$^+$] in the medullary interstitium, K$^+$ competes with NH$_4^+$ for uptake by basolateral Na-K pumps in the medullary collecting duct. The net effects are reduced NH$_4^+$ excretion and acidosis.

Both glucocorticoids and mineralocorticoids stimulate acid secretion

Chronic adrenal insufficiency (see Chapter 35) leads to acid retention and, potentially, to life-threatening metabolic acidosis. Both glucocorticoids and mineralocorticoids stimulate H$^+$ secretion, but at different sites along the nephron.

Glucocorticoids (e.g., cortisol) enhance the activity of Na-H exchange in the proximal tubule and thus stimulate H$^+$ secretion. In addition, they inhibit phosphate reabsorption and raise the luminal availability of buffer anions for titration by secreted H$^+$.

Mineralocorticoids (e.g., aldosterone) stimulate H$^+$ secretion by three coordinated mechanisms, one direct and two indirect. First, mineralocorticoids *directly* stimulate H$^+$ secretion in the collecting tubules and ducts by increasing the activity of the apical electrogenic H$^+$ pump and basolateral Cl-HCO$_3$ exchanger (Fig. 39-4D). Second, mineralocorticoids *indirectly* stimulate H$^+$ secretion by enhancing Na$^+$ reabsorption in the collecting ducts (see Chapter 35), thus increasing the lumen-negative voltage. This increased negativity may stimulate the apical electrogenic H$^+$ pump in α intercalated cells to secrete acid. Third, mineralocorticoids—particularly when administered for longer periods of time and accompanied by high Na$^+$ intake—cause K$^+$ depletion and *indirectly* increase H$^+$ secretion (see previous section).

Diuretics can increase or decrease H$^+$ secretion, depending on how they affect transepithelial voltage, extracellular fluid volume, and plasma [K$^+$]

The effects of diuretics on renal H$^+$ secretion vary substantially from one diuretic to another, depending both on the site and the mechanism of action. From the point of view of acid-base balance, diuretics fall broadly into two groups: those that promote the excretion of a relatively alkaline urine and those that have the opposite effect.

To the first group belong CA inhibitors and K^+-sparing diuretics. The **CA inhibitors** lead to excretion of an alkaline urine by inhibiting H^+ secretion. Their greatest effect is in the proximal tubule, but they also inhibit H^+ secretion by the TAL and DCT. **K^+-sparing diuretics**—including amiloride, triamterene, and the spironolactones—also alkalinize the urine. Both amiloride and triamterene inhibit the apical epithelial Na^+ channels (ENaCs) (see Chapter 35) in the collecting tubules and ducts and render the lumen more positive so that it is more difficult for the electrogenic H^+ pump to secrete H^+ ions into the lumen. Spironolactones decrease H^+ secretion by interfering with the action of aldosterone.

The second group of diuretics—which tend to *increase* urinary acid excretion and often induce alkalosis—includes **loop diuretics** such as furosemide (which inhibits the apical Na/K/Cl cotransporter in the TAL) and **thiazide diuretics** such as chlorothiazide (which inhibits the apical Na/Cl cotransporter in the DCT). These diuretics act by three mechanisms. First, all cause some degree of volume contraction and thus lead to increased levels of ANG II and aldosterone (see Chapter 40), both of which enhance H^+ secretion. Second, these diuretics enhance Na^+ delivery to the collecting tubules and ducts and consequently increase the electrogenic uptake of Na^+, thus raising the lumen-negative voltage and enhancing H^+ secretion. Third, this group of diuretics causes K^+ *wasting*; as discussed earlier, K^+ depletion enhances H^+ secretion.

REFERENCES

Books and Reviews

Alper SL: Genetic diseases of acid-base transporters. Annu Rev Physiol 2002; 64:899-923.

Alpern RJ: Endocrine control of acid-base balance. In Fray JCS, Goodman HM (eds): Handbook of Physiology: Endocrine, vol 3, sect 7: Endocrine Regulation of Water and Electrolyte Balance, pp 570-606. New York: Oxford University Press, 2000.

Good DW: Ammonium transport by the thick ascending limb of Henle's loop. Annu Rev Physiol 1994; 56:623-647.

Moe OW: Acute regulation of proximal tubule apical membrane Na/H exchanger NHE-3: Role of phosphorylation, protein, trafficking, and regulatory factors. J Am Soc Nephrol 1999; 10:2412-2425.

Rose BD, Post TW: Clinical Physiology of Acid-Base and Electrolyte Disorders, 5th ed. New York: McGraw-Hill, 2001.

Journal Articles

Alpern RJ, Cogan MG, Rector FC: Effects of extracellular fluid volume and plasma bicarbonate concentration on proximal acidification in the rat. J Clin Invest 1983; 71:736-746.

Aronson PS, Nee J, Suhm MA: Modifier role of internal H in activating the Na-H exchanger in renal microvillus membrane vesicles. Nature 1982; 299:161-163.

Boron WF, Boulpaep EL: Intracellular pH regulation in the renal proximal tubule of the salamander: Basolateral HCO_3^- transport. J Gen Physiol 1983; 81:53-94.

Karet FE, Finberg KE, Nelson RD, et al: Mutations in the gene encoding B1 subunit of H^+-ATPase cause renal tubular acidosis with sensorineural deafness. Nat Genet 1999; 21:84-90.

McKinney TD, Burg MB: Bicarbonate transport by rabbit cortical collecting tubules: Effect of acid and alkali loads in vivo on transport in vitro. J Clin Invest 1977; 60:766-768.

Pitts RF: Renal excretion of acid. Fed Proc 1948; 7:418-426.

Romero MF, Hediger MA, Boulpaep EL, Boron WF: Expression cloning of the renal electrogenic Na/HCO_3 cotransporter. Nature 1997; 387:409-413.

Royaux IE, Wall SM, Karniski LP, et al: Pendrin, encoded by the Pendred syndrome gene, resides in the apical region of renal intercalated cells and mediates bicarbonate secretion. Proc Natl Acad Sci U S A 2001; 98:4221-4226.

Wang T, Malnic G, Giebisch G, Chan YL: Renal bicarbonate reabsorption in the rat. IV. Bicarbonate transport mechanisms in the early and late distal tubule. J Clin Invest 1993; 91:2776-2784.

Zhou Y, Zhao J, Bouyer P, Boron WF: Evidence from renal proximal tubules that HCO_3^- and solute reabsorption are acutely regulated not by pH but by basolateral HCO_3^- and CO_2. Proc Natl Acad Sci U S A 2005; 102:3875-3880.

CHAPTER 40

INTEGRATION OF SALT AND WATER BALANCE

Gerhard Giebisch and Erich Windhager

Two separate but closely interrelated control systems regulate the volume and osmolality of the extracellular fluid (ECF). It is important to regulate the **ECF volume** to maintain blood pressure, which is essential for adequate tissue perfusion and function. The body regulates ECF volume by monitoring and adjusting the total body content of NaCl. It is important to regulate the **extracellular osmolality** because hypotonic or hypertonic osmolalities cause changes in cell volume (see Chapter 5) that seriously compromise cell function, especially in the central nervous system (CNS). The body regulates extracellular osmolality by monitoring and adjusting total body water content. These two homeostatic mechanisms—for ECF volume and osmolality—use different sensors, different hormonal transducers, and different effectors (Table 40-1). However, they have one thing in common: some of their effectors, although different, are located in the kidney. In the case of the ECF volume, the control system modulates the urinary excretion of Na^+. In the case of osmolality, the control system modulates the urinary excretion of water.

SODIUM BALANCE

The maintenance of the ECF volume, or Na^+ balance, depends on signals that reflect the adequacy of the circulation—the so-called effective circulating volume, discussed later. Low- and high-pressure baroreceptors send afferent signals to the brain (see Chapter 23), which translates this volume signal into several responses that can affect ECF over either the short term or the long term. The short-term effects (over a period of seconds to minutes) occur as the autonomic nervous system and humoral mechanisms modulate the heart and blood vessels to control blood pressure. The long-term effects (over a period of hours to days) consist of nervous, humoral, and hemodynamic mechanisms that modulate renal Na^+ excretion. In the first part of this chapter, we discuss the entire feedback loop, of which Na^+ excretion (see Chapter 35) is the effector.

Why is the Na^+ content of the body the main determinant of the ECF volume? Na^+, with its associated anions, Cl^- and HCO_3^-, is the main osmotic constituent of the ECF volume;

when Na salts move, water must follow. Because the body generally maintains ECF osmolality within narrow limits (e.g., ~290 mOsmol/kg or mOsm), it follows that whole-body Na^+ content—which the kidneys control—must be the major determinant of the ECF volume. A simple example illustrates the point. If the kidney were to enhance the excretion of Na^+ and its accompanying anions by 145 mEq each—the amount of solute normally present in 1 L of ECF—the kidneys would have to excrete an additional liter of urine to prevent a serious fall in osmolality. Alternatively, adding 145 mmol of "dry" NaCl to the ECF necessitates adding 1 L of water to the ECF; this addition can be accomplished by drinking water or by reducing renal excretion of solute-free water. Relatively small changes in Na^+ excretion lead to marked alterations in the ECF volume. Thus, precise and sensitive control mechanisms are needed to safeguard and regulate the body's content of Na^+.

WATER BALANCE

The maintenance of osmolality, or water balance, depends on receptors in the hypothalamus that detect changes in the plasma osmolality. These receptors send signals to areas of the brain that (1) control thirst and thus regulate water intake and (2) control the production of arginine vasopressin (AVP)—also known as antidiuretic hormone (ADH)—and thus regulate water excretion by the kidneys. We discuss renal water excretion in Chapter 37. In the second part of this chapter, we discuss the entire feedback loop, of which water excretion is merely the endpoint.

Why is the water content of the body the main determinant of osmolality? Total body osmolality is defined as the ratio of total body osmoles to total body water (see Chapter 5). Although the ECF-volume control system can regulate the amount of *extracellular* osmoles, it has little effect on *total body* osmoles. Total body osmoles are largely a function of the *intracellular* milieu because the intracellular compartment is larger than the ECF and its solute composition is highly regulated. Total body osmoles do not change substantially except during growth or during certain disease states, such as diabetes mellitus (in which excess glucose increases

Table 40-1 Comparison of the Systems Controlling Extracellular Fluid Volume and Osmolality

What Is Sensed?	REGULATION OF ECF VOLUME		REGULATION OF OSMOLALITY	
	Effective Circulating Volume		**Plasma Osmolality**	
Sensors	Carotid sinus, aortic arch, renal afferent arteriole, atria		Hypothalamic osmoreceptors	
Efferent Pathways	Renin-angiotensin-aldosterone axis, sympathetic nervous system, AVP, ANP		AVP	Thirst
Effector	*Short term:* Heart, blood vessels *Long term:* Kidney		Kidney	Brain: drinking behavior
What Is Affected?	*Short term:* Blood pressure *Long term:* Na⁺ excretion		Renal water excretion	Water intake

total body osmolality). Only by controlling water independent of Na⁺ control can the body control osmolality.

CONTROL OF EXTRACELLULAR FLUID VOLUME

In the steady state, Na⁺ intake through the gastrointestinal tract equals Na⁺ output from renal and extrarenal pathways

The two principal solutes in the ECF are Na⁺ and Cl⁻. **Sodium**, one of the most abundant ions in the body, totals ~58 mEq/kg body weight. Approximately 65% of the total Na⁺ is located in the ECF, and an additional 5% to 10% is found in the intracellular fluid. Extracellular and intracellular Na⁺, comprising 70% to 75% of the total body pool, is readily exchangeable, as defined by its ability to equilibrate rapidly with injected radioactive Na⁺. The remaining 25% to 30% of the body's Na⁺ pool is bound as Na⁺ apatites in bone. The concentration of Na⁺ in the plasma and interstitial fluid typically ranges between 135 and 145 mM.

Chloride totals ~33 mEq/kg body weight. Approximately 85% is extracellular, and the remaining 15% is intracellular. Thus, all Cl⁻ is readily exchangeable. The [Cl⁻] of plasma and interstitial fluid normally varies between 100 and 108 mM. Changes in total body Cl⁻ are usually influenced by the same factors, and in the same direction, as changes in total body Na⁺. Exceptions arise during acid-base disturbances, when Cl⁻ metabolism may change independently of Na⁺.

By definition, in the steady state, the total body content of water and electrolytes is constant. Focusing on Na⁺,

$$\text{Oral Na}^+ \text{ intake} = \text{Renal Na}^+ \text{ output} + \text{Extrarenal Na}^+ \text{ output} \qquad (40\text{-}1)$$

Under normal circumstances, extrarenal Na⁺ output is negligible. However, large fluid losses from the gastrointestinal tract (e.g., vomiting, diarrhea) or skin (e.g., excessive sweating, extensive burns) can represent substantial extrarenal Na⁺ losses. The kidney responds to such deficits by reducing

renal Na⁺ excretion. Conversely, in conditions of excessive Na⁺ intake, the kidneys excrete the surfeit of Na⁺.

The kidneys increase Na⁺ excretion in response to an increase in extracellular fluid volume, not an increase in extracellular Na⁺ concentration

In contrast to many other renal mechanisms of electrolyte excretion, the renal excretion of Na⁺ depends on the *amount* of Na⁺ in the body and not on the Na⁺ *concentration* in ECF. Because the amount of Na⁺ is the product of ECF volume and the extracellular Na⁺ concentration, and because the osmoregulatory system keeps plasma osmolality constant within very narrow limits, it is actually the *volume* of ECF that acts as the signal for Na⁺ homeostasis.

Figure 40-1A demonstrates the renal response to an abrupt step increase and a step decrease in Na⁺ intake. A subject weighing 70 kg starts with an unusually low Na⁺ intake of 10 mmol/day, matched by an equally low urinary output. When the individual abruptly increases dietary Na⁺ intake from 10 to 150 mmol/day—and maintains it at this level for several days—urinary Na⁺ output also increases, but at first it lags behind intake. This initial period during which Na⁺ intake exceeds Na⁺ output is a state of **positive Na⁺ balance**. After ~5 days, urinary Na⁺ output rises to match dietary intake, after which total body Na⁺ does not increase further. In this example, we assume that the cumulative retention of Na⁺ amounts to 140 mmol.

The abrupt increase in dietary Na⁺ initially elevates plasma osmolality, thus stimulating thirst and release of AVP. Because the subject has free access to water, and because the kidneys salvage water in response to AVP (see Chapter 38), the volume of solute-free water rises. This increase in free water not only prevents a rise in [Na⁺] and osmolality, but also it produces a weight gain that—in this example—is 1 kg (Fig. 40-1A). This weight gain corresponds, in our example, to the accumulation of 140 mmol of Na⁺ and the accompanying free water, which makes 1 L of isotonic saline. In the new steady state, only the *extracellular* compartment has increased in volume. *Intracellular* volume does not change because, in the end, no driving force exists for water to cross cell membranes (i.e., extracellular osmolality is normal). The

A EFFECT OF ABRUPT CHANGES IN Na⁺ INTAKE

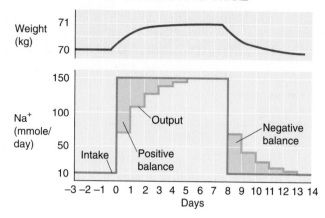

B EFFECT OF POSITIVE Na⁺ BALANCE ON Na⁺ EXCRETION

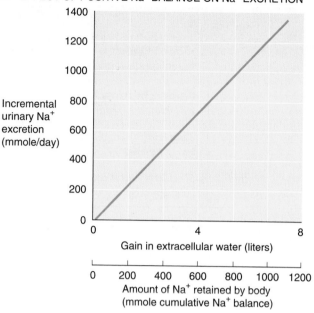

Figure 40-1   Na⁺ balance. In **A**, the *red curve* shows the time course of dietary Na⁺ intake, and the *green curve* shows Na⁺ excretion. The *golden area* between the two curves at the beginning of the experiment corresponds to the accumulated total body Na⁺ of 140 mmol. This additional Na⁺, dissolved in ~1 L of ECF, accounts for the 1-kg gain in body weight (*blue curve*). (**B**, Data from Walser M: Kidney Int 1985; 27:837-841.)

slight expansion of the extracellular volume signals the kidney to increase its rate of Na⁺ excretion. The extracellular Na⁺ *concentration* is unchanged during this period and thus cannot be the signal to increase Na⁺ excretion.

When the subject in our example later reduces Na⁺ intake to the initial level of 10 mmol/day (Fig. 40-1A), Na⁺ excretion diminishes until the initial balanced state (input = output) is re-established once again. Immediately after the reduction in Na⁺ intake, Na⁺ is temporarily out of balance. This time, it is a period of **negative Na⁺ balance**, in which output exceeds input. During this period, the ECF volume falls by 1 L, and body weight returns to normal. The extracellular Na⁺ *concentration* is unchanged during this transient period.

Ingesting increasingly larger amounts of Na⁺ results in *retaining* progressively larger amounts in the steady state and thus accumulating progressively more ECF volume. Urinary Na⁺ excretion increases linearly with this rise in ECF volume or body weight; the *slope* in Figure 40-1B is idealized for the subject in Figure 40-1A. The control system that so tightly links urinary Na⁺ excretion to ECF volume is extremely sensitive. In our example (Fig. 40-1A)—a 70-kg individual with an initial ECF volume of 17 L—expanding ECF volume by 1 L, or ~6%, triggers a 15-fold increase in steady-state urinary Na⁺ excretion (i.e., from 10 mmol/day to 150 mmol/day in Fig. 40-1A). Physiologically normal individuals can be in Na⁺ balance on a nearly Na⁺-free diet (1 to 2 mmol/day) without overt signs of ECF volume depletion. Conversely, even on a high Na⁺ diet (200 mmol/day versus the "normal" ~100 mmol/day for a Western diet), clinical signs of ECF volume excess, such as edema, are absent.

It is not the extracellular fluid volume as a whole, but the effective circulating volume, that regulates Na⁺ excretion

Although we have referred to the overall expansion of the ECF volume as the signal for increased urinary Na⁺ excretion, this is an oversimplification. Only certain regions of the extracellular compartment are important for this signaling. For an expansion in ECF volume to stimulate Na⁺ excretion, the expansion must make itself evident in the part of the ECF compartment where the ECF-volume sensors are located.

The thoracic blood vessels appear to be the site of greatest importance. For example, in congestive heart failure, particularly when edema is extensive, the total extracellular volume is greatly increased. However, the low cardiac output fails to expand the thoracic blood vessels. As a result, Na⁺ reabsorption by the renal tubules remains high (i.e., urinary Na⁺ excretion is inappropriately low compared with Na⁺ intake) and thus exacerbates the systemic congestion.

Another example of the importance of the thoracic vessels for regulating renal Na⁺ excretion is the effect of gravity in modulating venous return. Urinary Na⁺ excretion is lowest when one is standing (when thoracic perfusion is lowest), higher when one is lying down (recumbency), and highest when immersing one's self up to the chin for several hours in warm water. During immersion, the hydrostatic pressure of the water compresses the tissues—and thus the vessels, particularly the veins—in the extremities and abdomen and consequently enhances venous return to the thorax. The thoracic vessels are immune to this compression because their extravascular pressure (i.e., intrapleural pressure; see

Chapter 27) is unaffected by the water. Thus, the enhanced venous return alone stimulates vascular sensors to increase Na$^+$ excretion.

In the foregoing three examples of the effects of gravity, Na$^+$ excretion varies widely even though the total ECF volume is the same. Thus, *ECF volume* per se is not the critical factor in regulating renal Na$^+$ excretion. Recumbency—and, to a greater extent, water immersion—shifts blood into the thoracic vessels, increasing the so-called central blood volume (see Chapter 19). In contrast, the upright position depletes the intrathoracic blood volume. This example clearly demonstrates that only special portions within the ECF compartment play critical roles in the sensing of ECF volume.

The critical parameter that the body recognizes as an index of changes in Na$^+$ content is the **effective circulating volume**. The effective circulating volume cannot be identified anatomically. Rather, it is a *functional* blood volume that reflects the extent of tissue perfusion in specific regions, as evidenced by the fullness or pressure within their blood vessels. Normally, changes in the effective circulating volume parallel those in total ECF volume. However, this relationship may be distorted in certain diseases. For example, in patients with congestive heart failure (see earlier), nephrotic syndrome, or liver cirrhosis, *total* ECF volume is grossly expanded (e.g., edema or ascites). In contrast, the *effective* circulating volume is low, resulting in Na$^+$ retention.

Low- and high-pressure baroreceptors sense decreases in effective circulating volume and use four parallel effector pathways to decrease renal Na$^+$ excretion

Figure 40-2 summarizes the elements of the feedback loop that controls the effective circulating volume. As summarized in Table 40-2, sensors that monitor changes in effective circulating volume are **baroreceptors** located in both high-pressure and low-pressure areas of the circulation (see Chapter 23). Although most are located within the vascular tree of the thorax, additional baroreceptors are present in the kidney—particularly in the afferent arterioles (see Chapter 33)—CNS, and liver. These sensors generate four distinct hormonal or neural signals (Fig. 40-2, pathways 1 to 4).

In the first pathway, a reduced effective circulating volume directly stimulates a hormonal effector pathway, the **renin-angiotensin-aldosterone system**. The second and third effector pathways are neural. Baroreceptors detect decreases in effective circulating volume and communicate these through afferent neurons to the medulla of the brainstem. From the medulla, two types of efferent signals emerge that ultimately act on the kidney. In one, increased activity of the **sympathetic division** of the autonomic nervous system reduces renal blood flow and thus reduces Na$^+$ excretion. In the other effector pathway, the **posterior pituitary** increases its secretion of AVP and thus conserves water. This second mechanism becomes active only after large declines in effective circulating volume. The final pathway is hormonal. Reduced effective circulating volume decreases the release of **atrial natriuretic peptide** (ANP), thus reducing Na$^+$ excretion.

Volume Expansion and Contraction

When Na$^+$ intake persists in the presence of impaired renal Na$^+$ excretion (e.g., during renal failure), the body retains isosmotic fluid. The result is an expansion of plasma volume and of the interstitial fluid compartment. In the extreme, the interstitial volume increase can become so severe that the subepidermal tissues swell (e.g., around the ankles). When the physician presses with a finger against the skin, and then removes the finger, the finger imprint remains in the tissue (**pitting edema**). Not all cases of lower extremity edema reflect Na$^+$ and fluid retention. Particularly in elderly persons, peripheral vascular insufficiency is a common cause and does not reflect total body fluid overload, but rather a local malfunction, usually of the veins. These patients should elevate their feet whenever possible and should wear compression stockings.

Fluid can also accumulate in certain transcellular spaces (see Chapter 5), such as the pleural cavity (pleural effusion) or the peritoneal cavity (ascites), conditions reflecting derangements of local Starling forces (see Chapter 20 for the box titled Interstitial Edema) that determine the fluid distribution between the plasma and the ECF. In cases of abnormal Na$^+$ retention, a low-Na$^+$ diet can partially correct the edema. Diuretics can also reduce volume overload, as long as the kidney retains sufficient function to respond to them.

An excessive loss of Na$^+$ into the urine can be caused by disturbances of Na$^+$ reabsorption along the nephron, thus leading to a dramatic shrinkage of the ECF volume. Because the plasma volume is part of the ECF volume, significant reductions can severely affect the circulation and can culminate in **hypovolemic shock** (see Chapter 25). Renal causes of reduced ECF volume include the prolonged use of powerful loop and osmotic diuretics (see Chapter 35) and various renal tubule malfunctions, including proximal renal tubular acidosis and the recovery phase following acute renal failure.

All four parallel effector pathways modulate renal Na$^+$ excretion and correct the primary change in effective circulating blood volume. Thus, an increase in effective circulating volume promotes Na$^+$ excretion (thus reducing ECF volume), whereas a decrease in effective circulating volume inhibits Na$^+$ excretion (thus raising ECF volume). In addition to baroreceptors and the four parallel effector pathways, purely **hemodynamic/physical mechanisms** contribute to the regulation of Na$^+$ excretion thus of effective circulating volume.

An important feature of renal Na$^+$ excretion is the two-way redundancy of control mechanisms. First, efferent pathways may act in concert on a single effector within the kidney. For instance, both sympathetic input and hemodynamic/physical factors often act on proximal tubules. Second, one efferent pathway may act at different effector sites. For example, angiotensin II (ANG II) enhances Na$^+$ retention *directly* by stimulating apical Na-H exchange in tubule cells (see Fig. 35-4) and *indirectly* by lowering renal plasma flow (see Chapter 34).

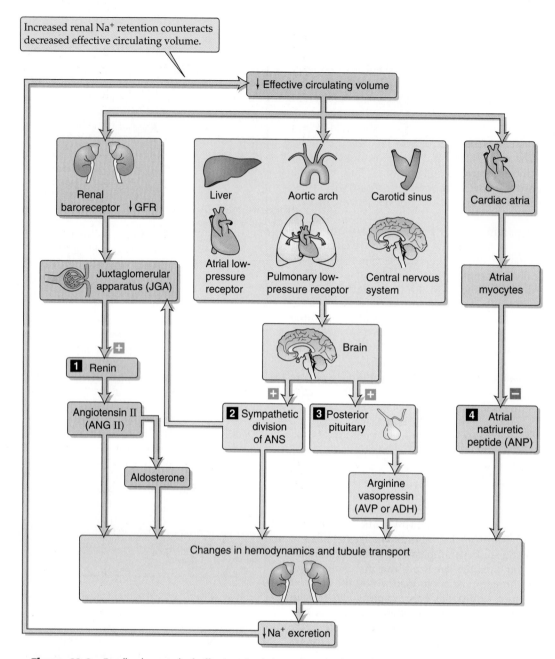

Figure 40-2 Feedback control of effective circulating volume. A low effective circulating volume triggers four parallel effector pathways (numbered 1 to 4) that act on the kidney, either by changing the hemodynamics or by changing Na⁺ transport by the renal tubule cells. ANS, autonomic nervous system.

Table 40-2   ECF Volume Receptors

"Central" Vascular Sensors
Low-Pressure Sensors (very important)
Cardiac atria
Pulmonary vasculature
High-Pressure Sensors (less important)
Carotid sinus
Aortic arch
Juxtaglomerular apparatus (renal afferent arteriole)

Sensors in the CNS (*less important*)

Sensors in the Liver (*less important*)

The next two sections focus on the four parallel effector pathways. In the third, we discuss how purely hemodynamic/physical factors modulate effective circulating volume.

Increased activity of the renin-angiotensin-aldosterone axis is the first of four parallel pathways that correct a low effective circulating volume

The **renin-angiotensin-aldosterone** axis (Fig. 40-3) promotes Na⁺ retention through the actions of both ANG II and aldosterone. In Chapter 50, we discuss this axis in the context of the physiology of the adrenal cortex.

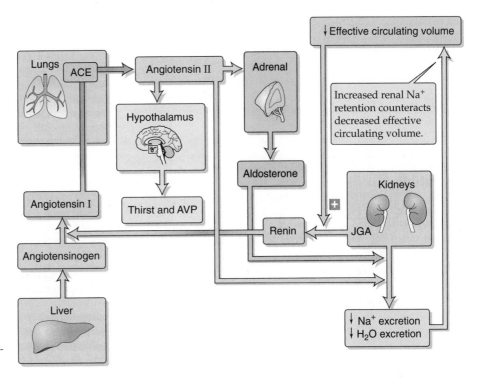

Figure 40-3 The renin-angiotensin-aldosterone axis.

Angiotensinogen, also known as renin substrate, is an α_2-globulin that is synthesized by the liver and released into the systemic circulation. The liver contains only small stores of angiotensinogen. Another protein, **renin**, is produced and stored in distinctive granules by the **granular cells** of the renal juxtaglomerular apparatus (JGA; see Chapter 33). As discussed later, decreases in effective circulating volume stimulate these cells to release renin, which is a protease that cleaves a peptide bond near the C terminus of angiotensinogen and thereby releases the decapeptide **ANG I**. **Angiotensin-converting enzyme (ACE)** rapidly removes the two C-terminal amino acids from the physiologically inactive ANG I to form the physiologically active octapeptide **ANG II**. ACE is present on the luminal surface of vascular endothelia throughout the body and is abundantly present in the endothelium-rich lungs. ACE in the kidney—particularly in the endothelial cells of the afferent and efferent arterioles—can produce enough ANG II to exert *local* vascular effects. Thus, the kidney receives ANG II from two sources: (1) systemic ANG II comes from the general circulation and originates largely from the pulmonary region, and (2) local ANG II forms from the renal conversion of systemic ANG I. In addition, the proximal tubule secretes ANG II into its lumen and thus achieves intraluminal concentrations in excess of those in the general circulation. ANG II in the circulation has a short half-life (~2 min) because aminopeptidases further cleave it to the heptapeptide **ANG III**, which is still biologically active.

The principal factor controlling plasma ANG II levels is renin release from JGA granular cells. A decrease in effective circulating volume manifests itself to the JGA—and thus stimulates renin release—in three ways (Fig. 40-2):

1. **Decreased systemic blood pressure (sympathetic effect on JGA).** A low effective circulating volume, sensed by baroreceptors located in the central arterial circulation (see Chapter 23), signals medullary control centers to increase sympathetic outflow to the JGA, thus increasing renin release. Renal denervation or β-adrenergic blocking drugs (e.g., propranolol) inhibit renin release.

2. **Decreased NaCl concentration at macula densa (NaCl sensor).** Independent of renal nerve activity (point 1) or renal perfusion pressure (point 3), decreased effective circulating volume decreases GFR and thus reduces luminal [NaCl] at the macula densa, thereby increasing renin release.

3. **Decreased renal perfusion pressure (renal baroreceptor).** Stretch receptors in the granular cells (see Chapter 33) of the *afferent* arterioles sense the decreased distention associated with low effective circulating volume. This decreased stretch lowers $[Ca^{2+}]_i$, thereby increasing renin release and initiating a cascade that tends to increase blood pressure. Conversely, increased distention (high extracellular volume) inhibits renin release.

The foregoing stimulation of renin release by a *decrease* in $[Ca^{2+}]_i$ stands in contrast to most Ca^{2+}-activated secretory processes, in which an *increase* in $[Ca^{2+}]_i$ stimulates secretion (see Chapter 8). Another exception is the chief cell of the parathyroid gland, in which an increase in $[Ca^{2+}]_i$ inhibits secretion of parathyroid hormone (see Chapter 52).

$[cAMP]_i$ also appears to be a second messenger for renin release. Agents that activate adenylyl cyclase enhance renin secretion, presumably through protein kinase A. The question whether the effects of $[cAMP]_i$ and $[Ca^{2+}]_i$ are independent or sequential remains open.

Additional factors also modulate renin release. Prostaglandins E_2 and I_2 and endothelin all activate renin release. Agents that blunt renin release include ANG II (which represents a short feedback loop), AVP, thromboxane A$_2$, high plasma levels of K$^+$, and NO.

ANG II has several important actions, as follows:

1. **Stimulation of aldosterone release from glomerulosa cells in the adrenal cortex** (see Chapter 50). In turn, aldosterone promotes Na$^+$ reabsorption in the collecting tubules and ducts (see Chapter 35).
2. **Vasoconstriction of renal and other systemic vessels.** ANG II increases Na$^+$ reabsorption by altering **renal** hemodynamics, probably in two ways (Fig. 40-4). First, at high concentrations, ANG II constricts the efferent more than the afferent arterioles, thus increasing filtration fraction and reducing the *hydrostatic pressure* in the downstream peritubular capillaries. The increased filtration fraction also increases the protein concentration in the downstream blood and hence raises the *colloid osmotic pressure* of the peritubular capillaries. The changes in each of these two Starling forces favor the uptake of reabsorbate from peritubular interstitium into peritubular capillaries (see Chapter 35) and hence enhance the reabsorption of Na$^+$ and fluid by the proximal tubule. Second, ANG II decreases medullary blood flow through vasa recta. Low blood flow decreases the medullary washout of NaCl and urea (see Chapter 38), a process that raises [urea] in the medullary interstitium and enhances Na$^+$ reabsorption along the thin ascending limb of Henle's loop (see Chapter 38).
3. **Enhanced tubuloglomerular feedback.** ANG II raises the sensitivity and lowers the set point of the tubuloglomerular feedback mechanism (see Chapter 34), so that an increase in Na$^+$ and fluid delivery to the macula densa elicits a more pronounced fall in the glomerular filtration rate (GFR).
4. **Enhanced Na-H exchange.** As noted in Chapter 34, ANG II promotes Na$^+$ reabsorption in the proximal tubule, thick ascending limb (TAL), and initial collecting tubule (see Chapter 35).
5. **Renal hypertrophy.** ANG II induces hypertrophy of renal tubule cells.
6. **Stimulated thirst and AVP release.** ANG II acts on the hypothalamus, where it increases the sensation of thirst

and stimulates secretion of AVP from the posterior pituitary, both of which increase total body free water. This ANG II effect represents an intersection between the systems for regulating effective circulating volume and osmolality.

Increased sympathetic nerve activity and arginine vasopressin, as well as decreased atrial natriuretic peptide, are the other three parallel pathways that correct a low effective circulating volume

Renal Sympathetic Nerve Activity The second of the four parallel effector pathways for the control of effective circulating volume is the sympathetic nervous system. As discussed in Chapter 35, enhanced activity of the renal sympathetic nerves has two *direct* effects on Na$^+$ reabsorption: (1) increased renal vascular resistance and (2) increased Na$^+$ reabsorption by tubule cells. In addition, increased sympathetic tone has an *indirect* effect—enhancing renin release from granular cells (see previous section). These multiple actions of sympathetic traffic to the kidney reduce GFR and enhance Na$^+$ reabsorption, thereby increasing Na$^+$ retention and increasing effective circulating volume.

In everyday life (i.e., the unstressed state), the role of sympathetic nerve activity in kidney function appears to be modest at best. However, sympathetic innervation may play a role during challenges to volume homeostasis. For example, low Na$^+$ intake triggers reduced renal Na$^+$ excretion; renal denervation blunts this response. Another example is hemorrhage, in which renal sympathetic nerves emerge as important participants in preserving ECF volume. Conversely, expansion of the intravascular volume increases renal Na$^+$ excretion; renal denervation sharply reduces this response as well.

Arginine Vasopressin (Antidiuretic Hormone) As discussed in the next major section, the posterior pituitary releases AVP primarily in response to increases in extracellular *osmolality*. Indeed, AVP mainly increases distal nephron water permeability and thus promotes water retention (see

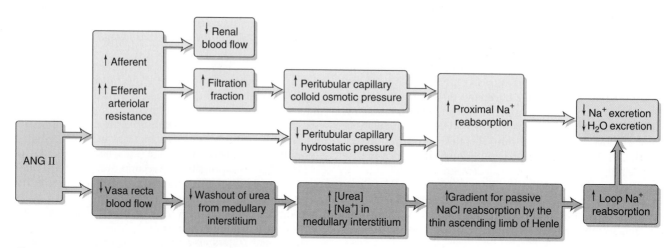

Figure 40-4 Hemodynamic actions of ANG II on Na$^+$ reabsorption.

Renal Hypertension

In the 1930s, Goldblatt produced hypertension experimentally in unilaterally nephrectomized animals by placing a surgical clip around the renal artery of the remaining kidney (**one-kidney Goldblatt hypertension**). The constriction can be adjusted so that it does not result in renal ischemia, but only in a reduction of the perfusion pressure distal to the clip. This maneuver stimulates the renal baroreceptors and leads to a rapid increase in synthesis and secretion of renin from the clipped kidney. The renin release reaches a peak after 1 hour. As renin cleaves ANG I from angiotensinogen, systemic ANG I levels rise quickly. ACE, present mainly in the lungs but also in the kidneys, then rapidly converts ANG I into ANG II. Thus, within minutes of clamping the renal artery, one observes a sustained rise in systemic arterial pressure. The newly established stable elevation in systemic pressure then normalizes the pressure in the renal artery downstream from the constriction. From this time onward, circulating renin and ANG II levels decline toward normal over 5 to 7 days, whereas the systemic arterial pressure remains abnormally high. The early rise in blood pressure is the result of the renin-angiotensin vasoconstrictor mechanism, which is activated by the experimentally induced reduction in pressure and flow in the renal artery distal to the constriction. The later phase of systemic hypertension is the result of aldosterone release and of the retention of salt and water.

Unilateral partial clamping of a renal artery in an otherwise healthy animal also produces hypertension (**two-kidney Goldblatt hypertension**). As in the one-kidney model, the clipped kidney increases its synthesis and secretion of renin. Renin then causes ANG II levels to increase systemically and will, in addition to the effect on the clamped kidney, cause the nonclamped, contralateral kidney to retain salt and water. As in the one-kidney model, the resulting hypertension has an early vasoconstrictive phase and a delayed volume-dependent phase.

In both types of Goldblatt hypertension, administration of ACE inhibitors can lower arterial blood pressure. However, inhibiting the converting enzyme is therapeutically effective even after circulating renin and ANG II levels have normalized. Maintaining the hypertension must involve an increased *intrarenal* conversion of ANG I to ANG II (through renal ACE), with the ANG II enhancing proximal Na^+ reabsorption. Indeed, direct measurements show that, even after *circulating* renin and ANG II levels have returned to normal, the *intrarenal* levels of ACE and ANG II are elevated.

These experimental models serve as paradigms for some forms of human hypertension, including renin-secreting tumors of the JGA and all cases of pathologic impairment of renal arterial blood supply. Thus, coarctation of the aorta, in which the aorta is constricted above the renal arteries but below the arteries to the head and upper extremities, invariably leads to hypertension. Renal hypertension also results from stenosis of a renal artery, caused, for example, by arteriosclerotic thickening of the vessel wall. However, the most common form of renal hypertension occurs, in parts of the kidney, when inflammatory or fibrotic lesions stenose preglomerular arteries or arterioles. Such local intrarenal vasoconstriction may lead to local ischemia, although some parts of the kidney remain entirely normal. This pattern therefore closely resembles the two-kidney Goldblatt hypertension model. In fact, high levels of ANG II may be encountered in such patients. The administration of ACE inhibitors is generally beneficial because they lower ANG II levels, systemically and within the kidney itself.

Chapter 38). However, the posterior pituitary also releases AVP in response to large reductions in effective circulating volume (e.g., hemorrhage), and a secondary action of AVP—promoting Na^+ retention (see Chapter 35)—is appropriate for this stimulus.

Atrial Natriuretic Peptide   Of the four parallel effectors that correct a low effective circulating volume (Fig. 40-2), AVP is the only one that does so by *decreasing* its activity. As its name implies, ANP promotes **natriuresis** (i.e., Na^+ excretion). Atrial myocytes synthesize and store ANP and release ANP in response to stretch (a low-pressure volume sensor) (see Chapter 23). Thus, reduced effective circulating volume inhibits ANP release and reduces Na^+ excretion. ANP plays a role in the diuretic response to the redistribution of ECF and plasma volume into the thorax that occurs during water immersion and space flight (see Chapter 61).

Acting through a receptor guanylyl cyclase (see Chapter 3), ANP has many synergistic effects on renal hemodynamics and on transport by renal tubules that promote renal Na^+ and water excretion. Although ANP directly inhibits Na^+ transport in the inner medullary collecting duct, its major actions are **hemodynamic**—increased GFR, increased cortical and medullary blood flow, and decreased release of renin and AVP. Thus, a decrease in effective circulating volume leads to a fall in ANP release and a net decrease in Na^+ and water excretion (see Chapter 35).

Elevations of arterial pressure increase Na^+ excretion by purely hemodynamic mechanisms, independent of changes in effective circulating volume

We have seen that expanding the effective circulating volume stimulates sensors that increase Na^+ excretion through four parallel effector pathways (Fig. 40-2). However, the kidney can also modulate Na^+ excretion in response to purely hemodynamic changes, as in the following two examples.

Large and Acute Decrease in Arterial Blood Pressure   If glomerulotubular (GT) balance were perfect, decreasing the GFR would cause Na^+ excretion to fall linearly (Fig. 40-5, blue line). However, acutely lowering GFR by partial clamping of the aorta causes a steep, nonlinear decrease in urinary Na^+ excretion (Fig. 40-5, red curve). When GFR falls sufficiently, the kidneys excrete only traces of Na^+ in a small volume of urine. This response primarily reflects the transport of the classical distal tubule, which continues to reabsorb Na^+ at a high rate despite the decreased Na^+ delivery (see Chapter 35).

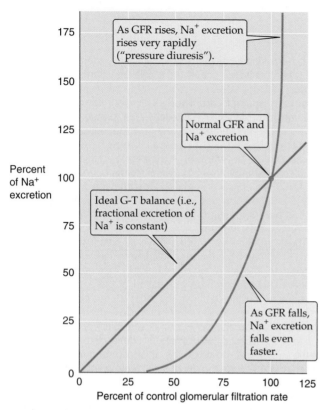

Figure 40-5 Effect of changes in GFR on urinary Na⁺ excretion. The *blue line* represents the ideal GT balance. The *red curve* summarizes data from dogs. The investigators reduced GFR by inflating a balloon in the aorta, above the level of the renal arteries. They increased GFR by compressing the carotid arteries, and thus increased blood pressure. *(Data from Thompson DD, Pitts RF: Am J Physiol 1952; 168:490-499.)*

Large Increase in Arterial Pressure In some cases, an increased effective circulating volume is accompanied by an increase in arterial pressure. An example is Liddle disease, a state of abnormally high distal Na⁺ reabsorption. The excess Na⁺ reabsorption leads to high blood pressure and compensatory pressure-induced natriuresis. One reason for this **pressure diuresis** is that hypertension increases GFR and raises the filtered load of Na⁺, which by itself would increase urinary Na⁺ excretion (Fig. 40-5, blue line). However, at least four other mechanisms contribute to the natriuresis (Fig. 40-5, red curve). First, the increased effective circulating volume inhibits the renin-angiotensin-aldosterone axis and thus reduces Na⁺ reabsorption (see Chapter 35). Second, the high blood pressure augments blood flow in the vasa recta, washes out medullary solutes and reduces interstitial hypertonicity in the medulla, and ultimately reduces passive Na⁺ reabsorption in the thin ascending limb (see Chapter 38). Third, an increase in arterial pressure leads, by an unknown mechanism, to prompt reduction in the number of apical Na-H exchangers in the proximal tubule. Normalizing the blood pressure rapidly reverses this effect. Finally, hypertension leads to increased pressure in the peritubular capillaries, thereby reducing proximal tubule reabsorption (physical factors; see Chapter 35).

CONTROL OF WATER CONTENT (EXTRACELLULAR OSMOLALITY)

Water accounts for half or more of body weight (~60% in men and 50% in women) and is distributed between the intracellular fluid and ECF compartments (see Chapter 5). Changes in whole-body water content lead to changes in osmolality, to which the CNS is extremely sensitive. Osmolality deviations of ±15% lead to severe disturbances of CNS function. Thus, osmoregulation is critical.

Two elements control water content and thus whole-body osmolality: (1) the kidneys, which control water excretion (see Chapter 38), and (2) thirst mechanisms, which control the oral intake of water. These two effector mechanisms are part of negative feedback loops that begin within the hypothalamus. An increase in osmolality stimulates separate osmoreceptors to secrete AVP (which reduces renal excretion of free water) and to trigger thirst (which, if fulfilled, increases intake of free water). As a result, the two complementary feedback loops stabilize osmolality and thus [Na⁺].

Increased plasma osmolality stimulates osmoreceptors in the hypothalamus that trigger the release of arginine vasopressin, which inhibits water excretion

An increase in the osmolality of the ECF is the primary signal for the secretion of AVP from the posterior pituitary gland. An elegant series of animal studies by Verney in the 1940s established that infusing a hyperosmotic NaCl solution into the *carotid artery* abruptly terminates an established water diuresis (Fig. 40-6A). Infusing hyperosmotic NaCl into the peripheral circulation has no effect because the hyperosmolar solution becomes diluted by the time it reaches the cerebral vessels. Therefore, the osmosensitive site is intracranial. Surgically removing the posterior pituitary abolishes the effect of infusing hyperosmotic NaCl into the carotid artery (Fig. 40-6B). However, injecting posterior pituitary extracts into the animal inhibits the diuresis, regardless of whether the posterior pituitary is intact. Later work showed that Verney's posterior pituitary extract contained an "antidiuretic hormone"—now known to be AVP—that the posterior pituitary secretes in response to increased plasma osmolality. Ingesting large volumes of water causes plasma osmolality to fall, thus leading to reduced AVP secretion.

In healthy individuals, plasma osmolality is ~290 mOsm. The **threshold** for AVP release is somewhat lower, ~280 mOsm (Fig. 40-7, red curve). Increasing the osmolality by only 1% higher than this level is sufficient to produce a detectable increase in plasma [AVP], which rises steeply with further increases in osmolality. Thus, hyperosmolality leads to increased levels of AVP, which completes the feedback loop by causing the kidneys to retain water (see Chapter 38).

Although a change in plasma [NaCl] is usually responsible for a change in plasma osmolality, other solutes can do the same. For example, hypertonic mannitol resembles NaCl

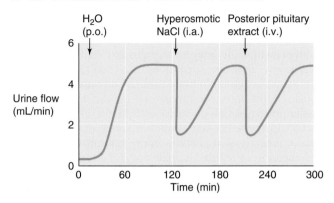

A BEFORE REMOVAL OF POSTERIOR PITUITARY

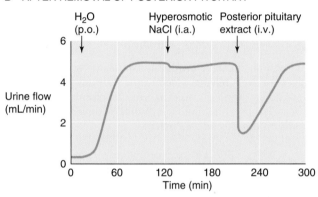

B AFTER REMOVAL OF POSTERIOR PITUITARY

Figure 40-6 Sensing of blood osmolality in the dog brain. i.a., intra-arterial (carotid) injection; i.v., intravenous injection; p.o., per os (by mouth). *(Data from Verney EG: Proc R Soc Lond B 1947;135:25-106.)*

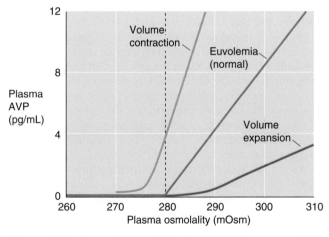

Figure 40-7 Dependence of AVP release on plasma osmolality. *(Data from Robertson GL, Aycinena P, Zerbe RL: Am J Med 1982; 72:339-353.)*

in stimulating AVP release. However, an equivalent increase in extracellular osmolality by urea has little effect on plasma AVP levels. The reason is that urea has a low effective osmolality or tonicity (see Chapter 5) and is thus ineffective in shrinking cells.

Hypothalamic neurons synthesize AVP and transport it along their axons to the posterior pituitary, where they store it in nerve terminals before release

Osmoreceptors of the CNS appear to be located in two areas that breech the blood-brain barrier: the organum vasculosum of the lamina terminalis (OVLT) and the subfornical organ (SFO), two of the circumventricular organs (see Chapter 11). Specific neurons in these regions (Fig. 40-8) are able to sense changes in *plasma* osmolality. Elevated osmolality increases the activity of mechanosensitive cation channels located in the neuronal membrane and results in depolarization and thus an increased frequency of action potentials. Hypo-osmolality causes a striking decrease of frequency. The osmosensitive neurons project to large-diameter neurons in the supraoptic and paraventricular nuclei of the anterior hypothalamus (Fig. 40-8). These neurons synthesize AVP, package it into granules, and transport the granules along their axons to nerve terminals in the posterior lobe of the pituitary, which is part of the brain (see Chapter 47). When stimulated by the osmosensitive neurons, these **magnocellular neurons** release the stored AVP into the posterior pituitary—an area that also lacks a blood-brain barrier—and AVP enters the general circulation.

In humans and most mammals, the antidiuretic hormone is AVP, which is encoded by the messenger RNA for **prepro-neurophysin** II. After cleavage of the signal peptide, the resulting prohormone contains AVP, neurophysin II (NpII), and a glycopeptide. Cleavage of the prohormone within the secretory granule yields these three components. AVP has nine amino acids, with a disulfide bridge connecting two cysteine residues. Mutations of NpII impair AVP secretion, a finding suggesting that NpII assists in the processing or secretion of AVP.

Levels of circulating AVP depend on both the rate of AVP release from the posterior pituitary and the rate of AVP degradation. The major factor controlling *AVP release* is plasma osmolality. However, as discussed later, other factors also can modulate AVP secretion.

Two organs, the liver and the kidney, contribute to the *breakdown of AVP* and the rapid decline of AVP levels when secretion has ceased. The half-life of AVP in the circulation is 18 minutes. Diseases of the liver and kidney may impair AVP degradation and may thereby contribute to water retention. For example, the congestion of the liver and impairment of renal function that accompany heart failure can compromise AVP breakdown and can lead to inappropriately high circulating levels of AVP.

Increased osmolality stimulates a second group of osmoreceptors that trigger thirst, which promotes water intake

The second efferent pathway of the osmoregulatory system is **thirst**, which regulates the oral intake of water. Like the osmoreceptors that trigger AVP release, the osmoreceptors that trigger thirst are located in two circumventricular organs, the OVLT and the SFO. Also like the osmoreceptors that trigger AVP release, those that trigger thirst respond to

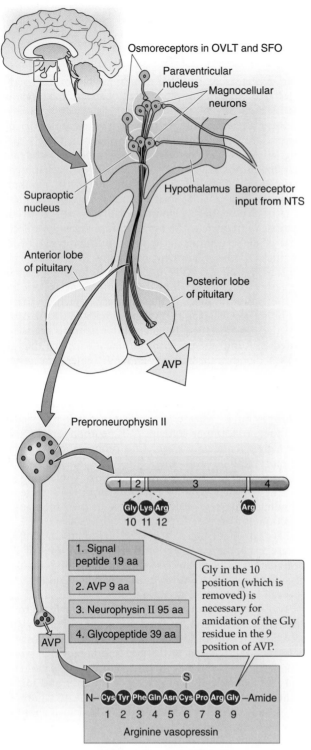

Figure 40-8 Control of AVP synthesis and release by osmoreceptors. Osmoreceptors are located in the OVLT and the SFO, two areas that breech the blood-brain barrier. Signals from atrial, low-pressure baroreceptors travel with the vagus nerve to the nucleus tractus solitarii (NTS); a second neuron carries the signal to the hypothalamus.

the cell shrinkage that is caused by hyperosmolar solutions. However, these thirst osmoreceptor neurons are distinct from the adjacent AVP osmoreceptor neurons in the OVLT and SFO.

Hyperosmolality triggers two parallel feedback control mechanisms that have a common endpoint (Fig. 40-9): an increase in whole-body free water. In response to hyperosmolality, the AVP osmoreceptors in the hypothalamus trigger other neurons to release AVP. The result is the insertion of aquaporin 2 (AQP2) water channels in the collecting duct of the kidney, an increase in the reabsorption of water, and, therefore, a reduced *excretion* of free water. In response to hyperosmolality, the thirst osmoreceptors stimulate an appetite for water that leads to the increased *intake* of free water. The net effect is an increase in whole-body free water and, therefore, a reduction in osmolality.

Several nonosmotic stimuli also enhance arginine vasopressin secretion

Although an increase in plasma osmolality is the primary trigger for AVP release, several other stimuli increase AVP release, including a decrease in **effective circulating volume** or arterial pressure and pregnancy. Conversely, volume expansion diminishes AVP release.

Reduced Effective Circulating Volume As noted earlier in Chapter 23, a mere 1% rise in plasma *osmolality* stimulates AVP release by a detectable amount. However, fairly large reductions in effective circulating volume (5% to 10%) are required to stimulate AVP release of similar amounts. However, once the rather high threshold for nonosmotic release of AVP is exceeded, AVP release rises steeply with further volume depletion. The interaction between osmotic and volume stimuli on AVP release is illustrated in Figure 40-7, which shows that the effective circulating volume modifies the **slope** of the relationship between plasma AVP levels and osmolality, as well as the osmotic **threshold** for AVP release. At a fixed osmolality, volume contraction (Fig. 40-7, green curve) increases the rate of AVP release. Therefore, during volume depletion, low plasma osmolality that would normally inhibit the release of AVP allows AVP secretion to continue. This leftward shift of the osmolality threshold for AVP release is accompanied by an increased slope, reflecting an increased sensitivity of the osmoreceptors to changes in osmolality.

Figure 40-9 summarizes the three pathways by which decreased effective circulating volume and low arterial pressure enhance AVP release. First, a reduction in left atrial pressure—produced by volume depletion—through low-pressure receptors in the left atrium decreases the firing rate of vagal afferents (see Chapter 23). These afferents signal brainstem neurons and cause magnocellular neurons in the hypothalamus to release AVP (Fig. 40-8). Indeed, at constant osmolality, AVP secretion varies inversely with left atrial pressure. Second, low effective circulating volume triggers granular cells in the JGA to release renin. This leads to the formation of ANG II, which acts on receptors in the OVLT and the SFO to stimulate AVP release. Third and more important, a fall in the arterial pressure similarly causes

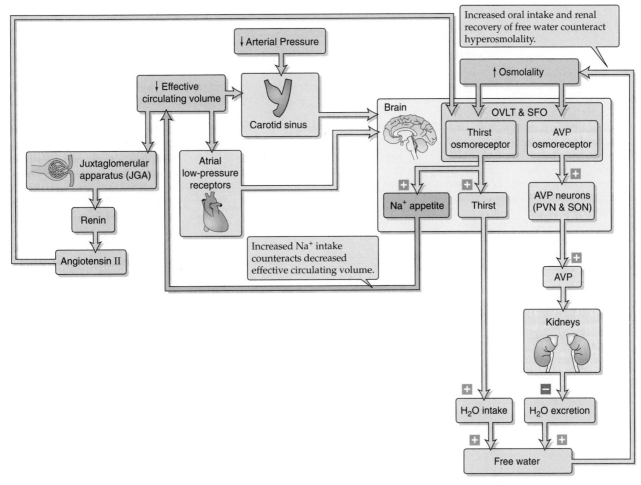

Figure 40-9   Feedback systems involved in the control of osmolality. PVN, paraventricular nucleus; SON, supraoptic nucleus of the hypothalamus.

high-pressure carotid sinus baroreceptors to stimulate AVP release (see Chapter 23).

Two clinical examples in which reduced effective circulating volume leads to increases in AVP are severe **hemorrhagic shock** and **hypovolemic shock** (e.g., shock resulting from excessive loss of ECF, as in cholera). In both cases, the water retention caused by AVP release accounts for the accompanying hyponatremia. In the first part of this chapter, we said that the appropriate renal response to decreased effective circulating volume is to retain Na+ (i.e., isotonic saline). Why is it that, in response to shock, the body also retains free water? Compared with isotonic saline, free water is less effective as an expander of the ECF volume (see Chapter 5). Nevertheless, in times of profound need, the body uses free water retention to help expand extracellular (and plasma) volume. Clearly, the body is willing to tolerate some hypo-osmolality of the body fluids as the price for maintaining an adequate blood volume.

A clinical example in which reduced effective circulating volume can lead to an *inappropriate* increase in AVP levels is **congestive heart failure**. In this situation, the water retention may be so severe that the patient develops **hyponatremia** (i.e., hypo-osmolality).

Volume Expansion   In contrast to volume contraction, chronic volume *expansion* reduces AVP secretion, as a consequence of the rightward shift of the threshold to higher osmolalities and of a decline in the slope (Fig. 40-7, blue curve). In other words, volume expansion decreases the sensitivity of the central osmoreceptors to changes in plasma osmolality. A clinical example is **hyperaldosteronism**. With normal thirst and water excretion, the chronic Na+ retention resulting from the hyperaldosteronism would expand the ECF volume isotonically, thus leaving plasma [Na+] unchanged. However, because chronic volume expansion downregulates AVP release, the kidneys do not retain adequate water, and **hypernatremia** (i.e., elevated plasma [Na+]) and hyperosmolality result.

Pregnancy   A leftward shift in the threshold for AVP release and thirst often occurs during pregnancy. These changes probably reflect the action of chorionic gonadotropin on the sensitivity of the osmoreceptors. Pregnancy is therefore often associated with a decrease of 8 to 10 mOsm in plasma osmolality. A similar but smaller change may also occur in the late phase of the menstrual cycle.

Diuretics

Diuretics reversibly inhibit Na$^+$ reabsorption at specific sites along the nephron, increase the excretion of Na$^+$ and water, create a state of negative Na$^+$ balance, and thereby reduce the volume of ECF. Clinicians use diuretics to treat hypertension as well as edema (see Chapter 20 for the box titled Interstitial Edema) caused by heart failure, cirrhosis of the liver, or nephrotic syndrome. Common to these edematous diseases is an abnormal shift of ECF away from the *effective* circulating volume, thereby activating the feedback pathways. The results are Na$^+$ retention and expansion of *total* extracellular volume. However, this expansion, which results in edema formation, falls short of correcting the underlying decrease in the *effective* circulating volume. The reason that most of this added extracellular volume remains ineffective—and does not restore the effective circulating volume—is not intuitive but reflects the underlying disorder that initiated the edema in the first place. Thus, treating these diseases requires generating a negative Na$^+$ balance, which can often be achieved by rigid dietary Na$^+$ restriction or the use of diuretics. Diuretics are also useful in treating hypertension. Even though the primary cause of the hypertension may not always be an increase in the effective circulating volume, enhanced Na$^+$ excretion is frequently effective in lowering blood pressure.

Classification

The site and mechanism of a diuretic's action determine the magnitude and nature of the response (Table 40-3). Both chemically and functionally, diuretics are very heterogeneous. For example, acetazolamide produces diuresis by inhibiting carbonic anhydrase and thus the component of proximal tubule Na$^+$ reabsorption that is coupled to HCO$_3^-$ reabsorption. The diuretic effect of hydrochlorothiazide is largely the result of its ability to inhibit Na/Cl cotransport in the distal convoluted tubule. Spironolactone (which resembles aldosterone) competitively inhibits mineralocorticoid receptors in principal cells of the initial and cortical collecting tubule. Mannitol (reduced fructose) is a powerful osmotic diuretic that reduces net Na$^+$ transport along water-permeable nephron segments by retaining water in the lumen (see Chapter 35 for the box titled Osmotic Diuretics).

An ideal diuretic should promote the excretion of urine whose composition resembles that of the ECF. Such diuretics do not exist. In reality, diuretics not only inhibit the reabsorption of Na$^+$ and its osmotically obligated water, but also interfere with the renal handling of Cl$^-$, H$^+$, K$^+$, and Ca^{2+}, as well as with urinary concentrating ability. Thus, many diuretics disturb the normal plasma electrolyte pattern. Table 40-4 summarizes the most frequent side effects of diuretic use on the electrolyte composition of the ECF. These electrolyte derangements are the predictable consequences of the mechanism of action of individual diuretics at specific tubule sites.

Delivery of Diuretics to Their Sites of Action

Diuretics generally inhibit transporters or channels at the apical membrane of tubule cells. How do the diuretics get there? Plasma proteins bind many diuretics so that the free concentration of the diuretic in plasma water may be fairly low. Thus,

glomerular filtration may deliver only a modest amount to the tubule fluid. However, organic anion or organic cation transporters in the S3 segment of the proximal tubule can secrete diuretics and can thereby produce high luminal concentrations. For example, the basolateral organic *anion* transporter system that carries PAH also secretes the diuretics furosemide, ethacrynic acid, and spironolactone. The organic *cation* transporter secretes amiloride (see Chapter 36). The subsequent reabsorption of fluid in the loop of Henle and downstream nephron segments further concentrates diuretics in the tubule lumen. Not surprisingly, renal disease may compromise the delivery of diuretics.

Response of Nephron Segments Downstream from a Diuretic's Site of Action

The proximal tubule reabsorbs the largest fraction of filtered Na$^+$; the loop of Henle, the distal convoluted tubule, and the collecting ducts retrieve smaller fractions. Thus, intuition could suggest that the proximal tubule would be the best target for diuretics. However, secondary effects in downstream nephron segments can substantially mitigate the primary effect of a diuretic. Inhibiting Na$^+$ transport by the proximal tubule raises Na$^+$ delivery to downstream segments and almost always stimulates Na$^+$ reabsorption there (see Chapter 35). As a result of this downstream Na$^+$ reclamation, the overall diuretic action of proximally acting diuretics (e.g., acetazolamide) is relatively weak.

A diuretic is most potent if it acts downstream of the proximal tubule, a condition met by loop diuretics, which inhibit Na$^+$ transport along the TAL. Although the TAL normally reabsorbs only 15% to 25% of the filtered load of Na$^+$, the reabsorptive capacity of the more distal nephron segments is limited. Thus, the loop diuretics are currently the most powerful diuretic agents. Because nephron segments distal to the TAL have only modest rates of Na$^+$ reabsorption, diuretics that target these segments are not as potent as loop diuretics. Nevertheless, distally acting diuretics are important because their effects are long lasting and because they are K$^+$ sparing (i.e., they tend to conserve body K$^+$).

It is sometimes advantageous to use two diuretics that act at different sites along the nephron, to generate a synergistic effect. Thus, if a loop diuretic alone is providing inadequate diuresis, one could complement its action with acetazolamide, which can deliver a larger Na$^+$ load to the inhibited loop.

Blunting of Diuretic Action with Long-Term Use

The prolonged administration of a diuretic may lead to sustained loss of body weight, but only transient natriuresis. Most of the decline in Na$^+$ excretion occurs because the drug-induced fall in effective circulating volume triggers Na$^+$ retention mediated by increased sympathetic outflow to the kidneys (which lowers GFR), increased secretion of aldosterone and AVP, and decreased secretion of ANP. Hypertrophy or increased activity of tubule segments downstream of the main site of action of the diuretic can also contribute to the diminished efficacy of the drug during long-term administration.

Other Factors Pain, nausea, and several drugs (e.g., morphine, nicotine, and high doses of barbiturates) *stimulate* AVP secretion. In contrast, alcohol and drugs that block the effect of morphine (opiate antagonists) inhibit AVP secretion and promote diuresis. Of great clinical importance is the hypersecretion of AVP that may occur postoperatively. In addition, ectopic metastases of some malignant tumors secrete large amounts of AVP. Such secretion of inappropriate amounts of "antidiuretic hormone" leads to pathologic retention of water with dilution of the plasma electrolytes, particularly Na^+. If progressive and uncorrected, this condition may lead to life-threatening deterioration of cerebral function (see Chapter 38 for the box titled Syndrome of Inappropriate Antidiuretic Hormone Secretion).

Decreased effective circulating volume and low arterial pressure also trigger thirst

Large decreases in effective circulating volume and blood pressure not only stimulate the release of AVP, they also profoundly stimulate the sensation of thirst. In fact, hemorrhage is one of the most powerful stimuli of hypovolemic thirst: "Thirst among the wounded on the battlefield is legendary" (Fitzsimons). Therefore, three distinct stimuli—hyperosmolality, profound volume contraction, and large decreases in blood pressure—lead to the sensation of thirst. Low effective circulating volume and low blood pressure stimulate thirst centers in the hypothalamus through the same pathways by which they stimulate AVP release (Fig. 40-9).

In addition to thirst, some of these hypothalamic areas are also involved in stimulating the desire to ingest salt (i.e., Na^+ appetite). In Chapter 58, we discuss the role of the hypothalamus in the control of appetite.

Defense of the effective circulating volume has priority over osmolality

Under physiological conditions, the body regulates plasma *volume* and plasma *osmolality* independently. However, as discussed earlier, this clear separation of defense mechanisms against volume and osmotic challenges breaks down when more dramatic derangements of fluid or salt metabolism occur. In general, the body defends volume at the expense of osmolality. Examples include severe reductions in absolute blood volume (e.g., hemorrhage) and decreases in effective circulating volume even when absolute ECF volume may be expanded (e.g., congestive heart failure, nephrotic syndrome, and liver cirrhosis). All are conditions that strongly stimulate both Na^+ *and* water retaining mechanisms. However, hyponatremia can be the consequence.

An exception to the rule of defending volume over osmolality occurs during severe water loss (i.e., dehydration). In this case, the hyperosmolality that accompanies the dehydration maximally stimulates AVP secretion and thirst (Fig. 40-9). Of course, severe dehydration also reduces total body volume. However, this loss of free water occurs at the expense of both intracellular water (60%) and extracellular water (40%). Thus, dehydration does not put the effective circulating volume at as great a risk as the acute loss of an equivalent

Table 40-3 Action of Diuretics

Site	Molecular Target	Drug	PHYSIOLOGICAL REGULATION OF "TARGET"	
			Stimulator	Inhibitor
PCT	Carbonic anhydrase	Acetazolamide		
PCT	Na-H exchanger	Dopamine	ANG II, sympathetic nerve activity, α-adrenergic agonists	Dopamine
TAL	Na/K/Cl cotransporter	Loop diuretics: Furosemide Bumetanide Ethacrynic acid	Aldosterone	PGE_2
DCT	Na/Cl cotransporter	Thiazides Metolazone	Aldosterone	DCT
CCT	Na^+ channel	Amiloride Triamterene Spironolactone	Aldosterone	
IMCD	cGMP-gated cation channel	Amiloride	Aldosterone	ANP
Water-permeable segments		Osmotic diuretics (mannitol)		

CCT, cortical collecting tubule; DCT, distal convoluted tubule; IMCD, inner medullary collecting duct; PCT, proximal convoluted tubule; PGE_2, prostaglandin E_2.

Table 40-4   Complications of Diuretic Therapy

Complication	Causative Diuretic	Symptoms	Causative Factors
Extracellular volume depletion	Loop diuretics and thiazides	Lassitude, thirst, muscle cramps, hypotension	Rapid reduction of plasma volume
K^+ depletion	Acetazolamide, loop diuretics, thiazides	Muscle weakness, paralysis, cardiac arrhythmias	Flow and Na^+-related stimulation of distal K^+ secretion
K^+ retention	Amiloride, triamterene, spironolactone	Cardiac arrhythmias, muscle cramps, and paralysis	Blocking ENaC in the collecting duct
Hyponatremia	Thiazides, furosemide	CNS symptoms, coma	Block of Na^+ transport in water-impermeable nephron segment
Metabolic alkalosis	Loop diuretics, thiazides	Cardiac arrhythmias, CNS symptoms	Excessive Cl^- excretion, secondary volume contraction
Metabolic acidosis	Acetazolamide, amiloride, triamterene	Hyperventilation, muscular and neurologic disturbances	Interference with H^+ secretion
Hypercalcemia	Thiazides	Abnormal tissue calcification, disturbances of nerve and muscle function	Increased Ca^{2+} reabsorption in distal convoluted tubule
Hyperuricemia	Thiazides, loop diuretics	Gout	Consequence of decreased ECV that activates proximal fluid and uric acid reabsorption

ECV, extracellular volume; ENaC, epithelial Na^+ channel.

volume of blood. Because dehydration reduces effective circulating volume, you would think that the renin-angiotensin-aldosterone axis would lead to Na^+ retention during dehydration. However, the opposite effect may occur, possibly because hyperosmolality makes the glomerulosa cells of the adrenal medulla less sensitive to ANG II, thereby reducing the release of aldosterone. Thus, the kidneys fail to retain Na^+ appropriately. Accordingly, in severe dehydration, the net effect is an attempt to correct hyperosmolality by both water intake and retention, as well as by the loss of Na^+ (i.e., natriuresis) that occurs because aldosterone levels are inappropriately low for the effective circulating volume. Therefore, in severe dehydration, the body violates the principle of defending volume over osmolality.

REFERENCES

Books and Reviews

Bonny O, Rossier BC: Disturbances of Na/K balance: Pseudohypoaldosteronism revised. J Am Soc Nephrol 2002; 13:2399-2414.

Bourque CW, Oliet SHR: Osmoreceptors in the central nervous system. Annu Rev Physiol 1997; 59:601-619.

DiBona GF, Kopp UC: Neural control of renal function. Physiol Rev 1997; 77:75-197.

Fitzsimons JT: Angiotensin, thirst and sodium appetite. Physiol Rev 1998; 78:583-686.

Gutkowska J, Antunes-Rodrigues J, McCann SM: Atrial natriuretic peptide in brain and pituitary gland. Physiol Rev 1997; 77:465-515.

Navar LG, Zou L, Von Thun A, et al: Unraveling the mystery of Goldblatt hypertension. News Physiol Sci 1998; 13:170-176.

Rose BD, Rennke HG (eds): Renal Pathophysiology: The Essentials. Baltimore: Lippincott Williams & Wilkins, 1994.

Sterns RH: Fluid, electrolyte and acid-base disturbances. In Glassock RJ (ed): Nephrology Self-Assessment Program (*NephSAP*) 3, pp 187-238. Philadelphia: Lippincott Williams & Wilkins, 2004.

Journal Articles

Chou CL, Marsh DJ: Role of proximal convoluted tubule in pressure diuresis in the rat. Am J Physiol 1986; 251:F283-F289.

Mason WT: Supraoptic neurones of rat hypothalamus are osmosensitive. Nature 1980; 287:154-157.

Oliet SHR, Bourque CW: Mechanosensitive channels transduce osmosensitivity in supraoptic neurons. Nature 1993; 364:341-343.

Robertson GL, Aycinena P, Zerbe RL: Neurogenic disorders of osmoregulation. Am J Med 1982; 72:339-353.

Thompson DD, Pitts RF: Effects of alterations of renal arterial pressure on sodium and water excretion. Am J Physiol 1952; 168:490-499.

Walser M: Phenomenological analysis of renal regulation of sodium and potassium balance. Kidney Int 1985; 27:837-841.

Verney EG: The antidiuretic hormone and the factors which determine its release. Proc R Soc London B Biol Sci 1947; 135:25-106.

Yang LE, Maunsbach AB, Leong PKK, McDonough AA: Differential traffic of proximal tubule Na^+ transporters during hypertension or PTH: NHE3 to base of microvilli vs. NaPi2 to endosomes. Am J Physiol 2004; 287:F896-F906.

THE GASTROINTESTINAL SYSTEM

CHAPTER 41

ORGANIZATION OF THE GASTROINTESTINAL SYSTEM

Henry J. Binder

OVERVIEW OF DIGESTIVE PROCESSES

The gastrointestinal tract is a tube that is specialized along its length for the sequential processing of food

The gastrointestinal (GI) tract consists of both the series of hollow organs stretching from the mouth to the anus and the several accessory glands and organs that add secretions to these hollow organs (Fig. 41-1). Each of these hollow organs, separated from each other at key locations by sphincters, has evolved to serve a specialized function. The mouth and oropharynx are responsible for chopping food into small pieces, lubricating it, initiating carbohydrate and fat digestion, and propelling the food into the esophagus. The esophagus acts as a conduit to the stomach. The stomach (see Chapter 42) temporarily stores food and also initiates digestion by churning and by secreting proteases and acid. The small intestine (see Chapters 44 and 45) continues the work of digestion and is the primary site for the absorption of nutrients. The large intestine (see Chapters 44 and 45) reabsorbs fluids and electrolytes and also stores the fecal matter before expulsion from the body. The accessory glands and organs include the salivary glands, pancreas, and liver. The pancreas (see Chapter 43) secretes digestive enzymes into the duodenum, in addition to secreting HCO_3^- to neutralize gastric acid. The liver secretes bile (see Chapter 46), which the gallbladder stores for future delivery to the duodenum during a meal. Bile contains bile acids, which play a key role in the digestion of fats.

Although the anatomy of the wall of the GI tract varies along its length, certain organizational themes are common to all segments. Figure 41-2, a cross section through a generic piece of stomach or intestine, shows the characteristic layered structure of mucosa, submucosa, muscle, and serosa.

The **mucosa** consists of the epithelial layer, as well as an underlying layer of loose connective tissue known as the **lamina propria**, which contains capillaries, enteric neurons, and immune cells (e.g., mast cells), as well as a thin layer of smooth muscle known as the *lamina muscularis mucosae* (literally, the muscle layer of the mucosa). The surface area of the epithelial layer is amplified by several mechanisms.

Most cells have microvilli on their apical surfaces. In addition, the layer of epithelial cells can be evaginated to form villi or invaginated to form glands (or crypts). Finally, on a macroscopic scale, the mucosa is organized into large folds.

The **submucosa** consists of loose connective tissue and larger blood vessels. The submucosa may also contain glands that secrete material into the GI lumen.

The **muscle layer**, the *muscularis externa*, includes two layers of smooth muscle. The inner layer is circular, whereas the outer layer is longitudinal. Enteric neurons are present between these two muscle layers.

The **serosa** is an enveloping layer of connective tissue that is covered with squamous epithelial cells.

Assimilation of dietary food substances requires digestion as well as absorption

The sedentary human body requires ~30 kcal/kg body weight each day (see Chapter 58). This nutrient requirement is normally acquired by the oral intake of multiple food substances that the GI tract then assimilates. Although antigenic amounts of protein enter the body through the skin and across the pulmonary epithelium, caloric uptake by routes other than the GI tract is not thought to occur. Both the small and large intestines absorb water and electrolytes, but only the small intestine absorbs lipids, carbohydrates, and amino acids. However, even without effective GI function, parenteral (i.e., intravenous) alimentation can provide sufficient calories to sustain adults and to support growth in premature infants. Total parenteral nutrition has been used successfully on a long-term basis in many clinical settings in which oral intake is impossible or undesirable.

Food substances are not necessarily—and often are—consumed in a chemical form that the small intestine can directly absorb. To facilitate absorption, the GI tract digests the food by both mechanical and chemical processes.

Mechanical disruption of ingested food begins in the mouth with chewing (mastication). Individuals without teeth usually require their solid food to be cut into smaller pieces before eating. The mechanical processes that alter

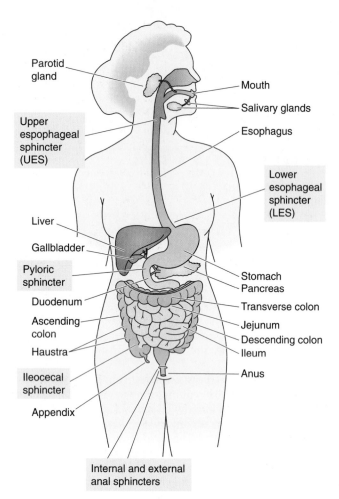

Figure 41-1 The major components of the human digestive system.

food composition to facilitate absorption continue in the stomach (see Chapter 42), both to initiate protein and lipid enzymatic digestion and to allow passage of gastric contents through the pylorus into the duodenum. This change in the size and consistency of gastric contents is necessary because solids that are greater than 2 mm in diameter do not pass through the pylorus.

The chemical form in which different nutrients are ingested and absorbed varies according to the specific nutrient in question. For example, although most lipids are consumed in the form of triglycerides, it is fatty acids and monoglycerides, *not* triglycerides, that are absorbed by the small intestine. Thus, complex series of chemical reactions (i.e., lipid digestion) are required to convert dietary triglycerides to these smaller lipid forms (see Chapter 45). Similarly, amino acids are present in food as proteins and large peptides, but only amino acids and small peptides—primarily dipeptides and tripeptides—are absorbed by the small intestine. Carbohydrates are present in the diet as starch, disaccharides, and monosaccharides (e.g., glucose). However, because the small intestine absorbs all carbohydrates as monosaccharides, most dietary carbohydrates require chemical digestion before their absorption.

Digestion requires enzymes secreted in the mouth, stomach, pancreas, and small intestine

Digestion involves the conversion of dietary food nutrients to a form that the small intestine can absorb. For carbohydrates and lipids, these digestive processes are initiated in the mouth by salivary and lingual enzymes: amylase for carbohydrates and lipase for lipids. Protein digestion is initiated in the stomach by gastric proteases (i.e., pepsins), whereas additional lipid digestion in the stomach occurs primarily as a result of the lingual lipase that is swallowed, although some gastric lipase is also secreted. Carbohydrate digestion does not involve any secreted gastric enzymes.

Digestion is completed in the small intestine by the action of both pancreatic enzymes and enzymes at the brush border of the small intestine. Pancreatic enzymes, which include lipase, chymotrypsin, and amylase, are critical for the digestion of lipids, protein, and carbohydrates, respectively. The enzymes on the luminal surface of the small intestine (e.g., brush border disaccharidases and dipeptidases) complete the digestion of carbohydrates and proteins. Digestion by these brush border enzymes is referred to as *membrane digestion*.

The material presented to the small intestine includes both dietary intake and secretory products. The food material entering the small intestine differs considerably from that of the ingested material because of the mechanical and chemical changes just discussed. The load to the small intestine is also significantly greater than that of the ingested material. Dietary fluid intake is 1.5 to 2.5 L/day, whereas the fluid load presented to the small intestine is 8 to 9 L/day. The increased volume results from substantial quantities of salivary, gastric, biliary, pancreatic, and small intestinal secretions. These secretions contain large amounts of protein, primarily in the form of the digestive enzymes discussed earlier.

Ingestion of food initiates multiple endocrine, neural, and paracrine responses

Digestion of food involves multiple secretory, enzymatic, and motor processes that are closely coordinated with one another. The necessary control is achieved by neural and hormonal processes that are initiated by dietary food substances; the result is a coordinated series of motor and secretory responses. For example, chemoreceptors, osmoreceptors, and mechanical receptors in the mucosa in large part generate the afferent stimuli that induce gastric and pancreatic secretions. These receptors sense the luminal contents and initiate a neurohumoral response.

Endocrine, neural, and paracrine mechanisms all contribute to digestion. All three include sensor and transmitter processes. An **endocrine** mechanism (see Chapter 3) involves the release of a transmitter (e.g., peptide) into the blood. For example, protein in the stomach stimulates the release of gastrin from antral G cells. Gastrin then enters the blood and stimulates H^+ release from parietal cells in the body of the stomach. A **neural** mechanism involves the activation of nerves and neurotransmitters that influence either secretory or motor activity. Neural transmission of these responses may involve the enteric nervous system (ENS; see later) or

Labels (Figure 41-1):
- Parotid gland
- Mouth
- Salivary glands
- Esophagus
- Upper esophageal sphincter (UES)
- Lower esophageal sphincter (LES)
- Liver
- Gallbladder
- Pyloric sphincter
- Duodenum
- Ascending colon
- Haustra
- Ileocecal sphincter
- Appendix
- Stomach
- Pancreas
- Transverse colon
- Jejunum
- Descending colon
- Ileum
- Anus
- Internal and external anal sphincters

A MACROSCOPIC VIEW OF THE WALL OF THE DUODENUM

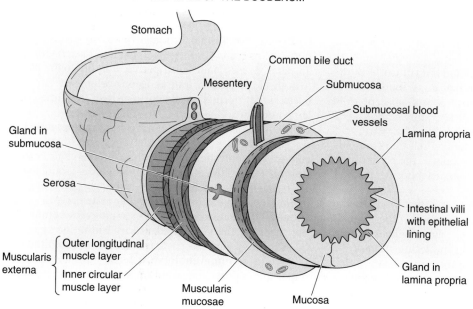

B MICROSCOPIC VIEW OF THE WALL OF THE COLON

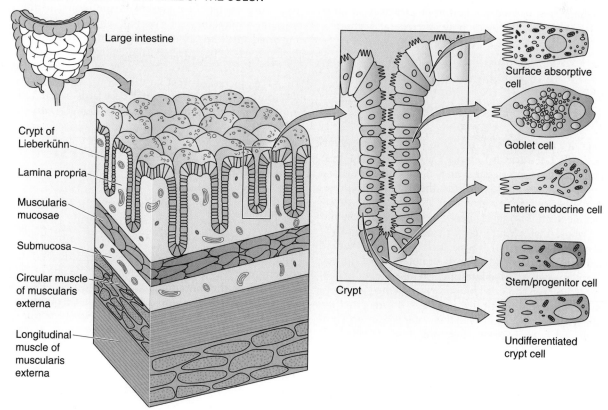

Figure 41-2   The wall of the gastrointestinal tract. **A,** The wall of a generic segment of the gastrointestinal tract consists of the following structures, from inside to outside: an epithelial layer with crypts, lamina propria, muscularis mucosae, submucosa, the circular and then the longitudinal layer of the muscularis externa, and serosa. **B,** The colon has the same basic structure as the small intestine. Some of the epithelial cells are on the surface, and others are in the crypts that penetrate into the wall of the colon.

the central nervous system (CNS). An example of neural control is activation of the vagus nerve in response to the smell of food. The resultant release of the neurotransmitter acetylcholine (ACh) also releases H^+ from parietal cells in the stomach.

The third mechanism of neurohumoral control is **paracrine** (see Chapter 3). In this mechanism, a transmitter is released from a sensor cell, and it affects adjacent cells without either entering the blood or activating neurons. For example, paracrine mechanisms help to regulate gastric acid secretion by parietal cells: the histamine released from so-called enterochromaffin-like (ECL) cells in the body of the stomach stimulates H^+ release from neighboring parietal cells.

In addition to the primary response that leads to the release of one or more digestive enzymes, other signals terminate these secretory responses. Enteric neurons are important throughout the initiation and termination of the responses.

Although the endocrine, neural, and paracrine responses are most often studied separately, with considerable effort made to isolate individual events, these responses do not occur as isolated events. Rather, each type is part of an integrated response to a meal that results in the digestion and absorption of food. This entire series of events that results from the ingestion of food can best be described as an integrated response that includes both afferent and efferent limbs.

In addition to its function in nutrition, the gastrointestinal tract plays important roles in excretion, fluid and electrolyte balance, and immunity

Although its primary roles are absorbing and digesting nutrients, the GI tract also excretes **waste material**. Fecal material includes nondigested and nonabsorbed dietary food products, colonic bacteria and their metabolic products, and several excretory products. These excretory products include the following: (1) heavy metals such as iron and copper, whose major route of excretion is in bile; and (2) several organic anions and cations, including drugs, that are excreted in bile but are either poorly or not at all reabsorbed by either the small or large intestine.

As noted earlier, the small intestine is presented with 8 to 9 L/day of fluid, an amount that includes ~1 L/day that the intestine itself secretes. Almost all this water is reabsorbed in the small and large intestine; therefore, stool has relatively small amounts of water (~0.1 L/day). Diarrhea (an increase in stool liquidity and weight, >200 g/day) results from either increased fluid secretion by the small or large intestine or decreased fluid reabsorption by the intestines. An important clinical example of diarrhea is cholera, especially in developing countries. Cholera can be fatal because of the water and electrolyte imbalance that it creates. Thus, the GI tract plays a crucial role in maintaining overall **fluid and electrolyte balance** (see Chapter 44).

The GI tract also contributes to **immune function**. The mucosal immune system, or **gut-associated lymphoid tissue (GALT)**, consists of both organized aggregates of lymphoid tissue (e.g., Peyer's patches; Fig. 41-2B) and diffuse populations of immune cells. These immune cells include lymphocytes that reside between the epithelial cells lining the gut, as well as lymphocytes and mast cells in the lamina propria. GALT has two primary functions: (1) to protect against potential microbial pathogens, including bacteria, protozoans, and viruses; and (2) to permit immunologic *tolerance* to both the potentially immunogenic dietary substances and bacteria that normally reside primarily in the lumen of the large intestine.

The mucosal immune system is important because the GI tract has the largest area of the body in potential direct contact with infectious, toxic, and immunogenic material. Approximately 80% of the immunoglobulin-producing cells are found in the small intestine. Although GALT has some interaction with the systemic immune system, GALT is operationally distinct. Finally, evidence indicates communication between the GALT and mucosal immune systems at other mucosal surfaces, such as the pulmonary epithelia.

Certain **nonimmunologic defense** processes are also important in protecting against potential luminal pathogens and in limiting the uptake of macromolecules from the GI tract. The nonimmunologic mechanisms that are critical in maintaining the ecology of intestinal flora include gastric acid secretion, intestinal mucin, peristalsis, and the epithelial cell permeability barrier. Thus, whereas relatively low levels of aerobic bacteria are present in the lumen of the small intestine of physiologically normal subjects, individuals with impaired small intestinal peristalsis often have substantially higher levels of both aerobic and anaerobic bacteria in their small intestine. A consequence may be diarrhea or steatorrhea (i.e., increased fecal fat excretion). The clinical manifestation of impaired intestinal peristalsis is referred to as either *blind loop syndrome* or *stagnant bowel syndrome*.

REGULATION OF GASTROINTESTINAL FUNCTION

The enteric nervous system is a "minibrain" with sensory neurons, interneurons, and motor neurons

The ENS is the primary neural mechanism that controls GI function and, as described in Chapter 14, is one of the three divisions of the autonomic nervous system (ANS), along with the sympathetic and parasympathetic divisions. One indication of the importance of the ENS is the number of neurons consigned to it. The ENS consists of ~100 million neurons, roughly the number in the spinal cord or in the rest of the entire ANS. The ENS is located solely within GI tissue, but it can be modified by input from the brain. Neurons of the ENS are primarily, but not exclusively, clustered in one of two collections of neurons (Fig. 41-3A): the submucosal plexus and the myenteric plexus. The **submucosal (or Meissner's) plexus** is found in the submucosa only in the small and large intestine. The **myenteric (or Auerbach's) plexus** is located between the circular and longitudinal muscle layers throughout the GI tract from the proximal end of the esophagus to the rectum.

The ENS is a complete reflex circuit and can operate totally within the GI tract, without the participation of either

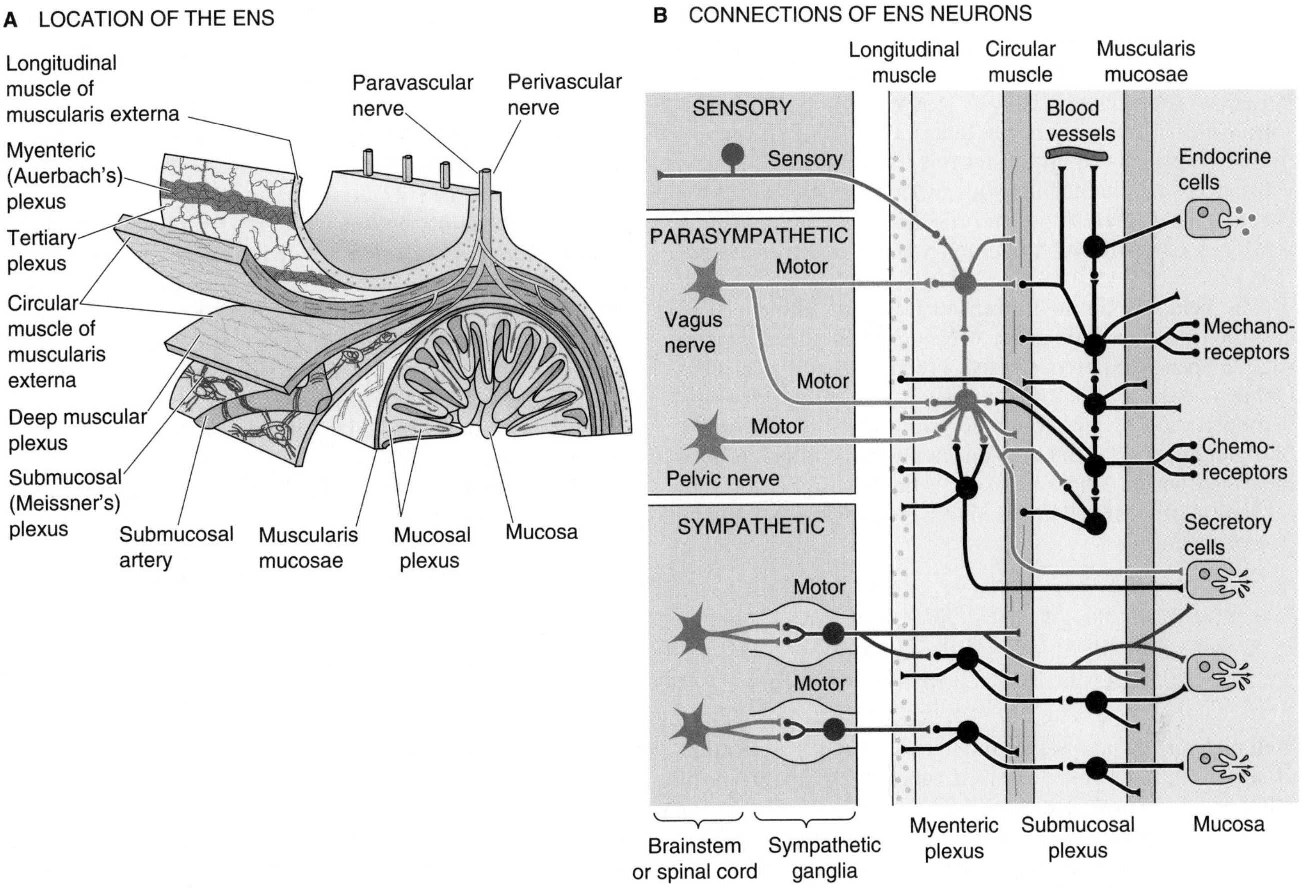

A LOCATION OF THE ENS

Longitudinal muscle of muscularis externa

Myenteric (Auerbach's) plexus

Tertiary plexus

Circular muscle of muscularis externa

Deep muscular plexus

Submucosal (Meissner's) plexus

Paravascular nerve

Perivascular nerve

Submucosal artery

Muscularis mucosae

Mucosal plexus

Mucosa

B CONNECTIONS OF ENS NEURONS

Longitudinal muscle   Circular muscle   Muscularis mucosae

SENSORY

Sensory

Blood vessels

Endocrine cells

PARASYMPATHETIC

Motor

Vagus nerve

Motor

Motor

Pelvic nerve

Mechano-receptors

Chemo-receptors

SYMPATHETIC

Motor

Motor

Secretory cells

Brainstem or spinal cord   Sympathetic ganglia   Myenteric plexus   Submucosal plexus   Mucosa

Figure 41-3 Schematic representation of the ENS. **A,** The submucosal (or Meissner's) plexus is located between the muscularis mucosae and the circular muscle of the muscularis externa. The myenteric (or Auerbach's) plexus is located between the circular and longitudinal layers of the muscularis externa. In addition to these two plexuses that have ganglia, three others—mucosal, deep muscular, and tertiary plexus—are also present. **B,** The ENS consists of sensory neurons, interneurons, and motor neurons. Some sensory signals travel centrally from the ENS. Both the parasympathetic and the sympathetic divisions of the ANS modulate the ENS. This figure illustrates some of the typical circuitry of ENS neurons.

the spinal cord or the cephalic brain. As with other neurons, the activity of the ENS is the result of the generation of action potentials by single neurons and the release of chemical neurotransmitters that affect either other neurons or effector cells (i.e., epithelial or muscle cells). The ENS consists of sensory circuits, interneuronal connections, and secretomotor neurons (Fig. 41-3B). Sensory (or **afferent**) neurons monitor changes in luminal activity, including distention (i.e., smooth muscle tension), chemistry (e.g., pH, osmolality, specific nutrients), and mechanical stimulation. These sensory neurons, in turn, activate **interneurons**, which relay signals that activate **efferent** secretomotor neurons. These efferent secretomotor neurons stimulate or inhibit a wide range of effector cells: smooth muscle cells, epithelial cells that secrete or absorb fluid and electrolytes, submucosal blood vessels, and enteric endocrine cells.

The largely independent function of the ENS has given rise to the concept of a GI "minibrain." Because the efferent response to several different stimuli is often quite similar, a generalized concept has developed that the ENS possesses multiple preprogrammed responses. For example, both mechanical distention of the jejunum and the presence of a

bacterial enterotoxin in the jejunum can elicit identical responses: stimulation of profuse fluid and electrolyte secretion, together with propagated, propulsive, coordinated smooth muscle contractions. Such preprogrammed efferent responses are probably initiated by sensory input to the enteric interneuronal connections. However, efferent responses controlled by the ENS may also be modified by input from autonomic ganglia, which are, in turn, under the influence of the spinal cord and brain (see Chapter 14). In addition, the ENS receives input directly from the brain through parasympathetic nerves (i.e., the vagus nerve).

Acetylcholine, peptides, and bioactive amines are the ENS neurotransmitters that regulate epithelial and motor function

ACh is the primary preganglionic and postganglionic neurotransmitter regulating both secretory function and smooth muscle activity in the GI tract. In addition, many other neurotransmitters are present in enteric neurons. Among the peptides, **vasoactive intestinal peptide (VIP)** has an important role in both inhibition of intestinal smooth muscle and stimulation of intestinal fluid and electrolyte secretion. Although VIP was first identified in the GI tract, it is now appreciated that VIP is also an important neurotransmitter in the brain (see Table 13-1). Other substances probably also play an important role in GI regulation. These substances include the following: other peptides, such as the enkephalins, somatostatin, and substance P; amines such as serotonin (5-hydroxytryptamine [5-HT]); and nitric oxide (NO).

The field of ENS neurotransmitters is rapidly evolving, and the list of agonists grows ever longer. In addition, substantial species differences exist. Frequently, chemical neurotransmitters are identified in neurons without a clear-cut demonstration of their physiological role in the regulation of organ function. More than one neurotransmitter has been identified within single neurons, a finding suggesting that regulation of some cell functions may require more than one neurotransmitter.

The brain-gut axis is a bidirectional system that controls gastrointestinal function through the autonomic nervous system, gastrointestinal hormones, and the immune system

Well recognized, but poorly understood, is the modification of several different aspects of GI function by the brain. In other words, neural control of the GI tract is a function not only of intrinsic nerves (i.e., the ENS), but also of nerves that are extrinsic to the GI tract. These extrinsic pathways are composed of both the parasympathetic—and, to a lesser extent, the sympathetic—nervous system and are under the control of autonomic centers in the brainstem (see Chapter 14).

Parasympathetic innervation of the GI tract from the pharynx to the distal colon is through the vagus nerve; the distal third of the colon receives its parasympathetic innervation from the pelvic nerves (see Fig. 14-4). The preganglionic fibers of the parasympathetic nerves use ACh as their neurotransmitter and synapse on some neurons of the ENS (Fig. 41-3B). These ENS neurons are thus postganglionic parasympathetic fibers, and their cell bodies are, in a sense, the parasympathetic ganglion. These postganglionic parasympathetic fibers use mainly ACh as their neurotransmitter; however, as noted in the previous section, many other neurotransmitters are also present. The results of parasympathetic stimulation are—after one or more synapses in a very complex ENS network—increased secretion and motility. The parasympathetic nerves also contain afferent fibers (see Chapter 14) that carry information to autonomic centers in the medulla from chemoreceptors, osmoreceptors, and mechanical receptors in the mucosa. The loop that is initiated by these afferents, integrated by central autonomic centers, and completed by the aforementioned parasympathetic efferents is known as a **vagovagal reflex**.

The preganglionic **sympathetic** fibers to the GI tract synapse on postganglionic neurons in the prevertebral ganglia (see Fig. 14-4); the neurotransmitter at this synapse is ACh (see Chapter 14). The postganglionic sympathetic fibers either synapse in the ENS or directly innervate effector cells (Fig. 41-3B).

In addition to the control that is entirely within the ENS, as well as control by autonomic centers in the medulla, the GI tract is also under the control of higher CNS centers. Examples of cerebral function that affects GI behavior include the flight-or-fight response, which reduces blood flow to the GI tract, and the sight and smell of food, which increase gastric acid secretion.

Communication between the GI tract and the higher CNS centers is bidirectional. For example, cholecystokinin from the GI tract mediates, in part, the development of food satiety in the brain. In addition, gastrin-releasing peptide, a neurotransmitter made in ENS cells (see Chapter 42), inhibits gastric acid secretion when it is experimentally injected into the ventricles of the brain. Table 41-1 summarizes peptide hormones made by the GI tract, as well as their major actions.

In addition to the "hard-wired" communications involved in sensory input and motor output, communication through the gut-brain axis also requires significant participation of the **immune system**. Neuroimmune regulation of both epithelial and motor function in the small and large intestine primarily involves **mast cells** in the lamina propria of the intestine. Because the mast cells are sensitive to neurotransmitters, they can process information from the brain to the ENS and can also respond to signals from interneurons of the ENS. In addition, mast cells monitor sensory input from the intestinal lumen by participating in the immune response to foreign antigens. In turn, chemical mediators released by mast cells (e.g., histamine) directly affect both intestinal smooth muscle cells and epithelial cells. Our understanding of how the immune system modulates the neural control of GI function is rapidly evolving.

In conclusion, three parallel components of the gut-brain axis—the ENS, GI hormones, and the immune system—control GI function, an arrangement that provides substantial redundancy. Such redundancy permits refinement of the regulation of digestive processes and provides backup or "fail-safe" mechanisms that ensure the integrity of GI function, especially at times of impaired function (i.e., during disease).

GASTROINTESTINAL MOTILITY

Tonic and rhythmic contractions of smooth muscle are responsible for churning, peristalsis, and reservoir action

The motor activity of the GI tract performs three primary functions. First, it produces segmental contractions that are associated with nonpropulsive movement of the luminal contents. The result is the increased mixing (or **churning**) that enhances the digestion and absorption of dietary nutrients. Second, GI motor activity produces **propulsion**, which is a progressive wave of relaxation, followed by contraction. Peristaltic contractions cause propulsion, or the propagated movement of food and its digestive products in a caudal direction. The result is elimination of nondigested, nonabsorbed material. We discuss churning and propulsion later in this chapter. Third, motor activity allows some hollow organs—particularly the stomach and large intestine—**to act**

Table 41-1   Gastrointestinal Peptide Hormones

Hormone	Source	Target	Action
Cholecystokinin	I cells in duodenum and jejunum and neurons in ileum and colon	Pancreas	↑ Enzyme secretion
		Gallbladder	↑ Contraction
Gastric inhibitory peptide	K cells in duodenum and jejunum	Pancreas	Exocrine: ↓ fluid absorption Endocrine: ↑ insulin release
Gastrin	G cells, antrum of stomach	Parietal cells in body of stomach	↑ H^+ secretion
Gastrin-releasing peptide	Vagal nerve endings	G cells in antrum of stomach	↑ Gastrin release
Guanylin	Ileum and colon	Small and large intestine	↑ Fluid absorption
Motilin	Endocrine cells in upper GI tract	Esophageal sphincter Stomach Duodenum	↑ Smooth muscle contraction
Neurotensin	Endocrine cells, widespread in GI tract	Intestinal smooth muscle	Vasoactive stimulation of histamine release
Peptide YY	Endocrine cells in ileum and colon	Stomach	↓ Vagally mediated acid secretion
		Pancreas	↓ Enzyme and fluid secretion
Secretin	S cells in small intestine	Pancreas	↑ HCO_3^- and fluid secretion by pancreatic ducts
		Stomach	↓ Gastric acid secretion
Somatostatin	D cells of stomach and duodenum, δ cells of pancreatic islets	Stomach	↓ Gastrin release
		Intestine	↑ Fluid absorption/ ↓ secretion ↑ Smooth muscle contraction
		Pancreas	↓ Endocrine/exocrine secretions
		Liver	↓ Bile flow
Substance P	Enteric neurons	Enteric neurons	Neurotransmitter
VIP	ENS neurons	Small intestine	↓ Smooth muscle relaxation ↑ Secretion by small intestine
		Pancreas	↑ Secretion by pancreas

as reservoirs for holding the luminal content. This reservoir function is made possible by **sphincters** that separate the organs of the GI tract. All these functions are primarily accomplished by the coordinated activity of **smooth muscle** (see Chapter 9).

The electrical and mechanical properties of intestinal smooth muscle needed for these functions include both tonic (i.e., sustained) contractions and rhythmic contractions (i.e., alternating contraction and relaxation) of individual muscle cells. The intrinsic rhythmic contractility is a function of the membrane voltage (V_m) of the smooth muscle cell. V_m can either oscillate in a subthreshold range at a low frequency (several per minute), referred to as **slow-wave activity**, or reach a threshold for initiating a true **action potential** (see Fig. 9-15). The integrated effect of the slow waves and action potentials determines the smooth muscle activity of the GI tract. Slow-wave activity apparently occurs as voltage-gated Ca^{2+} channels depolarize

the cell and increase $[Ca^{2+}]_i$, followed by the opening of Ca^{2+}-activated K^+ channels, which repolarize the cell (see Chapter 9).

These activities are regulated, in large part, by both neural and hormonal stimuli. Modulation of intestinal smooth muscle contraction is largely a function of $[Ca^{2+}]_i$ (see Chapter 9). Several agonists regulate $[Ca^{2+}]_i$ by one of the following two mechanisms: (1) activation of G protein–linked receptors, resulting in the formation of inositol 1,4,5-triphosphate (IP_3) and the release of Ca^{2+} from intracellular stores; or (2) opening and closing of plasma membrane Ca^{2+} channels. Both excitatory and inhibitory neurotransmitters can modulate smooth muscle $[Ca^{2+}]_i$ and thus contractility. In general, ACh is the predominant neurotransmitter of *excitatory* motor neurons, whereas VIP and NO are the neurotransmitters of *inhibitory* motor neurons. Different neural or hormonal inputs probably increase (or decrease) the frequency with which V_m exceeds threshold and produces an action potential and thus increases (or decreases) muscle contractility.

An additional, unique factor in the aforementioned regulatory control is that luminal food and digestive products activate mucosal chemical and mechanical receptors, as discussed earlier, thus inducing hormone release or stimulating the ENS and controlling smooth muscle function. For example, gastric contents with elevated osmolality or a high lipid content entering the duodenum activate mucosal osmoreceptors and chemoreceptors that increase the release of cholecystokinin and thus delay gastric emptying (see Chapter 42).

Segments of the gastrointestinal tract have both longitudinal and circular arrays of muscles and are separated by sphincters that consist of specialized circular muscles

The muscle layers of the GI tract consist almost entirely of smooth muscle. Exceptions are the striated muscle of the upper esophageal sphincter ([UES] which separates the hypopharynx from the esophagus), the upper third of the esophagus, and the external anal sphincter. As shown earlier in Figure 41-2, the two smooth muscle layers are arranged as an inner circular layer and an outer longitudinal layer. The myenteric ganglia of the ENS are located between the two muscle layers.

The segments of the GI tract through which food products pass are hollow, low-pressure organs that are separated by specialized circular muscles or **sphincters**. These sphincters function as barriers to flow by maintaining a positive **resting pressure** that serves to separate the two adjacent organs, in which lower pressures prevail. Sphincters thus regulate both antegrade (forward) and retrograde (reverse) movement. For example, the resting pressure of the pyloric sphincter controls, in part, the emptying of gastric contents into the duodenum. Conversely, the resting pressure of the lower esophageal sphincter (LES) serves to prevent gastric contents from refluxing back into the esophagus and causing gastroesophageal reflux disease (GERD). As a general rule, stimuli proximal to a sphincter cause sphincteric relaxation, whereas stimuli distal to a sphincter induce sphincteric contraction. Changes in sphincter pressure are coordinated with the smooth muscle contractions in the organs on either side. This coordination depends on both the intrinsic properties of sphincteric smooth muscle and neurohumoral stimuli.

Sphincters effectively serve as one-way valves. Thus, the act of deglutition (or swallowing) induces relaxation of the UES, whereas the LES remains contracted. Only when the UES returns to its initial pressure does the LES begin to relax, ~3 seconds after the start of deglutition. Disturbances in sphincter activity are often associated with alterations in one or more of these regulatory processes.

Location of a sphincter determines its function

Six sphincters are present in the GI tract (Fig. 41-1), each with different resting pressures and different responses to various stimuli. An additional sphincter, the sphincter of Oddi, regulates movement of the contents of the common bile duct into the duodenum.

Achalasia

Achalasia is a relatively uncommon condition associated with difficulty swallowing (dysphagia) and a dilated esophagus proximal to a narrowed, tapered area at the gastroesophageal junction. The term *achalasia* is derived from Greek words meaning "absence of relaxation." The distal narrowed area of the esophagus suggests the presence of a stricture. However, it is easy to introduce an esophagoscope into the stomach through the narrowed area. Subsequent studies of esophageal motility in which investigators measured intraesophageal pressure demonstrated the presence of two defects in patients with achalasia: (1) failure of the LES to relax and (2) impaired peristalsis in the distal two thirds of the body of the esophagus (i.e., the portion that consists of smooth muscle). Peristalsis is intact in the proximal third of the esophagus, which consists of striated muscle. In essence, the smooth muscle portions of the esophagus behave as a denervated structure. The fundamental defect in achalasia is unknown but is probably related to selective loss of inhibitory neurons that regulate the LES, the neurotransmitters of which are VIP and NO. Treatment is either physical distention (or stretching) of the LES with a pneumatic bag dilator or surgical cutting of the LES (i.e., an esophageal myotomy or Heller procedure).

Upper Esophageal Sphincter Separating the pharynx and the upper part of the esophagus is the UES, which consists of striated muscle and has the highest resting pressure of all the GI sphincters. Control of the swallowing mechanism, including the oropharynx and the UES, is largely under the control of the **swallowing center** in the medulla through cranial nerves V (trigeminal), IX (glossopharyngeal), X (vagus), and XII (hypoglossal). Respiration and deglutition are closely integrated (see Chapter 32). The UES is closed during inspiration, thereby diverting atmospheric air to the glottis and away from the esophagus. During swallowing, the situation reverses, with closure of the glottis and inhibition of respiration, but with relaxation of the UES (Fig. 41-4). These changes permit the entry of food contents into the esophagus and not into the airways of the respiratory tract.

Lower Esophageal Sphincter The esophagus is separated from the stomach by the LES, which is composed of specialized smooth muscle that is both anatomically and pharmacologically distinct from adjacent smooth muscle in the distal end of the esophagus and proximal portion of the stomach. The primary functions of the LES are (1) to permit coordinated movement of ingested food into the stomach from the esophagus after swallowing or deglutition and (2) to prevent reflux of gastric contents into the esophagus. Either deglutition or distention of the esophagus results in a reduction in LES pressure (Fig. 41-4) to that of intragastric pressure, thereby permitting entry of food into the stomach. Relaxation of the LES occurs after the UES has already returned to its resting pressure. The LES maintains a resting tone that is the result of both intrinsic myogenic properties of the sphincteric muscle and cholinergic regulation. Relaxation of the LES is mediated both by the vagus nerve and by

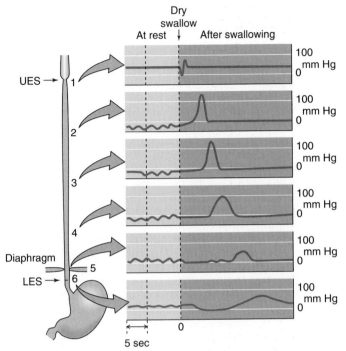

Figure 41-4 Esophageal pressures during swallowing. The swallowing center in the medulla that initiates deglutition includes the nucleus ambiguus (cranial nerves [CN] IX and X), the dorsal motor nucleus of the vagus (CN X), and others. Shown are recordings of intraluminal pressures at different sites along the esophagus, from the UES (*record 1*) to the LES (*record 6*). The *left side* of the graph shows the pressures at rest. As shown on the *right side*, after a dry swallow, the pressure wave of primary peristalsis moves sequentially down the esophagus. (*Data from Conklin JL, Christensen J: In Johnson LR [ed]: Physiology of the Gastrointestinal Tract, 3rd ed, pp 903-928. New York: Lippincott-Raven, 1994.*)

esophagus also produces such a local distention, without a swallow, and elicits the same response: peristaltic contractions that clear the esophagus of refluxed gastric material. Peristalsis that is initiated by swallowing is called **primary peristalsis**, whereas that elicited by distention of the esophagus is referred to as **secondary peristalsis**. Esophageal contractions after a swallow are regulated by the medullary swallowing center, intramural esophageal plexuses, the vagus nerve, and intrinsic myogenic processes.

Pyloric Sphincter The pylorus is the sphincter that separates the stomach from the duodenum. The pressure of the pyloric sphincter regulates, in part, gastric emptying and prevents duodenal-gastric reflux. However, although a specific pyloric sphincter is present, it is quite short and is a relatively poor barrier (i.e., it can resist only a small pressure gradient). The stomach, duodenum, biliary tract, and pancreas—which are closely related embryologically—function as a unit. Indeed, coordinated contraction and relaxation of the antrum, pylorus, and duodenum (which is sometimes referred to as the *antroduodenal cluster unit*) are probably more important than simply the pressure produced by the pyloric smooth muscle per se. Regulation of gastric emptying is discussed further in Chapter 42.

Ileocecal Sphincter The valve-like structure that separates the ileum and cecum is called the **ileocecal sphincter**. Similar to other GI sphincters, the ileocecal sphincter maintains a positive resting pressure and is under the control of the vagus nerve, sympathetic nerves, and the ENS. Distention of the ileum results in relaxation of the sphincter, whereas distention of the proximal (ascending) colon causes contraction of the ileocecal sphincter. As a consequence, ileal flow into the colon is regulated by luminal contents and pressure, both proximal and distal to the ileocecal sphincter.

Internal and External Anal Sphincters The "anal sphincter" actually consists of both an internal and an external sphincter. The **internal sphincter** has both circular and longitudinal smooth muscle and is under involuntary control. The **external sphincter**, which encircles the rectum, contains only striated muscle but is controlled by both voluntary and involuntary mechanisms. The high resting pressure of the overall anal sphincter predominantly reflects the resting tone of the *internal* anal sphincter. Distention of the rectum (Fig. 41-5A), either by colonic contents (i.e., stool) or experimentally by balloon inflation, initiates the **rectosphincteric reflex** by relaxing the internal sphincter (Fig. 41-5B). If defecation is not desired, continence is maintained by an involuntary reflex—orchestrated by the sacral spinal cord—that contracts the external anal sphincter (Fig. 41-5C). If defecation is desired, a series of both voluntary and involuntary events occur that include relaxation of the external anal sphincter, contraction of abdominal wall muscles, and relaxation of pelvic wall muscles. Flexure of the hips and descent of the pelvic floor then facilitate defecation by minimizing the angle between the rectum and anus. In contrast, if a delay in defecation is needed or desired, voluntary contraction of the external anal sphincter is usually sufficient to override the series of reflexes initiated by rectal distention.

intrinsic properties of the smooth muscle, including important inhibitory effects by VIP and by NO.

Abnormalities of both resting LES pressure and its relaxation in response to deglutition are often associated with significant symptoms. Thus, a reduced resting LES pressure often results in gastroesophageal reflux, which may cause esophagitis (i.e., inflammation of the esophageal mucosa). A defect in LES relaxation is a major component of a condition called **achalasia** (see the box titled Achalasia), which often results in dilatation of the esophagus (megaesophagus) and is associated with difficulty in swallowing (dysphagia).

Swallowing and the function of the UES and the LES are closely integrated into the function of the esophagus. Under normal circumstances, esophageal muscle contractions are almost exclusively peristaltic and are initiated by swallowing. Deglutition initiates relaxation of the UES and propagated contractions, first of the UES and then of the muscles along the esophagus (Fig. 41-4). In the meantime, the LES has already relaxed. The result of the advancing peristaltic wave is the caudad propulsion of a bolus toward the stomach.

Distention of the esophagus (in the absence of swallowing) also initiates propulsive esophageal contractions that are distal to the site of distention, as well as relaxation of the LES. Reflux of gastric contents into the lower part of the

A RECTUM

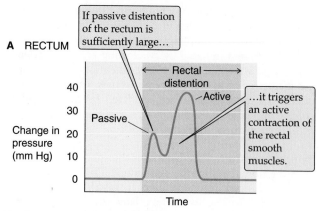

If passive distention of the rectum is sufficiently large…

…it triggers an active contraction of the rectal smooth muscles.

B INTERNAL ANAL SPHINCTER

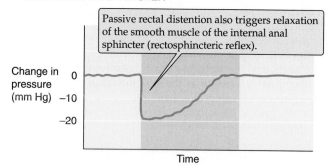

Passive rectal distention also triggers relaxation of the smooth muscle of the internal anal sphincter (rectosphincteric reflex).

C EXTERNAL ANAL SPHINCTER

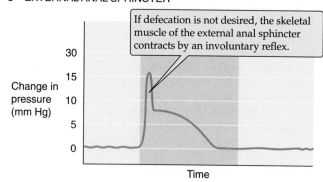

If defecation is not desired, the skeletal muscle of the external anal sphincter contracts by an involuntary reflex.

Figure 41-5 **A** to **C,** Pressure changes initiated by rectal distention. (*Data from Schuster MM: Johns Hopkins Med J 1965; 116:70-88.*)

Motility of the small intestine achieves both churning and propulsive movement, and its temporal pattern differs in the fed and fasted states

Digestion and absorption of dietary nutrients are the primary functions of the small intestine, and the motor activity of the small intestine is closely integrated with its digestive and absorptive roles. The two classes of small intestine motor activity are churning (or mixing) and propulsion of the bolus of luminal contents. **Churning**—which is accomplished by segmental, nonpropulsive contractions—mixes the luminal contents with pancreatic, biliary, and small intestinal secretions, thus enhancing the digestion of dietary nutrients in the lumen. These segmental contractions also decrease the unstirred water layer that is adjacent to the

Hirschsprung Disease

The anal sphincter controls defecation and consists of a smooth muscle internal sphincter and a striated muscle external sphincter. Distention of the rectum by inflation of a balloon—which simulates the effect of the presence of solid feces in the rectum—results in relaxation of the internal sphincter and contraction of the external sphincter (Fig. 41-5). Voluntary control of the external sphincter regulates the timing of defecation.

Hirschsprung disease is a congenital polygenic disorder. At least eight genes have been associated with Hirschsprung disease, including mutations in the endothelin-B receptor. Variable penetrance leads to variable manifestations of the disease. At the cellular level, the fundamental defect is arrest of the caudad migration of neural crest cells, which are the precursors of ganglion cells. Symptoms include constipation, megacolon, and a narrowed segment of colon in the rectum. Histologic examination of this narrowed segment reveals an absence of ganglion cells from both the submucosal (or Meissner's) and myenteric (or Auerbach's) plexuses (Fig. 41-3A). The patient's constipation and resulting megacolon are secondary to failure of this "aganglionic" segment to relax in response to proximal distention. Manometric assessment of the internal and external anal sphincters reveals that the smooth muscle internal sphincter does not relax after rectal distention (Fig. 41-5), but the external anal sphincter functions normally. Treatment of this condition is usually surgical, with removal of the narrowed segment that is missing the ganglia that normally regulate relaxation of the smooth muscle of the internal anal sphincter.

apical membranes of the small intestine cells, thus promoting absorption. Churning or mixing movements occur following eating and are the result of contractions of *circular* muscle in segments flanked at either end by receiving segments that relax. Churning, however, does not advance the luminal contents along the small intestine. In contrast, **propulsion**—which is accomplished by propagated, peristaltic contractions—results in caudad movement of the intestinal luminal contents, either for absorption at more distal sites of the small or large intestine or for elimination in stool. Peristaltic propulsion occurs as a result of contraction of the *circular* muscle and relaxation of the *longitudinal* muscle in the propulsive or upstream segment, together with relaxation of the *circular* muscle and contraction of the *longitudinal* muscle in the downstream receiving segment. Thus, circular smooth muscle in the small intestine participates in both churning and propulsion.

As noted earlier and in Chapter 9, the V_m changes of intestinal smooth muscle cells consist of both slow-wave activity and action potentials. The patterns of electrical and mechanical activity differ in the fasting and fed states. In the **fasting state**, the small intestine is relatively quiescent but exhibits synchronized, rhythmic changes in both electrical and motor activity (Fig. 41-6). The interdigestive myoelectric or **migrating motor complex (MMC)** is the term used to describe these rhythmic contractions of the small intestine that are observed in the fasting state. MMCs in humans

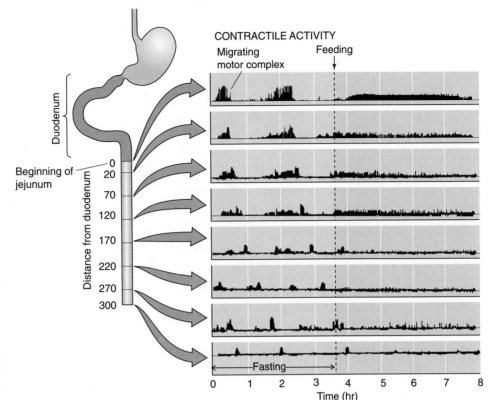

Figure 41-6 Mechanical activity in the fasting and fed states. Shown are records of intraluminal pressure along the small intestine of a conscious dog. Before feeding (*left side*), the pattern is one of MMCs. Feeding triggers a switch to a different pattern, characterized by both segmental contractions that churn the contents and peristaltic contractions that propel the contents along the small intestine. *(Data from Itoh Z, Sekiguchi T: Scand J Gastroenteral Suppl 1983; 82:121-134.)*

occur at intervals of 90 to 120 minutes and consist of four distinct phases: (1) a prolonged quiescent period, (2) a period of increasing action potential frequency and contractility, (3) a period of peak electrical and mechanical activity that lasts a few minutes, and (4) a period of declining activity that merges into the next quiescent period. During the interdigestive period, particles greater than 2 mm in diameter can pass from the stomach into the duodenum, thus permitting emptying of ingested material from the stomach (e.g., bones, coins) that could not be reduced in size to less than 2 mm. The slow propulsive contractions that characterize phases 2 to 4 of the MMCs clear the small intestine of its residual content, including undigested food, bacteria, desquamated cells, and intestinal and pancreatic biliary secretions. MMCs usually originate in the stomach and often travel to the distal end of the ileum, but ~25% are initiated in the duodenum and proximal part of the jejunum.

Feeding terminates MMCs and initiates the appearance of the fed motor pattern (Fig. 41-6). The latter is less well characterized than MMCs but, as noted earlier, consists of both segmental contractions (churning), which enhance digestion and absorption, and peristaltic contractions (propulsion).

Determination of the primary factors that regulate both MMCs and transition to the fed pattern has been hampered by both species differences and complex interactions among the multiple probable mediators. Nonetheless, clear evidence has been presented for a role of the ENS, one or more humoral factors, and extrinsic innervation. A major determinant of the MMC pattern is the hormone **motilin**, a 22–

amino acid peptide that is synthesized in the duodenal mucosa and is released just before the initiation of phase 3 of the MMC cycle. Motilin does not appear to have a role in the motor pattern that is observed in the fed state. Factors important in induction of the fed pattern include the vagus nerve (because sham feeding also both terminates MMCs and initiates a fed pattern) and the caloric content, as well as the type of food (e.g., fat more than protein) in the meal.

Motility of the large intestine achieves both propulsive movement and a reservoir function

The human large intestine has four primary functions. First, the colon absorbs large quantities of fluid and electrolytes and converts the liquid content of ileocecal material to solid or semisolid stool. Second, the colon avidly absorbs the short-chain fatty acids formed by the catabolism (or fermentation) of dietary carbohydrates that are not absorbed in the small intestine. The abundant colonic microflora accomplish this fermentation. Third, the storage of colonic content represents a reservoir function of the large intestine. Fourth, the colon eliminates its contents in a regulated and controlled fashion, largely under voluntary control. To accomplish these important activities, the large intestine functionally acts as two distinct organs. The proximal (or ascending and transverse) part of the colon is the site where most of the fluid and electrolyte absorption occurs and where bacterial fermentation takes place. The distal (or descending and rectosigmoid) portion of the colon provides final desiccation, as well as reservoir function, and serves as a storage organ for colonic material before defecation.

In contrast to the motor pattern in the small intestine, no distinct fasting and fed patterns of contractions are seen in the colon. Similar to small intestinal motor activity, colonic contractions are regulated by myogenic, neurogenic, and hormonal factors. Parasympathetic control of the proximal two thirds of the colon is mediated by the vagus nerve, whereas parasympathetic control of the descending and rectosigmoid colon is mediated by pelvic nerves originating from the sacral spinal cord.

The **proximal colon** has two types of motor activity: nonpropulsive segmentation and mass peristalsis. **Nonpropulsive segmentation** is generated by slow-wave activity that produces circular muscle contractions that churn the colonic contents and move them in an orad direction (i.e., toward the cecum). The segmental contractions that produce the churning give the colon its typical appearance of segments or haustra (Fig. 41-1). During this mixing phase, material is retained in the proximal portion of the large intestine for relatively long periods, and fluid and electrolyte absorption continues. One to three times a day, a so-called **mass peristalsis** occurs in which a portion of the colonic contents is propelled distally 20 cm or more. Such mass peristaltic contractions are the primary form of propulsive motility in the colon and may be initiated by eating. During mass peristalsis, the haustra disappear; they reappear after the completion of mass peristalsis.

In the **distal colon**, the primary motor activity is nonpropulsive segmentation that is produced by annular or segmental contractions. It is in the distal part of the colon that the final desiccation of colonic contents occurs. It is also here that these contents are stored before an occasional mass peristalsis that propels them into the rectum. The **rectum** itself is kept nearly empty by nonpropulsive segmentation until it is filled by mass peristalsis of the distal end of the colon. As described in Figure 41-5, filling of the rectum triggers a series of reflexes in the internal and external anal sphincters that lead to defecation.

REFERENCES

Books and Reviews

Andrews JM, Dent J: Small intestinal motor physiology. In Feldman J, Friedman LS, Sleisenger MH (eds): Gastrointestinal and Liver Disease, vol 2, 7th ed, pp 1665-1678. Philadelphia: WB Saunders, 2002.

Biancani P, Hartnett KM, Behar J: Esophageal motor function. In Yamada T (ed): Textbook of Gastroenterology, vol 1, 4th ed, pp 166-194. Philadelphia: Lippincott Williams & Wilkins, 2003.

Conklin JL, Christensen J: Motor functions of the pharynx and esophagus. In Johnson LR (ed): Physiology of the Gastrointestinal Tract, 3rd ed, pp 903-928. New York: Lippincott-Raven, 1994.

Cook IJ, Brookes SJ: Motility of the large intestine. In Feldman J, Friedman LS, Sleisenger MH (eds): Gastrointestinal and Liver Disease, vol 2, 7th ed, pp 1679-1691. Philadelphia: WB Saunders, 2002.

Maklouf GM: Smooth muscle of the gut. In Yamada T (ed): Textbook of Gastroenterology, vol 1, 4th ed, pp 92-116. Philadelphia: Lippincott Williams & Wilkins, 2003.

Rehfeld JF: The new biology of gastrointestinal hormones. Physiol Rev 1998; 78:1087-1108.

Surprenant A: Control of the gastrointestinal tract by enteric neurons. Annu Rev Physiol 1994; 56:117-140.

Wood JD: Enteric neuroimmunophysiology and pathophysiology. Gastroenterology 2004; 127:635-657.

Wood JD: The first Nobel prize for integrated systems physiology: Ivan Petrovich Pavlov, 1904. Physiology 2004; 19:326-330.

Journal Articles

Itoh Z, Sekiguchi T: Interdigestive motor activity in health and disease. Scand J Gastroenterol Suppl 1983; 82:121-134.

Schuster MM: Simultaneous manometric recording of internal and external anal sphincteric reflexes. Johns Hopkins Med J 1965; 116:70-88.

CHAPTER 42

GASTRIC FUNCTION

Henry J. Binder

The stomach plays several important roles in human nutrition and has secretory, motor, and humoral functions. These activities are not separate and distinct, but rather represent integrated functions that are required to initiate the normal digestive process.

The stomach has several specific **secretory** products. In addition to the stomach's best-known product—acid, these products include pepsinogen, mucus, bicarbonate, intrinsic factor, and water. These substances continue the food digestion that was initiated by mastication and the action of salivary enzymes in the mouth. In addition, they help protect the stomach from injury. The stomach also has several important **motor** functions that regulate the intake of food, its mixing with gastric secretions and reduction in particle size, and the exit of partially digested material into the duodenum. Moreover, the stomach produces two important **humoral agents**—gastrin and somatostatin—that have both endocrine and paracrine actions. These peptides are primarily important in the regulation of gastric secretion.

Although these functions are important in the maintenance of good health, the stomach is nevertheless not required for survival. Individuals who have had their entire stomach removed (i.e., total gastrectomy) for non-neoplastic reasons can maintain adequate nutrition and achieve excellent longevity.

FUNCTIONAL ANATOMY OF THE STOMACH

The mucosa is composed of surface epithelial cells and glands

The basic structure of the stomach wall is similar to that of other regions of the gastrointestinal (GI) tract (see Fig. 41-2); therefore, the wall of the stomach consists of both mucosal and muscle layers. The stomach can be divided, based on its gross anatomy, into three major **segments** (Fig. 42-1): (1) a specialized portion of the stomach called the **cardia** is located just distal to the gastroesophageal junction and is devoid of the acid-secreting parietal cells; (2) the body or **corpus** is the largest portion of the stomach; its most

proximal region is called the **fundus**; and (3) the distal portion of the stomach is called the **antrum**. The surface area of the gastric mucosa is substantially increased by the presence of **gastric glands**, which consist of a pit, a neck, and a base. These glands contain several cell types, including mucous, parietal, chief, and endocrine cells; endocrine cells also present in both corpus and antrum. The surface epithelial cells, which have their own distinct structure and function, secrete HCO_3^- and mucus.

Marked cellular heterogeneity exists not only *within* segments (e.g., glands versus surface epithelial cells) but also *between* segments of the stomach. For instance, as discussed later, the structure and function of the mucosal epithelial cells in the antrum and body are quite distinct. Similarly, although the smooth muscle in the proximal and distal portions of the stomach appear structurally similar, their functions and pharmacological properties differ substantially.

With increasing rates of secretion of gastric juice, the H^+ concentration rises, and the Na^+ concentration falls

The glands of the stomach typically secrete ~2 L/day of a fluid that is approximately isotonic with blood plasma. As a consequence of the heterogeneity of gastric mucosal function, early investigators recognized that gastric secretion consists of two distinct components: parietal cell and non-parietal cell secretion. According to this hypothesis, gastric secretion consists of (1) an Na^+-rich basal secretion that originates from nonparietal cells and (2) a stimulated component that represents a pure parietal cell secretion that is rich in H^+. This model helps to explain the inverse relationship between the luminal concentrations of H^+ and Na^+ as a function of the rate of gastric secretion (Fig. 42-2). Thus, at high rates of gastric secretion—for example, when gastrin or histamine stimulates parietal cells—intraluminal $[H^+]$ is high, whereas intraluminal $[Na^+]$ is relatively low. At low rates of secretion or in clinical situations in which maximal acid secretion is reduced (e.g., pernicious anemia; see Chapter 44 for the box on that topic), intraluminal $[H^+]$ is low but intraluminal $[Na^+]$ is high.

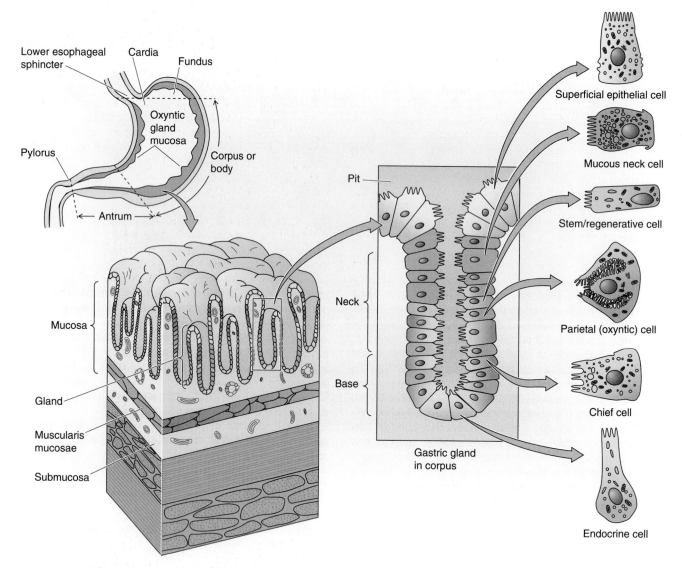

Figure 42-1 Anatomy of the stomach. Shown are the macroscopic divisions of the stomach, as well as two progressively magnified views of a section through the wall of the body of the stomach.

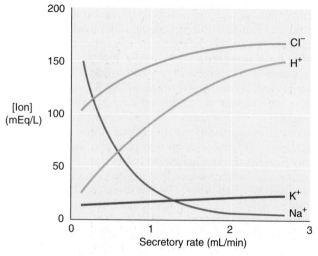

Figure 42-2 The effect of the gastric secretion rate on the composition of the gastric juice.

The proximal portion of the stomach secretes acid, pepsinogens, intrinsic factor, bicarbonate, and mucus, whereas the distal part releases gastrin and somatostatin

Corpus The primary secretory products of the proximal part of the stomach—acid (protons), pepsinogens, and intrinsic factor—are made by distinct cells from glands in the corpus of the stomach. The two primary cell types in the gastric glands of the body of the stomach are parietal cells and chief cells.

Parietal cells (or oxyntic cells) secrete both acid and intrinsic factor, a glycoprotein that is required for cobalamin (vitamin B_{12}) absorption in the ileum (see Chapter 45). The parietal cell has a very distinctive morphology (Fig. 42-1). It is a large, triangular cell with a centrally located nucleus, an abundance of mitochondria, intracellular tubulovesicular membranes, and canalicular structures. We discuss H^+ secretion in the next major section and intrinsic factor in Chapter 45.

Chief cells (or peptic cells) secrete pepsinogens, but not acid. These epithelial cells are substantially smaller than parietal cells. A close relationship exists among pH, pepsin secretion, and function. Pepsins are endopeptidases (i.e., they hydrolyze "interior" peptide bonds) and initiate protein digestion by hydrolyzing specific peptide linkages. The basal luminal pH of the stomach is 4 to 6; with stimulation, the pH of gastric secretions is usually reduced to less than 2. At pH values that are less than 3, pepsinogens are rapidly activated to pepsins. A low gastric pH also helps to prevent bacterial colonization of the small intestine.

In addition to parietal and chief cells, glands from the corpus of the stomach also contain **mucus-secreting cells**, which are confined to the neck of the gland (Fig. 42-1), and five or six **endocrine cells**. Among these endocrine cells are enterochromaffin-like (ECL) cells, which release histamine.

Antrum   The glands in the antrum of the stomach do not contain parietal cells. Therefore, the antrum does not secrete either acid or intrinsic factor. Glands in the antral mucosa contain **chief cells** and **endocrine cells**; the endocrine cells include the so-called G cells and D cells, which secrete gastrin and somatostatin, respectively (see Table 41-1). These two peptide hormones function as both endocrine and paracrine regulators of acid secretion. As discussed in more detail later, **gastrin** stimulates gastric acid secretion by two mechanisms and is also a major trophic or growth factor for GI epithelial cell proliferation. As discussed more fully later, **somatostatin** also has several important regulatory functions, but its primary role in gastric physiology is to inhibit both gastrin release and parietal cell acid secretion.

In addition to the cells of the gastric glands, the stomach also contains superficial epithelial cells that cover the gastric pits, as well as the surface in between the pits. These cells secrete HCO_3^-.

Gastric pH and Pneumonia

Many patients hospitalized in the intensive care unit (ICU) receive prophylactic antiulcer treatments (e.g., proton pump inhibitors, such as omeprazole) that either neutralize existing acid or block its secretion and thereby raise gastric pH. Patients in the ICU who are mechanically ventilated or who have coagulopathies are highly susceptible to hemorrhage from gastric stress ulcers, a complication that can contribute significantly to overall morbidity and mortality. These different antiulcer regimens do effectively lessen the risk of developing stress ulcers. However, by raising gastric pH, these agents also lower the barrier to gram-negative bacterial colonization of the stomach. Esophageal reflux and subsequent aspiration of these organisms are common in these very sick patients, many of whom are already immunocompromised or even mechanically compromised by the presence of a ventilator tube. If these bacteria are aspirated into the airway, pneumonia can result. The higher the gastric pH, the greater is the risk of pneumonia.

The stomach accommodates food, mixes it with gastric secretions, grinds it, and empties the chyme into the duodenum

In addition to its secretory properties, the stomach also has multiple motor functions. These functions are the result of gastric smooth muscle activity, which is integrated by both neural and hormonal signals. Gastric motor functions include both propulsive and retrograde movement of food and liquid, as well as a nonpropulsive movement that increases intragastric pressure.

Similar to the heterogeneity of gastric epithelial cells, considerable diversity is seen in both the regulation and contractility of gastric smooth muscle. The stomach has at least two distinct areas of motor activity; the proximal and distal portions of the stomach behave as separate, but coordinated, entities. At least four events can be identified in the overall process of gastric filling and emptying: (1) receiving and providing temporary storage of dietary food and liquids; (2) mixing of food and water with gastric secretory products, including pepsin and acid; (3) grinding of food so that particle size is reduced to enhance digestion and to permit passage through the pylorus; and (4) regulating the exit of retained material from the stomach into the duodenum (i.e., gastric emptying of chyme) in response to various stimuli.

The mechanisms by which the stomach receives and empties liquids and solids are significantly different. Emptying of *liquids* is primarily a function of the smooth muscle of the *proximal* part of the stomach, whereas emptying of *solids* is regulated by *antral* smooth muscle.

ACID SECRETION

The parietal cell has a specialized tubulovesicular structure that increases apical membrane area when the cell is stimulated to secrete acid

In the basal state, the rate of acid secretion is low. Tubulovesicular membranes are present in the apical portion of the resting, nonstimulated parietal cell and contain the H-K pump (or H,K-ATPase) that is responsible for acid secretion. On stimulation, cytoskeletal rearrangement causes the tubulovesicular membranes that contain the H-K pump to fuse into the canalicular membrane (Fig. 42-3). The result is a substantial increase (50- to 100-fold) in the surface area of the apical membrane of the parietal cell, as well as the appearance of microvilli. This fusion is accompanied by insertion of the H-K pumps, as well as K^+ and Cl^- channels, into the canalicular membrane. The large number of mitochondria in the parietal cell is consistent with the high rate of glucose oxidation and O_2 consumption that is needed to support acid secretion.

An H-K pump is responsible for gastric acid secretion by parietal cells

The parietal cell H-K pump is a member of the gene family of P-type ATPases (see Chapter 5) that includes the

A RESTING

Tubulovesicles

B ACTIVE

Canaliculus

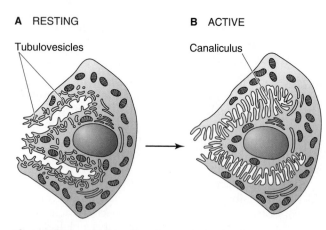

Figure 42-3   Parietal cell: resting and stimulated.

ubiquitous Na-K pump (Na,K-ATPase), which is present at the basolateral membrane of virtually all mammalian epithelial cells and at the plasma membrane of nonpolarized cells. Similar to other members of this ATPase family, the parietal cell H-K pump requires both an α subunit and a β subunit for full activity. The catalytic function of the H-K pump resides in the α subunit; however, the β subunit is required for targeting to the apical membrane. The two subunits form a heterodimer with close interaction at the extracellular domain.

The activity of these P-type ATPases, including the gastric H-K pump, is affected by inhibitors that are clinically important in the control of gastric acid secretion. The two types of gastric H-K pump inhibitors are as follows: (1) substituted benzimidazoles (e.g., omeprazole), which act by binding covalently to cysteines on the extracytoplasmic surface; and (2) substances that act as competitive inhibitors of the K+-binding site (e.g., the experimental drug Schering 28080). **Omeprazole** (see the box titled Gastrinoma or Zollinger-Ellison Syndrome) is a potent inhibitor of parietal cell H-K pump activity and is an extremely effective drug in the control of gastric acid secretion in both physiologically normal subjects and patients with hypersecretory states. In addition, H-K pump inhibitors have been useful in furthering understanding of the function of these pumps. Thus, ouabain, a potent inhibitor of the Na-K pump, does not inhibit the gastric H-K pump, whereas omeprazole does not inhibit the Na-K pump. The *colonic* H-K pump, whose α subunit has an amino acid sequence that is similar but not identical to that of both the Na-K pump and the parietal cell H-K pump, is partially inhibited by ouabain but not by omeprazole.

According to the model presented in Figure 42-4, the key step in gastric acid secretion is extrusion of H+ into the lumen of the gastric gland in exchange for K+. The K+ taken up into the parietal cells is recycled to the lumen through K+ channels. The final component of the process is passive movement of Cl− into the gland lumen. The apical membrane H-K pump energizes the entire process, the net result of which is the active secretion of HCl. Secretion of acid across the apical membrane by the H-K pump results in a rise in parietal cell pH. The adaptive response to this rise in pH includes passive uptake of CO_2 and H_2O, which the

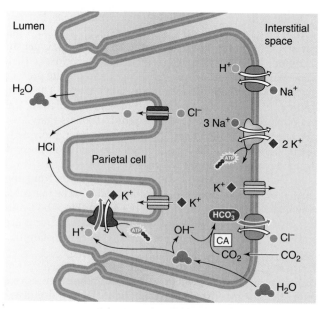

Figure 42-4   Acid secretion by parietal cells. When the parietal cell is stimulated, H-K pumps (fueled by ATP hydrolysis) extrude H+ into the lumen of the gastric gland in exchange for K+. The K+ recycles back into the lumen by K+ channels. Cl− exits through channels in the luminal membrane, thus completing the net process of HCl secretion. The H+ needed by the H-K pump is provided by the entry of CO_2 and H_2O, which are converted to H+ and HCO_3^- by carbonic anhydrase. The HCO_3^- exits across the basolateral membrane through the Cl-HCO3 exchanger.

enzyme **carbonic anhydrase** converts to HCO_3^- and H+. The H+ is the substrate of the H-K pump. The HCO_3^- exits across the basolateral membrane through the Cl-HCO3 exchanger. This process also provides the Cl− required for net HCl movement across the apical/canalicular membrane. The basolateral Na-H exchanger may participate in intracellular pH regulation, especially in the basal state.

Three secretagogues (acetylcholine, gastrin, and histamine) directly and indirectly induce acid secretion by parietal cells

The action of secretagogues on gastric acid secretion occurs through at least two parallel and perhaps redundant mechanisms (Fig. 42-5). In the first, acetylcholine (ACh), gastrin, and histamine bind **directly** to their respective membrane receptors on the parietal cell and synergistically stimulate and potentiate acid secretion. ACh (see Fig. 14-8) is released from endings of the vagus nerve (cranial nerve X), and as we see in the next section, gastrin is released from G cells. Histamine is synthesized from histidine (see Fig. 13-8). The documented presence of ACh, gastrin, and histamine receptors, at least on the canine parietal cell, provides the primary support for this view. In the second mechanism, ACh and gastrin **indirectly** induce acid secretion as a result of their stimulation of histamine release from ECL cells in the lamina propria. The central role of histamine and ECL cells is consistent with the observation that histamine-2 receptor antagonists (i.e., H2 blockers), such as cimetidine and ranitidine,

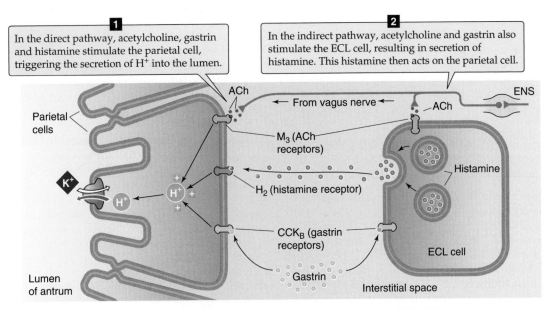

1 In the direct pathway, acetylcholine, gastrin and histamine stimulate the parietal cell, triggering the secretion of H^+ into the lumen.

2 In the indirect pathway, acetylcholine and gastrin also stimulate the ECL cell, resulting in secretion of histamine. This histamine then acts on the parietal cell.

Figure 42-5 The direct and indirect actions of the three acid secretagogues: ACh, gastrin, and histamine.

not only block the direct action of histamine on parietal cells but also substantially inhibit the acid secretion stimulated by ACh and gastrin. The effectiveness of H_2 blockers in controlling acid secretion after stimulation by most agonists is well established in studies of both humans and experimental animals. These drugs, but more importantly the proton pump inhibitors, are prescribed to treat active peptic ulcer disease.

The three acid secretagogues act through either Ca^{2+}/diacylglycerol or cAMP

Stimulation of acid secretion by ACh, gastrin, and histamine, is mediated by a series of intracellular signal transduction processes similar to those responsible for the action of other agonists in other cell systems. All three secretagogues bind to specific G protein–coupled receptors on the parietal cell membrane (Fig. 42-6).

ACh binds to an M_3 muscarinic receptor (see Chapter 14) on the parietal cell basolateral membrane. This ACh receptor couples to a GTP-binding protein (Ga_q) and activates phospholipase C (PLC), which converts phosphatidylinositol 4,5-biphosphate (PIP_2) to inositol 1,4,5-triphosphate (IP_3) and diacylglycerol (DAG; see Chapter 3). IP_3 causes internal stores to release Ca^{2+}, which then probably acts through calmodulin-dependent protein kinase (see Chapter 3). DAG activates protein kinase C (PKC). The M_3 receptor also activates a Ca^{2+} channel.

Gastrin binds to a specific parietal cell receptor that has been identified as the gastrin-cholecystokinin B (CCK_B) receptor. Two related CCK receptors have been identified: CCK_A and CCK_B. Their amino acid sequences are ~50% identical, and both are G protein coupled. The CCK_B receptor has equal affinity for both gastrin and CCK. In contrast, the CCK_A receptor's affinity for CCK is three orders of magnitude higher than its affinity for gastrin. These observations and the availability of receptor antagonists are beginning to

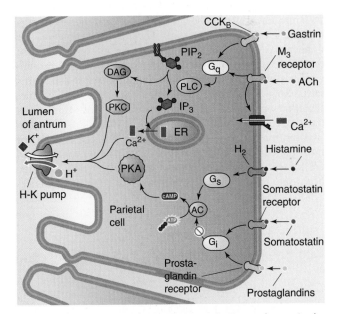

Figure 42-6 Receptors and signal transduction pathways in the parietal cell. The parietal cell has separate receptors for three acid secretagogues. ACh and gastrin each bind to specific receptors (M_3 and CCK_B, respectively) that are coupled to the G protein Ga_q. The result is activation of PLC, which ultimately leads to the activation of PKC and the release of Ca^{2+}. The histamine binds to an H_2 receptor, coupled through Ga_s to adenylyl cyclase (AC). The result is production of cAMP and activation of PKA. Two inhibitors of acid secretion also act directly on the parietal cell. Somatostatin and prostaglandins bind to separate receptors that are linked to Ga_i. These agents thus oppose the actions of histamine. ER, endoplasmic reticulum.

clarify the parallel, but at times opposite, effects of gastrin and CCK on various aspects of GI function. The CCK_B receptor couples to Ga_q and activates the same PLC pathway as does ACh, and this process leads to both an increase in $[Ca^{2+}]_i$ and activation of PKC.

The **histamine** receptor on the parietal cell is an H_2 receptor that is coupled to the Ga_s GTP-binding protein. Histamine activation of the receptor complex stimulates the enzyme adenylyl cyclase, which, in turn, generates cAMP. The resulting activation of protein kinase A leads to the phosphorylation of certain parietal cell–specific proteins, including the H-K pump.

Gastrin is released by both antral and duodenal G cells, and histamine is released by enterochromaffin-like cells in the corpus

The presence of a gastric hormone that stimulates acid secretion was initially proposed in 1905. Direct evidence of such a factor was obtained in 1938, and in 1964 Gregory and Tracey isolated and purified gastrin and determined its amino acid sequence. Gastrin has three major effects on GI cells: (1) stimulation of acid secretion by parietal cells (Fig. 42-5); (2) release of histamine by ECL cells; and (3) regulation of mucosal growth in the corpus of the stomach, as well as in the small and large intestine.

Gastrin exists in several different forms, but the two major forms are G-17, or "little gastrin," a 17–amino acid linear peptide (Fig. 42-7A), and G-34, or "big gastrin," a 34–amino acid peptide (Fig. 42-7B). A single gene encodes a peptide of 101 amino acids. Several cleavage steps and C-terminal amidation (i.e., addition of a $-NH_2$ to the C terminus) occur during gastrin's post-translational modification, a process that occurs in the endoplasmic reticulum, trans-Golgi apparatus, and both immature and mature secretory granules. The final product of this post-translational modification is either G-17 or G-34. The tyrosine residue may be either sulfated (so-called gastrin II) or nonsulfated (gastrin I); the two forms are equally active and are present in equal amounts. Gastrin and **CCK**, a related hormone, have identical C-terminal tetrapeptide sequences (Fig. 42-7C) that possess all the biological activities of both gastrin and CCK. Both G-17 and G-34 are present in blood plasma, and their plasma levels primarily reflect their degradation rates. Thus, although G-17 is more active than G-34, the latter is degraded at a substantially lower rate than G-17. As a consequence, the infusion of equal amounts of G-17 or G-34 produces comparable increases in gastric acid secretion.

Specialized endocrine cells (**G cells**) in both the antrum and duodenum make each of the two gastrins. Antral G cells are the primary source of G-17, whereas duodenal G cells are the primary source of G-34. Antral G cells are unusual in that they respond to both luminal and basolateral stimuli (Fig. 42-8). Antral G cells have microvilli on their apical membrane surface and are referred to as an *open-type* endocrine cell. These G cells release gastrin in response to luminal peptides and amino acids, as well as in response to **gastrin-releasing peptide** (GRP), a 27–amino acid peptide that is released by vagal nerve endings. As discussed later, gastrin release is inhibited by somatostatin, which is released from adjacent D cells.

Somatostatin, released by gastric D cells, is the central mechanism of inhibition of acid secretion

Gastric acid secretion is under close control of not only the stimulatory pathways discussed earlier but also the inhibitory pathways. The major inhibitory pathway involves the release of **somatostatin**, a polypeptide hormone made by D cells in the antrum and corpus of the stomach. Somatostatin is also made by the δ cells of the pancreatic islets (see Chapter 51) and by neurons in the hypothalamus (see Chapter 48). Somatostatin exists in two forms, SS-28 and SS-14, which have identical C termini. SS-28 is the predominant form in the GI tract.

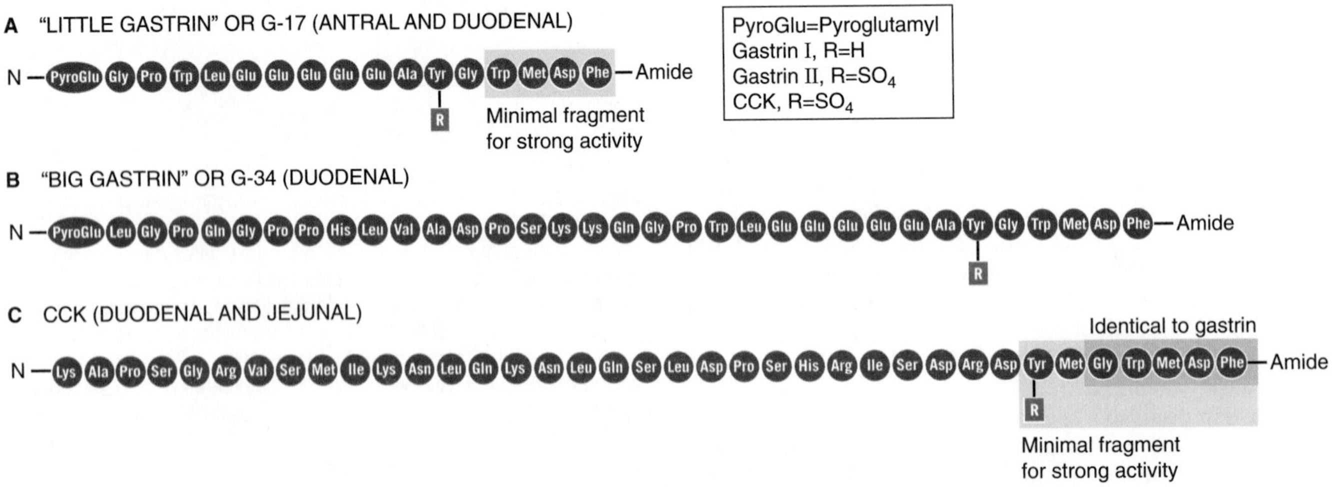

A "LITTLE GASTRIN" OR G-17 (ANTRAL AND DUODENAL)

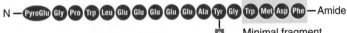

PyroGlu=Pyroglutamyl
Gastrin I, R=H
Gastrin II, R=SO₄
CCK, R=SO₄

Minimal fragment for strong activity

B "BIG GASTRIN" OR G-34 (DUODENAL)

C CCK (DUODENAL AND JEJUNAL)

Identical to gastrin

Minimal fragment for strong activity

Figure 42-7 Amino acid sequences of the gastrins and CCK. **A,** A single gene encodes a 101–amino acid peptide that is processed to both G-17 and G-34. The N-terminal glutamine is modified to create a pyroglutamyl residue. The C-terminal phenylalanine is amidated. These modifications make the hormone resistant to carboxypeptidases and aminopeptidases. **B,** The final 16 amino acids of G-34 are identical to the final 16 amino acids in G-17. Both G-17 and G-34 may be either *not sulfated* (gastrin I) or *sulfated* (gastrin II). **C,** The five final amino acids of CCK are identical to those of G-17 and G-34.

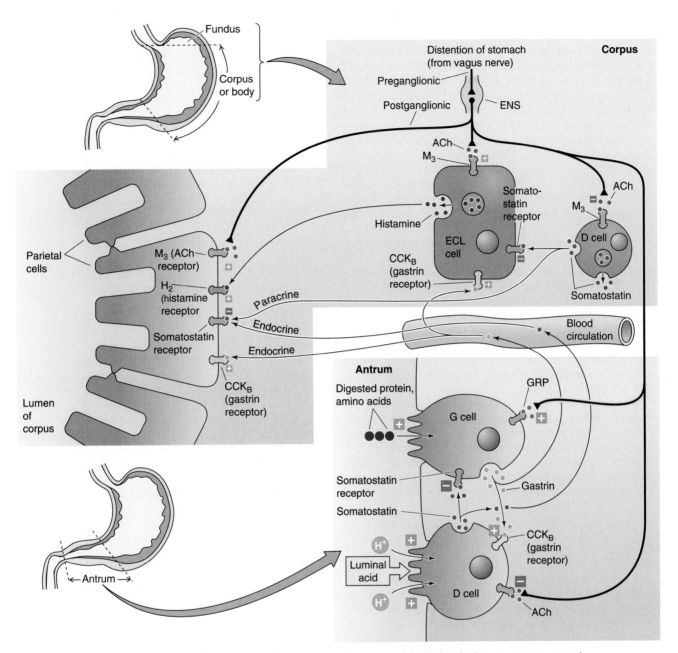

Figure 42-8 Regulation of gastric acid secretion. In the corpus of the stomach, the vagus nerve not only stimulates the parietal cell directly by releasing ACh but also stimulates both ECL and D cells. Vagal stimulation of the ECL cells enhances gastric acid secretion through increased histamine release. Vagal stimulation of the D cells also promotes gastric acid secretion by inhibiting the release of somatostatin, which would otherwise inhibit—by paracrine mechanisms—the release of histamine from ECL cells and the secretion of acid by parietal cells. In the antrum of the stomach, the vagus stimulates both G cells and D cells. The vagus stimulates the G cells through GRP, thus promoting gastrin release. This gastrin promotes gastric acid secretion by two endocrine mechanisms: directly through the parietal cell and indirectly through the ECL cell, which releases histamine. The vagal stimulation of D cells by ACh inhibits the release of somatostatin, which would otherwise inhibit—by paracrine mechanisms—the release of gastrin from G cells and—by an endocrine mechanism—acid secretion by parietal cells. Luminal H$^+$ directly stimulates the D cells to release somatostatin, which inhibits gastrin release from the G cells, thereby reducing gastric acid secretion (negative feedback). In addition, products of protein digestion (i.e., peptides and amino acids) directly stimulate the G cells to release gastrin, which stimulates gastric acid secretion (positive feedback).

Somatostatin inhibits gastric acid secretion by both direct and indirect mechanisms (Fig. 42-8). In the **direct pathway**, somatostatin coming from two different sources binds to a $G\alpha_i$-coupled receptor (SST) on the basolateral membrane of the parietal cell and inhibits adenylyl cyclase. The net effect is to antagonize the stimulatory effect of histamine and thus inhibit gastric acid secretion by parietal cells. The source of this somatostatin can either be *paracrine* (i.e., D cells present in the corpus of the stomach, near the parietal cells) or *endocrine* (i.e., D cells in the antrum). However, there is a major difference in what triggers the D cells in the corpus and antrum. Neural and hormonal mechanisms stimulate D cells in the *corpus* (which cannot sense intraluminal pH), whereas low intraluminal pH stimulates D cells in the *antrum*.

Somatostatin also acts through two **indirect pathways**, both of which are paracrine. In the corpus of the stomach, D cells release somatostatin that inhibits the release of *histamine* from ECL cells (Fig. 42-8). Because histamine is an acid secretagogue, somatostatin thus reduces gastric acid secretion. In the antrum of the stomach, D cells release somatostatin, which inhibits the release of *gastrin* from G cells. Because gastrin is another acid secretagogue, somatostatin also reduces gastric acid secretion by this route. The gastrin released by the G cell feeds back on itself by stimulating D cells to release the inhibitory somatostatin.

The presence of multiple mechanisms by which somatostatin inhibits acid secretion is another example of the *redundant regulatory pathways* that control acid secretion. An understanding of the regulation of somatostatin release from D cells is slowly evolving, but it appears that gastrin stimulates somatostatin release, whereas cholinergic agonists inhibit somatostatin release.

Several enteric hormones ("enterogastrone") and prostaglandins inhibit gastric acid secretion

Multiple processes in the duodenum and jejunum participate in the negative feedback mechanisms that inhibit gastric acid secretion. Fat, acid, and hyperosmolar solutions in the duodenum are potent inhibitors of gastric acid secretion. Of these inhibitors, lipids are the most potent, but acid is also quite important. Several candidate hormones have been suggested as the prime mediator of this acid inhibition (Table 42-1). These include CCK, secretin, and peptide YY (see Chapter 43), as well as vasoactive intestinal peptide (VIP), gastric inhibitory peptide (GIP), and neurotensin. Although each inhibits acid secretion after systemic administration, none has been *unequivocally* established as the sole physiological "enterogastrone."

Evidence suggests that **secretin**, which is released by duodenal S cells, may have a prime role in inhibiting gastric acid secretion after the entry of fat and acid into the duodenum. Secretin appears to reduce acid secretion by at least three mechanisms: (1) inhibition of antral gastrin release, (2) stimulation of somatostatin release, and (3) direct downregulation of the parietal cell H^+ secretory process.

The presence of luminal fatty acids causes enteroendocrine cells in the duodenum and the proximal part of the small intestine to release both GIP and CCK. **GIP** reduces acid secretion directly by inhibiting parietal cell acid secre-

Table 42-1   Enteric Hormones That Inhibit Gastric H^+ Secretion

Hormone	Source
CCK	I cells of duodenum and jejunum and neurons in ileum and colon
Secretin	S cells in small intestine
VIP	ENS neurons
GIP	K cells in duodenum and jejunum
Neurotensin	Endocrine cells in ileum
Peptide YY	Endocrine cells in ileum and colon
Somatostatin	D cells of stomach and duodenum, δ cells of pancreatic islets

tion and indirectly by inhibiting the antral release of gastrin. GIP also has the important function of stimulating insulin release from pancreatic islet cells in response to duodenal glucose and fatty acids and is therefore often referred to as glucose-dependent insulinotropic polypeptide (see Chapter 51). CCK participates in feedback inhibition of acid secretion by directly reducing parietal cell acid secretion. Finally, some evidence indicates that a neural reflex elicited in the duodenum in response to acid also inhibits gastric acid secretion.

Prostaglandin E_2 (PGE_2) inhibits parietal cell acid secretion, probably by inhibiting histamine's activation of parietal cell function at a site that is distal to the histamine receptor. PGE_2 appears to bind to an EP_3 receptor on the basolateral membrane of the parietal cell (Fig. 42-6) and stimulates $G\alpha_i$, which, in turn, inhibits adenylyl cyclase. In addition, prostaglandins also indirectly inhibit gastric acid secretion by reducing histamine release from ECL cells and gastrin release from antral G cells.

A meal triggers three phases of acid secretion

Basal State   Gastric acid secretion occurs throughout the day and night. Substantial increases in acid secretion occur after meals, whereas the rate of acid secretion between meals is low (i.e., the interdigestive phase). This interdigestive period follows a circadian rhythm; acid secretion is lowest in the morning before awakening and is highest in the evening. Acid secretion is a direct function of the number of parietal cells, which is also influenced, at least in part, by body weight. Thus, men have higher rates of basal acid secretion than do women. Considerable variability in basal acid secretion is also seen among physiologically normal individuals, and the resting intragastric pH can range from 3 to 7.

In contrast to the low rate of acid secretion during the basal or interdigestive period, acid secretion is enhanced several-fold by eating (Fig. 42-9). Regulation of gastric acid

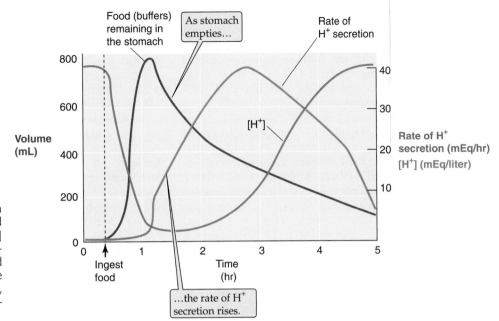

Food (buffers) remaining in the stomach

As stomach empties...

Rate of H^+ secretion

$[H^+]$

Rate of H^+ secretion (mEq/hr) $[H^+]$ (mEq/liter)

...the rate of H^+ secretion rises.

Volume (mL)

Ingest food

Time (hr)

Figure 42-9 Effect of eating on acid secretion. Ingesting food causes a marked fall in gastric $[H^+]$ because the food buffers the pre-existing H^+. However, as the food leaves the stomach and as the rate of H^+ secretion increases, $[H^+]$ slowly rises to its "interdigestive" level.

secretion is most often studied in the fasting state, a state in which intragastric pH is relatively low because of the basal H^+ secretory rate and the absence of food that would otherwise buffer the secreted gastric acid. Experimental administration of a secretagogue in the fasted state thus stimulates parietal cells and further lowers intragastric pH. However, the time course of intragastric pH after a meal can vary considerably despite stimulation of acid secretion. The reason is that intragastric pH depends not only on gastric acid secretion but also on the buffering power (see Chapter 28) of food and the rate of gastric emptying of both acid and partially digested material into the duodenum.

Regulation of acid secretion during a meal can be best characterized by three separate, but interrelated phases: the *cephalic*, the *gastric*, and the *intestinal* phases. The cephalic and gastric phases are of primary importance. Regulation of acid secretion includes both the stimulatory and inhibitory mechanisms that we discussed earlier (Fig. 42-8). ACh, gastrin, and histamine all promote acid secretion, whereas somatostatin inhibits gastric acid secretion.

Although dividing acid secretion during a meal into three phases has been used for decades, it is somewhat artificial because of considerable overlap in the regulation of acid secretion. For example, the vagus nerve is the central factor in the cephalic phase, but it is also important for the vago-vagal reflex that is part of the gastric phase. Similarly, gastrin release is a major component of the gastric phase, but vagal stimulation during the cephalic phase also induces the release of antral gastrin. Finally, the development of a consensus model has long been hampered by considerable differences in regulation of the gastric phase of acid secretion in humans, dogs, and rodents.

Cephalic Phase The smell, sight, taste, thought, and swallowing of food initiate the cephalic phase, which is primarily mediated by the vagus nerve (Fig. 42-8). Although the

cephalic phase has long been studied in experimental animals, especially dogs by Pavlov, more recent studies of sham feeding have confirmed and extended the understanding of the mechanism of the cephalic phase of acid secretion in humans. The aforementioned sensory stimuli activate the **dorsal motor nucleus of the vagus nerve** in the medulla (see Chapter 14) and thus activate parasympathetic preganglionic efferent nerves. Insulin-induced hypoglycemia also stimulates the vagus nerve and in so doing promotes acid secretion.

Stimulation of the vagus nerve results in four distinct physiological events (already introduced in Figure 42-8) that together result in enhanced gastric acid secretion. First, in the body of the stomach, vagal postganglionic muscarinic nerves release ACh, which stimulates parietal cell H^+ secretion directly. Second, in the lamina propria of the body of the stomach, the ACh released from vagal endings triggers histamine release from ECL cells, which stimulates acid secretion. Third, in the antrum, *peptidergic* postganglionic parasympathetic vagal neurons, as well as other enteric nervous system (ENS) neurons, release GRP, which induces gastrin release from antral G cells. This gastrin stimulates gastric acid secretion both directly by acting on the parietal cell and indirectly by promoting histamine release from ECL cells. Fourth, in both the antrum and the corpus, the vagus nerve inhibits D cells, thereby reducing their release of somatostatin and reducing the background inhibition of gastrin release. Thus, the cephalic phase stimulates acid secretion directly and indirectly by acting on the parietal cell. The cephalic phase accounts for ~30% of total acid secretion and occurs before the entry of any food into the stomach.

One of the surgical approaches for the treatment of peptic ulcer disease is cutting the vagus nerves (vagotomy) to inhibit gastric acid secretion. Rarely performed, largely because of the many effective pharmacological agents available to treat peptic ulcer disease, the technique has nevertheless proved effective in selected cases. Because vagus nerve stimulation affects several GI functions besides parietal cell acid secretion, the side effects of vagotomy include a delay in gastric emptying and diarrhea. To minimize these untoward events, successful attempts have been made to perform more selective vagotomies, severing *only those* vagal fibers leading to the parietal cell.

Gastric Phase   Entry of food into the stomach initiates the two primary stimuli for the gastric phase of acid secretion (Fig. 42-10). First, the food distends the gastric mucosa, which activates a vagovagal reflex as well as local ENS reflexes. Second, partially digested proteins stimulate antral G cells.

Distention of the gastric wall—both in the corpus and antrum—secondary to entry of food into the stomach elicits two distinct neurally mediated pathways. The first is activation of a **vagovagal reflex** (see Chapter 41), in which gastric wall distention activates a vagal *afferent* pathway, which, in turn, stimulates a vagal *efferent* response in the dorsal nucleus of the vagus nerve. Stimulation of acid secretion in response to this vagal efferent stimulus occurs through the same four parallel pathways that are operative when the vagus nerve is activated during the cephalic phase (Fig. 42-8). Second, gastric wall distention also activates a **local ENS pathway** that releases ACh, which, in turn, stimulates parietal cell acid secretion.

The presence of **partially digested proteins** (peptones) or amino acids in the antrum directly stimulates G cells to release gastrin (Fig. 42-8). Intact proteins have no effect. Acid secretion and activation of pepsinogen are linked in a positive feedback relationship. As discussed later, low pH

enhances the conversion of pepsinogen to pepsin. Pepsin digests proteins to peptones, which promote gastrin release. Finally, gastrin promotes acid secretion, which closes the positive feedback loop. Little evidence indicates that either carbohydrate or lipid participates in the regulation of gastric acid secretion. Components of wine, beer, and coffee stimulate acid secretion by this G cell mechanism.

In addition to the two stimulatory pathways acting during the gastric phase, a third pathway *inhibits* gastric acid secretion by a classic negative feedback mechanism, already noted earlier in our discussion of Figure 42-8. Low intragastric pH stimulates antral D cells to release somatostatin. Because somatostatin inhibits the release of gastrin by G cells, the net effect is a reduction in gastric acid secretion. The effectiveness of low pH in inhibiting gastrin release is emphasized by the following observation: Although peptones are normally a potent stimulus for gastrin release, they fail to stimulate gastrin release either when the intraluminal pH of the antrum is maintained at 1.0 or when somatostatin is infused. The gastric phase of acid secretion, which occurs primarily as a result of gastrin release, accounts for *50% to 60% of total gastric acid secretion*.

Intestinal Phase   The presence of amino acids and partially digested peptides in the proximal portion of the small intestine stimulates acid secretion by three mechanisms (Fig. 42-11). First, these peptones stimulate duodenal G cells to secrete gastrin, just as peptones stimulate antral G cells in the gastric phase. Second, peptones stimulate an unknown endocrine cell to release an additional humoral signal that has been referred to as entero-oxyntin. The chemical nature of this agent has not yet been identified. Third, amino acids absorbed by the proximal part of the small intestine stimulate acid secretion by mechanisms that require further definition.

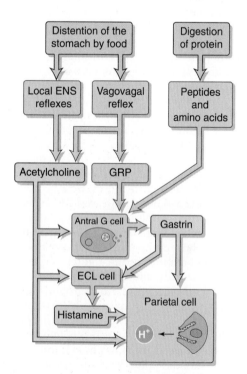

Figure 42-10   Gastric phase of gastric acid secretion. Food in the stomach stimulates gastric acid secretion by two major mechanisms: mechanical stretch and the presence of digested protein fragments (peptones).

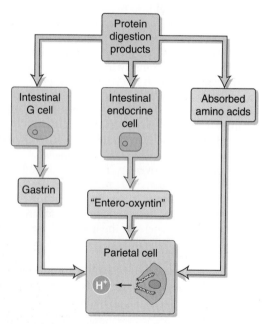

Figure 42-11   Intestinal phase of gastric acid secretion. Digested protein fragments (peptones) in the proximal small intestine stimulate gastric acid secretion by three major mechanisms.

Gastrinoma or Zollinger-Ellison Syndrome

On rare occasion, patients with one or more ulcers have very high rates of gastric acid secretion. The increased acid secretion in these patients is most often a result of elevated levels of serum gastrin, released from a pancreatic islet cell adenoma or gastrinoma (Table 42-2). This clinical picture is also known as the **Zollinger-Ellison syndrome**. Because gastrin released from these islet cell adenomas is not under physiological control, but rather is continuously released, acid secretion is substantially increased under basal conditions. However, the intravenous administration of pentagastrin—a synthetic gastrin consisting of the last four amino acids of gastrin plus β-alanine—produces only a modest increase in gastric acid secretion. Omeprazole, a potent inhibitor of the parietal cell H-K pump, is now an effective therapeutic agent to control the marked enhancement of gastric acid secretion in patients with gastrinoma and thus helps to heal their duodenal and gastric ulcers.

In contrast to patients with gastrinoma or Zollinger-Ellison syndrome, other patients with **duodenal ulcer** have serum gastrin levels that are near normal. Their basal gastric acid secretion rates are modestly elevated, but they increase markedly in response to pentagastrin. Patients with **pernicious anemia** (see Chapter 45 for the box on this topic) lack parietal cells and thus cannot secrete H^+. In the absence of a low luminal pH, the antral D cell is not stimulated by acid (Fig. 42-10). Consequently, the release of somatostatin from the D cell is low, and minimal tonic inhibition of gastrin release from G cells occurs. It is not surprising, then, that these patients have very high levels of serum gastrin, but virtually no H^+ secretion (Table 42-2).

Table 42-2 Serum Gastrin Levels and Gastric Acid Secretion Rates

	Serum Gastrin (pg/mL)	H^+ SECRETION (mEq/hr)	
		Basal	**After Pentagastrin**
Normal	35	0.5-2.0	20-35
Duodenal ulcer	50	1.5-7.0	25-60
Gastrinoma	500	15-25	30-75
Pernicious anemia	350	0	0

Gastric acid secretion mediated by the intestinal phase is enhanced after a portacaval shunt. Such a shunt—used in the treatment of portal hypertension caused by chronic liver disease—diverts the portal blood that drains the small intestine around the liver on its return to the heart. Thus, the signal released from the small intestine during the intestinal phase is probably—in normal individuals—removed in part by the liver before reaching its target, the corpus of the stomach. *Approximately 5% to 10% of total gastric acid secretion is a result of the intestinal phase.*

PEPSINOGEN SECRETION

Chief cells, triggered by both cAMP and Ca²⁺ pathways, secrete multiple pepsinogens that initiate protein digestion

The chief cells in gastric glands, as well as mucous cells, secrete **pepsinogens**, a group of proteolytic proenzymes (i.e., zymogens or inactive enzyme precursors) that belong to the general class of aspartic proteinases. They are activated to pepsins by cleavage of an N-terminal peptide. **Pepsins** are endopeptidases that initiate the hydrolysis of ingested protein in the stomach. Although eight pepsinogen isoforms were initially identified on electrophoresis, recent classifications are based on immunological identity, so pepsinogens are most often classified as group I pepsinogens, group II pepsinogens, and cathepsin E. Group I pepsinogens predominate. They are secreted from chief cells located at the base of glands in the corpus of the stomach. Group II pepsinogens are also secreted from chief cells but, in addition, are secreted from mucous neck cells in the cardiac, corpus, and antral regions.

Pepsinogen secretion in the basal state is ~20% of its maximal secretion after stimulation. Although pepsinogen secretion generally parallels the secretion of acid, the ratio of maximal to basal pepsinogen secretion is considerably less than that for acid secretion. Moreover, the cellular mechanism of pepsinogen release is quite distinct from that of H^+ secretion by parietal cells. Release of pepsinogen across the apical membrane is the result of a novel process called **compound exocytosis**, in which secretory granules fuse with both the plasma membrane and other secretory granules. This process permits rapid and sustained secretion of pepsinogen. After stimulation, the initial peak in pepsinogen secretion is followed by a persistent lower rate of secretion. This pattern of secretion has been interpreted as reflecting an initial secretion of *preformed* pepsinogen, followed by the secretion of *newly synthesized* pepsinogen. However, more recent in vitro studies suggested that a feedback mechanism may account for the subsequent reduced rate of pepsinogen secretion.

Two groups of agonists stimulate chief cells to secrete pepsinogen. One group acts through adenylyl cyclase and cAMP, and the other acts through increases in $[Ca^{2+}]_i$.

Agonists Acting Through cAMP Chief cells have receptors for **secretin/VIP**, **β₂-adrenergic** receptors, and **EP₂** receptors for **PGE₂** (see Chapter 3). All these receptors activate adenylyl cyclase. At lower concentrations than those required to *stimulate* pepsinogen secretion, PGE₂ can also *inhibit* pepsinogen secretion, probably by binding to another receptor subtype.

Agonists Acting Through Ca²⁺ Chief cells also have M₃ muscarinic receptors for **ACh**, as well as receptors for the **gastrin/CCK** family of peptides. Unlike gastric acid secretion, which is stimulated by the CCK_B receptor, pepsinogen secretion is stimulated by the CCK_A receptor, which has a much higher affinity for CCK than for gastrin. Activation of both the M_3 and CCK_A receptors causes Ca^{2+} release from intracellular stores by IP_3 and thereby raises $[Ca^{2+}]_i$. However, uncertainty exists about whether increased Ca^{2+} influx is also required and about whether PKC also has a role.

Of the agonists just listed, the most important for pepsinogen secretion is ACh released in response to vagal stimulation. Not only does ACh stimulate chief cells to release pepsinogen, but also it stimulates parietal cells to secrete acid. This gastric acid produces additional pepsinogen secretion by two different mechanisms. First, in the stomach, a fall in pH elicits a local cholinergic reflex that results in further stimulation of chief cells to release pepsinogen. Thus, the ACh that stimulates chief cells can come both from the vagus and from the local reflex. Second, in the duodenum, acid triggers the release of secretin from S cells. By an endocrine effect, this secretin stimulates the chief cells to release more pepsinogen. The exact role or roles of histamine and gastrin in pepsinogen secretion are unclear.

Low pH is required for both pepsinogen activation and pepsin activity

Pepsinogen is inactive and requires activation to a protease, pepsin, to initiate protein digestion. This activation occurs by spontaneous cleavage of a small N-terminal peptide fragment (the activation peptide), but only at a pH that is less than 5.0 (Fig. 42-12). Between pH 5.0 and 3.0, spontaneous activation of pepsinogen is slow, but it is extremely rapid at a pH that is less than 3.0. In addition, pepsinogen is also autoactivated; that is, newly formed pepsin itself cleaves pepsinogen to pepsin.

Once pepsin is formed, its *activity* is also pH dependent. It has optimal activity at a pH between 1.8 and 3.5; the precise optimal pH depends on the specific pepsin, type and concentration of substrate, and osmolality of the solution. pH values higher than 3.5 *reversibly* inactivate pepsin, and pH values higher than 7.2 *irreversibly* inactivate the enzyme. These considerations are sometimes useful for

establishing optimal antacid treatment regimens in peptic ulcer disease.

Pepsin is an endopeptidase that initiates the process of protein digestion in the stomach. Pepsin action results in the release of small peptides and amino acids (peptones) that, as noted earlier, stimulate the release of gastrin from antral G cells; these peptones also stimulate CCK release from duodenal I cells. As previously mentioned, the peptones generated by pepsin stimulate the very acid secretion required for pepsin activation and action. Thus, the peptides that pepsin releases are important in initiating a coordinated response to a meal. However, most protein entering the duodenum remains as large peptides, and nitrogen balance is not impaired after total gastrectomy.

Digestive products of both carbohydrates and lipid are also found in the stomach, although secretion of their respective digestive enzymes either does not occur or is not a major function of gastric epithelial cells. Carbohydrate digestion is initiated in the mouth by **salivary amylase**. However, after this enzyme is swallowed, the stomach becomes a more important site for starch hydrolysis than the mouth. No evidence indicates gastric secretion of enzymes that hydrolyze starch or other saccharides. Similarly, although lipid digestion is also initiated in the mouth by lingual lipase, significant lipid digestion occurs in the stomach as a result of both the **lingual lipase** that is swallowed and **gastric lipase**, both of which have an acid pH optimum (see Chapter 45).

PROTECTION OF THE GASTRIC SURFACE EPITHELIUM AND NEUTRALIZATION OF ACID IN THE DUODENUM

At maximal rates of H^+ secretion, the parietal cell can drive the intraluminal pH of the stomach to 1 or less (i.e., $[H^+] > 100$ mM) for long periods. The gastric epithelium must maintain an H^+ concentration gradient of more than a million-fold because the intracellular pH of gastric epithelial cells is ~7.2 (i.e., $[H^+] \cong 60$ nM) and plasma pH is ~7.4 (i.e., $[H^+] \cong 40$ nM). Simultaneously, a substantial plasma-to-lumen Na^+ concentration gradient of ~30 is present because plasma $[Na^+]$ is 140 mM, whereas intragastric $[Na^+]$ can reach values as low as 5 mM, but only at high secretory rates (Fig. 42-2). How is the stomach able to maintain these gradients? How is it that the epithelial cells are not destroyed by this acidity? Moreover, why do pepsins in the gastric lumen not digest the epithelial cells? The answer to all three questions is the so-called **gastric diffusion barrier**.

Although the nature of the gastric diffusion barrier had been controversial, it is now recognized that the diffusion barrier is both physiological and anatomical. Moreover, it is apparent that the diffusion barrier represents at least three components: (1) relative impermeability to acid of the apical membrane and epithelial cell tight junctions in the gastric glands, (2) a mucous gel layer varying in thickness between 50 and 200 μm overlying the surface epithelial cells, and (3) an HCO_3^--containing microclimate adjacent to the

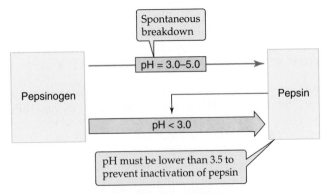

Figure 42-12 Activation of the pepsinogens to pepsins. At pH values from 5 to 3, pepsinogens spontaneously activate to pepsins by the removal of an N-terminal activation peptide. This spontaneous activation is even faster at pH values lower than 3. The newly formed pepsins themselves—which are active only at pH values lower than 3.5—also can catalyze the activation of pepsinogens.

surface epithelial cells that maintains a relatively high local pH.

Vagal stimulation and irritation stimulate gastric mucous cells to secrete mucin, a glycoprotein that is part of the mucosal barrier

The mucus layer is largely composed of mucin, phospholipids, electrolytes, and water. **Mucin** is the high-molecular-weight glycoprotein (see Chapter 2) that contributes to the formation of a protective layer over the gastric mucosa. Gastric mucin is a tetramer consisting of four identical peptides joined by disulfide bonds. Each of the four peptide chains is linked to long polysaccharides, which are often sulfated and are thus mutually repulsive. The ensuing high carbohydrate content is responsible for the viscosity of mucus, which explains, in large part, its protective role in gastric mucosal physiology.

Mucus is secreted by three different mucous cells: surface mucous cells (i.e., on the surface of the stomach), mucous neck cells (i.e., at the point where a gastric pit joins a gastric gland), and glandular mucous cells (i.e., in the gastric glands in the antrum). The type of mucus secreted by these cells differs; mucus that is synthesized and secreted in the glandular cells is a neutral glycoprotein, whereas the mucous cells on the surface and in the gastric pits secrete both neutral and acidic glycoproteins. Mucin forms a **mucous gel layer** in combination with phospholipids, electrolytes, and water. This mucous gel layer provides protection against injury from noxious luminal substances, including acid, pepsins, bile acids, and ethanol. Mucin also lubricates the gastric mucosa to minimize the abrasive effects of intraluminal food.

The mucus barrier is not static. Abrasions can remove pieces of mucus. When mucus comes in contact with a solution with a very low pH, the mucus precipitates and sloughs off. Thus, the mucous cells must constantly secrete mucus. Regulation of mucus secretion by gastric mucosal cells is less well understood than is regulation of the secretion of acid, pepsinogens, and other substances by gastric cells. The two primary stimuli for inducing mucus secretion are vagal stimulation and physical and chemical irritation of the gastric mucosa by ingested food. The current model of mucus secretion suggests that vagal stimulation induces the release of ACh, which leads to increases in $[Ca^{2+}]_i$ and thus stimulates mucus secretion. In contrast to acid and pepsinogen secretion, cAMP does not appear to be a second messenger for mucus secretion.

Gastric surface cells secrete HCO_3^-, stimulated by acetylcholine, acids, and prostaglandins

Surface epithelial cells both in the corpus and in the antrum of the stomach secrete HCO_3^-. Despite the relatively low rate of HCO_3^- secretion—in comparison with acid secretion—HCO_3^- is extremely important as part of the gastric mucosal protective mechanism. The mucus gel layer provides an unstirred layer under which the secreted HCO_3^- remains trapped and maintains a local pH of ~of 7.0 versus an intraluminal pH in the bulk phase of 1 to 3. As illustrated in Figure 42-13A, an electrogenic Na/HCO_3 cotransporter (NBC) appears to mediate the uptake of HCO_3^- across the basolateral membrane of surface epithelial cells. The mechanism of HCO_3^- exit from the cell into the apical mucus layer is unknown but may be mediated by a channel.

Similar to the situation for mucus secretion, relatively limited information is available about the regulation of HCO_3^- secretion. The present model suggests that *vagal stimulation* mediated by ACh leads to an increase in $[Ca^{2+}]_i$, which, in turn, stimulates HCO_3^- secretion. Sham feeding is a potent stimulus for HCO_3^- secretion through this pathway. A second powerful stimulus of gastric HCO_3^- secretion is *intraluminal acid*. The mechanism of stimulation by acid appears to be secondary to both activation of neural reflexes and local production of PGE_2. Finally, evidence suggests that a humoral factor may also be involved in the induction of HCO_3^- secretion by acid.

Mucus protects the gastric surface epithelium by trapping an HCO_3^--rich fluid near the apical border of these cells

Mucous cells on the surface of the stomach, as well as in the gastric pits and neck portions of the gastric glands, secrete both HCO_3^- and mucus. Why is this barrier so effective? First, the secreted mucus forms a mucous gel layer that is relatively impermeable to the *diffusion* of H^+ from the gastric lumen to the surface cells. Second, beneath this layer of mucus is a microclimate that contains fluid with a high pH and high $[HCO_3^-]$, the result of HCO_3^- secretion by gastric surface epithelial cells (Fig. 42-13A). Thus, this HCO_3^- neutralizes most acid that diffuses through the mucus layer. Mucosal integrity, including that of the mucosal diffusion barrier, is also maintained by PGE_2, which—as discussed in the previous section—stimulates mucosal HCO_3^- secretion.

Deep inside the gastric gland, where no obvious mucus layer protects the parietal, chief, and ECL cells, the impermeability of the cells' apical barrier appears to exclude H^+ even at pH values as low as 1. The paradox of how HCl secreted by the parietal cells emerges from the gland and into the gastric lumen may be explained by a process known as **viscous fingering**. Because the liquid emerging from the gastric gland is both extremely acidic and presumably under pressure, it can tunnel through the mucous layer covering the opening of the gastric gland onto the surface of the stomach. However, this stream of acid apparently does not spread laterally, but rather rises to the surface as a "finger" and thus does not neutralize the HCO_3^- in the microenvironment between the surface epithelial cells and the mucus.

The mucous gel layer and the trapped alkaline HCO_3^- solution protect the surface cells not only from H^+ but also from pepsin. The mucus per se acts as a pepsin diffusion barrier. The relative alkalinity of the trapped HCO_3^- inactivates any pepsin that penetrates the mucus. Recall that pepsin is reversibly inactivated at pH values higher than ~3.5 and is irreversibly inactivated by pH values higher than ~7.2. Thus, the mucus HCO_3^- layer plays an important role in preventing autodigestion of the gastric mucosa.

A NORMAL SURFACE EPITHELIUM

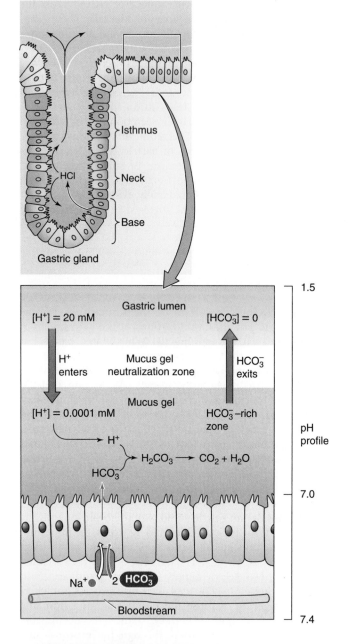

B DAMAGED MUCOSAL BARRIER

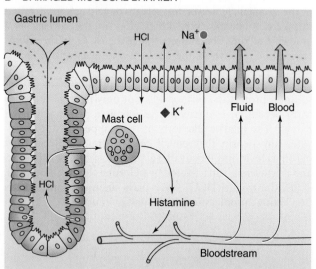

Figure 42-13 Diffusion barrier in the surface of the gastric mucosa. **A,** The mucus secreted by the surface cells serves two functions. First, it acts as a diffusion barrier for H^+ and also pepsins. Second, the mucus layer traps a relatively alkaline solution of HCO_3^-. This HCO_3^- titrates any H^+ that diffuses into the gel layer from the stomach lumen. The alkaline layer also inactivates any pepsin that penetrates into the mucus. **B,** If H^+ penetrates into the gastric epithelium, it damages mast cells, which release histamine and other agents, thereby setting up an inflammatory response. If the insult is mild, the ensuing increase in blood flow can promote the production of both mucus and HCO_3^- by the mucus cells. If the insult is more severe, the inflammatory response leads to a decrease in blood flow and thus to cell injury.

Breakdown of the Gastric Barrier

Integrity of the gastric-epithelial barrier can be conveniently judged by maintenance of a high lumen-negative transepithelial potential difference (PD) of ~−60 mV. Several agents that cause mucosal injury, including mucosal ulceration, can alter the mucosal diffusion barrier. Salicylates, bile acids, and ethanol all impair the mucosal diffusion barrier and result in H^+ (acid) backdiffusion, an increase in intraluminal $[Na^+]$, a fall in PD, and mucosal damage (Fig. 42-13B). Three decades ago, Davenport proposed an attractive model to explain how H^+, after having breached the mucosal diffusion barrier, produces injury to the gastric mucosa. Although several details of this original model have been modified during the ensuing years, it is still believed that entry of acid into the mucosa damages mast cells, which release histamine and other mediators of **inflammation**. The histamine and other agents cause local vasodilatation that increases blood flow. If the damage is not too severe, this response allows the surface cells to maintain their production of mucus and HCO_3^-. However, if the injury is more severe, inflammatory cells release a host of agents—including platelet-activating factor, leukotrienes, endothelins, thromboxanes, and oxidants—that reduce blood flow (ischemia) and result in tissue injury, including capillary damage.

Prostaglandins play a central role in maintaining mucosal integrity. For example, prostaglandins prevent or reverse mucosal injury secondary to salicylates, bile, and ethanol. This protective effect of prostaglandins is the result of several actions, including their ability to inhibit acid secretion, stimulate both HCO_3^- and mucus secretion, increase mucosal blood flow, and modify the local inflammatory response induced by acid.

Entry of acid into the duodenum induces the release of secretin from S cells, thus triggering the secretion of HCO_3^- by the pancreas and duodenum, which, in turn, neutralizes gastric acid

The overall process of regulating gastric acid secretion involves not only stimulation and inhibition of acid secretion (as discussed earlier), but also neutralization of the gastric acid that passes from the stomach into the duodenum. The amount of secreted gastric acid is reflected by a

Helicobacter pylori

During the past decade, our understanding of the etiology of duodenal and gastric ulcers has radically changed. Abundant evidence now indicates that most peptic ulcers are an infectious disease in that most (but not all) ulcers are caused by *Helicobacter pylori*, a gram-negative bacillus that colonizes the antral mucosa. Nonsteroidal anti-inflammatory drugs (NSAIDs) are responsible for ~20% of ulcers. Although almost all ulcers that are not associated with NSAID use are secondary to *H. pylori* infestation, many, if not most, individuals with evidence of *H. pylori* infestation do not have peptic ulcer disease. The factors responsible for *H. pylori*–induced inflammation or ulceration are not known. However, the increase in gastric acid secretion that is present in most patients with duodenal ulcers may occur because *H. pylori*–induced antral inflammation inhibits the release of somatostatin by antral D cells. Because somatostatin normally inhibits gastrin release by antral G cells, the result would be increased gastrin release and thus increased gastric acid secretion. Indeed, as noted in Table 42-2, serum gastrin levels are modestly elevated in patients with duodenal ulcers.

Inhibition of acid secretion heals, but does not cure *H. pylori*–induced peptic ulcers. However, antibiotic therapy that eradicates *H. pylori* cures peptic ulcer disease.

fall in intragastric pH. We have already seen that this fall in pH serves as the signal to antral D cells to release somatostatin and thus to inhibit further acid secretion, a classic negative feedback process. Similarly, low pH in the duodenum serves as a signal for the secretion of alkali to neutralize gastric acid in the duodenum.

The key factor in this neutralization process is **secretin**, the same secretin that inhibits gastric acid secretion and promotes pepsinogen secretion by chief cells. A low duodenal pH, with a threshold of 4.5, triggers the release of secretin from **S cells** in the duodenum. However, the S cells are probably not pH sensitive themselves but, instead, may respond to a signal from other cells that are pH sensitive. Secretin stimulates the secretion of fluid and HCO_3^- by the pancreas, thus leading to intraduodenal neutralization of the acid load from the stomach. Maximal HCO_3^- secretion is a function of the amount of acid entering the duodenum, as well as the length of duodenum exposed to acid. Thus, high rates of gastric acid secretion trigger the release of large amounts of secretin, which greatly stimulates pancreatic HCO_3^- secretion; the increased HCO_3^-, in turn, neutralizes the increased duodenal acid load.

In addition to *pancreatic* HCO_3^- secretion, the duodenal acid load resulting from gastric acid secretion is partially neutralized by *duodenal* HCO_3^- secretion. This duodenal HCO_3^- secretion occurs in the proximal—but not the distal—part of the duodenum under the influence of prostaglandins. Attention has been focused on duodenal epithelial cells (villus or crypt cells) as the cellular source of HCO_3^- secretion, but the possibility that duodenal HCO_3^- originates, at least in part, from duodenal submucosal Brunner's glands has not been excluded. The mechanism of duodenal HCO_3^-

secretion involves both $Cl-HCO_3$ exchange and cystic fibrosis transmembrane conductance regulator (CFTR) in the apical membrane (see Fig. 43-6). Patients with duodenal ulcer disease tend to have both increased gastric acid secretion and reduced duodenal HCO_3^- secretion. Thus, the increased acid load in the duodenum is only partially neutralized, so the duodenal mucosa has increased exposure to a low-pH solution.

FILLING AND EMPTYING OF THE STOMACH

Gastric motor activity plays a role in filling, churning, and emptying

Gastric motor activity has three functions. First, the receipt of ingested material represents the **reservoir function** of the stomach and occurs as smooth muscle relaxes. This response occurs primarily in the proximal portion of the stomach. Second, ingested material is **churned** and is thereby altered to a form that rapidly empties from the stomach through the pylorus and facilitates normal jejunal digestion and absorption. Thus, in conjunction with gastric acid and enzymes, the motor function of the stomach helps to initiate digestion. Third, the pyloric antrum, pylorus, and proximal part of the duodenum function as a single unit for **emptying** into the duodenum the modified gastric contents (chyme), consisting of both partially digested food material and gastric secretions. Gastric filling and emptying are accomplished by the coordinated activity of smooth muscle in the esophagus, lower esophageal sphincter, and proximal and distal portions of the stomach, as well as the pylorus and duodenum.

The pattern of gastric smooth muscle activity is distinct during fasting and after eating. The pattern during fasting is referred to as the **migrating myoelectric (or motor) complex (MMC)**, as discussed in Chapter 41 in connection with the small intestine. This pattern is terminated by eating, at which point it is replaced by the so-called **fed pattern**. Just as the proximal and distal regions of the stomach differ in secretory function, they also differ in the motor function responsible for storing, processing, and emptying liquids and solids. The proximal part of the stomach is the primary location for storage of both liquids and solids. The distal portion of the stomach is primarily responsible for churning the solids and generating smaller liquid-like material, which then exits the stomach in a manner similar to that of ingested liquids. Thus, the gastric emptying of liquids and of solids is closely integrated.

Filling of the stomach is facilitated by both receptive relaxation and gastric accommodation

Even a dry swallow relaxes both the lower esophageal sphincter and the proximal part of the stomach. Of course, the same happens when we swallow food. These relaxations facilitate the entry of food into the stomach. Relaxation in the fundus is primarily regulated by a vagovagal reflex and has been called **receptive relaxation**. In a **vagovagal reflex**, afferent fibers running with the vagus nerve carry information to the central nervous system (CNS), and efferent vagal fibers carry the signal from the CNS to the stomach and cause relaxation by a mechanism that is neither cholinergic nor adrenergic. The result is that intragastric volume increases *without* an increase in intragastric pressure. If vagal innervation to the stomach is interrupted, gastric pressure rises much more rapidly.

Quite apart from the receptive relaxation of the stomach that anticipates the arrival of food after swallowing and esophageal distention, the stomach can also relax in response to gastric filling per se. Thus, increasing intragastric volume, as a result of either entry of food into the stomach or gastric secretion, does not produce a proportionate increase in intragastric pressure. Instead, small increases in volume do not cause increases in intragastric pressure until a threshold is reached, after which intragastric pressure rises steeply (Fig. 42-14A). This phenomenon is the result of *active* dilatation of the fundus and has been called **gastric accommodation**. Vagotomy abolishes a major portion of gastric accommodation, so increases in intragastric volume produce greater increases in intragastric pressure. However, the role of the

vagus nerve in gastric accommodation is one of modulation. It is generally believed that the **ENS** (see Chapter 41) is the primary regulator permitting the storage of substantial amounts of solids and liquids in the proximal part of the stomach without major increases in intragastric pressure.

The stomach churns its contents until the particles are small enough to be gradually emptied into the duodenum

The substance most rapidly emptied by the stomach is isotonic saline or water. Emptying of these liquids occurs without delay and is faster the greater the volume of fluid. Acidic and caloric fluids leave the stomach more slowly, whereas fatty materials exit even more slowly (Fig. 42-14B).

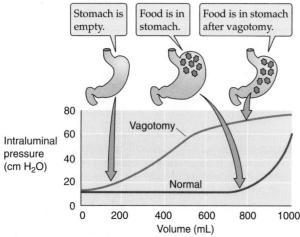

A   GASTRIC ACCOMMODATION

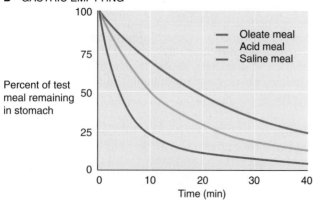

B   GASTRIC EMPTYING

Figure 42-14   Gastric filling and emptying. (***B,*** *Data from Dooley CP, Reznick JB, Valenzuela JE: Variations in gastric and duodenal motility during gastric emptying of liquid meals in humans. Gastroenterology 1984; 87:1114-1119.*)

Vomiting

Vomiting, a frequent sign and symptom in clinical medicine, represents a complex series of multiple afferent stimuli coordinated by one or more brain centers, leading to a coordinated neuromuscular response. **Nausea** is the sensation that vomiting may occur. The act of **emesis** involves several preprogrammed coordinated smooth and striated muscle responses. The initial event is the abolition of intestinal slow-wave activity that is linked to propulsive peristaltic contractions. As the normal peristaltic contractions of the stomach and small intestine wane, they are replaced by *retrograde* contractions, beginning in the ileum and progressing to the stomach. These retrograde contractions are accompanied by contraction of abdominal and inspiratory muscles (external intercostal muscles and diaphragm) against a closed glottis, thus resulting in an increase in intra-abdominal pressure. Relaxation of the diaphragmatic crural muscle and lower esophageal sphincter permits transmission of this increase in intra-abdominal pressure into the thorax, with expulsion of the gastric contents into the esophagus. Movement of the larynx upward and forward and relaxation of the upper esophageal sphincter are required for oral propulsion, whereas closure of the glottis prevents aspiration.

Three major categories of stimuli can potentially induce the foregoing series of events that lead to vomiting. First, gastric irritants and peritonitis, for example, probably act by vagal afferent pathways, presumably to rid the body of the irritant. Second, inner ear dysfunction or motion sickness acts through the vestibular nerve and vestibular nuclei. Third, drugs such as digitalis and certain cancer chemotherapeutic agents activate the *area postrema* in the brain (see Chapter 11). Pregnancy can also cause nausea and vomiting, by an unknown mechanism. Although several central loci receive these emetic stimuli, the primary locus is the *area postrema*, also called the *chemoreceptor trigger zone*. Although no single brainstem site coordinates vomiting, the nucleus tractus solitarii plays an important role in the initiation of emesis. Neurotransmitter receptors that are important in various causes of vomiting include neurokinin NK_1 and substance P receptors in the nucleus tractus solitarii, $5\text{-}HT_3$ receptors in vagal afferents, and dopamine D_2 receptors in the vestibular nucleus.

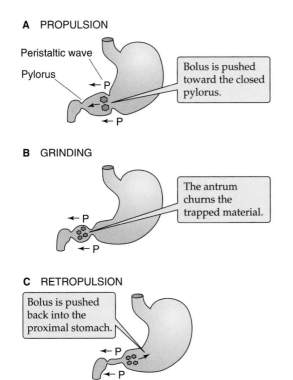

A PROPULSION

Peristaltic wave

Pylorus

← P

← P

Bolus is pushed toward the closed pylorus.

B GRINDING

← P

← P

The antrum churns the trapped material.

C RETROPULSION

Bolus is pushed back into the proximal stomach.

← P

← P

Figure 42-15 Mechanical actions of the stomach on its contents.

Solids do not leave the stomach as such, but must first be reduced in size (i.e., trituration). Particles larger than 2 mm do not leave the stomach during the immediate postprandial digestive period. The delay in gastric emptying of solids occurs because solids must be reduced to less than 2 mm; at that point, they are emptied by mechanisms similar to those of liquids.

Movement of solid particles toward the antrum is accomplished by the interaction of propulsive gastric contractions and occlusion of the pylorus, a process termed **propulsion** (Fig. 42-15A). Gastric contractions are initiated by the gastric pacemaker, which is located on the greater curvature, approximately at the junction of the proximal and middle portions of the stomach. These contractions propel the luminal contents toward the pylorus, which is partially closed by contraction of the pyloric musculature before delivery of the bolus. This increase in pyloric resistance represents the coordinated response of antral, pyloric, and duodenal motor activity. Once a bolus of material is trapped near the antrum, it is churned to help reduce the size of the particles, a process termed **grinding** (Fig. 42-15B). Only a small portion of gastric material—that containing particles smaller than 2 mm—is propelled through the pylorus to the duodenum. Thus, most gastric contents are returned to the body of the stomach for pulverization and shearing of solid

particles, a process known as **retropulsion** (Fig. 42-15C). These processes of propulsion, grinding, and retropulsion repeat multiple times until the gastric contents are emptied. Particles larger than 2 mm are initially retained in the stomach but are eventually emptied into the duodenum by MMCs during the interdigestive period that begins ~2 hours or more after eating.

Modification of gastric contents is associated with the activation of multiple feedback mechanisms. This feedback usually arises from the duodenum (and beyond) and almost always results in a delay in gastric emptying. Thus, as small squirts of gastric fluid leave the stomach, chemoreceptors and mechanoreceptors—primarily in the proximal but also in the distal portion of the small intestine—sense low pH, a high content of calories, lipid, or some amino acids (i.e., tryptophan), or changes in osmolarity. These signals all decrease the rate of gastric emptying by a combination of neural and hormonal signals, including the vagus nerve, secretin, CCK, and GIP released from duodenal mucosa. Delayed gastric emptying represents the following: the coordinated function of fundic relaxation; inhibition of antral motor activity; stimulation of isolated, phasic contractions of the pyloric sphincter; and altered intestinal motor activity.

REFERENCES

Books and Reviews

DelValle J, Todisco A: Gastric secretion. In Yamada T (ed): Textbook of Gastroenterology, vol 1, 4th ed, pp 266-307. Philadelphia: Lippincott Williams & Wilkins, 2003.

Dockray G, Dimaline, R, Varro A: Gastrin: Old hormone, new functions. Pflugers Arch 2005; 449:344-355.

Dockray G, Varro A, Dimaline R: Gastric endocrine cells: Gene expression, processing and targeting of active products. Physiol Rev 1996; 76:767-798.

Hasler WL: The physiology of gastric motility and gastric emptying. In Yamada T (ed): Textbook of Gastroenterology, vol 1, 4th ed, pp 266-307. Philadelphia: Lippincott Williams & Wilkins, 2003.

Hersey SJ, Sachs G: Gastric acid secretion. Physiol Rev 1995; 75:155-189.

Lichtenberger LM: The hydrophobic barrier properties of gastro-intestinal mucus. Annu Rev Physiol 1995; 57:565-583.

Sachs G, Prinz C: Gastric enterochromaffin-like cells and the regulation of acid secretion. News Physiol Sci 1996; 11:57-62.

Journal Articles

Dooley CP, Reznick JB, Valenzuela JE: Variations in gastric and duodenal motility during gastric emptying of liquid meals in humans. Gastroenterology 1984; 87:1114-1119.

Lambrecht NW, Yakubov I, Scott D, Sachs G: Identification of the efflux channel coupled to the gastric H,K-ATPase during acid secretion. Physiol Genomics 2005; 21:81-91.

Waisbren SJ, Geibel JP, Modlin IM, Boron WF: Unusual permeability properties of gastric gland cells. Nature 1994; 368:332-335.

PANCREATIC AND SALIVARY GLANDS

Christopher R. Marino and Fred S. Gorelick

OVERVIEW OF EXOCRINE GLAND PHYSIOLOGY

The pancreas and major salivary glands are compound exocrine glands

The exocrine pancreas and major salivary glands are compound exocrine glands—specialized secretory organs that contain a branching ductular system through which they release their secretory products. The principal function of these exocrine glands is to aid in the digestion of food. The saliva produced by the salivary glands lubricates ingested food and initiates the digestion of starch. Pancreatic juice, rich in HCO_3^- and digestive enzymes, neutralizes the acidic gastric contents that enter the small intestine and also completes the intraluminal digestion of ingested carbohydrate, protein, and fat. Each of these exocrine glands is under the control of neural and humoral signals that generate a sequential and coordinated secretory response to an ingested meal. We discuss the endocrine pancreas in Chapter 51.

Morphologically, the pancreas and salivary glands are divided into small but visible **lobules**, each of which represents a subdivision of the parenchyma and is drained by a single **intralobular duct** (Fig. 43-1A). Groups of lobules separated by connective tissue septa are drained by larger **interlobular ducts**. These interlobular ducts empty into a **main duct** that connects the entire gland to the lumen of the gastrointestinal tract.

Within the lobules reside the microscopic structural and functional secretory units of the gland. Each **secretory unit** is composed of an acinus and a small intercalated duct. The acinus represents a cluster of 15 to 100 acinar cells that synthesize and secrete proteins into the lumen of the epithelial structure. In the pancreas, acinar cells secrete ~20 different digestive zymogens (inactive enzyme precursors) and enzymes. In the salivary glands, the principal acinar cell protein products are α-amylase, mucins, and proline-rich proteins. Acinar cells from both the pancreas and salivary glands also secrete an isotonic, plasma-like fluid that accompanies the secretory proteins. In all, the final acinar secretion is a protein-rich product known as the *primary secretion*.

Each acinar lumen is connected to the proximal end of an **intercalated duct**. Distally, the intercalated ducts fuse with other small ducts to form progressively larger ducts that ultimately coalesce to form the intralobular duct that drains the lobule. Although the ducts provide a conduit for the transport of secretory proteins, the epithelial cells lining the ducts also play an important role in modifying the fluid and electrolyte composition of the primary secretion. Thus, the final exocrine gland secretion represents the combined product of two distinct epithelial cell populations, the acinar cell and the duct cell.

In addition to acini and ducts, exocrine glands contain a rich supply of nerves and blood vessels. Postganglionic **parasympathetic** and **sympathetic** fibers contribute to the autonomic regulation of secretion through the release of cholinergic, adrenergic, and peptide neurotransmitters that bind to receptors on the acinar and duct cells. Both central and reflex pathways contribute to the neural regulation of exocrine secretion. The autonomic nerves also carry afferent pain fibers that are activated by glandular inflammation and trauma. The vasculature not only provides oxygen and nutrients for the gland but also carries the hormones that help to regulate secretion.

Acinar cells are specialized protein-synthesizing cells

Acinar cells—such as those in the pancreas (Fig. 43-1B) and salivary glands—are polarized epithelial cells that are specialized for the production and export of large quantities of protein. Thus, the acinar cell is equipped with extensive rough endoplasmic reticulum (ER). However, the most characteristic feature of the acinar cell is the abundance of electron-dense secretory granules at the apical pole of the cell. These granules are storage pools of secretory proteins, and they are poised for releasing their contents after stimulation of the cell by neurohumoral agents. The secretory granules of pancreatic acinar cells contain the mixture of zymogens and enzymes required for digestion. The secretory granules of salivary acinar cells contain either α-amylase (in the parotid gland) or mucins (in the sublingual glands). Secretory granules in the pancreas appear uniform, whereas

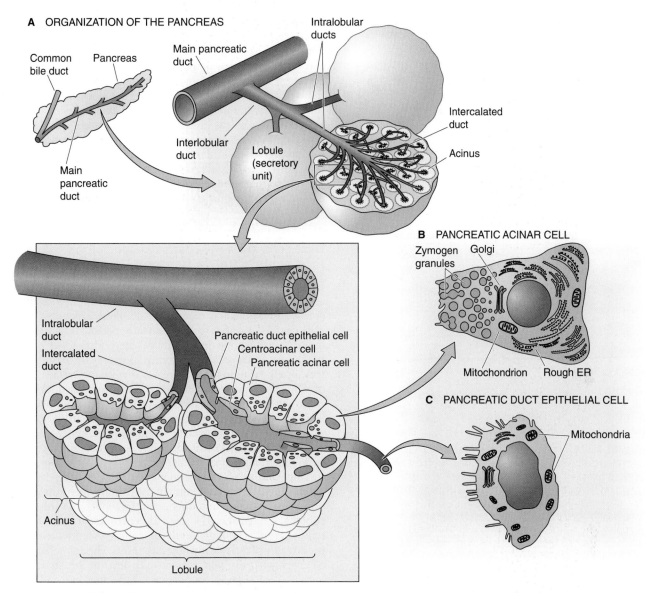

A ORGANIZATION OF THE PANCREAS

Common bile duct

Pancreas

Main pancreatic duct

Main pancreatic duct

Intralobular ducts

Interlobular duct

Lobule (secretory unit)

Intercalated duct

Acinus

Intralobular duct

Intercalated duct

Pancreatic duct epithelial cell
Centroacinar cell
Pancreatic acinar cell

Acinus

Lobule

B PANCREATIC ACINAR CELL

Zymogen granules   Golgi

Mitochondrion   Rough ER

C PANCREATIC DUCT EPITHELIAL CELL

Mitochondria

Figure 43-1 Acinus duct morphology. **A**, The fundamental secretory unit is composed of an acinus and an intercalated duct. Intercalated ducts merge to form intralobular ducts, which, in turn, merge to form interlobular ducts, and then the main pancreatic duct. **B**, The acinar cell is specialized for protein secretion. Large condensing vacuoles are gradually reduced in size and form mature zymogen granules that store digestive enzymes in the apical region of the acinar cell. **C**, The duct cell is a cuboidal cell with abundant mitochondria. Small microvilli project from its apical membrane.

those in the salivary glands often exhibit focal nodules of condensation within the granules known as *spherules*.

The pancreatic acinar cell has served as an important model for elucidating protein synthesis and export through the **secretory pathway**. Synthesis of secretory proteins (see Chapter 2) begins with the cellular uptake of amino acids and their incorporation into nascent proteins in the rough **ER** (Fig. 43-2). Vesicular transport mechanisms then shuttle the newly synthesized proteins to the Golgi complex.

Within the **Golgi complex**, secretory proteins are segregated away from lysosomal enzymes. Most lysosomal enzymes require the mannose 6-phosphate receptor for sorting to the lysosome (see Chapter 2). However, the signals

required to direct digestive enzymes into the secretory pathway remain unclear.

Secretory proteins exit the Golgi complex in **condensing vacuoles**. These large membrane-bound structures are acidic and maintain the lowest pH within the secretory pathway.

Maturation of the condensing vacuole to a secretory or zymogen granule is marked by condensation of the proteins within the vacuole and pinching off of membrane vesicles. The diameter of a **zymogen granule** is about two thirds that of a condensing vacuole, and its content is more electron dense. Secretory proteins are stored in zymogen granules that are located in the apical region of the acinar cell. The bottom portion of Figure 43-2 shows the results of a pulse-chase experiment that follows the cellular itinerary of radio-

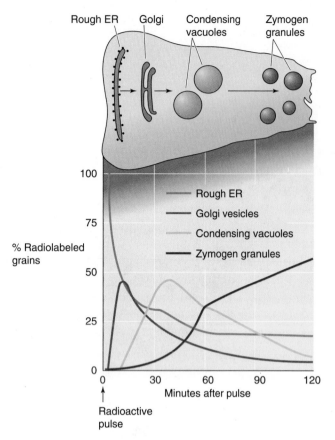

Figure 43-2 Movement of newly synthesized proteins through the secretory pathway. The cell model at the *top* illustrates the vectoral movement of nascent proteins through the compartments of the secretory pathway. The *four records* in the graph show the time course of secretory proteins moving through these compartments. To label newly synthesized proteins radioactively, the investigators briefly pulsed the pancreatic acinar cells with ³H-labeled amino acids. At specific times after the pulse, tissues were fixed, and the distribution of the radioactive amino acid was determined using autoradiography. Each of the four records shows the number of radiographic grains—as a fraction of all of the grains—found in each compartment at various times after the pulse. (*Data from Jamieson J, Palade G: J Cell Biol 1967; 34:597-615; and Jamieson J, Palade G: J Cell Biol 1971; 50:135-158.*)

labeled amino acids as they move sequentially through the four major compartments of the secretory pathway.

Exocytosis, the process by which secretory granules release their contents, is a complex series of events that involves the movement of the granules to the apical membrane, fusion of these granules with the membrane, and release of their contents into the acinar lumen. Secretion is triggered by either hormones or neural activity. At the onset of secretion, the area of the apical plasma membrane increases as much as 30-fold. Thereafter, activation of an apical endocytic pathway leads to retrieval of the secretory granule membrane for recycling and a decrease in the area of the apical plasma membrane back to its resting value. Thus, during the steady state of secretion, the secretory granule membrane is simultaneously delivered to and retrieved from the apical membrane.

The cytoskeleton of the acinar cell plays an important role in the regulation of exocytosis. A component of the actin network appears to be required for delivery of the secretory granules to the apical region of the cell. A second actin network, located immediately below the apical membrane, acts as a barrier that blocks fusion of the granules with the apical plasma membrane. On stimulation, this second network reorganizes and then releases the blockade to permit the secretory granules to approach the apical plasma membrane. Fusion of the granules with the plasma membrane probably requires the interaction of proteins on both the secretory granules and the apical plasma membrane, as well as various cytosolic factors (see Chapter 2). After fusion, the granule contents are released into the acinar lumen and are carried down the ducts into the gastrointestinal tract.

Duct cells are epithelial cells specialized for fluid and electrolyte transport

Pancreatic and salivary duct cells are polarized epithelial cells specialized for the transport of electrolytes across distinct apical and basolateral membrane domains. Duct epithelial cells contain specific membrane transporters and an abundance of mitochondria to provide energy for active transport, and they exhibit varying degrees of basolateral membrane infolding that increases membrane surface areas of pancreatic duct cells (Fig. 43-1C) and salivary duct cells. Although some duct cells contain prominent cytoplasmic vesicles, or storage granules—an indication of an additional protein secretory function, the synthetic machinery (i.e., ER and Golgi complex) of the duct cell is, in general, much less developed than that of the acinar cell.

Duct cells exhibit a considerable degree of morphologic heterogeneity along the length of the ductal tree. At the junction between acinar and duct cells in the pancreas are small cuboidal epithelial cells known as **centroacinar cells**. These cells express very high levels of carbonic anhydrase and presumably play a role in HCO_3^- secretion. The epithelial cells of the most proximal (intercalated) duct are squamous or low cuboidal, have an abundance of mitochondria, and tend to lack cytoplasmic vesicles. These features suggest that the primary function of these cells is fluid and electrolyte transport. Progressing distally, the cells become more cuboidal columnar and contain more cytoplasmic vesicles and granules. These features suggest that these cells are capable of both transport of fluid and electrolytes and secretion of proteins. Functional studies indicate that the types of solute transport proteins within duct cells differ depending on the cell's location in the ductal tree.

Ion transport in duct cells is regulated by neurohumoral stimuli that act through specific receptors located on the basolateral membrane. As is the case for cells elsewhere in the body, duct cells can increase transcellular electrolyte movement either by activating individual transport proteins or by increasing the number of transport proteins in the plasma membrane.

Goblet cells contribute to mucin production in exocrine glands

In addition to acinar and duct cells, exocrine glands contain varying numbers of goblet cells. These cells secrete high-molecular-weight glycoproteins known as **mucins**. When hydrated, mucins form **mucus** (see Chapter 2). Mucus has several important functions, including lubrication, hydration, and mechanical protection of surface epithelial cells. Mucins also play an important immunologic role by binding to pathogens and interacting with immune-competent cells. These properties may help to prevent infections. In the pancreas, mucin-secreting goblet cells are primarily found among the epithelial cells that line the large, distal ducts. They can account for as many as 25% of the epithelial cells in the distal main pancreatic duct of some species. In the salivary gland, goblet cells are also seen in the large distal ducts, although in less abundance than in the pancreas. However, in many salivary glands, mucin is also secreted by acinar cells.

PANCREATIC ACINAR CELL

The acinar cell secretes digestive proteins in response to stimulation

To study secretion at the cellular level, investigators use enzymes to digest pancreatic connective tissue and obtain single acini (small groups of 15 to 100 acinar cells), or they mechanically dissect single lobules (groups of 250 to 1000 cells). The measure of secretion is the release of digestive proteins into the incubation medium. The amount released over a fixed time interval is expressed as a percentage of the total content at the outset of the experiment. Because amylase is released in a fully active form, it is common to use the appearance of amylase activity as a marker for secretion by acinar cells.

When the acinar cells are in an unstimulated state, they secrete low levels of digestive proteins through a **constitu-tive secretory pathway**. Acinar cells stimulated by neurohumoral agents secrete proteins through a **regulated pathway**. Regulated secretion by acini and lobules in vitro is detected within 5 minutes of stimulation and is energy dependent. During a 30- to 60-minute stimulation period, acinar cells typically secrete 5 to 10 times more amylase than with constitutive release. However, during this period of regulated secretion, the cells typically secrete only 10% to 20% of the digestive proteins stored in their granules. Moreover, acinar cells are able to increase their rate of protein synthesis to replenish their stores.

The acinar cell may exhibit two distinct patterns of regulated secretion: monophasic and biphasic (Fig. 43-3A). An agonist that generates a *monophasic* dose-response relationship (e.g., gastrin-releasing peptide [GRP]) causes secretion to reach a maximal level that does not fall with higher concentrations of the agent. In contrast, a secretagogue that elicits a *biphasic* dose-response relationship (e.g., cholecystokinin [CCK] and carbachol) causes secretion to reach a maximal level that subsequently diminishes with higher concentrations of the agent. As discussed later, this biphasic response may reflect the presence of functionally separate high-affinity and low-affinity receptors and is related to the pathogenesis of acute pancreatitis (see the box entitled Acute Pancreatitis).

Regulated secretion of proteins by pancreatic acinar cells is mediated through cholecystokinin and muscarinic receptors

Although at least a dozen different receptors have been found on the plasma membrane of the pancreatic acinar cell, the most important in regulating protein secretion are the CCK receptors and the muscarinic acetylcholine (ACh) receptors. These receptors have many similarities: both are

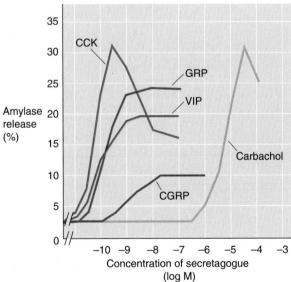

A PANCREATIC SECRETAGOGUES

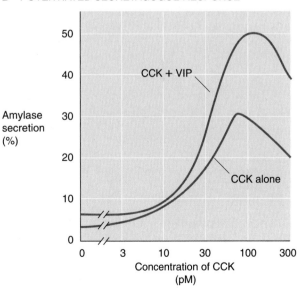

B POTENTIATED SECRETAGOGUE RESPONSE

Figure 43-3 Neurohumoral agents elicit different secretory responses from the pancreatic acinar cell. (**A**, Data from Jensen RT: In Johnson LR [ed]: Physiology of the Gastrointestinal Tract, pp 1377-1446. New York: Raven Press, 1994; **B**, Data from Burnham DB, McChesney DJ, Thurston KC, Williams JA: J Physiol 1984; 349:475-482.)

linked to the $G\alpha_q$ heterotrimeric G protein, both use the phospholipase C (PLC)/Ca^{2+} signal transduction pathway (see Chapter 3), and both lead to increased enzyme secretion from the acinar cell.

Two closely related CCK receptors are distinguished by their structure, affinity for ligands, and tissue distribution (see Chapter 42). Although both CCK receptors may be activated by CCK or gastrin, the CCK_A receptor has a much higher affinity for CCK than for gastrin, whereas the CCK_B receptor has approximately equal affinities for CCK and gastrin. In some species, both forms of the CCK receptor are present on the acinar cell.

An important feature of both CCK receptors is their ability to exist in both a high-affinity and a low-affinity state. Low (picomolar) concentrations of CCK activate the high-affinity forms of the CCK receptors and stimulate secretion. Conversely, supraphysiological (10- to 100-fold higher) concentrations of CCK activate the low-affinity forms of the receptors and inhibit secretion. As we explain in the next section, these two affinity states (i.e., activated by different concentrations of CCK) of each of the two CCK receptors generate distinct second-messenger signaling patterns. It is likely that, under physiological conditions, only the high-affinity states of the CCK or muscarinic receptor are activated. Stimulation of the lower-affinity states by supraphysiological concentrations of either CCK or ACh not only inhibits enzyme secretion but also may injure the acinar cell (see the box titled Acute Pancreatitis).

The muscarinic receptor on the acinar cell is probably of the M_3 subtype (see Chapter 14) found in many glandular tissues. Like the CCK receptor, the M_3 receptor is localized to the basolateral membrane of the cell. Numerous other receptors, including those for GRP, somatostatin, and vasoactive intestinal polypeptide (VIP; see Chapter 42); calcitonin gene–related peptide (CGRP; see Chapter 52), insulin (see Chapter 51), and secretin are also found on the pancreatic acinar cell. Although these other receptors may also play a role in regulating secretion, protein synthesis, growth, and transformation, their precise physiological functions remain to be clearly defined.

Activation of receptors that stimulate different signal transduction pathways may lead to an enhanced secretory response. For example, as shown in Figure 43-3B, simultaneous stimulation of the high-affinity CCK receptor (which acts through $[Ca^{2+}]_i$) and the VIP receptor (which acts through cAMP) generates an additive effect on secretion. Alternatively, acinar cells that have previously been stimulated may become temporarily refractory to subsequent stimulation. This phenomenon is known as *desensitization*.

Ca^{2+} is the major second messenger for the secretion of proteins by pancreatic acinar cells

Ca^{2+} Much of the pioneering work on the role of intracellular Ca^{2+} in cell signaling has been performed in the pancreatic acinar cell (Fig. 43-4A). Generation of a cytosolic Ca^{2+}

A SIGNAL-TRANSDUCTION PATHWAYS

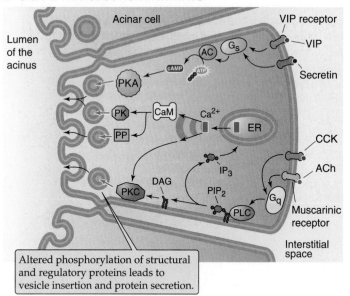

B CHANGES IN INTRACELLULAR $[Ca^{2+}]$

Altered phosphorylation of structural and regulatory proteins leads to vesicle insertion and protein secretion.

Figure 43-4 Stimulation of protein secretion from the pancreatic acinar cell. **A,** The pancreatic acinar cell has at least two pathways for stimulating the insertion of zymogen granules and thus releasing digestive enzymes. ACh and CCK both activate $G\alpha_q$, which stimulates PLC, which ultimately leads to the activation of PKC and the release of Ca^{2+}. Elevated $[Ca^{2+}]_i$ also activates calmodulin (CaM), which can activate protein kinases (PK) and phosphatases (PP). Finally, VIP and secretin both activate $G\alpha_s$, which stimulates adenylyl cyclase (AC), leading to the production of cAMP and the activation of PKA. **B,** Applying a physiological dose of CCK (i.e., 10 pM) triggers a series of $[Ca^{2+}]_i$ oscillations, as measured by a fluorescent dye. However, applying a supraphysiological concentration of CCK (1 nM) elicits a single large $[Ca^{2+}]_i$ spike and halts the oscillations. Recall that high levels of CCK also are less effective in causing amylase secretion. (**B,** *Data from Tsunoda Y, Stuenkel EL, Williams JA: Am J Physiol 1990; 259:G792-G801.*)

Chapter 43 • Pancreatic and Salivary Glands

signal is a complex summation of cellular events (see Chapter 3) that regulates cytosolic free Ca²⁺ levels ([Ca²⁺]ᵢ). Even when the acinar cell is in the resting state, [Ca²⁺]ᵢ oscillates slowly. In the presence of maximal stimulatory (i.e., physiological) concentrations of CCK or ACh, the frequency of the oscillations increases (Fig. 43-4B), but little change in their amplitude is noted. This increase in the frequency of [Ca²⁺]ᵢ oscillations is required for protein secretion by acinar cells. In contrast, supramaximal (i.e., hyperstimulatory) concentrations of CCK or ACh generate a sudden, large spike in [Ca²⁺]ᵢ and eliminate additional [Ca²⁺]ᵢ oscillations. This [Ca²⁺]ᵢ spike and the subsequent absence of oscillations are associated with an inhibition of secretion that appears to be mediated by disruption of the cytoskeletal components that are required for secretion.

cGMP Physiological stimulation of the acinar cell by either CCK or ACh also generates a rapid and prominent increase in [cGMP]ᵢ levels. The increase in [cGMP]ᵢ has been linked to nitric oxide metabolism; inhibition of nitric oxide synthase (see Chapter 3) blocks the increase in [cGMP]ᵢ after secretagogue stimulation. Some evidence suggests that cGMP may be involved in regulating Ca²⁺ entry and storage in the acinar cell.

cAMP Secretin, VIP, and CCK increase cAMP production and thus activate protein kinase A (PKA) activity in pancreatic acinar cells. Low concentrations of CCK cause transient stimulation of PKA, whereas supraphysiological concentrations of CCK cause a much more prominent and prolonged increase in [cAMP]ᵢ and PKA activity. ACh, however, has little, if any, effect on the cAMP signaling pathway.

Effectors As summarized in Figure 43-4A, the most important effectors of intracellular second messengers are the protein kinases. Stimulation of CCK and muscarinic receptors on the acinar cell leads to the generation of similar Ca²⁺ signals and activation of calmodulin-dependent protein kinases and members of the protein kinase C (PKC) family (see Chapter 3). Activation of secretin or VIP receptors increases [cAMP]ᵢ and thus activates PKA. These second messengers probably also activate protein phosphatases, as well as other protein kinases not depicted in Figure 43-4A. The protein targets of activated kinases and phosphatases in the pancreatic acinar cell are largely unknown. However, some are involved in regulating secretion, whereas others mediate protein synthesis, growth, transformation, and cell death.

In addition to proteins, the pancreatic acinar cell also secretes a plasma-like fluid

In addition to protein, acinar cells in the pancreas secrete an isotonic, plasma-like fluid (Fig. 43-5). This NaCl-rich fluid hydrates the dense, protein-rich material that the acinar cells secrete. The fundamental transport event is the secretion of Cl⁻ across the apical membrane. For transcellular (plasma to lumen) movement of Cl⁻ to occur, Cl⁻ must move into the cell across the basolateral membrane. As in many other Cl⁻-secreting epithelial cells (see Chapter 5), basolateral Cl⁻

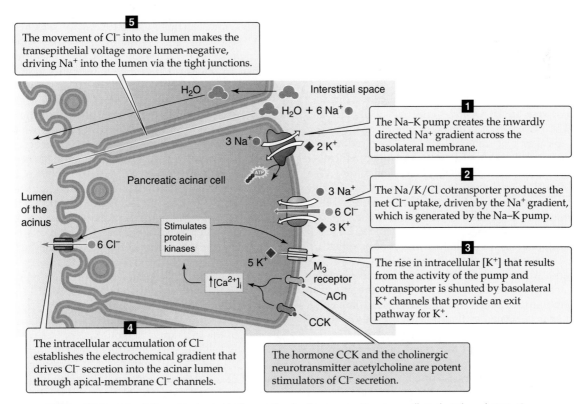

Figure 43-5 Stimulation of isotonic NaCl secretion by the pancreatic acinar cell. Both ACh and CCK stimulate NaCl secretion, probably through phosphorylation of basolateral and apical ion channels.

uptake by the acinar cell occurs through an Na/K/Cl cotransporter. The Na-K pump generates the Na^+ gradient that energizes the Na/K/Cl cotransporter. The K^+ entering through the Na-K pump and through the Na/K/Cl cotransporter exits through K^+ channels that are also located on the basolateral membrane. Thus, a pump, a cotransporter, and a channel are necessary to sustain the basolateral uptake of Cl^- into the acinar cell.

The rise in $[Cl^-]_i$ produced by basolateral Cl^- uptake drives the secretion of Cl^- down its electrochemical gradient through channels in the apical membrane. As the transepithelial voltage becomes more lumen negative, Na^+ moves through the cation-selective paracellular pathway (i.e., tight junctions) to join the Cl^- secreted into the lumen. Water also moves through this paracellular pathway, as well as through aquaporin water channels on the apical and basolateral membranes. Therefore, the net effect of these acinar cell transport processes is the production of an isotonic, NaCl-rich fluid that accounts for ~25% of total pancreatic fluid secretion.

Like the secretion of protein by acinar cells, secretion of fluid and electrolytes is stimulated by secretagogues that raise $[Ca^{2+}]_i$. In the pancreas, activation of muscarinic receptors by cholinergic neural pathways and activation of CCK receptors by humoral pathways increase the membrane conductance of the acinar cell. A similar effect is seen with GRP. Apical membrane Cl^- channels and basolateral membrane K^+ channels appear to be the effector targets of the activated Ca^{2+} signaling pathway. Phosphorylation of these channels by Ca^{2+}-dependent kinases is one likely mechanism that underlies the increase in open-channel probability that accompanies stimulation.

PANCREATIC DUCT CELL

The pancreatic duct cell secretes isotonic $NaHCO_3$

The principal physiological function of the pancreatic duct cell is to secrete an HCO_3^--rich fluid that alkalinizes and hydrates the protein-rich primary secretions of the acinar cell. The apical step of transepithelial HCO_3^- secretion (Fig. 43-6) is mediated in part by a **Cl-HCO₃ exchanger**, a member of the SLC26 family (see Chapter 5) that secretes intracellular HCO_3^- into the duct lumen. Luminal Cl^- must be available for this exchange process to occur. Although some luminal Cl^- is present in the primary secretions of the acinar cell, anion channels on the apical membrane of the duct cell provide additional Cl^- to the lumen in a process called *Cl⁻ recycling*. The most important of these anion channels is the **cystic fibrosis transmembrane conductance regulator (CFTR)**, a cAMP-activated Cl^- channel that is present on the apical membrane of pancreatic duct cells (see Chapter 5). Cl^- recycling is facilitated by the co-activation of CFTR and SLC26 exchangers through direct protein-protein interactions. In some species, such as the rat and mouse, pancreatic duct cells also contain a Ca^{2+}-activated Cl^- channel on the apical membrane; this channel also provides Cl^- to the lumen for recycling. Apical Cl^- channels may also directly serve as conduits for HCO_3^- movement from the duct cell to the lumen.

The intracellular HCO_3^- that exits the duct cell across the apical membrane arises from two pathways. The first is direct uptake of HCO_3^- through an electrogenic Na/HCO₃ cotransporter (NBCe1), which presumably operates with an Na^+/HCO_3^- stoichiometry of $1:2$. The second mechanism is the generation of intracellular HCO_3^- from CO_2 and OH^-, catalyzed by carbonic anhydrase. The OH^- in this reaction is derived, along with H^+, from H_2O. Thus, the H^+ that accumulates in the cell must be extruded across the basolateral membrane. One mechanism of H^+ extrusion is Na-H exchange. The second mechanism for H^+ extrusion across the basolateral membrane, at least in some species, is an ATP-dependent H^+ pump. Pancreatic duct cells contain acidic intracellular vesicles (presumably containing vacuolar-type H^+ pumps) that are mobilized to the basolateral membrane of the cell after stimulation by secretin, a powerful secretagogue (see later). Indeed, H^+ pumps are most active under conditions of neurohumoral stimulation. Thus, three basolateral transporters directly or indirectly provide the intracellular HCO_3^- that pancreatic duct cells need for secretion: (1) the electrogenic Na/HCO₃ cotransporter, (2) the Na-H exchanger, and (3) the H^+ pump. The physiological importance of these three acid-base transporters in humans has yet to be fully established. The pancreatic duct cell accounts for ~75% of total pancreatic fluid secretion.

Secretin (through cAMP) and acetylcholine (through Ca^{2+}) both stimulate HCO_3^- secretion by the pancreatic duct

When stimulated, the epithelial cells of the pancreatic duct secrete an isotonic $NaHCO_3$ solution. The duct cells have receptors for secretin, ACh, GRP (all of which stimulate HCO_3^- secretion) and substance P (which inhibits it). Although some evidence indicates that CCK modulates ductular secretory processes, CCK receptors have not been identified on these cells.

Secretin is the most important humoral regulator of ductal HCO_3^- secretion. Activation of the secretin receptor on the duct cell stimulates adenylyl cyclase, which raises $[cAMP]_i$. Because forskolin and cAMP analogues stimulate ductal HCO_3^- secretion, the secretin response has been attributed to its effect on $[cAMP]_i$ and activation of PKA. However, even low concentrations of secretin that do not measurably increase $[cAMP]_i$ can stimulate HCO_3^- secretion. This observation suggests that the secretin response may be mediated by (1) unmeasurably small increases in total cellular cAMP, (2) cAMP increases that are localized to small intracellular compartments, or (3) activation of alternative second-messenger pathways. Secretin acts by stimulating the apical CFTR Cl^- channel and the basolateral Na/HCO₃ cotransporter, without affecting the Na-H exchanger.

HCO_3^- secretion is also regulated by the parasympathetic division of the autonomic nervous system (see Chapter 14). The postganglionic parasympathetic neurotransmitter **ACh** increases $[Ca^{2+}]_i$ and activates Ca^{2+}-dependent protein kinases (PKC and the calmodulin-dependent protein kinases) in pancreatic duct cells. The ACh effect is inhibited by atropine, a finding indicating that this neurotransmitter is acting through **muscarinic receptors** on the duct cell. Although

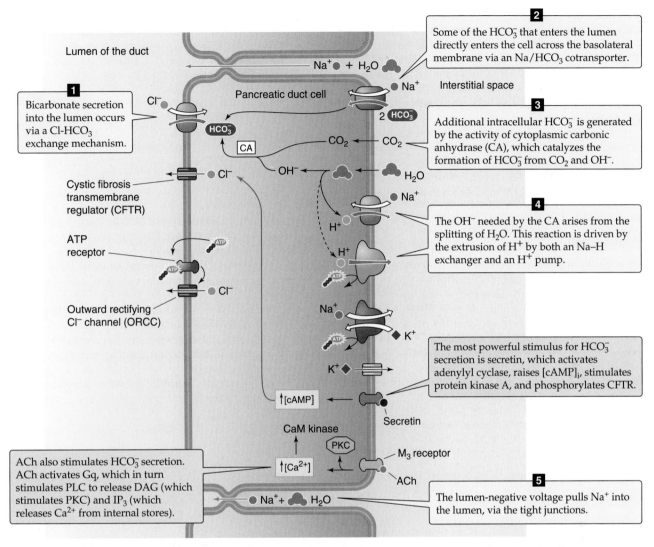

1 Bicarbonate secretion into the lumen occurs via a Cl-HCO₃ exchange mechanism.

2 Some of the HCO₃⁻ that enters the lumen directly enters the cell across the basolateral membrane via an Na/HCO₃ cotransporter.

3 Additional intracellular HCO₃⁻ is generated by the activity of cytoplasmic carbonic anhydrase (CA), which catalyzes the formation of HCO₃⁻ from CO₂ and OH⁻.

4 The OH⁻ needed by the CA arises from the splitting of H₂O. This reaction is driven by the extrusion of H⁺ by both an Na–H exchanger and an H⁺ pump.

The most powerful stimulus for HCO₃⁻ secretion is secretin, which activates adenylyl cyclase, raises [cAMP]ᵢ, stimulates protein kinase A, and phosphorylates CFTR.

ACh also stimulates HCO₃⁻ secretion. ACh activates Gq, which in turn stimulates PLC to release DAG (which stimulates PKC) and IP₃ (which releases Ca²⁺ from internal stores).

5 The lumen-negative voltage pulls Na⁺ into the lumen, via the tight junctions.

Cystic fibrosis transmembrane regulator (CFTR)

ATP receptor

Outward rectifying Cl⁻ channel (ORCC)

Figure 43-6 HCO₃⁻ secretion by the cells of the pancreatic duct. Secretin activates the cAMP signaling pathway and opens the CFTR Cl⁻ channels through phosphorylation. Cl⁻ movement out of the cell leads to basolateral membrane depolarization, thus generating the electrical gradient that favors NaHCO₃ cotransport.

ductular secretion in the rat is also stimulated by **GRP**, the second messenger mediating this effect is not known. Unlike the effect on the acinar cell, GRP does not increase [Ca²⁺]ᵢ in the duct cell. GRP also does not raise [cAMP]ᵢ.

In the rat, both basal and stimulated ductular HCO₃⁻ secretion is inhibited by **substance P**. The second messenger mediating this effect is also unknown. Because substance P inhibits HCO₃⁻ secretion regardless of whether the secretagogue is secretin, ACh, or GRP—which apparently act through three different signal transduction mechanisms—substance P probably acts at a site that is distal to the generation of second messengers, such as by inhibiting the Cl-HCO₃ exchanger.

Apical membrane chloride channels are important sites of neurohumoral regulation

In the regulation of pancreatic duct cells by the neurohumoral mechanisms just discussed, the only effector proteins that have been identified as targets of the protein kinases and phosphatases are the apical Cl⁻ channels, basolateral K⁺ channels, and the Na/HCO₃ cotransporter. CFTR functions as a low-conductance, apical Cl⁻ channel (see Chapter 5). CFTR has nucleotide-binding domains that control channel opening and closing as well as a regulatory domain with multiple potential PKA and PKC phosphorylation sites. Neurohumoral agents that control fluid and electrolyte secretion by the pancreatic duct cells act at this site. Agents that activate PKA are the most important regulators of CFTR function. PKC activation enhances the stimulatory effect of PKA on CFTR Cl⁻ transport, but alone it appears to have little direct effect on CFTR function. Thus, the CFTR Cl⁻ channel is regulated by ATP through two types of mechanisms: interaction with the nucleotide-binding domains and protein phosphorylation (see Fig. 5-10B).

In addition to CFTR, pancreatic duct cells in some species have an outwardly rectifying Cl⁻ channel (ORCC) on the apical membrane. This channel, which has been identified in a variety of epithelial cells, can be activated by increases in $[cAMP]_i$ or $[Ca^{2+}]_i$. Studies suggest that part of the effect of cAMP on ORCCs may be indirect and may occur through CFTR. The working hypothesis is that stimulation of CFTR somehow promotes ATP efflux from the cell to the lumen and that the ATP binds to an apical purinergic receptor to activate ORCCs in an autocrine/paracrine fashion (Fig. 43-6).

In rat pancreatic duct cells, Ca^{2+}-sensitive basolateral K^+ channels seem to be targets of neurohumoral stimulation. Activators of the cAMP pathway stimulate phosphorylation by PKA, thus enhancing the responsiveness of these channels to $[Ca^{2+}]_i$ and increasing their probability of being open.

Pancreatic duct cells may also secrete glycoproteins

Although the primary function of the pancreatic duct cells is to secrete HCO_3^- and water, these cells may also synthesize and secrete various high-molecular-weight proteoglycans. Some of these proteins are structurally distinct from the mucin that is produced by the specialized goblet cells in the duct. Unlike the proteins that are secreted by acinar cells, the glycoproteins synthesized in duct cells are not accumulated in large secretion granules. Rather, they appear to be continuously synthesized and secreted from small cytoplasmic vesicles. Secretin increases the secretion of glycoproteins

from these cells, but this action appears to result from stimulation of glycoprotein synthesis, rather than from stimulation of vesicular transport or exocytosis itself. The role of these proteins may be to protect against protease-mediated injury to mucosal cells.

COMPOSITION, FUNCTION, AND CONTROL OF PANCREATIC SECRETION

Pancreatic juice is a protein-rich, alkaline secretion

Humans produce ~1.5 L of pancreatic fluid each day. The pancreas has the highest rates of protein synthesis and secretion of any organ in the body. Each day, the pancreas delivers between 15 and 100 g of protein into the small intestine. The level of pancreatic secretion is determined by a balance between factors that stimulate secretion and those that inhibit it.

The human pancreas secretes more than 20 proteins, some of which are listed in Table 43-1. Most of these proteins are either inactive digestive enzyme precursors—**zymogens**—or active digestive enzymes. The secretory proteins responsible for digestion can be classified according to their substrates: **proteases** hydrolyze proteins, **amylases** digest carbohydrates, **lipases** and phospholipases break down

---

Cystic Fibrosis

CF is the most common lethal genetic disease in whites, in whom it affects ~1 in 2000. Approximately 1 in 20 whites carry the autosomal recessive genetic defect. Clinically, CF is characterized by progressive pancreatic and pulmonary insufficiency resulting from the complications of organ obstruction by thickened secretions. The disease results from mutations in the *CF* gene (located on chromosome 7) that alter the function of its product, CFTR (see Fig. 5-10). **CFTR** is a cAMP-activated Cl^- channel that is present on the apical plasma membrane of many epithelial cells. In the pancreas, CFTR has been localized to the apical membrane of duct cells, where it functions to provide the luminal Cl^- for Cl-HCO_3 exchange (Fig. 43-6).

Most *CF* gene mutations result in the production of a CFTR molecule that is abnormally folded after its synthesis in the ER. The ER quality control system recognizes these molecules as defective, and most mutant CFTR molecules are prematurely degraded before they reach the plasma membrane. Subsequent loss of CFTR expression at the plasma membrane disrupts the apical transport processes of the duct cell and results in decreased secretion of HCO_3^- and water by the ducts. As a result, protein-rich primary (acinar) secretions thicken within the duct lumen and lead to ductal obstruction and eventual tissue destruction. Pathologically, the ducts appear dilated and obstructed, and fibrotic tissue and fat gradually replace the pancreatic parenchyma—hence the original cystic fibrosis designation. The subsequent deficiency of pancreatic enzymes that occurs leads to the maldigestion of nutrients and thus the excretion of fat in the stool (steatorrhea) by patients with CF. Before the development of oral enzyme replacement therapy, many patients with CF died of complications of malnutrition.

Now, the major cause of morbidity and mortality in CF is progressive pulmonary disease. The pathophysiology of lung disease in CF is more complex than that of pancreatic disease. A major finding is that the airway mucus is thick and viscous as a result of insufficient fluid secretion into the airway lumen. The pulmonary epithelium probably both secretes fluid (in a mechanism that requires CFTR) and absorbs fluid (in a mechanism that requires apical ENaC Na^+ channels). In CF, the reduced activity of CFTR shifts the balance more toward absorption, and a thick mucous layer is generated that inhibits the ciliary clearance of foreign bodies (see Chapter 26). The results are increased rate and severity of infections and thus inflammatory processes that contribute to the destructive process in the lung.

The pulmonary symptoms most commonly bring the patient to the physician's attention in early childhood. Cough and recurrent respiratory infections that are difficult to eradicate are usually the first indications of the illness. The child's sputum is particularly thick and viscous. Pulmonary function progressively declines over the ensuing years, and patients may also experience frequent and severe infections, atelectasis (collapse of lung parenchyma), bronchiectasis (chronic dilatation of the bronchi), and recurrent pneumothoraces (air in the intrapleural space). In addition to the pancreatic and pulmonary manifestations, CF also causes a characteristic increase in the [NaCl] of sweat, which is intermediate in heterozygotes. Pharmacological approaches that bypass the Cl^- transport defect in a lung with CF are currently being evaluated, and considerable effort is being directed toward the development of in vivo gene transfer techniques to correct the underlying genetic defect.

Table 43-1 Pancreatic Acinar Cell Secretory Products

DIGESTIVE PROTEINS	
Zymogens	**Function**
Trypsinogens	Digestion
Chymotrypsinogen	Digestion
Proelastase	Digestion
Proprotease E	Digestion
Procarboxypeptidase A	Digestion
Procarboxypeptidase B	Digestion
ACTIVE ENZYMES	
α-Amylase	Digestion
Carboxyl ester lipase	Digestion
Lipase	Digestion
RNAase	Digestion
DNAase	Digestion
Colipase	Digestion
OTHERS	
Trypsin inhibitor	Blockade of trypsin activity
Lithostathine	Possible prevention of stone formation; constituent of protein plugs
GP2	Endocytosis?; formation of protein plugs
Pancreatitis-associated protein	Bacteriostasis?
Na^+, Cl^-, H_2O	Hydration of secretions
Ca^{2+}	?

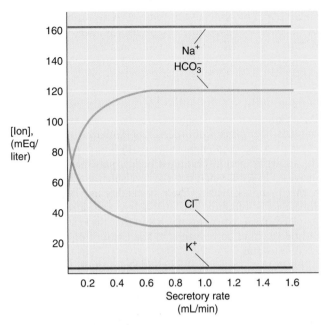

Figure 43-7 Flow dependence of the electrolyte composition of pancreatic fluid. In this experiment on a cat, increasing the level of secretin not only increases the rate at which fluids flow out of the pancreas but also changes the composition of the fluid. *(Data from Case RM, Harper AA, Scratcherd T: J Physiol 1969; 201:563-596.)*

lipids, and **nucleases** digest nucleic acids. The functions of other secretory proteins—such as glycoprotein II (GP2), lithostathine, and pancreatitis-associated protein—are less well defined.

GP2 is an unusual protein with an N-terminal glycosyl phosphatidylinositol moiety that links it to the inner leaflet of the zymogen granule membrane. GP2 has been implicated in the regulation of endocytosis. After exocytosis, luminal cleavage of the GP2 linkage to the zymogen granule membrane seems to be necessary for proper trafficking of the zymogen granule membrane back into the cell from the plasma membrane. Under certain circumstances, the released GP2—and also **lithostathine**—may form protein aggregates in the pancreatic juice. This finding is not surprising inasmuch as GP2 is structurally related to the Tamm-Horsfall protein, which is secreted by the renal thick ascending limb (see Chapter 33). The tendency of GP2 and lithostathine to form aggregates may have detrimental clinical consequences in that both proteins have been implicated in the pathologic formation of protein plugs that can obstruct the lumen of acini in patients with cystic fibrosis and chronic pancreatitis.

Pancreatitis-associated protein is a secretory protein that is present in low concentrations in the normal state. However, levels of this protein may increase up to several hundred-fold during the early phases of pancreatic injury. Pancreatitis-associated protein is a bacteriostatic agent that may help to prevent pancreatic infection during bouts of pancreatitis.

Pancreatic juice is also rich in Ca^{2+} and HCO_3^-. **Calcium** concentrations are in the millimolar range inside the organelles of the secretory pathway of the acinar cells. These high levels of Ca^{2+} may be required to induce the aggregation of secretory proteins and to direct them into the secretory pathway. **Bicarbonate** secreted by duct cells neutralizes the acidic gastric secretions that enter the duodenum and allows digestive enzymes to function properly; HCO_3^- also facilitates the micellar solubilization of lipids and mucosal cell function. The $[HCO_3^-]$ in pancreatic juice increases with increases in the secretory flow rate (Fig. 43-7). In the unstimulated state, the flow is low, and the electrolyte composition of pancreatic juice closely resembles that of blood plasma. As the gland is stimulated and flow increases, exchange of Cl^- in the pancreatic juice for HCO_3^- across the apical membrane of the duct cells produces a secretory product that is more alkaline (pH of ~8.1) and has a lower [Cl⁻]. Concentrations of Na⁺ or K⁺, however, are not significantly altered by changes in flow.

In the fasting state, levels of secreted pancreatic enzymes oscillate at low levels

Pancreatic secretion is regulated in both the fasted and fed states. Under basal conditions, the pancreas releases low levels of pancreatic enzymes (Fig. 43-8). However, during the digestive period (eating a meal), pancreatic secretion increases in sequential phases to levels that are 5- to 20-fold higher than basal levels. The systems that regulate secretion appear to be redundant; if one system fails, a second takes its place. These mechanisms ensure that the release of pancreatic enzymes corresponds to the amount of food in the small intestine.

Like other organs in the upper gastrointestinal tract, the pancreas has a basal rate of secretion even when food is not being eaten or digested. During this **interdigestive (fasting) period**, pancreatic secretions vary cyclically and correspond to sequential changes in the motility of the small intestine (see Chapter 41). Pancreatic secretion is minimal when intestinal motility is in its quiescent phase (phase I); biliary and gastric secretions are also minimal at this time. As duodenal motility increases (phase II), so does pancreatic secretion. During the interdigestive period, enzyme secretion is maximal when intestinal motility—the migrating motor complexes (MMCs; see Fig. 41-6)—is also maximal (phase III). However, even this maximal interdigestive secretory rate is only 10% to 20% of that stimulated by a meal. The peak phases of interdigestive intestinal motor activity and pancreatic secretory activity are followed by a declining period (phase IV). *Fluid and electrolyte secretion* rates during

the interdigestive phase are usually less than 5% of maximum levels.

The cyclic pattern of interdigestive pancreatic secretion is mediated by intrinsic and extrinsic mechanisms. The predominant mechanism of pancreatic regulation is through **parasympathetic** pathways. Telenzepine, an antagonist of the M_1 muscarinic ACh receptor, reduces interdigestive enzyme secretion by more than 85% during phases II and III. Although cholinergic pathways are the major regulators of interdigestive pancreatic secretion, CCK and adrenergic pathways also play a role. CCK appears to stimulate pancreatic enzyme secretion during phases I and II. In contrast, basal α-**adrenergic** tone appears to suppress interdigestive pancreatic secretion. Although human and canine pancreas denervated during transplantation exhibits cyclic secretion, this secretion is no longer synchronous with duodenal motor activity. These observations support a role for the autonomic nervous system in regulating basal (resting) pancreatic secretion.

Cholecystokinin from duodenal I cells stimulates enzyme secretion by the acini, and secretin from S cells stimulates HCO₃⁻ and fluid secretion by the ducts

CCK plays a central role in regulating pancreatic secretion. CCK is released from neuroendocrine cells (**I cells**; see Table 41-1) present in the duodenal mucosa and acts on pancreatic acinar cells to increase protein secretion (Fig. 43-4). In response to a meal, plasma CCK levels increase 5- to 10-fold within 10 to 30 minutes. Three lines of evidence show that CCK is a physiological mediator of pancreatic protein secretion: (1) CCK levels increase in the serum in response to a meal, (2) administration of exogenous CCK at the same

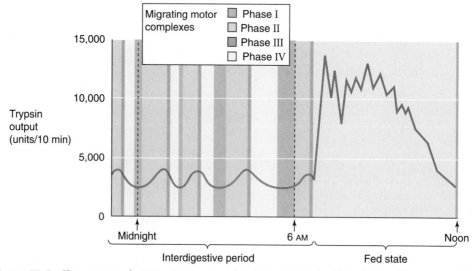

Figure 43-8 Time course of pancreatic secretion during fasting and feeding. The interdigestive output of secretory products (e.g., trypsin) by the pancreas varies cyclically and in rough synchrony with the four phases of motor activity (MMCs) of the small intestine, shown by *colored vertical bands*. During the fed state, one notes a massive and sustained increase in trypsin release by the pancreas, as well as a switch of small intestine motility to the fed state. *(Data from DiMagno EP, Layer P: In Go VLW, DiMagno EP, Gardner JD, et al [eds]: The Pancreas: Biology, Pathobiology and Disease, 2nd ed, pp 275-300. New York: Raven Press, 1993.)*

levels produced by a meal stimulates pancreatic protein secretion to higher levels than those generated by a meal (the meal may also stimulate the release of inhibitory factors in addition to CCK), and (3) a specific CCK inhibitor reduces pancreatic protein secretion by more than 50%.

The most potent stimulator of CCK release from I cells is **lipid**. Protein digestive products (i.e., peptones, amino acids) also increase CCK release, but carbohydrate and acid have little effect. CCK secretion may also be stimulated by **CCK-releasing factors**, which are peptides released by mucosal cells of the duodenum or secreted by the pancreas. The level of these releasing factors may reflect a balance between the relative amounts of nutrients and digestive enzymes that are present in the gut lumen at any one time, so the level of the factors reflects the digestive milieu of the duodenum. In the fasting state, luminal CCK releasing factors are degraded by digestive enzymes that accompany basal pancreatic secretion, so little releasing factor remains to stimulate the I cells. However, during a meal, the digestive enzymes are diverted to the digestion of ingested nutrients entering the gut lumen, and the CCK-releasing factors are spared degradation. Hence, the relative level of proteins to proteases in the small intestine determines the amount of CCK-releasing factor available to drive CCK release and thus pancreatic secretion.

CCK acts on the acinar cell through both direct and indirect pathways: it directly stimulates enzyme secretion through a CCK_A receptor on the acinar cell (Fig. 43-4), and it may indirectly stimulate enzyme secretion by activating the parasympathetic (cholinergic) nervous system. As we see later, the parasympathetic pathway plays a major role in mediating the intestinal phase of pancreatic secretion. Vagal stimulation can drive pancreatic secretion to nearly maximum levels. Atropine, an antagonist of muscarinic ACh receptors (see Chapter 14), reduces the secretion of enzymes and HCO_3^- during the intestinal phase of a meal. Atropine also inhibits secretion in response to stimulation by physiological levels of exogenous CCK. Together, these findings suggest that CCK somehow stimulates the parasympathetic pathway, which, in turn, stimulates muscarinic receptors on the acinar cell.

Like CCK, **GRP**—which is structurally related to bombesin—may also be a physiological regulator of pancreatic enzyme secretion. Stimulation of acinar cells with GRP leads to enzyme secretion. In contrast to the hormone CCK, the major source of GRP appears to be the vagal nerve terminals.

Secretin is the most potent humoral stimulator of fluid and HCO_3^- secretion by the pancreas (Fig. 43-6). Secretin is released from neuroendocrine cells (S cells) in the mucosa of the small intestine in response to duodenal acidification and, to a lesser extent, bile acids and lipids. To stimulate secretin secretion, duodenal pH must fall to less than 4.5. Like CCK, secretin levels increase after the ingestion of a meal. However, when these levels are reached experimentally by administration of exogenous secretin, pancreatic HCO_3^- secretion is less than that generated by a meal. These findings suggest that secretin is acting in concert with CCK, ACh, and other agents to stimulate HCO_3^- secretion.

In addition to hormones of intestinal origin, **insulin** and other hormones secreted by the islets of Langerhans within the pancreas (see Chapter 51) may also influence pancreatic exocrine secretion. Blood flow from the pancreatic islets moves to the exocrine pancreas through a portal system. This organization allows high concentrations of islet hormones to interact with pancreatic acinar cells. One result of this arrangement may be that insulin modifies the composition of digestive enzymes within the acinar cell and increases the relative levels of amylase.

Regulation of exocrine pancreatic secretion is complex, and understanding this process has been made difficult by the following: (1) tissue levels of an exogenously infused hormone may not match those generated physiologically; (2) because several neurohumoral factors are released in response to a meal, the infusion of a single agent may not accurately reflect its physiological role; (3) specific neurohumoral inhibitors are often unavailable; and (4) pancreatic responses may differ depending on the species.

A meal triggers cephalic, gastric, and intestinal phases of pancreatic secretion that are mediated by a complex network of neurohumoral interactions

The digestive period has been divided into three phases (Table 43-2) based on the site at which food acts to stimulate pancreatic secretion, just as for gastric secretion (see Chapter 42). These three phases (cephalic, gastric, and intestinal) are sequential and follow the progression of a meal from its initial smell and taste to its movement through the gastrointestinal tract (Fig. 43-9). These phases act in a coordinated fashion to maximize efficiency of the digestive process. For example, stimulation of secretion before the entry of food into the small intestine during the cephalic and gastric phases ensures that active enzymes are present when food arrives. Conversely, suppression of secretion during the late digestive phase suppresses the release of pancreatic enzymes when nutrients are no longer present in the proximal end of the small intestine.

The Cephalic Phase During the cephalic phase, the sight, taste, and smell of food usually generate only a modest

Table 43-2 The Three Phases of Pancreatic Secretion

Phase	Stimulant	Regulatory Pathway	Percentage of Maximum Enzyme Secretion
Cephalic	Sight Smell Taste Mastication	Vagal pathways	25%
Gastric	Distention Gastrin?	Vagal-cholinergic	10%-20%
Intestinal	Amino acids Fatty acids H+	Cholecystokinin Secretin Enteropancreatic reflexes	50%-80%

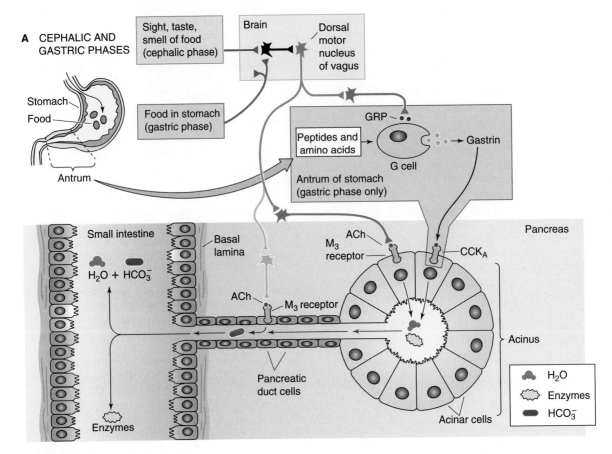

A CEPHALIC AND GASTRIC PHASES

Sight, taste, smell of food (cephalic phase)

Brain

Dorsal motor nucleus of vagus

Stomach

Food

Food in stomach (gastric phase)

Antrum

GRP

Peptides and amino acids

G cell

Gastrin

Antrum of stomach (gastric phase only)

Small intestine

Basal lamina

$H_2O + HCO_3^-$

ACh

M_3 receptor

CCK$_A$

ACh

M_3 receptor

Pancreas

Pancreatic duct cells

Acinus

Enzymes

Acinar cells

	H_2O
	Enzymes
	HCO_3^-

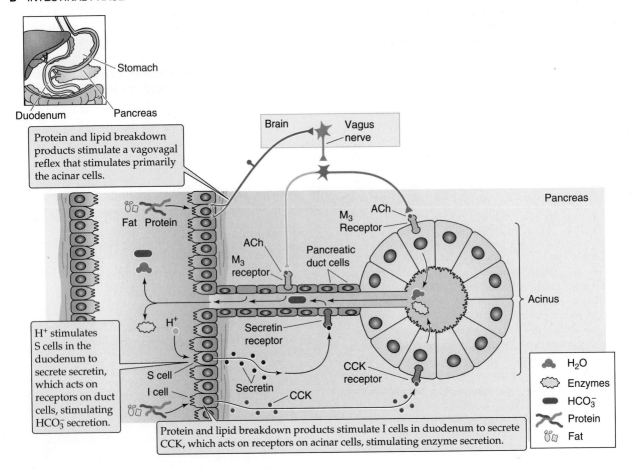

B INTESTINAL PHASE

Stomach

Duodenum

Pancreas

Protein and lipid breakdown products stimulate a vagovagal reflex that stimulates primarily the acinar cells.

Brain

Vagus nerve

Fat Protein

ACh

M_3 Receptor

ACh

M_3 receptor

Pancreatic duct cells

Pancreas

H^+

Secretin receptor

H^+ stimulates S cells in the duodenum to secrete secretin, which acts on receptors on duct cells, stimulating HCO_3^- secretion.

S cell

I cell

Secretin

CCK

CCK receptor

Acinus

Protein and lipid breakdown products stimulate I cells in duodenum to secrete CCK, which acts on receptors on acinar cells, stimulating enzyme secretion.

	H_2O
	Enzymes
	HCO_3^-
	Protein
	Fat

Figure 43-9 Three phases of pancreatic secretion. **A,** During the cephalic phase, the sight, taste, or smell of food stimulates pancreatic acinar cells, through the vagus nerve and muscarinic cholinergic receptors, to release digestive enzymes and, to a lesser extent, stimulates duct cells to secrete HCO_3^- and fluid. The release of gastrin from G cells is not important during this phase. During the gastric phase, the presence of food in the stomach stimulates pancreatic secretions—primarily from the acinar cells—through two routes. First, distention of the stomach activates a vagovagal reflex. Second, protein digestion products (peptones) stimulate G cells in the antrum of the stomach to release gastrin, which is a poor agonist of the CCK_A receptors on acinar cells. **B,** The arrival of gastric acid in the duodenum stimulates S cells to release secretin, which stimulates duct cells to secrete HCO_3^- and fluid. Protein and lipid breakdown products have two effects. First, they stimulate I cells to release CCK, which causes acinar cells to release digestive enzymes. Second, they stimulate afferent pathways that initiate a vagovagal reflex that primarily stimulates the acinar cells through M_3 cholinergic receptors.

increase in fluid and electrolyte secretion (Fig. 43-9A). However, these factors have prominent effects on enzyme secretion. In most animal species, enzyme secretion increases to 25% to 50% of the maximum rate evoked by exogenous CCK. In humans, the cephalic phase is short-lived and dissipates rapidly when food is removed. The cephalic phase is mediated by neural pathways. In the dog, stimulation of several regions of the hypothalamus (dorsomedial and ventromedial nuclei and the mammillary body) enhances pancreatic secretion. The efferent signal travels along vagal pathways to stimulate pancreatic secretion through ACh, an effect blocked by atropine. The cephalic phase does not depend on gastrin or CCK release, but it is probably mediated by the stimulation of muscarinic receptors on the *acinar* cell.

The Gastric Phase During the gastric phase (Fig. 43-9A), the presence of food in the stomach modulates pancreatic secretion by (1) affecting the release of hormones, (2) stimulating neural pathways, and (3) modifying the pH and availability of nutrients in the proximal part of the small intestine. The presence of specific peptides or amino acids (peptones) stimulates gastrin release from G cells in the antrum of the stomach and, to a much lesser extent, G cells in the proximal part of the duodenum. The gastrin/CCK_B receptor and the CCK_A receptor are closely related (see Chapter 42). Although in some species the gastrin/CCK_B receptor is not present on the pancreatic acinar cell, gastrin can still act—albeit not as well—through the CCK_A receptor. Although physiological concentrations of gastrin can stimulate pancreatic secretion in some species, the importance of gastrin in regulating secretion in the human pancreas remains unclear. As far as local neural pathways are concerned, gastric distention stimulates low levels of pancreatic secretion, probably through a vagovagal gastropancreatic reflex. Although the presence of food in the stomach affects pancreatic secretion, the most important role for chyme in controlling pancreatic secretion occurs after the gastric contents enter the small intestine.

The Intestinal Phase During the intestinal phase, chyme entering the proximal region of the small intestine stimulates a major pancreatic secretory response by three major mechanisms (Fig. 43-9B). First, gastric acid entering the duodenum and, to a lesser extent, bile acids and lipids stimulate duodenal **S cells** to release secretin, which stimulates duct cells to secrete HCO_3^- and fluid. The acid stimulates fluid and electrolyte secretion to a greater extent than it stimulates protein secretion. Second, lipids and, to a lesser degree, peptones stimulate duodenal I cells to release CCK, which stim-

ulates acinar cells to release digestive enzymes. Finally, the same stimuli that trigger I cells also activate a vagovagal enteropancreatic reflex that predominantly stimulates acinar cells.

The pattern of enzyme secretion—mediated by the CCK and vagovagal pathways—depends on the contents of the meal. For example, a *liquid meal* elicits a response that is only ~60% of maximal. In contrast, a solid meal, which contains larger particles and is slowly released from the stomach, elicits a prolonged response. Meals rich in *calories* cause the greatest response.

The *chemistry* of the ingested nutrients also affects pancreatic secretion through the CCK and vagovagal pathways. For example, perfusion of the duodenum with carbohydrates has little effect on secretion, whereas lipids are potent stimulators of pancreatic enzyme secretion. As far as *lipids* are concerned, triglycerides do not stimulate pancreatic secretion, but their hydrolytic products—monoglycerides and free fatty acids—do. The longer the chain length of the fatty acid, the greater is the secretory response; C-18 fatty acids generate protein secretion that is near the maximum produced by exogenous CCK. Some fatty acids also stimulate pancreatic HCO_3^- secretion. Because fatty acids also reduce gastric acid secretion and delay gastric emptying, they may play an important role in modulating pH conditions in the proximal part of the small intestine. *Protein* breakdown products are intermediate in their stimulatory effect. Nonessential amino acids have little effect on protein secretion, whereas some essential amino acids (see Chapter 58) stimulate secretion. The most potent amino acid stimulators are phenylalanine, valine, and methionine. Short peptides containing phenylalanine stimulate secretion to the same extent as the amino acid itself. Because gastric digestion generates more peptides than amino acids, it is likely that peptides provide the initial pancreatic stimulation during the intestinal phase.

The relative potency of the different nutrients in stimulating secretion is inversely related to the pancreatic reserves of digestive enzymes. Thus, the pancreas needs to release only a small portion of its amylase to digest the carbohydrate in a meal and to release only slightly greater portions of proteolytic enzymes to digest the proteins. However, a greater fraction of pancreatic lipase has to be released to efficiently digest the fat in most meals. The exocrine pancreas has the ability to respond to long-term changes in dietary composition by modulating the reserves of pancreatic enzymes. For example, a diet that is relatively high in carbohydrates may lead to a relative increase in pancreatic amylase content.

The pancreas has large reserves of digestive enzymes for carbohydrates and proteins, but not for lipids

The exocrine pancreas stores more enzymes than are required for digesting a meal. The greatest pancreatic reserves are those required for carbohydrate and protein digestion. The reserves of enzymes required for lipid digestion—particularly for triglyceride hydrolysis—are more limited. Even so, nutrient absorption studies after partial pancreatic resection show that maldigestion of dietary fat does not occur until 80% to 90% of the pancreas has been removed. Similar reserves exist for pancreatic endocrine function. These observations have important clinical implications because they indicate that individuals can tolerate large pancreatic resections for tumors without fear of developing maldigestion or diabetes postoperatively. When fat maldigestion or diabetes does develop because of pancreatic disease, the gland must have undergone extensive destruction.

Fat in the distal part of the small intestine inhibits pancreatic secretion

Once maximally stimulated, pancreatic secretion begins to decrease after several hours. Nevertheless, the levels of secretion remain adequate for digestion. Regulatory systems only gradually return secretion to its basal (interdigestive) state. The regulatory mechanisms responsible for this feedback inhibition are less well characterized than those responsible for stimulating pancreatic secretion. The presence of fat in the distal end of the small intestine reduces pancreatic secretion in most animals, including humans. This inhibition may be mediated by **peptide YY (PYY)**, which is present in neuroendocrine cells in the ileum and colon. PYY may suppress pancreatic secretion by acting on inhibitory neural pathways, as well as by decreasing pancreatic blood flow. **Somatostatin** (particularly SS-28; see Chapter 48), released from intestinal D cells, and **glucagon**, released from pancreatic islet α cells, may also be factors in returning pancreatic secretion to the interdigestive state after a meal.

Several mechanisms protect the pancreas from autodigestion

Premature activation of pancreatic enzymes within acinar cells may lead to autodigestion and could play a role in initiating pancreatitis. To prevent such injury, the acinar cell has certain mechanisms for preventing enzymatic activity (Table 43-3). First, many digestive proteins are stored in secretory granules as inactive precursors or zymogens. Under normal conditions, zymogens become activated only after entering the small intestine. There, the intestinal enzyme **enterokinase** converts trypsinogen to trypsin, which initiates the conversion of all other zymogens to their active forms (see Chapter 45). Second, the secretory granule membrane is impermeable to proteins. Thus, the zymogens and active digestive enzymes are sequestered from proteins in the cytoplasm and other intracellular compartments. Third, enzyme inhibitors such as **pancreatic trypsin inhibitor** are co-packaged in the secretory granule. Sufficient pancreatic

Acute Pancreatitis

Acute pancreatitis is an inflammatory condition that may cause extensive local damage to the pancreas, as well as compromise the function of other organs such as the lungs. The most common factors that initiate human acute pancreatitis are alcohol ingestion and gallstones. However, other insults may also precipitate acute pancreatitis. Hypertriglyceridemia, an inherited disorder of lipid metabolism, is one such culprit. Less commonly, toxins that increase ACh levels, such as cholinesterase inhibitors (some insecticides) or the sting of scorpions found in the Caribbean and South and Central America, may lead to pancreatitis. Supraphysiological levels of ACh probably cause pancreatitis by overstimulating the pancreatic acinar cell.

Experimental models of pancreatitis suggest a primary defect in protein processing and acinar cell secretory function. More than 100 years ago, it was found that treating animals with doses of ACh 10 to 100 times greater than those that elicited maximal enzyme secretion caused "hyperstimulation" pancreatitis. The same type of injury can be generated by CCK. The injury in this model appears to be linked to two events within the acinar cell: (1) zymogens, in particular proteases, are pathologically processed within the acinar cell into active forms; in this model, the protective mechanisms outlined in Table 43-3 are overwhelmed, and active enzymes are generated within the acinar cell; and (2) acinar cell secretion is inhibited, and the active enzymes are retained within the cell. Although premature activation of zymogens is probably an important step in initiating pancreatitis, other events are important for perpetuating injury, including inflammation, induction of apoptosis, vascular injury, and occlusion that results in decreased blood flow and reduced tissue oxygenation (ischemia).

Knowledge of the mechanisms of acute pancreatitis may lead to effective therapies. In experimental models, serine protease inhibitors that block the activation of pancreatic zymogens improve the course of the acute pancreatitis. In some clinical forms of pancreatitis, prophylactic administration of the protease inhibitor gabexate appears to reduce the severity of the disease.

Table 43-3 Mechanisms That Protect the Acinar Cell from Autodigestion

Protective Factor	Mechanism
Packaging of many digestive proteins as zymogens	Precursor proteins lack enzymatic activity
Selective sorting of secretory proteins and storage in zymogen granules	Restricts the interaction of secretory proteins with other cellular compartments
Protease inhibitors in the zymogen granule	Block the action of prematurely activated enzymes
Condensation of secretory proteins at low pH	Limits the activity of active enzymes
Nondigestive proteases	Degrade active enzymes

Table 43-4 Autonomic Control of Salivary Secretion

Autonomic Pathway	Neurotransmitter	Receptor	Signaling Pathway	Cellular Response
Parasympathetic	Acetylcholine Substance P	Muscarinic (M_3) Tachykinin NK-1	Ca^{2+} Ca^{2+}	Fluid > protein secretion Fluid > protein secretion
Sympathetic	Norepinephrine Norepinephrine	α-Adrenergic β-Adrenergic	Ca^{2+} cAMP	Fluid > protein secretion Protein > fluid secretion

trypsin inhibitor is present in the secretory granules to block 10% to 20% of the potential trypsin activity. Fourth, the condensation of zymogens, the low pH, and the ionic conditions within the secretory pathway may further limit enzyme activity. Fifth, enzymes that become prematurely active within the acinar cell may themselves be degraded by other enzymes or be secreted before they can cause injury.

Degradation of prematurely active enzymes may be mediated by other enzymes that are present within the secretory granule or by mixing secretory granule contents with lysosomal enzymes that can degrade active enzymes. Three mechanisms lead to the combination of digestive proteases and lysosomal enzymes: (1) lysosomal enzymes may be co-packaged in the secretory granule; (2) secretory granules may selectively fuse with lysosomes (a process called *crinophagy*); and (3) secretory granules, as well as other organelles, may be engulfed by lysosomes (a process called *autophagy*). Failure of these protective mechanisms may result in the premature activation of digestive enzymes within the pancreatic acinar cell and may initiate pancreatitis.

SALIVARY ACINAR CELL

Different salivary acinar cells secrete different proteins

The organizational structure of the salivary glands is similar to that of the pancreas (Fig. 43-1A); secretory acinar units drain into progressively larger ducts. Unlike the pancreas, the salivary glands are more heterogeneous in distribution and contain two distinct acinar cell populations that synthesize and secrete different protein products. The acinar cells of the parotid glands in most species secrete a serous (i.e., watery) product that contains an abundance of α-**amylase**. Many acinar cells of the sublingual glands secrete a mucinous product that is composed primarily of **mucin glycoproteins**. The morphologic appearance of these two acinar cell populations differs as well. The submandibular gland of many species contains both mucus-type and serous-type acinar cells. In some species, these two distinct cell types are dispersed throughout the submandibular gland, whereas in other species such as humans, distinct mucus and serous acinar units are the rule. In addition to α-amylase and mucin glycoproteins, salivary acinar cells also secrete many proline-rich proteins. Like mucin proteins, proline-rich proteins are highly glycosylated, and like other secreted salivary proteins,

they are present in the acinar secretory granules and are released by exocytosis.

Cholinergic and adrenergic neural pathways are the most important physiological activators of regulated secretion by salivary acinar cells

Unlike the pancreas, in which humoral stimulation plays an important role in stimulating secretion, the salivary glands are mostly controlled by the autonomic nervous system (see Chapter 14). The major agonists of salivary acinar secretion are ACh and norepinephrine, which are released from postganglionic parasympathetic and sympathetic nerve terminals, respectively (see Fig. 14-8; Table 43-4). The cholinergic receptor on the salivary acinar cell is the muscarinic M_3 glandular subtype. The adrenergic receptors identified on these cells include both the α and β subtypes. Other receptors identified in salivary tissue include those for substance P (NK1 receptors), VIP, purinergic agonists (P_{2z} receptors), neurotensin, prostaglandin, and epidermal growth factor (EGF). However, some of these other receptors are found only on specific salivary glands and may be present on duct cells rather than acinar cells. Significant species variation with regard to surface receptor expression is also seen. Thus, for the salivary glands, it is difficult to discuss the regulation of acinar cell secretion in general terms. It is fair to say, however, that both cholinergic and adrenergic neurotransmitters can stimulate exocytosis by salivary acinar cells.

Both cAMP and Ca^{2+} mediate salivary acinar secretion

Protein secretion by the salivary acinar cell, as in the pancreatic acinar cell, is associated with increases in both $[cAMP]_i$ and $[Ca^{2+}]_i$. Activation of cAMP through the β-adrenergic receptor is the most potent stimulator of amylase secretion in the rat parotid gland. Activation of Ca^{2+} signaling pathways through the α-adrenergic, muscarinic, and substance P receptors also stimulates amylase secretion by the parotid gland. Increases in $[Ca^{2+}]_i$ cause G protein–dependent activation of PLC and thus lead to the formation of inositol 1,4,5-trisphosphate (IP_3) and diacylglycerol (DAG). IP_3 releases Ca^{2+} from intracellular stores and stimulates Ca^{2+}-dependent protein kinases such as PKC and calmodulin kinase, whereas DAG directly activates PKC (see Chapter 3). The repetitive spikes in $[Ca^{2+}]_i$ in salivary acinar cells, as in pancreatic acinar cells, depend on Ca^{2+}-induced Ca^{2+} release from intracellular stores (see Chapter 9) and on the influx of extracellular Ca^{2+}. ATP co-released with norepinephrine (see Chapter 14) activates a P_{2z} receptor, which is a receptor-gated cation-selective channel that allows Ca^{2+} to enter across the plasma membrane and thus increase $[Ca^{2+}]_i$.

Fluid and electrolyte secretion is the second major function of salivary acinar cells, accounting for ~90% of total salivary volume output under stimulatory conditions. The mechanisms in salivary acinar cells are similar to those in pancreatic acinar cells (Fig. 43-5). The primary secretion of the salivary acinar cell is isotonic and results largely from the basolateral uptake of Cl^- through Na/K/Cl cotransporters, working in conjunction with Na-K pumps and basolateral K^+ channels. Secretion of Cl^- and water into the lumen is mediated by apical Cl^- and aquaporin water channels. Na^+ and some water reach the lumen through paracellular routes. The salivary acinar cells in some species express carbonic anhydrase as well as parallel basolateral Cl-HCO_3 and Na-H exchangers, a finding suggesting that other pathways may also contribute to the primary secretion.

Stimulation of fluid and electrolyte secretion by salivary acinar cells is largely mediated by cholinergic and α-adrenergic stimulation. Substance P, acting through its own receptor, also initiates conductance changes in the salivary acinar cell. All these effects seem to be mediated by rises in $[Ca^{2+}]_i$. Apical Cl^- channels and basolateral K^+ channels appear to be the effector targets of the activated Ca^{2+} signaling pathway. Phosphorylation of these channels by Ca^{2+}-dependent kinases may affect the probability that these channels will be open and may thus increase conductance.

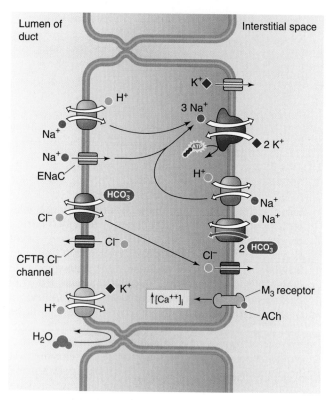

Figure 43-10 Salivary duct transporters.

SALIVARY DUCT CELL

Salivary duct cells produce a hypotonic fluid that is poor in NaCl and rich in KHCO₃

In the salivary glands, as in the pancreas, the duct modifies the composition of the isotonic, plasma-like primary secretion of the acinar cells (Fig. 43-10). The active transport activity of these cells is reflected by numerous basolateral membrane infoldings and abundant mitochondria, which give the basal portion of the cells a characteristic striated appearance—hence the term *striated* duct epithelial cell (Fig. 43-10C). In general, salivary duct cells absorb Na^+ and Cl^- and, to a lesser extent, secrete K^+ and HCO_3^-. Because the epithelium is not very water permeable, the lumen thus becomes hypotonic. However, significant differences are seen in the various types of salivary glands.

Reabsorption of Na$^+$ by salivary duct cells is a two-step transcellular process. First, Na^+ enters the cell from the lumen through apical epithelial Na^+ channels (ENaCs; see Chapter 5). Second, the basolateral Na-K pump extrudes this Na^+. Elevated $[Na^+]_i$ provides feedback inhibition by downregulating ENaC activity, presumably through the ubiquitin-protein ligase Nedd4 (see Chapter 2).

Reabsorption of Cl$^-$ is also a two-step transcellular process. Entry of Cl^- across the apical membrane occurs through a

Cl-HCO_3 exchanger. To a certain extent, apical Cl^- channels, including CFTR, recycle the Cl^- that is absorbed by the Cl-HCO_3 exchanger. Duct cells also have basolateral Cl^- channels that provide an exit pathway for Cl^-.

Secretion of HCO$_3^-$ occurs through the apical Cl-HCO_3 exchanger mentioned earlier. This process depends on functional CFTR, thereby confirming the coupling of CFTR to the Cl-HCO_3 exchanger in salivary duct cells. HCO_3^- accumulation inside the salivary duct cell may follow the same routes as in the pancreatic duct cell (Fig. 43-6). Indeed, Na/HCO_3 cotransporters in the identification of rat and human salivary duct epithelial cells support this possibility.

Secretion of K$^+$ occurs through the basolateral uptake of K^+ through the Na-K pump. The mechanism of the apical K^+ exit step is not well established, but it may involve K-H exchange or other pathways.

Parasympathetic stimulation decreases Na⁺ absorption, whereas aldosterone increases Na⁺ absorption by duct cells

Regulation of duct cell transport processes is less well understood in the salivary glands than in the pancreas. In the intact salivary gland (i.e., acini and ducts), secretion is stimulated primarily by *parasympathetic* input through ACh. In the duct cell, cholinergic agonists, acting through muscarinic receptors, increase $[Ca^{2+}]_i$ and presumably activate Ca^{2+}-

dependent regulatory pathways. The effector targets of this Ca^{2+} signaling pathway are not known. The role played by duct cells in the increased saliva production that occurs in response to cholinergic stimulation is limited and may reflect decreased Na-Cl absorption more than increased K-HCO_3 secretion.

The specific effects of *adrenergic* stimulation on duct cell transport activity are unclear. Nevertheless, activation of the β-adrenergic receptor increases [cAMP]$_i$ and activates the CFTR Cl^- channel.

Salivary duct cell function is also regulated by *circulating hormones*. The mineralocorticoid hormone **aldosterone** stimulates the absorption of Na-Cl and secretion of K^+ by salivary duct cells in several species. Although its role has not been well examined in salivary duct cells, aldosterone in other Na^+-absorbing epithelia (e.g., kidney and colon) stimulates Na^+ transport by increasing both ENaC and Na-K pump activity (see Chapter 35). Salivary duct cells may also have receptors for certain neuropeptides such as VIP, although their physiological significance remains unknown.

Salivary duct cells also secrete and take up proteins

Duct cells handle proteins in three ways. Some proteins that are synthesized by duct cells are secreted into the lumen, others are secreted into blood, and still others are reabsorbed from the lumen to the cell.

Intralobular duct epithelial cells in rodent submandibular glands synthesize various proteins that are stored in intracellular granules and are secreted in response to neurohumoral stimuli. EGF, nerve growth factor, and kallikrein are among the most abundant proteins that are packaged for secretion by these cells. Salivary duct cells may also synthesize, store, and secrete some digestive enzymes (α-amylase and ribonucleases). Degranulation of intralobular duct cells occurs primarily in response to α-adrenergic stimulation, a finding suggesting that protein secretion by duct cells is regulated primarily by the sympathetic division.

Although regulatory peptides (i.e., glucagon and somatostatin) have also been detected in salivary duct cells, no evidence indicates that they are stored in granules or are secreted into the lumen (i.e., they may be basolaterally secreted as peptide hormones). In addition, duct cells synthesize polymeric IgA receptors that are responsible for the basolateral endocytosis of IgA, and they also synthesize a secretory component that facilitates the apical release of IgA.

Salivary duct cells can also remove organic substances from the duct lumen. Endocytosis of acinar proteins and other materials (e.g., ferritin) at the apical pole of the duct cell has been demonstrated immunocytochemically. In addition, salivary duct cells express the transferrin receptor (see Chapter 2) on the apical membrane, a finding indicating that some regulated endocytosis also occurs in these cells. The latter process may function to take up specific luminal substances or to traffic ion transporters to and from the apical plasma membrane.

COMPOSITION, FUNCTION, AND CONTROL OF SALIVARY SECRETION

Depending on protein composition, salivary secretions can be serous, seromucous, or mucous

Most saliva (~90%) is produced by the major salivary glands: the parotid, the sublingual, and the submandibular glands. The remaining 10% of saliva comes from numerous minor salivary glands that are scattered throughout the submucosa of the oral cavity. Each salivary gland produces either a serous, a seromucous, or a mucous secretion; the definition of these three types of saliva is based on the glycoprotein content of the gland's final secretory product. In humans and most other mammals, the parotids produce a serous (i.e., low glycoprotein content) secretion, the sublingual and submandibular glands produce a seromucous secretion, and the minor salivary glands produce a mucous secretion.

Serous secretions are enriched in α-amylase, and mucous secretions are enriched in mucin. However, the most abundant proteins in parotid and submandibular saliva are members of the group of **proline-rich proteins**, in which one third of all amino acids are proline. These proteins exist in acidic, basic, and glycosylated forms. They have antimicrobial properties and may play an important role in neutralizing dietary tannins, which can damage epithelial cells. In addition to these protective functions, proline-rich salivary proteins contribute to the lubrication of ingested foods and may enhance tooth integrity through their interactions with Ca^{2+} and hydroxyapatite. Saliva also contains smaller amounts of lipase, nucleases, lysozyme, peroxidases, lactoferrin, secretory IgA, growth factors, regulatory peptides, and vasoactive proteases such as kallikrein and renin (Table 43-5).

Saliva functions primarily to prevent dehydration of the oral mucosa and to provide lubrication for the mastication and swallowing of ingested food. The sense of taste and, to a lesser extent, smell depend on an adequate supply of saliva. Saliva plays a very important role in maintaining proper oral hygiene. It accomplishes this task by washing away food particles, killing bacteria (lysozyme and IgA activity), and contributing to overall dental integrity. Although α-amylase is a major constituent of saliva and digests a significant amount of the ingested starch, salivary amylase does not appear to be essential for effective carbohydrate digestion in the presence of a normally functioning pancreas. The same can be said for lingual lipase. However, in cases of pancreatic insufficiency, these salivary enzymes can partially compensate for the maldigestion that results from pancreatic dysfunction.

At low flow rates, the saliva is hypotonic and rich in K^+, whereas at higher flow rates, its composition approaches that of plasma

The composition of saliva varies from gland to gland and from species to species. The primary secretion of the salivary acinar cell at rest is plasma-like in composition. Its osmolal-

Table 43-5 Major Organic Components of Mammalian Saliva

Components	Cell Type	Glands	Possible Function
Proline-rich proteins	Acinar	P, SM	Enamel formation Ca^{2+} binding Antimicrobial Lubrication
Mucin glycoproteins	Acinar	SL, SM	Lubrication
Enzymes			
α-Amylase	Acinar	P, SM	Starch digestion
Lipase	Acinar	SL	Fat digestion
Ribonuclease	Duct	SM	RNA digestion
Kallikrein	Duct	P, SM, SL	Unknown
Miscellaneous			
Lactoperoxidase	Acinar	SM	Antimicrobial
Lactoferrin	Acinar	Unknown	Antimicrobial
Lysozyme	Duct	SM	Antimicrobial
IgA receptor	Duct	Unknown	Antimicrobial
IgA secretory piece	Duct	Unknown	Antimicrobial
Growth factors	Duct	SM	Unknown

P, parotid; SL, sublingual; SM, submandibular.

Table 43-6 Electrolyte Components of Human Parotid Saliva

Component	Unstimulated or Basal State (mM)	Stimulated (Cholinergic Agonists) (mM)
Na^+	15	90
K^+	30	15
Cl^-	15	50
Total CO_2	15	60

Data from Thaysen JH, Thorn NA, Schwartz IL: Am J Physiol 1954; 178:155-159.

ity, which is mostly the result of Na^+ and Cl^-, is ~300 mosmol/kg. The only significant difference from plasma is that the $[K^+]$ of the salivary primary secretion is always slightly higher than that of plasma. In some species, acinar cells may help to generate a Cl^--poor, HCO_3^--rich primary secretion after salivary gland stimulation. In most species, however, salivary gland stimulation does not significantly alter acinar cell transport function or the composition of the primary secretion. The leakiness of the tight junctions between acinar cells contributes to the formation of a plasma-like primary secretory product (see Chapter 5).

The composition of the primary salivary secretion is subsequently modified by the transport processes of the duct cell (Fig. 43-10). At *low (basal) flow rates*, Na^+ and Cl^- are absorbed and K^+ is secreted by the duct cells of most salivary glands (Table 43-6). These transport processes generate a K^+-rich, hypotonic salivary secretion at rest. The tightness of the ductal epithelium inhibits paracellular water movement and therefore contributes to the formation of a hypotonic secretory product.

At *higher flow rates*, the composition of the final secretory product begins to approach that of the plasma-like primary secretion (Table 43-6). This observation suggests that, as in the case of the renal tubules, the ductular transport processes have limited capacity to handle the increased load that is presented to them as the flow rate accelerates. However, the extent to which the transporters are flow dependent varies from gland to gland and from species to species. Human saliva is always hypotonic, and salivary $[K^+]$ is always greater

than plasma $[K^+]$. In humans, increased salivary flow alkalinizes the saliva and increases its $[HCO_3^-]$. This salivary alkalinization and net HCO_3^- secretion in humans neutralize the gastric acid that normally refluxes into the esophagus.

Parasympathetic stimulation increases salivary secretion

Humans produce ~1.5 L of saliva each day. Under basal conditions, the salivary glands produce saliva at a rate of ~0.5 mL/min, with a much slower flow rate during sleep. After stimulation, flow increases 10-fold over the basal rate. Although the salivary glands respond to both cholinergic and adrenergic agonists in vitro, the parasympathetic nervous system is the most important physiological regulator of salivary secretion in vivo.

Parasympathetic Control Parasympathetic innervation to the salivary glands originates in the salivatory nuclei of the brainstem (see Fig. 14-5). Both local input and central input to the salivatory nuclei can regulate the parasympathetic signals transmitted to the glands. Taste and tactile stimuli from the tongue are transmitted to the brainstem, where their signals can excite the salivatory nuclei and stimulate salivary gland secretion. Central impulses triggered by the sight and smell of food also excite the salivatory nuclei and can induce salivation before food is ingested. These central effects were best illustrated by the classic experiments of Pavlov, who conditioned dogs to salivate at the sound of a bell. For his work on the physiology of digestion, Ivan Pavlov received the 1904 Nobel Prize in Physiology or Medicine.

Preganglionic parasympathetic fibers travel in cranial nerve (CN) VII to the submandibular ganglia, from which postganglionic fibers reach the sublingual and submandibular glands (see Fig. 14-4). Preganglionic parasympathetic fibers also travel in CN IX to the otic ganglia, from which postganglionic fibers reach the parotid glands. In addition, some parasympathetic fibers reach their final destination through the buccal branch of CN V to the parotid glands or through the lingual branches of CN V to the sublingual and submandibular glands. Postganglionic parasympathetic

Sjögren Syndrome

Sjögren syndrome is a chronic and progressive autoimmune disease that affects salivary secretion. Patients with Sjögren syndrome generate antibodies that react primarily with the salivary and lacrimal glands. Lymphocytes infiltrate the glands, and subsequent immunologic injury to the acini leads to a decrease in net secretory function. Expression of the Cl-HCO₃ exchanger is lost in the striated duct cells of the salivary gland. Sjögren syndrome can occur as a primary disease (salivary and lacrimal gland dysfunction only) or as a secondary manifestation of a systemic autoimmune disease, such as rheumatoid arthritis. The disease primarily affects women; systemic disease usually does not develop.

Individuals with Sjögren syndrome have *xerostomia* (dry mouth) and *keratoconjunctivitis sicca* (dry eyes). Loss of salivary function causes these patients to have difficulty tasting, as well as chewing and swallowing dry food. They also have difficulty with continuous speech and complain of a chronic burning sensation in the mouth. On physical examination, patients with Sjögren syndrome have dry, erythematous oral mucosa with superficial ulceration and poor dentition (dental caries, dental fractures, and loss of dentition). Parotid gland enlargement is commonly present.

The proteins that are the targets of the immunologic attack in Sjögren syndrome are not known. Therefore, no specific therapy for the disorder is available. Until the underlying cause of Sjögren syndrome is discovered, patients will have to rely on eyedrops and frequent oral fluid ingestion to compensate for their deficiencies in lacrimal and salivary secretion. Various stimulants of salivary secretion (sialogogues), such as methylcellulose and sour candy, can also be helpful. Patients with severe involvement and functional disability are sometimes treated with corticosteroids and immunosuppressants.

fibers from these ganglia directly stimulate the salivary glands through their release of ACh. The prominent role of the parasympathetic nervous system in salivary function can be readily appreciated by examining the consequences of cholinergic blockage. Disruption of the parasympathetic fibers to the salivary glands can lead to glandular atrophy. This observation suggests that parasympathetic innervation is necessary for maintaining the normal mass of salivary glands. Clinically, some medications (particularly psychiatric drugs) have "anticholinergic" properties that are most commonly manifested as "dry mouth." For some medications, this effect is so uncomfortable for the patient that use of the medication must be discontinued. Conversely, excessive salivation is induced by some anticholinesterase agents that can be found in certain insecticides and "nerve gases."

Sympathetic Control The salivary glands are also innervated by postganglionic sympathetic fibers from the superior cervical ganglia that travel along blood vessels to the salivary glands (see Fig. 14-4). Although sympathetic (adrenergic) stimulation increases saliva flow, interruption of sympathetic nerves to the salivary glands has no major effect on salivary gland function in vivo. However, the sympathetic nervous system is the primary stimulator of the **myoepithelial cells** that are closely associated with cells of the acini and proximal (intercalated) ducts. These stellate cells have structural features of both epithelial and smooth muscle cells. They support the acinar structures and decrease the flow resistance of the intercalated ducts during stimulated secretion. Thus, the net effect of myoepithelial cell activation is to facilitate secretory flow in the proximal regions of the gland, thus minimizing the extravasation of secretory proteins that could otherwise occur during an acute increase in secretory flow.

The sympathetic division can also indirectly affect salivary gland function by modulating blood flow to the gland. However, the relative contribution of this vascular effect to the overall secretory function of the salivary glands is difficult to determine.

In addition to cholinergic and adrenergic regulation of salivary secretion, some autonomic fibers that innervate the salivary glands contain VIP and substance P. Although acinar cells in vitro respond to stimulation by substance P, the physiological significance of these neurotransmitters in vivo has not been established. Salivary secretion is also regulated, in part, by mineralocorticoids. The adrenal hormone aldosterone produces saliva that contains relatively less Na⁺ and more K⁺. The opposite effect on saliva is seen in patients with adrenal insufficiency caused by **Addison disease**. The mineralocorticoid effect represents the only well-established example of a humoral (i.e., non-neural) agent regulating salivary secretion.

REFERENCES

Books and Reviews

Beger HG, Warshaw AL, Büchler M, et al. (eds): The Pancreas, 2nd ed. Cambridge, MA: Blackwell Publishing, 2008.

Dobrosielski-Vergona K (ed): Biology of the Salvary Glands. Boca Raton, FL: CRC Press, 1993.

Go VLW, DiMagno EP, Gardner JD, et al: The Pancreas: Biology, Pathobiology, and Disease, 2nd ed. New York: Raven Press, 1993.

Johnson LR, et al. (eds): Physiology of the Gastrointestinal Tract, 4th ed. New York: Raven Press, 2006.

Turner RJ, Sugiya H: Understanding salivary fluid and protein secretion. Oral Diseases 2002; 8:3-11.

Williams JA: Intracellular signaling mechanisms activated by cholecystokinin-regulating synthesis and secretion of digestive enzymes in pancreatic acinar cells. Annu Rev Physiol 2001; 63:77-97.

Journal Articles

Ishiguro H, Naruse S, Steward MC, et al: Fluid secretion in interlobular ducts isolated from guinea pig pancreas. J Physiol 1998; 511:407-422.

Jamieson J, Palade G: Synthesis, intracellular transport, and discharge of secretory proteins in stimulated pancreatic exocrine cells. J Cell Biol 1971; 50:135-158.

Petersen OH: Stimulus-secretion coupling: Cytoplasmic calcium signals and the control of ion channels in exocrine acinar cells. J Physiol 1992; 448:1-51.

Sohma Y, Gray MA, Imai Y, Argent BE: HCO_3^- transport in a mathematical model of the pancreatic ductal epithelium. J Membr Biol 2000; 176:77-100.

Thaysen JH, Thorn NA, Schwartz IL: Excretion of sodium, potassium, chloride, and carbon dioxide in human parotid saliva. Am J Physiol 1954; 178:155-159.

Zhao H, Xu X, Diaz J, Muallem S: Na^+, K^+, and H^+/HCO_3^- transport in submandibular salivary ducts. J Biol Chem 1995; 270: 19599-19605.

CHAPTER 44

INTESTINAL FLUID AND
ELECTROLYTE MOVEMENT

Henry J. Binder

FUNCTIONAL ANATOMY

The small intestine and large intestine have many similarities in structure and function. In some cases, different regions of the intestinal tract carry out certain functions in much the same manner. In other cases, however, substantial heterogeneity exists between different intestinal segments (e.g., ileum versus jejunum) or between different mucosal areas (i.e., villus versus crypt) in one intestinal segment.

As discussed in Chapter 41, the basic structure of the intestine is a hollow cylinder with columnar epithelial cells lining the lumen, with circular and longitudinal layers of smooth muscle in the wall, and with endocrine and neural elements (see Fig. 41-2). Enteric neurons, as well as endocrine and paracrine agonists, regulate both epithelial transport and motor activity during both the interdigestive and the postprandial periods. As a result, the intestines propagate their contents in a caudad direction while either removing fluid and electrolytes from the intestinal lumen (i.e., absorption) or adding these substances to the lumen (i.e., secretion).

Both the small intestine and large intestine absorb and secrete fluid and electrolytes, whereas only the small intestine absorbs nutrients

Among mammals, **absorption** of dietary nutrients is an exclusive function of the small intestine. Only during the neonatal period does significant nutrient absorption take place in the large intestine. The small intestine absorbs non-electrolytes after extensive digestion of dietary nutrients by both luminal and brush border enzymes, as discussed in Chapter 45. In contrast, *both* the small intestine and the large intestine absorb fluid and electrolytes by several different cellular transport processes, which may differ between the small intestine and the large intestine and are the subject of this chapter.

Another vitally important function of the intestinal epithelium is the **secretion** of intestinal fluid and electrolytes. Teleologically, fluid secretion may be considered an adaptive mechanism used by the intestinal tract to protect itself from noxious agents, such as bacteria and bacterial toxins. In general, the cellular mechanisms of intestinal electrolyte secretion in the small intestine and colon are similar, if not identical. Frequently, the adaptive signal that induces the secretory response also stimulates a simultaneous motor response from the intestinal muscle; together, these factors result in a propagated propulsive response in an attempt to dilute and eliminate the offending toxin.

The small intestine has a villus crypt organization, whereas the colon has surface epithelial cells with interspersed crypts

Both the small intestine and the large intestine have a specialized epithelial structure that correlates well with epithelial transport function. The small intestine (Fig. 44-1A) consists of finger-like projections—**villi**—surrounded by the openings of glandular structures called **crypts of Lieberkühn**, or simply crypts. Both villi and crypts are covered by columnar epithelial cells. The cells lining the villi are considered to be the primary cells responsible for both nutrient and electrolyte *absorption*, whereas the crypt cells primarily participate in *secretion*.

The colon (Fig. 44-1B) does not have villi. Instead, the cells lining the large intestine are surface epithelial cells, and interspersed over the colonic surface are numerous apertures of colonic crypts (or glands) that are similar in function and structure to the small intestinal crypts. Not surprisingly, the surface epithelial cells of the colon are the primary cells responsible for colonic electrolyte *absorption*, whereas colonic gland cells are generally believed to mediate ion *secretion*.

The intestinal mucosa is a dynamic organ with continuous cell proliferation and migration. The zone of cell proliferation is at the base of the crypt in both the small and large intestine, and the program of events is similar in both organs. The **progenitor cell** is a stem cell that differentiates into several specialized cells (e.g., vacuolated, goblet, and Paneth cells) that line the villi and crypts in the small intestine and the surface and glands in the colon. The vacuolated cell migrates along the crypt-villus axis and becomes a villous absorptive cell after undergoing substantial changes in its

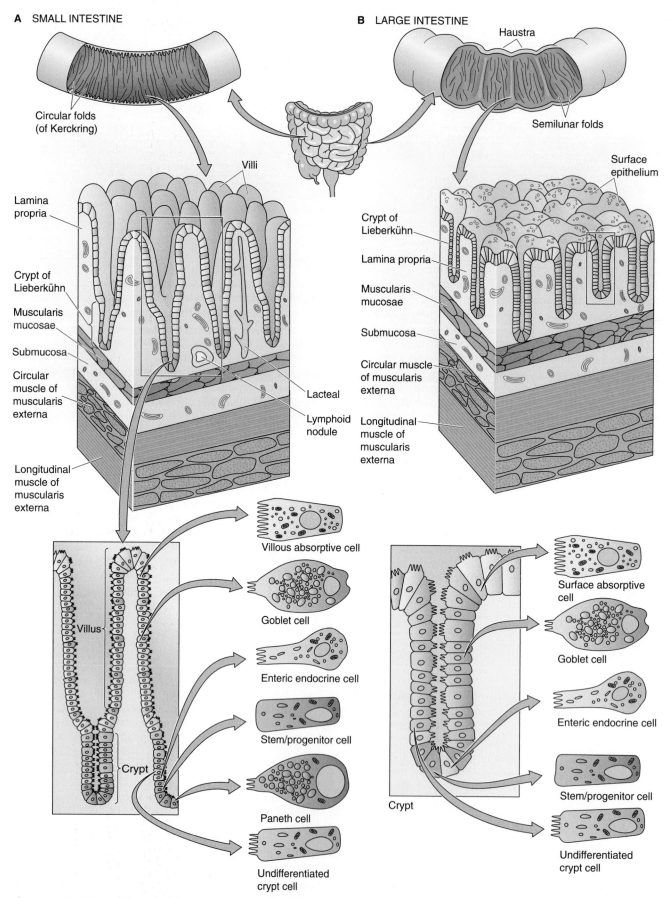

Figure 44-1 Microscopic view of the anatomy of small and large intestine. **A**, The surface area of the small intestine is amplified at three levels: (1) macroscopic folds of Kerckring, (2) microscopic villi and crypts of Lieberkühn, and (3) submicroscopic microvilli. **B**, The surface area of the colon is amplified at the same three levels as the small intestine: (1) macroscopic semilunar folds, (2) crypts (but not villi), and (3) microvilli.

morphologic and functional characteristics. In the small intestine, these villous cells migrate until they reach the tips of the villi and then slough into the lumen of the intestine. The overall period from the initiation of cell proliferation to sloughing is ~48 to 96 hours. The overall rate of cell migration may increase or decrease: decreased cell turnover occurs during starvation, whereas increased cell turnover occurs during feeding and lactation, as well as after intestinal resection. The compensatory response that follows intestinal resection involves both luminal and hormonal factors.

The surface area of the small intestine is amplified by folds, villi, and microvilli; amplification is less marked in the colon

An additional hallmark of both the small and large intestine is the presence of structures that amplify function by increasing the luminal surface area. These structures exist at three levels. In the small intestine, the first level consists of the macroscopic **folds of Kerckring**. The second level consists of the microscopic **villi** and **crypts** that we have already discussed. The third level is the submicroscopic **microvilli** on the apical surfaces of the epithelial cells. Thus, if the small intestine is thought of as a hollow cylinder, the net increase in total surface area of the small intestine (versus that of a smooth cylinder) is 600-fold. The total surface area of the human small intestine is ~200 m², or the surface area of a doubles tennis court (Table 44-1). The colonic surface area is also amplified, but to a more limited extent. Because the colon lacks villi, amplification is a result of only the presence of colonic folds, crypts, and microvilli. Amplification is an effective means of increasing the surface area that is available for intestinal absorption, the primary function of the small and large intestine.

Table 44-1 Structural and Functional Differences Between the Small and the Large Intestine

	Small Intestine	Large Intestine
Length (m)	6	2.4
Area of apical plasma membrane (m²)	~200	~25
Folds	Yes	Yes
Villi	Yes	No
Crypts or glands	Yes	Yes
Microvilli	Yes	Yes
Nutrient absorption	Yes	No
Active Na⁺ absorption	Yes	Yes
Active K⁺ secretion	No	Yes

OVERVIEW OF FLUID AND ELECTROLYTE MOVEMENT IN THE INTESTINES

The small intestine absorbs ~6.5 L/day of an ~8.5-L fluid load that is presented to it, and the colon absorbs ~1.9 L/day

The fluid content of the average diet is typically 1.5 to 2.5 L/day. However, the fluid load to the small intestine is considerably greater—8 to 9 L/day. The difference between these two sets of figures is accounted for by salivary, gastric, pancreatic, and biliary secretions, as well as the secretions of the small intestine itself (Fig. 44-2). Similarly, the total quantity of electrolytes (Na^+, K^+, Cl^-, and HCO_3^-) that enter the lumen of the small intestine also consists of dietary sources in addition to endogenous secretions from the salivary glands, stomach, pancreas, liver, and small intestine.

We can calculate the absorption of water and electrolytes from the small intestine by comparing the total load that is presented to the lumen of the small intestine (i.e., 7.5 L/day entering from other organs +1.0 L/day secreted by the small intestine = 8.5 L/day) with that leaving the small intestine (i.e., ileocecal flow). The latter is ~2.0 L/day in normal subjects. Thus, overall small intestinal water absorption is 8.5 to 2.0, or ~6.5 L/day. Na^+ absorption is ~600 mEq/day. Maximal small intestinal fluid absorption has not been directly determined but has been estimated to be as great as 15 to 20 L/day.

Colonic fluid absorption is the difference between ileocecal flow (~2.0 L/day) and stool water, which is usually less than 0.2 L/day (~0.1 L/day). Thus, colonic water absorption is ~2.0 to 0.1, or 1.9 L/day. In contrast, the maximal colonic water **absorptive capacity** is between 4 and 5 L/day. As a result, a significant increase in ileocecal flow (e.g., up to perhaps 5 L/day, as occurs with a decrease in small intestinal fluid absorption) will not exceed the absorptive capacity of the large intestine. Thus, a compensatory increase in colonic fluid absorption can prevent an increase in stool water (i.e., diarrhea) despite substantial decreases in fluid absorption by the small intestine.

The small intestine absorbs net amounts of water, Na⁺, Cl⁻, and K⁺ and secretes HCO₃⁻, whereas the colon absorbs net amounts of water, Na⁺, and Cl⁻ and secretes both K⁺ and HCO₃⁻

Net ion movement represents the summation of several events. At the level of the entire small or large intestine, substantial movement of ions occurs from the intestinal lumen into the blood and from the blood into the lumen. The *net* ion movement across the entire epithelium is the difference between these two unidirectional fluxes.

Fluid and electrolyte transport in the intestine varies considerably in two different axes, both along the length of the intestines (*segmental heterogeneity*) and from the bottom of a crypt to the top of a villus or to the surface cells (*crypt-villus/surface heterogeneity*). A comparison of two different segments of intestine (e.g., duodenum versus ileum) shows that they differ substantially in function. These differences

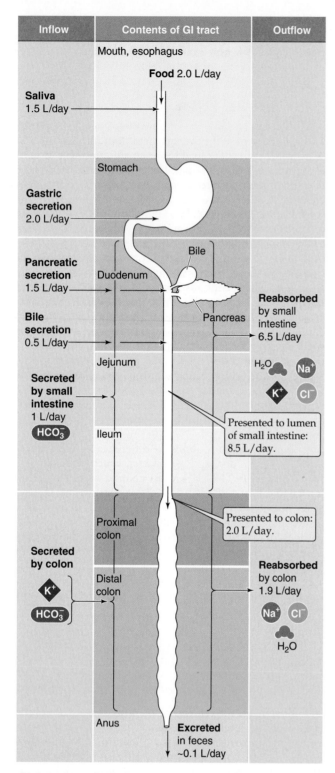

Inflow	Contents of GI tract	Outflow
	Mouth, esophagus	
Saliva 1.5 L/day	**Food** 2.0 L/day	
	Stomach	
Gastric secretion 2.0 L/day		
Pancreatic secretion 1.5 L/day	Bile / Duodenum	**Reabsorbed** by small intestine 6.5 L/day
Bile secretion 0.5 L/day	Pancreas	
	Jejunum	H_2O Na^+ K^+ Cl^-
Secreted by small intestine 1 L/day HCO_3^-	Ileum	Presented to lumen of small intestine: 8.5 L/day.
		Presented to colon: 2.0 L/day.
	Proximal colon	
Secreted by colon K^+ HCO_3^-	Distal colon	**Reabsorbed** by colon 1.9 L/day Na^+ Cl^- H_2O
	Anus	**Excreted** in feces ~0.1 L/day

Figure 44-2 Fluid balance in the gastrointestinal (GI) tract. For each segment of the GI tract, the figure shows substances flowing into the lumen on the left and substances flowing out of the lumen on the right. Of the ~8.5 L/day presented to the small intestine, the small intestine removes ~6.5 L/day, delivering ~2 L/day to the colon. The large intestine removes ~1.9 L/day, leaving ~0.1 L/day in the feces.

in function reflect **segmental heterogeneity** of ion transport processes along the longitudinal axis of the intestine in different macroscopic regions of both the small and the large intestine; these differences are both qualitative and quantitative. For example, HCO_3^- stimulation of Na^+ absorption occurs only in the proximal part of the small intestine. In contrast, the so-called electrogenic Na^+ absorption (i.e., absorption associated with the development of a transepithelial potential difference) is restricted to the rectosigmoid segment of the colon.

Within an intestinal segment (e.g., a piece of ileum), **crypt-villus/surface heterogeneity** leads to differences in transport function along the radial axis of the intestine wall. For example, it is generally believed that absorptive function is located in villous cells in the small intestine (and surface epithelial cells in the large intestine), whereas secretory processes reside in the crypt cells. Finally, at a certain level within a single villus or crypt—or within a very small area of the colonic surface epithelium—individual cells may demonstrate further heterogeneity (**cellular heterogeneity**), with specific transport mechanisms restricted to different cells.

Overall ion movement in any segment of the intestine represents the summation of these various absorptive and secretory events. These events may be paracellular or transcellular, may occur in the villus or crypt, and may be mediated by a goblet cell or an absorptive cell.

Despite the segmental heterogeneity of small intestinal electrolyte transport, overall water and ion movement in the proximal and distal portions of the small intestine is similar: in health, the small intestine is a net absorber of water, Na^+, Cl^-, and K^+, but it is a net secretor of HCO_3^- (Fig. 44-2). Fluid absorption is isosmotic in the small intestine, similar to that observed in the renal proximal tubule (see Chapter 35). In general, absorptive processes in the small intestine are enhanced in the postprandial state. The human colon carries out net absorption of water, Na^+, and Cl^- with few exceptions, but it carries out net secretion of K^+ and HCO_3^-.

The intestines absorb and secrete solutes by both active and passive mechanisms

As discussed in Chapter 5, intestinal epithelial cells are polar; that is, they have two very different membranes—an apical membrane and a basolateral membrane—separated from one another by tight junctions. The transport processes present in the small and large intestine are quite similar to those present in other epithelia, such as the renal tubules, with only some organ-specific specialization to distinguish them. The transepithelial movement of a solute across the entire epithelium can be either absorptive or secretory. In each case, the movement can be either transcellular or paracellular. In transcellular movement, the solute must cross the two cell membranes in series. In general, movement of the solute across at least one of these membranes must be active (i.e., against an electrochemical gradient). In paracellular movement, the solute moves passively between adjacent epithelial cells through the tight junctions.

All transcellular Na^+ absorption is mediated by the Na-K pump (i.e., Na,K-ATPase) located at the basolateral membrane. This enzyme is responsible for Na^+ extrusion across the basolateral membrane and results in a relatively low [Na$^+$]$_i$ (~15 mM) and an intracellular-negative membrane potential. This Na$^+$ gradient serves as the driving force, in large part, for Na$^+$ entry into the epithelial cell across the luminal (apical) membrane, a process mediated either by Na$^+$ channels or by Na$^+$-coupled transporters (e.g., Na/glucose cotransport, Na-H exchange). The epithelial cell may also use this Na$^+$ gradient to energize other transport processes at the apical or basolateral membrane.

Intestinal fluid movement is always coupled to solute movement, whereas solute movement may be coupled to fluid movement by "solvent drag"

Fluid movement is always coupled to active solute movement. The model of the osmotic coupling of fluid movement to solute movement in the intestine is similar to that in all or most epithelial cells (see Chapter 5). It is likely that the water movement occurs predominantly by a paracellular route rather than by a transcellular route.

Solute movement is the driving force for fluid movement. However, the converse may also be true: solute movement may be coupled to fluid movement by **solvent drag**, a phenomenon in which the dissolved solute is swept along by bulk movement of the solvent (i.e., water). Solvent drag accounts for a significant fraction of the Na$^+$ and urea absorbed in the human jejunum (but not in the more distal segments of the small intestine or the large intestine). For all intents and purposes, solvent drag occurs through the paracellular route, and it depends on the permeability properties of the tight junctions (reflection coefficient; see Chapter 20) and the magnitude of the convective water flow. Thus, solvent drag contributes primarily to the absorption of relatively small, water-soluble molecules, such as urea and Na$^+$, and it does so mainly in epithelia with relatively high permeability. The transepithelial permeability of the jejunum is considerably greater than that of the ileum or colon, as evidenced by its lower spontaneous transepithelial voltage difference (V_{TE}), higher passive movement of NaCl, and larger apparent pore size.

The resistance of the tight junctions primarily determines the transepithelial resistance of intestinal epithelia

Epithelial permeability is an inverse function of transepithelial resistance. In epithelial structures such as the small and large intestine, transepithelial resistance is determined by cellular resistance and paracellular resistance, which are arranged in parallel (see Chapter 5). Paracellular resistance is considerably lower than transcellular resistance; therefore, overall mucosal resistance depends mainly on paracellular resistance, which, in turn, depends primarily on the properties of the tight junctions. Therefore, intestinal permeability is essentially a function of tight junction structure. Just as transport function varies greatly throughout the intestine, major differences in transepithelial permeability and the properties of tight junctions are also present throughout the intestinal tract. In general, resistance increases in the aboral direction (i.e., moving away from the mouth). Thus, the resistance of the jejunum is considerably lower than that of the distal end of the colon. Evidence also indicates that the permeability of the tight junctions in the crypt is greater than that in the villus.

CELLULAR MECHANISMS OF NA$^+$ ABSORPTION

Both the small intestine and the large intestine absorb large amounts of Na$^+$ and Cl$^-$ daily, but different mechanisms are responsible for this extremely important physiological process in different segments of the intestine. The villous epithelial cells in the small intestine and the surface epithelial cells in the colon are responsible for absorbing most of the Na$^+$. Absorption of Na$^+$ is the result of a complex interplay of both apical and basolateral membrane transport processes. Figure 44-3 summarizes the four fundamental mechanisms by which Na$^+$ may enter the cell across the apical membrane. In each case, the Na-K pump is responsible, at least in part, for the movement of Na$^+$ from cell to blood. Also in each case, the driving force for apical Na$^+$ entry is provided by the large, inwardly directed electrochemical gradient for Na$^+$, which, in turn, is provided by the Na-K pump. The following four sections describe these four apical membrane transport processes.

Na/glucose and Na/amino acid cotransport in the small intestine is a major mechanism for postprandial Na$^+$ absorption

Nutrient-coupled Na$^+$ absorption (Fig. 44-3A) occurs throughout the small intestine. Although glucose- and amino acid–coupled Na$^+$ absorption also takes place in the colon of the newborn, it disappears during the neonatal period. Glucose- and amino acid–coupled Na$^+$ absorption occurs only in villous epithelial cells and not in crypt epithelial cells (Fig. 44-3A). This process is the primary mechanism for Na$^+$ absorption after a meal, but it makes little contribution during the interdigestive period, when only limited amounts of glucose and amino acids are present in the intestinal lumen.

Glucose- and amino acid–coupled Na$^+$ absorption is mediated by specific apical membrane transport proteins. The Na/glucose cotransporter SGLT1 (see Chapter 5) is responsible for glucose uptake across the apical membrane, as discussed in Chapter 45. Several distinct Na/amino acid cotransporters, each specific for a different class of amino acids (see Table 36-1), are responsible for the Na$^+$-coupled uptake of amino acids across the apical membrane. Because these transporters couple the energetically downhill movement of Na$^+$ to the uphill movement of glucose or an amino acid, the transporter processes are examples of **secondary active transport** (see Chapter 5). The glucose- and amino acid–coupled uptake of Na$^+$ entry across the apical membrane increases [Na$^+$]$_i$, which, in turn, increases Na$^+$ extrusion across the basolateral membrane through the Na-K pump. Because the apical Na/glucose and Na/amino acid cotransporters are electrogenic, as is the Na-K pump, the overall transport of Na$^+$ carries net charge and makes V_{TE} more lumen negative. Thus, glucose- and

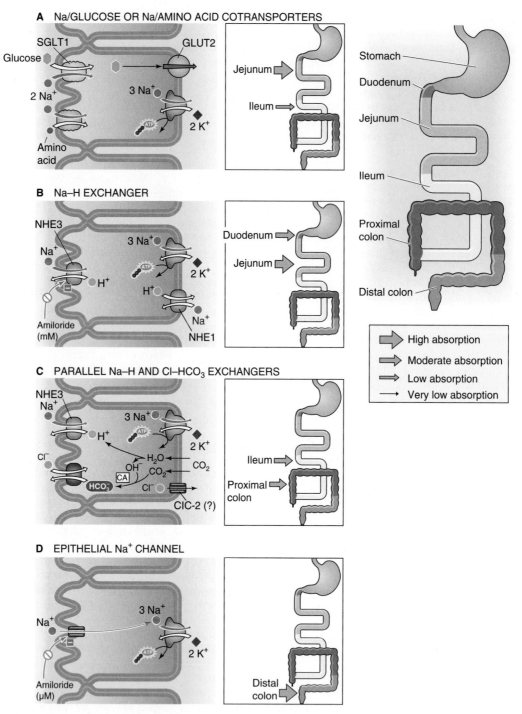

Figure 44-3 Modes of active Na⁺ absorption by the intestine. **A**, Nutrient-coupled Na⁺ absorption occurs in the villous cells of the jejunum and ileum and is the primary mechanism for postprandial Na⁺ absorption. The thickness of the arrows in the inset indicates the relative magnitude of the Na⁺ absorptive flux through this pathway. **B**, Electroneutral Na-H exchange at the apical membrane, in the absence of Cl-HCO₃ exchange, is stimulated by the high pH of the HCO₃⁻-rich luminal contents. **C**, Na-H and Cl-HCO₃ exchange is coupled by a change in intracellular pH that results in electroneutral NaCl absorption, which is the primary mechanism for interdigestive Na⁺ absorption. **D**, In electrogenic Na⁺ absorption, the apical step of Na⁺ movement occurs through the ENaC. CA, carbonic anhydrase.

amino acid–stimulated Na$^+$ absorption is an **electrogenic** process. As discussed later, the increase in the lumen-negative V_{TE} provides the driving force for the parallel absorption of Cl$^-$.

Nutrient-coupled Na$^+$ transporters, unlike other small intestinal Na$^+$ absorptive mechanisms, are not inhibited by either cAMP or [Ca^{2+}]$_i$. Thus, agonists that increase [cAMP]$_i$ (i.e., *Escherichia coli* or cholera enterotoxin) or [Ca^{2+}]$_i$ (i.e., serotonin) do not inhibit glucose- or amino acid–stimulated Na$^+$ absorption.

Electroneutral Na-H exchange in the duodenum and jejunum is responsible for Na$^+$ absorption that is stimulated by luminal alkalinity

Luminal HCO$_3^-$—the result of pancreatic, biliary, and duodenal secretion—increases Na$^+$ absorption in the proximal portion of the small intestine by stimulating apical membrane Na-H exchange (Fig. 44-3B). The Na-H exchanger couples Na$^+$ uptake across the apical membrane to proton extrusion into the intestinal lumen, a process that is enhanced by both decreases in intracellular pH (pH$_i$) and increases in luminal pH. The energy for Na-H exchange comes from the Na$^+$ gradient, a consequence of the ability of the Na-K pump to extrude Na$^+$, thereby lowering [Na$^+$]$_i$. This process is characteristically inhibited by *millimolar* concentrations of the diuretic amiloride.

Several isoforms of the Na-H exchanger exist (see Chapter 5), and different isoforms are present on the apical and basolateral membranes. Intestinal epithelial cells also have Na-H exchangers on their basolateral membranes. However, this NHE1 isoform, like its counterpart in nonepithelial cells, regulates pH$_i$ (a "housekeeping" function) and does not contribute to the transepithelial movement of Na$^+$. In contrast, both the NHE2 and NHE3 exchanger isoforms present on the apical membrane are responsible for both transepithelial Na$^+$ movement *and* pH$_i$ regulation. Although Na-H exchangers are present on the apical membrane of villous epithelial cells throughout the entire intestine, only in the duodenum and jejunum (i.e., the proximal part of the small intestine) is Na-H exchange present without the parallel presence of Cl-HCO$_3$ exchangers (see next section). Thus, in the proximal portion of the small intestine, the Na-H exchanger solely mediates the Na$^+$ absorption that is stimulated by the alkalinity of the HCO$_3^-$-rich intraluminal contents.

Parallel Na-H and Cl-HCO$_3$ exchange in the ileum and proximal part of the colon is the primary mechanism of Na$^+$ absorption during the interdigestive period

Electroneutral NaCl absorption occurs in portions of both the small and large intestine (Fig. 44-3C). Electroneutral NaCl absorption is not the result of an Na/Cl cotransporter, but rather of parallel apical membrane Na-H and Cl-HCO$_3$ exchangers that are closely linked by small changes in pH$_i$. In the human colon, DRA (downregulated-in-adenoma; SLC26A3; see Chapter 5) mediates this Cl-HCO$_3$ exchange. This mechanism of NaCl absorption is the primary method of Na$^+$ absorption between meals (i.e., the interdigestive

Oral Rehydration Solution

The therapeutic use of **oral rehydration solution (ORS)** provides an excellent demonstration of applied physiology. Many diarrheal illnesses (see the box titled Secretory Diarrhea) are caused by bacterial exotoxins that induce fluid and electrolyte secretion by the intestine. Hence such a toxin is referred to as an **enterotoxin**. Despite the massive toxin-induced fluid secretion, both intestinal morphology and nutrient-coupled Na$^+$ absorption are normal. Because nutrient-coupled (e.g., glucose or amino acid) fluid absorption is intact, therapeutically increasing the concentration of glucose or amino acids in the intestinal lumen can enhance absorption. ORS contains varying concentrations of glucose, Na$^+$, Cl$^-$, and HCO$_3^-$ and is extremely effective in enhancing fluid and electrolyte absorption in secretory diarrhea when the intestine secretes massive amounts of fluid. Administration of ORS can reverse the dehydration and metabolic acidosis that may occur in severe diarrhea and that are often the primary cause of morbidity and mortality, especially in children younger than 5 years. ORS is the major advance of the past half century in the treatment of diarrheal disease, especially in developing countries. The development of ORS was a direct consequence of research on the physiology of glucose- and amino acid–stimulated Na$^+$ absorption.

period), but it does not contribute greatly to postprandial Na$^+$ absorption, which is mediated primarily by the nutrient-coupled transporters described previously. Electroneutral NaCl absorption occurs in the ileum and throughout the large intestine, with the exception of the most distal segment. It is not affected by either luminal glucose or luminal HCO$_3^-$. However, aldosterone inhibits electroneutral NaCl absorption.

The overall electroneutral NaCl absorptive process is regulated by both cAMP and cGMP, as well as by intracellular Ca^{2+}. Increases in each of these three intracellular messengers *reduce* NaCl absorption. Conversely, decreases in [Ca^{2+}]$_i$ *increase* NaCl absorption. Decreased NaCl absorption is important in the pathogenesis of most diarrheal disorders. For example, one of the common causes of traveler's diarrhea (see the box titled Secretory Diarrhea) is the heat-labile enterotoxin produced by the bacterium *E. coli*. This toxin activates adenylyl cyclase and increases [cAMP]$_i$, which, in turn, decreases NaCl absorption and stimulates active Cl$^-$ secretion, as discussed later. This toxin does not affect glucose-stimulated Na$^+$ absorption.

Epithelial Na$^+$ channels are the primary mechanism of electrogenic Na$^+$ absorption in the distal part of the colon

In electrogenic Na$^+$ absorption (Fig. 44-3D), Na$^+$ entry across the apical membrane occurs through epithelial Na$^+$ channels (ENaCs) that are highly specific for Na$^+$ (see Chapter 5). Like the Na-H exchanger, these ENaCs are blocked by the diuretic amiloride, but at *micro*molar rather than *milli*molar concentrations. Na⁺ absorption in the distal part of the colon is highly efficient. Because this segment of the colon is capable of absorbing Na⁺ against large concentration gradients, it plays an important role in Na⁺ conservation. Na⁺ movement through electrogenic Na⁺ absorption is not affected by luminal glucose or by HCO_3^-, nor is it regulated by cyclic nucleotides. However, it is markedly enhanced by mineralo-corticoids (e.g., aldosterone).

Mineralocorticoids increase Na⁺ absorption in the colon—as in other aldosterone-responsive epithelia, notably the renal collecting duct (see Chapter 35)—through multiple mechanisms. Aldosterone increases electrogenic Na⁺ absorption by increasing Na⁺ entry through the apical Na⁺ channel and by stimulating activity of the Na-K pump. The increase in apical Na⁺ uptake can occur (1) rapidly (i.e., within seconds) as a consequence of an increase in the opening of apical Na⁺ channels, (2) more gradually (within minutes) because of the insertion of preformed Na⁺ channels from subapical epithelial vesicle pools into the apical membrane, or (3) very slowly (within hours) as a result of an increase in the synthesis of both new apical Na⁺ channels and Na-K pumps.

CELLULAR MECHANISMS OF CL⁻ ABSORPTION AND SECRETION

Cl⁻ absorption occurs throughout the small and large intestine and is often closely linked to Na⁺ absorption. Cl⁻ and Na⁺ absorption may be coupled through either an electrical potential difference or by pH_i. However, sometimes *no* coupling takes place, and the route of Cl⁻ movement may be either paracellular or transcellular.

Voltage-dependent Cl⁻ absorption represents coupling of Cl⁻ absorption to electrogenic Na⁺ absorption in both the small intestine and the large intestine

Cl⁻ absorption can be a purely passive process (Fig. 44-4A), driven by the electrochemical gradient for Cl⁻ either across the tight junctions (paracellular route) or across the individual membranes of the epithelial cell (transcellular route). In either case, the driving force for Cl⁻ absorption derives from either of the two electrogenic mechanisms of Na⁺ absorption described previously (namely, nutrient-coupled transport in the small intestine and the ENaCs in the distal end of the colon), which, in turn, are energized by the Na-K pump. This process is referred to as *voltage-dependent Cl⁻ absorption;* it is not an active transport process.

Within the *small intestine,* induction of a lumen-negative potential difference by glucose- and amino acid–induced Na⁺ absorption (Fig. 44-3A) provides the driving force for Cl⁻ absorption that occurs following a meal. As noted earlier, nutrient-coupled Na⁺ absorption primarily represents a villous cell process that occurs in the postprandial period and is insensitive to cyclic nucleotides and changes in $[Ca^{2+}]_i$. Voltage-dependent Cl⁻ absorption shares these properties. It is most likely that the route of voltage-dependent Cl⁻ absorption is paracellular.

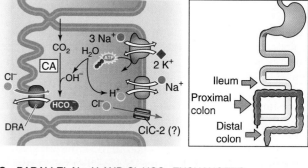

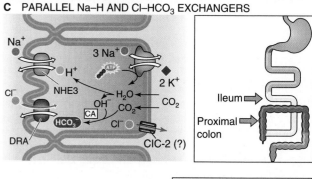

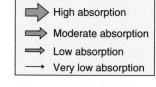

Figure 44-4 Modes of Cl⁻ absorption by the intestine. **A,** In voltage-dependent Cl⁻ absorption, Cl⁻ may passively diffuse from lumen to blood across the tight junctions, driven by the lumen-negative transepithelial voltage (paracellular route). Alternatively, Cl⁻ may diffuse through apical and basolateral Cl⁻ channels. The thickness of the arrows in the inset indicates the relative magnitude of the Cl⁻ absorptive flux through this pathway. **B,** In the absence of a parallel Na-H exchanger, electroneutral Cl-HCO_3 exchange at the apical membrane results in Cl⁻ absorption and HCO_3^- secretion. **C,** Electro-neutral NaCl absorption (see Fig. 44-3C) can mediate Cl⁻ absorption in the interdigestive period. pH_i couples the two exchangers. CA, carbonic anhydrase.

In the *large intestine,* especially in the distal segment, elec-trogenic Na⁺ absorption through the ENaC (Fig. 44-3D) also induces a lumen-negative potential difference that provides the driving force for colonic voltage-dependent Cl⁻ absorp-tion. Factors that increase or decrease the voltage difference similarly affect Cl⁻ absorption.

Congenital Chloridorrhea

The congenital absence of an apical Cl-HCO₃ exchanger (which mediates the Cl-HCO₃ involved in electroneutral NaCl absorption) is an autosomal recessive disorder known as **congenital chloridorrhea** or **congenital Cl⁻ diarrhea (CLD)**. Affected children have diarrhea with an extremely high stool [Cl⁻], a direct consequence of absence of the apical membrane Cl-HCO₃ exchanger. In addition, because HCO₃⁻ secretion is reduced, patients are alkalotic (i.e., have an increased plasma [HCO₃⁻]). The gene for congenital chloridorrhea is located on chromosome 7q31. The gene product is the same as that of the *DRA* gene. DRA (SLC26A3; see Chapter 5) and mediates Cl-HCO₃ exchange. In addition, DRA transports sulfate and other anions. However, DRA is distinct from the AE (anion exchanger) gene family that encodes the Cl-HCO₃ exchangers in erythrocytes and several other tissues. Indeed, Cl-HCO₃ exchange in the renal tubule, erythrocytes, and other cells is unaffected in individuals with CLD, as are other intestinal transport processes.

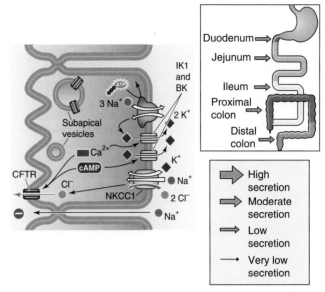

Figure 44-5 Cellular mechanism of electrogenic Cl⁻ secretion by crypt cells. The basolateral Na/K/Cl cotransporter brings Cl⁻ into the crypt cell; the Cl⁻ exits across the apical Cl⁻ channel. Secretagogues may open preexisting Cl⁻ channels or may cause subapical vesicles to fuse with the apical membrane, thus delivering new Cl⁻ channels. The paracellular pathway allows Na⁺ movement from blood to lumen, driven by the lumen-negative transepithelial voltage. The thickness of the *arrows in the inset* indicates that the magnitude of the Cl⁻ secretory flux through this pathway is the same throughout the intestine.

Electroneutral Cl-HCO₃ exchange results in Cl⁻ absorption and HCO₃⁻ secretion in the ileum and colon

Electroneutral Cl-HCO₃ exchange, in the absence of parallel Na-H exchange, occurs in villous cells in the ileum and in surface epithelial cells in the large intestine (Fig. 44-4B). It is not known whether this process occurs in the cells lining the crypts. A Cl-HCO₃ exchanger in the apical membrane is responsible for the 1:1 exchange of apical Cl⁻ for intracellular HCO₃⁻. In humans, this Cl-HCO₃ exchanger is DRA (see Chapter 5). The details of Cl⁻ movement across the *basolateral* membrane are not well understood, but the process may involve a ClC-2 Cl⁻ channel (see Chapter 6).

Parallel Na-H and Cl-HCO₃ exchange in the ileum and the proximal part of the colon mediates Cl⁻ absorption during the interdigestive period

Electroneutral NaCl absorption, discussed in connection with Na⁺ absorption (Fig. 44-3C), also mediates Cl⁻ absorption in the ileum and proximal part of the colon (Fig. 44-4C). The apical step of Cl⁻ absorption by this mechanism is mediated by parallel Na-H exchange (NHE3 or SLC9A3) and Cl-HCO₃ exchange (DRA or SLC26A3), which are coupled through pH$_i$.

Electrogenic Cl⁻ secretion occurs in crypts of both the small intestine and the large intestine

In the previous three sections, we saw that intestinal Cl⁻ *absorption* occurs through three mechanisms. The small intestine and the large intestine are also capable of active Cl⁻ secretion, although Cl⁻ secretion is believed to occur mainly in the crypts rather than in either the villi or surface cells.

A small amount of Cl⁻ secretion probably occurs in the "basal" state but is masked by the higher rate of the three Cl⁻ absorptive processes that are discussed earlier in this subchapter. However, Cl⁻ secretion is markedly stimulated by secretagogues such as acetylcholine and other neurotransmitters. Moreover, Cl⁻ secretion is the major component of the ion transport events that occur during most clinical and experimental diarrheal disorders.

The cellular model of active Cl⁻ secretion is outlined in Figure 44-5 and includes three transport pathways on the basolateral membrane: (1) an Na-K pump, (2) an Na/K/Cl cotransporter (NKCC1 or SLC12A2), and (3) two types of K⁺ channels (IK1 and BK). In addition, a Cl⁻ channel (cystic fibrosis transmembrane regulator [CFTR]) is present on the apical membrane. This complex Cl⁻ secretory system is energized by the Na-K pump, which generates a low [Na⁺]$_i$ and provides the driving force for Cl⁻ entry across the basolateral membrane through Na/K/Cl cotransport. As a result, [Cl⁻]$_i$ is raised sufficiently that the Cl⁻ electrochemical gradient favors the passive efflux of Cl⁻ across the apical membrane. One consequence of these many transport processes is that the transepithelial voltage becomes more lumen negative, thereby promoting voltage-dependent Na⁺ secretion. This Na⁺ secretion that accompanies active Cl⁻ secretion presumably occurs through the tight junctions (paracellular pathway). Thus, the net result is stimulation of NaCl and fluid secretion.

Normally (i.e., in the unstimulated state), the crypts secrete little Cl⁻ because the apical membrane Cl⁻ channels are either closed or not present. Cl⁻ secretion requires activation by cyclic nucleotides or [Ca^{2+}], which are increased by any of several **secretagogues**, including (1) bacterial exotoxins (i.e., enterotoxins), (2) hormones and neurotransmitters, (3) products of cells of the immune system (e.g., histamine), and (4) laxatives (Table 44-2).

Some secretagogues initially bind to membrane receptors and stimulate the activation of adenylyl cyclase (vasoactive intestinal peptide [VIP]), guanylyl cyclase (the heat-stable toxin of *E. coli*), or phospholipase C (acetylcholine). Others increase [Ca^{2+}]$_i$ by opening Ca^{2+} channels at the basolateral membrane. The resulting activation of one or more protein kinases—by any of the aforementioned pathways—increases the Cl^- conductance of the apical membrane either by activating preexisting Cl^- channels or by inserting into the apical membrane Cl^- channels that—in the unstimulated state—are stored in subapical membrane vesicles. In either case, Cl^- is now able to exit the cell through apical Cl^- channels. The resulting decrease in [Cl^-]$_i$ leads to increased uptake of Na^+, Cl^-, and K^+ across the basolateral membrane through the Na/K/Cl cotransporter (NKCC1). The Na^+ is recycled out of the cell through the Na-K pump. The K^+ is recycled through basolateral K^+ channels that are opened by the same protein kinases that increase Cl^- conductance. The net result of all these changes is the initiation of active Cl^- secretion across the epithelial cell.

The induction of apical membrane Cl^- channels is extremely important in the pathophysiology of many diarrheal disorders. The box titled Secretory Diarrhea discusses the changes in ion transport that occur in secretory diarrheas such as cholera. A central role in **cystic fibrosis** has been posited for the CFTR Cl^- channel in the apical membrane (see Chapter 43). However, more than one (and possibly several) Cl^- channels are present in the intestine, and CFTR may not be the only Cl^- channel associated with active Cl^- secretion.

Table 44-2 Mode of Action of Secretagogues

Category	Secretagogue	Second Messenger
Bacterial enterotoxins	Cholera toxin	cAMP
	Escherichia coli toxins: heat labile	cAMP
	E. coli toxins: heat stable	cGMP
	Yersinia toxin	cGMP
	Clostridium difficile toxin	Ca^{2+}
Hormones and neurotransmitters	VIP	cAMP
	Guanylin	cGMP
	Acetylcholine	Ca^{2+}
	Bradykinin	Ca^{2+}
	Serotonin (5-HT)	Ca^{2+}
Immune cell products	Histamine	cAMP
	Prostaglandins	cAMP
Laxatives	Bile acids	Ca^{2+}
	Ricinoleic acid	?

CELLULAR MECHANISMS OF K^+ ABSORPTION AND SECRETION

Overall net transepithelial K^+ movement is absorptive in the small intestine and is secretory in the colon

The gastrointestinal tract participates in overall K^+ balance, although when compared with the role of the kidneys, the small intestine and large intestine play relatively modest roles, especially in healthy individuals. The pattern of intestinal K^+ movement parallels that of the kidney: (1) the intestines have the capacity for both K^+ absorption and secretion, and (2) the intestines absorb K^+ in the proximal segments but secrete it in the distal segments.

Dietary K^+ furnishes 80 to 120 mmol/day, whereas stool K^+ output is only ~10 mmol/day. The kidney is responsible for disposal of the remainder of the daily K^+ intake (see Chapter 37). Substantial quantities of K^+ are secreted in gastric, pancreatic, and biliary fluid. Therefore, the total K^+ load presented to the small intestine is considerably greater than that represented by the diet. The concentration of K^+ in stool is frequently more than 100 mM. This high stool [K^+] is the result of several factors, including both colonic K^+ secretion and water absorption, especially in the distal part of the colon.

K^+ absorption in the small intestine probably occurs through solvent drag

Studies in which a plasma-like solution is perfused through segments of the intestine established that K^+ is absorbed in the jejunum and ileum of the small intestine and is secreted in the large intestine. Although the small intestine absorbs substantial amounts of K^+, no evidence has been presented to suggest that K^+ absorption in the jejunum and ileum is an active transport process or even carrier mediated. Thus, K^+ absorption in the small intestine is probably passive, most likely a result of **solvent drag** (i.e., pulled along by bulk water movement), as illustrated in Figure 44-6A. Although changes in dietary Na^+ and K^+ and alterations in hydration influence K^+ movement in the *colon*, similar physiological events do not appear to affect K^+ absorption in the *small intestine*.

Passive K^+ secretion is the primary mechanism for net colonic secretion

In contrast to the small intestine, the human colon is a net *secretor* of K^+. This secretion occurs by two mechanisms: a passive transport process that is discussed in this section and an active process that is discussed in the next. Together, these two K^+ secretory pathways are greater than a modest component of active K^+ absorption in the distal part of the colon and thus account for the overall secretion of K^+ by the colon.

Passive K^+ secretion, which is the pathway that is primarily responsible for overall net colonic K^+ secretion, is driven by the lumen-negative V_{TE} of 15 to 25 mV. The route of passive K^+ secretion is predominantly paracellular, not transcellular (Fig. 44-6B). Because V_{TE} is the primary determinant

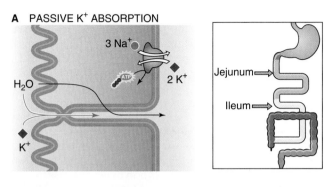

A PASSIVE K⁺ ABSORPTION

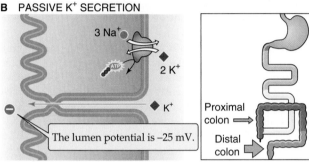

B PASSIVE K⁺ SECRETION

The lumen potential is –25 mV.

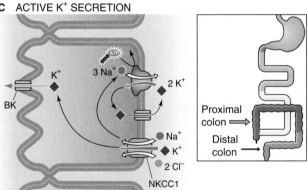

C ACTIVE K⁺ SECRETION

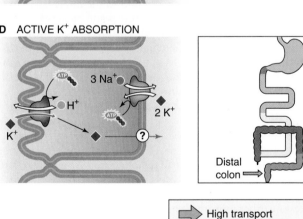

D ACTIVE K⁺ ABSORPTION

⟹ High transport
⟹ Moderate transport
⟹ Low transport
→ Very low transport

Figure 44-6 Cellular mechanisms of K⁺ secretion and absorption. **A,** This mechanism pertains only to the small intestine, which is a net absorber of K⁺ through solvent drag across tight junctions. The thickness of the arrows in the inset indicates the relative magnitude of the K⁺ flux through this pathway. **B,** The colon is a net secretor of K⁺. The primary mechanism is passive K⁺ secretion through tight junctions, which occurs throughout the colon. The driving force is a lumen-negative transepithelial voltage. **C,** Another mechanism of K⁺ secretion throughout the colon is a transcellular process that involves the basolateral uptake of K⁺ through the Na-K pump and the Na/K/Cl cotransporter, followed by the efflux of K⁺ through apical K⁺ channels. **D,** Confined to the distal colon is a transcellular mechanism of K⁺ absorption that is mediated by an apical H-K pump.

of passive K⁺ secretion, it is not surprising that passive K⁺ secretion is greatest in the distal end of the colon, where V_{TE} difference is most negative. Similarly, increases in the lumen-negative V_{TE} that occur as an adaptive response to dehydration—secondary to an elevation in aldosterone secretion (see the next section)—result in an enhanced rate of passive K⁺ secretion. Information is not available regarding the distribution of passive K⁺ secretion between surface epithelial and crypt cells.

Active K⁺ secretion is also present throughout the large intestine and is induced both by aldosterone and by cAMP

In addition to *passive* K⁺ secretion, *active* K⁺ transport processes—both secretory and absorptive—are also present in the colon. However, active transport of K⁺ is subject to considerable segmental variation in the colon. Whereas active K⁺ *secretion* occurs throughout the colon, active K⁺ *absorption* is present only in the distal segments of the large intestine. Thus, in the rectosigmoid colon, active K⁺ absorption and active K⁺ secretion are both operative and appear to contribute to total body homeostasis.

The model of active K⁺ secretion in the colon is quite similar to that of active Cl⁻ secretion (Fig. 44-5) and is also parallel to that of active K⁺ secretion in the renal distal nephron (see Chapter 37). The general paradigm of active K⁺ transport in the colon is a pump-leak model (Fig. 44-6C). Uptake of K⁺ across the basolateral membrane is a result of both the Na-K pump and the Na/K/Cl cotransporter (NKCC1), which is energized by the low $[Na^+]_i$ that is created by the Na-K pump. Once K⁺ enters the cell across the basolateral membrane, it may exit either across the apical membrane (K⁺ secretion) or across the basolateral membrane (K⁺ recycling). The cell controls the extent to which secretion occurs, in part by K⁺ channels present in both the apical and the basolateral membranes. When apical K⁺ channel activity is less than basolateral channel activity, K⁺ recycling dominates. Indeed, in the basal state, the rate of active K⁺ secretion is low because the apical K⁺ channel activity is minimal in comparison with the K⁺ channel activity in the basolateral membrane.

It is likely that aldosterone stimulates active K⁺ secretion in surface epithelial cells of the large intestine, whereas cAMP enhances active K⁺ secretion in crypt cells. In both cases, the rate-limiting step is the apical BK K⁺ channel, and both secretagogues act by increasing K⁺ channel activity.

Aldosterone This mineralocorticoid enhances overall net K^+ secretion by two mechanisms. First, it increases **passive** K^+ secretion by increasing Na-K pump activity and thus increasing electrogenic Na^+ absorption (Fig. 44-3D). The net effects are to increase the lumen-negative V_{TE} and to enhance passive K^+ secretion (Fig. 44-6B). Second, aldosterone stimulates **active** K^+ secretion by increasing the activity of both apical K^+ channels and basolateral Na-K pumps (Fig. 44-6C).

cAMP and Ca^{2+} VIP and cholera enterotoxin both increase $[cAMP]_i$ and thus stimulate K^+ secretion. Increases in $[Ca^{2+}]_i$—induced, for example, by serotonin (or 5-hydroxytryptamine [5-HT])—also stimulate active K^+ secretion. In contrast to aldosterone, neither of these second messengers has an effect on the Na-K pump; rather, they increase the activity of both the apical and the basolateral K^+ channels. Because the stimulation of K^+ channels is greater at the apical than at the basolateral membrane, the result is an increase in K^+ exit from the epithelial cell across the apical membrane (i.e., secretion). Stimulation of K^+ secretion by cAMP and Ca^{2+}, both of which also induce active Cl^- secretion (Fig. 44-5), contributes to the significant fecal K^+ losses that occur in many diarrheal diseases.

Active K^+ absorption is located only in the distal portion of the colon and is energized by an apical H-K pump

As noted earlier, not only does the distal end of the colon actively secrete K^+, but also it actively absorbs K^+. The balance between the two processes plays a role in overall K^+ homeostasis. Increases in dietary K^+ enhance both passive and active K^+ *secretion* (Fig. 44-6B, C). However, dietary K^+ depletion enhances active K^+ absorption (Fig. 44-6D). The mechanism of active K^+ absorption appears to be an exchange of luminal K^+ for intracellular H^+ across the apical membrane, mediated by an H-K pump (see Chapter 5). The colonic H-K pump is ~60% identical at the amino acid level to both the Na-K pump and the gastric parietal cell H-K pump. Thus, colonic K^+ movement through the active K^+ absorption process occurs through a transcellular route, in contrast to the paracellular route that characterizes K^+ absorption in the small intestine (Fig. 44-6A). The mechanism of K^+ exit across the basolateral membrane may involve K/Cl cotransport. Not known is whether active K^+ secretion (Fig. 44-6C) and active K^+ absorption (Fig. 44-6D) occur in the same cell or in different cells.

REGULATION OF INTESTINAL ION TRANSPORT

Chemical mediators from the enteric nervous system, endocrine cells, and immune cells in the lamina propria may be either secretagogues or absorptagogues

Numerous chemical mediators from several different sources regulate intestinal electrolyte transport. Some of these agonists are important both in health and in diarrheal disorders, and at times only quantitative differences separate normal regulatory control from the pathophysiology of diarrhea. These mediators may function in one or more modes: neural, endocrine, paracrine, and perhaps autocrine (see Chapter 3). Most of these agonists (i.e., secretagogues) promote secretion, whereas some others (i.e., absorptagogues) enhance absorption.

The **enteric nervous system** (ENS), discussed in Chapters 14 and 41, is important in the normal regulation of intestinal epithelial electrolyte transport. Activation of enteric secretomotor neurons results in the release of acetylcholine from mucosal neurons and in the induction of active Cl^- secretion (Fig. 44-5). Additional neurotransmitters, including VIP, 5-HT, and histamine, mediate ENS regulation of epithelial ion transport.

An example of regulation mediated by the **endocrine system** is the release of aldosterone from the adrenal cortex and the subsequent formation of angiotensin II; both dehydration and volume contraction stimulate this renin-angiotensin-aldosterone axis (see Chapter 40). Both angiotensin and aldosterone regulate total body Na^+ homeostasis by stimulating Na^+ absorption, angiotensin in the small intestine and aldosterone in the colon. Their effects on cellular Na^+ absorption differ. In the small intestine, angiotensin enhances electroneutral NaCl absorption (Fig. 44-3C), probably by upregulating apical membrane Na-H exchange. In the colon, aldosterone stimulates electrogenic Na^+ absorption (Fig. 44-3D).

The response of the intestine to angiotensin and aldosterone represents a classic endocrine feedback loop: dehydration results in increased levels of angiotensin and aldosterone, the primary effects of which are to stimulate fluid and Na^+ absorption by both the renal tubules (see Chapter 35) and the intestines, thus restoring total body fluid and Na^+ content.

Regulation of intestinal transport also occurs by **paracrine effects**. Endocrine cells constitute a small fraction of the total population of mucosal cells in the intestines. These endocrine cells contain several peptides and bioactive amines that are released in response to various stimuli. Relatively little is known about the biology of these cells, but gut distention can induce the release of one or more of these agonists (e.g., 5-HT). The effect of these agonists on adjacent surface epithelial cells represents a paracrine action.

Another example of paracrine regulation of intestinal fluid and electrolyte transport is the influence of **immune cells** in the *lamina propria* (Fig. 44-1). Table 44-3 presents these immune cells and a partial list of the agonists that they release. The same agonist may be released from more than one cell, and individual cells produce multiple agonists. These agonists may activate epithelial cells directly or may activate other immune cells or enteric neurons. For example, reactive oxygen radicals released by mast cells affect epithelial cell function by acting on enteric neurons and fibroblasts, and they also have direct action on surface and crypt epithelial cells.

A single agonist usually has multiple sites of action. For example, the histamine released from mast cells can induce fluid secretion as a result of its interaction with receptors on surface epithelial cells (Fig. 44-7). However, histamine can also activate ENS motor neurons, which can, in turn, alter epithelial cell ion transport, as well as intestinal smooth muscle tone and blood flow. As a consequence, the effects of histamine on intestinal ion transport are multiple and amplified.

Secretagogues can be classified by their type and by the intracellular second-messenger system they stimulate

Several agonists induce the accumulation of fluid and electrolytes in the intestinal lumen (i.e., net secretion). These secretagogues are a diverse, heterogeneous group of compounds, but they can be effectively classified in two different ways: by the type of secretagogue and by the intracellular second messenger that these agonists activate.

Grouped according to type, the secretagogues fall into four categories: (1) bacterial exotoxins (i.e., enterotoxins), (2) hormones and neurotransmitters, (3) products of cells of the immune system, and (4) laxatives. Table 44-2 provides

Table 44-3 Products of Lamina Propria Cells That Affect Intestinal Ion Transport

Cell	Product
Macrophages	Prostaglandins O_2 radicals
Mast cells	Histamine
Neutrophils	Eicosanoids Platelet-activating factor
Fibroblasts	Eicosanoids Bradykinin

a partial list of these secretagogues. A **bacterial exotoxin** is a peptide that is produced and excreted by bacteria that can produce effects independently of the bacteria. An **enterotoxin** is an exotoxin that induces changes in intestinal fluid and electrolyte movement. For example, *E. coli* produces two distinct enterotoxins (the so-called heat-labile and heat-stable toxins) that induce fluid and electrolyte secretion through two distinct receptors and second-messenger systems.

We can also classify secretagogues according to the signal transduction system that they activate after binding to a specific membrane receptor. As summarized in Table 44-2, the second messengers of these signal transduction systems include cAMP, cGMP, and Ca^{2+}. For example, the **heat-labile** toxin of *E. coli* binds to apical membrane receptors, becomes internalized, and then activates basolateral adenylyl cyclase. The resulting increase in $[cAMP]_i$ activates protein kinase A. VIP also acts by this route (Fig. 44-8). The **heat-stable** toxin of *E. coli* binds to and activates an apical receptor guanylyl cyclase, similar to the atrial natriuretic peptide (ANP) receptor (see Chapter 3). The newly produced cGMP activates protein kinase G and may also activate protein kinase A. The natural agonist for this pathway is guanylin, a 15–amino acid peptide secreted by mucosal cells of the small and large intestine. Still other secretory agonists (e.g., 5-HT) produce their effects by increasing $[Ca^{2+}]_i$ and thus activating protein kinase C or Ca^{2+}-calmodulin–dependent protein kinases. One way that secretagogues can increase $[Ca^{2+}]_i$ is by stimulating phospholipase C, which leads to the production of inositol 1,4,5-triphosphate (IP_3) and the release of Ca^{2+} from intracellular stores (see Chapter 3). Secretagogues can also increase $[Ca^{2+}]_i$ by activating protein kinases, which may stimulate basolateral Ca^{2+} channels.

Although the secretagogues listed in Table 44-2 stimulate fluid and electrolyte secretion through one of three distinct second messengers (i.e., cAMP, cGMP, and Ca^{2+}), the *end*

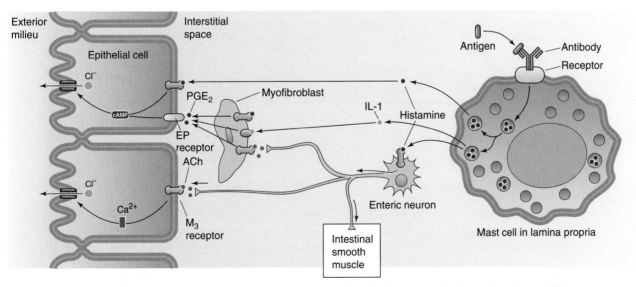

Figure 44-7 Mast cell activation. Activation of mast cells in the lamina propria triggers the release of histamine, which directly affects epithelial cells, or which stimulates an enteric neuron and thus has an indirect effect. The neuron modulates the epithelium (secretion), intestinal smooth muscle (motility), or vascular smooth muscle (blood flow). ACh, acetylcholine.

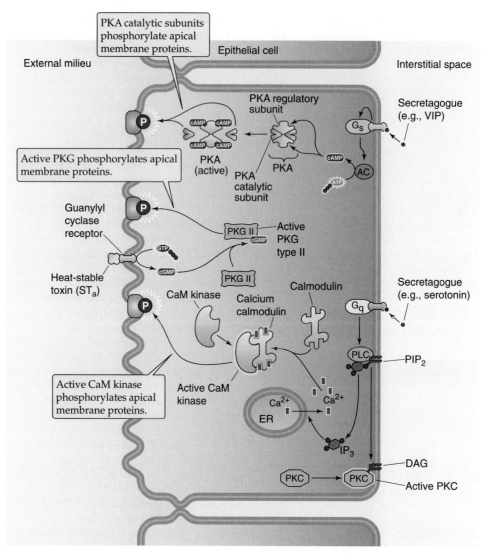

Figure 44-8 Action of secretagogues. Secretagogues (agents that stimulate the net secretion of fluid and electrolytes into the intestinal lumen) act by any of three mechanisms. Some (e.g., VIP, heat-labile toxin) activate adenylyl cyclase, which, in turn, generates cAMP and thus stimulates protein kinase A (PKA). Others (e.g., a heat-stable toxin, also known as ST_a) bind to the guanylin receptor, which is a receptor guanylyl cyclase that generates cGMP and results in the stimulation of protein kinase G (PKG). Others (e.g., serotonin) stimulate the phospholipase C (PLC) pathway, which leads to the generation of IP_3 and diacylglycerol (DAG). The DAG activates protein kinase C (PKC). The increased $[Ca^{2+}]_i$ stimulates PKC and Ca^{2+}-calmodulin–dependent protein kinase (CaM kinase). These activated kinases stimulate net secretion by phosphorylating apical membrane transporters or other proteins. AC, adenylyl cyclase; G_q and G_s, a-subunit types of G proteins; PIP_2, phosphatidylinositol 4,5-biphosphate.

effects are quite similar. As summarized in Table 44-4, all three second-messenger systems stimulate active Cl⁻ secretion (Fig. 44-5) and inhibit electroneutral NaCl absorption (Fig. 44-3C). The abilities of cAMP and Ca^{2+} to stimulate Cl⁻ secretion and to inhibit electroneutral NaCl absorption are almost identical. In contrast, cGMP's ability to stimulate Cl⁻ secretion is somewhat less, although its effects on electroneutral NaCl absorption are quantitatively similar to those of cAMP and Ca^{2+}. Both stimulation of Cl⁻ secretion and inhibition of electroneutral NaCl absorption have the

Table 44-4 End Effects of Second Messengers on Intestinal Transport

Second Messenger	Increased Anion Secretion	Inhibited NaCl Absorption
cAMP	+++	+++
cGMP	+	+++
Ca^{2+}	+++	+++

same overall effect: *net secretion of fluid and electrolytes*. It is uncertain whether the observed decrease in electroneutral NaCl absorption is the result of inhibiting Na-H exchange, Cl-HCO₃ exchange, or both, inasmuch as electroneutral NaCl absorption represents the coupling of separate Na-H and Cl-HCO₃ exchange processes through pH_i (Fig. 44-3C).

Mineralocorticoids, glucocorticoids, and somatostatin are absorptagogues

Although multiple secretagogues exist, relatively few agonists can be found that *enhance* fluid and electrolyte *absorption*. The cellular effects of these absorptagogues are less well understood than those of the secretagogues. Those few absorptagogues that have been identified increase intestinal fluid and electrolyte absorption by either a paracrine or an endocrine mechanism.

Secretory Diarrhea

Diarrhea is a common medical problem and can be defined as a symptom (i.e., an increase in the number of bowel movements or a decrease in stool consistency) or as a sign (i.e., an increase in stool volume of more than 0.2 L/24 hours). Diarrhea has many causes and can be classified in various ways. One classification divides diarrheas by the causative factor. The causative factor can be a dietary nutrient that is not absorbed, in which case the result is **osmotic diarrhea**. An example of osmotic diarrhea is primary lactase deficiency. Alternatively, the causative factor may *not* be a dietary nutrient, but rather endogenous secretions of fluid and electrolytes from the intestine, in which case the result is **secretory diarrhea**.

The leading causes of secretory diarrhea include infections with *E. coli* (the major cause of traveler's diarrhea) and cholera (a substantial cause of morbidity and mortality in developing countries). In these infectious diarrheas, an enterotoxin produced by one of many bacterial organisms raises $[cAMP]_i$, $[cGMP]_i$, or $[Ca^{2+}]_i$ (see Table 44-2).

A second group of secretory diarrheas includes those produced by different, although relatively uncommon, hormone-producing tumors. Examples include tumors that produce VIP (the Verner-Morrison syndrome), glucagon (glucagonomas), and serotonin (the carcinoid syndrome). These secretagogues act by raising either $[cAMP]_i$ or $[Ca^{2+}]_i$ (Table 44-2). When a tumor produces these secretagogues in abundance, the resulting diarrhea can be copious and explosive.

As we have seen, the secretory diarrheas have in common their ability to increase $[cAMP]_i$, $[cGMP]_i$, or $[Ca^{2+}]_i$. Table 44-4 summarizes the mechanisms by which these second messengers produce the secretory diarrhea. Because the second messengers do not alter the function of nutrient-coupled Na⁺ absorption, administration of an ORS containing glucose and Na⁺ is effective in the treatment of enterotoxin-mediated diarrhea (see the earlier box titled Oral Rehydration Solution).

Corticosteroids are the primary hormones that enhance intestinal fluid and electrolyte absorption. **Mineralocorticoids** (e.g., aldosterone) stimulate Na⁺ absorption and K⁺ secretion in the distal end of the colon; they do not affect ion transport in the small intestine. Their cellular actions are outlined in Chapter 50. Aldosterone induces both apical membrane Na⁺ channels (a process that is inhibited by the diuretic amiloride) and basolateral Na-K pumps; this action results in substantial enhancement of colonic electrogenic Na⁺ absorption. Although the effects of glucocorticoids on ion transport have most often been considered a result of crossover binding to the mineralocorticoid receptor (see Chapter 35), it is now evident that glucocorticoids also have potent actions on ion transport through their own receptor and that these changes in ion transport are distinct from those of the mineralocorticoids. **Glucocorticoids** stimulate electroneutral NaCl absorption (Fig. 44-3C) throughout the large and small intestine without any effect on either K⁺ secretion or electrogenic Na⁺ absorption. Both corticosteroids act, at least in part, by genomic mechanisms (see Chapter 4).

Other agonists appear to stimulate fluid and electrolyte absorption by stimulating electroneutral NaCl absorption and inhibiting electrogenic HCO₃⁻ secretion; both these changes *enhance fluid absorption*. Among these absorptagogues are **somatostatin**, which is released from endocrine cells in the intestinal mucosa (see Chapter 42), and the enkephalins and norepinephrine, which are neurotransmitters of enteric neurons. The limited information available suggests that these agonists affect ion transport by *decreasing* $[Ca^{2+}]_i$, probably by blocking Ca^{2+} channels. Thus, it appears that fluctuations in $[Ca^{2+}]_i$ regulate Na⁺ and Cl⁻ transport in both the absorptive (low $[Ca^{2+}]_i$) and secretory (high $[Ca^{2+}]_i$) directions. Therefore, Ca^{2+} is clearly a critical modulator of intestinal ion transport.

REFERENCES

Books and Reviews

Binder HJ, Sandle GI: Electrolyte transport in the mammalian colon. In Johnson LR (ed): Physiology of the Gastrointestinal Tract, 3rd ed, pp 2133-2172. New York: Raven Press, 1994.

Greger R, Bleich M, Leipziger J, et al: Regulation of ion transport in colonic crypts. News Physiol Sci 1997; 12:62-66.

Montrose MH, Keely SJ, Barrett KE: Electrolyte secretion and absorption: Small intestine and colon. In Yamada T (ed): Textbook of Gastroenterology, vol 1, 4th ed, pp 308-340. Philadelphia: Lippincott Williams & Wilkins, 2003.

Palacin M, Estevez R, Bertran J, Zorzano A: Molecular biology of mammalian plasma membrane amino acid transporters. Physiol Rev 1998; 78:969-1054.

Rao MC: Oral rehydration therapy: New explanations for an old remedy. Annu Rev Physiol 2004; 66: 385-417.

Zachos NC, Tse M, Donowitz M: Molecular physiology of intestinal Na/H exchange. Annu Rev Physiol 2005; 67: 411-443.

Journal Articles

Canessa CM, Horisberger J-D, Rossier BC: Epithelial sodium channel related to proteins involved in neurodegeneration. Nature 1993; 361:467-470.

Knickelbein RG, Aronson PS, Schron CM, et al: Sodium and chloride transport across rabbit ileal brush border. II. Evidence for

Cl-HCO$_3$ exchange and mechanism of coupling. Am J Physiol 1985; 249:G236-G245.

Moseley RH, Hoglund P, Wu GD, et al: Downregulated in adenoma gene encodes a chloride transporter defective in congenital chloride diarrhea. Am J Physiol 1999; 276:G185-G192.

Schulz S, Green CK, Yuen PST, Garbers DL: Guanylyl cyclase is a heat-stable enterotoxin receptor. Cell 1990; 63:941-948.

Singh SK, Binder HJ, Boron WF, Geibel JP: Fluid absorption in isolated perfused colonic crypts. J Clin Invest 1995; 96: 2373-2379.

CHAPTER 45

NUTRIENT DIGESTION AND ABSORPTION

Henry J. Binder and Adrian Reuben

In general, the digestive-absorptive processes for most of the constituents of our diet are highly efficient. For example, normal adult intestine absorbs ~95% of dietary lipid. However, we ingest most of the constituents of dietary food in a form that the intestine cannot readily absorb. Multiple digestive processes convert dietary food to a form that can be absorbed, primarily in the small intestine, but also, to a much smaller extent, in the colon.

The **digestive process**—the enzymatic conversion of complex dietary substances to a form that can be absorbed—is initiated by the sight, smell, and taste of food. Although some digestion (that of carbohydrates) begins in the mouth and additional digestion may occur within the lumen of the stomach, most digestive processes occur in the small intestine. Digestion within the small intestine occurs either in the *lumen*, mediated by pancreatic enzymes, or at the small intestine *brush border membrane* (membrane digestion), mediated by brush border enzymes. Several different patterns of luminal, brush border, and cytosolic digestion exist (Fig. 45-1). Some of the dietary carbohydrate and protein that escape digestion and absorption in the small intestine are altered in the large intestine by bacterial enzymes to short-chain fatty acids that are absorbed by the colon.

The digestive processes for carbohydrates, proteins, and lipids result in the conversion of dietary nutrients to a chemical form for which intestinal **absorptive processes** exist. As a consequence, the digestive-absorptive processes for the several dietary constituents are closely integrated and regulated biological events that ensure survival. Multiple diseases can alter these digestive-absorptive processes and can thereby impair nutrient **assimilation** (i.e., the overall process of digestion and absorption). Because of the substantial segmental distribution of nutrient absorption along the gastrointestinal tract (Fig. 45-2), the clinical manifestations of disease (Table 45-1) often reflect these segmental differences.

CARBOHYDRATE DIGESTION

Carbohydrates, which provide ~45% of the total energy needs of Western diets, require hydrolysis to monosaccharides before absorption

We classify dietary carbohydrates into two major groups: (1) the **monosaccharides** (monomers) and (2) the **oligosac-** **charides** (short polymers) and **polysaccharides** (long polymers). The small intestine can directly absorb the monomers but not the polymers. Some polymers are **digestible**, that is, the body can digest them to form the monomers that the small intestine can absorb. Other polymers are **nondigestible**, or "fiber." The composition of dietary carbohydrate is quite varied and is a function of culture. The diet of so-called developed countries contains considerable amounts of "refined" sugar and, compared with most developing countries, less fiber. Such differences in the fiber content of the Western diet may account for several diseases that are more prevalent in these societies (e.g., colon carcinoma and atherosclerosis). As a consequence, the consumption of fiber by the health-conscious public in the United States has increased during the past 2 decades. In general, increased amounts of fiber in the diet are associated with increased stool weight and frequency.

Approximately 45% to 60% of dietary carbohydrate is in the form of **starch**, which is a polysaccharide. Starch is a storage form for carbohydrates that is primarily found in plants, and it consists of both amylose and amylopectin. In contrast, the storage form of carbohydrates in animal tissues is glycogen, which is consumed in much smaller amounts. **Amylose** is a straight-chain glucose polymer that typically contains multiple glucose residues, connected by α-1,4 linkages. In contrast, **amylopectin** is a massive branched glucose polymer that may contain 1 million glucose residues. In addition to the α-1,4 linkages, amylopectin has frequent α-1,6 linkages at the branch points. Amylopectins are usually present in much greater quantities (perhaps 4-fold) than amylose. Glycogen—the "animal starch"—also has α-1,4 and α-1,6 linkages like amylopectin. However, glycogen is more highly branched (i.e., α-1,6 linkages).

Most dietary oligosaccharides are the disaccharides sucrose and lactose, which represent 30% to 40% of dietary carbohydrates. **Sucrose** is table sugar, derived from sugar cane and sugar beets, whereas **lactose** is the sugar found in milk. The remaining carbohydrates are the monosaccharides **fructose** and **glucose**, which make up 5% to 10% of total carbohydrate intake. There is no evidence of any intestinal absorption of either starches or disaccharides. Because the small intestine can absorb only *monosaccharides*, all dietary carbohydrate must be digested to monosaccharides before absorption. The colon cannot absorb monosaccharides.

Dietary fiber consists of both soluble and insoluble forms and includes lignins, pectins, and cellulose. These fibers are primarily present in fruits, vegetables, and cereals. Cellulose

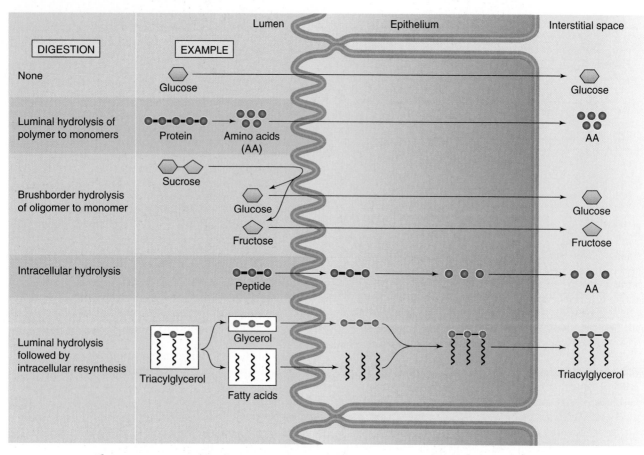

Figure 45-1 General mechanisms of digestion and absorption. Digestion-absorption can follow any of five patterns. First, the substance (e.g., glucose) may not require digestion; the intestinal cells may absorb the nutrient as ingested. Second, a polymer (e.g., protein) may be digested in the lumen to its constituent monomers (e.g., amino acids) by pancreatic enzymes before absorption. Third, an oligomer (e.g., sucrose) is digested into its constituent monomers (e.g., monosaccharides) by brush border enzymes before absorption. Fourth, an oligomer (e.g., oligopeptide) may be directly absorbed by the cell and then broken down into monomers (e.g., amino acids) inside the cell. Finally, a substance (e.g., TAG) may be broken down into its constituent components before absorption; the cell may then resynthesize the original molecule.

is a glucose polymer connected by β-1,4 linkages, which cannot be digested by mammalian enzymes. However, enzymes from colonic bacteria may degrade fiber. This process is carried out with varying efficiency; pectins, gum, and mucilages are metabolized to a much greater degree than either cellulose or hemicellulose. In contrast, lignins, which are aromatic polymers and not carbohydrates, are not altered by microbial enzymes in the colonic lumen and are excreted unaltered in stool.

As we discuss later, the digestive process for dietary carbohydrates has two steps: (1) **intraluminal hydrolysis** of starch to oligosaccharides by salivary and pancreatic amylases (Fig. 45-3) and (2) so-called **membrane digestion** of oligosaccharides to monosaccharides by brush border disaccharidases. The resulting carbohydrates are absorbed by transport processes that are specific for certain monosaccharides. These transport pathways are located in the apical membrane of the small intestine villous epithelial cells.

Luminal digestion begins with the action of salivary amylase and finishes with pancreatic amylase

Both salivary and pancreatic acinar cells (see Chapter 43) synthesize and secrete α-amylases. Salivary and pancreatic amylases, unlike most of the pancreatic proteases that we discuss later, are secreted not in an inactive proenzyme form, but rather in an active form. Salivary and pancreatic α-amylases have similar enzymatic function, and their amino acid sequences are 94% identical. **Salivary amylase** in the mouth initiates starch digestion; in healthy adults, this step is of relatively limited importance. Salivary amylase is inactivated by gastric acid, but it can be partially protected by complexing with oligosaccharides.

Pancreatic α-amylase completes starch digestion in the lumen of the small intestine. Although amylase binds to the apical membrane of enterocytes, this localization does not provide any kinetic advantage for starch hydrolysis. Chole-

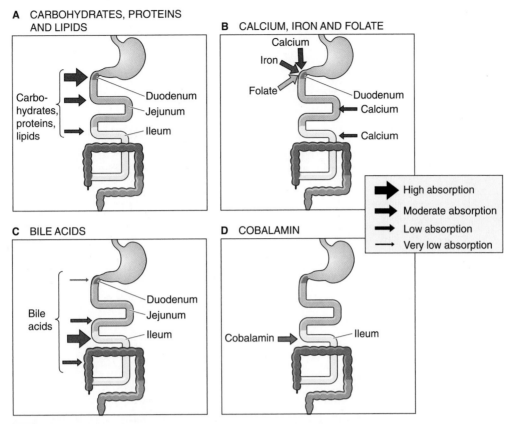

Figure 45-2 Sites of nutrient absorption. **A**, The entire small intestine absorbs carbohydrates, proteins, and lipids. However, the absorption is greatest in the duodenum, somewhat less in the jejunum, and much less in the ileum. The thickness of the *arrows in the inset* indicates the relative magnitude of total absorption at the indicated site in vivo. The maximal absorptive capacity of a specific segment under *optimized* experimental conditions (e.g., substrate concentrations) may be greater. **B**, Some substances are actively absorbed only in the duodenum. **C**, Bile acids are absorbed along the entire small intestine, but active absorption occurs only in the ileum. **D**, The vitamin cobalamin is absorbed only in the ileum.

Table 45-1 Major Gastrointestinal Diseases and Nutritional Deficiencies

Disease	Organ Site of Predominant Disease	Defects in Nutrient Digestion/Absorption
Celiac sprue	Duodenum and jejunum	Fat absorption, lactose hydrolysis
Chronic pancreatitis	Exocrine pancreas	Fat digestion
Surgical resection of ileum; Crohn disease of ileum	Ileum	Cobalamin and bile acid absorption
Primary lactase deficiency	Small intestine	Lactose hydrolysis

cystokinin (CCK) stimulates the secretion of pancreatic α-amylase by pancreatic acinar cells (see Chapter 43).

α-Amylase is an **endoenzyme** that hydrolyzes *internal* α-1,4 linkages (Fig. 45-3A). α-Amylase does not cleave terminal α-1,4 linkages, α-1,6 linkages (i.e., branch points), or

α-1,4 linkages that are immediately adjacent to α-1,6 linkages. As a result, starch hydrolysis products are maltose, maltotriose, and α-limit dextrins. Because α-amylase has no activity against terminal α-1,4 linkages, glucose is *not* a product of starch digestion. The intestine cannot absorb these products of amylase digestion of starch, and thus further digestion is required to produce substrates (i.e., monosaccharides) that the small intestine can absorb by specific transport mechanisms.

Membrane digestion involves hydrolysis of oligosaccharides to monosaccharides by brush border disaccharidases

The human small intestine has three brush border oligosaccharidases: lactase, glucoamylase (most often called maltase), and sucrase-isomaltase. These enzymes are all integral membrane proteins whose catalytic domains face the intestinal lumen (Fig. 45-3B). Sucrase-isomaltase is actually two enzymes—sucrase and isomaltase (also known as α-dextrinase or debranching enzyme)—bound together. Thus, four oligosaccharidases are present at the brush border. **Lactase** has only one substrate; it breaks lactose into glucose and galactose. The other three enzymes have more complicated

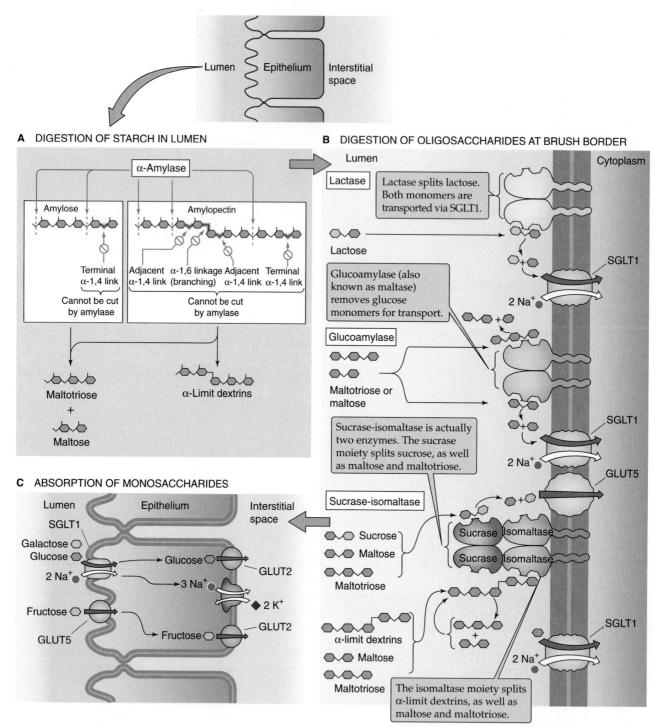

Figure 45-3 Digestion of carbohydrates to monosaccharides. **A**, Salivary and pancreatic α-amylase are endoenzymes. They can digest the linear internal α-1,4 linkages between glucose residues, but they cannot break terminal α-1,4 linkages (i.e., between the last two sugars in the chain). They also cannot split the α-1,6 linkages at the branch points of amylopectin or the adjacent α-1,4 linkages. As a result, the products of α-amylase action are linear glucose oligomers, maltotriose (a linear glucose trimer), maltose (a linear glucose dimer), and α-limit dextrins (which contain an α-1,6 branching linkage). **B**, The brush border oligosaccharidases are intrinsic membrane proteins with their catalytic domains facing the lumen. The sucrase-isomaltase is actually two enzymes, and, therefore, four oligosaccharidases split the oligosaccharides produced by α-amylase into monosaccharides. **C**, SGLT1 is the Na⁺-coupled transporter that mediates the uptake of glucose or galactose from the lumen of the small intestine into the enterocyte. GLUT5 mediates the facilitated diffusion of fructose into the enterocyte. Once the monosaccharides are inside the enterocyte, GLUT2 mediates their efflux across the basolateral membrane into the interstitial space.

substrate spectra. All cleave the terminal α-1,4 linkages of maltose, maltotriose, and α-limit dextrins. In addition, each of these three enzymes has at least one other activity. **Maltase** can also degrade the α-1,4 linkages in straight-chain oligosaccharides up to nine monomers in length. However, maltase cannot split either sucrose or lactose. The **sucrase** moiety of sucrase-isomaltase is required to split sucrose into glucose and fructose. The **isomaltase** moiety of sucrase-isomaltase is critical; it is the only enzyme that can split the branching α-1,6 linkages of α-limit dextrins.

The action of the four oligosaccharidases generates several monosaccharides. Maltose is hydrolyzed to two glucose residues, whereas the hydrolysis products of sucrose are glucose and fructose. The hydrolysis of lactose by lactase yields glucose and galactose. The activities of the hydrolysis reactions of sucrase-isomaltase and maltase are considerably greater than the rates at which the various transporters can absorb the resulting monosaccharides. Thus, uptake, not hydrolysis, is the rate-limiting step. In contrast, lactase activity is considerably less than that of the other oligosaccharidases and is rate limiting for overall lactose digestion-absorption.

The oligosaccharidases have a varying spatial distribution throughout the small intestine. In general, peak oligosac-

charidase distribution and activity occur in the proximal jejunum (i.e., at the ligament of Treitz). Considerably less activity is noted in the duodenum and distal ileum, and none is reported in the large intestine. The distribution of oligosaccharidase activity parallels that of active glucose transport.

These oligosaccharidases are affected by developmental and dietary factors in different ways. In many nonwhite ethnic groups, as well as in almost all other mammals, lactase activity markedly decreases after weaning in the postnatal period. The regulation of this decreased lactase activity is genetically determined. The other oligosaccharidases do not decrease in the postnatal period. In addition, long-term feeding of sucrose upregulates sucrase activity. In contrast, sucrase activity is greatly reduced much more by fasting than is lactase activity. In general, lactase activity is both more susceptible to enterocyte injury (e.g., following viral enteritis) and is slower to recover from damage than is other oligosaccharidase activity. Thus, reduced lactase activity (as a consequence of both genetic regulation and environmental effects) has substantial clinical significance in that lactose ingestion may result in a range of symptoms in affected individuals (Fig. 45-4).

A   PRESENCE OF LACTASE ACTIVITY

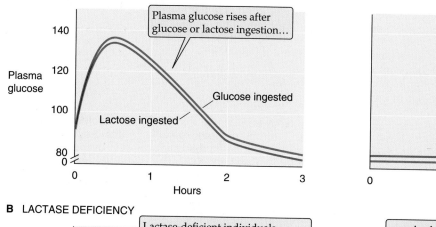

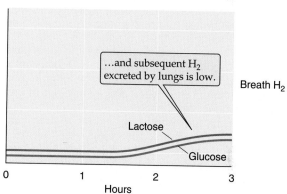

B   LACTASE DEFICIENCY

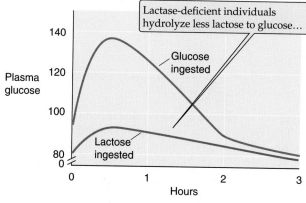

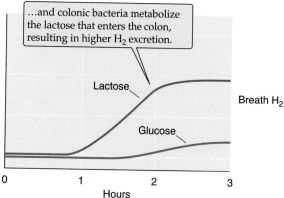

Figure 45-4   Effects of lactase deficiency on levels of glucose in the plasma and H_2 in the breath. **A,** In an individual with normal lactase activity, blood glucose levels rise after the ingestion of either glucose or lactose. Thus, the small intestine can split the lactose into glucose and galactose and can absorb the two monosaccharides. At the same time, H_2 in the breath is low. **B,** In an adult with low lactase activity, the rise in blood levels is less pronounced after ingesting lactose. Because the rise is normal after ingesting glucose, we can conclude that the difference is the result of lactase activity. Conversely, the individual with lactase deficiency excretes large amounts of H_2 into the breath. This H_2 is the product of lactose catabolism by colonic bacteria.

Lactase Deficiency

Primary lactase deficiency is extremely common in non-whites, and it also occurs in some whites. Lactase activity decreases after weaning; the time course of its reduction is determined by hereditary factors. Ingestion of lactose in the form of milk and milk products by individuals with decreased amounts of small intestinal lactase activity may be associated with a range of gastrointestinal symptoms, including diarrhea, cramps, and flatus, or with no discernible symptoms. Several factors determine whether individuals with lactase deficiency experience symptoms after ingestion of lactose, including rate of gastric emptying, transit time through the small intestine, and, most importantly, the ability of colonic bacteria to metabolize lactose to short-chain fatty acids, CO_2, and H_2. Figure 45-4A shows the rise of plasma [glucose] following the ingestion of either lactose or glucose in adults *with* normal lactase levels. This figure also shows that the [H_2] in the breath rises only slightly following the ingestion of either lactose or glucose in these individuals with normal lactase levels. Figure 45-4B shows that in individuals with primary lactase deficiency, the ingestion of lactose leads to a much smaller rise in plasma [glucose], although the ingestion of glucose itself leads to a normal rise in plasma [glucose]. Thus, no defect in glucose absorption per se is present, but simply a markedly reduced capacity to hydrolyze lactose to glucose and galactose. In lactase-deficient individuals, breath H_2 is increased after lactose ingestion, because nonabsorbed lactose is metabolized by colonic bacteria to H_2, which is absorbed into the blood and is subsequently excreted by the lungs. In contrast, the rise in breath H_2 is normal after the ingestion of glucose in these individuals.

Treatment for symptomatic individuals with primary lactase deficiency is reduction or elimination of milk and milk products or the use of milk products treated with a commercial lactase preparation. No other defects in intestinal function or structure are associated with primary lactase deficiency.

A STRUCTURE OF SGLT1

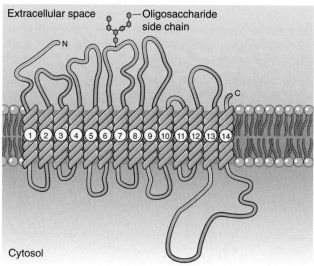

B STRUCTURAL REQUIREMENTS OF SUGAR

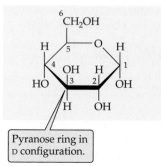

Pyranose ring in D configuration.

Figure 45-5 SGLT1. **A,** The SGLT family of proteins is believed to have 12 membrane-spanning segments. The deduced amino acid sequence has an open reading frame of 662 amino acids, predicting a molecular mass of 73 kDa. SGLT1 has a Na⁺-sugar stoichiometry of 2:1. **B,** SGLT1 transports only hexoses in a D-configuration and with a pyranose ring. This figure shows D-glucose; D-galactose is identical, except the H and OH on C-4 are inverted.

CARBOHYDRATE ABSORPTION

The three monosaccharide products of carbohydrate digestion—**glucose, galactose**, and **fructose**—are absorbed by the small intestine in a two-step process involving their uptake across the apical membrane into the epithelial cell and their coordinated exit across the basolateral membrane (Fig. 45-3C). The Na/glucose transporter 1 (SGLT1) is the membrane protein responsible for glucose and galactose uptake at the *apical membrane*. The exit of all three monosaccharides across the *basolateral membrane* uses a facilitated sugar transporter (GLUT2). Because SGLT1 cannot carry fructose, the apical step of fructose absorption occurs by the facilitated diffusion of fructose through GLUT5. Thus, although two different apical membrane transport mechanisms exist for glucose and fructose uptake, a single transporter (GLUT2) is responsible for the movement of both monosaccharides across the basolateral membrane.

SGLT1 is responsible for the Na⁺-coupled uptake of glucose and galactose across the apical membrane

The uptake of glucose across the apical membrane through SGLT1 (Fig. 45-5A) represents active transport, because the glucose influx occurs against the glucose concentration gradient (see Chapter 5). Glucose uptake across the apical membrane is energized by the electrochemical Na⁺ gradient, which, in turn, is maintained by the extrusion of Na⁺ across the basolateral membrane by the Na-K pump. This type of Na⁺-driven glucose transport is an example of *secondary active transport* (see Chapter 5). Inhibition of the Na-K pump reduces active glucose absorption by decreasing the apical membrane Na⁺ gradient and thus decreasing the driving force for glucose entry.

The affinity of SGLT1 for glucose is markedly reduced in the absence of Na⁺. The varied affinity of SGLT1 for

Glucose-Galactose Malabsorption

Molecular studies have been performed with jejunal mucosa from patients with so-called glucose-galactose malabsorption (or monosaccharide malabsorption). These individuals have diarrhea when they ingest dietary sugars that are normally absorbed by SGLT1. This diarrhea results from both reduced small intestine Na$^+$ and fluid absorption (as a consequence of the defect in Na$^+$-coupled monosaccharide absorption) and fluid secretion secondary to the osmotic effects of nonabsorbed monosaccharide. Eliminating the monosaccharides glucose and galactose, as well as the disaccharide lactose (i.e., glucose + galactose), from the diet eliminates the diarrhea. The monosaccharide fructose, which crosses the apical membrane through GLUT5, does not induce diarrhea. Early studies identified the abnormality in this hereditary disorder as a defect at the apical membrane that is presumably related to defective or absent SGLT1. Molecular studies of SGLT1 have revealed multiple mutations that result in single amino acid substitutions in SGLT1, each of which prevents the transport of glucose by SGLT1 in affected individuals. Patients with glucose-galactose malabsorption do not have glycosuria (i.e., glucose in the urine), because glucose reabsorption by the proximal tubule normally occurs through both SGLT1 and SGLT2 (see Chapter 36).

different monosaccharides reflects its preference for specific molecular configurations. SGLT1 has two structural requirements for monosaccharides: (1) a hexose in a D-configuration and (2) a hexose that can form a six-membered pyranose ring (Fig. 45-5B). SGLT1 does not absorb L-glucose, which has the wrong stereochemistry, and it does not absorb D-fructose, which forms a five-membered ring.

The GLUT transporters mediate the facilitated diffusion of fructose at the apical membrane and of all three monosaccharides at the basolateral membrane

Early work showed that fructose absorption is independent of Na$^+$ but has characteristics of both a carrier-mediated and a passive process. These observations show that the small intestine has separate transport systems for glucose and fructose. Subsequent studies established that *facilitated diffusion* is responsible for fructose absorption. Fructose uptake across the *apical membrane* is mediated by **GLUT5** (see Chapter 5), a member of the GLUT family of transport proteins. GLUT5 is present mainly in the jejunum.

The efflux of glucose, fructose, and galactose across the *basolateral membrane* also occurs by facilitated diffusion. The characteristics of the basolateral sugar transporter, identified as **GLUT2**, are similar to those of other sugar transport systems in erythrocytes, fibroblasts, and adipocytes. GLUT2 has no homology to SGLT1 but is 41% identical to GLUT5, which is responsible for the uptake of fructose from the lumen.

PROTEIN DIGESTION

Proteins require hydrolysis to oligopeptides or amino acids before absorption in the small intestine

With the exception of antigenic amounts of dietary protein that are absorbed intact, proteins must first be digested into their constituent oligopeptides and amino acids before being taken up by the enterocytes. Digestion-absorption occurs through four major pathways. First, several *luminal* enzymes (i.e., proteases) from the stomach and pancreas may hydrolyze proteins to peptides and then to amino acids, which are then absorbed (Fig. 45-6). Second, *luminal* enzymes may digest proteins to peptides, but enzymes present at the *brush border* digest the peptides to amino acids, which are then absorbed. Third, *luminal* enzymes may digest proteins to peptides, which are themselves taken up as oligopeptides by

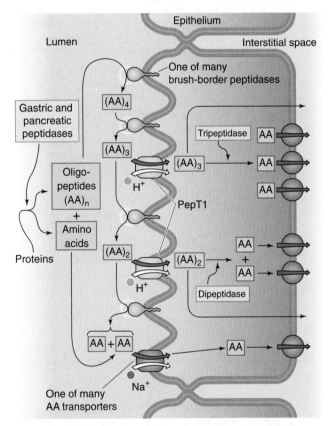

Figure 45-6 Action of luminal, brush border, and cytosolic peptidases. Pepsin from the stomach and the five pancreatic proteases hydrolyze proteins—both dietary and endogenous—to single amino acids, AA, or to oligopeptides, (AA)$_n$. These reactions occur in the lumen of the stomach or small intestine. Various peptidases at the brush borders of enterocytes then progressively hydrolyze oligopeptides to amino acids. The amino acids are directly taken up by any of several transporters. The enterocyte directly absorbs some of the small oligopeptides through the action of the H$^+$/oligopeptide cotransporter (PepT1). These small peptides are digested to amino acids by peptidases in the cytoplasm of the enterocyte. Several Na$^+$-independent amino acid transporters move amino acids out of the cell across the basolateral membrane.

the enterocytes. Further digestion of the oligopeptides by cytosolic enzymes yields intracellular amino acids, which are moved by transporters across the basolateral membrane into the blood. Fourth, luminal enzymes digest dietary proteins to oligopeptides, which are taken up by enterocytes and moved directly into the blood. Overall protein digestion-absorption is very efficient; less than 4% of ingested nitrogen is excreted in the stool.

The protein that is digested and absorbed in the small intestine comes from both dietary and endogenous sources. Dietary protein in developed countries amounts to 70 to 100 g/day. This amount is far in excess of minimum daily requirements and represents 10% to 15% of energy intake. In contrast, dietary protein content in developing countries in Africa is often 50 g/day. Deficiency states are rare unless intake is markedly reduced.

Proteins are encoded by mRNA and consist of 20 amino acids. Nine of these amino acids are essential (see Chapter 58); that is, they are not synthesized in adequate amounts by the body and thus must be derived from either animal or plant protein sources. In addition, cells synthesize additional amino acids by post-translational modifications: γ-carboxyglutamic acid, hydroxylysine, 4-hydroxyproline, and 3-hydroxyproline. Protein digestion is influenced by the amino acid composition of the protein, by the source of protein, and by food processing. Thus, proteins rich in proline and hydroxyproline are digested relatively less completely. Cooking, storage, and dehydration also reduce the completeness of digestion. In general, protein derived from animal sources is digested more completely than plant protein.

In addition to dietary sources of protein, significant amounts of endogenous protein are secreted into the gastrointestinal tract, then conserved by protein digestion and absorption. Such endogenous sources represent ~50% of the total protein entering the small intestine and include enzymes, hormones, and immunoglobulins present in salivary, gastric, pancreatic, biliary, and jejunal secretions. A second large source of endogenous protein is desquamated intestinal epithelial cells as well as plasma proteins that the small intestine secretes.

Neonates can absorb substantial amounts of *intact protein* from colostrum (see Chapter 57) through the process of endocytosis. This mechanism is developmentally regulated and in humans remains active only until ~6 months of age.

In adults, proteins are almost exclusively digested to their constituent amino acids and dipeptides and tripeptides or tetrapeptides before absorption. However, even adults absorb small amounts of intact proteins. These absorbed proteins can be important in inducing immune responses to dietary proteins.

Luminal digestion of protein involves both gastric and pancreatic proteases, thus yielding amino acids and oligopeptides

Both gastric and pancreatic proteases, unlike the digestive enzymes for carbohydrates and lipids, are secreted as **proenzymes** that require conversion to their active form for protein hydrolysis to occur. The gastric chief cells secrete **pepsinogen**. We discuss the pH-dependent activation of pepsinogen in Chapter 42. The hydrolytic activity of **pepsin** is maximal at a pH of 1.8 to 3.5, and pepsin is irreversibly inactivated at a pH of less than 7. Pepsin is an endopeptidase with primary specificity for peptide linkages of aromatic and larger neutral amino acids. Although pepsin in the stomach partially digests 10% to 15% of dietary protein, pepsin hydrolysis is not absolutely necessary; patients with either total gastrectomies or pernicious anemia (who do not secrete acid and thus whose intragastric pH is always >7) do not have increased fecal nitrogen excretion.

Five pancreatic enzymes (Table 45-2) participate in protein digestion and are secreted as inactive proenzymes. Trypsinogen is initially activated by a jejunal brush border enzyme, enterokinase (enteropeptidase), by the cleavage of a hexapeptide, thereby yielding trypsin. Trypsinogen is also autoactivated by trypsin. Trypsin also activates the other pancreatic proteolytic proenzymes. The secretion of proteolytic enzymes as proenzymes, with subsequent luminal activation, prevents pancreatic **autodigestion** before enzyme secretion into the intestine.

Pancreatic proteolytic enzymes are either exopeptidases or endopeptidases and function in an integrated manner. Trypsin, chymotrypsin, and elastase are **endopeptidases** with affinity for peptide bonds adjacent to specific amino acids, thus resulting in the production of oligopeptides with two to six amino acids. In contrast, the **exopeptidases**—carboxypeptidase A and carboxypeptidase B—hydrolyze peptide bonds adjacent to the carboxy terminus, thereby resulting in the release of individual amino acids. The coordinated action

Table 45-2 Pancreatic Peptidases

Proenzyme	Activating Agent	Active Enzyme	Action	Products
Trypsinogen	Enteropeptidase (i.e., enterokinase from jejunum) and trypsin	Trypsin	Endopeptidase	Oligopeptides (2-6 amino acids)
Chymotrypsinogen	Trypsin	Chymotrypsin	Endopeptidase	Oligopeptides (2-6 amino acids)
Proelastase	Trypsin	Elastase	Endopeptidase	Oligopeptides (2-6 amino acids)
Procarboxypeptidase A	Trypsin	Carboxypeptidase A	Exopeptidase	Single amino acids
Procarboxypeptidase B	Trypsin	Carboxypeptidase B	Exopeptidase	Single amino acids

of these pancreatic proteases converts ~70% of luminal amino nitrogen to oligopeptides and ~30% to free amino acids.

Brush border peptidases fully digest some oligopeptides to amino acids, whereas cytosolic peptidases digest oligopeptides that directly enter the enterocyte

Small peptides present in the small intestinal lumen after digestion by gastric and pancreatic proteases undergo further hydrolysis by peptidases at the brush border (Fig. 45-6). Multiple peptidases are present on both the brush border and in the cytoplasm of villous epithelial cells. This distribution of cell-associated peptidases stands in contrast to that of the oligosaccharidases, which are found only at the brush border. Because each peptidase recognizes only a limited repertoire of peptide bonds, and because the oligopeptides to be digested contain 24 different amino acids, large numbers of peptidases are required to ensure the hydrolysis of peptides.

As we discuss later, a transporter on the apical membrane of enterocytes can take up small oligopeptides, primarily dipeptides and tripeptides. Once inside the cell, these oligopeptides may be further digested by *cytoplasmic* peptidases. The brush border and cytoplasmic peptidases have substantially different characteristics. For example, the brush border peptidases have affinity for relatively larger oligopeptides (three to eight amino acids), whereas the cytoplasmic peptidases primarily hydrolyze dipeptides and tripeptides. Because the brush border and cytoplasmic enzymes often have different biochemical properties (e.g., heat lability and electrophoretic mobility), it is evident that the peptidases in the brush border and cytoplasm are distinct, independently regulated molecules.

Like the pancreatic proteases, each of the several brush border peptidases is an endopeptidase, an exopeptidase, or a dipeptidase and has affinity for specific peptide bonds. The exopeptidases are either carboxypeptidases, which release carboxy-terminal amino acids, or aminopeptidases, which hydrolyze the amino acids at the amino-terminal end. **Cytoplasmic peptidases** are relatively less numerous.

PROTEIN, PEPTIDE, AND AMINO ACID ABSORPTION

Absorption of whole protein by apical pinocytosis occurs primarily during the neonatal period

During the postnatal period, intestinal epithelial cells absorb protein by endocytosis, a process that provides a mechanism for transfer of passive immunity from mother to child. The uptake of intact protein by the epithelial cell ceases by the sixth month; the cessation of this protein uptake, called *closure*, is hormonally mediated. For example, administration of corticosteroids during the postnatal period induces closure and reduces the time that the intestine can absorb significant amounts of whole protein.

The adult intestine can absorb finite amounts of intact protein and polypeptides. Uncertainty exists regarding the cellular route by which these substances are absorbed, as well as the relationship of the mechanism of protein uptake in adults to that in neonates. Enterocytes can take up by endocytosis a small amount of intact protein, most of which is degraded in lysosomes (Fig. 45-7). A small amount of intact protein appears in the interstitial space. The uptake of intact proteins also occurs through a second, more specialized route. In the small intestine, immediately overlying **Peyer's patches** (follicles of lymphoid tissue in the lamina propria), **M cells** replace the usual enterocytes on the surface of the gut. M cells have few microvilli and are specialized for protein uptake. They have limited ability for lysosomal protein degradation; rather, they package ingested proteins (i.e., antigens) in clathrin-coated vesicles, which they secrete at their basolateral membranes into the lamina propria. There, immunocompetent cells process the target antigens and transfer them to lymphocytes to initiate an immune response. Although protein uptake in adults may not have nutritional value, such uptake is clearly important in mucosal immunity and probably is involved in one or more disease processes.

The apical absorption of dipeptides, tripeptides, and tetrapeptides occurs through an H⁺-driven cotransporter

Virtually all absorbed protein products exit the villous epithelial cell and enter the blood as individual amino acids.

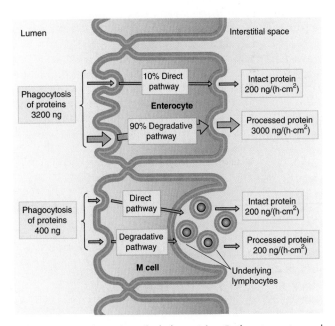

Figure 45-7 Absorption of whole proteins. Both enterocytes and specialized M cells can take up intact proteins. The more abundant enterocytes can endocytose far more total protein than can the M cells. However, the lysosomal proteases in the enterocytes degrade ~90% of this endocytosed protein. The less abundant M cells take up relatively little intact protein, but approximately half of this emerges intact at the basolateral membrane. There, immunocompetent cells process the target antigens and then transfer them to lymphocytes, thus initiating an immune response.

Substantial portions of these amino acids are released in the lumen of the small intestine by luminal proteases and brush border peptidases and, as we discuss later, move across the apical membranes of enterocytes through several amino acid transport systems (Fig. 45-6). However, substantial amounts of protein are absorbed from the intestinal lumen as dipeptides, tripeptides, or tetrapeptides and are then hydrolyzed to amino acids by intracellular peptidases.

The transporter responsible for the uptake of luminal oligopeptides (Fig. 45-8A) is distinct from the various amino acid transporters. Furthermore, administering an amino acid as a peptide (e.g., the dipeptide glycylglycine) results in a higher blood level of the amino acid than administering an equivalent amount of the same amino acid as a monomer (e.g., glycine; Fig. 45-8B). One possible explanation for this effect is that the oligopeptide cotransporter, which carries multiple amino acids rather than a single amino acid into the cell, may simply be more effective than amino acid transporters in transferring amino acid monomers into the cell. This accelerated peptide absorption has been referred to as a *kinetic advantage* and raises the question of the usefulness of the enteral administration of crystalline amino acids to patients with impaired intestinal function or catabolic deficiencies. The evidence for a specific transport process for dipeptides, tripeptides, and tetrapeptides comes from direct measurements of oligopeptide transport, molecular identification of the transporter, and studies of the hereditary disorders of amino acid transport, cystinuria, and Hartnup disease.

Oligopeptide uptake is an active process driven not by a Na^+ gradient, but by a proton gradient. Oligopeptide uptake occurs through an **H^+/oligopeptide cotransporter** known as PepT1 (SLC15A1; see Chapter 5), which is also present in the renal proximal tubule. PepT1 also appears to be responsible for the intestinal uptake of certain dipeptide-like antibiotics (e.g., oral amino-substituted cephalosporins). As noted earlier, after their uptake, dipeptides, tripeptides, and tetrapeptides are usually hydrolyzed by cytoplasmic peptidases to their constituent amino acids, the forms in which they are transported out of the cell across the basolateral membrane. Because peptides are almost completely hydrolyzed to amino acids intracellularly, few peptides appear in the portal vein. Proline-containing dipeptides, which are relatively resistant to hydrolysis, are the primary peptides present in the circulation.

Amino acids enter enterocytes through one or more group-specific apical membrane transporters

Multiple amino acid transport systems have been identified and characterized in various nonepithelial cells. The absorption of amino acids across the small intestine requires sequential movement across both the apical and basolateral membranes of the villous epithelial cell. Although the amino acid transport systems have overlapping affinities for various amino acids, the general consensus is that at least seven distinct transport systems are present at the apical membrane (see Table 36-1); we discuss the basolateral amino acid transporters in the next section. Whereas many apical amino acid transporters are probably unique to epithelial cells, some of those at the basolateral membrane are probably the same as in nonepithelial cells.

The predominant apical amino acid transport system is **system B^0** (SLC6A19; see Table 36-1), and it results in Na^+-dependent uptake of neutral amino acids. As is the case for

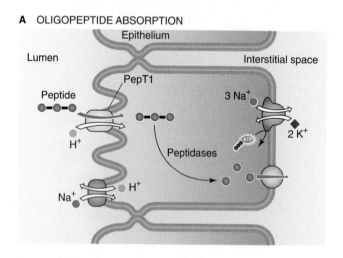

A OLIGOPEPTIDE ABSORPTION

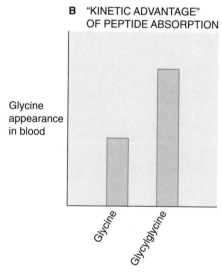

B "KINETIC ADVANTAGE" OF PEPTIDE ABSORPTION

Figure 45-8   Absorption of oligopeptides. **A,** The H^+/oligopeptide cotransporter PepT1 moves dipeptides, tripeptides, and tetrapeptides into the enterocyte, across the apical membrane. Peptidases in the cytoplasm hydrolyze the oligopeptides into their constituent amino acids, which then exit across the basolateral membrane through one of three Na^+-independent amino acid transporters. **B,** If glycine is present in the lumen only as a free amino acid, then the enterocyte absorbs it only through apical amino acid transporters. However, if the same amount of glycine is present in the lumen in the form of the dipeptide glycylglycine, the rate of appearance of glycine in the blood is about twice as high. Thus, PepT1, which moves several amino acid monomers for each turnover of the transporter, is an effective mechanism for absorbing "amino acids."

glucose uptake, uphill movement of neutral amino acids is driven by an inwardly directed Na$^+$ gradient that is maintained by the basolateral Na-K pump. The uptake of amino acids by system B^0 is an electrogenic process and represents another example of *secondary active transport*. It transports amino acids with an L-stereo configuration and an amino group in the α position. System B^{0+} (SLC6A14) is similar to system B^0 but has broader substrate specificity. System b^{0+} (SLC7A9/SLC3A1 dimer) differs from B^{0+} mainly in being independent of Na$^+$.

Other carrier-mediated transport mechanisms exist for anionic (i.e., acidic), cationic (i.e., basic), β amino acids, and imino acids (see Table 36-1). Because the apical amino acid transporters have overlapping affinities for amino acids, and because of species differences as well as segmental and developmental differences among the transporters, it has been difficult to establish a comprehensive model of apical membrane amino acid transport in the mammalian small intestine.

At the basolateral membrane, amino acids exit enterocytes through Na$^+$-independent transporters and enter through Na$^+$-dependent transporters

Amino acids appear in the cytosol of intestinal **villous cells** as the result either of their uptake across the apical membrane or of the hydrolysis of oligopeptides that had entered the apical membrane (Fig. 45-6). The enterocyte subsequently uses ~10% of the absorbed amino acids for intracellular protein synthesis.

Movement of amino acids across the basolateral membrane is bidirectional; the movement of any one amino acid can occur through one or more amino acid transporters. At least five amino acid transporters are present in the basolateral membrane (see Table 36-1). Three amino acid transport

processes on the basolateral membrane mediate amino acid *exit* from the cell into the blood and thus complete the process of protein assimilation. Two other amino acid transporters mediate *uptake* from the blood for the purposes of cell nutrition. The three Na$^+$-independent amino acid transport systems appear to mediate amino acid movement *out* of the epithelial cell into blood. One of these, system y$^+$ (SLC7A1), is also present on the apical membrane. The two Na$^+$-dependent processes facilitate their movement *into* the epithelial cell. Indeed, these two Na$^+$-dependent transporters resemble those that are also present in nonpolar cells.

In general, the amino acids incorporated into protein within villous cells are derived more from those that enter across the apical membrane than from those that enter across the basolateral membrane. In contrast, **epithelial cells in the intestinal crypt** derive almost all their amino acids for protein synthesis from the circulation; crypt cells do not take up amino acids across their apical membrane.

LIPID DIGESTION

Natural lipids are organic compounds of biological origin that are sparingly soluble in water

Lipids in the diet are derived from animals or plants and are composed of carbon, hydrogen, and a smaller amount of oxygen. Some lipids also contain small but functionally important amounts of nitrogen and phosphorus (Fig. 45-11). Lipids are typified by their preferential solubility in organic solvents, compared with water. A widely used indicator of the lipidic nature of a compound is its octanol-water partition coefficient, which for most lipids is between 10^4 and 10^7. The biological fate of lipids depends critically on their chemical structure as well as on their interactions with

---

Defects in Apical Amino Acid Transport: Hartnup Disease and Cystinuria

Hartnup disease and cystinuria are hereditary disorders of amino acid transport across the apical membrane. These autosomal recessive disorders are associated with both small intestine and renal tubule abnormalities (see Chapter 36 for the box on hyperaminoacidurias) in the absorption of neutral amino acids in the case of Hartnup disease and of cationic (i.e., basic) amino acids and cystine in the case of cystinuria.

The clinical signs of **Hartnup disease** are most evident in children and include the skin changes of pellagra, cerebellar ataxia, and psychiatric abnormalities. In Hartnup disease, the absorption of neutral amino acids by system B^0 (SLC6A19) in the small intestine is markedly reduced, whereas that of cationic amino acids is intact (Fig. 45-9).

The principal manifestation of **cystinuria** is the formation of kidney stones. In cystinuria, the absorption of cationic amino acids by system b^{0+} (SLC7A9/SLC3A1 dimer) is abnormal—as a result of mutations in *SLC7A9* or *SLC3A1*—but absorption of neutral amino acids is normal.

Because neither of these diseases involves the oligopeptide cotransporter, the absorption of oligopeptides containing either neutral or cationic amino acids is normal in both diseases. Only 10% of patients with Hartnup disease have clinical evidence of protein deficiency (i.e., pellagra) commonly associated with defects in protein or amino acid absorption. The lack of evidence of protein deficiency is a consequence of the presence of more than one transport system for different amino acids, as well as a separate transporter for oligopeptides. Thus, oligopeptides containing neutral amino acids are absorbed normally in Hartnup disease, and oligopeptides with cationic amino acids are absorbed normally in cystinuria.

These two genetic diseases also emphasize the existence of amino acid transport mechanisms on the basolateral membrane that are distinct and separate from the apical amino acid transporters. Thus, in both Hartnup disease and cystinuria, oligopeptides are transported normally across the apical membrane and are hydrolyzed to amino acids in the cytosol, and the resulting neutral and cationic amino acids are readily transported out of the cell across the basolateral membrane.

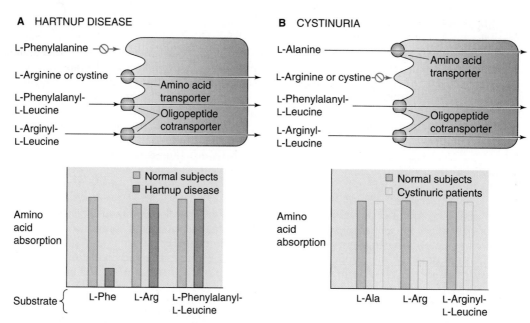

Figure 45-9   Genetic disorders of apical amino acid transport. **A**, In Hartnup disease, an autosomal recessive disorder, the apical system B⁰ (SLC6A19) is defective. As a result, the absorption of neutral amino acids such as L-phenylalanine, is reduced. (However, the absorption of L-cystine (i.e., Cys-S-S-Cys) and cationic (i.e., basic) amino acids (e.g., L-arginine) remains intact.) The enterocyte can absorb L-phenylalanine normally if the amino acid is present in the form of the dipeptide L-phenylalanyl-L-leucine, inasmuch as the oligopeptide cotransporter PepT1 is normal. **B**, In cystinuria, an autosomal recessive disorder, the apical system b⁰⁺ (SLC7A9/SLC3A1 dimer) is defective. As a result, the absorption of L-cystine (i.e., Cys-S-S-Cys) and cationic (i.e., basic) amino acids (e.g., L-arginine) is reduced. However, the absorption of amino acids that use system B⁰ (e.g., L-Ala) is normal. The enterocyte can absorb L-arginine normally if the amino acid is present in the form of the dipeptide L-arginyl-L-leucine.

Basolateral Amino Acid Transport Defects: Lysinuric Protein Intolerance

Lysinuric protein intolerance is a rare autosomal recessive disorder of amino acid transport across the basolateral membrane (Fig. 45-10). Evidence indicates impaired cationic amino acid transport and symptoms of malnutrition. It appears that the defect is in system y⁺L, which is located solely on the basolateral membrane. System y⁺L has two subtypes, y⁺LAT1 (SLC7A7/SLC3A2 dimer) and y⁺LAT2 (SLC7A6/SLC3A2 dimer). Mutations in the *SLC7A7* gene (subtype y⁺LAT1) cause the disease lysinuric protein intolerance. Cationic amino acids are absorbed normally across the apical membrane in these patients. Unlike in Hartnup disease or cystinuria, in which the enterocytes can absorb the amino acid normally if it is presented as an oligopeptide, in lysinuric protein intolerance the enterocytes cannot absorb the amino acid regardless of whether the amino acid is "free" or is part of an oligopeptide. These observations are best explained by hypothesizing that the patients hydrolyze intracellular oligopeptides properly but have a defect in the transport of cationic amino acids across the basolateral membrane. This defect is present not only in the small intestine, but also in hepatocytes and kidney cells, and perhaps in nonepithelial cells as well.

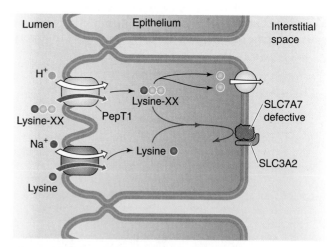

Figure 45-10   A genetic disorder of basolateral amino acid transport, lysinuric protein intolerance is an autosomal recessive defect in which the Na⁺-independent y⁺L amino acid transporter on the apical and basolateral membranes is defective. However, the absence of apical y⁺L (SLC7A6/SLC3A2 or SLC7A7/SLC3A2 dimers) does not present a problem because Na⁺-dependent amino acid transporters can take up lysine, and PepT1 can take up lysine-containing oligopeptides (lysine-XX). However, no other mechanism exists for moving lysine out of the enterocyte across the basolateral membrane.

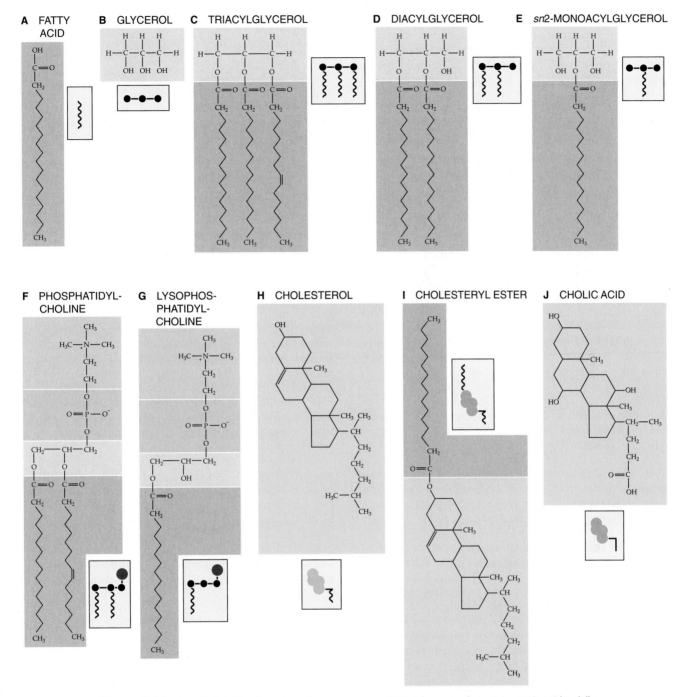

Figure 45-11 **A** to **J**, Chemical formulas of some common lipids. The example in **A** is stearic acid, a fully saturated fatty acid with 18 carbon atoms. **B** shows glycerol, a trihydroxy alcohol, with hydroxyl groups in positions *sn*1-, *sn*2-, and *sn*3-. In **C**, the left *sn*1- and center *sn*2- fatty acids are palmitic acid, a fully saturated fatty acid with 16 carbon atoms. The rightmost *sn*3- fatty acid is palmitoleic acid, which is also a 16-carbon structure, but with a double bond between carbons 9 and 10. In **F**, the left *sn*1- fatty acid is palmitic acid (16 carbons, fully saturated), and the right *sn*2- fatty acid is palmitoleic acid (16 carbons, double bond between carbons 9 and 10). In **I**, the example is the result of esterifying cholesterol and palmitic acid (16 carbons, fully saturated).

water and other lipids in aqueous body fluids (e.g., intestinal contents and bile). Thus, lipids have been classified according to their physicochemical interactions with water. Lipids may be either **nonpolar** and completely insoluble in water (e.g., cholesteryl esters and carotene) or **polar** and amphi-philic, that is, having both polar (hydrophilic) and nonpolar (hydrophobic) groups. Added in small amounts, polar lipids form stable or unstable monolayers on the surface of water (see Fig. 2-1C), whereas in bulk their physicochemical behavior varies from insolubility (as is the case with triacylglycerols [TAGs] and cholesterol) to the formation of various macroaggregates, such as liquid crystals and micelles. Less-soluble lipids are incorporated into the macroaggregates of the more-polar lipids and are thus stably maintained in aqueous solutions. The term **fat** is generally used to refer to TAG—formerly called triglyceride—but it is also used loosely to refer to lipids in general.

Dietary lipids are predominantly TAGs, but food also contains membrane lipids, vitamins, and chemicals from the environment

Typical adult Western diets contain ~140 g of fat (providing ~55% of the energy), which is more than the recommended intake of less than 30% of total dietary calories (<70 g of fat). Of this fat, more than 90% is **TAGs**, which are commonly long-chain fatty acyl esters of glycerol, a trihydroxyl alcohol. The three esterification (i.e., acylation) positions on the glycerol backbone that are occupied by hydroxyl groups, are designated *sn1*-, *sn2*- and *sn3*-, according to a *stereochemical numbering* system adopted by an international committee on biochemical nomenclature (Fig. 45-11A-C). At body temperature, fats are usually liquid droplets. Newborn infants consume three to five times more lipid than adults, relative to body weight. Dietary fat is the body's only source of essential fatty acids, and it acts as a vehicle for the absorption of fat-soluble vitamins (the handling of which is discussed in Chapter 46). Fat is also the major nutrient responsible for postprandial satiety. The ratio of **saturated** to **unsaturated** fatty acids in TAGs is high in animal fats and low in plant fats. Evidence indicates that in so-called developed countries, average fat intake is falling, as is the proportion of fat contributed by saturated fatty acids. Conversely, the proportion of polyunsaturated fats has risen. Milk and milk products contain 7% short-chain, 15% to 20% *sn3*-medium-chain, and 73% to 77% long-chain fatty acids. Fish contains unusual but metabolically important fatty acids (e.g., omega fatty acids), as well as wax esters.

Approximately 5% (4 to 6 g/day) of dietary lipids come from cell membranes and are **phospholipids**. Most phospholipids are *glycerophospholipids*. They consist of a glycerol backbone that is esterified at the first two positions to fatty acids and at the third position to a phosphate that, in turn, is esterified to a head group (see Fig. 2-2). One of the *glycerophospholipids*, phosphatidylcholine (lecithin), is the predominant phospholipid (Fig. 45-11F). The other major class of membrane phospholipid is the *sphingolipid*, which has a serine rather than a glycerol backbone.

The diet contains ~0.5 g of unesterified **cholesterol** (also derived from animal cell membranes; Fig. 45-11H), whereas esterified cholesterol (Fig. 45-11I) is usually found only in liver or food made from blood products. Traces of lipovitamins and provitamins (e.g., carotene) are present in dietary fat, which may also contain lipid-soluble toxins and carcinogens from the environment. These undesirable lipid-soluble chemicals—which include nitrosamines, aflatoxins, and polycyclic hydrocarbons such as benzo(a)pyrene—are all found in margarine, vegetable oils, and other dietary fats. The diet also may contain skin lipids, which are chemically diverse and complex and are difficult to digest.

Endogenous lipids are predominantly lecithin and cholesterol from bile and membrane lipids from desquamated intestinal epithelial cells

The bile secreted into the intestine (see Chapter 46) plays a key role in the assimilation of dietary lipids, as we explain later. This bile contains phospholipid (10 to 15 g/day)—also predominantly lecithin—and unesterified cholesterol (1 to 2 g/day). Quantitatively, these biliary lipids exceed those present in the diet by 2- to 4-fold. Membrane lipids from desquamated intestinal cells account for a further 2 to 6 g of lipid for digestion. Investigators have estimated that ~10 g/day of lipids are derived from dead bacteria. Most bacterial lipids are added in the colon.

Dietary lipids are disrupted mechanically in the mouth and stomach, and the resulting lipid particles are stabilized as an emulsion

The central process in the digestion of lipids is their hydrolysis in the aqueous milieu of the intestinal lumen. Lipid hydrolysis is catalyzed by **lipases** secreted by the glands and cells of the upper gastrointestinal tract. The products of lipolysis diffuse through the aqueous content of the intestinal lumen, traverse the so-called unstirred water layer and mucus barrier that line the intestinal epithelial surface, and enter the enterocyte for further processing. Because dietary lipids are insoluble in water, digestive lipases have evolved to act more efficiently at oil-water interfaces than on water-soluble substrates.

A key step preliminary to lipid digestion is the transformation of ingested solid fat and oil masses into an emulsion of fine oil droplets in water. The **emulsification** of dietary fats begins with food preparation (grinding, marinating, blending, and cooking), followed by chewing and gastric churning (see Chapter 42) caused by antral peristalsis against a closed pylorus. Emulsification of ingested lipids is enhanced when muscular movements of the stomach intermittently squirt the gastric contents into the duodenum and, conversely, when peristalsis of the duodenum propels the duodenal contents in retrograde fashion into the stomach through the narrow orifice of a contracted pylorus. The grinding action of the antrum also mixes food with the various digestive enzymes derived from the mouth and stomach. Intestinal peristalsis mixes luminal contents with pancreatic and biliary secretions. Together, these mechanical processes that reduce the size of the lipid droplets also dramatically increase their ratio of surface area to volume, thereby increasing the area of the oil-water interface.

The emulsion, produced by the mechanical processes just outlined, is stabilized by preventing the dispersed lipid particles from coalescing. This is achieved by coating the emulsion droplets with membrane lipids, denatured protein, dietary polysaccharides, certain products of digestion (e.g., fatty acids released by gastric lipase, and fatty acids and monoacylglycerols [MAGs] from intestinal and pancreatic digestion), and biliary phospholipids and cholesterol. Phospholipids and cholesterol are well suited as emulsion stabilizers because they dissolve neither in oil nor in water, but they have excellent interfacial solubilities at oil-water interfaces. Thus, they form a surface monomolecular layer on emulsion particles. The polar groups of the phospholipids project into the water; the charges of the polar groups and their high degree of hydration prevent coalescence of the emulsion particles. The core of the emulsion particle is composed of TAG, which also contains cholesteryl esters and other nonpolar or weakly polar lipids. A very small fraction of the TAG in the lipid particle localizes to the particle surface. The fat in breast milk is already emulsified by proteins and phospholipids incorporated into the surface of fat droplets during lactation. Foods such as sauces, ice cream, and puddings are stably emulsified during their preparation.

Lingual and gastric (acid) lipase initiate lipid digestion

In some species, but not in humans, a small amount of lipid digestion begins in the mouth, mediated by lingual lipase. In the stomach, both **lingual lipase** that is swallowed and a gastric lipase secreted by gastric chief cells digest substantial amounts of lipid. Human **gastric lipase** is a 42-kDa glycoprotein whose secretion is stimulated by gastrin. Gastric lipase secretion is already well established in the neonatal period (unlike pancreatic lipase secretion), and thus gastric lipolysis is important for fat digestion in newborn infants. Gastric and lingual—as well as pharyngeal—lipases belong to a family of serine hydrolases that have acidic pH optima (pH 4), are stable in the acidic environment of the stomach, are resistant to digestion by pepsin, and are not inhibited by the surface layer of membrane lipids (emulsifiers) that envelopes TAG droplets. However, acid lipases are inactive at neutral pH and also are readily inactivated by pancreatic proteases (especially in the presence of bile salts) once they reach the small intestine.

In vivo, gastric lipase releases a single *sn3*-**fatty acid** from **TAGs**, thus leaving behind intact **diacyclglycerols** (Fig. 45-11D). The carboxyl groups of long-chain fatty acids, released from TAGs in the stomach, are protonated and insoluble at the acidic pH prevailing in the stomach. These fatty acids are not absorbed in the stomach, but rather they remain in the core of the TAG droplets, in whose emulsification they participate in the small intestine. Medium- and short-chain fatty acids are mainly protonated in gastric juice during feeding and passively move across the gastric mucosa into portal blood.

In healthy adult humans, ~15% of fat digestion occurs in the stomach. In patients with pancreatic insufficiency, however, the lack of pancreatic proteases and HCO_3^- in the duodenal lumen may permit the continued action of gastric lipase after the gastric contents leave the stomach and enter the duodenum. Extended gastric lipase activity partly alleviates fat malabsorption resulting from pancreatic disease and pancreatic lipase deficiency.

Pancreatic (alkaline) lipase, colipase, milk lipase, and other esterases—aided by bile salts—complete lipid hydrolysis in the duodenum and jejunum

The process of fat digestion that begins in the stomach is completed in the proximal small intestine, predominantly

by enzymes synthesized and secreted by pancreatic acinar cells (see Chapter 43), and is carried into the duodenum in the pancreatic juice. In humans, a lipase found in human milk—the so-called **bile salt**–stimulated milk lipase—also digests fat. A similar lipase is found in the milk of relatively few other animal species. Milk lipase is stable during passage through the acid environment of the stomach, yet it is active at the alkaline pH of the duodenum and jejunum, where it hydrolyzes diacylglycerols, MAGs, cholesteryl esters, and fat-soluble vitamin esters, as well as TAGs. Bile salts not only stimulate milk lipase activity but also protect the enzyme from proteolysis in the small intestine. Like gastric lipase, milk lipase is important for fat digestion in breast-fed infants.

Once the fatty acids generated in the stomach reach the duodenum, they trigger the release of **CCK** and gastric inhibitory polypeptide (GIP) from the duodenal mucosa. CCK stimulates the *flow of bile* into the duodenum by causing the gallbladder to contract and the sphincter of Oddi to relax (see Chapter 46). CCK also stimulates the *secretion of pancreatic enzymes*, including lipases and esterases (see Chapter 43). As we discuss later, long-chain fatty acids also facilitate the lipolytic action of pancreatic lipase.

The major lipolytic enzyme of pancreatic juice is a 48-kDa carboxylic esterase known as **pancreatic lipase**, sometimes referred to as TAG lipase or as colipase-dependent pancreatic lipase. In adults but not in infants, this enzyme, which is secreted into the duodenum in its active form in 1000-fold excess, is thought to effectively digest all dietary TAGs not hydrolyzed in the stomach. Full lipolytic activity of pancreatic lipase requires the presence of a small (10-kDa) protein cofactor called **colipase**, as well as an alkaline pH, Ca^{2+}, bile salts, and fatty acids. The pancreas secretes colipase in the proform (i.e., procolipase), which has no intrinsic lipolytic activity. Trypsin cleaves procolipase into colipase and an N-terminal pentapeptide, enterostatin. This cleavage is important because the newly formed colipase is a cofactor of pancreatic lipase, as we discuss later. In addition, the N-terminal pentapeptide may partially control satiety.

Pancreatic lipase is active only at the oil-water interface of a TAG droplet. However, surface emulsifier components (e.g., phospholipids, protein) present at that interface inhibit lipase action. Bile salt micelles also inhibit lipolysis by displacing the lipase from the oil-droplet surface. Binding of colipase reverses this inhibition either by attaching first to the interface and serving as an anchor for the binding of the lipase or by first forming a colipase-pancreatic-lipase complex that then binds to the lipid interface. Colipase also can penetrate the phospholipid coating of the TAG emulsion. Bile salt micelles bring the colipase closer to the interface. Because bile salts are nearby, they can participate in the solubilization and removal of the products of lipolysis released from the emulsion droplet. Fatty acids have a biphasic effect. They enhance emulsification and augment lipolysis (probably by enhancing the binding of the colipase-lipase complex to the lipid interface). In contrast, their buildup causes product inhibition of lipase.

Studies of the crystal structure of pancreatic lipase have shown that when the enzyme is free in solution, the catalytic site of the lipase—located in a cleft in the molecule—is partly covered by a lid formed of loops of its peptide chain.

The interaction of the colipase and lipase with the interface causes a conformational change in the lipase molecule that opens the lid, thereby allowing lipid substrate to diffuse to the now-exposed catalytic site of the enzyme.

Pancreatic lipase mainly hydrolyzes the ester bonds of TAGs at the first and third positions of the glycerol backbone. The end products of such reactions are two fatty acids and a single sn2-MAG (2-MAG) (Fig. 45-11E).

The pancreas secretes other enzymes that hydrolyze lipid esters. **Carboxyl ester hydrolase** is a pancreatic enzyme that is the same protein as bile salt–stimulated milk lipase. Like milk lipase, carboxyl ester hydrolase lacks substrate specificity and is active against a wide range of esters. Carboxyl ester hydrolase is probably the same enzyme as "pancreatic esterase," "cholesterol esterase," "lysophospholipase," and others. Among the many products of reactions catalyzed by this enzyme are free cholesterol and free glycerol.

The pancreas also secretes **phospholipase A$_2$** (PLA$_2$), which is active against glycerophospholipids (but not sphingolipids), from which it releases a single sn2-fatty acid to yield lysophospholipids (Fig. 45-11G). Pancreatic PLA$_2$, secreted as a proenzyme, is effective at alkaline pH and requires bile salts for activity. PLA$_2$ in the small intestine may also be derived from Paneth's cells, whereas phospholipase found in the colon probably comes from anaerobic flora there. In contrast to the human intestinal lipases, bacterial lipases are nonspecific with respect to substrates, have neutral or slightly acidic pH optima, are not inhibited by bile acids, and do not require cofactors. In the human colon, both TAGs and phospholipids are totally hydrolyzed by bacteria. Fecal fat is thus generally present as **fatty acid soaps** and sterols. Even in severe fat malabsorption, intact acylglycerols are rarely found in the stools. The chemical test for stool fat, Sudan III staining, must be done in an acid environment because it depends on the property of Sudan III dye to partition into "oils" that contain protonated fatty acids.

LIPID ABSORPTION

Products of lipolysis enter the bulk water phase of the intestinal lumen as vesicles, mixed micelles, and monomers

After their secretion in pancreatic juice and bile, respectively, the various activated pancreatic lipases and biliary bile salts, lecithin, and cholesterol adsorb to the surface of the **emulsion droplets** arriving from the stomach (Fig. 45-12A). The lipolytic products—MAGs, fatty acids (including long-chain species from gastric lipolysis) that are now ionized at duodenal pH 5.5 to 6.5, lysolecithin, and cholesterol—act as additional emulsifiers. As surface TAGs are hydrolyzed, they are replaced by TAGs from the core of the emulsion particle. As the emulsion droplets become progressively smaller, their surface area increases, thereby increasing the rate of hydrolysis. Initially, a crystalline Ca^{2+}-fatty acid soap phase forms near the surface of the TAG droplet, until the local free Ca^{2+} is depleted. At the same time, a multilamellar liquid crystalline layer of fatty acids, MAGs, lysolecithins, cholesterol, and possibly bile salts builds up on the surface of the emulsion particle. This liquid crystalline layer buds off as a **multilamellar liquid crystal vesicle** (Fig. 45-12B), which consists of several lipid bilayers. Bile salt micelles transform these multilamellar vesicles into **unilamellar vesicles** (Fig. 45-12C), which are single-lipid bilayers, and then into **mixed micelles** (Fig. 45-12D) composed of bile salts and mixed lipids (i.e., fatty acids, MAGs, lysophospholipids, and cholesterol).

Continued digestion by PLA$_2$ and other esterases can still occur on the mixture of aggregates now present. If intestinal contents taken from humans during fat digestion are centrifuged, three phases separate. An oily layer floats on top and contains fat droplets and lipolytic products that have not been solubilized by bile salts. A middle layer contains lipid vesicles, mixed lipid-bile salt micelles, simple bile salt micelles, and lipid monomers. Finally, a pellet contains debris and precipitated Ca^{2+} soaps of fatty acids. Whereas most fat absorption in health is from the micellar phase of digested lipid, in situations in which intraluminal bile salt concentrations are low (e.g., in newborns and patients with obstructive jaundice), lipid absorption can occur from vesicles.

Lipids, as mixed micelles and monomers, diffuse across the unstirred water layer on the surface of the jejunal mucosa and cross the enterocyte brush border

To reach the interior of the enterocyte, lipolytic products must cross several barriers. These include (1) the mucous gel layer that lines the intestinal epithelial surface, (2) the unstirred water layer (disequilibrium zone) contiguous with the enterocyte's apical membrane, and (3) the apical membrane itself. Although the mucous gel that lines the intestine is 95% water, its interstices provide a barrier to the free diffusion—from the bulk phase to the unstirred water layer—of lipid macroaggregates, particularly the various vesicles that exist in equilibrium with the mixed micelles and monomers. Because of this diffusion barrier, the unstirred water lying adjacent to the enterocyte's apical membrane is not in equilibrium with the bulk phase of water in the lumen. According to calculations based on the diffusion of various probes under different experimental conditions and luminal fluid flow rates, it was originally estimated that the unstirred water layer was several hundred microns thick and posed a significant barrier to the diffusion of lipid nutrients to the enterocyte brush border. It is now thought that the unstirred water layer is likely only ~40 μm thick and does not constitute a major absorptive barrier. For short- and medium-chain fatty acids, which are readily soluble in water, diffusion of these monomers through the unstirred water layer to the enterocyte is efficient. As fatty acid chain length increases, the monomer's solubility in water decreases, whereas its partitioning into micelles increases. It is true that the diffusion of a single monomer through the aqueous barriers is speedier than that of a single micelle or vesicle. However, mixed-lipid micelles act as a reservoir to give the aqueous solution such a high *effective concentration* of fatty acids and other lipid products that the diffusion of these micelles is the most efficient mechanism for bringing lipolytic products to the enterocytes. Calculations suggest that, compared with monomers dissolved in water, vesicular solubilization increases the

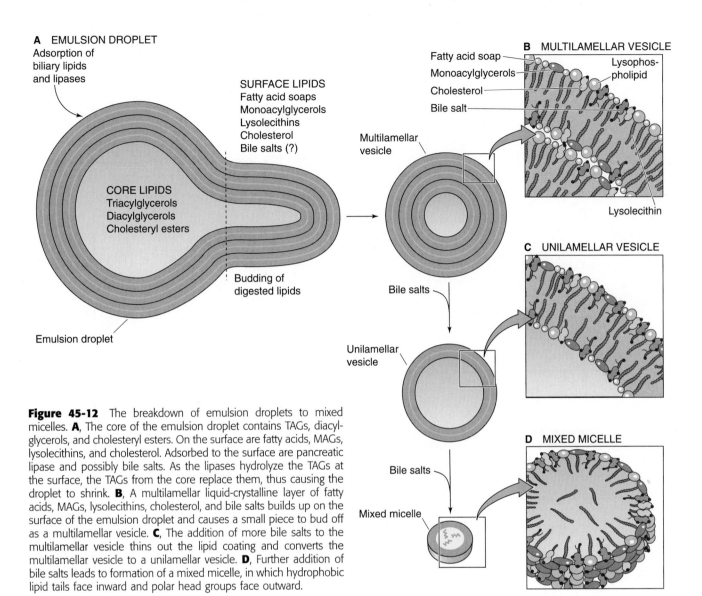

Figure 45-12 The breakdown of emulsion droplets to mixed micelles. **A,** The core of the emulsion droplet contains TAGs, diacylglycerols, and cholesteryl esters. On the surface are fatty acids, MAGs, lysolecithins, and cholesterol. Adsorbed to the surface are pancreatic lipase and possibly bile salts. As the lipases hydrolyze the TAGs at the surface, the TAGs from the core replace them, thus causing the droplet to shrink. **B,** A multilamellar liquid-crystalline layer of fatty acids, MAGs, lysolecithins, cholesterol, and bile salts builds up on the surface of the emulsion droplet and causes a small piece to bud off as a multilamellar vesicle. **C,** The addition of more bile salts to the multilamellar vesicle thins out the lipid coating and converts the multilamellar vesicle to a unilamellar vesicle. **D,** Further addition of bile salts leads to formation of a mixed micelle, in which hydrophobic lipid tails face inward and polar head groups face outward.

"concentration" of long-chain fatty acids near the enterocyte's brush border membrane by a factor of 100,000 and micellar solubilization by a factor of 1,000,000.

When the fatty acid/bile salt mixed micelles reach the enterocyte surface, they encounter an acidic microclimate generated by Na-H exchange at the brush border membrane. It is postulated that fatty acids now become protonated and leave the mixed micelle to enter the enterocyte, either by nonionic diffusion (see Chapter 36) of the uncharged fatty acid, or by collision and incorporation of the fatty acid into the cell membrane, or by carrier-mediated transport through fatty acid translocase (FAT/CD36) (Fig. 45-13). A plasma membrane fatty acid–binding protein (FABPpm) appears to enhance the translocation. Similarly, unesterified cholesterol and lysophospholipids must leave the micelle carrier to enter the enterocyte as monomers. Investigators have suggested that cholesterol derived from bile is better absorbed than is dietary cholesterol. After the entry of lipids into enterocytes, the remaining bile salts return to the lumen and are then absorbed passively throughout the small intestine and through active transport in the distal ileum (see Chapter 46). As with fatty acids, 2-MAGs, lysophospholipids, and cholesterol traditionally were assumed to enter the enterocyte by simple diffusion across the apical plasma membrane of the brush border villi. More recently, however, in addition to carriers for fatty acids, membrane proteins have been identified in both enterocytes and hepatocytes that may be responsible for the transfer of fatty acids, phospholipids, and cholesterol across their respective cell membranes. As well as providing a mechanism for facilitated or active absorption of the various products of lipid digestion, such carriers may yet be therapeutic targets for inhibiting lipid absorption. The drug ezetimibe, which lowers plasma cholesterol by interfering with its absorption and not its synthesis, appears to impede cholesterol uptake by enterocytes by inhibiting the brush border **Niemann-Pick C-1–like-1 (NPC1L1) protein.** NPC1L1 may yet prove to be the putative intestinal cholesterol transporter.

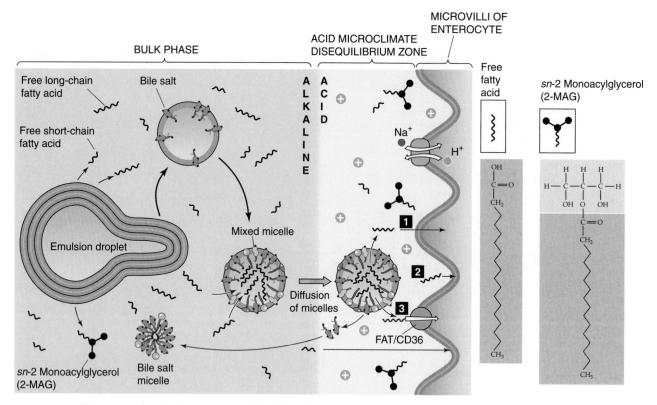

Figure 45-13 Micellar transport of lipid breakdown products to the surface of the enterocyte. Mixed micelles carry lipids through the acidic unstirred layer to the surface of the enterocyte. 2-MAG, fatty acids, lysophospholipids, and cholesterol leave the mixed micelle and enter an acidic microenvironment created by an apical Na-H exchanger. The acidity favors the protonation of the fatty acids. The lipids enter the enterocyte by (1) nonionic diffusion, (2) incorporation into the enterocyte membrane (collision), or (3) carrier-mediated transport.

The enterocyte re-esterifies lipid components and assembles them into chylomicrons

The assimilation of fats, thus far, has been a process of disassembly of energy-dense, water-insoluble lipid macromolecular aggregates into monomers for intestinal absorption. The enterocyte elegantly reverses this process (Fig. 45-14). After absorbing long-chain fatty acids, MAGs, lysophospholipids, and cholesterol, the enterocyte re-esterifies them and assembles the products with specific apolipoproteins (or simply apoproteins) into emulsion-like particles called *chylomicrons*. The enterocyte then exports the chylomicrons to the lymph (chyle) for ultimate delivery to other organs through the bloodstream.

Chylomicrons are the largest of the five lipoprotein particles in the bloodstream. (The other lipoprotein particles—very-low-density lipoproteins (VLDLs), intermediate-density lipoproteins (IDLs), low-density lipoproteins (LDLs), and high-density lipoproteins (HDLs)—are discussed in Chapter 46 and Table 46-5). With an average diameter of ~250 nm (range, 75 to 1200 nm), chylomicrons consist primarily of TAGs, with smaller amounts of phospholipids, cholesteryl esters, cholesterol, and various apolipoproteins.

The first step in the enterocyte's reformation of TAGs is for long-chain fatty acids to bind to a 12-kDa cytosolic protein called **fatty acid–binding protein**. The concentra-

tion of fatty acid–binding protein in the intestine is highest in regions that absorb fats, namely, the villi of the proximal jejunal enterocytes. Fatty acid–binding protein preferentially binds long-chain (rather than medium- or short-chain) fatty acids, thus minimizing both reflux back into the intestinal lumen and toxic damage to the enterocyte. Fatty acid–binding protein also ensures transfer of fatty acids to the smooth endoplasmic reticulum (SER) of the enterocyte. The re-esterification to form TAGs occurs within the SER. After a meal, enterocytes mainly use the **MAG pathway** to re-esterify absorbed fatty acids to absorbed 2-MAG. During fasting, enterocytes mainly use the phosphatidic acid pathway to esterify fatty acids that enter from the bloodstream. The necessary phosphatidic acid may arise either from glycerol-3-phosphate—itself derived from the metabolism of glucose or amino acids—or from the breakdown of bile lecithin that enters from the intestinal lumen. Both the MAG and the phosphatidic acid pathways depend on the activation of the fatty acid to acyl coenzyme A (acyl CoA), catalyzed by acyl CoA synthase. Long-chain fatty acids are the preferred substrate for this enzyme. The net effect of this series of reactions is the very rapid formation of TAGs in the SER, which maintains low fatty acid concentrations in the enterocyte. TAGs and fat droplets may be seen in the cisternae of the SER on electron microscopy. The enterocyte also esterifies both **cholesterol** and **lysolecithin**.

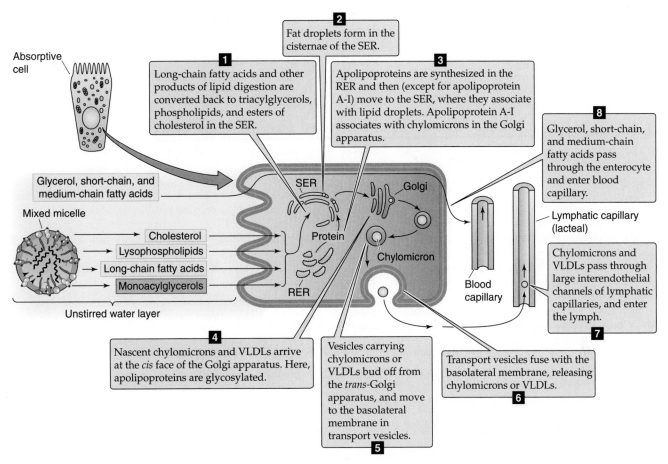

Figure 45-14 Re-esterification of digested lipids by the enterocyte and the formation and secretion of chylomicrons. The enterocyte takes up short- and medium-chain fatty acids and glycerol and passes them unchanged into the blood capillaries. The enterocyte also takes up long-chain fatty acids and 2-MAG and resynthesizes them into TAG in the SER. The enterocyte also processes cholesterol into cholesteryl esters and lysolecithin into lecithin. The fate of these substances, and the formation of chylomicrons, is illustrated by steps 1 to 8.

Besides the lipids, the other components of the chylomicron are the various apolipoproteins (see Table 46-5), which the enterocyte synthesizes in the rough endoplasmic reticulum (RER). These apolipoproteins, with the exception of apolipoprotein A-I, move to the lumen of the SER, where they associate with newly synthesized TAGs (Fig. 45-14). Apolipoprotein A-I associates with chylomicrons in the Golgi apparatus. Besides incorporating apolipoproteins, the packaging of nascent chylomicrons involves adding esterified cholesterol and a surface coating of lecithin and other phospholipids. It is thought that vesicles derived from the SER carry nascent chylomicrons to the *cis* face of the Golgi apparatus, where they fuse and deliver their contents internally. Enzymes in the Golgi apparatus glycosylate the apolipoproteins. Vesicles carrying processed chylomicrons bud off from the *trans* face of the Golgi and move toward the basolateral plasma membrane of the enterocyte. There they fuse with the basolateral membrane and leave the enterocyte.

The foregoing discussion focused on the digestion and absorption of *long-chain* TAGs. The handling of TAGs with **medium-length fatty acid chains** is very different. In the first place, the uptake into the enterocyte of fatty acids and MAGs derived from medium-chain TAGs does not depend on the presence of either mixed micelles or bile salts. Moreover, the enterocyte does not re-esterify the medium-chain fatty acids but instead transfers them directly into the portal blood. As a result, medium-chain TAGs are suitable fat substitutes for feeding patients with fat malabsorption.

The enterocyte secretes chylomicrons into the lymphatic circulation during feeding and secretes very-low-density lipoproteins during fasting

As we have described, vesicles carrying mature chylomicrons discharge their contents outside the enterocyte through exocytosis at the basolateral membrane. Chylomicrons are too large to pass through the fenestrae of blood capillaries, and thus they enter **lymph** through the larger interendothelial channels of the lymphatic capillaries. In both the fed and fasted states, the intestine secretes **VLDLs**, which are smaller (30 to 80 nm) than chylomicrons. These lipoprotein particles are of similar protein and lipid composition to chylomicrons (see Table 46-5), but they are synthesized independently and carry mainly endogenous (as opposed to dietary) lipids. The lymph lacteals originate in the tips of the villi and discharge their contents into the cisternae chyli. Lymph flows from the cisternae chyli to the thoracic duct, to enter the blood circulation through the left subclavian vein. The protein and lipid composition of both chylomicrons and VLDLs are modified during their passage through lymph and on entry into the blood.

The process of lipid digestion and absorption has great reserve capacity and many redundancies. For example, the mechanical disruption of food is accomplished in several ways by the mouth, stomach, and proximal intestine. Many of the digestive lipases have overlapping functions, and pancreatic lipase, in particular, is secreted in great excess. Much of the small intestine is not used for fat absorption in healthy individuals. Nonetheless, fat malabsorption does occur in many disease states. A logical classification for these disorders can be devised based on knowledge of the normal physiology. Thus, fat malabsorption may occur because of impairments in intraluminal digestion, intraluminal dispersion, mucosal penetration, or transport from enterocyte to the blood circulation. Within each major category are subdivisions. Frequently, the pathophysiology of these disorders is mixed (i.e., more than one step in the digestive or absorptive process is deranged), but nonetheless the defective components can be identified, and appropriate therapy can be given.

DIGESTION AND ABSORPTION OF VITAMINS AND MINERALS

Intestinal absorption of fat-soluble vitamins follows the pathways of lipid absorption and transport

Table 45-3 summarizes the fat-soluble vitamins A (see Chapter 15), D (see Chapter 52), E, and K (see Chapter 17). As a class, these vitamins rely on the lipid absorption process discussed in the preceding subchapter. Although individual fat-soluble vitamins, once digested and absorbed, have somewhat specific fates according to their chemical nature, they have numerous overlapping physical properties that determine their similar handling in the intestinal lumen, and uptake and processing by enterocytes. In contrast to their water-soluble counterparts (discussed later), fat-soluble vitamins do not form classical coenzyme structures or prosthetic groups with soluble apoproteins. Fat-soluble vitamins can also be stored in fat depots in the body. Each of the fat-soluble vitamins is really a family of related compounds, some of which are esters.

After ingestion, fat-soluble vitamins are released from their association with proteins by the acidity of gastric juice or by proteolysis. In addition, carboxyl ester hydrolases (found in pancreatic juice and in the mucosal brush border) liberate free vitamins from their esters. In the proximal small intestine, fat-soluble vitamins incorporate with other lipid products into emulsion droplets, vesicles, and mixed micelles, which ferry them to the enterocyte surface for uptake. The absorption efficiency of fat-soluble vitamins varies from 50% to 80% for A, D, and K to only 20% to 30% for vitamin E. Other ingestants—including dietary components and drugs and their carrier vehicles—can modify the absorption of fat-soluble vitamins. For example, high doses of vitamin A impair the absorption of vitamins E and K, whereas high doses of vitamin E enhance the absorption of vitamin A.

Enterocytes take up fat-soluble vitamins by simple diffusion or through transporters. After entry into the enterocyte, fat-soluble vitamins diffuse to the SER either as free molecules or attached to carrier proteins, such as a **cellular retinol-binding protein** in the case of vitamin A or retinol. In the SER, the vitamins associate with lipid droplets that form nascent chylomicrons and VLDLs, which then translocate through the Golgi and secretory vesicles for exocytosis into lymph. During passage through the enterocyte, vitamin A and tiny amounts of vitamin D are esterified with long-chain fatty acids, but vitamin E and K are not. Once in the systemic blood circulation, the fat-soluble vitamins A, D, E, and K enter the liver by receptor-mediated endocytosis of chylomicrons or remnant chylomicrons, as discussed in Chapter 46.

Fat-soluble vitamin deficiency occurs in various fat malabsorption states, including those induced by malabsorptive bariatric surgery, drugs (e.g., orlistat) that impair TAG hydrolysis, drugs (e.g., cholestyramine) that bind bile acids, and reduction of bile acids by impaired hepatobiliary function or by unabsorbable dietary fat substitutes. Fat-soluble vitamin deficiency can also result from impaired hepatic function. The consequences can include blindness and other irreversible eye disorders (vitamin A), bone demineralization and resorption (vitamin D), neurologic, neuromuscular and erythrocyte aberrations (vitamin E), and both hemorrhagic and hypercoagulable states (vitamin K).

Treatment of fat-soluble vitamin deficiency includes water-miscible emulsions of vitamins A and E, which can enter enterocytes without special handling in the intestinal lumen. These compounds then move into portal blood together with small amounts of the more polar forms of some of the vitamins, such as retinoic acid in the case of vitamin A and menadione in the case of vitamin K.

Dietary folate (PteGlu7) must be deconjugated by a brush border enzyme before absorption by an anion exchanger at the apical membrane

Folate is also referred to as folic acid, or pteroylmonoglutamate (PteGlu1). As we discuss later, the reduced form of folate—tetrahydrofolate (THF)—is a cofactor in biochemical reactions involving the transfer of 1-carbon fragments. The recommended dietary allowance (RDA) for folate is 200 μg for men and 180 μg for women (Table 45-3), but it is more than doubled in pregnant women (see Chapter 56). THF is essential for the synthesis of thymine and purines, which are critical components of DNA. Thus, folate deficiency compromises DNA synthesis and cell division, an effect that is most clinically noticeable in the bone marrow, where the turnover of cells is rapid. Because RNA and protein synthesis are not impaired, large red blood cells called *megaloblasts* are produced. The resultant *megaloblastic anemia* can become quite severe if untreated. Megaloblastic cells also

Table 45-3 Vitamins

Vitamin	Role	Recommended Dietary Allowance	Deficiency
A (retinol)	Retinal pigment	Male: 1000 µg Female: 800 µg	Follicular hyperkeratosis, night blindness
B_1 (thiamine)	Coenzyme in decarboxylation of pyruvate and α-keto acids	Male: 1.5 mg Female: 1.1 mg	Beriberi
B_2 (riboflavin)	Coenzymes flavin adenine dinucleotide and flavin mononucleotide, H carriers in mitochondria	Male: 1.7 mg Female: 1.3 mg	Hyperemia of nasopharyngeal mucosa, normocytic anemia
B_3 niacin (nicotinic acid)	Coenzymes NAD and NADP, H carriers in mitochondria	Male: 19 mg Female: 15 mg	Pellagra
B_6 (pyridoxine)	Coenzyme in transamination for synthesis of amino acids	Male: 2 mg Female: 1.6 mg	Stomatitis, glossitis, normocytic anemia
B_{12} (cobalamin)	Coenzyme in reduction of ribonucleotides to deoxyribonucleotides; promotion of formation of erythrocytes, myelin	2 µg	Pernicious anemia (megaloblastic anemia)
C (ascorbic acid)	Coenzyme in formation of hydroxyproline used in collagen	60 mg	Scurvy
D (1,25-cholecalciferol)	Ca^{2+} absorption	5-10 µg	Rickets
E (α-tocopherol)	Antioxidant: thought to prevent oxidation of unsaturated fatty acids	Male: 10 mg Female: 8 mg	Peripheral neuropathy
K (K_1 = phylloquinone, K_2 = various menaquinones)	Clotting: necessary for synthesis by liver of prothrombin and factors VII, IX, and X	Male: 70-80 µg Female: 60-65 µg	Hemorrhagic disease
Folate	Backbone used to synthesize purines and thymine	Male: 200 µg Female: 180 µg Pregnancy: 400 µg	Megaloblastic anemia
Biotin	Coenzyme in carboxylation reactions	30-100 µg*	Neurologic changes
Pantothenic acid	CoA; necessary for carbohydrate and fat metabolism involving acetyl-CoA amino acid synthesis	4-7 mg*	Abdominal pain, vomiting, neurologic signs

*Safe and allowable range.
NAD, nicotinamide adenine dinucleotide; NADP, nicotinamide adenine dinucleotide phosphate.

may be seen in other organs with rapid cell turnover, such as the small intestine. Folic acid supplementation during pregnancy also reduces the risk of neural tube defects.

The medicinal form of folate is PteGlu1, a **monoglutamate**. Figure 45-15A shows the structure of PteGlu1 and also illustrates how folate can act as a methyl acceptor or donor in the interconversion of serine to glycine. Dietary folate exists in several forms, much of it as **folate polyglutamate**, or PteGlu7 (Fig. 45-15B), which is widely available in the diet, particularly in spinach, beans, and liver. The intestinal absorption of PteGlu7 requires deconjugation by a brush border peptidase to PteGlu1, which then enters the enterocyte through a transporter (Fig. 45-15C). This deconjuga-

tion is catalyzed by folate conjugase, a zinc-activated exopeptidase present in the brush border. This enzyme removes glutamate residues from PteGlu7 in a stepwise fashion before absorption of PteGlu1. This stepwise hydrolysis of the polyglutamate chain of PteGlu7 is the rate-limiting step in folate digestion-absorption. Both folate deconjugation and absorption occur only in the proximal small intestine and are maximally active at a pH of 5.

PteGlu1 absorption is saturable, shows substrate specificity, and is markedly enhanced at an acid pH. Folate absorption represents an apical membrane anion exchange process, in which folate uptake is linked to the efflux of OH^- across the apical membrane (i.e., folate-OH exchange). The mecha-

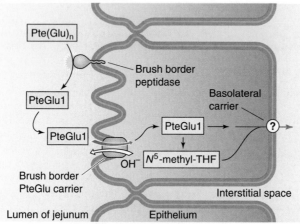

A MEDICINAL FOLATE (PteGlu1)

Pteridine

p-Aminobenzoate   **Glutamate**

"R"

B FOOD FOLATE (PteGlu7)

Pteroylpolyglutamate

C FOLATE ABSORPTION

Pte(Glu)$_n$

Brush border peptidase

Basolateral carrier

PteGlu1

PteGlu1

PteGlu1

?

Brush border PteGlu carrier

OH$^-$ N^5-methyl-THF

Interstitial space

Lumen of jejunum   Epithelium

D METHYLATION OF REDUCED FOLATE

Reactive

Reactive

Ser   Gly

H$^+$ + NADH   NAD$^+$

5,10-methylene-THF

dUMP

dTMP → DNA

DHF

Tetrahydrofolate (THF)

N^5-methyl-tetrahydrofolate

Figure 45-15 Folate deconjugation and absorption. **A,** Tetrahydrofolate has three parts: the biologically active pteridine moiety, a p-aminobenzoate, and a glutamate. PteGlu1 is the oxidized form of folate and is biologically inactive. **B,** Dietary folate is similar to medicinal folate but has several glutamate residues. PteGlu7 is also oxidized and inactive. **C,** In the proximal small intestine, a brush border peptidase sequentially removes all but the last of the glutamate residues from dietary folate. The enterocyte then absorbs the resulting PteGlu1 using a folate-OH exchanger. Once inside the enterocyte, the PteGlu1 exists across the basolateral membrane through an unknown transporter. The enterocyte may reduce some of the PteGlu1 to DHF and then to THF, the biologically active form of folate. The enterocyte may then methylate some of the THF to form N^5-methyl-THF. **D,** After the cell has reduced PteGlu1 to THF by adding the four highlighted hydrogens, it first converts THF to 5,10-methylene-THF, thus breaking down serine to glycine in the process. This 5,10-methylene-THF is the methyl donor in the conversion of the nucleotide deoxyuridine monophosphate (dUMP) to deoxythymidine monophosphate (dTMP) in the synthesis of DNA. A second reaction converts this 5,10-methylene-THF to N^5-methyl-THF, which can then act as a methyl donor in the synthesis of methionine (see Fig. 45-16B). NAD, nicotinamide adenine dinucleotide; NADH, nicotinamide adenine dinucleotide (reduced form).

nism of folate movement out of the epithelial cell across the basolateral membrane is not understood.

The PteGlu1 taken up by the enterocyte is not biologically active. The enzyme difolate reductase acts on PteGlu1 to first form dihydrofolate (DHF) and then the biologically active derivative THF. The cell then converts THF to 5,10-methylene THF (Fig. 45-15D), the form of folate needed for DNA synthesis. The cell also can transform this 5,10-methylene THF to N^5-methyl THF, which—as we discuss in the next section—can act as a methyl donor in the synthesis of methionine. The circulating, storage, and active forms of folate constitute various reduced (DHF and THF) and methylated derivatives of THF. The liver is the primary site at which dietary pteroylglutamates are reduced and methylated, although the intestinal epithelium may make a small contribution to these reactions.

Vitamin B₁₂ (cobalamin) binds to haptocorrin in the stomach, and then to intrinsic factor in the small intestine, before endocytosis by enterocytes in the ileum

Cobalamin, or vitamin B_{12} (Fig. 45-16A), is synthesized only by microorganisms, not by mammalian cells. The primary source of cobalamin in humans is the ingestion of animal products—meat, fish, shellfish, eggs, and (to a limited extent) milk. Cobalamin is not present in vegetables or fruit. Therefore, strict vegetarians are at risk of developing dietary cobalamin deficiency.

Cobalamin's primary function is to serve as a coenzyme for homocysteine:methionine methyltransferase (Fig. 45-16B), which transfers a methyl group from methyltetrafolate to homocysteine, thereby converting homocysteine to methionine. Methionine is an essential amino acid and in an altered form serves as an important donor of methyl groups in several important enzymatic reactions. If cobalamin is deficient and methionine levels fall, then the body converts its stores of intracellular folate (e.g., PteGlu1, THF, 5,10-methylene THF) into N^5-methyl THF (Fig. 45-15D) in an effort to produce more methionine. As a result, 5,10-methylene THF (the form of folate needed for DNA synthesis) falls, an effect that explains why folate and cobalamin deficiencies cause identical hematologic abnormalities (i.e., megaloblastic anemia). In addition, cobalamin deficiency causes various neurologic and psychological abnormalities that are not part of the syndrome of folate deficiency. Some of these abnormalities may be linked to deficient activity of methylmalonyl CoA mutase, another cobalamin-dependent coenzyme.

Cobalamin reaches the stomach bound to proteins in ingested food. In the stomach, pepsin and the low gastric pH release the cobalamin from the ingested proteins (Fig. 45-16C). The now-free cobalamin binds to **haptocorrin** (formerly known as "R" type binder), a glycoprotein secreted by the salivary and gastric glands. The parietal cells of the stomach secrete a second protein, **intrinsic factor** (IF), crucial for the absorption of cobalamin. However cobalamin and IF do not interact in the acidic milieu of the stomach. Rather, gastric acidity enhances the binding of cobalamin to haptocorrin. When this cobalamin-haptocorrin complex reaches the duodenum, the haptocorrin is degraded by pancreatic proteases (Fig. 45-16C).

After the release of cobalamin from the cobalamin-haptocorrin complex in the proximal small intestine—made alkaline by the secretion of HCO_3^- from the pancreas and duodenum—both dietary cobalamin and cobalamin derived from bile bind to IF. The cobalamin-IF complex is highly resistant to enzyme degradation. As noted earlier, the gastric parietal cells secrete IF, a 45-kDa glycoprotein. Histamine, acetylcholine, and gastrin stimulate gastric acid secretion (see Chapter 42), and they also stimulate IF secretion. Although IF secretion parallels proton secretion, three important differences exist. First, similar to pepsinogen secretion, histamine triggers an IF release that peaks within minutes and then continues at a reduced rate. This secretory pattern is related to the secretion of preformed IF; histamine has no effect on IF synthesis. Second, although cAMP is important in IF secretion, a role for intracellular Ca^{2+} has not yet been established. Third, H_2 histamine-receptor antagonists block IF secretion, but omeprazole, an inhibitor of the parietal cell H-K pump, does not affect IF secretion.

The next step in the absorption of cobalamin is the binding of the cobalamin-IF complex to specific receptors on the apical membranes of enterocytes in the ileum. Cobalamin without IF neither binds to ileal receptors nor is absorbed. The binding of the cobalamin-IF complex is selective and rapid and requires Ca^{2+}, but it is not energy dependent. The enterocyte next internalizes the cobalamin-IF complex in a process that is energy dependent but has not been well characterized. Inside the cell, cobalamin and IF dissociate; lysosomal degradation may play a role here. Within the enterocyte, cobalamin binds to another transport protein—transcobalamin II—which is required for cobalamin's exit from the enterocyte. The cobalamin exits the ileal enterocyte across the basolateral membrane bound to transcobalamin II, possibly by an exocytotic mechanism. The transcobalamin II-cobalamin complex enters the portal circulation, where it is delivered to the liver for storage and for secretion into the bile.

Total body cobalamin stores are large (~5 mg), particularly when compared with the daily rate of cobalamin absorption and loss. (The daily cobalamin requirement for normal adults is only 2 *micrograms*.) The load of cobalamin presented to the small intestine is derived about equally from two sources: the diet and biliary secretions. The latter is the result of the enterohepatic circulation (see Chapter 46) of cobalamin; after its absorption, cobalamin is delivered throughout the body, and the excess is secreted by the liver into the bile, where it once again can be reabsorbed by the small intestine and recirculated.

Cobalamin deficiency has many possible causes. As already mentioned, a strict vegetarian diet is deficient in cobalamin. In **pernicious anemia**, a disorder seen primarily in elderly persons, the absence of gastric parietal cells results in the absence of gastric acid and IF secretion. Consequently, cobalamin absorption is markedly reduced, and cobalamin deficiency develops. Other causes of cobalamin deficiency include related problems in the intestine. Bacterial overgrowth in the small intestine as a result of stasis (e.g., multiple jejunal diverticulosis) can be associated with cobalamin deficiency as a consequence of bacterial binding and metabolism of cobalamin. Crohn disease affecting the ileum and ileal resection are other possible causes of cobalamin

A CYANOCOBALAMIN

B METHYLATION CYCLE

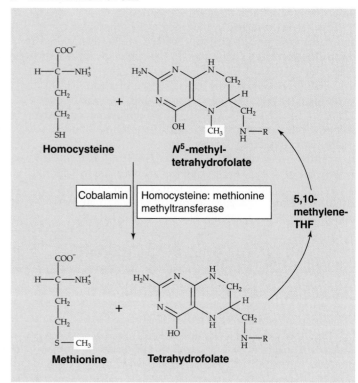

C COBALAMIN HANDLING BY THE STOMACH AND PROXIMAL SMALL INTESTINE

D COBALAMIN ABSORPTION BY ILEAL ENTEROCYTE

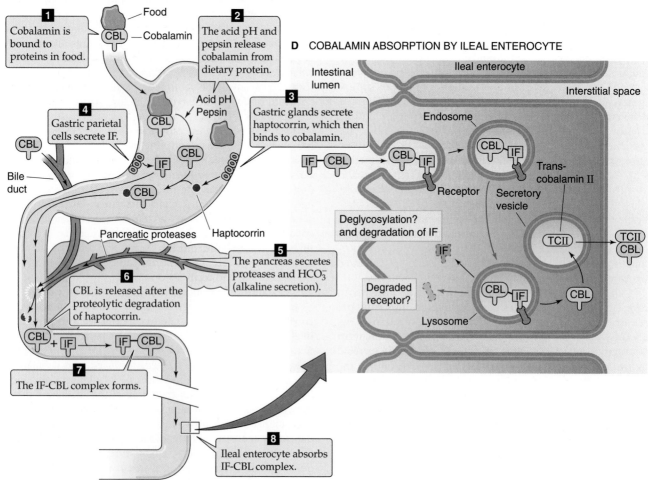

Figure 45-16 Cobalamin and the role of IF in the absorption of cobalamin. **A**, Cyanocobalamin. **B**, Methylation cycle. Cobalamin is the coenzyme for the enzyme homocysteine:methionine methyltransferase, which transfers a methyl group from N^5-methyltetrafolate to homocysteine, thereby forming methionine and tetrahydrofolate. **C**, Steps 1 to 8 show the fate of dietary cobalamin (CBL). Steps 4 to 8 show the role of IF. In addition, bile carries cobalamin into the duodenum. **D**, The intrinsic-factor/cobalamin complex is thought to be endocytosed. The cobalamin is liberated within the enterocyte by mechanisms that have not been established. Within the enterocyte, cobalamin binds to transcobalamin II (TCII), which is required for cobalamin's exit from the enterocyte.

Pernicious Anemia

The close relationship between acid and gastrin release is clearly manifested in individuals with impaired acid secretion. In **pernicious anemia**, atrophy of the gastric mucosa in the corpus and an absence of parietal cells result in the lack in the secretion of both gastric acid and IF. Many patients with pernicious anemia exhibit antibody-mediated immunity against their parietal cells, and many of these patients also produce anti-IF autoantibodies.

Because IF is required for cobalamin absorption in the ileum, the result is impaired cobalamin absorption. In contrast, the antrum is normal. Moreover, plasma gastrin levels are markedly elevated as a result of the absence of intraluminal acid, which normally triggers gastric D cells to release somatostatin (see Chapter 42), which, in turn, inhibits antral gastrin release (see Chapter 42 for the box titled Gastrinoma or Zollinger-Ellison Syndrome). Because parietal cells are absent, the elevated plasma gastrin levels are not associated with enhanced gastric acid secretion.

The clinical complications of cobalamin deficiency evolve over a period of years. Patients develop **megaloblastic anemia** (in which the circulating red blood cells are enlarged), a distinctive form of glossitis, and neuropathy. The earliest neurologic findings are those of peripheral neuropathy, as manifested by paresthesias and slow reflexes, as well as impaired senses of touch, vibration, and temperature. If untreated, the disease will ultimately involve the spinal cord, particularly the dorsal columns, thus producing weakness and ataxia. Memory impairment, depression, and dementia can also result. Parenteral administration of cobalamin reverses and prevents the manifestations of pernicious anemia, but it does not influence parietal cells or restore gastric secretion of either IF or intraluminal acid.

malabsorption and deficiency as a result of an absence of ileal receptors for the cobalamin-IF complex.

Ca^{2+} absorption, regulated primarily by vitamin D, occurs by active transport in the duodenum and by diffusion throughout the small intestine

The physiological importance and complex regulation of Ca^{2+} and vitamin D are discussed in Chapter 52. The Ca^{2+} load presented to the small intestine comprises dietary sources and digestive secretions. Most of the dietary Ca^{2+} (~1000 mg/day) comes from milk and milk products (see Fig. 52-1), but not all of it is bioavailable. For example, only very little of the Ca^{2+} present in leafy vegetables is absorbed because of the concomitant presence of oxalate, a salt that

binds Ca^{2+} and reduces its availability for absorption. The small intestine absorbs ~500 mg/day of Ca^{2+}, but it also secretes ~325 mg/day of Ca^{2+}. Thus the net uptake is ~175 mg/day.

Active, transcellular uptake of Ca^{2+} occurs only in the epithelial cells of the duodenum, but Ca^{2+} is absorbed by passive, paracellular diffusion throughout the small intestine. More Ca^{2+} is absorbed in the jejunum and ileum by diffusion than in the duodenum by active transport; this difference arises largely because the duodenum has a smaller total surface area and because the flow of Ca^{2+}-containing fluid through the duodenum is faster (Fig. 45-17).

The *active* transport of Ca^{2+} across the villous epithelial cells of the duodenum is transcellular and is under the control of vitamin D—primarily through genomic effects (see Chapter 4). Transcellular Ca^{2+} absorption involves three steps. The uptake of Ca^{2+} across the apical membrane occurs through **Ca^{2+} channels**, driven by the electrochemical gradient between the lumen and the cell. Cytosolic Ca^{2+} then binds to a protein called **calbindin**, which buffers intracellular Ca^{2+}. This step is important because it allows unbound (i.e., free) intracellular Ca^{2+} to remain rather low despite large transcellular fluxes of Ca^{2+}. A **Ca^{2+} pump** and an **Na-Ca exchanger** on the basolateral membrane then extrude the Ca^{2+} from the cell into the interstitial fluid. The active form of vitamin D—1,25-dihydroxyvitamin D—stimulates all three steps of the transcellular pathway, but its most important effect is to enhance the second step by increasing the synthesis of calbindin.

The passive absorption of Ca^{2+} throughout the small intestine occurs through the paracellular pathway, which is *not* under the control of vitamin D. Ca^{2+} absorption is also enhanced by low plasma [Ca^{2+}] and during pregnancy and lactation. Absorption tends to diminish with aging.

Vitamin D itself is a fat-soluble vitamin that is absorbed mainly in the jejunum. Of course, the skin synthesizes vitamin D$_3$ from cholesterol in a process that requires ultraviolet light (see Chapter 52). Thus, dietary vitamin D (both vitamin D$_2$ and D$_3$) is most important in regions of the world that do not receive much sunlight and during long, dark winters.

Mg^{2+} absorption occurs by an active process in the ileum

Mg^{2+} is an important intracellular ion that is required as an enzyme cofactor—many enzymes using ATP actually require that the ATP be complexed with Mg^{2+}—and is critical for neurotransmission and muscular contractions. Mg^{2+} deficiency can affect neuromuscular, cardiovascular, and gastrointestinal function. Mg^{2+} is also important for the

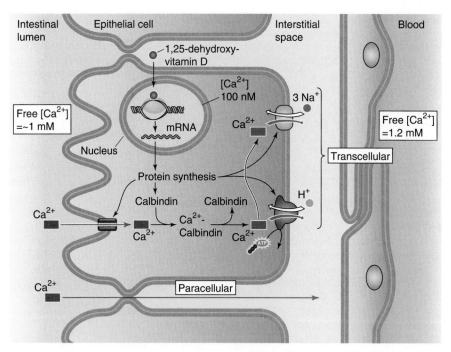

Figure 45-17 Active Ca^{2+} uptake in the duodenum. The small intestine absorbs Ca^{2+} by two mechanisms. The passive, paracellular absorption of Ca^{2+} occurs throughout the small intestine. This pathway predominates, but it is *not* under the control of vitamin D. The second mechanism—the active, transcellular absorption of Ca^{2+}—occurs only in the duodenum. Ca^{2+} enters the cell across the apical membrane through a channel. Inside the cell, the Ca^{2+} is buffered by binding proteins, such as calbindin, and is also taken up into intracellular organelles, such as the endoplasmic reticulum. The enterocyte then extrudes Ca^{2+} across the basolateral membrane through a Ca^{2+} pump and an Na-Ca exchanger. Thus, the net effect is Ca^{2+} absorption. The active form of vitamin D (1,25 dihydroxyvitamin D) stimulates all three steps of transcellular Ca^{2+} absorption.

Hemochromatosis

Hereditary hemochromatosis (HH) is a relatively common inherited disorder (3 to 5 persons per 1000 of northwestern European ancestry are homozygous) in which the body absorbs excessive iron from the diet. This autosomal recessive disease becomes clinically significant only in homozygotes. If left untreated, HH can be fatal. The excess iron is stored in the liver, where it reaches toxic concentrations. Cirrhosis eventually results, and the risk of hepatoma is greatly increased. Iron also ultimately accumulates in other organ systems, where it causes pancreatic damage (diabetes mellitus), bronze pigmentation of the skin, pituitary and gonadal failure, arthritis, and cardiomyopathy. The disease hardly ever becomes apparent before the individual enters the third decade of life. Women are relatively protected as long they are premenopausal, because their monthly menstrual flow keeps total body iron stores relatively normal.

The diagnosis can be made by detection of elevated iron and transferrin-saturation levels and elevated ferritin. A liver biopsy is confirmatory.

Treatment, reminiscent of the medieval approach to disease, is to remove (phlebotomize) one or even several units of blood (1 unit = 500 mL) from the patient on a regular basis until the iron overload is corrected, as evidenced by normal plasma ferritin levels. Afterward, most patients require phlebotomy only once every few months to maintain their low iron stores.

The **HFE gene** that is associated with HH is related to the major histocompatibility complex (MHC) class I family. More than 80% of patients with HH are homozygous for a *missense* mutation (C282Y) in *HFE*. However, the role of this mutated gene in hemochromatosis is not yet clear because the penetrance of hemochromatosis in individuals with the C282Y allele is very low (<5%). Attention has also focused on hepcidin, a recently identified hepatic protein that appears to play a critical role in the regulation, by body iron stores, of duodenal iron absorption.

Because increased body iron stores reduce iron absorption, hemochromatosis represents an inappropriately high rate of iron absorption relative to body iron stores. Because hepcidin downregulates both DMT1 expression and iron absorption, hemochromatosis may represent a defect in the regulation of hepcidin, but the relationship between the *HFE* gene and hepcidin is not known. It is possible that a mutated *HFE* gene causes an inappropriately low hepatic hepcidin expression, thus resulting in hemochromatosis.

The relationship between hepcidin and iron absorption has also been identified in **the anemia of inflammation**, caused by a reduction in duodenal iron absorption. In this setting, the cytokine interleukin-6 stimulates hepcidin expression, which, in turn, results in decreased DMT1 expression, ferroportin activity, and iron absorption.

proper secretion of, and end-organ response to, parathyroid hormone. Thus, Mg^{2+} depletion is typically associated with hypocalcemia.

Mg^{2+} is widely available in different foods but is present in particularly large amounts in green vegetables, cereals, and meats. The RDA for Mg^{2+} (Table 45-3) in young adults is ~350 mg/day for men and ~280 mg/day for women. The Mg^{2+} load to the small intestine is derived from both dietary sources and digestive secretions.

Mg^{2+} absorption by the gastrointestinal tract is not yet well understood, but it appears to differ substantially from the absorption of the other key divalent cation, Ca^{2+}, in three important respects. First, an active transport process for Mg^{2+} absorption appears to exist in the ileum, rather than in the duodenum, as is the case for Ca^{2+}. Second, 1,25-dihydroxyvitamin D does not consistently increase Mg^{2+} absorption. Third, patients with increased intestinal Ca^{2+} absorption (e.g., absorptive hypercalciuria) have normal Mg^{2+} absorption. Along with active Mg^{2+} absorption in the ileum, the rest of the small intestine absorbs Mg^{2+} passively.

Heme and nonheme iron are absorbed in the duodenum by distinct cellular mechanisms

Iron plays several critical roles in human physiology, both in the heme groups of the cytochromes and as a key component of the oxygen-carrying heme moieties of hemoglobin and myoglobin. The most important complication of iron depletion is anemia. Iron overload produces **hemochromatosis**, a not uncommon genetic disease (see the box titled Hemochromatosis).

Dietary iron takes two major forms: iron that is part of a heme moiety and iron that is not. These two types of dietary iron are absorbed by distinctly different mechanisms (Fig. 45-18). Overall iron absorption is low; 10% to 20% of ingested iron is absorbed. Heme iron is absorbed more efficiently than nonheme iron. Body stores of iron depend almost exclusively on iron absorption because no regulated pathway for iron excretion exists. Except in menstruating women, who require ~50% more iron in their diets, very little iron is lost from the body. Dietary iron comes primarily

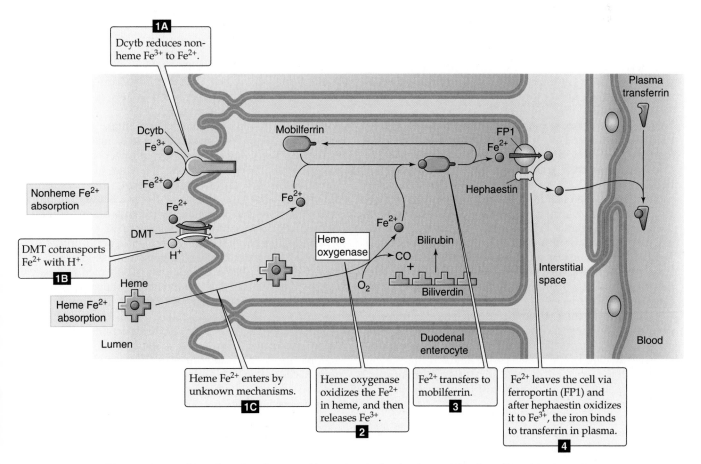

Figure 45-18 Absorption of nonheme and heme iron in the duodenum. The absorption of nonheme iron occurs almost exclusively as Fe^{2+}, which crosses the duodenal apical membrane through DMT1, driven by a H^+ gradient, which is maintained by Na-H exchange. Heme enters the enterocyte by an unknown mechanism. Inside the cell, heme oxygenase releases Fe^{3+}, which is then reduced to Fe^{2+}. Cytoplasmic Fe^{2+} then binds to mobilferrin for transit across the cell to the basolateral membrane. Fe^{2+} probably exits the enterocyte through basolateral ferroportin. The ferroxidase activity of hephaestin converts Fe^{2+} to Fe^{3+} for carriage in the blood plasma bound to transferrin.

from meat—especially liver and fish—as well as vegetables. The RDA for iron (Table 45-3) in young adults is ~10 mg/day for men and ~15 mg/day for women.

Nonheme Iron   Nonheme iron may be either ferric (Fe^{3+}) or ferrous (Fe^{2+}). Ferric iron tends to form salt complexes with anions quite easily and thus is not readily absorbed; it is not soluble at pH values higher than 3. Ferrous iron does not complex easily and is soluble at pH values as high as 8. Ascorbic acid (vitamin C) forms soluble complexes with iron and reduces iron from the ferric to the ferrous state, thereby enhancing iron absorption. Tannins, present in tea, form insoluble complexes with iron and lower its absorption.

Iron movement does not occur passively but requires one or more proteins to facilitate its movement into and out of cells (especially enterocytes, hepatocytes, and macrophages), as well as for intracellular binding. The absorption of nonheme iron is restricted to the duodenum. The enterocyte takes up nonheme iron across the apical membrane through the **divalent metal transporter DMT1** (SLC11A2), which cotransports Fe^{2+} and H^+ into the cell (see Chapter 5). DMT1, as well as the oligopeptide cotransporter that we discussed earlier, is unusual in being energized by the inwardly directed H^+ gradient. DMT1 also efficiently absorbs a host of other divalent metals, including several that are highly toxic (e.g., Cd^{2+}, Pb^{2+}). In the case of dietary ferric iron, the **ferric reductase Dcytb**—which is related to cytochrome b—presumably reduces Fe^{3+} to Fe^{2+} at the extracellular surface of the apical membrane before uptake through DMT1.

Fe^{2+} moves into the cytoplasm of the enterocyte, where it binds to **mobilferrin**, an intracellular protein that ferries the Fe^{2+} to the basolateral membrane. The enterocyte then translocates the Fe^{2+} across the basolateral membrane, possibly through **ferroportin transporter** (**FP1**, also known as IREG1). The mRNA encoding FP1 has an iron-responsive element (see Chapter 4) in its 5′ untranslated region; thus, an increase in intracellular iron levels would be expected to decrease FP1 synthesis. Following the exit of Fe^{2+} from the enterocyte through FP1, the **ferroxidase hephaestin**—a homologue of the plasma protein ceruloplasmin, which carries copper (see Chapter 46)—apparently oxidizes the Fe^{2+} to Fe^{3+}, which then binds to plasma **transferrin** (see Chapter 2) for carriage in the blood.

Once in the circulation, nonheme iron bound to transferrin is ultimately deposited in all the tissues of the body, but it has a particular predilection for the liver and reticuloendothelial system. Inside these cells, it binds to the protein apoferritin to form **ferritin**, the major storage form of iron. Smaller amounts of storage iron exist in an insoluble form called *hemosiderin*.

Heme Iron   Derived from myoglobin and hemoglobin, heme iron is also absorbed by duodenal epithelial cells. Heme iron enters the cells either by binding to a brush border protein or through an endocytotic mechanism. Inside the cell, **heme oxygenase** enzymatically splits the heme iron, thus releasing free Fe^{3+}, CO, and biliverdin (see Fig. 46-6). The cell reduces the biliverdin to bilirubin, which the liver eventually excretes in bile (see Chapter 46 for the box on jaundice). The enterocyte reduces the Fe^{3+} to Fe^{2+}, which it then handles in the same manner as nonheme iron.

Iron absorption is tightly regulated by the size of existing body iron stores. In physiologically normal subjects, iron absorption is limited but is markedly *increased* in states of iron deficiency, caused most often by gastrointestinal bleeding or excessive menstrual flow. For example, the expressions of DMT1 and FP1 increase in iron deficiency. Conversely, an increase in iron stores modestly reduces iron absorption.

The molecular mechanisms by which iron stores regulate iron absorption are incompletely understood but play a role in the pathophysiology of hemochromatosis. Recent attention has focused on a 25–amino acid peptide secreted by hepatic Kupffer's cells, **hepcidin**, which appears to down-regulate duodenal iron absorption by regulating DMT1 activity as well as other proteins in the iron-responsive pathways (e.g., FP1). Hepcidin likely is a negative regulator of iron absorption because mice that fail to express hepcidin have elevated body iron stores, whereas mice with enhanced hepcidin expression have profound iron deficiency.

NUTRITIONAL REQUIREMENTS

No absolute daily requirement for carbohydrate or fat intake exists

Nutritionists recommend that the daily intake of carbohydrate versus fat should not differ with age, gender, or activity level. Of the total caloric intake in a Western diet, 55% to 60% is typically carbohydrate, 25% to 30% is fat, and the remaining 10% to 15% is protein.

The requirements for **total** caloric intake vary among individuals and depend on certain factors, including a person's ability to use and store energy (efficiency) and the daily activity level. Differences in the efficiency of energy use among individuals are the result, in part, of variations in muscle mass but also of genetic factors. Because adipose tissue has a low metabolic rate, people with a large fat mass require less caloric intake per kilogram of body weight. Stated differently, the requirement for energy intake is greater per kilogram of *lean* body mass than per kilogram of *total* body mass (which includes fat). Thus, men generally require a greater daily caloric intake per kilogram of body weight than do women, who have relatively less muscle and more fat.

Activity level is the primary factor determining the daily energy requirement, assuming a stable body weight. For example, in a steady state, athletes must consume more than nonathletes not only because of a higher muscle-to-fat ratio but also because of a higher energy expenditure. Manual labor necessitates greater energy intake than does sedentary activity, again to maintain energy balance and body weight. Excess intake over output causes weight gain over time. Using the conversion of 9.4 kcal/g, 1 kg of fat stores 9400 kcal, sufficient energy to carry the BMR for 4 days.

Eating a low-carbohydrate diet (e.g., the Atkins diet) leads to an accelerated breakdown of tissue protein and thus to the wasting of muscle and other vital tissues, as well as the breakdown of fat. The breakdown of both protein and fat leads to an accumulation of ketone bodies in the blood (from the conversion of amino acids and fatty acids to acetyl CoA).

In addition to serving as a source of energy, fatty acids are also important for membrane structure (see Chapter 2), as well as signal transduction by pathways such as those involving diacylglycerols and arachidonic acid (see Chapter 3). In mammalian cells, fatty acid synthase produces two major fatty acids: palmitic and oleic acids. Palmitic acid, which has 16 carbons and is fully saturated, is referred to as $16:0$. Oleic acid has 18 carbons and a single *cis* double bond between carbons 9 and 10. This unsaturated fatty acid is referred to as $18:1$ *cis*-Δ^9. Because mammals cannot insert double bonds beyond carbon 9, they need two fatty acids in the diet: linoleate ($18:2$ *cis*-$\Delta^9\Delta^{12}$) and linolenate ($18:3$ *cis*-$\Delta^9\Delta^{12}\Delta^{15}$). These **essential fatty acids** serve as precursors for other unsaturated fatty acids, including arachidonic acid, which is a precursor to prostaglandins, leukotrienes, and thromboxanes.

The current recommendations favoring low fat intake are based on the view that a high fat intake is associated with chronic diseases such as atherosclerosis and non–insulin-dependent diabetes (see Chapter 51 for the box on sulfonylureas). However, fats have a positive side. In addition to the roles we have discussed in this chapter, fats enhance satiety and aid in the absorption of certain vitamins. Finally, the so-called ω-3 polyunsaturated fatty acids—in which the first double bond is three carbons from the terminal methyl group (or "ω carbon")—appear to protect against cardiovascular disease and some forms of cancer.

The daily protein requirement for adult humans is typically 0.8 g/kg body weight, but is higher in pregnant women, postsurgical patients, and athletes

The diet must contain the nine essential amino acids (see Table 58-2) because the body cannot synthesize them (see Chapter 46). Eleven other amino acids are necessary for protein synthesis, but the body can synthesize their carbon skeletons from intermediates of carbohydrate metabolism. **Vegetarian diets** can meet the protein needs of the body, provided the protein contains adequate amounts of essential amino acids. Food protein is "scored" based on its content of essential amino acids, compared with that of a reference protein, usually egg protein, which is given a score of 100. For example, a food containing protein with a score of 40 for threonine, 80 for phenylalanine, and 100 for lysine—all three of which are essential amino acids—receives a protein score of 40 because, relative to the standard, threonine is present in the lowest amount.

Protein intake is most important to meet the needs for tissue maintenance and repair, for muscle and neural function, and to maintain host defense mechanisms. The daily requirement for protein intake depends on one's nutritional status. The average human needs ~0.6 g of protein per kilogram of body weight per day to maintain nitrogen balance. The RDA of protein is ~0.8 g/kg of body weight for adults, ~1 g/kg for adolescents, and ~2 g/kg in the first 6 months of life. Pregnant and lactating women require extra protein intake to ensure adequate fetal development and milk production. Athletes require more than 1 g/kg to maintain a greater lean body mass and to fuel a highly active metabolism. Well-balanced but larger meals usually provide adequate protein for those with a greater need. Burn victims,

patients recovering from surgery, and patients with disorders of protein absorption all require increased daily protein intake.

The distribution of amino acids required for protein accretion by growing infants and children is different than that for tissue maintenance. Moreover, the requirements change throughout development. The child uses 25% of amino acid intake for protein accretion at 6 months of age but only 10% by 18 months of age. More than 40% of a child's protein intake must consist of essential amino acids versus only 20% for an adult.

Proteins play a key role in host defenses. For example, proteins provide the structural backbone for skin and mucus. Protein synthesis is essential for phagocytes and lymphocytes that are responsible for antibody and cell-mediated immunity. The skin, lungs, and intestinal tract are the main structural defenses against invading organisms. In both the lungs and the gastrointestinal tract, mucus (containing glycoproteins) coats the surface of these passageways and aids in defending against disease by catching most foreign particles. Protein-depleted individuals, regardless of age, have impaired immune competence. Protein depletion limits the availability of amino acids for synthesis of the cellular proteins of the immune system, including glutathione, mucus glycoproteins, and metallothreonine. The acute-phase response to invading organisms is suboptimal in a protein-deficient state.

The impaired immune competence of patients with AIDS is a function of poor nutrition in addition to the effects of the virus itself. During infection, the body mobilizes amino acids to synthesize proteins for defense against invading organisms. Thus, improving protein and energy intake may be beneficial for some patients with AIDS.

Aside from being the backbone of proteins, amino acids play a variety of physiological roles. For example, arginine is a precursor to **nitric oxide** (see Chapter 3). Glutamate is a major **excitatory neurotransmitter** in the brain, whereas glycine is a major **inhibitory neurotransmitter** (see Chapter 13). Glutamine is a major source of NH_3 **production** in the kidney (see Chapter 39), and it also regulates **protein turnover** in muscle. The decrease in muscle glutamine concentration that occurs during trauma and infection is associated with a general decline of muscle function. Research on anorectic patients shows that the most important factor affecting muscle function is insufficient nutrient intake. Increasing total nutrient intake in these subjects by total parenteral nutrition increases muscle function before having a measurable effect on muscle mass.

Minerals and vitamins are not energy sources, but are necessary for certain enzymatic reactions, for protein complexes, or as precursors for biomolecules

Vitamins and minerals do not provide energy but are essential for such functions as metabolism, immune competence, muscle force production, and blood clotting.

Minerals Table 45-4 lists the essential minerals. The current recommendations for daily mineral intake are based on a mix of *balance studies* and usual dietary intakes in the United States. The recommendation for copper, for example,

Table 45-4 Essential Minerals

Mineral	Role	Recommended Dietary Allowance
Ca	Bone, intracellular signaling	800-1200 mg
Cr	Possibly a cofactor in metabolism of carbohydrates, protein, lipids	50-200 μg
Cu	Enzyme cofactor (e.g., superoxide dismutase)	1.5-3 mg
Fe	Hemoglobin and cytochromes	Male: 10 mg Female (childbearing age): 15 mg
I	Thyroid hormones	150 μg
Mg	Complexes with ATP	Male: ~350 mg Female: ~280 mg
Mn	Antioxidant	2-5 mg
Mo	Cofactor in carbon, nitrogen, and sulfur metabolism	75-250 μg
P	Bone	800-1000 mg
Se	Antioxidant	Male: 70 μg Female: 55 μg
Zn	Antioxidant Enzyme cofactor	Male: 15 mg Female: 12 mg

is based on balance studies, whereas those for manganese, chromium, and molybdenum are based on dietary intakes.

Assigning daily mineral intakes is problematic because some methods of determining mineral status do not always expose functional deficiencies. For example, a frank deficiency in Ca^{2+} intake leads to bone loss even though blood Ca^{2+} levels remain normal. Iron deficiency is difficult to detect because no clinical signs appear until iron stores are depleted. It is difficult to base recommendations simply on absorption because, for some minerals, absorption varies with intake. For example, copper deficiency or toxicity is unlikely in humans because absorption is *inversely* related to intake. Furthermore, interactions among minerals must be taken into account when establishing recommendations.

The goal is to base recommendations on scientific evidence. Radioisotopes can be used to monitor storage, absorption, and excretion. Another approach is to establish the physiological role of the mineral and then determine the mineral intake required for maintaining that physiological role. However, because of redundancy in function, it is often difficult to assess which mineral is deficient when function is compromised. For example, both iron and copper are involved in energy metabolism at the level of the electron transport chain. The blood clotting cascade involves Ca^{2+}, copper, and vitamin K. Zinc, selenium, and manganese all have antioxidant activities.

Vitamins Even though vitamins are not energy sources themselves, they play an integral role as cofactors in many metabolic processes. Some vitamins are involved in group transfer reactions, such as decarboxylations and carboxylations in fatty acid and glucose metabolism and transaminations in amino acid metabolism. Vitamins act as oxidizing and reducing agents in the generation of ATP, as well as antioxidants to quench free radicals produced as a byproduct of oxidation.

Of the 13 identified vitamins, RDAs have been established for 11 (Table 45-3). Safe and allowable ranges are estimated for the remaining two—biotin and pantothenic acid. Recommendations differ widely among countries. Lower recommendations are generally based on scientific evidence. For each vitamin, a person's nutritional *status* falls into one of five categories: deficient, marginal, satisfactory, excessive, and toxic. Although "marginal" and "excessive" are not usually associated with overt clinical signs, people whose vitamin status falls into one of these categories are at increased risk of various diseases.

In the past, recommendations for the intake of vitamins and minerals were based largely on levels necessary to promote normal growth and development. However, the role of vitamins and minerals in optimizing body function and in promoting longevity is becoming an area of intense interest both to researchers and to the general public. Older people generally have a less vigorous immune response than do young people, in large part because of deficiencies in iron, zinc, and vitamin C. Correcting these deficiencies improves immune competence significantly. In addition, older people with poor dietary habits may have inadequate intake of Ca^{2+}, vitamin D, and other nutrients involved in bone deposition and strength (see Chapter 52), thus putting them at greater risk for hip fracture.

Mineral deficiencies usually do not occur without extreme abnormalities in diet, and even then, a mineral deficiency may not impair function (Table 45-4). However, deficiencies of almost every vitamin can cause functional impairment (Table 45-3).

Excessive intake of vitamins and minerals has mixed effects on bodily function

A current controversy surrounds the use of so-called mega-doses of certain vitamins and minerals. Such excessive intake has mixed effects. Slight excesses of vitamins A and E, zinc, and selenium are associated with an enhanced immune response, especially for patients with burns, trauma, and sepsis. In these conditions, "excess" intake may not be an excess at all but rather the intake that meets the greater need. Increased intake of fruits and vegetables—which contain a variety of vitamins as well as "fiber"—clearly decreases the risk of various cancers. However, efforts to link these effects specifically to dietary carotenoid levels have failed to show a correlation; indeed, the excessive intake of β-carotene supplements may even increase the risk of some cancers. Antioxidants (e.g., β-carotene, vitamins C and E) quench peroxyl radicals, suppress tumor growth, and decrease atherosclerotic lesions in rabbits. Enhanced vitamin E intake lowers the risk of coronary heart disease, by nearly one half.

The excessive intake of certain minerals and vitamins may compromise the immune response. Excess vitamin E intake in infants may increase the risk of infection, possibly by quenching superoxide radicals that are important for killing bacteria. Excess lipids can impair the immune response, too. High intake of saturated and polyunsaturated fatty acids leads to decreases in cell-mediated immunity. Excessive Ca^{2+} intake interferes with the ability to use iron, zinc, and Mg^{2+}, whereas high dietary copper affects zinc absorption and excretion.

Because the kidneys readily excrete water-soluble vitamins in the urine, toxicity from excessive intake is not common. Because fat-soluble vitamins are not easily excreted in the urine, it is easier to develop toxicity for these vitamins. In particular, polar bear liver, a component of the Inuit diet, contains extraordinarily high levels of vitamin A (35,000 IU/g versus the RDA of 5000 IU), which can lead to acute hypervitaminosis A and death.

REFERENCES

Books and Reviews

Daniel H: Molecular and integrative physiology of intestinal peptide transport. Annu Rev Physiol 2004; 66:361-384.

Farrell JJ: Digestion and absorption of nutrients and vitamins. In Feldman M, Friedman LS, Sleisenger MH (ed): Gastrointestinal and Liver Disease, vol 2, 7th ed. Philadelphia: WB Saunders, 2002, pp 1715-1750.

Hentze MW, Muckenthaler MU, Andrews NC: Balancing acts: Molecular control of mammalian iron metabolism. Cell 2004; 117:285-297.

Palacin M, Estevez R, Bertran J, Zorzano A: Molecular biology of mammalian plasma membrane amino acid transporters. Physiol Rev 1998; 78:969-1054.

Verrey F, Ristic Z, Romeo E, et al: Novel renal amino acid transporters. Annu Review Physiol 2005; 67:557-572.

Wright EM: The intestinal Na^+/glucose cotransporter. Annu Rev Physiol 1993; 55:575-589.

Journal Articles

Clarke DC, Miskovic D, Han XX, et al: Overexpression of membrane-associated fatty acid binding protein (FABPpm) in vivo increases fatty acid sarcolemmal transport and metabolism. Physiol Genomics 2004; 17:31-37.

Feder JN, Gnirke A, Thomas W, et al: A novel MHC class I–like gene is mutated in patients with hereditary haemochromatosis. Nat Genet 1996; 13:399-408.

Fei YJ, Kanai Y, Nussberger S, et al: Expression cloning of a mammalian proton-coupled oligopeptide transporter. Nature 1994; 368:563-566.

Gunshin H, Mackenzie B, Berger UV, et al: Cloning and characterization of a proton-coupled mammalian metal ion transporter. Nature 1997; 388:482-488.

Shiau YF: Mechanisms of intestinal fatty acid uptake in the rat: The role of an acidic microclimate. J Physiol 1990; 421:463-474.

CHAPTER 46

HEPATOBILIARY FUNCTION

Frederick J. Suchy

OVERVIEW OF LIVER PHYSIOLOGY

After the skin, the liver and the brain (see Chapter 11) are the largest organs in the human body. The liver weighs between 1200 and 1500 g, representing 2% to 5% of body weight in the adult and ~4% to 5% in the newborn. The liver is strategically situated in the circulatory system to receive the portal blood that drains the stomach, small intestine, large intestine, pancreas, and spleen (see Fig. 17-3). In this position, the liver plays a key role in handling foodstuffs assimilated by the small intestine. However, the liver's role is far more diverse; it serves as a chemical factory, an excretory system, an exocrine gland, and an endocrine gland.

The liver biotransforms and degrades substances taken up from blood and either returns them to the circulation or excretes them into bile

A major function of the liver is to metabolize, detoxify, and inactivate both endogenous compounds (e.g., steroids and other hormones) and exogenous substances (e.g., drugs and toxins). In addition, by virtue of its large vascular capacity and abundance of phagocytes (Kupffer's cells), the liver provides an important filtering mechanism for the circulation by removing foreign particulate matter, including bacteria, endotoxins, parasites, and aging red blood cells. Kupffer's cells constitute 80% to 90% of the fixed macrophages of the reticuloendothelial system.

The liver has the capacity to convert important hormones and vitamins into a more active form. Examples include the initial hydroxylation of vitamin D and the deiodination of the thyroid hormone thyroxine (T_4) to triiodothyronine (T_3). Moreover, numerous enzymes in the liver process lipophilic chemicals into more polar, water-soluble metabolites, which are more readily excreted into bile.

Bile is a complex secretory product produced by the liver. Biliary secretion has two principal functions: (1) elimination of many endogenous and exogenous waste products from the body, such as bilirubin and cholesterol; and (2) promotion of digestion and absorption of lipids from the intestine. The composition of bile is modified significantly as a result of the absorptive and secretory properties of epithelial cells that line the intrahepatic and extrahepatic bile ducts. Moreover, bile solutes are further concentrated as bile is stored in the gallbladder.

The liver stores carbohydrates, lipids, vitamins, and minerals; it synthesizes carbohydrates, protein, and intermediary metabolites

The products of digested food, including carbohydrates, peptides, vitamins, and some lipids, are avidly extracted from portal blood by the liver. Depending on the metabolic requirements of the body, these substrates may be stored by the hepatocytes or released into the bloodstream either unbound (e.g., glucose) or associated with a carrier molecule (e.g., a triglyceride molecule complexed to a lipoprotein).

The liver also synthesizes—in a highly regulated fashion—many substances that are essential to the metabolic demands of the body. These substances include albumin and other plasma proteins, glucose, cholesterol, fatty acids for triglyceride biosynthesis, and phospholipids. The liver must provide a supply of substrates as fuels for other organs, particularly in the fasted state. For example, the liver produces ketone bodies, which can be used by the central nervous system during periods of fasting, thereby sparing ~50% of the amount of glucose that would otherwise be used by this tissue. Thus, the liver has a critical and unique role in the energy metabolism of all nonhepatic organs.

FUNCTIONAL ANATOMY OF THE LIVER AND BILIARY TREE

Hepatocytes are secretory epithelial cells that separate the lumen of the bile canaliculi from the fenestrated endothelium of the vascular sinusoids

One way of looking at the organization of the liver is to imagine that a classic lobule is a hexagon in cross section (Fig. 46-1A), with a branch of the hepatic vein at its center and, at each of the six corners, triads composed of branches

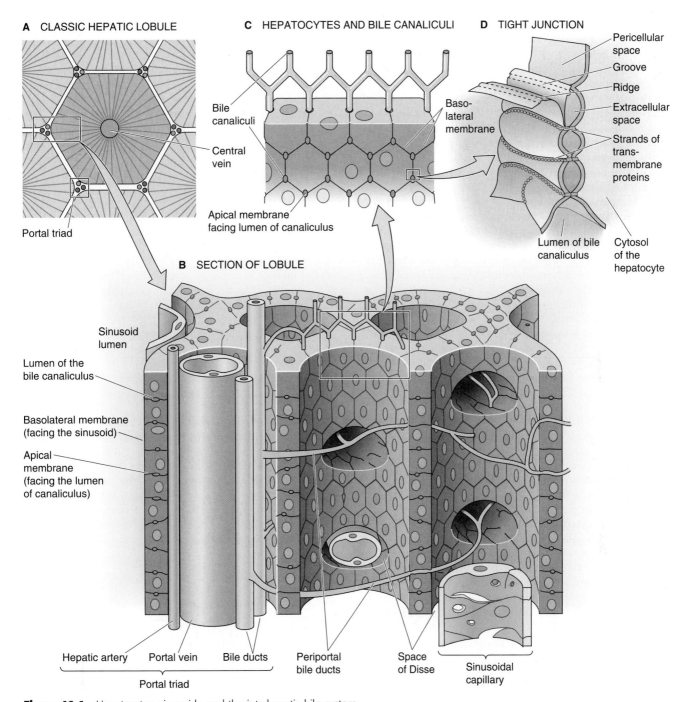

A   CLASSIC HEPATIC LOBULE

Central vein

Portal triad

C   HEPATOCYTES AND BILE CANALICULI

Bile canaliculi

Baso-lateral membrane

Apical membrane facing lumen of canaliculus

D   TIGHT JUNCTION

Pericellular space

Groove

Ridge

Extracellular space

Strands of trans-membrane proteins

Lumen of bile canaliculus

Cytosol of the hepatocyte

B   SECTION OF LOBULE

Sinusoid lumen

Lumen of the bile canaliculus

Basolateral membrane (facing the sinusoid)

Apical membrane (facing the lumen of canaliculus)

Hepatic artery   Portal vein   Bile ducts

Portal triad

Periportal bile ducts

Space of Disse

Sinusoidal capillary

Figure 46-1   Hepatocytes, sinusoids, and the intrahepatic bile system.

of the hepatic artery, portal vein, and bile duct. Hepatocytes account for ~80% of the parenchymal volume in human liver. Hepatocytes form an epithelium, one cell thick, that constitutes a functional barrier between two fluid compartments with differing ionic compositions: the tiny **canalicular lumen** containing bile and the much larger **sinusoid** containing blood (Fig. 46-1B). Moreover, hepatocytes significantly alter the composition of these fluids by vectorial transport of solutes across the hepatocyte. This vectorial transport depends critically on the polarized distribution of specific transport mechanisms and receptors that are local-

ized to the **apical membrane** that faces the canalicular lumen and the **basolateral membrane** that faces the pericellular space between hepatocytes and the blood-filled sinusoid (Fig. 46-1B,C). As in other epithelia, the apical and basolateral membrane domains of hepatocytes are structurally, biochemically, and physiologically distinct.

The **space of Disse**, or perisinusoidal space, is the extracellular gap between the endothelial cells lining the sinusoids and the basolateral membranes of the hepatocytes. These basolateral membranes have microvilli that project into the space of Disse to facilitate contact with the solutes in sinusoidal blood. The microvilli greatly amplify the basolateral membrane, which accounts for ~85% of the total surface area of the hepatocyte.

The bile canaliculi, into which bile is initially secreted, are formed by the apical membranes of adjoining hepatocytes. The apical membrane of the hepatocyte runs as a narrow belt that encircles and grooves into the polygonal hepatocyte (Fig. 46-1B,C). Two adjacent hepatocytes form a canaliculus that is ~1 μm in diameter by juxtaposing their groove-like apical membranes along their common face (i.e., one side of the polygon). Because a hepatocyte has many sides and a different neighbor on each side, the canaliculi form a chicken wire–like pattern along the contiguous surfaces of hepatocytes and communicate to form a three-dimensional tubular network. Although the apical membrane belt is very narrow (i.e., ~1 μm), its extensive microvillous structure amplifies its surface area so that the canalicular membrane constitutes as much as 15% of the total membrane surface area. Because of this high surface-to-volume ratio, the total apical surface area available for the movement of water and solutes in the human liver is in excess of 10.5 m².

The seal that joins the apical membranes of two juxtaposed hepatocytes and that separates the canalicular lumen from the pericellular space—which is contiguous with the space of Disse—comprises several elements, including **tight junctions** (Fig. 2-25) and desmosomes (see Chapter 2). By virtue of their permeability and morphology, hepatic junctions can be classified as having an intermediate tightness, somewhat between tight epithelia (e.g., toad bladder) and leaky epithelia (e.g., proximal tubule). Specialized structures called *gap junctions* (see Chapter 4) allow functional communication between adjacent hepatocytes.

Hepatocytes do not have a true basement membrane, but rather they rest on complex scaffolding provided by the **extracellular matrix** in the space of Disse, which includes several types of collagens (I, III, IV, V, and VI), fibronectin, undulin, laminin, and proteoglycans. Cells are linked to the matrix through specific adhesion proteins on the cell surface. The extracellular matrix not only provides structural support for liver cells but also seems to influence and maintain the phenotypic expression of hepatocytes and sinusoidal lining cells.

The liver contains endothelial cells, macrophages (Kupffer's cells), and stellate cells (Ito's cells) within the sinusoidal spaces

Slightly more than 6% of the volume of the liver parenchyma is made up of cells other than hepatocytes, including endothelial cells (2.8%), Kupffer's cells (2.1%), and stellate cells (fat-storing or Ito's cells, 1.4%). The **endothelial cells** that line the vascular channels or sinusoids form a fenestrated structure with their bodies and cytoplasmic extensions. Plasma solutes, but not blood cells, can move freely into the space of Disse through pores, or fenestrae, in the endothelial cells. Some evidence indicates that the fenestrae may regulate access into the perisinusoidal space of Disse by means of their capacity to contract.

 Kupffer's cells are present within the sinusoidal vascular space. This population of fixed macrophages removes par-

ticulate matter from the circulation. **Stellate cells** are in the space of Disse and are characterized morphologically by the presence of large fat droplets in their cytoplasm. These cells play a central role in the storage of vitamin A, and evidence suggests that they can be transformed into proliferative, fibrogenic, and contractile myofibroblasts. On liver injury, these activated cells participate in fibrogenesis through remodeling of the extracellular matrix and deposition of type I collagen, which can lead to cirrhosis.

The liver has a dual blood supply, but a single venous drainage system

The blood supply to the liver has two sources. The **portal vein** contributes ~ 75% of the total circulation to the liver; the **hepatic artery** contributes the other 25% (Fig. 46-2A). Blood from portal venules and hepatic arterioles combines in a complex network of hepatic sinusoids (Fig. 46-2B). Blood from these sinusoids converges on terminal hepatic venules (or **central veins**), which, in turn, join to form the **hepatic veins** (Fig. 46-2C). Branches of the portal vein, hepatic artery, and a bile duct (i.e., the triad), as well as lymphatics and nerves, travel together as a **portal tract**.

The arterial supply for the bile ducts arises mainly from the right hepatic artery (Fig. 46-2C). These arterioles give rise to an extraordinarily rich plexus of capillaries that surround the bile ducts as they pass through the portal tracts. Blood flowing through this peribiliary plexus empties into the sinusoids by way of branches of the portal vein so that this blood may pick up solutes from the bile ducts and cycle them back to the hepatocytes. Thus, the peribiliary plexus may provide the means for modifying biliary secretions through the bidirectional exchange of compounds such as proteins, inorganic ions, and bile acids between the bile and blood within the portal tract.

Hepatocytes can be thought of as being arranged as classic hepatic lobules, portal lobules, or acinar units

The complex structure of the liver makes it difficult to define a single unit—something analogous to the nephron in the kidney—that is capable of performing the functions of the entire liver. One way of viewing the organization of the liver is depicted in Figures 46-1 and 46-2, in which we regard the central vein as the core of the **classic hepatic lobule**. Thus, the classic hepatic lobule (Fig. 46-3A) includes all hepatocytes drained by a single central vein, and it is bounded by two or more portal triads. Alternatively, we can view the liver as though the triad is the core of a **portal lobule** (Fig. 46-3B). Thus, the portal lobule includes all hepatocytes drained by a single bile ductule and is bounded by two or more central veins. A third way of viewing the liver is to group the hepatocytes according to their supply of arterial blood (Fig. 46-3C). Thus, the **portal acinus** is a small, three-dimensional mass of hepatocytes that are irregular in size and shape, with one axis formed by a line between two triads (i.e., high P_{O_2}) and another axis formed by a line between two central veins (i.e., low P_{O_2}).

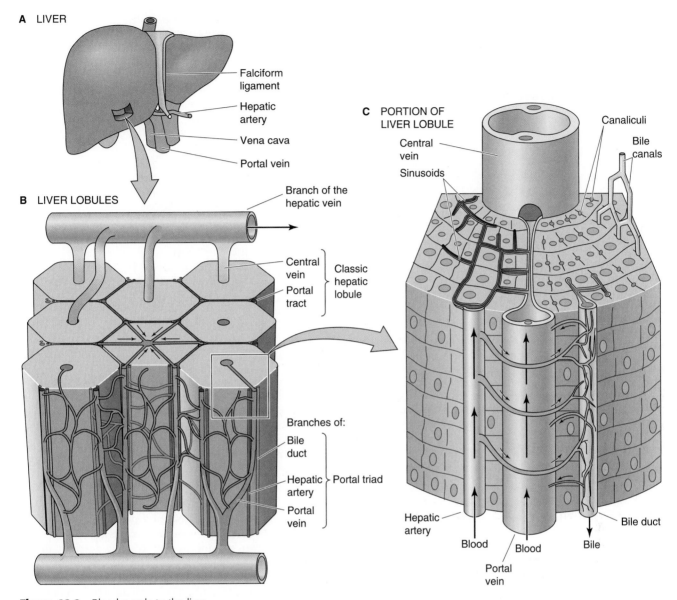

Figure 46-2 Blood supply to the liver.

Periportal hepatocytes specialize in oxidative metabolism, whereas pericentral hepatocytes detoxify drugs

Rappaport first proposed that a zonal relationship exists between cells that constitute the portal acini and their blood supply (Fig. 46-3C). Hepatocytes close to the vascular core formed by the terminal portal venule and terminal hepatic arteriole are perfused first and thus receive the highest concentrations of oxygen and solutes. These **periportal** hepatocytes are said to reside in **zone I**, and as a consequence of their location, they are the most resistant to the effects of circulatory compromise or nutritional deficiency. These cells are also more resistant to other forms of cellular injury and are the first to regenerate. Hepatocytes in the intermediate **zone II** and the most distal population of **pericentral** hepatocytes located near the terminal hepatic venule (central

vein) in **zone III** are sequentially perfused with blood that is already modified by the preceding hepatocytes; thus, they are exposed to progressively lower concentrations of nutrients and oxygen. The exact boundaries of these zones are difficult to define.

The concept of zonal heterogeneity of liver function has evolved as a result of these differences in access to substrate. Because of the specialized microenvironments of cells in different zones, some enzymes are preferentially expressed in one zone or another (Table 46-1). For example, in zone I, oxidative energy metabolism with β oxidation, amino acid metabolism, ureagenesis, gluconeogenesis, cholesterol synthesis, and bile formation is particularly important. Localized in zone III are glycogen synthesis from glucose, glycolysis, liponeogenesis, ketogenesis, xenobiotic metabolism, and glutamine formation. Molecular techniques have allowed an even more precise definition of which hepato-

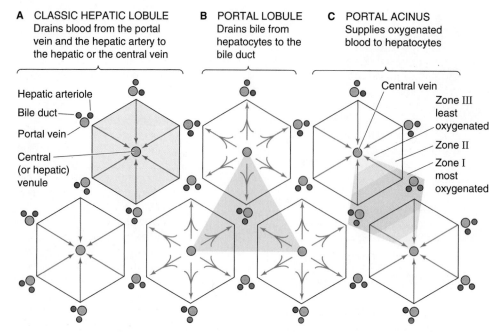

Figure 46-3 Zones in the acinus. **A,** The classic lobule includes all hepatocytes drained by a single central vein. At each corner of the hexagon are triads composed of branches of the hepatic artery, portal vein, and bile duct. **B,** The portal lobule includes all hepatocytes drained by a bile ductule. **C,** This organization emphasizes the arterial blood supply to the hepatocytes and thus the oxygenation gradient between a branch of the hepatic artery and branches of the hepatic vein (i.e., central vein). The periportal hepatocytes of zone I immediately surround the portal tract and thus have the highest P_{O_2} and the most nutrients. They specialize in oxidative metabolism and certain other functions. The pericentral hepatocytes of zone III surround the central vein and have the lowest P_{O_2}. The zone III hepatocytes specialize in biotransformations and drug detoxification. Zone II is an intermediate zone between zones I and III.

Table 46-1 Zonal Heterogeneity of Preferential Hepatocyte Function

Zone 1	Zone III
Amino acid catabolism	Glycolysis
Gluconeogenesis	Glycogen synthesis from glucose
Glycogen degradation	Liponeogenesis
HMG-CoA reductase (cholesterol synthesis)	Cholesterol 7α-hydroxylase (bile acid biosynthesis)
Ureagenesis (all hepatocytes with exception of the last one or two rows encircling the hepatic venules)	Ketogenesis
Bile acid–dependent canalicular bile flow	Glutamine synthesis
Oxidative energy metabolism and probably β oxidation of fatty acids	Bile acid–independent canalicular bile flow Biotransformation of drugs

cytes express particular mRNA and proteins. For example, the enzyme glutamine synthetase is expressed exclusively in only one or two hepatocytes immediately adjacent to the hepatic venules. Hepatocytes of zone III also seem to be important for general detoxification mechanisms and the biotransformation of drugs. The zonal distribution of drug-induced toxicity manifested as cell necrosis may be attributed to zone III localization of the enzymatic pathways involved in the biotransformation of substrates by oxidation, reduction, or hydrolysis. Although it appears that each hepatocyte is potentially capable of multiple metabolic functions, the predominant enzymatic activity appears to result from adaptation to the microenvironment provided by the hepatic microcirculation. In some cases, it has been possible to reverse the zone I–to–zone III gradient of hepatocyte function by experimentally reversing the direction of blood supply (i.e., nutrient flow).

Bile drains from its site of secretion in the canaliculi into small terminal ductules, then into progressively larger ducts of the biliary tree, and eventually into the duodenum through a single large common duct

The adult human liver has more than 2 km of bile ductules and ducts, with a volume of ~20 cm³ and a macroscopic surface area of ~400 cm^2. Microvilli at the apical surface magnify this area by ~5.5 fold.

As noted earlier, the **canaliculi** into which bile is secreted form a three-dimensional polygonal meshwork of tubes between hepatocytes, with many anastomotic interconnections (Fig. 46-1). From the canaliculi, the bile enters the small terminal bile **ductules** (i.e., **canals of Hering**), which have a basement membrane and in cross section are surrounded by three to six ductal epithelial cells or hepatocytes (Fig. 46-4A). The canals of Hering then empty into a system of **perilobular ducts**, which, in turn, drain into interlobular bile ducts. The **interlobular bile ducts** form a richly anastomosing network that closely surrounds the branches of the portal vein. These bile ducts are lined by a layer of cuboidal or columnar epithelium that has microvillous architecture on its luminal surface. The cells have a prominent Golgi apparatus and numerous vesicles, which probably participate in the exchange of substances among the cytoplasm, bile, and blood plasma through exocytosis and endocytosis.

The interlobular bile ducts unite to form larger and larger ducts, first the septal ducts and then the lobar ducts, two

hepatic ducts, and finally a common hepatic duct (Fig. 46-4B). Along the biliary tree, the biliary epithelial cells, or **cholangiocytes**, are similar in their fine structure except for size and height. However, emerging evidence suggests that they differ in their complement of transporters and receptors. Increasing emphasis has been placed on the absorptive and secretory properties of the biliary epithelial cells, properties that contribute significantly to the process of bile formation. As with other epithelial cells, cholangiocytes are highly cohesive, with the lateral plasma membranes of contiguous cells forming tortuous interdigitations. Tight junctions seal contacts between cells that are close to the luminal region and thus limit the exchange of water and solutes between plasma and bile.

The **common hepatic duct** emerges from the porta hepatis after the union of the right and left hepatic ducts. It merges with the cystic duct emanating from the gallbladder to form the common bile duct. In adults, the **common bile duct** is quite large, ~7 cm in length and ~0.5 to 1.5 cm in diameter. In most individuals, the common bile duct and the pancreatic duct merge before forming a common antrum known as the **ampulla of Vater**. At the point of transit

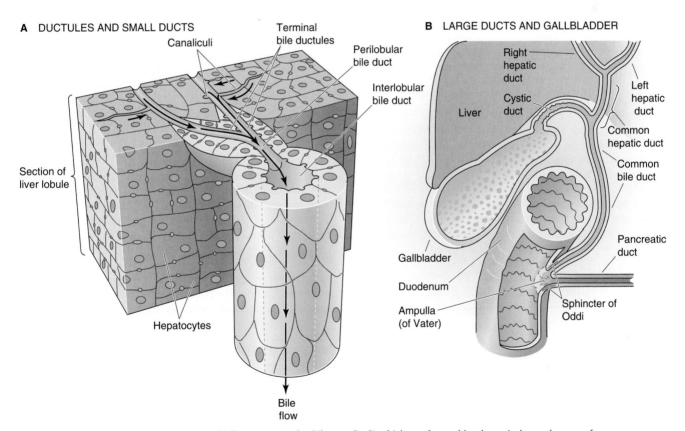

A DUCTULES AND SMALL DUCTS

Canaliculi
Terminal bile ductules
Perilobular bile duct
Interlobular bile duct
Section of liver lobule
Hepatocytes
Bile flow

B LARGE DUCTS AND GALLBLADDER

Liver
Right hepatic duct
Cystic duct
Left hepatic duct
Common hepatic duct
Common bile duct
Pancreatic duct
Gallbladder
Duodenum
Ampulla (of Vater)
Sphincter of Oddi

Figure 46-4   Structure of biliary tree. **A**, The bile canaliculi, which are formed by the apical membranes of adjacent hepatocytes, eventually merge with terminal bile ductules (canals of Hering). The ductules eventually merge into perilobular ducts, and then interlobular ducts. **B**, The interlobular ducts merge into septal ducts, lobar ducts, and eventually the right and left hepatic ducts, which combine as the common hepatic duct. The confluence of the common hepatic and the cystic ducts gives rise to the common bile duct. The common bile duct may merge with the pancreatic duct and form the ampulla of Vater before entering the duodenum, as shown in the figure, or it may have a completely independent lumen. In either case, a common sphincter—the sphincter of Oddi—simultaneously regulates flow out of the common bile duct and the pancreatic duct.

through the duodenal wall, this common channel is surrounded by a thickening of both the longitudinal and the circular layers of smooth muscle, the so-called **sphincter of Oddi**. This sphincter constricts the lumen of the bile duct and thus regulates the flow of bile.

The gallbladder is a concentrative and storage reservoir that can deliver bile acid in high concentration and in a controlled manner to the duodenum for the solubilization of dietary lipid

The gallbladder lies in a fossa beneath the right lobe of the liver. This distensible, pear-shaped structure has a capacity of 30 to 50 mL in adults. The absorptive surface of the gallbladder is enhanced by numerous prominent folds that are important for concentrative transport activity, as discussed later. The gallbladder is connected at its neck to the **cystic duct**, which empties into the common bile duct (Fig. 46-4B). The cystic duct maintains continuity with the surface columnar epithelium, lamina propria, muscularis, and serosa of the gallbladder. Instead of a sphincter, the gallbladder has, at its neck, a spiral valve (the valve of Heister) formed by the mucous membrane. This valve regulates flow into and out of the gallbladder.

UPTAKE, PROCESSING, AND SECRETION OF COMPOUNDS BY HEPATOCYTES

The liver metabolizes an enormous variety of compounds that are brought to it by the portal and systemic circulations. These compounds include endogenous molecules (e.g., bile salts and bilirubin, which are key ingredients of bile) and exogenous molecules (e.g., drugs and toxins). The hepatocyte handles these molecules in four major steps (Fig. 46-5A): (1) the hepatocyte imports the compound from the blood across its basolateral (i.e., sinusoidal) membrane, (2) the hepatocyte transports the material within the cell, (3) the hepatocyte may chemically modify or degrade the compound intracellularly, and (4) the hepatocyte excretes the molecule or its product or products into the bile across the apical (i.e., canalicular) membrane. Thus, compounds are secreted in a vectorial manner through the hepatocyte.

An Na-K pump at the basolateral membrane of hepatocytes provides the energy for transporting a wide variety of solutes through channels and transporters

Like other epithelial cells, the hepatocyte is endowed with a host of transporters that are necessary for basic housekeeping functions. To the extent that these transporters are restricted to either the apical or basolateral membrane, they have the potential of participating in net transepithelial transport. For example, the Na-K pump (see Chapter 3) at the basolateral membrane of hepatocytes maintains a low $[Na^+]_i$ and high $[K^+]_i$ (Fig. 46-5B). A basolateral, ATP-dependent Ca^{2+} pump maintains $[Ca^{2+}]_i$ at an extremely low level, ~100 nM, as in other cells. The hepatocyte uses the inwardly directed Na^+ gradient to fuel numerous active

transporters, such as the Na-H exchanger, the Na/HCO_3 cotransporter, and Na^+-driven amino acid transporters. As discussed later, the Na^+ gradient also drives one of the bile acid transporters. The hepatocyte takes up glucose through the GLUT2 facilitated diffusion mechanism (see Chapters 3 and 50), which is insensitive to regulation by insulin.

The resting basolateral membrane has a voltage (V_m) of −30 to −40 mV and is endowed with both K^+ and Cl^- channels. Basolateral K^+ conductance helps to maintain a negative V_m; the resting V_m is considerably more positive than the equilibrium potential for K^+ (E_K) because of the presence of numerous "leak" pathways, such as the aforementioned electrogenic Na^+-driven transporters, as well as channels for ions other than K^+. For example, Cl^- is passively distributed (i.e., $E_{Cl} = V_m$).

Hepatocytes take up bile acids, other organic anions, and organic cations across their basolateral (sinusoidal) membranes

Bile Acids and Salts The primary bile acids are cholic acid and chenodeoxycholic acid, both of which are synthesized by hepatocytes, as described later in Figure 46-9. Other "secondary" bile acids form in the intestinal tract as bacteria dehydroxylate the primary bile acids. Because the pK values of the primary bile acids are near neutrality, most of the bile acid molecules are neutral; that is, they are *bile acids* (H · BA) and thus are not very water soluble. Of course, some of these molecules are deprotonated and hence are *bile salts* (BA⁻). The liver may conjugate the primary bile acids and salts to glycine or taurine (Z in Fig. 46-5C), as well as to sulfate or glucuronate (Y in Fig. 46-5C). Most of the bile acids that the liver secretes into the bile are conjugated, such as taurocholate (the result of conjugating cholic acid to taurine). These conjugated derivatives have a negative charge, and hence they, too, are *bile salts* (BA-Z⁻ and BA-Y⁻). Bile salts are far more water soluble than the corresponding bile acids.

Because the small intestine absorbs some bile acids and salts, they appear in the blood plasma, mainly bound to albumin, and are presented to the hepatocytes for re-uptake. This recycling of bile acids, an example of **enterohepatic circulation**, is discussed later in Figure 46-13. Dissociation from albumin occurs before uptake. Surprisingly, the presence of albumin actually stimulates Na^+-dependent taurocholate uptake, perhaps by increasing the affinity of the transporter for taurocholate.

Uptake of bile acids has been studied extensively and is mediated predominantly by an Na^+-coupled transporter known as **Na-taurocholate cotransporting polypeptide** or **NTCP** (a member of the SLC10A1 family) (Fig. 46-5C). This transporter is a 50-kDa glycosylated protein, and it appears to have seven membrane-spanning segments. NTCP handles unconjugated bile acids, but it has a particularly high affinity for conjugated bile acids. In addition, NTCP can also transport other compounds, including neutral steroids (e.g., progesterone, 17β-estradiol sulfate), cyclic oligopeptides (e.g., amantadine and phalloidin), and a wide variety of drugs (e.g., verapamil, furosemide). As is the case for other transporters, NTCP activity is low in the fetus and neonate and increases with development.

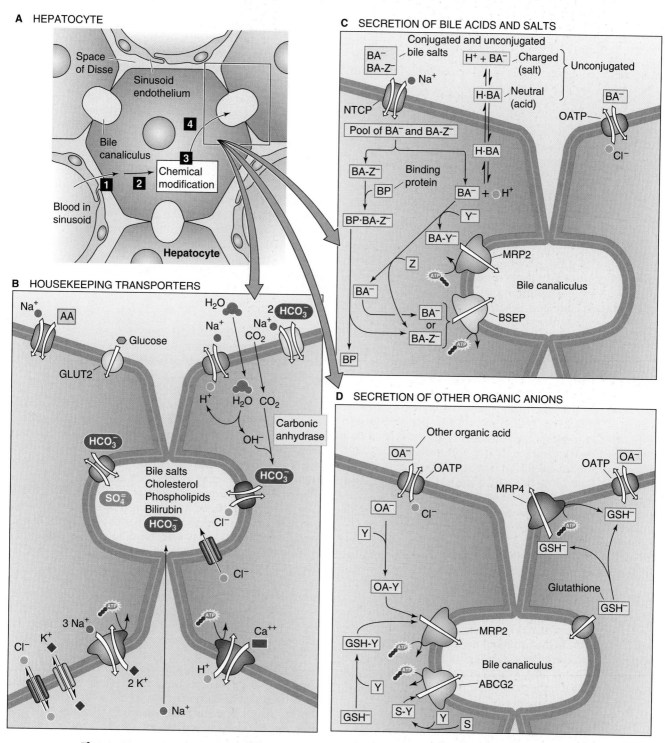

Figure 46-5 Transporters in hepatocyte. **A**, The hepatocyte can process compounds in four steps: (1) uptake from blood across the basolateral (i.e., sinusoidal) membrane, (2) transport within the cell, (3) control chemical modification or degradation, and (4) export into the bile across the apical (i.e., canalicular) membrane. **B**, The hepatocyte has a full complement of housekeeping transporters. **C**, Bile acids can enter the hepatocyte in any of several forms: the unconjugated salt (BA$^-$); the neutral, protonated bile acid (H·BA); the bile salt conjugated to taurine or glycine (BA-Z$^-$, where Z represents taurine or glycine). The three pathways for bile acid entry across the basolateral membrane are as follows: the Na$^+$-driven transporter NTCP, which prefers BA-Z$^-$, but also carries BA$^-$; nonionic diffusion of H·BA; and an OATP. Binding proteins (BP) may ferry conjugated bile acids across the cytoplasm. Some bile acids are conjugated to sulfate or glucuronate (Y); these exit the cell across the canalicular membrane through the MRP2 transporter. Most bile acids are conjugated to glycine or taurine (Z) before their extrusion into the bile through the BSEP. **D**, Organic anions (including bile acids) may enter across the basolateral membrane through an OATP. After conjugation with sulfate or glucuronate (Y), these compounds may be extruded into the bile by MRP2. GSH synthesized in the hepatocyte, after conjugation to Y, can enter the canaliculus through MRP2. Unconjugated GSH can enter the canaliculus through an unidentified transporter. GSH can exit the hepatocyte across the basolateral membrane through an OATP. ABCG2, G2 member of ABC protein family.

Although NTCP also carries unconjugated bile acids, as much as 50% of these *unconjugated* bile acids may enter the hepatocyte by passive nonionic diffusion (Fig. 46-5B). Because unconjugated bile acids are weak acids of the form

$$H \cdot BA \leftrightarrow H^+ + BA^- \qquad (46\text{-}1)$$

the neutral $H \cdot BA$ form can diffuse into the cell. Conjugation of bile acids enhances their hydrophilicity (taurine more so than glycine) and promotes dissociation of the proton from the side chain (i.e., lowering the pK_a), thus raising the concentration of BA^-. Both properties decrease the ability of bile acid to traverse membranes through passive nonionic diffusion.

Organic Anions The **organic anion transporting polypeptides** or **OATPs** (members of the SLC21 family) are a group of polyspecific membrane carriers (Fig. 46-5D) with partially overlapping substrate specificities for a wide range of amphipathic solutes, including bile salts, organic dyes, steroid conjugates, thyroid hormone, anionic oligopeptides, numerous drugs, toxins, and other xenobiotics. The driving force for OATP-mediated transport appears to be anion exchange for intracellular Cl^-, glutathione, and possibly other substrates. Several human OATPs—including OATP-A, OATP-C, and OATP8—appear to be liver specific and transport bile acids and many other amphipathic substrates. Others—OATP-B, OATP-E, and OATP-F—are widely distributed and multispecific. Another ubiquitous OATP—PGT—transports prostanoids (e.g., prostaglandins E_2 and $F_{2\alpha}$ and thromboxane B_2, but not arachidonic acid). Thus, basolateral uptake of **bile acids** into the hepatocyte is a complex process that involves both an Na^+-dependent transporter (NTCP) and Na^+-*in*dependent transporters (OATPs), as well as nonionic diffusion of unconjugated bile acids.

Bilirubin Senescent erythrocytes are taken up by macrophages in the reticuloendothelial system, where the degradation of hemoglobin leads to the release of bilirubin into the blood (Fig. 46-6A; see the box titled Jaundice). The mechanism by which hepatocytes take up unconjugated bilirubin remains controversial. As evidenced by yellow staining of the sclerae and skin in the jaundiced patient, bilirubin can leave the circulation and enter cells by diffusion. However, uptake of albumin-bound bilirubin by the isolated, perfused rat liver and isolated rat hepatocytes is faster than can occur by diffusion and is consistent with a carrier-mediated process. Electroneutral, electrogenic, and Cl^--dependent transport have been proposed (Fig. 46-6B). However, although one of the OATPs may account for a minor portion of uptake, the majority of transport occurs through proteins that have not been convincingly identified.

Organic Cations The major organic cations transported by the liver are aromatic and aliphatic amines, including such important drugs as cholinergics, local anesthetics, and antibiotics, as well as endogenous solutes such as choline, thiamine, and nicotinamide (Fig. 46-7). The basolateral membrane of the hepatocyte contains several well-characterized transporters for organic cations. The polyspecific **organic cation transporters OCT1** and **OCT2** mediate

electrogenic, facilitated diffusion (see Chapter 3) of small (type 1) organic cations, including many drugs, toxins, and endogenous compounds. These Na^+-independent transporters, also expressed in the intestine and kidney, may reverse direction, depending on transmembrane concentration and voltage gradients. OATP-A mediates the uptake of bulky (type 2) organic cations. Physiological studies have identified proton-organic cation exchangers at both the basolateral and the canalicular membranes; however, the molecular identities of these transporters are currently unknown.

Neutral Organic Compounds This group of molecules is also taken up by an Na^+-independent, energy-dependent process, but the nature of the driving force is not known. The best characterized substrate is ouabain, uptake of which is inhibited by other neutral steroids, such as cortisol, aldosterone, estradiol, and testosterone. OATP8 transports some of these compounds. We return to Figures 46-5, 46-6, and 46-7 later, when we discuss the movement of solutes into the bile canaliculus.

Inside the hepatocyte, the basolateral-to-apical movement of many compounds occurs by vesicular or protein-bound routes

Bile Salts Some compounds traverse the cell while bound to **intracellular "binding" proteins** (Fig. 46-5C). The binding may serve to trap the molecule within the cell, or it may be involved in intracellular transport. For bile salts, three such proteins have been identified. In humans, the main bile acid–binding protein appears to be the hepatic **dihydrodiol dehydrogenase**, one of a large family of dehydrogenases, the catalytic and binding properties of which are organ and species specific. The two others are **glutathione-S-transferase B** and **fatty acid–binding protein**. Intracellular sequestration of bile salts by these proteins may serve an important role in bile acid transport or regulation of bile acid synthesis. Transcellular diffusion of bile salts bound to proteins can be detected within seconds after bile salts are applied to hepatocytes; this mechanism may be the primary mode of cytoplasmic transport under basal conditions. Free, unbound bile salts may also traverse the hepatocyte by rapid diffusion.

At high sinusoidal concentrations, hydrophobic bile acids may partition into membranes of intracellular vesicles. These conditions may also cause increased targeting of the vesicles to the canalicular membrane—that is, transcellular bile acid transport by a **vesicular pathway**.

Bilirubin After uptake at the basolateral membrane, unconjugated bilirubin is transported to the endoplasmic reticulum (ER), where it is conjugated to glucuronic acid (Fig. 46-6). Because the resulting bilirubin glucuronide is markedly hydrophobic, it was thought that intracellular transport was mediated by binding proteins such as glutathione transferase B. More recently, however, spontaneous transfer of bilirubin between phospholipid vesicles was observed to occur by rapid movement through the aqueous phase, in the absence of soluble proteins. Therefore, investigators have suggested that direct membrane-to-membrane

A HEME METABOLISM

B BILIRUBIN SECRETION

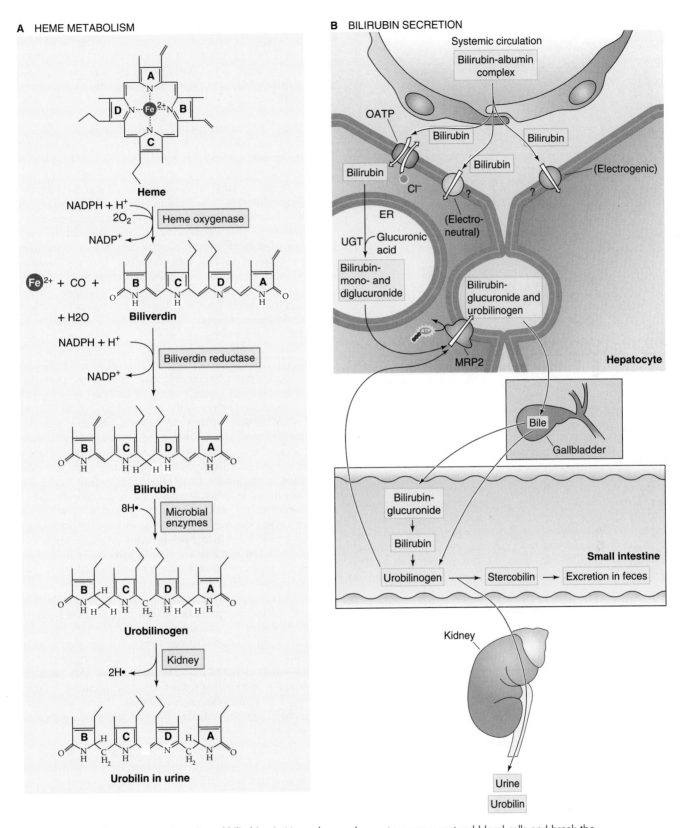

Figure 46-6 Excretion of bilirubin. **A,** Macrophages phagocytose senescent red blood cells and break the heme down to bilirubin, which travels in the blood, linked to albumin, to the liver. The conversion to the colorless urobilinogen occurs in the terminal ileum and colon, whereas the oxidation to the yellowish urobilin occurs in the urine. **B,** The hepatocyte takes up bilirubin across its basolateral membrane through an OATP and other unidentified mechanisms. The hepatocyte then conjugates the bilirubin with one or two glucuronic acid residues and exports this conjugated form of bilirubin into the bile. Bacteria in the terminal ileum and colon convert some of this bilirubin glucuronide back to bilirubin. This bilirubin is further converted to the colorless urobilinogen. If it remains in the colon, the compound is further converted to stercobilin, which is the main pigment of feces. If the urobilinogen enters the plasma and is filtered by the kidney, it is converted to urobilin and gives urine its characteristic yellow color.

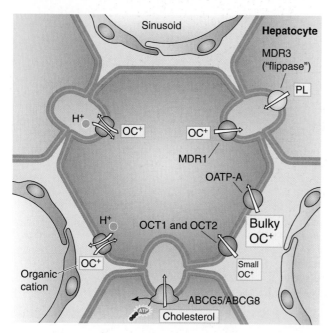

Figure 46-7 Excretion of organic cations and lipids. Small organic cations (type 1) enter the hepatocyte across the basolateral (i.e., sinusoidal) membrane through OCT1 and OCT2. Bulky organic cations (type 2) enter through OATP-A. Organic cations may also enter through a proton–organic cation exchanger. The organic cations exit the hepatocyte across the apical (i.e., canalicular) membrane through MDR1. MDR3 transports phospholipids (PL), and ABCG5/ABCG8 heterodimer transports cholesterol (C).

transfer is the principal mode of bilirubin transport within the hepatocyte. In addition, the membrane-to-membrane flux of bilirubin is biased toward the membrane with the higher cholesterol/phospholipid ratio. Hence, the inherent gradient for cholesterol from the basolateral membrane to the ER membrane may direct the flux of bilirubin to the ER.

In phase I of the biotransformation of organic anions and other compounds, hepatocytes use mainly cytochrome P-450 enzymes

The liver is responsible for the metabolism and detoxification of many endogenous and exogenous compounds. Some compounds (e.g., proteins and other ligands) taken up by hepatocytes are completely digested within lysosomes. Specific carriers exist for the lysosomal uptake of sialic acid, cysteine, and vitamin B_{12}. Clinical syndromes resulting from an absence of these carriers have also been identified. The lysosomal acid hydrolases cleave sulfates, fatty acids, and sugar moieties from larger molecules.

Hepatocytes handle other compounds by biotransformation reactions that usually occur in two phases. Phase I reactions represent oxidation or reduction reactions in large part catalyzed by the P-450 cytochromes. The diverse array of phase I reactions includes hydroxylation, dealkylation, and dehalogenation, among others. The common feature of all these reactions is that one atom of oxygen is inserted into the substrate. Hence these monooxygenases make the sub-

strate a more polar compound, poised for further modification by a phase II reaction. For example, when the phase I reaction creates a hydroxyl group, the phase II reaction may increase the water solubility of ROH by conjugating it to a highly hydrophilic compound such as glucuronate, sulfate, or glutathione:

$$RH \xrightarrow{\text{Phase I}} ROH \xrightarrow{\text{Phase II}} RO\text{-Conjugate} \quad (46\text{-}2)$$

Finally, the conjugated compound is secreted into the blood or bile.

The major enzymes involved in phase I reactions are the **P-450 cytochromes**. Cytochromes are colored proteins that contain heme for use in the transfer of electrons. Some cytochromes—not the P-450 system—are essential for the electron transport events that culminate in oxidative phosphorylation in the mitochondria. The P-450 cytochromes, so named because they absorb light at 450 nm when bound to CO, are a diverse, but related group of enzymes that reside mainly in the ER and typically catalyze **hydroxylation** reactions. More than 150 P-450 isoforms have been characterized.

In this text, we encounter P-450 oxidases in two sets of organs. In cells that synthesize steroid hormones—the adrenal cortex (see Chapter 49), testes (see Chapter 53), and ovary and placenta (see Chapters 54 and 55)—P-450 oxidases are localized either in the mitochondria or in the ER, where they catalyze various steps in steroidogenesis. In the liver, these enzymes are located in the ER, where they catalyze a vast array of hydroxylation reactions involving the metabolism of drugs and chemical carcinogens, bile acid synthesis, and the activation and inactivation of vitamins. The same reactions occur in other tissues, such as the intestines and the lungs.

Hepatic microsomal P-450 enzymes have similar molecular weights (48 to 56 kDa). The functional protein is a holoenzyme that consists of an apoprotein and a heme prosthetic group. The apoprotein region confers substrate specificity, which differs among the many P-450 enzymes. These substrates include RH moieties that are as wide ranging as the terminal methyl group of fatty acids, carbons in the rings of steroid molecules, complex heterocyclic compounds, and phenobarbital. In general, phase I processes add or expose a functional group, a hydroxyl group in the case of the P-450 oxidases, which renders the molecule reactive with phase II enzymes. The metabolic products of phase I may be directly excreted, but more commonly, because of only a modest increment in solubility, further metabolism by phase II reactions is required.

In phase II of biotransformation, hepatocytes conjugate the products of phase I to make them more water soluble for secretion into blood or bile

In phase II, the hepatocyte conjugates the metabolites generated in phase I to produce more hydrophilic compounds, such as glucuronides, sulfates, and mercapturic acids. These phase II products are readily secreted into the blood or bile. Conjugation reactions are generally considered to be the critical step in detoxification. Either a defect in a particular

Jaundice

Jaundice denotes a yellowish discoloration of body tissues, most notable in the skin and sclera of the eyes. The condition is caused by an accumulation of bilirubin in extracellular fluid, either in free form or after conjugation. Bilirubin is a yellow-green pigment that is the principal degradation product of heme (Fig. 46-6A), the iron-binding portion of hemoglobin. The metabolism of hemoglobin of senescent red cells accounts for 65% to 80% of total bilirubin production. Because of avid extraction and conjugation by the liver, the normal plasma concentration of bilirubin, which is mostly of the unconjugated variety, is ~0.5 mg/dL or lower. The skin or eyes may begin to appear jaundiced when the bilirubin level rises to 1.5 to 3 mg/dL.

Hemoglobin released into the circulation is phagocytized by macrophages throughout the body and is split into globin and heme. Cleavage of the heme ring releases both free iron, which travels in the blood by transferrin, and a straight chain of 4-pyrrole nuclei called **biliverdin** (Fig. 46-6A), which the cell rapidly reduces to free bilirubin. This form of bilirubin is often referred to as free or **unconjugated bilirubin** (we discuss its conjugation later). After it enters the circulation, unconjugated bilirubin binds reversibly to albumin and travels to the liver, which avidly removes it from the plasma (Fig. 46-6B). The hepatocyte esterifies the bilirubin, which is extremely insoluble, with glucuronic acid to form the monoconjugated and diconjugated derivatives. **Conjugated bilirubin** is more soluble and thus is suitable for excretion into bile, but it cannot be absorbed by the biliary or intestinal epithelia.

Jaundice occurs under several circumstances. Increased destruction of red blood cells or hemolysis may occur with rapid release of free, unconjugated bilirubin into the circulation. **Unconjugated hyperbilirubinemia** occurs commonly in neonates not only because of increased production of heme but also because of the immaturity of the pathways for glucuronidation in the liver. Obstruction of the bile ducts or damage to the liver may also result in jaundice. In this setting, **conjugated bilirubin** produced by the liver cannot be excreted in bile and consequently refluxes back into the systemic circulation. Therefore, most of the bilirubin in plasma is the highly soluble conjugated bilirubin, a small amount of which can be filtered by the kidneys, rather than the poorly soluble free form of bilirubin, which is mostly bound to albumin and is not excreted by the kidneys. Thus, in obstructive jaundice, conjugated bilirubin imparts a dark yellow color to the urine. Measurement of free and conjugated bilirubin in serum serves as a sensitive test for detecting liver disease.

Under normal conditions, approximately half of the bilirubin reaching the intestinal lumen is metabolized by bacteria into the colorless **urobilinogen** (Fig. 46-6A). The intestinal mucosa reabsorbs ~20% of this soluble compound into the portal circulation. The liver then extracts most of the urobilinogen and re-excretes it into the gastrointestinal tract. The kidneys excrete a small fraction (~20% of daily urobilinogen production) into the urine. Urobilinogen may be detected in urine by using a clinical dipstick test. Oxidation of urobilinogen yields **urobilin**, which gives urine its yellow color. In the feces, metabolism of urobilinogen yields **stercobilin**, which contributes to the color of feces. In obstructive jaundice, no bilirubin reaches the intestine for conversion into urobilinogen, and therefore no urobilinogen appears in the blood for excretion by the kidney. As a result, tests for urobilinogen in urine are negative in obstructive jaundice. Because of the lack of stercobilin and other bile pigments in obstructive jaundice, the stool becomes clay colored.

---

enzyme, which may result from a genetic defect, or saturation of the enzyme with excess substrate may result in a decrease in the overall elimination of a compound. One example is the *gray syndrome*, a potentially fatal condition that occurs after the administration of chloramphenicol to newborns who have low glucuronidation capacity. Infants have an ashen gray appearance and become weak and apathetic, and complete circulatory collapse may ensue.

Hepatocytes use three major conjugation reactions, as follows:

1. **Conjugation to glucuronate.** The uridine diphosphate glucuronosyl transferases (UGTs), which reside in the smooth ER (SER) of the liver, are divided into two families based on their substrate specificity. Family 1 consists of at least four members and is encoded by genes that are located on chromosome 2. These UGTs catalyze the conjugation of glucuronic acid with phenols or bilirubin (Fig. 46-6B). Family 2 contains at least five UGTs that are encoded by genes on chromosome 4. These UGTs catalyze the glucuronidation of steroids or bile acids. Because family 1 UGTs are essential for the dual conjugation of bilirubin (Fig. 46-6B) and because only *conjugated* bilirubin can be excreted in bile, congenital absence of bilirubin UGT activity results in jaundice from birth and

bilirubin encephalopathy, as seen in patients with Crigler-Najjar type I syndrome.

2. **Conjugation to sulfate.** The **sulfotransferases**—which are located in the cytosol rather than in the SER—catalyze the sulfation of steroids, catechols, and foreign compounds such as alcohol and metabolites of carcinogenic hydrocarbons. Their substrate specificity is greater than that of the UGTs. The different cellular localization of these two groups of enzymes suggests that they act cooperatively rather than competitively. In general, sulfates are not toxic and are readily eliminated, with the exception of sulfate esters of certain carcinogens.

3. **Conjugation to glutathione.** Hepatocytes also conjugate a range of compounds to reduced glutathione (GSH) for excretion and later processing in either the bile ducts or kidney (Fig. 46-8). **Glutathione** is a tripeptide composed of glutamate γ-linked to cysteine, which, in turn, is α-linked to glycine. The liver has the highest concentration of glutathione (~5 mM), with ~90% found in the cytoplasm and 10% in the mitochondria. **Glutathione-S-transferases**, which are mainly cytosolic, catalyze the conjugation of certain substrates to the cysteine moiety of GSH. Substrates include the electrophilic metabolites of lipophilic compounds (e.g., epoxides of polycyclic aromatic hydrocarbons), products of lipid peroxidation, and

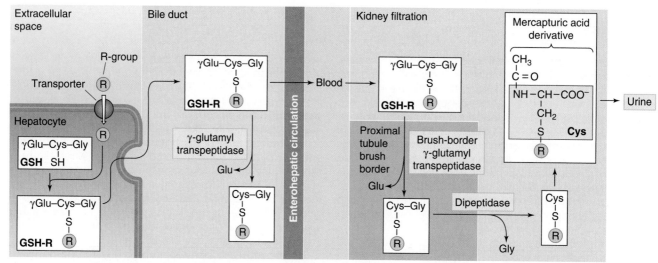

Figure 46-8 Conjugation to GSH and formation of mercapturic acids. The hepatocyte detoxifies compounds by chemically linking (conjugating) them to small molecules, such as GSH, which is a tripeptide. The first step is for glutathione-*S*-transferase to couple the target compound (R) to the S on the cysteine residue of GSH. After MRP2 transports this GSH conjugate into the canalicular lumen (see Fig. 46-5D), a γ-glutamyl transpeptidase may remove the terminal glutamate residue. Alternatively, the conjugate may reach the blood and may be filtered by the kidney, where a γ-glutamyl transpeptidase at the brush border and a dipeptidase generate a cysteine derivative of R. Acetylation yields the mercapturic acid derivative, which appears in the urine.

alkyl and aryl halides. In some cases, the conjugates are then secreted into bile and are further modified by removing the glutamyl residue from the glutathione by γ-glutamyl transpeptidase on the bile duct epithelial cell. The fate of glutathione-*S*-conjugates in bile is largely unknown. Some (e.g., the leukotrienes) undergo enterohepatic circulation. In other cases, the glutathione conjugates are secreted into plasma and are filtered by the kidney, where a γ-glutamyl transpeptidase on the proximal tubule brush border again removes the glutamyl residue. Next, a dipeptidase removes the glycine residue to produce a cysteine-*S*-conjugate. The cysteine-*S*-conjugate is either excreted in the urine or is acetylated in the kidney or liver to form a mercapturic acid derivative, which is also excreted in the urine.

Although glutathione conjugation is generally considered a detoxification reaction, several such conjugates undergo activation into highly reactive intermediates.

Other Conjugations   Other forms of conjugation include methylation (e.g., catechols, amines, and thiols), acetylation (e.g., amines and hydrazines), and conjugation (e.g., bile acids) with amino acids such as taurine, glycine, or glutamine. The involvement of multiple enzyme systems in these detoxification reactions facilitates the rapid removal of toxic species and provides alternative pathways in the event of failure of the preferred detoxification mechanism.

The interactions of xenobiotics with the nuclear receptors SXR and CAR control the phase I and II reactions

The liver and intestine express a nuclear receptor (see Chapter 4) called the **steroid and xenobiotic receptor (SXR)**. A chemically diverse array of substances binds to this relatively "promiscuous" transcription factor, which then binds to response elements on DNA and alters the expression of multiple drug-metabolizing enzymes as well as transporters that excrete drug metabolites. Thus, SXR serves as a master regulator of xenobiotic metabolism. Enzymes upregulated by SXR include the phase I drug-metabolizing enzymes of the P-450 family, such as CYP3A, which metabolizes more than 50% of all drugs in humans. SXR also activates the phase II enzyme glutathione-*S*-transferase, which is critical for catalyzing conjugation of many substrates to glutathione. SXR also upregulates the multidrug resistance transporter MDR1 (see later). Although these pathways are for the most part hepatoprotective, a particular compound may elicit SXR-mediated alterations in CYP3A activity that may profoundly influence the metabolism of another drug—perhaps thereby compromising the therapeutic efficacy of that drug or enhancing the production of a toxic metabolite. Another nuclear receptor—the **constitutive androstane receptor (CAR)**—is also an important regulator of drug metabolism. CAR regulates all the components of bilirubin metabolism, including uptake (possibly through OATP), conjugation (UTG1A1), and excretion (through multidrug resistance-associated protein 2 [MRP2], as discussed later).

Hepatocytes secrete bile acids, organic anions, organic cations, and lipids across theirapical (canalicular) membrane

At the apical membrane, the transport of compounds is generally unidirectional, from cell to canalicular lumen. An exception is certain precious solutes, such as amino acids and adenosine, which are reabsorbed from bile by Na+-dependent secondary active transport systems.

Bile Salts   Bile salt transport from hepatocyte to canalicular lumen (Fig. 46-5C) occurs through an ATP-dependent transporter called the **bile salt export pump (BSEP)**. The ABCB11 member of the ABC (ATP-binding cassette) protein family (see Table 5-6 on p. 124), BSEP has a very high affinity for bile salts (taurochenodeoxycholate > taurocholate > tauroursodeoxycholate > glycocholate). The electrical charge of the side chain is an important determinant of canalicular transport inasmuch as only negatively charged bile salts are effectively excreted. Secretion of bile salts occurs against a significant cell-to-canaliculus concentration gradient, which may range from 1:100 to 1:1000. Mutations in the **BSEP** gene can, in children, cause a form of progressive intrahepatic cholestasis that is characterized by extremely low bile acid concentrations in the bile.

Organic Anions   Organic anions that are *not bile salts* move from the cytoplasm of the hepatocyte to the canalicular lumen through **MRP2**, the ABCC2 member of the ABC protein family (see Table 5-6) (Fig. 46-5D). MRP2 is electrogenic, ATP dependent, and has a broad substrate specificity—particularly for divalent, amphipathic, phase II conjugates with glutathione, glucuronide, glucuronate, and sulfates. Its substrates include bilirubin diglucuronide, sulfated bile acids, glucuronidated bile acids, and several xenobiotics. In general, transported substrates must have a hydrophobic core and at least two negative charges separated by a specific distance. MRP2 is critical for the transport of GSH conjugates across the canalicular membrane into bile. Although MRP2 has a low affinity for GSH, functional studies suggest that other mechanisms for GSH transport exist. Animal models of defective MRP2 exhibit hyperbilirubinemia, which corresponds phenotypically to the Dubin-Johnson syndrome in humans. Another canalicular efflux pump for sulfated conjugates is the human ABC protein **ABCG2**, which transports estrone-3-sulfate (see Fig. 55-10) and dehydroepiandrosterone sulfate (see Fig. 54-5)—breakdown products of sex steroids. Other anions, such as HCO_3^- and SO_4^{2-}, are excreted by anion exchangers.

Organic Cations   Biliary excretion of organic cations is poorly understood. With the exception of transport that is mediated by the MDR proteins such as BSEP (discussed earlier), the hepatic MDR proteins belong to the ABC family of transporters (see Table 5-6). **MDR1** (ABCB1) is present in the canalicular membrane, where it mediates the excretion of some organic cations into the bile canaliculus (Fig. 46-7). The nomenclature of the MDRs is especially confusing because different and conflicting numbering systems have been used for different species; we use the human numbering system. MDR1 secretes bulky organic cations, including xenobiotics, cytotoxins, anticancer drugs, and other drugs (e.g., colchicine, quinidine, verapamil, cyclosporine).

Other organic cations appear to be secreted into the canaliculus by a transport process driven by a pH gradient (Fig. 46-7). The presence of an electroneutral H-organic cation exchanger has been demonstrated at the canalicular membrane. However, the importance of this process is uncertain because major H^+ gradients probably do not exist in the bile canaliculus. In some cases, it appears that organic cations passively move across the apical membrane into the canaliculus, where they are sequestered by biliary micelles.

Biliary Lipids   Phospholipid is a major component of bile. **MDR3** (ABCB4) is a "flippase" that promotes the active translocation of phosphatidylcholine (PC) from the inner to the outer leaflet of the canalicular membrane. Bile salts then extract the PC from the outer leaflet so that the PC becomes a component of bile, where it participates in micelle formation. Indeed, in humans with an inherited deficiency of MDR3, progressive liver disease develops, characterized by extremely low concentrations of phospholipids in the bile.

Bile is also the main pathway for elimination of **cholesterol**. A heterodimer composed of the "half" ABC transporters **ABCG5 and ABCG8** is located on the canalicular membrane. This transporter is responsible for the secretion of cholesterol into bile. Although the mechanism is uncertain, the ABCG5/ABCG8 complex may form a channel for cholesterol translocation or alternatively may undergo a conformational change following ATP hydrolysis, thus flipping a cholesterol molecule into the outer membrane leaflet in a configuration favoring release into the canalicular lumen. Mutations in the genes encoding either of the two ABC monomers lead to sitosterolemia, a disorder associated with defective secretion into the bile of dietary sterols, increased intestinal absorption of plant and dietary sterols, hypercholesterolemia, and early-onset atherosclerosis.

Hepatocytes take up proteins across their basolateral membrane both by specific receptor-mediated endocytosis and by nonspecific fluid-phase endocytosis

The hepatocyte takes up macromolecules, such as plasma proteins, from the blood plasma through endocytosis, transports these molecules across the cytoplasm, and then secretes them into the bile through exocytosis. Three forms of endocytosis have been identified in the basolateral (sinusoidal) membrane: fluid-phase endocytosis, adsorptive endocytosis, and receptor-mediated endocytosis.

Fluid-phase endocytosis involves the uptake of a small amount of extracellular fluid, with its solutes, and is a result of the constitutive process of membrane invagination and internalization (see Chapter 2). The process is nondiscriminatory and inefficient. **Adsorptive endocytosis** involves nonspecific binding of the protein to the plasma membrane before endocytosis, and it results in more efficient protein uptake. **Receptor-mediated endocytosis** is quantitatively the most important mechanism for the uptake of macromolecules (see Chapter 2). After endocytosis, the receptor recycles to the plasma membrane, and the ligand may be excreted directly into bile by exocytosis or delivered to lysosomes for degradation. Receptor-mediated endocytosis is involved in the hepatic removal from the blood of proteins such as insulin, polymeric immunoglobulin A (IgA), asialoglycoproteins, and epidermal growth factor.

BILE FORMATION

The secretion of canalicular bile is active and isotonic

The formation of bile occurs in three discrete steps. First, the hepatocytes actively secrete bile into the bile canaliculi.

Second, intrahepatic and extrahepatic bile ducts not only transport this bile but also secrete into it a watery, HCO_3^--rich fluid. These first two steps may produce ~900 mL/day of so-called hepatic bile (Table 46-2). Third, between meals, approximately half the hepatic bile—perhaps 450 mL/day—is diverted to the gallbladder, which stores the bile and isosmotically removes salts and water. The result is that the gallbladder concentrates the key remaining solutes in bile fluid—bile salts, bilirubin, cholesterol, and lecithin—by 10- to 20-fold. The 500 mL/day of bile that reaches the duodenum through the ampulla of Vater is thus a mixture of relatively "dilute" hepatic bile and "concentrated" gallbladder bile.

The first step in bile formation cannot be ultrafiltration because the hydrostatic pressure in the canaliculi is significantly higher than the sinusoidal perfusion pressure. This situation is in marked contrast to glomerular filtration by the kidney (see Chapter 33), which relies predominantly on passive hydrostatic forces for producing the fluid in Bowman's space. Instead, bile formation is an *active process*. It is sensitive to changes in temperature and to metabolic inhibitors. Bile formation by hepatocytes requires the active, energy-dependent secretion of inorganic and organic solutes into the canalicular lumen, followed by the passive movement of water. This movement of water through the tight junctions between hepatocytes carries with it other solutes by solvent drag (see Chapter 19). Canalicular bile is an isosmotic fluid; thus, the intercellular junctions allow the passage

of water and small ions. The canalicular membrane expresses the water channel aquaporin 8 (AQP8). Under basal conditions, AQP8 is predominantly localized to intracellular vesicles but redistributes to the canalicular domain with stimulation by the secretagogue cAMP, thereby increasing apical water permeability. Thus, water transport into the bile canaliculus follows both paracellular and transcellular pathways. Further down the biliary tree (i.e., ducts and gallbladder), where the pore size of paracellular junctions is significantly smaller, solvent drag is not as important. Organic solutes do not readily enter bile distal to the canaliculi.

Major organic molecules in bile include bile acids, cholesterol, and phospholipids

Bile has two important functions: (1) bile provides the sole excretory route for many solutes that are not excreted by the kidney, and (2) secreted bile salts and acids are required for normal lipid digestion and absorption (see Chapter 44).

Both hepatic bile and gallbladder bile are complex secretions that are isosmotic with plasma (~300 mosmol/kg) and consist of water, inorganic electrolytes, and a variety of organic solutes, including bilirubin, cholesterol, fatty acids, and phospholipid (Table 46-2). The predominant cation in bile is Na^+, and the major inorganic anions are Cl^- and HCO_3^-. Solutes whose presence in bile is functionally important include micelle-forming bile acids, phospholipids, and IgA.

Bile acids promote dietary lipid absorption through their micelle-forming properties (see Chapter 45). As shown in Figure 45-9, hepatocytes synthesize the so-called **primary bile acids**—cholic acid and chenodeoxycholic acid—from cholesterol. Indeed, biliary excretion of cholesterol and conversion of **cholesterol** to bile acids are the principal routes of cholesterol excretion and catabolism, thus making bile formation pivotal for total body cholesterol balance. The first step in this conversion is catalyzed by **cholesterol 7α-hydroxylase ($CYP7\alpha1$)**, a specific cytochrome P-450 enzyme located in the SER. As we see later, **secondary bile acids** are the products of bacterial dehydroxylation in the terminal ileum and colon. After being absorbed and returning to the liver (enterohepatic circulation, discussed later), these secondary bile acids may also undergo conjugation. Figure 46-9 shows typical examples of conjugation reactions. **Phospholipids** in bile help to solubilize cholesterol as well as diminish the cytotoxic effects of other bile acids on hepatocytes and bile duct cells. **IgA** inhibits bacterial growth in bile.

Excretory or **waste products** found in bile include cholesterol, bile pigments, trace minerals, plant sterols, lipophilic drugs and metabolites, antigen-antibody complexes, and oxidized glutathione. Bile is also the excretory route for compounds that do not readily enter the renal glomerular filtrate, either because they are associated with proteins such as albumin or because they are associated with formed elements in blood. Although these compounds are generally lipophilic, they also include the heavy metals. Some bile acids (e.g., the trihydroxy bile acid cholic acid) are only partly bound to serum albumin and may therefore enter the glomerular filtrate. However, they are actively reabsorbed by the renal tubule. In health, bile acids are virtually absent from the urine.

Table 46-2 Composition of Bile

Parameter	Hepatic Bile	Gallbladder Bile
pH	7.5	6.0
Na^+ (mM)	141-165	220
K^+ (mM)	2.7-6.7	14
Ca^{2+} (mM)	1.2-3.2	15
Cl^- (mM)	77-117	31
HCO_3^- (mM)	12-55	19
Total phosphorus (g/L)	0.15	1.4
Bile acids (g/L)	3-45	32
Total fatty acids (g/L)	2.7	24
Bilirubin (g/L)	1-2	3
Phospholipids (g/L)	1.4-8.1	34
Cholesterol (g/L)	1-3.2	6.3
Proteins (g/L)	2-20	4.5

Data from Boyer JL: In Andreoli TE, Hoffman JF, Fanestil DD, Schultz SG (eds): Physiology of Membrane Disorders. New York: Plenum, 1986.

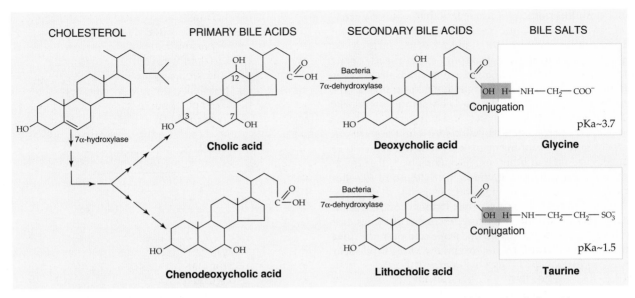

Figure 46-9 Synthesis of bile acids. The liver converts cholesterol to the primary bile acids—cholic acid and chenodeoxycholic acid—in a series of 14 reactions occurring in four different cellular organelles. The first reaction is the 7α-hydroxylation of cholesterol. In addition, the action of bacteria in the terminal ileum and colon may *de*hydroxylate bile acids, thus yielding the secondary bile acids deoxycholic acid and lithocholic acid. The hepatocytes conjugate most of the primary bile acids to small molecules such as glycine and taurine (not shown) before secreting them into the bile. In addition, those secondary bile acids that return to the liver through the enterohepatic circulation may also be conjugated to glycine or taurine, as shown in the figure. The liver may also conjugate some primary and secondary bile acids to sulfate or glucuronate (not shown).

Canalicular bile flow has a constant component driven by the secretion of small organic molecules and a component driven by the secretion of bile acids

Total bile flow is the sum of the bile flow from hepatocytes into the canaliculi (canalicular flow) and the additional flow from cholangiocytes into the bile ducts (ductular flow). In most species, the rate of **canalicular bile secretion** (i.e., milliliters per minute) increases more or less linearly with the rate of bile acid secretion (i.e., moles per minute). Canalicular bile flow is the sum of two components (Fig. 46-10): (1) a "constant" component that is independent of bile acid secretion (bile acid–*in*dependent flow) and (2) a rising component that increases linearly with bile acid secretion (bile acid–*dependent* flow). In humans, most of the canalicular bile flow is bile acid dependent. If we now add the **ductular secretion**, which is also "constant," we have the **total bile flow** in Figure 46-10. We discuss the canalicular secretion in the remainder of this section and ductular secretion in the following section.

Bile Acid–Independent Flow in the Canaliculi The secretion of *organic* compounds probably provides the major driving force for bile acid–independent flow. For example, glutathione, present in bile in high concentrations, may generate a potent osmotic driving force for canalicular bile formation.

Bile Acid–Dependent Flow in the Canaliculi The negatively charged bile salts in bile are in a micellar form and

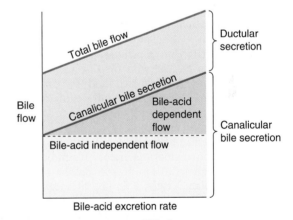

Figure 46-10 Components of bile flow.

are—in a sense—large polyanions. Thus, they are effectively out of solution and have a low **osmotic activity coefficient**. However, the positively charged counter ions accompanying these micellar bile acids are still in aqueous solution and may thus represent the predominant osmotic driving force for water movement in bile acid–dependent flow. If one infuses an animal with a nonphysiological bile acid that does not form micelles or one that forms micelles only at a rather high concentration, the osmotic activity will be higher, and thus the exogenous bile acid will be more effective in producing bile acid–dependent flow. In other words, the slope of the blue bile acid–dependent line in Figure 46-10 would be steeper than for physiological bile acids.

Bile flow does not always correlate with the osmotic activity of the bile acid. In some cases, bile acids increase electrolyte and water flux by other mechanisms, such as by stimulating Na^+-coupled cotransport mechanisms or by modulating the activity of other solute transporters. For example, the bile acid ursodeoxycholic acid produces a substantial increase in bile flow by markedly stimulating biliary HCO_3^- excretion.

Bile acids in the lumen may also stimulate the secretion of other solutes by trapping them in the lumen. These solutes include bilirubin and other organic anions, as well as lipids such as cholesterol and phospholipids. The mixed micelles formed by the bile acids apparently sequester these other solutes, thus lowering their effective luminal concentration and favoring their entry. Therefore, excretion of cholesterol and phospholipid is negligible when bile acid output is low, but it increases and approaches maximum values as bile acid output increases.

Secretin stimulates the cholangiocytes of ductules and ducts to secrete a watery, HCO_3^--rich fluid

As discussed in the previous section, biliary epithelial cells, or **cholangiocytes**, are the second major source of the fluid in hepatic bile. Experimentally, one can isolate cholangiocytes from normal liver or from the liver of experimental animals in which ductular hyperplasia has been induced by ligating the bile duct. These cholangiocytes have numerous transporters (Fig. 46-11), including the apical Cl-HCO_3 exchanger AE2, 6 of the 11 known human aquaporins (AQPs), and several apical Cl^- channels, including the cystic fibrosis transmembrane regulator (CFTR). In a mechanism that may be similar to that in pancreatic duct cells, the Cl-HCO_3 exchanger, in parallel with the Cl^- channels for Cl^- recycling, can secrete an HCO_3^--rich fluid (see Chapter 42). AQP1, CFTR, and AE2 co-localize to intracellular vesicles in cholangiocytes; secretory agonists cause all three to co-redistribute to the apical membrane.

A complex network of hormones, mainly acting through cAMP, regulates cholangiocyte secretory function. Secretin receptors (see Chapter 42) are present on the basolateral membranes of cholangiocytes, a finding that explains why **secretin** produces water-rich choleresis—that is, bile rich in HCO_3^- (i.e., alkaline) but diluted in bile acids. Similarly, the hormones **glucagon** (see Chapter 50) and **vasoactive intestinal peptide** (VIP; see Chapter 43) also produce HCO_3^--rich choleresis at the level of the ducts. These hormones raise $[cAMP]_i$ and thus stimulate apical Cl^- channels and the Cl-HCO_3 exchanger. A Ca^{2+}-activated Cl^- channel is also present in the apical membrane.

Cholangiocytes are also capable of reabsorbing fluid and electrolytes, as suggested by the adaptation that occurs after removal of the gallbladder (i.e., cholecystectomy). Bile found within the common bile duct of cholecystectomized, fasting animals is similar in composition to the concentrated bile typically found in the gallbladder. Thus, the ducts have partially taken over the function of the gallbladder (see later).

The hormone **somatostatin** inhibits bile flow by lowering $[cAMP]_i$, an effect opposite that of secretin. This inhibition may be caused by enhancing fluid reabsorption by bile ducts

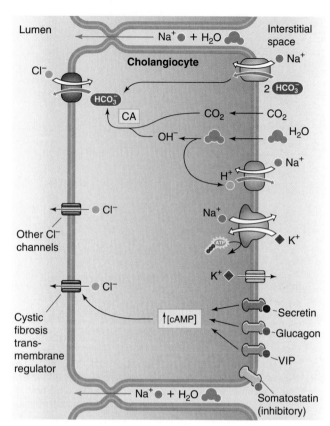

Figure 46-11   Secretion of an HCO_3^--rich fluid by cholangiocytes. The apical step of HCO_3^- secretion by the duct cell is mediated by a Cl-HCO_3 exchanger. The Cl^- recycles back to the lumen through Cl^- channels, such as CFTR. The basolateral step of HCO_3^- secretion probably is mediated in part by the uptake of HCO_3^- through an electrogenic Na/HCO_3 cotransporter. The uptake of CO_2, combined with the extrusion of H^+ through an Na-H exchanger and an H^+ pump, generates the rest of the HCO_3^- through carbonic anhydrase (CA). Secretin, glucagon, VIP, and gastrin-releasing peptide (GRP) all are choleretics. Somatostatin either enhances fluid absorption or inhibits secretion.

or by inhibiting ductular secretion of the HCO_3^--rich fluid discussed earlier.

Solutes reabsorbed from bile by cholangiocytes can be returned to the hepatocyte for repeat secretion. As shown earlier in Figure 46-2, the intralobular bile ducts are endowed with a rich peribiliary vascular plexus that is supplied by the hepatic artery. The blood draining this plexus finds its way into the hepatic sinusoids. This plexus is analogous to the capillaries of the gut, which, through the portal vein, also find their way into the hepatic sinusoids. Thus, some solutes, such as the hydrophilic bile acid ursodeoxycholic acid, may be absorbed by the cholangiocytes from bile and returned to the hepatocytes for repeat secretion, thus inducing significant choleresis.

The gallbladder stores and concentrates bile and delivers it to the duodenum during a meal

The gallbladder is not an essential structure of bile secretion, but it does serve to concentrate bile acids up to 10- or even 20-fold during interdigestive periods. Tonic contraction of the sphincter of Oddi facilitates gallbladder filling by maintaining a positive pressure within the common bile duct. As we noted earlier, up to 50% of hepatic bile—or ~450 mL/day—is diverted to the gallbladder during fasting. The remaining ~450 mL/day passes directly into the duodenum. Periods of gallbladder filling between meals are interrupted by brief periods of partial emptying of concentrated bile and probably aspiration of dilute hepatic bile in a process analogous to the function of a bellows.

Bile salts and certain other components of bile are concentrated up to 20-fold within the gallbladder lumen because they are left behind during the isotonic reabsorption of NaCl and $NaHCO_3$ by the leaky gallbladder epithelium (Fig. 46-12). The apical step of NaCl uptake and transport is electroneutral and is mediated by parallel Na-H and Cl-HCO_3 exchangers. At the basolateral membrane, Na^+ exits through the Na-K pump, whereas Cl^- most likely exits by Cl^- channels. Both water and HCO_3^- move passively from lumen to blood through the tight junctions, which are rather leaky. Water can also move through the cell. The net transport is isotonic, which leaves behind gallbladder bile that is also isotonic but has a higher concentration of bile salts, K^+, and Ca^{2+}. Net fluid and electrolyte transport across the gallbladder epithelium is under hormonal regulation. Both VIP (released from neurons innervating the gallbladder) and serotonin inhibit net fluid and electrolyte absorption. Conversely, α-adrenergic blockade of neuronal VIP release increases fluid absorption.

Although the gallbladder reabsorbs NaCl by parallel Na-H and Cl-HCO_3 exchange at the apical membrane, Na-H exchange outstrips Cl-HCO_3 exchange; the end result is net secretion of **H^+ ions**. This action neutralizes the HCO_3^- and acidifies the bile. The H^+ secreted by the gallbladder protonates the intraluminal contents. This action greatly increases the solubility of calcium salts in bile and reduces the likelihood of calcium salt precipitation and **gallstone formation**.

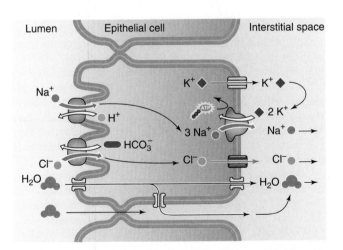

Figure 46-12 Isotonic fluid reabsorption by the gallbladder epithelium. The gallbladder epithelium performs the isotonic absorption of NaCl. The apical step is parallel Na-H exchange and Cl-HCO_3 exchange. Because Na-H exchange is somewhat faster, net secretion of acid into the lumen occurs. The basolateral step of NaCl absorption is mediated by the Na-K pump and by Cl^- channels. K^+ channels provide a route for basolateral K^+ recycling. Water follows passively through the tight junctions and through the basolateral membrane.

Common pigment gallstones contain one or more of several calcium salts, including carbonate, bilirubinate, phosphate, and fatty acids. The solubility of each of these compounds is significantly increased by the acidification of bile.

Mucus secretion by gallbladder epithelial cells results in the formation of a polymeric gel that protects the apical surface of the gallbladder epithelium from the potentially toxic effects of bile salts. However, excessive mucin synthesis can be deleterious. For example, in animal models of cholesterol cholelithiasis (i.e., formation of gallstones made of cholesterol), a marked increase in mucin release precedes crystal and stone formation.

The relative tone of the gallbladder and sphincter of Oddi determines whether bile secreted by the liver flows from the common hepatic duct into the gallbladder or into the duodenum

Bile exiting the liver and flowing down the common hepatic duct reaches a bifurcation that permits flow either into the cystic duct and then into the gallbladder or into the common bile duct, through the sphincter of Oddi, and into the duodenum (Fig. 46-4). The extent to which bile takes either path depends on the relative resistance of the two pathways.

The sphincter of Oddi—which also controls the flow of pancreatic secretions into the duodenum—corresponds functionally to a short (4- to 6-mm) zone within the wall of the duodenum. The basal pressure within the lumen of the duct at the level of the sphincter is 5 to 10 mm Hg. The pressure in the lumen of the resting common bile duct is also 5 to 10 mm Hg, compared with a pressure of ~0 mm Hg inside the duodenum.

The basal contraction of the sphincter prevents reflux of the duodenal contents into the common bile duct. In its basal state, the sphincter exhibits high-pressure, phasic contractions several times per minute. These contractions are primarily peristaltic and directed in antegrade fashion to provide a motive force toward the duodenum. Thus, the sphincter of Oddi acts principally as an adjustable occluding mechanism and a regulator of bile flow.

Both hormonal and cholinergic mechanisms appear to be involved in gallbladder emptying. Dietary lipid stimulates the release of cholecystokinin (CCK) from duodenal I cells (see Chapter 44). This CCK not only stimulates pancreatic secretion but also causes smooth muscle contraction and evacuation of the gallbladder. The coordinated response to CCK also includes relaxation of the sphincter of Oddi, thus enhancing bile flow into the duodenum.

ENTEROHEPATIC CIRCULATION OF BILE ACIDS

The enterohepatic circulation of bile acids is a loop consisting of secretion by the liver, reabsorption by the intestine, and return to the liver in portal blood for repeat secretion into bile

Bile acids are important for promoting the absorption of dietary lipids in the intestine. The quantity of bile acid that

Cholestasis

The term *cholestasis* refers to the suppression of bile secretion. Biliary constituents may therefore be retained within the hepatocyte and regurgitated into the systemic circulation. Cholestasis causes three major groups of negative effects: first, regurgitation of bile components (bile acids, bilirubin) into the systemic circulation gives rise to the symptoms of jaundice and pruritus (itching). Second, cholestasis damages hepatocytes, as evidenced by the release of liver enzymes (e.g., alkaline phosphatase) into the plasma. Third, because the bile acids do not arrive in the duodenum, lipid digestion and absorption may be impaired.

Many acute and chronic liver diseases produce cholestasis by mechanically obstructing the **extrahepatic** bile ducts or by impairing bile flow at the level of the hepatocytes or **intrahepatic** bile ducts. The mechanisms underlying the obstructive and functional forms of cholestasis are complex and have not been completely defined. Experimental models of cholestasis have produced multiple abnormalities: (1) altered plasma membrane composition and fluidity; (2) inhibition of membrane proteins, including the Na-K pump; (3) reduced expression of genes encoding transporters for bile acids and other organic anions; (4) increased permeability of the paracellular pathway, with backdiffusion of biliary solutes into the plasma; (5) altered function of microfilaments, with decreased contractions of bile canaliculi; and (6) loss of the polarized distribution of some plasma membrane proteins. Cholestatic conditions, such as bile duct obstruction, markedly increase the basolateral expression of MRP3—which normally is expressed only minimally. This induction of MRP3 allows the efflux of bile acids and other cholephilic anions from the hepatocyte into sinusoidal blood.

the liver normally *secretes* in a day varies with the number of meals and the fat content of these meals, but it typically ranges between 12 and 36 g. The liver's basal rate of *synthesis* of bile acids from cholesterol (Fig. 46-9) is only ~600 mg/day in healthy humans, sufficient to replace the equivalent losses of bile acid in the feces. Obviously, the gastrointestinal tract must have an extremely efficient mechanism for recycling the bile acids secreted by the liver (Fig. 46-13). This recycling, known as the **enterohepatic circulation**, occurs as the terminal ileum and colon reabsorb bile acids and return them to the liver in the portal blood. The total pool of bile acids in the gastrointestinal tract is ~3 g. This pool must recirculate ~ 4 to 12 times per day, or as many as 5 or more times for a single fat-rich meal. If reabsorption of bile acids is defective, as can happen after resection of the ileum, de novo synthesis of bile acids by the liver can be as high as 4 to 6 g/day.

The intestinal conservation of bile acids is extremely efficient and is mediated both by active apical absorption in the terminal ileum and by passive absorption throughout the intestinal tract

Most of the bile secreted into the duodenum is in the conjugated form. Very little of these bile salts are reabsorbed

into the intestinal tract until they reach the terminal ileum, an arrangement that allows the bile salts to remain at high levels throughout most of the small intestine, where they can participate in lipid digestion and absorption (see Chapter 44). However, the enterohepatic circulation must eventually reclaim 95% or more of these secreted bile salts. Some of the absorption of bile acids by the intestines is passive and occurs along the entire small intestine and colon. Nevertheless, the major component of bile acid absorption is active and occurs only in the terminal ileum (Fig. 46-13).

Passive absorption of bile acids occurs along the entire small intestine and colon (Fig. 46-13), but it is less intensive than active absorption. The mechanism of bile acid uptake across the apical membrane may consist of either **ionic** or **nonionic diffusion**. Nonionic diffusion—or passive diffusion of the protonated or neutral form of the bile acid—is 10-fold greater than ionic diffusion. The extent of nonionic diffusion for a given bile acid depends on the concentration of its neutral, protonated form, which is maximized when the luminal pH is low and the pK of the bile acid is high. At the normal intestinal pH of 5.5 to 6.5, few of the taurine-conjugated bile salts are protonated, a small amount of the glycine-conjugated bile salts are protonated, and ~50% of unconjugated bile acids are protonated. Thus, the unconjugated bile acids are in the best position to be reabsorbed by nonionic diffusion, followed by the glycine-conjugated bile acids and then finally by the taurine-conjugated bile acids. Among these unconjugated bile acids, more lipophilic bile acids, such as chenodeoxycholate and deoxycholate, diffuse more readily through the apical membrane than do hydrophilic bile acids such as cholic acid. Nonionic diffusion also depends on the total concentration of the bile acid (i.e., neutral plus charged form), which, in turn, depends on the maximum solubilizing capacity of bile salt micelles for that bile acid.

Active absorption of bile acids in the intestine is restricted to the *terminal ileum*. This active process preferentially absorbs the negatively charged *conjugated* bile salts—the form *not* well absorbed by the passive mechanisms. Active uptake of bile salts involves saturation kinetics, competitive inhibition, and a requirement for Na^+ (Fig. 46-13). The Na^+-dependent transporter responsible for the apical step of active absorption is known as the apical **Na^+/bile salt transporter ASBT** (SLC10A2), a close relative of the hepatocyte transporter NTCP (Fig. 46-5C). Once bile salts have entered ileal enterocytes across the apical membrane, they exit across the basolateral membrane via a heteromeric **organic solute transporter (Ostα/Ostβ)**.

Because the most polar bile salts are poorly absorbed by nonionic diffusion, it is not surprising that the ASBT in the apical membrane of the enterocytes of the terminal ileum has the highest affinity and maximal transport rates for these salts. For example, the ASBT is primarily responsible for absorbing the ionized, taurine-conjugated bile salts in the ileum. Conversely, the ASBT in the ileum is relatively poor at absorbing the more lipophilic bile acids, which tend to be absorbed passively in the upper intestine.

On their entry into portal blood, the bile acids are predominantly bound to albumin and, to a lesser extent, lipoproteins. The liver removes or clears these bile acids from portal blood by the transport mechanisms

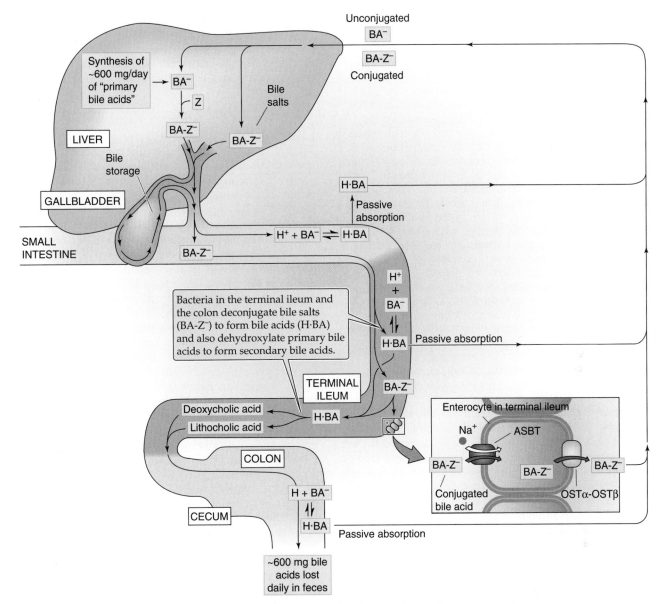

Figure 46-13 Enterohepatic circulation of bile acids. The bile acids that the liver delivers to the duodenum in the bile are primarily conjugated to taurine or glycine (BA-Z⁻). Most bile acids are reabsorbed as conjugated bile salts (BA-Z⁻) in the terminal ileum through an Na⁺-coupled cotransporter (ASBT). Also in the terminal ileum and colon, bacteria deconjugate a small amount of these bile salts to form unconjugated bile acids (H·BA ↔ H⁺ + BA⁻), thereby allowing H·BA to be passively absorbed by nonionic diffusion. In addition, bacteria in the terminal ileum and colon dehydroxylate primary bile acids to form secondary bile acids (see Fig. 46-9). Some of these are passively absorbed, and the rest are excreted in the feces. The absorbed bile acids return to the liver through the portal blood and are then taken up into the hepatocyte for secretion again.

outlined earlier in Figure 46-5C. Hepatic clearance of bile acids is often expressed as the percentage of bile acids removed during a single pass through the liver. The hepatic extraction of bile acids is related to bile acid structure and the degree of albumin binding. It is greatest for hydrophilic bile acids and is least for protein-bound, hydrophobic bile acids.

The small fraction of bile acids that escapes active or passive absorption in the small intestine is subject to *bacterial modification* in the *colon*. This bacterial modification takes two forms. First, the bacteria deconjugate the bile. Second, the bacteria perform a 7α-dehydroxylation reaction

with the formation of *secondary bile acids*. These secondary bile acids include **deoxycholate** and **lithocholate** (Fig. 46-9). The deconjugated secondary bile acids may then be either absorbed passively in the colon or excreted in the feces; their fate depends on their physicochemical properties and their binding to luminal contents. Up to one third of the deoxycholate formed in the colon may be reabsorbed by nonionic diffusion. Lithocholate, which is relatively insoluble, is absorbed to a much lesser extent. The secondary bile acids formed by colonic bacteria and recycled back to the liver may undergo biotransformation through conjugation to glycine and taurine.

Gallstones

Most gallstones (~80%) consist mainly of cholesterol. Thus, **cholelithiasis** may be regarded as a disturbance of bile secretion and cholesterol elimination. When cholesterol and phospholipids are secreted together into the bile, they form unilamellar bilayered vesicles. These vesicles become incorporated into mixed micelles that form because of the amphiphilic properties of bile acids. Micellation allows cholesterol to remain in solution in its passage through the biliary tree. However, if the concentration of bile acids is insufficient to maintain all the cholesterol in the form of mixed micelles, the excess cholesterol is left behind as vesicles in the aqueous phase. These cholesterol-enriched vesicles are relatively unstable and are prone to aggregate and form large multilamellar vesicles, from which cholesterol crystals nucleate. Growth of crystals may result in the formation of gallstones. An excess of biliary cholesterol in relation to the amount of phospholipids and bile acids can result from hypersecretion of cholesterol, inadequate secretion of bile acids, or both. Cholelithiasis may be further promoted by other factors, such as gallbladder mucin and other nonmucous glycoproteins, as well as by stasis of bile in the gallbladder.

Thus, the enterohepatic circulation of bile acids is driven by two *mechanical* pumps: (1) the motor activity of the gallbladder and (2) peristalsis of the intestines to propel the bile acids to the terminal ileum and colon. It is also driven by two *chemical* pumps: (1) energy-dependent transporters located in the terminal ileum and (2) energy-dependent transporters in the hepatocyte.

The **bile acid receptor FXR**, a member of the nuclear receptor family, controls multiple components of the enterohepatic circulation of bile acids. Primary bile acids are potent agonists of FXR, which transcriptionally regulates several genes involved in bile acid homeostasis. Four examples of negative feedback by activated FXR are as follows: (1) FXR inhibits the expression of cholesterol 7α-hydroxylase (Fig. 46-9), the rate-limiting enzyme for bile acid synthesis; (2) FXR induces the expression of an *inhibitory* transcription factor—the small heterodimer partner (SHP)—which controls the activity of another nuclear receptor, the liver receptor homologue-1 (LRH-1), which is required for CYP7a1 expression; (3) FXR upregulates BSEP (*increasing* bile acid secretion; Fig. 46-5C) and downregulates NTCP (*decreasing* bile acid uptake; Fig. 46-5C) by SHP-dependent mechanisms; and (4) FXR, through SHP, downregulates ASBT and thereby reduces ileal bile acid uptake. Thus, FXR coordinates bile acid synthesis and transport by the liver and intestine.

THE LIVER AS A METABOLIC ORGAN

The liver is a metabolically active and highly aerobic organ. It receives ~28% of the total blood flow and extracts ~20% of the oxygen used by the body. The liver is responsible for the synthesis and degradation of carbohydrates, proteins, and lipids. The small molecules that are products of digestion are efficiently sorted in the liver for metabolism, storage, or distribution to extrahepatic tissues for energy. The liver provides energy to other tissues mainly by exporting two substrates that are critical for oxidization in the peripheral tissues, glucose and ketone bodies (e.g., acetoacetate).

The liver can serve as either a source or a sink for glucose

The liver is one of the key organs that maintain blood glucose concentrations within a narrow range, in a dynamic process involving endogenous glucose production and glucose utilization. The fasting blood [glucose] is normally 4 to 5 mM. Between meals, when levels of insulin are relatively low and levels of glucagon are high (see Chapter 50), the liver serves as a source of plasma glucose, both by synthesizing glucose and by generating it from the breakdown of glycogen. The de novo synthesis of glucose, or **gluconeogenesis** (see Fig. 51-12), is one of the liver's most important functions; it is essential for maintaining a normal plasma concentration of glucose, which is the primary energy source for most tissues (see Chapter 57). Glucose is synthesized in the lumen of the ER, principally from amino acids and lactate. Dietary fructose and galactose are also largely converted to glucose. Glucose exits the ER by facilitated diffusion (mediated by GLUT7) and then passes into the blood through another facilitated diffusion mechanism (GLUT2), which has a low affinity and high capacity and is located in the hepatocyte's basolateral membrane.

The second way in which the liver delivers glucose to blood plasma is by **glycogenolysis**. Stored glycogen may account for as much as 7% to 10% of the total weight of the liver. Glycogenolysis in the *liver* yields glucose as its major product, whereas glycogen breakdown in *muscle* produces lactic acid (see Chapter 59).

After a meal, when levels of insulin are relatively high, the liver does just the opposite: it acts as a sink for glucose by taking it up from the portal blood and either breaking it down to pyruvate or using it to synthesize glycogen (see Fig. 50-8). Glucose oxidation has two phases. In the anaerobic phase, glucose is broken down to pyruvic acid (**glycolysis**). In the aerobic phase, pyruvic acid is completely oxidized to H_2O and CO_2 through the citric acid cycle.

The liver also consumes glucose by using it for **glycogen synthesis**. Carbohydrate that is not stored as glycogen or oxidized is metabolized to **fat**.

All the aforementioned processes are regulated by hormones such as insulin and glucagon (see Chapter 50), which enable rapid responses to changes in the metabolic requirements of the body.

The liver synthesizes a variety of important plasma proteins (e.g., albumin, coagulation factors, and carriage proteins) and metabolizes dietary amino acids

Protein Synthesis One of the major functions of the liver is to produce a wide array of proteins for export to the blood plasma (Table 46-3). These products include major **plasma proteins** that are important for maintaining the colloid

Table 46-3 Proteins Made by the Liver for Export

Major Plasma Proteins
Albumin
α_1-Fetoprotein
Plasma fibronectin (an α_2-glycoprotein)
C-reactive protein
α_2-Microglobulin
Various other globulins

Factors Involved in Hemostasis/Fibrinolysis
Coagulation: fibrinogen and all others except factor VIII
Inhibitors of coagulation: α_1-antitrypsin and antithrombin III, α_2-macroglobulin, protein S, protein C
Fibrinolysis: plasminogen
Inhibitors of fibrinolysis: α_2-antiplasmin
Complement C3

Carriage Proteins (Binding Proteins)
Ceruloplasmin
Corticosteroid-binding globulin (CBG; also called transcortin)
GH-binding protein (low-affinity form)
Haptoglobin
Hemopexin
IGF-binding proteins
Retinol-binding protein
Sex hormone–binding globulin (SHBG)
Thyroid-binding globulin (TBG)
Transferrin
Transthyretin
Vitamin D–binding protein

Prohormones
Angiotensinogen

Apolipoproteins
Apo A-I
Apo A-II
Apo A-IV
Apo B-100
Apo C-II
Apo D
Apo E

GH, growth hormone; IGF, insulin-like growth factor.

osmotic pressure of plasma (see Chapter 19). Other products include factors involved in **hemostasis** (blood clotting) and **fibrinolysis** (breakdown of blood clots), **carriage proteins** that bind and transport hormones and other substances in the blood, **prohormones**, and **lipoproteins** (Table 46-4). The liver synthesizes plasma proteins at a maximum rate of 15 to 50 g/day.

Amino Acid Uptake A major role of the liver is to take up and metabolize dietary amino acids that are absorbed by the gastrointestinal tract (see Chapter 44) and are transported to the liver in portal blood. These amino acids are taken up by both Na$^+$-*dependent* and Na$^+$-*in*dependent transporters that are identical to some of the amino acid transporters in the kidney, small intestine, and other tissues (see Table 35-1). An unusual feature of the liver is that, with few exceptions, the same amino acid transporter may be located on

both the basolateral and apical membranes. For example, Na$^+$-dependent glutamate uptake by the excitatory amino acid transporters SLC1A1 (EAAT3) and SLC1A2 (EAAT2) occurs primarily at the apical membrane, but dexamethasone (corticosteroid) treatment can induce their expression at the basolateral membrane. In general, hepatic amino acid transporters are highly regulated at the transcriptional and post-translational levels.

Amino Acid Metabolism Under physiological conditions, total and individual plasma concentrations of amino acids are tightly regulated. The liver controls the availability of amino acids in the systemic blood, activating ureagenesis after a high protein meal and repressing it during fasting or low protein intake. Unlike glucose, which can be stored, amino acids must either be used immediately (e.g., for the synthesis of proteins) or broken down. The breakdown of α-amino acids occurs by **deamination** to α-keto acids and NH$_4^+$ (Fig. 46-14). The α-keto acids ("carbon skeleton"), depending on the structure of the parent amino acid, are metabolized to pyruvate, various intermediates of the citric acid cycle (see Fig. 57-9), acetyl coenzyme A (acetyl CoA), or acetoacetyl CoA. The liver detoxifies ~95% of the NH$_4^+$ through a series of reactions known as the **urea cycle** (Fig. 46-14); the liver can also use NH$_4^+$—together with glutamate—to generate glutamine. Individual deficiencies in each of the enzymes involved in the urea cycle have been described and result in life-threatening hyperammonemia. The urea generated by the urea cycle exits the hepatocyte through a urea channel, which is, in fact, AQP9. The urea then enters the blood and is ultimately excreted by the kidneys (see Chapter 37). The glutamine synthesized by the liver also enters the blood. Some of this glutamine is metabolized by the kidney to yield glutamate and NH$_4^+$, which is exported in the urine (see Chapter 37).

The liver is also the main site for the synthesis and secretion of **glutathione**. GSH is critical for detoxification (in conjugation reactions in the liver) and for protection against oxidative stress in multiple organs. Thus, erythrocytes that have low levels of GSH are more prone to hemolysis. Because more than 90% of the GSH in the circulation is synthesized in the liver, GSH efflux across the basolateral membrane from the hepatocyte to the sinusoid is important. Bidirectional transport of glutathione across the *basolateral membrane* may occur in part by one of the OATPs as well as MRP4 by cotransport with bile acids. In addition, MRP2 exports some conjugated GSH across the *canalicular membrane* into bile, as stated earlier, and an unidentified transporter can similarly export smaller amounts of unconjugated GSH.

The liver obtains dietary triglycerides and cholesterol by taking up remnant chylomicrons through receptor-mediated endocytosis

As discussed in Chapter 44, enterocytes in the small intestine process fatty acids consumed as dietary triglycerides and secrete them into the lymph primarily in the form of extremely large proteolipid aggregates called chylomicrons (Fig. 46-15). These **chylomicrons**—made up of triglycerides (80% to 90%), phospholipids, cholesterol, and several apo-

Table 46-4 Major Classes of Lipoproteins

	Chylomicrons	VLDLs	IDLs	LDLs	HDLs
Density (g/cm³)	<0.95	<1.006	1.006-1.019	1.019-1.063	1.063-1.210
Diameter (nm)	75-1200	30-80	25-35	18-25	50-120
Mass (kDa)	400,000	10,000-80,000	5000-10,000	2300	175-360
Protein (surface) (%)	1.5-2.5	5-10	15-20	20-25	40-55
Phospholipid (surface) (%)	7-9	15-20	22	15-20	20-35
Free cholesterol (surface) (%)	1-3	5-10	8	7-10	3-4
Triglycerides (core) (%)	84-89	50-65	22	7-10	3-5
Cholesteryl esters (core) (%)	3-5	10-15	30	35-40	12
Major apolipoproteins	A-I, A-II, B-48, C-I, C-II, C-III, E	B-100, C-I, C-II, C-III, E	B-100, C-III, E	B-100	A-I, A-II, C-I, C-II, C-III, D, E

Data from Voet D, Voet JG: Biochemistry, 2nd ed. New York: John Wiley, 1995, p 317.

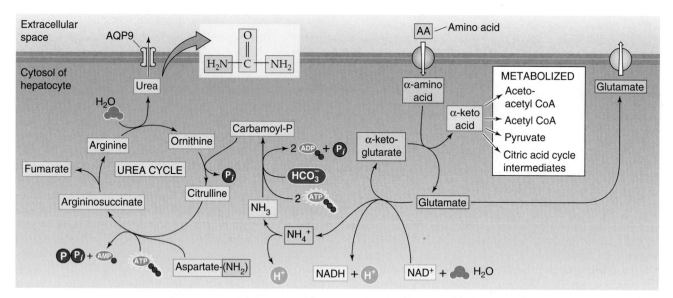

Figure 46-14 Amino acid metabolism and urea formation in hepatocytes. When a hepatocyte takes up an α-amino acid, it either must use it immediately in protein synthesis or deaminate it. The deamination reaction transfers the amino group of the α-amino acid to α-ketoglutarate, thus yielding glutamate and the corresponding α-keto acid. Depending on the backbone of the α-keto acid, it may be metabolized into acetoacetyl CoA, acetyl CoA, pyruvate, or a variety of citric acid cycle intermediates. The NH_4^+ results from the regeneration of the α-ketoglutarate consumed in the urea cycle. The other amino group of the urea is derived from the amino group of aspartate. The C = O moiety of urea is derived from CO_2. The liver then exports the urea, which exits the hepatocyte through AQP9.

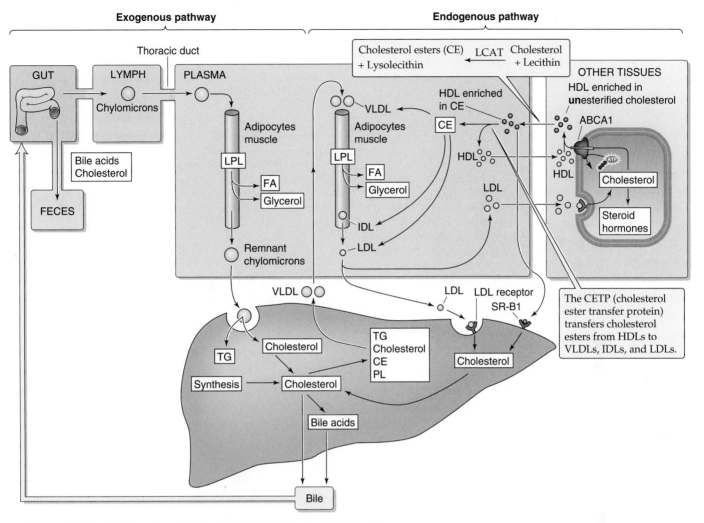

Figure 46-15 Cholesterol metabolism. CE, cholesteryl ester; FA, fatty acid.

proteins (Chapter 44)—pass from the lymph to the blood through the thoracic duct. As discussed later in Chapter 58, lipoprotein lipase (LPL) on the walls of the capillary endothelium in adipose tissue and muscle then partially digests the triglycerides in these chylomicrons. The results of this digestion are glycerol, fatty acids, and smaller or "remnant" chylomicrons, which are triglyceride depleted and thus enriched in cholesterol. The glycerol and fatty acids generated by LPL enter adipocytes and muscle cells. The cholesterol-rich **remnant chylomicrons**, conversely, remain in the blood and make their way to the liver, where they enter hepatocytes by a process that is saturable, specific, and of high affinity. Although low-density lipoprotein (LDL) receptors can recognize chylomicron remnants, another member of the LDL receptor gene family, the LDL-related receptor, is of greater importance. The chylomicron remnant binds to this receptor on the basolateral membrane, enters the hepatocyte through receptor-mediated endocytosis (see Chapter 2), and is degraded in lysosomes. Thus, chylomicrons transport dietary triglycerides to adipose tissue and muscle, whereas their remnants transport dietary triglycerides and cholesterol to hepatocytes.

The hepatocyte can also take up across its basolateral membrane the **long-chain fatty acids** liberated by LPL but not used by other tissues. Fatty acid uptake occurs by at least two different mechanisms: facilitated uptake and a nonspecific "flip-flop" across the lipid bilayer.

To extract energy from the neutral fats derived from the remnant chylomicrons, hepatocytes must first split the triglycerides into glycerol and fatty acids. The fatty acids thus derived from remnant chylomicrons, as well as those that enter the hepatocyte directly, are metabolized by β oxidation into two-carbon acetyl intermediates that then form acetyl CoA. Acetyl CoA can enter the citric acid cycle, where it is oxidized to produce large amounts of energy. The acetyl CoA that is not used by the liver is converted by the condensation of two molecules of acetyl CoA to yield acetoacetic acid. The liver is the only organ that produces **acetoacetate** for metabolism by muscle, brain, and kidney, but it does not use this substrate for its own energy needs. In fasting or in poorly controlled diabetes, in which the supply of acetyl CoA is in excess, the acetyl CoA is diverted to produce acetoacetate, which, in turn, can yield β-hydroxybutyrate and acetone. Together, acetoacetate, β-hydroxybutyrate, and acetone are referred to as **ketone bodies**. Another fate of fatty acids in the liver is that they can be re-esterified to glycerol, with the formation of triglycerides that can either be stored or exported as **very-low-density lipoproteins** (**VLDLs**) and released into the circulation for use by peripheral tissues.

Cholesterol, synthesized primarily in the liver, is an important component of cell membranes and serves as a precursor for bile acids and steroid hormones

The body's major pools of cholesterol include the cholesterol and cholesterol derivatives in bile, cholesterol in membranes, cholesterol carried as lipoproteins in blood (Table 46-4), and cholesterol-rich tissues. Cholesterol is present in membranes and bile mainly as free cholesterol. In plasma and in some tissues, cholesterol is esterified with long-chain fatty acids. The major *sources* of cholesterol are dietary uptake of cholesterol and de novo synthesis of cholesterol by various cells (Table 46-5). The major *fates* of cholesterol are secretion into bile, excretion in the feces when intestinal cells are sloughed, sloughing of skin, and synthesis of steroid hormones. However, in mammals, the most important route for the elimination of cholesterol is the hepatic conversion of cholesterol into bile acids. In the steady state, the liver must excrete an amount of sterol (as cholesterol and bile acids) that equals the amount of cholesterol that is synthesized in the various organs and absorbed from the diet.

The liver is the major organ for controlling cholesterol metabolism (Fig. 46-15). The liver obtains cholesterol from three major sources. First, the intestine packages dietary cholesterol as chylomicrons, which travel through the lymph to blood vessels in adipocytes and muscle, where LPL hydrolyzes triglycerides to fatty acids and glycerol. The resultant cholesterol-enriched remnant chylomicrons are then delivered as cholesterol to the liver. Second, the liver synthesizes cholesterol de novo. Third, the liver takes up cholesterol in the guise of **LDLs**. However, the liver exports cholesterol in two major ways: (1) the liver uses cholesterol to synthesize bile acids and also includes cholesterol and cholesteryl esters in the bile, and (2) the liver also exports cholesterol to the blood in the form of VLDLs.

Table 46-5 Sources and Fates of Cholesterol in Humans

Process	Flow (g/day for a 70-kg Human)
Intestinal absorption	0.1-0.5
Synthesis	1.05
Biliary secretion	0.9
Cholesterol consumed in synthesis of bile acids	0.5
Cholesterol secreted in VLDLs by the liver	0.25-1.75

Data from Cooper AD, Ellsworth JL: In Zakim D, Boyer TD (eds): Hepatology. Philadelphia: WB Saunders, 1996.

Synthesis of Cholesterol The de novo synthesis of cholesterol occurs in many extrahepatic tissues, as well as in the intestine and liver. The synthesis of cholesterol proceeds from acetyl CoA in a multistep process that takes place in the SER and cytosol (Fig. 46-16). The hepatic synthesis of cholesterol is inhibited by dietary cholesterol and by fasting and is increased with bile drainage (fistula) and bile duct obstruction. The rate-limiting step in cholesterol synthesis is the conversion of 3-hydroxy-3-methylglutaryl-CoA (HMG-CoA) to mevalonate by **HMG-CoA reductase**, the level of which is decreased—in typical negative feedback fashion—by cholesterol levels in the cell. The most potent cholesterol-lowering agents that are clinically available today—the "statins"—are inhibitors of HMG-CoA reductase.

The liver is the organ principally responsible for cholesterol homeostasis in the body, as well as for the synthesis and degradation of low-density lipoprotein

The liver is the hub of cholesterol metabolism. It is the central feature of an exogenous loop in which the liver takes up dietary cholesterol as remnant chylomicrons and exports cholesterol and cholesterol metabolites into bile. The liver is also the central feature of an endogenous loop in which the

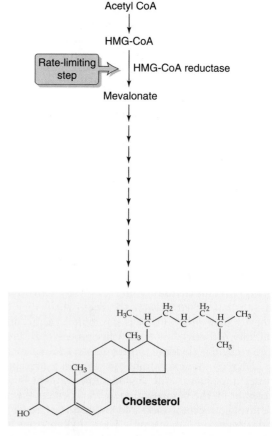

Figure 46-16 Cholesterol synthesis. The liver synthesizes cholesterol de novo from acetyl CoA in a multistep process that occurs in the SER and cytosol. The rate-limiting step is the conversion of HMG-CoA to mevalonate by HMG-CoA reductase.

liver exports cholesterol and other lipids as VLDLs and takes them up from the blood as LDLs. Table 46-4 summarizes the properties of these lipoproteins, as well as two others: the intermediate-density lipoproteins (IDLs) and the **high-density lipoproteins** (HDLs). As we move from left to right in Table 46-4, the size of the particles decreases, the density increases (because the fractional mass of protein increases), the fractional amount of triglycerides decreases, and the fractional amount of phospholipids increases.

Regardless of the source of the cholesterol, the liver can package cholesterol along with other lipids and apoproteins as **VLDLs**. The VLDLs are large—and therefore less dense—when the availability of triglycerides is high (e.g., obesity, diabetes), but they are small when triglyceride availability is low. VLDLs enter the bloodstream (Fig. 46-15) and eventually make their way to the blood vessels of adipose tissue and muscle, where the same LPL that degrades chylomicrons degrades the VLDLs on the luminal surface of blood vessel endothelial cells. In the process, fatty acids are released to the tissues. Thus, VLDLs act as lipid shuttles that transport endogenous triglycerides to adipose tissue for storage as fat or to muscle for immediate use. As a result of the LPL activity, the large, buoyant VLDLs rapidly shrink to become the smaller **IDLs** and the even smaller LDLs. The half-life of VLDLs is less than an hour. In plasma, only minute amounts of IDLs are present.

Both the liver and extrahepatic tissue can take up LDLs—and to a lesser extent, IDLs—by the process of receptor-mediated endocytosis (see Chapter 2). **LDLs** are the major carriers of cholesterol in plasma. The half-life of LDLs is 2 to 3 days. Of course, uptake of LDL by the liver is a major pathway of cholesterol input to the liver. The liver degrades ~40% to 60% of LDLs, and no other tissue takes up more than ~10%. LDL uptake by other tissues provides a mechanism for the delivery of cholesterol that can be used for the synthesis of cell membranes and steroid hormones or for storage as cholesteryl ester droplets.

The other major player in cholesterol metabolism is **HDL**, which is composed of cholesterol, phospholipids, triglycerides, and apoproteins (Table 46-4). The two major apoproteins of HDLs, A-I and A-II, are made by the intestines as part of chylomicrons, as well as by the liver. As LPL digests VLDLs on endothelial cells, some excess surface material (i.e., cholesterol and phospholipids) of these rapidly shrinking particles is transferred to the HDLs. In peripheral cells such as macrophages, the cholesterol transporter ABCA1 facilitates the efflux of cholesterol, which then combines with lipid-poor HDLs. An enzyme that is associated with HDL, lecithin **cholesterol acyltransferase (LCAT)**—synthesized in the liver, then takes an acyl group from lecithin and esterifies it to cholesterol to produce a cholesterol ester (CE).

When the CE-enriched HDL (HDL-CE) reaches the liver, it binds to the **scavenger receptor class B type 1 (SR-B1)**, which mediates selective uptake of HDL-CE. The cholesterol moiety is targeted for biliary excretion. This pathway may also process LDL-CE and free cholesterol. In contrast to the LDL receptor, the selective uptake of CE by **SR-B1** does not involve endocytosis. Instead, a poorly defined mechanism first moves CE to a reversible plasma membrane pool and then to an irreversible pool within the cell.

In addition to traveling to the liver for handling through SR-B1, HDL-CE can transfer its CE to apolipoprotein B–containing lipoproteins (i.e., VLDL, IDLs, LDLs) through the action of **CE transfer protein (CETP)**. These less-dense lipoproteins can now move to the liver for uptake by the LDL receptor. The HDL-mediated removal of cholesterol from peripheral tissues—through both SR-B1 and CETP—for transport to the liver and excretion in bile is known as **reverse cholesterol transport**. This process is thought to protect against atherosclerosis.

The liver is the prime site for metabolism and storage of the fat-soluble vitamins A, D, E, and K

We discuss the intestinal uptake of the fat-soluble vitamins in Chapter 45.

Vitamin A Vitamin A (retinol and its derivatives)—like dietary vitamin D, as well as vitamins E and K—is absorbed from the intestine and is then transported in newly synthesized chylomicrons or VLDLs. After some peripheral hydro-

---

Control of Cholesterol Synthesis

HMG-CoA reductase, the rate-limiting enzyme in cholesterol biosynthesis, is a 97-kDa enzyme intrinsic to the ER. The protein is anchored in the ER by a 339–amino acid domain that spans the membrane eight times and is required for activity of the protein. In the short term, decreased intracellular levels of ATP lead to phosphorylation of HMG-CoA reductase, which reduces the activity of the enzyme, presumably preserving energy stores in the cell.

Far more important than the short-term regulation of HMG-CoA reductase is the long-term control of the amount of the enzyme, which can increase as much as 200-fold. The amount of HMG-CoA reductase protein increases after cells are depleted of mevalonate or when the demand for mevalonate-derived metabolites is increased. HMG-CoA reductase activity is upregulated by a combination of enhanced gene transcription, increased mRNA translation, and increased stability of the enzyme. These changes are reversed by the addition of cholesterol or mevalonate to the cells. The transmembrane domain of HMG-CoA reductase may serve as a receptor for the regulatory effects of sterols.

Sterol repression of HMG-CoA reductase gene expression—as well as the expression of LDL and HMG-CoA synthase genes—is mediated by specific transcription factors and specific sequence elements within the 5′ upstream region to which *trans*-acting proteins bind. Several related sterol regulatory elements whose activities mediate sterol repression of gene expression, such as SRE-1, provide a specific sequence required for the recognition of DNA-binding proteins. These SRE-binding proteins (SREBPs; see Chapter 5) are membrane-bound basic helix-loop-helix transcriptional activators (see Chapter 5) that control genes involved in the synthesis and receptor-mediated uptake of cholesterol and fatty acids.

lysis of its triglyceride, the remnant chylomicrons are taken up by the liver. In the hepatocyte, retinyl esters may be hydrolyzed to release free retinol, which can then be transported into the sinusoids bound to **retinol-binding protein** (RBP) and prealbumin. Alternatively, retinyl esters may be stored in the hepatocyte or transported as RBP-bound retinol to **stellate (Ito) cells**, the storage site of more than 80% of hepatic vitamin A under normal conditions. Retinol may also undergo oxidation to **retinal** and conversion to **retinoic acid**, which plays a key role in phototransduction (see Chapter 13). Retinoic acid is conjugated to glucuronide and is secreted into bile, where it undergoes enterohepatic circulation and excretion. Liver disease resulting in cholestasis may lead to a secondary vitamin A deficiency by interfering with absorption in the intestine (lack of the bile needed for digestion/absorption of vitamin A) or by impairing delivery to target tissues because of reduced hepatic synthesis of RBP.

Vitamin D   Skin cells—under the influence of ultraviolet light—synthesize vitamin D_3 (see Chapter 52). Dietary vitamin D can come from either animal sources (D_3) or plant sources (D_2). In either case, the first step in activation of vitamin D is the 25-hydroxylation of vitamin D, catalyzed by a hepatic cytochrome P-450 enzyme. This hydroxylation is followed by 1-hydroxylation in the kidney to yield a product (1,25-dihydroxyvitamin D) with full biological activity. Termination of the activity of 1,25-dihydroxyvitamin D also occurs in the liver by hydroxylation at carbon 24, mediated by another cytochrome P-450 enzyme.

Vitamin E   This fat-soluble vitamin is absorbed from the intestine primarily in the form of α- and γ-tocopherol. It is incorporated into chylomicrons and VLDLs with other products of dietary lipid digestion. As noted earlier, these particles reach the systemic circulation through the lymphatics and undergo some triglyceride hydrolysis. In the process, some vitamin E is transferred to other tissues. The α- and γ-tocopherol remaining in the remnant chylomicrons is transported into the liver, which is the major site of discrimination between the two forms. The α-tocopherol is secreted again as a component of hepatically derived VLDL and perhaps HDL. The γ-tocopherol appears to be metabolized or excreted by the liver. A hepatic tocopherol-binding protein may play a role in this discriminatory process.

Vitamin K   Vitamin K is a fat-soluble vitamin produced by intestinal bacteria. This vitamin is essential for the γ-carboxylation—by the ER enzyme γ-glutamyl carboxylase—of certain glutamate residues in coagulation factors II, VII, IX, and X as well as anticoagulants protein C and protein S and certain other proteins. Intestinal absorption and handling of vitamin K—which is present in two forms, K_1 and K_2—are similar to those of the other fat-soluble vitamins: A, D, and E. Common causes of vitamin K deficiency, which can lead to a serious bleeding disorder, include extrahepatic or intrahepatic cholestasis, fat malabsorption, biliary fistulas, and dietary deficiency, particularly in association with antibiotic therapy.

The liver stores copper and iron

Copper   The trace element copper is essential for the function of cuproenzymes such as cytochrome c oxidase and superoxide dismutase (see Chapter 57). Approximately half the copper in the diet (recommended dietary allowance, 1.5 to 3 mg/day) is absorbed in the jejunum and reaches the liver in the portal blood, mostly bound to albumin. A small fraction is also bound to amino acids, especially histidine. More than 80% of the copper absorbed by the jejunum each day is excreted in bile, for a total of 1.2 to 2.4 mg/day.

The **copper-transport protein Ctr1** imports copper across the hepatocyte basolateral membrane. Copper then binds to a family of intracellular metallochaperones that direct the metal to the appropriate pathway for incorporation into cuproenzymes or for biliary excretion. The copper chaperone **Atox1** moves copper to the secretory pathway and directly interacts with ATP7B, a member of the P_{1B} subfamily of P-type ATPases (see Chapter 5). **ATP7B**, which is mutated in **Wilson disease**, is located predominantly in the *trans*-Golgi network and delivers copper either for incorporation into ceruloplasmin (which is released into the blood; see later) or for excretion into bile. Another chaperone, **Murr1**, appears to be involved in transport of copper to the canalicular membrane for excretion into the bile, complexed to large proteins, such as metallothioneins. The biliary copper-protein complexes cannot be reabsorbed by the small intestine, and hence represent a pathway for copper excretion. Processes that impair the biliary excretion of copper result in the accumulation of copper, initially in the lyso-

---

Wilson Disease

Wilson disease is inherited as an autosomal recessive illness caused by a mutation in ATP7B, the pump responsible for copper accumulation in the *trans*-Golgi network. The impaired biliary excretion of copper causes a buildup of copper in cells, which produces toxic effects in the liver, brain, kidney, cornea, and other tissues. The disease is rare, but it must be considered in the differential diagnosis of anyone younger than 30 years with evidence of significant liver disease. Patients most often have neuropsychiatric complications, including ataxia, tremors, increased salivation, and behavioral changes. Slit-lamp examination of the cornea reveals the diagnostic Kayser-Fleischer rings at the limbus of the cornea.

Because of the lack of functional ATP7B, the apoceruloplasmin in the trans-Golgi network cannot bind copper to form ceruloplasmin. As a result, the hepatocytes secrete **apoceruloplasmin**, which lacks the ferroxidase activity of ceruloplasmin. Moreover, the serum concentrations of ceruloplasmin are low. Indeed, the best way to confirm the diagnosis of Wilson disease is the detection of a low serum ceruloplasmin level and elevated urinary copper excretion. A few affected patients have normal ceruloplasmin levels, and the diagnosis must then be sought with liver biopsy. The disease can be treated by chelating the excess copper with penicillamine.

somal fraction of hepatocytes, with subsequent elevation of plasma copper levels.

Ceruloplasmin, an α_2-globulin synthesized by the liver, binds 95% of copper present in the systemic circulation. Ceruloplasmin has ferroxidase activity but has no critical role in the membrane transport or metabolism of copper.

Iron Dietary iron is absorbed by the duodenal mucosa and is then transported through the blood bound to **transferrin** (see Chapter 45), a protein synthesized in the liver. The liver also takes up, secretes, and stores iron. Entry of iron into hepatocytes is mediated through specific cell surface transferrin receptors (see Chapter 2). Within the cell, a small pool of soluble iron is maintained for intracellular enzymatic reactions, primarily for those involved in electron transport. However, iron is also toxic to the cell. Hence, most intracellular iron is complexed to **ferritin**. The toxicity of iron is clearly evident when normal storage mechanisms become overwhelmed, as occurs in hemochromatosis (see the box on hereditary hemochromatosis in Chapter 45), an autosomal recessive disease in which regulation of iron absorption is uncoupled from total body storage levels.

REFERENCES

Books and Reviews

Boyer JL: Mechanisms of bile secretion and hepatic transport. In Andreoli TE, Hoffman JF, Fanestil DD, Schultz SG (eds): Physiology of Membrane Disorders. New York: Plenum, 1986.

Cooper AD, Ellsworth JL: Lipoprotein metabolism. In Zakim D, Boyer TD (eds): Hepatology. Philadelphia: WB Saunders, 1996.

Kipp H, Arias IM: Trafficking of canalicular ABC transporters in hepatocytes. Annu Rev Physiol 2002; 64:595-608.

Kullak-Ublick GA, Stieger B, Meier PJ: Enterohepatic bile salt transporters in normal physiology and liver disease. Gastroenterology 2004; 126:322-342.

Rhainds D, Brissette L: The role of scavenger receptor class B type I (SR-BI) in lipid trafficking: Defining the rules for lipid traders. Int J Biochem Cell Biol 2004; 36:39-77.

Small DM: Role of ABC transporters in secretion of cholesterol from liver into bile. Proc Natl Acad Sci U S A 2003; 100:4-6.

Tao TY, Gitlin JD: Hepatic copper metabolism: Insights from genetic disease. Hepatology 2003; 37:1241-1247.

Journal Articles

Bull LN, van Eijk MJT, Pawlikowska L: A gene encoding a P-type ATPase mutated in two forms of hereditary cholestasis. Nat Genet 1998; 18:219-224.

Hagenbuch B, Meier PJ: Molecular cloning, chromosomal localization and functional characterization of a human liver Na$^+$/bile acid cotransporter. J Clin Invest 1994; 93:1326-1331.

Kullak-Ublick GA, Hagenbuch B, Stieger B: Molecular and functional characterization of an organic anion transporting polypeptide cloned from human liver. Gastroenterology 1995; 109:1274-1282.

Oude Elferink RPJ, Meijer DKF, Kuipers F, et al: Hepatobiliary secretion of organic compounds: Molecular mechanisms of membrane transport. Biochim Biophys Acta 1995; 1241:215-268.

THE ENDOCRINE SYSTEM

CHAPTER 47

ORGANIZATION OF ENDOCRINE CONTROL

Eugene J. Barrett

With the development of multicellular organisms that have specialized tissues and organs, two major systems evolved to communicate and coordinate body functions:

1. The **nervous system** integrates tissue functions by a network of cells and cell processes that constitute the nervous system and all its subdivisions, as discussed in Chapters 10 through 14.
2. The **endocrine system** integrates organ function through chemicals that are secreted from endocrine tissues or "glands" into the extracellular fluid. These chemicals, called **hormones**, are then carried through the blood to distant target tissues, where they are recognized by specific, high-affinity receptors. As discussed in Chapter 3, these receptors may be located either on the surface of the target tissue, within the cytosol, or in the target cell's nucleus. These receptor molecules allow the target cell to recognize a unique hormonal signal from among the numerous chemicals that are carried through the blood and bathe the body's tissues. The accuracy and sensitivity of this recognition are remarkable in view of the very low concentration (10^{-9} to 10^{-12} M) at which many hormones circulate.

Once a hormone is recognized by its target tissue or tissues, it can exert its biological action by a process known as **signal transduction** (see Chapter 3). In this chapter, we discuss how the signal transduction cascades couple the hormone to its appropriate end responses (see Chapter 3). Some hormones elicit responses within seconds (e.g., the increased heart rate provoked by epinephrine or the stimulation of hepatic glycogen breakdown caused by glucagon), whereas others may require many hours or days (e.g., the changes in salt retention elicited by aldosterone or the increases in protein synthesis caused by growth hormone [GH]). We also examine the principles underlying the feedback mechanisms that control endocrine function. In Chapters 48 to 52, we see how the principles introduced in this chapter apply to specific endocrine systems.

PRINCIPLES OF ENDOCRINE FUNCTION

Chemical signaling can occur through endocrine, paracrine, or autocrine pathways

As shown in Figure 3-1A, in classic **endocrine** signaling, a hormone carries a signal from a secretory gland across a large distance to a target tissue. Hormones secreted into the extracellular space can also regulate nearby cells without ever passing through the systemic circulation. This regulation is referred to as **paracrine** action of a hormone (see Fig 3-1B). Finally, chemicals can also bind to receptors on or in the cell that is actually secreting the hormone and can thus affect the function of the hormone-secreting cell itself. This action is referred to as **autocrine** regulation (see Fig 3-1C). All three mechanisms are illustrated for individual endocrine systems in subsequent chapters. At the outset, it can be appreciated that summation of the endocrine, paracrine, and autocrine actions of a hormone can provide the framework for a complex regulatory system.

Endocrine Glands   The major hormones of the human body are produced by one of seven classic endocrine glands or gland pairs: the pituitary, the thyroid, the parathyroids, the testes, the ovary, the adrenal (cortex and medulla), and the endocrine pancreas. In addition, other tissues that are not classically recognized as part of the endocrine system produce hormones and play a vital role in endocrine regulation. These tissues include the central nervous system (CNS), particularly the hypothalamus, and the gastrointestinal tract, liver, heart, kidney, and others. In some circumstances, particularly with certain neoplasms, nonendocrine tissues can produce hormones that are usually thought to be made only by endocrine glands (see the box titled Neoplastic Hormone Production).

Paracrine Factors   Numerous specialized tissues that are not part of the classic endocrine system release "factors" into the extracellular fluid that can signal neighboring cells to effect a biological response. The interleukins, or lymphokines, are an example of such paracrine factors, as are several of the growth factors, such as platelet-derived growth factor (PDGF), fibroblast growth factor, and others. These factors are not hormones in the usual sense. They are not secreted by glandular tissue, and their sites of action are usually (but not always) within the local environment. However, these signaling molecules share many properties of the classic peptide and amine hormones in that they bind to surface receptors and regulate one or more of the specific intracellular signaling mechanisms described in Chapter 3.

The distinction between the hormones of the classic endocrine systems and other biologically active secreted peptides blurs even further in the case of neuropeptides. For example, the hormone somatostatin is a 28–amino acid peptide secreted by the Δ cells of the pancreatic islet, in which it can exert a paracrine action in the regulation of insulin and glucagon secretion (see Chapter 51). However, somatostatin is also made by hypothalamic neurons. Nerve terminals in the hypothalamus release somatostatin into the pituitary portal bloodstream (see Chapter 48). This specialized segment of the circulatory system then carries the somatostatin from the hypothalamus to the **anterior pituitary**, where it inhibits the secretion of GH. Somatostatin in the hypothalamus is one of several neuropeptides that bridge the body's two major communication systems.

Hormones may be peptides, metabolites of single amino acids, or metabolites of cholesterol

Although the chemical nature of hormones is diverse, most commonly recognized mammalian hormones can be grouped into one of several classes. Table 47-1 is a list of many of the recognized classic mammalian hormones, which are divided into three groups based on their chemical structure and how they are made in the body.

Peptide hormones include a large group of hormones made by a variety of endocrine tissues. Insulin, glucagon, and somatostatin are made in the pancreas. The pituitary gland makes the following: GH; the two gonadotropin hormones, luteinizing hormone (LH) and follicle-stimulating hormone (FSH); adrenocorticotropic hormone (ACTH); thyrotropin (also called thyroid-stimulating hormone or TSH); and prolactin (PRL). Parathyroid hormone (PTH) is made in the parathyroid, and calcitonin is made in the thyroid glands.

In addition, other peptide hormones, such as somatostatin and several releasing hormones (e.g., GH-releasing hormone [GHRH]), are made by the hypothalamus. Secretin, cholecystokinin, and other hormones are made by the gastrointestinal tract, yet these tissues are not considered classic endocrine glands.

More restricted numbers of tissues make **catecholamines** and **steroid hormones**. Synthesis of these hormones (from tyrosine and cholesterol, respectively) necessitates certain enzymatic steps. Only very specialized tissues are capable of the series of enzymatic conversions necessary to make active hormone from the starting materials. Synthesis of thyroid hormone is even more complex and is essentially entirely restricted to the thyroid gland.

Several glands make two or more hormones. Examples are the pituitary, the pancreatic islets, and the adrenal

---

Neoplastic Hormone Production

The ability of nonendocrine tissue to produce hormones first became apparent with the description of clinical syndromes in which some patients with lung cancer were found to make excessive amounts of AVP, a hormone usually made by the hypothalamus. Shortly afterward, people with other lung or gastrointestinal tumors were found to make ACTH, which is normally made only in the pituitary. Subsequently, many hormone-secreting neoplastic tissues were described. As the ability to measure hormones in tissues has improved and, in particular, as the capability of measuring mRNA that codes for specific peptide hormones has developed, it has become clear that hormone production by neoplastic tissue is quite common, although most tumors produce only small amounts that may have no clinical consequence.

The production of hormones by nonendocrine neoplastic cells has been most clearly defined for cancers of the lung. Several different types of lung cancer occur, each deriving from a different cell line, and yet each is capable of producing one or several hormones. The clinical syndromes that result from secretion of these hormones are often called **paraneoplastic syndromes**. Thus, lung cancers arising from squamous cells are sometimes associated with hypercalcemia, which results from the secretion of a protein—PTH-related peptide—that can mimic the activity of PTH (see Chapter 52). Small cell lung cancers are notorious for their ability to secrete numerous hormones, including AVP or ADH (with resultant hyponatremia; see Chapter 38 for the box on Syndrome of Inappropriate Antidiuretic Hormone Secretion), ACTH (with resultant Cushing syndrome; see Chapter 50), and many others. Still other types of lung cancer produce other paraneoplastic syndromes.

Nearly all these ectopic, neoplastic sources of hormone produce *peptide* hormones. Other sources of hormone production, in addition to lung cancer, include gastrointestinal tumors, renal and bladder cancer, neural tumors, unique tumors called **carcinoid tumors** that can arise almost anywhere in the body, and even lymphomas and melanomas. In some patients, the symptoms and signs resulting from ectopic hormone production may appear before any other reason exists to suspect an underlying neoplasm, and these symptoms may be the key clues to the correct diagnosis.

---

medulla. However, for the most part, individual cells within these glands are specialized to secrete a single hormone. One exception is the gonadotropin-producing cells of the pituitary, which secrete both FSH and LH.

Hormones can circulate either free or bound to carrier proteins

Once secreted, many hormones circulate freely in the blood until they reach their target tissue. Others form complexes with circulating **binding proteins**; this use of binding proteins is particularly true for thyroid hormones (thyroxine [T_4] and triiodothyronine [T_3]), steroid hormones, insulin-

Table 47-1   Chemical Classification of Selected Hormones

Peptide Hormones
ACTH
Atrial natriuretic peptide (ANP)
AVP (ADH)
Calcitonin
Cholecystokinin (CCK)
CRH
FSH
Glucagon
GnRH
GH
GHRH
Inhibin
Insulin
IGFs
LH
Oxytocin
PTH
PRL
Secretin
Somatostatin
TSH
TRH
Vasoactive intestinal peptide (VIP)

Amino Acid–Derived Hormones
DA
Epinephrine (adrenaline)
Norepinephrine (noradrenaline)
Serotonin (5-HT)
T_4
T_3

Steroid Hormones
Aldosterone
Cortisol
Estradiol (E2)
Progesterone
Testosterone

like growth factor types 1 and 2 (IGF-1 and IGF-2), and GH.

Forming a complex with a circulating binding protein serves several functions. First, it provides the blood with a reservoir or pool of the hormone, thus minimizing minute-to-minute fluctuations in hormone concentration. Second, it extends the half-life of the hormone in the circulation. For example, more than 99.99% of T_4 circulates bound to one of three binding proteins (see Chapter 49); the half-life of circulating T_4 is 7 to 8 days, whereas the half-life of free T_4 is only several minutes. The hormones bound to plasma binding proteins appear to be those whose actions are *long term*—in particular, those involving induction of the synthesis of new protein in target tissues. Hormones that play a major *short-term* role in the regulation of body metabolism (e.g., catecholamines, many peptide hormones) circulate freely without associated binding proteins.

The presence of plasma binding proteins can affect the total circulating concentration of a hormone without neces-

sarily affecting the concentration of unbound or **free hormone** in the blood. For example, during pregnancy, the liver's synthesis of T_4-binding globulin increases. Because this protein avidly binds T_4, the free T_4 concentration would fall. However, the pituitary senses the small decline in free T_4 levels and secretes more TSH. As a result, the thyroid makes more T_4, so plasma levels of total T_4 rise. However, the free T_4 level is unchanged.

Immunoassays allow measurement of circulating hormones

In the late 1950s, Solomon Berson and Rosalyn Yalow demonstrated that in patients who receive insulin, the body forms antibodies directed against the insulin molecule. This observation was important in two respects:

1. It advanced the principle that the body's immune system can react to endogenous compounds; therefore, autoimmunity or reaction to self-antigens does occur. This notion is a fundamental tenet of our current understanding of many autoimmune diseases, among which are endocrine diseases such as type 1 diabetes mellitus, autoimmune hypothyroidism, and Graves disease, a common form of autoimmune hyperthyroidism. Before the description of insulin autoantibodies, it was thought that the immune system simply did not react to self-antigens.

2. Because antibodies with a high affinity for insulin were induced in patients who were treated with insulin, Berson and Yalow reasoned that these antibodies could be used to measure the amount of insulin in serum. Figure 47-1 illustrates the principle of a **radioimmunoassay** and how it is used to measure the concentration of a hormone (or many other chemicals). If we incubate increasing amounts of a radiolabeled hormone with an antibody to that hormone, the quantity of labeled hormone that is bound to the antibody will yield a saturation plot (Fig. 47-1A). If we now add unlabeled hormone to the incubation mixture, less radioactively labeled hormone will remain complexed to the antibody as unlabeled hormone takes its place. The more unlabeled hormone we add, the less labeled hormone is bound to the antibody (Fig. 47-1B). A **displacement curve** is created by plotting the amount of radioactively labeled hormone complexed to the antibody as a function of the concentration of unlabeled hormone that is added (Fig. 47-1C). This displacement curve can then be used as a standard curve to estimate the amount of hormone present in unknown samples. This estimate is accurate only if two assumptions hold true: first, that nothing else in the unknown mixture binds with the antibody other than the hormone under study, and second, that nothing in the unknown sample interferes with normal binding of the hormone to the antibody.

Antibodies that are highly specific for the chemical structure of interest can frequently be obtained. Moreover, these antibodies are of sufficiently high affinity to bind even the often minute amounts of hormone that is circulating in blood. Thus, radioimmunoassays—and recent adaptations

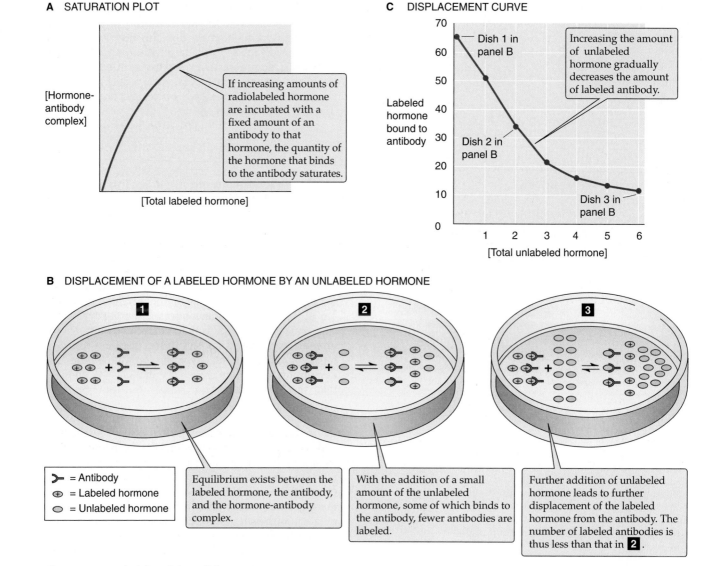

Figure 47-1 Principles of the radioimmunoassay.

that substitute chemiluminescent or enzymatic detection for radioactivity—have emerged as a potent and popular tool. Radioimmunoassays are now used for the measurement of virtually all hormones, as well as many drugs, viruses, and toxins. Much of our understanding of the physiology of hormone secretion and action has been gained by the use of immunoassay methodology. Yalow shared the 1977 Nobel Prize in Medicine or Physiology for the discovery of the radioimmunoassay (Berson died before the honor was bestowed).

Hormones can have complementary and antagonistic actions

Regulation of certain complex physiological functions necessitates the **complementary action** of several hormones. This principle is true both for minute-to-minute homeostasis and for more long-term processes. For example, epinephrine (adrenaline), cortisol, and glucagon each contribute to the body's response to a short-term period of exercise (e.g., swimming the 50-m butterfly or running the 100-m dash). If any of these hormones is missing, exercise performance is adversely affected, and even more seriously, severe hypoglycemia and hyperkalemia (elevated plasma $[K^+]$) may develop. On a longer time scale, GH, insulin, IGF-1, thyroid hormone, and sex steroids are all needed for normal growth. Deficiency of GH, IGF-1, or thyroid hormone results in dwarfism. Deficiency of sex steroids, cortisol, or insulin produces less severe disturbances of growth.

Integration of hormone action can also involve hormones that exert **antagonistic actions**. In this case, the overall effect on an end organ depends on the balance between opposing influences. One example is the counterpoised effects of insulin and glucagon on blood glucose levels. Insulin lowers glucose levels by *inhibiting* glycogenolysis and gluconeogenesis in the liver and by stimulating glucose uptake into muscle and adipose tissue. Glucagon, in contrast, *stimulates* hepatic glycogenolysis and gluconeogenesis. Whereas glucagon does not appear to antagonize glucose uptake directly, epinephrine (which, like glucagon, is released in response to hypoglycemia) does. Balancing of tissue function by opposing humoral effector mechanisms appears to be an important regulatory strategy for refining the control of many cellular functions.

Endocrine regulation occurs through feedback control

The key to any regulatory system is its ability to sense when it should increase or decrease its activity. For the endocrine system, this function is accomplished by feedback control of hormone secretion (Fig. 47-2A). The hormone-secreting cell functions as a sensor that continually monitors the circulating concentration of some regulated variable. This variable may be a metabolic factor (e.g., glucose concentration) or the activity of another hormone. When the endocrine gland

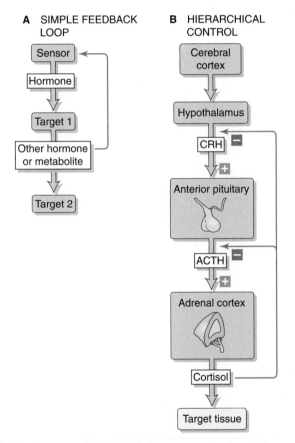

A   SIMPLE FEEDBACK LOOP

B   HIERARCHICAL CONTROL

senses that too much (or too little) of the regulated variable is circulating in blood, it responds by decreasing (or increasing) the rate of hormone secretion. This response, in turn, affects the metabolic or secretory behavior of the target tissue, which may either directly feed back to the sensing cell or stimulate some other cell that eventually signals the sensor regarding whether the altered function of the endocrine gland has been effective.

A simple example is insulin secretion by the β cells of the pancreas. Increases in plasma [glucose] are sensed by the β cell, which secretes insulin in response. The rise in plasma [insulin] acts on the liver to decrease the synthesis of glucose and on the muscle to promote the storage of glucose. As a result, plasma [glucose] falls, and this decrease is sensed by the β cell, which reduces the rate of insulin secretion. This arrangement represents a very simple feedback system. Other systems can be quite complex; however, even this simple system involves the recognition of two circulating signals. The liver and muscle recognize the increase in plasma [insulin] as one signal, and the pancreatic β cell (the cell responsible for insulin secretion) recognizes the signal of a rise or decline in blood [glucose] as the other signal. In each case, the sensing system within a particular tissue is linked to an effector system that transduces the signal to the appropriate biological response.

Endocrine regulation can involve hierarchic levels of control

Faced with a stressor (e.g., a severe infection or extensive blood loss), the cerebral cortex stimulates the hypothalamus to release a neuropeptide called corticotropin-releasing hormone (CRH; Fig. 47-2B). Carried by the pituitary portal system (blood vessels that connect the hypothalamus to the anterior pituitary), CRH stimulates the anterior pituitary to release another hormone, ACTH, which, in turn, stimulates the adrenal cortical cells to synthesize cortisol. Cortisol regulates vascular tone as well as metabolic and growth functions in a variety of tissues.

This *stress response* therefore involves two glands, the pituitary and the adrenal cortex, as well as specialized neuroendocrine tissue in the hypothalamus and the CNS. This hierarchic control is regulated by feedback, just as in the simple feedback between plasma [glucose] and insulin. Within this CRH-ACTH-cortisol axis, feedback can occur at several levels. Cortisol inhibits the production of CRH by the hypothalamus, as well as the sensitivity of the pituitary to a standard dose of CRH, which directly reduces ACTH release.

Feedback in hierarchic endocrine control systems can be quite complex and frequently involves interaction between the CNS and the endocrine system. Other examples are regulation of the female menstrual cycle (see Chapter 55) and regulation of GH secretion (see Chapter 48).

Among the classic endocrine tissues, the **pituitary** (also known as the hypophysis) plays a special role (Fig. 47-3). Located at the base of the brain, just below the hypothalamus, the pituitary resides within a saddle-shaped cavity called the *sella turcica* (from the Latin *sella* [saddle] + *turcica* [Turkish]), which has bony anterior, posterior, and inferior borders and fibrous tissue that separate it from venous

Figure 47-2   Feedback control of hormone secretion. **A**, A sensor (e.g., a β cell in a pancreatic islet) detects some regulated variable (e.g., plasma [glucose]) and responds by modulating its secretion of a hormone (e.g., insulin). This hormone, in turn, acts on a target (e.g., liver or muscle) to modulate its production of another hormone or a metabolite (e.g., glucose), which may affect a second target (e.g., making glucose available to the brain). In addition, the other hormone or metabolite feeds back on the original sensor cell. **B**, Under the influence of the cerebral cortex, the hypothalamus releases CRH, which stimulates the anterior pituitary to release ACTH, which, in turn, stimulates the adrenal cortex to release cortisol. The cortisol acts on certain effector organs. In addition, the cortisol feeds back on both the anterior pituitary and the hypothalamus.

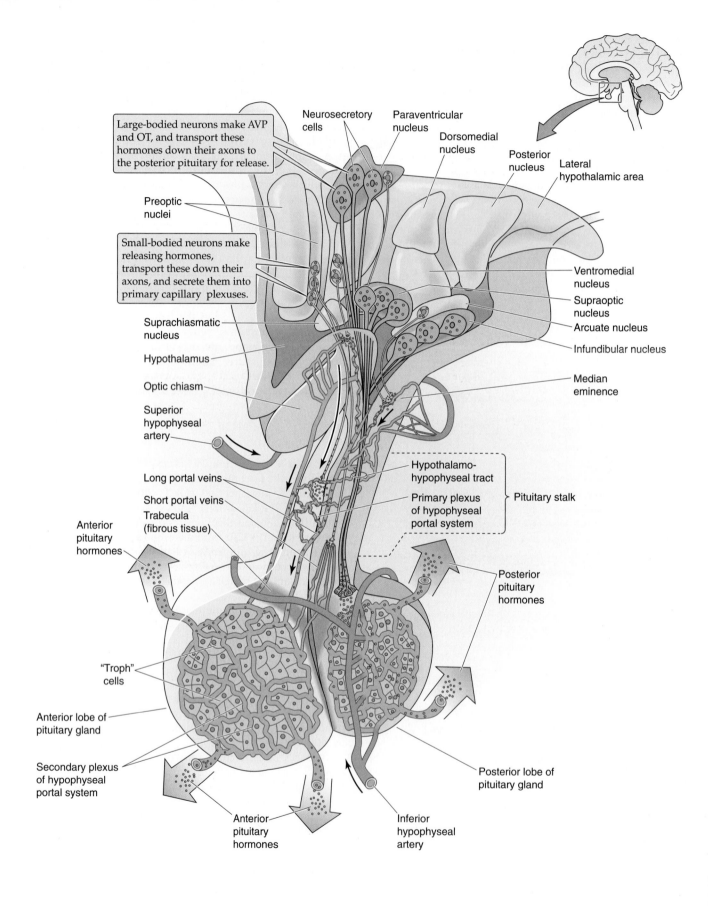

Large-bodied neurons make AVP and OT, and transport these hormones down their axons to the posterior pituitary for release.

Neurosecretory cells

Paraventricular nucleus

Dorsomedial nucleus

Posterior nucleus

Lateral hypothalamic area

Preoptic nuclei

Small-bodied neurons make releasing hormones, transport these down their axons, and secrete them into primary capillary plexuses.

Ventromedial nucleus

Supraoptic nucleus

Arcuate nucleus

Suprachiasmatic nucleus

Infundibular nucleus

Hypothalamus

Optic chiasm

Median eminence

Superior hypophyseal artery

Hypothalamo-hypophyseal tract

Long portal veins

Primary plexus of hypophyseal portal system

Pituitary stalk

Short portal veins

Trabecula (fibrous tissue)

Anterior pituitary hormones

Posterior pituitary hormones

"Troph" cells

Anterior lobe of pituitary gland

Secondary plexus of hypophyseal portal system

Posterior lobe of pituitary gland

Anterior pituitary hormones

Inferior hypophyseal artery

Figure 47-3 The hypothalamopituitary axis. The pituitary (or hypophysis) is actually two glands—an anterior pituitary and a posterior pituitary (or neurohypophysis). Although in both cases the hypothalamus controls the secretion of hormones by the pituitary, the mechanisms are very different. **Anterior pituitary:** Small-bodied neurons in the hypothalamus secrete *releasing* and *inhibitory factors* into a rich, funnel-shaped plexus of capillaries that penetrates the median eminence and surrounds the infundibular recess. The cell bodies of these neurons are found in several nuclei that surround the third ventricle. These include the arcuate, the paraventricular and ventromedial nuclei, and the medial preoptic and periventricular regions. The capillaries (primary plexus), which are outside of the blood-brain barrier, coalesce into *long* portal veins that carry the releasing and inhibitory factors down the pituitary stalk to the anterior pituitary. Other neurons secrete their releasing factors into a capillary plexus that is much farther down the pituitary stalk; *short* portal veins carry these releasing factors to the anterior pituitary. There, the portal veins break up into the secondary capillary plexus of the anterior pituitary and deliver the releasing and inhibitory factors to the "troph" cells that actually secrete the anterior pituitary hormones (TSH, ACTH, PRL) that enter the systemic bloodstream and distribute throughout the body. **Posterior pituitary:** Large neurons in the paraventricular and supraoptic nuclei of the hypothalamus actually synthesize the hormones AVP and oxytocin (OT). These hormones travel down the axons of the hypothalamic neurons to the posterior pituitary where the nerve terminals release the hormones, like neurotransmitters, into a rich plexus of vessels.

sinuses on either side. The human pituitary is composed of both an anterior lobe and a posterior lobe. Through vascular and neural connections, the pituitary bridges and integrates the neural and endocrine mechanisms of homeostasis. The pituitary is a highly vascular tissue. The posterior pituitary receives arterial blood, whereas the anterior pituitary receives only portal venous inflow from the median eminence. The **pituitary portal system** is particularly important in its function of carrying neuropeptides from the hypothalamus and pituitary stalk to the anterior pituitary.

The anterior pituitary regulates reproduction, growth, energy metabolism, and stress response

Glandular tissue in the anterior lobe of the pituitary synthesizes and secretes six peptide hormones: GH, TSH, ACTH, LH, FSH, and PRL. In each case, secretion of these hormones is under the control of hypothalamic **releasing hormones** (Table 47-2). The sources of these releasing hormones are small-diameter neurons located mainly in the periventricu-

Table 47-2 Hypothalamic and Pituitary Hormones

ANTERIOR PITUITARY			
Releasing (Inhibitory) Factor Made by Hypothalamus	**Target Cell in Anterior Pituitary**	**Hormone Released by Anterior Pituitary**	**Target of Anterior Pituitary Hormone**
GHRH (inhibited by somatostatin)	Somatotroph	GH	Stimulates IGF-1 production by multiple somatic tissues, especially liver
TRH	Thyrotroph	TSH	Thyroid follicular cells, stimulated to make thyroid hormone
CRH	Corticotroph	ACTH	Fasciculata and reticularis cells of the adrenal cortex, to make corticosteroids
GnRH	Gonadotroph	FSH	Ovarian follicular cells, to make estrogens and progestins Sertoli cells, to initiate spermatogenesis
GnRH	Gonadotroph	LH	Leydig cells, to make testosterone
(inhibited by dopamine)	Lactotroph	PRL	Mammary glands, to initiate and maintain milk production
POSTERIOR PITUITARY			
Hormone Synthesized in Hypothalamus	**Hormone Released into Posterior Pituitary**	**Target of Posterior Pituitary**	
AVP	AVP	Collecting duct, to increase water permeability	
OT	OT	Uterus and breast	

OT, oxytocin.

lar portion of the hypothalamus that surrounds the third ventricle. These small-diameter neurons synthesize the releasing hormones and discharge them into the median eminence and neural stalk, where they enter leaky capillaries—which are not part of the blood-brain barrier (see Chapter 11). The releasing hormones then travel through the pituitary portal veins to the anterior pituitary. Once in the anterior pituitary, a releasing factor stimulates specialized cells to release a particular peptide hormone into the systemic bloodstream. The integrative function of the anterior pituitary can be appreciated by realizing that the main target for four of the anterior pituitary hormones (i.e., TSH, ACTH, and LH/FSH) is other endocrine tissue. Thus, these four anterior pituitary hormones are themselves releasing hormones that trigger the secretion of specific hormones. For example, TSH causes the follicular cells in the thyroid gland to synthesize and release thyroid hormones. The mechanism by which the pituitary regulates these endocrine glands is discussed in detail in Chapters 48 to 52.

GH also acts as a releasing factor in that it regulates the production of another hormone, IGF-1. IGF-1 is made in principally *non*endocrine tissues (e.g., liver, kidney, muscle, and cartilage). Nevertheless, IGF-1 in the circulation feeds back on the hypothalamus and on the pituitary to inhibit GH secretion. In this respect, the GH–IGF-1 axis is similar to axes involving classic pituitary pathways, such as the thyrotropin-releasing hormone (TRH)–TSH axis.

Regulation of PRL secretion differs from that of other anterior pituitary hormones in that no endocrine feedback mechanism has yet been identified. The pituitary secretes **PRL** at relatively low levels throughout life both in boys and men and in girls and women. However, its major biological action, promotion of lactation, is important only in women and only at specific times in a woman's life. Although PRL is not part of an identified feedback system, its release is controlled. Left to its own devices, the anterior pituitary would secrete high levels of PRL. However, secretion of PRL is normally inhibited by the release of dopamine (DA) from the hypothalamus (see Chapter 56). During breast stimulation, neural afferents inhibit hypothalamic DA release, thus inhibiting release of the inhibitor and permitting lactation to proceed. PRL receptors are present on multiple tissues other than the breast. However, other physiological actions beyond lactation have not been well characterized.

The posterior pituitary regulates water balance and uterine contraction

Unlike the anterior pituitary, the posterior lobe of the pituitary is actually part of the brain. The posterior pituitary (or neurohypophysis) contains the nerve endings of *large*-diameter neurons whose cell bodies are in the supraoptic and paraventricular nuclei of the hypothalamus (Fig. 47-3). Recall that the hypothalamic neurons that produce releasing factors, which act on "troph" cells in the anterior pituitary, are *small*-diameter neurons. The large-diameter hypothalamic neurons synthesize arginine vasopressin (AVP) and oxytocin and then transport these hormones along their axons to the site of release in the posterior pituitary. Thus, like the anterior pituitary, the posterior pituitary releases peptide hormones. Also as in the anterior pituitary, release

of these hormones is under ultimate control of the hypothalamus. However, the hypothalamic axons traveling to the posterior pituitary replace both the transport of releasing factors by the portal system of the anterior pituitary and the synthesis of hormones by the anterior pituitary "troph" cells. Although the posterior pituitary is part of the brain, it is one of the so-called *circumventricular organs* (see Chapter 11) whose vessels breach the blood-brain barrier and allow the secreted AVP and oxytocin to reach the systemic circulation.

AVP, or antidiuretic hormone (ADH), is a neuropeptide hormone that acts on the collecting duct of the kidney to increase water reabsorption (see Chapter 38). **Oxytocin** is the other neuropeptide secreted by the posterior pituitary. However, its principal biological action relates to stimulation of smooth muscle contraction by the uterus during parturition and by the mammary gland during suckling (see Chapter 56).

These two posterior pituitary hormones appear to have a common ancestor—vasotocin—in amphibians and other submammalian species. The two peptide hormones secreted by the posterior pituitary are each made by hypothalamic neurons as a precursor molecule that is transported along the axons of the hypothalamic neurons to the posterior pituitary. For AVP, this precursor protein is proneurophysin II, as detailed in Chapter 40 and illustrated in Figure 40-8, whereas for oxytocin it is proneurophysin I. In each case, cleavage of the precursor occurs during transport along the axons from the hypothalamus to the posterior pituitary. When the active neurohormone is secreted (e.g., AVP), its residual neurophysin is co-secreted stoichiometrically. Defects in the processing of the neurophysin precursor can lead to impaired and secretion of active hormone. In the case of AVP, the result is partial or complete diabetes insipidus.

PEPTIDE HORMONES

Specialized endocrine cells synthesize, store, and secrete peptide hormones

Organisms as primitive as fungi secrete proteins or peptides in an effort to respond to and affect their environment. In more complex organisms, peptide hormones play important developmental and other regulatory roles. Transcription of peptide hormones is regulated by both *cis*- and *trans*-acting elements (see Chapter 4). When transcription is active, the mRNA is processed in the nucleus, and the capped message moves to the cytosol, where it associates with ribosomes on the rough endoplasmic reticulum. These peptides are destined for secretion because an amino acid *signal sequence* present near the N terminus targets the protein to the endoplasmic reticulum while the protein is still associated with the ribosome (see Fig. 2-15).

With minor modification, the **secretory pathway** that is illustrated in Figure 2-18 describes the synthesis, processing, storage, and secretion of peptides by a wide variety of endocrine tissues. Once the protein is in the lumen of the endoplasmic reticulum, processing (e.g., glycosylation or further proteolytic cleavage) yields the mature, biologically active hormone. This processing occurs in a very dynamic setting.

The protein is first transferred to the *cis*-Golgi domain, then through to the *trans*-Golgi, and finally to the mature, membrane-bound secretory vesicle or granule in which the mature hormone is stored before secretion. This pathway is referred to as the **regulated pathway** of hormone synthesis because external stimuli can trigger the cell to release hormone that is stored in the secretory granule, as well as to promote the synthesis of additional hormone. For example, binding of GHRH to somatotrophs causes them to release GH.

A second pathway of hormone synthesis is the **constitutive pathway**. Here, secretion occurs more directly from the endoplasmic reticulum or vesicles formed in the *cis*-Golgi. Secretion of hormone, both mature and partially processed, by the constitutive pathway is less responsive to secretory stimuli than is secretion by the regulated pathway.

In both the regulated and constitutive pathways, fusion of the vesicular membrane with the plasma membrane—exocytosis of the vesicular contents—is the final common pathway for hormone secretion. In general, the regulated pathway is capable of secreting much larger amounts of hormone—on demand—than is the constitutive pathway. However, even when stimulated to secrete its peptide hormone, the cell typically secretes only a very small amount of the total hormone present in the secretory granules. To maintain this secretory reserve, many endocrine cells increase the synthesis of peptide hormones in response to the same stimuli that trigger secretion.

Peptide hormones bind to cell surface receptors and activate a variety of signal transduction systems

Once secreted, most peptide hormones exist free in the circulation. As noted earlier, this lack of binding proteins contrasts with the situation for steroid and thyroid hormones, which circulate bound to plasma proteins. IGF-1 and IGF-2 are an exception to this rule: at least six plasma proteins bind these peptide growth factors.

While traversing the circulation, peptide hormones encounter receptors on the surface of target cells. These receptors are intrinsic membrane proteins that bind the hormone with very high affinity (typically, K_D ranges from 10^{-8} to 10^{-12} M). Examples of several types of peptide hormone receptors are shown in Figure 47-4. Each of these receptors has already been introduced in Chapter 3. The primary sequence of most peptide hormone receptors is known from molecular cloning, mutant receptors have been synthesized, and the properties of native and mutant receptors have been compared to assess primary structural requirements for receptor function. Despite this elegant work, too little information is available on the three-dimensional structure of these membrane proteins for us to know just how the message that a hormone has bound to the receptor is transmitted to the internal surface of the cell membrane. However, regardless of the details, occupancy of the receptor can activate many different intracellular signal transduction systems (Table 47-3) that transfer the signal of cell activation from the internal surface of the membrane to intracellular targets. The receptor provides the link between a specific extracellular hormone and the activation of a specific signal transduction system. We discussed each of these signal transduction systems in Chapter 3. Here, we briefly review the various signal transduction systems through which peptide hormones act.

G Proteins Coupled to Adenylyl Cyclase cAMP, the prototypic second messenger, was discovered during an investigation of the action of glucagon on glycogenolysis in the liver. In addition to playing a role in hormone action, cAMP is involved in such diverse processes as lymphocyte activation, mast cell degranulation, and even slime mold aggregation.

As summarized in Figure 47-4A, binding of the appropriate hormone (e.g., PTH) to its receptor initiates a cascade of events (see Chapter 3): (1) activation of a heterotrimeric G protein (α_s or α_i); (2) activation (by α_s) or inhibition (by α_i) of a membrane-bound adenylyl cyclase; (3) formation of intracellular cAMP from ATP, catalyzed by adenylyl cyclase; (4) binding of cAMP to the enzyme protein kinase A (PKA); (5) separation of the two catalytic subunits of PKA from the two regulatory subunits; (6) phosphorylation of *serine* and *threonine* residues on a variety of cellular enzymes and other proteins by the free catalytic subunits of PKA that are no longer restrained; and (7) modification of cellular function by these phosphorylations. The activation is terminated in two ways. First, phosphodiesterases in the cell degrade cAMP. Second, *serine/threonine*-specific protein phosphatases can dephosphorylate enzymes and proteins that had previously been phosphorylated by PKA.

G Proteins Coupled to Phospholipase C As summarized in Figure 47-4B, binding of the appropriate peptide hormone (e.g., AVP) to its receptor initiates the following cascade of events (see Chapter 3): (1) activation of $G\alpha_q$; (2) activation of a membrane-bound phospholipase C (PLC); and (3) cleavage of phosphatidylinositol 4,5-biphosphate (PIP_2) by this PLC, with the generation of *two* signaling molecules, inositol 1,4,5-triphosphate (IP_3) and diacylglycerol (DAG); (4) the first step in the IP_3 fork of the pathway is binding of IP_3 to a receptor on the cytosolic surface of the endoplasmic reticulum; (5) release of Ca^{2+} from internal stores, which causes $[Ca^{2+}]_i$ to rise by several-fold; (6) activation of Ca^{2+}-dependent kinases (e.g., Ca^{2+}-calmodulin–dependent protein kinases, protein kinase C [PKC]) by the increases in $[Ca^{2+}]_i$; and (7) alteration of cell function.

The first step in the DAG fork of the pathway is (4) allosteric activation of PKC by DAG (the activity of this enzyme is also stimulated by the increased $[Ca^{2+}]_i$) and (5) phosphorylation of a variety of proteins by PKC, which is activated in the plane of the cell membrane. An example of a hormone whose actions are in part mediated by DAG is TSH.

G Proteins Coupled to Phospholipase A₂ As summarized in Figure 47-4C, some peptide hormones (e.g., TRH) activate phospholipase A_2 (PLA_2) through the following cascade (see Chapter 3): (1) activation of $G\alpha_q$ or $G\alpha_{11}$, (2) stimulation of membrane-bound PLA_2 by the activated $G\alpha$, (3) cleavage of membrane phospholipids by PLA_2 to produce lysophospholipid and arachidonic acid, and (4) conversion—by certain enzymes—of arachidonic acid into

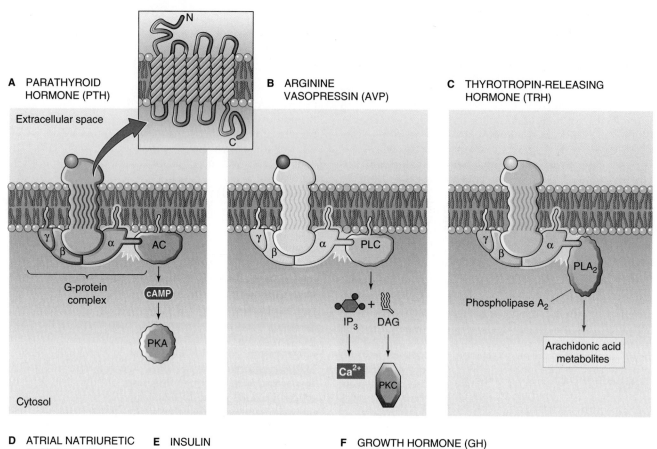

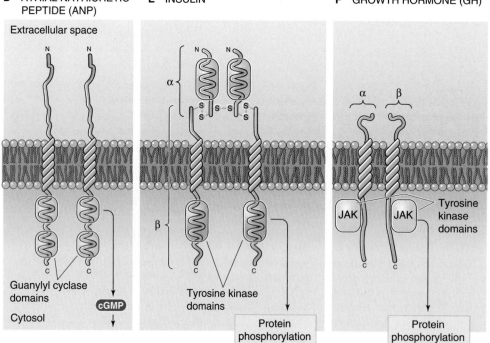

Figure 47-4 **A** to **F**, Receptors and downstream effectors for peptide hormones. AC, adenylyl cyclase; JAK, Janus kinase or just another kinase.

Table 47-3 Peptide Hormones and Their Signal Transduction Pathways

Agonists	Receptor	Linked Enzyme	Second Messenger
PTH	Coupled to $G\alpha_s$	Adenylyl cyclase	cAMP
ANG II	Coupled to $G\alpha_i$	Adenylyl cyclase (inhibited)	cAMP
AVP, ANG II, TRH	Coupled to $G\alpha_q$	PLC	IP_3 and DAG
ANG II	Coupled to G_i/G_o	PLA_2	Arachidonic acid metabolites
ANP	Guanylyl cyclase	Guanylyl cyclase	cGMP
Insulin, IGF-1, IGF-2, EGF, PDGF	Tyrosine kinase	Tyrosine kinase	Phosphoproteins
GH, erythropoietin, LIF	Associated with tyrosine kinase	JAK-STAT family of tyrosine kinases	Phosphoproteins

ANG II, angiotensin II; ANP, atrial natriuretic peptide; EGF, epidermal growth factor; JAK-STAT, Janus kinase/signal transducer and activator of transcription; LIF, leukemia inhibitory factor.

Pseudohypoparathyroidism

Inasmuch as G proteins are part of the signaling system involved in large numbers of hormone responses, molecular alterations in G proteins could be expected to affect certain signaling systems. In the disorder **pseudohypoparathyroidism**, the key defect is an abnormality in a stimulatory α subunit (α_s) of a heterotrimeric G protein. The result is an impairment in the ability of PTH to regulate body calcium and phosphorus homeostasis (see Chapter 52). Patients with this disorder have a low serum $[Ca^{2+}]$ and high serum phosphate level, just like patients whose parathyroid glands have been surgically removed. However, patients with pseudohypoparathyroidism have **increased** circulating concentrations of PTH; the hormone simply cannot act normally on its target tissue, hence the term *pseudohypoparathyroidism*. These individuals also have an increased risk of hypothyroidism, as well as of gonadal dysfunction in women. These additional endocrine deficiencies arise from the same defect in signaling.

a variety of biologically active eicosanoids (e.g., prostaglandins, prostacyclins, thromboxanes, and leukotrienes).

Guanylyl Cyclase Other peptide hormones (e.g., atrial natriuretic peptide) bind to a receptor (Fig. 47-4D) that is itself a guanylyl cyclase that converts cytoplasmic guanosine triphosphate to cGMP (see Chapter 3). In turn, cGMP can activate cGMP-dependent kinases, phosphatases, or ion channels.

Receptor Tyrosine Kinases For some peptide hormones, notably insulin and IGF-1 and IGF-2, the hormone receptor (Fig. 47-4E) itself possesses tyrosine kinase activity (see Chapter 3). This property is also true for other growth factors, including PDGF and epidermal growth factor. Occupancy of the receptor by the appropriate hormone increases kinase activity. For the insulin and IGF-1 receptor, as well as for others, this kinase autophosphorylates tyrosines within the hormone receptor, as well as substrates within the cytosol, thus initiating a cascade of phosphorylation reactions.

Tyrosine Kinase–Associated Receptors Some peptide hormones (e.g., GH) bind to a receptor that, when occupied, activates a cytoplasmic tyrosine kinase (Fig. 47-4F), such as a member of the JAK (Janus kinase) family of kinases (see Chapter 3). As for the receptor tyrosine kinases, activation of these receptor-associated kinases initiates a cascade of phosphorylation reactions.

AMINE HORMONES

Amine hormones are made from tyrosine and tryptophan

Four major amine hormones are recognized. The adrenal medulla makes the catecholamine hormones **epinephrine** and **norepinephrine** from the amino acid tyrosine (see Fig. 13-8C). These hormones are the principal active amine hormones made by the endocrine system. In addition to its role as a hormone, norepinephrine also serves as a neurotransmitter by the CNS (see Chapter 13) and by postganglionic sympathetic neurons (see Chapter 14). **DA**, which is also synthesized from tyrosine, acts as a neurotransmitter (see Chapter 13); it is synthesized in certain other tissues, but its functional role outside the nervous system is not well clarified. Finally, the hormone **serotonin** is made from tryptophan (see Fig. 12-8B) by endocrine cells that are located within the gut mucosa. Serotonin appears to act locally to regulate both motor and secretory function of the gut.

The human **adrenal medulla** secretes principally epinephrine (see Chapter 50). The final products are stored in vesicles called **chromaffin granules**. Secretion of catecholamines by the adrenal medulla appears to be mediated entirely by stimulation of the sympathetic division of the autonomic nervous system (see Chapter 14). Unlike the situation for many peptide hormones, in which the circulating concentration of the hormone (e.g., TSH) negatively feeds back on secretion of the releasing hormone (e.g., TRH), the amine hormones do not have such a hierarchic feedback system. Rather, the feedback of amine hormones is indirect. The higher control center does not sense circulating levels of the amine hormones (e.g., epinephrine), but rather a physiological end effect of that amine hormone (e.g., blood pressure; see Chapter 23). The sensor of the end effect may be a peripheral receptor (e.g., stretch receptor) that communicates to the higher center (e.g., the CNS), and the efferent limb is the sympathetic outflow that determines release of the amine.

Serotonin (5-hydroxytryptamine [5-HT]), in addition to being an important neurotransmitter in the CNS (see Fig. 13-7B), is a hormone made by **neuroendocrine cells**, principally located within the lining of the small intestine and larger bronchi. Unlike the other hormones that we discuss in this chapter, serotonin is not made by a specific gland. Little is known about feedback regulation or even regulation of secretion of this hormone. Serotonin arouses considerable clinical interest because of the dramatic clinical presentation of patients with unusual tumors—called **carcinoid tumors**—of serotonin-secreting cells. These individuals frequently present with a *carcinoid syndrome* characterized by episodes of spontaneous, intense flushing in a typical pattern involving the head and neck, associated with diarrhea, bronchospasm, and occasionally right-sided valvular heart disease. The primary tumors involved can occur within the intestinal tract, in the bronchial tree, or more rarely at other sites.

Amine hormones act through surface receptors

Once secreted, circulating epinephrine is free to associate with specific adrenergic receptors or **adrenoceptors** located on the surface membranes of target cells. Numerous types of adrenoceptors exist and are generically grouped as α or β, each of which has several subtypes (see Table 15-2). All adrenoceptors, isolated from a variety of tissues and species, are classic G protein–coupled receptors. As indicated in Figure 47-5, the intracellular action of a specific catecholamine is determined by the complement of receptors present on the surface of a specific cell. For example, when epinephrine binds to the β_1-adrenergic receptor, it activates a $G\alpha_s$ protein, which stimulates adenylyl cyclase, promotes increases in $[cAMP]_i$, and thus enhances the activity of PKA (see Table 15-2). In contrast, when the same hormone binds to a cell displaying principally α_2 receptors, it activates a $G\alpha_i$ protein, which inhibits adenylyl cyclase, diminishes $[cAMP]_i$, and therefore reduces PKA activity. Thus, the response of a specific tissue to adrenergic stimulation (whether through circulating epinephrine or through norepinephrine released locally by sympathetic neurons) is determined by the receptor repertoire displayed by the cell. The same is true for DA; the DA-1 (D_1) receptor is coupled to $G\alpha_s$ and the DA-2 (D_2) receptor is linked to $G\alpha_i$.

Epinephrine has a greater affinity for β-adrenergic receptors than for α-adrenergic receptors, whereas norepinephrine acts predominantly through α-adrenergic receptors. The various signal transduction systems linked to these receptors are discussed in Chapter 3. β-Adrenergic stimulation occurs through the adenylyl cyclase system. The α_2-adrenergic receptor also usually acts through adenylyl cyclase. However, α_1-adrenergic stimulation is linked to $G\alpha_q$, which activates a membrane-associated PLC that liberates IP_3 and DAG. IP_3 can release Ca^{2+} from intracellular stores, and DAG directly enhances the activity of PKC. Combined, these actions enhance the cellular activity of Ca^{2+}-dependent kinases, which produce a metabolic response that is characteristic of the specific cell. The response to adrenergic agonists may be, for example, glycogenolysis in the liver or muscle (predominantly a β effect), contraction (an α_1 effect) or relaxation (a β_2 effect) of vascular smooth muscle, a change in the inotropic or chronotropic state of the heart (a β_1 effect), or various other effects.

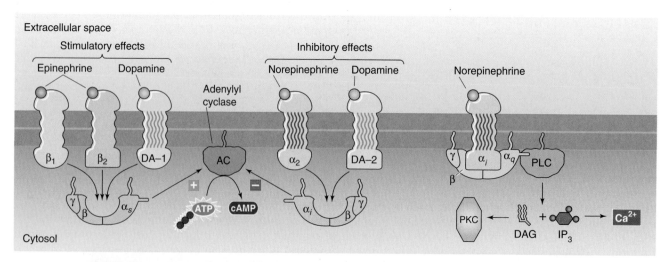

Figure 47-5   Catecholamine receptors. The β_1, β_2, and D_1 receptors all interact with $G\alpha_s$, which activates AC and raises levels of cAMP. The α_2 and D_2 receptors interact with $G\alpha_i$, which inhibits AC. Additionally, the α_1 receptor interacts with $G\alpha_q$, which activates PLC, which, in turn, converts phosphoinositides in the cell membrane to IP_3 and DAG.

STEROID AND THYROID HORMONES

Cholesterol is the precursor for the steroid hormones: cortisol, aldosterone, estradiol, progesterone, and testosterone

The family of hormones called *steroids* shares a common biochemical parentage: all are synthesized from cholesterol. Only two tissues in the body possess the enzymatic apparatus to convert cholesterol to active hormones. The **adrenal cortex** makes cortisol (the main glucocorticoid hormone), aldosterone (the principal mineralocorticoid in humans), and androgens. The **gonads** make either estrogen and progesterone (ovary) or testosterone (testes). In each case, production of steroid hormones is regulated by trophic hormones released from the pituitary. For aldosterone, the renin-angiotensin system also plays an important regulatory role.

The pathways involved in steroid synthesis are summarized in Figure 47-6. Cells that produce steroid hormones can use, as a starting material for hormone synthesis, the cholesterol that is circulating in the blood in association with low-density lipoprotein (LDL; see Chapter 46). Alternatively, these cells can synthesize cholesterol de novo from acetate (see Fig. 46-16). In humans, LDL cholesterol appears to furnish ~80% of the cholesterol used for steroid synthesis (Fig. 47-6). An LDL particle contains both free cholesterol and cholesteryl esters, in addition to phospholipids and protein. The cell takes up this LDL particle through the LDL receptor and receptor-mediated endocytosis (see Chapter 2)

into clathrin-coated vesicles. Lysosomal hydrolases then act on the cholesteryl esters to release free cholesterol. The cholesterol nucleus, whether taken up or synthesized de novo, subsequently undergoes a series of reactions that culminate in the formation of **pregnenolone**, the common precursor of all steroid hormones. Through divergent pathways, pregnenolone is then further metabolized to the major steroid hormones: the mineralocorticoid aldosterone and the glucocorticoid cortisol (see Fig. 50-2), the estrogen estradiol (see Fig. 55-10), and the androgen testosterone (see Fig. 54-5).

Unlike the peptide and amine hormones considered earlier, steroid hormones are not stored in secretory vesicles before their secretion (Table 47-4). For these hormones, synthesis and secretion are very closely linked temporally. Steroid-secreting cells are capable of increasing the secretion of steroid hormones many-fold within several hours. The lack of a preformed storage pool of steroid hormone does not appear to limit the effectiveness of these cells as an endocrine regulatory system. Furthermore, steroid hormones, unlike peptide and amine hormones, mediate nearly all their actions on target tissues by regulating gene transcription. As a result, the response of target tissues to steroids typically occurs over hours to days.

Like cholesterol itself, steroid hormones are poorly soluble in water. On their release into the circulation, steroid hormones associate with specific binding proteins (e.g., sex hormone–binding globulin) that transport the steroid hormones through the circulatory system to their target tissues. The presence of these binding proteins, whose concentration in the circulation can change in response to

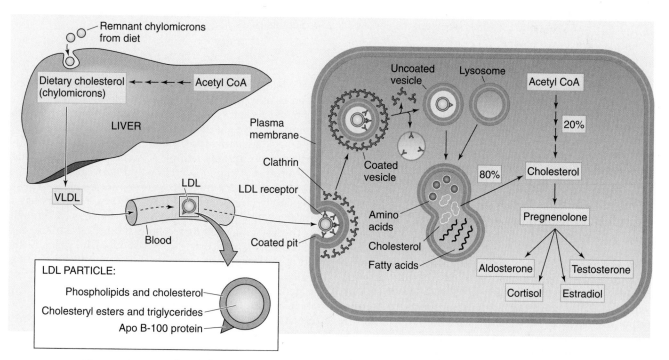

Figure 47-6 Uptake of cholesterol and synthesis of steroid hormones from cholesterol. The cholesterol needed as the starting material in the synthesis of steroid hormones comes from two sources. Approximately 80% is taken up as LDL particles through receptor-mediated endocytosis. The cell synthesizes the remaining cholesterol de novo from acetyl coenzyme A (acetyl CoA). VLDL, very-low-density lipoprotein.

Table 47-4 Differences Between Steroid and Peptide Amine Hormones

Property	Steroid Hormones	Peptide Amine Hormones
Storage pools	None	Secretory vesicles
Interaction with cell membrane	Diffusion through cell membrane	Binding to receptor on cell membrane
Receptor	In cytoplasm or nucleus	On cell membrane
Action	Regulation of gene transcription (primarily)	Signal transduction cascades affecting a variety of cell processes
Response time	Hours to days (primarily)	Seconds to minutes

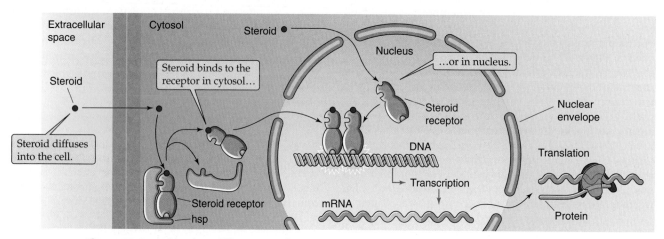

Figure 47-7 Action of steroid hormones. The activated steroid hormone receptor binds to specific stretches of DNA called SREs, thus stimulating the transcription of appropriate genes. hsp, heat shock protein.

a variety of physiological conditions, can complicate efforts to measure the amount of active steroid hormone in the circulation.

Steroid hormones bind to intracellular receptors that regulate gene transcription

Steroid hormones appear to enter their target cell by simple diffusion across the plasma membrane (Fig. 47-7). Once within the cell, steroid hormones are bound with high affinity (K_D in the range of 1 nM) to receptor proteins located in the cytosol or the nucleus. As detailed in Chapter 4, binding of steroid hormone to its receptor results in a change in the receptor conformation so that the active receptor-hormone complex now binds with high affinity to specific DNA sequences called **hormone response elements** or **steroid response elements** (SREs). These sequences are within the 5′ region of target genes whose transcription is regulated by the specific steroid hormone–receptor complex. *Termination* of gene regulation by the steroid hormone–receptor complex is not as well understood as *initiation* of the signal. The receptor protein may be modified in a manner that permits dissociation of the hormone and DNA. The receptor

itself could then be recycled and the steroid molecule metabolized or otherwise cleared from the cell.

Steroid receptors are monomeric phosphoproteins with a molecular weight that is between 80 and 100 kDa. A remarkable similarity is seen among receptors for the glucocorticoids, sex steroids, retinoic acid, the steroid-like vitamin 1,25-dihydroxyvitamin D, and thyroid hormone. The receptors for these diverse hormones are considered part of a gene superfamily (see Chapter 3). Each of these receptors has a similar modular construction with six domains (A through F). The homology among receptors is especially striking for the C domain, particularly the C1 subdomain, which is the part of the receptor molecule that is responsible for binding to DNA.

Steroid hormone receptors dimerize on binding to their target sites on DNA. Dimerization appears essential for the regulation of gene transcription. Within the C1 DNA-binding domain of the steroid receptor monomer are two zinc fingers that are involved in binding of the receptor to DNA (see Chapter 4). Even receptors with very different biological actions have a striking sequence similarity in this domain of the receptor. Because the specificity with which genes are regulated by a specific steroid receptor arises from the specificity of the DNA-binding domain, mutations in this region can greatly alter hormone function. For example, substitution of two amino acids in the *glucocorticoid* receptor causes the mutated glucocorticoid receptor to bind to DNA to which the *estrogen* receptor normally binds. In such a system, a glucocorticoid could have an estrogen-like effect.

The activated steroid receptor, binding as a dimer to SREs in the 5′ region of a gene, regulates the rate of transcription of that gene. Each response element is identifiable as a consensus sequence of nucleotides, or a region of regulatory DNA in which the nucleotide sequences are preserved through different cell types. The effect of gene regulation by activated steroid receptors binding to an SRE is dramatically illustrated by the chick ovalbumin gene. Chicks that are not exposed to estrogen have approximately four copies of the ovalbumin mRNA per cell in the oviduct. A 7-day course of estrogen treatment increases the number of copies of message 10,000-fold. This increase in message is principally the result of an increased rate of gene transcription. However, steroid hormones can also stabilize specific mRNA molecules and increase their half-life.

The 5′ flanking region of the gene typically has one or more SREs upstream of the TATA box, a nucleotide sequence rich in adenine and thymine that is located near the starting point for transcription (see Chapter 4). The activated steroid hormone receptors recognize these SREs from their specific consensus sequences. For example, one particular consensus sequence designates a site as a *glucocorticoid* response element if the SRE is in a cell with a glucocorticoid receptor. This same consensus sequence in a cell of the endometrium would be recognized by the activated *progesterone* receptor or, in the renal distal tubule, by the activated *mineralocorticoid* receptor. The specificity of the response thus depends on the cell's expression of particular steroid receptors, not simply the consensus sequence. For example, the renal distal tubule cell expresses relatively more mineralocorticoid receptors than it does progesterone receptors when compared with the endometrium. As a result, changes in plasma aldosterone regulate Na^+ reabsorption in the kidney with greater sensitivity than does circulating progesterone. However, very high levels of progesterone can, like aldosterone, promote salt reabsorption.

From the foregoing, it should be apparent that the specificity of response of a tissue to steroid hormones depends on the abundance of specific steroid receptors expressed within a cell. Because all somatic cells have the full complement of DNA with genes possessing SREs, whether a cell responds to circulating estrogen (e.g., breast), androgen (e.g., prostate), or mineralocorticoid (e.g., renal collecting duct) depends on the receptors present in the cell. This specificity raises the obvious, but as yet unanswered question of what regulates the expression of specific steroid receptors by specific tissues.

Within a given tissue, certain factors control the concentration of steroid hormone receptors. In the cytosol of all steroid-responsive tissues, steroid receptor levels usually drop dramatically immediately after exposure of the tissue to the agonist hormone. This decrease in receptor level is the result of net movement of the agonist-receptor complex to the nucleus. Eventually, the cytosolic receptors are repopulated. Depending on the tissue, this repopulation may involve new synthesis of steroid hormone receptors or simply recycling of receptors from the nucleus after dissociation of the agonist from the receptor. In addition, some steroids reduce the synthesis of their own receptor in target tissues. For example, progesterone reduces the synthesis of progesterone receptor by the uterus, thus leading to an overall net reduction or downregulation of progesterone receptor concentration in a target tissue. An interesting observation in this regard is that the genes for steroid receptor proteins do *not* appear to have SREs in their 5′ flanking region. Thus, this regulation of receptor number probably involves *trans*-acting transcriptional factors (see Chapter 4) other than the steroid hormones themselves.

Other factors that affect the concentration of steroid receptors in target tissues include the state of differentiation of the tissue, the presence of other hormones that affect steroid receptor synthesis, and whether the steroid hormone has previously stimulated the tissue. For example, estrogen receptor concentrations are low in an unstimulated uterus but rise dramatically in an estrogen-primed uterus (receptor upregulation). Regulation of steroid receptor number is clearly one factor that alters overall tissue sensitivity to these hormones.

Thyroid hormones bind to intracellular receptors that regulate metabolic rate

In many respects, the thyroid gland and thyroid hormone are unique among the classic endocrine axes. In Chapter 49, in which thyroid physiology is discussed in more detail, this uniqueness begins with the structure of the thyroid gland, which is composed of follicles. Each follicle is an epithelial layer of cells encircling a lake of fluid that contains very protein-rich follicular fluid. The principal protein component of the follicular fluid is an extremely large protein, thyroglobulin. Neither of the two thyroid hormones—T_4 and T_3—is free in the follicular fluid. Rather, these hormones are formed by the iodination of tyrosine residues on the thyroglobulin molecule and are thus part of the primary structure of the thyroglobulin molecule.

T_4 and T_3 remain part of the thyroglobulin molecule in the follicle lumen until thyroid secretion is stimulated. The entire thyroglobulin molecule then undergoes endocytosis by the follicular cell and is degraded within the lysosomes of these cells. Finally, the follicular cell releases the free T_4 and T_3 into the circulation. Once secreted, T_4 is tightly bound to one of several binding proteins. It is carried to its sites of action, which include nearly all the cells in the body. In the process of this transport, the liver and other tissues take up some of the T_4 and partially deiodinate it to T_3; this T_3 can then re-enter the circulation.

Both T_3 and T_4 enter target cells and bind to cytosolic and nuclear receptors. These receptors are similar to those for steroid hormones (see Chapter 3). T_3 has higher affinity than T_4 for the thyroid hormone receptor. Even though it accounts for only ~5% of the circulating thyroid hormone, T_3 is probably the main effector of thyroid hormone signaling. The activated thyroid hormone receptor binds to thyroid hormone response elements in the 5′ region of responsive genes and regulates the transcription of multiple target genes.

Quantitation of Steroid Receptors in Patients with Cancer

The affinity of steroid molecules for their receptors can be studied in vitro in a manner analogous to that described for the radioimmunoassay of peptide hormones (Fig. 47-8). In a typical immunoassay, an antibody with high affinity for a hormone or other compound binds to a radioactively labeled hormone or other molecule. A sample containing an unknown amount of the compound to be measured is added to the antibody-labeled hormone mixture and displaces the radioisotope from the antibody in proportion to the concentration of the unknown. The amount of unknown can be quantitated by comparison to the displacing activity of known standards.

For quantitating *steroid receptors*, cell extracts containing an unknown amount of steroid receptors are incubated with increasing concentrations of labeled steroid hormone. At each concentration, hormone that is bound by the receptor is separated from that remaining free in the extract. The result is a saturation curve (Fig. 47-8A), provided the tissue extract has a finite number of specific hormone receptors. This saturation curve can often be linearized by a simple arithmetic manipulation called a *Scatchard plot* (Fig. 47-8B). This analysis allows quantitation of the affinity of the receptor for the hormone and provides an estimate of the number of receptors (actually, the *concentration* of receptors) for that particular hormone.

The technique of quantitating receptor number has found an important application in determining the number of estrogen and progesterone receptors present in breast cancer cells. The number of estrogen and progesterone receptors per milligram of breast cancer tissue (obtained by biopsy of the breast or involved lymph node) is quantitated with radiolabeled estrogen (or progesterone). For postmenopausal women with estrogen receptor–positive breast cancer (i.e., a tumor with a high level of estrogen receptors), treatment with an antiestrogen (e.g., tamoxifen) is effective therapy. For premenopausal women, an antiestrogen may be used as well, or the ovaries can be removed surgically. The woman may also be given a long-acting gonadotropin-releasing hormone (GnRH) agonist, which paradoxically blocks both LH and FSH production by the anterior pituitary, thereby reducing estradiol production and accomplishing a medical oophorectomy. The continuous (as opposed to the normally pulsatile) administration of GnRH downregulates GnRH receptors in the anterior pituitary.

These therapies are not effective in patients with cancers that do not express significant numbers of estrogen receptors. The presence of abundant estrogen and progesterone receptors in breast tumors correlates with a more favorable prognosis, possibly because of the relatively advanced state of differentiation of the tumor, as well as the tumor's responsiveness to manipulation by estrogen or progesterone therapy.

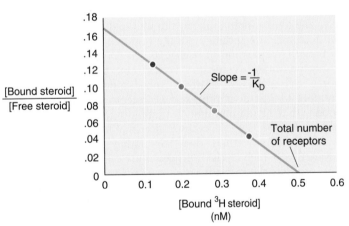

A SATURATION CURVE

B SCATCHARD PLOT

Figure 47-8   Quantitating receptor affinity and number of receptors. **A,** The plot of bound hormone (i.e., hormone-receptor complex) on the y-axis versus that of free steroid concentration on the x-axis. In this example, we have assumed that the K_D for hormone binding is 3 nM and that the maximal bound hormone concentration is 0.5 nM. **B,** This plot is a transformation of the data in **A.** The colored points in this plot match the points of like color in **A.** Plotted on the y-axis is the ratio of [Bound hormone]/[Free hormone]. Plotted on the x-axis is [Bound hormone]. The slope of this relationship gives the $-1/K_D$, where K_D is the dissociation constant (3 nM). The x-axis intercept gives the total number of receptors (0.5 nM).

Thyroid hormone receptors are present in many tissues, including the heart, vascular smooth muscle, skeletal muscle, liver, kidney, skin, and CNS. A major role for thyroid hormone is overall regulation of metabolic rate. Because T_4 affects multiple tissues, individuals affected by disorders involving oversecretion or undersecretion of thyroid hormone manifest a host of varied symptoms that reflect the involvement of multiple organ systems.

Steroid and thyroid hormones can also have nongenomic actions

A central dogma of steroid hormone and thyroid hormone action has been that all their diverse actions are secondary to genomic regulation. However, evidence accumulating over the past decade demonstrated that these receptors can also bind to and modulate the activity of cytosolic proteins and can thereby regulate their activity or behavior through a nongenomic action. The quest to explain some of the very rapid onset of steroid and thyroid hormone actions (occurring within 2 to 15 minutes) which appeared incompatible with a mechanism requiring new protein synthesis led to the discovery of their nongenomic actions.

An example of the foregoing is the association of the estrogen receptor (ERα) with **phosphatidylinositol-3-kinase** (PI3K; see Chapter 58). In the absence of estradiol, ERα binds weakly, if at all, to PI3K. However, in the presence of estradiol, ERα binds strongly to the 85-kDa regulatory subunit of PI3K, thus stimulating the 110-kDa catalytic subunit to phosphorylate PIP_2 to phosphatidylinositol 3,4,5-trisphosphate (PIP_3). In vascular endothelial cells, PIP_3 increases the activity of downstream protein kinases that phosphorylate and regulate NO synthase, which is itself an important regulator of vascular function (see Chapter 20). In addition to estrogen, thyroid hormones, testosterone, glucocorticoids, and aldosterone may also have nongenomic actions, some of which also appear to be mediated by binding to PI3K.

REFERENCES

Books and Reviews

Berson SA, Yalow RS: Peptide hormones in plasma. Harvey Lect 1966-1967; 62:107-163.

Farfel Z, Bourne HR, Iiri T: The expanding spectrum of G protein diseases. N Engl J Med 1999; 340:1012-1020.

Larsen PR, Kronenberg HM, Melmed S, Polonsky KS (eds): Williams Textbook of Endocrinology, 10th ed. Philadelphia: WB Saunders, 2003.

Losel RM, Falkenstein E, Feuring M, et al: Nongenomic steroid action: Controversies, questions, and answers. Physiol Rev 2003; 83:965-1016.

Missale C, Nash SR, Robinson SW, et al: Dopamine receptors: From structure to function. Physiol Rev 1998; 78:189-225.

Scatchard G: The attraction of proteins for small molecules and ions. Ann N Y Acad Sci 1949; 51:660-672.

Journal Articles

Berson SA, Yalow RS: Assay of insulin in human subjects by immunological methods. Nature 1959; 184:1948-1949.

Elgin RC, Busby WL, Clemmons DR: An insulin-like growth factor binding protein enhances the biological response to IGF-1. Proc Natl Acad Sci U S A 1987; 84:3254-3258.

Upton GV, Amatruda TT Jr: Evidence for the presence of tumor peptides with corticotropin-releasing-factor–like activity in the ectopic ACTH syndrome. N Engl J Med 1971; 285:419-424.

Yu D, Yu S, Schuster V, et al: Identification of two novel deletion mutations within the Gs alpha gene (GNAS1) in Albright hereditary osteodystrophy. J Clin Endocrinol Metab 1999; 84:3254-3259.

CHAPTER 48

ENDOCRINE REGULATION OF GROWTH AND BODY MASS

Eugene J. Barrett

GENES, NUTRITION, ACTIVITY, AND HORMONES REGULATE SOMATIC GROWTH AND BODY MASS

Growth from the fertilized ovum to the adult is an exceedingly complex process involving both **hyperplasia** (an increase in the number of cells) and **hypertrophy** (an increase in the size of cells) of the cellular elements of body tissues. The timing and capacity for cell division vary among tissues. In the human central nervous system (CNS), neuronal division is essentially complete by the age of 1 year, whereas bone, muscle, and fat cells continue to divide until later in childhood. Other tissues retain the capacity for hyperplasia throughout life; these include the skin, gastrointestinal epithelial cells, and liver.

In humans, the genetic contribution to growth is evident from the observation that midparental height (i.e., the average of paternal and maternal height) is one of the better predictors of a child's ultimate stature. For domestic animals, breeding based on desired growth characteristics has been a mainstay of animal husbandry for millennia. For humans, in whom such planned breeding does not occur, body height differences among different populations suggest a genetic contribution. Even more striking are some of the differences seen with specific genetic mutations that affect skeletal growth (e.g., achondroplasia). The basis of these population height differences and of those related to genetic syndromes is beyond the scope of this chapter. Rather, I focus on nutritional and hormonal processes in which physiological regulation appears to play an important role across individuals. The impact of environmental and nutritional factors, such as emotional or nutritional deprivation, on growth is most profound when it occurs during periods of tissue hyperplasia, most critically during the first 2 years of life.

The first two major sections of this chapter deal with factors that affect **linear growth**, whereas the third section deals with factors that regulate **body mass**. This division is somewhat artificial because changes in linear growth and body mass often occur simultaneously. The control of linear growth in humans depends on multiple hormones, including growth hormone (GH), insulin-like growth factors 1 and 2 (IGF-1 and IGF-2), insulin, thyroid hormones, glucocor-

ticoids, androgens, and estrogens. Among these, GH and IGF-1 have been implicated as the major determinants of growth in normal postuterine life. However, deficiencies (or excesses) of each of the other hormones can seriously affect the normal growth of the musculoskeletal system as well as the growth and maturation of other tissues. The control of body mass depends on many newly discovered humoral factors made in adipose, intestine, hypothalamus, and other tissues that regulate appetite and energy expenditure.

GROWTH HORMONE

Growth hormone, secreted by somatotrophs in the anterior pituitary, is the principal endocrine regulator of growth

Individuals with excessive GH secretion during childhood develop **gigantism**, and those with a deficiency of GH develop **pituitary dwarfism**. It is thus quite clear that GH profoundly affects somatic size. Dramatic examples of the somatotrophic action of GH can be found in the descriptions of Tom Thumb and the Alton giant. GH deficiency resulted in Tom Thumb's achieving an adult height of approximately 0.9 m. In contrast, the Alton giant had a GH-secreting pituitary tumor present from early childhood and reached an adult height of more than 2.7 m. It is important that, in both cases, the abnormality of GH secretion was present from early life. Children with GH deficiency are of normal size at birth and only subsequently fall behind their peers in stature.

A deficiency of GH beginning in adult life does not result in any major clinical illness. However, it is now appreciated that *replacement* of GH (clinically available as a recombinant protein) in adults with **GH deficiency** leads to increased lean body mass, decreased body fat, and perhaps an increased sense of vigor or well-being. An *excess* of GH after puberty results in the clinical syndrome of **acromegaly** (from the Greek *akron* [top] + *megas* [large]). This condition is characterized by the growth of bone and many other somatic tissues, including skin, muscle, heart, liver, and the gastrointestinal tract. The lengthening of long bones is not part of the syndrome because the epiphyseal growth plates close at the end of puberty. Thus, acromegaly causes progressive thickening of bones and soft tissues of the head, hands, feet, and other parts of the body. If untreated, these somatic changes cause significant morbidity and shorten life as a result of joint deformity, hypertension, pulmonary insufficiency, and heart failure.

GH is made in the **somatotrophs** throughout the anterior pituitary (see Chapter 47). Like other peptide hormones, GH is synthesized as a larger prehormone (Fig. 48-1). During processing through the endoplasmic reticulum and Golgi system, several small peptides are removed. GH exists in at least three molecular forms. The predominant form is a 22-kDa polypeptide with two intramolecular sulfhydryl bonds. Alternative splicing generates a 20-kDa form of GH. Other GH forms include a 45-kDa protein, which is a dimer of the 22-kDa form, as well as larger forms that are multimers of monomeric GH. There is little information to suggest that the different principal forms of GH (i.e., the 20- and 22-kDa versions) vary in their activity, but the 20-kDa form may exert fewer of the acute metabolic actions of GH. Once synthesized, GH is stored in secretory granules in the cytosol of the somatotrophs until it is secreted.

Growth hormone is one of a family of homologous hormones that exhibit overlap of activity

GH appears to be a single-copy gene, but four other hormones have significant homology to GH. Most striking are three hormones made by the placenta: placental-variant GH (pvGH) and human chorionic somatomammotropins 1 and 2 (hCS1 and hCS2) (Table 48-1). Human genes for these hormones are also located in the GH gene cluster on the long arm of chromosome 17. The multiple genes in this cluster have an identical intron structure and code for proteins of similar size. Substantial amino acid sequence homology occurs among GH and these three other proteins. **pvGH**, like the 22-kDa GH, is a 191–amino acid peptide. It has a 93% primary sequence homology with GH and virtually the same affinity for the hepatic GH receptor as GH. It appears able to mimic some of the biological actions of GH and may be an important modulator of systemic IGF-1 production during pregnancy. (As discussed later, a major action of GH is to stimulate secretion of IGF-1.) The **hCSs** are also called human placental lactogens (hPLs). The affinity of the two forms of hCS for the GH receptor is 100- to 1000-fold less than that of either GH or pvGH. As a result, the hCSs are less effective in promoting IGF-1 or IGF-2 production. The somatomammotropins are primarily lactogenic, priming the breast for lactation after birth (see Table 56-7).

The pituitary hormone **prolactin** (PRL; Table 48-1) is the fourth hormone with homology to GH. It has a 16% amino acid homology with pituitary GH. The principal physiological role of PRL involves promoting milk production in lactating women (see Chapter 56). PRL is made by *lactotrophs* in the anterior pituitary. Its homology to GH suggests that the two hormones, despite their divergent actions, arose from some common precursor by a gene-duplication event. The sequence homology between these proteins is underscored by the observation that GH and PRL have similar

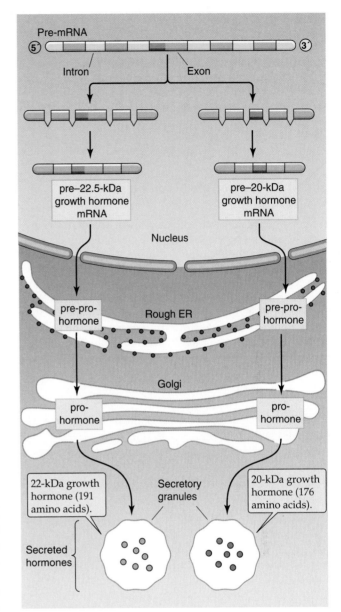

Figure 48-1 Synthesis of GH. Somatotrophic cells in the anterior pituitary are responsible for the synthesis of GH. The cell transcribes five exons to form GH messenger RNA (mRNA) for either the 22-kDa protein (191 amino acids) or the 20-kDa protein (176 amino acids). Alternative splicing in the third exon, which removes the RNA-encoding amino acids 32 to 46, is responsible for the two isoforms found in the pituitary. Both mRNAs have a signal sequence that causes them to be translated in the rough endoplasmic reticulum (ER) and enter the secretory pathway. Subsequent processing converts the two pre–pro-GHs first to the pro-GHs and then to the mature GHs. The cleavage of the pro-sequence and disulfide bond formation occur during transit through the Golgi bodies. The somatotroph stores mature GH in granules until GHRH stimulates the somatotroph to secrete the hormones. The 22-kDa version is the dominant form of GH.

affinities for the PRL receptor. The converse is not true—that is, PRL has no significant affinity for the GH receptor and thus has no growth-promoting activity. As discussed later, the PRL and GH receptors are coupled to an intracellular signaling system that involves stimulation of the JAK family of tyrosine kinases (see Chapter 3) as an early post-receptor event.

Men, like women, make PRL throughout their lives. However, no physiological role for PRL in boys or men has been defined. Both men and women with disorders involving hypersecretion of GH or PRL can develop galactorrhea (breast milk secretion). Although GH and PRL are normally secreted by distinct cell populations in the anterior pituitary, some benign, GH-producing pituitary adenomas (i.e., tumors) secrete PRL along with GH.

Somatotrophs secrete growth hormone in pulses

It remains a paradox that whereas growth occurs slowly over months and years, the secretion of GH is highly episodic, varying on a minute-to-minute basis. Most physiologically normal children experience episodes or bursts of GH secretion throughout the day, most prominently within the first several hours of sleep. Underlying each peak in plasma levels of GH, illustrated for an adult in Figure 48-2, are bursts of many hundreds of pulses of GH secretion by the somatotrophs in the anterior pituitary. With the induction of slow-wave sleep, several volleys of GH pulses may occur; it is estimated that more than 70% of total daily GH secretion

Table 48-1 Homology of Growth Hormone to Chorionic Hormones and Prolactin

Hormone	Number of Amino Acids	Homology	Chromosome
Human GH (hGH)	191	100%	17
pvGH	191	93%	17
Human CS1 (hCS1)	191	84%	17
Human CS2 (hCS2)	191	84%	17
Human PRL (hPRL)	199	16%	6

occurs during these periods. This pulsatile secretion underlines the prominent role of the CNS in the regulation of GH secretion and growth. The circulating GH concentrations may be up to 100-fold higher during the bursts of GH secretion (i.e., the peaks in Fig. 48-2) than during intervening periods. The pattern of bursts depends on sleep-wake patterns, not on light-dark patterns. Exercise, stress, high-protein meals, and fasting also cause a rise in the mean GH level in humans. In circumstances in which GH secretion is stimulated (e.g., fasting or a high-protein diet), the increased GH output results from an increase in the frequency, rather than the amplitude, of pulses of GH that the somatotrophs secrete.

Growth hormone secretion is under hierarchical control from growth hormone–releasing hormone and somatostatin

The coordination of GH secretion by the somatotrophs during a secretory pulse presumably occurs in response to both positive and negative hypothalamic control signals.

Growth Hormone–Releasing Hormone Small-diameter neurons in the arcuate nucleus of the hypothalamus secrete **GH-releasing hormone** (GHRH), a 43–amino acid peptide that reaches the somatotrophs in the anterior pituitary through the hypophyseal portal blood (Fig. 48-3). As the name implies, this neuropeptide promotes GH secretion by the somatotrophs. GHRH is made principally in the hypothalamus, but it can also be found in neuroectodermal tissue outside the CNS; it was first isolated and purified from a pancreatic islet cell tumor of a patient with acromegaly.

Growth Hormone–Releasing Hormone Receptor GHRH binds to a G protein–coupled receptor (GPCR) on the somatotrophs and activates $G_{\alpha s}$, which, in turn, stimulates adenylyl cyclase (see Chapter 3). The subsequent rise in $[cAMP]_i$ causes increased gene transcription and synthesis of GH. In addition, the rise in $[cAMP]_i$ opens Ca^{2+} channels in the plasma membrane and causes $[Ca^{2+}]_i$ to rise. This increase in $[Ca^{2+}]_i$ stimulates the release of preformed GH.

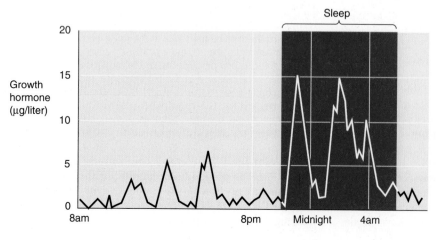

Figure 48-2 Bursts in plasma levels of GH, sampled in the blood plasma of a 23-year-old woman every 5 minutes over a 24-hour period. Each peak in the plasma GH concentration reflects bursts of hundreds of GH secretory pulses by the somatotrophs of the anterior pituitary. These bursts are most common during the first few hours of sleep. The integrated amount of GH secreted each day is higher during pubertal growth than in younger children or in adults. (*Data from Hartman ML, Veldhuis JD, Vance ML, et al: J Clin Endocrinol Metab 1990; 70:1375.*)

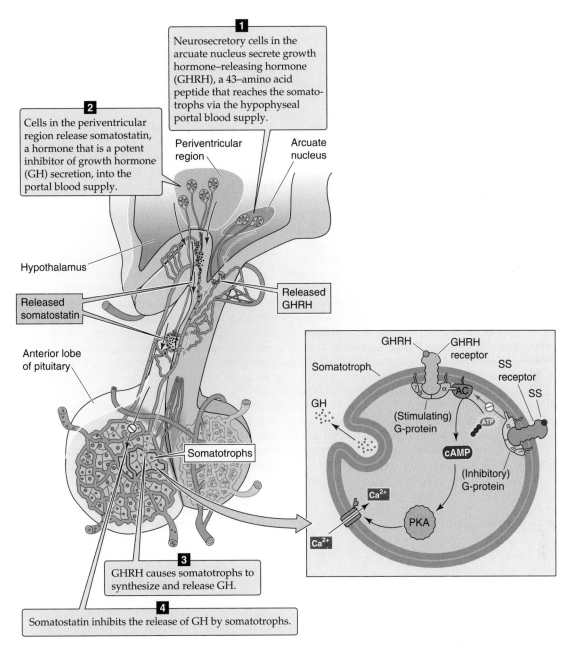

1 Neurosecretory cells in the arcuate nucleus secrete growth hormone–releasing hormone (GHRH), a 43–amino acid peptide that reaches the somatotrophs via the hypophyseal portal blood supply.

2 Cells in the periventricular region release somatostatin, a hormone that is a potent inhibitor of growth hormone (GH) secretion, into the portal blood supply.

Periventricular region

Arcuate nucleus

Hypothalamus

Released somatostatin

Released GHRH

Anterior lobe of pituitary

Somatotrophs

3 GHRH causes somatotrophs to synthesize and release GH.

4 Somatostatin inhibits the release of GH by somatotrophs.

GHRH   GHRH receptor

Somatotroph   SS receptor

GH   SS

(Stimulating) G-protein   ATP

cAMP   (Inhibitory) G-protein

Ca²⁺   PKA

Ca²⁺

Figure 48-3 Synthesis and release of GHRH and SS and the control of GH release. Small-bodied neurons in the arcuate nucleus of the hypothalamus secrete GHRH, a 43–amino acid peptide that reaches the somatotrophs in the anterior pituitary through the long portal veins. GHRH stimulates the somatotrophs to release GH stored in secretory granules by raising $[cAMP]_i$ and $[Ca^{2+}]_i$. Neurons in the *periventricular region* of the hypothalamus synthesize SS, a 14–amino acid neuropeptide. SS, which also travels to the anterior pituitary through the long portal vessels, is a potent inhibitor of GH secretion. SS acts by inhibiting adenylyl cyclase (AC) and thus lowering $[Ca^{2+}]_i$. PKA, protein kinase A.

Ghrelin A relatively newly discovered hormone, ghrelin consists of 28 amino acids. One of the serine residues is linked to an octanol group, and only this acylated form of the peptide is biologically active. Distinct endocrine cells within the mucosal layer of the stomach release ghrelin in response to fasting. Endocrine cells throughout the gastrointestinal tract also make ghrelin, although the highest ghrelin concentrations are in the fundus of the stomach. The arcuate nucleus of the hypothalamus also makes small amounts of ghrelin. Infusion of ghrelin either into the bloodstream or into the cerebral ventricles markedly increases growth hormone secretion. Indeed, ghrelin appears to be involved in the postmeal stimulation of growth hormone secretion. It has been more difficult to define the extent to which ghrelin—versus GHRH and somatostatin (SS)—contributes to the changes in normal growth hormone secretion in response to fasting, amino acid feeding, and carbohydrate feeding. Ghrelin also appears to stimulate appetite, thereby contributing to body mass regulation as well as linear growth.

Ghrelin Receptor The hormone binds to a GPCR designated the GH secretagogue receptor (GHSR). This receptor was first identified because it binds synthetic peptide ligands that stimulate GH secretion. In this regard, GHSR is like the GHRH receptor (GHRHR); however, GHRH is not a ligand for GHSR.

Somatostatin The hypothalamus also synthesizes **SS**, a 14–amino acid neuropeptide. SS is made in the periventricular region of the hypothalamus and is secreted into the hypophyseal portal blood supply. It is a potent inhibitor of GH secretion. SS is also made elsewhere in the brain and in selected tissues outside the CNS, such as the pancreatic islet Δ cells (see Chapter 51) and D cells in the gastrointestinal tract (see Chapter 42). Within the CNS, the 14–amino acid form of SS (SS-14) dominates. The gastrointestinal tract predominantly expresses a 28–amino acid splice variant; the N-terminal 14 amino acids of SS-28 are identical to those of SS-14.

It appears that the primary regulation of GH secretion is stimulatory, because sectioning the pituitary stalk, thereby interrupting the portal blood flow from the hypothalamus to the pituitary, leads to a decline in GH secretion. Conversely, sectioning of the stalk leads to a *rise* in PRL levels, presumably because dopamine made in the hypothalamus inhibits PRL secretion in the anterior pituitary (see Chapter 47). It also appears that the pulses of GH secretion are entrained by the pulsatile secretion of GHRH (as opposed to the periodic loss of SS inhibition). Such a relationship between releasing factors and pulses of pituitary hormone secretion has been directly documented in primates for the secretion of gonadotropin-releasing hormone (GnRH) and luteinizing hormone (LH), but not yet for GHRH.

Somatostatin Receptor SS binds to a GPCR on the somatotrophs and activates $G_{\alpha i}$, which inhibits adenylyl cyclase. As a result, $[Ca^{2+}]_i$ decreases, thereby diminishing the responsiveness of the somatotroph to GHRH. When somatotrophs are exposed to both GHRH and SS, the inhibitory action of SS prevails.

Both growth hormone and insulin-like growth factor 1, whose secretion is stimulated by growth hormone, negatively feed back on growth hormone secretion by somatotrophs

In addition to being controlled by GHRH and SS released from the hypothalamus, somatotroph secretion of GH is regulated by a negative feedback loop involving IGF-1. As discussed later, GH triggers the secretion of IGF-1 from GH target tissues throughout the body. Indeed, IGF-1 appears to mediate many of the growth-promoting actions of GH. The circulating levels of IGF-1, which produce its **endocrine** effects, largely reflect its hepatic synthesis. IGF-1 synthesized in tissues such as muscle, cartilage, and bone may act more in a **paracrine** or **autocrine** fashion to promote local tissue growth. An increase in the circulating concentration of IGF-1 suppresses GH secretion through both direct and indirect mechanisms (Fig. 48-4). First, circulating IGF-1 exerts a *direct* action on the pituitary to suppress GH secretion by the somatotrophs, probably inhibiting GH secretion by a

mechanism different from that of SS. In its peripheral target cells, IGF-1 acts through a receptor tyrosine kinase (see Chapter 3), and not by either the Ca^{2+} or cAMP messenger systems. IGF-1 presumably acts by this same mechanism to inhibit GH secretion in somatotrophs.

Second, evidence also points to two *indirect* feedback pathways by which circulating IGF-1 inhibits GH secretion. IGF-1 appears to suppress GHRH release in the hypothalamus and to increase SS secretion. Yet another feedback system, independent of IGF-1, reduces GH secretion; GH itself appears to inhibit GH secretion in a short-loop feedback system.

Growth hormone has acute anti-insulin metabolic effects and chronic growth-promoting effects mediated by insulin-like growth factor 1

Once secreted, most GH circulates free in the plasma. However, a significant fraction (~40% for the 22-kDa GH) is complexed to a **GH-binding protein** formed by proteolytic cleavage of the extracellular domain of GH receptors in GH target tissues. This protein fragment binds to GH with high affinity, thereby increasing the half-life of GH and competing with GH target tissues for GH. In the circulation, GH has a half-life of ~25 minutes.

Growth Hormone Receptor GH binds to specific receptors on the surface of multiple target tissues. The monomeric GH receptor is a 620–amino acid protein with a single membrane spanning segment. The molecular weight of the purified receptor (~130 kDa) greatly exceeds that predicted from the amino acid composition (~70 kDa) as a result of extensive glycosylation. The receptor does not resemble any of the GPCRs or receptors with intrinsic tyrosine kinase activity, but rather is a **tyrosine kinase–*associated* receptor** that is related to several cytokine receptors (see Chapter 3). The GH receptor forms a dimer when one GH molecule simultaneously binds to sites on two monomers and acts as a bridge. Receptor occupancy increases the activity of a tyrosine kinase (JAK 2 family) that is associated with, but is not an integral part of, the GH receptor. This tyrosine kinase triggers a series of protein phosphorylations that modulate target cell activity.

Acute Effects of Growth Hormone GH has certain acute (minutes to hours) actions on muscle, adipose tissue, and liver that may not necessarily be related to the more long-term growth-promoting actions of GH. These acute metabolic effects (Table 48-2) include stimulation of lipolysis in adipose tissue, inhibition of glucose uptake by muscle, and stimulation of gluconeogenesis by hepatocytes. These actions oppose the normal effects of insulin (see Chapter 56) on these same tissues and have been termed the **anti-insulin** or **diabetogenic** actions of GH. Chronic oversecretion of GH, such as occurs in patients with GH-producing tumors in acromegaly, is accompanied by insulin resistance and often by glucose intolerance or frank diabetes.

Long-Term Effects of Growth Hormone Through IGF-1 Distinct from these short-term actions of GH is its action to promote tissue growth by stimulating target tissues

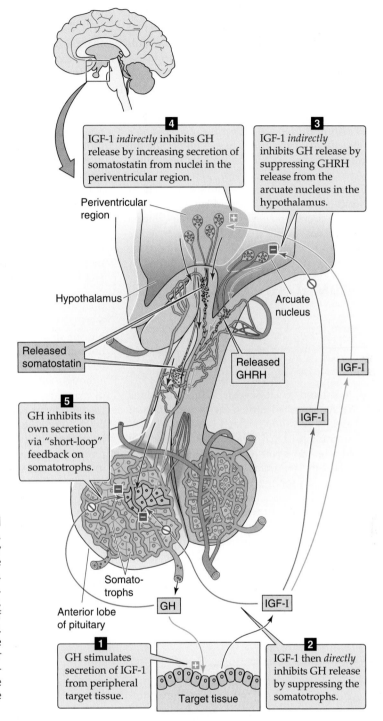

Figure 48-4 GH and IGF-1 (also called somatomedin C) negative feedback loops. Both GH and IGF-1 feed back—either directly or indirectly—on the somatotrophs in the anterior pituitary to decrease GH secretion. GH itself inhibits GH secretion (short loop). IGF-1, whose release is stimulated by GH, inhibits GH release by three routes, one of which is direct and two of which are indirect. The direct action is for IGF-1 to inhibit the somatotroph. The first indirect pathway is for IGF-1 to suppress GHRH release in the hypothalamus. The second is for IGF-1 to increase secretion of SS, which, in turn, inhibits the somatotroph.

Within the figure:

4 IGF-1 *indirectly* inhibits GH release by increasing secretion of somatostatin from nuclei in the periventricular region.

3 IGF-1 *indirectly* inhibits GH release by suppressing GHRH release from the arcuate nucleus in the hypothalamus.

Periventricular region

Hypothalamus

Arcuate nucleus

Released somatostatin

Released GHRH

IGF-I

IGF-I

5 GH inhibits its own secretion via "short-loop" feedback on somatotrophs.

Somato-trophs

Anterior lobe of pituitary

GH

IGF-I

IGF-I

1 GH stimulates secretion of IGF-1 from peripheral target tissue.

Target tissue

2 IGF-1 then *directly* inhibits GH release by suppressing the somatotrophs.

Table 48-2 Diabetogenic Effects of Growth Hormone

Target	Effect
Muscle	↓ Glucose uptake
Fat	↑ Lipolysis
Liver	↑ Gluconeogenesis
Muscle, fat, and liver	Insulin resistance

to produce IGFs. In 1957, Salmon and Daughaday reported that GH itself does not have growth-promoting action on epiphyseal cartilage (the site where longitudinal bone growth occurs). In those experiments, the addition of serum from normal animals, but not from hypophysectomized (GH-deficient) animals, stimulated cartilage growth in vitro (assayed as incorporation of radiolabeled sulfate into cartilage). The addition of GH to GH-deficient serum did not restore the growth-promoting activity seen with normal serum. However, when the GH-deficient animals were treated in vivo with GH, their plasma promoted cartilage growth in vitro. This finding led to the hypothesis that, in animals, GH provokes the secretion of another circulating factor that "mediates" the action of GH. Initially called "sulfation factor" because of how it was assayed, this intermediate was subsequently termed **somatomedin** because it mediates the somatic effects of GH. The responsible proteins were isolated and purified and were found to be identical to two peptides with a primary structure much like that of proinsulin, and they were termed IGFs (Fig. 48-5). These peptide hormones are made in various tissues, including the liver, kidney, muscle, cartilage, and bone. They are called "insulin-like" growth factors because they exert insulin-like actions in isolated adipocytes and can produce hypoglycemia in animals and humans. The liver produces most of the IGF-1 present in the circulation. IGF-1 production appears to be more closely related to GH secretion than does IGF-2 production.

GROWTH-PROMOTING HORMONES

Insulin-like growth factor 1, which interacts with a receptor similar to the insulin receptor, is the principal mediator of the growth-promoting action of growth hormone

The synthesis of IGF-1 and, to a lesser extent, IGF-2 depends on circulating GH. As described earlier, the periodic nature of GH secretion results in a wide range of plasma GH concentrations. In contrast, plasma [IGF-1] does not vary by more than ~2-fold over a 24-hour period. The plasma [IGF-1] in effect integrates the pulsatile, highly fluctuating GH concentration. The reason for the relatively steady plasma levels of IGF-1 is that like GH—but unlike most peptide hormones—IGF-1 circulates bound to several **IGF-1–binding proteins**. These binding proteins are made principally in the liver, but they are also manufactured by other tissues. More than 90% of IGF-1 measured in the serum is bound to these proteins. At least six distinct IGF-binding proteins have been identified. In addition to providing a buffer pool in plasma of bound IGF, these proteins may also aid the transfer of IGF to the tissue receptors, thereby facili-

tating the action of these hormones. The local free fraction of IGF-1 is probably the more biologically active component that binds to the receptor and stimulates tissue growth.

Like other peptide hormones, IGF-1 and IGF-2 are synthesized through the secretory pathway (see Chapter 2) and are secreted into the extracellular space, where they may act locally in a paracrine fashion. In the extracellular space, the IGFs encounter binding proteins that may promote local retention of the secreted hormone by increasing the overall molecular size of the complex. This action inhibits the entry of the IGFs into the vascular system. Thus, local concentrations of the IGFs are likely to be much higher than plasma concentrations.

Whether made locally or reaching tissue through the circulation, IGF-1 acts through a specific **receptor tyrosine kinase** (see Chapter 3), a heterotetramer that is structurally related to the insulin receptor (Fig. 48-6). Like the insulin receptor (see Chapter 51), the IGF-1 receptor has two completely extracellular α chains and two transmembrane β chains. Also like in the insulin receptor, the β chains have the intrinsic tyrosine kinase activity. Binding of IGF-1 to its receptor enhances receptor autophosphorylation as well as phosphorylation of downstream effectors. The structural homology between the insulin and IGF-1 receptors is sufficiently high that insulin can bind to the IGF-1 receptor, although with an affinity that is approximately two orders of magnitude less than that for IGF-1. The same is true for the binding of IGF-1 to insulin receptors. In fact, the homology between the insulin and IGF-1 receptors is so strong that hybrid receptors containing one α-β chain of the insulin receptor and one α-β chain of the IGF-1 receptor are present in many tissues. These hybrid receptors bind both insulin and IGF-1, but their affinity for IGF-1 is greater.

Given the structural similarity between insulin and IGFs and between the insulin receptor and the IGF-1 receptor, it is not surprising that IGFs can exert insulin-like actions in vivo. This effect has been particularly well studied for IGF-1, which, like insulin, induces hypoglycemia when it is injected into animals. This action is largely the result of the increased uptake of glucose into muscle tissue. IGF-1 is less effective in mimicking insulin's action on adipose and liver tissue; in humans, these tissues have few IGF-1 receptors. In muscle,

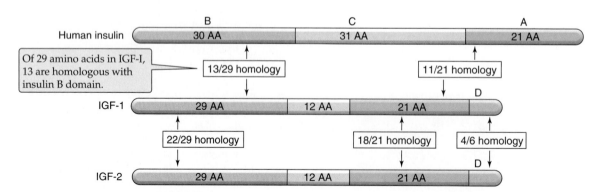

Figure 48-5 Structure of the IGFs. Insulin, IGF-1, and IGF-2 share three domains (A, B, and C), which have in common a high degree of amino acid sequence homology. The C region is cleaved from insulin (as the C peptide) during processing, but it is not cleaved from either IGF-1 or IGF-2. In addition, IGF-1 and IGF-2 also have a short D domain.

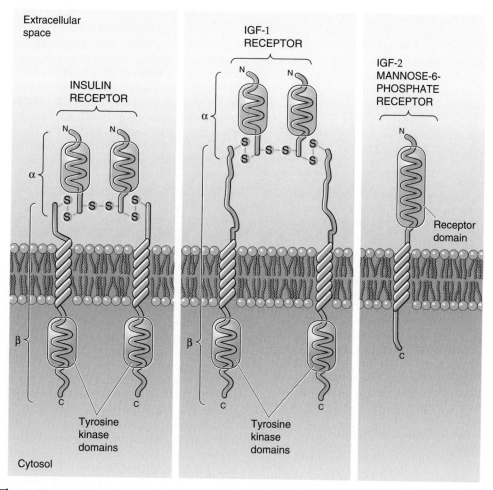

Figure 48-6 Comparison of insulin, IGF-1, and IGF-2 receptors. Both the insulin and IGF-1 receptors are heterotetramers joined by disulfide bonds. For both, the cytoplasmic portions of the β subunits have tyrosine kinase domains as well as autophosphorylation sites. The IGF-2 receptor (also called M6P receptor) is a single polypeptide chain with no kinase domain.

IGF-1 promotes the uptake of radiolabeled amino acids and stimulates protein synthesis at concentrations that do not stimulate glucose uptake, findings indicating that the growth-promoting actions of IGF-1 are expressed at lower circulating concentrations than those required to produce hypoglycemia.

Insulin-like growth factor 2 has actions similar to those of insulin-like growth factor 1 but is less dependent on growth hormone

The physiology of IGF-2 differs from that of IGF-1 in certain important respects. First, as noted earlier, the synthesis of IGF-2 depends less on circulating GH than does that of IGF-1. In pituitary dwarfism secondary to GH deficiency, the circulating concentration of IGF-1 is decreased, but that of IGF-2 is not. In states of excessive GH secretion, plasma IGF-1 is reliably elevated, whereas plasma IGF-2 is not.

Although IGF-2 also binds to the IGF-1 receptor, it preferentially binds to its own so-called IGF-2 receptor. This IGF-2 receptor consists of a single-chain polypeptide and is structurally very distinct from the IGF-1 receptor (Fig.

48-6). The IGF-2 receptor lacks a tyrosine kinase domain and does not undergo autophosphorylation in response to the binding of either IGF-2 or IGF-1. The IGF-2 receptor also binds mannose-6-phosphate (M6P), but at a site different from that for IGF-2 binding, and the receptor's physiological role appears to be in processing mannosylated proteins by targeting them for lysosomal degradation. Thus, the term *IGF-2 receptor* is somewhat of a misnomer; the IGF-2 receptor's role in the physiological action of IGF-2 is not clear.

Despite these differences, IGF-2 does share with IGF-1 (and also with insulin) the ability to promote tissue growth and to cause acute hypoglycemia. These properties appear to result from IGF-2's structural similarity to proinsulin and its ability to bind to the IGF-1 receptor.

Although growth rate usually parallels plasma levels of insulin-like growth factor 1, the two diverge both early and late in life

Illustrated in Figure 48-7 is the mean concentration of total IGF-1 (both free and bound) found in human serum as a function of age. Also shown is the normal rate of height increase (cm/yr). During puberty, the greatest growth rates are observed at times when plasma [IGF-1] is highest. A similar comparison can be made using GH, provided care is taken to obtain multiple measurements at each age and thereby account for the pulsatile secretion and marked diurnal changes that occur in plasma [GH].

Plasma Level of IGF-1 as a Measure of Growth Hormone Secretion

The plasma concentration of IGF-1 is a valuable measure of GH secretion. The wide swings in plasma [GH] that result from the pulsatile secretion of this hormone have confounded efforts to use GH measurements to diagnose disorders of GH deficiency or excess. However, an increased circulating concentration of IGF-1 is one of the most useful clinical measures of the excess GH secretion that occurs in acromegaly (i.e., GH excess in adults) and gigantism (i.e., GH excess in children). Measurement of plasma [IGF-1] has also helped to explain the genesis of a particular type of dwarfism known as *Laron dwarfism*. These patients were initially identified as persons with growth failure mimicking that of typical pituitary dwarfism; however, plasma [GH] is normal or elevated, and treatment with GH is ineffective in reversing the growth failure. It was subsequently demonstrated that these individuals have mutations of their GH receptors that make the receptors nonfunctional. Thus, the mutant GH receptors cannot trigger the production of IGFs. With the availability of recombinant IGF-1, it is possible that effective treatment of these children will restore growth.

Despite the structural similarity of their receptors, IGF-1 and insulin exert different actions on tissues. IGF-1 has a more marked effect on growth, and insulin has a more significant effect on glucose and lipid metabolism. However, the differences in the postreceptor signaling pathways triggered by the two hormones have not been well defined.

Whereas good general concordance exists between growth rate and the plasma [IGF-1] during puberty, the two diverge at both younger and older ages. First, during adulthood, longitudinal growth essentially ceases, yet secretion of GH and of IGF-1 continues to be highly regulated. As both men and women age, the circulating concentrations of both hormones decline. For many years, the continued secretion of these hormones in adults was considered to be largely vestigial. This belief was reinforced by the observation that cessation of GH secretion and the consequent decline of IGF-1 after trauma, tumor, or surgical removal of the pituitary did not result in any clear clinical syndrome. However, with the availability of recombinant human GH, replacement of GH in GH-deficient adults has led to remarkable increases in body muscle mass, decreases in fat mass, and improved nitrogen balance (a measure of protein nutrition). These findings support the conclusion that—even after linear growth ceases after puberty—GH and IGF-1 remain important regulators of body composition and appear to promote anabolic actions in muscle. Indeed, some investigators have suggested that supplementing physiologically normal adults with GH or IGF-1 may reverse some of the effects of aging, including loss of muscle mass, negative nitrogen balance, and osteoporosis.

A second period of life during which divergence between longitudinal growth and IGF-1 occurs is very early childhood (Fig. 48-7). This period is characterized by a very rapid growth rate, but quite low IGF-1 levels. If this time frame is extended back to intrauterine life, then the discordance is even greater. Indeed, children with complete GH deficiency have very low plasma [IGF-1] levels but are of normal length and weight at birth. This observation suggests that during intrauterine life, factors other than GH and IGF-1 are important regulators of growth. One of these additional factors may be insulin, as discussed later.

Another explanation for the divergence between growth rate and IGF-1 levels may be IGF-2, which may be an important mediator of intrauterine growth. The plasma concentra-

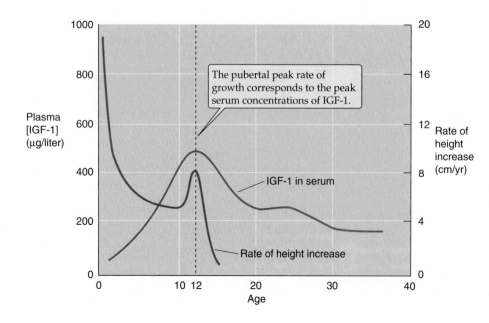

Figure 48-7 Serum IGF-1 levels and height velocity as a function of age. The *red curve* shows the mean plasma concentrations of IGF-1 as a function of age in female humans. The curve for male humans is similar, but the peak is shifted to an older age by 3 to 4 years. The *brown curve* indicates mean female height velocity—the rate at which height increases (cm/yr). The *pubertal* peak rate of growth corresponds to the peak serum concentrations of IGF-1. *(Data from Reiter EO, Rosenfeld RG: Normal and aberrant growth. In Wilson JD, Foster DW, Kronenberg HM, Larsen PR [eds]: Williams Textbook of Endocrinology, 9th ed, pp 1427-1507. Philadelphia: WB Saunders, 1998.)*

The pubertal peak rate of growth corresponds to the peak serum concentrations of IGF-1.

IGF-1 in serum

Rate of height increase

tion of IGF-2 is greater during fetal life than later, and it peaks just before birth. Plasma [IGF-2] plummets soon after birth, but then it gradually doubles between birth and age 1 year and remains at this level until at least the age of 80 years. Thus, IGF-2 levels are at adult levels during the first several years of life, when IGF-1 levels are low but growth is rapid. However, several other hormones may also contribute to somatic growth during the first several years of life.

By age 3 or 4 years, GH and IGF-1 begin to play major roles in the regulation of growth. The concentrations of these hormones rise throughout childhood and peak during the time of the pubertal growth spurt. The rate of long bone growth in the pubertal growth spurt is exceeded only during intrauterine life and early childhood. The frequency of pituitary GH secretory pulses increases markedly at puberty. The factors responsible for this acceleration are not clear. However, the accompanying sexual maturation likely plays some role, because both estradiol and testosterone appear to promote GH secretion.

In addition to these humoral influences, nutritional factors also modulate both GH secretion and IGF-1 production. In both children and adults, GH secretion is triggered by high dietary protein intake. Teleologically, this is intriguing in that it may provide linkage between the availability of amino acids to serve as substrates for body protein synthesis (growth) and the endocrine stimulus of cells to grow. This relationship is not simple, however, because the rise in GH levels in the setting of protein intake is not sufficient to stimulate IGF-1 production fully. This principle is well illustrated by **fasting**, which is associated with a decline in IGF-1 even with increased GH. During fasting, insulin levels are low. Increased insulin appears to be required, at least in some tissues, for GH to stimulate IGF-1 effectively.

Thyroid hormones, steroids, and insulin also promote growth

Although the discussion to this point emphasizes the action of GH and the GH-induced growth factors as modulators of somatic growth, we could regard them as necessary but not sufficient agents for normal growth. Certain other hormones, as well as receptive growth-responsive cartilage, are required. Because growth is a difficult phenomenon to study, especially in humans (few scientists want to follow an experiment over 10 to 20 years), much of our understanding of endocrine regulation of normal growth derives from observations of abnormal growth as it occurs in clinical syndromes of endocrine excess or deficiency. Several of the more important of these endocrine influences are illustrated here. The exact mechanism by which growth is regulated by these agents is not always well understood.

Thyroid Hormones   Next to GH, perhaps the most prominent among the growth-promoting hormones are the thyroid hormones thyroxine and triiodothyronine, which are discussed in Chapter 49. In many nonhuman species, thyroid hormone plays a major role in tissue growth and remodeling. For example, resorption of the tadpole tail during morphogenesis requires thyroid hormone. In humans, deficiency of thyroid hormones early in life can cause dwarfism or cretinism (see Chapter 49). In children with normal thyroid

function at birth, development of hypothyroidism at any time before epiphyseal fusion leads to growth retardation or arrest. Much of the loss in height that occurs can be recovered through thyroid hormone treatment, a phenomenon called *catch-up growth*. However, because the diagnosis of hypothyroidism may elude detection for many months or years, delays in initiating treatment can lead to some loss of potential growth. A child's growth curve can provide a particularly sensitive early indicator of hypothyroidism.

Sex Steroids   As with thyroid hormones, the importance of sex steroids for growth is most readily understood by considering the effects of deficiency or excess of these hormones. Androgen or estrogen excess occurring before the pubertal growth spurt accelerates bone growth. However, the sex steroids also accelerate the rate at which the skeleton matures and thus shorten the time available for growth before epiphyseal closure occurs. Most of the time, the dominant effect of sex steroids is to narrow the growth window, thereby diminishing ultimate longitudinal bone growth. This effect is well illustrated in settings in which children are exposed to excessive sex steroid at an early age. The sex steroids can come from endogenous sources (e.g., early maturation of the hypothalamic-pituitary-gonadal axis that produces premature puberty, or tumors that secrete estrogen or androgen) or from exogenous sources (e.g., children who take sex steroids prescribed for others). Again, the growth curve is useful in that it typically shows an increase in growth rate, followed by an early leveling off of growth associated with the development of secondary sexual characteristics.

Glucocorticoids   An *excess* of adrenal glucocorticoids inhibits growth. In children who produce too much cortisol, as a result of either adrenal or pituitary tumors (which produce adrenocorticotropic hormone [ACTH] and cause secondary increases in plasma cortisol), growth ceases. The use of synthetic glucocorticoids in treating various serious illnesses (e.g., asthma, organ transplantation, various chronic autoimmune processes) also arrests growth. Restoration of normal growth does not occur until the glucocorticoid levels return toward normal. Neither GH nor IGF-1 concentrations drop significantly during glucocorticoid treatment. The failure of GH administration to correct the growth retardation that occurs in glucocorticoid-treated children further confirms that GH deficiency cannot account for the growth failure associated with glucocorticoid excess. Because linear growth is related to cartilage and bone synthesis at the growth plates, glucocorticoids presumably are acting at least in part at these sites to impair growth. However, the specific biochemical locus at which glucocorticoids act remains unclear. In adults, as in children, glucocorticoid excess impairs tissue anabolism and thus may manifest as wasting in some tissues (e.g., bone, muscle, subcutaneous connective tissue), rather than growth failure. This tissue wasting results in some of the major clinical morbidity of glucocorticoids (i.e., osteoporosis, muscle weakness, and bruising).

In glucocorticoid *deficiency*, growth is not substantially affected. However, other deleterious effects of cortisol deficiency (e.g., hypoglycemia; see Chapter 51) dominate.

Insulin This hormone is also an important growth factor, particularly in utero. For example, women with diabetes frequently have high blood levels of glucose during pregnancy and deliver babies of high birth weight (fetal **macrosomy**). The developing fetus, exposed to glucose concentrations that are higher than normal, secretes additional insulin. Hyperinsulinemia results in increased fetal growth. Fetal macrosomy can create significant obstetric difficulties at the time of delivery.

Conversely, infants born with pancreatic agenesis or with one of several forms of severe insulin resistance are very small at birth. One form of this condition, **leprechaunism**, is the result of a defect in the insulin receptor (see Chapter 51 for the box on this topic). Thus, it appears that insulin, acting through its own receptor, is an intrauterine growth factor.

Severe insulin deficiency produces a marked catabolic effect associated with wasting of lean body mass in both children and adults. The acute adverse effects of such deficiency (dehydration and acidosis) dominate the clinical picture. Milder degrees of insulin deficiency, seen in patients with chronically undertreated diabetes, diminish growth in affected children. Improved diabetes management may allow restoration of normal growth rates and possibly even some transient accelerated or catch-up growth. Thus, with good care, children with diabetes can expect to achieve normal adult height.

The musculoskeletal system responds to growth stimuli of the GHRH-GH–IGF-1 axis

Longitudinal growth involves lengthening of the somatic tissues (including bone, muscle, tendons, and skin) through a combination of tissue hyperplasia and hypertrophy. Each of these tissues remodels its structure throughout life. For bone, **longitudinal growth** occurs by the hyperplasia of chondrocytes at the growth plates of the long bones, fol-

lowed by endochondral ossification. The calcified cartilage is remodeled as it moves toward the metaphyses of the bone, where it is eventually replaced by true lamellar and trabecular bone (see Chapter 52). This process continues until epiphyseal closure occurs toward the completion of puberty.

The process of cartilage formation and longitudinal bone growth begins as the cellular elements capable of forming cartilage divide along the growth plate and then migrate toward the more mature bone. These cells synthesize the extracellular matrix of cartilage, which include type II collagen, hyaluronic acid, and mucopolysaccharides. These cells appear to respond directly to GH by proliferating and increasing production of the extracellular matrix. This response involves local generation of IGF-1 within the cartilage as an early event in the growth process. As the cells more closely approach the already formed cortical and trabecular bone, ossification of the extracellular matrix begins, and eventually the cellular elements become isolated by the calcifying cartilage. However, this calcified cartilage is not structurally the same as normal bone, and soon after formation, it begins to be remodeled by an ingrowth of cellular elements (osteoclasts and osteoblasts) from adjacent bone. Eventually, it is replaced by normal bone and becomes part of the metaphysis of the long bone.

In most children, growth ceases within several years after completion of puberty, when the chondrocytes at the growth plates of the long bones stop dividing and calcify the previously cartilaginous surrounding matrix. After puberty, **radial growth** occurs as bones increase their *diameter* through a process of endosteal bone resorption and periosteal bone deposition. This process is not strictly compartmentalized; that is, resorption and deposition of bone occur at both the periosteal and endosteal surfaces. However, during periods of growth, the rate of periosteal deposition exceeds the rate of endosteal resorption, and the bone shafts grow in width and thickness.

As may be expected, numerous disorders disrupt the complex process of endochondral bone growth on a genetic or congenital basis (e.g., defects in collagen or mucopolysaccharide synthesis) and lead to genetic forms of dwarfism. In these settings, the GHRH-GH–IGF-1 axis is entirely intact and appears to regulate normally. No apparent compensation occurs for the short stature by increased GH secretion, a finding suggesting that the axis is not sensitive to the growth process per se, but simply to the intermediate chemical mediator IGF-1.

GH and IGF-1 clearly play important roles in mediating longitudinal bone growth and also modulate growth of other tissues. Thus, proportional growth of muscle occurs as bones elongate, and the visceral organs enlarge as the torso increases in size. The mechanisms by which GH and IGF-1 coordinate this process and the way in which other hormones or growth factors may be involved continue to be investigated. It is clear that, whereas GH and, more recently, IGF-1 have been considered the major hormones responsible for somatic growth, other tissue growth factors play an important, albeit incompletely defined, role. Table 48-3 lists some of these growth factors. In general, the tissue growth factors have more tissue-specific actions on organogenesis and their

Anabolic-Androgenic Steroids

We are all unfortunately familiar with the potential for abuse of anabolic-androgenic steroids by bodybuilders and competitive athletes. Illicit use of these agents appears to be widespread in sports, where strength is closely linked to overall performance. In addition to naturally occurring androgens such as testosterone, dihydrotestosterone, androstenedione, and dehydroepiandrosterone, many different synthetic androgenic steroids—as well as GH—serve as performance enhancers. In addition to the sought after "beneficial" effects of increasing muscle mass and strength, each of these agents carries with it a plethora of adverse side effects. Some—such as oily skin, acne, and hair growth—are principally cosmetic. Others—including liver function abnormalities, mood changes with aggressive behavior, and hepatocellular carcinoma—are much more serious. Illicit use of these agents by younger athletes, especially teenagers, is also problematic with regard to alterations in growth and sexual maturation.

Table 48-3 Other Growth Factors Affecting Growth

Nerve growth factor (NGF)
Fibroblast growth factor (FGF)
Angiogenesis factor
Vascular endothelial growth factor (VEGF)
Epidermal growth factor (EGF)
Hepatocyte growth factor (HGF)

growth-promoting activity than the IGFs, and they appear to act largely in a paracrine or autocrine fashion.

REGULATION OF BODY MASS

The multiple hormonal factors that influence longitudinal growth—discussed in the previous two sections—are themselves responsive to the nutritional intake of a growing individual. For example, amino acids and carbohydrates promote insulin secretion, and amino acids stimulate GH secretion. In addition, the availability of an adequate, balanced nutrient supply likely exerts both direct and indirect influences to promote tissue growth. Independent of any hormonal factors, glucose, fatty acids, and amino acids can each influence the transcription of specific genes. Similarly, amino acids can directly activate the signaling pathways involved in regulating mRNA translation.

Beyond the effects of macronutrients, micronutrients can be similarly important in regulating cell growth and, by extension, growth of the organism. An example is iodine, a deficiency of which can produce dwarfism (see Chapter 49). In a more global fashion, the effect of nutrient limitation on height can be appreciated by considering the differences in mean height between men in North Korea (165 cm) and South Korea (171 cm). As mentioned in Chapter 49, nutritional deprivation early in life can markedly limit longitudinal growth. Perhaps equally fascinating, and only recently appreciated, is that nutritional deprivation early in life also appears to predispose affected individuals to *obesity* when they reach middle age. This phenomenon was first noted in epidemiologic studies from several European countries that revealed a positive correlation between middle-aged obesity and being born during periods of deprivation during and immediately following the Second World War. Such findings suggest that some level of genetic programming occurs early in life that both diminishes longitudinal growth and predisposes persons to body mass accretion.

The balance between energy intake and expenditure determines body mass

At any age or stage of life, the factors that govern body mass accretion relate specifically to the energy balance between intake and expenditure. If energy intake exceeds expenditure over time—**positive energy balance** (see Chapter 58)—body mass will increase, assuming the diet is not deficient in essential macronutrients or micronutrients. Small positive deviations from a perfect energy balance, over time, contribute to the major increase in body weight—the "obesity epidemic"—that afflicts many middle-aged adults, and increasingly adolescents, in developed societies. For example, if energy intake in the form of feeding exceeds energy expenditure by only 20 kcal (1 tsp of sugar) daily, over 1 year a person would gain ~1 kg of fat and, over 2 decades, ~20 kg.

Indeed, it is remarkable that many adults maintain a consistent body weight for decades essentially in the absence of conscious effort. Thus, a finely tuned regulatory system must in some manner monitor one or more aspect of body mass, direct the complex process of feeding (appetite and satiety) to replete perceived deficiencies, and yet avoid excesses.

Energy expenditure comprises resting metabolic rate, activity-related energy expenditure, and diet-induced thermogenesis

We can group energy expenditure into three components:

1. **Resting metabolic rate (RMR).** The metabolism of an individual who is doing essentially nothing (e.g., sleeping) is known as the RMR (see Chapter 58), which amounts to ~2100 kcal/day for a 70-kg adult. The RMR supports maintenance of body temperature, the basal functioning of multiple body systems (e.g., heartbeat, gastrointestinal motility, ventilation), and basic cellular processes (e.g., synthesizing and degrading proteins, maintaining ion gradients, metabolizing nutrients).

2. **Activity-related energy expenditure.** As we wake up in the morning and begin to move about, we do more than resting metabolism. Exercise or physical work can have a major impact on total daily energy expenditure and varies widely across individuals and within an individual on a day-to-day basis. We also expend energy in activities not classically regarded as exercise or heavy work—tapping our foot while sitting in a chair, looking about the room during physiology lecture, typing at a keyboard—activities dubbed non–exercise-associated thermogenesis or **NEAT**. Such energy expenditures can vary 3- to 10-fold across individuals and can account for 500 kcal or more of daily energy expenditure. NEAT differences, over time, could considerably contribute to differences in weight gain by individuals consuming identical caloric intake.

3. **Diet-induced thermogenesis.** Eating requires an additional component of energy expenditure for digesting, absorbing, and storing food. Typically, diet-induced thermogenesis accounts for 10% of energy expenditure. Proteins have a higher *thermic effect* than either carbohydrates or fats.

Each of these three components of energy expenditure can vary considerably from day to day and is subject to regulation. For example, thyroid hormone is a major regulator of thermogenesis (see Chapter 49). Overproduction of thyroid hormone increases both RMR and NEAT, whereas thyroid hormone deficiency has the opposite effect.

Hypothalamic centers control the sensations of satiety and hunger

Classic studies—in which investigators made lesions in, or electrically stimulated, specific brain regions—identified two areas in the hypothalamus that are important for controlling eating. A **satiety center** is located in the ventromedial nucleus (VMN; see Fig. 47-3). Electrical stimulation of the satiety center elicits sensations of satiety, even when an animal is in the presence of food. Conversely, a lesion of the satiety center causes continuous food intake *(hyperphagia)* even in the absence of need. A **hunger** (or feeding) **center** is located in the lateral hypothalamic area (LHA; see Fig. 47-3). Electrical stimulation of this center elicits a voracious appetite, even after an animal has ingested adequate amounts of food. A lesion of the hunger center causes complete and lasting cessation of food intake *(aphagia)*.

Leptin tells the brain how much fat is stored

Only in the last decade have we begun to understand regulatory mechanisms that maintain body mass, made possible by the study of mouse models of obesity. One monogenic model is the Ob/Ob strain of hyperphagic mice that develop morbid obesity; affected mice typically weigh > 100% more than unaffected animals of the same strain. In parabiosis experiments, in which an Ob/Ob mouse was surgically connected to a wild-type mouse (Fig. 48-8A), the Ob/Ob mouse lost weight, a finding suggesting that such mice lack a blood-borne factor. Another model of monogenic obesity is the (Db/Db) mouse, named Db because it secondarily develops type 2 diabetes. These mice are hyperphagic, with adult body weights ~100% higher than those of lean littermates. In parabiosis experiments connecting a Db/Db and a wild-type

mouse (Fig. 48-8B), the wild-type mouse starved. Finally, in parabiosis experiment connecting an Ob/Ob to a Db/Db mouse (Fig. 48-8C), the Ob mouse lost weight, but the Db mouse remained obese. These results indicate that (1) the Db mouse makes an excess of the blood-borne factor that cures the Ob mouse, (2) the Db mouse lacks the receptor for this factor, and (3) the absence of the receptor in the Db mouse removes the negative feedback, thus leading to high levels of the blood-borne factor.

In 1994, Jeffrey Friedman and his colleagues used positional cloning to identify **leptin** (from the Greek *leptos* [thin]), the blood-borne factor lacked by Ob mice. Leptin is a 17-kDa protein made almost exclusively in adipocytes. The replacement of leptin in Ob/Ob mice leads to rapid weight loss. In 1995, Tepper and collaborators cloned the **leptin receptor** (Ob-r). The deficiency of this receptor in Db mice makes them leptin resistant. Ob-r is a tyrosine kinase–associated receptor (see Fig. 3-11D) that signals through JAK-2 and STAT (see Fig. 4-15).

Although leptin acts on numerous tissues within the body, most importantly it somehow crosses the blood-brain barrier (see Chapter 11) and modulates specific neurons in the arcuate nucleus of the hypothalamus that control feeding behavior. These same neurons also have insulin receptors. Plasma leptin levels in humans appear to rise in proportion to the mass of adipose tissue. Conversely, the absence of leptin produces extreme hyperphagia, as in Ob/Ob mice. Plasma leptin has a half-time of ~75 minutes, and acute changes in food intake or fasting do not appreciably affect leptin levels. In contrast, **insulin** concentrations change dramatically throughout the day in response to dietary intake. Thus, it appears that leptin in some fashion acts as a *long-term regulator* of CNS feeding behavior, whereas insulin (in addition to multiple other factors) is a *short-term regulator* of the activity of hypothalamic feeding centers.

In addition to its actions in controlling appetite, leptin promotes fuel utilization. Indeed, leptin-deficient humans paradoxically exhibit some characteristics of starvation (e.g., fuel conservation).

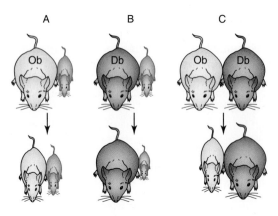

Figure 48-8 Parabiosis experiments. In parabiotically coupled mice, ~ 1% of the cardiac output of one mouse goes to the other, and vice versa, so that the animals exchange blood-borne factors.

A = Ob mouse + Wt mouse
B = Db mouse + Wt mouse
C = Ob mouse + Db mouse

Leptin and insulin are anorexigenic (i.e., satiety) signals for the hypothalamus

At least two classes of neurons within the arcuate nucleus contain receptors for both leptin and insulin. These neurons, in turn, express neuropeptides. One class of neurons produces pro-opiomelanocortin (POMC), whereas the other produces neuropeptide Y (NPY) and agouti-related protein (AgRP).

POMC Neurons Both insulin and leptin stimulate the **POMC-secreting neurons** (Fig. 48-9), which produce POMC (see Fig. 50-4). At their synapses, POMC neurons release a POMC cleavage product, the melanocortin α-melanocyte–stimulating hormone (α-MSH), which, in turn, binds to MC3R and MC4R **melanocortin receptors** on second-order neurons. Stimulation of these receptors not only produces satiety and decreases food intake—that is, α-MSH is **anorexigenic** (from the Greek *a* [not] + *orexis* [appetite])—but also increases energy expenditure through activation of descending sympathetic pathways. An indica-

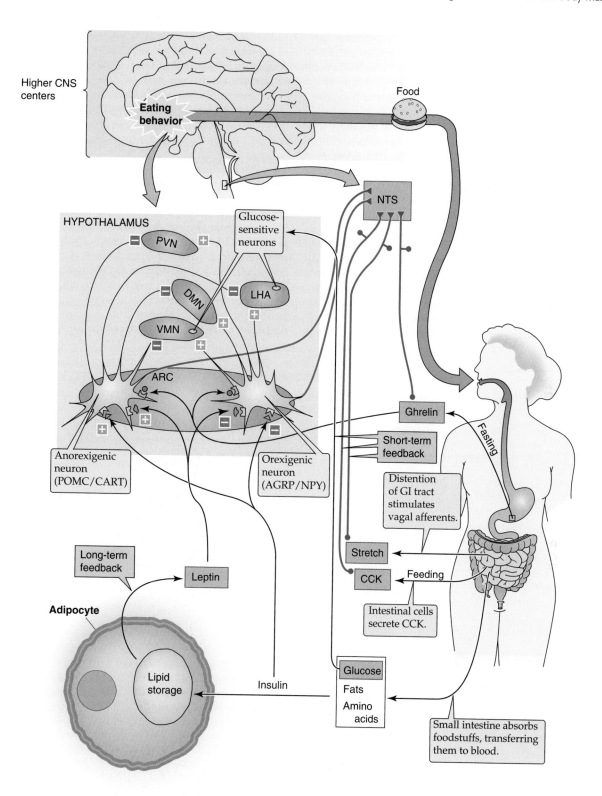

Figure 48-9   Control of appetite. ARC, arcuate nucleus.

tion of the importance of this pathway is that ~4% of individuals with severe, early-onset obesity have mutations in MC3R or MC4R. POMC neurons also synthesize another protein—**CART** or cocaine-amphetamine–related transcript, which, like α-MSH, is anorexigenic.

NPY/AgRP Neurons   In addition to stimulating POMC neurons, both insulin and leptin also suppress neurons in the arcuate nucleus that release **NPY** and **AgRP** at their synapses (Fig. 48-9). NPY activates NPY receptors—predominantly Y_1R and Y_5R, which are GPCRs—on secondary neurons, thus *stimulating* eating behavior. AgRP binds to and *inhibits* MC4R melanocortin receptors on the secondary neurons in the POMC pathway, thereby inhibiting the anorexigenic effect of α-MSH. In other words, both NPY and AgRP are **orexigenic**. The yellow obese or **agouti mouse** overexpresses the agouti protein, which inhibits melanocortin receptors. Overinhibition of MC1R on melanocytes inhibits the dispersion of pigment granules (leading to yellow rather than dark fur). Overinhibition of MC3R and MC4R on anorexigenic neurons blocks the action of α-MSH (leading to obesity).

The secondary neurons to which the POMC and NPY/AgRP neurons project are in five major locations (Fig. 48-9 and also see Fig. 47-3):

1. **LHA.** In this hunger center, NPY/AgRP neurons stimulate—but POMC neurons *inhibit*—secondary neurons producing the orexigenic peptides **melanin-concentrating hormone** (MCH) or **orexins** A and B.
2. **VMN.** This nucleus is a satiety center.
3. **Dorsomedial hypothalamic nucleus (DMN).**

4. **Paraventricular nucleus (PVN).** This nucleus contains neurons that, in turn, project to both cerebral cortex and areas of the brainstem (see Fig. 47-3).
5. **Nucleus tractus solitarii (NTS).** This nucleus integrates sensory information from the viscera (see Chapter 2) and also receives input from paraventricular neurons.

Ghrelin is an orexigenic signal for the hypothalamus

Signals originating from the periphery can be not only *anorexigenic* (i.e., promoting satiety)—as in the case of leptin (from adipose tissue) and insulin (from the pancreas)—but also *orexigenic* (i.e., promoting appetite). One of these is **ghrelin**, made in response to fasting by specialized endocrine cells in the gastric mucosa. Indeed, systemically administered ghrelin acutely increases food intake when it is given at physiological doses in both animals and humans. Circulating ghrelin concentrations, however, appear to be lower in obese than lean humans, a finding suggesting that ghrelin does not drive the increased caloric intake in the obese.

Human Obesity

One approach for gauging the extent to which human body mass is appropriate for body height is to compute the **body mass index (BMI)**:

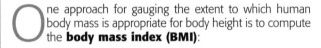

$$BMI = \frac{\text{Weight in kg}}{(\text{Height in m})^2}$$

BMIs fall into four major categories:

1. Underweight: less than 18.5
2. Normal weight: 18.5 to 24.9
3. Overweight: 25 to 29.9
4. Obesity: 30 or more

Although a BMI of 30 or more is an indication of obesity, it is not a direct measure of adipose tissue fat mass. Obesity is an area of intense investigation driven in part by the "obesity epidemic" that is adversely affecting the health of a large fraction of the population of developed nations.

The demonstration that replacement of leptin in Ob/Ob mice led to rapid weight loss raised considerable enthusiasm for the potential of leptin as a pharmacological agent in the treatment of human obesity. Indeed, several extremely rare individuals had been identified with autosomal recessive monogenic obesity secondary to leptin deficiency, like the Ob/Ob mouse. As expected, these individuals respond to exogenous leptin administration with a marked reduction in body weight. However, investigators soon appreciated that most obese persons are *not* leptin deficient. Quite the contrary, human plasma leptin concentrations increase proportionately to BMI, which is a rough estimate of adipose tissue fat mass.

Although obese persons generally are not leptin deficient, approximately one third of obese persons lose weight in response to exogenous leptin. These individuals are **leptin resistant**, but they eventually respond to sufficiently high

levels of the hormone. In the other two thirds of obese persons, the leptin resistance is so severe that they fail to respond even to the exogenous hormone. Lean persons lose weight in response to leptin.

In addition to mutations to the leptin gene, two other extremely rare mutations cause monogenic human obesity. One is mutation of the leptin receptor gene (analogous to the Db mouse) and the other is mutation of the POMC gene (leading to loss of the anorexigenic α-MSH). A more common—although rare—cause of monogenic human obesity is a mutation in the melanocortin MC4 receptor, the target of α-MSH.

Currently, no satisfactory pharmacological approaches are available to treat obesity. Of the two agents currently approved in the United States by the Food and Drug Administration, one is a serotonin re-uptake inhibitor and one blocks fat digestion and therefore absorption within the gastrointestinal tract. Neither agent directly intervenes at targets within the hypothalamic neuroendocrine control system (Fig. 48-9). More importantly, each is limited by side effects, and each is only minimally effective in decreasing weight. Perhaps more promising, but still being tested, are antagonists of the cannabinoid receptors (CB-1 and CB-1), which are GPCRs. These drugs decrease body weight by blocking access of endogenously produced arachidonic acid derivatives known as **endocannabinoids**, which are ligands of CB-1 and CB-2. These receptors are located in many areas throughout the brain, as well as in peripheral tissues. They are richly represented in the basal hypothalamus as well as within the nucleus accumbens in the limbic system. CB blockers appear to be effective in achieving and maintaining meaningful weight reduction (10 to 20 kg) for more than 1 year. The same agents are also effective in decreasing smoking behavior. Investigators are still unraveling how blocking the cannabinoid receptor affects the output of hypothalamic neurons that regulate appetite.

However, gastric bypass procedures in morbidly obese patients cause ghrelin levels to decline dramatically along with decreases in body weight and food consumption.

As discussed previously, ghrelin binds to GHSR, which is present in neurons of the arcuate nucleus as well as vagal afferents. Some hypothalamic neurons themselves contain ghrelin, and injection of ghrelin into the cerebral ventricles stimulates feeding. It is not clear to what extent circulating ghrelin promotes appetite through vagal afferents versus hypothalamic receptors. As noted earlier, ghrelin also promotes the secretion of GH and thus appears to have a role in both longitudinal growth and body mass accretion.

Plasma nutrient levels and enteric hormones are short-term factors that regulate feeding

Investigators have proposed various theories to explain the *short-term* regulation of food intake, including models focusing on the regulation of levels of blood glucose (glucostatic), amino acid (aminostatic), or lipid (lipostatic). For example, hypoglycemia produces hunger and also increases the firing rate of glucose-sensitive neurons in the hunger center in the LHA, but it decreases the firing rate of glucose-sensitive neurons in the satiety center in the VMN. Hypoglycemia also activates orexin-containing neurons in the LHA.

Feedback from the gastrointestinal tract also controls the short-term desire for food (Fig. 48-9). Gastrointestinal distention triggers vagal afferents that, through the NTS, suppress the hunger center. Peripherally administering any of several gastrointestinal peptide hormones normally released in response to a meal—glucagon; gastrin-releasing peptide (GRP), SS, and peptide YY (PYY) (see Chapter 41); cholecystokinin (CCK, see Chapter 43); and glucagon-like peptide 1 (GLP-1; see Chapter 51)—reduces meal size (i.e., these substances are anorexigenic). The most important is CCK, which is more effective when it is injected directly into the peritoneal cavity; this effect requires an intact vagus nerve. Therefore, CCK—like gastric distention—may act through vagal afferents. Additionally, an oropharyngeal reflex responds to chewing and swallowing; it may meter food intake, thus inhibiting further eating after a threshold.

An important aspect of our increasing understanding of the neuroendocrine control systems that regulate appetite, satiety, and energy expenditure and thereby body mass is the further affirmation that these processes have a genetic and biochemical basis. Two other factors that influence body mass are cortical control (e.g., "will power") and environment (e.g., the availability of high-calorie foods). Our emerging appreciation of the biological basis of obesity may allow a more scientific and clinical approach to therapeutic interventions—rather than simply blaming affected patients for their obesity.

REFERENCES

Books and Reviews

Argetsinger LS, Carter-Su C: Mechanism of signaling by growth hormone receptor. Physiol Rev 1996; 76:1089-1107.

Etherton TD, Bauman DE: Biology of somatotropin in growth and lactation of domestic animals. Physiol Rev 1998; 78:745-761.

Flier JS: Obesity wars: Molecular progress confronts an expanding epidemic. Cell 2004; 116:337-350.

Kojima M, Kangawa K: Ghrelin: Structure and function. Physiol Rev 2005; 85:495-522.

Mayo KE, Godfrey PA, Suhr ST, et al: Growth hormone–releasing hormone: Synthesis and signaling. Recent Prog Horm Res 1995; 50:35-73.

Reiter EO, Rosenfeld RG: Normal and aberrant growth. In Wilson JD, Foster DW, Kronenberg HM, Larsen PR (eds): Williams Textbook of Endocrinology, 9th ed, pp 1427-1507. Philadelphia: WB Saunders, 1998.

Stewart CEH, Rotwein P: Growth, differentiation, and survival: Multiple physiological functions for insulin-like growth factors. Physiol Rev 1996; 76:1005-1026.

Journal Articles

Coleman DL: Effects of parabiosis of obese with diabetes and normal mice. Diabetologia 1973; 9:294-298.

Daughaday WH, Trivedi B: Absence of serum growth hormone binding protein in patients with growth hormone receptor deficiency (Laron dwarfism). Proc Natl Acad Sci USA 1987; 84:4636-4640.

Hartman ML, Clayton PE, Johnson ML, et al: A low-dose euglycemic infusion of recombinant human insulin-like growth factor I rapidly suppresses fasting-enhanced pulsatile growth hormone secretion in humans. J Clin Invest 1993; 91:2453-2462.

Hartman ML, Veldhuis JD, Vance ML, et al: Somatotropin pulse frequency and basal concentrations are increased in acromegaly and are reduced by successful therapy. J Clin Endocrinol Metab 1990; 70:1375.

Tartaglia LA, Dembski M, Weng X, et al: Identification and expression cloning of a leptin receptor, OB-R. Cell 1995; 83:1263-1271.

Zhang Y, Proenca R, Maffie M, et al: Positional cloning of the mouse *obese* gene and its human homologue. Nature 1994; 372:425-432.

CHAPTER 49

THE THYROID GLAND

Eugene J. Barrett

The thyroid gland is located in the anterior neck, lying like a small bow tie across the front of the trachea. In adults, the normal thyroid weighs ~20 g. It is composed of left and right lobes and a small connecting branch, or isthmus.

The thyroid gland possesses many features unique among endocrine glands, not the least of which is that it is the only endocrine gland that can be easily seen and palpated in the course of a routine clinical examination. At the biochemical level, the thyroid hormones are the only ones that require an essential trace element, iodine, for the production of active hormone. One of the rather unusual features of thyroid hormone physiology is that the hormone is stored in an extracellular site within a highly proteinaceous material called *thyroid colloid*. The major protein within this material is thyroglobulin, which contains—as part of its primary structure—the thyroid hormones **thyroxine (tetraiodothyronine or T$_4$)** and **triiodothyronine (T$_3$)**. These sequestered hormones are entirely surrounded by thyroid follicular cells, which are responsible for the synthesis of thyroid hormones (Fig. 49-1).

The physiological actions of thyroid hormones also display several unique aspects. Although, like most peptide hormones, T$_4$ and T$_3$ are made as part of a larger protein, unlike peptide hormones, no cell-membrane receptors exist for these hormones. Instead, like the steroid hormones, thyroid hormones act by binding to *nuclear* receptors (see Chapter 3) and regulate the transcription of cell proteins. The hormones secreted by the thyroid act on multiple tissues and are essential for normal development, growth, and metabolism. The thyroid makes another hormone, calcitonin, which is synthesized by thyroid **C cells** (parafollicular cells); these C cells are not part of the follicular unit (Fig. 49-1). Calcitonin may play a role in Ca^{2+} and phosphate homeostasis. The physiology of calcitonin is discussed along with that of parathyroid hormone in Chapter 52.

SYNTHESIS OF THYROID HORMONES

Thyroid hormones are made by iodinating tyrosine residues on thyroglobulin and are stored as part of thyroglobulin molecules in thyroid follicles

The structures of T$_4$ and T$_3$, the two active thyroid hormones, are shown in Figure 49-2. T$_3$ is far more active than

T$_4$. Also shown is **reverse T$_3$ (rT$_3$)**, which has no known biological activity. It has two iodines on its *outer* benzyl ring, rather than two on its *inner* ring, as is the case for T$_3$. All three compounds derive from the ether linkage of a tyrosine molecule to the benzyl group of a second tyrosine molecule; one or two iodine atoms are attached to each benzyl group. The bottom panel of Figure 49-2 shows T$_4$ as part of the thyroglobulin molecule.

The synthesis of thyroid hormones begins with the trapping of iodide by the thyroid gland. Iodine is essential for the formation of thyroid hormones. It exists in nature as a trace element in soil and is incorporated into many foods. The iodide anion (I$^-$) is rapidly absorbed by the gastrointestinal tract and is actively taken up by the thyroid gland. A specialized Na/I cotransporter (NIS) is located at the basolateral membrane (i.e., facing the blood) of the thyroid **follicular cell** (Fig. 49-3). **NIS** (for Na Iodide Symporter) is a 65-kDa integral membrane protein that is believed to have 12 membrane-spanning segments. NIS moves I$^-$ into the follicular cell against the I$^-$ electrochemical gradient, fueled by the energy of the Na$^+$ electrochemical gradient (see Chapter 5). Several other anions (e.g., perchlorate, pertechnetate, and thiocyanate) can compete with I$^-$ for uptake by the thyroid. Iodide leaves the follicular cell and enters the lumen of the follicle across the apical membrane. **Pendrin**, a member of the SLC26 family of anion exchangers (see Chapter 5), is present on the apical membrane and may contribute to I$^-$ secretion. Mutations in this protein can lead to a congenital syndrome typically characterized by a large thyroid gland (goiter) and hearing loss. The thyroid enlarges because of deficient I$^-$ uptake, just as it would with an I$^-$-deficient diet (see the box titled Iodine Deficiency).

In parallel with the secretion of I$^-$ into the follicle lumen, the follicular cell secretes **thyroglobulin** into the lumen; thyroglobulin contains the tyrosyl groups to which the I$^-$ will ultimately attach. The thyroglobulin molecule is a glycoprotein synthesized inside the follicular cell, following the secretory pathway (see Chapter 2). Thyroglobulin is a very large protein (>600 kDa), and it accounts for approximately half of the protein content of the thyroid gland. It has relatively few tyrosyl residues (~100/molecule of thyroglobulin), and only a few of these (<20) are subject to iodination. The secretory vesicles that contain thyroglobulin also carry the enzyme **thyroid peroxidase** on their intravesicular surfaces. As the secretory vesicles fuse with the apical membrane, this enzyme faces the follicular lumen and catalyzes the oxidation of I$^-$ to

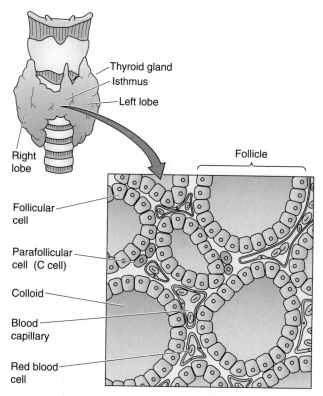

Figure 49-1 Structure of the thyroid gland. The thyroid gland is located anterior to the cricoid cartilage in the anterior neck. The gland comprises numerous follicles, which are filled with colloid and lined by follicular cells. These follicular cells are responsible for the trapping of iodine, which they secrete along with thyroglobulin—the major protein of the thyroid colloid—into the lumen of the follicle.

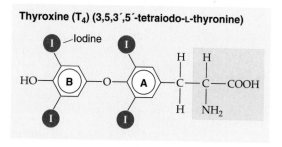

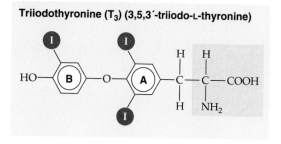

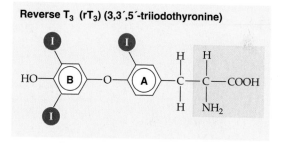

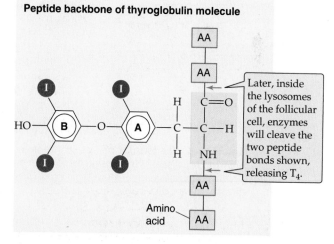

Figure 49-2 The structure of T_4, T_3, and rT_3. T_4, T_3, and rT_3 all are products of the coupling of two iodinated tyrosine derivatives. Only T_4 and T_3 are biologically active, and T_3 is far more active than T_4 because of a higher affinity for TRs. rT_3 forms as an iodine is removed from the inner benzyl ring (labeled A) of T_4; rT_3 is present in approximately equal molar amounts with T_3. However, rT_3 is essentially devoid of biological activity. As shown in the bottom panel, T_4 is part of the peptide backbone of the thyroglobulin molecule, as are T_3 and rT_3. Cleavage of the two indicated peptide bonds would release T_4.

I^0. As the thyroglobulin is entering the lumen of the thyroid follicle by the process of exocytosis, its tyrosyl groups react with I^0.

One or two oxidized iodine atoms incorporate selectively into specific tyrosyl residues of thyroglobulin. Within the thyroglobulin molecule, an internal rearrangement occurs, resulting in the conjugation of two iodinated tyrosyl residues to form a single iodothyronine, as well as a remnant dehydroalanine. Both remain as part of the primary structure of the iodinated thyroglobulin until it is later degraded inside the follicular cell. This coupling of two tyrosines, catalyzed by thyroid peroxidase, does not occur unless they are iodinated. Because only a few tyrosyl groups become iodinated, something specific about the structure of the protein near these residues probably facilitates both iodination and conjugation. The thyroid hormones, although still part of the thyroglobulin molecule, are stored as colloid in the thyroid follicle.

Follicular cells take up iodinated thyroglobulin, hydrolyze it, and release T_4 and T_3 into the blood for binding to thyroid-binding globulin and other proteins

While they are attached to thyroglobulin in the thyroid follicular lumen (Fig. 49-1), thyroid hormones remain inactive until the iodinated thyroglobulin is hydrolyzed. Before this

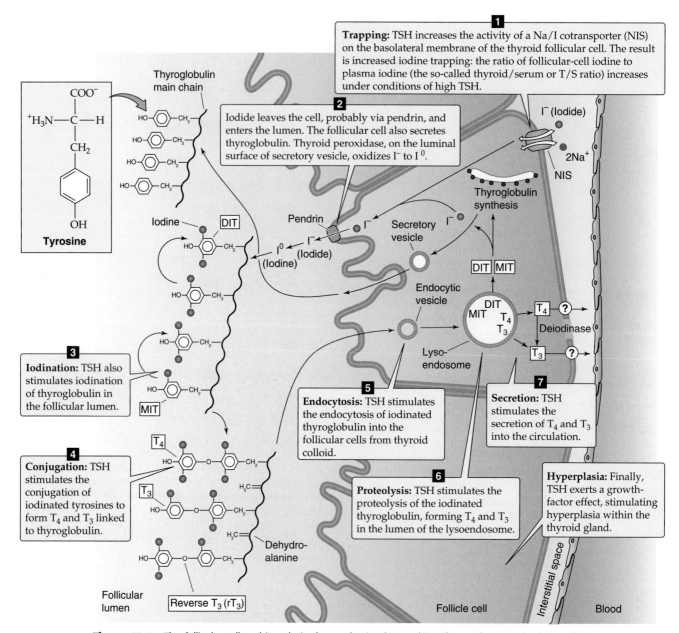

Figure 49-3 The follicular cell and its role in the synthesis of T_4 and T_3. The synthesis and release of T_4 and T_3 occurs in seven steps. Inside the follicular cell, a deiodinase converts some of the T_4 to T_3. Thyrotropin (or TSH) stimulates each of these steps except step 2. In addition, TSH exerts a growth factor or hyperplastic effect on the follicular cells.

proteolysis can begin, the follicular cells must resorb thyroglobulin from the follicular lumen by fluid-phase endocytosis (see Chapter 2). As the endocytic vesicle containing the colloid droplet moves from the apical toward the basolateral membrane, it fuses with lysosomes to form a lysoendosome. Inside this vesicle, lysosomal enzymes hydrolyze the thyroglobulin and form T_4 and T_3, as well as diiodothyronine (DIT) and monoiodothyronine (MIT). The vesicle releases both T_4 and T_3 near the basolateral membrane, and these substances exit the cell into the blood by an unknown mechanism. Approximately 90% of the thyroid hormone secreted by the thyroid is released as T_4, and 10% is released as T_3. The thyroid releases very little reverse T_3 into the blood. As

discussed in the next section, nonthyroidal tissues metabolize the T_4 released by the thyroid into T_3 and rT_3. Approximately three fourths of circulating T_3 arises from the peripheral conversion of T_4, which occurs principally in the liver and kidneys.

In the circulation, both T_4 and T_3 are highly bound to plasma proteins. **Thyroid-binding globulin (TBG)**, albumin, and **transthyretin (TTR)** account for most of this binding. The affinity of these binding proteins is sufficiently high that, for T_4, more than 99.98% of the hormone circulates tightly bound to protein. T_3 is bound only slightly less: ~99.5% is protein bound. Because the free or unbound hormone in the circulation is responsible for the actions of the thyroid hor-

Iodine Deficiency

In areas where soil is relatively iodine deficient, human iodine deficiency is common. Because seawater and seafood contain large amounts of iodide, iodine deficiency is more common in inland areas, particularly in locales that rely on locally grown foods. For example, in inland areas of South America along the Andes Mountains, in central Africa, and in highland regions of Southeast Asia, iodine deficiency is common. In the early 1900s, investigators first recognized that iodide was present in high concentrations in the thyroid and that iodine deficiency promoted goiter formation. These observations led to efforts to supplement dietary iodine. Iodine deficiency causes thyroid hormone deficiency. The pituitary responds to this deficit by increasing the synthesis of thyrotropin (or TSH), which, in turn, increases the activity of the iodine-trapping mechanism in the follicular cell in an effort to overcome the deficiency. The increased TSH also exerts a trophic effect that increases the *size* of the thyroid gland. If this trophic effect persists for sufficient time, the result is an iodine-deficient **goiter**. The word *goiter* is simply a generic term for an enlarged thyroid. If this effort at compensation is not successful (i.e., if insufficient thyroid hormone levels persist), the person will develop signs and symptoms of goitrous **hypothyroidism**. When iodine deficiency occurs at critical developmental times in infancy, the effects on the CNS are particularly devastating and produce the syndrome known as **cretinism**. Persons so affected have a characteristic facial appearance and body habitus, as well as severe mental retardation. Dietary supplementation of iodine in salt and bread has all but eliminated iodine deficiency from North America. In many nations, especially in mountainous and landlocked regions of developing nations, iodine deficiency remains a major cause of preventable illness.

Free Versus Bound Thyroxine

Most of the T_4 and T_3 in the serum is bound to proteins, the most important of which is TBG. For the binding of T_4 to TBG, the reaction is as follows:

$$T_4 + TBG \xleftrightarrow{K} T_4 TBG$$

$$K = \frac{[T_4 TBG]}{[T_4][TBG]}$$

The binding constant K is ~2×10^{10} M^{-1} for T_4. The comparable binding constant for T_3 is ~5×10^8 M^{-1}. Approximately one third of TBG's binding sites are occupied by T_4. Therefore, we have all the information we need to compute the concentration of free T_4:

$$[T_4]_{FREE} = \frac{[T_4 TBG]}{K[TBG]}$$

A reasonable value for $[T_4 TBG]$ would be 100 nM, and for $[TBG]$, 250 nM. Thus,

$$[T_4]_{FREE} = \frac{(100\ nM)}{(2 \times 10^{10}\ M^{-1}) \cdot (250\ nM)}$$
$$= 0.20 \times 10^{-10}\ M$$
$$= 20\ pM$$

Because the bound T_4 in this example is 100 nM, and the free T_4 is only 20 pM, we can conclude that only ~0.02% of the total T_4 in the plasma is free. Because 99.98% of the total T_4 in the plasma is bound, moderate fluctuations in the rate of T_4 release from the thyroid have only tiny effects on the level of free T_4. To simplify, we have not included the minor contribution of albumin and TTR in this sample calculation.

mones on their target tissues, the large amount of bound hormone has considerably confounded our ability to use simple measurements of the total amount of either T_4 or T_3 in the plasma to provide a reliable index of the adequacy of thyroid hormone secretion. For example, the amount of TBG in the serum can change substantially in different physiological states. Pregnancy, oral estrogen therapy, hepatitis, and chronic heroin abuse can all elevate the amount of TBG and hence the *total* concentration of T_4 and T_3. Decreased levels of TBG, associated with diminished concentration of *total* T_4 and T_3, can accompany steroid usage and the nephrotic syndrome. However, despite the marked increases or decreases in the amounts of circulating TBG, the concentrations of *free* T_4 and T_3 do not change in the aforementioned examples. The box titled Free Versus Bound Thyroxine indicates how one can calculate levels of free T_4 or T_3, knowing the concentration of TBG and the concentration of total T_4 or total T_3.

The liver makes each of the thyroid-binding proteins. TBG is a 54-kDa glycoprotein consisting of 450 amino acids. It has the highest affinity for T_4 and T_3 and is responsible for most of the thyroid-binding capacity in the plasma. The extensive binding of thyroid hormones to plasma proteins serves several functions. It provides a large buffer pool of

thyroid hormones in the circulation, so that the active concentrations of hormone in the circulation change very little on a minute-to-minute basis. The binding to plasma proteins markedly prolongs the half-lives of both T_4 and T_3. T_4 has a half-life of 8 days, and T_3 has a half-life of ~24 hours; each is longer than the half-life of the steroid or peptide hormones. Finally, because much of the T_3 in the circulation is formed by the conversion of T_4 to T_3 in extrathyroidal tissues, the presence of a large pool of T_4 in the plasma provides a reserve of prohormone available for synthesis of T_3. This reserve may be of particular importance because T_3 is responsible for most of the biological activity of thyroid hormones.

Peripheral tissues deiodinate T_4 to produce T_3

The thyroid synthesizes and stores much more T_4 than T_3, and this is reflected by the ~10:1 ratio of T_4/T_3 secreted by the thyroid. However, certain tissues in the body have the capacity to selectively deiodinate T_4, thereby producing either T_3 or rT_3. T_3 and rT_3 can each be further deiodinated to various DITs and MITs (Fig. 49-4); both DITs and MITs are biologically inactive. Both iodine atoms on the inner ring, and at least one iodine atom on the outer ring, appear essential for biological activity. Similarly, the loss of the amino group renders T_4 or T_3 inactive. The importance of the peripheral deiodination of T_4 to T_3 can be readily appreciated from the observation that persons whose thyroids have been removed have normal circulating concentrations of T_3 when they receive oral T_4 supplementation.

Inasmuch as T_3 is biologically much more active than the far more abundant T_4, the regulation of the conversion of T_4 to T_3 in peripheral tissues assumes considerable importance. Two distinct deiodinases convert T_4 to T_3 (Fig. 49-4): The 5'/3'-deiodinase removes an I from the *outer* ring, thus producing T_3, whereas the 5/3-deiodinase removes an I from the *inner* ring, thereby producing the inactive rT_3. Because the 3' and 5' positions in T_4 are equivalent stereochemically, removal of either of these yields T_3. Similarly, removing the I from either the 3 or the 5 position of the inner ring of T_4 yields rT_3. Further deiodination by these two enzymes ultimately yields T_0 (i.e., thyronine).

The 5'/3'-deiodinase, which acts on the outer ring, comes in two forms. Type 1 is present in high concentrations in the liver, kidneys, and thyroid. It appears to be responsible for generating most of the T_3 that reaches the circulation. Type 2 is found predominantly in the pituitary, central nervous system (CNS), and placenta and is involved in supplying those tissues with T_3 by local generation from plasma-derived T_4. As shown later, the type 2 enzyme in the pituitary is of particular importance because the T_3 that is generated there is responsible for the feedback inhibition of the release of thyrotropin (or thyroid-stimulating hormone, TSH).

The relative activity of the deiodinases changes in response to physiological and pathologic stimuli. Caloric restriction or severe stress inhibits the *type 1* outer ring deiodinase; this process decreases the conversion of T_4 to T_3—and thus reduces the levels of T_3. In contrast, levels of rT_3 rise by default in these situations, in part because of reduced conversion to DITs. These decreases in T_3 levels are accompanied by a decline in metabolic rate. You may think that because plasma levels of T_3 *fall*, there would be a compensatory *rise* in TSH, the secretion of which is inhibited by T_3. However, because *type 2* deiodinase mediates the conversion of T_4 to T_3 within the pituitary and CNS, and because caloric restriction does not affect this enzyme, local T_3 levels in the pituitary are normal. Thus, the thyrotrophs in the pituitary continue to have adequate amounts of T_3, and no compensatory rise in TSH occurs. Teleologically, the rationale to restrain calorie expenditure in settings of decreased caloric intake is appealing.

ACTION OF THYROID HORMONES

Thyroid hormones act through nuclear receptors in target tissues

Thyroid hormones act on many body tissues to exert both metabolic and developmental effects. Most, if not all, of the actions of thyroid hormones occur as thyroid hormones bind to and activate **nuclear receptors** (see Chapter 3). These receptors, in turn, are bound to chromatin and alter the transcription of specific genes. The multitude of thyroid hormone actions is mirrored by the ubiquitous expression of thyroid hormone receptors (TRs) throughout the body's tissues. Once T_4 and T_3 leave the plasma, they enter the cell either by diffusing through the lipid of the cell membrane or by carrier-mediated transport (Fig. 49-5). Once in the cytoplasm, T_4 and T_3 bind to sites in the cytosol, microsomes, and mitochondria, as well as the nucleus. This observation has prompted speculation that thyroid hormones may exert actions through mechanisms not involving

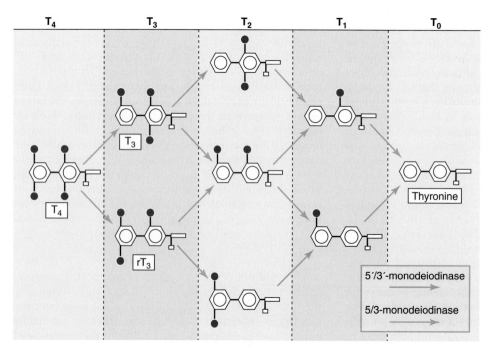

Figure 49-4 Peripheral metabolism of T_4. A 5'/3'-monodeiodinase (*green arrows*) removes I from the outer benzyl ring, whereas a 5/3-monodeiodinase (*orange arrows*) removes I from the inner benzyl ring. Thus, the action of the 5'/3'-monodeiodinase on T_4 yields T_3, whereas the action of the 5/3-monodeiodinase yields rT_3. Sequential deiodination yields T_0 (thyronine).

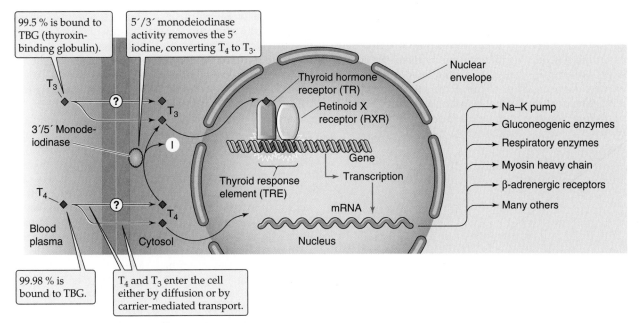

Figure 49-5 Action of thyroid hormones on target cells. Free extracellular T_4 and T_3 enter the target cell. Once T_4 is inside the cell, a cytoplasmic 5'/3'-monodeiodinase converts much of the T_4 to T_3, so cytoplasmic levels of T_4 and T_3 are about equal. TRs bind to nuclear DNA at thyroid response elements in the promoter region of genes regulated by thyroid hormones. The binding of T_3 or T_4 to the receptor regulates the transcription of these genes. Of the total thyroid hormone bound to receptor, ~90% is T_3. The receptor that binds to the DNA is preferentially a heterodimer of the TR and RXR.

transcriptional regulation. However, current evidence suggests that if these nongenomic mechanisms are operative, they are exceptions to the general schema shown in Figure 49-5, which appears to account for most of the actions of thyroid hormones.

Biologically, T_3 is much more important than T_4. This statement may be surprising inasmuch as the *total* concentration of T_4 in the circulation is 50-fold or higher than that of T_3. T_3 has greater biological activity for three reasons. First, T_4 is bound (only 0.02% is *free*) more tightly to plasma proteins than is T_3 (0.50% is *free*; i.e., a 25-fold higher ratio of free to bound). The net effect is that the amount of free T_4 in the circulation is only ~2-fold greater than the amount of free T_3. Second, because the target cell converts T_4—once it has entered the cell—to T_3, it turns out that T_4 and T_3 are present at similar concentrations in the cytoplasm of target cells. Finally, the TR in the nucleus has ~10-fold greater affinity for T_3 than T_4, so that T_3 is more potent on a molar basis. As a result, T_3 is responsible for ~90% of the occupancy of TRs in the euthyroid state.

When T_3 or T_4 binds to the TR in the nucleus, the hormone-bound receptors either activate or repress the transcription of specific genes. As discussed earlier in Chapter 4, TR preferentially binds to DNA as a heterodimer of TR and the retinoid X receptor (RXR). TR belongs to the superfamily of nuclear receptors that contains domains A through F (see Chapter 3). Three regions are especially important for TR: (1) The amino-terminal A/B region contains the first of two transactivation domains, which are responsible for transducing receptor binding into a conformational change in the DNA, thereby initiating transcription; (2) the middle or C region is responsible for DNA binding through two zinc

fingers (see Chapter 4), as well as dimerization between receptors; and (3) the E region, toward the carboxyl terminus, is responsible for binding the ligand (T_3 or T_4), and also for dimerization.

Actually, two TR genes—α and β—are present on chromosomes 17 and 3, respectively. The expression of these receptor genes is tissue specific and varies with time of development. The liver expresses principally the β isoform, whereas the α isoform predominates in the brain. During development, the amount of α expressed may vary 10-fold or more.

Thyroid hormones can also act by nongenomic pathways

Nongenomic actions of thyroid hormone have been observed in several tissues, including heart, muscle, fat, and pituitary. Early on, it was thought that thyroid hormone could act through nongenomic pathways to enhance mitochondrial oxidative phosphorylation—or at least energy expenditure as measured by O_2 consumption. More recent data support this hypothesis as well as actions on ion channels, second messengers, and protein kinases. It is less clear whether these actions are mediated through the classical TR, as they are for nongenomic actions of the estradiol receptor (see Chapter 47), or another high-affinity thyroid-binding protein.

Thyroid hormones increase basal metabolic rate by stimulating futile cycles of catabolism/anabolism

Investigators have long observed that excess thyroid hormone raises the **basal metabolic rate** (BMR) as measured by either heat production (direct calorimetry) or O_2 consumption (indirect calorimetry). Conversely, thyroid hormone deficiency is accompanied by a decreased BMR. Figure 49-6 illustrates the effect of thyroid hormone levels on BMR, and Table 49-1 summarizes the effect of the thyroid hormones on several parameters. Thyroid hormones increase the BMR by stimulating both catabolic and anabolic reactions in pathways affecting fats, carbohydrates, and proteins.

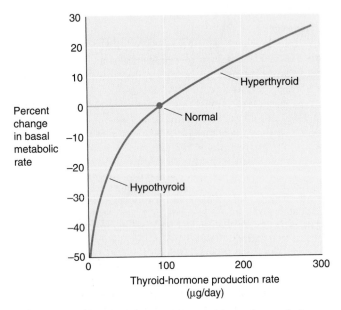

Figure 49-6 Effect of thyroid hormone on BMR. This graph shows the dependence of BMR on the daily rate of thyroid hormone secretion (T_4 and T_3). We use the secretion rate because it is difficult to know whether to use free T_4 or free T_3. Thus, the secretion rate is a crude measure of effective thyroid hormone levels. (*Data from Guyton AC, Hall JE: Textbook of Medical Physiology, 9th ed. Philadelphia: WB Saunders, 1996.*)

Carbohydrate Metabolism Thyroid hormones raise the rate of hepatic glucose production, principally by increasing hepatic gluconeogenic activity. This effect generally does not result in increases in plasma [glucose], provided the pancreas responds by augmenting insulin secretion. Thyroid hormones also enhance the availability of the starting materials required for increased gluconeogenic activity (i.e., amino acids and glycerol), and they specifically induce the expression of several key gluconeogenic enzymes, including phosphoenolpyruvate carboxykinase, pyruvate carboxylase, and glucose-6-phosphatase.

Protein Metabolism The amino acids required for increased hepatic gluconeogenesis, stimulated by thyroid hormones, come from increased proteolysis, predominantly in muscle. Thyroid hormones also increase protein synthesis. Because the increases in protein degradation usually outweigh the increases in synthesis, a net loss of muscle protein occurs. The catabolic effect is exaggerated when T_3 is present in great excess, so that muscle wasting and weakness, as well as increased nitrogen loss in the urine as urea (see Chapters 36 and 46), can be prominent features of clinical thyrotoxicosis (hyperthyroidism).

Lipid Metabolism The glycerol required for increased hepatic gluconeogenesis, stimulated by thyroid hormones, comes from increased degradation of stored triglycerides in adipose tissue. The fatty acids released along with the glycerol provide fuel for the liver to support the energy demand of gluconeogenesis. Thyroid hormones not only increase lipolysis but also enhance lipogenesis. Indeed, modest amounts of thyroid hormones are needed for the normal synthesis of fatty acid by liver. Very high levels of T_3 shift the balance in favor of lipolysis, with resulting generalized fat mobilization and loss of body fat stores.

By accelerating the rates of glucose production, protein synthesis, and degradation, as well as of lipogenesis and

Table 49-1 Physiological Effects of the Thyroid Hormones (T_3 and T_4)

Parameter	Low Level of Thyroid Hormones (Hypothyroid)	High Level of Thyroid Hormones (Hyperthyroid)
Basal metabolic rate	↓	↑
Carbohydrate metabolism	↓ Gluconeogenesis ↓ Glycogenolysis Normal serum [glucose]	↑ Gluconeogenesis ↑ Glycogenolysis Normal serum [glucose]
Protein metabolism	↓ Synthesis ↓ Proteolysis	↑ Synthesis ↑ Proteolysis Muscle wasting
Lipid metabolism	↓ Lipogenesis ↓ Lipolysis ↑ Serum [cholesterol]	↑ Lipogenesis ↑ Lipolysis ↓ Serum [cholesterol]
Thermogenesis	↓	↑
Autonomic nervous system	Normal levels of serum catecholamines	↑ Expression of β adrenoceptors (increased sensitivity to catecholamines, which remain at normal levels)

lipolysis, the thyroid hormones stimulate energy consumption. Therefore, to the extent that thyroid hormones stimulate both synthesis and degradation, they promote **futile cycles** that contribute significantly to the increased O_2 consumption seen in thyrotoxicosis (hyperthyroidism).

How, at the molecular level, thyroid hormones affect the BMR in states of both spontaneous and experimentally induced thyroid hormone excess or deficiency has been a difficult question to answer. The changes in metabolic rate do not appear to be determined by changes in the expression of a single gene. Several specific examples of the effects of thyroid hormones on target tissues serve to illustrate their general mechanism of action.

Na-K Pump Activity   In muscle, liver, and kidney, thyroid hormone–induced increases in O_2 consumption are paralleled by increases in the activity of the **Na-K pump** in the plasma membrane (see Chapter 5). This increase in transport is the result, at least in part, of an increase in the synthesis of new transporter units that are inserted into the plasma membrane. At least in some tissues, blockade of the increases in Na-K pump activity with ouabain also blocks the increase in O_2 consumption. T_3 stimulates the transcription of the genes for both the α and β subunits of the Na-K pump. In addition, T_3 increases translation by stabilizing the mRNA that encodes the Na-K pump. Increases in the activity of this transporter use additional ATP and thereby consume O_2 and generate heat. Inasmuch as states of thyroid hormone excess are not accompanied by any noticeable derangement of plasma electrolyte levels, presumably the increase in Na-K pump activity is compensated in some manner by a leak of Na^+ and K^+, although such pathways have not yet been defined. Overall, the increased activity of the Na-K pump (with an accompanying cation leak) would result in a futile cycle whereby energy was consumed without useful work.

Thermogenesis   In rodents, thyroid hormones may affect metabolic rate and thermogenesis through another futile cycle mechanism. Brown fat in these animals expresses a mitochondrial **uncoupling protein** (UCP), or **thermogenin**, that dissociates **oxidative phosphorylation** from ATP generation. Thus, mitochondria consume O_2 and produce heat without generating ATP. Both T_3 and β-adrenergic stimulation (acting through the β_3 receptor) enhance respiration in brown adipose tissue by stimulating this uncoupling mechanism. We discuss thermogenin—and the vital role it plays in helping to keep newborn humans warm—in Chapter 57.

Thyroid hormones also increase the BMR by increasing the thermogenic effects of other processes. An example is the effect of adrenergic stimulation on thermogenesis, discussed earlier. In humans, plasma *concentrations* of catecholamines are normal in states of both excess and deficient T_3 and T_4. However, excess thyroid hormone raises the *sensitivity* of tissues to the action of adrenergic hormones. In heart, skeletal muscle, and adipose tissue, this effect is the result, at least in part, of increased expression of β-**adrenergic receptors** by these tissues. In patients who are acutely thyrotoxic, treatment with β-receptor antagonists is one of the first priorities. This treatment blunts the hypersympathetic state induced by the excess of thyroid hormones. Thyroid hor-

mones may also exert postreceptor effects that enhance adrenergic tone. In the heart, thyroid hormones also regulate the expression of specific forms of **myosin heavy chain**. Specifically, in rodents, thyroid hormone increases the expression of the myosin α chain, thereby favoring the α/α isoform of myosin heavy chain (see Chapter 9). This isoform is associated with greater activity of both actin and Ca^{2+}-activated ATPase, faster fiber shortening, and greater contractility.

Thyroid hormones are essential for normal growth and development

In amphibians, thyroid hormone regulates the process of metamorphosis. Removing the thyroid gland from tadpoles causes development to arrest at the tadpole stage. Early administration of excess thyroid hormone can initiate premature metamorphosis. Iodothyronines are present even farther down the phylogenetic tree, at least as far as primitive chordates, although these animals lack a thyroid gland per se. However, the biological actions of iodothyronines in many species are not known.

Thyroid hormones are essential for normal human development as well, as starkly illustrated by the unfortunate condition of cretinism in regions of endemic iodine deficiency. **Cretinism** is characterized by profound mental retardation, short stature, delay in motor development, coarse hair, and a protuberant abdomen. Correction of iodine deficiency has essentially eliminated endemic cretinism in developed nations. Sporadic cases continue to occur, however, as a result of congenital defects in thyroid hormone synthesis. If hypothyroidism is recognized and corrected within a few days of birth, development—including mental development—can proceed almost normally. For this reason, many localities have initiated laboratory screening of newborns for hypothyroidism because clinical recognition of the full syndrome often occurs only after the developmental abnormalities in the CNS are irreversible.

Typically overshadowed by the impaired cognitive development that occurs in cretinism is the **dwarfism** that results from the effects of thyroid hormone deficiency on human growth (Fig. 49-7). In children with normal thyroid function at birth, development of hypothyroidism at any time before the fusion of the epiphyses of the long bones leads to growth retardation or arrest. Much of the loss in height that occurs can be recovered after thyroid hormone treatment is begun, a phenomenon called *catch-up growth*. If the diagnosis and treatment of hypothyroidism are delayed, loss of potential growth may occur. As indicated in Figure 49-7, catch-up growth may not apply to mental development unless the treatment is begun very early, certainly within a few days of birth. In general, the longer the duration of congenital hypothyroidism, the more profound is the mental retardation. The growth curve (i.e., a plot of the child's height and weight versus age) can provide a particularly sensitive early indicator of hypothyroidism. An overactive thyroid is much less a problem than is an underactive thyroid with regard to its effect on growth; other signs and symptoms of an overactive thyroid predominate.

Cellular explanations of the effects of thyroid hormones on human development are incomplete. In rats, thyroid hormone induces the secretion of pituitary growth hormone

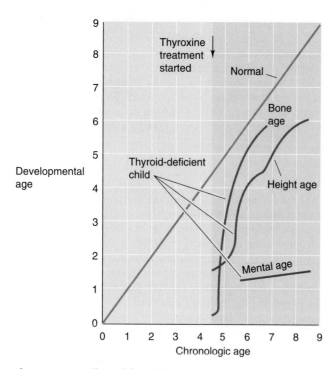

Figure 49-7 Effect of thyroid hormone on growth and development. This is a graph of developmental age—that is, the age that the child appears based on height, bone radiograph, and mental function—versus chronological age. For a normal child, the relationship is the *straight line in red*, for which developmental and chronological age are identical. The *three green curves* are growth curves for a child with thyroid hormone deficiency. At age 4.5 years, before initiation of therapy, height age, bone age, and mental age are all substantially lower than normal. Initiating replacement therapy with thyroid hormone at age 4.5 years causes a rapid increase in both height age and bone age (catch-up growth) but has no effect on mental age, which remains infantile. Treatment can help mental development only if the therapy is begun within a few days of birth. *(Data from Wilkins L: The Diagnosis and Treatment of Endocrine Disorders of Childhood and Adolescence. Springfield, IL: Charles C Thomas, 1965.)*

(GH); thus, the growth retardation in thyroid-deficient rats may be partly the result of decreased GH secretion. However, in humans, who have no thyroid hormone response element in the promoter region of the GH gene, plasma [GH] is normal in hypothyroidism. Thus, the growth failure of hypothyroid human infants is not as readily explained. In humans, changes in the growth of long bones are more or less characteristic of thyroid hormone deficiency. These changes include a delay in formation of centers of ossification at the growth plate, followed by the appearance of several ossification centers, which eventually merge. Short stature in human juvenile or infantile hypothyroidism may be in part related to these abnormalities of cartilage growth and development as well as to resistance to the normal action of GH to promote growth. In rodents, thyroid hormone regulates the induction of expression of several neural proteins, including myelin basic protein. How deficiencies in these proteins may result in the generalized cortical atrophy seen in infantile hypothyroidism is not clear.

THE HYPOTHALAMIC-PITUITARY-THYROID AXIS

The pituitary regulates the synthesis and secretion of thyroid hormones through the release of **thyrotropin**—also known as thyroid stimulating hormone (TSH)—from the anterior pituitary. The hypothalamus, in turn, stimulates the release of TSH through **thyrotropin-releasing hormone (TRH)**. Finally, circulating thyroid hormones exert feedback control on both TRH and TSH secretion.

Thyrotropin-releasing hormone from the hypothalamus stimulates the thyrotrophs of the anterior pituitary to secrete thyrotropin, which, in turn, stimulates T_4/T_3 synthesis

Thyrotropin-Releasing Hormone   TRH is a tripeptide pyro-Glu-His-Pro containing the modified amino acid pyro-Glu. It is found in many tissues, including the cerebral cortex, multiple areas of the gastrointestinal tract, and the β cells of the pancreas. However, the arcuate nucleus and the median eminence of the **hypothalamus** appear to be the major sources of the TRH that stimulates TSH synthesis and secretion (Fig. 49-8). TRH released by neurons in the hypothalamus travels to the anterior pituitary through the hypophyseal portal system (see Chapter 47). Hypothalamic lesions that interrupt TRH release or delivery cause a fall in basal TSH levels. Conversely, administering TRH intravenously can cause a rapid, dose-dependent release of TSH from the anterior pituitary. However, it is not clear that such bursts of TRH release and TSH secretion occur physiologically.

Thyrotropin-Releasing Hormone Receptor   Once it reaches the thyrotrophs in the anterior pituitary, TRH binds to the TRH receptor, a G protein–coupled receptor on the cell membranes of the thyrotrophs. TRH binding triggers the phospholipase C pathway (see Chapter 3). The formation of diacylglycerols (DAGs) stimulates protein kinase C and leads to protein phosphorylation. The simultaneous release of inositol triphosphate (IP_3) triggers Ca^{2+} release from internal stores, thus raising $[Ca^{2+}]_i$. The result is an increase in both the synthesis and release of TSH, which is stored in secretory granules. TRH produces some of its effects by activating phospholipase A_2, a process leading to the release of arachidonic acid and the formation of a variety of biologically active eicosanoids (see Chapter 3). In healthy persons, administering TRH also raises plasma [prolactin] by stimulating lactotrophs in the anterior pituitary (see Chapter 52). However, no evidence indicates a regulatory role for TRH in prolactin secretion or action.

Thyrotropin   The thyrotrophs represent a relatively small number of cells in the **anterior pituitary**. The TSH that they release is a 28-kDa glycoprotein with α and β chains. The α chain of TSH is identical to that of the other glycoprotein hormones: the gonadotropins luteinizing hormone (LH), follicle-stimulating hormone (FSH), and human chorionic

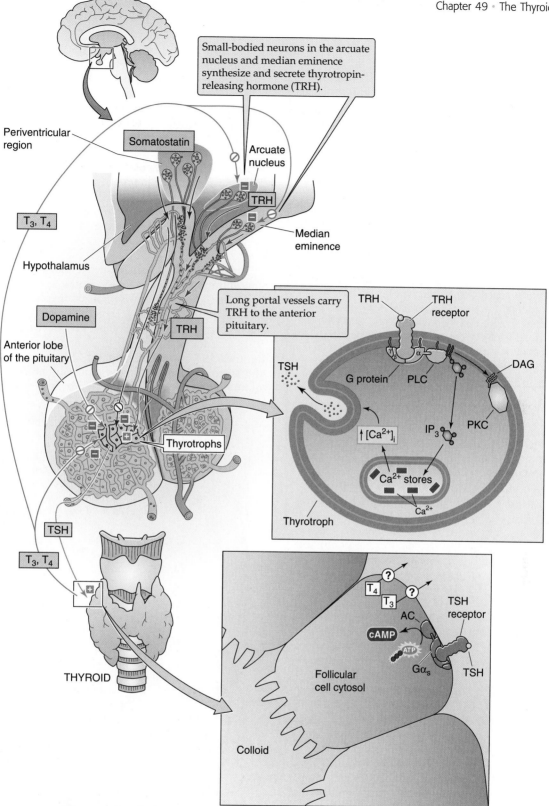

Figure 49-8 The hypothalamic-pituitary-thyroid axis. Small-bodied neurons in the arcuate nucleus and median eminence of the hypothalamus secrete TRH, a tripeptide that reaches the thyrotrophs in the anterior pituitary through the long portal veins. TRH binds to a G protein–coupled receptor on the thyrotroph membrane, thus triggering the DAG/IP_3 pathway, leading to protein phosphorylation, and raising $[Ca^{2+}]_i$. These pathways stimulate the thyrotrophs to synthesize and release thyrotropin (or TSH), which is a 28-kDa glycoprotein stored in secretory granules. The TSH binds to receptors on the basolateral membrane of thyroid follicular cells, thereby stimulating $G\alpha_s$. This process, in turn, activates adenylyl cyclase (AC) and raises $[cAMP]_i$. As outlined in Figure 49-3, TSH stimulates certain steps in the synthesis and release of T_4 and T_3. Inside the pituitary, the type 2 form of 5′/3′-monodeiodinase converts T_4 to T_3, which negatively feeds back on the thyrotrophs as well as on the TRH-secreting neurons. Somatostatin and dopamine—released by hypothalamic neurons—inhibit TSH release and thus can influence the set point at which TSH is released in response to a given amount of T_3 in the pituitary. PKC, protein kinase C; PLC, phospholipase C.

Graves Disease

Surprisingly, it is not uncommon for B lymphocytes to synthesize immune globulins that bind to and activate the TSH receptor, thereby reproducing all the actions of TSH on the thyroid. Unfortunately, these errant lymphocytes do not regulate the production of these immunoglobulins in a manner analogous to the regulated secretion of TSH by the pituitary. As a result, iodide trapping by the thyroid increases, the synthesis and secretion of both T_3 and T_4 increase, and the thyroid enlarges to produce a goiter. Untreated, the affected individual becomes increasingly hyperthyroid. The clinical manifestations of hyperthyroidism include an increased metabolic rate with associated weight loss, sweating and heat intolerance, a rapid and more forceful heartbeat, muscle weakness and wasting, tremulousness, difficulty concentrating, and changes in hair growth and skin texture. Because TSH stimulates all areas of the thyroid, the thyroid is symmetrically enlarged, and even the isthmus is frequently palpable on clinical examination.

The abnormal immunoglobulin is designated TSI for **thyroid-stimulating immunoglobulin**. The constellation of symptoms noted previously, together with a symmetrically enlarged **goiter**, is called Graves disease, after Robert Graves, who provided one of the first detailed descriptions of the disorder in the early 19th century. These antibodies are also able to stimulate connective tissue in the extraocular muscles and in the dermis of the lower extremity to synthesize mucopolysaccharides, thus leading to thickening of both the muscle and the dermis. Therefore, in addition to the abnormalities of thyroid growth and hyperfunction, a few individuals with Graves disease develop a peculiar infiltrative abnormality in the extraocular muscles. When severe, this *infiltrative ophthalmopathy* impairs muscle function and causes diplopia (double vision) and forward protrusion of the eyes **(exophthalmos)**. Even less frequently, patients with Graves disease develop infiltrating dermopathy in the skin over the lower legs called *pretibial myxedema*. This thickening of the skin occurs in localized patches and is pathologically distinct from the generalized thickening and coarsening of the skin seen in hypothyroidism *(generalized myxedema)*.

gonadotropin (hCG). The β chain is unique to TSH and confers the specificity of the hormone. Once secreted, TSH acts on the thyroid follicular cell through a specific receptor.

Thyrotropin Receptor The TSH receptor on the thyroid follicular cells is a member of the family of G protein–coupled receptors. Like receptors for the other glycoprotein hormones (LH, FSH, and hCG), the TSH receptor activates adenylyl cyclase through $G\alpha_s$ (see Chapter 3). This activation of the TSH receptor stimulates a diverse range of physiological processes or events, summarized in Figure 49-3:

1. Iodide uptake by the **NIS** on the basolateral membrane of the thyroid follicular cell. Stimulation of this cotransporter allows for trapping of dietary iodine within the thyroid gland. The ratio of follicular cell iodine to serum iodine (the so-called thyroid/serum or T/S ratio) is 30:1

in euthyroid individuals. The T/S ratio decreases under conditions of low TSH (e.g., hypophysectomy) and increases under conditions of high TSH (e.g., a TSH-secreting pituitary adenoma);
2. **Iodination** of thyroglobulin in the follicular lumen;
3. **Conjugation** of **iodinated** tyrosines to form T_4 and T_3 linked to thyroglobulin;
4. **Endocytosis** of iodinated thyroglobulin into the follicular cells from thyroid colloid;
5. **Proteolysis** of the iodinated thyroglobulin in the follicular cell;
6. **Secretion** of T_4 and T_3 into the circulation; and
7. **Hyperplasia** of the thyroid gland because of the growth factor effects of TSH.

Figure 49-9 illustrates the goiter that occurs when TSH concentrations are elevated for a prolonged period of time and stimulates an otherwise normal thyroid gland (see the box on Iodine Deficiency). Hyperplasia of the thyroid gland also occurs in Graves disease because of stimulation of the TSH receptor by a thyroid-stimulating immunoglobulin. In contrast, the chronic elevation of TSH typically seen when the thyroid gland undergoes autoimmune *injury* (Hashimoto thyroiditis) does not respond by hypertrophy.

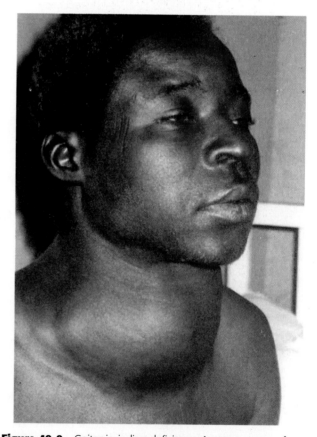

Figure 49-9 Goiter in iodine deficiency. A young woman from a region in Central Africa where iodine deficiency is prevalent exhibits a large goiter secondary to iodine deficiency and the growth-promoting effects of TSH, the levels of which as part of a feedback mechanism for achieving a sufficient amount of thyroid hormone.

T₃ exerts negative feedback on thyrotropin secretion

Circulating *free* T₄ and T₃ inhibit both the synthesis of TRH by hypothalamic neurons and the release of TSH by the thyrotrophs in the anterior pituitary. Plasma [TSH] is very sensitive to alteration in the levels of free T₄ and T₃; a 50% decline in free T₄ levels can cause plasma [TSH] to increase 50- to 100-fold. Conversely, as may be expected of a well-functioning feedback system, an excess of thyroid hormone leads to a decrease in plasma [TSH].

At the level of the thyrotroph, the sensor in this feedback system monitors the concentration of T₃ *inside* the thyrotroph (Fig. 49-8). As noted earlier, T₃ either can enter directly from the blood plasma or can form inside the thyrotroph by deiodination of T₄. The negative feedback of T₄ and T₃ on TSH release occurs at the level of the pituitary thyrotroph by both indirect and direct mechanisms. In the **indirect feedback pathway**, intracellular T₃ decreases the number of TRH receptors on the surface of the thyrotroph. As a result, thyroid hormones *indirectly* inhibit TSH release by reducing the sensitivity of the thyrotrophs to TRH. In the **direct feedback pathway**, intracellular T₃ inhibits the synthesis of both the α and the β chains of TSH. Indeed, both the α and β TSH genes have T₃ response elements in their promoter regions. These response elements, which are *inhibitory*, differ from those found in genes that are *positively* regulated by T₃ (e.g., Na-K pump).

Hypothyroidism

Hypothyroidism is one of the most common of all endocrine illnesses—even more common than Graves disease. Hypothyroidism affects between 1% and 2% of all adults at some time in their lives. Women are much more commonly affected than men. Although hypothyroidism has several causes, the most common cause worldwide is iodine deficiency. In the United States, by far the most common cause is an autoimmune disorder called *Hashimoto thyroiditis*. Like Graves disease, Hashimoto thyroiditis is caused by an abnormal immune response that includes the production of antithyroid antibodies, in this case, antibodies against the thyroid follicular cells, microsomes, and TSH receptors. Unlike in Graves disease, the antibodies in Hashimoto thyroiditis are not stimulatory, but rather are part of an immune process that blocks and destroys thyroid function. The titers of these autoantibodies can reach colossal proportions.

Typically, hypothyroidism in Hashimoto thyroiditis is an insidious process that develops slowly; indeed, many patients are diagnosed, long before striking clinical manifestations are apparent, by routine blood tests revealing an elevated TSH despite normal levels of T₃ and T₄. These individuals, although not yet clinically hypothyroid, are sometimes treated with thyroid hormone replacement, so the clinical manifestations of hypothyroidism are never given a chance to develop.

In patients in whom the disease does evolve, the classical presentation consists of painless goiter, skin changes, peripheral edema, constipation, headache, joint aches, fatigue, and, in women, anovulation. The TSH level should be checked in any female patient with secondary amenorrhea. In time, some of these patients also develop other autoimmune disorders, such as pernicious anemia, myasthenia gravis, Addison disease, diabetes mellitus, and ovarian failure.

Like patients with hyperthyroidism, who may be threatened by thyroid storm, those with hypothyroidism also have their severe, life-threatening variant, in this case called **myxedema coma**. This malady is quite rare and occurs most commonly in elderly patients with established hypothyroidism. Hypothermia and coma evolve slowly in these patients, and the usual causes are failure to take prescribed thyroid hormone replacement, cold exposure, sepsis, heart failure, and alcohol abuse.

Clinical Assessment of Thyroid Function

Plasma thyrotropin levels. Direct measurements of T₄/T₃ provide a measure of *total* circulating hormone (i.e., the sum of *free* T₄ and T₃, as well as T₄ and T₃ *bound* to TBG, TTR, and albumin). However, these direct measurements do not allow one to distinguish between bound and free T₄/T₃. The sensitive response of TSH to changes in thyroid hormone levels provides an extremely valuable tool for assessing whether the free T₄/T₃ levels in the circulation are deficient, sufficient, or excessive. Indeed, the level of TSH reflects the amount of free, biologically active thyroid hormone in the target tissue. As a result, in recent years, measurements of plasma TSH using very sensitive immune assay methods have come to be regarded as the single best determinants of thyroid hormone status. Obviously, this approach is valid only if the thyrotrophs themselves are able to respond to T₃/T₄—that is, if patients have no evidence of pituitary dysfunction.

The health of the thyrotrophs themselves can be tested by injecting a bolus of synthetic TRH and monitoring changes in plasma [TSH]. In hypothyroid patients, the subsequent rise in plasma [TSH] is more dramatic than in physiologically normal individuals. This test was of great value in confirming the diagnosis of hypothyroidism before the advent of today's sensitive assays, but it has largely been abandoned.

Radioactive iodine uptake. Measuring the amount of a standard bolus of radioactive iodine that the thyroid can take up was also once widespread as a measure of thyroid function. A hyperactive gland would take up increased amounts of the tracer, whereas an underactive gland would take up subnormal amounts. Today, the test is mostly used for three other purposes. First, radioactive iodine uptake can show whether a solitary thyroid nodule, detected on physical examination, is "hot" (functioning) or "cold" (nonfunctioning). Cold nodules are more likely than hot ones to harbor a malignancy. Second, radioactive iodine uptake can show whether hyperthyroidism is the result of thyroid inflammation (i.e., thyroiditis), in which tracer uptake is minimal, or Graves disease, in which tracer uptake is increased. Third, high doses of radioactive iodine are commonly used to treat patients with hyperthyroidism.

Free T_4 and T_3 concentrations in the plasma, which determine intracellular T_3 levels in the thyrotroph, are relatively constant over the course of 24 hours, a finding reflecting the long half-lives of both T_4 and T_3. Given that the levels of T_4 and T_3 are the primary triggers in the afferent limb of the negative feedback for the hypothalamic-pituitary-thyroid axis, the feedback regulation of TSH secretion by thyroid hormones appears to be a slow process—essentially integrating thyroid hormone levels over time. Indeed, T_3 feeds back on the thyrotroph by modulating *gene transcription*, which by its very nature is a slow process.

The feedback of T_4 and T_3 on the release of TSH may also be under the control of somatostatin and dopamine, which travel from the hypothalamus to the thyrotrophs through the portal vessels (Fig. 49-8). Somatostatin and dopamine both inhibit TSH secretion, apparently by making the thyrotroph more sensitive to inhibition by intracellular T_3—that is, shifting the set point for T_3. Thus, somatostatin and dopamine appear to counterbalance the stimulatory effect of TRH. Although these inhibitory effects are readily demonstrated with pharmacological infusion of these agents, their physiological role in the regulation of TSH secretion appears small. In particular, with long-term administration of somatostatin or dopamine, compensatory mechanisms appear to override any inhibition.

A special example of feedback between T_3 and TSH is seen in neonates of mothers with abnormal levels of T_3. If the mother is *hyper*thyroid, both she and the fetus will have low TSH levels because T_3 crosses the placenta. After birth, the newborn rapidly metabolizes T_3, but TSH remains suppressed, so the infant temporarily becomes *hypo*thyroid. Conversely, if the mother's thyroid gland has been removed and she is *hypo*thyroid because she is not receiving sufficient thyroid hormone replacement therapy, both she and the fetus will have high levels of circulating TSH. Immediately after birth, the newborn will be temporarily *hyper*thyroid.

REFERENCES

Books and Reviews

Bassett JH, Harvey CB, Williams GR: Mechanisms of thyroid hormone receptor–specific nuclear and extra nuclear actions. Mol Cell Endocrinol 2003; 213:1-11.

Cavalieri RR: Iodine metabolism and thyroid physiology: Current concepts. Thyroid 1997; 7:177-181.

Dumont JE, Lamy F, Roger P, Maenhaut C: Physiological and pathological regulation of thyroid cell proliferation and differentiation by thyrotropin and other factors. Physiol Rev 1992; 72:667-697.

Gershengorn MC, Osman R: Molecular and cellular biology of thyrotropin-releasing hormone receptors. Physiol Rev 1996; 76:175-191.

Guyton AC, Hall JE: Textbook of Medical Physiology, 9th ed. Philadelphia: WB Saunders, 1996.

Larsen PR: Update on the human iodothyronine selenodeiodinases, the enzymes regulating the activation and inactivation of thyroid hormone. Biochem Soc Trans 1997; 25:588-592.

Orban Z, Bornstein SR, Chrousos GP: The interaction between leptin and the hypothalamic-pituitary-thyroid axis. Horm Metab Res 1998; 30:231-235.

Samuels HH, Forman BM, Horowitz ZD, Ye Z-S: Regulation of gene expression by thyroid hormone. Annu Rev Physiol 1989; 51:623-639.

Wilkins L: The Diagnosis and Treatment of Endocrine Disorders of Childhood and Adolescence. Springfield, IL, Charles C Thomas, 1965.

Journal Articles

Arvan P, Kim PS, Kuliawat R, et al: Intracellular protein transport to the thyrocyte plasma membrane: Potential implications for thyroid physiology. Thyroid 1997; 7:89-105.

Dai G, Levy O, Carrasco N: Cloning and characterization of the thyroid iodide transporter. Nature 1996; 379:458-460.

Koenig RJ: Thyroid hormone receptor coactivators and corepressors. Thyroid 1998; 8:703-713.

CHAPTER 50

THE ADRENAL GLAND

Eugene J. Barrett

The human adrenal glands, each weighing only ~4 g, are located above the upper pole of each kidney in the retroperitoneal space. They produce four principal hormones: cortisol, aldosterone, epinephrine (adrenaline), and norepinephrine. Each adrenal gland is composed of an inner medulla and an outer cortex (Fig. 50-1). Embryologically, the cortex is derived from mesoderm, whereas the medulla is derived from neural crest cells (see Chapter 10) that migrate into the developing cortex. The cortex produces two principal steroid hormones, cortisol and aldosterone, as well as several androgenic steroids. The medulla produces epinephrine and norepinephrine.

The **adrenal cortex** can be further divided into three cellular layers: the *glomerulosa* layer near the surface, the *fasciculata* layer in the midcortex, and the *reticularis* layer near the cortical-medullary junction. **Aldosterone**, the main mineralocorticoid in humans, is made in the glomerulosa cell layer. **Cortisol**, the principal glucocorticoid, is made in the fasciculata and reticularis layers. Although both cortisol and aldosterone are made by enzymatic modification of cholesterol and are structurally quite similar, their actions on the body differ dramatically. Cortisol is considered a **glucocorticoid** because it was recognized early on to increase plasma glucose levels; deficiency of cortisol can result in hypoglycemia. Aldosterone is considered a **mineralocorticoid** because it promotes salt and water retention by the kidney. The activities of these two hormones overlap, particularly at high hormone levels, but this distinction is still very useful in identifying their most obvious functions. The adrenal cortex also synthesizes and secretes **androgenic steroids**, which to a large extent appear to be byproducts of cortisol production.

In the **adrenal medulla**, chromaffin cells produce **epinephrine** or adrenaline, a catecholamine that is synthesized from the amino acid tyrosine. Although the primary product of the medulla is epinephrine, it also produces variable amounts of the epinephrine precursor **norepinephrine**. These catecholamines are distinct from the steroid hormones both structurally and functionally.

THE ADRENAL CORTEX: CORTISOL

Cortisol is the primary glucocorticoid hormone in humans

Steroid hormones are divided into three major classes based on their actions: glucocorticoids, mineralocorticoids, and sex steroids. **Cortisol** is the prototypical, naturally occurring glucocorticoid. The ability of cortisol to increase plasma [glucose] largely results from its ability to enhance mobilization of amino acids from proteins in many tissues and to enhance the ability of the liver to convert these amino acids into glucose and glycogen by activating gluconeogenesis.

Only a small difference can be seen in the structures of cortisol and aldosterone (Fig. 50-2): aldosterone lacks the –OH group at position 17 but has an aldehyde (aldo) group at position 18. Despite the seemingly minor chemical difference, aldosterone at physiological concentrations has virtually no glucocorticoid activity.

Target Tissues Although classified as a glucocorticoid, cortisol affects more than the principal glucose regulatory tissues, namely, the liver, fat, and muscle. Most body tissues, including bone, skin, other viscera, hematopoietic and lymphoid tissue, and the central nervous system (CNS), are target sites for glucocorticoid action. Although cortisol is the primary glucocorticoid in humans, in other species (e.g., the rat), corticosterone is the major glucocorticoid.

Actions Glucocorticoids have numerous actions other than their ability to raise plasma glucose levels. These actions are described later but include potent immunosuppressive and anti-inflammatory activity, effects on protein and fat metabolism, behavioral effects on the CNS, and important effects on calcium and bone metabolism. Some of the diverse physiological effects of the glucocorticoids can be appreciated from studies of clinical states of excess glucocorticoid secretion (Cushing syndrome) and glucocorticoid deficiency (Addison disease). The multiple actions of glucocorticoids, in particular, their "anti-inflammatory" action on leuko-

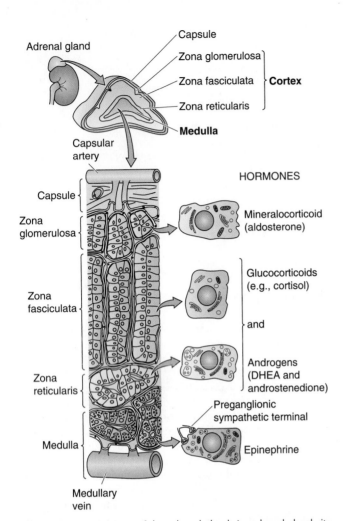

Figure 50-1 Anatomy of the adrenal gland. An adrenal gland sits on each kidney. The adrenal gland is actually two glands—the cortex and the medulla. The **adrenal cortex** comprises three layers that surround the medulla. The outermost layer contains the glomerulosa cells that secrete aldosterone, and the two inner layers of cortex (fasciculata and reticularis) synthesize cortisol and sex steroids. The blood supply enters the cortex in the subcapsular region and flows through anastomotic capillary beds while coursing through both the cortex and the medulla. The **adrenal medulla** contains chromaffin cells that secrete epinephrine and a small amount of norepinephrine.

Cushing Syndrome and Addison Disease

Glucocorticoid excess is most commonly seen clinically in individuals receiving glucocorticoids for treatment of a chronic inflammatory or neoplastic disorder. Less commonly, individuals overproduce cortisol either because of a primary cortisol-producing adrenal tumor or secondary to a pituitary tumor that produces ACTH, which, in turn, stimulates excess cortisol production from normal adrenal glands. In either case, the cortisol excess causes a constellation of symptoms and signs including truncal adiposity (abdomen, neck, facies), hypertension, loss of subcutaneous adipose and connective tissue in the extremities with associated easy bruising, loss of bone mineral, muscle weakness and wasting, and hyperglycemia. This constellation is referred to as **Cushing syndrome** after the famous American neurosurgeon who characterized this disorder. Specific therapy is based on identifying whether the clinical picture arises from a tumor in the adrenal or the pituitary gland and then removing the culprit. When the pituitary gland is responsible, the disorder is referred to as **Cushing disease**. In the case of patients receiving glucocorticoid therapy, the signs and symptoms of Cushing syndrome are carefully monitored, and efforts made to minimize these side effects. Unfortunately, all glucocorticoid drugs with anti-inflammatory actions also produce these other side effects.

Like glucocorticoid excess, glucocorticoid deficiency—or more accurately adrenal insufficiency (which includes both glucocorticoid and mineralocorticoid)—can produce an array of symptoms and signs. Although tuberculosis was once a common cause of primary adrenal insufficiency, today autoimmune adrenal disease is the most common cause. Failure of adrenal cortical hormone secretion leads to increases in circulating concentrations of ACTH as well as other products of POMC. Two of these products (α-MSH and γ-MSH) cause skin hyperpigmentation. The lack of glucocorticoid predisposes to hypoglycemia. The combined absence of glucocorticoid and mineralocorticoid leads to hypotension, whereas aldosterone deficiency leads to hyperkalemia. Before the development of glucocorticoid and mineralocorticoid therapy, this disorder was uniformly fatal.

The fasciculata and reticularis layers of the adrenal cortex convert cholesterol to cortisol

Synthesis of cortisol, as with all steroid hormones, starts with cholesterol (Fig. 50-2). Like other cells producing steroid hormones, the adrenal gland has two sources of cholesterol (see Chapter 47): (1) it can import cholesterol from circulating cholesterol-containing low-density lipoprotein (LDL cholesterol) by means of LDL receptor–mediated endocytosis (see Chapter 2), or (2) it can synthesize cholesterol de novo from acetate (see Fig. 46-16). Although both pathways provide the steroid nucleus needed for cortisol and aldosterone synthesis, circulating LDL is quantitatively more important.

In the adrenal gland, cholesterol is metabolized through a series of five reactions to make either cortisol or aldosterone. Except for 3β-hydroxysteroid dehydrogenase (3β-

cytes, led to the development of numerous synthetic analogues that are more potent, have a longer half-life, and are more selective in their specific glucocorticoid actions than are cortisol or corticosterone. Table 50-1 lists some of these compounds and indicates their relative potency as mineralocorticoids and glucocorticoids.

As discussed in Chapter 47, most of the well-characterized actions of glucocorticoids result from their genomic actions to influence (either positively or negatively) the transcription of a variety of genes through GREs. However, glucocorticoids also exert nongenomic actions (see Chapter 47) that occur promptly (0 to 3 hours) and are not inhibited by blockade of gene transcription.

Table 50-1 Relative Potency* of Glucocorticoid and Mineralocorticoid Analogues

Compound	Glucocorticoid Effect	Mineralocorticoid Effect
Cortisol	1	1.5
Prednisone	3-4	0.5
Methylprednisone	10	0.5
Dexamethasone	20	1
Fludrocortisone	12	125

*Relative potency is determined by a combined consideration of the compound's biological half-life and its affinity for the glucocorticoid or mineralocorticoid receptor.

Table 50-2 Cytochrome P-450 Enzymes Involved in Steroidogenesis*

Enzyme	Synonym	Gene
Cholesterol side chain cleavage	$P-450_{SSC}$	*CYP11A1*
11β-Hydroxylase	$P-450_{c11}$	*CYP11B1*
17α-Hydroxylase	$P-450_{c17}$	*CYP17*
17,20-Desmolase	$P-450_{c17}$	*CYP17*
21α-Hydroxylase	$P-450_{c21}$	*CYP21A2*
Aldosterone synthase	$P-450_{aldo}$	*CYP11B2*
Aromatase	$P-450_{arom}$	*CYP19*

*$P-450_{arom}$ catalyzes a reaction essential for the production of estrogens (see Chapter 55).

HSD), the enzymes responsible belong to the family of cytochrome P-450 oxidases (Table 50-2) and are located within the cells in either the mitochondria or the smooth endoplasmic reticulum (SER).

1. The pathway for cortisol and aldosterone synthesis begins in the mitochondria, where the cytochrome P-450 side chain–cleavage (SCC) enzyme (also called 20,22-desmolase or $P-450_{SSC}$) removes the long side chain (carbons 22 to 27) from the carbon at position 20 of the **cholesterol** molecule (27 carbon atoms). This enzyme, or the supply of substrate to it, appears to be the rate-limiting step for the overall process of steroid hormone synthesis.
2. The product of the SCC-catalyzed reaction is **pregnenolone** (21 carbon atoms), which exits the mitochondrion. The SER enzyme 3β-HSD (*not* a P-450 enzyme) oxidizes the hydroxyl group at position 3 of the A-ring to a ketone to form **progesterone**.
3. A P-450 enzyme in the SER, 17α-hydroxylase ($P-450_{c17}$), then adds a hydroxyl group at position 17 to form **17α-hydroxyprogesterone**. However, as shown in Figure 50-2, an alternative path to 17α-hydroxyprogesterone may be used: the 17α-hydroxylase may first add a hydroxyl group at position 17 of *pregnenolone* and form **17α-hydroxypregnenolone**, which can then be converted to 17α-hydroxyprogesterone by the aforementioned 3β-HSD.
4. In the SER, 21α-hydroxylase ($P-450_{c21}$) adds a hydroxyl at carbon 21 to produce **11-deoxycortisol**.
5. In the mitochondria, 11β-hydroxylase ($P-450_{c11}$) adds yet another hydroxyl, this time at position 11, to produce **cortisol**.

The enzymes represented by the *vertical bars* in Figure 50-2, as well as SCC, are present in all three cellular layers of the adrenal cortex. However, 17α-hydroxylase is not substantially present in the glomerulosa layer. Thus, only the fasciculata and reticularis layers can synthesize cortisol.

The cells of the fasciculata and reticularis layers of the adrenal cortex can synthesize androgens. These cells convert 17α-hydroxypregnenolone and 17α-hydroxyprogesterone into the adrenal androgens **dehydroepiandrosterone** and **androstenedione**. The enzyme that catalyzes this reaction is called 17,20-desmolase; however, it turns out to be the same SER enzyme as the 17α-hydroxylase that produced the 17α-hydroxypregnenolone and 17α-hydroxyprogesterone in the first place. The androgens formed by the adrenal are far less potent than either testosterone or dihydrotestosterone. However, peripheral tissue can use 17-ketosteroid reductase to convert androstenedione to testosterone (see Chapter 54). In this manner, the adrenal can contribute significant amounts of circulating androgen.

The cortisol synthesized by the adrenal cortex diffuses out of the cells and into the blood plasma. There, ~90% of the cortisol is transported bound to **corticosteroid-binding globulin** (CBG), also known as transcortin, which is made in the liver. Transcortin is a 383–amino acid glycoprotein whose affinity for cortisol is ~30-fold higher than for aldosterone. An additional ~7% of the circulating cortisol is bound to albumin. Thus, only 3% to 4% of the circulating cortisol is free.

The clearance of cortisol from the body depends principally on the liver and kidney. An early step is the formation of an inactive metabolite, cortisone, by the action of **11β-hydroxysteroid dehydrogenase** (11β-HSD). This 11β-HSD pathway (Fig. 50-2) is not part of the adrenal's normal formation of cortisone. Rather, one of the two 11β-HSD isozymes (11β-HSD1) is highly expressed in certain glucocorticoid *target tissues*, including liver and both subcutaneous and visceral adipose tissue. The enzyme is quite *reversible*. Indeed, when glucocorticoids were first developed as pharmaceutical agents, it was cortisone that was used to treat patients suffering from a variety of inflammatory disorders (e.g., rheumatoid arthritis). For some time, investigators thought that cortisone was the active principle. Only later did it become apparent that the body must convert the administered cortisone to cortisol, which is the biologically active agent. Because excess cortisol produces insulin resistance and many features of the metabolic syndrome (e.g., glucose intolerance, hypertension, dyslipidemia; see Chapter 51)—and 11β-HSD1 is expressed abundantly in adipose tissue—an interesting hypothesis is that increased 11β-HSD1 activity in adipose tissue locally produces cortisol and thus promotes the development of insulin resistance.

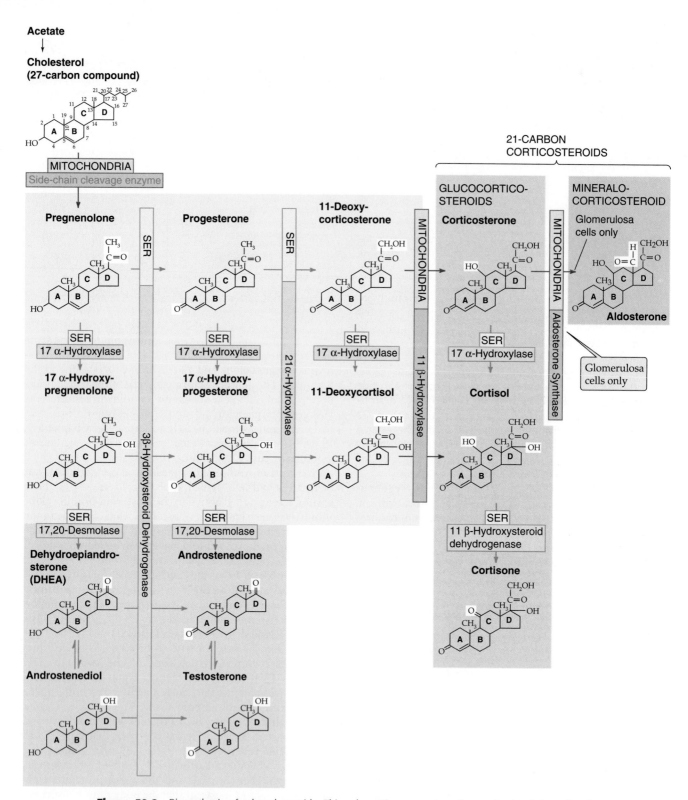

Figure 50-2 Biosynthesis of adrenal steroids. This schematic summarizes the synthesis of the adrenal steroids—the mineralocorticoid *aldosterone* and the glucocorticoid *cortisol*—from cholesterol. The individual enzymes are shown in the horizontal and vertical boxes; they are located in either the SER or the mitochondria. The SCC enzyme that produces pregnenolone is also known as 20,22-desmolase. The chemical groups modified by each enzyme are highlighted in the reaction product. If the synthesis of cortisol is prevented by any one of several dysfunctional enzymes, other steroid products may be produced in excess. For example, a block in 21α-hydroxylase diminishes production of both cortisol and aldosterone and increases production of the sex steroids. Certain of these pathways are shared in the biosynthesis of the androgens (see Fig. 54-5) and estrogens (see Fig. 55-9).

21α-Hydroxylase Deficiency

Mutations can affect one or more of the enzyme steps in steroid hormone synthesis and can produce unique clinical syndromes that are a direct result of failure to manufacture a particular hormone, accumulation of excessive amounts of precursor steroids, or both. The most common of these enzymatic disorders is 21α-hydroxylase deficiency. From Figure 50-2, we would predict that deficiency of this enzyme would lead to inadequate production of both glucocorticoid and mineralocorticoid hormones, which is indeed what occurs. Affected infants are ill with symptoms of "salt losing" (hypotension, dehydration) and glucocorticoid deficiency (hypoglycemia). The natural reaction of the body is to attempt to overcome this deficiency by increasing the secretion of pituitary ACTH, which stimulates the synthesis of cortisol and aldosterone. ACTH also causes growth of the adrenal gland. However, if the mutant enzyme is totally inactive, no cortisol or aldosterone synthesis will occur, although all other enzymes of the pathway involved in glucocorticoid and mineralocorticoid synthesis will be expressed in increased amounts. The result is greater than normal activity of the SCC enzyme, 3β-HSD, 17α-hydroxylase, and 11β-hydroxylase, and the net effect is increased synthesis of both precursor molecules and adrenal androgens. The combination of inadequate production of glucocorticoids and mineralocorticoids, excessive production of androgens, and enhanced growth of the adrenal gland is the classical clinical syndrome of salt-losing, virilizing congenital adrenal hyperplasia. In female patients, the presence of excessive adrenal androgen in utero results in ambiguous genitalia at birth, a condition that should alert the pediatrician to the potential diagnosis.

The second 11β-HSD isozyme (11β-HSD2) is expressed highly in the renal distal tubule and collecting duct (see Fig. 35-13B). The 11-βHSD2 in these cells catalyzes an essentially *irreversible* conversion of cortisol to cortisone. This breakdown of cortisol allows aldosterone to regulate the relatively nonspecific mineralocorticoid receptor (MR) without interference from cortisol.

Cortisol binds to a cytoplasmic receptor that translocates to the nucleus and modulates transcription in multiple tissues

The multiple hydroxylation reactions that convert cholesterol to cortisol result in a hydrophilic compound that, unlike cholesterol, is soluble in plasma, yet lipophilic enough to cross the plasma membrane of target tissue without requiring a membrane transporter. Cortisol, like all steroid hormones, binds to intracellular receptors within target cells (see Chapter 3). Virtually all nucleated tissues in the body contain receptors for glucocorticoids. The glucocorticoid receptor (GR) is primarily located in the cytoplasm, where in its unbound form it is complexed to a chaperone protein (i.e., the heat shock protein hsp90, among others; see Fig. 4-16A). Binding of cortisol causes the chaperone to dissociate from the GR and thus allows the cortisol-GR complex to translocate to the nucleus. There, the cortisol-receptor complex associates with **glucocorticoid response elements** (GREs) on the 5′ untranslated region of multiple genes to either enhance or diminish gene expression (see Chapter 4).

GRs are structurally similar to the receptors for mineralocorticoids, sex steroids, vitamin D, vitamin A, and thyroid hormone. These receptors, either homodimers or heterodimers, belong to the superfamily of nuclear receptors that contains domains A through F (see Chapter 3). The middle, or C, region is responsible for DNA binding through two "zinc fingers" (see Chapter 4), whereas the E region, located toward the C terminus, binds cortisol. Activity of the glucocorticoid-receptor complex requires dimerization of two identical receptor complexes (i.e., the GR functions as a *homodimer*) at the near-palindromic nucleotide site of the GRE on the chromatin. Most actions of glucocorticoids are expressed by modulation of gene transcription. One exception is the acute feedback effect of cortisol to block the release of preformed adrenocorticotropic hormone (ACTH) in the secretory granules of pituitary corticotrophs. This glucocorticoid effect is demonstrable within seconds to minutes and may relate to an as yet undefined effect of glucocorticoid on membrane trafficking.

Although glucocorticoids are named for their ability to increase hepatic glucose and glycogen synthesis, they affect many somatic tissues. In **liver**, cortisol induces the synthesis of enzymes that are involved in the metabolism of amino acids, thus facilitating their conversion to carbohydrates through gluconeogenesis. In **muscle**, cortisol stimulates the breakdown of muscle protein, thus providing amino acid substrate to the circulation and subsequently to the liver. Similarly, cortisol induces mobilization of fat from subcutaneous **adipose tissue**. Fatty acids supplied to the circulation afford an alternative fuel to glucose and increase the availability of glucose. For unknown reasons, although fat is mobilized from the extremities, some is also deposited centrally (see the description of moon facies in the box titled Therapy with Glucocorticoids).

Cortisol has other actions that are not clearly related to its glucocorticoid action, including effects on the **immune system**, among which is an acute action to promote neutrophil release from the bone marrow into the systemic circulation. In humans, cortisol also diminishes the circulating lymphocyte count, partly as a result of sequestration of lymphocytes in the reticuloendothelial system (spleen, thymus, and bone marrow). At high concentrations, glucocorticoids cause the lysis of lymphocytes in some species. Glucocorticoids also act on the cellular elements of trabecular bone (see Chapter 52) in that they decrease the ability of osteoblasts to synthesize new bone. They also interfere with absorption of Ca^{2+} from the gastrointestinal tract. In addition, glucocorticoids act on the CNS and can cause a variety of effects, including alterations in mood and cognition.

Corticotropin-releasing hormone from the hypothalamus stimulates the corticotrophs of the anterior pituitary to secrete ACTH, which, in turn, stimulates the adrenal cortex to synthesize and secrete cortisol

As summarized in Figure 50-3, regulation of the synthesis and secretion of cortisol begins with the release of cortico-

Therapy with Glucocorticoids

The variety of glucocorticoid actions on body tissue is well illustrated by considering some of the clinically observed effects of hypercortisolism in patients receiving glucocorticoid drugs. Most strikingly, the entire body habitus changes. Body fat is centripetally distributed from the extremities to the face and trunk. This change is apparent on the trunk by an increase in supraclavicular and dorsal interscapular fat. It also causes a rounding of the face called the **moon facies**, which is a result of increasing subcutaneous fat in the cheeks and submandibular region. Conversely, the wasting of fat (and some supporting tissues) in the extremities produces thinning of the skin and fragility of cutaneous blood vessels. Direct effects of glucocorticoids on bone, as well as their inhibition of intestinal Ca^{2+} absorption, produce osteopenia, which can be manifested as osteoporosis, frequently with pathologic fractures. The interference with normal immune function increases both the frequency and severity of infections. Rare malignancies can develop. Wasting of muscle tissue results in generalized weakness that is usually most prominent in the proximal muscles of the lower extremities. Finally, as would be expected from a glucocorticoid, patients are glucose intolerant. After an oral glucose challenge (see Chapter 51), blood glucose levels become higher than normal because glucocorticoid antagonizes the action of insulin. Not infrequently, frank diabetes develops (see Chapter 51 for the box on diabetes mellitus). When cortisol is overproduced endogenously (from tumors producing either ACTH or cortisol), hypertension is common. The hypertension most likely results from the weak mineralocorticoid action of cortisol. Exogenous synthetic glucocorticoid therapy rarely produces hypertension because most of these drugs lack the mineralocorticoid activity of the endogenous hormone.

---

tropin-releasing hormone (CRH) from hypothalamic neurons, as part of either a normal, daily circadian rhythm or a centrally driven stress response. CRH stimulates the release of ACTH, also called corticotropin, from the anterior pituitary. ACTH directly stimulates the adrenal fasciculata and reticularis layers to produce and secrete cortisol. Circulating cortisol exerts negative feedback control on the release of both ACTH and CRH.

CRH CRH is a 41–amino acid neuropeptide made by small-bodied neurons in the paraventricular nucleus of the **hypothalamus** (see Chapter 47). The structure of CRH is highly conserved among species. In humans, in addition to

the hypothalamus, CRH is present in several tissues, including the pancreas and the testes, as well as throughout the CNS, where it serves as a neurotransmitter. The hypothalamic neurons synthesize and release CRH through the classic secretory pathway (see Chapter 2). Neurons store CRH in secretory vesicles located in synaptic terminals in the median eminence of the hypothalamus and can release CRH acutely in the absence of new synthesis. After release into the interstitial fluid of the median eminence, CRH enters the hypophyseal portal venous plexus and travels to the anterior pituitary.

CRH Receptor CRH arriving in the anterior pituitary binds to a G protein–coupled receptor (GPCR) on the cell membrane of corticotroph cells. Hormone binding activates $G\alpha_s$, which, in turn, stimulates adenylyl cyclase and raises $[cAMP]_i$ (see Chapter 3). Subsequent stimulation of protein kinase A (PKA) activates L-type Ca^{2+} channels and thus leads to an increase in $[Ca^{2+}]_i$. This rise in $[Ca^{2+}]_i$ rapidly leads to the exocytosis of preformed ACTH. Over a much longer time, CRH receptor activation also leads to increased gene transcription and synthesis of the ACTH precursor (discussed later).

Arginine Vasopressin Although CRH is the major regulator of ACTH secretion, the paraventricular nuclei also make another hormone, arginine vasopressin (AVP; see Chapter 47). AVP is also a potent ACTH secretagogue. AVP probably plays a physiological role in the regulation of ACTH secretion in various stress states.

ACTH A 39–amino acid peptide hormone secreted by the corticotroph cells of the anterior pituitary, ACTH can also be produced by ectopic sources, particularly by small cell carcinomas of the lung. Pituitary corticotrophs synthesize ACTH by complex post-translational processing of a large precursor protein (i.e., a preprohormone) called **proopiomelanocortin** (POMC). POMC is the precursor not only for ACTH but also for a variety of peptide hormones (Fig. 50-4). In the anterior pituitary, POMC yields a long N-terminal peptide, a joining (J) peptide, ACTH, and β-**lipotropin** (β-LPH). During fetal life and pregnancy, the intermediate pituitary lobe—a small wedge of tissue between the more familiar anterior and posterior lobes—processes the same POMC in a very different manner to yield a different array of peptides: a short N-terminal peptide, γ-melanocyte–stimulating hormone (γ-**MSH**), J peptide, α-**MSH**, corticotropin-like intermediate lobe peptide (CLIP), γ-LPH, and β-endorphin. Other cells—such as the appetite-controlling POMC neurons in the hypothalamus (see Chapter 48)—

Figure 50-3 The hypothalamic-pituitary-adrenocortical axis. Small-bodied neurons in the paraventricular nucleus of the hypothalamus secrete CRH, a 41–amino acid peptide that reaches the corticotrophs in the anterior pituitary through the long portal veins. CRH binds to a GPCR on the corticotroph membrane, triggering the adenylyl cyclase/cAMP/PKA (AC/cAMP/PKA) pathway. The activation of L-type Ca^{2+} channels leads to an increase in $[Ca^{2+}]_i$ that rapidly leads to the release of preformed ACTH. CRH also increases gene transcription and synthesis of the ACTH precursor, POMC. After its release by corticotrophs, ACTH binds to **MC2Rs** on the cell membranes in all three layers of the adrenal cortex. This receptor triggers the AC/cAMP/PKA pathway, thus rapidly enhancing the conversion of cholesterol to pregnenolone and more slowly increasing the synthesis of several proteins that are needed for cortisol synthesis. The cerebral cortex can stimulate the hypothalamic neurons to increase their secretion of CRH. Cortisol exerts negative feedback at the level of both the pituitary and hypothalamus. In addition, ACTH produced by the corticotrophs negatively feeds back on the hypothalamic neurons in a short loop.

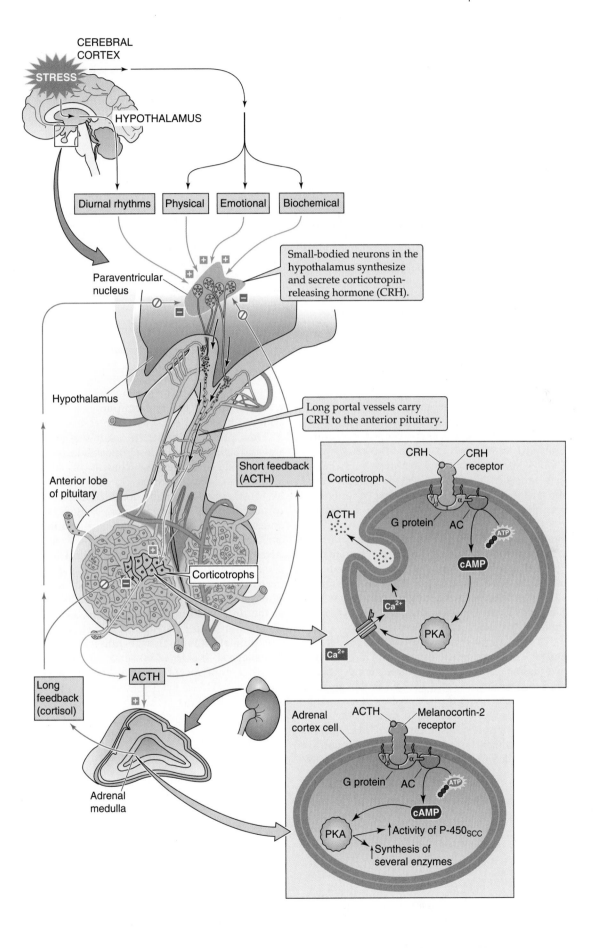

CEREBRAL CORTEX

STRESS

HYPOTHALAMUS

Diurnal rhythms | Physical | Emotional | Biochemical

Paraventricular nucleus

Small-bodied neurons in the hypothalamus synthesize and secrete corticotropin-releasing hormone (CRH).

Hypothalamus

Long portal vessels carry CRH to the anterior pituitary.

Anterior lobe of pituitary

Short feedback (ACTH)

Corticotrophs

Long feedback (cortisol)

ACTH

Adrenal medulla

CRH | CRH receptor
Corticotroph
ACTH
G protein | AC
ATP
cAMP
Ca²⁺
PKA
Ca²⁺

Adrenal cortex cell
ACTH | Melanocortin-2 receptor
G protein | AC
ATP
cAMP
PKA | ↑Activity of P-450$_{SCC}$
↑Synthesis of several enzymes

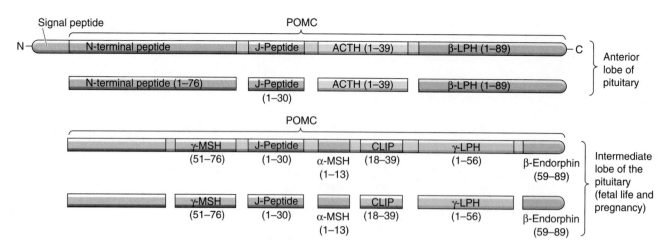

Figure 50-4 The primary gene transcript is the preprohormone POMC. The processing of POMC yields a variety of peptide hormones. This processing is different in the anterior and intermediate lobes of the pituitary. In the anterior pituitary, POMC yields a long N-terminal peptide, a joining (J) peptide, ACTH, and β-LPH. In the intermediate pituitary, the same POMC yields a short N-terminal peptide, γ-MSH, J peptide, α-MSH, CLIP, γ-LPH, and β-endorphin. Metabolism by the intermediate lobe is only important during fetal life and pregnancy. *(Data from Young JB, Landsberg L: Catecholamines and the adrenal medulla. In Wilson JD, Foster DW, Kronenberg HM, Larsen PR (eds): Williams Textbook of Endocrinology, 9th ed, pp 665-728. Philadelphia: WB Saunders, 1998.)*

can also synthesize POMC. The **melanocortins** include ACTH as well as α-, β-, and γ-MSH. The melanocortins bind to a family of five GPCRs, the **melanocortin receptors** (MC1R to MC5R).

α-MSH and γ-MSH act on MC1R receptors in melanocytes to increase the dispersion of pigment granules. In some patients who greatly overproduce ACTH, hyperpigmentation is a prominent clinical finding. Whether this hyperpigmentation is the result of increased production of MSH, increased production of β-LPH (which also has MSH activity), or the melanotropic action of ACTH per se remains uncertain. β-**LPH** and γ-**LPH** mobilize lipids from adipocytes in animals, although their physiological role in humans is unclear. β-**Endorphin** has potent opioid actions in the CNS (see Chapter 13), but its physiological actions (if any) in the systemic circulation are not known.

ACTH Receptor In the adrenal cortex, ACTH binds to **MC2R** on the plasma membranes of all three steroid-secreting cell types. However, because only the cells in the fasciculata and reticularis layers have the 17α-hydroxylase needed for synthesizing cortisol (Fig. 50-2), these cells are the only ones that secrete cortisol in response to ACTH. ACTH appears to have few other actions at physiological concentrations. MC2R is coupled to a heterotrimeric G protein and stimulates adenylyl cyclase (see Chapter 3). The resulting increase in $[cAMP]_i$ activates PKA, which phosphorylates a variety of proteins. A rapid effect of ACTH is to stimulate the rate-limiting step in cortisol formation, that is, the conversion of cholesterol to pregnenolone through the SCC enzyme. In addition, ACTH—over a longer time frame—increases the synthesis of several proteins needed for cortisol synthesis: (1) each of the P-450 enzymes involved in cortisol synthesis (Fig. 50-2), (2) the LDL receptor required for the uptake of cholesterol from blood (see Chapter 2), and (3) the 3-hydroxy-3-methylglutaryl–coenzyme A (HMG-CoA)

reductase that is the rate-limiting enzyme for cholesterol synthesis by the adrenal (see Chapter 45).

Thus, ACTH promotes the acute synthesis of cortisol—and as discussed later, aldosterone to a lesser extent—by the adrenal and increases the content of adrenal enzymes involved in steroidogenesis. In the absence of pituitary ACTH, the fasciculata and reticularis layers of the adrenal cortex atrophy. The glomerulosa layer does not atrophy under these conditions because in addition to ACTH, angiotensin II (ANG II) and high levels of K^+ are trophic factors that act on the glomerulosa layer. The atrophy of the fasciculata and reticularis layers occurs routinely in people treated with glucocorticoid drugs and leaves the person with an iatrogenic form of adrenal insufficiency when use of the drug is abruptly discontinued. Conversely, chronic stimulation of the adrenal by ACTH, such as can occur with pituitary tumors (Cushing disease) or with the simple physiological ACTH excess that can occur with chronic stress, can increase the weight of the adrenals several-fold.

Cortisol exerts negative feedback on CRH and ACTH secretion, whereas stress acts through higher CNS centers to stimulate the axis

Cortisol exerts negative feedback control on the very axis that stimulates its secretion (Fig. 50-3), and it does so at the level of both the anterior pituitary and hypothalamus.

Feedback to the Anterior Pituitary In the corticotrophs of the anterior pituitary, cortisol acts by binding to a cytosolic receptor, which then moves to the nucleus, where it binds to GREs and modulates gene expression and thus inhibits the synthesis of both the CRH receptor and ACTH. Even though, as seen earlier, the POMC gene yields multiple secretory products, *cortisol* is the main regulator of the transcription of POMC. In addition, elevated levels of cortisol in plasma inhibit the release of presynthesized ACTH stored in vesicles.

Feedback to the Hypothalamus   The negative feedback of cortisol on the CRH-secreting neurons of the hypothalamus is less important than that on the corticotrophs discussed earlier. Plasma cortisol decreases the mRNA and peptide levels of CRH in paraventricular hypothalamic neurons. Cortisol also inhibits the release of presynthesized CRH. Synthetic glucocorticoids have a similar action.

Control by a Higher CNS Center   CRH-secreting neurons in the hypothalamus are under higher CNS control, as illustrated by two important features of the hypothalamic-pituitary-adrenocortical axis: (1) the circadian and pulsatile nature of ACTH and cortisol secretion and (2) integration of signals from higher cortical centers that modulate the body's responses to a variety of stressors.

The pituitary secretes ACTH with a **circadian rhythm**. The suprachiasmatic nucleus of the hypothalamus, which lies above the optic chiasm and receives input from the retina, controls the circadian rhythms of the body. Indeed, blind people lose their circadian rhythms. Input from hypothalamic nuclei to the corticotrophs—through both CRH and ADH—appears to modulate the circadian secretion of ACTH and thus the circadian secretion of cortisol as well. As is the case for other hypothalamic releasing hormones, CRH is released in pulses. As a result, superimposed on the circadian rhythm of ACTH is the **pulsatile secretion** of ACTH, as shown in Figure 50-5. The greatest ACTH secretory activity occurs in the early morning and diminishes late in the afternoon and early evening. The mechanism by which hypothalamic neurons generate pulses of secretory activity is not understood.

Other evidence of higher CNS control is the enhanced CRH secretion—and thus the enhanced ACTH secretion—that occurs in response to physical, psychological, and biochemical stress. An example of biochemical stress is hypoglycemia, which stimulates the secretion of both CRH and ACTH and thus leads to an increased release of cortisol that tends to raise blood glucose levels.

The increase in ACTH secretion that occurs nocturnally and with stress appears to be the result of an increased amplitude of the secretory CRH burst, rather than an increased frequency of secretion episodes. Because the half-life of cortisol is much longer than that of ACTH, the period of the pulsatile changes in cortisol is longer and the magnitude of the excursions is damped in comparison with those of ACTH.

THE ADRENAL CORTEX: ALDOSTERONE

The mineralocorticoid aldosterone is the primary regulator of salt balance and extracellular volume

Aldosterone determines extracellular volume by controlling the extent to which the kidney excretes or reabsorbs the Na^+ filtered at the renal glomerulus. Na^+ in the extracellular space retains water—it is the primary osmotically active particle in the extracellular space—and thus the amount of Na^+ that is present determines the volume of extracellular fluid (see Chapter 5). The extracellular volume is itself a prime determinant of arterial blood pressure (see Chapter 23), and therefore aldosterone plays an important role in the maintenance of blood pressure.

The effects of aldosterone on salt balance determine the extracellular volume and should not be confused with the

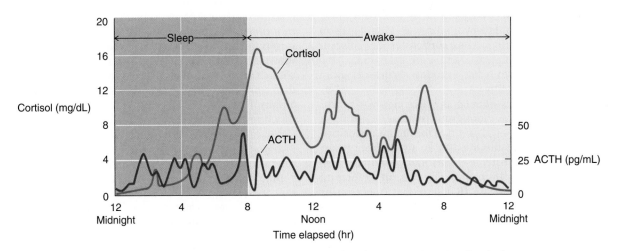

Figure 50-5   Rhythm of ACTH and cortisol. The corticotrophs release ACTH in a circadian rhythm, greater in the early morning hours and less late in the afternoon and early evening. Superimposed on the circadian rhythm is the effect on the corticotrophs of the pulsatile secretion of CRH by the hypothalamus. Thus, ACTH levels exhibit both circadian and pulsatile behavior. Although both ACTH and cortisol are secreted episodically, the duration of the ACTH bursts is briefer, reflecting the shorter half-life of ACTH in plasma. *(Data from Young JB, Landsberg L: Catecholamines and the adrenal medulla. In Wilson JD, Foster DW, Kronenberg HM, Larsen PR (eds): Williams Textbook of Endocrinology, 9th ed, pp 665-728. Philadelphia: WB Saunders, 1998.)*

effects of AVP (also known as antidiuretic hormone or ADH). AVP regulates the *free water* balance of the body (see Chapter 40). Water freely passes across cell membranes and thus affects the *concentration* of Na^+ and other solutes throughout the body (see Chapter 5). Unlike aldosterone, AVP makes only a small contribution to the maintenance of extracellular volume; instead, AVP regulates serum osmolality and hence the Na^+ concentration. Thus, to a first approximation, one can think of aldosterone as the primary regulator of extracellular volume because of its effect on renal Na^+ reabsorption and AVP as the primary regulator of plasma osmolality because of its effect on free water balance.

The glomerulosa cells of the adrenal cortex synthesize aldosterone from cholesterol, through progesterone

As is the case for cortisol, the adrenal cortex synthesizes aldosterone from cholesterol by using P-450 enzymes in a series of five steps. The initial steps in the synthesis of aldosterone from cholesterol follow the same synthetic pathway that cortisol-secreting cells use to generate **progesterone** (Fig. 50-2). Because glomerulosa cells are the only ones that contain aldosterone synthase, these cells are the exclusive site of aldosterone synthesis.

1. The cytochrome P-450 **SCC enzyme** (P-450$_{SCC}$) produces pregnenolone from cholesterol. This enzyme—or the supply of substrate to it—appears to be the rate-limiting step for the overall process of steroid hormone synthesis.
2. The SER enzyme 3β-HSD, which is *not* a P-450 enzyme, oxidizes pregnenolone to form **progesterone**.
3. Because *glomerulosa* cells have minimal 17α-hydroxylase (P-450$_{c17}$), they do not convert progesterone to 17α-hydroxyprogesterone. Instead, glomerulosa cells use a 21α-hydroxylase (P-450$_{c21}$) in the SER to hydroxylate the progesterone further at position 21 and to produce **11-deoxycorticosterone** (DOC).
4. In the mitochondria, 11β-hydroxylase (P-450$_{c11}$) adds an —OH at position 11 to produce **corticosterone**. This pair of hydroxylations in steps 3 and 4 are catalyzed by the same two enzymes that produce cortisol from 17α-hydroxyprogesterone.
5. The glomerulosa cells—but *not* the fasciculata and reticularis cells—also have aldosterone synthase (P-450$_{aldo}$), which first adds an —OH group to the methyl at position 18 and then oxidizes this hydroxyl to an *aldehyde* group, hence the name **aldosterone**. This mitochondrial P-450 enzyme, also called 18-methyloxidase, is an isoform of the same 11β-hydroxylase (P-450$_{c11}$) that catalyzes the DOC-to-corticosterone step. In fact, aldosterone synthase can catalyze all three steps between DOC and aldosterone: 11β-hydroxylation, 18-methyl hydroxylation, and 18-methyl oxidation.

As with cortisol, no storage pool of presynthesized aldosterone is available in the glomerulosa cell for rapid secretion. Thus, secretion of aldosterone by the adrenal is limited by the rate at which the glomerulosa cells can synthesize the hormone. Although ACTH also stimulates the production

of aldosterone in the glomerulosa cell, increases in extracellular $[K^+]$ and the peptide hormone ANG II are physiologically more important secretagogues. These secretagogues enhance secretion by increasing the activity of enzymes acting at rate-limiting steps in aldosterone synthesis. These enzymes include the SCC enzyme, which is common to all steroid-producing cells, and aldosterone synthase, which is unique to glomerulosa cells and is responsible for formation of the C-18 aldehyde.

Once secreted, ~37% of circulating aldosterone remains free in plasma. The rest weakly binds to CBG (~21%) and albumin (~42%).

Aldosterone stimulates Na^+ reabsorption and K^+ excretion by the renal tubule

The major action of aldosterone is to stimulate the kidney to reabsorb Na^+ and water and to enhance K^+ secretion. Aldosterone has similar actions on salt and water transport in the colon, salivary glands, and sweat glands. MRs are also present in the myocardium, liver, brain, and other tissues, but the physiological role of mineralocorticoids in these latter tissues is unclear.

Aldosterone, like cortisol and all the other steroid hormones (see Chapter 4), acts by modulating gene transcription. In the kidney, aldosterone binds to both low- and high-affinity receptors. The low-affinity receptor appears to be identical to the **GR**. The high-affinity receptor is a distinct **MR**; it has homology to the GR, particularly in the zinc finger region involved in DNA binding. Surprisingly, MR in the kidney has a similar affinity for aldosterone and cortisol. Because cortisol normally circulates at much higher concentrations than does aldosterone (5 to 20 μg/dL versus 2 to 8 ng/dL), the biological effect of aldosterone on any potential target would be expected to be greatly overshadowed by that of cortisol. (Conversely, aldosterone has essentially no significant glucocorticoid action because aldosterone binds only weakly to its low-affinity receptor—that is, the GR.)

How then do the renal tubule cells avoid sensing cortisol as a *mineralocorticoid*? As noted earlier, the cells that are targets for aldosterone, particularly the distal convoluted tubule and the initial cortical collecting duct of the kidney, contain an enzyme (**11β-hydroxysteroid dehydrogenase 2**) that converts cortisol to cortisone, which has a very low affinity for the MR (see Fig. 35-13B). Unlike 11β-HSD1, which reversibly interconverts cortisone with cortisol, 11β-HSD2 cannot convert cortisone back to cortisol. As a result, locally within the target cell, the ratio of cortisol to aldosterone is much smaller than the cortisol dominance seen in plasma. In other words, 11β-HSD2 is so effective at removing cortisol from the cytosol of aldosterone target tissues that cortisol behaves as only a weak mineralocorticoid despite the high affinity of cortisol for the so-called MR. Thus, the presence of 11β-HSD2 effectively confers aldosterone specificity on the MR.

In the target cells of the renal tubule, aldosterone increases the activity of several key proteins involved in Na^+ transport (see Chapter 35). It increases transcription of the Na-K pump, thus augmenting distal Na^+ reabsorption. Aldosterone also raises the expression of apical Na^+ channels and an Na/K/Cl cotransporter. The net effect of these actions is to increase Na$^+$ reabsorption and K$^+$ secretion. The enhanced K$^+$ secretion (see Chapter 37) appears to occur as a secondary effect to the enhanced Na$^+$ reabsorption. However, the stoichiometry between Na$^+$ reabsorption and K$^+$ secretion in the distal tubule is not fixed.

Aldosterone regulates only that small fraction of renal Na$^+$ reabsorption that occurs in the distal tubule and collecting duct. Although most Na$^+$ reabsorption occurs in the proximal tubule by aldosterone-independent mechanisms, loss of aldosterone-mediated Na$^+$ reabsorption can result in significant electrolyte abnormalities, including life-threatening hyperkalemia and, in the absence of other compensatory mechanisms, hypotension. Conversely, excess aldosterone secretion produces hypokalemia and hypertension.

Hyperaldosteronism is an uncommon cause of hypertension. Primary aldosteronism can result from either an isolated adrenal adenoma or bilateral adrenal hyperplasia; even more rarely, adrenal carcinoma can produce excess aldosterone.

Renin-angiotensin, potassium, and ACTH all stimulate aldosterone secretion

Three secretagogues are known for the aldosterone synthesized in the glomerulosa cells of the adrenal cortex. The most important is ANG II, which is a product of the renin-angiotensin cascade. An increase in plasma [K$^+$] is also a powerful stimulus for aldosterone secretion. Third, just as ACTH promotes cortisol secretion, it also promotes the secretion of aldosterone, although this effect is weak.

Renin-Angiotensin The renin-angiotensin-aldosterone axis is introduced in the discussion of the control of extracellular fluid volume in Chapter 40. The liver synthesizes and secretes a very large protein called **angiotensinogen**, which is an α_2-globulin (Fig. 50-6). **Renin**, which is synthesized by the granular cells (or juxtaglomerular cells) of the juxtaglomerular apparatus (JGA) in the kidney (see Chapter 33), is the enzyme that cleaves this angiotensinogen to form **ANG I**, a decapeptide. Finally, angiotensin-converting enzyme (ACE) cleaves the ANG I to form the octapeptide **ANG II**. ACE is present in both the vascular endothelium of the lung (~40%) and elsewhere (~60%). In addition to its role as a potent secretagogue for aldosterone, ANG II exerts powerful vasoconstrictor actions on vascular smooth muscle (see Chapter 23). ANG II has a short half-life (<1 minute) because plasma aminopeptidases further cleave it to the heptapeptide ANG III.

On the plasma membrane of the glomerulosa cell, ANG II binds to the **AT$_1$ receptor** (type 1 ANG II receptor), which couples through the Gα_q-mediated pathway to phospholipase C (PLC). Stimulation of PLC leads to the formation of diacylglycerol (DAG) and inositol 1,4,5-triphosphate (IP$_3$; see Chapter 3). DAG activates protein kinase C (PKC). IP$_3$ triggers the release of Ca^{2+} from intracellular stores, thus causing a rise in [Ca^{2+}]$_i$, which activates Ca^{2+}-dependent enzymes such as PKC and Ca^{2+}–calmodulin-dependent protein kinases. These changes lead to depolarization of the glomerulosa cell's plasma membrane, opening of voltage-activated Ca^{2+} channels, and a *sustained* increase in Ca^{2+} influx from the extracellular space. This rise in [Ca^{2+}]$_i$ is

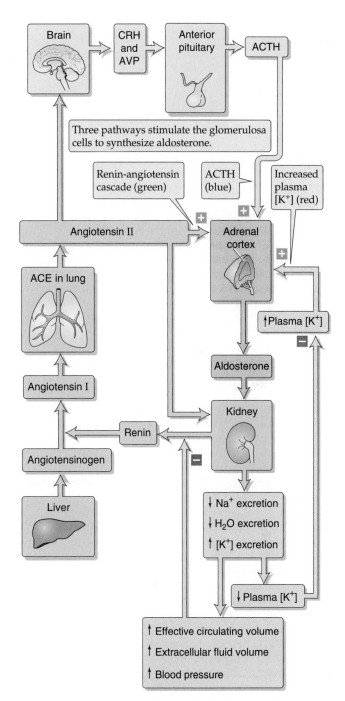

Figure 50-6 Control of aldosterone secretion. Three pathways, shown in three different colors, stimulate the glomerulosa cells of the adrenal cortex to secrete aldosterone.

primarily responsible for triggering the synthesis (i.e., secretion) of aldosterone. Aldosterone secretion increases because the rise in [Ca^{2+}]$_i$ facilitates the production of pregnenolone either by directly increasing the activity of SCC or by enhancing the delivery of cholesterol to the SCC enzyme in the mitochondria (Fig. 50-2). In addition, increased [Ca^{2+}]$_i$ also stimulates aldosterone synthase and in this manner enhances the conversion of corticosterone to aldosterone.

Potassium An increase in extracellular K^+ ($[K^+]_o$) has a more direct action on the glomerulosa cell (Fig. 50-6). High $[K^+]_o$ depolarizes the plasma membrane and opens voltage-gated Ca^{2+} channels. The result is an influx of Ca^{2+} and a rise in $[Ca^{2+}]_i$ that stimulates the same two steps as ANG II—production of pregnenolone from cholesterol and conversion of corticosterone to aldosterone. Unlike the situation for ANG II, the $[Ca^{2+}]_i$ increase induced by high $[K^+]_o$ does not require activation of PLC or release of Ca^{2+} from the intracellular stores. Because increased $[K^+]_o$ and ANG II both act by raising $[Ca^{2+}]_i$, they act synergistically on the glomerulosa cell.

ACTH ACTH has only a minor effect on aldosterone secretion by glomerulosa cells (Fig. 50-6). ACTH regulates aldosterone secretion by a pathway that is distinct from that of ANG II or high $[K^+]_o$. As noted earlier for the fasciculata and reticularis cells, MC2R in the glomerulosa cell is coupled through a heterotrimeric G protein to adenylyl cyclase. Increases in ACTH raise $[cAMP]_i$ and activate PKA, which phosphorylates large numbers of cytosolic proteins. At some as yet undefined level, these changes stimulate Ca^{2+} influx across the plasma membrane and enhance the synthesis and secretion of aldosterone. ACTH also enhances mineralocorticoid activity by a second mechanism: stimulation of the fasciculata cells to secrete cortisol, corticosterone, and DOC, all of which have weak mineralocorticoid activity. The hypertension seen in individuals who oversecrete ACTH appears to be mediated by the excess synthesis of these weak mineralocorticoids. Neither ANG II nor hyperkalemia affects the cAMP pathway triggered by ACTH.

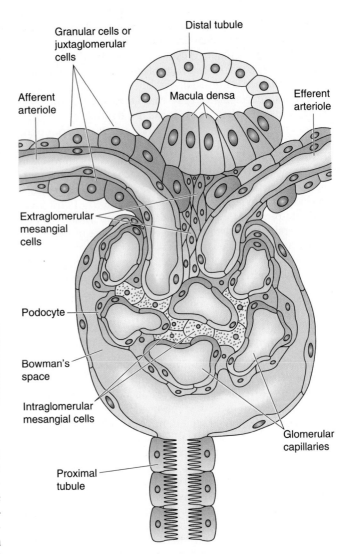

Figure 50-7 Structure of the JGA.

Aldosterone exerts indirect negative feedback on the renin-angiotensin axis by increasing effective circulating volume and by lowering plasma $[K^+]$

The feedback regulation exerted by aldosterone is indirect and occurs through its effects of both increasing salt retention (i.e., extracellular volume) and decreasing $[K^+]_o$.

Renin-Angiotensin Axis As discussed in Chapter 40, a decrease in effective circulating volume stimulates the granular cells of the JGA of the kidney to increase their synthesis and release of renin, which increases the generation of ANG II and, therefore, aldosterone (Fig. 50-6). The **JGA** is located at the glomerular pole of the nephron, between the afferent and efferent arterioles, where the early distal tubule comes in close proximity with its own glomerulus (Fig. 50-7). Histologically, the JGA comprises specialized epithelial cells of the distal tubule called macula densa cells, as well as specialized smooth muscle cells of the *afferent* arteriole, which are called granular cells or juxtaglomerular cells. Macula densa cells and granular cells communicate by means of an extracellular matrix.

Decreases in effective circulating volume—or the associated decreases in systemic arterial pressure—stimulate renin release from the JGA in two ways (see Chapter 40): first, decreased systemic arterial blood pressure stimulates the baroreceptor reflex, which triggers medullary control centers to increase sympathetic outflow to the JGA. The result of both α- and β-adrenergic stimulation is enhanced renin secretion. Second, "renal" baroreceptors in the afferent arteriole—possibly the **granular cells** themselves—respond to a fall in pressure of the afferent arteriole (i.e., decreased stretch in the arteriolar wall) by increasing the secretion of renin. Thus, both mechanisms enhance renin release and lead to increased levels of ANG II and aldosterone. ANG II negatively feeds back on renin release by directly inhibiting renin release by the kidney (short-loop feedback). ANG II also negatively feeds back on renin release by acutely increasing blood pressure (see Chapter 23), a process that reduces the stimuli to the aforementioned two baroreceptor pathways. Finally, aldosterone negatively feeds back on renin release more slowly by enhancing renal Na^+ reabsorption (see Chapter 35) and thus increasing effective circulating blood volume and blood pressure. Therefore, ANG II and aldosterone complete the regulatory feedback circuit that governs the secretion of aldosterone.

Potassium High plasma $[K^+]$ stimulates the glomerulosa cell in the adrenal cortex to synthesize and release aldosterone, which, in turn, stimulates the principal cells of the renal collecting duct to reabsorb more Na^+ and excrete more K^+ (Fig. 50-6). This excretion of K^+ causes plasma $[K^+]$ to fall toward normal. As a result, stimulation of glomerulosa cells declines, aldosterone secretion falls, and the negative feedback loop is completed. This sequence of events (i.e., hyperkalemia → aldosterone secretion → K^+ excretion) probably plays a vital role in preventing wide swings in plasma $[K^+]$ in response to episodic dietary intake of large K^+ loads.

Role of Aldosterone in Normal Physiology What, then, is the role of aldosterone in normal physiology? Presumably, the salt- and water-retaining properties of aldosterone are of greatest value in meeting the environmental stresses associated with limited availability of salt, water, or both. Such conditions are not prevalent in most Western societies, but they still exist in many developing countries and were probably universal in previous periods of human evolutionary history. In healthy, normotensive humans, blockade of aldosterone generation with ACE-inhibiting drugs reduces ANG II production and markedly decreases plasma aldosterone, but it causes only slight decreases in total body Na^+ and blood pressure. Redundant mechanisms for maintaining blood pressure probably prevent a larger blood pressure decrease. The reason for the mild effect on Na^+ balance is probably an adaptive increase in salt intake; indeed, patients with adrenal cortical insufficiency frequently crave dietary salt. In contrast to the minor effects of low aldosterone on blood pressure and Na^+ balance in physiologically normal people, the effects of blocking aldosterone production can

be catastrophic for K^+ balance; low aldosterone can result in life-threatening hyperkalemia.

Role of Aldosterone in Disease Aldosterone does play important roles in several pathologic conditions. For example, in many patients with *hyper*tension, ACE inhibitors are effective in reducing blood pressure, a finding implying that their renin-angiotensin-aldosterone axis was overactive. In *hypo*tension, as occurs with hemorrhage or dehydration, aldosterone secretion increases, thus increasing effective circulating volume and blood pressure.

Aldosterone secretion also increases in congestive heart failure. However, the increased salt retention in this setting is inappropriate because it results in worsening edema formation. In this case, the increase in circulating aldosterone occurs *despite* preexisting volume overload. The problem in congestive heart failure is that the JGA does not perceive the very real volume overload as an increase in *effective* circulating volume. Indeed, the reduced cardiac output in heart failure diminishes renal glomerular filtration, partly because of decreased arterial blood pressure and partly because of enhanced sympathetic nervous system activity, which constricts the afferent arterioles of the kidney. As a result, the kidney inappropriately assumes that the extracellular volume is decreased and stimulates the renin-angiotensin-aldosterone system.

Spontaneous increases in aldosterone synthesis can occur in patients with tumors of the glomerulosa cell, a disorder called hyperaldosteronism or **Conn syndrome**. Hypertension and hypokalemia frequently develop in these patients. As would be expected from feedback regulation of the renin-angiotensin-aldosterone system, the plasma renin concentration is characteristically suppressed in this form of hypertension.

In addition to its renal effects, aldosterone increases fibrosis within certain tissues, including myocardium and blood vessel wall. Agents that block the aldosterone receptor (e.g., spironolactone or eplerenone) have been used successfully to antagonize these actions of aldosterone and to improve clinical outcomes in patients with heart failure. This effect appears to be independent of any diuretic effect of these agents.

THE ADRENAL MEDULLA

The adrenal medulla bridges the endocrine and sympathetic nervous systems

In Chapter 47, I describe cells of the hypothalamus as neuroendocrine because they are part of the CNS and appear anatomically as neural tissue, yet they release peptide hormones (e.g., CRH) into the blood that act downstream on the pituitary—a classic endocrine function. The adrenal medulla is similar in many ways. The cells of the medulla, termed **chromaffin cells** because the catecholamines that they contain stain avidly with chromium, derive from neural crest cells (see Chapter 10) and migrate into the center of the adrenal cortex, which is derived from the mesoderm. The adrenomedullary cells synthesize and secrete epinephrine and—to a lesser extent—norepinephrine. Norepinephrine is the neurotransmitter of the sympathetic division of the autonomic nervous system (see Chapter 14). Both the norepinephrine and epinephrine made in the adrenal medulla enter the circulation and act on distal tissues just like other hormones.

Chromaffin cells are the structural and functional equivalents of the **postganglionic** neurons in the sympathetic nervous system (see Chapter 14). The preganglionic sympathetic fibers of the splanchnic nerves, which release acetylcholine (ACh), are the principal regulators of adrenomedullary hormone secretion.

The vascular supply to the adrenal medulla is also unusual. The medulla receives vascular input from vessels that begin in a subcapsular plexus of the adrenal cortex. The vessels then branch into a capillary network in the cortex only to merge into small venous vessels that branch into a second capillary network within the medulla. This **portal blood supply** (originating at the entrance to the adrenal) exposes the adrenal medulla to the highest concentrations of glucocorticoids and mineralocorticoids of all somatic tissues.

Chromaffin cells of the adrenal medulla are the only ones that have the enzyme for synthesizing epinephrine

Investigators first appreciated nearly a century ago that extracts of the adrenal medulla have a powerful pressor effect. Subsequent work showed that the **catecholamines**—dopa, dopamine, norepinephrine, and epinephrine—are all made in the adrenal medulla. **Norepinephrine** is found in many other somatic tissues in amounts that roughly parallel the extent of sympathetic innervation of the tissue. In other words, the norepinephrine in these other tissues is not made there but is derived from the sympathetic nerve endings in them. **Epinephrine**, the principal product of the adrenal medulla, is made *only* in the adrenal medulla.

Dopamine, norepinephrine, and epinephrine are all synthesized from the amino acid tyrosine. Figure 50-8A summarizes the reactions involved in the synthesis of epinephrine. Figure 50-9 illustrates the cellular localization of the four enzymatic reactions, as well as the three critical transport steps that shuttle the reactants and products to their proper location:

1. The activity of the first enzyme in the pathway, **tyrosine hydroxylase**, which converts tyrosine to L-dopa, is rate limiting for overall synthesis. This enzyme is located within the *cytosol* of adrenal medullary cells, as well as in sympathetic nerve terminals and in specific cells within the CNS.
2. The *cytosolic* enzyme **amino acid decarboxylase** converts L-dopa to dopamine in numerous tissues, including the adrenal medulla.

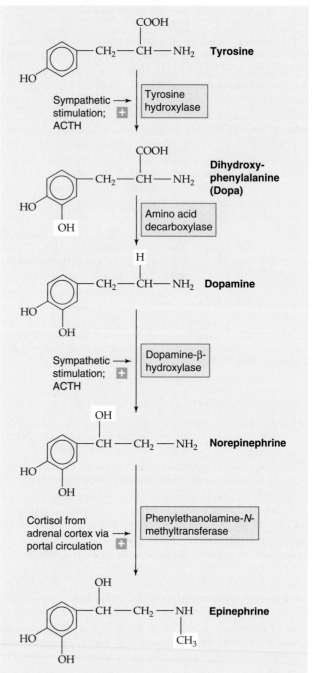

A CATECHOLAMINE SYNTHESIS

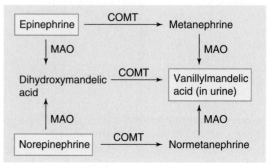

B DEGRADATIVE METABOLISM OF CATECHOLAMINES

Figure 50-8 A and **B**, Synthesis and degradation of catecholamines. In **A**, the *horizontal arrows* indicate enhancement of the reaction. MAO, monoamine oxidase.

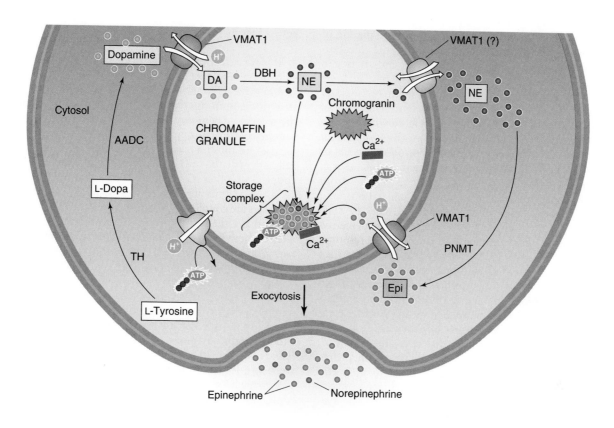

Figure 50-9 Cellular view of catecholamine synthesis. The chromaffin cell synthesizes and stores epinephrine in a sequence of four enzymatic and three transport steps. AADC, amino acid decarboxylase; DA, dopamine; DBH, dopamine β-hydroxylase; Epi, epinephrine; NE, norepinephrine; TH, tyrosine hydroxylase.

3. A catecholamine-H$^+$ exchanger (VMAT1) moves the dopamine into membrane-enclosed dense-core vesicles called **chromaffin granules**.

4. **Dopamine β-hydroxylase** converts dopamine to norepinephrine by hydroxylating the β carbon. This β-hydroxylase is localized to the inner surface of the membrane of granules within the adrenal medulla and sympathetic nerves. In the nerve terminals of postganglionic sympathetic neurons, the synthetic pathway terminates at this step, and the granules store the norepinephrine for later secretion. However, the cells of the adrenal medulla convert the norepinephrine to epinephrine in three final steps.

5. Norepinephrine formed in the secretory granules moves out into the cytosol.

6. The cytosolic enzyme **phenylethanolamine-N-methyltransferase** (PNMT) transfers a methyl group from *S*-adenosylmethionine to norepinephrine, thus creating epinephrine. This enzyme is present only in the cytosol and the adrenal medulla.

7. The secretory granules in the adrenal medulla take up the newly synthesized epinephrine. The same VMAT1 catecholamine-H$^+$ exchanger noted in step 3 appears to mediate this uptake of epinephrine. The proton gradient is maintained by an H$^+$ pump (i.e., a vacuolar-type H-ATPase) within the secretory vesicle membrane (see Chapter 5). Thus, in the adrenal medulla, the secretory granules store both epinephrine and norepinephrine before secretion.

Epinephrine synthesis is under control of the CRH-ACTH-cortisol axis at two levels. First, ACTH stimulates the synthesis of dihydroxyphenylalanine (Dopa) and norepinephrine. Second, cortisol transported from the adrenal cortex by the portal circulation to the medulla upregulates PNMT in chromaffin cells. The result is synergy between the CRH-ACTH-cortisol axis and the sympathetic-epinephrine axis. Thus, the stress that is sensed and propagated by the CRH-ACTH-cortisol axis sustains the epinephrine response.

Similar to the secretory granules that are present in the postganglionic sympathetic neurons, the secretory granules of the adrenal medulla contain very high concentrations of catecholamines (≤0.5 M). These catecholamines—along with ATP and Ca^{2+}—bind to granular proteins called **chromogranins** and thus are not osmotically active in these storage vesicles. Chromogranins are what make dense-core vesicles dense. In humans, the dominant chromogranin is chromogranin B. The release of catecholamines is initiated by CNS control. ACh released from preganglionic neurons in the splanchnic nerves acts on nicotinic ACh receptors to depolarize the postganglionic chromaffin cells. This depolarization triggers the opening of voltage-gated Ca^{2+} channels, a process that raises [Ca^{2+}]$_i$ and triggers the exocytotic release of epinephrine. The secretion of adrenal catecholamines is accompanied by the release of ATP and the granule proteins.

The release of chromogranin A has been used as a marker of adrenal medullary activity. In the circulation, the catecholamines dissociate from the binding complex and are free to act on target tissues.

The early description of the fight-or-flight response to stress (see Chapter 14) exemplifies the central control of adrenomedullary function. An organism faced with a severe external threat responds with centrally driven release of adrenal hormones, as well as activation of other aspects of the sympathetic division. This response includes increases in heart rate and contractility, mobilization of fuel stores from muscle and fat, piloerection, pupillary dilatation, and increased sphincter tone of the bowel and bladder. Each response is in some way adapted to deal with the perceived threat successfully. This combined neuroendocrine response is activated within seconds. The secreted catecholamines act very quickly after reaching their target tissues.

The biological actions of catecholamines are very brief, lasting only ~10 seconds in the case of epinephrine. Circulating catecholamines are degraded first by the enzyme **catecholamine-O-methyltransferase** (COMT), which is present in high concentrations in endothelial cells and the heart, liver, and kidneys (Fig. 50-8B). COMT converts epinephrine to metanephrine, as well as norepinephrine to normetanephrine. A second enzyme, **monoamine oxidase**, converts these metabolites to vanillylmandelic acid (VMA). The liver and also the gut then conjugate these compounds to sulfate or glucuronide (see Chapter 46) to form derivatives that the kidney excretes in the urine. Measurement of the concentration of catecholamines, metanephrines, and VMA in the urine provides a measure of the total adrenal catecholamine production by both the adrenal medulla and the sympathetic system.

Catecholamines bind to α and β adrenoceptors on the cell surface and act through heterotrimeric G proteins

Many of the hormones already discussed have a unique receptor on the cell surface (e.g., insulin, parathyroid hormone, growth hormone, thyroid-stimulating hormone) or within the cell (e.g., thyroid hormones or cortisol). Other hormones (e.g., AVP) and neurotransmitters (e.g., ACh and glutamate) may bind to more than one type of receptor, each acting through a different signal transduction process. The situation for the catecholamines is even more complex. Epinephrine and norepinephrine can each bind to more than one type of adrenergic receptor or **adrenoceptor**, all of which are GPCRs. Conversely, individual adrenoceptors can generally bind both epinephrine and norepinephrine—albeit with different affinities.

About a half century ago, investigators found that epinephrine could stimulate both vasodilatory and vasoconstrictor responses in the same vascular bed, depending on the epinephrine concentration. This property, together with the observation that certain drugs could selectively block one or the other of these effects, led to the designation of α- and β-adrenergic receptors. This dichotomy proved too simple when it was observed that the actions of some drugs that have pure α or pure β activity could be blocked in some tissues but not in others; this variability in response suggested that the tissue response is determined by a *subtype* of α or β receptor.

It is now clear that at least three types of β and two types of α receptors exist (see Table 14-2), as well as subtypes within these major classes. These receptors differ in primary structure and in the types of G proteins that associate with the receptor. The several β receptors are coupled to stimulatory heterotrimeric G proteins ($G\alpha_s$) that *stimulate* adenylyl cyclase and thus increase levels of cAMP, the principal intracellular mediator of β activation. The α_2 adrenoceptors are coupled to other G proteins ($G\alpha_i$) that *inhibit* adenylyl cyclase and thus lower [cAMP]$_i$ in target tissues. The α_1 receptors are coupled to yet another heterotrimeric G protein ($G\alpha_q$) that either activates PLC or, in some cases, appears to alter the activity of a plasma membrane ion channel directly (see Chapter 3). The net effect of α_1 stimulation is to increase the concentration of IP$_3$ and [Ca^{2+}]$_i$ in target tissues.

Recognition of the diversity of adrenoceptor subtypes has led to a panoply of pharmacological agents that block or stimulate one or the other of these receptor subtypes. Some drugs are nonspecific and affect several receptor subtypes; others specifically block only a single subtype. The clinical value of a particular drug depends on its spectrum of activity. Thus, for example, an agent that selectively blocks the vasoconstrictor response to norepinephrine could be a very useful antihypertensive agent, but its utility would be compromised if it also blocked the ability of bladder smooth muscle to contract.

The CNS-epinephrine axis provides integrated control of multiple functions

The actions of the autonomic nervous system (see Chapter 14) in the control of blood pressure and heart rate (see Chapter 22), sweating (see Chapter 59), micturition (see Chapter 32), and airway resistance (see Chapter 27) are discussed in more detail in other chapters, as indicated. Here, I mention only some of the unique actions attributed to adrenal catecholamine release that integrate several bodily functions as part of the stress response. These adrenally mediated activities do not occur in isolation but are usually accompanied by generalized noradrenergic sympathetic discharge.

In response to the stress of simple **exercise** (see Chapters 25 and 60), blood flow to muscle is increased; circulating epinephrine appears to be important in this response. Circulating epinephrine also relaxes bronchial smooth muscle to meet the demand for increased ventilation and, when combined with the increased blood flow, increases oxygen delivery to the exercising muscle. Similarly, to sustain muscular activity, particularly early in exercise, epinephrine acting through the β adrenoceptor activates the degradation of muscle glycogen to provide a ready fuel source for the contracting muscle (see Chapter 3). Epinephrine also activates lipolysis in adipose tissue to furnish free fatty acids for more sustained muscular activity if needed. In liver, as in muscle, epinephrine activates glycogenolysis, thus maintaining the supply of glucose in the blood.

In addition to enhancing blood flow and ventilation, the integrated response to exercise increases fuel availability by decreasing insulin levels. Circulating epinephrine, acting through a β adrenoceptor, *stimulates* the secretion of insulin (see Chapter 51). However, during exercise, local autonomic innervation, acting by means of an α adrenoceptor of the pancreas, *inhibits* this effect, so insulin levels fall. The net effects are to promote glycogenolysis and to allow muscle to increase its work while maintaining glycemia so that brain function is not impaired. The fleeing human must not only run, but know *where* to run.

Unlike other glandular tissue, no endocrine feedback loop governs the secretion of adrenal medullary hormones. Control of catecholamine secretion resides within the CNS. This principle can be illustrated by the changes in epinephrine secretion that occur with even mild **hypoglycemia**.

Decreases in blood glucose to less than ~3.5 mM (normally, ~5.5 mM) are sensed by the CNS, which triggers a central sympathetic response that increases the firing of preganglionic fibers in the celiac plexus. This sympathetic outflow suppresses endogenous insulin secretion by the α-adrenergic mechanism noted earlier, thus promoting an increase in plasma [glucose]. This sympathetic outflow to the adrenal medulla also triggers a major release of epinephrine that, through β adrenoreceptors in the liver, stimulates increased hepatic glycogenolysis. This response helps to restore plasma [glucose] to normal. Restoration of normoglycemia diminishes central sympathetic outflow.

Pheochromocytoma

The dramatic biological effects of catecholamines are well illustrated by patients with pheochromocytoma. A **pheochromocytoma** is a relatively uncommon tumor caused by hyperplasia of either adrenal medullary tissue or extra-adrenal chromaffin tissue that failed to involute after birth. These tumors can be benign or malignant. They make catecholamines, just like the normal medulla, except in an unregulated fashion. Patients with pheochromocytomas typically have a plethora of symptoms, as would be expected from such a wide-ranging hormonal system. Paroxysmal (sudden outburst) hypertension, tachycardia, headache, episodes of sweating, anxiousness, tremor, and glucose intolerance usually dominate the clinical findings. The key to the diagnosis of this disorder is a careful history, evidence on physical examination of excessive adrenergic tone, and laboratory detection of increased amounts of urinary catecholamines and their metabolites. When chemical evaluation of the urinary metabolites confirms the presence of a pheochromocytoma, it is often possible to localize the tumor to one or the other adrenal gland and to resect the tumor. Rarely, both glands are affected, and bilateral adrenalectomy is necessary. Such patients must subsequently receive glucocorticoid and mineralocorticoid replacement. No therapy is routinely given to replace the adrenal *medullary* function. It is not clear whether these individuals react less well to external stimuli that would trigger the fight-or-flight response.

REFERENCES

Books and Reviews

Autelitano DJ, Lundblad JR, Blum M, Roberts JL: Hormonal regulation of POMC gene expression. Annu Rev Physiol 1989, 51:715-726.

Burnstein KL, Cidlowski JA: Regulation of gene expression by glucocorticoids. Annu Rev Physiol 1989; 51:683-699.

Fitzsimons JT: Angiotensin, thirst, and sodium appetite. Physiol Rev 1998; 78:583-686.

Funder JW: Glucocorticoid and mineralocorticoid receptors: Biology and clinical relevance. Annu Rev Med 1997; 48:231-240.

Young JB, Landsberg L: Catecholamines and the adrenal medulla. In Wilson JD, Foster DW, Kronenberg HM, Larsen PR (eds): Williams Textbook of Endocrinology, 9th ed, pp 665-728. Philadelphia: WB Saunders, 1998.

Journal Articles

Fevold HR: Regulation of the adrenal cortex secretory pattern by adrenocorticotropin. Science 1967; 156:1753-1755.

Gordon RD: Primary aldosteronism. J Endocrinol Invest 1995; 18:495-511.

Smith GW, Aubry JM, Dellu F, et al: Corticotropin releasing factor receptor 1–deficient mice display decreased anxiety, impaired stress response, and aberrant neuroendocrine development. Neuron 1998; 20:1093-1102.

Turnbull AV, Rivier C: Corticotropin-releasing factor (CRF) and endocrine responses to stress: CRF receptors, binding protein, and related peptides. Proc Soc Exp Biol Med 1997; 215:1-10.

Weitzman ED, Fukushima D, Nogeire C, et al: Twenty-four hour pattern of the episodic secretion of cortisol in normal subjects. J Clin Endocrinol Metab 1971; 33:14-22.

CHAPTER 51

THE ENDOCRINE PANCREAS

Eugene J. Barrett

ENDOCRINE AND PARACRINE TISSUES

The pancreas contains two types of glands: (1) exocrine glands, which secrete digestive enzymes and HCO_3^- into the intestinal lumen (see Chapter 43); and (2) endocrine glands, called the *islets of Langerhans*.

The normal human pancreas contains between 500,000 and several million islets. Islets can be oval or spherical and measure between 50 and 300 μm in diameter. Islets contain at least four types of secretory cells—α cells, β cells, Δ cells, and F cells—in addition to various vascular and neural elements (Fig. 51-1 and Table 51-1). **β Cells** secrete insulin, proinsulin, C peptide, and a recently described protein, amylin. β cells are the most numerous type of secretory cell within the islets; they are located throughout the islet but are particularly numerous in the center. **α Cells** principally secrete glucagon, **δ cells** secrete somatostatin, and **F cells** (also called pancreatic polypeptide cells) secrete pancreatic polypeptide.

The cells within an islet receive information from the world outside the islet. These cells also can communicate with each other and influence each other's secretion. We can group these communication links into three categories:

1. **Humoral communication.** The blood supply of the islet courses outward from the center of the islet toward the periphery, carrying glucose and other secretagogues. In the rat—and less strikingly in humans—β cells are more abundant in the center of the islet, whereas α and Δ cells are more abundant in the periphery. Cells within a given islet can influence the secretion of other cells as the blood supply courses outward through the islet carrying the secreted hormonal product of each cell type with it. For example, glucagon is a potent insulin secretagogue, insulin modestly inhibits glucagon release, and somatostatin potently inhibits the secretion of both insulin and glucagon (as well as the secretion of growth hormone and other non-islet hormones).
2. **Cell-cell communication.** Both gap and tight junctional structures connect islet cells with one another. Cells within an islet can communicate through gap junctions,

which may be important for the regulation of both insulin and glucagon secretion.
3. **Neural communication.** Another level of regulation of islet secretion occurs through innervation from both the sympathetic and the parasympathetic divisions of the autonomic nervous system (ANS). Cholinergic stimulation augments insulin secretion. Adrenergic stimulation can have either a stimulatory or inhibitory effect, depending on whether β-adrenergic (stimulatory) or α-adrenergic stimulation (inhibitory) dominates (see Chapter 50).

These three communication mechanisms allow for tight control over the synthesis and secretion of islet hormones.

INSULIN

The discovery of insulin was among the most exciting and dramatic events in the history of endocrine physiology and therapy. In the United States and Europe, insulin-dependent diabetes mellitus (IDDM), or type 1 diabetes, develops in ~1 in every 600 children in their lifetime. However, the prevalence is only ~1 in 10,000 in eastern Asia. Before 1922, all children with diabetes died within 1 or 2 years of diagnosis. It was an agonizing illness; the children lost weight despite eating well, became progressively weaker and cachectic, were soon plagued by infections, and eventually died of overwhelming acidosis. No effective therapy was available, and few prospects were on the horizon. It was known that the blood sugar was elevated in this disease, but beyond that, there was little understanding of its pathogenesis.

In 1889, Minkowski and von Mering demonstrated that removing the pancreas from dogs caused hyperglycemia, excess urination, thirst, weight loss, and death—in short, a syndrome closely resembling type 1 diabetes. Following this lead, a group of investigators in the Department of Physiology at the University of Toronto prepared extracts of pancreas and tested the ability of these extracts to lower plasma [glucose] in pancreatectomized dogs. Despite months of failures, these investigators persisted in their belief that such extracts could be beneficial. Finally, by the winter of 1921,

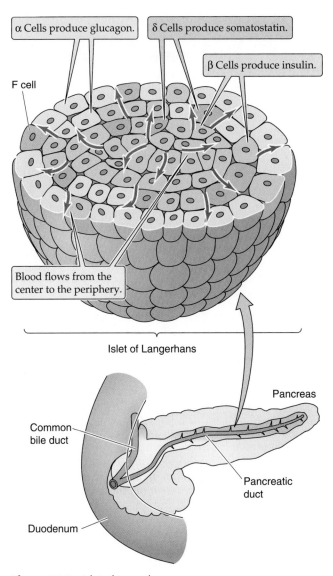

α Cells produce glucagon.

δ Cells produce somatostatin.

β Cells produce insulin.

F cell

Blood flows from the center to the periphery.

Islet of Langerhans

Pancreas

Common bile duct

Pancreatic duct

Duodenum

Figure 51-1 Islet of Langerhans.

Table 51-1 Products of Pancreatic Islet Cells

Cell Type	Product
α	Glucagon
β	Insulin Proinsulin C peptide Amylin
δ	Somatostatin
F	Pancreatic polypeptide

Banting and Best were able to demonstrate that an aqueous extract of pancreas could lower blood glucose and prolong survival in a pancreatectomized dog. Within 2 months, a more purified extract was shown to lower blood glucose in a young man with diabetes. By the end of 1923, insulin (as the islet hormone was named) was being prepared from beef and pork pancreas on an industrial scale, and patients from around the world were receiving effective treatment of their diabetes.

Since that time, the physiology of insulin synthesis, secretion, and action has been more extensively studied than that of any other hormone. Now, more than 85 years later, much is known about the metabolic pathways through which insulin regulates carbohydrate, lipid, and protein metabolism in its major targets: the liver, muscle, and adipose tissue. However, the sequence of intracellular signals that triggers insulin secretion by pancreatic β cells, the signal transduction process triggered when insulin binds to a plasma membrane receptor on target tissues, and the process by which the immune system recognizes and targets β cells for destruction remain areas of intense study.

Insulin replenishes fuel reserves in muscle, liver, and adipose tissue

What does insulin do? Succinctly put, insulin efficiently integrates body fuel metabolism both during periods of fasting and during feeding (Table 51-2). When an individual is *fasting*, the β cell secretes less insulin. When insulin levels decrease, lipids are mobilized from adipose tissue, and amino acids are mobilized from body protein stores within muscle and other tissues. These lipids and amino acids provide fuel for oxidation and serve as precursors for hepatic ketogenesis and gluconeogenesis, respectively. During *feeding*, insulin secretion increases. Elevated levels of insulin diminish the mobilization of endogenous fuel stores and stimulate carbohydrate, lipid, and amino acid uptake by specific, insulin-sensitive target tissues. In this manner, insulin directs tissues to replenish the fuel reserves that were used during periods of fasting.

As a result of its ability to regulate the mobilization and storage of fuels carefully, insulin maintains the concentration of glucose in the plasma within narrow limits. Such regulation provides the central nervous system (CNS) with a constant supply of glucose for fuel to maintain cortical function. In higher organisms, if the plasma glucose concentration declines to less than 2 to 3 mM (hypoglycemia) for even a brief period, confusion, seizures, and coma may result. Conversely, persistent elevations of plasma [glucose] are characteristic of the diabetic state. Severe *hyper*glycemia (plasma glucose levels >30 to 40 mM) produces osmotic diuresis (see Chapter 35 for the box on this topic) and can lead to severe dehydration, hypotension, and vascular collapse.

β cells synthesize and secrete insulin

The Insulin Gene Insulin is made only in the β cells of the pancreatic islet. It is encoded by a single gene on the short arm of chromosome 11. Insulin synthesis and secretion are

Table 51-2 Effects of Nutritional States

Parameter	After a 24-Hr Fast	2 Hr After a Mixed Meal
Plasma [glucose], mg/dL mM	60-80 3.3-4.4	100-140 5.6-7.8
Plasma [insulin], μU/mL	3-8	50-150
Plasma [glucagon], pg/mL	40-80	80-200
Liver	↑ Glycogenolysis ↑ Gluconeogenesis	↓ Glycogenolysis ↓ Gluconeogenesis ↑ Glycogen synthesis
Adipose tissue	Lipids mobilized for fuel	Lipids synthesized
Muscle	Lipids metabolized Protein degraded and amino acids exported	Glucose oxidized or stored as glycogen Protein preserved

Clinical Manifestations of Hypoglycemia and Hyperglycemia

Hypoglycemia

Early manifestations include palpitations, tachycardia, diaphoresis, anxiety, hyperventilation, shakiness, weakness, hunger, and nausea. For prolonged or severe hypoglycemia, manifestations include confusion, unusual behavior, hallucinations, seizures, hypothermia, focal neurologic deficits, and coma.

Hyperglycemia

Early manifestations include weakness, polyuria, polydipsia, altered vision, weight loss, and mild dehydration. For prolonged or severe hyperglycemia (accompanied by metabolic acidosis or diabetic ketoacidosis), manifestations include Kussmaul hyperventilation (deep, rapid breathing), stupor, coma, hypotension, and cardiac arrhythmias.

stimulated when islets are exposed to glucose. These effects require that glucose be metabolized. However, the molecular mechanisms by which glucose metabolites regulate insulin synthesis are not known.

Insulin Synthesis Transcription of the insulin gene product and subsequent processing result in production of the full-length mRNA that encodes **preproinsulin**. Starting from its 5′ end, this mRNA encodes a leader sequence and then peptide domains B, C, and A. Insulin is a *secretory protein* (see Chapter 2). As the preprohormone is synthesized, the leader sequence of ~24 amino acids is cleaved from the nascent peptide as it enters the rough endoplasmic reticulum. The result is **proinsulin** (Fig. 51-2), which consists of domains B, C, and A. As the *trans*-Golgi packages the proinsulin and creates secretory granules, proteases slowly begin to cleave the proinsulin molecule at two spots and thus excise the 31–amino acid C peptide. The resulting insulin molecule has two peptide chains, designated the **A and B chains**, that are joined by two disulfide linkages. The mature insulin molecule has a total of 51 amino acids, 21 on the A

chain and 30 on the B chain. In the secretory granule, the insulin associates with zinc. The secretory vesicle contains this insulin, as well as proinsulin and C peptide. All three are released into the portal blood when glucose stimulates the β cell.

Secretion of Insulin, Proinsulin, and C Peptide C peptide has no established biological action. However, because it is secreted in a 1:1 molar ratio with insulin, it is a useful marker for insulin secretion. Proinsulin does have modest insulin-like activities; it is ~1/20th as potent as insulin on a molar basis. In addition, the β cell secretes only ~5% as much proinsulin as insulin. As a result, proinsulin does not play a major role in the regulation of blood glucose.

Most of the insulin (~60%) that is secreted into the portal blood is removed in a first pass through the liver. In contrast, C peptide is not extracted by the liver at all. As a result, whereas measurements of the insulin concentration in systemic blood do not quantitatively mimic the secretion of insulin, measurements of C peptide do. C peptide is eventually excreted in the urine, and measurements of the quantity of C peptide excreted in a 24-hour period therefore reflect— on a molar basis—the amount of insulin made during that time. Measurements of urinary C peptide can be used clinically to assess a person's insulin secretory capability.

Glucose is the major regulator of insulin secretion

In healthy individuals, plasma [glucose] remains within a remarkably narrow range. After an overnight fast, it typically runs between 4 and 5 mM; the plasma [glucose] rises after a meal, but even with a very large meal it does not exceed 10 mM. Modest increases in plasma [glucose] provoke marked increases in insulin secretion and hence marked increases in the plasma [insulin], as illustrated in Figure 51-3A by an oral glucose tolerance test. Conversely, a decline in plasma [glucose] of only 20% markedly lowers plasma [insulin]. The change in the concentration of plasma glucose

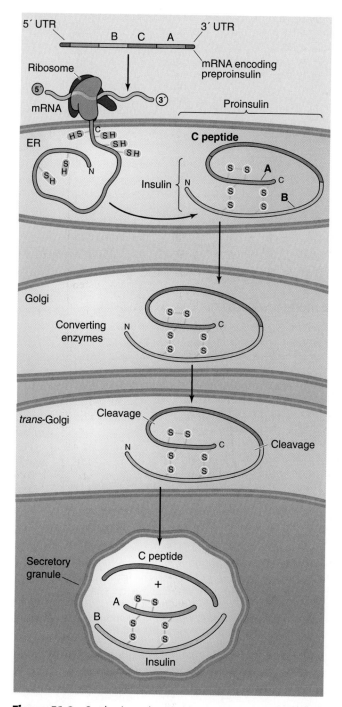

Figure 51-2 Synthesis and processing of the insulin molecule. The mature mRNA of the insulin gene product contains the following: a 5′ untranslated region (UTR); nucleotide sequences that encode a 24–amino acid leader sequence, as well as B, C, and A peptide domains; and a 3′ UTR. Together, the leader and the B, C, and A domains constitute preproinsulin. During translation of the mRNA, the leader sequence is cleaved in the lumen of the rough endoplasmic reticulum (ER). What remains is proinsulin, which consists of the B, C, and A domains. Beginning in the *trans*-Golgi, proteases cleave the proinsulin at two sites and release the C peptide as well as the mature insulin molecule, which consists of the B and A chains that are connected by two disulfide bonds. The secretory granule contains equimolar amounts of insulin and the C peptide, as well as a small amount of proinsulin. These components all are released into the extracellular space during secretion.

Nonhuman and Mutant Insulin

Cloning of the insulin gene has led to an important therapeutic advance, namely, the use of recombinant human insulin for the treatment of diabetes. Human insulin was the first recombinant protein available for routine clinical use. Before the availability of human insulin, either pork or beef insulin was used to treat diabetes. Pork and beef insulin differ from human insulin by one and three amino acids, respectively. The difference, although small, is sufficient to be recognized by the immune system, and antibodies to the injected insulin develop in most patients treated with beef or pork insulin; occasionally, the reaction is severe enough to cause a frank allergy to the insulin. This problem is largely avoided by using human insulin.

Sequencing of the insulin gene has not led to a major understanding of the genesis of the common forms of human diabetes. However, we have learned that rare patients with diabetes make a mutant insulin molecule. In these patients, the abnormal insulin possesses a single amino acid substitution in either the A or B chain. In each case that has been described, these changes lead to a less active insulin molecule (typically only ~1% as potent as insulin on a molar basis). These patients have either glucose intolerance or frank diabetes, but very high concentrations of immunoreactive insulin in their plasma. In these individuals, the immunoreactivity of insulin is not affected to the same extent as the bioactivity.

In addition to identifying these mutant types of insulin, sequencing of the insulin gene has allowed identification of a flanking polymorphic site upstream of the insulin gene that contains one of several common alleles. In some populations, one of these alleles is associated with an increased risk for the development of type 1 diabetes mellitus. The mechanism by which this increased risk is conferred is not known.

that occurs in response to feeding or fasting is the main determinant of insulin secretion. In a patient with type 1 diabetes mellitus caused by destruction of pancreatic islets, an oral glucose challenge evokes either no response or a much smaller insulin response, but a much larger increment in plasma [glucose] that lasts for a much longer time (Fig. 51-3B).

A glucose challenge of 0.5 g/kg body weight given *as an intravenous bolus* raises the plasma glucose concentration more rapidly than if given *orally*. Such a rapid rise in plasma glucose leads to two distinct phases of insulin secretion (Fig. 51-3C). The acute-phase or first-phase insulin response lasts only 2 to 5 minutes; the duration of the second insulin response persists as long as the blood glucose level remains elevated. The insulin released during the acute-phase insulin response to intravenous glucose arises from preformed insulin that has been packaged in secretory vesicles in the cytosol of the β cell. The late-phase insulin response also comes from preformed insulin with some contribution from newly synthesized insulin. One of the earliest detectable metabolic defects that occurs in diabetes is loss of the first phase of insulin secretion, which can be detected experimen-

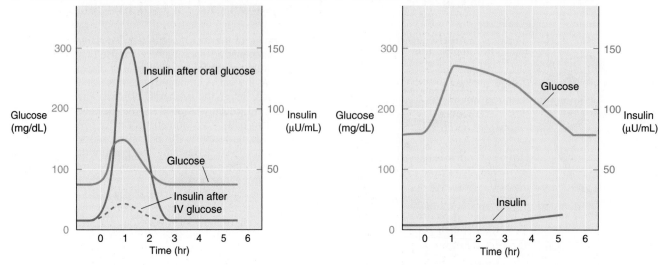

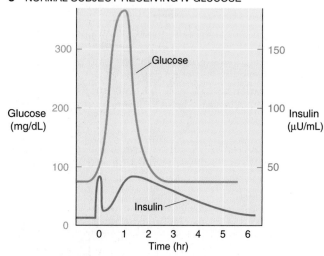

Figure 51-3 Glucose tolerance test. **A**, When a person ingests a glucose meal (75 g), plasma [glucose], shown by the *green curve*, rises slowly, reflecting the intestinal uptake of the glucose. In response, the pancreatic β cells secrete insulin, and plasma [insulin], shown by the *solid red curve*, rises sharply. When the glucose is given intravenously rather than orally—but in a manner that exactly reproduces the time course of plasma [glucose] in response to oral glucose in the green curve—the time course of plasma [insulin] follows the *dashed red curve*. The difference between the insulin responses in the solid and dashed red lines is the result of the incretin effect of oral glucose ingestion. **B**, In a patient with type 1 diabetes, the same glucose load as that in **A** causes plasma [glucose] to rise to a higher level and to remain there longer. The reason is that plasma [insulin] rises very little in response to the glucose challenge, so the tissues fail to dispose of the glucose load as rapidly as normal. The diagnosis of diabetes is made if the plasma glucose is higher than 200 mg/dL at the second hour. **C**, If the glucose challenge (0.5 g glucose/kg body weight given as a 25% glucose solution) is given intravenously, then the plasma [glucose] rises much more rapidly than it does with an oral glucose load. Sensing a rapid rise in [glucose], the β cells first secrete some of their stores of presynthesized insulin. Following this acute phase, the cells secrete both presynthesized and newly manufactured insulin in the chronic phase, which lasts as long as the glucose challenge. IV, intravenous.

tally by an intravenous glucose tolerance test. If a subject consumes glucose or a mixed meal, plasma [glucose] rises much more slowly—as in Figure 51-3A—because the appearance of glucose depends on intestinal absorption. Given that plasma [glucose] rises so slowly, the acute-phase insulin response can no longer be distinguished from the chronic response, and only a single phase of insulin secretion is apparent. However, the total insulin response to an oral glucose challenge exceeds the response observed when comparable changes in plasma [glucose] are produced by intravenously administered glucose (Fig. 51-3A). This difference is referred to as the *incretin effect*.

Metabolism of glucose by the β cell triggers insulin secretion

The pancreatic β cells take up and metabolize glucose, galactose, and mannose, and each can provoke insulin secretion by the islet. Other hexoses (e.g., 3-O-methylglucose or 2-deoxyglucose) that are transported into the β cell but that cannot be metabolized do not stimulate insulin secretion. Although glucose itself is the best secretagogue, some amino acids (especially arginine and leucine) and small keto acids (α-ketoisocaproate), as well as ketohexoses (fructose), can also weakly stimulate insulin secretion. The amino acids and keto acids do not share any metabolic pathway with hexoses other than *terminal oxidation through the citric acid cycle* (see Chapter 58). These observations have led to the suggestion that the ATP generated from the metabolism of these varied substances may be involved in insulin secretion. In the laboratory, depolarizing the islet cell membrane by raising extracellular $[K^+]$ provokes insulin secretion. In addition, glucagon has long been known to be a strong insulin secretagogue.

From these data has emerged a relatively unified picture of how various secretagogues trigger insulin secretion. Key to this picture is the presence in the islet of an ATP-sensitive K^+ channel and a **voltage-gated Ca^{2+} channel** in the plasma membrane (Fig. 51-4). The **K^+ channel (K_{ATP})** is an octamer of four Kir 6.2 channels and four **sulfonylurea receptors (SURs)**; see Chapter 7. Glucose triggers insulin release in a seven-step process:

1. Glucose enters the β cell through the GLUT2 glucose transporter by facilitated diffusion (see Chapter 5). Amino acids enter through a different set of transporters.
2. In the presence of glucokinase (the rate-limiting enzyme in glycolysis), the entering glucose undergoes glycolysis and raises $[ATP]_i$ by phosphorylating ADP. Some amino acids also enter the citric acid cycle and produce similar changes in $[ATP]_i$ and $[ADP]_i$. In both cases, the $NADH/NAD^+$ ratio (see Chapter 58) also would increase.
3. The increased $[ATP]_i$, the increased $[ATP]_i/[ADP]_i$ ratio, or the elevated $[NADH]_i/[NAD^+]_i$ ratio causes K_{ATP} channels (see Chapter 7) to close.
4. Reducing the K^+ conductance of the cell membrane causes the β cell to depolarize (i.e., the membrane potential is less negative).
5. This depolarization activates voltage-gated Ca^{2+} channels (see Chapter 7).
6. The increased Ca^{2+} permeability leads to increased Ca^{2+} influx and increased intracellular free Ca^{2+}. This rise in $[Ca^{2+}]_i$ additionally triggers Ca^{2+}-induced Ca^{2+} release (see Chapter 9).
7. The increased $[Ca^{2+}]_i$, perhaps by activation of a Ca^{2+}-calmodulin phosphorylation cascade, ultimately leads to insulin release.

In addition to the pathway just outlined, other secretagogues can also modulate insulin secretion through the phospholipase C pathway or through the adenylyl cyclase pathway (see Chapter 3). For example, glucagon, which stimulates insulin release, may bypass part or all of the glucose/$[Ca^{2+}]_i$ pathway by stimulating the adenylyl cyclase, thus raising cAMP levels and activating protein kinase A (PKA). Conversely, somatostatin, which inhibits insulin release, may act by inhibiting adenylyl cyclase.

Neural and humoral factors modulate insulin secretion

The islet is richly innervated by both the sympathetic and the parasympathetic divisions of the ANS. Neural signals appear to play an important role in the β-cell response in several settings. **β-Adrenergic** stimulation augments islet insulin secretion, whereas **α-adrenergic** stimulation inhibits it (Fig. 51-4). Isoproterenol, a synthetic catecholamine that is a specific agonist for the β-adrenergic receptor, potently stimulates insulin release. In contrast, norepinephrine and synthetic α-adrenergic agonists suppress insulin release both basally and in response to hyperglycemia. Because the post-synaptic sympathetic neurons of the pancreas release norepinephrine, which stimulates α more than β adrenoceptors, sympathetic stimulation through the celiac nerves inhibits insulin secretion. In contrast to α-adrenergic stimulation, **parasympathetic** stimulation through the vagus nerve, which releases acetylcholine, causes an increase in insulin release.

Exercise The effect of the sympathetic division on insulin secretion may be particularly important during exercise, when adrenergic stimulation of the islet increases. The major role for α-adrenergic *inhibition* of insulin secretion during exercise is to prevent hypoglycemia. Exercising muscle tissue uses glucose even when plasma [insulin] is low. If insulin levels were to rise, glucose use by the muscle would increase even further and promote hypoglycemia. Furthermore, an increase in [insulin] would inhibit lipolysis and fatty acid release from adipocytes and would thus diminish the availability of fatty acids, which the muscle can use as an alternative fuel to glucose (see Chapter 60). Finally, a rise in [insulin] would decrease glucose production by the liver. Suppression of insulin secretion during exercise may thus serve to prevent excessive glucose uptake by muscle, which if it were to exceed the ability of the liver to produce glucose, would lead to severe hypoglycemia, compromise the brain, and abruptly end any exercise.

Feeding Another important setting in which neural and humoral factors regulate insulin secretion is during feeding. Food ingestion triggers a complex series of neural, endocrine, and nutritional signals to many body tissues. The *cephalic phase* (see Chapters 42, 43, and 45) of eating, which occurs before food is ingested, results in stimulation of gastric acid secretion and a small rise in plasma insulin. This response appears to be mediated by the vagus nerve in both cases. If no food is forthcoming, blood [glucose] declines slightly and insulin secretion is again suppressed. If food ingestion does occur, the acetylcholine released by postganglionic vagal fibers in the islet augments the insulin response of the β cell to glucose.

As already discussed, after a subject drinks a glucose solution, the total amount of insulin secreted is greater than when the same amount of glucose is administered

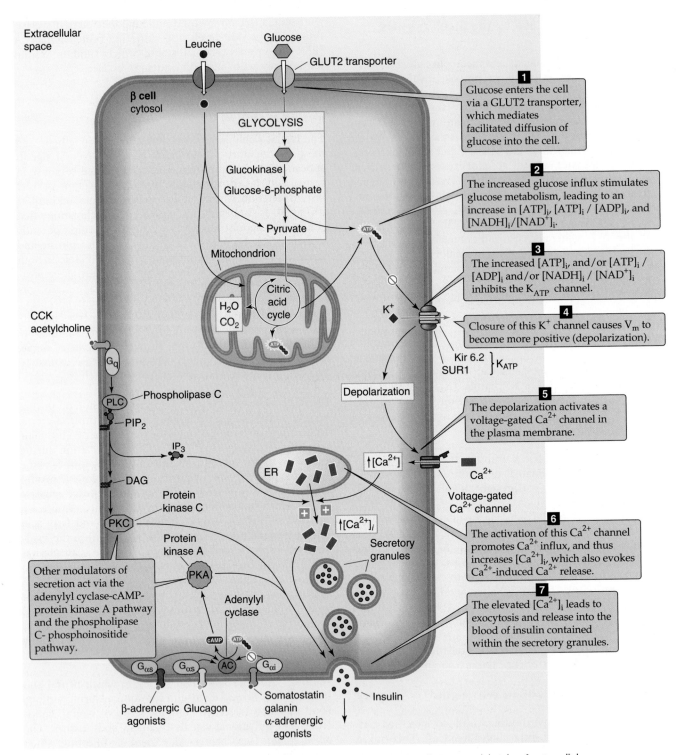

Figure 51-4 Mechanism of insulin secretion by the pancreatic β cell. Increased levels of extracellular glucose trigger the β cell to secrete insulin in the seven steps outlined in this figure. Metabolizable sugars (e.g., galactose and mannose) and certain amino acids (e.g., arginine and leucine) can also stimulate the fusion of vesicles that contain previously synthesized insulin. In addition to these fuel sources, certain hormones (e.g., glucagon, somatostatin, cholecystokinin [CCK]) can also modulate insulin secretion. DAG, diacylglycerol; ER, endoplasmic reticulum; IP_3, inositol 1,4,5-triphosphate; PIP_2, phosphatidylinositol 4,5-biphosphate.

Sulfonylureas

An entire class of drugs—the sulfonylurea agents—is used in the treatment of patients with adult-onset diabetes, also called type 2 diabetes or non–insulin-dependent diabetes mellitus (NIDDM). Patients with type 2 diabetes have two defects: (1) although their β cells are capable of making insulin, they do not respond normally to increased blood glucose levels; and (2) the target tissues are less sensitive to insulin.

The sulfonylurea agents were discovered accidentally. During the development of sulfonamide antibiotics after the Second World War, investigators noticed that the chemically related sulfonylurea agents produced hypoglycemia. These drugs turned out to have no value as antibiotics, but they did prove effective in treating the hyperglycemia of NIDDM. The sulfonylureas enhance insulin secretion by β cells by binding to the SUR subunits (see Chapter 7) of K_{ATP} channels, thereby decreasing the likelihood that these channels will be open. This action enhances glucose-stimulated insulin secretion (Fig. 51-4). By increasing insulin secretion and decreasing blood glucose, the sulfonylureas decrease the insulin resistance that is seen in these patients.

Unlike insulin, which must be injected, sulfonylureas can be taken orally and are therefore preferred by many patients. However, they have a therapeutic role only in NIDDM; the β cells in patients with type 1 or juvenile-onset diabetes (i.e., IDDM) are nearly all destroyed, and these patients must be treated with insulin replacement therapy.

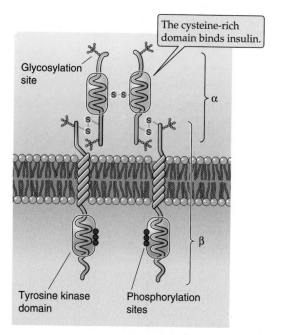

Figure 51-5 The insulin receptor. The insulin receptor is a heterotetramer that consists of two extracellular α chains and two membrane-spanning β chains. Insulin binding takes place on the cysteine-rich region of the α chains.

intravenously (Fig. 51-3A versus C). This observation has led to a search for enteric factors or *incretins* that could augment the islet β-cell response to an oral glucose stimulus. Currently, three peptides, cholecystokinin, glucagon-like intestinal peptide 1 (GLP-1), and gastric inhibitory polypeptide (GIP)—all of which are released by gut tissues in response to feeding—have been found to enhance insulin secretion. GLP-1, discussed later, may be the most important incretin yet discovered. A peptide analogue of GLP-1 that is found in the salivary secretion of the Gila monster has been approved for use in treating diabetic patients, based on the ability of this agent to enhance insulin secretion and to ameliorate hyperglycemia.

In the laboratory, incretins stimulate insulin secretion by isolated islets of Langerhans, and glucose increases this secretion even further. The presence of these incretins in the gut mucosa gives the islets advance notice that nutrients are being absorbed, and it primes the β cells to amplify their response to glucose. In addition, vagal stimulation of the β cells primes the islets for an amplified response.

The insulin receptor is a receptor tyrosine kinase

Once insulin is secreted into the portal blood, it first travels to the liver, where more than half is bound and removed from the circulation. The insulin that escapes the liver is available to stimulate insulin-sensitive processes in other tissues. At each target tissue, the first action of insulin is to bind to a specific receptor tyrosine kinase (see Chapter 3) on the plasma membrane (Fig. 51-5).

As discussed in Chapter 3, the insulin receptor—as well as the closely related insulin-like growth factor 1 (IGF-1) receptor—is a heterotetramer, with two identical α chains and two identical β chains. The α and β chains are synthesized as a single polypeptide that is subsequently cleaved. The two chains are joined by disulfide linkage (reminiscent of the synthesis of the A and B chains of insulin itself) in the sequence β-α-α-β. The insulin receptor shares considerable structural similarity with the IGF-1 receptor (see Chapter 48). The overall sequence homology is ~50%, and this figure rises to more than 80% in the tyrosine kinase region. This similarity is sufficient that very high concentrations of insulin can stimulate the IGF-1 receptor, and, conversely, high levels of IGF-1 can stimulate the insulin receptor.

The insulin receptor's extracellular α chains have multiple *N*-glycosylation sites. The β chains have an extracellular, a membrane spanning, and an intracellular portion. The β subunit of the receptor is glycosylated on its extracellular domains; receptor glycosylation is required for insulin binding and action. The intracellular domain of the β chain possesses tyrosine kinase activity, which increases markedly when insulin binds to sites on the α chains of the receptor. The insulin receptor can phosphorylate both itself and other intracellular substrates at tyrosine residues. The targets of tyrosine phosphorylation include a family of cytosolic proteins known as **insulin-receptor substrates (IRS-1, IRS-2, IRS-3, and IRS-4)** as well as *Src homology C terminus* (**SHC**), as illustrated in Figure 51-6. This phosphorylation mechanism appears to be the major one by which insulin transmits its signal across the plasma membrane of insulin target tissues.

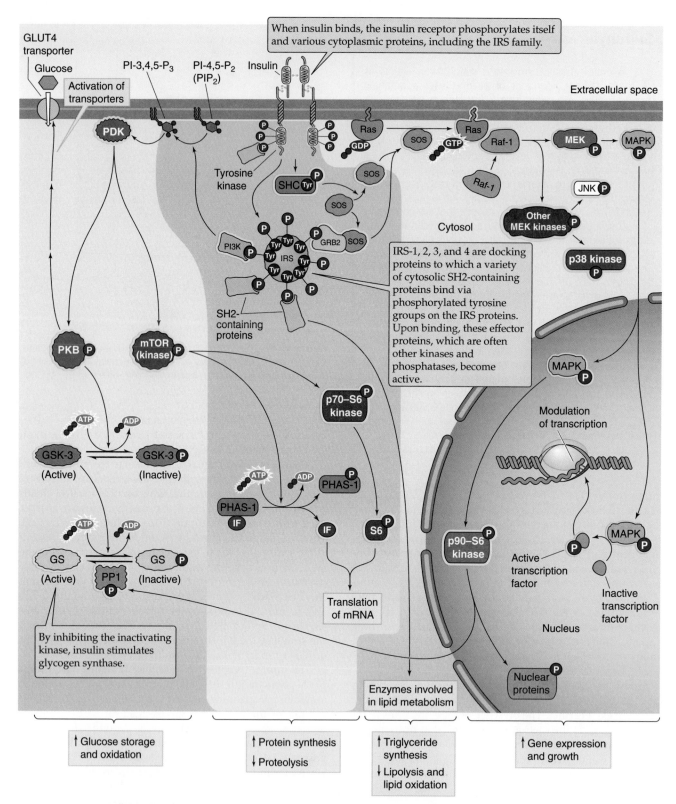

Figure 51-6 The insulin signal transduction system. When insulin binds to its receptor—which is a receptor tyrosine kinase (RTK)—tyrosine kinase domains on the intracellular portion of the β chains become active. The activated receptor transduces its signals to downstream effectors by phosphorylating at tyrosine residues the receptor itself, the insulin-receptor substrate family (IRS-1, IRS-2, IRS-3, IRS-4), and other cytosolic proteins (e.g., SHC). SH2-containing proteins dock onto certain phosphorylated tyrosine groups on the IRSs and thus become activated. Not all the signaling pathways are active in all of insulin's target cells. For example, the liver cell does not rely on the GLUT4 transporter to move glucose in and out of the cell. Similarly, the liver is a very important target for regulation by insulin of the gluconeogenic enzymes, whereas muscle and adipose tissue are not. MAPK, MAP kinase.

The IRS proteins are *docking proteins* to which various downstream effector proteins bind and thus become activated. IRS-1 has at least eight tyrosines within specific motifs that generally bind proteins containing SH2 (Src homology domain 2) domains, so that a single IRS molecule simultaneously activates multiple pathways. The IGF-1 receptor, which is closely related to the insulin receptor, also acts through IRS proteins.

Figure 51-6 illustrates three major signaling pathways triggered by the aforementioned tyrosine phosphorylations. The first begins when **phosphatidylinositol 3-kinase (PI3K)** binds to phosphorylated IRS and becomes activated. PI3K phosphorylates a membrane lipid phosphatidylinositol 4,5-bisphosphate (PIP_2) to form PIP_3, and it leads to major changes in glucose and protein metabolism.

The second signaling pathway begins in one of two ways: (1) the insulin receptor phosphorylates SHC, or (2) GRB2 binds to an IRS and becomes activated. As illustrated in Figure 51-6, both phosphorylated SHC and activated GRB2 trigger the Ras signaling pathway, leading through MEK and MAP kinases to increased gene expression and growth (see Chapter 4). Gene deletion studies in mice show that IRS-1 deletion does not cause diabetes, but it results in small mice. In contrast, IRS-2 deletion does cause diabetes, in part because of *impaired insulin secretion* by the pancreatic β cell.

The Insulin Receptor and Rare Forms of Diabetes

The ability of insulin to act on a target cell depends on three things: the number of receptors present on the target cell, the receptor's affinity for insulin, and the receptor's ability to transduce the insulin signal.

Several disorders have been described in which a mutation of the insulin receptor blunts or prevents insulin's actions. One such mutation markedly affects growth in utero, as well as after birth. This rare disorder is called **leprechaunism**, and it is generally lethal within the first year of life. Other mutations of the receptor have less devastating consequences.

Some individuals make antibodies to their own insulin receptors. Insulin, produced either endogenously or administered to these patients, does not work well because it must compete with these antibodies for sites on the receptor; as a result, these patients are hyperglycemic. Other antibodies can be insulin mimetic; that is, not only do the antibodies bind to the receptor, but they also actually mimic insulin's action. This mimicry causes severe *hypo*glycemia in affected individuals.

Neither receptor mutations nor antireceptor antibodies appear to be responsible for any of the common forms of diabetes seen clinically. However, abnormal function of the insulin receptor may be involved. Indeed, activation of inflammatory pathways involving p38 MAP kinase and nuclear factor-κβ can lead to phosphorylation of the insulin receptor (and of IRS proteins), principally at *serine* residues. This serine phosphorylation occurs commonly in animal models of insulin resistance and type 2 diabetes, as well as in human diabetes.

The third signaling pathway begins with the binding of SH2-containing proteins—other than PI3K and GRB2, already discussed—to specific phosphotyrosine groups on either the insulin receptor or IRS proteins. This binding activates the SH2-containing protein.

High levels of insulin lead to downregulation of insulin receptors

The number of insulin receptors expressed on the cell surface is far greater than that needed for the maximal biological response to insulin. In fact, in a physiologically normal individual, the glucose response to insulin is maximal when only ~5% of the receptors are occupied; that is, the target cells have many "spare" receptors for insulin.

The number of insulin receptors present on a target cell is determined by the balance among three factors: (1) receptor synthesis, (2) endocytosis of receptors followed by recycling of receptors back to the cell surface, and (3) endocytosis followed by degradation of receptors. Cells chronically exposed to high concentrations of insulin have fewer receptors than do those exposed to lower concentrations. This dynamic ability of cells to decrease the number of specific receptors on their surface is called *downregulation*. Insulin downregulates insulin receptors by decreasing receptor synthesis and increasing degradation. Such downregulation is one mechanism by which target tissues modulate their response to hormones. Downregulation of insulin receptors results in a decrease in the sensitivity of the target tissue to insulin without diminishing insulin's maximal effect.

One example of how downregulation can affect insulin's action is shown in Figure 51-7, which illustrates the effect of increases in insulin concentration on glucose uptake in adipocytes from normal individuals or type 2 diabetics. Adipocytes from patients with type 2 diabetes (see box on Diabetes Mellitus) have fewer insulin receptors per unit of surface area than do adipocytes from normal individuals. The markedly lower glucose transport across the entire physiological

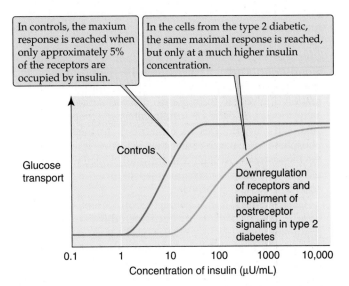

Figure 51-7 Response to insulin of normal and downregulated adipocytes.

range of insulin concentrations in diabetic adipocytes is characteristic of *insulin resistance.* In healthy controls, glucose transport is maximal when only a few (~5%) of the receptors are occupied. In diabetic adipocytes, a much higher concentration of insulin is required, and a larger *fraction* of the insulin receptors is occupied. However, the major effects in type 2 diabetes are apparently not the result of a decrease in receptor number, but rather are caused by impairment in signaling downstream from the receptor. This impairment includes diminished activity of the insulin receptor tyrosine kinase, PI3K activity, and perhaps other steps along the pathway to GLUT4 recruitment to the plasma membrane (Fig. 51-6). The summation of these multiple defects, only some of which have been identified, leads to insulin resistance.

In liver, insulin promotes storage of glucose as glycogen, as well as conversion of glucose to triglycerides

Insulin's actions on cellular targets frequently involve numerous different enzymatic and structural processes. These effects are illustrated as I consider—in this and the next two sections—the three principal targets for insulin action: the liver, muscle, and adipose tissue.

Because the pancreatic veins drain into the portal venous system, all hormones secreted by the pancreas must traverse the liver before entering the systemic circulation. For insulin, the liver is both a target tissue for hormone action and a major site of degradation.

The concentration of insulin in portal venous blood before extraction by the liver is three to four times greater than its concentration in the systemic circulation. The hepatocyte is therefore bathed in a relatively high concentration of insulin and is thus well positioned to respond acutely to changes in plasma [insulin].

After feeding, the plasma [insulin] rises, triggered by glucose and by neural and incretin stimulation of β cells. In the liver, this insulin rise acts on four main processes involved in fuel metabolism (Fig. 51-7). These divergent effects of insulin entail the use of multiple enzymatic control mechanisms.

Glycogen Synthesis and Glycogenolysis Physiological increases in plasma [insulin] decrease the breakdown and utilization of glycogen and—conversely—promote the formation of glycogen from plasma glucose. Although moderately increased levels of insulin allow gluconeogenesis to persist, the hepatocytes store the newly formed glucose 6-phosphate as glycogen rather than releasing it as glucose to the bloodstream. At high concentrations, insulin can inhibit the gluconeogenic conversion of lactate/pyruvate and amino acids to glucose 6-phosphate.

Glucose enters the hepatocyte from the blood through GLUT2, which mediates the facilitated diffusion of glucose (numbered boxes in Fig. 51-8). GLUT2 is present in abundance in the liver plasma membrane, even in the absence of insulin, and its activity is not influenced by insulin. Insulin stimulates glycogen synthesis from glucose by activating **glucokinase** (1) and **glycogen synthase** (2). The latter enzyme contains multiple serine phosphorylation sites. Insulin

causes a net dephosphorylation of the protein, thus increasing the enzyme's activity. At the same time that glycogen synthase is being activated, increases in both insulin and glucose diminish **glycogen phosphorylase** activity (3). This enzyme is rate limiting for the breakdown of glycogen. The same enzyme that dephosphorylates (and thus *activates*) glycogen synthase also dephosphorylates (and thus *inhibits*) phosphorylase. Thus, insulin has opposite effects on the opposing enzymes, with the net effect that it promotes glycogen formation. Insulin also inhibits **glucose-6-phosphatase (G6Pase)** (4), which converts glucose 6-phosphate to glucose and thus completes the conversion of glycogen to glucose. Glycogen is an important storage form of carbohydrate in both liver and muscle. The glycogen stored during the postprandial period is then available for use many hours later as a source of glucose.

Glycolysis and Gluconeogenesis Insulin promotes the conversion of some of the glucose taken up by the liver into pyruvate and—conversely—diminishes the use of pyruvate and other three-carbon compounds for gluconeogenesis (numbered boxes in Fig. 51-8). Insulin induces transcription of the **glucokinase** gene (1) and thus results in increased synthesis of this enzyme, which is responsible for phosphorylating glucose to glucose 6-phosphate and initiating the metabolism of glucose. In acting to promote glycolysis and diminish gluconeogenesis, insulin induces the synthesis of a glucose metabolite, fructose 2,6-bisphosphate. This compound is a potent allosteric activator of **phosphofructokinase** (5), a key regulatory enzyme in glycolysis. Insulin also stimulates **pyruvate kinase** (6), which forms pyruvate, and stimulates **pyruvate dehydrogenase** (8), which catalyzes the first step in pyruvate oxidation. Finally, insulin promotes glucose breakdown by the hexose monophosphate shunt (7).

In addition, insulin also inhibits gluconeogenesis at several steps. Insulin diminishes transcription of the **phosphoenolpyruvate carboxykinase (PEPCK)** gene (9), thus reducing the synthesis of a key regulatory enzyme required to form phosphoenolpyruvate from oxaloacetate early in the gluconeogenic pathway. The increased levels of fructose 2,6-bisphosphate also inhibit the activity of **fructose-1,6-bisphosphatase (FBPase)** (10), which is also part of the gluconeogenic pathway.

Lipogenesis Insulin promotes the storage of fats and inhibits the oxidation of fatty acids (see Fig. 58-9) through allosteric and covalent modification of key regulatory enzymes, as well as by transcription of new enzymes (numbered boxes in Fig. 51-8). The pyruvate that is now available from glycolysis can be used to synthesize fatty acids. Insulin promotes dephosphorylation of **acetyl coenzyme A (CoA) carboxylase 2 (ACC2)** (11), the first committed step in fatty acid synthesis in the liver. This dephosphorylation leads to increased synthesis of malonyl CoA, which allosterically inhibits **carnitine acyltransferase I (CAT I)**. This enzyme (13) converts acyl CoA and carnitine to acyl carnitine. Thus, malonyl CoA inhibits fatty acid transport into the mitochondria, where fat oxidation occurs. At the same time, insulin stimulates **fatty acid synthase** (12), which generates fatty acids. Thus, because insulin promotes the formation of

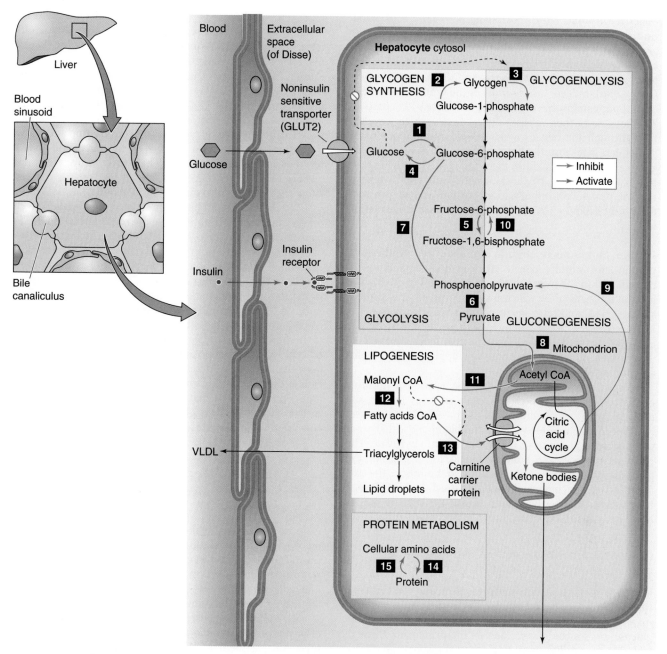

Figure 51-8 Effect of insulin on hepatocytes. Insulin has four major effects on liver cells. First, insulin promotes glycogen synthesis from glucose by enhancing the transcription of **glucokinase** (*1*) and by activating **glycogen synthase** (*2*). Additionally, insulin together with glucose inhibits glycogen breakdown to glucose by diminishing the activity of **G6Pase** (*4*). Glucose also inhibits **glycogen phosphorylase** (*3*). Second, insulin promotes glycolysis and carbohydrate oxidation by increasing the activity of **glucokinase** (*1*), **phosphofructokinase** (*5*), and **pyruvate kinase** (*6*). Insulin also promotes glucose metabolism through the **hexose monophosphate shunt** (*7*). Finally, insulin promotes the oxidation of pyruvate by stimulating **pyruvate dehydrogenase** (*8*). Insulin also inhibits gluconeogenesis by inhibiting the activity of **PEPCK** (*9*), **FBPase** (*10*), and **G6Pase** (*4*). Third, insulin promotes the synthesis and storage of fats by increasing the activity of **acetyl CoA carboxylase** (*11*) and **fatty acid synthase** (*12*) as well as the synthesis of several apoproteins packaged with VLDL. Insulin also indirectly inhibits fat oxidation because the increased levels of malonyl CoA inhibit **CAT I** (*13*). The inhibition of fat oxidation helps shunt fatty acids to esterification as triglycerides and storage as VLDL or lipid droplets. Fourth, by mechanisms that are not well understood, insulin promotes protein synthesis (*14*) and inhibits protein breakdown (*15*).

malonyl CoA and fatty acids but inhibits fatty acid oxidation, this hormone favors esterification of the fatty acids with glycerol within the liver, thus forming triglycerides. The liver can either store these triglycerides in lipid droplets or export them as very-low-density lipoprotein (VLDL) particles (see Chapter 46). Indeed, insulin induces the synthesis of several of the **apoproteins** that are packaged with the VLDL particle. The hepatocyte then releases these VLDLs, which leave the liver through the hepatic vein. Muscle and adipose tissue subsequently take up the lipids in these VLDL particles and either store them or oxidize them for fuel. Thus, by regulation of transcription, by allosteric activation, and by regulation of protein phosphorylation, insulin acts to promote the synthesis and storage of fat and diminish its oxidation in liver.

Protein Metabolism Insulin stimulates the synthesis of protein and simultaneously reduces the degradation of protein within the liver (numbered boxes in Fig. 51-8). The general mechanism by which insulin stimulates net protein synthesis (14) and restrains proteolysis (15) by the liver has not been nearly as well defined as have its effects on the enzymes involved in carbohydrate and lipid metabolism. The regulatory steps in these pathways appear more complex and are less well understood.

In summary, insulin modulates the activity of multiple regulatory enzymes, which are responsible for the hepatic metabolism of carbohydrates, fat, and protein. Insulin causes the liver to take up glucose from the blood and either store the glucose as glycogen or break it down into pyruvate. The pyruvate provides the building blocks for storage of the glucose carbon atoms as fat. Insulin also diminishes the oxidation of fat, which normally supplies much of the ATP used by the liver. As a result, insulin causes the liver, as well as other body tissues, to burn carbohydrates preferentially.

In muscle, insulin promotes the uptake of glucose and its storage as glycogen

Muscle is a major insulin-sensitive tissue and the principal site of insulin-mediated glucose disposal. Insulin has four major effects on muscle. First, in muscle, unlike the liver, glucose crosses the plasma membrane principally through GLUT4, an *insulin-sensitive* glucose transporter. GLUT4, which is found virtually exclusively in striated muscle and adipose tissue, belongs to a family of proteins that mediate the facilitated diffusion of glucose (see Chapter 5). Insulin markedly stimulates GLUT4 in both muscle and fat (see later) by a process involving recruitment of preformed transporters from a membranous compartment in the cell cytosol out to the plasma membrane (Fig. 51-9). Recruitment places additional glucose transporters in the plasma membrane, thus increasing the V_{max} of glucose transport into muscle and increasing the flow of glucose from the interstitial fluid to the cytosol. As discussed earlier, a different glucose transporter, GLUT2, mediates glucose transport into hepatocytes (Fig. 51-8), and insulin does *not* increase the activity of that transporter.

The second effect of insulin on muscle (Fig. 51-9) is to enhance the conversion of glucose to glycogen by activating **hexokinase** ([1] different from the glucokinase in liver) and

glycogen synthase (2). Third, insulin increases glucose breakdown and oxidation by increasing **phosphofructokinase** (3) and **pyruvate dehydrogenase** (4) activity. Fourth, insulin also stimulates the synthesis of protein in skeletal muscle (5) and slows the degradation of existing proteins (6). The result is preservation of muscle protein mass, which has obvious beneficial effects in preserving strength and locomotion. The insulin-induced increase in glucose utilization permits the muscle to diminish fat utilization and allows it to store as triglycerides some of the fatty acid that it removes from the circulation. The stored triglycerides and glycogen are major sources of energy that muscle can use later when called on to exercise or generate heat.

Exercise and insulin have some interesting parallel effects on skeletal muscle. Both increase the recruitment of GLUT4 transporters to the sarcolemma, and both increase glucose oxidation; therefore, both increase glucose uptake by muscle. Additionally, exercise and insulin appear to have synergistic effects on the foregoing processes. Clinically, this synergism is manifested as a marked increase in insulin sensitivity induced by exercise and is exploited as part of the treatment of patients with diabetes mellitus.

In muscle, as in the liver, insulin directs the overall pattern of cellular fuel metabolism by acting at multiple sites. In both tissues, insulin increases the oxidation of carbohydrate, thus preserving body protein and fat stores. Carbohydrate ingested in excess of that used immediately as an oxidative fuel is either stored as glycogen in liver and muscle or is converted to lipid in the liver and exported to adipose tissue and muscle.

In adipocytes, insulin promotes uptake of glucose and its conversion to triglycerides for storage

Adipose tissue is the third major insulin-sensitive tissue involved in the regulation of body fuel. Again, insulin has several sites of action in adipocytes. All begin with the same receptor-mediated action of insulin to stimulate several cellular effector pathways. Insulin has four major actions on adipocytes. First, like muscle, adipose contains the insulin-sensitive GLUT4 glucose transporter. In insulin-stimulated cells, preformed transporters are recruited from an intracellular compartment to the cell membrane, thus markedly accelerating the entry of glucose into the cell.

Second, insulin promotes the breakdown of glucose to metabolites that will eventually be used to synthesize triglycerides (Fig. 51-10). Unlike muscle or liver, little of the glucose taken up is stored as glycogen. Instead, the adipocyte glycolytically metabolizes much of the glucose to α-glycerol phosphate, which it will use in the synthesis of triglycerides. The glucose that is not converted to α-glycerol phosphate goes on to form acetyl CoA and then malonyl CoA and fatty acids. Insulin enhances this flow of glucose to fatty acids by stimulating **pyruvate dehydrogenase** (1) and **acetyl CoA carboxylase** (2).

Third, insulin promotes the formation of triglycerides by simple mass action; the increased levels of α-glycerol phosphate increase its esterification with fatty acids (principally C-16 and C-18) to yield triglycerides. Some of the fatty acids are a result of the glucose metabolism noted earlier. Most of

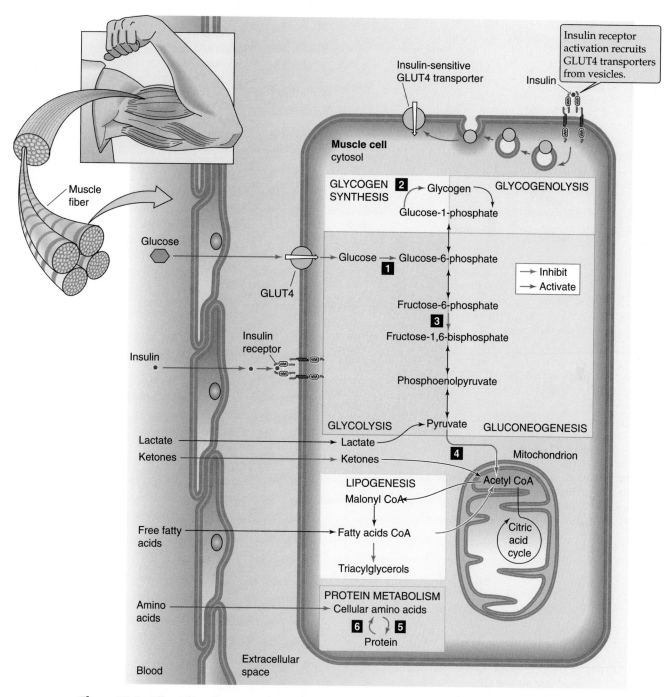

Figure 51-9 Effect of insulin on muscle. Insulin has four major effects on muscle cells. First, insulin promotes glucose uptake by recruiting GLUT4 transporters to the plasma membrane. Second, insulin promotes glycogen synthesis from glucose by enhancing the transcription of **hexokinase** (*1*) and by activating **glycogen synthase** (*2*). Third, insulin promotes glycolysis and carbohydrate oxidation by increasing the activity of **hexokinase** (*1*), **phosphofructokinase** (*3*), and **pyruvate dehydrogenase** (*4*). These actions are similar to those in liver; little or no gluconeogenesis occurs in muscle. Fourth, insulin promotes protein synthesis (*5*) and inhibits protein breakdown (*6*).

the fatty acids, however, enter the adipocyte from chylomicrons and VLDLs (see Table 46-5) in the blood (see later). The cell sequesters these triglycerides in lipid droplets, which form most of the mass of the adipose cell. Conversely, insulin restrains the activity of a **hormone-sensitive triglyceride lipase (HSL)** (3). In fat, this enzyme mediates the conversion of stored triglyceride to fatty acids and glycerol for export to other tissues.

Fourth, insulin induces the synthesis of a different enzyme—**lipoprotein lipase (LPL)**. This lipase does not act

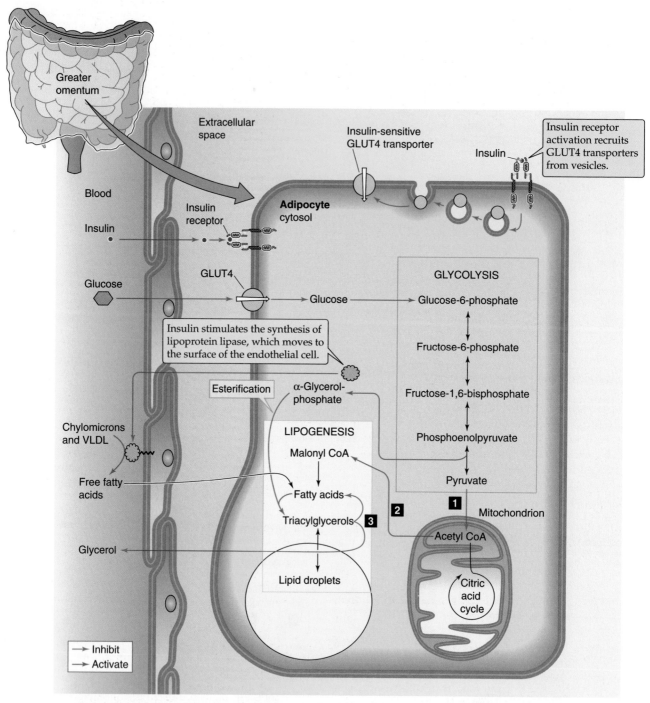

Figure 51-10 Effect of insulin on adipocytes. Insulin has four major effects on adipocytes. First, insulin promotes glucose uptake by recruiting GLUT4 transporters to the plasma membrane. Second, insulin promotes glycolysis, leading to the formation of α-glycerol phosphate. Insulin also promotes the conversion of pyruvate to fatty acids by stimulating **pyruvate dehydrogenase** (*1*) and **acetyl CoA carboxylase** (*2*). Third, insulin promotes the esterification of α-glycerol phosphate with fatty acids to form triglycerides, which the adipocyte stores in fat droplets. Conversely, insulin inhibits **hormone-sensitive triglyceride lipase** (*3*), which would otherwise break the triglycerides down into glycerol and fatty acids. Fourth, insulin promotes the synthesis of LPL in the adipocyte. The adipocyte then exports this enzyme to the endothelial cell, where it breaks down the triglycerides contained in chylomicrons and VLDL, thus yielding fatty acids. These fatty acids then enter the adipocyte for esterification and storage in fat droplets as triglycerides.

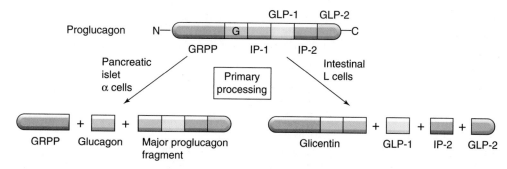

Figure 51-11 The synthesis of the glucagon molecule. The proglucagon molecule includes amino acid sequences that, depending on how the peptide chain is cleaved, can yield glucagon-related polypeptide (GRPP), glucagon, IP-1, GLP-1, IP-2, and GLP-2. Proteases in the pancreatic α cells cleave proglucagon at points that yield GRPP, glucagon, and a C-terminal fragment. Proteases in neuroendocrine cells in the intestine cleave proglucagon to yield glicentin, GLP-1, IP-2, and GLP-2.

on the lipid stored within the adipose cell. Rather, the adipocyte exports the LPL to the endothelial cell, where it resides on the extracellular surface of the endothelial cell, facing the blood and anchored to the plasma membrane. In this location, the LPL acts on triglycerides in chylomicrons and VLDLs and cleaves them into glycerol and fatty acids. These fatty acids are then available for uptake by nearby adipocytes, which esterify them with glycerol phosphate to form triglycerides. This mechanism provides an efficient means by which insulin can promote the storage of lipid in adipose tissue.

GLUCAGON

Glucagon is the other major pancreatic islet hormone that is involved in the regulation of body fuel metabolism. Ingestion of protein appears to be the major stimulus to secretion of glucagon. Glucagon's principal target tissue is the liver. Like insulin, glucagon is secreted first into the portal blood and is therefore anatomically well positioned to regulate hepatic metabolism.

Although the *amino acids* released by digestion of a protein meal appear to be the major glucagon secretagogue, glucagon's main actions on the liver appear to involve the regulation of *carbohydrate* and *lipid* metabolism. Glucagon is particularly important in stimulating glycogenolysis, gluconeogenesis, and ketogenesis. Glucagon does not act solely on the liver, but also has glycogenolytic action on cardiac and skeletal muscle and lipolytic action on adipose tissue, and it promotes the breakdown of protein by several tissues. However, these effects on protein tissue breakdown appear to be more prominent when tissues are exposed to pharmacological concentrations of glucagon. At more physiological concentration, the liver appears to be the major target tissue.

In many circumstances, the actions of glucagon antagonize those of insulin. Unlike the cellular mechanism of action of insulin, the mechanism of glucagon action is understood in considerable detail.

Pancreatic α cells secrete glucagon in response to ingested protein

Glucagon is a 31–amino acid peptide (molecular weight, ~3500 Da) synthesized by α cells in the islets of Langerhans. In humans, the glucagon gene is located on chromosome 2. The initial gene product is the mRNA encoding preproglucagon. As is the case for insulin, a peptidase removes the signal sequence of preproglucagon during translation of the mRNA in the rough endoplasmic reticulum to yield proglucagon. Proteases in the α cells subsequently cleave the proglucagon (molecular weight, ~9000 Da) into the mature glucagon molecule and several biologically active peptides (Fig. 51-11). Neuroendocrine cells (i.e., L cells) within the gut process the proglucagon differently to yield not glucagon, but GLP-1—a potent incretin—and other peptides.

Pancreatic α Cells The mature glucagon molecule is the major secretory product of the α cell. As in insulin, the fully processed glucagon molecule is stored in secretory vesicles within the cell's cytosol. Although amino acids are the major secretagogues, the concentrations of amino acids required to provoke secretion of glucagon in vitro are higher than those generated in vivo. This observation suggests that other neural or humoral factors amplify the response in vivo, analogous to the effects of incretin on insulin secretion. Whereas glucose and several amino acids both stimulate insulin secretion by β cells, only amino acids stimulate glucagon secretion by α cells; glucose inhibits glucagon secretion. The signaling mechanism by which α cells recognize either amino acids or glucose is not known.

Glucagon, like the incretins, is a potent insulin secretagogue. Because most of the α cells are located downstream from the β cells (recall that the circulation of blood proceeds from the β cells and then out past the α cells), however, it is unlikely that glucagon exerts an important paracrine effect on insulin secretion.

Intestinal L Cells Proteases in neuroendocrine cells in the intestine process proglucagon differently than do α cells. L cells produce a peptide fragment called *glicentin* that contains the amino acid sequence of glucagon but does not bind to glucagon receptors. Downstream from the glucagon-coding region, the L cells generate two peptides from proglucagon: **GLP-1 and GLP-2**. Both are glucagon-like in that they cross-react with some antisera directed to glucagon, but GLP-1 and GLP-2 have very weak biological activity as glucagon analogues. However, GLP-1 is one of the most potent incretins, and it stimulates insulin secretion. GLP-1 is released by the gut into the circulation in response to carbohydrate or protein ingestion. GLP-2 is not an incretin, and its biological actions are not known.

Glucagon, acting through cAMP, promotes the synthesis of glucose by the liver

Glucagon is an important regulator of hepatic glucose production and ketogenesis in the liver. As shown in Figure 51-12, glucagon binds to a receptor that activates the heterotrimeric G protein $G\alpha_s$, which stimulates membrane-bound adenylyl cyclase (see Chapter 3). The cAMP formed by the cyclase, in turn, activates PKA, which phosphorylates numerous regulatory enzymes and other protein substrates, thus altering glucose and fat metabolism in the liver. Whereas insulin leads to the *dephosphorylation* of certain key enzymes (i.e., glycogen synthase, acetyl CoA carboxylase, phosphorylase), glucagon leads to their *phosphorylation*.

A particularly clear example of the opposing actions of insulin and glucagon involves the activation of **glycogenolysis**, which is discussed in Chapter 3 (see Fig 3-7). PKA phosphorylates the enzyme **phosphorylase kinase** (see Fig. 59-8), thus increasing the activity of phosphorylase kinase and allowing it to increase the phosphorylation of its substrate, **glycogen phosphorylase *b***. The addition of a single phosphate residue to phosphorylase *b* converts it to phosphorylase *a*. Liver phosphorylase *b* has little activity in breaking the 1 to 4 glycosidic linkages of glycogen, but phosphorylase *a* is very active. In addition to converting phosphorylase *b* to the active phosphorylase *a* form, PKA also phosphorylates a peptide called **inhibitor I**. In its phosphorylated form, inhibitor I decreases the activity of protein phosphatase 1 (PP1) that otherwise would dephosphorylate both phosphorylase kinase and phosphorylase *a* (converting them to their *inactive* forms). PP1 also activates glycogen synthase. Thus, through inhibitor I, glucagon modulates several of the enzymes involved in hepatic glycogen metabolism to provoke *net glycogen breakdown*. As a result of similar actions on the pathways of gluconeogenesis and lipid oxidation, glucagon also stimulates these processes. Conversely, glucagon restrains glycogen synthesis, glycolysis, and lipid storage.

The effects of the glucagon—as well as the effect of glucocorticoids—to enhance gluconeogenesis involve activation of the transcription factor CBP as well as PGC-1 (PPAR-γ coactivator-1), which enhances the transcription factor PPAR-γ (see Chapter 4). The net effect is an increase in the synthesis of such key regulatory enzymes as G6Pase and PEPCK—both of which promote the release of glucose. Insulin restrains the transcription of these two enzymes in two ways, both through the PI3K/protein kinase B pathway (Fig. 51-6). First, insulin increases the release of the transcription factor domain of SREBP-1 (see Chapter 3), which antagonizes the transcription of mRNA encoding the two enzymes. Second, insulin increases the phosphorylation of several transcription factors of the Foxo family, thereby promoting their movement out of the nucleus and preventing them from binding to the promoter regions of the two enzymes.

These actions of glucagon can be integrated with our understanding of insulin's action on the liver in certain physiological circumstances. For example, after an overnight fast, when insulin concentrations are low, glucagon stimulates the liver to produce the glucose that is required by the brain and other tissues for their ongoing function. With ingestion of a protein meal, absorbed amino acids provoke insulin secretion, which can inhibit hepatic glucose production and promote glucose storage by liver and muscle (see earlier). If the meal lacked carbohydrate, the secreted insulin could cause hypoglycemia. However, glucagon secreted in response to a protein meal balances insulin's action on the liver and thus maintains glucose production and avoids hypoglycemia.

Glucagon promotes the oxidation of fat in the liver, which can lead to the formation of ketone bodies

Glucagon plays a major regulatory role in hepatic lipid metabolism. As shown in the earlier discussion of insulin (Fig. 51-8), the liver can esterify fatty acids with glycerol to form triglycerides, which it can store or export as VLDL particles. Alternatively, the liver can partially oxidize fatty acids—and form ketones—or can fully oxidize them to CO_2 (see Chapter 58). Whereas fatty acid esterification and storage occur in the liver cytosol, oxidation and ketogenesis occur within the mitochondria.

Glucagon stimulates fat oxidation indirectly by increasing the activity of the **CAT** system, which mediates the transfer of fatty acids across the mitochondrial membrane. Glucagon produces this stimulation by inhibiting acetyl CoA carboxylase, which generates malonyl CoA, the first committed intermediate in the synthesis of fatty acids by the liver. Malonyl CoA is also an inhibitor of the CAT system. By inhibiting acetyl CoA carboxylase, glucagon lowers the concentration of malonyl CoA, releases the inhibition of CAT, and allows fatty acids to be transferred into the mitochondria. These fatty acids are oxidized to furnish ATP to the liver cell. If the rate of fatty acid transport into the mitochondria exceeds the need of the liver to phosphorylate ADP, the fatty acids will be only *partially oxidized*, and the keto acids (or "ketone bodies") β-**hydroxybutyric acid** and **acetoacetic acid** will accumulate. These keto acids can exit the mitochondria and the liver to be used by other tissues as oxidative fuel.

During fasting, the decline in insulin and the increase in glucagon promote ketogenesis; this process is of vital importance to the CNS, which can use keto acids but not fatty acids as fuel. In the adaptation to fasting, glucagon therefore plays the important role of stimulating the conversion of fatty acids to ketones and provides the brain with the fuel

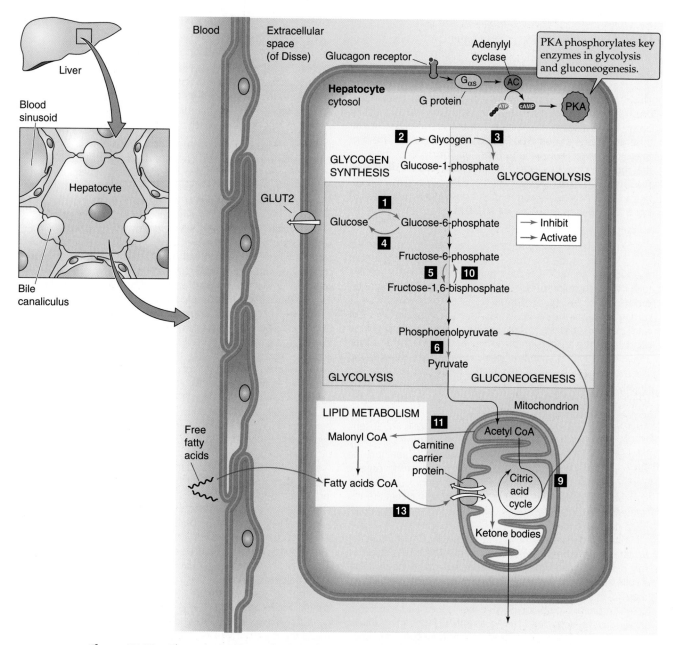

Figure 51-12 Glucagon signal transduction. Glucagon generally antagonizes the effects of insulin in the liver. Glucagon binds to a $G_{\alpha s}$-coupled receptor, thereby activating the adenylyl cyclase/cAMP/PKA cascade. Glucagon has three major effects on liver cells. First, glucagon promotes net glycogen breakdown. Glucagon inhibits glycogen synthesis by reducing the activity of **glucokinase** (*1*) and **glycogen synthase** (*2*). However, glucagon promotes glycogen breakdown by activating **glycogen phosphorylase** (*3*) and **G6Pase** (*4*). Second, glucagon promotes net gluconeogenesis. The hormone inhibits glycolysis and carbohydrate oxidation by reducing the activity **glucokinase** (*1*), **phosphofructokinase** (*5*), and **pyruvate kinase** (*6*). Glucagon also stimulates gluconeogenesis by increasing the transcription of **PEPCK** (*9*), **FBPase** (*10*), and **G6Pase** (*4*). Third, glucagon promotes the oxidation of fats. The hormone inhibits the activity of **acetyl CoA carboxylase** (*11*). Glucagon indirectly stimulates fat oxidation because the decreased levels of malonyl CoA relieve the inhibition of malonyl CoA on **CAT** (*13*). The numbering scheme for these reactions is the same as that in Figure 51-8.

Diabetes Mellitus

Diabetes is the most common serious metabolic disease in humans. The hallmark of diabetes is an elevated blood glucose concentration, but this abnormality is just one of many biochemical and physiological alterations that occur in the disease. Diabetes is not one disorder, but it can arise as a result of numerous defects in regulation of the synthesis, secretion, and action of insulin. The type of diabetes that most commonly affects children is called **type 1 diabetes mellitus** or **IDDM**. The diabetes that generally begins in adulthood and is particularly common in obese individuals is called **type 2 diabetes mellitus or NIDDM**.

Type 1 Diabetes

IDDM is caused by an immune-mediated selective destruction of the β cells of the pancreas. The other cell types present in the islet are spared. The consequence of the loss of insulin, with the preservation of glucagon, can be viewed as an accelerated form of fasting or starvation. A healthy person who is fasting for several days continues to secrete insulin at a low rate that is sufficient to balance the action of glucagon in modulating the production of glucose and ketones by the liver. However, in type 1 diabetes, insulin deficiency is severe, and glucose and ketone production by the liver occur at a rate that greatly exceeds the rate at which they are being used. As a result, the concentration of these substances in blood begins to rise. Even when glucose concentrations reach levels 5 to 10 times normal, no insulin is secreted because β cells are absent. The increased glucose and ketones provide an immense solute load to the kidney that causes osmotic diuresis. In addition, the keto acids that are produced are moderately strong organic acids (pK < 4.0), and their increased production causes severe metabolic acidosis (see Chapter 28). If these patients are not treated with insulin, the acidosis and dehydration lead to death from **diabetic ketoacidosis**.

With appropriate diagnosis and the availability of insulin as an effective treatment, persons with type 1 diabetes can lead full, productive lives. Indeed, some patients have been taking insulin successfully for treatment of type 1 diabetes for more than 75 years. As technology has improved, patients have been able to monitor their blood glucose themselves and adjust their insulin doses accordingly using specifically designed insulin analogues that have either short or very long half-lives. Thus, individuals with type 1 diabetes can avoid not only severe life-threatening episodes of ketoacidosis but also the chronic consequences of diabetes, namely, blood vessel injury that can lead to blindness, kidney failure, and accelerated atherosclerosis.

Type 2 Diabetes

In type 2 diabetes, the cause of hyperglycemia is more complex. These individuals continue to make insulin. β Cells not only are present but also are frequently hyperplastic (at least early in the course of the disease). For reasons still being defined, the β cells do not respond normally to increases in plasma glucose by increasing insulin secretion. However, altered insulin secretion is only part of the problem. If we administered identical doses of insulin to the liver, muscle, and adipose tissue of a person with type 2 diabetes and a healthy control, we would find that the patient with type 2 diabetes was resistant to the action of insulin. Thus, both the metabolism of glucose in response to insulin and the secretion of insulin are abnormal in type 2 diabetes. Which problem—decreased insulin release or insulin resistance—is more important in provoking development of the diabetic state likely varies among individuals. Usually, these subjects make enough insulin—and it is sufficiently active—that the severe ketoacidosis described earlier in patients with type 1 diabetes does not develop.

The insulin resistance seen in individuals with type 2 diabetes appears to bring with it an increase in the prevalence of hypertension, obesity, and a specific dyslipidemia characterized by elevated triglycerides and a low high-density cholesterol (see Fig. 46-15). Insulin resistance (along with one or more of these other metabolic abnormalities) is frequently found in individuals before the development of type 2 diabetes and is referred to as the **metabolic syndrome**. This constellation of abnormalities is estimated to affect more than 45 million individuals in the United States alone. Because each component of this syndrome has adverse effects on blood vessels, these individuals are at particularly increased risk for early atherosclerosis.

Studies have now shown that tight control of glucose concentrations in both type 1 and type 2 diabetes, together with careful management of blood pressure and plasma lipids, can retard the development of many of the chronic complications of diabetes.

---

that is needed to allow continued function during a fast. We discuss fasting in more depth beginning in Chapter 58.

In addition to its effects on hepatic glucose and lipid metabolism, glucagon also has the extrahepatic actions of accelerating **lipolysis** in adipose tissue and **proteolysis** in muscle. However, these effects are generally demonstrable only with high concentrations of glucagon, and although they may be important in certain pathologic situations associated with greatly elevated glucagon concentrations (e.g., ketoacidosis or sepsis), they appear less important in the day-to-day actions of glucagon.

SOMATOSTATIN

Somatostatin inhibits the secretion of growth hormone, insulin, and other hormones

Somatostatin is made in the δ cells of the pancreatic islets (Fig. 51-1), as well as in the D cells of the gastrointestinal tract (see Chapter 42), in the hypothalamus, and in several other sites in the CNS (see Chapter 48). Somatostatin was first described as a hypothalamic peptide that *suppressed* the release of growth hormone—which had also been called somatotropin, thus accounting for the name somatostatin.

In both pancreatic δ cells and the hypothalamus, somatostatin exists as both 14– and 28–amino acid peptides. In the hypothalamus, the 14–amino acid form is predominant, whereas in the gastrointestinal tract (including the δ cells), the 28–amino acid form predominates. The 14–amino acid form is the C-terminal portion of the 28–amino acid form. The biological activity of somatostatin resides in these 14 amino acids.

Somatostatin inhibits the secretion of multiple hormones, including growth hormone, insulin, glucagon, gastrin, vasoactive intestinal peptide (VIP), and thyroid-stimulating hormone. This property has led to therapeutic use of a long-acting somatostatin analogue (octreotide) in some difficult-to-treat endocrine tumors, including those that produce growth hormone (acromegaly), insulin (insulinoma), serotonin (carcinoid), among others. The concentrations of somatostatin found in pancreatic venous drainage are sufficiently high to inhibit basal insulin secretion. Recall that blood flows from the center of each islet—which is where the bulk of the β cells are—to the periphery of the islet—which is where the δ cells tend to be located (Fig. 51-1). This spatial arrangement minimizes the effect of somatostatin on the islet from which it is secreted. Whether somatostatin has important paracrine actions on some β cells or on α cells remains controversial.

The islet cells also make other peptides, for example, pancreatic polypeptide formed in the F cells of the pancreas. As with insulin and glucagon, the secretion of pancreatic polypeptide is altered by dietary intake of nutrients. However, whether pancreatic polypeptide has any actions in mammalian fuel metabolism is not clearly understood.

Occasionally, islet cell tumors may develop and secrete gastrin, VIP, growth hormone–releasing factor, or other hormones. Although these individual instances prove that these peptides can be made by islet tissue, they have no known normal function in the islet.

REFERENCES

Books and Reviews

Alberti KG, Zimmet P, DeFronzo RA: International Textbook of Diabetes Mellitus, 2nd ed. New York: Wiley, 1997.

Cryer PE, Polonsky KS: Glucose homeostasis and hypoglycemia. In Wilson JD, Foster DW, Kronenberg HM, Larsen PR (eds): Williams Textbook of Endocrinology, 9th ed, pp 939-971. Philadelphia: WB Saunders, 1998.

Jones PM, Persaud SJ: Protein kinases, protein phosphorylation, and the regulation of insulin secretion from pancreatic beta-cells. Endocr Rev 1998; 19:429-461.

Kimball SR, Vary TC, Jefferson LS: Regulation of protein synthesis by insulin. Annu Rev Physiol 1994; 56:321-348.

Poitout V, Robertson RP: An integrated view of beta-cell dysfunction in type-II diabetes. Annu Rev Med 1996; 47:69-83.

Journal Articles

Araki E, Lipes MA, Patti ME, et al: Alternative pathway of insulin signalling in mice with targeted disruption of the IRS-1 gene. Nature 1994; 372:186-190.

Bell GI, Pictet RL, Rutter WJ, et al: Sequence of the human insulin gene. Nature 1980; 284:26-32.

Cherrington AD: Banting lecture 1997: Control of glucose uptake and release by the liver in vivo. Diabetes 1999; 48:1198-1214.

Gribble FM, Tucker SJ, Haug T, Ashcroft FM: MgATP activates the beta cell K_{ATP} channel by interaction with its SUR1 subunit. Proc Natl Acad Sci U S A 1998; 95:7185-7190.

Miki T, Nagashima K, Tashiro F, et al: Defective insulin secretion and enhanced insulin action in K_{ATP} channel–deficient mice. Proc Natl Acad Sci U S A 1998; 95:10402-10406.

Pilch PF, Czech MP: Hormone binding alters the conformation of the insulin receptor. Science 1980; 210:1152-1153.

CHAPTER 52

THE PARATHYROID GLANDS AND VITAMIN D

Eugene J. Barrett and Paula Barrett

CALCIUM AND PHOSPHATE BALANCE

Calcium plays a critical role in many cellular processes, including hormone secretion, muscle contraction, nerve conduction, exocytosis, and the activation and inactivation of many enzymes. As described in Chapter 3 and elsewhere, Ca^{2+} also serves as an intracellular second messenger by carrying information from the cell membrane into the interior of the cell. It is therefore not surprising that the body very carefully regulates the plasma concentration of free ionized Ca^{2+} ($[Ca^{2+}]$), the physiologically active form of the ion, and maintains plasma $[Ca^{2+}]$ within a narrow range (between 1.0 and 1.3 mM, or between 4.0 and 5.2 mg/dL).

Phosphate is no less important. Because it is part of the ATP molecule, PO_4^{3-} plays a critical role in cellular energy metabolism. It also plays crucial roles in the activation and deactivation of enzymes. However, unlike Ca^{2+}, the plasma PO_4^{3-} concentration is not very strictly regulated, and its levels fluctuate throughout the day, particularly after meals.

Calcium homeostasis and PO_4^{3-} homeostasis are intimately tied to each other for two reasons. First, Ca^{2+} and PO_4^{3-} are the principal components of hydroxyapatite crystals $[Ca_{10}(PO_4)_6(OH)_2)]$, which by far constitute the major portion of the mineral phase of bone. Second, they are regulated by the same hormones, primarily parathyroid hormone (PTH) and 1,25-dihydroxyvitamin D (calcitriol) and, to a lesser extent, the hormone calcitonin. These hormones act on three organ systems—the bone, the kidneys, and the gastrointestinal (GI) tract—to control the levels of these two ions in plasma. However, the actions of these hormones on Ca^{2+} and PO_4^{3-} are typically opposed in that a particular hormone may elevate the level of one ion while lowering that of the other. Figures 52-1 and 52-2 depict the overall daily balance of Ca^{2+} and PO_4^{3-} for a subject in a steady state.

Calcium balance

Most Ca^{2+} is located within bone, ~1 kg (Fig. 52-1). The total amount of Ca^{2+} in the extracellular pool is only a fraction of this amount, ~1 g or 1000 mg. The typical daily dietary intake of Ca^{2+} is ~800 to 1200 mg. Dairy products are the major dietary source of Ca^{2+}. Although the intestines absorb approximately one half the dietary Ca^{2+} (~500 mg/day), they also secrete Ca^{2+} for removal from the body (~325 mg/day), and, therefore, the *net* intestinal uptake of Ca^{2+} is only ~175 mg/day. The second major organ governing Ca^{2+} homeostasis is bone, in which Ca^{2+} deposition of ~280 mg/day is matched by an equal amount of Ca^{2+} resorption in the steady state. The third organ system involved, the kidney, filters ~10 times the total extracellular pool of Ca^{2+} per day, ~10,000 mg/day. More than 98% of this Ca^{2+} is reabsorbed, and, therefore, the net renal excretion of Ca^{2+} is less than 2% of the filtered load (see Chapter 36). In a person in Ca^{2+} balance, urinary excretion (~175 mg/day) is the same as net absorption by the GI tract.

In plasma, Ca^{2+} exists in three physicochemical forms: (1) as a free ionized species, (2) bound to (more accurately, associated with) anionic sites on serum proteins (especially albumin), and (3) complexed with low-molecular-weight organic anions (e.g., citrate and oxalate). The **total concentration** of all three forms in the plasma is normally 2.2 to 2.6 mM (8.8 to 10.6 mg/dL). In healthy individuals, ~45% of Ca^{2+} is free, 45% is bound to protein, and 10% is bound to small anions (e.g. PO_4^{3-}, citrate, and sulfate). The ionized form is the most important with regard to regulating the secretion of PTH and is involved in most of the biological actions of Ca^{2+}.

Phosphate balance

Most PO_4^{3-} is also present in bone, ~0.6 kg of elemental phosphorus (Fig. 52-2). A smaller amount of phosphorus (0.1 kg) exists in the soft tissues, mainly as organic phosphates such as phospholipids, phosphoproteins, nucleic acids, and nucleotides. An even smaller amount (~500 mg) is present in the extracellular fluid as inorganic phosphate (P_i). The daily dietary intake of phosphorus is typically 1400 mg, mostly as P_i. Again, dairy products are the major source. The net absorption of PO_4^{3-} by the intestines is ~900 mg/day. In the steady state, bone has relatively small PO_4^{3-} turnover, ~210 mg/day. The kidneys filter ~14 times the total extracellular pool of PO_4^{3-} per day (~7000 mg/day) and reabsorb ~6100 mg/day. Hence, the net renal excretion of phosphorus

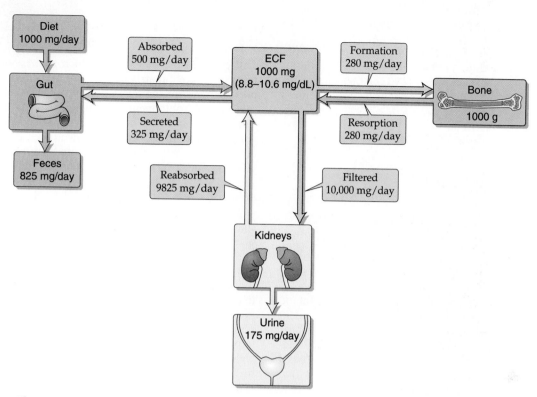

Figure 52-1 Calcium distribution and balance. All values are examples for a 70-kg human, expressed in terms of elemental calcium. These values can vary depending on factors such as diet. ECF, extracellular fluid.

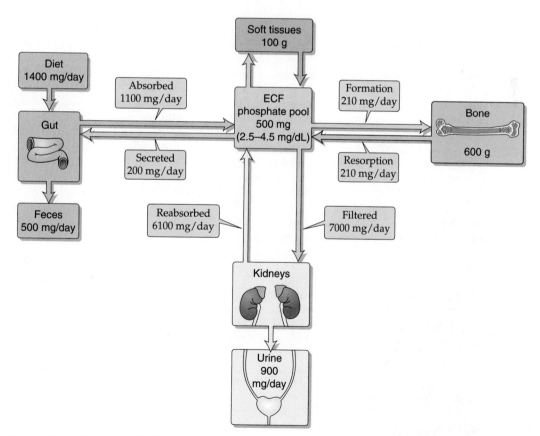

Figure 52-2 Phosphate distribution and balance. All values are examples for a 70-kg human, expressed in elemental phosphorus. These values can vary depending on factors such as diet. ECF, extracellular fluid.

is ~900 mg/day, the same as the net absorption by the GI tract.

The concentration of total PO_4^{3-} in plasma ranges from 0.8 to 1.5 mM (or 2.5 to 4.5 mg/dL of elemental phosphorus), a variation of 80%. Between 85% and 90% of the circulating PO_4^{3-} is filterable by the kidneys, either ionized (50%) or complexed to Na^+, Ca^{2+} or Mg^{2+} (40%), and only a small proportion (10% to 15%) is protein bound.

PHYSIOLOGY OF BONE

Dense cortical bone and the more reticulated trabecular bone are the two major bone types

Bone consists largely of an extracellular matrix composed of proteins and hydroxyapatite crystals, in addition to a small population of cells. The matrix provides strength and stability. The cellular elements continually remodel bone to accommodate growth and allow bone to reshape itself in response to varying loading stresses. Basically, bone has three types of bone cells. **Osteoblasts** promote bone formation. **Osteoclasts** promote bone resorption and are found on the growth surfaces of bone. **Osteocytes** are found within the bony matrix and are derived from osteoblasts that have encased themselves within bone. These cells sense mechanical stress on bone and secrete growth factors that stimulate both osteoblasts and lining cells. They also appear to play a role in the transfer of mineral from the interior of bone to the growth surfaces. Bone remodeling consists of a carefully coordinated interplay of osteoblastic, osteocytic, and osteoclastic activity.

As shown in Figure 52-3, bone consists of two types of bone tissue. **Cortical** (also called compact) bone represents ~80% of the total bone mass. Cortical bone is the outer layer (the cortex) of all bones and forms the bulk of the interior of the long bones of the body. It is a dense tissue composed mostly of bone mineral and extracellular matrix elements, interrupted only by penetrating blood vessels and a sparse population of osteocytes nested within the bone. These osteocytes are interconnected with one another and with the osteoblasts on the surface of the bone by canaliculi, through which the osteocytes extend cellular processes. These connections permit the transfer of Ca^{2+} from the interior of the bone to the surface, a process called *osteocytic osteolysis*. Dense cortical bone provides much of the strength for weight bearing by the long bones.

Trabecular (or **cancellous** or **medullary**) bone constitutes ~20% of the total bone mass. It is found in the interior of bones and is especially prominent within the vertebral bodies. It is composed of thin spicules of bone that extend from the cortex into the medullary cavity. The lacework of bone spicules is lined in many areas by osteoblasts and osteoclasts, the cells involved in bone remodeling. Trabecular bone is constantly being synthesized and resorbed by these cellular elements. Similar bone turnover occurs in cortical bone, but the fractional rate of turnover is much lower. When the rate of bone resorption exceeds that of synthesis over time, the loss of bone mineral produces the disease osteoporosis.

The extracellular matrix forms the nidus for the nucleation of hydroxyapatite crystals

Collagen and the other extracellular matrix proteins that form the protein matrix of bone are called *osteoid*. **Osteoid** provides sites for the nucleation of hydroxyapatite crystals, the mineral component of bone. Osteoid is not a single compound, but rather is a highly organized matrix of proteins synthesized principally by osteoblasts. Type I collagen accounts for ~90% of the protein mass of osteoid. It comprises a triple helix of two α1 monomers and one α2 collagen monomer. While they are still within the osteoblast, the monomers self-associate into the helical structure. After secretion from the osteoblast, the helices associate into collagen fibers; cross-linking of collagen occurs both within a fiber and between fibers. These collagen fibers are arranged in the osteoid in a highly ordered manner. The organization of collagen fibers is important for the tensile strength (i.e., the ability to resist stretch or bending) of bone. In addition to providing tensile strength, collagen also acts as a nidus for nucleation of bone mineralization. Within the collagen fibers, the crystals of hydroxyapatite are arranged with their long axis aligned with the long axis of the collagen fibers.

Several other osteoblast-derived proteins are important to the mineralization process, including osteocalcin and osteonectin. **Osteocalcin** is a 6-kDa protein synthesized by osteoblasts at sites of new bone formation. 1,25-Dihydroxyvitamin D induces the synthesis of osteocalcin. Osteocalcin has an unusual structure in that it possesses three γ-carboxylated glutamic acid residues. These residues are formed by post-translation modification of glutamic acid by vitamin K–dependent enzymes. Like other proteins with γ-carboxylated glutamic acid, osteocalcin binds Ca^{2+} avidly. It binds hydroxyapatite, the crystalline mineral of bone, with even greater avidity. This observation has led to the suggestion that osteocalcin participates in the nucleation of bone mineralization at the crystal surface. **Osteonectin**, a 35-kDa protein, is another osteoblast product that binds to hydroxyapatite. It also binds to collagen fibers and facilitates the mineralization of collagen fibers in vitro. Additional proteins have been identified that appear likely to participate in the mineralization process. Some evidence indicates that the glycoproteins present extracellularly in bone may act to inhibit mineralization; removal of these glycoproteins may be necessary for bone formation to occur.

Bone remodeling depends on the closely coupled activities of osteoblasts and osteoclasts

In addition to providing the proteins in osteoid, osteoblasts promote mineralization by exporting Ca^{2+} and PO_4^{3-} from intracellular vesicles that have accumulated these minerals. Exocytosis of Ca^{2+} and PO_4^{3-} raises the local extracellular concentration of these ions around the osteoblast to levels that are higher than in the bulk extracellular fluid, thus promoting crystal **nucleation** and growth (Fig. 52-4). Bone formation along spicules of trabecular bone appears to occur exclusively at sites of previous resorption by osteoclasts. The processes of bone resorption and synthesis are thus spatially coupled.

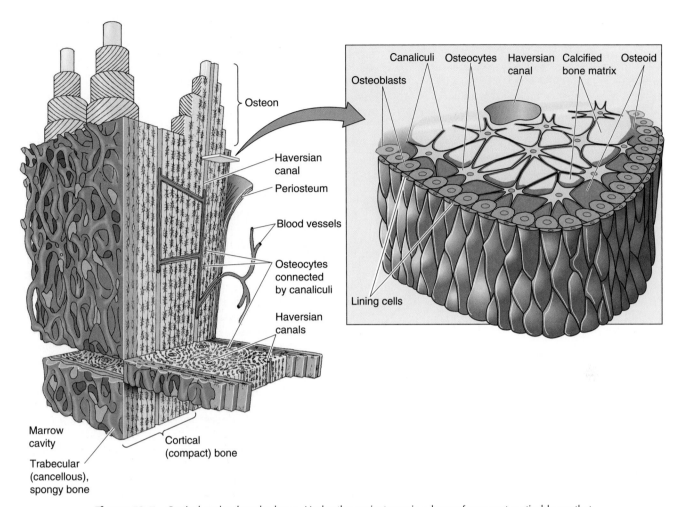

Figure 52-3 Cortical and trabecular bone. Under the periosteum is a layer of compact cortical bone that surrounds the more reticulated trabecular bone. The fundamental unit of cortical bone is the osteon, which is a tube-like structure that consists of a haversian canal, surrounded by ring-like lamellae. The *inset* shows a cross section through an osteon. The superficial lining cells surround the osteoblasts, which secrete osteoid, a matrix of proteins that are the organic part of bone. The lining cells are formed from osteoblasts that become quiescent. Osteocytes are osteoblasts that have become surrounded by matrix. Canaliculi allow the cellular processes of osteocytes to communicate, through gap junctions, with each other and with osteoblasts on the surface. Trabecular bone has both osteoblasts and osteoclasts on its surface; this is where most bone remodeling takes place.

Vitamin D and PTH stimulate osteoblastic cells to secrete factors—such as macrophage colony-stimulating factor (M-CSF)—that cause osteoclast precursors to proliferate (Fig. 52-4). These precursors differentiate into mononuclear osteoclasts and then fuse to become multinucleated osteo-clasts. **Osteoclasts** resorb bone in discrete areas in contact with the ruffled border of the cell (Fig. 52-5). The osteoclast closely attaches to the bone matrix when integrins on its membrane attach to vitronectin in the bone matrix. The osteoclast—in reality a one-cell epithelium—then secretes acid and proteases across its ruffled border membrane into a confined resorption space (the lacuna). The acid secretion is mediated by a V-type H^+ pump (see Chapter 2) at the ruffled border membrane. Abundant carbonic anhydrase provides the H^+. Cl-HCO_3 exchangers, located in the membrane on the opposite side of the osteoclast, remove the HCO_3^- formed by carbonic anhydrase as a byproduct. The acidic environment beneath the osteoclast dissolves bone mineral, and acid proteases hydrolyze the matrix proteins. Having reabsorbed some of the bone in a very localized area, the osteoclast moves away from the pit or trough in the bone that it has created. Osteoblastic cells replace the osteoclast and now build new bone matrix and promote its mineralization.

A newly described protein called **osteoprotegerin ligand** or **RANK ligand** appears to be a major stimulator both of the differentiation of preosteoclasts to osteoclasts and of the activity of mature osteoclasts. RANK ligand is a member of the tumor necrosis factor (TNF) cytokine family and exists both as a membrane-bound form on the surface of stromal cells and osteoblasts and as a soluble protein secreted by these same cells. RANK ligand binds to and stimulates a membrane-bound receptor of the osteoclast called **RANK** (receptor for activation of nuclear factor-κB), a member of

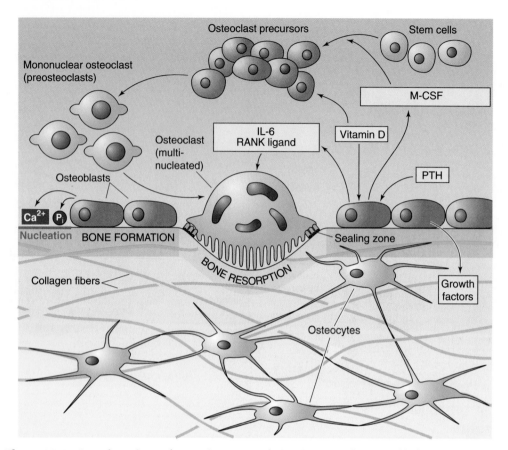

Figure 52-4 Bone formation and resorption. PTH and vitamin D stimulate osteoblastic cells to secrete factors such as M-CSF. This and other agents induce stem cells to differentiate into osteoclast precursors, mononuclear osteoclasts, and, finally, mature, multinucleated osteoclasts. Osteoblasts also secrete Ca²⁺ and P_i, which nucleate on the surface of bone. PTH indirectly stimulates bone resorption by osteoclasts. Osteoclasts do not have PTH receptors. Instead, the PTH binds to receptors on osteoblasts and stimulates the release of factors, such as IL-6 and RANK ligand, and the expression of membrane-bound RANK ligand. These factors promote bone resorption by osteoclasts.

the TNF receptor family. Osteoblastic and stromal cells also produce a soluble member of the TNF receptor family called **osteoprotegerin** (from the Latin *osteo* [bone] + *protegere* [protect]). By binding RANK ligand, osteoprotegerin protects the bone from osteoclastic activity. **Glucocorticoids** increase the production of RANK ligand by osteoblastic cells but decrease the production of osteoprotegerin. The net result is that more free RANK ligand is available to bind to RANK and thus to promote bone loss. The precise role of these proteins in the development of various forms of osteoporosis and osteopetrosis is only beginning to be understood. However, the balance between the amounts of osteoprotegerin and RANK ligand produced by the osteoblast/stromal cell appears to be a very important factor.

PARATHYROID HORMONE

Plasma Ca²⁺ regulates the synthesis and secretion of PTH

We have four parathyroid glands, two located on the posterior surface of the left lobe of the thyroid and two more on

the right. Combined, these four glands weigh less than 500 mg. They are composed largely of **chief cells**, which are responsible for the synthesis and secretion of PTH. These cells, like cells that secrete other peptide hormones, are highly specialized to synthesize, process, and secrete their product. The major regulator of PTH secretion is ionized plasma Ca²⁺, although vitamin D also plays a role. Both inhibit the synthesis or release of PTH. In contrast, an increase in plasma phosphorus concentration stimulates PTH release.

PTH Synthesis and Vitamin D The PTH gene possesses upstream regulatory elements in the 5′ region, including both vitamin D and vitamin A response elements (see Chapter 4). The vitamin D response element binds a vitamin D receptor (VDR) when the receptor is occupied by a vitamin D metabolite, usually 1,25-dihydroxyvitamin D. The VDR is a member of the family of nuclear receptors, like the steroid hormone and thyroid hormone receptors. Like the thyroid hormone receptor, VDR forms a heterodimer with the retinoic acid X receptor (RXR) and acts as a transcription factor (see Table 4-2). The receptor has a very high affinity for the 1,25-dihydroxylated form of vitamin D ($K_D \cong 10^{-10}$ M), less

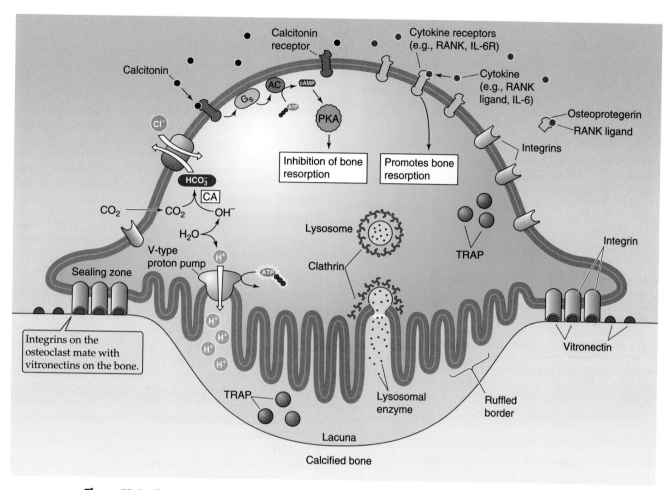

Figure 52-5 Bone resorption by the osteoclast. The osteoclast moves along the surface of bone and settles down, sealing itself to the bone through integrins that bind to vitronectins on the bone surface. The osteoclast reabsorbs bone by secreting H$^+$ and acid proteases into the lacuna. Thus, the osteoclast behaves as a one-cell epithelium. The acid secretion is mediated by a V-type H$^+$ pump at the ruffled border membrane facing the lacuna. Carbonic anhydrase (CA) in the cytosol supplies the H$^+$ to the H$^+$ pump and also produces HCO$_3^-$ as a byproduct. Cl-HCO$_3$ exchangers—located on the membrane opposite the ruffled border—remove this HCO$_3^-$. AC, adenylyl cyclase; PKA, protein kinase A; TRAP, tartrate-resistant acid phosphatase.

affinity for the 25-hydroxy form (K$_D$ ≅ 10^{-7} M), and little affinity for the parent vitamin (either D$_2$ or D$_3$; see later). Binding of the vitamin D–VDR complex to the VDR response element *decreases* the rate of PTH transcription.

Processing of PTH   After transport of the mature PTH mRNA to the cytosol, PTH is synthesized on ribosomes of the rough endoplasmic reticulum and begins its journey through the secretory pathway. PTH is transcribed as a prepro-PTH of 115 amino acids (Fig. 52-6). The 25–amino acid "pre" fragment targets PTH for transport into the lumen of the endoplasmic reticulum. This signal sequence appears to be cleaved as the PTH enters the rough endoplasmic reticulum (see Chapter 2). During transit through the secretory pathway, the 90–amino acid pro-PTH is further processed to the mature, active 84–amino acid PTH. This cleavage appears quite efficient, and no pro-PTH appears in the storage granules. Conversely, the breakdown of 1-84 PTH or "intact" PTH into its N- and C-terminal frag-

ments—as discussed later—already starts in the secretory granules.

Metabolism of PTH   Once secreted, PTH circulates free in blood plasma and is rapidly metabolized; the half-life of 1-84 PTH is ~4 minutes. Beginning in the secretory granules inside the parathyroid chief cells and continuing in the circulation—predominantly in the liver—PTH is cleaved into two principal fragments, a 33– or 36–amino acid N-terminal peptide and a larger C-terminal peptide (Fig. 52-6). Virtually all the known biological activity of PTH resides in the N-terminal fragment, which is rapidly hydrolyzed, especially in the kidney. However, the half-life of the C-terminal fragment is much longer than that of either the N-terminal peptide or the intact 84–amino acid PTH molecule. An estimated 70% to 80% of the PTH-derived peptide in the circulation is represented by the biologically inactive C-terminal fragment. The presence of a significant amount of antigenically recognized, but biologically inactive C-terminal frag-

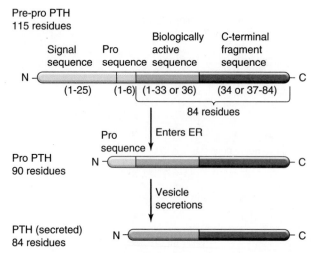

Figure 52-6 PTH synthesis. The synthesis of PTH begins with the production of pre-pro-PTH (115 amino acids) in the rough endoplasmic reticulum (ER). Cleavage of the signal sequence in the ER lumen yields pro-PTH (90 amino acids). During transit through the vesicular pathway, enzymes in the Golgi cleave the "pro" sequence, thus yielding the mature or "intact" PTH (84 amino acids), which is stored in secretory granules. Beginning in the secretory granule, enzymes cleave PTH into two fragments. The N-terminal fragment is either 33 or 36 amino acids in length and contains all the biological activity.

ments in the circulation has complicated the use of the usual radioimmunoassay methods for measuring PTH in both clinical and experimental settings. This problem has been solved by the development of sensitive enzyme-linked immunosorbent assays that use two antibodies that react with two distinct sites on the PTH molecule. This method measures only the **intact PTH hormone** (i.e., 84 amino acids). These assays are invaluable in the diagnosis of disorders of PTH secretion, particularly when kidney function is impaired (a circumstance that further prolongs the half-life of the inactive C-terminal metabolites).

High plasma [Ca^{2+}] inhibits the synthesis and release of PTH

To a first approximation, and ignoring the contributions of vitamin D that are discussed later, regulation of PTH secretion by plasma Ca^{2+} appears to be a simple negative feedback loop. The major stimulus for PTH secretion is a *decline* in the concentration of Ca^{2+} in the blood (hypocalcemia) and extracellular fluid. Hypocalcemia also stimulates synthesis of new PTH, which is necessary because the parathyroid gland contains only enough PTH to maintain a stimulated secretory response for several hours.

The mechanism by which the parathyroid gland senses extracellular [Ca^{2+}] and signals both the synthesis and secretion of PTH has only recently been clarified. Studies with cultured parathyroid chief cells showed that these cells respond to very small decreases in the concentration of ionized Ca^{2+} in the bathing medium, similar to the way the parathyroid gland acts in vivo. Using an expression cloning approach, investigators identified a Ca^{2+}-sensing receptor

(CaSR) that resides in the plasma membrane of the parathyroid cell (Fig. 52-7). This receptor binds Ca^{2+} in a saturable manner, with an affinity profile that is similar to the concentration dependence for PTH secretion. CaSR is a member of the G protein–coupled receptor family. Coupling of this Ca^{2+} receptor to Gα_q activates phospholipase C, thus generating inositol 1,4,5-triphosphate (IP$_3$) and diacylglycerol (DAG) and resulting in the release of Ca^{2+} from internal stores and the activation of protein kinase C (PKC) (see Chapter 3). Unlike most endocrine tissues, in which activation of these signaling systems promotes a secretory response, in the parathyroid, the rise in [Ca^{2+}]$_i$ and activation of PKC *inhibit* hormone secretion. (Another example is the granular cell of the juxtaglomerular apparatus, in which an increase in [Ca^{2+}]$_i$ inhibits secretion of renin; see Chapter 40.) Thus, increasing levels of plasma [Ca^{2+}] decrease PTH secretion (Fig. 52-7B).

The PTH receptor couples through G proteins to either adenylyl cyclase or phospholipase C

The action of PTH to regulate plasma [Ca^{2+}] appears to be secondary to its binding to the PTH 1R receptor. A second PTH receptor, PTH 2R, has been identified. However, its role, if any, in the regulation of plasma [Ca^{2+}] is uncertain. Kidney and bone have the greatest abundance of PTH 1R receptors. Within the kidney, PTH 1R receptors are most abundant in the proximal and distal convoluted tubules. In bone, the osteoblast appears to be the important target cell. The PTH 1R receptor is a G protein–linked receptor (see Chapter 3). The PTH 1R receptor binds some N-terminal fragments of PTH (Fig. 52-6), as well as the 1-84 intact PTH molecule. The PTH 1R receptor also binds PTH-related peptide (PTHrP), which is discussed later. In contrast, the PTH 2R receptor is selectively activated by PTH.

The PTH 1R receptor appears to be coupled to two heterotrimeric G proteins and thus to two signal transduction systems. Binding of PTH to the receptor stimulates Gα_s, which, in turn, activates **adenylyl cyclase** and thus releases cAMP and stimulates protein kinase A. The activated PTH receptor also stimulates Gα_q, which, in turn, stimulates **phospholipase C** to generate IP$_3$ and DAG (see Chapter 3). The IP$_3$ releases Ca^{2+} from internal stores, thus increasing [Ca^{2+}]$_i$ and activating Ca^{2+}-dependent kinases. In humans, the bone PTH receptor on osteoblastic cells is identical to that present in renal cortical cells. As discussed in the next two sections, the net effects of PTH on the kidney and bone are to increase plasma [Ca^{2+}] and to lower plasma [PO$_4^{3-}$].

In the kidney, PTH promotes Ca^{2+} reabsorption, PO$_4^{3-}$ loss, and 1-hydroxylation of 25-hydroxyvitamin D

PTH exerts a spectrum of actions on target cells in the kidney (Fig. 52-8). In the renal proximal tubule, PTH receptors are located on the basolateral membrane of the polarized epithelial cell. Binding of PTH to its receptors activates dual intracellular signaling systems and in this manner modifies several properties of the cell related to transepithelial transport.

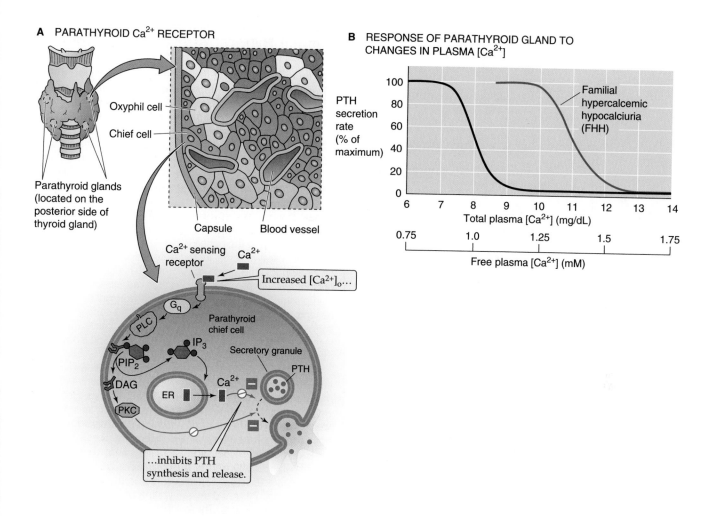

Figure 52-7 PTH secretion and its dependence on ionized Ca^{2+} in the plasma. **A,** Four parathyroid glands lie on the posterior side of the thyroid. The chief cells synthesize, store, and secrete PTH. Increases in extracellular $[Ca^{2+}]$ inhibit PTH secretion in the following manner: Ca^{2+} binds to a receptor that is coupled to a heterotrimeric G protein, $G\alpha_q$, which activates phospholipase C (PLC). This enzyme converts phosphoinositides (PIP_2) to IP_3 and DAG. The IP_3 causes the release of Ca^{2+} from internal stores, whereas the DAG stimulates PKC. Paradoxically, both the elevated $[Ca^{2+}]_i$ and the stimulated PKC inhibit release of granules containing PTH. Increased $[Ca^{2+}]_o$ also inhibits PTH synthesis. Thus, increased levels of plasma Ca^{2+} lower PTH release and thus tend to lower plasma $[Ca^{2+}]$. **B,** Small decreases in *free* plasma $[Ca^{2+}]$ greatly increase the rate of PTH release. About half of the total plasma Ca^{2+} is free. In patients with familial hypocalciuric hypercalcemia (FHH), the curve is shifted to the right; that is, plasma $[Ca^{2+}]$ must rise to higher levels before inhibiting PTH secretion. As a result, the patients have normal PTH levels, but elevated plasma $[Ca^{2+}]$.

Stimulation of Ca^{2+} Reabsorption **A key action of PTH is to promote the reabsorption of Ca^{2+}** in the thick ascending limb and distal convoluted tubule of the kidney (see Chapter 36). Most of the ~250 mmol of Ca^{2+} filtered each day is reabsorbed in the proximal tubule (~65%) and thick ascending limb (~25%). The distal nephron is responsible for reabsorbing an additional 5% to 10% of the filtered load of Ca^{2+}, with ~0.5% of the filtered load left in the urine. Thus, when PTH stimulates distal Ca^{2+} reabsorption, it greatly decreases the amount of Ca^{2+} excreted in the urine (usually 4 to 5 mmol/day) and tends to raise plasma $[Ca^{2+}]$ (Fig. 52-8).

Greater fractional Ca^{2+} excretion occurs when either proximal or distal Ca^{2+} reabsorption is impaired, as occurs with osmotic diuresis and hypoparathyroidism, respectively. As discussed later, vitamin D has a synergistic action of promoting Ca^{2+} reabsorption in the distal convoluted tubule.

Inhibition of PO_4^{3-} Reabsorption Most strikingly, PTH reduces the reabsorption of PO_4^{3-} in both the proximal and distal tubule. Because most of the PO_4^{3-} reabsorption occurs in the proximal tubule and because the effect of PTH is greatest on the proximal tubule, PTH produces characteristic phosphaturia and tends to decrease plasma PO_4^{3-} levels (Fig. 52-8). This phosphaturia results from a PTH-induced redistribution of the Na/PO cotransporter (NaPi) away from the apical membrane of the renal proximal tubule and into

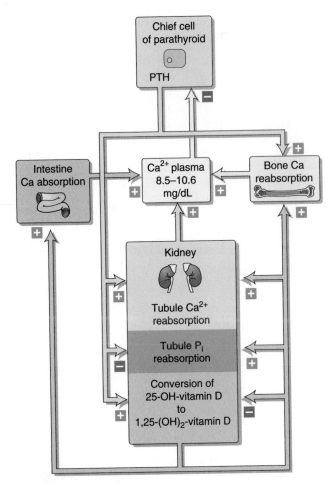

Figure 52-8 Feedback loops in the control of plasma Ca^{2+} levels. PTH released from the parathyroid glands acts through receptors in both bone and kidney. In **kidney**, PTH has three effects. First, PTH promotes Ca^{2+} reabsorption and thus an increase in plasma $[Ca^{2+}]$. Second, PTH inhibits PO_4^{3-} reabsorption. Third, PTH promotes the hydroxylation of 25-hydroxyvitamin D, thereby creating the active metabolite 1,25-dihydroxyvitamin D. This metabolite further promotes renal Ca^{2+} reabsorption. In **bone**, PTH promotes net bone reabsorption and hence increases plasma $[Ca^{2+}]$. In **intestine**, the 1,25-dihydroxyvitamin D (produced indirectly as the result of PTH) enhances Ca^{2+} absorption. Thus, net effect on bone, kidney, and gut, as far as Ca^{2+} is concerned, is to increase plasma $[Ca^{2+}]$. The increased plasma $[Ca^{2+}]$ feeds back on the parathyroid glands and inhibits the release of PTH.

Familial Hypocalciuric Hypercalcemia

The Ca^{2+} receptor on the parathyroid cell is mutated in patients with the disorder **familial hypocalciuric hypercalcemia (FHH)**. Serum Ca^{2+} in these patients is typically elevated 10% to 30% higher than the normal range. These patients generally tolerate this elevated plasma $[Ca^{2+}]$ very well, and the finding of a total plasma Ca^{2+} of 3.0 to 3.3 mM (12 to 13 mg/dL)—the normal range is 2.2 to 2.7 mM (8.8 to 10.6 mg/dL)—is frequently more alarming to the physician than to the patient. Despite a plasma $[Ca^{2+}]$ that would make most people symptomatic with kidney stones, fatigue, or loss of mental concentration, these patients have remarkably few symptoms. The amount of Ca^{2+} present in their urine is typically less than that seen in physiologically normal individuals (hence the designation *hypocalciuric*) and much lower than that encountered in persons with hypercalcemia of other causes. Despite the high plasma $[Ca^{2+}]$, the serum PTH concentrations in these patients are typically normal. The normal PTH concentration suggests that regulation of PTH secretion is intact, but the set-point at which the Ca^{2+} turns off PTH secretion is shifted toward higher plasma $[Ca^{2+}]$ (see Fig. 52-7B).

Only one allele for CaSR appears to be present. FHH is an autosomal dominant disorder, and several different point mutations have been identified in different families. *Heterozygotes* express both normal and mutated Ca^{2+} receptors. Rarely, infants are born with the *homozygous* disorder (i.e., both copies of the receptor are defective). These infants have very severe hypercalcemia ($[Ca^{2+}]$, >15 mg/dL) and severe hyperparathyroidism. The condition is life threatening and is characterized by markedly elevated plasma $[Ca^{2+}]$, neuronal malfunction, demineralization of bone, and calcification of soft tissues. These infants die unless the inappropriately regulated parathyroid glands are removed.

As in the parathyroid gland, the distal convoluted tubule of the kidney has abundant plasma membrane Ca^{2+} receptors. Investigators have suggested that serum Ca^{2+} binds to this renal Ca^{2+} receptor and inhibits Ca^{2+} reabsorption (see Chapter 36). Thus, with a mutated receptor, renal Ca^{2+} reabsorption may not be inhibited until plasma $[Ca^{2+}]$ rises to abnormally high levels. The result would be the increased Ca^{2+} reabsorption and hypocalciuria characteristic of FHH.

The discovery of CaSR led to the development of a CaSR agonist that mimics Ca^{2+} (a *calcimetic*). This drug has now come into clinical use for treating patients with parathyroid cancer or hyperparathyroidism secondary to chronic renal disease. Calcimetics decrease the secretion of PTH and secondarily decrease plasma $[Ca^{2+}]$.

a pool of subapical vesicles (see Chapter 36). As discussed later, PTH stimulates bone to resorb Ca^{2+} and PO_4^{3-} from the hydroxyapatite crystals of bone mineral. Thus, PTH stimulates both steps in the movement of PO_4^{3-} from bone to blood to urine.

Elimination of PO_4^{3-} through urine plays an important role when elevated levels of PTH liberate Ca^{2+} and PO_4^{3-} from bone. At normal plasma Ca^{2+} and phosphorus concentrations, the Ca/PO ion product approaches the solubility product. Further PTH-induced increases in $[Ca^{2+}]$—if accompanied by a rise in PO_4^{3-} levels—could cause Ca/PO salts to precipitate out of the soluble phase, thereby at least partly negating the action of PTH to raise plasma $[Ca^{2+}]$.

Thus, PTH-induced phosphaturia diminishes the Ca/PO ion product and prevents precipitation when Ca^{2+} mobilization is needed. The body tightly regulates plasma $[Ca^{2+}]$ but allows plasma levels of PO_4^{3-} to vary rather widely.

In addition to affecting PO_4^{3-} reabsorption, PTH causes a decrease in proximal tubule reabsorption of HCO_4^{3-} (see Chapter 39) and of several amino acids. These actions appear to play a relatively minor role in whole-body acid-base and nitrogen metabolism, respectively.

Stimulation of the Last Step of Synthesis of 1,25-Dihydroxyvitamin D   A third important renal action of PTH is to stimulate the 1-hydroxylation of 25-hydroxyvitamin D in the mitochondria of the proximal tubule. The resulting 1,25-dihydroxyvitamin D is the most biologically active metabolite of dietary or endogenously produced vitamin D. Its synthesis by the kidney is highly regulated, and PTH is the primary stimulus to increase 1-hydroxylation. Hypophosphatemia, either spontaneous or induced by the phosphaturic action of PTH, also promotes the production of 1,25-dihydroxyvitamin D. As discussed later, the 1,25-dihydroxyvitamin D formed in the proximal tubule has three major actions: (1) enhancement of renal Ca^{2+} reabsorption, (2) enhancement of Ca^{2+} absorption by the small intestine, and (3) modulation of the movement of Ca^{2+} and PO_4^{3-} in and out of bone.

In bone, PTH can promote net resorption or net deposition

The second major target tissue for PTH is bone, in which PTH promotes both bone resorption and bone synthesis.

Bone Resorption by Indirect Stimulation of Osteoclasts   The net effect of *persistent* increases of PTH on bone is to stimulate bone *resorption*, thus increasing plasma $[Ca^{2+}]$. Osteoblasts express abundant surface receptors for PTH; osteoclasts do not. Because osteoclasts lack PTH receptors, PTH by itself cannot regulate the coupling between osteoblasts and osteoclasts. Rather, it appears that PTH acts on osteoblasts and osteoclast precursors to induce the production of several cytokines that increase both the number and the activity of bone-resorbing osteoclasts. Precisely which cytokines are involved in the physiological signaling of osteoclasts by PTH-stimulated osteoblasts in vivo is not clear. PTH causes osteoblasts to release agents such as M-CSF and stimulates the expression of RANK ligand (i.e., osteoprotegerin ligand), actions that promote the development of osteoclasts (Fig. 52-4). In addition, PTH and vitamin D stimulate osteoblasts to release interleukin 6 (IL-6), which stimulates existing osteoclasts to resorb bone (Fig. 52-5).

One of the initial clues that cytokines are important mediators of osteoclastic bone resorption came from observations on patients with multiple myeloma—a malignancy of plasma cells, which are of B-lymphocyte lineage. The tumor cells produce several proteins that activate osteoclasts and enhance bone resorption. These proteins were initially called "osteoclast-activating factors." We now know that certain lymphocyte-derived proteins strongly activate osteoclastic bone resorption; these proteins include lymphotoxin, IL-1, and TNF-α.

Bone Resorption by Reduction in Bone Matrix   PTH also changes the behavior of osteoblasts in a manner that can promote net loss of bone matrix. For example, PTH inhibits collagen synthesis by osteoblasts and also promotes the production of proteases that digest bone matrix. Digestion of matrix is important because osteoclasts do not easily reabsorb bone mineral if the bone has an overlying layer of unmineralized osteoid.

Bone Deposition   Whereas persistent increases in PTH favor net resorption, *intermittent* increases in plasma [PTH] have predominantly bone synthetic effects. PTH can promote bone synthesis by two mechanisms. First, PTH promotes bone synthesis *directly* by activating Ca^{2+} channels in osteocytes, a process that leads to a net transfer of Ca^{2+} from bone fluid to the osteocyte. The osteocyte then transfers this Ca^{2+} through gap junctions to the osteoblasts at the bone surface. This process is called *osteocytic osteolysis*. The osteoblasts then pump this Ca^{2+} into the extracellular matrix, thus contributing to mineralization. Second, PTH stimulates bone synthesis *indirectly* in that osteoclastic bone resorption leads to the release of growth factors such as insulin-like growth factor 1 (IGF-1), IGF-2, and transforming growth factor β.

The PTH–1-34 peptide is now available as a pharmacological agent for the treatment of osteoporosis. Clinical data show marked increases in bone density—particularly within the axial skeleton—in response to injections of PTH–1-34 once or twice daily. The effects on trabecular bone are striking, with less positive responses seen in cortical bone—particularly in the limbs.

VITAMIN D

The active form of vitamin D is its 1,25-dihydroxy metabolite

By the 1920s, investigators recognized that dietary deficiency of a fat-soluble vitamin was responsible for the childhood disease **rickets**. This disorder is characterized clinically by hypocalcemia and multiple skeletal abnormalities. Dietary replacement of vitamin D corrects this disorder and has led to the practice of adding vitamin D to milk, bread, and other products. This practice has greatly reduced the prevalence of this previously common disorder.

Our understanding of the involvement of vitamin D in the regulation of plasma $[Ca^{2+}]$ and skeletal physiology has been clarified only over the past 2 decades. Vitamin D exists in the body in two forms, vitamin D_3 and vitamin D_2 (Fig. 52-9). **Vitamin D_3** can be synthesized from the 7-dehydrocholesterol that is present in the skin, provided sufficient ultraviolet light is absorbed. This observation explains why nutritional rickets had been a much more prevalent problem in northern countries, where clothing covers much of the skin and where individuals remain indoors much more of the year. Vitamin D_3 is also available from several natural sources, including cod and halibut liver, eggs, and fortified milk. **Vitamin D_2** is obtained only from the diet, largely from vegetables. Vitamins D_3 (Fig. 52-9A) and vitamin D_2 (Fig. 52-9B) differ only in the side chains of ring D. The side chain in vitamin D_3 (cholecalciferol) is characteristic of cholesterol, whereas that of vitamin D_2 (ergocalciferol) is characteristic of plant sterols.

Vitamin D (i.e., either D_2 or D_3) is fat soluble but water insoluble. Its absorption from the intestine depends on its solubilization by bile salts (see Chapter 45). In the circulation, vitamin D is found either solubilized with chylomicrons (see Chapter 46) or associated with a plasma binding

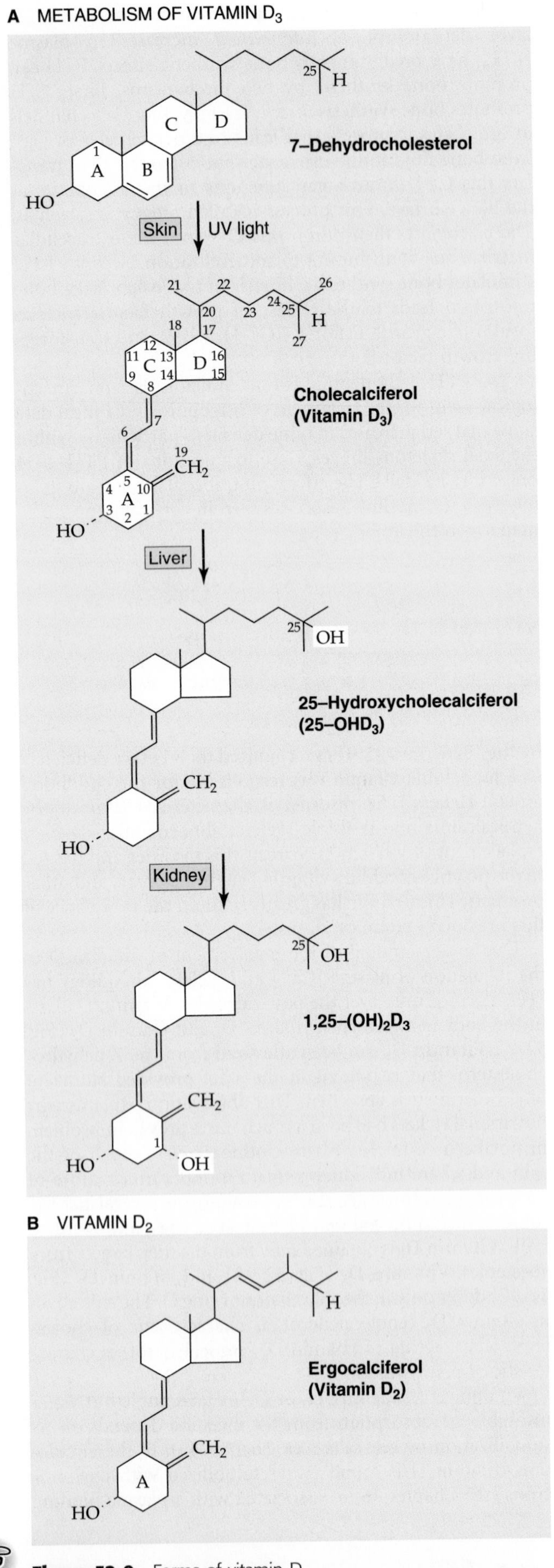

A   METABOLISM OF VITAMIN D₃

7–Dehydrocholesterol

Skin ↓ UV light

**Cholecalciferol
(Vitamin D₃)**

Liver ↓

**25–Hydroxycholecalciferol
(25–OHD₃)**

Kidney ↓

1,25–(OH)₂D₃

B   VITAMIN D₂

**Ergocalciferol
(Vitamin D₂)**

Figure 52-9   Forms of vitamin D.

protein. Most of the body stores of vitamin D are located in body fat. The body's pools of vitamin D are large, and only 1% to 2% of the body's vitamin D is turned over each day. Therefore, several years of very low dietary intake (as well as diminished endogenous synthesis) is required before the endogenous pools are depleted and deficiency develops.

The principal active form of vitamin D is not vitamin D_2 or D_3, but rather a dihydroxylated metabolite of either. Hydroxylation of vitamin D proceeds in two steps (Fig. 52-9A). When circulating levels of 25-hydroxyvitamin D are low, adipocytes release vitamin D into the blood plasma. A cytochrome P-450 mixed-function oxidase, principally in the liver, creates the first hydroxyl group at carbon 25. The 25-hydroxylation of vitamin D does not appear to be highly regulated, but rather it depends on the availability of vitamin D_2 or D_3. The second hydroxylation reaction occurs in the renal proximal tubule under the tight control of PTH, vitamin D itself, and PO_4^{3-}. PTH stimulates this 1-hydroxylation, whereas PO_4^{3-} and 1,25-dihydroxyvitamin D (the reaction product) both inhibit the process (Fig. 52-8).

In addition to vitamins D_2 and D_3 and their respective 25-hydroxy and 1,25-dihydroxy metabolites, more than 15 other metabolites of vitamin D have been identified in plasma. However, the specific physiological function of these metabolites, if any, is unclear.

Although considered a vitamin because of its dietary requirement, vitamin D can also be considered a hormone, both because it is endogenously synthesized and because even the fraction that arises from the diet must be metabolized to a biologically active form.

Vitamin D and its metabolites, like the steroid hormones, circulate bound to a globulin binding protein, in this case a 52-kDa vitamin D–binding protein. This binding protein appears particularly important for the carriage in the blood of vitamins D_2 and D_3, which are less soluble than their hydroxylated metabolites. Vitamin D and its metabolites arrive at target tissues and, once in the cytosol, associate with the VDR, a transcription factor that is in the family of nuclear receptors (see Chapter 3). Like the thyroid hormone receptor (see Table 4-2), VDR forms a heterodimer with RXR. The VDR specifically recognizes the 1,25-dihydroxyvitamin D with an affinity that is three orders of magnitude higher than that for 25-hydroxyvitamin D. However, because the circulating concentration of 25-hydroxyvitamin D is ~1000-fold higher than that of 1,25-dihydroxyvitamin D, both species probably contribute to the biological actions of the hormone.

The biological actions of 1,25-dihydroxyvitamin D appear to be expressed principally, but not exclusively, through regulation of the transcription of a variety of proteins. The VDR/RXR complex associates with a regulatory site in the promoter region of the genes coding for certain vitamin D–regulated proteins. Thus, the occupied VDR alters the synthesis of these vitamin D–dependent proteins. An example is PTH, which stimulates the formation of 1,25-dihydroxyvitamin D. The 5′ regulatory region of the PTH gene has a VDR consensus sequence; when occupied by the VDR complex, this element *diminishes* transcription of the PTH gene.

Vitamin D, by acting on the small intestine and kidney, raises plasma [Ca²⁺] and thus promotes bone mineralization

The actions of vitamin D can be grouped into two categories: actions on classic target tissues involved in regulating body mineral and skeletal homeostasis and a more general action that regulates cell growth. The actions of vitamin D on the small intestine, bone, and kidney serve to prevent any abnormal decline or rise in plasma [Ca²⁺].

Small Intestine In the duodenum, 1,25-dihydroxyvitamin D increases the production of several proteins that enhance Ca²⁺ absorption. Figure 52-10A summarizes the intestinal absorption of Ca²⁺ (see Chapter 45), which moves from the intestinal lumen to the blood by both paracellular and transcellular routes. In the paracellular route, which occurs throughout the small intestine, Ca²⁺ moves *passively* from the lumen to the blood; 1,25-dihydroxyvitamin D does *not* regulate this pathway. The transcellular route, which occurs only in the duodenum, involves three steps. First, Ca²⁺ enters the cell across the apical membrane through Ca²⁺ channels and possibly endocytosis. Second, the entering Ca²⁺ binds to several high-affinity binding proteins, particularly **calbindin**. These proteins, together with the exchangeable Ca²⁺ pools in the endoplasmic reticulum and mitochondria, effectively buffer the cytosolic Ca²⁺ and maintain a favorable gradient for Ca²⁺ entry across the apical membrane of the enterocyte. Thus, the intestinal cell solves the problem of absorbing relatively large amounts of Ca²⁺ while keeping its free, cytosolic [Ca²⁺] low. Third, the enterocyte extrudes Ca²⁺ across the basolateral membrane by means of both a Ca²⁺ pump and an Na-Ca exchanger.

Vitamin D promotes Ca²⁺ absorption primarily by genomic effects that involve induction of the synthesis of epithelial Ca²⁺ channels and pumps and Ca²⁺-binding proteins, as well as other proteins (e.g., alkaline phosphatase). Although these actions probably facilitate Ca²⁺ transport by the intestine, not all steps involved in the action of vitamin D to enhance transcellular Ca²⁺ transport have been well defined experimentally. The effect of PTH to stimulate intestinal Ca²⁺ absorption is thought to be entirely indirect and mediated by increasing the renal formation of 1,25-dihydroxyvitamin D (Fig. 52-8), which then enhances Ca²⁺ absorption.

Vitamin D also stimulates PO_4^{3-} absorption by the small intestine (Fig. 52-10B). The initial step is mediated by the NaPi cotransporter (see Chapter 36) and appears to be rate limiting for transepithelial transport and subsequent delivery of PO_4^{3-} to the circulation. 1,25-Dihydroxyvitamin D stimulates the synthesis of this transport protein and thus promotes PO_4^{3-} entry into the mucosal cell.

Kidney In the kidney, vitamin D appears to act synergistically with PTH to enhance *Ca²⁺ reabsorption* in the distal convoluted tubule (see Chapter 36). High-affinity Ca²⁺-binding proteins, similar to those found in the intestinal mucosa, have been specifically localized to this region of the kidney. It appears that PTH is a more potent regulator of Ca²⁺ reabsorption than vitamin D is (Fig. 52-8). Indeed, parathyroidectomy increases the fractional excretion of Ca²⁺,

Rickets and Osteomalacia

Deficiency of vitamin D in *children* produces the disease **rickets**, in which bone has abnormal amounts of unmineralized osteoid. Both cortical bone and trabecular bone are involved. The lack of mineralization diminishes bone rigidity and leads to a characteristic bowing of the long bones of the legs. In *adults*, vitamin D deficiency produces a disorder called **osteomalacia**. Microscopically, the bone looks very much the same in adult and childhood vitamin D deficiency. However, because the longitudinal growth of the long bones has been completed in adults, bowing of weight-bearing bones does not occur. Instead, the increased unmineralized osteoid content of bone causes a decline in bone strength. Affected individuals are more prone to the development of bone fractures. These fractures may be very small and difficult to see radiographically. As more and more of the bone surface is covered by osteoid and as recruitment of new osteoclasts is diminished, osteoclastic bone resorption is impaired, and hypocalcemia develops. Hypocalcemia causes nerves to become more sensitive to depolarization. In sensory nerves, this effect leads to sensations of numbness, tingling, or burning; in motor nerves, it leads to increased spontaneous contractions, or tetany.

Whereas rickets and osteomalacia are very uncommon in developed countries because of vitamin D supplementation, milder degrees of vitamin D deficiency are increasingly recognized, particularly in the elderly population, in whom milk consumption and sunlight exposure are frequently inadequate. The resulting fall in plasma [Ca²⁺] can lead to mild, secondary hyperparathyroidism. Such *continuous* elevations of PTH can lead to further bone resorption and worsening osteoporosis.

Rickets or osteomalacia also can occur with impaired ability of the kidney to 1-hydroxylate the 25-hydroxyvitamin D previously synthesized in the liver. An acquired version is seen in many patients with chronic renal failure, in which the activity of 1α-hydroxylase is reduced. The genetic form of the 1α-hydroxylase deficiency is a rare autosomal recessive disorder. Either form is called vitamin D–dependent rickets because it can be successfully treated with either 1,25-dihydroxyvitamin D or higher doses of dietary vitamin D₂ or vitamin D₃ (~10- to 100-fold) than the 400 U/day used to prevent nutritional rickets.

and even high doses of vitamin D cannot correct this effect. In addition, as in the intestine, vitamin D promotes PO_4^{3-} *reabsorption* in the kidney. The effects of vitamin D on PO_4^{3-} reabsorption, like its effects on Ca²⁺, are less dramatic than those of PTH. Finally, 1,25-dihydroxyvitamin D directly inhibits the *1-hydroxylation* of vitamin D.

Bone The actions of vitamin D on bone are complex and are the result of both indirect and direct actions. The overall effect of vitamin D replacement in animals with dietary-induced vitamin D deficiency is to increase the flux of Ca²⁺ into bone. However, as we see later, these major effects of vitamin D on bone are *indirect*: the action of vitamin D on both the small intestine and the kidneys makes more Ca²⁺

A INTESTINAL Ca²⁺ ABSORPTION

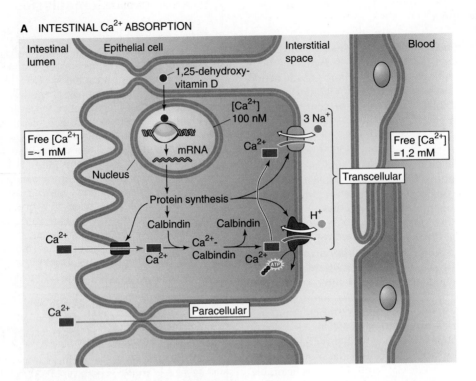

B INTESTINAL PHOSPHATE ABSORPTION

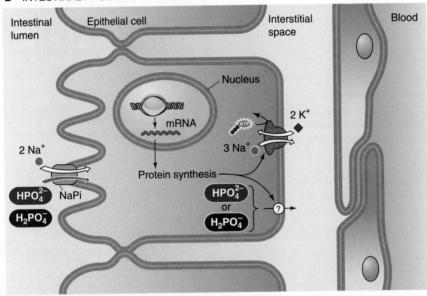

Figure 52-10 Intestinal absorption of Ca^{2+} and PO_4^{3-}. **A,** The small intestine absorbs Ca^{2+} by two mechanisms. The passive, paracellular absorption of Ca^{2+} occurs throughout the small intestine. This pathway predominates but is *not* under the control of vitamin D. The second mechanism—the active, transcellular absorption of Ca^{2+}—occurs only in the duodenum. Ca^{2+} enters the cell across the apical membrane through a channel. Inside the cell, the Ca^{2+} is buffered by binding proteins, such as calbindin, and is also taken up into intracellular organelles, such as the endoplasmic reticulum. The enterocyte then extrudes Ca^{2+} across the basolateral membrane through a Ca^{2+} pump and an Na-Ca exchanger. Thus, the net effect is Ca^{2+} absorption. The active form of vitamin D—25-dihydroxyvitamin D—stimulates all three steps of transcellular Ca^{2+} absorption. **B,** P_i enters the enterocyte across the apical membrane through an Na/P_i (NaPi) cotransporter. Once inside the cell, the P_i is extruded across the basolateral membrane. Thus, the net effect is P_i absorption.

available to mineralize previously unmineralized osteoid. The *direct* effect of vitamin D on bone is to *mobilize* Ca^{2+} out of bone. Both osteoblasts and osteoclast precursor cells have VDRs. In response to vitamin D, osteoblasts produce certain proteins, including alkaline phosphatase, collagenase, and plasminogen activator. In addition, as noted earlier (Fig. 52-4), vitamin D and PTH promote the development of osteoclasts from precursor cells. Thus, because vitamin D directly increases the number of mature osteoclasts, supplying vitamin D to bone obtained from vitamin D–deficient animals in in vitro experiments mobilizes Ca^{2+} from bone into the medium. Additional evidence that vitamin D directly promotes bone resorption comes from experiments on rachitic animals who are maintained on a Ca^{2+}-deficient diet. Treating these animals with vitamin D causes plasma $[Ca^{2+}]$ to rise, an indication of net bone resorption. At the same time, however, the elevated plasma $[Ca^{2+}]$ promotes the mineralization of previously unmineralized osteoid—at the expense of bone resorption from other sites.

The direct effects of vitamin D on bone, which are to mobilize Ca^{2+}, seem to be contrary to the overall effect of vitamin D on bone, which is to promote mineralization. These observations, as well as others, have led to the hypothesis, now generally accepted, that the antirachitic action of vitamin D is largely indirect. By enhancing the absorption of Ca^{2+} and PO_4^{3-} from the intestine and by enhancing the reabsorption of Ca^{2+} and PO_4^{3-} from the renal tubules, vitamin D raises the concentrations of both Ca^{2+} and PO_4^{3-} in the blood and extracellular fluid. This increase in the Ca/PO ion product results in net bone mineralization. These indi-

rect effects overshadow the direct effect of vitamin D to increase bone mobilization.

Ca^{2+} ingestion lowers levels of PTH and 1,25-dihydroxyvitamin D, whereas PO_4^{3-} ingestion raises levels of both PTH and 1,25-dihydroxyvitamin D

Consider a situation in which a subject ingests a meal containing Ca^{2+}. The rise in plasma $[Ca^{2+}]$ inhibits PTH secretion. The decline in PTH causes a decrease in the resorption of Ca^{2+} and phosphorus from bone, thus limiting the postprandial increase in plasma Ca^{2+} and PO_4^{3-} levels. In addition, the decrease in PTH diminishes Ca^{2+} reabsorption in the kidney and thus facilitates a calciuric response. If dietary Ca^{2+} intake remains high, the lower PTH will result in decreased 1-hydroxylation of 25-hydroxyvitamin D, which will eventually diminish the fractional absorption of Ca^{2+} from the GI tract.

If dietary Ca^{2+} intake is deficient, the body will attempt to restore Ca^{2+} toward normal by increasing plasma [PTH]. This response will help to mobilize Ca^{2+} from bone, to promote renal Ca^{2+} retention, and over time, to increase the level of 1,25-dihydroxyvitamin D, which will enhance gut absorption of Ca^{2+}.

If one ingests phosphorus much in excess of Ca^{2+} (e.g., after drinking several colas), the rise in plasma $[PO_4^{3-}]$ will lower plasma $[Ca^{2+}]$ because the increased plasma Ca/PO ion product will promote the deposition of mineral in bone. The resultant decrease in plasma $[Ca^{2+}]$ will, in turn, increase

Osteoporosis

Approximately 25 million Americans, mostly elderly women, are afflicted with **osteoporosis**, and between 1 and 2 million of these individuals experience a fracture related to osteoporosis every year. The cost in economic and human terms is immense. Hip fractures are responsible for much of the morbidity associated with osteoporosis, but even more concerning is the observation that as many as 20% of women with osteoporotic hip fractures die within 1 year of their fracture.

The major risk factor for osteoporosis is the declining estrogen levels in aging women. Rarely, other endocrine disorders such as hyperthyroidism, hyperparathyroidism, and Cushing disease (hypercortisolism) are responsible. Other risk factors include inadequate dietary Ca^{2+} intake, alcoholism, cigarette smoking, and a sedentary lifestyle.

Strategies to prevent the development of osteoporosis begin in the premenopausal years. High Ca^{2+} intake and a consistent program of weight-bearing exercises are widely recommended.

Pharmacological agents are now available for preventing or at least retarding the development of osteoporosis or for treating the disease once it has become established. These agents can be broadly classified into two groups: antiresorptive drugs and agents that are able to stimulate bone formation.

Among the former, estrogen is by far the most widely used therapy. It is most effective when started at the onset of meno-

pause, although it may offer benefits even in patients who are 20 or more years past menopause. Calcitonin is generally offered to women who cannot or are unwilling to take estrogen. However, it is expensive and must be given parenterally; an intranasal spray is also available. Another class of drugs, the bisphosphonates, is becoming popular. These drugs are powerful inhibitors of bone resorption, but some of the first agents of this class have also been found to impair mineralization. The newer bisphosphonates can be safely given in doses that decrease bone resorption without affecting mineralization.

Among the drugs that can stimulate bone formation, vitamin D—often given as 1,25-dihydroxyvitamin D (calcitriol)—is combined with Ca^{2+} therapy to increase the fractional absorption of Ca^{2+} and to stimulate the activity of osteoblasts. PTH, recently available as an injectable treatment for osteoporosis, potently stimulates osteoblast formation and increases bone mass. PTH also appears to decrease the rate of vertebral fractures.

Calcitriol and the bisphosphonates have also been used successfully to treat **Paget disease of bone**, a disorder characterized by localized regions of bone resorption and reactive sclerosis. The level of bone turnover can be extremely high. Although it remains asymptomatic in many individuals, the disease can cause pain, deformity, fractures, and vertigo and hearing loss if bony overgrowth occurs in the region of the eighth cranial nerve. The cause of Paget disease is not known.

PTH secretion. This rise in PTH will provoke phosphaturia that will act to restore plasma $[PO_4^{3-}]$ toward normal while Ca^{2+} and PO_4^{3-} are mobilized from bone by the action of PTH. Over longer periods, the action of PTH to modulate the 1-hydroxylation of 25-hydroxyvitamin D plays an increasingly important role in defending the plasma $[Ca^{2+}]$ by increasing intestinal Ca^{2+} absorption.

CALCITONIN AND OTHER HORMONES

Calcitonin inhibits osteoclasts, but its effects are transitory

Calcitonin is a 32–amino acid peptide hormone made by the clear or C cells of the thyroid gland. C cells (also called parafollicular cells) are derived from neural crest cells of the fifth branchial pouch, which in humans migrate into the evolving thyroid gland. Although it is located within the thyroid, calcitonin's major, if not sole, biological action relates to the regulation of mineral metabolism and bone turnover. The incidental nature of its relationship with the major functions of the thyroid is emphasized by the finding that in many nonhuman species, C cells are found in a body called the ultimobranchial gland and not in the thyroid at all.

Calcitonin is synthesized in the secretory pathway (see Chapter 2) by post-translational processing of a large procalcitonin. As illustrated in Figure 52-11, alternative splicing of the calcitonin gene product gives rise to several biologically active peptides. In the C cells, calcitonin is the only peptide made in biologically significant amounts. Within the central nervous system, calcitonin gene–related peptide (CGRP) is the principal gene product, and it appears to act as a neurotransmitter in peptidergic neurons (see Table 13-1). Calcitonin is stored in secretory vesicles within the C cells, and its release is triggered by raising the extracellular $[Ca^{2+}]$ to levels higher than normal. Conversely, lowering the extracellular $[Ca^{2+}]$ diminishes calcitonin secretion. The threshold $[Ca^{2+}]$ for enhancing calcitonin secretion is in the midphysiological range. In principle, this secretory profile would leave calcitonin well poised to regulate body Ca^{2+} homeostasis.

The precise role for calcitonin in body Ca^{2+} homeostasis has been difficult to define. This difficulty was first apparent from the simple clinical observation that after complete thyroidectomy with removal of all calcitonin-secreting tissue, plasma $[Ca^{2+}]$ remains normal (provided the parathyroid glands are not injured). Conversely, patients with a rare calcitonin-secreting tumor of the C cells frequently have plasma calcitonin concentrations that are 50 to 100 times normal, yet they maintain normal plasma levels of Ca^{2+}, vitamin D, and PTH. Nevertheless, several lines of evidence suggest that calcitonin does have biologically important actions. First, although calcitonin appears to have a minimal role in the minute-to-minute regulation of plasma $[Ca^{2+}]$ in humans, it does serve an important role in many nonmammalian species. This role is particularly clear for teleost fish. Faced with the relatively high $[Ca^{2+}]$ in sea water (and therefore in food), calcitonin, secreted in response to a rise in plasma $[Ca^{2+}]$, decreases bone resorp-

tion, thus returning the plasma $[Ca^{2+}]$ toward normal. Salmon calcitonin, which differs from human calcitonin in 14 of its 32 amino acid residues, is roughly 10-fold more potent on a molar basis in inhibiting osteoclast function than is the human hormone.

The second line of evidence that calcitonin may have biologically important actions is the presence of calcitonin receptors. Like PTH receptors, the **calcitonin receptor** is a G protein–coupled receptor that, depending on the target cell, may activate either adenylyl cyclase or phospholipase C (see Chapter 3). Within bone, the osteoclast—which lacks PTH receptors—appears to be the principal target of calcitonin. Indeed, the presence of calcitonin receptors may be one of the most reliable methods of identifying osteoclasts. In the osteoclast, calcitonin appears to work by raising $[cAMP]_i$ and then presumably acting through one or more protein kinases. Calcitonin inhibits the resorptive activity of the osteoclast and slows the rate of bone turnover. It also appears to diminish osteocytic osteolysis, and this action—together with calcitonin's effect on the osteoclast—is responsible for the hypocalcemic effect after the short-term administration of pharmacological doses of calcitonin. The hypocalcemic action of calcitonin is particularly effective in circumstances in which bone turnover is accelerated, as occurs in rapidly growing young animals and in human patients with hyperparathyroidism. The antiosteoclastic activity of calcitonin is also useful in treating Paget disease of bone (see the box titled Osteoporosis). However, within hours of exposure of osteoclasts to high concentrations of calcitonin, the antiresorptive action of calcitonin begins to wane. This "escape" from the hypocalcemic effect of calcitonin has limited the use of calcitonin in the clinical treatment of hypercalcemia. The transitory nature of the action of calcitonin appears partly to result from rapid downregulation of calcitonin receptors.

In the kidney, calcitonin, like PTH, causes mild phosphaturia by inhibiting proximal tubule PO_4^{3-} transport. Calcitonin also causes mild natriuresis and calciuresis. These actions may contribute to the acute hypocalcemic and hypophosphatemic actions of calcitonin. However, these renal effects are of short duration and do not appear to be important in the overall renal handling of Ca^{2+}, PO_4^{3-}, or Na^+.

Sex steroid hormones promote bone deposition, whereas glucocorticoids promote resorption

Although PTH and 1,25-dihydroxyvitamin D are the principal hormones involved in modulating bone turnover, other hormones participate in this process. For example, the sex steroids **testosterone** and **estradiol** are needed for maintaining normal bone mass in male and female subjects, respectively. The decline in estradiol that occurs postmenopausally exposes women to the risk of **osteoporosis**, that is, a decreased mass of both cortical and trabecular bone caused by a decrease in bone matrix (see the box titled Osteoporosis). Osteoporosis is less common in men because their skeletal mass tends to be greater throughout adult life and because testosterone levels in men decline slowly as they age, unlike the abrupt menopausal decline of estradiol in women.

Glucocorticoids also modulate bone mass. This action is most evident in circumstances of glucocorticoid excess,

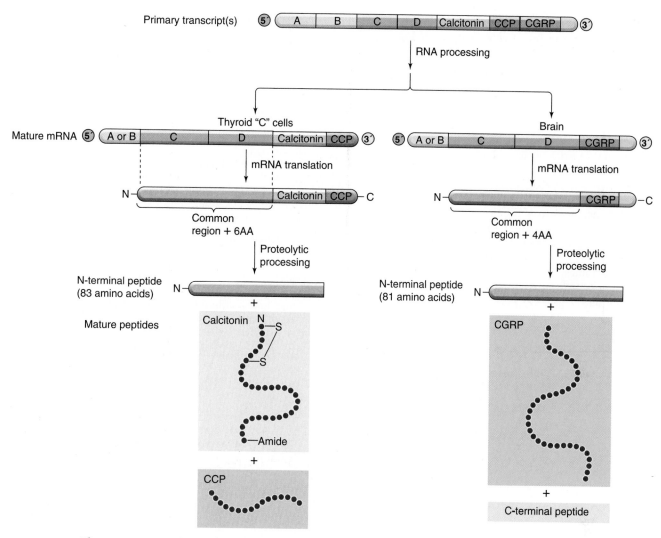

Figure 52-11   Synthesis of calcitonin and CGRP. A common primary RNA transcript gives rise to both calcitonin and CGRP. In the thyroid gland, C cells produce a mature mRNA that they translate to procalcitonin. They then process this precursor to produce an N-terminal peptide, calcitonin (a 32–amino acid peptide), and CCP. In the brain, neurons produce a different mature mRNA and a different "pro" hormone. They process the peptide to produce an N-terminal peptide, CGRP, and a C-terminal peptide.

which leads to osteoporosis, as suggested by the effects of glucocorticoids on the production of osteoprotegerin and osteoprotegerin ligand.

The precise cellular mechanisms that mediate the action of androgens, estrogens, or glucocorticoids on bone have not been well defined. Despite the loss of bone that occurs with androgen or estrogen deficiency or glucocorticoid excess, in each case, the coupling of bone synthesis to degradation is *qualitatively* preserved. Synthesis of new bone continues to occur at sites of previous bone resorption, and no excess of unmineralized osteoid is present. Presumably, the decline in bone mass reflects a *quantitative* shift whereby the amount of new bone formed at any site is less than what was resorbed. Because this shift occurs at multiple sites, the result is a decline in overall bone mass.

PTH-related peptide, encoded by a gene that is entirely distinct from that for PTH, can cause hypercalcemia in certain malignancies

Unlike PTH, which is synthesized exclusively by the parathyroid gland, a peptide called PTHrP appears to be made in many different normal and malignant tissues. The PTH 1R receptor in kidney and bone recognizes PTHrP with an affinity similar to that for intact PTH. PTHrP mimics each of the actions of PTH on kidney and bone. Thus, when present in sufficient concentrations, PTHrP causes hypercalcemia. PTHrP exists in three alternatively spliced isoforms of a single gene product. The gene encoding PTHrP is completely distinct from that for PTH. The similar actions of PTHrP and PTH arise from homology within the first 13 amino acids of PTHrP with native PTH. Only weak homology is seen between amino acids 14 and 34 (three amino acids are identical) and essentially no homology beyond amino acid 34. This situation is an unusual example of mimicry among peptides that are structurally quite diverse.

The normal physiological function of PTHrP is still largely undefined. The lactating breast secretes PTHrP, and this hormone is present in very high concentrations in milk. PTHrP may promote the mobilization of Ca^{2+} from maternal bone during milk production. In nonlactating humans, the plasma PTHrP concentration is very low, and PTHrP does not appear to be involved in the day-to-day regulation of plasma $[Ca^{2+}]$. It appears likely that under most circumstances, PTHrP acts in a paracrine or autocrine, rather than an endocrine, regulatory fashion.

Many tumors are capable of manufacturing and secreting PTHrP, among them the following: squamous cell tumors of the lung, head, and neck; renal and bladder carcinomas; adenocarcinomas; and lymphomas. Patients with any of these tumors are subject to severe hypercalcemia of fairly abrupt onset.

REFERENCES

Books and Reviews

Bringhurst FR, Demay MB, Kronenberg HM: Hormones and disorders of mineral metabolism. In Wilson JD, Foster DW, Kronenberg HM, Larsen PR (eds): Williams Textbook of Endocrinology, 9th ed, pp 1155-1209. Philadelphia: WB Saunders, 1998.

DeLuca HF: The transformation of a vitamin into a hormone: The vitamin D story. Harvey Lect 1979-1980; 75:333-379.

Habener JF, Rosenblatt M, Potts JT Jr: Parathyroid hormone: Biochemical aspects of biosynthesis, secretion, action, and metabolism. Physiol Rev 1984; 64:985-1053.

Jones G, Strugnell SA, DeLuca HD: Current understanding of the molecular actions of vitamin D. Physiol Rev 1998; 78:1193-1231.

Murer H, Forster I, Hilfiker H, et al: Cellular/molecular control of renal Na/Pi-cotransport. Kidney Int Suppl 1998; 65:2-10.

Stein GS, Lian JB, Stein JL, et al: Transcriptional control of osteoblast growth and differentiation. Physiol Rev 1996; 76:593-629.

Journal Articles

Broadus AE, Mangin M, Ikeda K, et al: Humoral hypercalcemia of cancer: Identification of a novel parathyroid hormone–like peptide. N Engl J Med 1988; 319:556-563.

Brown EM, Gamba G, Riccardi D, et al: Cloning and characterization of an extracellular Ca^{2+}-sensing receptor from bovine parathyroid. Nature 1993; 366:575-580.

Burgess TL, Qian Y, Kaufman S, et al: The ligand for osteoprotegerin (OPGL) directly activates mature osteoclasts. J Cell Biol 1999; 145:527-538.

THE REPRODUCTIVE SYSTEM

CHAPTER 53

SEXUAL DIFFERENTIATION

Ervin E. Jones

One of nature's primary goals is perpetuation of the species. All living organisms must reproduce in some manner. Nature also favors those species that are able to produce diversification among members, an attribute critical to species survival as the nature of environmental (and other) stresses changes through time. One solution to this problem is sexual differentiation, that is, the evolution of two sexually dissimilar individuals belonging to the same species, one male and one female, and each equipped with its own specific attributes necessary for its particular contribution to the process of procreation. Each sex produces its own type of sex cell (**gamete**), and the union of male and female gametes generates species-specific progeny. In addition, mechanisms, some simple, some complex, have evolved to ensure the proximity and union of the sex cells (*syngamy*). Thus, within each species, the relevant sexual characteristics of each partner have adapted differently to achieve the most efficient union of these progenitor cells. These differences between the sexes of one species are called **sexual dimorphism**. For example, oviparous species such as frogs release their eggs into a liquid medium only when they are in relative proximity to sperm. As effective as this approach is, it also typifies the wastefulness of reproduction among higher species inasmuch as most gametes go unfertilized.

Even among species that normally reproduce sexually, sexual dimorphism is not universal. For example, monoecious (i.e., hermaphroditic) species, such as cestodes and nematodes, have the capacity to produce both sperm and eggs. By definition, the ability to produce just one kind of gamete depends on sexually dimorphic differentiation.

Throughout evolution, conservation and expression of genes involved in the perpetuation of a species have clearly followed a process of *adaptation*, which is an advantageous change in structure or function of an organ or tissue to meet the challenges of new conditions. Higher mammals normally have a single pair of **sex chromosomes** that are morphologically distinguishable from other chromosomes, the **autosomes**. Each of the sex chromosomes carries genetic information that determines the primary and secondary sexual characteristics of an individual, that is, whether the individual functions and appears as male or female. It has also become abundantly clear that genes determine gender,

sexual expression, and as a result, mechanisms and patterns of reproduction.

The functional and spatial organization of all organ systems during development is genetically determined. Thus, the sex of the gonad is genetically programmed: Will a female gonad (ovary) or a male gonad (testis) develop? Although germ cells of the early embryonic gonad are totipotent, these cells develop into female gametes (ova) if the gonad becomes an ovary, but they develop into male gametes (sperm) if the gonad becomes a testis. These two anatomically and functionally distinct gonads determine either "maleness" or "femaleness" and dictate the development of both primary and secondary sexual characteristics. Endocrine and paracrine modulators that are specific for either the ovary or the testis are primarily responsible for female or male sexual differentiation and behavior and therefore the individual's role in procreation.

GENETIC ASPECTS OF SEXUAL DIFFERENTIATION

Meiosis, which occurs only in germ cells, gives rise to male and female gametes

Mitosis is the only kind of cell division that occurs in somatic cells. Mitosis results in the formation of two identical daughter cells (Fig. 53-1A), each having the same number of chromosomes (i.e., 46 in humans) and same DNA content as the original cell. Mitosis is a continuum consisting of five phases: prophase, prometaphase, metaphase, anaphase, and telophase. One reason for the genetic identity of the two daughter cells is that no exchange of genetic material occurs between homologous chromosomes, so sister **chromatids** (i.e., the two copies of the same DNA on a chromosome) are identical. A second reason for the genetic identity is that the sister chromatids of each chromosome split, one going to each daughter cell during anaphase of the single mitotic division.

Meiosis occurs only in germ cells. After having undergone several mitotic divisions, the germ cells (spermatogonia in males and oogonia in females)—still with a complement

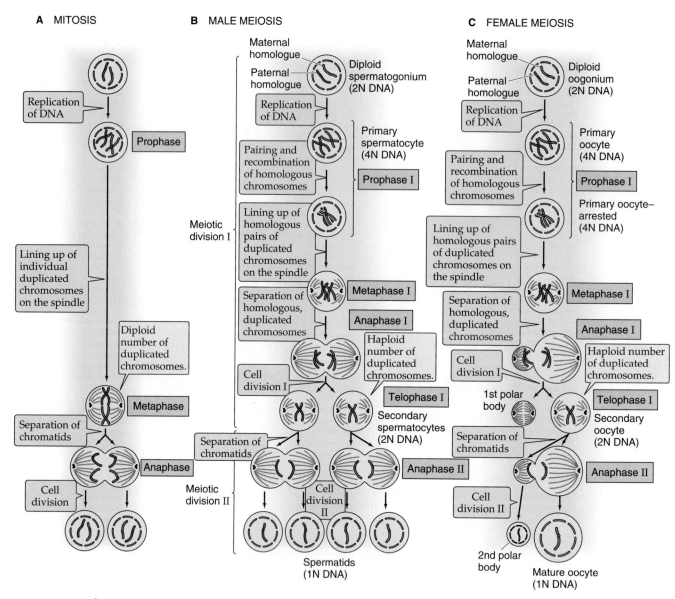

Figure 53-1 Mitosis and meiosis. **A**, In mitosis, the two daughter cells are genetically identical to the mother cell. **B**, In male meiosis, the four daughter cells are haploid. Cell division I produces both recombination (i.e., crossing over of genetic material between homologous chromosomes) and the reduction to the haploid number of chromosomes. Cell division II separates the chromatids of each chromosome, just as in mitosis. **C**, Female meiosis is similar to male meiosis. A major difference is that instead of producing four mature gametes, it produces only one mature gamete and two polar bodies.

of 2N DNA (N = 23)—undergo two meiotic divisions in both males (Fig. 53-1B) and females (Fig. 53-1C) to reduce the number of chromosomes from the diploid number (2N = 46) to the haploid number (N = 23). Because of this halving of the diploid number of chromosomes, meiosis is often referred to as a *reduction division*. Meiosis is a continuum composed of two phases: the homologous *chromosomes* separate during meiosis I, and the *chromatids* separate during meiosis II. At the start of meiosis I, the chromosomes duplicate so that the cells have 23 pairs of duplicated chromosomes (i.e., each chromosome has two chromatids)—or 4N DNA. During prophase of the first meiotic division, homol-

ogous pairs of chromosomes—22 pairs of autosomal chromosomes (autosomes) in addition to a pair of sex chromosomes—exchange genetic material. This genetic exchange is the phenomenon of *crossing over* that is responsible for the *recombination* of genetic material between maternal and paternal chromosomes. At the completion of meiosis I, the daughter cells have a haploid number (23) of duplicated, crossed-over chromosomes—or 2N DNA. During meiosis II, no additional duplication of DNA takes place. The chromatids simply separate so that each daughter receives a haploid number of unduplicated chromosomes—1 N DNA. A major difference between male and female gametogenesis is that one spermatogonium yields four spermatids (Fig. 53-1B), whereas one oogonium yields one mature oocyte and two polar bodies (Fig. 53-1C). The details emerge for spermatogenesis in Chapters 54 and 55. When two haploid gametes fuse, a mature spermatozoon from the father and a mature oocyte from the mother, a new individual is formed, a diploid zygote—2 N DNA.

When an X- or Y-bearing sperm fertilizes an oocyte, it establishes the zygote's genetic sex

The sex chromosomes that the parents contribute to the offspring determine the **genotypic sex** of that individual. The genotypic sex determines the **gonadal sex**, which, in turn, determines the **phenotypic sex** that becomes fully established at puberty. Thus, sex-determining mechanisms established at fertilization direct all later ontogenetic processes (processes that lead to the development of an organism) involved in male-female differentiation.

The process of fusion of a sperm and an ovum is referred to as **fertilization**, which is discussed in Chapter 55. Fusion of a sperm and egg—two haploid germ cells—results in a **zygote**, which is a diploid cell containing 46 chromosomes (Fig. 53-2), 22 pairs of somatic chromosomes (autosomes) and a single pair of sex chromosomes. In the female, these sex chromosomes are both X chromosomes, whereas males have one X and one Y chromosome.

When the karyotypes of normal females and males are compared, two differences are apparent. First, among the 23 pairs of chromosomes in the female, 8 pairs—including the 2 X chromosomes—are of similar size, whereas males have only $7\frac{1}{2}$ such pairs. Second, instead of a second X chromosome, males have a Y chromosome that is small and acrocentric (i.e., the centromere is located at one end of the chromosome); this chromosome is the only such chromosome that is not present in the female.

In the offspring, 23 of the chromosomes—including 1 of the sex chromosomes—are from the mother, and 23—including the other sex chromosome—come from the father. Thus, the potential offspring has a unique complement of chromosomes differing from those of both the mother and father. The ovum provided by the mother (XX) always provides an X chromosome. Because the male is the heterogenetic (XY) sex, half the spermatozoa are X bearing, whereas the other half are Y bearing. Thus, the type of sperm that fertilizes the ovum determines the sex of the zygote. X-bearing sperm produce XX zygotes that develop into females with a 46,XX karyotype, whereas Y-bearing sperm produce XY zygotes that develop into males with a 46,XY karyotype. The genetic sex of an individual is therefore determined at the time of fertilization. The Y chromosome appears to be the fundamental determinant of sexual development. When a Y chromosome is present, the individual develops as a male; when the Y chromosome is absent, the individual develops as a female. In embryos with abnormal sex chromosome complexes, the number of X chromosomes is apparently of little significance.

Differentiation of the indifferent gonad into an ovary requires two intact X chromosomes

The primary sex organs of an individual are the gonads. Gene complexes on sex chromosomes determine whether the indifferent gonad differentiates into a testis or an ovary. As discussed later, the Y chromosome exerts a powerful testis-determining effect on the indifferent gonad. The primary sex cords differentiate into seminiferous tubules under the influence of the Y chromosome. In the absence of a Y chromosome, the indifferent gonad develops into an ovary. The differentiated gonads, in turn, determine the sexual differentiation of the genital ducts and external genitalia.

The indifferent gonad is composed of an outer cortex and an inner medulla. In embryos with an XX sex chromosome complement, the cortex develops into an ovary, and the medulla regresses. Conversely, in embryos with an XY chromosome complex, the medulla differentiates into a testis, and the cortex regresses. Loss of a sex chromosome causes abnormal gonadal differentiation or gonadal dysgenesis. Loss of one of the X chromosomes of the XX pair results in an individual with an XO sex chromosome constitution and ovarian dysgenesis (see the box titled Gonadal Dysgenesis). Thus, two X chromosomes are necessary for normal ovarian development. In an XO individual, the gonads appear only as streaks on the pelvic sidewall in the adult. Because these streak gonads of XO individuals may contain germ cells, germ cell migration apparently can occur during development. The absence of only some genetic material from one

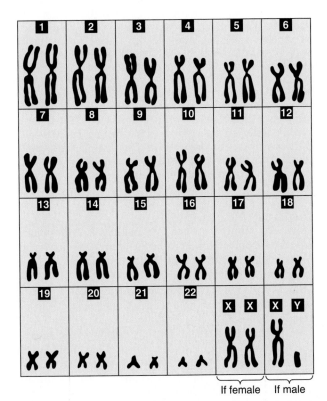

Figure 53-2 Normal human karyotype. The normal human has 22 pairs of autosomal chromosomes (autosomes) as well as a pair of sex chromosomes. Females have two X chromosomes, whereas males have one X and one Y chromosome.

Gonadal Dysgenesis

The best known example of gonadal dysgenesis is a syndrome referred to as **Turner syndrome**, a disorder of the female sex characterized by short stature, primary amenorrhea, sexual infantilism, and certain other congenital abnormalities. The cells in these individuals have a total number of 45 chromosomes and a normal karyotype, except they lack a second sex chromosome. The karyotype is 45,XO. Examination of the gonads of individuals with Turner syndrome reveals so-called streak gonads, which are firm, flat, glistening streaks lying below the fallopian tubes. These glands generally do not show evidence of either germinal or secretory elements but, instead, are largely composed of connective tissue arranged in whorls suggestive of ovarian stroma. Individuals with Turner syndrome have normal female differentiation of both the internal and external genitalia, although these genitalia are usually small and immature for the patient's age.

Partial deletion of the X chromosome may also result in the full Turner phenotype, particularly if the entire short arm of the X chromosome is missing.

The so-called **ring chromosome** is an example of an abnormality of the second sex chromosome. A ring chromosome is a small round or oval chromosome that often appears as a single black dot without a central hole. It forms as a result of a deletion and subsequent joining of the two free ends of the chromosome. Formation of a ring chromosome is, in effect, a deletion of the X chromosome and produces the same characteristics as gonadal dysgenesis.

The aforementioned defects result from disordered meiosis. A central genetic lesion is an abnormality of the second sex chromosome in some or all of the cells of the person. In at least half of affected individuals, this abnormality appears to be total absence of the second X chromosome. In others, the lesion is structural, as shown by the presence of ring chromosomes that have lost some genetic material. In at least a third of cases, these lesions appear as parts of a mosaicism; that is, *some* of the germ cells carry the aberrant or absent chromosome, whereas the rest are normal.

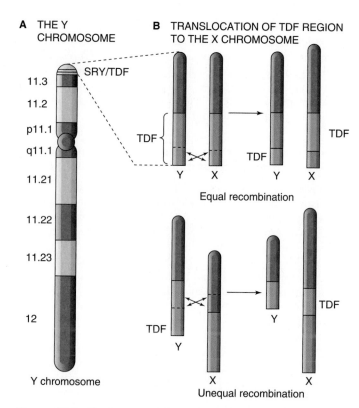

Figure 53-3 The location of the testis-determining region of the Y chromosome and an example of translocation. **A**, The Y chromosome is much smaller than the X chromosome. Giemsa staining of the chromosome results in alternating light and dark bands, some of which are shown here. The short or p arm of the Y chromosome is located above the centromere, whereas the long or q arm is located below it. The numbers to the left of the chromosome indicate the position of bands. The TDF is the *SRY* gene. **B**, Crossing-over events between normal X and Y chromosomes of the father can generate an X chromatid that contains a substantial portion of the TDF region and a Y chromatid that lacks its TDF. The figure shows both an equal and an unequal recombination event. If a sperm cell bearing an X chromosome with a translocated TDF fertilizes an ovum, the result is a male with a 46,XX karyotype, because one of the X chromosomes contains the TDF. Conversely, if the sperm cell carries a Y chromosome lacking its TDF, the result can be a 46,XY individual that appears to be female.

X chromosome in an XX individual—for example, as may occur as a result of breakage or deletion—may also cause abnormal sexual differentiation.

The testis-determining gene is located on the Y chromosome

Investigators have clearly established that a Y chromosome (Fig. 53-3A), with rare exception (see later), is necessary for normal testicular development. Thus, it stands to reason that the gene that determines organogenesis of the testis is normally located on the Y chromosome. This so-called **testis-determining factor** (TDF) has been mapped to the short arm of the Y chromosome and, indeed, turns out to be a single gene called *SRY* (for *Sex-determining Region Y*). The *SRY* gene encodes a transcription factor that belongs to the high-mobility group (HMG) superfamily of transcription factors. The family to which *SRY* belongs is evolutionarily ancient. One portion of *SRY*, the 80–amino acid HMG box, which actually binds to the DNA—is highly conserved among members of the family.

Rarely, the TDF may also be found translocated on other chromosomes. One example is an XX male (Fig. 53-3B), an individual whose sex chromosome complement is XX but whose phenotype is male. During normal male meiosis, human X and Y chromosomes pair and recombine at the distal end of their short arms. It appears that most XX males arise as a result of an aberrant exchange of genetic material between X and Y chromosomes in the father; in such cases, the TDF is transferred from a Y chromatid to an X chromatid. If the sperm cell that fertilizes the ovum contains such an X chromosome with a TDF, the resultant individual will be an XX male.

Endocrine and paracrine messengers modulate phenotypic differentiation

Just as an individual's genes determine whether the indifferent gonad develops into an ovary or a testis, so does the sex of the gonad dictate the gonad's endocrine and paracrine functions. Normally, chemical messengers—both endocrine and paracrine—produced by the gonad determine the primary and secondary sexual phenotypes of the individual. However, if the gonads fail to produce the proper messengers, if other organs (e.g., the adrenal glands) produce abnormal levels of sex steroids, or if the mother is exposed to chemical agents (e.g., synthetic progestins, testosterone) during pregnancy, sexual development of the fetus may deviate from that programmed by the genotype. Therefore, genetic determination of sexual differentiation is not irrevocable; numerous internal and external influences during development may modify or completely reverse the phenotype of the individual, whatever the genotypic sex.

An abnormal chemical environment can affect sexual differentiation at the level of either the genital ducts or the development of secondary sex characteristics. Higher vertebrates, including humans, have evolved highly elaborate systems of glands and ducts for transporting gametes. This system of glands and conduits collectively comprises the **accessory sex organs**. Together with the gonads, these accessory sex organs constitute the primary sex characteristics. The gonads produce and secrete hormones that condition and develop these accessory sex organs and, to a large extent, influence phenotypic sexual differentiation; that is, they induce either "maleness" or "femaleness" and influence the psychobiological phenomena involved in sex behavior.

Secondary sex characteristics are external specializations that are not essential for the production and movement of gametes; instead, they are primarily concerned with sex behavior and with the birth and nutrition of offspring. Examples include the development of pubic hair and breasts. Not only do the sex steroids produced by the gonads affect the accessory sex organs, but they also modulate the physiological state of the secondary sex characteristics toward "maleness" in the case of the testes and "femaleness" in the case of the ovaries.

DIFFERENTIATION OF THE GONADS

After migration of germ cells from the yolk sac, the primordial gonad develops into either a testis or an ovary

The **primordial germ cells** do not originate in the gonad; instead, they migrate to the gonad from the yolk sac along the mesentery of the hindgut at about the fifth week of embryo development (Fig. 53-4A, B). The primordial germ cells of humans are first found in the endodermal epithelium of the yolk sac in the vicinity of the allantoic stalk, and from there the germ cells migrate into the adjoining mesenchyme. They eventually take up their position embedded in the gonadal ridges. Gonadal development fails to progress normally in the absence of germ cells. Thus, any event that

---

Discordance Between Genotype and Gonadal Phenotype

A group of individuals has been reported to have no recognizable Y chromosome but do have testes. Some of these individuals are 46,XX and are **true hermaphrodites**; that is, they possess both male and female sex organs. Other patients have **mixed gonadal dysgenesis**—a testis in addition to a streak ovary—and a 45,XO karyotype. Some are **pseudohermaphrodites**; that is, affected individuals have only one type of gonadal tissue, but morphological characteristics of both sexes. All these patterns can result from mosaicisms (e.g., 46,XY/46,XX) or from translocation of the *SRY* gene (Fig. 53-3B)—which normally resides on the Y chromosome—to either an X chromosome or an autosome. A "normal" testis in the absence of a Y chromosome has never been reported.

Another group of individuals with a sex chromosome complex of 46,XY has **pure gonadal dysgenesis**—streak gonads, but no somatic features of XO. In the past, investigators assumed that these individuals possessed an abnormal Y chromosome. Perhaps the *SRY* gene is absent, or its expression is somehow blocked.

---

interferes with germ cell migration may cause abnormal gonadal differentiation.

The gonad forms from a portion of the coelomic epithelium, the underlying mesenchyme, and the primordial germ cells that migrate from the yolk sac. At 5 weeks' development, a thickened area of coelomic epithelium develops on the medial aspect of the urogenital ridge as a result of proliferation of both the coelomic epithelium and cells of the underlying mesenchyme. This prominence, which forms on the medial aspect of the mesonephros, is known as the **gonadal ridge** (Fig. 53-4B, C).

Migration of the primordial germ cells to the gonadal ridge establishes the *anlagen* for the primordial gonad. The primordial gonad at this early stage of development consists of both a peripheral cortex and a central medulla (Fig. 53-4C) and has the capacity to develop into either an ovary or a testis. As discussed later, the cortex and medulla have different fates in the male and female. The germ cells themselves seem to direct the sexual development of the gonad. An embryo with an XY chromosome complement undergoes development of the medullary portion of the gonad to become a testis, and the cortex regresses. Conversely, XX germ cells appear to stimulate development of the cortex of the early gonad to become an ovary, and the medulla regresses.

Development of the Primitive Testis   In male embryos, primordial germ cells migrate from the cortex of the gonad, in which they were originally embedded, into the primitive sex cords of the medulla (Fig. 53-4D). The primitive sex cords become hollowed out and develop into the **seminiferous tubules**. The primordial germ cells give rise to spermatogonia, the first cells in the pathway to mature sperm (see Chapter 54). The sex cords give rise to the Sertoli cells.

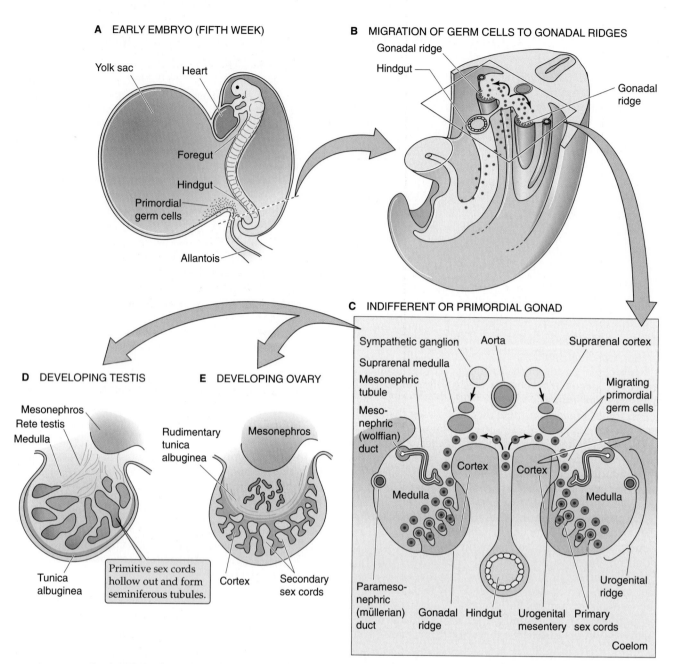

Figure 53-4   The early gonad and germ cell migration. **A**, The primordial germ cells originate in the endodermal endothelium of the yolk sac. **B**, The primordial germ cells migrate along the mesentery of the hindgut and reach the region of the urogenital ridge called the gonadal ridge. **C**, The indifferent gonad consists of an outer cortex and an inner medulla. **D**, The testis develops from the medulla of the indifferent gonad; the cortex regresses. **E**, The ovary develops from the cortex of the indifferent gonad; the medulla regresses.

The **rete testis** is a system of thin, interconnected tubules that develop in the dorsal part of the gonad; they drain the seminiferous tubules. The contents of the rete testis flow into the **efferent ductules**, which—as discussed later—develop from the adjoining tubules of the mesonephros. These tubular structures establish a pathway from the male gonad to the mesonephric duct, which—as also discussed later—evolves into the outlet for sperm. The cortex of the primordial gonad is a thin epithelial layer covering the coelomic surface of the testis.

Development of the Primitive Ovary   In female embryos, the medulla of the gonad regresses, the primary sex cords are resorbed, and the interior of the gonad is filled with a loose mesenchyme that is highly permeated by blood vessels. However, the cortex greatly increases in thickness, and the primordial germ cells remain embedded within it (Fig. 53-4E). Masses of cortical cells are split up on the inner surface of the cortex into groups and strands of cells, or secondary sex cords, surrounding one or several primordial germ cells, or oogonia, during growth of the gonad. These germ cells become primary oocytes that enter the initial stages of oogenesis.

The embryonic gonad determines the development of the internal genitalia and the external sexual phenotype

As discussed in the next section of this chapter, several products of the developing male or female gonad have profound effects on differentiation of the internal sex ducts, as well as on development of the external genitalia. Thus, just as genetic sex determines the gonadal phenotype, so also products of the gonad primarily determine the sexual phenotype. Androgens produced by the developing testis cause development of the mesonephric or **wolffian ducts**. The paramesonephric or müllerian ducts degenerate in the male under the influence of antimüllerian hormone (AMH). In the female embryo, the **müllerian ducts** develop, whereas the wolffian ducts degenerate. In the absence of a functioning testis, the left and right müllerian ducts develop according to the female phenotype, that is, as the fallopian tubes (oviducts), the uterus, and the upper third of the vagina (see the next section).

Just as the absence of male hormones or androgens causes the *internal* genital ducts to follow a female pattern of differentiation, so also the absence of androgens causes the *external* genital development to be female. Conversely, testosterone and dihydrotestosterone (DHT) cause masculinization of the external genitalia (see the later section on differentiation of the external genitalia).

DIFFERENTIATION OF THE INTERNAL GENITAL DUCTS

The genital ducts are an essential part of the genital organs and are the means by which the sex cells—ova and spermatozoa—are transported to a location where fertilization occurs. As discussed in the previous section, embryos of both sexes have a double set of genital ducts (Fig. 53-5A): the mesonephric or **wolffian ducts**, which in males develop into the vas deferens and other structures; and the paramesonephric or **müllerian ducts**, which in females become the oviducts, uterus, and upper third of the vagina.

During mammalian development, three sets of kidneys develop, two of which are transient. The **pronephric kidney**, which develops first, is so rudimentary that it never functions. However, the duct that connects the pronephric kidney to the urogenital sinus—the pronephric duct—eventually serves the same purpose for the second kidney, the **mesonephric kidney** or mesonephros, as it develops embryologically. Unlike the pronephric kidney, the mesonephros functions transiently as a kidney. It has glomeruli and renal tubules; these tubules empty into the mesonephric duct (Fig. 53-5A), which, in turn, carries fluid to the urogenital sinus. As discussed later, the mesonephros and its mesonephric duct will—depending on the sex of the developing embryo—either degenerate or develop into other reproductive structures. In addition to the mesonephric ducts, a second pair of genital ducts, the paramesonephric or müllerian ducts, will develop as invaginations of the coelomic epithelium on the lateral aspects of the mesonephros. These parameso-

nephric ducts run caudally and parallel to the mesonephric ducts. In the caudal region, they cross ventral to the mesonephric ducts and fuse to form a cylindrical structure, the uterovaginal canal. The third or **metanephric kidney** becomes the permanent mammalian kidney. Its excretory duct is the ureter.

In males, the mesonephros becomes the epididymis, and the mesonephric (wolffian) ducts become the vas deferens, seminal vesicles, and ejaculatory duct

During development, the **mesonephros** ceases to be an excretory organ in both sexes. The only part that remains functional is the portion—in males—that develops into the most proximal end of the epididymis, the **efferent ductules**. As the mesonephros degenerates, persisting mesonephric tubules develop into many parallel efferent ductules that connect the upstream rete testis to the head of the epididymis, which serves as a reservoir for sperm.

The **mesonephric ducts** develop into the channels through which the spermatozoa exit the testes (Fig. 53-5B). The most proximal portion of the mesonephric duct becomes the head, the body, and the tail of the epididymis. The tail of the epididymis connects to the **vas deferens**, which also arises from the wolffian duct. A lateral outgrowth from the distal end of the mesonephric duct forms the **seminal vesicle**. The portion of the mesonephric duct between the seminal vesicle and the point where the mesonephric duct joins the urethra becomes the **ejaculatory duct**. At about the level where the ejaculatory duct joins with the urethra, multiple outgrowths of the urethra grow into the underlying mesenchyme and form the **prostate gland**. The mesenchyme of the prostate gives rise to the stroma of the prostate, whereas the prostatic glands develop from endodermal cells of the prostatic urethra.

In females, the paramesonephric (müllerian) ducts become the fallopian tubes, the uterus, and the upper third of the vagina

In female embryos, both the mesonephros and the wolffian (mesonephric) ducts degenerate. The müllerian ducts establish three functional regions (Fig. 53-5C). The cranial portions of the müllerian ducts remain separate and give rise to the fallopian tubes. The upper end of the duct gains a fringe, which will become the fimbria, by adding a series of minor pits or müllerian tunnels. The midportions of the left and right müllerian ducts fuse and give rise to the fundus and corpus of the uterus. The most distal portions of the bilateral müllerian ducts had previously fused as the **uterovaginal primordium**. The cranial portion of this common tube gives rise to the cervix and remains the longest portion of the uterus until puberty. The caudal portion of this common tube becomes the upper third of the vagina.

In males, development of the wolffian ducts requires testosterone

As already noted, the developing embryo has two precursor duct systems (Fig. 53-6A). In a normal male embryo (Fig. 53-6B), the wolffian ducts develop, whereas the müllerian

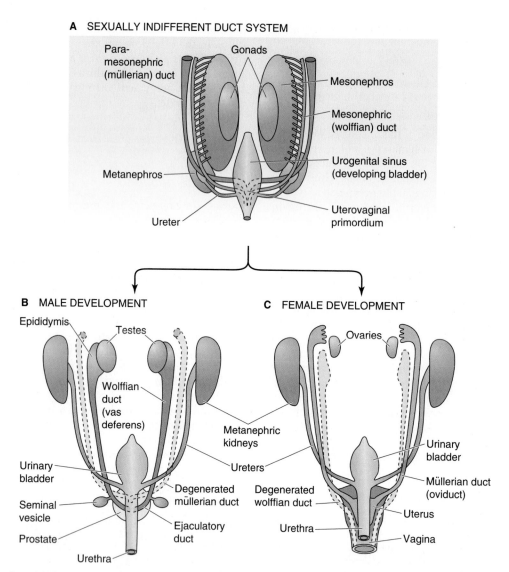

A SEXUALLY INDIFFERENT DUCT SYSTEM

Para-mesonephric (müllerian) duct

Gonads

Mesonephros

Mesonephric (wolffian) duct

Urogenital sinus (developing bladder)

Metanephros

Ureter

Uterovaginal primordium

B MALE DEVELOPMENT

Epididymis

Testes

Wolffian duct (vas deferens)

Urinary bladder

Seminal vesicle

Prostate

Urethra

Metanephric kidneys

Ureters

Degenerated müllerian duct

Ejaculatory duct

C FEMALE DEVELOPMENT

Ovaries

Degenerated wolffian duct

Urethra

Urinary bladder

Müllerian duct (oviduct)

Uterus

Vagina

Figure 53-5 Transformation of the genital ducts. **A**, At the time the gonad is still indifferent, it is closely associated with the mesonephros, as well as the excretory duct (mesonephric or wolffian duct) that leads from the mesonephros to the urogenital sinus. Parallel to the wolffian ducts are the paramesonephric or müllerian ducts, which merge caudally to form the uterovaginal primordium. **B**, In males, the mesonephros develops into the epididymis. The wolffian duct develops into the vas deferens, seminal vesicles, and ejaculatory duct. The müllerian ducts degenerate. **C**, In females, the mesonephros and the wolffian (mesonephric) ducts degenerate. The paramesonephric or müllerian ducts develop into the fallopian tubes, the uterus, the cervix, and the upper one third of the vagina.

ducts regress. In a normal female embryo (Fig. 53-6C), the müllerian ducts develop, whereas the wolffian ducts regress. It appears that maturation of one of these systems and degeneration of the other depend on local factors produced by the developing gonad.

A classic series of experiments performed by Alfred Jost in 1953 revealed that masculine genital development requires factors produced by fetal testicular tissue. The experimental approach was to castrate rabbit fetuses at various stages of development and allow the pregnancies to continue. Castrating a male fetus before maturation of the wolffian ducts caused the müllerian ducts to persist (i.e., fail to regress) and

induced the development of female internal and external genitalia (Fig. 53-6D). However, castrating female fetuses at a comparable stage in development had no appreciable effect, and müllerian development continued along normal female lines (Fig. 53-6E). Thus, although normal male development requires the testes, development of the fallopian tubes and uterus does *not* require the ovaries.

Unilateral removal of the testis resulted in female duct development on the same (ipsilateral) side as the castration, but virilization of the external genitalia proceeded normally (Fig. 53-6F). Removing both testes—and administering testosterone—resulted in essentially normal development of

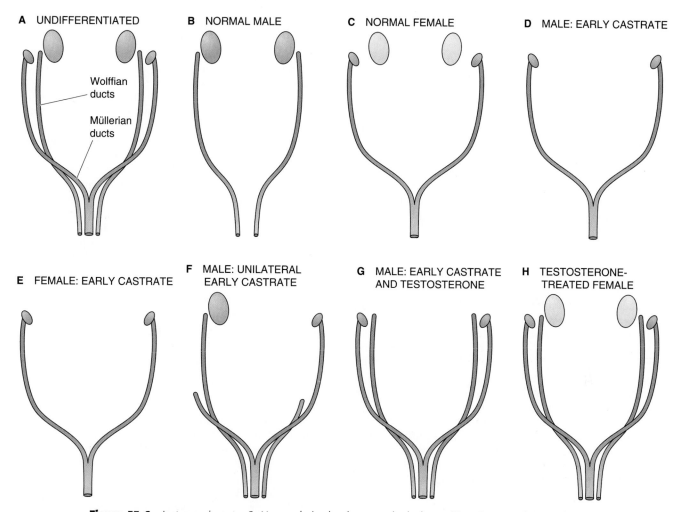

Figure 53-6 Jost experiments. **A**, Very early in development, both the wolffian (mesonephric) and the müllerian (paramesonephric) ducts are present in parallel. **B**, The wolffian duct develops into the vas deferens, the seminal vesicles, and the ejaculatory duct. The müllerian ducts degenerate. **C**, The paramesonephric or müllerian ducts develop into the fallopian tubes, the uterus, the cervix, and the upper one third of the vagina. The wolffian (mesonephric) ducts degenerate. **D**, Bilateral removal of the testes deprives the embryo of both AMH (also known as MIS) and testosterone, which are both testicular products. As a result of the absence of AMH, the müllerian ducts follow the female pattern of development. In the absence of testosterone, the wolffian ducts degenerate. Thus, the genetically male fetus develops female internal and external genitalia. **E**, After bilateral removal of the ovaries, müllerian development continues along normal female lines. Thus, the ovary is not required for female duct development. **F**, Unilateral removal of the testis results in female duct development on the same (ipsilateral) side as the castration. Duct development follows the male pattern on the side with the remaining testis. Virilization of the external genitalia proceeds normally. **G**, In the absence of both testes, administering testosterone preserves development of the wolffian ducts. However, because of the absence of AMH—which is a product of the testis—no müllerian regression occurs. **H**, In the presence of both ovaries, the testosterone promotes development of the wolffian ducts. Because there are no testes—and therefore no AMH—the müllerian ducts develop normally.

the wolffian ducts, but no müllerian regression was seen (Fig. 53-6G). Thus, although testosterone can support wolffian development, it is unable to cause müllerian regression. It became clear that a testicular product other than testosterone is necessary for regression of the müllerian ducts. Thus, one would predict that treating a normal female with testosterone would lead to preservation of the wolffian ducts, as well as the müllerian ducts. This pattern of dual ducts is indeed observed (Fig. 53-6H).

In males, antimüllerian hormone causes regression of the müllerian ducts

After Jost, other investigators performed experiments indicating that the Sertoli cells of the testis produce a nonsteroid macromolecule—**AMH** or **müllerian-inhibiting substance (MIS)**—that causes müllerian degeneration in the male fetus. AMH, a growth-inhibitory glycoprotein, is a member of the transforming growth factor β (TGF-β) superfamily of glycoproteins involved in the regulation of growth and differentiation (see Chapter 3). Besides TGF-β, this gene super-family includes the inhibins and activins (see Chapter 55). The proteins produced by this gene family are all synthesized as dimeric precursors and undergo post-translational processing for activation. AMH is glycosylated and is secreted as a 140-kDa dimer consisting of two identical disulfide-linked subunits. The antimitogenic activity and müllerian duct bioactivity of AMH reside primarily in its C-terminal domain.

The human AMH gene is located on chromosome 19, and AMH is one of the earliest sexually dimorphic genes expressed during development. The transcription factor SRY, which represents the TDF, may be involved in initiating the transcription of AMH. The sequential timing of SRY and AMH expression is consistent with activation of AMH by SRY, a series of events that may control sexual dimorphism.

Although the exact mechanism of AMH action has not been completely clarified, it is thought to involve receptor-mediated *de*phosphorylation. AMH appears to act directly on mesenchymal cells of the müllerian duct and, indirectly through the mesenchyme, on müllerian duct epithelial cells. AMH binding has been localized to the mesenchymal cells surrounding the müllerian duct and to the developing oocytes in preantral follicles.

During embryogenesis in males, AMH—which is secreted by the Sertoli cells in the testis—causes involution of the müllerian ducts, whereas testosterone—which is secreted by the Leydig cells of the testis—stimulates differentiation of the wolffian ducts. In females, the müllerian ducts differentiate spontaneously in the absence of AMH, and the wolffian ducts involute spontaneously in the absence of testosterone.

DIFFERENTIATION OF THE EXTERNAL GENITALIA

The urogenital sinus develops into the urinary bladder, the urethra, and, in females, the vestibule of the vagina

Early in embryologic development, a tubular structure called the cloaca is the common termination of the urogenital and gastrointestinal systems (Fig. 53-7A). The cloacal membrane separates the cloaca from the amniotic fluid. Eventually, a wedge of mesenchymal tissue separates the cloaca into a dorsal and a ventral cavity (Fig. 53-7B). The dorsal cavity is the rectum. The ventral compartment is the **urogenital sinus**. Both the wolffian and the müllerian ducts empty into this urogenital sinus (Fig. 53-5A).

The urogenital sinus can be divided into three regions: the vesicle part, the pelvic part, and the phallic part. In the male (Fig. 53-7C), the vesicle part becomes the urinary bladder, the pelvic part becomes the prostatic part of the urethra, and the phallic part becomes the initial portion of the penile urethra.

In the female (Fig. 53-7D), the vesicle part of the urogenital sinus also develops into the urinary bladder. The pelvic part becomes the entire female urethra. The phallic portion of the urogenital sinus develops into the vestibule of the

vagina; into this vestibule empty the urethra, the vagina, and the ducts of the greater vestibular glands of Bartholin.

As noted earlier, fusion of the caudal portion of the müllerian ducts produces the uterovaginal primordium. As this primordium contacts the dorsal wall of the urogenital sinus, it induces the development of paired sinovaginal bulbs, which grow into the urogenital sinus and then fuse to form a solid core of tissue called the **vaginal plate**. This plate grows caudally to the phallic portion of the urogenital sinus. Resorption of the center of the vaginal plate creates the vaginal lumen. The remaining cells of the vaginal plate appear to form the vaginal epithelium. During early fetal development, a thin membrane, the **hymen**, separates the lumen of the vagina from the cavity of the urogenital sinus. Usually, the hymen partially opens during the prenatal period. Occasionally, the hymenal membrane persists completely, does not allow escape of the menstrual effluvium at menarche, and gives rise to a condition known clinically as hematocolpos.

In the male, the vagina disappears when the müllerian ducts are resorbed. However, remnants of the vagina sometimes persist as a prostatic utricle.

The external genitalia of both sexes develop from common anlagen

Although anatomically separate precursors give rise to the internal genitalia, common anlagen give rise to the external genitalia of the two sexes (Fig. 53-8A). Knowledge of the common origins of the external genitalia during normal development facilitates understanding of the ambiguities of abnormal sexual development.

The **genital tubercle** (Fig. 53-8B) develops during the fourth week on the ventral side of the cloacal membrane. As a result of elongation of the genital tubercle, a phallus develops in both sexes. The genital tubercle of the primitive embryo develops into the **glans penis** in the male (Fig. 53-8C) and the **clitoris** in the female (Fig. 53-8D). Until about the end of the first trimester of pregnancy, the external genitalia of males and females are anatomically difficult to distinguish. The phallus undergoes rapid growth in the female initially, but its growth slows, and in the absence of androgens, the phallus becomes the relatively small clitoris in the female.

The paired **urogenital folds** give rise to the ventral aspect of the penis in the male (Fig. 53-8C) and the labia minora in the female (Fig. 53-8D). After formation of the urogenital opening, a groove—the urethral groove—forms on the ventral side of the phallus; this groove is continuous with the urogenital opening. The bilateral urogenital folds fuse over the urethral groove to form an enclosed spongy urethra; the line of fusion is the penile raphe. As the urogenital folds fuse to form the ventral covering of the penis, they do so in a posterior-to-anterior direction, thus displacing the urethral orifice to the tip of the penis. Elongation of the genital tubercle and fusion of the genital folds occur at the 12th to the 14th week of gestation. However, in the female, the urogenital folds normally remain separate as the labia minora.

In the male, the **genital** or **labioscrotal swellings** fuse to give rise to the scrotum. In females, however, the labioscrotal swellings fuse anteriorly to give rise to the mons pubis and

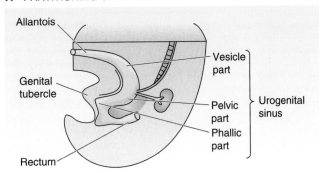

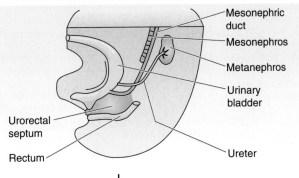

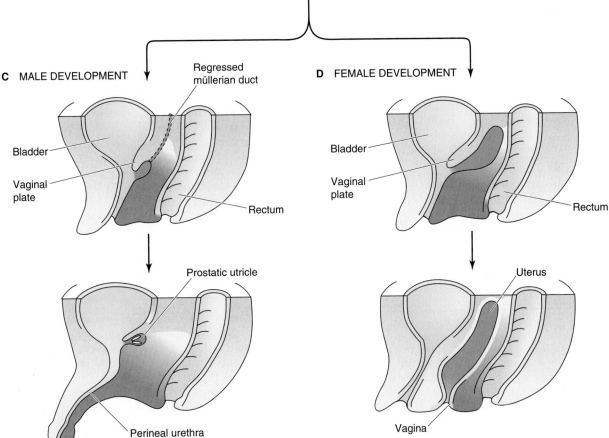

Figure 53-7 Differentiation of the urogenital sinus. **A**, The urorectal septum begins to separate the rectum (dorsal) from the urogenital sinus (ventral). The urogenital sinus is divided into a vesicle (i.e., urinary bladder) part, a pelvic part, and a phallic part. The common space into which the rectum and urogenital sinus empty—the cloaca—is closed by the cloacal membrane. **B**, At this stage, the rectum and the urogenital sinus are fully separated. The urogenital membrane separates the urogenital sinus from the outside of the embryo. **C**, The male has a common opening for the reproductive and urinary tracts. The prostatic utricle, which is the male homologue of the vagina, empties into the prostatic urethra. **D**, A solid core of tissue called the *vaginal plate* grows caudally from the posterior wall of the urogenital sinus. The lumen of the vagina forms as the center of this plate resorbs. Thus, the female has separate openings for the urinary and reproductive systems.

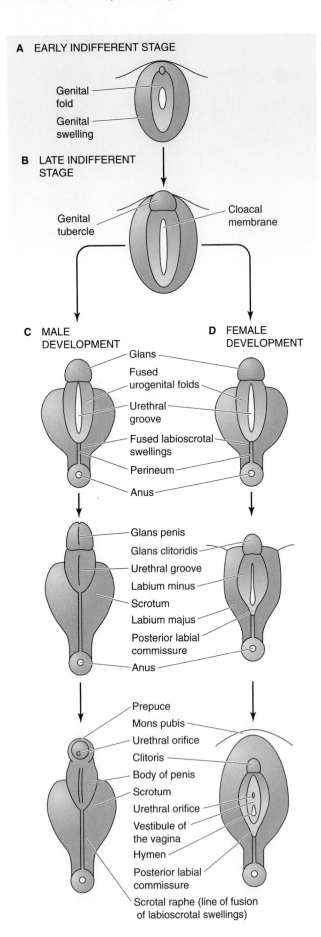

A EARLY INDIFFERENT STAGE

Genital fold
Genital swelling

B LATE INDIFFERENT STAGE

Genital tubercle
Cloacal membrane

C MALE DEVELOPMENT

Glans
Fused urogenital folds
Urethral groove
Fused labioscrotal swellings
Perineum
Anus

Glans penis
Urethral groove
Scrotum
Anus

Prepuce
Urethral orifice
Clitoris
Body of penis
Scrotum

Scrotal raphe (line of fusion of labioscrotal swellings)

D FEMALE DEVELOPMENT

Glans clitoridis
Labium minus
Labium majus
Posterior labial commissure

Mons pubis
Urethral orifice
Vestibule of the vagina
Hymen
Posterior labial commissure

Figure 53-8 Development of the external genitalia. **A**, Genital folds and genital swellings surround the cloacal membrane. **B**, Early in the fourth week of development—in both sexes—the genital tubercle begins to enlarge to form the phallus. **C**, In males, the genital tubercle becomes the glans penis. The urogenital folds fuse to form the shaft of the penis. The labioscrotal swellings become the scrotum. **D**, In females, the genital tubercle becomes the clitoris. The urogenital folds remain separate as the labia minora. The labioscrotal swellings become the labia majora where they remain unfused. Ventrally, the labioscrotal swellings fuse to form the mons pubis. Dorsally they fuse to form the posterior labial commissure.

posteriorly to form the posterior labial commissure. The unfused labioscrotal swellings give rise to the labia majora.

ENDOCRINE AND PARACRINE CONTROL MECHANISMS IN SEXUAL DIFFERENTIATION

The *SRY* gene triggers development of the testis, which makes the androgens and AMH necessary for male sexual differentiation

I already noted that the female pattern of sexual differentiation occurs in the absence of testes. In fact, the embryo follows the female pattern even in the absence of all gonadal tissue. It thus appears that the male pattern of sexual differentiation is directed by endocrine and paracrine control mechanisms. Therefore, I successively examine the control of testicular development, the development of the male internal system of genital ducts, and the development of the male urogenital sinus and external genitalia.

Testicular development proceeds in the presence of TDF—the gene product of the *SRY* gene—before 9 weeks of gestation. If TDF is not present or if TDF is present only after the critical window of 9 weeks has passed, an ovary will develop instead of a testis. Further male-pattern sexual differentiation depends on the presence of three hormones, testosterone, DHT, and AMH. The testis directly produces both testosterone and AMH. Peripheral tissues convert testosterone to DHT.

Testosterone Production The primary sex steroid produced by both the fetal and the postnatal testis is testosterone. The testes also produce DHT and estradiol, although in lesser amounts. The **Leydig cells** are the source of sex steroid production in the testes. The Leydig cells differentiate from mesenchymal tissue that surround the testicular cords. This tissue makes up more than half the testicular volume by 60 days of gestation. The early increase in the number of Leydig cells and secretion of testosterone in humans could depend on either maternal human chorionic gonadotropin (hCG) or fetal luteinizing hormone (LH). The human testis has its greatest abundance of side-chain–cleavage enzyme—which catalyzes the first committed step in steroid synthesis (see Fig. 50-2)—at 14 to 15 weeks of gestation and low values by 26 weeks of gestation. Because hCG follows a similar temporal pattern, it may be hCG that supports *early* testosterone production. Late regulation of testosterone production by fetal LH is supported by the finding that the testes of anencephalic fetuses (see the box in Chapter 10 on abnormalities of neural tube closure) at term have few Leydig cells.

The Androgen Receptor Androgens diffuse into target cells and act by binding to androgen receptors, which are present in genital tissues. In the absence of adequate androgen production or functioning androgen receptors, sexual ambiguity occurs. The androgen receptor functions as a homodimer (AR/AR) and is a member of the family of nuclear receptors (see Chapter 3). The AR/AR receptor complex is a transcription factor that binds to hormone-response elements on DNA located 5′ from the genes controlled by the androgens (see Table 4-2). Interaction between the receptor-steroid complex and nuclear chromatin causes increased transcription of structural genes, the appearance of mRNA, and subsequent translation and production of new proteins. Congenital absence of the androgen receptor, or the production of abnormal androgen receptor, leads to a syndrome known as testicular feminization (see the box on Impaired Androgen Action in Target Tissues).

Dihydrotestosterone Formation In certain target tissues, cytoplasmic 5α-reductase converts testosterone to DHT (see Fig. 54-5), which binds to the same androgen receptor as does testosterone. However, DHT binds to the androgen receptor with an affinity that is ~100-fold greater than the binding of testosterone to the androgen receptor. Moreover, the DHT-receptor complex binds to chromatin more tightly than does the testosterone-receptor complex.

Antimüllerian Hormone As noted earlier, the Sertoli cells of the testis produce AMH, also known as MIS. AMH is a homodimer of two monomeric glycoprotein subunits that are linked by disulfide bonds.

Androgens direct the male pattern of sexual differentiation of the internal ducts, the urogenital sinus, and the external genitalia

Androgens play two major roles in male phenotypic differentiation: (1) they trigger conversion of the wolffian ducts to the male ejaculatory system, and (2) they direct the differentiation of the urogenital sinus and external genitalia. The wolffian phase of male sexual differentiation is regulated by testosterone itself and does not require conversion of testosterone to DHT. In contrast, virilization of the urogenital sinus, the prostate, the penile urethra, and the external genitalia during embryogenesis requires DHT, as does sexual maturation at puberty.

Differentiation of the Duct System After formation of the testicular cords, the Sertoli cells produce AMH, which causes the müllerian ducts to regress. The cranial end of the müllerian duct becomes the vestigial appendix testis at the superior pole of the testis. Shortly after the initiation of AMH production, the fetal Leydig cells begin producing testosterone. The embryonic mesenchyme contains androgen receptors and is the first site of androgen action during for-

---

Congenital Adrenal Hyperplasia

Ambiguous genitalia in genotypic females may result from disorders of adrenal function. Several forms of **congenital adrenal hyperplasia** have been described, including the deficiency of several enzymes involved in steroid synthesis (see Fig. 50-2): the side chain–cleavage enzyme, 17α-hydroxylase, 21α-hydroxylase, 11β-hydroxylase, and 3β-hydroxysteroid dehydrogenase. Deficiencies in 21α-hydroxylase, 11β-hydroxylase, and 3β-hydroxysteroid dehydrogenase all lead to virilization in females—and thus ambiguous genitalia—as a result of the hypersecretion of adrenal androgens. **21α-Hydroxylase deficiency**, by far the most common, accounts for ~95% of cases. Some of the consequences of this deficiency are discussed in the box on 21α-hydroxylase deficiency in Chapter 50.

As summarized in Figure 50-2, 21α-hydroxylase deficiency reduces the conversion of progesterone to 11-deoxycorticosterone—which goes on to form aldosterone—and also reduces the conversion of 17α-hydroxyprogesterone to 11-deoxycortisol—which is the precursor of cortisol. As a result, adrenal steroid precursors are shunted into androgen pathways. In female infants, the result is sometimes called the *adrenogenital syndrome*. The external genitalia are difficult to distinguish from male genitalia on visual inspection. The clitoris is enlarged and resembles a penis, and the labioscrotal folds are enlarged and fused and resemble a scrotum. The genitalia thus have a male phenotype in an otherwise normal female infant.

---

mation of the male urogenital tract. The Sertoli cells also produce a substance referred to as **androgen-binding protein (ABP)**. It is possible that ABP binds and maintains a high concentration of testosterone locally. These high local levels of testosterone stimulate growth and differentiation of the medulla of the gonad into the rete testes, as well as differentiation of the wolffian ducts into the epididymis, the vas deferens, the seminal vesicles, and the ejaculatory duct. Testosterone also promotes development of the prostate from a series of endodermal buds located at the proximal aspect of the urethra. Cells of the wolffian ducts lack 5α-reductase and therefore cannot convert testosterone to DHT. Thus, the internal male ducts respond to testosterone per se and do not require the conversion of testosterone to DHT. In the absence of testosterone, the wolffian system remains rudimentary, and normal male internal ductal development does not occur.

Differentiation of the Urogenital Sinus and External Genitalia The cells of the urogenital sinus and external genitalia, unlike those of the wolffian duct, contain 5α-reductase and are thus capable of converting testosterone to DHT. Indeed, conversion of testosterone to DHT is required for normal male development of the external genitalia. Congenital absence of 5α-reductase (see the box titled Impaired Androgen Action in Target Tissues) is associated with normal development of the wolffian duct system but impaired virilization of the external genitalia.

At ~9 weeks' gestation, soon after virilization of the internal genital ducts of the male, development of the external genitalia commences. It is completed by 13 weeks of gestation. In the presence of high intracellular concentrations of DHT, the genital tubercle, the bipotential predecessor to either a clitoris or a penis, elongates to become the glans penis, the corpus spongiosum, and the two corpora cavernosa. Formation of the penis and scrotum is complete by ~13 weeks, and even extremely high concentrations of testosterone after this time fail to cause midline fusion of the urethral groove or scrotum, although the clitoris will enlarge. The urogenital sinus gives rise to the prostate and the bulbourethral glands, also under the influence of DHT.

In the absence of androgen secretion by the fetal testis—or abnormal extragonadal sources—the indifferent external genitalia remain unfused and follow the female pattern of differentiation.

Androgen Dependence of Testicular Descent

In preparation for descent, the testes enlarge. In addition, the mesonephric kidneys and wolffian (mesonephric) ducts atrophy. This process frees the testes for their future move down the posterior abdominal wall and across the abdomen to the deep inguinal rings. Testicular descent occurs in three phases during the last two thirds of gestation. During the first stage of testicular descent, rapid growth of the abdominopelvic region causes *relative* movement of the testes down to the inguinal region (Fig. 53-9A). The role of the gubernaculum—the ligament attaching the inferior part of the testes to the lower segment of the labioscrotal fold—is uncertain. However, the gubernaculum shortens and appears to guide the testis to its place of ultimate functional residence in the scrotum. The second stage of testicular descent is herniation of the abdominal wall adjacent to the gubernaculum (Fig. 53-9B). This herniation, which occurs as a result of increasing abdominal pressure, forms the processus vaginalis; the processus vaginalis then folds around the gubernaculum and creates the inguinal canal. In the third stage, the gubernaculum increases to the approximate diameter of the testis. As its proximal portion degenerates, the gubernaculum draws the testis into the scrotum through the processus vaginalis (Fig. 53-9C).

The testes usually complete their descent by the seventh month of gestation; ~97.5% of full-term infants and 79% of premature infants have fully descended testes at birth. At 9 months of age, only 0.8% of male infants have undescended testes. The incidence of undescended testes in young men is 0.2%.

Testicular descent is an androgen-dependent process, and development of the structures involved in testicular descent depends on testosterone. Thus, in testosterone-deficient states caused by inadequate secretion or disordered androgen action, the testes of genetic males often fail to descend. This abnormality can be seen in individuals with both 5α-reductase deficiency and complete androgen resistance (i.e., testicular feminization syndrome).

Androgens and estrogens influence sexual differentiation of the brain

Anatomically sexually dimorphic nuclei have been identified in the diencephalons of rodents and lower primates. Gonadal steroids influence the development of these sexually dimorphic nuclei. Androgens do not act directly on the hypothalamus and other areas of the brain having to do with sex behavior and control of gonadotropin secretion. Rather, aromatase—which catalyzes the formation of estrone and estradiol (see Fig. 55-10)—converts androgens to estrogens in the brain. Thus, androgens in the brain serve as prohormones for estrogens. Therefore, estrogens are derived from androgens that appear to masculinize sexually dimorphic nuclei directly in the brain. It is not clear why, in females, estrogens do not *masculinize* the brain.

Gonadal steroids affect sex behavior in both males and females. In rodents, lordosis behavior in females and mounting behavior in males are examples of sex behavior. An example of functional sexual dimorphism in the human brain is the manner in which gonadotropin is released. Gonadotropin release has been described as *cyclic* in the female and *tonic* in the male inasmuch as females have mid-cycle cyclic release of gonadotropin before ovulation, whereas males seem to have a continuous tonic pattern of gonadotropin release. Although controversy continues over the role of prenatal virilization in the determination of sexual dimorphism, sex steroids clearly have an impact on sexual behavior and sexual reference in humans.

The appearance of secondary sex characteristics at puberty completes sexual differentiation and development

Although at birth humans have the primary and secondary sex organs necessary for procreation, final sexual maturity occurs only at puberty. Profound alterations in hormone

---

Impaired Androgen Action in Target Tissues

As already discussed, in the absence of androgens, male embryos follow a typically female pattern of sexual development. However, such a female developmental pattern can occur even if testosterone levels are normal or elevated. Any defect in the mechanisms by which androgens *act* on target tissues—in genotypic males—may lead to a syndrome of **male pseudohermaphroditism**. Affected individuals have a normal male karyotype (46,XY) and unambiguous male gonads but ambiguous external genitalia, or they may phenotypically appear as female. In principle, impaired androgen action could result from a deficiency of the enzyme that converts testosterone to DHT in target tissues, absent androgen receptors, qualitatively abnormal receptors, a quantitative deficiency in receptor levels, or postreceptor defects. The two major forms that have been identified clinically are defects in the conversion of testosterone to DHT (5α-reductase deficiency) and androgen receptor defects.

A MOVEMENT OF TESTES TO THE INGUINAL REGION

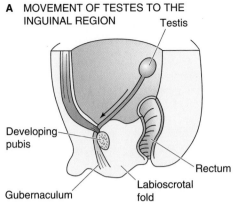

B HERNIATION OF THE ABDOMINAL WALL

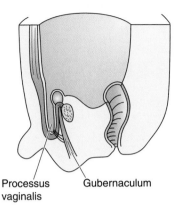

C DESCENT OF TESTES INTO THE SCROTUM

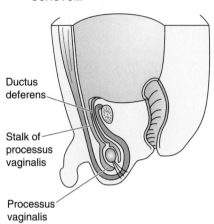

Figure 53-9 Testicular descent.

secretion during the peripubertal period cause changes in the primary and secondary sex organs. The events occurring in puberty are discussed in more detail for both males (see Chapter 54) and females (see Chapter 55).

Female The vagina reflects the effects of estrogens on the vaginal mucosa. The uterus and cervix enlarge, and their secretory functions increase under the influence of estrogen. The uterine glands increase in number and length, and the endometrium and stroma proliferate in response to estrogen secretion. The cervical glands produce increasing quantities of cervical mucus, which serves to lubricate the vaginal vault. The mucous membranes of the female urogenital tract are made of stratified squamous epithelium; these membranes respond to hormones, particularly estrogens. Estrogen levels increase and cause increased epithelial proliferation with the formation of successive intermediate and superficial layers. The cells of the vaginal mucosa are transformed into superficial cells, and the thickness of the vaginal mucosa increases.

Development of the breasts occurs under the influence of a complex of hormones. Progesterone is primarily responsible for development of the alveoli, which are analogous to the acini of other exocrine glands. Estrogen is the primary stimulus for development of the duct system that connects the alveoli to the exterior. Insulin, growth hormone, glucocorticoids, and thyroxine contribute to breast development, but they are incapable of causing breast growth by themselves. Lactation is discussed in Chapter 56.

Male The penis undergoes rapid growth under the influence of testosterone secreted by the testes. The testes also increase dramatically in size in response to increasing androgen secretion at puberty.

REFERENCES

Books and Reviews

Donahoe PK, Budzik GP, Trelstad R, et al: Müllerian-inhibiting substance: An update. Recent Prog Horm Res 1982; 38:279.

Grumbach MM, Conte FA: Disorders of sex differentiation. In Wilson JD, Foster DW, Kronenberg HM, Larsen PR (eds): Williams Textbook of Endocrinology, 9th ed, pp 1303-1425. Philadelphia: WB Saunders, 1998.

Haqq CM, Donahoe PK: Regulation of sexual dimorphism in mammals. Physiol Rev 1998; 78:1-33.

Jost A, Vigier B, Prepin J, Perchellet JP: Studies on sex differentiation in mammals. Recent Prog Horm Res 1973; 29:1-41.

Lee MM, Donahoe PK: Müllerian inhibiting substance: A gonadal hormone with multiple functions. Endocr Rev 1993; 14:152-164.

Naftolin F, Ryan KJ, Davie KJ, et al: The formation of estrogens by central neuroendocrine tissues. Recent Prog Horm Res 1975; 31:295-319.

Rebar RW: Normal and abnormal sexual differentiation and pubertal development. In Moore TR, Reiter RC, Rebar RW, Baker VV (eds): Gynecology and Obstetrics: A Longitudinal Approach, pp 97-146. New York: Churchill Livingstone, 1993.

Journal Articles

Griffin JE, Wilson JD: The syndromes of androgen resistance. N Engl J Med 1980; 302:198-209.

Judd HL, Hamilton CR, Barlow JJ, et al: Androgen and gonadotropin dynamics in testicular feminization syndrome. J Clin Endocrinol Metab 1972; 34:229-234.

New MI, Dupont B, Pang S, et al: An update of congenital adrenal hyperplasia. Recent Prog Horm Res 1981; 37:105-181.

Sinclair AH, Berta P, Palmer MS, et al: A gene from the human sex-determining region encodes a protein with homology to a conserved DNA-binding motif. Nature 1990; 346:240-244.

Turner HH: A syndrome of infantilism, congenital webbed neck, and cubitus valgus. Endocrinology 1938; 23:566-574.

Wilkins L: Masculinization of the female fetus due to the use of orally given progestins. JAMA 1960; 172:1028-1032.

CHAPTER 54

THE MALE REPRODUCTIVE SYSTEM

Ervin E. Jones

The male reproductive system (Fig. 54-1A) consists of two essential elements: the *gonads* and the complex array of glands and conduits that constitute the **sex accessories**. The **gonads** in males are the testes, and they are responsible for the production of gametes, the haploid cells (spermatozoa) necessary for sexual reproduction. The gonads also synthesize and secrete the hormones that are necessary for functional conditioning of the sex organs, control of gonadotropin secretion, and modulation of sexual behavior.

The testis (Fig. 54-1B, C) is largely composed of seminiferous tubules and the interstitial cells of Leydig, located in the spaces between the tubules. The seminiferous tubules are lined by seminiferous epithelium, which rests on the inner surface of a basement membrane (Fig. 54-1D). The basement membrane is supported by a thin lamina propria externa.

The **sex accessories** in the male include the paired epididymides, the vas deferens, the seminal vesicles, and the ejaculatory ducts. Also included among the sex accessories are the prostate, the bulbourethral glands (Cowper's glands), the urethra, and the penis. The primary role of the male sex accessory glands and ducts is to store and transport spermatozoa to the exterior at the proper time, thus enabling spermatozoa to come in contact with and fertilize female gametes.

PUBERTY

Puberty occurs in five defined stages

During the final month of fetal life, the testes descend (see the box titled Androgen Dependence of Testicular Descent in Chapter 53) into an integumentary pouch called the scrotum. The inguinal canals through which the testes descend are sealed off shortly after birth. Because the internal temperature of the testicle must be closely regulated for optimum function, localization of the testes within the scrotum appears to be a necessary adaptation for testicular function. Aberrant retention of the testes in the abdominal cavity (cryptorchidism) causes marked damage to the seminiferous tubules and diminished testicular function.

Puberty is the transition between the juvenile and adult states, during which time the individual develops secondary sexual characteristics, experiences the adolescent growth spurt, and achieves the ability to procreate. The range of onset of normal male puberty extends from 9 to 14 years. Boys complete pubertal development within 2 to $4\frac{1}{2}$ years. In a normal boy, the first sign of puberty (stage 2) is enlargement of the testes to greater than 2.5 cm. Testicular enlargement is mainly a result of growth of the seminiferous tubules, but enlargement of the Leydig cells contributes as well. Androgens from the testes are the driving force behind secondary sexual development, although adrenal androgens play a role in normal puberty. The Tanner method of describing the stages of pubertal development is widely accepted. Genital development and growth of pubic hair are best described separately, as indicated by the two columns in Table 54-1. Thus, it is possible for an adolescent boy to be at genital stage 3, pubic hair stage 2.

Testicular size is generally determined by using a ruler or calipers. It is expected that a length greater than 2.5 cm is compatible with the onset of normal pubertal development. The **testicular volume index** is defined as the sum of the length times width product for the left and right testes. An orchidometer allows direct comparison of the patient's testes with an oval of measured volume. A popular method uses the Prader orchidometer, a set of solid or hollow ovals encompassing the range from infancy to adulthood (1 to 25 mL). The volumes of the testes are then recorded; a volume of 3 mL closely correlates with the onset of pubertal development.

Spermarchy, or the first appearance of spermatozoa in early morning urine, occurs at a mean age of ~13.4 years and corresponds to genital stages 3 to 4 and pubic hair stages 2 to 4. The **pubertal spurt**, a marked increase in growth rate (total body size), occurs late in puberty in boys, at genital stages 3 to 4. The acceleration of growth appears to be partly a result of increased secretion of growth hormone at puberty and partially a result of testosterone production. Boys experience, on average, 28 cm of growth during the pubertal spurt. The 10-cm mean difference in adult stature between men and women is the result of a greater pubertal growth spurt in boys and to greater height at the onset of peak height

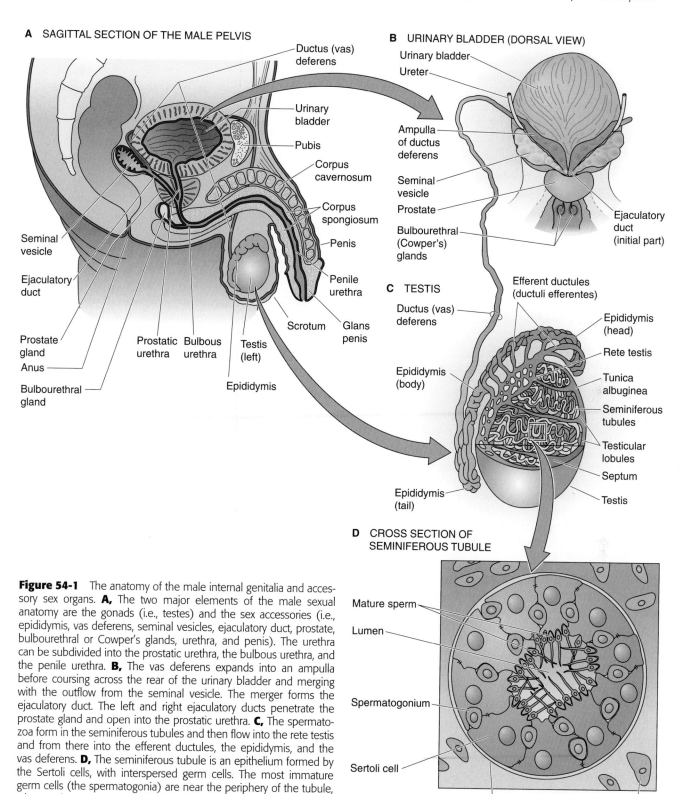

A SAGITTAL SECTION OF THE MALE PELVIS

- Ductus (vas) deferens
- Urinary bladder
- Pubis
- Corpus cavernosum
- Corpus spongiosum
- Penis
- Penile urethra
- Scrotum
- Glans penis
- Seminal vesicle
- Ejaculatory duct
- Prostate gland
- Anus
- Bulbourethral gland
- Prostatic urethra
- Bulbous urethra
- Testis (left)
- Epididymis

B URINARY BLADDER (DORSAL VIEW)

- Urinary bladder
- Ureter
- Ampulla of ductus deferens
- Seminal vesicle
- Prostate
- Bulbourethral (Cowper's) glands
- Ejaculatory duct (initial part)

C TESTIS

- Ductus (vas) deferens
- Epididymis (body)
- Epididymis (tail)
- Efferent ductules (ductuli efferentes)
- Epididymis (head)
- Rete testis
- Tunica albuginea
- Seminiferous tubules
- Testicular lobules
- Septum
- Testis

D CROSS SECTION OF SEMINIFEROUS TUBULE

- Mature sperm
- Lumen
- Spermatogonium
- Sertoli cell
- Basal lamina surrounding seminiferous tubule
- Leydig cell

Figure 54-1 The anatomy of the male internal genitalia and accessory sex organs. **A,** The two major elements of the male sexual anatomy are the gonads (i.e., testes) and the sex accessories (i.e., epididymis, vas deferens, seminal vesicles, ejaculatory duct, prostate, bulbourethral or Cowper's glands, urethra, and penis). The urethra can be subdivided into the prostatic urethra, the bulbous urethra, and the penile urethra. **B,** The vas deferens expands into an ampulla before coursing across the rear of the urinary bladder and merging with the outflow from the seminal vesicle. The merger forms the ejaculatory duct. The left and right ejaculatory ducts penetrate the prostate gland and open into the prostatic urethra. **C,** The spermatozoa form in the seminiferous tubules and then flow into the rete testis and from there into the efferent ductules, the epididymis, and the vas deferens. **D,** The seminiferous tubule is an epithelium formed by the Sertoli cells, with interspersed germ cells. The most immature germ cells (the spermatogonia) are near the periphery of the tubule, whereas the mature germ cells (the spermatozoa) are near the lumen of the tubule. The Leydig cells are interstitial cells that lie between the tubules.

Table 54-1 Stages in Male Puberty

Stage	Genital Development	Pubic Hair
1	Preadolescent: the penis, scrotum, and testes are the same size—relative to body size—as in a young child	Preadolescent: no pubic hair is present, only vellus hair, as on the abdomen
2	Scrotum and testes are enlarged	Pubic hair is sparse, mainly at the base of the penis
3	Penis is enlarged, predominantly in length; scrotum and testes are further enlarged	Pubic hair is darker, coarser, and curlier and spreads above the pubis
4	Penis is further enlarged in length and also in diameter; scrotum and testes are further enlarged	Pubic hair is of the adult type, but covers an area smaller than in most adults
5	Adult pattern	Adult pattern

velocity in boys versus girls. Before puberty, boys and girls have the same mean body mass, skeletal mass, and body fat. However, men have 150% of the average woman's lean and skeletal body mass, and women have 200% of the body fat of men. Men have twice the number of muscle cells that women have and 1.5 times the muscle mass.

Androgens determine male secondary sexual characteristics

The male sex steroids, which are known as androgens, affect nearly every tissue in the body, including the brain. The development of both the external and the internal genitalia depends on male sex hormones (see Chapter 53). Androgens stimulate adult maturation of the external genitalia and accessory sexual organs, including the penis, the scrotum, the prostate, and the seminal vesicles. Androgens also determine the male secondary sexual characteristics, which include deepening of the voice, as well as evolving male patterns of hair growth. The effects on the voice are a result of androgen-dependent effects on the size of the larynx, as well as the length and thickness of the vocal cords. In boys, the length of the vocal cords increases by ~50% during puberty, whereas girls have little increase in vocal cord length. The surfaces of the human body that bear secondary sexual hair include the face (particularly the upper lip, chin, and the sideburn areas), the axilla, and the pubic region. Temporal hair recession and male-pattern balding are also androgen-dependent phenomena.

Muscle development and growth are androgen-dependent processes

Androgens have anabolic effects, including stimulation of linear body growth, nitrogen retention, and muscular development in adolescent boys and in men. The biological effects of testosterone and its metabolites have been classified according to their tissue sites of action. Effects that relate to growth of the male reproductive tract or development of secondary sexual characteristics are referred to as **androgenic**, whereas the growth-promoting effects on somatic tissue are called **anabolic**. These androgenic and anabolic effects are two independent biological actions of the same class of steroids. Experimental evidence, however, indicates that these responses are organ specific and that the molecular mechanisms that initiate androgenic responses are the same as those that stimulate anabolic activity.

HYPOTHALAMIC-PITUITARY-GONADAL AXIS AND CONTROL OF MALE SEXUAL FUNCTION

The male hypothalamic-pituitary-gonadal axis (Fig. 54-2) controls two primary functions: (1) production of male gametes (spermatogenesis) in the seminiferous tubules and (2) androgen biosynthesis in the Leydig cells in the testes. The hypothalamus produces gonadotropin-releasing hormone (GnRH), which stimulates the gonadotrophs in the anterior pituitary to secrete the two gonadotropins, luteinizing hormone (LH) and follicle-stimulating hormone (FSH). As discussed in Chapter 55, the names of these hormones reflect their function in the female reproductive system. LH and FSH control, respectively, the Leydig and Sertoli cells of the testes.

The hypothalamus secretes GnRH, which acts on gonadotrophs in the anterior pituitary

GnRH, which is synthesized by small-bodied peptidergic neurons in the hypothalamus, stimulates the synthesis, storage, and secretion of gonadotropins by gonadotroph cells in the anterior pituitary. The hypothalamic-pituitary-portal system (see Chapter 47) describes the route by which GnRH and other releasing hormones emanating from the hypothalamus reach the anterior pituitary gland. The neurons that synthesize, store, and release GnRH are dispersed throughout the hypothalamus but are principally located in the arcuate nucleus and preoptic area. Studies involving both rats and primates showed that sites other than the hypothalamus (e.g., the limbic system) of GnRH production can also participate in the control of sex behavior. Neuronal systems originating from other areas of the brain impinge on the hypothalamic GnRH-releasing neurons and thus form a functional neuronal network.

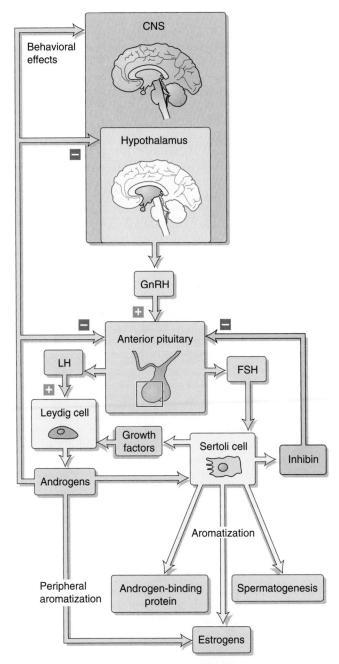

Figure 54-2 The hypothalamic-pituitary-testicular axis. Small-bodied neurons in the arcuate nucleus and preoptic area of the hypothalamus secrete GnRH, a decapeptide that reaches the gonadotrophs in the anterior pituitary through the long portal veins. Stimulation by GnRH causes the gonadotrophs to synthesize and release FSH and LH. The LH binds to receptors on the Leydig cells, thus stimulating the transcription of several proteins involved in the biosynthesis of testosterone. FSH binds to receptors on the basolateral membrane of the Sertoli cells, thereby stimulating gene transcription and protein synthesis. These proteins include ABP, aromatase, growth factors, and inhibin. Negative feedback on the hypothalamic-pituitary-testicular axis occurs by two routes. First, testosterone inhibits the pulsatile release of GnRH by the hypothalamic neurons and the release of LH by the gonadotrophs in the anterior pituitary. Second, inhibin inhibits the release of FSH by the gonadotrophs in the anterior pituitary.

GnRH is a decapeptide hormone synthesized by aforementioned hypothalamic neurons in the secretory pathway (see Chapter 2). Like many other peptide hormones, GnRH is synthesized as a prohormone—69 amino acids long in this case—from which the mature GnRH is generated by enzymatic cleavage. The synthesis of GnRH is discussed in more detail in Chapter 55. The neurons release GnRH into the extracellular space, to be carried to the anterior pituitary through the long portal vessels.

GnRH stimulates the release of both FSH and LH from the gonadotroph cells of the anterior pituitary. FSH and LH are the primary gonadotropins; in males, they stimulate testicular function. The cell surface of the pituitary gonadotrophs is the site of high-affinity membrane receptors for GnRH. These receptors are coupled to the G protein $G\alpha_q$, which activates phospholipase C (PLC; see Chapter 3). PLC acts on membrane phosphoinositides to liberate inositol 1,4,5-triphosphate (IP_3), which triggers Ca^{2+} release from internal stores, and diacylglycerol (DAG), which stimulates protein kinase C. The results are the synthesis and release of both LH and FSH from the gonadotrophs. Because secretion of GnRH into the portal system is pulsatile, secretion of both LH and FSH by the gonadotrophs is also episodic. The frequency of pulsatile LH discharge in men is ~8 to 14 pulses over a 24-hour period. FSH pulses are not as prominent as LH pulses, both because of their lower amplitude and because of the longer half-life of FSH in the circulation.

Although pulsatile GnRH discharge elicits a corresponding pulsatile release of LH and FSH, *continuous* administration of GnRH—or intermittent administration of high doses of GnRH analogues—suppresses the release of gonadotropins. As described in the box titled Therapeutic Uses of GnRH in Chapter 55, the mechanism is inhibition of the replenishment of GnRH receptors so that insufficient receptors are available for GnRH function. A clinical application of this principle is in prostatic cancer, in which the administration of GnRH analogues lowers LH and FSH levels and thereby reduces testosterone production (i.e., chemical castration).

Products of the testes, particularly sex steroids and inhibin (see later), exert negative feedback control on hypothalamic and anterior pituitary function. Neural elements in the arcuate nucleus respond to sex steroids. Sex steroids alter the frequency and amplitude of the LH secretory pulses in both men and women. Androgens also exert powerful influences on higher brain function, as evidenced by alterations in sex behavior.

Under the control of GnRH, gonadotrophs in the anterior pituitary secrete LH and FSH

LH and FSH, which are secreted by the gonadotrophs of the anterior pituitary, are the primary regulators of testicular function. LH and FSH are members of the same family of hormones as human chorionic gonadotropin (hCG; see Chapter 56) and thyroid-stimulating hormone (TSH; see Chapter 49). All these glycoprotein hormones are composed of two polypeptide chains designated α and β. Both subunits, α and β, are required for full biological activity. The α subunits of LH and FSH, as well as the α subunits of hCG and TSH, are identical. In humans, the common α subunit has 92 amino acids and a molecular weight of ~20 kDa. The β subunits differ among these four hormones and thus confer specific functional and immunologic characteristics to the intact molecules.

Each of the unique β subunits of FSH and LH is 115 amino acids in length. The β subunits of LH and hCG are identical, except the β subunit of hCG has an additional 24 amino acids and additional glycosylation sites at the C terminus. hCG is secreted by the placenta, and some reports have described that small amounts of this substance are made in the testes, pituitary gland, and other nonplacental tissue. The biological activities of LH and hCG are very similar. Indeed, in most clinical uses (e.g., in an attempt to initiate spermatogenesis in oligospermic men), hCG is substituted for LH because hCG is much more readily available.

The specific gonadotropin and the relative proportions of each gonadotropin released from the anterior pituitary depend on the developmental age, as well as the existing hormonal milieu. The pituitary gland of the male fetus contains functional gonadotrophs by the end of the first trimester of gestation. Thereafter, gonadotropin secretion rises rapidly and then plateaus. Gonadotropin secretion begins to decline in utero during late fetal life and increases again during the early postnatal period.

Male primates release LH in response to GnRH administration at 1 to 3 months of age, a finding indicative of functional competence of the anterior pituitary gland. Also during this time, a short-lived postnatal surge of LH and testosterone secretion occurs in males. Although the cause of this short-lived surge of gonadotropins remains to be understood, it is clearly independent of sex steroids. The sensitivity of the gonadotrophs to stimulation subsequently diminishes, and the system remains quiescent until just before puberty.

Release of FSH is greater than that of LH during the prepubertal period, a pattern that is reversed after puberty. GnRH preferentially triggers LH release in men. This preferential release of LH may reflect maturation of the testes, which secrete inhibin, a specific inhibitor of FSH secretion at the level of the anterior pituitary gland. Increased sensitivity of the pituitary to increasing gonadal steroid production may also be responsible for the diminished secretion of FSH.

Luteinizing hormone stimulates the Leydig (interstitial) cells of the testis to produce testosterone

LH derives its name from effects observed in the female, that is, from the ability to stimulate luteal function. The comparable substance in the male was originally referred to as interstitial cell–stimulating hormone (ICSH). Subsequently, investigators realized that LH and ICSH are the same substance, and the common name became LH.

Testosterone production decreases in males after hypophysectomy. This observation led to our current understanding that LH secreted by the anterior pituitary gland is essential for testosterone production by the testis. The interstitial cells of the testis, the **Leydig cells**, are the primary source of testosterone production in the male. Leydig cells synthesize

androgens from cholesterol by using a series of enzymes that are part of the steroid biosynthetic pathways (see later).

LH binds to specific high-affinity cell surface receptors on the plasma membrane of Leydig cells (Fig. 54-3). Binding of LH to this G protein–coupled receptor on the Leydig cell stimulates membrane-bound adenylyl cyclase (see Chapter 3), which catalyzes the formation of cAMP and thus activates protein kinase A (PKA). Activated PKA modulates gene transcription (see Chapter 4) and increases the synthesis of enzymes and other proteins necessary for the biosynthesis of testosterone. Two of these other proteins are the sterol-carrier protein (SCP-2) and the steroidogenic acute regulatory protein or (StAR or STARD1). **SCP** is a 13.5-kDa protein that appears to transport cholesterol from the plasma membrane or organellar membranes to other organellar membranes, including the outer mitochondrial membrane.

StAR belongs to a large family of proteins that contain a ~210-residue START domain and are involved in lipid trafficking and metabolism. The 37-kDa **pro-StAR** protein—the precursor to StAR—may participate in ferrying cholesterol from the endoplasmic reticulum (ER) to the outer mitochondrial membrane. The 30-kDa **mature StAR protein** resides in the mitochondrial intermembrane space (see Fig. 58-10) and extracts cholesterol from the mitochondrial outer membrane, ferries it across the space to the mitochondrial inner membrane, and then deposits the cholesterol in the mitochondrial inner membrane where the cytochrome P-450 side-chain–cleavage (SCC) (P-450$_{scc}$) enzyme is located. As discussed later, the P-450$_{scc}$–mediated conversion of cholesterol to pregnenolone is the rate-limiting step in steroidogenesis—including testosterone synthesis. Thus, the net effect of LH on Leydig cells is to stimulate testosterone synthesis.

Follicle-stimulating hormone stimulates the sertoli cells to synthesize certain products needed by both the Leydig cells and the developing spermatogonia

The Sertoli cells seem to be the primary testicular site of FSH action (Fig. 54-3), as clearly shown by experiments involving suppression of LH secretion. FSH also regulates Leydig cell physiology through effects on the Sertoli cells. The early biochemical events after FSH binding are similar to those described for LH on the Leydig cell. Thus, binding of FSH to a G protein–coupled receptor initiates a series of reactions involving stimulation of adenylyl cyclase, increase in [cAMP]$_i$, stimulation of PKA, transcription of specific genes, and increased protein synthesis. Several proteins are synthesized in response to FSH. Some are important for steroid action:

1. FSH leads to the synthesis of **androgen-binding protein (ABP)**, which is secreted into the luminal space of the seminiferous tubule, near the developing sperm cells. ABP helps to keep local testosterone levels high (see Chapter 53).
2. FSH causes the synthesis of a **P-450 aromatase** (P-450$_{arom}$; see Chapter 55). Inside the Sertoli cells, this enzyme converts testosterone, which diffuses from the Leydig cells to the Sertoli cells, into estradiol.

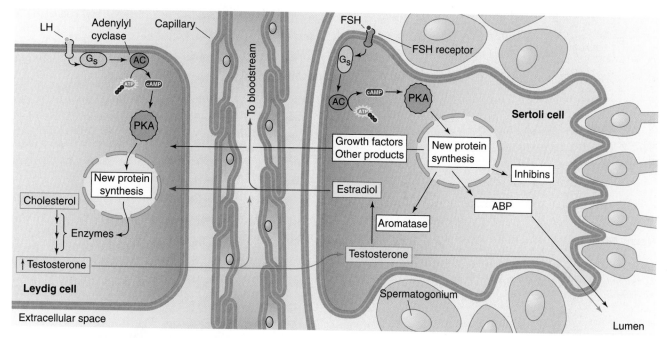

Figure 54-3 Physiology of the Leydig and Sertoli cells. The Leydig cell *(left)* has receptors for LH. The binding of LH increases testosterone synthesis. The Sertoli cell *(right)* has receptors for FSH. (Useful mnemonics: "L" for LH and Leydig, "S" for FSH and Sertoli.) FSH promotes the synthesis of ABP, aromatase, growth factors, and inhibin. Crosstalk occurs between the Leydig cells and the Sertoli cells. The Leydig cells make testosterone, which acts on the Sertoli cells. Conversely, the Sertoli cells convert some of this testosterone to estradiol (because of the presence of aromatase), which can act on the Leydig cells. The Sertoli cells also generate growth factors that act on the Leydig cells.

3. FSH leads to the production of certain **growth factors** and other products by the Sertoli cells that support sperm cells and spermatogenesis. These substances significantly increase the number of spermatogonia, spermatocytes, and spermatids in the testis. Therefore, it appears that the stimulatory effect of FSH on spermatogenesis is not a direct action of FSH on the spermatogonia; instead, stimulation of spermatogenesis occurs through the action of FSH on the Sertoli cells. FSH may also increase the fertility potential of sperm; it appears that this effect of FSH results from stimulation of motility, rather than from an increase in the absolute number of sperm.

4. FSH causes the Sertoli cells to synthesize **inhibins**. The inhibins are members of the so-called transforming growth factor β (TGF-β) gene family, which also includes the activins and antimüllerian hormone (see Chapter 53). Inhibins are glycoprotein heterodimers consisting of one α and one β subunit that are covalently linked. The granulosa cells in the ovary and the Sertoli cells in the testis are the primary sources of inhibin in humans, other primates, and the lower vertebrates. I discuss the biology of inhibins and activins in more detail in Chapter 55. Inhibins are secreted into the seminiferous tubule fluid and into the interstitial fluid of the testicle. Inhibins have both paracrine and endocrine actions. Locally, the inhibins are some of the growth factors secreted by the Sertoli cells that are thought to act on the Leydig cells. More importantly, inhibins in the male play an important feedback role in the hypothalamic-pituitary-testicular axis (see later).

The Leydig cells and the Sertoli cells engage in **crosstalk**. For example, the Leydig cells make testosterone, which acts on the Sertoli cells. In the rat, β endorphin produced by the fetal Leydig cells binds to opiate receptors in the Sertoli cells and inhibits their multiplication. Synthesis of β endorphins could represent a local feedback mechanism by which the Leydig cells modulate the Sertoli cell numbers. Conversely, the Sertoli cells also have an effect on the Leydig cells. For example, the Sertoli cells convert testosterone—manufactured by the Leydig cells—to estradiol, which then acts on the Leydig cells. In addition, FSH acting on the Sertoli cells produces growth factors that may increase the number of LH receptors on the Leydig cells during development and may thus result in an increase in steroidogenesis (i.e., an increase in testosterone production).

What, then, is required for optimal spermatogenesis to occur? It appears that two testicular cell types (the Leydig cells and the Sertoli cells) are required, as well as two gonadotropins (LH and FSH) and one androgen (testosterone). First, LH and the Leydig cells are required to produce testosterone. Thus, LH, or rather its substitute hCG, is used therapeutically to initiate spermatogenesis in azoospermic or oligospermic men. Second, FSH and the Sertoli cells are important for the nursing of developing sperm cells and for the production of inhibin and growth factors, which affect the Leydig cells. Thus, FSH plays a primary role in regulating development of the appropriate number of the Leydig cells such that adequate testosterone levels are available for spermatogenesis. During early puberty in boys, both FSH and LH levels increase while, simultaneously, the Leydig cells

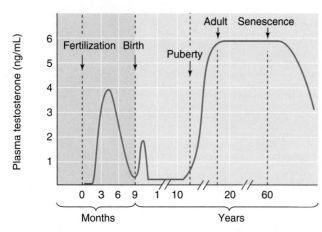

Figure 54-4 Plasma testosterone versus age in male humans. *(Data from Griffin JE, et al: In Bondy PK, Rosenberg LE: Metabolic Control and Disease. Philadelphia: WB Saunders, 1980; and Winter JS, Hughes IA, Reyes FI, Faiman C: J Clin Endocrinol Metab 1976; 42:679-686.)*

proliferate and plasma levels of testosterone increase (Fig. 54-4).

The hypothalamic-pituitary-testicular axis is under reciprocal inhibition by testicular hormones and inhibin

The hypothalamic-pituitary-testicular axis not only generates testosterone and inhibin but also receives negative feedback from these substances (Fig. 54-2). Normal circulating levels of both testosterone and estradiol exert inhibitory effects on LH secretion in males. Testosterone inhibits the pulsatile release of LH, presumably by inhibiting the pulsatile release of GnRH by the hypothalamus. Testosterone also appears to have negative feedback action on LH secretion at the level of the pituitary gonadotrophs.

A testicular hormone also feeds back on FSH secretion. Evidence for negative feedback by a testicular substance on FSH secretion is that plasma FSH concentrations increase in proportion to the loss of germinal elements in the testis. The FSH-inhibiting substance—inhibin—is a nonsteroid present in both the testis and cultures of Sertoli cells. Thus, FSH specifically stimulates the Sertoli cells to produce inhibin, and inhibin "inhibits" FSH secretion. The preponderance of evidence indicates that inhibin diminishes FSH secretion by acting at the level of the anterior pituitary gland (not at the level of the hypothalamus).

TESTOSTERONE

The Leydig cells of the testis synthesize and secrete testosterone

Cholesterol is the obligate precursor for androgens, as well as for other steroids produced by the testis. The Leydig cell can synthesize cholesterol de novo from acetyl coenzyme A or can take it up as low-density lipoproteins from the extracellular fluid by receptor-mediated endocytosis (see Chapter 1). The two sources appear to be equally important in humans.

The **Leydig cell** uses a series of five enzymes to convert cholesterol to testosterone. Three of these enzymes are P-450 enzymes (see Table 50-2). As summarized in Figure 54-5, because 3β-hydroxysteroid dehydrogenase (3β-HSD) can oxidize the A ring of four intermediates, testosterone synthesis from cholesterol can take four pathways. The following is the "preferred" pathway:

1. The pathway for testosterone synthesis begins in the mitochondria, where P-450$_{scc}$ (also called 20,22-desmolase) removes the long side chain (carbons 22 to 27) from the carbon at position 20 of the **cholesterol** molecule (27 carbon atoms). The rate-limiting step in the biosynthesis of testosterone, as for other steroid hormones, is the conversion of cholesterol to pregnenolone. LH stimulates this reaction and is the primary regulator of the overall rate of testosterone synthesis by the Leydig cell. LH appears to promote pregnenolone synthesis in two ways. First, it increases the affinity of the enzyme for cholesterol. Second, LH has long-term action in which it increases steroidogenesis in the testis by stimulating synthesis of the SCC enzyme.
2. The product of the SCC-catalyzed reaction is **pregnenolone** (21 carbon atoms). In the smooth ER (SER), 17α-hydroxylase (P-450$_{c17}$) then adds a hydroxyl group at position 17 to form **17α-hydroxypregnenolone**.
3. In the SER, the 17,20-desmolase (a different activity of the *same* P-450$_{c17}$ whose 17α-hydroxylase activity catalyzes the previous step) removes the side chain from carbon 17 of 17α-hydroxypregnenolone. That side chain begins with carbon 20. The result is a 19-carbon steroid called **dehydroepiandrosterone (DHEA)**.
4. In the SER of the Leydig cell, a 17β-hydroxysteroid dehydrogenase (17β-HSD, which is *not* a P-450 enzyme) converts the ketone at position 17 to a hydroxyl group to form **androstenediol**.
5. Finally, 3β-HSD (*not* a P-450 enzyme) oxidizes the hydroxyl group at position 3 of the A ring to a ketone to form **testosterone**.

In addition, the testis can also use 5α-reductase, which is located in the SER, to convert testosterone to dihydrotestosterone (DHT). However, extratesticular tissue is responsible for most of the production of DHT. The conversion of testosterone to DHT is especially important in certain testosterone target cells (see Chapter 53).

The Leydig cells of the testes make ~95% of the circulating testosterone. Although testosterone is the major secretory product, the testis also secretes pregnenolone, progesterone, 17-hydroxyprogesterone, androstenedione, androsterone, and DHT. Androstenedione is of major importance because it serves as a precursor for extraglandular estrogen formation.

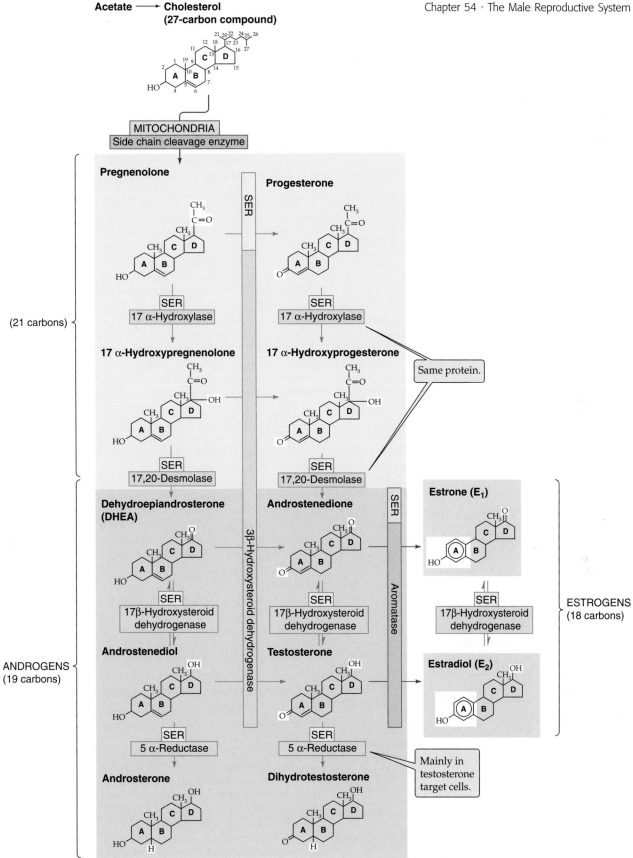

Figure 54-5 Biosynthesis of testosterone. This scheme summarizes the synthesis of the androgens from cholesterol. The individual enzymes are shown in the *horizontal and vertical boxes*; they are located in either the SER or the mitochondria. The SCC enzyme that produces pregnenolone is also known as 20,22 desmolase. The chemical groups modified by each enzyme are *highlighted* in the reaction product. Four possible pathways from pregnenolone to testosterone are recognized; the preferred pathway in the human testis appears to be the one along the *left edge of the figure* to androstenediol, followed by oxidation of the A ring to testosterone. Some of these pathways are shared in the biosynthesis of the glucocorticoids and mineralocorticoids (see Fig. 50-2) as well as estrogens (see Fig. 55-9).

Table 54-2 Androgen Production and Turnover

Steroid	Blood Production Rate: Hormone Delivered to the Blood (µg/day)	Plasma Concentration (µg/L)
Testosterone	6500	6.5
Androstenedione	2000-6000	1.5
Dihydrotestosterone	300	0.5

Other organs—such as adipose tissue, skin, and the adrenal cortex—also produce testosterone and other androgens

In men between the ages of 25 and 70 years, the rate of testosterone production remains relatively constant (Table 54-2). Figure 54-4 summarizes the changes in plasma testosterone levels as a function of age in male humans.

Several tissues besides the testes—including adipose tissue, brain, muscle, skin, and adrenal cortex—produce testosterone and several other androgens. These substances may be synthesized de novo or produced by peripheral conversion of precursors. Moreover, the peripheral organs and tissues may convert sex steroids to less active forms (Fig. 54-5). Notable sites of extragonadal conversion include the skin and adipose tissue. Androstenedione is converted to testosterone in peripheral tissues. In this case, **androstenedione** is the precursor for the hormone testosterone. Testosterone can be converted to estradiol or DHT or go "backward" by reversible interconversion to androstenedione. Thus, a potent hormone such as testosterone may also serve as a precursor for a weaker hormone (androstenedione), a hormone with different activities (estradiol), or a more potent hormone having similar activities (DHT). This last example may be illustrated by the effects of DHT on hair follicles, sebaceous glands, and the sex accessories.

The adrenal gland (see Chapter 50) is another source of androgen production in both males and females. Normal human adrenal glands synthesize and secrete the androgens DHEA, conjugated DHEA sulfate, and androstenedione. Essentially, all the DHEA in male plasma is of adrenal origin. However, less than 1% of the total testosterone in plasma is derived from DHEA. As summarized in Table 54-2, the plasma concentration of androstenedione in males is only ~25% that of testosterone. About 20% of androstenedione is generated by peripheral metabolism of other steroids. Although the adrenal gland contributes significantly to the total androgen milieu in males, it does not appear to have significant effects on stimulation and growth of the male accessory organs.

Testosterone acts on target organs by binding to a nuclear receptor

Most testosterone in the circulation is bound to specific binding proteins. About 45% of plasma testosterone is bound to **sex hormone–binding globulin (SHBG)**—also called testosterone-binding globulin (TeBG), whereas ~55% is bound to serum albumin and corticosteroid-binding globulin

(CBG) (see Chapter 50). A small fraction (~2%) of the total circulating testosterone circulates free, or unbound, in plasma. The free form of testosterone enters the cell by passive diffusion and subsequently exerts biological actions or undergoes metabolism by other organs such as the prostate, liver, and intestines (see the next section). The quantity of testosterone entering a cell is determined by the plasma concentration and by the intracellular milieu of enzymes and binding proteins.

Once it diffuses into the cell, testosterone either binds to a high-affinity androgen receptor in the nucleus or is converted to DHT, which also binds to the androgen receptor. The androgen receptor functions as a homodimer (AR/AR) and is a member of the family of nuclear receptors (see Table 4-2) that includes receptors for glucocorticoids, mineralocorticoids, progestins, estrogens, vitamin D, thyroid hormone, and retinoic acid. The gene coding for the androgen receptor is located on the X chromosome. The androgen receptor is a protein with a molecular weight of ~110 kDa. The androgen-AR complex is a transcription factor that binds to hormone response elements on DNA located 5′ from the genes that the androgens control. Interaction between the androgen-AR complex and nuclear chromatin causes marked increases in transcription, ultimately leading to the synthesis of specific proteins. As a result of these synthetic processes, specific cell functions ensue, including growth and development. The presence of the androgen receptor in a cell or tissue determines whether that tissue can respond to androgens.

Whether the active compound in any tissue is DHT or testosterone depends on the presence or absence in that tissue of the microsomal enzyme **5α-reductase**, which converts testosterone to DHT. The biological activity of DHT is 30 to 50 times higher than that of testosterone. Some tissues, including the brain, aromatize testosterone to estradiol, and thus the action of this metabolite occurs through the estrogen receptor.

Some of the effects of androgens may be nongenomic. For example, androgens may stimulate hepatic microsomal protein synthesis by a mechanism independent of binding to the androgen receptor. Other evidence indicates that the action of androgens on the prostate gland may occur through

Testosterone and the Aging Man

For a long time, the abrupt hormonal alterations that signal the dramatic changes of female menopause were believed to have no correlate in men. We now know that men do experience a gradual decline in their serum testosterone levels (Fig. 54-4) and that this decline is closely correlated with many of the changes that accompany aging: decreases in bone formation, muscle mass, growth of facial hair, appetite, and libido. The blood hematocrit also decreases. Testosterone replacement can reverse many of these changes by restoring muscle and bone mass and correcting the anemia.

Although the levels of both total and free testosterone decline with age, levels of LH are frequently not elevated. This finding is believed to indicate that some degree of hypothalamic-pituitary dysfunction accompanies aging.

the adenylyl cyclase/PKA system (see Chapter 4) and could result in gene activation under some circumstances.

Metabolism of testosterone occurs primarily in the liver and prostate

Only small amounts of testosterone enter the urine without metabolism; this urinary testosterone represents less than 2% of the daily testosterone production. The large remaining balance of testosterone and other androgens is converted in the liver to 17-ketosteroids and in the prostate to DHT. The degradation products of testosterone are primarily excreted in the urine as water-soluble conjugates of either sulfuric acid or glucuronic acid. These conjugated testosterone metabolites are also excreted in the feces.

BIOLOGY OF SPERMATOGENESIS AND SEMEN

Spermatogenesis includes the mitotic divisions of spermatogonia, the meiotic divisions of spermatocytes to haploid spermatids, and maturation to spermatozoa

Mature spermatozoa are derived from germ cells through a series of complex transformations. When seminiferous tubules are viewed in cross section (Fig. 54-1D), the least mature cells are located adjacent to the basement membrane, whereas the most differentiated germ cells are located nearest the lumen.

As discussed in Chapter 53, the primordial germ cells migrate into the gonad during embryogenesis; these cells become immature germ cells, or **spermatogonia** (Fig. 54-6). Beginning at puberty and continuing thereafter throughout life, these spermatogonia, which lie next to the basement membrane of the stratified epithelium lining the seminiferous tubules, divide mitotically (Fig. 54-7). The spermatogonia have the normal diploid complement of 46 chromosomes (2N): 22 pairs of autosomal chromosomes plus 1 X and 1 Y chromosome.

Some of the spermatogonia enter into their first meiotic division and become **primary spermatocytes**. At the prophase of this first meiotic division, the chromosomes undergo crossing over (see Fig. 53-1). At this stage, each cell has a duplicated set of 46 chromosomes (4N): 22 pairs of duplicated autosomal chromosomes, a duplicated X chromosome, and a duplicated Y chromosome. After completing this first meiotic division, the daughter cells become **secondary spermatocytes**, which have a haploid number of duplicated chromosomes (2N): 22 duplicated autosomal chromosomes and either a duplicated X or a duplicated Y chromosome. These secondary spermatocytes enter their second meiotic division almost immediately. This division results in smaller cells called spermatids, which have a *haploid* number of *unduplicated* chromosomes (1N). **Spermatids** form the inner layer of the epithelium and are found in rather discrete aggregates inasmuch as the cells derived from a single spermatogonium tend to remain together—with cytoplasm linked in a syncytium—and differentiate synchronously. Spermatids transform into **spermatozoa** in

a process called **spermiogenesis**, which involves cytoplasmic reduction and differentiation of the tail pieces. Thus, as maturation progresses, developing male gametes decrease in volume. Conversely, maturation leads to an increase in cell number, with each primary spermatocyte producing four spermatozoa, two with an X chromosome and two with a Y chromosome.

As additional generations of spermatogonia mature, the advanced cells are displaced toward the lumen of the tubule. Groups of spermatogonia at comparable stages of development undergo mitosis simultaneously. Transformation of spermatogonia into functional spermatozoa requires ~74 days. Each stage of spermatogenesis has a specific duration. In humans, the life span of the germ cells is 16 to 18 days for spermatogonia, 23 days for primary spermatocytes, 1 day for secondary spermatocytes, and ~23 days for spermatids. The rate of spermatogenesis is constant and cannot be accelerated by hormones such as gonadotropins or androgens. Germ cells must move forward in their differentiation; if the environment is unfavorable and makes it impossible for them to pursue their differentiation at the normal rate, they degenerate and are eliminated.

The most reliable expression of the sperm production rate is the daily number of sperm cells produced per gram of testicular parenchyma. In 20-year-old men, the production rate is ~6.5 million sperm per gram per day. The rate falls progressively with age and averages ~3.8 million sperm per gram per day in men 50 to 90 years old. This decrease is probably related to the high rate of degeneration of germ cells during meiotic prophase. Among fertile men, those aged 51 to 90 years exhibit a significant decrease in the percentage of morphologically normal and motile spermatozoa.

In summary, three processes occur concurrently in the seminiferous epithelium: (1) an increase in the number of cells by mitosis, (2) a reduction in the number of chromosomes by meiosis, and (3) the production of mature sperm from spermatids by spermiogenesis. Thus, spermatogenesis is a regular, ordered, sequential process resulting in the production of mature male gametes.

It is instructive to consider how spermatogenesis in the male differs from oogenesis in the female. In fact, the two processes differ in each of the three steps just noted: (1) in the female, the *mitotic* proliferation of germ cells takes place entirely before birth, whereas in the male, spermatogonia proliferate only after puberty and then throughout life; (2) the *meiotic* divisions of a primary oocyte in the female produce only one mature ovum, whereas in the male, the meiotic divisions of a primary spermatocyte produce four mature spermatozoa; and (3) in the female, the second meiotic division is completed only on fertilization (see Chapter 56) and thus no further development of the cell takes place after the completion of meiosis, whereas in the male, the products of meiosis (the spermatids) undergo substantial further differentiation to produce mature spermatozoa.

The Sertoli cells support spermatogenesis

The Sertoli cells are generally regarded as support or nurse cells for the spermatids (Fig. 54-7). The **Sertoli cells** are

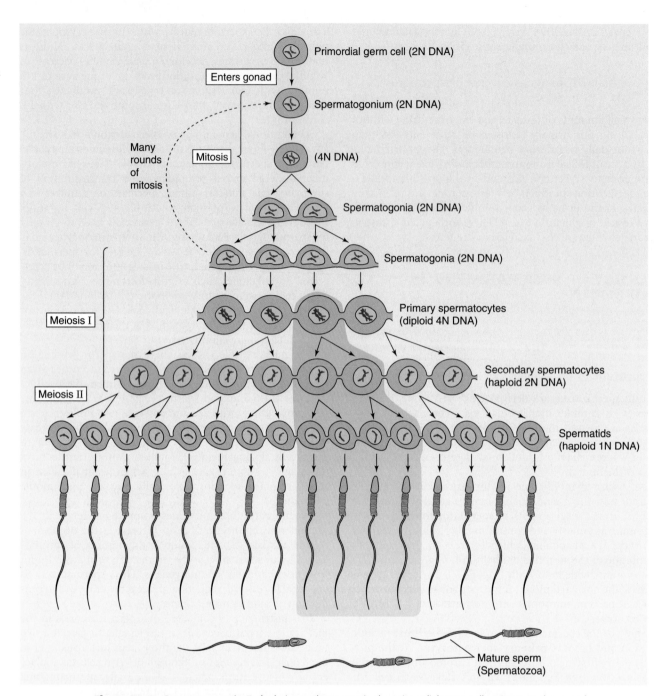

Figure 54-6 Spermatogenesis. Early during embryogenesis, the primordial germ cells migrate to the gonad, where they become spermatogonia. Beginning at puberty, the spermatogonia undergo many rounds of mitotic division. Some of these spermatogonia (2N DNA) enter the first meiotic division, at which time they are referred to as *primary spermatocytes*. During prophase, each primary spermatocyte has a full complement of duplicated chromosomes (4N DNA). Each primary spermatocyte divides into two secondary spermatocytes, each with a haploid number of duplicated chromosomes (2N DNA). The secondary spermatocyte enters the second meiotic division, producing two spermatids, each of which has a haploid number of unduplicated chromosomes (1N DNA). Further maturation of the spermatids yields the spermatozoa (mature sperm). One primary spermatocyte yields four spermatozoa.

large, polyhedral cells extending from the basement membrane toward the lumen of the seminiferous tubule. Spermatids are located adjacent to the lumen of the seminiferous tubules during the early stages of spermiogenesis and are surrounded by processes of Sertoli cell cytoplasm. Tight

junctions connect the adjacent Sertoli cells, to forming a blood-testis barrier—analogous to the blood-brain barrier (see Chapter 11)—that presumably provides a protective environment for developing germ cells. In addition, gap junctions between the Sertoli cells and developing sperma-

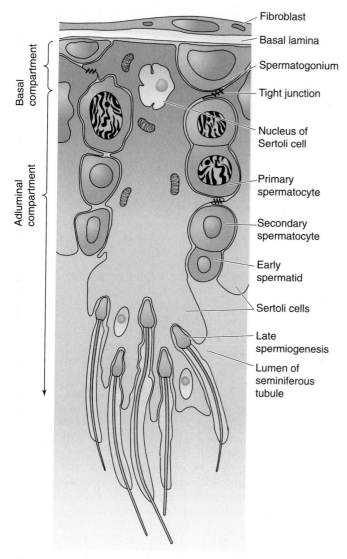

Fibroblast
Basal lamina
Spermatogonium
Tight junction
Nucleus of Sertoli cell
Primary spermatocyte
Secondary spermatocyte
Early spermatid
Sertoli cells
Late spermiogenesis
Lumen of seminiferous tubule

Basal compartment

Adluminal compartment

Figure 54-7 Interaction of the Sertoli cells and sperm. This figure is an idealized high-magnification view of a portion of the wall of a seminiferous tubule (see Fig. 54-1C). A single Sertoli cell spans from the basal lamina to the lumen of the seminiferous tubule. The adjacent Sertoli cells are connected by tight junctions and surround developing germ cells. From the basal lamina to the lumen of the tubule, gradual maturation of the germ cells occurs.

tozoa may represent a mechanism for transferring material between these two types of cells. Release of the spermatozoa from the Sertoli cell has been called **spermiation**. Spermatids progressively move toward the lumen of the tubule and eventually lose all contact with the Sertoli cell after spermiation.

Sperm maturation occurs in the epididymis

The seminiferous tubules open into a network of tubules, the **rete testes**, which serve as a reservoir for sperm. The rete testes are connected to the epididymis through the **efferent ductules** (see Chapter 53), which are located near the superior pole of the testicle. The **epididymis** is a highly convoluted single long duct, 4 to 5 m in total length, on the

The Sertoli Cell–Only Syndrome

Investigators have described a group of normally virilized men whose testes are small bilaterally and whose ejaculates contain no sperm cells (azoospermia). The seminiferous tubules of these men are lined by the Sertoli cells, but the tubules show a complete absence of germ cells. The Sertoli cell–only syndrome (or germinal cell aplasia) accounts for 10% to 30% of male infertility secondary to azoospermia and can either be caused by a single-gene defect or be acquired (e.g., as a result of orchitis, alcoholism, toxic agents). The Leydig cell function is usually preserved. Plasma testosterone and LH levels are usually normal, whereas FSH levels are often, but not always, elevated. It is not entirely clear why FSH levels are elevated in these men. This elevation may result from the absence of germ cells or from suboptimal secretion of inhibin by the Sertoli cells, inasmuch as inhibin is a powerful inhibitor of FSH secretion at the level of the anterior pituitary gland. Segments of Sertoli cell–only tubules may be observed in conditions such as orchitis or exposure to other agents that are toxic to the gonads. However, these individuals generally have functional spermatogenesis in the other seminiferous tubules.

posterior aspect of the testis. The epididymis can be divided anatomically into three regions: the head (the segment closest to the testis), the body, and the tail.

Spermatozoa are essentially immotile on completion of spermiogenesis. Thus, transfer of spermatozoa from the seminiferous tubule to the rete testes is passive. Secretions flow from the testes through the epididymis, with assistance by ciliary action of the luminal epithelium and contractility of the smooth muscle elements of the efferent duct wall. Thus, sperm transport through this ductal system is also primarily passive. As noted earlier, ~74 days is required to produce spermatozoa, ~50 days of which is spent in the seminiferous tubule. After leaving the testes, sperm take 12 to 26 days to travel through the epididymis and appear in the ejaculate. The epididymal transit time for men between the ages of 20 and 80 years does not differ significantly.

Sperm are stored in the epididymis, where they undergo a process of maturation before they are capable of progressive motility and fertilization (Table 54-3). Spermatozoa released at ejaculation are fully motile and capable of fertilization, whereas spermatozoa obtained directly from the testis are functionally immature insofar as they cannot penetrate an ovum. However, these immature spermatozoa can fertilize if they are injected into an ovum. During maturation in the epididymis, spermatozoa undergo changes in motility, metabolism, and morphology. Spermatozoa derived from the head (caput) of the epididymis (Fig. 54-1C) are often unable to fertilize ova, whereas larger proportions of spermatozoa captured from the body (corpus) are fertile. Spermatozoa obtained from the tail (cauda) of the epididymis, or from the vas deferens, are almost always capable of fertilization.

The epididymis empties into the **vas deferens**, which is responsible for the movement of sperm along the tract. The

Table 54-3 Sperm Maturation in the Epididymis

Progressive increase in forward motility
Increased ability to fertilize
Maturation of acrosome
Molecular reorganization of the plasma membrane: Lipids (stabilization of plasma membrane) Proteins (shedding as well as acquisition of new proteins)
Ability to bind to zona pellucida
Acquisition of receptors for proteins of the zona pellucida
Increased disulfide bonds between cysteine residues in sperm nucleoproteins
Topographic regionalization of glycosidic residues
Accumulation of mannosylated residues on the periacrosomal plasma membrane
Decreased cytoplasm and cell volume

Table 54-4 Normal Values for Semen

Parameter	Value
Volume	2-6 mL
Viscosity	Liquefaction in 1 hr
pH	7-8
Count	≥20 million/mL
Motility	≥50%
Morphology	60% normal

vas deferens contains well-developed muscle layers that facilitate sperm movement. The vas deferens passes through the inguinal canal, traverses the ureter, and continues medially to the posterior and inferior aspect of the urinary bladder, where it is joined by the duct arising from the **seminal vesicle**; together, they form the ejaculatory duct. The **ejaculatory duct** enters the prostatic portion of the urethra after passing through the prostate. Sperm are stored in the epididymis as well as in the proximal end of the vas deferens. All these accessory structures depend on androgens secreted by the testis for full functional development.

The accessory male sex glands—the seminal vesicles, prostate, and bulbourethral glands—produce the seminal plasma

Only 10% of the volume of **semen** (i.e., seminal fluid) is sperm cells. The normal concentration of sperm cells is greater than 20 million/mL, and the typical ejaculate volume is greater than 2 mL. The typical ejaculate content varies between 150 and 600 million spermatozoa.

Aside from the sperm cells, the remainder of the semen (i.e., 90%) is **seminal plasma**, the extracellular fluid of semen (Table 54-4). Very little seminal plasma accompanies the spermatozoa as they move through the testes and epididymis. The seminal plasma originates primarily from the accessory glands (the seminal vesicles, prostate gland, and the bulbourethral glands). The seminal vesicles contribute ~70% of the volume of semen. Aside from the sperm, the remaining ~20% represents epididymal fluids, as well as secretions of the prostate gland and bulbourethral glands. However, the composition of the fluid exiting the urethral meatus during ejaculation is not uniform. The first fluid to exit is a mixture of prostatic secretions and spermatozoa with epididymal fluid. Subsequent emissions are composed of mainly secretions derived from the seminal vesicle. The

first portion of the ejaculate contains the highest density of sperm; it also usually contains a higher percentage of motile sperm cells.

The seminal plasma is isotonic. The pH in the lumen of the epididymis is relatively acidic (6.5 to 6.8) as the result of H⁺ secretion by clear cells that are analogous to intercalated cells in the nephron. Addition of the relatively alkaline secretions of the seminal vesicles raises the final pH of seminal plasma to between 7.3 and 7.7. The quiescence of epididymal sperm is not well correlated with pH. Spermatozoa generally tolerate alkalinity better than acidity. A pH near neutrality or slightly higher is optimal for the motility and survival of sperm cells in humans and in other species as well.

Seminal plasma contains a plethora of sugars and ions. Fructose and citric acid are contributed to the seminal plasma by the accessory glands, and their concentrations vary with the volume of semen ejaculated. The **fructose** is produced in the seminal vesicles. In a man with oligospermia (i.e., a low daily sperm output) and a low ejaculate volume (recall that more than half of the ejaculate comes from the seminal vesicles), the absence of fructose suggests obstruction or atresia of the seminal vesicles. Ascorbic acid and traces of B vitamins are also found in human seminal plasma. The prostate gland releases a factor—which contains sugars, sulfate, and a vitamin E derivative—that acts to prevent the clumping of sperm heads. In addition, human semen also contains high concentrations of choline and spermine, although their roles remain to be clarified.

Seminal plasma is also rich in Ca^{2+}, Na^+, Mg^{2+}, K^+, Cl^-, and phosphate. Concentrations of Zn^{2+} and Ca^{2+} are higher in semen than in any other fluid and most other tissues. Calcium ions stimulate the motility of immature epididymal spermatozoa, but they inhibit the motility of spermatozoa in ejaculates obtained from humans. It appears that the diminished response of sperm to Ca^{2+} and the acquisition of progressive motility are functions of epididymal maturation.

Semen also contains low-molecular-weight polypeptides and proteins. The free amino acids probably arise from the breakdown of protein after the semen is ejaculated. The amino acids may protect spermatozoa by binding heavy metals, which may be toxic, or by preventing the agglutination of proteins.

Human semen coagulates immediately after ejaculation. Coagulation is followed by liquefaction, which is apparently caused by proteolytic enzymes, which are contained in

Congenital and Acquired Ductal Obstruction

Genital duct obstruction may be congenital and may result from ductal absence or structural abnormality, or it may be acquired as a result of stricture, infection, or vasectomy. Genital duct obstruction is found in ~7% of infertile men. An uncommon cause of male infertility is congenital **absence of the vas deferens**, which accounts for as many as 50% of cases of congenital ductal obstruction. These patients generally have azoospermic ejaculates with low volume. Congenital absence of the vas deferens is common in male patients with cystic fibrosis (CF) and is sometimes the only manifestation of CF.

Epididymal abnormalities range from the presence of an incomplete epididymis to the presence of only small portions of the epididymis; in addition, the seminal vesicles are often absent. Spermatogenesis is thought to be normal inasmuch as testicular biopsy specimens demonstrate germ cells in several stages of development. Obstruction of the epididymis may also occur as a result of gonococcal or tuberculous epididymitis. Smallpox and filariasis are common causes of ductal obstruction in areas where these diseases are endemic. Inspissated secretions may occlude the epididymis in men with Young syndrome or CF.

Elective vasectomy, a simple surgical procedure in which a small segment of the vas deferens is removed to ensure male infertility, is currently the leading cause of ductal obstruction.

Azoospermia in men with normal testes is the hallmark of genital duct obstruction. However, when specimens of testicles from men who have had vasectomies are examined microscopically, interstitial fibrosis has been found in as many as 20% of cases. This group exhibits low fertility after elective reversal of vasectomy. When the seminiferous tubules are examined, increased thickness of the tubule wall, an increase in cross-sectional tubular area, and decreased numbers of the Sertoli cells are usually noted. Testosterone and gonadotropin levels are normal in most patients with ductal obstruction.

---

prostatic secretions. Prostatic secretion is rich in acid phosphatase. The natural substrate for acid phosphatase is phosphorylcholine, which is contributed by the seminal vesicles. Hyaluronidase is also present in human semen, although its functional role remains to be clarified. Hyaluronidase is not a product of the accessory glands; rather, it is contained within the sperm cell cytoplasm and is rapidly released into the seminal plasma. Hyaluronidase may perform a role in facilitating penetration of the oocyte by the sperm cell because of the ability of hyaluronidase to depolymerize hyaluronic acid.

MALE SEX ACT

Sex steroids influence the central nervous system, even in utero, and play important roles in determining and regulating complex patterns of sexual behavior. However, reproductive behavior is extraordinarily complex and is influenced by numerous factors other than sex steroids, such as one's genetic constitution, social contacts, and the age at which hormones exert their effects. In this section, I describe the neurophysiology of the male sex act.

The sympathetic and parasympathetic divisions of the autonomic nervous system control the male genital system

The testes, epididymis, male accessory glands, and erectile tissue of the penis receive dual innervation from the sympathetic and parasympathetic branches of the autonomic nervous system (ANS). The penis also receives both somatic efferent (i.e., motor) and afferent (i.e., sensory) innervation through the pudendal nerve (S2 through S4).

Sympathetic Division of the ANS   As described in Chapter 15, the preganglionic **sympathetic neurons** originate in the thoracolumbar segments of the spinal cord (T1 through T12, L1 through L3; see Fig. 14-4). For the lower portion of the sympathetic chain (T5 and lower), the preganglionic fibers may pass through the paravertebral sympathetic trunk and then pass through splanchnic nerves to a series of prevertebral plexuses and ganglia (see later). Once within one of these plexuses or ganglia, the preganglionic fiber may either (1) synapse with the postganglionic fiber or (2) pass on to a more caudal plexus or ganglion without synapsing.

The sympathetic efferent (motor) nerve fibers that are supplied to the male sex organs emanate from five primary prevertebral nerve plexuses (Fig. 54-8): the celiac, superior mesenteric, inferior mesenteric, superior hypogastric, and inferior hypogastric or pelvic plexuses. The **celiac plexus** is of interest in a discussion of male sex organs only because preganglionic sympathetic fibers pass through this plexus on their way to more caudal plexuses. The **superior mesenteric** plexus lies on the ventral aspect of the aorta. Preganglionic fibers from the celiac plexus pass through the superior mesenteric plexus on their way to more caudal plexuses.

Most of the preganglionic sympathetic fibers pass from the superior mesenteric plexus to the **inferior mesenteric** plexus, although some of the nerves pass directly to the hypogastric plexus. The **superior hypogastric plexus** is a network of nerves located distal to the bifurcation of the aorta. The **inferior hypogastric** or **pelvic plexus** receives sympathetic supply from the hypogastric nerve.

In addition to these five plexuses, two other small ganglia are of interest. The **spermatic ganglion** is located near the origin of the testicular artery from the aorta. The spermatic ganglion receives fibers directly from the lumbar sympathetic nerves and from branches of several other ganglia. The **hypogastric (or pelvic) ganglion** is located at the junction of the hypogastric and pelvic nerve trunks.

Parasympathetic Division of the ANS   The preganglionic **parasympathetic neurons** relating to the male reproductive system originate in the sacral segments of the spinal cord (S2 through S4; see Fig. 14-4). These fibers pass through the pelvic nerve to the pelvic plexus, where they synapse with the postganglionic parasympathetic neurons.

Visceral Afferents   Sensory fibers are present in all the nerve tracts described (see Fig. 14-2). These fibers travel (1) with the pelvic nerves to the dorsal root of the spinal cord,

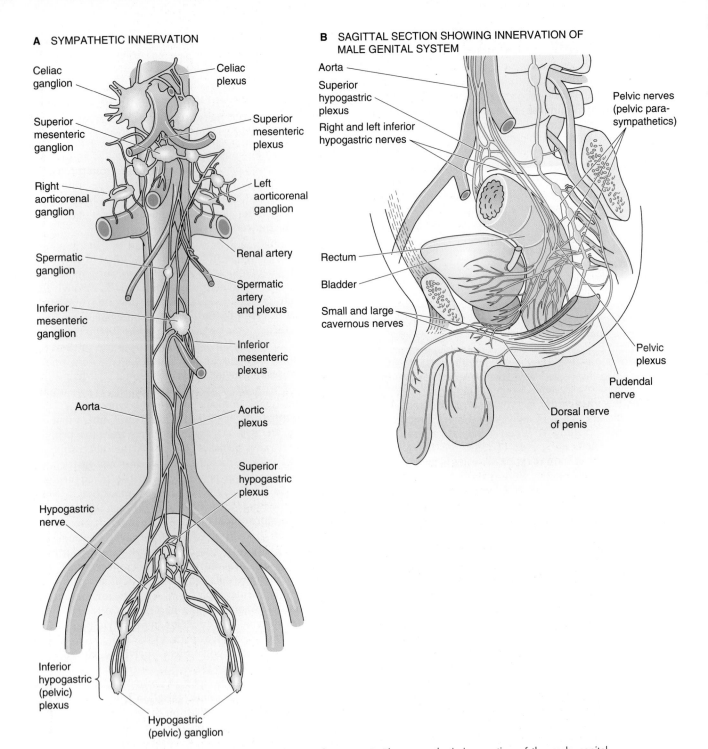

A SYMPATHETIC INNERVATION

Celiac ganglion
Celiac plexus
Superior mesenteric ganglion
Superior mesenteric plexus
Right aorticorenal ganglion
Left aorticorenal ganglion
Renal artery
Spermatic ganglion
Spermatic artery and plexus
Inferior mesenteric ganglion
Inferior mesenteric plexus
Aorta
Aortic plexus
Superior hypogastric plexus
Hypogastric nerve
Inferior hypogastric (pelvic) plexus
Hypogastric (pelvic) ganglion

B SAGITTAL SECTION SHOWING INNERVATION OF MALE GENITAL SYSTEM

Aorta
Superior hypogastric plexus
Right and left inferior hypogastric nerves
Pelvic nerves (pelvic parasympathetics)
Rectum
Bladder
Small and large cavernous nerves
Pelvic plexus
Pudendal nerve
Dorsal nerve of penis

Figure 54-8 Innervation of the male genital system. **A,** The sympathetic innervation of the male genital system involves a series of prevertebral nerve plexuses and ganglia. **B,** Three motor pathways as well as a sensory pathway are involved in erection: (1) parasympathetic innervation: preganglionic parasympathetic fibers arise from the sacral spinal cord and from the pelvic nerve, and they synapse in the pelvic plexus; the postganglionic parasympathetic fibers follow the cavernous nerve to the penile corpora and vasculature; (2) sympathetic innervation: preganglionic sympathetic fibers exit the thoracolumbar cord and synapse in one of several prevertebral ganglia; postganglionic fibers reach the genitalia through the hypogastric nerve, the pelvic plexus, and the cavernous nerves; and (3) somatic innervation: somatic (i.e., not autonomic) motor fibers originate in the sacral spinal cord and form the motor branch of the pudendal nerve; the fibers innervate the striated penile muscles. In addition to these three motor pathways, there is also an afferent pathway from the penis. The dorsal nerve of the penis is the main terminus of the sensory pudendal nerve and is the sole identifiable root for tactile sensory information from the penis.

(2) with the sacral nerves to the sympathetic trunk and then rising in the sympathetic trunk to the spinal cord, or (3) with the hypogastric nerve and ascending to more rostral prevertebral plexuses and then to the spinal cord. The principal functions of motor innervation to the male accessory glands include control of smooth muscle contraction, vascular tone, and epithelial secretory activity.

Erection is primarily under parasympathetic control

The two corpora cavernosa and the corpus spongiosum are usually coordinated in their erection (i.e., tumescence) and detumescence. However, they may act independently inasmuch as their vascular and neuroeffector systems are relatively independent. During erection, relaxation of the smooth muscles of the corpora allows increased inflow of blood to fill the corporal interstices and results in an increase in volume and rigidity. Vascular actions of the smooth muscles of the corpora and the perineal striated muscles are coordinated. For example, contraction of the striated muscles overlying the vascular reservoirs of the penile bulb increases the pressure of the blood in the corpora and promotes increased rigidity. The three major efferent (i.e., motor) pathways for the regulation of penile erection are parasympathetic (pelvic nerve), sympathetic (hypogastric nerve), and somatic (pudendal nerve).

Parasympathetic Innervation   The first and most important pathway for erection is the parasympathetic division of the ANS. These fibers derive from the lumbar and sacral portions of the spinal cord and travel through the *pelvic nerve*, the *pelvic plexus*, and the *cavernous nerve* to the penile corpora and vasculature (Fig. 54-8). This pathway is almost entirely parasympathetic, but apparently it also carries some sympathetic fibers (see later). The parasympathetic activity results in vasodilatation of the penile blood vessels, thus increasing blood flow to the cavernous tissue and engorging the organ with blood. In erectile tissue, parasympathetic postganglionic terminals release acetylcholine (ACh) and nitric oxide (NO), similar to the system discussed in Chapter 14 (see Fig. 14-11). First, ACh may bind to M_3 muscarinic receptors on endothelial cells. Through $G\alpha_q$, these receptors would then lead to stimulation of PLC, increased $[Ca^{2+}]_i$, activation of NO synthase, and local release of NO (see Chapter 3). Second, the nerve terminals may also directly release NO. Regardless of the source of NO, this gas diffuses to the vascular smooth muscle cell, where it stimulates guanylyl cyclase to generate cGMP, which, in turn, causes vasodilation (see Chapter 23). See the box titled Erectile Dysfunction.

Sympathetic Innervation   The second pathway, which is thought to be entirely **sympathetic**, exits the thoracolumbar spinal cord. The preganglionic fibers then course through the least splanchnic nerve, the sympathetic chain, and the inferior mesenteric ganglion. The postganglionic fibers reach the genitalia through the *hypogastric nerve*, the *pelvic plexus*, and the *cavernous nerves* (see earlier). Tonic sympathetic activity contributes to penile *flaccidity*. During erection, a decrease in this sympathetic tone allows relaxation of the corpora and thus contributes to tumescence.

Somatic Innervation   The third pathway is the motor branch of the pudendal nerve. It has primarily **somatic** (i.e., not autonomic) fibers, originates in the sacral spinal cord, and innervates the striated penile muscles. Contraction of the striated ischiocavernosus muscle during the final phase of erection increases pressure inside the corpora cavernosa to values that are even higher than systemic arterial pressure. Contraction of the striated bulbospongiosus muscle increases engorgement of the corpus spongiosum, and thus the glans penis, by pumping blood up from the penile bulb underlying this muscle. Humans are apparently less dependent on their striated penile muscle for achieving and maintaining erection. However, these muscles are active during ejaculation and contribute to the force of seminal expulsion. Postganglionic neurons release other so-called nonadrenergic, noncholinergic neurotransmitters (see Chapter 23)—including NO—that also contribute to the erectile process.

Afferent Innervation   The penis also has an afferent pathway. The dorsal nerve of the penis is the main terminus of the sensory pudendal nerve and is the sole identifiable root for tactile sensory information from the penis.

Emission is primarily under sympathetic control

The term **seminal emission** refers to movement of the ejaculate into the prostatic or proximal part of the urethra. Under some conditions, seminal fluid escapes episodically or continuously from the penile urethra; this action is also referred to as **emission**. Emission is the result of peristaltic contractions of the ampullary portion of the vas deferens, the seminal vesicles, and the prostatic smooth muscles. These actions are accompanied by constriction of the internal sphincter of the bladder, which is under sympathetic control (see Chapter 33), thus preventing retrograde ejaculation of sperm into the urinary bladder (see the box on Ejaculatory Dysfunction: Retrograde Ejaculation).

The rhythmic contractions involved in emission result from contraction of smooth muscle. In contrast to other visceral organ systems, the smooth muscle cells of the male ducts and accessory glands fail to establish close contact with one another and show limited electrotonic coupling. In the male accessory glands, individual smooth muscle cells are directly innervated and have only limited spontaneous activity (i.e., multiunit smooth muscle; see Chapter 9). This combination allows a fast, powerful, and coordinated response to neural stimulation.

Motor Activity of the Duct System   A gradation between two forms of smooth muscle activity occurs along the male duct system. The efferent ducts and proximal regions of the epididymis are sparsely innervated, but they display spontaneous contractions that can be increased through adrenergic agents acting on α-adrenergic receptors. In contrast, the distal end of the epididymis and the vas deferens are normally quiescent until neural stimulation is received during the ejaculatory process. Contraction of the smooth muscle of the distal epididymis, vas deferens, and accessory sex

Erectile Dysfunction

Sildenafil (Viagra), vardenafil (Levitra), and tadalafil (Cialis) are reasonably well tolerated oral medications used to treat erectile dysfunction. Men with erectile dysfunction experience significant improvement in rigidity and duration of erections after treatment with these medications.

As indicated in the text, the smooth muscle tone of the human corpus cavernosum is regulated by the synthesis and release of NO, which raises $[cGMP]_i$ in vascular smooth muscle cells, thereby relaxing the smooth muscle and leading to vasodilatation and erection. Breakdown of cGMP by cGMP-specific phosphodiesterase type 5 limits the degree of vasodilation and, in the case of the penis, limits erection. Sildenafil, vardenafil, and tadalafil are highly selective, high-affinity inhibitors of cGMP-specific phosphodiesterase type 5 and thereby raise $[cGMP]_i$ in smooth muscle and improve erection in men with erectile dysfunction.

The new medications are attractive because they have established efficacy that benefit most men with insufficient erection. These medications stimulate erection only during sexual arousal and thus have a rather natural effect. They can be taken as little as 1 hour before planned sexual activity.

One of the side effects of sildenafil is "blue vision," a consequence of the effect of inhibiting cGMP-specific phosphodiesterase in the retina. In individuals taking other vasodilators, sildenafil can lead to sudden death. In women, sildenafil may improve sexual function by increasing blood flow to the accessory secretory glands (see Chapter 55).

Ejaculatory Dysfunction: Retrograde Ejaculation

As noted in the text, emission is normally accompanied by constriction of the internal urethral sphincter. Retrograde ejaculation occurs when this sphincter fails to constrict. As a result, the semen enters the urinary bladder rather than passing down the urethra. Retrograde ejaculation should be suspected in patients who report absent or small-volume ejaculation after orgasm. The presence of more than 15 sperm per high-power field in urine specimens obtained after ejaculation confirms the presence of retrograde ejaculation.

Lack of emission or retrograde ejaculation may result from any process that interferes with innervation of the vas deferens and bladder neck. Several medical illnesses, such as diabetes mellitus (which can cause peripheral neuropathy) and multiple sclerosis, or the use of pharmaceutical agents that interfere with sympathetic tone can lead to retrograde ejaculation. Retrograde ejaculation may also occur as a result of nerve damage associated with certain surgical procedures, including bladder neck surgery, transurethral resection of the prostate, colorectal surgery, and retroperitoneal lymph node dissection. Retrograde ejaculation from causes other than surgery involving the bladder neck may be treated with pharmacological therapy. Sympathomimetic drugs such as phentolamine (an α-adrenergic agonist), ephedrine (which enhances norepinephrine release), and imipramine (which inhibits norepinephrine re-uptake by presynaptic terminals) may promote normal (i.e., anterograde) ejaculation by increasing the tone of the vas deferens (propelling the seminal fluid) and the internal sphincter (preventing retrograde movement).

glands occurs in response to stimulation of the *sympathetic* fibers in the hypogastric nerve and release of norepinephrine. Indeed, an intravenous injection of epinephrine or norepinephrine can induce seminal emission, whereas selective chemical sympathectomy or an adrenergic antagonist can inhibit seminal emission. The role of *parasympathetic* innervation to the musculature of these ducts and accessory glands in the male is not entirely clear. Parasympathetic fibers may be preferentially involved in basal muscular activity during erection (i.e., before ejaculation) and during urination.

Secretory Activity of the Accessory Glands
The effect of autonomic innervation on the secretory activity of the epithelia of the male accessory glands has been studied extensively. Electrical stimulation of the pelvic nerves (parasympathetic) induces copious secretions. The secretory rate depends on the frequency of stimulation and can be blocked with atropine, a competitive inhibitor of muscarinic ACh receptors. Cholinergic drugs induce the formation of copious amounts of secretions when these drugs are administered systemically. Secretions from the bulbourethral glands also contribute to the ejaculate. The bulbourethral glands do not store secretions but produce them during coitus. The secretory activity of the bulbourethral glands also appears to be under cholinergic control inasmuch as administration of atropine causes marked inhibition of secretion from these glands.

Control of the motor activity of the ducts and of the secretory activity of the accessory glands is complex and involves both the sympathetic and the parasympathetic divisions of the ANS. The central nervous system initiates and coordinates all these activities.

Ejaculation is under control of a spinal reflex

As discussed, seminal emission transports semen to the proximal (posterior) part of the urethra. **Ejaculation** is the forceful expulsion of this semen from the urethra. Ejaculation is normally a reflex reaction triggered by the entry of semen from the prostatic urethra into the bulbous urethra. Thus, emission sets the stage for ejaculation. The ejaculatory process is a spinal cord reflex, although it is also under considerable cerebral control. The afferent (i.e., sensory) impulses reach the sacral spinal cord (S2 through S4) and trigger efferent activity in the somatic motor neurons that travel through the pudendal nerve. The resulting rhythmic contractions of the striated muscles of the perineal area—including the muscles of the pelvic floor, as well as the ischiocavernosus and bulbospongiosus muscles—forcefully propel the semen through the urethra through the external meatus. In addition, spasmodic contractions of the muscles of the hips and the anal sphincter generally accompany ejaculation.

Neuronal Lesions Affecting Erection and Ejaculation

Erectile dysfunction is often associated with disorders of the central and peripheral nervous systems. Spinal cord disease and peripheral neuropathies are of particular interest, and spinal cord injuries have been studied in some detail. Erectile capacity is usually preserved in men with lesions of the premotor neurons (neurons that project from the brain to the spinal cord; Table 54-5). In these men, reflexogenic erections occur in 90% to 100% of cases, whereas psychogenic erections do not occur because the pathways from the brain are blocked. Ejaculation is more significantly impaired in upper than in lower motor neuron lesions, presumably because of loss of the psychogenic component.

A clinically important feature of the spinal segmentation of nerve roots for generating erection (i.e., thoracolumbar and lumbosacral) is that spinal or peripheral nerve damage may affect only one of the effector systems. Because the lumbosacral system also carries most of the penile afferents, erection in response to penile stimulation (reflexogenic) is most affected by damage to the lower spinal cord or the nerves that project there. Evidence from men with spinal injuries in the T10 through T12 region has implicated the sympathetic thoracolumbar pathway in mediating erections resulting from sexual stimuli received through the cranial nerves or generated within the brain as memories, fantasies, or dreams. In men with lower motor neuron lesions, reflexogenic erections are absent. However, psychogenic erections still occur in most men with incomplete lesions and in about one fourth of men with complete lesions. It remains uncertain whether this sympathetic pathway is normally the principal route for psychogenic erections or whether it just assumes the role when lumbosacral parasympathetic pathways are damaged.

Table 54-5 Effects of Neural Lesions on Erection and Ejaculation

Lesion	Reflexogenic Erection	Psychogenic Erection	Effect on Ejaculation
Upper motor neuron	Present	Absent	Significantly impaired
Lower motor neuron	Absent	Present	Less impaired

Orgasm is a term best restricted to the culmination of sexual excitation, as generally applied to both men and women. Orgasm is the cognitive correlation of ejaculation in the male human. Although orgasm, the pleasurable sensation that accompanies ejaculation, is not well understood, clearly, it is as much a central phenomenon as it is a peripheral one.

REFERENCES

Books and Reviews
Ackland JF, Schwartz NB, Mayo KE, Dodson RE: Nonsteroidal signals originating in the gonads. Physiol Rev 1992; 72:731-787.

Andersson K-E, Wagner G: Physiology of penile erection. Physiol Rev 1995; 75:191-236.

Griffin JE, et al: The testis. In Bondy PK, Rosenberg LE: Metabolic Control and Disease. Philadelphia: WB Saunders, 1980.

Hecht NB: Molecular mechanisms of male germ cell differentiation. Bioessays 1998; 20:555-561.

Mather JP, Moore A, Li RH: Activins, inhibins, and follistatins: Further thoughts on a growing family of regulators. Proc Soc Exp Biol Med 1997; 215:209-222.

Skinner MK: Cell-cell interaction in the testis. Endocr Rev 1991; 12:45-77.

Wilson JD, Foster DW, Kronenberg HM, Larsen PR (eds): Williams Textbook of Endocrinology, 9th ed. Philadelphia: WB Saunders, 1998.

Journal Articles
Beitins IZ, Padmanabhan V, Kasa-Vubu J, et al: Serum bioactive follicle-stimulating hormone concentrations from prepuberty to adulthood: A cross-sectional study. J Clin Endocrinol Metab 1990; 71:1022-1027.

Carter AJ, Ballard SA, Naylor AM: Effect of the selective phosphodiesterase type 5 inhibitor sildenafil on erectile dysfunction in the anesthetized dog. J Urol 1998; 160:242-246.

Koraitim M, Schafer W, Melchior H, Lutzeyer W: Dynamic activity of bladder neck and external sphincter in ejaculation. Urology 1977; 10:130-132.

Ludwig DG: The effect of androgen on spermatogenesis. Endocrinology 1950; 46:453-481.

Reiter EO, Beitins IZ, Ostrea TR, Gutai JP: Bioassayable luteinizing hormone during childhood and adolescence and in patients with delayed pubertal development. J Clin Endocrinol Metab 1982; 54:155-161.

Winter JS, Hughes IA, Reyes FI, Faiman C: Pituitary-gonadal relations in infancy: 2. Patterns of serum gonadal steroid concentrations in man from birth to two years of age. J Clin Endocrinol Metab 1976; 42:679-686.

CHAPTER 55

THE FEMALE REPRODUCTIVE SYSTEM

Ervin E. Jones

REPRODUCTIVE FUNCTION IN THE FEMALE HUMAN

Reproductive function in female humans is controlled by hormones that emanate from the hypothalamic-pituitary-gonadal axis (see Chapter 47). The release of a mature ovum from an ovary, known as **ovulation**, is the dominant event of the **menstrual cycle**. Whereas ovulation in some mammals is triggered by mating, ovulation in the female human is spontaneous and is regulated by *cyclic functional interactions* among signals coming from the hypothalamus, the anterior pituitary, and the ovaries. Although many aspects of female reproduction are cyclic, maturation and demise (i.e., atresia) of the functional units of the ovaries—the ovarian follicles—are continuous processes that occur throughout reproductive life.

The ovaries are not the only female organs that undergo rhythmic changes. Alterations in cervical and uterine function are controlled by changes in the circulating concentrations of ovarian hormones, that is, the estrogens and progestins. For example, the uterine lining or endometrium thickens under the influence of ovarian hormones and deteriorates and sloughs at the end of the cycle when ovarian estrogen and progestin secretion diminishes. Menstruation reflects this periodic shedding of the endometrium. Menstrual cycles are generally repetitive unless they are interrupted by pregnancy or terminated by menopause. All the cyclic physiological changes prepare the female reproductive tract for sperm and ovum transport, fertilization, implantation, and pregnancy.

Female reproductive organs include the ovaries and accessory sex organs

The ovaries lie on the sides of the pelvic cavity (Fig. 55-1A). A layer of mesothelial cells covers the surface of the ovary. The ovary itself consists of an inner medulla and an outer zone, or cortex, that surrounds the medulla except at the hilar area. The **cortex** of the ovary in a mature woman contains developing follicles and corpora lutea in various stages of development (Fig. 55-1B). These elements are interspersed throughout the stroma, which includes connective tissue, interstitial cells, and blood vessels. The **medulla** comprises large blood vessels and other stromal elements.

The female **accessory sex organs** include the fallopian tubes, the uterus, the vagina, and the external genitalia. The **fallopian tube** provides a pathway for the transport of ova from the ovary to the uterus. The distal end of the fallopian tube expands as the infundibulum, which ends in multiple fimbriae. The infundibulum is lined with epithelial cells that have cilia that beat toward the uterus. The activity of these cilia and the contractions of the wall of the fallopian tube, particularly around the time of ovulation, facilitate transport of the ovum.

The **uterus** is a complex, pear-shaped, muscular organ that is suspended by a series of supporting ligaments. It is composed of a fundus, a corpus, and a narrow caudal portion called the **cervix**. The external surface of the uterus is covered by serosa, whereas the interior, or **endometrium**, of the uterus consists of complex glandular tissue and stroma. The uterus is continuous with the vagina through the cervical canal. The cervix is composed of dense fibrous connective tissue and muscle cells. The cervical glands lining the cervical canal produce a sugar-rich secretion, the viscosity of which is conditioned by estrogen and progesterone.

The human **vagina** is ~10 cm in length and is a single, expandable tube. The vagina is lined by stratified epithelium and is surrounded by a thin muscular layer. During development, the lower end of the vagina is covered by the membranous hymen, which is partially perforated during fetal life. In some instances, the hymen remains continuous. The **external genitalia** include the clitoris, the labia majora, and the labia minora, as well as the accessory secretory glands (including the glands of Bartholin), which open into the vestibule. The **clitoris** is an erectile organ, which is homologous to the penis (see Chapter 53) and mirrors the cavernous ends of the glans penis.

PUBERTY

Puberty marks the transition to cyclic, adult reproductive function

Puberty is the transition from a noncyclic, relatively quiescent reproductive endocrine system to a state of cyclic reproductive function that allows procreation. *Puberty* is the transition between the juvenile state and adulthood during

A OBLIQUE VIEW OF THE INTERNAL FEMALE SEX ORGANS

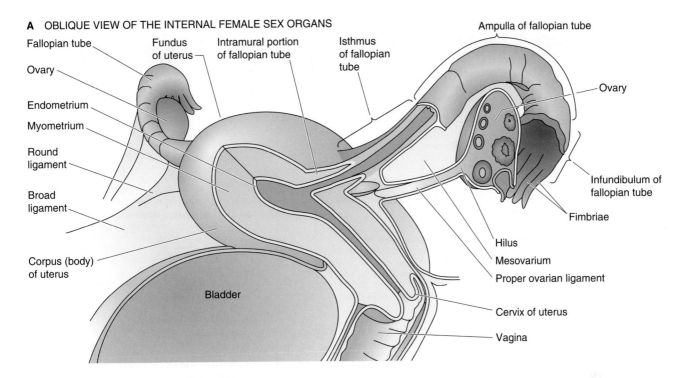

B CROSS SECTION THROUGH AN OVARY

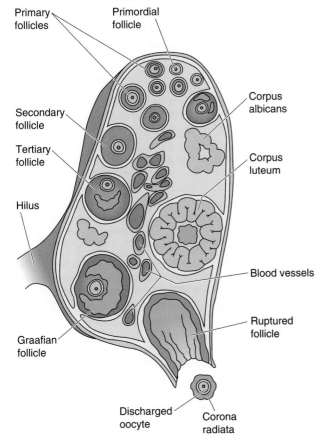

Figure 55-1 The anatomy of the female internal genitalia and accessory sex organs.

Table 55-1 Stages in Female Puberty

Stage	Breast Development	Pubic Hair
1	Preadolescent: only papillae are elevated	Preadolescent: no pubic hair is present, only vellus hair, as on the abdomen
2	Breasts and papillae are both elevated, and the diameter of the areolae increases	Pubic hair is sparse, mainly along the labia majora
3	The breasts and areolae further enlarge	Pubic hair is darker, coarser, and curlier and spreads over the pubis
4	The areolae and papillae project out beyond the level of the expanding breast tissue	The pubic hair is of adult type, but covers an area smaller than in most adults
5	With further enlargement of the breast, the areolae are now on the same level as the rest of the breast; only the papillae project; adult pattern	Adult pattern

which time secondary sexual characteristics appear, the adolescent growth spurt occurs, and the ability to procreate is achieved. Table 55-1 summarizes the stages of puberty in the female. Puberty in girls involves the beginning of menstrual cycles (**menarche**), breast development (**thelarche**), and an increase in adrenal androgen secretion (**adrenarche**).

The precise cause of the onset of puberty is not completely understood, although multiple intrinsic and extrinsic factors play a role. Genetic factors are major determinants of pubertal onset. Other factors, such as nutrition, geographic location, and exposure to light, also play a role. Over the last century, the age of girls at menarche in the United States and Europe has gradually decreased. Although the reason that menarche now occurs at a younger age remains incompletely understood, it is probably because of improved nutritional status. However, better nutritional status alone cannot completely explain the decreased age of pubertal onset. Distance from the equator and lower altitudes are associated with early onset of puberty. A loose correlation is also seen between the onset of menarche in the mother and the onset of menarche in the daughter. The onset of puberty is also related to body composition and to fat deposition. Severe obesity and heavy exercise delay puberty.

Gonadotropin levels are low during childhood

As shown in Figure 55-2A, a surge in the levels of the pituitary gonadotropins, luteinizing hormone (LH) and follicle-stimulating hormone (FSH), occurs during intra-uterine life. A second peak takes place in the immediate postnatal period. However, gonadotropin levels tend to decrease at ~4 months of age; thereafter, they decline further and remain low until just before puberty. Gonadotropin levels are lowest between 6 and 8 years of age. Although the reason for low gonadotropin secretion by the pituitary in childhood remains unknown, it was once thought to result from feedback inhibition by *high levels* of gonadal steroids. However, an experiment of nature has revealed that such is not the case. Indeed, girls with gonadal dysgenesis, like physiologically normal girls, have low levels of LH and FSH, even though their

ovaries produce *low levels* of steroids. Thus, it is likely that the low levels of gonadotropins in the prepubertal period do not reflect high levels of steroids, but rather a *high sensitivity* to feedback inhibition of the hypothalamic-pituitary system by these steroids. I discuss this feedback mechanism in the next section.

During puberty, gonadotropin-releasing hormone secretion becomes pulsatile, and the sensitivity of the gonadotrophs to feedback inhibition by estrogens decreases

As shown by the insets to Figure 55-2A, one of the earliest events of puberty is the onset of pulsatile gonadotropin secretion from the pituitary during rapid eye movement (REM) sleep; this pulsatile gonadotropin secretion reflects the pulsatile release of gonadotropin-releasing hormone (GnRH) from the hypothalamus. The development of secondary sexual characteristics follows the onset of sleep-associated pulsatility. With maturation, these pulses occur throughout the day. It is not understood why pulsatile behavior should occur initially only during REM sleep. The precipitating event that is responsible for initiating pulsatile GnRH release is also unknown, although it may reflect the maturation of hypothalamic neurons. Once a pulsatile pattern of gonadotropin secretion is established, it continues throughout reproductive life into menopause.

The increased pulsatility of GnRH release eventually leads to a marked increase in plasma LH levels—the **LH surge** that marks the initiation of the first menstrual cycle. During early pubescence, the LH surges do not occur in a regular pattern, so menstrual cycles are generally irregular. As the reproductive system matures, the LH surges gradually come at regular intervals, and cyclic reproductive function becomes firmly established.

The appearance of GnRH pulsatility early in puberty is associated with decreased sensitivity of the hypothalamic-pituitary system to circulating sex steroids. In young girls, even low levels of sex steroids are sufficient to feed back on the hypothalamic-pituitary system and to block the release

A PATTERNS OF GONADOTROPIN LEVELS THROUGHOUT THE LIFE OF A FEMALE

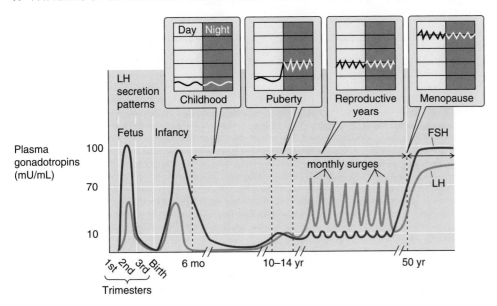

B NEGATIVE FEEDBACK OF ESTROGENS ON GONADOTROPIN RELEASE

C AGE DEPENDENCE OF FEEDBACK SENSITIVITY

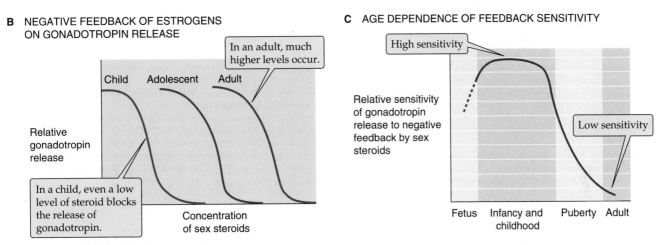

Figure 55-2 Gonadotropin function during life. **A,** The levels of both LH and FSH peak during fetal life and again during early infancy, before falling to low levels throughout the rest of childhood. At the onset of puberty, LH and FSH levels slowly rise and then begin to oscillate at regular monthly intervals. At menopause, gonadotropin levels rise to very high levels. The *four insets* show daily changes in gonadotropin levels. **B,** This is a highly schematic plot of how estrogen levels negatively feed back on gonadotropin secretion by the gonadotroph cells of the anterior pituitary. In childhood, even very low estrogen levels are sufficient to suppress gonadotropin output fully. In adolescence, higher levels of estrogens are required. In the adult woman, estrogens must be at very high levels to suppress gonadotropin release. **C,** This is a plot—versus age—of the midpoints of curves such as those in **B**.

of gonadotropins (Fig. 55-2B). As a girl goes through puberty, the levels of steroids required to block gonadotropin release progressively become higher and higher. At about the same time, the levels of sex steroids also rise. Eventually, a situation is reached in which the monthly oscillations in sex steroid levels produce the full range of feedback inhibition of gonadotropin release. Thus, during maturation, the sensitivity of the hypothalamic-pituitary system to inhibition by sex steroids falls to reach the low level that is characteristic

of the adult (Fig. 55-2C). As discussed later, in addition to the negative feedback of sex steroids on gonadotropin release, *positive* feedback also occurs near the midpoint of the menstrual cycle.

During puberty, basal levels of LH and FSH increase (Fig. 55-2A). Concentrations of androgens and estrogens also increase many-fold as a result of gonadal stimulation by FSH and LH. The LH surge that occurs at midcycle is thus superimposed on an already high basal level of circulating LH.

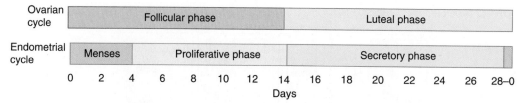

Figure 55-3 The ovarian and endometrial cycles. The menstrual cycle comprises parallel ovarian and endometrial cycles. The follicular phase of the ovarian cycle and the menses start on day 0. In this idealized example, ovulation occurs on day 14, and the entire cycle lasts 28 days.

HYPOTHALAMIC-PITUITARY-GONADAL AXIS AND CONTROL OF THE FEMALE MENSTRUAL RHYTHM

The menstrual cycle includes both the ovarian and endometrial cycles

The menstrual cycle actually involves cyclic changes in two organs: the ovary and the uterus (Fig. 55-3). The **ovarian cycle** includes the follicular phase and the luteal phase, separated by ovulation. The **endometrial cycle** includes the menstrual, the proliferative, and the secretory phases.

Although menstrual cycles are generally regular during the reproductive years, the length of the menstrual cycle may be highly variable because of disturbances in neuroendocrine function. The mean menstrual cycle is 28 days long, but considerable variation occurs during both the early reproductive years and the premenopausal period. Irregular menses during adolescence and the premenopausal period occur primarily because of the increased frequency of anovulatory cycles.

The first phase of the *ovarian cycle* is the **follicular phase**—during which FSH stimulates a follicle to complete its development (i.e., folliculogenesis). The follicular phase begins with the initiation of menstruation and averages ~14 days in length. The duration of the follicular phase is the most variable of the cycle. During folliculogenesis, the granulosa cells of the follicles increase production of the estrogen **estradiol**, which stimulates the endometrium to undergo rapid and continuous growth and maturation. This period is the **proliferative phase** of the *endometrial cycle*. A rapid rise in ovarian estradiol secretion eventually triggers a surge in LH, which causes **ovulation**.

After releasing its ovum, the follicle transforms into a corpus luteum, which is why the second half of the *ovarian cycle* is called the **luteal phase**. The luteal cells produce **progesterone** and estrogen, which stimulate further endometrial growth and development. This period is the **secretory phase** of the *endometrial cycle*. For unknown reasons, the corpus luteum rapidly diminishes its production of estrogens and progestins, thereby resulting in a catastrophic degeneration of the endometrium that leads to menstrual bleeding. This period is the **menstrual phase** of the *endometrial cycle*.

The hypothalamic-pituitary-ovarian axis drives the menstrual cycle

Neurons in the hypothalamus synthesize, store, and release **GnRH**. Long portal vessels carry the GnRH to the anterior pituitary, where the hormone binds to receptors on the surface of gonadotrophs. The results are the synthesis and release of both **FSH** and **LH** from the gonadotrophs.

These trophic hormones, LH and FSH, stimulate the ovary to synthesize and secrete the sex steroids **estrogens** and **progestins**. The ovaries also produce peptides called **inhibins** and **activins**. Together, these ovarian steroids and peptides exert both negative and positive feedback on both the hypothalamus and the anterior pituitary. This complex interaction is unique among the endocrine systems of the body inasmuch as it generates a monthly pattern of hormone fluctuations. Because the cyclic secretion of estrogens and progestins primarily controls endometrial maturation, menstruation reflects these cyclic changes in hormone secretion.

Neurons in the hypothalamus release GnRH in a pulsatile fashion

At the rostral end of the hypothalamic-pituitary-ovarian axis (Fig. 55-4), neurons in the arcuate nucleus and the preoptic area of the hypothalamus synthesize GnRH. They transport GnRH to their nerve terminals for storage and subsequent release. As discussed later, each of the aforementioned two groups of neurons is responsible for a very different kind of rhythm of GnRH secretion. Axons of the GnRH neurons project directly to the median eminence, the extreme basal portion of the hypothalamus, and terminate near portal vessels. These vessels carry GnRH to the gonadotrophs in the anterior pituitary.

The gene encoding GnRH is located on chromosome 9 (Fig. 55-5). The mature mRNA for GnRH encodes a preprohormone composed of 92 amino acids. After removing the 23–amino acid signal sequence (residues −23 to −1), the neuron produces a prohormone (residues 1 to 69). Cleavage of this prohormone yields the decapeptide GnRH (residues 1 to 10), a 56–amino acid peptide (residues 14 to 69) referred to as **GnRH-associated peptide (GAP)**, and three amino acids that link the two. The neuron transports both GnRH and GAP down the axon for secretion into the portal circulation. The importance of GAP is unknown, but it may inhibit prolactin secretion.

GnRH is present in the hypothalamus at 14 to 16 weeks' gestation, and its target, the gonadotropin-containing cells (gonadotrophs), are present in the anterior pituitary gland as early as 10 weeks' gestation. The hypothalamic-pituitary system is functionally competent by ~23 weeks' gestation, at which time fetal tissues release GnRH.

The GnRH neurons do not release GnRH continuously, but rather in rhythmic pulses (Fig. 55-6). GnRH is released

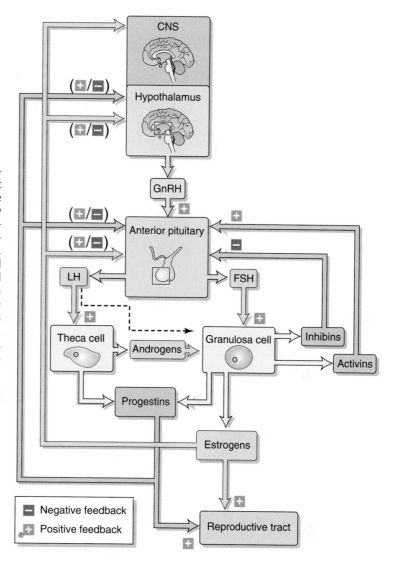

Figure 55-4 Hypothalamic-pituitary-ovarian axis. Small-bodied neurons in the arcuate nucleus and the preoptic area of the hypothalamus secrete GnRH, a decapeptide that reaches the gonadotrophs in the anterior pituitary through the long portal veins. GnRH binds to a G-protein-coupled receptor on the gonadotroph membrane, triggering the IP_3/DAG pathway, raising $[Ca^{2+}]_i$ and phosphorylation. Stimulation causes the gonadotrophs to synthesize and release two gonadotropins—FSH and LH—that are stored in secretory granules. Both FSH and LH are glycoprotein heterodimers comprising common α subunits and unique β subunits. The LH binds to receptors on theca cells, thus stimulating $G\alpha_s$, which, in turn, activates adenylyl cyclase. The resultant rise in $[cAMP]_i$ stimulates protein kinase A (PKA), which increases the transcription of several proteins involved in the biosynthesis of progestins and androgens. The androgens enter granulosa cells, which convert the androgens to estrogens. The *dashed arrow* indicates that the granulosa cells also have LH receptors. FSH binds to receptors on the basolateral membrane of granulosa cells, also activating PKA, thereby stimulating gene transcription and synthesis of the relevant enzymes (e.g., aromatase), activins, and inhibins. Negative feedback on the hypothalamic-pituitary-ovarian axis occurs by several routes. The activins and inhibins act only on the anterior pituitary. The estrogens and progestins act on both the anterior pituitary and on the hypothalamic neurons, by exerting both positive and negative feedback controls. CNS, central nervous system.

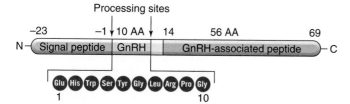

Figure 55-5 Map of the gonadotropin-releasing-hormone gene. The mature mRNA encodes a preprohormone with 92 amino acids. Removal of the 23–amino acid signal sequence yields the 69–amino acid prohormone. Cleavage of this prohormone yields GnRH.

in bursts into the portal vessels about once per hour, thereby intermittently stimulating the gonadotrophs in the anterior pituitary. Because the half-life of GnRH in blood is only 2 to 4 minutes, these hourly bursts of GnRH cause clearly discernible oscillations in portal plasma GnRH levels that result in hourly surges in release of the gonadotropins LH and FSH. Early in the follicular phase of the cycle, when the gonadotrophs are not very GnRH sensitive, each burst of GnRH elicits only a small rise in LH (Fig. 55-6A). Later in

the follicular phase, when the gonadotrophs in the anterior pituitary become much more sensitive to the GnRH in the portal blood, each burst of GnRH triggers a much larger release of LH (Fig. 55-6B).

Although the mechanisms controlling the hourly pulses of GnRH remain unclear, the pulse generator for GnRH is thought to be located in the **arcuate nucleus** of the medial basal hypothalamus, where one group of GnRH neurons resides. In rodents, bursts of nerve impulses from neurons in these nuclei correspond in time with the pulsatile release of GnRH from the hypothalamus and with the episodic release of LH from the anterior pituitary. These data suggest that a built-in system within the hypothalamus controls the pulsatile discharge of GnRH from nerve terminals. The pulse-generating mechanism is key to control of cyclic reproductive function and to regulation of the menstrual cycle. The *frequency* of GnRH release, and thus LH release, determines the specific response of the gonad. Pulses spaced 60 to 90 minutes apart upregulate the gonadotrophs' GnRH receptors and thus stimulate the release of gonadotropins. However, continuous administration of GnRH (or an analogue) causes downregulation of the gonadotrophs' GnRH

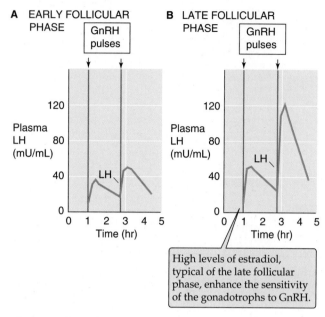

A EARLY FOLLICULAR PHASE

B LATE FOLLICULAR PHASE

High levels of estradiol, typical of the late follicular phase, enhance the sensitivity of the gonadotrophs to GnRH.

Figure 55-6 Pulsatile release of GnRH and pulsatile secretion of LH. (*Data from Wang CF, Lasley BL, Lein A, Yen SS: J Clin Endocrinol Metab 1976; 42:718-728.*)

receptors and thus suppresses gonadotropin release and gonadal function (see the box titled Therapeutic Uses of GnRH).

In addition to the hourly rhythm of GnRH secretion, orchestrated by the arcuate nucleus, a monthly rhythm of GnRH secretion also occurs—in rhesus monkeys. A massive increase in GnRH secretion at midcycle is, in part, responsible for the LH surge, which, in turn, leads to ovulation. Which neurons produce the massive surge in GnRH that leads to the LH surge? These are not the GnRH neurons in the arcuate nucleus but, rather, those in the preoptic area. The preoptic GnRH neurons have inhibitory γ-aminobutyric acid (GABA) receptors, whereas the arcuate GnRH neurons have inhibitory opioid receptors. Later in this chapter, I discuss how these two sets of GnRH neurons may underlie the negative and positive feedback produced by estrogens.

GnRH stimulates gonadotrophs in the anterior pituitary to secrete FSH and LH, which stimulate ovarian cells to secrete estrogens and progestins

GnRH enters the anterior pituitary through the portal system and binds to GnRH receptors on the surface of the gonadotroph, thus initiating a series of cellular events that result in the synthesis and secretion of gonadotropins (Fig. 55-7). GnRH binds to a G protein–linked receptor coupled to $G\alpha_q$. The result is activation of phospholipase C (PLC), which, in turn, hydrolyzes phosphatidylinositol 4,5-biphosphonate (PIP_2) to inositol 1,4,5-triphosphate (IP_3), and diacylglycerol (DAG) (see Chapter 3). Both IP_3 and DAG are second messengers. Release of Ca^{2+} from the endo-

Therapeutic Uses of GnRH

Continuous administration of GnRH leads to downregulation (suppression) of gonadotropin secretion, whereas pulsatile release of GnRH causes upregulation (stimulation) of FSH and LH secretion. Clinical problems requiring upregulation of gonadotropin secretion, which leads to stimulation of the gonads, are therefore best treated by a *pulsatile* mode of GnRH administration. In contrast, when the patient requires gonadal inhibition, a *continuous* mode of administration is necessary.

An example of a disease requiring *pulsatile* GnRH administration is **Kallmann syndrome**. Disordered migration of GnRH cells during embryologic development causes Kallmann syndrome, which in adults results in **hypogonadotropic hypogonadism** and **anosmia** (loss of sense of smell). Normally, primordial GnRH cells originate in the nasal placode during embryologic development. These primitive cells then migrate through the forebrain to the diencephalon, where they become specific neuronal groups within the medial basal hypothalamus and preoptic area. In certain individuals, both male and female, proper migration of GnRH cells fails to occur. The cause of Kallmann syndrome was confirmed in humans when researchers studied a fetus at 19 weeks' gestation that had complete deletion of the X-linked Kallmann locus. The GnRH cells were found along their known migration route, but not in the brain. Girls and women with Kallmann syndrome generally have amenorrhea (no menstrual cycles). However, the pituitary and gonads of these individuals can function properly when appropriately stimulated. Thus, women treated with exogenous gonadotropins or GnRH analogues—*pulsatile administration* with a programmed infusion pump—can have normal folliculogenesis, ovulation, and pregnancy.

An example of a disease requiring *continuous* GnRH administration to downregulate gonadal function is endometriosis. **Endometriosis** is a common condition caused by the aberrant presence of endometrial tissue outside the uterine cavity. This tissue responds to estrogens during the menstrual cycle and is a source of pain and other problems, including infertility. In patients with endometriosis, *continuous administration* of GnRH analogue inhibits replenishment of the receptor for GnRH in the gonadotrophs in the anterior pituitary. As a result, insufficient numbers of GnRH receptors are available for optimum GnRH action, thereby diminishing gonadotropin secretion and producing relative hypoestrogenism. Because estrogen stimulates the endometrium, continuous administration of GnRH or GnRH analogues causes involution and diminution of endometriotic tissue.

Leiomyomas (smooth muscle tumors) of the uterus (also called a uterine fibroid) are also estrogen dependent. When estrogen levels are decreased, the proliferation of these lesions is decreased. Therefore, leiomyomas of the uterus can also be effectively treated by *continuous* administration of GnRH analogues.

plasmic reticulum by IP_3 causes an increase in $[Ca^{2+}]_i$. This Ca^{2+} induces the Ca^{2+} channels at the cell membrane to open and allows an influx of extracellular Ca^{2+} that sustains the elevated $[Ca^{2+}]_i$. The rise in $[Ca^{2+}]_i$ triggers exocytosis and gonadotropin release.

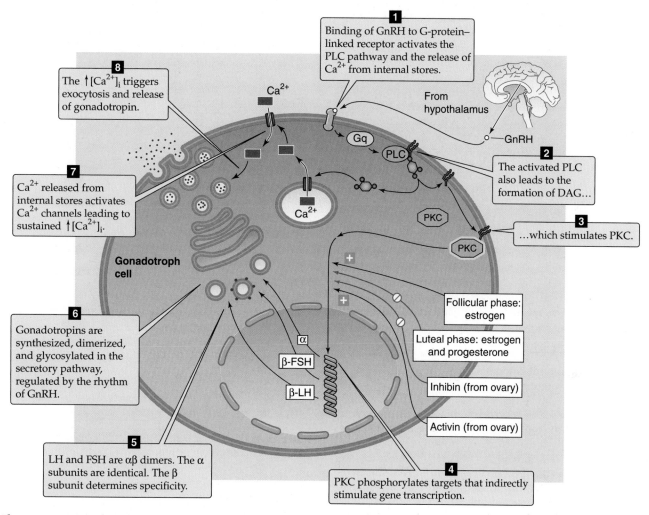

1 Binding of GnRH to G-protein–linked receptor activates the PLC pathway and the release of Ca^{2+} from internal stores.

8 The $\uparrow[Ca^{2+}]_i$ triggers exocytosis and release of gonadotropin.

From hypothalamus

GnRH

2 The activated PLC also leads to the formation of DAG…

7 Ca^{2+} released from internal stores activates Ca^{2+} channels leading to sustained $\uparrow[Ca^{2+}]_i$.

3 …which stimulates PKC.

Gonadotroph cell

Follicular phase: estrogen

Luteal phase: estrogen and progesterone

6 Gonadotropins are synthesized, dimerized, and glycosylated in the secretory pathway, regulated by the rhythm of GnRH.

Inhibin (from ovary)

Activin (from ovary)

5 LH and FSH are αβ dimers. The α subunits are identical. The β subunit determines specificity.

4 PKC phosphorylates targets that indirectly stimulate gene transcription.

Figure 55-7 Gonadotropin secretion. PKC, protein kinase C.

In addition to the IP₃ pathway, GnRH also acts through the DAG pathway. The DAG formed by PLC stimulates protein kinase C, which indirectly leads to increases in gene transcription. The net effect is an increase in synthesis of the gonadotropins FSH and LH. In addition, GnRH increases mRNA levels for certain immediate early response genes (e.g., *c-Fos*, *c-Jun*, and *JunB*).

The GnRH receptor is internalized and partially degraded in the lysosomes. However, a portion of the GnRH receptor is shuttled back to the cell surface. Return of the GnRH receptor to the cell membrane is referred to as **receptor replenishment** and is related to the upregulation of receptor activity discussed earlier. The mechanism through which GnRH receptor replenishment occurs remains unclear.

FSH and LH are in the same family as thyroid-stimulating hormone (TSH; see Chapter 49) and **human chorionic gonadotropin** (hCG; see Chapter 56). All four are glycoprotein hormones with α and β chains. The α chains of all four of these hormones are identical; in humans, they have 92 amino acids and a molecular weight of ~20 kDa. The β chains of FSH and LH are unique and confer the specificity of the hormones. The rhythm of GnRH secretion influences the relative rates of expression for genes encoding the syn-

thesis of the α, β_{FSH}, and β_{LH} subunits of FSH and LH. GnRH pulsatility also determines the dimerization of the α and β_{FSH} subunits, or α and β_{LH}, as well as their glycosylation.

Differential secretion of FSH and LH is also affected by several other hormonal mediators, including ovarian steroids, inhibins, and activins. I discuss the role of these agents in the section on feedback control of the hypothalamic-pituitary-ovarian axis. Thus, depending on the specific hormonal milieu produced by different physiological circumstances, the gonadotroph produces and secretes the α and β subunits of FSH and LH at different rates. The secretion of LH and FSH is further modulated by neuropeptides, amino acids such as aspartate, neuropeptide Y, corticotropin-releasing hormone (CRH), and endogenous opioids.

Before ovulation, the LH and FSH secreted by the gonadotrophs act on cells of the developing follicle. The **theca cells** of the follicle have LH receptors, whereas the **granulosa cells** have both LH and FSH receptors. Both LH and FSH are required for estrogen production because neither the theca cell nor the granulosa cell can carry out all the required steps. After ovulation, LH acts on the cells of the corpus luteum; recall that after ovulation, the cells of the follicle give rise to the corpus luteum.

LH and FSH bind to specific receptors on the surface of their target cells. Both the LH and the FSH receptors are coupled through $G\alpha_s$ to adenylyl cyclase (see Chapter 3), which catalyzes the conversion of ATP to cAMP. cAMP stimulates protein kinase A, which not only stimulates the enzymes involved in steroid biosynthesis but also induces the synthesis of certain proteins and increases cell division. Among the proteins whose synthesis is promoted by gonadotropins is the low-density lipoprotein (LDL) receptor required for cholesterol uptake and the aromatase required for estrogen synthesis.

Ovaries also produce peptide hormones: inhibins, which inhibit FSH secretion, and activins, which activate it

The inhibins and the activins are peptides that modulate FSH secretion by the gonadotrophs. The transforming growth factor β (TGF-β) supergene family is a group of molecules that are structurally related and include TGF-β, antimüllerian hormone (AMH; see Chapter 53), the activins, the inhibins, and other glycoproteins. These growth factors modulate growth and differentiation during development. The inhibins and activins are dimers constructed from a related set of building blocks: a glycosylated 20-kDa α subunit and two nonglycosylated 12-kDa β subunits, one called $β_A$ and the other called $β_B$ (Fig. 55-8). The *inhibins* are always composed of one α subunit and either a $β_A$ or a $β_B$ subunit; the α and β subunits are linked by disulfide bridges. The $α$-$β_A$ dimer is called inhibin A, whereas the $α$-$β_B$ dimer is called inhibin B. The *activins*, however, are composed of two β-type subunits. Thus, three kinds of activins are recognized: $β_A$-$β_A$, $β_B$-$β_B$, and the heterodimer $β_A$-$β_B$.

The **inhibins** are produced by the granulosa cells of the follicle, as well as other tissues, including the pituitary, the brain, the adrenal gland, the kidney, the bone marrow, the corpus luteum, and the placenta. FSH specifically stimulates the granulosa cells to produce inhibins. Also involved in the regulation of inhibin production are certain other factors, including hormones and growth-stimulating factors. Estradiol may stimulate inhibin production through an intraovarian mechanism. Just before ovulation, after the granulosa cells acquire LH receptors, LH also stimulates the production of inhibin by granulosa cells. The biological action of the inhibins is primarily confined to the reproductive system. As discussed later, the inhibins inhibit FSH production by gonadotrophs. The **activins** are produced in the same tissues as the inhibins, but they *stimulate*—rather than inhibit—FSH release from pituitary cells.

Both the ovarian steroids (estrogens and progestins) and peptides (inhibins and activins) feed back on the hypothalamic-pituitary axis

As summarized in Figure 55-4, the ovarian steroids—the estrogens and progestins—exert both negative and positive feedback on the hypothalamic-pituitary axis. Whether the feedback is negative or positive depends on both the concentration of the gonadal steroids and the duration of the exposure to these steroids (i.e., the time in the menstrual cycle).

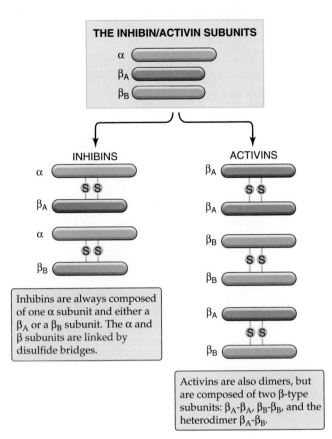

Figure 55-8 The inhibins and activins. The inhibins and activins are peptide hormones that are made up of a common set of building blocks. For both the inhibins and the activins, disulfide bonds link the two subunits.

In addition, the ovarian peptides—the inhibins and activins—also feed back on the anterior pituitary.

Negative Feedback by Ovarian Steroids   Throughout most of the menstrual cycle, the estrogens and progestins that are produced by the ovary feed back negatively on both the hypothalamus and the gonadotrophs of the anterior pituitary. The net effect is to reduce the release of both LH and FSH. The estrogens exert negative feedback at both low and high concentrations, whereas the progestins are effective only at high concentrations.

Although estrogens inhibit the GnRH neurons in the arcuate nucleus and preoptic area of the hypothalamus, this inhibition is not direct. Rather, the estrogens stimulate interneurons that inhibit the GnRH neurons. In the arcuate nucleus, these inhibitory neurons exert their inhibition through opiates. However, in the preoptic area, the inhibitory neurons exert their inhibitory effect through GABA, a classic inhibitory neurotransmitter (see Chapter 13).

Positive Feedback by Ovarian Steroids   Although ovarian steroids feed back *negatively* on the hypothalamic-pituitary axis during most of the menstrual cycle, they have the opposite effect at the end of the follicular phase. Levels of **estrogen**, mainly estradiol, rise gradually during the first half of the follicular phase of the ovarian cycle and then steeply during the second half (Fig. 55-9). After the estradiol

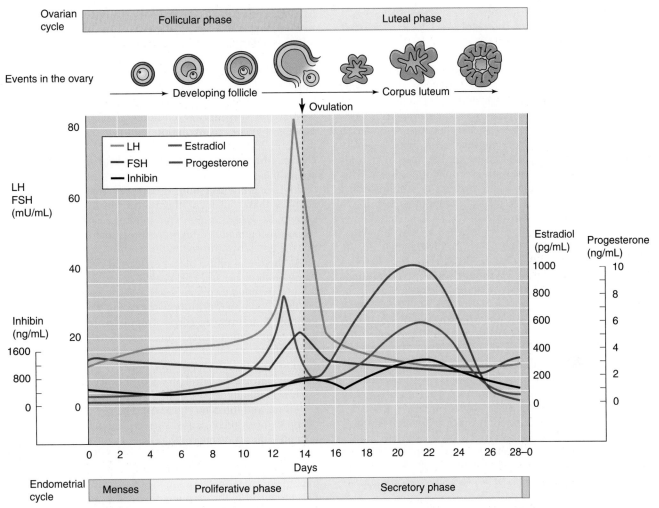

Figure 55-9   Hormonal changes during the menstrual cycle. The menstrual cycle is a cycle of the hypothalamic-pituitary-ovarian axis, as well as a cycle of the targets of the ovarian hormones: the endometrium of the uterus. Therefore, the menstrual cycle includes both an ovarian cycle—which includes the follicular phase, ovulation, and the luteal phase—and an endometrial cycle—which includes the menstrual, the proliferative, and the secretory phases.

levels reach a certain threshold for a minimum of 2 days—and perhaps because of the accelerated rate of estradiol secretion—the hypothalamic-pituitary axis reverses its sensitivity to estrogens; that is, estrogens now feed back *positively* on the axis. One manifestation of this positive feedback is that estrogens now *increase* the sensitivity of the gonadotrophs in the anterior pituitary gland to GnRH. As discussed in the next section, this switch to positive feedback promotes the LH surge. Indeed, pituitary cells that are cultured in the absence of estrogen have suboptimal responses to GnRH. Once high levels of estrogens have properly conditioned the gonadotrophs, rising levels of **progesterone** during the late follicular phase also produce a positive feedback response and thus facilitate the LH surge.

Negative Feedback by the Inhibins   The inhibins inhibit FSH secretion by the gonadotrophs of the anterior pituitary (hence the name inhibin) in a classic negative feedback arrangement. The initial action of inhibin appears to be

beyond the Ca^{2+}-mobilization step in FSH secretion. In cultured pituitary cells, even very small amounts of inhibin markedly reduce mRNA levels for both the $\alpha_{LH/FSH}$ and the β_{FSH} subunits. As a result, inhibins suppress FSH secretion. In contrast, inhibins have no effect on the mRNA levels of β_{LH}. In addition to their actions on the anterior pituitary, the inhibins also have the intraovarian effect of decreasing androgen production, which can have secondary effects on intrafollicular estrogen production.

Positive Feedback by the Activins   Activins promote marked increases in β_{FSH} mRNA and FSH release, with no change in β_{LH} formation. The stimulatory effect of activins on FSH release is independent of GnRH action. Like the inhibins, the activins also have the intraovarian action of stimulating the synthesis of estrogens. Thus, by their actions on both the gonadotrophs and the ovaries, the activins and inhibins regulate the activity of the follicular cells during the menstrual cycle.

Modulation of gonadotropin secretion by positive and negative ovarian feedback produces the normal menstrual rhythm

We already saw in Figure 55-6 that the pulsatile release of GnRH from the hypothalamus, generally occurring every 60 to 90 minutes, triggers a corresponding pulsatile release of LH and FSH from the gonadotrophs of the anterior pituitary. Because the gonadotropins elicit the release of ovarian steroids, and these steroids modulate the hypothalamic-pituitary axis, the interaction between the ovarian steroids and gonadotropin release is an example of feedback. This feedback is especially interesting because it is bidirectional in that it elicits *negative* feedback throughout most of the menstrual cycle but *positive* feedback immediately before ovulation.

Figure 55-9 illustrates the cyclic hormonal changes during the menstrual cycle. The time-averaged records of LH and FSH levels mask their hour-by-hour pulsatility. The **follicular phase** is characterized by a relatively high frequency of GnRH—and thus LH—pulses. Early in the follicular phase, when levels of estradiol are low but rising, the frequency of LH pulses remains unchanged, but their amplitude gradually *increases* with time. We see this increase in amplitude in Figure 55-6, in which the early and late follicular phases are compared. Later in the follicular phase of the menstrual cycle, the higher estrogen levels cause both the frequency and the amplitude of the LH pulses to increase gradually. During this time of high estradiol levels, the ovarian steroids are beginning to feed back positively on the hypothalamic-pituitary axis. Late in the follicular phase, the net effect of this increased frequency and amplitude of LH and FSH pulses is an increase in their time-averaged circulating levels (Fig. 55-9).

The **LH surge** is an abrupt and dramatic rise in the LH level that occurs around the 13th to 14th day of the follicular phase in the average woman. The LH surge peaks ~12 hours after its initiation and lasts for ~48 hours. The peak concentration of LH during the surge is ~3-fold greater than the concentration before the surge (Fig. 55-9). The LH surge is superimposed on the smaller FSH surge. Positive feedback of estrogens, progestins, and activins on the hypothalamic-pituitary axis is involved in the induction of this LH surge. The primary trigger of the gonadotropin surge is a rise in **estradiol** to very high threshold levels just before the LH surge. The rise in estrogen levels has two effects. First, the accelerated rate of increase in estradiol levels in the preovulatory phase sensitizes the gonadotrophs in the anterior pituitary to GnRH pulses (Fig. 55-6). Second, the increasing estrogen levels also modulate hypothalamic neuronal activity and induce a GnRH surge, presumably through GnRH neurons in the preoptic area of the hypothalamus. Thus, the powerful *positive* feedback action of estradiol induces the midcycle surge of LH and, to a lesser extent, FSH. Gradually rising levels of the activins—secreted by granulosa cells—also act in a positive feedback manner to contribute to the FSH surge. In addition, gradually increasing levels of LH trigger the preovulatory follicle to increase its secretion of progesterone. These increasing—but still "low"—levels of **progesterone** also have a positive feedback effect on the

hypothalamic-pituitary axis that is synergistic with the positive feedback effect of the estrogens. Thus, although progesterone is not the primary trigger for the LH surge, it augments the effects of estradiol.

The gonadotropin surge causes ovulation and luteinization. The ovarian follicle ruptures, probably because of weakening of the follicular wall, and expels the oocyte and with it the surrounding cumulus and corona cells. This process is known as **ovulation**, and it is discussed in more detail in Chapter 56. As discussed later, a physiological change—**luteinization**—in the granulosa cells of the follicle causes these cells to secrete progesterone rather than estradiol. The granulosa and theca cells undergo structural changes that transform them into luteal cells, a process known as *luteinization*. The pulsatile rhythm of GnRH release and gonadotropin secretion is maintained throughout the gonadotropin surge.

As the **luteal phase** of the menstrual cycle begins, circulating levels of LH and FSH rapidly decrease (Fig. 55-9). This fall-off in gonadotropin levels reflects *negative* feedback by three ovarian hormones—estradiol, progesterone, and inhibin. Moreover, as gonadotropin levels fall, so do the levels of ovarian steroids. Thus, immediately after ovulation we see more or less concurrent decreases in the levels of both gonadotropins and ovarian hormones.

Later, during the luteal phase, the luteal cells of the corpus luteum gradually increase their synthesis of estradiol, progesterone, and inhibin (Fig. 55-9). The rise in concentration of these hormones causes—in typical negative feedback fashion—the continued decrease of gonadotropin levels midway through the luteal phase. One of the mechanisms of this negative feedback is the effect of progesterone on the hypothalamic-pituitary axis. Recall that at the peak of the LH surge, both the frequency and the amplitude of LH pulses are high. Progesterone levels rise, and high levels stimulate inhibitory opioidergic interneurons in the hypothalamus, thus inhibiting the GnRH neurons. This inhibition decreases the frequency of LH pulses, although the amplitude remains rather high.

By ~48 hours before onset of the menses, the pulsatile rhythm of LH secretion has decreased to one pulse every 3 to 4 hours. As a result, circulating levels of LH slowly fall during the luteal phase. During the late luteal phase, the gradual demise of the corpus luteum leads to decreases in the levels of progesterone, estradiol, and inhibin (Fig. 55-9). After the onset of menstruation, the hypothalamic-pituitary axis returns to a follicular-phase pattern of LH secretion (i.e., a gradual increase in the frequency of GnRH pulses).

OVARIAN STEROIDS

Starting from cholesterol, the ovary synthesizes estradiol, the major estrogen, and progesterone, the major progestin

Estrogens in female humans are derived from the ovary and the adrenal gland and from peripheral conversion in adipose tissue. In a *nonpregnant* woman, estradiol, the primary cir-

Table 55-2 Benefits and Risks of Oral Contraceptives

Oral Contraceptives Decrease the Risk of
Ovarian cancer
Endometrial cancer
Ovarian retention cysts
Ectopic pregnancy
Pelvic inflammatory disease
Benign breast disease

Oral Contraceptives Increase the Risk of
Benign liver tumors
Cholelithiasis (gallstones)
Hypertension
Heart attack
Stroke
Deep vein thrombosis
Pulmonary embolus

culating estrogen, is secreted principally by the ovary. The precursor for the biosynthesis of the ovarian steroids, as it is for all other steroid hormones produced elsewhere in the body, is cholesterol. Cholesterol is a 27-carbon sterol that is both ingested in the diet and synthesized in the liver from acetate (see Chapter 46). Ovarian cells can synthesize their own cholesterol de novo. Alternatively, cholesterol can enter cells in the form of LDL cholesterol and can bind to LDL receptors.

As shown in Figure 55-10, a cytochrome P-450 enzyme (see Table 50-2) known as the side-chain–cleavage enzyme (or 20,22-desmolase) catalyzes the conversion of cholesterol to **pregnenolone**. This reaction is the rate-limiting step in estrogen production. Ovarian cells then convert pregnenolone to progestins and estrogens. The initial steps of estrogen biosynthesis from pregnenolone follow the same steps as synthesis of the two so-called adrenal androgens **dehydroepiandrosterone** (**DHEA**) and **androstenedione**, both of which have 19 carbon atoms. These steps are discussed in connection with both substances (see Figs. 50-2 and 54-5). The Leydig cells in the testis can use either of two pathways to convert these weak androgens to **testosterone**. Cells in the ovaries are different because, as shown in Figure 55-10, they have an aromatase that can convert androstenedione to estrone and testosterone to estradiol. This aromatization also results in loss of the 19-methyl group (thus, the estrogens have only 18 carbons), as well as conversion of the ketone at position 3 to a hydroxyl in the A ring of the androgen precursor. Once formed, **estrone** can be converted into the more powerful estrogen **estradiol**, and vice versa, by 17β-hydroxysteroid dehydrogenase (17β-HSD). Finally, the liver can convert both estradiol and estrone into the weak estrogen **estriol**.

The two major **progestins**, **progesterone** and **17α-hydroxyprogesterone**, are formed even earlier in the biosynthetic pathway than the adrenal androgens. Functionally, progesterone is the more important progestin, and it has higher circulating levels.

Estrogen biosynthesis requires two ovarian cells and two gonadotropins, whereas progestin synthesis requires only a single cell

In the follicular phase of the menstrual cycle, the follicle synthesizes estrogens, whereas in the luteal phase, the corpus luteum does the synthesis. A unique aspect of estradiol synthesis is that it requires the contribution of two distinct cell types: the theca and granulosa cells within the follicle and the theca-lutein and granulosa-lutein cells within the corpus luteum (Fig. 55-11). I discuss these cells—as well as development of the follicle and corpus luteum—in the next major section.

The superficial **theca cells** and theca-lutein cells can take up cholesterol and produce the adrenal androgens, but they do not have the aromatase necessary for estrogen production. However, the deeper **granulosa cells** and granulosa-lutein cells have the aromatase, but they lack the 17α-hydroxylase and 17,20-desmolase (which are the same protein) necessary for making the adrenal androgens. Another difference between the two cell types is that—in the follicle—the superficial theca cell is near blood vessels and is hence a source of LDL cholesterol. The granulosa cell, conversely, is far from blood vessels and instead is surrounded by LDL-poor follicular fluid. Thus, in the follicular stage, the granulosa cells obtain most of their cholesterol by de novo synthesis. However, after formation of the corpus luteum, the accompanying vascularization makes it possible for the granulosa-lutein cell to take up LDL cholesterol from the blood and to thus synthesize large amounts of progesterone. A final difference between the two cell types is that theca cells have LH receptors, and granulosa cells have both LH and FSH receptors.

Because of their unique physiological properties, neither the theca/theca-lutein cells nor the granulosa/granulosa-lutein cells can make estrogens by themselves. According to the **two-cell, two-gonadotropin hypothesis**, estrogen synthesis occurs in the following steps:

Step 1. LH stimulates the theca cell, through the adenylyl cyclase pathway, to increase its synthesis of LDL receptors and the side-chain–cleavage enzyme.

Step 2. Thus stimulated, the theca cell increases its synthesis of androstenedione.

Step 3. The androstenedione synthesized in the theca cells freely diffuses to the granulosa cells.

Step 4. FSH, also acting through the adenylyl cyclase pathway, stimulates the granulosa cell to produce aromatase.

Step 5. The aromatase converts androstenedione to estrone (Fig. 55-10). 17β-HSD then converts the estrone to estradiol. Alternatively, 17β-HSD can first convert the same androstenedione to testosterone, and then the aromatase can convert this product to estradiol. By these pathways, theca-derived androgens are converted to estrogens in the granulosa cell.

Step 6. The estradiol diffuses into the blood vessels.

At low concentrations, the weak androgens produced by the theca cells are substrates for estrogen synthesis by the

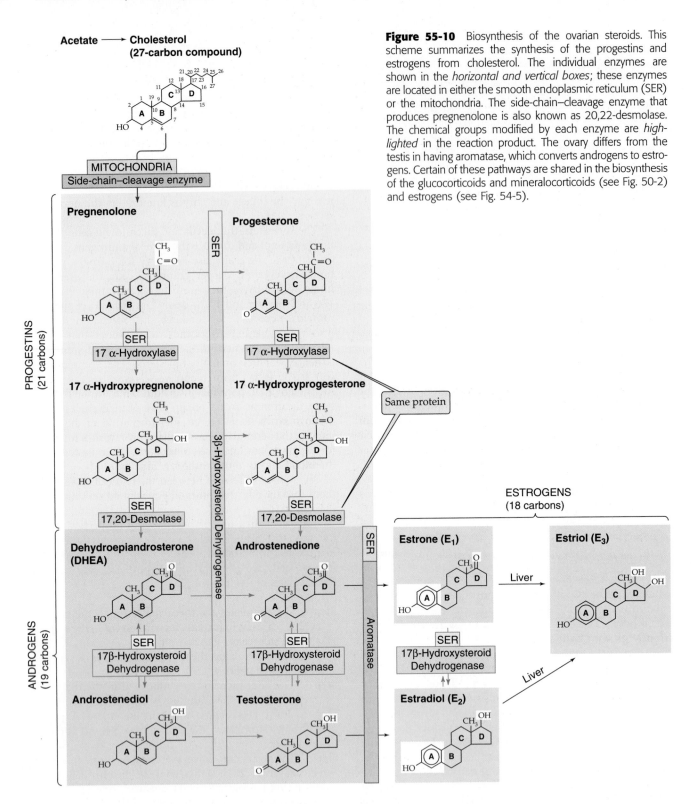

Figure 55-10 Biosynthesis of the ovarian steroids. This scheme summarizes the synthesis of the progestins and estrogens from cholesterol. The individual enzymes are shown in the *horizontal and vertical boxes*; these enzymes are located in either the smooth endoplasmic reticulum (SER) or the mitochondria. The side-chain–cleavage enzyme that produces pregnenolone is also known as 20,22-desmolase. The chemical groups modified by each enzyme are *highlighted* in the reaction product. The ovary differs from the testis in having aromatase, which converts androgens to estrogens. Certain of these pathways are shared in the biosynthesis of the glucocorticoids and mineralocorticoids (see Fig. 50-2) and estrogens (see Fig. 54-5).

granulosa cells, in addition to enhancing the aromatase activity of granulosa cells. However, at high concentrations, conversion of androgens to estrogens is diminished. Instead, the weak androgens are preferentially converted by 5α-reductase (see Fig. 54-5) to more potent androgens, such as **dihydrotestosterone**, a substance that cannot be converted to estrogen. Furthermore, these 5α-reduced androgens

inhibit aromatase activity. Thus, the net effect of a high-androgen environment in the follicle is to decrease estrogen production. These androgens also inhibit LH receptor formation on follicular cells.

In the luteal phase of the cycle, luteinization of the follicle substantially changes the biochemistry of the theca and granulosa cells. As part of the formation of the corpus

The Birth Control Pill

Hormonal contraception is the most commonly used method of contraception in the United States; ~30% of sexually active women take the oral contraceptive pill (OCP). Numerous combination (i.e., estrogen and progestin) oral contraceptives and progestin-only pills are available. The estrogens and progestins used in OCPs have varying potencies. In the United States, two estrogen compounds are approved for oral contraceptive use: ethinyl estradiol and mestranol. The progestins used in OCPs are modified steroids in which the methyl at position 19 (Fig. 55-10) is removed; these progestins include norethindrone, norgestrel, norethynodrel, norethindrone acetate, and ethynodiol diacetate. A new generation of progestins—including gestodene and norgestimate—have reduced androgenic effects.

The woman takes the OCP daily for 21 days out of the 28-day cycle; she takes no pill, a placebo, or an iron pill during days 22 to 28. No medication is usually given during this fourth week, to allow withdrawal bleeding to occur. Three regimens of contraceptive steroid administration are used:

1. **Monophasic or fixed-combination OCPs.** The pills taken for the first 21 days of the cycle are identical.
2. **Multiphasic or varying-dose OCPs.** The pills contain two or three different amounts of the same estrogen and progestin, the dosages of which vary at specific intervals during the 21-day medication period. Multiphasic OCPs generally maintain a low dose of estrogen throughout the cycle, combined with varying amounts of progestin. The rationale for this type of formulation is that the woman takes a lower total dose of steroid but is not at increased risk of breakthrough endometrial bleeding.
3. **Progestin-only OCPs** ("minipill"). The woman takes these estrogen-free OCPs daily for 3 weeks of a 4-week cycle. This regimen may be associated with irregular, low-grade, breakthrough endometrial bleeding. The progestin-only OCP is a good option for nursing mothers, as well as women for whom estrogens are contraindicated (e.g., those with thromboembolic disease, cerebral vascular incidents, and hypertension).

Biological Action of Oral Contraceptives

The contraceptive effectiveness of OCPs accrues from several actions. Like natural ovarian steroids, contraceptive steroids feed back both directly at the level of the hypothalamus (decreasing secretion of GnRH) and at the level of the gonadotrophs in the anterior pituitary (Fig. 55-4). The net effect is suppressed secretion of the gonadotropins, FSH and LH. The low FSH levels are insufficient to stimulate normal folliculogenesis; the low LH levels obviate the LH surge and therefore inhibit ovulation. However, in the commonly used doses, contraceptive steroids do not completely abolish either gonadotropin secretion or ovarian function.

The progestin effect of the OCP causes the cervical mucus to thicken and become viscid and scant. These actions inhibit sperm penetration into the uterus. The progestins also impair the motility of the uterus and oviducts and therefore decrease transport of both ova and sperm to the normal site of fertilization in the distal fallopian tube (see Chapter 56). Progestins also produce changes in the endometrium that are not conducive for implantation of the embryo. These changes include decreased glandular production of glycogen and thus diminished energy for the blastocyst to survive in the uterus.

Progestin-only OCPs do not effectively inhibit ovulation, as do the combination pills. However, they do produce the other actions: mucus thickening, reduced motility, and impaired implantation. Because they are inconsistent inhibitors of ovulation, the progestin-only OCPs have a substantially higher failure rate than does the combined type of OCP.

Side effects of the compounds in OCPs are those associated with estrogens and progestins and include nausea, edema, headaches, and weight gain. Side effects of progestins include depression, mastodynia, acne, and hirsutism. Many of the side effects associated with the progestin component of the pill are the result of the androgenic actions of the progestins used, particularly the acne and hirsutism. The potential benefits of the newer progestins include decreased androgenic effects, such as increased sex hormone–binding globulin, improved glucose tolerance (see Chapter 51), and increased high-density lipoprotein and decreased LDL cholesterol (see Chapter 46). The clinical impact of these changes remains to be determined. Table 55-2 lists the major benefits and risks of OCPs.

luteum, blood vessels invade deep toward the granulosa-lutein cells. Recall that in the follicle, the granulosa cells had been surrounded by follicular fluid, which is poor in LDL cholesterol. The increased vascularity facilitates the delivery of LDL cholesterol to the granulosa-lutein cells. In addition, LH stimulates the granulosa-lutein cell to take up and process cholesterol—as it does in theca cells. The net effect is the increased progesterone biosynthesis that is characteristic of the midluteal phase. Indeed, the major products of the corpus luteum are **progesterone** and 17α-hydroxyprogesterone, although the corpus luteum also produces estradiol. As indicated in Figure 55-11, the granulosa-lutein cells cannot make either 17α-hydroxyprogesterone or estradiol directly because these cells lack the protein that has dual activity for 17α-hydroxylase and 17,20-desmolase (Fig. 55-10). Thus, 17α-hydroxyprogesterone synthesis necessi-

tates that progesterone first moves to the theca-lutein cell (Fig. 55-11), which can convert progesterone to **17α-hydroxyprogesterone**, as well as androstenedione. Furthermore, estradiol synthesis necessitates that androstenedione from the theca-lutein cell moves to the granulosa-lutein cell for aromatization and formation of **estradiol**.

The principal functions of estrogens are stimulation of cellular proliferation and growth of sex organs and other tissues related to reproduction

Most estrogens in blood plasma are bound to carrier proteins, as are testosterone and other steroid hormones. In the case of estradiol, 60% is bound to **albumin** and 38% to **sex hormone–binding globulin (SHBG)**—also known as

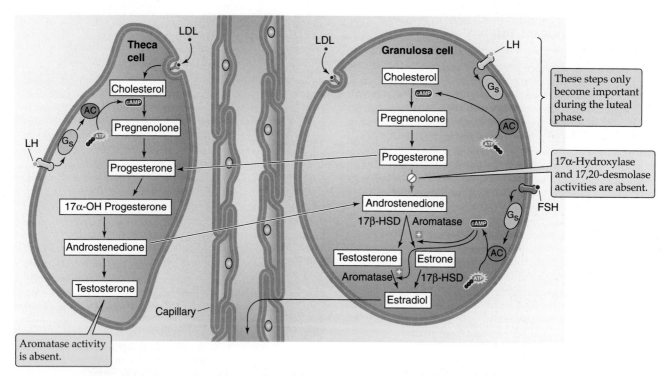

Figure 55-11   Two-cell, two-gonadotropin model. During the follicular phase, the major product of the follicle is estradiol, whereas during the luteal phase, the major products of the corpus luteum are the progestins, although estradiol synthesis is still substantial. In the follicular phase, LH primes the theca cell to convert cholesterol to androstenedione. Because the theca cell lacks aromatase, it cannot generate estradiol from this androstenedione. Instead, the androstenedione diffuses to the granulosa cell, whose aromatase activity has been stimulated by FSH. The aromatase converts the androstenedione to estradiol. In the luteal phase, the vascularization of the corpus luteum makes low LDL available to the granulosa-lutein cells. Thus, both the theca-lutein and the granulosa-lutein cells can produce progesterone, the major product of the corpus luteum. For production of 17α-hydroxyprogesterone (17α-OH progesterone), some of the progesterone diffuses into the theca-lutein cell, which has the 17α-hydroxylase activity needed for converting the progesterone to 17α-hydroxyprogesterone. The theca-lutein cell can also generate the androstenedione, which diffuses into the granulosa-lutein cell for estradiol synthesis. AC, adenylyl cyclase.

testosterone-binding globulin (TeBG; see Chapter 54). The latter name is doubly a misnomer; not only does TeBG bind estradiol, but also TeBG levels are twice as high in women as they are in men. At least one reason for the higher levels in women is that estrogens (including birth control pills) stimulate the synthesis of SHBG. Only 2% of total plasma estradiol circulates as the free hormone. Because of their lipid solubility, estrogens readily cross cell membranes. Although it was once believed that estrogens bound to cytoplasmic receptors, more recently it became clear that the receptor for estradiol resides in the cell nucleus (see Chapter 3). The **estrogen receptor (ER)** functions as a homodimer (see Table 4-2). The estrogen–estrogen receptor complex interacts with steroid response elements on chromatin and rapidly induces the transcription of specific genes to produce mRNA. The RNA enters the cytoplasm and increases protein synthesis, which modulates numerous cellular functions. Over the next several hours, DNA synthesis increases, and the mitogenic action of estrogens becomes apparent. Estrogens almost exclusively affect particular target sex organs that have the estrogen receptor. These organs include the uterus and the breasts.

The **progestins**, particularly progesterone, stimulate glandular secretion in reproductive tissue and promote the maturation of certain estrogen-stimulated tissue. One of the most prominent actions of progesterone, which binds to the dimeric **progesterone receptor** (PR; see Table 4-2), is the induction of secretory changes in the endometrium. The endometrium must be conditioned by estrogen for progesterone to act effectively. During the latter half of the menstrual cycle, progesterone induces final maturation of the uterine endometrium for reception and implantation of the fertilized ovum.

THE OVARIAN CYCLE: FOLLICULOGENESIS, OVULATION, AND FORMATION OF THE CORPUS LUTEUM

Follicles mature in stages from primordial to graafian (or preovulatory) follicles

Oocyte maturation—the production of a haploid female gamete capable of fertilization by a sperm—begins in the fetal ovary. The **primordial germ cells** migrate from the hind gut to the gonadal ridge. These primordial germ cells develop into **oogonia**, or immature germ cells, which, in turn, proliferate in the fetal ovary by *mitotic* division (see Chapter 53). By 6 to 7 weeks of intrauterine life, ~10,000 oogonia are present. This figure is the result of migration and rapid mitotic division; up until this time, no atresia occurs. By ~8 weeks' gestation, ~600,000 oogonia are present, and they may enter prophase of the first meiosis and become **primary oocytes**. From this point onward, the number of germ cells is determined by three ongoing processes: mitosis, meiosis, and atresia. By middle fetal life, all the mitotic divisions of the female germ cells have been completed, and the number of germ cells peaks at 6 to 7 million around 20 weeks' gestation. At this point, oogonia enter their first *meiotic* division. During prophase of the first meiosis, when the primary oocytes have a duplicated set of 23 chromosomes (4N DNA)—22 duplicated pairs of autosomal chromosomes and 1 pair of duplicated X chromosomes)—crossing over occurs (see Fig. 53-1C). Meiosis arrests in prophase I. This prolonged state of meiotic arrest is known as the **dictyotene stage**. During the remainder of fetal life and childhood, the number of primary oocytes gradually declines to ~2 to 2.5 million at birth and to ~400,000 just before puberty. As we shall see, they remain primary oocytes—arrested in prophase I of meiosis—until just before ovulation, many years later, when meiosis is completed and the first polar body is extruded. Oocyte maturation is complete when the resulting haploid oocyte is capable of fertilization by a sperm.

The few primary oocytes that survive are those that are surrounded by flat, spindle-shaped follicular or **pregranulosa cells** (Fig. 55-12). This oocyte-pregranulosa cell complex is enclosed by a basement lamina. At this stage of development, the primary oocyte with its surrounding single layer of pregranulosa cells is called a **primordial follicle**. Primordial follicles are 30 to 60 μm in diameter. The first primordial follicle usually appears ~6 weeks into intrauterine life, and the generation of primordial follicles is complete by ~6 months after birth.

The ovarian follicle is the primary functional unit of the ovary. Throughout reproductive life, some 90% to 95% of all follicles are the primordial (i.e., "nongrowing") follicles discussed earlier. The growing follicles that are recruited from this pool of primordial follicles undergo a striking series of changes in size, morphology, and physiology. This follicular development, as well as the subsequent ovulation, is central to control of the menstrual cycle.

The first step in follicular growth is that a primordial follicle becomes a primary follicle. The **primary follicle** (Fig. 55-12) forms as the spindle cells of the primordial follicle become cuboidal cells. In addition, the oocyte enlarges. Thus, the primary follicle contains a larger primary oocyte that is surrounded by a single layer of cuboidal **granulosa cells**.

The **secondary follicle** (Fig. 55-12) contains a primary oocyte surrounded by *several* layers of cuboidal granulosa cells. The granulosa cells of a primary follicle proliferate and give rise to several layers of cells. In addition, stromal cells differentiate, surround the follicle, and become the theca cells. These **theca cells** are on the outside of the follicle's

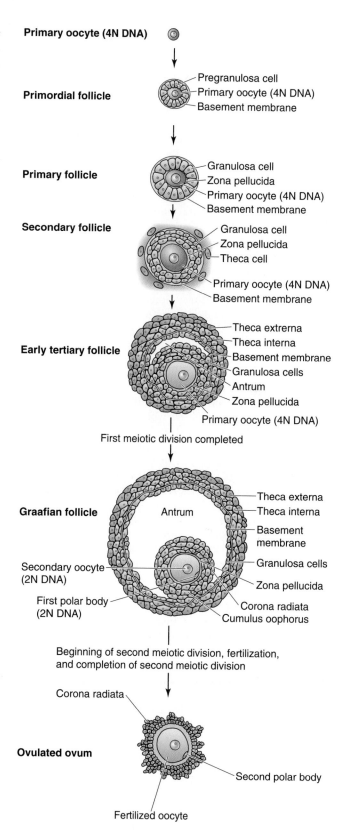

Figure 55-12 The maturation of the ovarian follicle.

basement membrane. The oocyte increases in size to a diameter of ~120 µm. As the developing follicle increases in size, the number of granulosa cells increases to ~600, and the theca cells show increasing differentiation. The progression to secondary follicles also entails the formation of capillaries and an increase in the vascular supply to developing follicular units.

As the increasingly abundant granulosa cells secrete fluid into the center of the follicle, they create a fluid-filled space called the **antrum**. At this stage, the follicle is now a **tertiary follicle** (Fig. 55-12), the first of the two antral stages. In contrast to this tertiary follicle, the primordial, primary, and secondary follicles are solid masses of cells that lack an antrum; they are therefore referred to as *preantral* follicles. In tertiary follicles, gap junctions are located among both theca cells and granulosa cells. In addition, tight junctions and desmosomes exist between adjacent cells. Gap junctions may also exist between the oocyte and the granulosa cells closest to the oocyte and may function as thoroughfares to transport nutrients and information from the granulosa cells to the oocyte and vice versa. The granulosa cells closest to the oocyte also secrete the mucopolysaccharides that form the **zona pellucida** immediately surrounding the oocyte.

As the antrum enlarges, it nearly encircles the oocyte, except for a small mound or cumulus that attaches the oocyte to the rest of the follicle, whose diameter increases to 20 to 33 mm. This preovulatory or **graafian follicle** (Fig. 55-12) is the second of the two antral stages.

The granulosa cells of the tertiary and graafian follicles are of three types: (1) **mural granulosa cells**, which are the farthest from the center of the follicle, are the most metabolically active, and contain large quantities of LH receptors and enzymes that are necessary for the synthesis of steroids; (2) **cumulus granulosa cells** are shed with the oocyte at the time of ovulation; and (3) **antral granulosa cells**, which face the antrum, are left behind within the follicle to become the large luteal cells of the corpus luteum. The capacity of the three types of granulosa cells to generate steroids differs. Cumulus cells contain neither the side-chain–cleavage enzyme (P-450$_{scc}$) nor aromatase (P-450$_{arom}$) and therefore cannot generate estrogens. Moreover, cumulus cells respond less to LH and have a low overall LH receptor content. The exact role of the cumulus layer has not been definitively established, although investigators have postulated that the cumulus layer may function as a feeder layer and may provide stem cells that differentiate into other follicular cell types.

Both FSH and LH stimulate follicular growth

Even in fetal life and childhood, some primordial follicles can develop all the way to the antral stage. However, these follicles all undergo **atresia** (death of the ovum, followed by collapse of the follicle and scarring) at some stage in their development. At the time of puberty, the increase in levels of gonadotropins and ovarian steroids produces a marked increase in the rate of follicular development. During the luteal phase of each cycle, a cohort of primordial follicles is recruited for further development into graafian follicles, a process that occurs during the follicular phase of the next cycle. Thus, primordial follicles may remain in a nongrowing state for 50 years before they develop into primary follicles. All along the course of this development, follicular units undergo atresia until only one dominant graafian follicle remains at the time of ovulation. Some controversy exists about the length of this developmental process. Some investigators believe that the entire developmental process takes three to four monthly cycles. However, the predominant view is that a cohort of primary follicles is recruited during the end of one cycle, and one of these follicles develops into the dominant graafian follicle.

Primary Follicles   Appropriate structural and functional development of the follicle necessitates that the follicle is exposed to the appropriate sequence of three hormones: FSH, estradiol, and LH. FSH secretion occurs during early fetal life, and FSH can be detected as early as 5 months into gestation (Fig. 55-2). Three pieces of evidence suggest that gonadotropins and estrogens are essential for early follicular growth, that is, for the progression from *primordial* to *primary follicles*. First, hypophysectomy (i.e., removal of the pituitary) causes depletion of *primordial* follicular units in primates. Thus, with the absence of gonadotropins—as well as other pituitary hormones—and a reduction in estrogens, no follicular development takes place in females. Second, patients with *resistant ovary syndrome* have a normal complement of *primordial* follicles, but the follicles do not develop beyond the primordial stage. Although these patients have high circulating levels of FSH, they have no receptors for FSH and LH in their ovaries. Thus, FSH or LH must be able to act on the ovary for follicular development to occur. Third, in individuals with 17α-hydroxylase deficiency—and thus low estrogen levels—follicular development does not progress beyond the *primordial* stage. Circulating levels of LH in these individuals are normal or high. These three lines of evidence suggest that removal of the gonadotropins, the gonadotropin receptors, or the estrogens halts early follicular growth.

Secondary Follicles   As primary follicles form secondary follicles, the theca cells proliferate and acquire LH receptors, as well as the ability to synthesize steroids. Moreover, the granulosa cells acquire receptors for FSH, androgens, and estrogens. When the granulosa cells acquire FSH receptors, the follicular unit becomes a functional steroid-producing entity.

Tertiary Follicles   Formation of the antrum, which leads to the development of a tertiary follicle, also requires gonadotropins. FSH, acting in concert with estrogens, causes the proliferation of granulosa cells after development of the antrum, and as a result, the total number of receptors for FSH is increased. FSH, along with estradiol, also induces the proliferation of LH receptors in granulosa cells.

Graafian Follicles   When human granulosa cells from graafian follicles are studied in vitro, the mitotic and steroid-synthesizing characteristics of these cells reflect the hormonal condition of the follicle from which they came. Both FSH and estradiol are needed for mitosis to occur in granulosa cells. FSH, LH, and estradiol are necessary for maximum progesterone production by granulosa cells. Premature exposure of developing follicles to LH *inhibits* mitosis, as well as steroidogenesis. Therefore, the follicle must be exposed to the appropriate sequence of hormones (e.g., FSH, followed by estradiol and then LH) for appropriate maturational and functional development.

Each month, a cohort of follicles is recruited, one of which achieves dominance

The consensus is that the monthly cycle of folliculogenesis actually begins from the primary follicle stage 2 to 3 days before onset of the menses of the previous cycle. At this time, FSH levels begin to increase (Fig. 55-9) because of decreasing inhibin concentrations, thus inducing folliculogenesis, which is completed in the next cycle.

Although we do not understand why some primordial follicles—and not others—join a developing cohort of follicles, FSH is thought to be at least partly responsible for continued development of a cohort of follicles each cycle. The number of follicles in a cohort depends on the residual pool of remaining follicles in the ovary. As the cycle continues, only some of the cohort of follicles continue to develop in response to gonadotropin secretion. The other members of the cohort of follicles undergo atresia.

The one follicle destined to ovulate is recruited during the early days of the current menstrual cycle and eventually achieves dominance. Although the mechanism of selection of the dominant follicle is not completely understood, it is thought to be caused by estrogen-induced events within the follicles. As estrogen levels rise during the follicular phase of the cycle, the pituitary gradually lowers its secretion of FSH (Fig. 55-9). Rising inhibin levels also feed back on the anterior pituitary to decrease FSH secretion. Peak inhibin levels correlate with the number of follicles present and rise in parallel with circulating estradiol levels.

Decreased levels of FSH cause a decline in FSH-dependent aromatase activity in granulosa cells. As a result, estrogen production decreases in the less mature follicles. Conversely, estrogen *increases* the effectiveness of FSH in the more mature follicles by increasing the number of FSH receptors. Although the dominant follicle continues to be dependent on FSH, it has more FSH receptors, a greater rate of granulosa cell proliferation, more FSH-dependent aromatase activity, and more estrogen production than the less dominant follicles. Because the less dominant follicles have less aromatase activity, the androstenedione in the theca cells cannot be converted as readily to estrogens in the granulosa cell. Instead, the androstenedione either builds up or is converted to other androgens. The less dominant follicles consequently undergo atresia under the influence of androgens in their local environment. In contrast, the production of estrogens and inhibins allows the dominant follicle to become prominent and to gain an even greater edge over its competitors. The vascular supply to the thecal layer of the dominant follicle increases rapidly, so that during the late follicular phase, the vasculature of the dominant follicle is several-fold greater than that of other follicles in the cohort. Increased vascularity may allow greater FSH delivery to the dominant follicle and may thus help to maintain dominance of the follicle selected for ovulation.

Estradiol secretion by the dominant follicle triggers the LH surge, which, in turn, signals ovulation

Ovulation occurs at the midpoint of every normal menstrual cycle and is triggered by the LH surge, which, in turn, is stimulated by rapidly rising levels of estradiol. Estradiol secretion by the dominant follicle increases rapidly near the end of the late follicular phase (Fig. 55-9). This dramatic rise in circulating estradiol exerts positive feedback on the anterior pituitary and sensitizes it to GnRH. The net effect of a rising estradiol level is induction of the LH surge. The LH surge is generally initiated 24 to 36 hours after peak estradiol secretion is achieved, and ovulation usually occurs ~36 hours after onset of the LH surge and ~12 hours after its peak. Thus, it appears that the developing follicle, through its increased estradiol secretion, signals the hypothalamic-pituitary system that follicular maturation is complete and that the hypothalamic-pituitary axis can now release a bolus of gonadotropin to induce ovulation. The LH surge appears to terminate in part as a result of rising levels of progesterone, through negative feedback, and in part as a result of loss of the positive feedback that is derived from estradiol. Depletion of gonadotropin stores in the anterior pituitary gland may also contribute to termination of the LH surge.

At the time of the LH surge, the primary oocyte (4N DNA), which had been arrested in the prophase of its first meiotic division since fetal life (see Chapter 53), now resumes meiosis and completes its first meiotic division several hours before ovulation. The result of this first meiotic division is a small **first polar body**, which degenerates or divides to form nonfunctional cells, and a much larger **secondary oocyte**. Both the first polar body and the secondary oocyte, like secondary spermatocytes (see Chapter 54), have a haploid number of duplicated chromosomes (2N DNA): 22 duplicated somatic chromosomes and 1 duplicated X chromosome. This secondary oocyte begins its second meiotic division, but it becomes arrested in metaphase until the time of fertilization (see Chapter 56). The secondary oocyte is surrounded by the zona pellucida and one or more layers of follicular cells, the **corona radiata**. Before ovulation, the **cumulus oophorus** expands under the influence of LH, and eventually a complex consisting of the cumulus, the oocyte, and its surrounding cells breaks free with its "stalk" and floats inside the antrum, surrounded by follicular fluid. Breaking away of the oocyte-cumulus complex is probably facilitated by increased hyaluronidase synthesis that is stimulated by FSH.

Release of the oocyte from the follicle—**ovulation**—follows thinning and weakening of the follicular wall, probably under the influence of both LH and progesterone. Both LH and progesterone enhance the activity of proteolytic enzymes (e.g., collagenase) within the follicle and thus lead to the digestion of connective tissue in the follicular wall. Prostaglandins, particularly those in the E and F series, may also contribute to ovulation, perhaps by triggering the release of lysosomal enzymes that digest the follicular wall. Ultimately, a **stigma**—or spot—forms on the surface of the dominant follicle. As this stigma balloons out and forms a vesicle, it ruptures, and the oocyte is expelled. Ovulation is apparently facilitated by increased intrafollicular pressure and contraction of smooth muscle in the theca as a result of prostaglandin stimulation.

The expelled oocyte, with its investment of follicular cells, is picked up by the fimbriae of the fallopian tube (Fig. 55-1) as they move over the surface of the ovary. The oocyte is then transported through the infundibulum into the ampulla by means of ciliary movement of the tubal epithelium, as well as by muscular contractions of the tube. Fertilization, if it occurs, takes place in the ampullary portion of the fallopian tube. The resulting zygote subsequently resides there for ~72 hours, followed by rapid transport through the isthmus to the uterine cavity, where it floats free for an additional 2 to 3 days before attaching to the endometrium.

After ovulation, the theca and granulosa cells of the follicle differentiate into the theca-lutein and granulosa-lutein cells of the highly vascularized corpus luteum

After expulsion of the oocyte, the granulosa and theca cells are thrown up into folds that occupy the follicular cavity and form the **corpus luteum**, a temporary endocrine organ whose major product is progesterone. The corpus luteum is highly vascularized, and surrounding blood vessels penetrate the theca and granulosa layers. Blood accumulates in the resealed antral cavity of the corpus luteum soon after ovulation. Formation of the corpus luteum occurs as a result of transformation of the granulosa and theca cells under the influence of LH (Fig. 55-12). The theca cells at the periphery of the follicle differentiate into stroma and give rise to **theca-lutein cells**—also known as small luteal cells. The granulosa cells, in contrast, enlarge and give rise to **granulosa-lutein cells**—also known as large luteal cells. Therefore, the mature corpus luteum is composed of two cell types: theca-lutein and granulosa-lutein cells.

During the luteal phase of the menstrual cycle, estrogens and progestins inhibit folliculogenesis. Luteal function begins to decrease ~11 days after ovulation. The mechanisms responsible for luteal regression—or **luteolysis**—remain open to speculation. One school of thought postulates that withdrawal of trophic support results in demise of the corpus luteum, whereas the second school maintains that local factors induce luteal regression. For example, prostaglandin $F_{2\alpha}$ inhibits luteal function and terminates the life of the corpus luteum.

Growth and involution of the corpus luteum produce the rise and fall in progestins and estrogens during the luteal phase of the menstrual cycle

Although the corpus luteum produces both estrogen and progesterone, the luteal phase is primarily dominated by progesterone secretion. Estrogen production by the corpus luteum is largely a function of the theca-lutein or the small cells, which also produce androgens. Progestin production in the corpus luteum is primarily a function of the granulosa-lutein or large cells (Fig. 55-11), which also produce estrogens.

As shown earlier in Figure 55-9, **progesterone** production rises before follicular rupture. After ovulation, proges-

terone levels rise sharply and peak in ~7 days. Progesterone acts locally to inhibit follicular growth during the luteal phase. In addition, progesterone may act centrally by inhibiting gonadotropin secretion. Progestins are also antiestrogens. As a result, progestins acting locally may downregulate ERs and may reduce the effectiveness of estradiol. Therefore, increasing progesterone production may have adverse effects on folliculogenesis.

Estradiol levels also rise during the luteal phase (Fig. 55-9) and reflect production by the corpus luteum. The estradiol produced during the luteal phase is necessary for the occurrence of progesterone-induced changes in the endometrium.

Unless rescued by hCG (see Chapter 56)—produced by the syncytial trophoblasts of the blastocyst—luteal production of progesterone ceases toward the end of the menstrual cycle. hCG produced by the developing conceptus maintains steroidogenic function of the corpus luteum until approximately the ninth week of gestation, at which time placental function is well established. If not rescued by pregnancy, the hormone-producing cells of the corpus luteum degenerate and leave behind a fibrotic **corpus albicans**.

THE ENDOMETRIAL CYCLE

In the human female fetus, the uterine mucosa is capable of responding to steroid hormones by 20 weeks' gestation. Indeed, some of the uterine glands begin secreting material by the 22nd week of gestation. Endometrial development in utero apparently occurs in response to estrogens derived from the maternal placenta. At ~32 weeks' gestation, glycogen deposition and stromal edema are present in the endometrium. As estrogenic stimulation is withdrawn after delivery, the endometrium regresses, and at ~4 weeks after birth, the glands are atrophic and lack vascularization. The endometrium remains in this state until puberty.

The ovarian hormones drive the morphological and functional changes of the endometrium during the monthly cycle

The ovarian steroids—estrogens and progestins—control the cyclic monthly growth and breakdown of the endometrium. The three major phases in the endometrial cycle are the menstrual, proliferative, and secretory phases.

The Menstrual Phase If the oocyte was not fertilized and pregnancy did not occur in the previous cycle, a sudden diminution in estrogen and progesterone secretion will signal the demise of the corpus luteum. As hormonal support of the endometrium is withdrawn, the vascular and glandular integrity of the endometrium degenerates, the tissue breaks down, and menstrual bleeding ensues; this moment is defined as day 1 of the menstrual cycle (Fig. 55-13). After menstruation, all that remains on the inner surface of most of the uterus is a thin layer of *nonepithelial* stromal cells and some remnant glands. However, epithelial cells remain in the lower uterine segments, as well as regions close to the fallopian tubes.

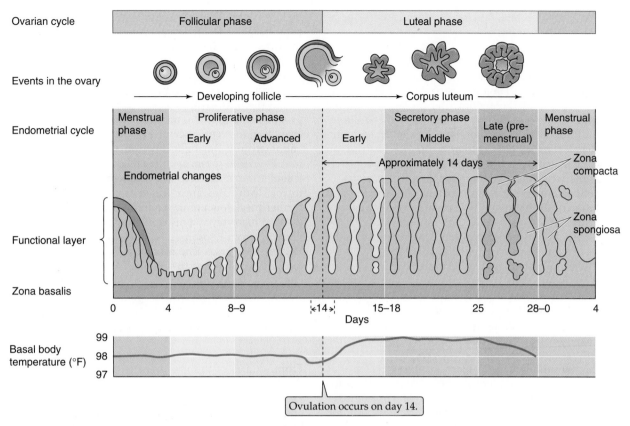

Figure 55-13 The endometrial cycle. The ovarian cycle includes the follicular phase—in which the follicle develops—and the luteal phase—in which the remaining follicular cells develop into the corpus luteum. The endometrial cycle has three parts: the menstrual, the proliferative, and the secretory phases.

The Proliferative Phase After menstruation, the endometrium is restored by about the fifth day of the cycle (Fig. 55-13) as a result of proliferation of the basal stromal cells on the denuded surface of the uterus (the *zona basalis*), as well as the proliferation of epithelial cells from other parts of the uterus. The stroma gives rise to the connective tissue components of the endometrium. Increased mitotic activity of the stromal and glandular epithelium continues throughout the follicular phase of the cycle and beyond, until ~3 days after ovulation. Cellular hyperplasia and increased extracellular matrix result in thickening of the endometrium during the late proliferative phase. The thickness of the endometrium increases from ~0.5 to as much as 5 mm during the proliferative phase.

Proliferation and differentiation of the endometrium are stimulated by estrogen that is secreted by the developing follicles. Levels of estrogen rise early in the follicular phase and peak just before ovulation (Fig. 55-9). *ER* levels in the endometrium also increase during the follicular phase of the menstrual cycle. Levels of endometrial ER are highest during the proliferative phase and decline after ovulation in response to changing levels of progesterone. As already discussed, estradiol binds to a nuclear receptor on the endometrial cell, and the activated receptor interacts with the hormone response elements of specific genes and modulates their transcription rates.

Estrogen is believed to act on the endometrium in part through its effect on the expression of proto-oncogenes (see Chapter 3) that are involved in the expression of certain genes. Part of the effect of estrogens is to induce the synthesis of growth factors such as the insulin-like growth factors (IGFs, also called **somatomedins**; see Chapter 48), TGFs, and epidermal growth factor (EGF). These autocrine and paracrine mediators are necessary for maturation and growth of the endometrium. Estrogen causes the stromal components of the endometrium to become highly developed. Estrogen also induces the synthesis of progestin receptors in endometrial tissue. Levels of progestin receptors peak at ovulation, when estrogen levels are highest, to prepare the cells for the high progestin levels of the luteal phase of the cycle.

Progesterone, in contrast, opposes the action of estrogen on the epithelial cells of the endometrium and functions as an antiestrogen. Although progesterone inhibits *epithelial* cell proliferation, it promotes proliferation of the endometrial *stroma*. Progesterone exerts its primary antiestrogen effects by stimulating 17β-HSD and sulfotransferase, enzymes that convert estradiol to weaker compounds. Thus, 17β-HSD may convert the estradiol captured from the extracellular environment to estrone (Fig. 55-10), and sulfotransferase may conjugate estrogens to sulfate and produce derivatives such as estradiol 3-sulfate. Estrone is far less active than estradiol, and sulfated estrogens are by themselves biologically inactive.

The Secretory Phase During the early luteal phase of the ovarian cycle, progesterone further stimulates the 17β-HSD and sulfation reactions. These antiestrogenic effects halt the proliferative phase of the endometrial cycle. Progesterone also stimulates the glandular components of the endometrium and thus induces secretory changes in the endometrium. The epithelial cells exhibit a marked increase in secretory activity, as indicated by increased amounts of endoplasmic reticulum and mitochondria. These increases in synthetic activity occur in anticipation of the arrival and implantation of the blastocyst. The **early secretory phase** of the menstrual cycle (Fig. 55-13) is characterized by the development of a network of interdigitating tubes within the nucleolus of the endometrial epithelial cells. These tubes are referred to as the **nucleolar channel system**, and progesterone apparently stimulates their development. The cytoplasm invaginates near the nucleolar channel system, although it remains unclear whether actual connections exist between the channel system and the cytoplasm. The nucleolar channel system may provide a route of transport for mRNA to the cytoplasm.

During the **middle to late secretory phase**, evidence of increased secretory capacity of the endometrial glands becomes more apparent. Vascularization of the endometrium increases, the glycogen content increases, and the thickness of the endometrium increases to 5 to 6 mm. The endometrial glands become engorged with secretions. They are no longer straight; instead, they become tortuous and achieve maximal secretory activity at approximately day 20 or 21 of the menstrual cycle.

The changes in the endometrium are not limited to the glands; they also occur in the stromal cells between the glands. Beginning 9 to 10 days after ovulation, stromal cells that surround the spiral arteries of the uterus enlarge and develop eosinophilic cytoplasm, with a prominent Golgi complex and endoplasmic reticulum. This process is referred to as **predecidualization**. The rounded **decidual cells** differentiate from spindle-shaped fibroblast-like stromal cells under the influence of progesterone. As the stromal cells differentiate into decidual cells, their biochemical activity changes, and they form secretory products typical of decidual cells. Laminin, fibronectin, heparin sulfate, and type IV collagen surround matrices of decidualizing cells. Multiple foci of these decidual cells spread throughout the upper layer of the endometrium and form a dense layer called the **zona compacta** (Fig. 55-13). This spreading is so extensive that the glandular structures of the zona compacta become inconspicuous. Inflammatory cells accumulate around glands and blood vessels. Edema of the midzone of the endometrium distinguishes the compact area from the underlying **zona spongiosa**, where the endometrial glands become more prominent.

Together, the superficial *zona compacta* and the midlevel *zona spongiosa* make up the so-called **functional layer** of the endometrium. This functional layer is the region that proliferates early in the monthly endometrial cycle, that later interacts with the embryo during pregnancy, that is shed after pregnancy, and that is also shed each month during menstruation. The deepest layer of the endometrium—the **zona basalis**—is the layer left behind after parturition or menstruation. The cells of the zona basalis give rise to the proliferation at the beginning of the next endometrial cycle.

During the late luteal phase of the menstrual cycle, just before the next menstruation, levels of both estrogens and progestins diminish, and these decreased ovarian steroid levels lead to eventual demise of the upper two thirds of the endometrium. During this period, the spiral arteries rhythmically go into spasm and then relax. This period of the cycle is sometimes referred to as the **ischemic phase**. As cells begin to die, hydrolases are released from lysosomes and cause further breakdown of the endometrium. Prostaglandin production increases as a result of the action of phospholipases liberated from lysosomes. Necrosis of vascular cells leads to microhemorrhage. The average loss of blood, tissues, and serous fluid amounts to ~30 mL. Menstrual blood does not clot because of the presence of fibrolysins released from necrotic endometrial tissue.

The effective implantation window is 3 to 4 days

From studies of embryo transfer to recipient mothers in oocyte donation programs (see the box in Chapter 56 on in vitro fertilization), when both the age of the donated embryo and the time of the endometrial cycle of the recipient are known, the period of endometrial receptivity for implantation of the embryo is estimated to extend from as early as day 16 to as late as day 19 of the menstrual cycle. Of course, because implantation must normally follow the ovulation that occurs on day 14 and because fertilization normally occurs within 1 day of ovulation, the effective window is less than 4 days, from day 16 to day 19. In contrast, when embryos are transferred on cycle days 20 through 24, no pregnancies are achieved.

Although the mechanisms underlying endometrial receptivity remain unclear, several changes in the endometrium are believed to be associated with increased receptivity of the endometrium for the embryo. The formation of microvilli and pinopods (i.e., protrusions of endometrial cells near gland openings) during the midluteal phase and the secretion of extracellular matrix composed of such materials as glycoproteins, laminin, and fibronectin may provide a surface that facilitates attachment of the embryo (see Chapter 56).

THE FEMALE SEX ACT

Female sexual desire—**libido**—is a complex phenomenon that consists of physical and psychological effects, all modulated by circulating sex steroids. Libido varies during the ovarian cycle, and the frequency of female sexual activity increases around the time of ovulation. There may also be an increase in the rate of initiation of sexual activity by women around the time of ovulation. These changes may, in part, reflect the increased secretion of androgenic steroids that occurs just before and during ovulation secondary to the LH surge.

The female sex response, which is elicited by physical, psychic, and hormonal stimuli, occurs in four distinct phases

Although sexual function has a strong physiological basis, it is not possible to separate sexual response from the other emotional and contributing factors involved in sexual relationships. Masters and Johnson published, in their now classic work *Human Sexual Response*, a discussion of data obtained on the sexual cycles of 700 subjects. Our current understanding of the female sexual response is based on their findings. Masters and Johnson described four stages of the sex response in women: the excitement or seduction phase, plateau, orgasm, and resolution. Following is a brief description of each phase.

Excitement   The excitement or arousal phase of the female sex response may be initiated by a multitude of internal or external stimuli, including psychological factors, such as thoughts and emotions, and physical factors, such as sight and tactile stimuli. Table 55-3 summarizes the responses of the excitement phase, many of which reflect activity of the parasympathetic division of the autonomic nervous system (ANS). Sexual intensity rises in crescendo fashion.

Plateau   The plateau stage is the culmination of the excitement phase as it reaches its peak. It is associated with a marked degree of vasocongestion throughout the body.

Orgasm   During orgasm, the sexual tension that has built up in the entire body is released. The climax, or orgasm, is intense and includes a myotonic response throughout the body. Muscle contractions start 2 to 4 seconds after the woman begins to experience orgasm, and they repeat at 0.8-second intervals. The actual number of contractions, as well as their intensity, varies from woman to woman. Some women observed to have orgasmic contractions are not aware that they are having an orgasm. Masters and Johnson suggested that prolonged stimulation during the excitement phase leads to more pronounced orgasmic activity. Whereas the excitement phase is under the influence of the parasympathetic division of the ANS, as is the erection phase in men, orgasm seems to be related to the sympathetic division, as is the emission phase in men (see Chapter 54).

Resolution   The last phase of the female sex response is a return of the woman's physiological state to the pre-excitement level. During the resolution phase, the woman generally experiences a feeling of personal satisfaction, well-being, and relaxation of sexual desire. A new sexual excitement cycle may be initiated at any time after orgasm without the refractory phase that occurs in men.

Both the sympathetic and the parasympathetic divisions control the female sex response

Much of the response in the excitement phase results from stimulation of the **parasympathetic fibers** of the ANS. In some cases, anticholinergic drugs may interfere with a full

Table 55-3   Female Sexual Response Cycle

Excitement
Warmth and erotic feelings
Increased sexual tension
Deep breathing
Increased heart rate
Increased blood pressure
Generalized vasocongestion
Skin flush
Breast engorgement
Nipple erection (myotonic effect)
Engorgement of labia and clitoris
Vaginal "sweating" (transudative lubrication)
Secretions from Bartholin glands
Uterine tenting into pelvis
Plateau
Marked vasocongestion
"Sex flush" (maculopapular rash on breasts, chest, and epigastrium)
Nipple erection
Engorgement of the labia
Engorgement of lower third of the vagina, with narrowing of diameter
Dilation of upper two thirds of vagina
Clitoral swelling and erection
Vaginal "sweating"
Uterine tenting
Orgasm
Release of tension
Generalized, rhythmic myotonic contractions
Contractions of perivaginal muscles and anal sphincter
Uterine contractions
Resolution
Return to pre-excitement state
Personal satisfaction and well-being
New excitement cycles may be initiated

response in this stage. Dilatation of blood vessels in the erectile tissues causes engorgement with blood and erection of the clitoris, as well as distention of the peri-introital tissues and subsequent narrowing of the lower third of the vagina. Parasympathetic fibers emanating from the sacral plexus (see Chapter 14) innervate these erectile tissues, just as in men (see Chapter 54). In addition, the parasympathetic system innervates Bartholin's glands, which empty into the introitus, as well as the vaginal glands. Adequate lubrication is necessary to minimize the friction of intercourse and thus maximize the stimulation to achieve orgasm.

Both physical stimulation and psychic stimuli are important for female orgasm. Psychic stimuli are coordinated through the cerebrum, which causes the generalized tension throughout the body, as discussed earlier, and also modulates the autonomic response. The female orgasm is also coordinated through a spinal cord reflex that results in rhythmic contractions of the perineal muscles. The afferent pathways for this spinal cord reflex follow the pudendal nerves, which emanate through sacral segments 2 to 4 and are the primary innervation to the perineum and the female external genitalia. This spinal cord reflex is similar to that observed in men.

Table 55-4 The Menopausal Syndrome and Physical Changes in Menopause

Menopausal Syndrome	Physical Changes in Menopause
Vasomotor instability	Atrophy of the vaginal epithelium
Hot flashes	Changes in vaginal pH
Night sweats	Decrease in vaginal secretions
Mood changes	Decrease in circulation to vagina and uterus
Short-term memory loss	Pelvic relaxation
Sleep disturbances	Loss of vaginal tone
Headaches	
Loss of libido	Cardiovascular disease Osteoporosis Alzheimer disease

The female sex response facilitates sperm transport through the female reproductive tract

The spinal reflexes previously discussed may also increase uterine and cervical activity and may thus promote transport of gametes. The cervix dilates during orgasm, thereby facilitating sperm transport into the upper part of the reproductive tract. The release of oxytocin at the time of orgasm stimulates uterine contractility, which also facilitates gamete transport. Although 150 to 600 million sperm cells (see Chapter 54) are normally deposited in the vagina during sexual intercourse, ~100,000 reach the cavity of the uterus, and only 50 to 100 viable sperm reach the distal fallopian tube where fertilization occurs. Aside from the one or more sperm that will fertilize the ovum (or ova), most sperm degenerate, to be disposed of by the female genital tract. Sperm transport is accomplished by swimming movements of the sperm tail through the mucus of the cervical canal. The sperm reach the ampulla of the fallopian tubes within 5 minutes of ejaculation. Clearly, this rapid rate of transport could not be achieved by the swimming activity of the sperm alone. Therefore, uterine or tubal activity must serve a major role in sperm transport.

MENOPAUSE

Menopause, or the **climacteric**, signals the termination of reproductive function in women. Cyclic reproductive function ceases, menstruation comes to an end, and childbearing is generally no longer possible. Also occurring are significant physiological changes (Table 55-4) that have a major impact on health.

Only a few functioning follicles remain in the ovaries of a menopausal woman

Progressive loss of ovarian follicular units occurs throughout life. Approximately 6 to 7 million germ cells are present in the two ovaries of the developing female fetus at 20 weeks' gestation. At birth, only ~1 to 2 million follicular units remain in the ovaries. At puberty ~400,000 remain, a finding again reflecting the continued process of atresia during the prepubertal years. Puberty generally occurs in American girls at ~12.5 years of age. The average age of menopause in American women is 51.5 years. Thus, it is estimated that more than 400 oocytes are ovulated during the reproductive life of a woman. At menopause and during the ensuing 5 years, the ovary contains only an occasional secondary follicle and a few primary follicles in a prominent stroma. The massive loss of oocytes over the reproductive life of a woman—from 400,000 at puberty to virtually none at menopause—is the result of the rapid, continuous process of atresia during reproductive life. During each cycle, a large cohort (~10 to 30) of follicles is recruited, but only one follicle reaches dominance and ovulates. The others become atretic. However, even if we multiply the number of follicles in a cohort by the total number of menstrual cycles, we cannot account for all 400,000 of the prepubertal units. Thus, most of the primordial and primary ovarian follicles are lost as a result of atresia during the reproductive life of the individual.

During menopause, levels of the ovarian steroids fall, whereas gonadotropin levels rise

The loss of functional ovarian follicles is primarily responsible for menopause in primates. Even before the onset of meno-

Hormone Replacement Therapy During Menopause

Although the mean age at menopause is ~51.5 years, changes in hormone secretion patterns are seen much earlier. Increases in levels of FSH occur as early as 35 years of age. The mechanisms responsible for this change remain to be elucidated. However, it is clear that ovarian function begins to diminish far in advance of a woman's last menstrual period. The increase in gonadotropin secretion is probably a result of decreased folliculogenesis leading to decreased secretion of sex steroids and inhibin and thus lowered negative feedback on the gonadotrophs during the perimenopausal period.

The characteristic changes associated with menopause are primarily the result of low circulating estrogen levels. Estrogen is a very important regulatory hormone in girls and women. In addition to the role of estrogen in reproductive processes, this hormone has profound effects on several other physiological systems (Table 55-4).

Hormone replacement therapy is indicated during menopause to alleviate the menopausal syndrome and to prevent or diminish the physical changes that occur as a result of estrogen deficiency. Menopausal hormone replacement therapy consists of estrogen and progestin administration. The reason for administering progestins is that the endometrium is at significant risk of neoplasia from the unopposed actions of estrogens. Thus, progestins are not generally administered to women who have had hysterectomies. Estrogen replacement is very effective against the menopausal syndrome, as well as against osteoporosis and cardiovascular disease. However, because of side effects (e.g., menstruation) and concern about endometrial and breast cancer, compliance with hormone replacement therapy is often compromised.

The **selective ER modulators (SERMS)** comprise a group of structurally dissimilar compounds that interact with ERs. However, these agents act as either estrogen agonists or estrogen antagonists, depending on the target tissue and hormonal status of the individual. The exact mechanisms through which SERMS elicit their effects in specific tissues remain unclear and constitute an area of active research. The estrogen antagonist effects of SERMS may be mediated by classic competition for the ER. SERMS such as tamoxifen and raloxifene have beneficial effects, similar to those of estrogens, on bone and the cardiovascular system, whereas they antagonize estrogen in reproductive tissue. Clearly, the ideal SERM would have all the beneficial effects of estrogen without the negative and potentially dangerous side effects. For example, the perfect SERM would alleviate the menopausal syndrome, protect against cardiovascular and Alzheimer disease, and act as estrogen agonists in certain reproductive tissues and as antagonists in others.

pause, significant hormonal changes occur very early during reproductive life. Because of a gradual decline in the number of follicles, the decreased ovarian production of estrogen reduces the negative feedback to the anterior pituitary and leads to increased levels of FSH. Increased levels of FSH are seen as early as 35 years of age, even though cyclic reproductive function continues. When compared with younger women, older—but premenopausal—women have diminished estradiol production and decreased luteal function during natural cycles. Diminished inhibin production by the aging ovary may also contribute to the sharp rise in FSH levels that occurs in the perimenopausal period of life.

During menopause, estradiol levels are generally less than 30 pg/mL, and progesterone levels are often less than 1 ng/mL of plasma. Both these values are somewhat less than the lowest levels seen during the menstrual cycle of a younger woman (Fig. 55-9). Ovarian production of androstenedione is minimal during menopause, although androstenedione production by the adrenal cortex remains normal.

Because the output of estrogens, progestins, and inhibins from the ovaries falls to very low levels during menopause, negative feedback on the hypothalamic-pituitary-ovarian axis (Fig. 55-4) becomes minimal. As a result, levels of FSH and LH may be higher than those seen during the midcycle surge in premenopausal women—the futile attempt of the axis to stimulate follicular development and production of the female sex steroids. During menopause, the anterior pituitary still secretes FSH and LH in pulses, presumably after cyclic release of GnRH from the hypothalamus (Fig. 55-2A). Although gonadotropins cannot generally stimulate the postmenopausal ovary, it appears that the gonadotrophs in the anterior pituitary can respond to exogenous GnRH.

REFERENCES

Books and Reviews

Adashi EY, Rock JA, Rosenwaks Z (eds): Reproductive Endocrinology, Surgery and Technology. Philadelphia: Lippincott-Raven, 1996.

de Kretser DM, Robertson DM, Risbridger GP: Recent advances in the physiology of human inhibin. J Endocrinol Invest 1990; 13:611-624.

Dufau ML: The luteinizing hormone receptor. Annu Rev Physiol 1998; 60:461-496.

Marshall WA, Tanner JM: Puberty. In Falkner F, Tanner JM (eds): Human Growth, vol 2, pp 171-209. New York: Plenum, 1986.

Masters WH, Johnson VE: Human Sexual Response. Boston: Little, Brown, 1966.

Wilson JD, Foster DW, Kronenberg HM, Larsen PR (eds): Williams Textbook of Endocrinology, 9th ed. Philadelphia: WB Saunders, 1998.

Woodruff TK, Mather JP: Inhibin, activin and the female reproductive axis. Annu Rev Physiol 1995; 57:214-244.

Journal Articles

Erickson GF, Wang C, Hsueh AJW: FSH induction of functional LH receptors in granulosa cells cultured in a chemically defined medium. Nature 1979; 279:336-338.

Fiddes JC, Goodman HM: The gene encoding the common alpha subunit of the four human glycoprotein hormones. J Mol Appl Genet 1981; 1:3-18.

Ryan KJ: Granulosa-thecal cell interaction in ovarian steroidogenesis. J Steroid Biochem 1979; 11:799-800.

Schwanzel-Fukuda M, Pfaff DW: Origin of luteinizing hormone-releasing hormone neurons. Nature 1989; 338:161-164.

Veldhuis JD, Dufau ML: Estradiol modulates the pulsatile secretion of bioactive luteinizing hormone in vivo. J Clin Invest 1987; 80:631-638.

Wang CF, Lasley BL, Lein A, Yen SS: The functional changes of the pituitary gonadotrophs during the menstrual cycle. J Clin Endocrinol Metab 1976; 42:718-728.

CHAPTER 56

FERTILIZATION, PREGNANCY, AND LACTATION

Ervin E. Jones

TRANSPORT OF GAMETES AND FERTILIZATION

Cilia and smooth muscle transport the egg and sperm within the female genital tract

Following ovulation, the fimbriae of the fallopian tube sweep over the ovarian surface and pick up the oocyte—surrounded by its complement of granulosa cells, the cumulus oophorus, and corona radiata (see Chapter 55)—and deposit it in the fallopian tube. Shortly after ovulation, movements of the cilia and the smooth muscle of the fallopian tube propel the oocyte-cumulus complex toward the uterus.

A man normally deposits 150 to 600 million sperm into the vagina of a woman at the time of ejaculation. Only 50 to 100 of these sperm actually reach the ampullary portion of the fallopian tube, where fertilization normally occurs. However, the sperm get there very quickly, within ~5 minutes of ejaculation. The swimming motion of the sperm alone cannot account for such rapid transport. Forceful contractions of the uterus, cervix, and fallopian tubes propel the sperm into the upper reproductive tract during female orgasm. Prostaglandins in the seminal plasma may induce further contractile activity.

The capacitation of the spermatozoa that occurs in the female genital tract enhances the ability of the sperm cell to fertilize the ovum

As discussed in Chapter 54, maturation of sperm continues while they are stored in the epididymis. In most species, neither freshly ejaculated sperm cells nor sperm cells that are removed from the epididymis are capable of fertilizing the egg until these cells have undergone further maturation (*capacitation*) in the female reproductive tract or in the laboratory. **Capacitation** is a poorly understood physiological process by which spermatozoa acquire the ability to penetrate the zona pellucida of the ovum. The removal or modification of a protective protein coat from the sperm cell membrane appears to be an important molecular event in the process of capacitation.

In women, sperm do not need to pass through the cervix and uterus to achieve capacitation. Successful pregnancy can occur with gamete intrafallopian transfer (GIFT), in which spermatozoa and oocytes are placed directly into the ampulla of the fallopian tube, and also with direct ultrasound-guided intraperitoneal insemination, in which the sperm are deposited in the peritoneal cavity, near the fimbria. Thus, capacitation of sperm in the reproductive tract is not strictly organ specific. As evidenced by the success of in vitro fertilization and embryo transfer (IVF-ET; see the box titled In Vitro Fertilization and Embryo Transfer), capacitation is feasible even if the sperm does not make contact with the female reproductive tract.

Fertilization begins as the sperm cell attaches to the zona pellucida and undergoes the acrosomal reaction, and it ends with the fusion of the male and female pronuclei

After ovulation, the egg in the fallopian tube is in a semidormant state. If it remains unfertilized, the ripe egg will remain quiescent for some time and eventually degenerates. In the case of fertilization, the sperm normally comes into contact with the oocyte in the ampullary portion of the tube, usually several hours after ovulation. Fertilization causes the egg to awaken (**activation**), thus initiating a series of morphological and biochemical events that lead to cell division and differentiation. **Fertilization** occurs in eight steps:

Step 1. The sperm head weaves its way past the follicular cells and attaches to the *zona pellucida* that surrounds the oocyte (Fig. 56-1). The zona pellucida is composed of three glycoproteins; ZP1 cross-links the filamentous ZP2 and ZP3 into a latticework. Receptors on the plasma membrane of the sperm cell bind to **ZP3**, thereby initiating a signal transduction cascade.

Step 2. As a result of the sperm-ZP3 interaction, the sperm cell undergoes the **acrosomal reaction**, a prelude to the migration of the sperm cell through the mucus-like zona pellucida. The acrosome is a unique sperm organelle, essentially a large secretory vesicle, that originates from the Golgi complex in the spermatid (see Chapter 54). The

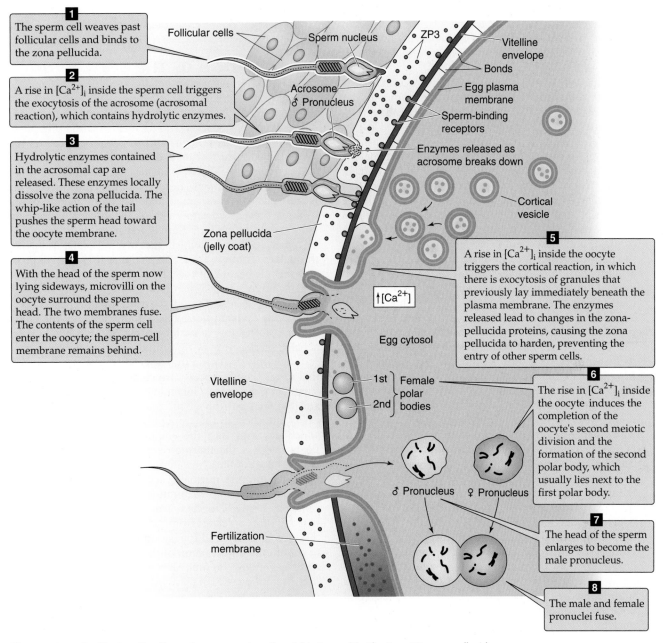

1 The sperm cell weaves past follicular cells and binds to the zona pellucida.

2 A rise in $[Ca^{2+}]_i$ inside the sperm cell triggers the exocytosis of the acrosome (acrosomal reaction), which contains hydrolytic enzymes.

3 Hydrolytic enzymes contained in the acrosomal cap are released. These enzymes locally dissolve the zona pellucida. The whip-like action of the tail pushes the sperm head toward the oocyte membrane.

4 With the head of the sperm now lying sideways, microvilli on the oocyte surround the sperm head. The two membranes fuse. The contents of the sperm cell enter the oocyte; the sperm-cell membrane remains behind.

5 A rise in $[Ca^{2+}]_i$ inside the oocyte triggers the cortical reaction, in which there is exocytosis of granules that previously lay immediately beneath the plasma membrane. The enzymes released lead to changes in the zona-pellucida proteins, causing the zona pellucida to harden, preventing the entry of other sperm cells.

6 The rise in $[Ca^{2+}]_i$ inside the oocyte induces the completion of the oocyte's second meiotic division and the formation of the second polar body, which usually lies next to the first polar body.

7 The head of the sperm enlarges to become the male pronucleus.

8 The male and female pronuclei fuse.

Labels in figure: Follicular cells; Sperm nucleus; ZP3; Vitelline envelope; Bonds; Egg plasma membrane; Sperm-binding receptors; Enzymes released as acrosome breaks down; Acrosome; ♂ Pronucleus; Cortical vesicle; Zona pellucida (jelly coat); $\uparrow[Ca^{2+}]$; Egg cytosol; Vitelline envelope; 1st / 2nd Female polar bodies; ♂ Pronucleus; ♀ Pronucleus; Fertilization membrane

Figure 56-1 Fertilization. The illustration summarizes the eight steps of fertilization. ZP, zona pellucida.

acrosome contains hydrolyzing enzymes that are necessary for the sperm to penetrate the zona pellucida. The acrosome lies in front of and around the anterior two thirds of the sperm nucleus, much like a motorcycle helmet fits over one's head. During the acrosomal reaction, an increase in $[Ca^{2+}]_i$ triggers fusion of the *outer* acrosomal membrane with the sperm cell's plasma membrane and results in the exocytosis of most of the acrosomal contents.

Step 3. The spermatozoon penetrates the zona pellucida. One mechanism of this penetration is the action of the acrosomal enzymes. Protease inhibitors can block the penetration of spermatozoa through the zona pellucida. The sperm cell also penetrates the zona pellucida by

mechanical action. The sperm head rapidly oscillates about a fulcrum that is situated in the neck region. This rapid, vigorous, rocking action occurs with a frequency of approximately six to eight oscillations per second. The sperm penetrates the zona pellucida at an angle, thus creating a tangential cleavage slit and leaving the sperm head lying sideways against the oocyte membrane.

Step 4. The cell membranes of the sperm and the oocyte fuse. Microvilli on the oocyte surface envelop the sperm cell, which probably binds to the oocyte membrane through specific proteins on the surfaces of the two cells. The posterior membrane of the acrosome—which remains part of the sperm cell after the acrosomal reaction—is the first portion of the sperm to fuse with the plasma membrane of the egg. The sperm cell per se does not enter the oocyte. Rather, the cytoplasmic portions of the head and tail enter the oocyte and leaving the sperm cell plasma membrane behind, similar to a snake's crawling out of its skin.

Step 5. The oocyte undergoes the cortical reaction. As the spermatozoon penetrates the oocyte's plasma membrane, it initiates formation of inositol 1,4,5-triphosphate (IP_3) and causes Ca^{2+} release from internal stores (see Chapter 3) and an increase in $[Ca^{2+}]_i$ and $[Ca^{2+}]_i$ waves. This rise in $[Ca^{2+}]_i$, in turn, triggers the oocyte's second meiotic division—discussed later—and the cortical reaction. In the **cortical reaction**, small electron-dense granules that lie just beneath the plasma membrane fuse with the oocyte's plasma membrane. Exocytosis of these granules releases enzymes that act on glycoproteins in the zona pellucida and cause them to harden. In the process, polysaccharides are liberated from these glycoproteins. From a teleological perspective, the cortical granule reaction prevents **polyspermy**. Polyspermic embryos are abnormal because they are polyploid. They do not develop beyond the early cleavage stages.

Step 6. The oocyte completes its second meiotic division. The oocyte, which had been arrested in the prophase of its first meiotic division since fetal life (see Chapter 53), completed its first meiotic division at the time of the surge of luteinizing hormone (LH), which occurred several hours before ovulation (see Chapter 55). The results were the first polar body and a secondary oocyte with a haploid number of duplicated chromosomes (see Fig. 53-1). Before fertilization, this secondary oocyte had begun a second meiotic division, which was arrested in metaphase. The rise in $[Ca^{2+}]_i$ inside the oocyte—which the sperm cell triggers, as noted earlier—causes not only the cortical reaction but also the completion of the oocyte's second meiotic division. One result is the formation of the **second polar body**, which contains a haploid number of unduplicated maternal chromosomes. The oocyte extrudes the chromosomes of the second polar body, together with a small amount of ooplasm, into a space immediately below the zona pellucida; the second polar body usually lies close to the first polar body. The nucleus of the oocyte also contains a haploid number of unduplicated chromosomes. As its chromosomes decondense, the nucleus of this mature ovum becomes the **female pronucleus**.

Step 7. The sperm nucleus decondenses and transforms into the **male pronucleus**, which, like the female pronucleus, contains a haploid number of unduplicated chromosomes (see Fig. 54-6). The cytoplasmic portion of the sperm's tail degenerates.

Step 8. The male and female pronuclei fuse, to form a new cell, the **zygote**. The mingling of chromosomes (syngamy) can be considered as the end of fertilization and the beginning of embryonic development. Thus, fertilization results in a conceptus that bears 46 chromosomes, 23 from the maternal gamete and 23 from the paternal gamete. As noted in Chapter 53, fertilization of the ovum by a sperm bearing an X chromosome produces a zygote with XX sex chromosomes; this develops into a female. Fertilization with a Y-bearing sperm produces an XY

zygote, which develops into a male. Therefore, chromosomal sex is established at fertilization.

IMPLANTATION OF THE DEVELOPING EMBRYO

As discussed, the ovum is fertilized in the ampullary portion of the fallopian tube several hours after ovulation (Fig. 56-2), and the conceptus remains in the fallopian tube for ~72 hours, during which time it develops to the **morula** stage (i.e., a mulberry-shaped solid mass of 12 or more cells), receiving nourishment from fallopian tube secretions. During these 3 days, smooth muscle contractions of the isthmus prevent advancement of the conceptus into the uterus while the endometrium is preparing for implantation. The mechanisms by which the ovum is later propelled through the isthmus of the fallopian tube to the uterus probably include beating of the cilia of the tubal epithelium and contraction of the fallopian tube.

After the morula rapidly moves through the isthmus to the uterine cavity, it floats freely in the lumen of the uterus and transforms into a blastocyst (Fig. 56-2). A **blastocyst** is a ball-like structure with a fluid-filled inner cavity. Surrounding this cavity is a thin layer of **trophoectoderm** cells that forms the trophoblast, which develops into a variety of supporting structures, including the amnion, the yolk sac, and the fetal portion of the placenta. On one side of the cavity, attached to the trophoblast, is an **inner cell mass**, which develops into the embryo proper. The conceptus floats freely in the uterine cavity for ~72 hours before it attaches to the endometrium. Thus, implantation of the human blastocyst normally occurs 6 to 7 days following ovulation. Numerous maturational events occur in the conceptus as it travels to the uterus. The embryo must be prepared to draw nutrients from the endometrium on arrival in the uterine cavity, and the endometrium must be prepared to sustain the implantation of the blastocyst. Because of the specific window in time during which implantation can occur, temporal relationships between embryonic and endometrial maturation assume extreme importance.

The presence of an embryo leads to decidualization, a completion of the predecidualization of the endometrium that was initiated during the late secretory phase of the endometrial cycle

During the middle to late secretory phase of the normal endometrial cycle, the endometrium becomes more vascularized and thickened, and the endometrial glands become tortuous and engorged with secretions. These changes, driven by progesterone from the corpus luteum, peak at ~7 days after ovulation. Additionally, beginning 9 to 10 days after ovulation, a process known as **predecidualization** begins near the spiral arteries (see Chapter 55). During predecidualization, stromal cells transform into rounded decidual cells, and these cells spread across the superficial layer of the endometrium to make it more compact (zona compacta) and to separate it from the deeper, more spongy layer (zona spongiosa; see Fig. 55-13). If conception fails to occur, the

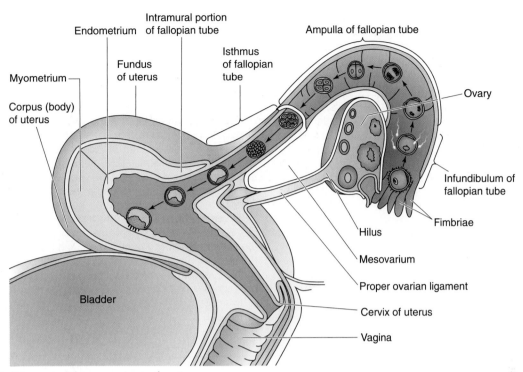

Figure 56-2 Transport of the conceptus to the uterus.

secretory activity of the endometrial glands decreases, followed by regression of the glands 8 to 9 days after ovulation, which is ultimately followed by menstruation.

When pregnancy occurs, the predecidual changes in the endometrium are sustained and extended, thus completing the process of **decidualization**. The **decidua** is the specialized endometrium of pregnancy. Its original name was *membrana decidua*, a term referring to the membranes of the endometrium that are shed following pregnancy, like the leaves of a deciduous tree. Because the degree of decidualization is considerably greater in conception cycles than in nonconception cycles, it is likely that the blastocyst itself promotes decidualization. Indeed, either the presence of the embryo or a traumatic stimulus that mimics the embryo's invasion of the endometrium induces changes in the endometrium.

The area underneath the implanting embryo becomes the **decidua basalis** (Fig. 56-3). Other portions of the decidua that become prominent later in pregnancy are the **decidua capsularis**, which overlies the embryo, and the **decidua parietalis**, which covers the remainder of the uterine surface. The upper zona compacta layer and the middle zona spongiosa layer of the nonpregnant endometrium are still recognizable in the decidualized endometrium of pregnancy. The glandular epithelium within the zona spongiosa continues its secretory activity during the first trimester. Some of the glands take on a hypersecretory appearance in what has been referred to as the *Arias-Stella* phenomenon of early pregnancy—named after the pathologist Javier Arias-Stella. Although the decidualized endometrium is most prominent during the first trimester, before the establishment of the definitive placenta, elements of decidualization persist throughout gestation.

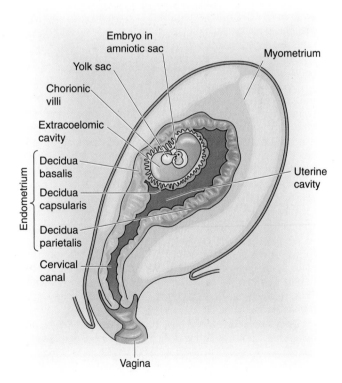

Figure 56-3 The three decidual zones during early embryonic development (~13 to 14 days after fertilization). The figure shows a sagittal section through a pregnant uterus, with the anterior side to the right.

In Vitro Fertilization and Embryo Transfer

IVF is a procedure in which an oocyte is or oocytes are **removed** from a woman and are then fertilized with sperm under laboratory conditions. Early development of the embryo also proceeds under laboratory conditions. Finally, the physician transfers one or more embryos to the uterine cavity, where the embryo will, one hopes, implant and develop.

Indications. Indications for IVF-ET include disorders that impair the normal meeting of the sperm and the egg in the distal portion of the fallopian tube. In addition to ovulatory dysfunction, these disorders include tubal occlusion, tubal-peritoneal adhesions, endometriosis, or other disease processes of the female peritoneal cavity. In addition, IVF-ET is indicated in some cases of male-factor infertility (abnormalities in male reproductive function) or unexplained infertility.

Ovarian stimulation. Because the success rates are less than 100% for each of the stages of IVF-ET, the physician needs several oocytes, all obtained in a single ovarian cycle. However, a woman normally develops a single dominant follicle each cycle (see Chapter 55). Thus, to obtain the *multiple* oocytes for IVF-ET, the physician must stimulate the development of multiple follicles in the woman by controlled ovarian hyperstimulation. Although this procedure qualitatively mimics the hormonal control of the normal cycle, the high dose of gonadotropins triggers the development of *many* follicles. The physician administers some combination of FSH and LH or pure FSH preparation, either intramuscularly or subcutaneously. Because exogenous gonadotropins stimulate the ovaries directly, GnRH analogues (see box in Chapter 55 on therapeutic uses of GnRH) are often used to downregulate the hypothalamic-pituitary axis during controlled ovarian stimulation. One usually administers these GnRH analogues before initiating gonadotropin therapy, primarily to prevent a premature LH surge and ovulation.

Cycle monitoring. After administering the gonadotropins, the physician monitors the simulated follicular growth in the ovaries with sonographic imaging. Size, number, and serial growth of ovarian follicles may be assessed daily or at other appropriate intervals. Serum estradiol levels provide an additional measure of follicular growth and function. When estradiol levels and follicular growth indicate—by established criteria—appropriate folliculogenesis, the physician simulates a natural LH surge by injecting hCG, which is a close relative of LH (see Chapter 55). However, in this case, the simulated LH surge completes the final maturation of *multiple* follicles and oocytes. As we already know, ovulation usually occurs 36 to 39 hours following the beginning of the LH surge. Thus, the physician plans oocyte retrieval in such a way to allow maximal follicular maturation, but still to harvest the oocytes *before* ovulation. Thus, retrievals are scheduled for 34 to 36 hours following the administration of hCG.

Oocyte retrieval. The physician retrieves oocytes by aspirating them from individual follicles, under sonographic guidance. With the patient under conscious or unconscious sedation, and after applying a local anesthetic to the posterior vaginal wall, the physician inserts a probe, equipped with a needle guide, into the vagina. After inserting a 16- to 18-gauge needle through the vaginal wall, the specialist aspirates the follicular fluid from each mature follicle and collects it in a test tube containing a small amount of culture medium. The eggs are identified in the follicular fluid, are separated from the fluid and other follicular cells, and are then washed and prepared for insemination. This procedure normally yields 8 to 15 oocytes.

Insemination. The sperm sample is subjected to numerous washes, followed by column chromatography to separate the sperm cells from the other cells and from debris found in the ejaculate. Each egg is inseminated with 50,000 to 300,000 motile sperm in a drop of culture medium and is incubated overnight. Fertilization can usually be detected by the presence of two pronuclei in the egg cytoplasm after 16 to 20 hours. Fertilization rates generally range from 60% to 85%. Embryo development is allowed to continue in vitro for another 48 to 120 hours until embryos are transferred to the uterus.

Among couples whose male partner has very low numbers of motile sperm, high fertilization rates can be achieved using **intracytoplasmic sperm injection (ICSI)**. Micromanipulation techniques are used to inject a sperm cell into the cytoplasm of each egg in vitro. Fertilization rates after ICSI are generally 60% to 70%, or approximately equivalent to conventional insemination in vitro.

Embryo transfer. After culturing the cells for 48 to 120 hours, the physician transfers three to four embryos to the uterus at the four- to eight-cell stage (after 2 days) or fewer embryos at the blastocyst stage (after 5 days). Embryos are selected and are loaded into a thin, flexible catheter, which is inserted into the uterine cavity to the desired depth under ultrasonic guidance. The woman usually receives supplemental progesterone to support implantation and pregnancy. In certain cases, the embryos are transferred to the fallopian tube during laparoscopy. This procedure is referred to as **tubal embryo transfer (TET)**. The rationale for this procedure is that the fallopian tube contributes to the early development of the embryo as it travels down the tube to the uterus.

Success rates. Implantation rates usually range from 8% to 15% per embryo transferred. In the United States, the mean live birth rate per ET procedure is ~33%. Success rates in IVF-ET depend on numerous factors, including age as well as the type and severity of the disease causing infertility.

GIFT. In certain cases of infertility, the physician collects the oocytes and sperm cells in much the same way as described earlier for IVF-ET, but directly transfers the gametes to the fallopian tube, where fertilization occurs. GIFT is accomplished using laparoscopic techniques.

Uterine secretions nourish the preimplantation embryo, promote growth, and prepare it for implantation

Before the embryo implants in the endometrium and establishes an indirect lifeline between the mother's blood and its own, it must receive its nourishment from uterine secretions. Following conception, the endometrium is primarily controlled by progesterone, which initially comes from the corpus luteum (see Chapter 55). The uterine glandular epithelium synthesizes and secretes several steroid-dependent proteins (Table 56-1) that are thought to be important for

Table 56-1 Endometrial Proteins, Glycoproteins, and Peptides Secreted by the Endometrial Glands During Pregnancy

Mucins
Prolactin
Insulin-like growth factor–binding protein 1 (IGFBP-1)
Placental protein 14 (PP14) or glycodelin
Pregnancy-associated endometrial α_2-globulin (α_2-PEG)
Endometrial protein 15
Fibronectin
Laminin
Entactin
Collagen type IV
Heparan sulfate
Proteoglycan
Integrins
Albumin
β Lipoprotein
Relaxin
Acidic fibroblast growth factor
Basic fibroblast growth factor
Pregnancy-associated plasma protein A (PAPP-A)
Stress response protein 27 (SRP-27)
CA-125
β Endorphin
Leu-enkephalin
Diamine oxidase
Plasminogen activator (PA)
Plasminogen activator inhibitor
Renin
Progesterone-dependent carbonic anhydrase
Lactoferrin

Table 56-2 Substances Secreted by the Blastocyst

Immunoregulatory Agents
Platelet-activating factor (PAF)
Early pregnancy factor
Immunosuppressive factor
PGE_2
Interleukins 1α, 6, and 8
Interferon α
Leukemia inhibitory factor
Colony-stimulating factor
Human leukocyte antigen 6
Fas ligand

Metalloproteases (facilitate invasion of trophoblast into the endometrium)
Collagenases: digest collagen types I, II, III, VII, and X
Gelatinases: two forms, digest collagen type IV and gelatin
Stromelysins: digest fibronectin, laminin, and collagen types IV, V, and VII

Serine Proteases (facilitate invasion of trophoblast into the endometrium)

Other Factors or Actions
hCG: autocrine growth factor
Ovum factor
Early pregnancy factor
Embryo-derived histamine-releasing factor
Plasminogen activator and its inhibitors
Insulin-like growth factor 2 (IGF-2): promotes trophoblast invasiveness
Estradiol
β_1 Integrin
Fibroblast growth factor (FGF)
Transforming growth factor α (TGF-α)
Inhibins

dependent, and it is inhibited by estrogens. Pinopods endocytose macromolecules and uterine fluid and absorb most of the fluid in the lumen of the uterus during the early stages of embryo implantation. By removing uterine luminal fluid, the pinopods may allow the embryo and the uterine epithelium to approximate one another more closely. Because apposition and adhesion of the embryo to the uterus are the first events of implantation, the presence and action of pinopods may determine the extent of the implantation window.

The blastocyst secretes substances that facilitate implantation

If the blastocyst is to survive, it must avoid rejection by the maternal cellular immune system. It does so by releasing immunosuppressive agents (Table 56-2). The embryo also synthesizes and secretes macromolecules that promote implantation, the development of the placenta, and the maintenance of pregnancy.

Both short-range and long-range embryonic signals may be necessary for implantation, although the nature of some of these signals remains enigmatic. One short-range signal from the blastocyst may stimulate local changes in the endo-

the nourishment, growth, and implantation of the embryo. The endometrium secretes cholesterol, steroids, and various nutrients, including iron and fat-soluble vitamins. It also synthesizes matrix substances, adhesion molecules, and surface receptors for matrix proteins, all of which may be important for implantation.

Pinopods appear as small, finger-like protrusions on endometrial cells between day 19 (about the time the embryo would arrive in the uterus) and day 21 (about the time of implantation) of the menstrual cycle; they persist for only 2 to 3 days. Pinopod formation appears to be progesterone

metrium at the time of its apposition to the endometrium. A long-range signal that is secreted by the early blastocyst is **human chorionic gonadotropin (hCG)**, which is closely related to LH (see Chapter 55) and sustains the corpus luteum in the presence of rapidly falling levels of maternal LH.

hCG is one of the most important of the factors secreted by the trophoblast of the blastocyst, both before and after implantation. Besides rescuing the corpus luteum, hCG is an autocrine growth factor that promotes trophoblast growth and placental development. hCG levels are high in the area where the trophoblast faces the endometrium. hCG may have a role in the adhesion of the trophoblast to the epithelia of the endometrium, and it also has protease activity.

During implantation, the blastocyst apposes itself to the endometrium, adheres to epithelial cells, and then finally breaks through the basement membrane and invades the stroma

As noted earlier, the conceptus lies unattached in the uterine cavity for ~72 hours. About halfway through this period (i.e., 5 to 6 days after ovulation), the morula transforms into the blastocyst (Fig. 56-4A). Before the initiation of implantation, the zona pellucida that surrounds the blastocyst degenerates. This process, known as **hatching** of the embryo, occurs 6 to 7 days after ovulation. Lytic factors in the endometrial cavity appear to be essential for the dissolution of the zona pellucida. The blastocyst probably also participates in the process of zona lysis and hatching; when an *unfertil*ized egg is placed in the uterus under the same conditions, its zona pellucida remains intact. A factor produced by the blastocyst may activate a lytic factor that is derived from a uterine precursor. Plasmin, produced from plasminogen, is a plausible candidate for this uterine factor, because plasmin exhibits a lytic effect on the zona pellucida in vitro, and inhibitors of plasmin block in vitro hatching of rat blastocysts. Implantation occurs in three stages: (1) apposition, (2) adhesion, and (3) invasion.

Apposition   The earliest contact between the blastocyst wall, the trophoectoderm, and the endometrial epithelium is a loose connection called *apposition* (Fig. 56-4B). Apposition usually occurs in a crypt in the endometrium. From the standpoint of the blastocyst, it appears that apposition occurs at a site where the zona pellucida is ruptured or lysed and where it is possible for the cell membranes of the trophoblast to make direct contact with the cell membranes of the endometrium. Although the preimplantation blastocyst is asymmetric, it seems that the entire trophoectoderm has the potential to interact with the endometrium, and the final correct orientation—with the inner cell mass pointing toward the endometrium—occurs by free rotation of the inner cell mass within the sphere of overlying trophoectoderm cells.

Adhesion   The trophoblast appears to attach to the uterine epithelium through the microvilli of the trophoblast; ligand-receptor interactions are probably involved in adhesion (Fig. 56-4C). The receptors for these ligand-receptor interactions are often members of the **integrin family** (see Chapter 2)

and can be either on the blastocyst or on the endometrium. Integrins are bifunctional integral membrane proteins; on their intracellular side, they interact with the cytoskeleton, whereas on their extracellular side, they have receptors for **matrix proteins** such as collagen, laminin, fibronectin, and vitronectin. Therefore, ligand-receptor interactions have two possible orientations. For the first, the extracellular surface of the *trophoblast* has integrins for binding fibronectins, laminin, and collagen type IV. Thus, during implantation, the trophoblast binds to the laminin that is distributed around the stromal (decidual) cells of the endometrium. Fibronectin, a component of the basement membrane, probably guides the implanting embryo (see later) and is subsequently broken down by the trophoblast.

For the second orientation of matrix-integrin interactions, the extracellular surface of the *glandular epithelium* also expresses integrins on days 20 to 24 of the menstrual cycle, the implantation window (see Chapter 55). The expression of receptors for fibronectin and vitronectin (i.e., integrins) may serve as markers of the endometrial capacity for implantation. Small peptides containing sequences that are homologous to specific sequences of fibronectin block blastocyst attachment and outgrowth on fibronectin.

In addition to the integrin-matrix interactions, another important class of ligand-receptor interactions appears to be between heparin or heparan sulfate proteoglycans (see Chapter 2), which are attached to the surface of the blastocyst and surface receptors on the uterine epithelial cell. These endometrial proteoglycan receptors increase as the time of implantation approaches.

Any of the foregoing ligand-receptor interactions can lead to cytoskeletal changes. Thus, adhesion of the trophoblast through ligand-receptor interactions may dislodge the uterine epithelial cells from their basal lamina and may thereby facilitate access of the trophoblast to the basal lamina for penetration.

Invasion   As the blastocyst attaches to the endometrial epithelium, the trophoblastic cells rapidly proliferate, and the trophoblast differentiates into two layers: an inner **cytotrophoblast** and an outer syncytiotrophoblast (Fig. 56-4D). The **syncytiotrophoblast** is a multinucleated mass without cellular boundaries. During implantation, long protrusions from the syncytiotrophoblast extend among the uterine epithelial cells. The protrusions dissociate these endometrial cells by secreting tumor necrosis factor α (TNF-α), which interferes with the expression of cadherins (cell adhesion molecules; see Chapter 2) and β-catenin (an intracellular protein that helps to anchor cadherins to the cytoskeleton). The syncytiotrophoblast protrusions then penetrate the basement membrane of the uterine epithelial cells and ultimately reach the uterine stroma.

The trophoblast secretes several autocrine factors, which appear to stimulate invasion of the endometrial epithelium, as well as proteases (Table 56-2). By degrading the extracellular matrix, metalloproteases and serine proteases may control both the proliferation and the invasion of the trophoblast into the endometrium.

Around the site of penetration of the syncytiotrophoblast, uterine stromal cells take on a polyhedral shape and become laden with lipids and glycogen. These are the **decidual cells**

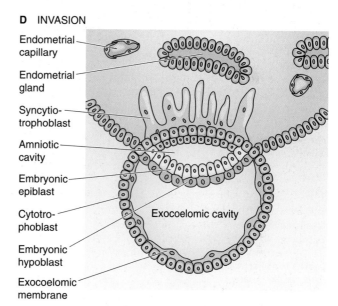

A HATCHING

Degenerating zona pellucida

Blastocyst cavity

Inner cell mass

Trophoblast

Lytic factors break down the zona pellucida.

B APPOSITION

Endometrial capillary

Endometrial gland

Endometrial epithelium

Inner cell mass

Trophoblast

Embryonic pole

Blastocyst cavity

C ADHESION

Endometrial stroma

Glandular secretion

Inner cell mass

Trophoblast

Uterine cavity

Blastocyst cavity

D INVASION

Endometrial capillary

Endometrial gland

Syncytiotrophoblast

Amniotic cavity

Embryonic epiblast

Cytotrophoblast

Embryonic hypoblast

Exocoelomic membrane

Exocoelomic cavity

Figure 56-4 Embryo hatching, apposition, adhesion, and invasion.

discussed earlier. The decidual cells degenerate in the region of the invading syncytiotrophoblast and thus provide nutrients to the developing embryo. The blastocyst superficially implants in the zona compacta of the endometrium and eventually becomes completely embedded in the decidua. As the finger-like projections of the syncytiotrophoblast invade the endometrium, they reach the maternal blood supply and represent a primordial form of the chorionic villus of the mature placenta, as discussed in the next section.

PHYSIOLOGY OF THE PLACENTA

Eventually, almost all the materials that are necessary for fetal growth and development move from the maternal circulation to the fetal circulation across the placenta, either by passive diffusion or by active transport. Except for CO_2, waste products are largely excreted through the amniotic fluid.

At the placenta, the space between the fetus's chorionic villi and the mother's endometrial wall contains a continuously renewed pool of extravasated maternal blood

Within the syncytium of the invading syncytiotrophoblast, fluid-filled holes called **lacunae** develop 8 to 9 days after fertilization (Fig. 56-5A). Twelve to 15 days after fertilization, the finger-like projections of the syncytiotrophoblast finally penetrate the endothelial layer of small veins of the endometrium. Later, these projections also penetrate the small spiral arteries. The result is free communication between the lacunae of the syncytiotrophoblast and the lumina of maternal blood vessels (Fig. 56-5B). Within 12 to 15 days after fertilization, some cytotrophoblasts proliferate and invade the syncytiotrophoblast, to form finger-like projections that are the **primary chorionic villi**.

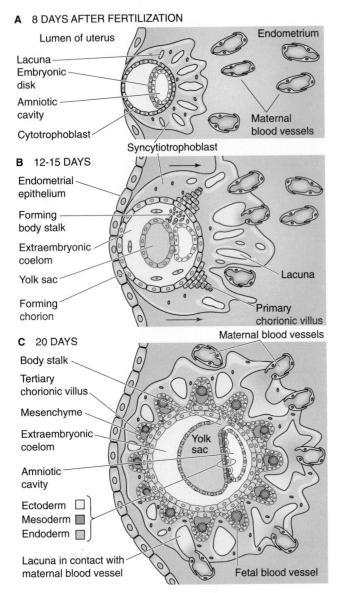

A 8 DAYS AFTER FERTILIZATION

Lumen of uterus
Endometrium
Lacuna
Embryonic disk
Amniotic cavity
Maternal blood vessels
Cytotrophoblast
Syncytiotrophoblast

B 12-15 DAYS

Endometrial epithelium
Forming body stalk
Extraembryonic coelom
Yolk sac
Lacuna
Forming chorion
Primary chorionic villus

C 20 DAYS

Maternal blood vessels
Body stalk
Tertiary chorionic villus
Mesenchyme
Extraembryonic coelom
Yolk sac
Amniotic cavity
Ectoderm ☐
Mesoderm ◼
Endoderm ☐
Lacuna in contact with maternal blood vessel
Fetal blood vessel

Figure 56-5 Development of the placenta. **A,** Shortly after the blastocyst has implanted (6 to 7 days after fertilization), the syncytiotrophoblast invades the stroma of the uterus (i.e., the decidua). Within the syncytiotrophoblast are lacunae. **B,** The invading syncytiotrophoblast breaks through into endometrial veins first, and then later into the arteries, thus creating direct communication between lacunae and maternal vessels. In addition, the proliferation of cytotrophoblasts creates small mounds known as *primary chorionic villi.* **C,** The primary chorionic villus continues to grow with the proliferation of cytotrophoblastic cells. In addition, mesenchyme from the extraembryonic coelom invades the villus, to form the secondary chorionic villus. Eventually, these mesenchymal cells form fetal capillaries; at this time, the villus is known as a *tertiary chorionic villus.* The lacunae also enlarge by merging with one another.

With further development, mesenchymal cells from the extraembryonic mesoderm invade the primary chorionic villi, which now are known as **secondary chorionic villi.** Eventually, these mesenchymal cells form fetal blood vessels de novo, at which point the villi are known as **tertiary chorionic villi** (Fig. 56-5C). Continued differentiation and amplification of the surface area of the fetal tissue protruding into the maternal blood create mature chorionic villi. The outer surface of each villus is lined with a very thin layer of syncytiotrophoblast, which has prominent microvilli (brush border) that face the maternal blood. Under the syncytiotrophoblast lie sparse cytotrophoblasts, mesenchyme, and fetal blood vessels. The lacunae, filled with maternal blood, eventually merge with one another, to create one massive, intercommunicating **intervillous space** (Fig. 56-6). The fetal villi protruding into this space resemble a thick forest of trees arising from the chorionic plate, which is the analogue of the soil from which the trees sprout. Thus, in the mature placenta, fetal blood is separated from maternal blood only by the fetal capillary endothelium, some mesenchyme and cytotrophoblasts, and a thin layer of syncytiotrophoblast.

Maternal Blood Flow The maternal arterial blood is discharged from ~120 spiral arteries; these arteries may have multiple openings, not all of which need be open at the same time. Blood enters in pulsatile spurts through the wall of the uterus and moves in discrete streams into the intervillous space toward the chorionic plate (Fig. 56-6). Small lakes of blood near the chorionic plate dissipate the force of the arterial spurts and reduce blood velocity. The maternal blood spreads laterally and then reverses direction and cascades over the closely packed villi. Blood flow slows even more, to allow adequate time for exchange. After bathing the chorionic villi, the maternal blood drains through venous orifices in the basal plate, enters the larger maternal placental veins, and ultimately flows into the uterine and other pelvic veins. No capillaries are present between the maternal arterioles and venules; the intervillous space is the functional capillary. Because the intervillous spaces are very narrow, and the arterial and venous orifices are randomly scattered over the entire base of the placenta, the maternal blood moves efficiently among the chorionic villi and avoids arteriovenous shunts.

The spiral arteries are generally perpendicular, and the veins are generally parallel to the uterine wall. Thus, because of both the geometry of the maternal blood vessels and the difference between maternal arterial and venous pressure, the uterine contractions that occur periodically during pregnancy, as well as during delivery, attenuate arterial inflow and completely interrupt venous drainage. Thus, the volume of blood in the intervillous space actually increases, to provide continual, albeit reduced, exchange. The principal factors that regulate the flow of maternal blood in the intervillous space are maternal arterial blood pressure, intra-uterine pressure, and the pattern of uterine contraction.

Fetal Blood Flow The fetal blood originates from two **umbilical arteries.** Unlike *systemic* arteries after birth, umbilical arteries carry *deoxygenated* blood. As these umbilical arteries approach the placenta, they branch repeatedly beneath the amnion, penetrate the chorionic plate, and then branch again within the chorionic villi, to form a capillary network. Blood that has obtained a significantly higher O_2 and nutrient content returns to the fetus from the placenta through the single **umbilical vein.**

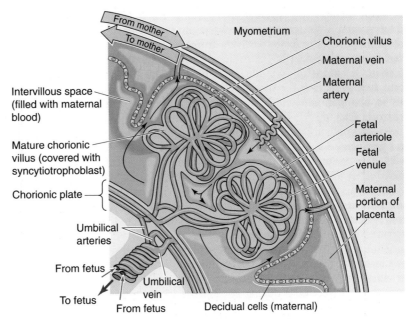

Figure 56-6 The mature placenta. With further development beyond that shown in Figure 56-5C, the outer surface of the mature chorionic villus is covered with a thin layer of syncytiotrophoblast. Under this are cytotrophoblasts, mesenchyme, and fetal blood vessels. The lacunae into which the villi project gradually merge into one massive intervillous space. Maternal blood is trapped in this intervillous space, between the endometrium on the maternal side and the villi on the fetal side. In the mature placenta, as shown here, "spiral" arteries from the mother empty directly into the intervillous space, which is drained by maternal veins. The villi look like a thick forest of trees arising from the chorionic plate, which is the analogue of the soil from which the trees sprout.

The **amniotic fluid** that fills the amniotic cavity serves two important functions. First, it serves as a mechanical buffer and thus protects the fetus from external, physical insults. Second, it serves as a mechanism by which the fetus excretes many waste products. The water in the amniotic fluid turns over at least once a day. After the fetal kidneys mature (10 to 12 weeks), the renal excretions of the fetus are the major source of amniotic fluid production (~75%); pulmonary secretions account for the rest. Fluid removal occurs through the actions of the fetal gastrointestinal tract (~55%), amnion (~30%), and lungs (~15%).

Gases and other solutes move across the placenta through simple diffusion, facilitated diffusion, secondary active transport, and endocytosis

The placenta is the major lifeline between the mother and the fetus. It provides nutrients and O_2 to the fetus, and it removes CO_2 and certain waste products from the fetus.

O_2 and CO_2 Transport The maternal blood coming into the intervillous space has a gas composition similar to that of systemic arterial blood: a P_{O_2} of ~100 mm Hg (Table 56-3), a P_{CO_2} of ~40 mm Hg, and a pH of 7.40. However, the diffusion of O_2 from the maternal blood into the chorionic villi of the fetus causes the P_{O_2} of blood in the intervillous space to fall, so the average P_{O_2} is 30 to 35 mm Hg. Given the O_2 dissociation curve of maternal (i.e., adult) hemoglobin (Hb), this P_{O_2} translates to an O_2 saturation of ~65%. The P_{O_2} of blood in the umbilical vein is even less. Despite the relatively low P_{O_2} of the maternal blood in the intervillous space, the fetus does not suffer from a lack of O_2. Because fetal Hb has a much higher affinity for O_2 than does maternal Hb, the fetal Hb can extract O_2 from the maternal Hb (see Chapter 29). Thus, a P_{O_2} of 30 to 35 mm Hg, which yields an Hb saturation of ~65% in the intervillous space in the mother's blood, produces an Hb saturation of ~85% in the umbili-

Table 56-3 Maternal and Fetal Oxygen Levels

Site	P_{O_2} (mm Hg)	Hemoglobin Saturation
Maternal Values		
Uterine artery	100	97.5%
Intervillous space	30-35	57%-67%
Uterine vein	30	57%
Fetal Values		
Umbilical arteries	23	60.5%
Umbilical vein	30	85.5%

cal vein of the fetus (Table 56-3), assuming that the O_2 fully equilibrates between intervillous and fetal blood. Other mechanisms of ensuring adequate fetal oxygenation include the relatively high cardiac output per unit body weight of the fetus and the increasing O_2-carrying capacity of fetal blood late in pregnancy as the Hb concentration rises to a level 50% higher than that of the adult.

The transfer of CO_2 from the fetus to the mother is driven by a concentration gradient between the blood in the umbilical arteries and that in the intervillous space. Near the end of pregnancy, the P_{CO_2} in the umbilical arteries is ~48 mm Hg, and the P_{CO_2} in the intervillous space is ~43 mm Hg, a gradient of ~5 mm Hg. The fetal blood also has a somewhat lower affinity for CO_2 than does maternal blood, thus favoring the transfer of CO_2 from the fetus to mother.

Other Solutes Various other solutes besides O_2 and CO_2 move across the placenta between the mother and the fetus and avail themselves of numerous transport mechanisms. Some of these solutes, such as the waste products urea and creatinine, probably move passively from fetus to mother. The lipid-soluble steroid hormones shuttle among the mother, the placenta, and the fetus by simple diffusion. Glucose moves from the mother to the fetus by facilitated diffusion, and amino acids move by secondary active transport (see Chapter 5). The placenta also transports several other essential substances, such as vitamins and minerals, that are needed for fetal growth and development. Many substances are present in the fetal circulation at concentrations higher than in the maternal blood, and they must be actively transported against concentration or electrochemical gradients. The necessary energy (i.e., ATP) is derived from glycolysis and the citric acid cycle, for which the enzymes are present in the human placenta at term. Also present are the enzymes for the pentose phosphate pathway, an alternative pathway for the oxidation of glucose, which provides the NADPH that is necessary for several synthetic pathways that require reducing equivalents in the human placenta at term.

The placenta takes up large molecules from the mother through receptor-mediated endocytosis (see Chapter 2). The uptake of substances such as low-density lipoproteins (LDL), transferrin, hormones (e.g., insulin), and antibodies (e.g., immunoglobulin G) increases throughout gestation until just before birth.

The placenta makes a variety of peptide hormones, including human chorionic gonadotropin and human chorionic somatomammotropin

The placenta plays a key role in steroid synthesis, which is discussed in the next major section. In addition, the placenta manufactures numerous amines, polypeptides (including peptide hormones and neuropeptides), proteins, glycoproteins, and steroids (Table 56-4). Among these peptides are the placental variants of all known releasing hormones, which are produced by the hypothalamus (see Chapter 47). These placental releasing hormones may act in a paracrine fashion, controlling the release of local placental hormones, or they may enter the maternal or fetal circulations. In addition, several proteases are also present in the placenta. Although the placenta synthesizes a wide variety of substances, the significance of many of these substances is not clear.

The most important placental peptide hormone is **hCG**. In the developing blastocyst, and later in the mature placenta, the syncytiotrophoblast cells synthesize hCG, perhaps under the direction of progesterone and estrogens. The placenta also produces two **human chorionic somatomammotropins**, hCS1 and hCS2, also called *human placental lactogen* (hPL). hCS1 and hCS2 are polypeptide hormones structurally related to growth hormone (GH) and placental-variant GH, as well as to prolactin (PRL; see Table 48-1). They play a role in the conversion of glucose to fatty acids and ketones, thus coordinating the fuel economy of the feto-placental unit. The fetus and placenta use fatty acids and ketones as energy sources and store them as fuels in preparation for the early neonatal period, when a considerable reservoir of energy is necessary for the transition from intra-

Table 56-4 Hormones Made by the Placenta

Peptide Hormones and Neuropeptides
- hCG
- Thyrotropin (thyroid-stimulating hormone [TSH])
- Placental-variant growth hormone
- hCS1 and hCS2, also known as hPL (hPL1 and hPL2)
- Placental proteins PP12 and PP14
- TRH
- Corticotropin-releasing hormone (CRH)
- Growth hormone–releasing hormone (GHRH)
- GnRH
- Substance P
- Neurotensin
- Somatostatin
- Neuropeptide Y
- ACTH-related peptide
- The inhibins

Steroid Hormones
- Progesterone
- Estrone
- Estradiol
- Estriol

uterine life to life outside the uterus. hCS1 and hCS2 also promote the development of maternal mammary glands during pregnancy.

In addition to its secretory functions, the placenta also stores vast amounts of proteins, polypeptides, glycogen, and iron. Many of these stored substances can be used at times of poor maternal nutrition and also during the transition from intrauterine to extrauterine life.

THE MATERNAL-PLACENTAL-FETAL UNIT

During pregnancy, progesterone and estrogens rise to levels that are substantially higher than their peaks in a normal cycle

Following ovulation during a normal or nonconception cycle, the cells of the ovarian follicle functionally transform into luteal cells, which produce mainly progesterone, but also estrogens (see Chapter 55). However, the corpus luteum has a finite life span, which lasts only ~12 days before it begins its demise in the presence of declining LH levels. As a consequence of luteal demise, levels of both progesterone and estrogens decline.

In contrast, during pregnancy, maternal levels of progesterone and estrogens (estradiol, estrone, estriol) all increase and reach concentrations substantially higher than those achieved during a normal menstrual cycle (Fig. 56-7). These elevated levels are necessary for maintaining pregnancy. For example, progesterone reduces uterine motility and inhibits propagation of contractions. How are these elevated levels of female steroids achieved? Early in the first trimester, hCG that is manufactured by the syncytiotrophoblast rescues the corpus luteum, which is the major source of progesterone and estrogens. This function of the corpus luteum in the ovary continues well into early pregnancy. However, by itself, the corpus luteum is not adequate to generate the very high steroid levels characteristic of late pregnancy. The developing placenta itself augments its production of progesterone and estrogens, so by 8 weeks of gestation, the placenta has become the major source of these steroids. The placenta continues to produce large quantities of estrogens, progestins, and other hormones throughout gestation. **Estriol**, which is not important in nonpregnant women, is a major estrogen during pregnancy (Fig. 56-7).

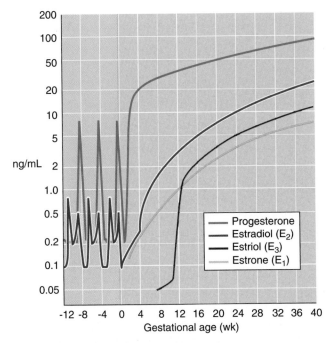

Figure 56-7 Maternal levels of progesterone and the estrogens just before and during pregnancy. The y-axis scale is logarithmic. The zero point on the x-axis is the time of fertilization. The progesterone spikes near −8 and −4 weeks refer to the two menstrual cycles before the one that resulted in the pregnancy. *(Data from Wilson JD, Foster DW, Kronenberg HM, Larsen PR [eds]: Williams Textbook of Endocrinology, 9th ed. Philadelphia: WB Saunders, 1998.)*

After 8 weeks of gestation, the coordinated biosynthetic activity of the maternal-placental-fetal unit maintains high levels of progesterone and estrogens

Although it emerges as the major source of progesterone and estrogens (Table 56-5), the placenta cannot synthesize these hormones by itself; it requires the assistance of both mother and fetus. This joint effort in steroid biosynthesis has led to the concept of the **maternal-placental-fetal unit**. Figure 56-8—which resembles the maps describing the synthesis of glucocorticoids, mineralocorticoids (see Fig. 50-2), male steroids (see Fig. 54-5), and female steroids (see Fig. 55-10, later)—illustrates the pathways used by the maternal-placental-fetal unit to synthesize progesterone and the estrogens. Figure 56-9 summarizes the exchange of synthetic intermediates among the three members of the maternal-placental-fetal unit.

Unlike the corpus luteum, which manufactures progesterone, estrone, and estradiol early in pregnancy (see Chapter 55), the placenta is an imperfect endocrine organ. First, the placenta cannot manufacture adequate cholesterol, the precursor for steroid synthesis. Second, the placenta lacks two crucial enzymes that are needed for synthesizing estrone and estradiol. Third, the placenta lacks a third enzyme that is needed to synthesize estriol. The enzymes missing from the placenta are listed in Table 56-5, and they also are indicated with a brown background in Figures 56-8 and 56-9.

The maternal-placental-fetal unit overcomes these placental shortcomings in two ways. First, the mother supplies most of the cholesterol as LDL particles (see Chapter 46). With this supply of maternal cholesterol, the placenta can

Table 56-5 Roles of the Mother, Placenta, and Fetus in Steroid Biosynthesis

	Needs	Contributes	Lacks
Mother	Progesterone Estrone Estradiol Estriol	LDL cholesterol	Adequate synthetic capacity for progesterone and estrogens
Placenta		3β-Hydroxysteroid dehydrogenase aromatase (P-450$_{arom}$)	Adequate cholesterol synthesizing capacity 17α-Hydroxylase (P-450$_{c17}$; needed to synthesize estrone and estradiol) 17,20-Desmolase (P-450$_{c17}$; needed to synthesize estrone and estradiol) 16α-Hydroxylase (needed to synthesize estriol)
Fetus		17α-Hydroxylase (P450$_{c17}$; needed to synthesize estrone and estradiol) 17,20-Desmolase (P450$_{c17}$; needed to synthesize estrone and estradiol) 16α-Hydroxylase (needed to synthesize estriol)	3β-Hydroxysteroid dehydrogenase aromatase (P450$_{arom}$)

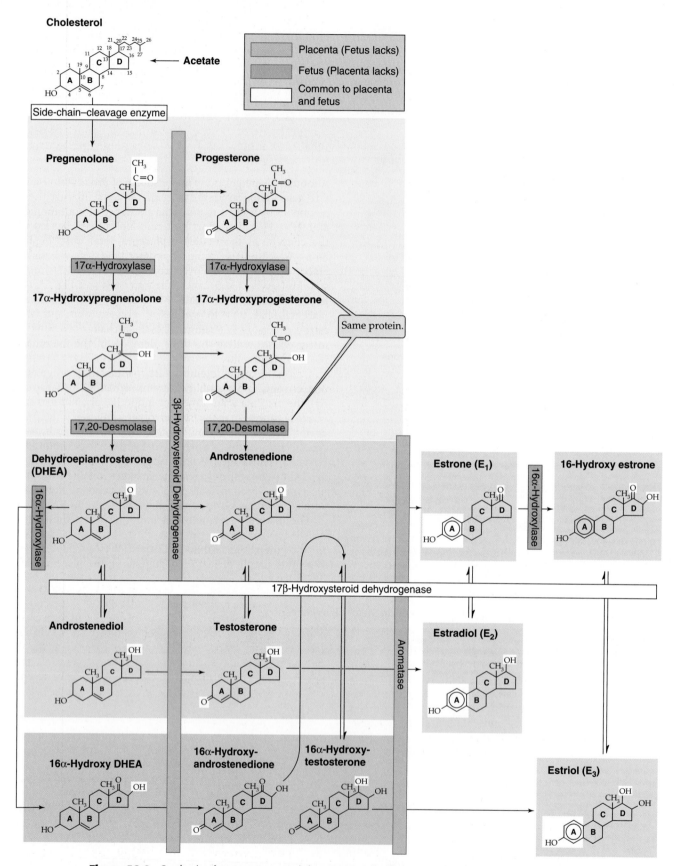

Figure 56-8 Synthesis of progesterone and the estrogens by the maternal-placental-fetal unit. Individual enzymes are shown in the *horizontal and vertical boxes*. See Figures 50-2, 54-5, and 55-9 for cellular localizations of enzymes. Chemical groups modified by each enzyme are *highlighted* in the reaction products. The fetus lacks 3β-hydroxysteroid dehydrogenase (3β-HSD) and aromatase (P-450arom), shown on the blue background. Placenta lacks 17α-hydroxylase and 17,20-desmolase activity (contributed by the same protein, P-450c17) and 16α-hydroxylase, shown on the brown background. The blue and brown color coding of enzymes distinguishes fetus from placenta, whereas color coding in previous steroidogenesis figures indicates subcellular localization.

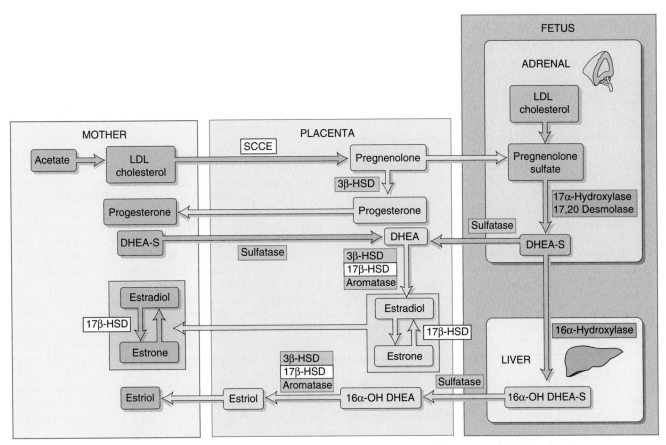

Figure 56-9 The interactions of the maternal-placental-fetal unit. The details of the enzymatic reactions are provided in Figure 56-8. SCCE is the side-chain–cleavage enzyme; the S in DHEA-S and 16α-OH DHEA-S represents sulfate. 17β-HSD, 17β-hydroxysteroid dehydrogenase.

generate large amounts of progesterone and can export it to the mother, thus solving the problem of maintaining maternal progesterone levels after the corpus luteum becomes inadequate. Second, the fetal adrenal gland and liver supply the three enzymes lacking in the placenta. The fetal adrenal glands are up to this metabolic task; at term, these glands are as large as those of an adult.

The fetus does not synthesize estrogens without assistance, for two reasons. First, it *cannot*, because the fetus lacks the enzymes that catalyze the last two steps in the production of estrone, the precursor of estradiol. These two enzymes are also necessary to synthesize estriol. The enzymes missing from the fetus are listed in Table 56-5, and they also are indicated with a blue background in Figures 56-8 and 56-9. Second, the fetus *should not* synthesize estrogens without assistance. If the fetus were to carry out the complete, classic biosynthesis of progesterone and the estrogens, it would expose itself to dangerously high levels of hormones that are needed not by the fetus, but by the mother.

The fetus and its placenta use three strategies to extricate themselves from this conundrum. First, because the fetus lacks the two enzymes noted earlier, it never makes anything beyond dehydroepiandrosterone (DHEA) and 16α-hydroxy-DHEA (Fig. 56-8). In particular, the fetus cannot make progesterone or any of the three key estrogens. Second, the placenta is a massive sink for the weak androgens that the

fetus does synthesize, thus preventing the masculinization of female fetuses. Third, the fetus conjugates the necessary steroid intermediates to sulfate, which greatly reduces their biological activity (Fig. 56-9). Thus, as pregnenolone moves from the placenta to the fetus, it is sulfated. The products of fetal pregnenolone metabolism are also sulfated (DHEA-S and 16α-hydroxy-DHEA-S) as long as they reside inside the fetus. It is only when DHEA-S and 16α-hydroxy-DHEA-S finally move to the placenta that a sulfatase removes the sulfate groups, and thus the placenta can complete the process of steroidogenesis and can export the hormones to the mother.

RESPONSE OF THE MOTHER TO PREGNANCY

The mean duration of pregnancy is ~266 days (38 weeks) from the time of ovulation or 280 days (40 weeks) from the first day of the last menstrual period. During this time, the mother experiences numerous and profound adaptive changes in her cardiovascular system, fluid volume, respiration, fuel metabolism, and nutrition. These orderly changes reflect the effects of various hormones, as well as the increase in the size of the pregnant uterus.

Both maternal cardiac output and blood volume increase during pregnancy

The maternal **blood volume** starts to increase during the first trimester, expands rapidly during the second trimester, rises at a much lower rate during the third trimester, and finally achieves a plateau during the last several weeks of pregnancy. Maternal blood volume may have increased by as much as 45% near term in singleton pregnancies and up to 75% to 100% in twin or triplet pregnancies. The ultimate increase in blood volume results from an increase in the volume of both the plasma and erythrocytes. However, the rise in plasma volume begins earlier and is ultimately greater (~50%) than the rise in total erythrocyte volume (~33%). A proposed mechanism for the increase in plasma volume is that elevated progesterone and estrogens cause a vasodilation that decreases peripheral vascular resistance and thus renal perfusion. One mechanism of the vasodilation is refractoriness to the pressor effects of angiotensin II. The renin-angiotensin-aldosterone axis responds by increasing aldosterone, which augments renal reabsorption of salt and water. In addition, pregnancy causes a leftward shift of the relationship between arginine vasopressin (AVP) release and plasma osmolality (see Chapter 41). Immediately after the delivery of the placenta, with the attendant decreases in progesterone and estrogen levels, the mother commences vigorous diuresis.

The increase in blood volume is needed to meet the demands of the enlarged pregnant uterus with its greatly hypertrophied vascular system. It also protects mother and fetus against the deleterious effects of impaired venous return in the supine and erect positions, and it safeguards the mother against the adverse effects of the blood loss associated with parturition.

Cardiac output increases appreciably during the first trimester of pregnancy (by 35% to 40%), but it increases only slightly during the second and third trimesters (~45% at term). The increase in cardiac output, which reflects mainly an increase in stroke volume but also heart rate, is highly targeted. Renal blood flow increases 40%. Uterine blood flow rises from just 1% to 15% of cardiac output. Blood flow to the heart (to support increased cardiac output), skin (to increase heat radiation), and breasts (to support mammary development) also increases. However, no change occurs in blood flow to the brain, gut, or skeleton. The increase in cardiac output with physical activity is greater in pregnant women (for most of the pregnancy) than it is in nonpregnant women.

Despite the large increase in plasma volume, **mean arterial pressure (MAP)** usually decreases during midpregnancy and then rises during the third trimester, although it normally remains at or lower than normal. The reason for this initial fall in MAP is a decrease in peripheral vascular resistance, possibly reflecting—in part—the aforementioned vasodilating effects of progesterone and estradiol.

Posture has a major effect on cardiac output (see Chapter 25). In late pregnancy, cardiac output is typically higher when the mother is in the lateral recumbent position than when she is in the supine position. In the supine position, the fundus of the enlarged uterus rests on the inferior vena cava near L5, thereby impeding venous return to the heart.

Increased levels of progesterone during pregnancy increase alveolar ventilation

During pregnancy, hormonal and mechanical factors lead to several anatomical changes that have the net effect of increasing alveolar ventilation. The level of the diaphragm rises ~4 cm, probably reflecting the relaxing effects of progesterone on the diaphragm muscle and fascia. At the same time, the costovertebral angle widens appreciably as the transverse diameter of the thoracic cage increases ~2 cm. Although these two changes have opposite effects on the residual volume (RV) of air in the lungs (see Chapter 27), the elevation of the diaphragm dominates, thus causing a net decrease in RV and functional residual capacity (FRC). Vital capacity (VC), maximal pulmonary ventilation, and pulmonary compliance do not change appreciably. Total pulmonary resistance falls, thereby facilitating airflow. Because of the increased size of the abdominal contents during pregnancy, the abdominal muscles are less effective in aiding forced expirations.

Although pregnancy has little effect on respiratory rate, it increases tidal volume (V_T) markedly—by ~40%—and thereby increases **alveolar ventilation** ($\dot{V}_A$; see Chapter 30). These increases in V_T and $\dot{V}_A$ are some of the earliest physiological changes during pregnancy, beginning 6 weeks after fertilization. They may reflect, at least in part, a direct stimulatory effect of progesterone and, to a lesser extent, estrogen on the medullary respiratory centers. The physiological effect of the increased $\dot{V}_A$ during pregnancy is a fall in maternal arterial P_{CO_2}, which typically decreases from a value before pregnancy of ~40 to ~32 mm Hg, despite the net increase in CO_2 production that reflects fetal metabolism. A side effect is mild respiratory alkalosis for which the kidneys compensate by lowering plasma $[HCO_3^-]$ modestly (see Chapter 28).

Pregnancy increases the demand for dietary protein, iron, and folic acid

During pregnancy, an additional 30 g of protein will be needed each day to meet the demand of the growing fetus, placenta, uterus, and breasts, as well as the increased maternal blood volume. Most protein should come from animal sources, such as meat, milk, eggs, cheese, poultry, and fish, because these foods furnish amino acids in optimal combinations.

Almost any diet that includes iodized salt and adequate caloric intake to support the pregnancy also contains enough minerals, except **iron** (see Table 45-3). Pregnancy necessitates a net gain of ~800 mg of circulating iron to support the expanding maternal Hb mass, the placenta, and the fetus. Most of this iron is used during the latter half of pregnancy. A *nonpregnant* woman of reproductive age needs to *absorb* ~1.5 mg/day of iron in a diet that contains 15 to 20 mg/day (see Chapter 45). In contrast, during pregnancy, the average required iron uptake rises to ~7 mg/day. Very few women have adequate iron stores to supply this amount of iron, and a typical diet seldom contains sufficient iron. Thus, the recommended supplementation of elemental iron is 60 mg/day, taken in the form of a simple ferrous iron salt.

Maternal **folate** requirements increase significantly during pregnancy, in part reflecting an increased demand for producing blood cells. This increased demand can lead to lowered plasma folate levels or, in extreme cases, to maternal megaloblastic anemia (see Chapter 45). Folate deficiency may cause neural tube defects in the developing fetus. Because oral supplementation of 400 to 800 μg/day of folic acid produces a vigorous hematologic response in pregnant women with severe megaloblastic anemia, this dose would almost certainly provide very effective prophylaxis.

Less than one third of the total maternal weight gain during pregnancy represents the fetus

The recommended weight gain during a singleton pregnancy for a woman with a normal ratio of weight to height (i.e., body mass index) is 11.5 to 16 kg. This number is higher for women with a low body mass index. A weight gain of 14 kg would include 5 kg for intrauterine contents—the fetus (3.3 kg), placenta and membranes (0.7 kg), and amniotic fluid (1 kg). The maternal contribution of 9 kg would include increases in the weight of the uterus (0.7 kg), the blood (1.3 kg), and the breasts (2.0 kg), as well as adipose tissue and interstitial fluid (5.0 kg). The interstitial fluid expansion may be partly the result of increased venous pressure created by the large pregnant uterus and, as noted earlier, partly caused by aldosterone-dependent Na^+ retention.

For a woman whose weight is normal before pregnancy, a weight gain in the recommended range correlates well with a favorable outcome of the pregnancy. Most pregnant women can achieve an adequate weight gain by eating—according to appetite—a diet adequate in calories, protein, minerals, and vitamins. Seldom, if ever, should maternal weight gain be deliberately restricted to less than this level. Failure to gain weight is an ominous sign; birth weight parallels maternal weight, and neonatal mortality rises with low birth weight, particularly for babies weighing less than 2500 g.

PARTURITION

Throughout most of pregnancy, the uterus is quiescent. Both progesterone and relaxin may promote this inactivity.

Weak and irregular uterine contractions occur throughout the last month of pregnancy. Eventually, a series of regular, rhythmic, and forceful contractions develops to facilitate thinning and dilation of the cervix—the obstetric definition of labor (Table 56-6). These contractions may last for several hours, a day, or even longer and may eventually result in the expulsion of the fetus, placenta, and membranes. Although not all the factors leading to the initiation of labor are known, endocrine, paracrine, and mechanical stretching of the uterus all play a role. Once labor is initiated, it is sustained by a series of positive feedback mechanisms.

Signals from the placenta or fetus may initiate labor

In rabbits, withdrawal of progesterone, made primarily in the *placenta*, results in prompt evacuation of the uterus; administration of progesterone delays the onset of labor. However, most human studies have failed to provide evidence that progesterone levels fall *before* the onset of labor. Nonetheless, it appears that progesterone plays an important role in maintaining the length of gestation in primates.

Other studies point to the importance of the *fetal* hypothalamic-pituitary-adrenal axis in the preparation for, or initiation of, parturition. In the fetal lamb, transection of the hypothalamic portal vessels prolongs gestation. In the human, an equivalent disruption of the fetal hypothalamic-pituitary-adrenal axis occurs in anencephalic fetuses, in which the cerebral hemispheres are absent and the rest of the brain is severely malformed. Indeed, gestation is prolonged in human pregnancies with anencephalic fetuses.

Infusing adrenocorticotropic hormone (ACTH) into fetal lambs with intact adrenal glands, or directly infusing cortisol, causes premature parturition. Although the theory that cortisol plays a role in initiating parturition remains attractive, several naturally occurring instances of failure of cortisol production in the human fetus do not prolong gestation. As discussed in the next section, prostaglandins appear to play a crucial role in the initiation of labor.

Table 56-6 Stages of Labor

Stage	Characteristics	Physiological Changes
0	Uterine tranquility and refractoriness to contraction	
1	Uterine awakening, initiation of parturition, extending to complete cervical dilatation	Increase in the number of gap junctions between myometrial cells; increase in the number of OT receptors
2	Active labor, from complete cervical dilatation to delivery of the newborn	
3	From delivery of the fetus to expulsion of the placenta and final uterine contraction	

Data from Casey ML, MacDonald PC: In Wilson JD, Foster DW, Kronenberg HM, Larsen PR (eds): Williams Textbook of Endocrinology. Philadelphia: WB Saunders, 1998.

Prostaglandins initiate uterine contractions, and both prostaglandins and oxytocin sustain labor

Whereas hormones (particularly oxytocin [OT]) and paracrine factors (particularly prostaglandins) play an important role in stimulating the uterine contractions that sustain labor, only the prostaglandins are believed to have a key role in the initiation of labor.

Prostaglandins   The uterus, the placenta, and the fetal membranes synthesize and release prostaglandins (see Chapter 3). Prostaglandins from the uterine decidual cells, particularly prostaglandins F_2 and E_2 ($PGF_{2\alpha}$ and PGE_2), act by a paracrine mechanism on uterine smooth muscle cells. OT (see later) stimulates uterine decidual cells to increase their $PGF_{2\alpha}$ synthesis. Arachidonic acid, the precursor of prostaglandins, is present in very high concentrations in the fetal membranes near term.

Prostaglandins have three major effects. First, prostaglandins strongly stimulate the contraction of uterine smooth muscle cells. Second, $PGF_{2\alpha}$ potentiates the contractions induced by OT by promoting formation of **gap junctions** between uterine smooth muscle cells; estradiol also increases the number of gap junctions (see Chapter 9). These gap junctions permit synchronous contraction of the uterine smooth muscle cells, reminiscent of the contraction of the ventricles of the heart. Third, prostaglandins also cause softening, dilatation, and thinning (*effacement*) of the cervix, which occurs early during labor. This softening is akin to an inflammatory reaction in that it is associated with an invasion by polymorphonuclear leukocytes (e.g., neutrophils). Because of these effects, prostaglandins are used to induce labor and delivery in certain clinical settings.

Prostaglandins may physiologically initiate labor. Both $PGF_{2\alpha}$ and PGE_2 evoke myometrial contractions at *any* stage of gestation, regardless of the route of administration. The levels of prostaglandins or their metabolic products naturally increase in the blood and amniotic fluid just before and during labor. Arachidonic acid instilled into the amniotic cavity causes the uterus to contract and to expel its contents. Aspirin, which inhibits the enzyme cyclooxygenase (see Chapter 3), reduces the formation of $PGF_{2\alpha}$ and PGE_2, thus inhibiting labor and prolonging gestation.

Oxytocin   The nonapeptide OT is closely related to AVP (Fig. 56-10). The two hormones apparently evolved from vasotocin, the single neurohypophyseal hormone in nonmammalian vertebrates. OT and AVP, which both differ from vasotocin by a single amino acid, are synthesized in the cell bodies of the neurons in the supraoptic and paraventricular nuclei of the hypothalamus. Both OT and AVP then move by fast axonal transport to the posterior pituitary gland, where they are stored in the nerve terminals until they are released in response to the appropriate stimuli. Both OT and AVP are closely associated with—and released with—peptides known as neurophysins.

Circulating OT binds to $G\alpha_q$-coupled **OT receptors** on the plasma membrane of uterine smooth muscle cells; this process triggers the phospholipase C cascade (see Chapter 3). Presumably, formation of IP_3 leads to Ca^{2+} release from

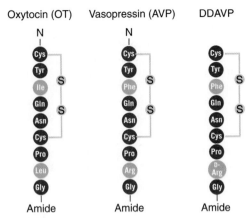

Figure 56-10   Comparison of structures of OT and AVP. DDAVP is a synthetic AVP in which the N-terminal Cys is deaminated and L-Arg at position 8 is replaced with D-Arg (see the box on diabetes insipidus in Chapter 38).

internal stores and to an increase in $[Ca^{2+}]_i$. The rise in $[Ca^{2+}]_i$ activates calmodulin, which stimulates myosin light-chain kinase to phosphorylate the regulatory light chain and to cause contraction of uterine smooth muscle cells (see Chapter 9) and increased intrauterine pressure. OT also binds to a receptor on decidual cells, thereby stimulating $PGF_{2\alpha}$ production, as discussed earlier.

Estrogen increases the *number* of OT receptors in the myometrial and decidual tissue of pregnant women. The uterus actually remains *insensitive* to OT until ~20 weeks' gestation, at which time the number of OT receptors increases progressively to 80-fold higher than baseline values by ~36 weeks' gestation, plateaus just before labor, then rises again to 200-fold during early labor. The time course of the expression of OT receptors may account for the increase in spontaneous myometrial contractions even in the absence of increased plasma OT levels. Whereas the uterus is sensitive to OT only at the end of pregnancy, it is susceptible to prostaglandins throughout pregnancy.

Although the prevailing view is that OT of *maternal* origin is not involved in initiating labor in humans, maternal OT may help to maintain labor. OT of *fetal* origin, which moves to the maternal circulation, could be involved in the onset of labor, because fetal plasma OT levels rise during the first stage of labor (Table 56-6). However, infusing OT at pharmacological doses into the circulation of the fetal lamb only stimulates uterine contractions. Therefore, normal levels of fetal OT probably have little influence on labor.

Once labor is initiated (stage 1), **maternal OT** is released in bursts, and the frequency of these bursts increases as labor progresses. The primary stimulus for the release of maternal OT appears to be distention of the cervix; this effect is known as the **Ferguson reflex**. OT is an important stimulator of myometrial contraction late in labor. During the second stage of labor, OT release may play a synergistic role in the expulsion of the fetus by virtue of its ability to stimulate prostaglandin release.

During the third stage of labor, uterine contractions induced by OT are also important for constricting uterine blood vessels at the site where the placenta used to be, thus promoting hemostasis (i.e., blood coagulation). Basal maternal plasma OT levels are unchanged after delivery. Fetal plasma OT levels are higher after vaginal delivery than after delivery by cesarean section, presumably because the maternal OT triggered by the Ferguson reflex crosses the placenta into the fetus.

Relaxin   This 48–amino acid polypeptide hormone, structurally related to insulin, is produced by the corpus luteum, the placenta, and the decidua. Relaxin may play a role in keeping the uterus in a quiet state during pregnancy. Production and release of relaxin increase during labor, when relaxin may soften and may thus help to dilate the cervix.

Mechanical Factors   Mechanical stretch placed on the uterine muscle may lead to the rhythmic contractions of labor. Thus, the increase in the size of the uterine contents to a critical level may stimulate uterine contractions, thereby leading to initiation of labor.

Positive Feedback   Once labor is initiated, several positive feedback loops involving prostaglandins and OT help to sustain it. First, uterine contractions stimulate prostaglandin release, which itself increases the intensity of uterine contractions. Second, uterine activity stretches the cervix, thus stimulating OT release through the Ferguson reflex. Because OT stimulates further uterine contractions, these contractions become self-perpetuating.

Involution of the uterus is primarily the result of a changing endocrine milieu

Almost immediately following delivery of the newborn, marked changes occur in the endocrine status of the mother. During pregnancy, many hormones are secreted in massive quantities. Estrogens are mitogenic, causing considerable hypertrophy of the uterine muscle cells during gestation. As the levels of these hormones fall abruptly, stimulation ceases, and uterine smooth muscle cells decrease in size. The vasculature of the uterus regresses, and blood flow to the uterus is significantly curtailed, thus leading to further involution of this organ.

LACTATION

The fundamental secretory unit of the breast (Fig. 56-11A) is the alveolus (Fig. 56-11B, C), which is surrounded by contractile myoepithelial cells and adipose cells. These alveoli are organized into lobules, each of which drains into a ductule. Groups of 15 to 20 ductules drain into a duct, which widens at the ampulla—a small reservoir. The lactiferous duct carries the secretions to the outside.

Breast development at puberty depends on several hormones, but primarily on the estrogens and progesterone. During pregnancy, gradual increases in levels of PRL and hCS, as well as very high levels of estrogens and progesterone, lead to full development of the breasts.

Table 56-7   Hormones Affecting the Mammary Gland During Pregnancy and Breast-Feeding

Mammogenic Hormones (promote cell proliferation)
Lobuloalveolar Growth
Estrogen
Growth hormone (IGF-1)
Cortisol
Prolactin
Relaxin?
Ductal Growth
Estrogen
Growth hormone
Cortisol
Relaxin

Lactogenic Hormones (promote initiation of milk production by alveolar cells)
Prolactin
hCS (or hPL)
Cortisol
Insulin (IGF-1)
Thyroid hormones
Growth hormone?
Withdrawal of estrogens and progesterone

Galactokinetic Hormones (promote contraction of myoepithelial cells and thus milk ejection)
OT
AVP (1% to 20% as powerful as OT)

Galactopoietic Hormones (maintain milk production after it has been established)
PRL (primary)
Cortisol and other metabolic hormones (permissive)

IGF-1, insulin-like growth factor type 1.

As summarized in Table 56-7, hormones affecting the breast are **mammogenic** (promoting the proliferation of alveolar and duct cells), **lactogenic** (promoting initiation of milk production by alveolar cells), **galactokinetic** (promoting contraction of myoepithelial cells, and thus milk ejection), or **galactopoietic** (maintaining milk production after it has been established).

The epithelial alveolar cells of the mammary gland secrete the complex mixture of sugars, proteins, lipids, and other substances that constitute milk

Milk is an emulsion of fats in an aqueous solution containing sugar (lactose), proteins (lactalbumin and casein), and several cations (K^+, Ca^{2+}, and Na^+) and anions (Cl^- and phosphate). The composition of human milk differs from that of human **colostrum** (the thin, yellowish, milk-like substance secreted during the first several days after parturition) and cow's milk (Table 56-8). Cow's milk has nearly three times more protein than human milk, almost exclusively a result of its much higher casein concentration. It also has a higher electrolyte content. The difference in composition between human milk and cow's milk is important because a newborn,

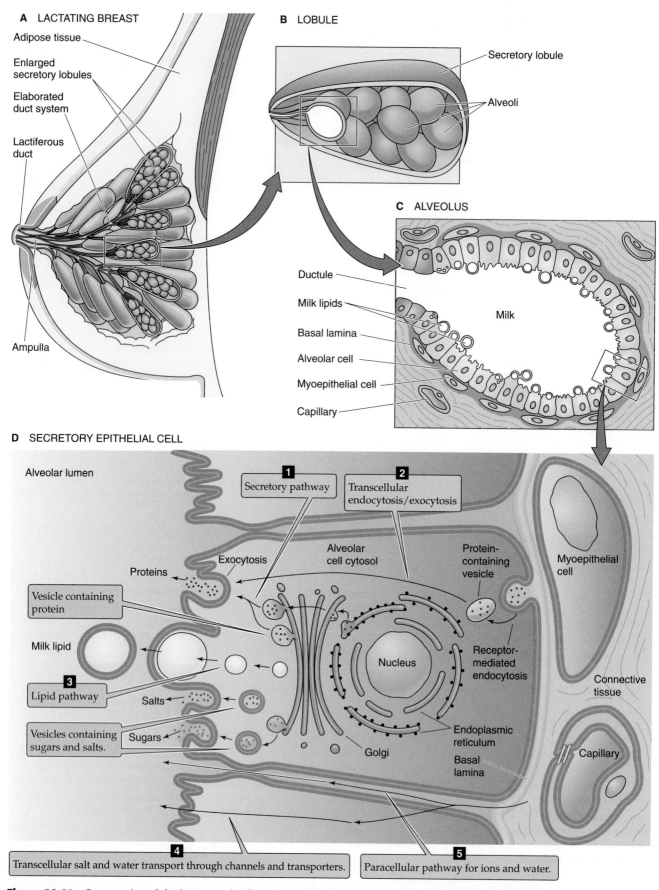

Figure 56-11 Cross section of the breasts and milk production. **A,** The breast consists of a series of secretory lobules, which empty into ductules. The ductules from 15 to 20 lobules combine into a duct, which widens at the ampulla—a small reservoir. The lactiferous duct carries the secretions to the outside. **B,** The lobule is made up of many alveoli, the fundamental secretory units. **C,** Each alveolus consists of secretory epithelial cells (alveolar cells) that actually secrete the milk, as well as contractile myoepithelial cells, which are, in turn, surrounded by adipose cells. **D,** The alveolar cell secretes the components of milk through five pathways.

Table 56-8 Composition of Human Colostrum, Human Milk, and Cow's Milk (per Deciliter of Fluid)

Component	Human Colostrum	Human Milk	Cow's Milk
Total protein (g)	2.7	0.9	3.3
Casein (% of total protein)	44	44	82
Total fat (g)	2.9	4.5	3.7
Lactose (g)	5.7	7.1	4.8
Caloric content (kcal)	54	70	69
Calcium (mg)	31	33	125
Iron (μg)	10	50	50
Phosphorus (mg)	14	15	96
Cells (macrophages, neutrophils, and lymphocytes)	$7\text{-}8 \times 10^6$	$1\text{-}2 \times 10^6$	—

with his or her delicate gastrointestinal tract, may not tolerate the more concentrated cow's milk.

The epithelial cells in the alveoli of the mammary gland secrete the complex mixture of constituents that make up milk by five major routes (Fig. 56-11D):

1. **Secretory pathway.** The milk proteins **lactalbumin** and **casein** are synthesized in the endoplasmic reticulum and are sorted to the Golgi apparatus (see Chapter 2). Here alveolar cells add Ca^{2+} and **phosphate** to the lumen. Lactose synthetase in the lumen of the Golgi catalyzes synthesis of **lactose**, the major carbohydrate. Lactose synthetase has two components, a galactosyl transferase and lactalbumin, both made in the endoplasmic reticulum. Water enters the secretory vesicle by osmosis. Finally, exocytosis discharges the contents of the vesicle into the lumen of the alveolus.

2. **Transcellular endocytosis and exocytosis.** The basolateral membrane takes up maternal immunoglobulins by receptor-mediated endocytosis (see Chapter 2). Following transcellular transport of these vesicles to the apical membrane, the cell secretes these immunoglobulins (primarily IgA) by exocytosis. The gastrointestinal tract of the infant takes up these immunoglobulins (see Chapter 45), which are important for conferring immunity before the infant's own immune system matures.

3. **Lipid pathway.** Epithelial cells synthesize short-chain fatty acids. However, the longer chain fatty acids (>16 carbons) that predominate in milk originate primarily from the diet or from fat stores. The fatty acids form into lipid droplets and move to the apical membrane. As the apical membrane surrounds the droplets and pinches off, it secretes the **milk lipids** into the lumen in a membrane-bound sac.

4. **Transcellular salt and water transport.** Various transport processes at the apical and basolateral membranes move small electrolytes from the interstitial fluid into the lumen of the alveolus. Water follows an osmotic gradient

generated primarily by lactose (present at a final concentration of ~200 mM) and, to a lesser extent, by the electrolytes.

5. **Paracellular pathway.** Salt and water can also move into the lumen of the alveolus through the tight junctions (see Chapter 5). In addition, cells, primarily leukocytes, squeeze between cells and enter the milk.

Prolactin is essential for milk production, and suckling is a powerful stimulus for prolactin secretion

PRL is a polypeptide hormone that is structurally related to GH, placental-variant GH, and hCS1 and hCS2 (see Table 48-1). Like GH, PRL is made and released in the anterior pituitary; however, lactotrophs rather than somatotrophs, are responsible for PRL synthesis. Another difference is that whereas GH-releasing hormone *stimulates* somatotrophs to release GH, dopamine (DA) *inhibits* the release of PRL from lactotrophs. Thus, the removal of inhibition promotes PRL release.

The actions of PRL on the mammary glands (Table 56-7) include the promotion of mammary growth (mammogenic effect), the initiation of milk secretion (lactogenic effect), and the maintenance of milk production once it has been established (galactopoietic effect). Although the initiation of lactation requires the coordinated action of several hormones, PRL is the classic lactogenic hormone. Initiating milk production also necessitates the abrupt fall in estrogens and progesterone that accompanies parturition. PRL is also the primary hormone responsible for maintaining milk production once it has been initiated.

PRL binds to a tyrosine kinase–associated receptor (see Chapter 3) in the same family of receptors as the GH receptor. PRL receptors, which have equal affinities for GH, are present in tissues such as breast, ovary, and liver. Presumably through pathways initiated by protein phosphorylation at tyrosine residues, PRL stimulates transcription of the genes

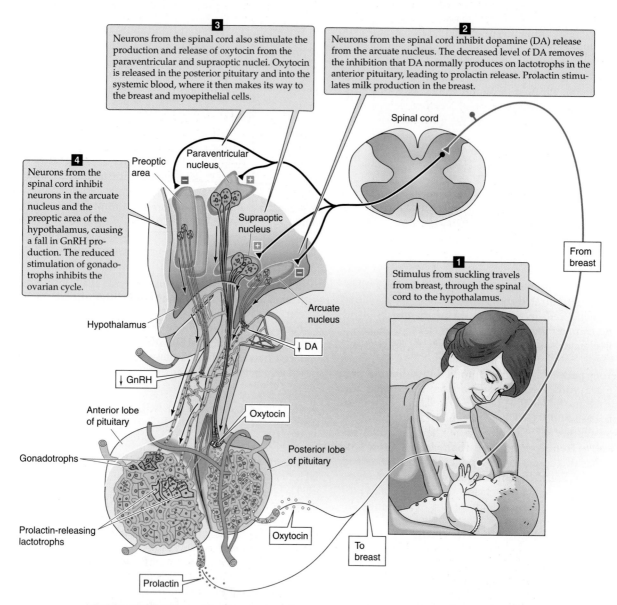

3 Neurons from the spinal cord also stimulate the production and release of oxytocin from the paraventricular and supraoptic nuclei. Oxytocin is released in the posterior pituitary and into the systemic blood, where it then makes its way to the breast and myoepithelial cells.

2 Neurons from the spinal cord inhibit dopamine (DA) release from the arcuate nucleus. The decreased level of DA removes the inhibition that DA normally produces on lactotrophs in the anterior pituitary, leading to prolactin release. Prolactin stimulates milk production in the breast.

4 Neurons from the spinal cord inhibit neurons in the arcuate nucleus and the preoptic area of the hypothalamus, causing a fall in GnRH production. The reduced stimulation of gonadotrophs inhibits the ovarian cycle.

1 Stimulus from suckling travels from breast, through the spinal cord to the hypothalamus.

Spinal cord

Preoptic area

Paraventricular nucleus

Supraoptic nucleus

Arcuate nucleus

From breast

Hypothalamus

↓ DA

↓ GnRH

Anterior lobe of pituitary

Oxytocin

Posterior lobe of pituitary

Gonadotrophs

Prolactin-releasing lactotrophs

Oxytocin

To breast

Prolactin

Figure 56-12 Effect of suckling on the release of PRL, OT, and GnRH. Suckling has four effects. First, it stimulates sensory nerves, which carry the signal from the breast to the spinal cord, where the nerves synapse with neurons that carry the signal to the brain. Second, in the arcuate nucleus of the hypothalamus, the afferent input from the nipple inhibits neurons that release DA. DA normally travels through the hypothalamic-portal system to the anterior pituitary, where it inhibits PRL release by lactotrophs. Thus, inhibition of DA release leads to an increase in PRL release. Third, in the supraoptic and paraventricular nuclei of the hypothalamus, the afferent input from the nipple triggers the production and release of OT in the posterior pituitary. Fourth, in the preoptic area and arcuate nucleus, the afferent input from the nipple inhibits GnRH release. GnRH normally travels through the hypothalamic-portal system to the anterior pituitary, where it stimulates the synthesis and release of FSH and LH. Thus, inhibiting GnRH release curbs FSH and LH release and thereby inhibits the ovarian cycle.

that encode several milk proteins, including lactalbumin and casein.

Suckling is the most powerful physiological stimulus for PRL release. Nipple stimulation triggers PRL secretion through an afferent neural pathway through the spinal cord, thereby inhibiting dopaminergic neurons in the median eminence of the hypothalamus (Fig. 56-12). Because **DA** normally inhibits PRL release from the lactotrophs, it is called a **PRL-inhibitory factor (PIF)**. Thus, because suckling decreases DA delivery through the portal vessels, it relieves the inhibition on the lactotrophs in the anterior pituitary and stimulates bursts of PRL release. Treating women with DA-receptor agonists rapidly inhibits PRL secretion and milk production.

Several factors act as **PRL-releasing factors (PRFs)**: thyrotropin-releasing hormone (TRH), angiotensin II, substance P, β endorphin, and AVP. In the rat, suckling stimulates the release of **TRH** from the hypothalamus. In lactating women, TRH leads to increased milk production. **Estradiol** modulates PRL release in two ways. First, estradiol increases the sensitivity of the lactotroph to stimulation by TRH. Second, estradiol decreases the sensitivity of the lactotroph to inhibition by DA.

During the first 3 weeks of the neonatal period, maternal PRL levels remain tonically elevated. Thereafter, PRL levels decrease to a constant baseline level higher than that observed in women who are not pregnant. If the mother does *not* nurse her young, PRL levels generally fall to nonpregnant levels after 1 to 2 weeks. If the mother *does* breast-feed, increased PRL secretion is maintained for as long as suckling continues. Suckling causes episodic increases in PRL secretion with each feeding, thus producing peaks in PRL levels superimposed on the elevated baseline PRL levels. After the infant completes a session of nursing, PRL levels return to their elevated baseline and remain there until the infant nurses again.

Oxytocin and psychic stimuli initiate milk ejection ("let-down")

OT, which can promote uterine contraction, also enhances milk ejection by stimulating the contraction of the network of myoepithelial cells surrounding the alveoli and ducts of the breast (galactokinetic effect). Nursing can sometimes cause uterine cramps. During nursing, suckling stimulates nerve endings in the nipple and triggers rapid bursts of OT release (Fig. 56-12). This neurogenic reflex is transmitted through the spinal cord, the midbrain, and the hypothalamus, where it stimulates neurons in the paraventricular and supraoptic nuclei that release OT from their nerve endings in the *posterior pituitary*. From the posterior pituitary, OT enters the systemic circulation and eventually reaches the myoepithelial cells arranged longitudinally on the lactiferous ducts and around the alveoli in the breast (Fig. 56-11C, D). Because these cells have OT receptors, OT causes them to contract by mechanisms similar to those for the contraction of uterine smooth muscle, described earlier. The result is to promote the release of pre-existing milk after 40 to 60 seconds, a process known as the **let-down reflex**.

In addition to the suckling stimulus, many different psychic stimuli emanating from the infant, as well as neuro-endocrine factors, also promote OT release. The site or sound of an infant may trigger milk let-down, a phenomenon observed in many mammals. Thus, the posterior pituitary releases OT episodically even in anticipation of suckling. This psychogenic reflex is suppressed when fear, anger, or other stresses are encountered, and the results are inhibition of OT release and suppression of milk outflow.

Suckling inhibits the ovarian cycle

Lactation generally inhibits cyclic ovulatory function. Suckling likely reduces the release of gonadotropin-releasing hormone (GnRH) by neurons in the arcuate nucleus and the preoptic area of the hypothalamus (Fig. 56-12). Normally, GnRH travels through the portal vessels to the gonadotrophs in the anterior pituitary. Thus, the decreased GnRH release induced by suckling reduces the secretion of follicle-stimulating hormone (FSH) and LH and has a negative effect on ovarian function. As a result, breast-feeding delays ovulation and normal menstrual cycles. However, if the mother continues to nurse her infant for a prolonged period, ovulatory cycles will eventually resume. Suckling intensity and frequency, which decrease with the introduction of supplementary foods to the infant, determine the duration of anovulation and amenorrhea in well-nourished women. In breast-feeding women in Bangladesh, the period of anovulation averages 18 to 24 months. If the mother does *not* nurse her child after delivery, ovulatory cycles resume, on average, 8 to 10 weeks after delivery, with a range of up to 18 weeks.

REFERENCES

Books and Reviews

Casey ML, MacDonald PC: Endocrine changes of pregnancy. In Wilson JD, Foster DW, Kronenberg HM, Larsen PR (eds): Williams Textbook of Endocrinology. Philadelphia: WB Saunders, 1998.

Fuchs A-R: Physiology and endocrinology of lactation. In Gabbe SG, Niebyl JR, Simpson JL (eds): Obstetrics: Normal and Problem Pregnancies, 3rd ed. New York: Churchill Livingstone, 1996, pp 137-157.

Lamberts SWJ, Macleod RM: Regulation of prolactin secretion at the level of the lactotroph. Physiol Rev 1990; 70:279-318.

Moore TR, Reiter RC, Rebar RW, Baker VV (eds): Gynecology and Obstetrics: A Longitudinal Approach. New York: Churchill Livingstone, 1993.

Ramsey EM, Eonner MW: Placental Vasculature and Circulation. Philadelphia: WB Saunders, 1980.

Stulc J: Placental transfer of inorganic ions and water. Physiol Rev 1997; 77:805-836.

Vonderhaar BK, Ziska SE: Hormonal regulation of milk protein gene expression. Annu Rev Physiol 1989; 51:641-652.

Wilson JD, Foster DW, Kronenberg HM, Larsen PR (eds): Williams Textbook of Endocrinology, 9th ed. Philadelphia: WB Saunders, 1998.

Yen SSC, Jaffe RB (eds): Reproductive Endocrinology. Philadelphia: WB Saunders, 1986.

Journal Articles

Fuch AR, Fuchs F, Husslein P, et al: Oxytocin receptors and human parturition: A dual role for oxytocin in the initiation of labor. Science 1982; 215:1396-1398.

Goebelsmann U, Jaffe RB: Oestriol metabolism in pregnant women. Acta Endocrinol 1971; 66:679-693.

Liggins GC: Initiation of parturition. Br Med Bull 1979; 35:145-150.

Perez A, Vela P, Masnick GS, Potter RG: First ovulation after childbirth: The effect of breast feeding. Am J Obstet Gynecol 1972; 114:1041-1047.

Tabibzadeh S, Babaknia A: The signals and molecular pathways involved in implantation, a symbiotic interaction between blastocyst and endometrium involving adhesion and tissue invasion. Hum Reprod 1995; 10:1579-1602.

Wigglesworth JS: Vascular organization of the human placenta. Nature 1967; 216:1120-1121.

Wilkening RB, Meschia G: Fetal oxygen uptake, oxygenation, and acid-base balance as a function of uterine blood flow. Am J Physiol 1983; 244:H749-H755.

CHAPTER 57

FETAL AND NEONATAL PHYSIOLOGY

Ervin E. Jones

Growth of the fetus begins soon after fertilization, when the first cell division occurs. Cell division, hypertrophy, and differentiation are highly coordinated events that result in the growth and development of specialized organ systems. The fetus, fetal membranes, and placenta develop and function as a unit throughout pregnancy, and their development is interdependent. The growth trajectory of fetal mass is relatively flat during the first trimester, increases linearly at the beginning of the second trimester, and rises rapidly during the third trimester.

BIOLOGY OF FETAL GROWTH

Growth occurs by hyperplasia and hypertrophy

The growth of an organ occurs as a result of an increase in cell number (**hyperplasia**), an increase in cell size (**hypertrophy**), or both. We can define three sequential phases of growth: (1) pure hyperplasia, (2) hyperplasia and concomitant hypertrophy, and (3) hypertrophy alone. The time courses of the three phases of growth are organ specific. For example, the **placenta** goes through all three phases of growth, but these phases are compressed because the placental life span is relatively short. Moreover, simple hypertrophy is the primary form of placental growth. Thus, the weight, RNA content, and protein content of the human placenta increase linearly until term, but cell number does not increase during the third trimester.

In contrast to placental growth and development, growth of the **fetus** occurs almost entirely by hyperplasia. Thus, DNA content increases linearly in all fetal organs beginning early in the second trimester. Stimuli that either increase or decrease cell number, cell size, or both may accelerate or retard the growth of the whole fetus or of individual organs. The phase of growth during which the stimulus acts determines the response of the organ. For example, malnutrition occurring during the period of *hyperplasia* retards cell division and causes a deficiency in cell number. Therefore, adequacy of nutrition early in life may determine the number of cells in any organ. This effect on cell number may be irreversible, even if normal nutrition is restored later. Con-

versely, malnutrition occurring during the period of *hypertrophy* causes a reduction in cell size. However, this effect can be reversed, and normal cell size can be achieved if adequate nutrition is restored. Thus, reversibility depends on the timing of the stimulus.

Genetic factors primarily determine growth during the first half of gestation, and epigenetic factors determine growth during the second half

The fertilized egg contains the genetic material that directs cell multiplication and differentiation and guides development of the human phenotype. For specific developmental events to occur at precise times (Table 57-1), a programmed sequence of gene activation and suppression is necessary. Ignoring apoptosis, the fertilized egg must undergo an average of ~42 divisions to reach newborn size. A fertilized ovum, weighing less than 1 ng, gives rise to a newborn weighing slightly more than 3 kg (an increase of more than 10^{12} fold). Not only must the total cell number in a term fetus lie within relatively narrow limits, but also the developmental program must trigger cell differentiation after a specified number of cell divisions. After birth, only approximately five additional divisions are necessary for the net increase in mass that is necessary to achieve adult size. Obviously, many tissues (e.g., gastrointestinal tract, skin, blood cells) must continually undergo cell division to replenish cells lost by apoptosis.

Although the genetic makeup of the fetus principally determines its growth and development, other influences—both stimulatory and inhibitory—are superimposed on the genetic program. During the first half of pregnancy, the fetus' own genetic program is the primary determinant of growth, thus constraining patterns of growth. During the second half of pregnancy, the patterns of growth and development are more variable. The four primary epigenetic factors at work during the second half of pregnancy are placental, hormonal, environmental (e.g., maternal nutrition, disease, drugs, altitude), and metabolic (e.g., diabetes). We discuss the first two factors (placental and hormonal) in the next two sections.

Table 57-1   Chronologic Development of Organs, Systems, and Body Form

Organ	Chronology of Development
Bronchial apparatus and pharyngeal pouches	4th week, ridges and grooves appear over the future neck region
Thyroid gland	4th week, endoderm appears over the floor of the pharynx
Tongue	4th week, primordia appear in the floor of the pharynx
Face	End of 4th week, primordia appear
Palate	Begins in the 5th week
Upper respiratory system	4th week, laryngotracheal groove appears
Digestive system 　Foregut derivatives 　　Pharynx and its derivatives 　　Lower respiratory tract 　　Esophagus, stomach, proximal duodenum (from stomach to entry of the common bile duct) 　　Liver, biliary tract, gallbladder, pancreas 　Midgut derivatives 　　Small intestine, except proximal duodenum 　　Cecum, appendix 　　Ascending colon and proximal half of transverse colon 　Hindgut derivatives 　　Distal half of transverse colon 　　Descending and sigmoid colon 　　Rectum and upper portion of anal canal 　　Part of the urogenital system	4th week, primitive gut forms 4th week, formation of midgut derivatives begins 6th week, primordia appear, midgut elongates End of 7th week, anal canal has formed
Kidneys, urinary bladder, urethra	5th week, permanent adult kidney begins to develop
Adrenal glands	5th week, primordia of adrenal glands develop
Gonads, genital ducts, external genitalia	5th week, gonadal ridges form
Heart	3rd week, development of the heart begins
Atria	5th week, the atria are formed
Ventricles	5th week, the ventricles form
Fetal circulation	3rd week, embryonic blood vessels develop
Brain and spinal cord	End of 4th week, primary vesicles form and walls of the neural tube thicken to form the spinal cord
Pituitary	6th week, connection of Rathke's with oral cavity disappears
Limbs	End of 4th week, limb buds appear
Skull	7th week, paired cartilages begin to fuse to form the cranium

Table 57-2 Determinants of Birth Weight

Factor	Contribution to Final Birth Weight
Maternal environment	30%
Maternal genotype	20%
Paternal genotype	20%
Fetal genotype (excluding gender)	15%
Fetal gender	2%
Multifactorial (e.g., gestational age at delivery, multiple gestation)	13%

Studies of birth weights in families reveal that both parental and fetal genotypes affect birth weight (Table 57-2). The mother contributes to birth weight both through her influence on the environment that she provides for the fetus (~30%) and through the genes that she passes on to the fetus (~20%). The mother's contribution to the fetal environment includes maternal health and nutritional status, environment, lifestyle, age (e.g., adolescents and older women have infants with lower birth weight), parity, prepregnancy weight and prenatal weight gain, early fat deposition, height, chronic diseases, infection, and stress. The father contributes to birth weight only through the genes that he passes on to his child (~20%). The unique fetal genotype—the interaction of the alleles provided by the parents (e.g., dominant versus recessive genes) considered apart from the individual contributions of the two parents—contributes ~15%. The gender of the fetus contributes ~2%. The remaining ~13% of the contribution to birth weight is multifactorial and may include variations in such factors as gestational age at delivery and multiple gestation (e.g., twinning).

Increases in placental mass parallel periods of rapid fetal growth

The placenta plays several important roles in fetal growth and development. In addition to its transport and storage functions, the placenta is involved in numerous biosynthetic activities. These include the synthesis of steroids, such as estrogen and progesterone, and protein hormones, such as human chorionic gonadotropin (hCG) and the human chorionic somatomammotropins (hCSs) (see Chapter 56).

Fetal growth closely correlates with placental weight. During periods of rapid fetal growth, placental weight increases. As the placental mass increases, the total surface area of the placental villi (see Chapter 56) increases to sustain gas transport and fetal nutrition. Moreover, maternal blood flow to the uterus and fetal blood flow to the placenta also increase in parallel with the increase in placental mass. Placental growth increases linearly until ~4 weeks before birth. **Intrauterine growth restriction** (**IUGR**; see the box titled Growth Restriction) may occur as a result of decreased *pla-*

cental reserve caused by any insult. Adequate placental reserve is particularly important during the third trimester, when fetal growth is very rapid. For example, mothers who smoke during pregnancy tend to have small placentas and are at high risk of delivering a low birth weight baby.

Insulin, the insulin-like growth factors, and thyroxine stimulate fetal growth

Chapter 48 includes a discussion of several hormones—including glucocorticoids, insulin, growth hormone (GH), the insulin-like growth factors (IGFs), and thyroid hormones—that are important for achieving final adult mass.

Glucocorticoids and Insulin As its major energy source, the growing fetus uses glucose, which moves across the placenta by facilitated diffusion. Unlike the adult, who uses sophisticated hormonal systems to control blood glucose levels (see Chapter 51), the fetus is passive: the exchange of glucose across the placenta controls fetal blood glucose levels. The fetus normally has little need for gluconeogenesis, and the levels of gluconeogenic enzymes in the fetal liver are low. **Glucocorticoids** in the fetus promote the storage of glucose as glycogen in the fetal liver, a process that increases greatly during the final month of gestation in preparation for the increased glycolytic activity required during and immediately after delivery. Near term, when fetal glucose metabolism becomes sensitive to **insulin**, this hormone contributes to the storage of glucose as glycogen, as well as to the uptake and utilization of amino acids, and lipogenesis (see Chapter 51). Transient increases in maternal blood glucose levels after meals are closely mirrored by increases in fetal blood glucose levels. This transient fetal hyperglycemia leads to increased fetal production of insulin. Maternal insulin cannot cross the placenta.

In a mother with poorly controlled diabetes (see the box on diabetes mellitus in Chapter 51), sustained maternal hyperglycemia leads to sustained fetal hyperglycemia and therefore fetal hyperinsulinemia. The resulting high levels of fetal insulin, which is a growth factor (see Chapter 48), increase both the size of fetal organs (organomegaly) and fetal body mass (macrosomia). During the last half of the third trimester, fetal weight in poorly controlled diabetic pregnancies generally exceeds that in normal pregnancies. In some cases, large fetal size leads to problems at delivery. Indeed, the frequency of cesarean section is much higher in deliveries of fetuses born to diabetic mothers.

Insulin-Like Growth Factors Postnatally, **GH** acts by binding to GH receptors, primarily in the liver, and triggering the production of somatomedin or IGF-1. IGF-2 is not so much under the control of GH. The IGF-1 receptor is similar, but not identical, to the insulin receptor and can bind both IGF-1 and IGF-2, as well as insulin (see Chapter 48). In the fetus, both IGF-1 and IGF-2, which are mitogenic peptides, are extremely important for growth. IGF-1 and IGF-2 are present in the fetal circulation from the end of the first trimester, and their levels increase thereafter in both mother and fetus. Birth weight correlates positively with IGF levels. However, both relative levels of the IGFs and control of the IGFs are very different in the fetal stage than they are postnatally. First, fetal IGF-2 levels are much higher than IGF-1 levels; IGF-1 and IGF-2 levels resemble those in adults soon after birth. Second, in the fetus, IGF-1 and IGF-2 levels correlate poorly with GH levels. Indeed, it appears that GH may have only a minimal effect on fetal growth. For example, anencephalic fetuses (see Chapter 10 for the box on abnormalities of neural tube closure), which have low GH levels, generally grow normally. Moreover, unlike the adult liver, the fetal liver has relatively few GH receptors.

Epidermal Growth Factor   The fetus has abundant epidermal growth factor (EGF) receptors (see Chapter 3), and EGF is well known for its mitogenic properties, especially with regard to development of ectodermal and mesodermal structures. However, the fetus has no detectable mRNA encoding EGF. Thus, transforming growth factor α (TGF-α), another potent mitogen, which binds to EGF receptors on target cells, may act as a ligand for the EGF receptor.

Thyroid Hormones   The thyroid hormones are obligatory for normal growth and development (see Chapter 49). Before the second trimester, most of the thyroxine (T_4) in the fetus is maternal. Fetal production of thyrotropin (thyroid-stimulating hormone [TSH]) and the thyroid hormone T_4 begin to increase in the second trimester, concurrent with development of the hypothalamic-pituitary portal system. Hypothyroidism has adverse effects on fetal growth, generally reflected as a reduction in the size of organs such as the heart, kidney, liver, muscle, and spleen.

Peptide Hormones   Peptide hormones secreted by the placenta (see Table 56-4) can act through endocrine, paracrine, and autocrine mechanisms to stimulate growth and differentiation in several organ systems.

Many fetal tissues produce red blood cells early in gestation

Early during gestation, production of red blood cells (erythropoiesis) occurs in many tissues not normally thought of as erythropoietic in the adult. Erythropoiesis begins during the third week of fetal development in the yolk sac and placenta. At approximately the fourth week of gestation, the endothelium of blood vessels and the mesenchyme also begin to contribute to the erythrocyte pool, shortly followed by the liver. The bone marrow, spleen, and other lymphoid tissues begin to produce red blood cells only near the end of the first trimester. All these organ systems except bone marrow gradually lose their ability to manufacture blood

---

Growth Restriction

IUGR is an abnormality of fetal growth and development. IUGR has been variously defined as a birth weight lower than the 3rd, 5th, or 10th percentile for gestational age or a birth weight that is more than two standard deviations lower than the mean for gestational age.

The growth-restricted fetus is at substantial risk of morbidity and mortality. Specific risks include birth asphyxia, neonatal hypoglycemia, hypocalcemia, meconium aspiration, persistent pulmonary hypertension of the newborn, pulmonary hemorrhage, thrombocytopenia, polycythemia, delayed neurologic development, and hypothermia. Ultrasound methods offer objective, reliable means for identifying IUGR. Intrauterine measurements of biparietal diameter (distance between the two parietal eminences of the head) and abdominal circumference predict IUGR in as many as 90% of the cases.

The three recognized categories of IUGR are related to the time of onset of the pathologic process, as follows:

Type I or **symmetrical IUGR** refers to the infant with decreased growth potential. Type I IUGR accounts for 20% to 30% of growth-restricted fetuses. The entire fetus is small for gestational age. Length, weight, and abdominal and head circumferences are all less than the 10th percentile for gestational age. Type I IUGR results from growth inhibition during early fetal development (4 to 20 weeks' gestation), a period referred to as the *hyperplastic stage* of fetal development. Thus, the pathologic result is fewer cells in the fetus. Causes include intrauterine infections (e.g., rubella, cytomegalovirus), chromosomal disorders, congenital malformations, maternal drug ingestion, and maternal smoking. Of fetuses with severe, early onset of growth retardation, ~25% have aneuploidy (i.e., abnormal number of chromosomes). Uniformly (or symmetrically) diminished growth of these fetuses may result from inhibition of mitosis during early development.

Type II or **asymmetric IUGR** refers to the infant with restricted growth, most frequently caused by uteroplacental insufficiency. This type accounts for 70% to 80% of growth-restricted fetuses. This type of growth restriction results from an insult that occurs later in gestation than type I IUGR, usually after 28 weeks' gestation. Late in the second trimester, hypertrophy dominates. A rapid increase in cell size and increases in the formation of fat, muscle, bone, and other tissues occur. Fetuses with type II IUGR have a normal total number of cells, but these cells are smaller than normal. The distinguishing feature of the fetus with asymmetric IUGR is that the fetus has a normal length and head circumference (brain-sparing effect), but abdominal growth slows during the late second and early third trimesters. Redistribution of fetal CO occurs, with increased flow to the brain, heart, and adrenals and decreased glycogen storage and liver mass. This form of IUGR is most often associated with maternal disease such as kidney disease, chronic hypertension, and severe diabetes mellitus, among others.

Intermediate IUGR is a combination of types I and II IUGR and accounts for 5% to 10% of all growth-restricted fetuses. It probably occurs during the middle phase of fetal growth (20 to 28 weeks' gestation), between the hyperplastic and hypertrophic phases. During this middle period, mitotic rate decreases and overall cell size increases progressively. Chronic hypertension, lupus nephritis, or other maternal vascular diseases that are severe and begin early in the second trimester may result in intermediate IUGR, with symmetric growth and no significant brain-sparing effect.

cells, and by the third trimester, the bone marrow becomes the dominant source of blood cells.

The erythrocytes formed early in gestation are nucleated, but as fetal development progresses, more and more of the circulatory erythrocytes are non-nucleated. The blood volume in the common circulation of the fetoplacental unit increases as the fetus grows. The fraction of total erythrocytes that are reticulocytes (immature, non-nucleated erythrocytes with residual polyribosomes) is high in the young fetus, but it decreases to only ~5% at term. In the adult, the reticulocyte count is normally less than 1%. The life span of fetal erythrocytes depends on the age of the fetus; in a term fetus, it is ~80 days, or two thirds that in an adult. The life span of erythrocytes of less mature fetuses is much shorter.

The hemoglobin (Hb) content of the fetal blood rises to ~15 g/dL by midgestation, equivalent to the level in normal men. The Hb concentration of fetal blood at term is higher than the Hb concentration of maternal blood, which may be only ~12 g/dL. Embryonic Hb with different combinations of α-type and β-type chains (see Table 29-1) is present very early in gestation. A genetic program of development governs the eventual transition to fetal Hb (HbF), which predominates at birth. HbA and a small amount of HbA_2 gradually replace HbF during the first 12 months of life, thus culminating in the adult pattern of Hb expression (see Table 29-2).

The fetal gastrointestinal and urinary systems excrete products into the amniotic fluid by midpregnancy

The fetus imbibes considerable quantities of amniotic fluid by 20 weeks' gestation. However, not until the final 12 weeks of gestation is fetal gastrointestinal function similar to that of the normal infant at term. The fetal gastrointestinal tract continuously excretes small amounts of meconium into the amniotic fluid. **Meconium** consists of excretory products from the gastrointestinal mucosa and glands, along with unabsorbed residua from the imbibed amniotic fluid.

By the beginning of the second trimester, the fetus also begins to urinate. Fetal urine constitutes ~75% of amniotic fluid production (see Chapter 56). The fetal renal system does not acquire the capacity to regulate fluid, electrolyte, and acid-base balance until the beginning of the third trimester. Full development of the renal system does not occur until several months following delivery.

A surge in protein synthesis, with an increase in muscle mass, is a major factor in the rapid fetal weight gain during the third trimester

Fetal tissues constantly synthesize and break down proteins. Protein synthesis predominates throughout gestation, especially during the third trimester, when fetal protein synthesis—primarily in muscle and liver—increases 3- to 4-fold. The number of ribosomes per cell increases throughout gestation and early postnatal life. The efficiency of ribosomes at translating mRNA may also improve during gestation. Substrate availability (i.e., amino acids) and modulation of the synthetic apparatus by endocrine and other factors play important roles in regulating protein synthesis during gestation.

The formation of each peptide bond requires four molecules of ATP, so the energy cost of protein synthesis is 0.86 kcal/g. Protein synthesis comprises 15% to 20% of fetal metabolic expenditure in the third trimester. At equivalent phases of development, fetuses across several species invest similar fractions of total energy in protein synthesis. Because glucose is the major metabolic fuel, a shortfall of oxidized metabolic substrates (e.g., glucose and lactate) has a direct, negative impact on protein synthesis.

Increases in skeletal muscle mass account for 25% to 50% of fetal weight gain during the second half of gestation, when the number of muscle cells increases 8-fold and cell volume increases ~2.6-fold. Although skeletal muscle fibers are not differentiated in the first half of gestation, distinct type I and type II muscle fibers (see Chapter 9) appear in equal amounts between 20 and 26 weeks of gestation.

Fetal lipid stores increase rapidly during the third trimester

Fetal fat stores account for only 1% of fetal body weight during the first trimester. By the third trimester, as much as 15% of fetal body weight is fat. At birth, humans have more fat than other warm-blooded animals (e.g., the newborn cat has 2%; the guinea pig, 9.5%; the rat, 11%), with the exception of hibernating mammals and migratory birds.

Approximately half the increase in body fat reflects increased lipid transport across the placenta, and the other half reflects increased fatty acid (FA) synthesis in the fetal liver. Blood levels of fetal lipids (i.e., triglycerides, FAs, and ketone bodies) remain low before 32 weeks' gestation. In the last 2 months, the fetus increases its lipid storage as triglycerides in white and brown adipose tissue as well as in liver. During this period, both subcutaneous fat (i.e., white fat) and deep fat (i.e., white and brown) increase exponentially. The stored fat ensures adequate fuel stores for postnatal survival, and it also provides thermal insulation to the newborn. In addition, brown fat is important for thermogenesis in the postnatal period.

Several factors are responsible for increased lipid stores in the near-term fetus. Increases in fetal albumin facilitate FA transfer across the placenta. Insulin acts on fetal hepatocytes to stimulate lipogenesis. Insulin also promotes the availability of substrates, including glucose and lactate, which, in turn, increase the synthesis of fat (see Chapter 51).

DEVELOPMENT AND MATURATION OF THE CARDIOPULMONARY SYSTEM

Fetal lung development involves repetitive branching of both the bronchial tree and the pulmonary arterial tree

The fetal lung begins as an outpouching of the foregut at ~24 days' gestation. Several days later, this lung bud branches into two tubular structures, the precursors of the main bronchi. At 4 to 6 weeks' gestation, the bronchial tree begins to branch repetitively. The further maturation of the lungs occurs in four overlapping phases: (1) the pseudoglandular period, (2) the canalicular period, (3) the terminal sac period, and (4) the alveolar period.

During the **pseudoglandular period** (5 to 17 weeks), the lung "airways" resemble branching exocrine glands. The **canalicular period** is characterized by canalization of the airways (16 to 25 weeks) and is complete when ~17 generations of airways have formed, including the respiratory bronchioles. Each respiratory bronchiole gives rise to as many as six alveolar ducts, which give rise to the primitive alveoli during the second trimester. The branching of the pulmonary *arterial* tree parallels, both temporally and spatially, the branching of the *bronchial* tree. However, at ~24 weeks' gestation, considerable interstitial tissue separates the capillaries from the respiratory epithelium. Thus, if the fetus were born at this stage of its development, the premature infant would have a very low diffusing capacity (see Chapter 30), owing to the great distance between the edge of the alveolar lumen and the edge of the capillary lumen.

During the **terminal sac period** (24 weeks' gestation to birth), the respiratory epithelium thins greatly, and the capillaries push into the alveolar sacs. The potential for gas exchange improves after ~24 weeks' gestation, when capillaries proliferate and come into closer proximity to the thin type I alveolar pneumocytes (see Chapter 26). During this period, surfactant synthesis and storage begin (although not extensively) in the differentiated type II cells.

In the **alveolar period** of lung development (late fetal life to 8 years of age), final alveolar growth occurs. Alveolar-like structures are present at ~32 weeks' gestation, and at 34 to 36 weeks' gestation, 10% to 15% of the adult number of alveoli will be present. Alveolar number continues to increase until as late as 8 years of age.

An increase in cortisol, in conjunction with other hormones, triggers production of surfactant by type II alveolar pneumocytes in the third trimester

Hormones play a major role in controlling fetal lung growth and development in preparation for ex utero function. A key target is surfactant (see Chapter 27), which increases lung compliance. Numerous hormones stimulate surfactant biosynthesis, including glucocorticoids, thyroid hormones, thyrotropin-releasing hormone, and prolactin, as well as growth factors such as EGF. Glucocorticoids in particular play an essential role in stimulating fetal lung maturation by increasing the number of both type II alveolar pneumocytes and lamellar bodies (see Chapter 27) within these cells. Glucocorticoid receptors are probably present in lung tissue at midterm. Fetal cortisol levels rise steadily during the third trimester and surge just before birth. Two thirds of this cortisol is of fetal origin; the rest crosses the placenta from the mother.

The predominant phospholipid in surfactant is **dipalmitoylphosphatidylcholine (DPPC)**. Glycogen serves as a primary energy and carbon source for the FAs involved in phospholipid synthesis (Fig. 57-1). The FAs used in the synthesis of surfactant enter the type II cells directly from the bloodstream. The condensation of diacylglycerol with cyto-

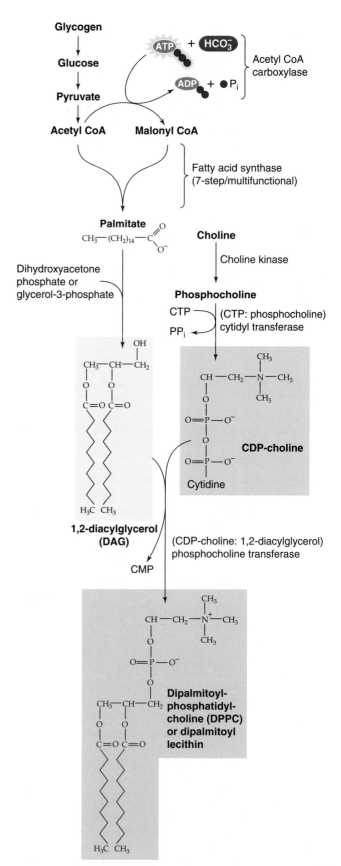

Figure 57-1 Synthesis of DPPC. Before birth, cortisol upregulates several enzymes that are important for the synthesis of surfactant, including FA synthase and phosphocholine transferase. CoA, coenzyme A.

Respiratory Distress Syndrome

Respiratory distress syndrome (RDS) affects 10% to 15% of infants born prematurely. In very immature infants, delivered before 30 weeks of gestation, cyanosis, tachypnea, nasal flaring, intercostal and subcostal retractions, the use of accessory musculature, and grunting may be immediately apparent in the delivery room. In more mature preterm infants, these symptoms may evolve over several hours. A chest radiograph reveals atelectasis with air bronchograms (i.e., air-filled bronchi standing out against the white background of collapsed lung tissue). Infants with severe RDS may develop edema and respiratory failure that requires mechanical ventilation. Uncomplicated cases usually resolve spontaneously. Because RDS occurs in premature infants, the course is often confounded by the coexistence of a patent ductus arteriosus. This combination of problems raises the risk for short- and long-term complications, such as alveolar rupture with pneumothorax and pulmonary interstitial emphysema, necrotizing enterocolitis, intraventricular hemorrhage, and bronchopulmonary dysplasia.

RDS is caused by a deficiency of pulmonary surfactant. Although prematurity is by far the single most important risk factor for developing RDS, others include male sex, cesarean section, perinatal asphyxia, second twin pregnancy, and maternal diabetes. Surfactant insufficiency can result from abnormalities of surfactant synthesis, secretion, or reutilization. Decreased lung compliance and atelectasis result from both structural immaturity and surfactant deficiency, thus promoting airway collapse. The consequent right-to-left shunting of blood past poorly ventilated alveoli results in hypoxemia, which—at the level of the alveoli—causes capillary damage and leakage of plasma proteins into the alveolar space. These proteins may inactivate surfactant, thus exacerbating the underlying condition.

The discovery that a deficiency of surfactant is the underlying problem in infants with RDS led investigators to look for ways of assessing fetal lung maturity and adequacy of surfactant production before delivery, so elective induction or cesarean section could be timed successfully in infants who need to be delivered prematurely. Clinical tests for assessing lung maturity exploit the knowledge that the major surfactant lipids are phosphatidyl cholines (i.e., lecithins) and that phosphatidylglycerol (PG) is also overrepresented (see Chapter 27). A ratio of lecithin to sphingomyelin (L/S ratio) greater than 2.0 in the amniotic fluid is consistent with mature lungs, as is a positive PG assay. The 2000 National Institutes of Health Antenatal Steroid Consensus Conferences recommended antenatal steroid therapy for pregnant women with fetuses between 24 and 34 weeks' gestational ages who are at risk of preterm delivery within 7 days. This treatment accelerates lung maturation and surfactant production.

In the newborn who develops signs of RDS soon after birth, surfactant is instilled into the trachea, preferably within the first hour after delivery. The administration of antenatal steroids and postnatal surfactant has markedly reduced the mortality from RDS and has improved the clinical course described earlier.

sine diphosphate choline ultimately leads to the production of DPPC. At ~32 weeks' gestation, increases in cortisol and in the other hormones mentioned previously stimulate several regulatory enzymes, including **FA synthase** and **phosphocholine transferase**. Thus, the net effect is vastly increased production of pulmonary surfactant late in gestation. Coincident with increased surfactant synthesis are large increases in lung distensibility and stability on inflation.

Fetal respiratory movements begin near the end of the first trimester but wane just before birth

Fetal breathing movements have been confirmed in humans by both Doppler ultrasound and tocodynamometer (an external device that records uterine movements) studies, commencing near the end of the first trimester. It appears that hypoxia and tactile stimulation of the fetus promote these breathing movements, which occupy less than half of any 24-hour period. Near term, breathing movements are regular, similar to those found after birth. However, just before labor, fetal breathing decreases.

The fetal lung undergoes many changes in preparation for birth. In utero, the alveoli and airways of the fetal lung are filled with a volume of fluid approximating the functional residual capacity (see Chapter 27) of the neonatal lung. The onset of labor is accompanied by increases in catecholamines and arginine vasopressin, which decrease fluid production by the fetal lung and initiate its active reabsorption. The pulmonary circulation absorbs the majority of the fluid, and the pulmonary lymphatics absorb some as well. A small portion of the lung fluid is forced out of the trachea as the fetus passes through the birth canal.

The fetal circulation has four unique shunts: the placenta, the ductus venosus, the foramen ovale, and the ductus arteriosus

The circulatory system differentiates from the mesoderm of the embryo. The fetal heart begins to beat in the fourth week of gestation. The major difference between the circulatory system of the fetus and that of the adult is the presence of the placenta. The placenta performs for the fetus functions that—at least in part—are performed by four organ systems in extrauterine life: (1) the lungs (gas exchange), (2) the gastrointestinal tract (nutrition), (3) the liver (nutrition, waste removal), and (4) the kidneys (fluid and electrolyte balance, waste removal). Thus, the fetal heart pumps large quantities of blood through the placenta and smaller amounts of blood through the other four organ systems. The key principle governing the unique pattern of blood flow in the fetus is the presence of four **shunts**, that is, pathways that allow blood to bypass the future postnatal route.

These shunts are illustrated in Figure 57-2. Because, to a large extent, the right and left sides of the fetal heart pump in *parallel* rather than in *series*, and because the inputs and outputs of these two sides mix, we define the **combined cardiac output (CCO)** as the sum of the outputs of the right and left ventricles. Figure 57-2A shows the fraction of the CCO that flows through the fetal circulatory system at important checkpoints. Figure 57-2B shows values for P_{O_2}

Fetal Asphyxia

Any insult that interferes with the ability of the placenta to exchange O_2 and CO_2 between the maternal and fetal circulations may lead to *fetal asphyxia*. Common causes include **maternal hypotension**, **abruptio placentae** (i.e., breaking away of a portion of the placenta from the uterine wall), and a **prolapsed umbilical cord** (i.e., the umbilical cord falls into the birth canal in front of the head or other part of the fetus). The results are low fetal P_{O_2}, high P_{CO_2}, and acidosis. These effects can decrease myocardial function, lead to lowering of CO and further compromise of O_2 delivery to the tissues, and thereby create a vicious cycle.

In the brain, asphyxia produces substantial alterations in cerebral intracellular metabolism. As the brain is forced to shift from aerobic to anaerobic metabolism, high-energy phosphate compounds (e.g., ATP) decrease in concentration, and their breakdown products (e.g., ADP and inorganic phosphate) increase. Lactic acid accumulates. Changes in P_{O_2}, P_{CO_2}, pH, and metabolism can profoundly affect neurotransmitter release and re-uptake and hence concentrations of various ions in neurons, glia, and brain extracellular fluid (see Chapter 11). Asphyxia also may lead to accumulation of prostaglandins and leukotrienes, vasoactive compounds that can dilate microvessels in critical areas of the brain, thus permitting the generation of free radicals that, in turn, lead to cell damage.

Fetuses experiencing chronic O_2 deficiency in utero are at increased risk of delayed breathing immediately after birth, in part because their energy reserves are already low. Therefore, fetal hypoxia can lead to neonatal hypoxia. The metabolic derangements of asphyxia remain evident for as long as 24 hours after birth.

and the percentage of saturation of HbF at these same checkpoints. The numeric values in Figure 57-2 are reasonable values for a healthy fetus.

Placenta The first of these shunts is the placenta itself. Of the CCO late in gestation, ~69% reaches the thoracic aorta (Fig. 57-2A). Half of the CCO enters the placenta as deoxygenated blood through the *paired* umbilical arteries, which arise from the two common iliac arteries. This massive blood flow to the placenta not only shunts blood away from the lower trunk, but also lowers effective blood flow to all abdominal viscera, including the kidneys. The umbilical arteries branch repeatedly under the amnion and ultimately form dense capillary networks within the terminal villi (see Chapter 56). The *single* umbilical vein returns oxygenated blood (which has a P_{O_2} of 30 to 35 mm Hg) back to the fetus from the placenta. This blood enters the ductus venosus, which then merges with the inferior vena cava.

Ductus Venosus This second shunt bypasses the liver, which is largely nonfunctional. The ductus venosus allows blood from the umbilical vein, ~50% of CCO, to enter the inferior vena cava directly, without ever entering the liver. In addition, some blood from the portal circulation may enter the ductus venosus. Blood from the ductus venosus then combines with blood from the inferior vena cava, ~19% of CCO, which drains the lower body and liver. Thus, ~69% of the CCO ($P_{O_2} \cong 27$ mm Hg) enters the right atrium.

Foramen Ovale The third major shunt is blood entering the right atrium and then crossing the foramen ovale to enter the *left* atrium. The foramen ovale is an oval hole in the septum dividing the atria, located in the posterior aspect of the right atrium. Of the 69% of the CCO that enters the right atrium through the inferior vena cava, ~27% shunts through the foramen ovale directly into the left atrium. This movement represents a **right-to-left shunt**. Therefore, the left side of the heart receives relatively well oxygenated blood ($P_{O_2} \cong 27$ mm Hg) from the inferior vena cava. In addition, the left atrium receives 7% of the CCO as poorly oxygenated blood ($P_{O_2} \cong 20$ mm Hg) from the nonfunctional lungs. Thus, the left ventricle pumps a total of 27% + 7% = 34% of the CCO ($P_{O_2} \cong 25$ mm Hg). Because this blood enters the aorta upstream from the ductus arteriosus, it primarily flows to the head and forelimbs.

Returning now to the *right* atrium, 69% − 27% = 42% of the CCO entering the right atrium from the inferior vena cava does not shunt through the foramen ovale. This relatively well-oxygenated blood ($P_{O_2} \cong 27$ mm Hg) joins the relatively poorly oxygenated 21% of the CCO ($P_{O_2} \cong 17$ mm Hg) that enters the right atrium from the superior vena cava and another 3% from the coronary vessels—a total of 24% of CCO. Because of the valve-like nature of the septum surrounding the foramen ovale, none of the incoming blood from the superior vena cava or coronary vessels shunts through the foramen ovale. Rather, it goes through the tricuspid valve to the right ventricle. Thus, the right ventricle receives 42% + 21% + 3% = 66% of the CCO (P_{O_2} = 18 to 22 mm Hg). The P_{O_2} in the fetal right ventricle is somewhat lower than that in the left ventricle. The blood from the right ventricle then enters the trunk of the pulmonary artery.

Ductus Arteriosus The fourth major shunt, also a right-to-left shunt, directs blood from the pulmonary artery to the aorta through the **ductus arteriosus**. The ductus arteriosus contains substantial smooth muscle in its vessel wall. The patency of this vessel is due to *active relaxation* of this smooth muscle, mediated by prostaglandins, particularly prostaglandin E_2 (PGE_2). Fetal PGE_2 levels are as much as 5-fold higher than adult levels are. Administering prostaglandin inhibitors to an experimental fetal animal causes the ductus arteriosus to vasoconstrict.

Although 66% of the CCO enters the pulmonary artery, only 7% of the CCO perfuses the unventilated fetal lungs, reflecting the high resistance of the pulmonary vasculature in the fetus. This high resistance is the result of hypoxic vasoconstriction and acidosis (see Chapter 31), the collapsed state of the airways, and perhaps leukotrienes (particularly leukotriene D_4 [LTD_4]). The rest of the blood entering the pulmonary artery, 66% − 7% = 59% of the CCO ($P_{O_2} \cong 22$ mm Hg), enters the descending aorta through the ductus arteriosus and mixes with the blood from the aortic arch, 10% of CCO, that did not perfuse the head and upper body ($P_{O_2} \cong 25$ mm Hg). Thus, the descending aorta receives 59%

A BLOOD FLOW EXPRESSED AS PERCENT
OF COMBINED CARDIAC OUTPUT

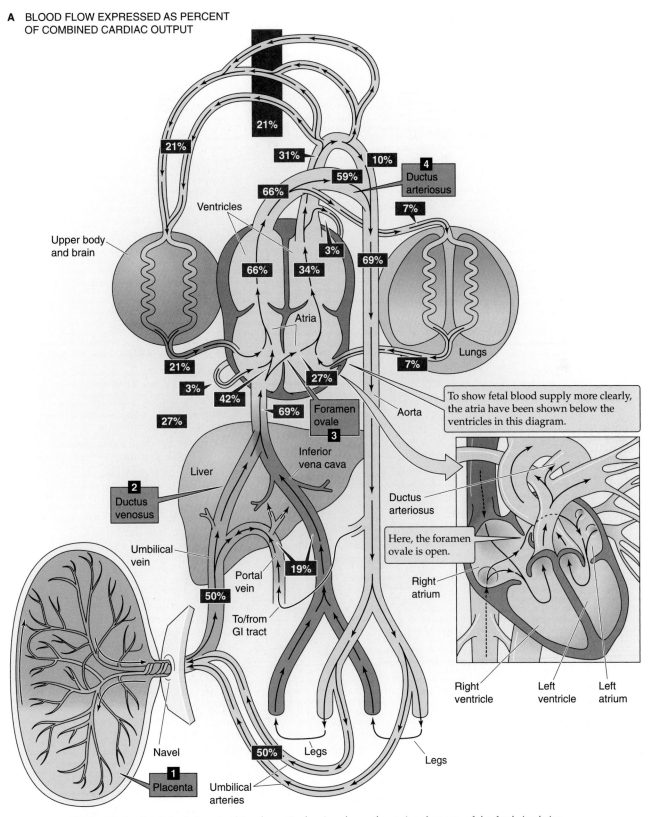

Figure 57-2 Fetal circulation. **A,** This schematic drawing shows the major elements of the fetal circulation. Note that—in the *main drawing*—the heart is upside down, for the sake of presenting the blood flow as simply as possible. The heart is right side up in the *inset*. Because the inputs and outputs of the right and left hearts mix, we define the CCO as the sum of the outputs of the right and left ventricles. The percentage of the CCO that passes various checkpoints is represented as a *number in a black box*. The CCOs of the right ventricle (66%) and the left ventricle (34%) add up to 100%. The fetal circulation has four major shunts: the placenta, the ductus venosus, the foramen ovale, and the ductus arteriosus.

Continued

B OXYGEN SATURATION / P$_{O_2}$

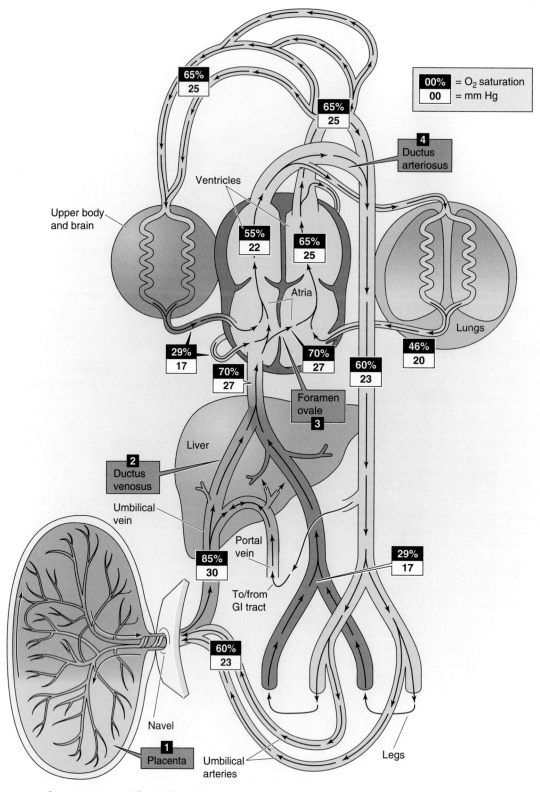

Figure 57-2, cont'd   B, The schematic drawing is the same as in **A,** except—at each checkpoint—we show the O$_2$ saturation of HbF against a *black background* and the P$_{O_2}$ (in mm Hg) against a *white background*. The relationship between the O$_2$ saturation and P$_{O_2}$ figures is based on the O$_2$ saturation curve for HbF (similar to the curve labeled Hb + CO$_2$ in Fig. 29-7).

+ 10% = 69% of the CCO ($P_{O_2} \cong 23$ mm Hg). The placenta receives blood with a P_{O_2} of 23 mm Hg, and returns blood to the fetus with a P_{O_2} of 30 to 35 mm Hg.

CARDIOPULMONARY ADJUSTMENTS AT BIRTH

As the newborn exits the birth canal, it takes its first breath, which not only expands the lungs, but also triggers a series of changes in the circulatory system. At the same time, the newborn loses its nutritional connection to the mother and apprehends a cold new world. Three major changes in metabolism accompany birth: *hypoxia*, *hypoglycemia*, and *hypothermia*. We discuss the adaptations of the respiratory and cardiovascular systems in this major section and adjustments of other organ systems in the next.

Loss of the placental circulation requires the newborn to breathe on its own

Although separation of the placenta does not occur until several minutes after birth, vasoconstriction in the umbilical *arteries* terminates the ability of the placenta to deliver oxygenated blood to the newborn immediately upon birth. Thus, even though the newborn may remain attached to its placenta during the first few moments of life, it is essential that the baby begins to breathe immediately. Umbilical vasoconstriction has two origins. First, stretching the umbilical arteries during delivery stimulates them to constrict. Second, the sudden rise in the systemic arterial P_{O_2} in the newborn also stimulates and maintains vasoconstriction in the umbilical arteries. Birth may also be associated with an "autotransfusion" as blood in the placental circulation preferentially moves into the body of the emerging baby. Because the umbilical *veins* do not constrict, as do the umbilical arteries, blood flows from placenta to newborn if the newborn is below the level of the placenta, and if the umbilical cord is not clamped. This autotransfusion may constitute 75 to 100 mL, which is a substantial fraction of the newborn's total blood volume of ~300 mL.

At birth, the newborn must transform its circulatory system from one that supports gas exchange in the placenta to one that supports O_2 and CO_2 exchange in the lungs. In addition, other circulatory adjustments must occur as the gastrointestinal tract, liver, and kidneys assume their normal roles. As the lungs become functional at birth, the pulmonary and systemic circulations shift from interconnected and *parallel* systems to separate entities that function in *series*.

Mild hypoxia and hypercapnia, as well as tactile stimuli and cold skin, trigger the first breath

The first breath is the defining event for the newborn. Not only does it inflate the lungs, but also—as discussed later—it triggers circulatory changes that convert the fetal pattern of blood flow to the adult pattern. The functional capabilities of the lungs depend on their surface area available for gas exchange, the ability of surfactant to maximize lung compli-

ance, neural mechanisms that control breathing, and the aforementioned circulatory changes.

The first breath is normally also the most difficult inspiration of a lifetime. A considerable negative pressure within the intrapleural space is necessary to overcome the effects of surface tension. The infant's first inspiratory effort requires a transpulmonary pressure (P_{TP})—the pressure difference between the intrapleural space and alveolar air spaces—of 60 cm H_2O to increase the lung volume by ~40 mL. In contrast, a typical adult only needs to change P_{TP} by ~2.5 cm H_2O during a typical tidal volume of 500 mL (see Chapter 27). The newborn's first ventilatory effort creates an air-water interface for the first time, opening the alveoli. Breathing becomes far easier once the alveoli are open and the type II alveolar pneumocytes deliver surfactant to the air-water interface. Thus, the second inspiration may require a P_{TP} of only 40 cm H_2O. The newborn may not achieve the adult level of relative lung compliance until 1 hour after birth. Very immature neonates, who lack adequate surfactant (see the box titled Respiratory Distress Syndrome), may have difficulty expanding the lungs.

The rapid onset of breathing immediately after delivery appears to be induced by a temporary state of **hypoxia** and **hypercapnia**. In most normal deliveries, these changes in P_{O_2} and P_{CO_2} result from the partial occlusion of the umbilical cord. Tactile stimulation and decreased skin temperature also promote the onset of breathing. When newborns do not begin to breathe immediately, hypercapnia and hypoxia increase and provide further simulation for the infant to breathe.

The peripheral and central chemoreceptors are responsible for sensing the blood gas parameters (i.e., low P_{O_2}, high P_{CO_2}, and low pH) characteristic of the asphyxia that accompanies birth. In addition, increased sympathetic tone may stimulate breathing at the time of birth by constricting vessels to the peripheral chemoreceptors, thereby lowering the local P_{O_2} in the microenvironment of the glomus cells and mimicking even more severe hypoxia (see Chapter 32). Finally, independent of the initial stimuli that trigger breathing, other central nervous system mechanisms may help to sustain breathing in the newborn.

The neonate's ability to control the blood gas parameters depends on the sensitivity of the lung's mechanical (i.e., stretch) reflexes, the sensitivity of the central and peripheral chemoreceptors, the gestational and postnatal age, the ability of the respiratory muscles to resist fatigue, and the effects of the sleep state.

Sleeping newborn infants, especially premature newborns, tend to have increased respiratory variability from breath to breath. For example, they exhibit **periodic breathing**, which consists of breaths with intermittent respiratory pauses (generally of a few to several seconds' duration) and varying tidal volumes. Periodic breathing and increased respiratory variability, including periodic breathing, occur more frequently in rapid eye movement sleep than during quiet sleep, a state characterized by regular breathing. In human adults and in adult experimental animals, periodic breathing may reflect an exaggerated ventilatory response to CO_2—which causes arterial P_{CO_2} to fall, thus lowering respiratory drive. However, the mechanisms underlying periodic breathing in the newborn may not be the same.

At birth, removal of the placental circulation increases systemic vascular resistance, whereas pulmonary expansion decreases pulmonary vascular resistance

As noted earlier, the fetal circulation has four unique shunts absent in the adult: the placental circulation, the ductus venosus, the foramen ovale, and the ductus arteriosus. At or around birth, these shunts disappear. In addition, the pulmonary circulation, which received only ~7% of the CCO in the fetus, now accepts the entire cardiac output (CO). In this and the next three sections, closure of each of these four shunts is discussed.

Closure of the Placental Circulation   In the fetus, the placental circulation receives ~50% of the CCO (Fig. 57-2A). Thus, the placental circulation represents a major parallel path in the systemic circulation and accounts for the low vascular resistance of the fetal systemic circulation. As the placental circulation disappears at birth, the total peripheral resistance doubles. Because blood flow through the descending aorta is essentially unchanged, aortic pressure must increase, thereby causing upstream pressure in the left ventricle to increase as well.

Opening of the Pulmonary Circulation   As noted earlier, during fetal life, pulmonary vascular resistance is high as the result of hypoxic vasoconstriction, acidosis, the collapsed state of the airways, and perhaps agents such as LTD₄ (see earlier). As a result, only ~7% of the CCO of the term fetus flows through the lungs, a figure corresponding to ~11% of the right ventricular output. At birth, expansion of the lungs by itself markedly decreases pulmonary vascular resistance, perhaps by triggering the release of prostaglandin I₂ (PGI₂ or prostacyclin). In addition, the increase in P_{O_2} and pH that occurs with breathing leads to pulmonary vasodilation. Together, these changes reduce pulmonary vascular resistance more than 5-fold (Fig. 57-3). Because the blood flow through the pulmonary vasculature increases by a slightly smaller factor, pressure in the pulmonary artery decreases. As a result, upstream pressure in the right ventricle also falls.

Closure of the ductus venosus within the first 3 hours of life forces portal blood to perfuse the liver

During fetal life, a large fraction of the blood in the portal vein bypasses the liver by entering the ductus venosus and merging with blood from the umbilical vein (Fig. 57-2A). Although blood flow through the umbilical vein ceases soon after birth, the majority of the portal blood continues to flow through the ductus venosus. Thus, immediately after birth, portal flow through the liver remains low. Within ~3 hours after term birth, however, constriction of the vascular smooth muscle within the ductus venosus completely occludes this shunt pathway. As a result, pressure in the portal vein increases markedly, thereby diverting blood into the liver. The mechanisms underlying the contraction of the muscular walls of the ductus venosus remain unknown.

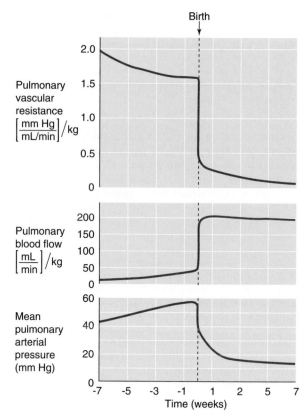

Figure 57-3   Effect of birth on pulmonary vascular resistance, blood flow, and mean arterial pressure. In the fetus, pulmonary vascular resistance is high, pulmonary blood flow is low, and mean pulmonary arterial pressure is high. At birth, each of these three situations rapidly reverses. The primary event is the fall in resistance, which occurs because of the following: (1) the pulmonary blood vessels are no longer being crushed; (2) breathing causes increased P_{O_2}, which, in turn, causes vasodilation; and (3) local prostaglandins cause vasodilation. The reason that pressure falls after birth is that the fall in pulmonary vascular resistance is greater than the rise in blood flow. *(Data from Rudolf AM: Congenital Diseases of the Heart: Clinical-Physiological Considerations. Armonk, NY: Futura, 2001.)*

At birth, left atrial pressure begins to exceed right atrial pressure, thus causing the foramen ovale to close

In the fetus, blood from the inferior vena cava moves preferentially from the right atrium across the **foramen ovale** into the left atrium (Fig. 57-2A). After entering the left ventricle, this well-oxygenated blood moves into the ascending aorta and primarily perfuses the head, neck, and coronary arteries. At birth, the decrease in the pulmonary vascular resistance increases blood flow through the lungs; the results are increased venous return to the left atrium and elevated **left atrial pressure**. At the same time, the venous return to the right atrium falls from 69% + 21% + 3% = 93% of the CCO of *both* ventricles in the fetus to 100% of the CO of a *single* ventricle at birth. Thus, **right atrial pressure** falls. The net effect is a reversal of the pressure gradient across the atrial septum, pushing the foramen ovale's "valve"—

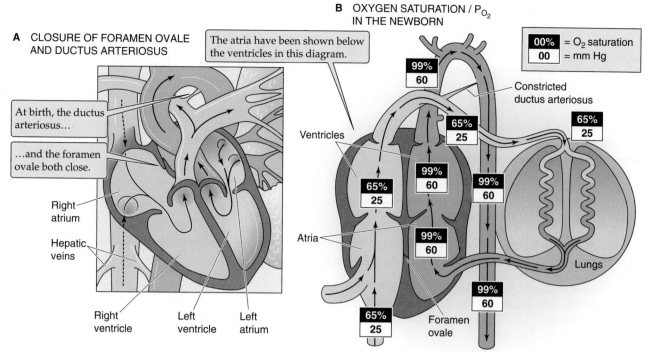

Figure 57-4 Changes in the circulation at and around birth. **A,** Closure of these two shunts establishes separate right and left circulatory systems. As the pressure in the left atrium rises higher than the pressure in the right atrium—owing to the large decrease in pulmonary vascular resistance—the flap of the foramen ovale pushes against the septum, thus preventing blood flow from the left to the right atrium. Eventually, this flap seals shut. As aortic pressure exceeds the pressure of the pulmonary artery, blood flow through the ductus arteriosus reverses. Well-oxygenated aortic blood now flows through the ductus arteriosus. This high P_{O_2} causes vasoconstriction, which functionally closes the ductus arteriosus within a few hours. Falling prostaglandin levels also contribute to the rapid closure. Eventually, the lumen of the ductus becomes anatomically obliterated. **B,** The elimination of the fetal shunts and the oxygenation of blood in the lungs lead to major increases in the O_2 saturation and P_{O_2} in the circulation.

situated on the "left" side of the septum—against the opening of the foramen ovale (Fig. 57-4A). Closing this valve usually prevents what would otherwise be movement of blood from the left to the right atrium of the newborn. The left side of the heart now receives blood only from the lungs.

Gradually, a *permanent seal* forms between the valve and the wall of the septum, a process that can take as little as a few months or as long as a few years. In some newborns, the valve does not completely seal to the septum, thus leaving a remnant potential pathway between the two atria. However, the 15% to 20% of adults with this condition do not have left-to-right shunting, because the valve of the foramen ovale is effective even if it is not completely sealed. However, if right atrial pressure should increase to more than left atrial pressure for some pathologic reason (e.g., pulmonary hypertension), then a right-to-left shunt between the atria would occur.

Closure of the ductus arteriosus completes the separation between the pulmonary and systemic circulations

During fetal life, blood flows from the pulmonary artery, through the ductus arteriosus, and into the aorta (Fig. 57-2A). Prostaglandins maintain the patency of the ductus

arteriosus during fetal life. Immediately after birth, the ductus arteriosus remains open. However, it now conducts blood in the direction *opposite* from that of the fetus: from the aorta to the pulmonary artery. This reversal of blood flow is the result of the increased systemic resistance (which elevates aortic pressure) and decreased pulmonary vascular resistance (which lowers pulmonary arterial pressure).

Obviously, the open ductus arteriosus during the first few hours of postnatal life constitutes an undesirable left-to-right shunt. Fortunately, within a few hours after term birth, the ductus arteriosus closes *functionally* because its muscular wall constricts (Fig. 57-4A). Usually, all blood flow through the ductus arteriosus ceases within 1 week after birth. Within a month or so, the lumen becomes obliterated *anatomically* because of thrombosis (i.e., blood clot within the lumen), proliferation of the vessel's intimal layer, and growth of fibrous tissue. Occasionally, the ductus arteriosus fails to close. The incidence of patent ductus arteriosus is one in several thousand.

The relatively rapid *functional* closure of the ductus arteriosus is primarily the result of the increased P_{O_2} of the blood perfusing this vessel immediately after birth. As the P_{O_2} of blood flowing through the ductus arteriosus rises from 18 to 22 mm Hg in utero to ~60 mm Hg a few hours after birth, the smooth muscle in the wall of the ductus arteriosus contracts. In newborns who are hypoxemic, the low P_{O_2} has three effects: (1) pulmonary vascular resistance and pressure remain high, (2) the ductus arteriosus remains patent, and (3) the patent ductus arteriosus maintains a right-to-left shunt. In these infants, raising the inspired P_{O_2} closes the ductus arteriosus. If these infants are allowed to breathe room air again too quickly, the ductus arteriosus will reopen.

Other factors, in addition to a high P_{O_2}, contribute to the rapid functional closure of the ductus arteriosus. Shortly after birth, circulating levels of *prostaglandins* fall quickly, thus relieving the ductus arteriosus of the vasodilating influence of these substances. Preterm infants tend to maintain high circulating prostaglandin levels, a feature that may account for their tendency to patent ductus arteriosus. Treating such infants with indomethacin (a nonsteroidal anti-inflammatory drug that inhibits cyclooxygenase and thereby reduces prostaglandin synthesis) (see Chapter 3 for the box on inhibition of cyclooxygenase isoforms by aspirin) induces closure of the ductus arteriosus, even at a low P_{O_2}. Norepinephrine, acetylcholine, and bradykinin also produce constrictor responses.

The closure of the ductus arteriosus completes the separation of the right and left circulations initiated with closure of the foramen ovale. Whereas the ventricles functioned in *parallel* in the fetus, now they function in *series* in the neonate. As a result, the O_2 saturation of the newborn's Hb is similar to the adult's (Fig. 57-4B). However, because the O_2 saturation curve of *HbF* is shifted relatively leftward (see Chapter 29), the newborn achieves these O_2 saturations at lower P_{O_2} values. In the neonate, the sum of the ventricular outputs of the two ventricles (i.e., twice the CO) is larger than the CCO in the fetus, a result primarily of a marked rise in the output of the left ventricle, which doubles its stroke volume. Compared with the adult, the newborn has a markedly lower systemic vascular resistance and thus can achieve a relatively high blood flow with a relatively low perfusion pressure.

NEONATAL PHYSIOLOGY

In humans, the **neonatal period** is defined as the first 4 weeks of life. The newborn's ability to survive during this period depends on the adequate development and maturation of various fetal organ systems, as well as on adaptations of these organ systems to extrauterine life. As the newborn loses the nutritional link with the placenta, the infant must now rely on his or her own gastrointestinal tract. Moreover, other functions normally carried out by the placenta are now entrusted to the liver and kidneys. Finally, on exiting its uterine "incubator," the newborn must stabilize his or her body temperature.

Although the newborn is prone to hypothermia, nonshivering thermogenesis in brown fat helps to keep the neonate warm

The body loses heat to the environment by radiation, conduction, convection, and evaporation (see Chapter 59). The relative importance of these processes depends on the cir-

cumstances. For instance, at birth, the infant moves from a warm and liquid environment to cool and dry surroundings. Hence, evaporation is the main source of heat loss immediately after delivery. However, even after the newborn's skin is dry, the infant is at risk for losing body heat by each of the previously discussed mechanisms. The major reasons are as follows: (1) the large skin surface area of the newborn relative to the small body mass (i.e., large surface-to-volume ratio), (2) the limited ability of the newborn to generate heat through muscle contraction (e.g., shivering thermogenesis), (3) the newborn's poor thermal insulation from the environment by adipose tissue, and (4) the inability of the newborn to adjust his or her own protection (e.g., put on warmer clothes) from the thermal stress of the environment or to modify that environment (e.g., turn up the thermostat). Premature and growth-retarded infants are at an even higher risk for heat loss and hypothermia.

Fortunately, the newborn has one important asset for fighting hypothermia: **nonshivering thermogenesis**, a process that occurs primarily in liver, brain, and brown fat (Fig. 57-5). Cold stress triggers an increase in the levels of epinephrine and TSH. **TSH** stimulates the release of the thyroid hormones, predominantly T_4 (see Chapter 49). Working in parallel, **epinephrine** activates, particularly in brown fat, the 5'/3'-monodeiodinase responsible for the peripheral conversion of circulating T_4 to the far more active triiodothyronine (T_3). T_3 acts locally in brown fat to uncouple mitochondrial oxidation from phosphorylation and thereby to increase heat production.

Brown fat differs from white fat in having a high density of mitochondria; the cytochromes in these mitochondria give the brown fat cells their color. Newborns have particularly high levels of brown fat in the neck and midline of the upper back. In brown fat, the locally generated T_3 upregulates a protein called uncoupling protein **UCP1**, originally called thermogenin. This protein is an H^+ channel located in the inner mitochondrial membrane. Normally, intracellular purine nucleotides (e.g., ATP, GDP) inhibit UCP1. However, epinephrine, acting through a cAMP pathway, activates the lipase that liberates FAs from triglycerides. These FAs relieve the inhibition of the H^+ channel and increase its conduction of protons. Consequently, the protons generated by electron transport enter the mitochondrion through UCP1, which dissipates the H^+ gradient needed by the H^+-translocating ATP synthase (see Chapter 5). Thus, the mitochondria in brown fat can produce heat without producing useful energy in the form of ATP. The oxidation of FAs in brown fat generates ~27 kcal/kg of body weight each day and contributes a large fraction of the neonate's high metabolic rate.

The neonate mobilizes glucose and fatty acids soon after delivery

Carbohydrate Metabolism
Elimination of the placental circulation at birth means that the newborn now has to forage for his or her own food. However, the newborn may not start suckling for ~6 hours. During late fetal life, glucocorticoids promote rapid accumulation of glycogen through their action on glycogen synthase. In its first few hours, the

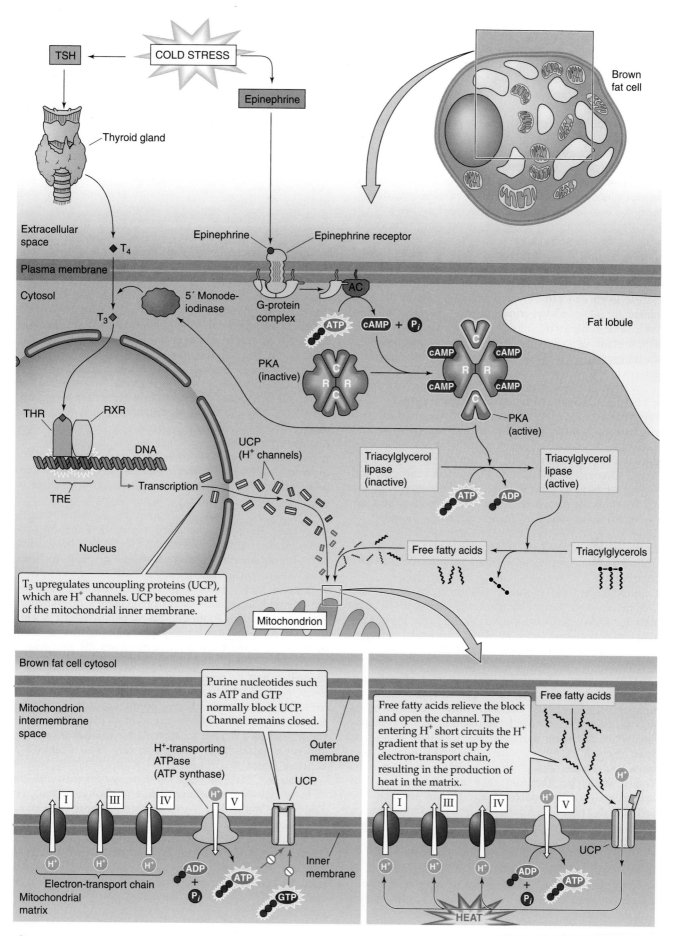

Figure 57-5 Nonshivering thermogenesis in brown fat. AC, adenylyl cyclase; RXR, retinoid X receptor; THR, thyroid hormone receptor; TRE, thyroid response element.

neonate uses glycogenolysis to mobilize hepatic glycogen stores, thereby releasing glucose into the bloodstream. The two enzymes needed for breaking down hepatic glycogen, phosphorylase, and glucose-6-phosphatase (G6Pase; see Chapter 58) are present in the fetus but do not become active until soon after birth.

The newborn depletes his or her hepatic glycogen stores in the first 12 hours of life. Stores of glycogen in cardiac muscle are 10 times those in the adult, and those in the skeletal muscle are 3 to 5 times those in the adult, but the fetus mainly uses the glycogen stored in these tissues to provide glucose for local use. The net effect is that, during the first day of life, blood glucose levels may decline to 40 to 50 mg/dL, although they soon rise to near adult values once nutrition becomes adequate.

Infants born of **diabetic mothers** run a very high risk of having pathologic hypoglycemia (i.e., <35 mg/dL). The high maternal blood glucose levels translate to high fetal blood glucose levels and cause hyperplasia of β cells in the fetal pancreatic islets and hyperinsulinism in the fetus. Insulin levels remain high after birth, thereby producing extreme symptomatic hypoglycemia. Blood glucose levels tend to reach their low point within a few hours after birth and begin to recover spontaneously within 6 hours.

Even in the physiologically normal newborn, low levels of blood glucose in the immediate postnatal period lead to a decrease in blood levels of **insulin** and a reciprocal increase of **glucagon** (see Chapter 51). This hormonal milieu promotes the net release of glucose by the liver. In the liver, glucagon acts through cAMP to stimulate glycogenolysis, inhibit glycogen synthesis, stimulate gluconeogenesis, and initiate synthesis of some gluconeogenic enzymes. All these actions promote formation of glucose for release into the bloodstream (see Fig. 51-12). In contrast to the adult, in whom phosphorylation is the main mechanism for regulating the enzymes involved in glycogen metabolism, in the fetus, the relative *concentration* of the enzymes may be more important.

Epinephrine also promotes glucose mobilization (see Chapter 3) in the immediate postnatal period, and it uses the same cAMP pathway as glucagon. Hypoxia, hypoglycemia, and hypothermia all stimulate the release of epinephrine from the adrenal medulla.

Fat Metabolism During the final 2 months of gestation, the fetus stores ~500 g of fat (i.e., ~15% of body weight), an important source of energy for the neonate. Decreased blood glucose just after birth raises levels of glucagon and epinephrine, which stimulate hormone-sensitive lipase in adipose tissue through cAMP (see Chapter 58). This lipase breaks down triglycerides into glycerol and FAs, which enter the bloodstream. The liver can take up glycerol and can ultimately synthesize glucose (i.e., gluconeogenesis). The liver can also take up FAs and can generate ketone bodies, which are important as the newborn deals with glycogen depletion.

Metabolic Rate The neonate's metabolic rate—expressed per kilogram of body weight—is much higher than that of the adult. Through the first year of life, the growing infant has a daily resting metabolic rate of ~55 kcal/kg, which is nearly double the value of ~30 kcal/kg for a healthy young adult. At birth, the growing infant has a daily caloric requirement of 100 to 120 kcal/kg, a requirement that falls to 90 to 100 kcal/kg by the end of the first year. The difference between the caloric requirement and resting metabolic rate represents physical activity and growth.

Breast milk from a mother with a balanced diet satisfies all the infant's nutritional requirements during the first several months of life

Provided the mother's diet is adequate during pregnancy, the newborn is in complete nutritional balance at birth. The newborn's natural nutrition for the first few days of life is **colostrum** (a milk-like substance secreted by the mammary glands), and thereafter it is **breast milk** (see Table 56-8 for compositions), both of which the newborn's gastrointestinal tract is prepared to digest. The American Academy of Pediatrics recommends breast-feeding until an infant is 1 year old. If the infant is breast-fed, and if the mother's nutritional status is good, colostrum and breast milk will meet all the newborn's nutritional needs. Moreover, colostrum and breast milk make important contributions to the newborn's immune status. Both contain high concentrations of immunoglobulin A (or secretory) antibodies directed against bacteria and viruses, and they also contain macrophages. Breast milk contains factors that promote the growth of lactobacilli, which colonize the colon and may protect the infant from some virulent strains of *Escherichia coli*.

If the mother's dietary intake of iron was adequate during pregnancy, the infant's hepatic stores of **iron** will be adequate for hematopoiesis for 6 to 9 months following delivery. Administering medicinal iron or providing iron-fortified milk can prevent iron-deficiency anemia.

The **calcium** in breast milk can meet the infant's needs for the rapid calcification of bones and teeth. However, fluoride for minimizing tooth decay must be provided as a supplement. Although the supply of calcium per se is unlikely to be a problem, **vitamin D** is necessary for the proper absorption of calcium by the intestines. Vitamin D supplementation may be necessary if the newborn or the mother is not exposed to sufficient sunlight to generate vitamin D in the skin (see Chapter 52). Supplementation may also be required in formula-fed infants and in infants born prematurely. **Rickets** (also see Chapter 52 for the box on rickets and osteomalacia) can develop rapidly in a vitamin D–deficient infant.

Vitamin C (ascorbic acid) is necessary for the synthesis of hydroxyproline in collagen and chondroitin sulfate (see Table 45-3) in cartilage, bone, and other connective tissues. The neonate is normally born with sufficient stores of vitamin C and receives adequate amounts of this vitamin in breast milk. If the breast milk or formula is vitamin C deficient, the infant may develop **scurvy**, which can be prevented with vitamin C supplements for the mother or infant.

Because of high rates of fluid turnover and acid production, the neonate is at special risk to develop fluid and acid-base imbalances

The newborn normally loses 6% to 10% of his or her body weight during the first week of life, a finding reflecting a decrease in interstitial and intravascular volume. After ~1 week, the rate of fluid intake begins to exceed that rate of loss, and term infants return close to birth weight by 1½ weeks.

The newborn's total body water is ~75% of body weight compared with 60% for men and 50% for women (see Table 5-1). Once the newborn is in a steady state, daily turnover of body water is 100 to 120 mL/kg, a rate that is 3- to 4-fold higher than in adults. Thus, even small changes in the balance between fluid intake and loss can lead to rapid and profound disturbances in body fluid compartments. The sick newborn can have a very difficult time maintaining fluid status and requires very careful management.

The immaturity of the neonate's **kidneys** further complicates matters. For example, the glomerular filtration rate (GFR; see Chapter 35) is extremely low at birth and increases rapidly during the first 2 weeks of life. However, even when normalized for body weight, the GFR does not reach adult levels until ~1 year of age. Moreover, the concentrating ability of the newborn kidney (i.e., a maximal urine osmolality of ~450 mOsm) is substantially less than that of an adult (~1200 mOsm).

Because of its relatively high metabolic rate, the neonate's CO and ventilation are also correspondingly higher than those of the adult. Metabolism generates fixed acids (see Chapter 39), and the newborn's relative acid load is also greater. The immature state of neonatal kidneys with respect to acid excretion puts the neonate at risk for developing metabolic acidosis (see Chapter 28).

Humoral and cellular immune responses begin at early stages of development in the fetus

Maternal **antibodies** play a key role in protecting the infant from infection both in utero and during the first several months after birth.

Fetus The placenta actively transports the small IgG immunoglobulins from mother to fetus, so that fetal IgG levels are even higher than those in the mother. These maternal IgG antibodies ward off infection by viruses and some bacteria. However, maternal IgA (which is primarily present in secretions), IgE, and IgM antibodies generally do not cross the placenta in appreciable amounts, and the baby is generally born with very low levels of these other immunoglobulins.

The fetus begins to develop its own immune capabilities at very early stages of development. However, because the fetus is isolated from antigens, the fetal immune system normally does not make large amounts of antibodies. Nevertheless, the fetus can respond to intrauterine infections by generating IgM antibodies. In addition, the fetus also begins to produce other proteins that help to protect against bacterial and viral infections. Among these are the following: (1)

the components of the **complement** pathway; (2) **lysozyme**, an enzyme found in secretions such as tears and mucus, which digests the cell walls of bacteria and fungi; and (3) **interferon γ**, which is produced by T lymphocytes and which activates B lymphocytes, macrophages, and endothelial cells.

Neonate In addition to high prenatal levels of maternal IgG, the newborn receives copious amounts of secretory IgA antibodies in colostrum and breast milk. However, the blood levels of *maternal* IgG antibodies progressively fall, and IgG levels in the infant's blood reach a nadir at ~3 months of age. After that time, the infant's own production of IgG antibodies causes total IgG levels to increase gradually. However, even at 1 year of age, IgG levels—as well as the levels of IgA, IgM, and IgE—are still only half of adult levels.

Antibodies obtained in utero from the mother protect against most childhood diseases, including **diphtheria**, **measles**, and **poliomyelitis**. The persistence of antibodies—at levels high enough for protection—varies considerably from one disease to another. For example, maternal measles antibodies are so persistent that vaccinations against measles often fail if they are attempted before 15 months of age. In contrast, maternal antibodies against **whooping cough** (pertussis) are generally inadequate to protect the infant beyond 1 to 2 months. The infant normally receives a first DTP immunization (diphtheria, tetanus, and pertussis), as well as a first poliomyelitis immunization, at 2 months of age.

The premature newborn has especially immature organ systems and homeostatic control mechanisms that exacerbate postnatal risks

According to the World Health Organization, a **premature infant** is defined as one born sooner than 37 weeks after the mother's last menstrual period, compared with the normal 40 weeks (see Chapter 50). For the premature infant whose birth weight is *appropriate for gestational age*, the only problem is that the uterus was unable to retain the fetus for the appropriate term for any of a variety of reasons (e.g., premature rupture of the membranes, incompetent cervix). The concept of **IUGR** (see the box titled Growth Restriction) describes a newborn who not only has a low birth weight, but also is *small for gestational age*. Virtually all the challenges to the health of the neonate are made more severe in prematurity or IUGR, conditions that are therefore associated with reduced chances of survival. These problems generally reflect immaturity either of certain organ systems (e.g., lungs, intestines, liver, kidneys) or of homeostatic mechanisms (e.g., thermoregulation).

REFERENCES

Books and Reviews
Ballard PL: Hormonal regulation of pulmonary surfactant. Endocr Rev 1989; 10:165-181.
Benirschke K: Normal embryologic development. In Moore TR, Reiter RC, Rebar RW, Baker VV (eds): Gynecology and

Obstetrics: A Longitudinal Approach, pp 37-53. New York: Churchill Livingstone, 1993.

Furon J-C, Skoll A: Fetal cardiovascular physiology and response to stress conditions. In Reece A, Hobbins J (eds): Medicine of the Fetus and Mother, pp 115-130. Philadelphia: WB Saunders, 1998.

Polin RA, Fox WW, Abman SH: Fetal and Neonatal Physiology, 3rd ed. Philadelphia: WB Saunders, 2004.

Strang LB: Fetal lung liquid: Secretion and reabsorption. Physiol Rev 1991; 71:991-1016.

Journal Articles

Avery ME, Mead J: Surface properties in relation to atelectasis and hyaline membrane disease. Am J Dis Child 1959; 97:517.

Gluck K, Kulovich M: Lecithin/sphingomyelin ratios in amniotic fluid in normal and abnormal pregnancy. Am J Obstet Gynecol 1973; 115-539.

Goldenberg RL, Cutter GR, Hoffman HJ, et al: Intrauterine growth retardation: Standards for diagnosis. Am J Obstet Gynecol 1989; 161:271-277.

Gross I: Regulation of fetal lung maturation. Am J Physiol 1990; 259:L337-L344.

Kari MA, Hallman M, Eronen M, et al: Prenatal dexamethasone treatment in conjunction with human surfactant therapy: A randomized placebo-controlled multicenter study. Pediatrics 1994; 94:730-736.

Wilkening RB, Meschia G: Fetal oxygen uptake, oxygenation, and acid-base balance as a function of uterine blood flow. Am J Physiol 1983; 244:H749-H755.

PHYSIOLOGY OF EVERYDAY LIFE

CHAPTER 58

METABOLISM

Gerald I. Shulman and Kitt Falk Petersen

The body's metabolism encompasses all the chemical processes involved in energy production, energy release, and growth. These processes can be **anabolic** (formation of substances) or **catabolic** (breakdown). Ultimately, all energy contained in ingested nutrients manifests as heat, work done on the environment, or growth. A healthy young man requires ~30 kcal/kg body weight to sustain resting metabolism for 1 day. Thus, a 70-kg human requires 2100 kcal/day, an amount known as the **resting metabolic rate (RMR)**. The number of calories rises with increased activity, illness, or other stress. For example, the metabolic rate can rise 2- to 3-fold with exposure to a cold environment or during the performance of heavy exercise. The **basal metabolic rate (BMR)** is a clinical definition for metabolism that is measured under standardized conditions in which the subject (1) has had a full night of restful sleep, (2) has been fasting for 12 hours, (3) is in a neutral thermal environment (see Chapter 59), (4) has been resting physically for 1 hour, and (5) is free of psychic and physical stimuli. The BMR (*units: kcal per hour and per square meter of body surface area*) in adults is ~5% higher for male than for female subjects and falls with age. The BMR is less than the RMR.

Regulation of energy metabolism in humans involves a complex interplay among ingested nutrients, hormones, and interorgan exchanges of substrates to maintain a constant and adequate supply of fuel for all organs of the body. Because energy acquisition by the body is intermittent, whereas energy expenditure is continuous, the body needs to store and then parcel out energy in a carefully coordinated fashion. Insulin (see Chapter 51) is the key hormone that orchestrates this exchange and distribution of substrates between tissues under fed and fasting conditions. Glucagon and catecholamines (see Chapter 51), cortisol (see Chapter 50), and growth hormone (see Chapter 48) play major roles in energy regulation at times of acute energy needs, which occur during exercise, in conditions of stress, or in response to hypoglycemia. The major organs involved in fuel homeostasis are as follows: (1) the liver, which is normally the only major producer of glucose; (2) the brain, which in the fed state or early in the fasted state is a near-obligate glucose consumer; and (3) the muscle and adipose tissue, which respond to insulin and store energy in the form of glycogen

and fat, respectively. The purpose of this chapter is to review how humans use energy and the means by which the body manages its energy stores during times of feeding, fasting, and exercise.

FORMS OF ENERGY

Virtually all energy that sustains human life is derived directly or indirectly from breaking of carbon-carbon bonds, which are created in plants during photosynthesis. Cellulose, the principal form of this stored energy in the biosphere, consists of polymers of glucose joined by β-1,4 linkages that we cannot digest (see Chapter 45). However, ruminants can degrade cellulose to glucose because they have cellulose-producing bacteria in their digestive tracts. Humans obtain their energy from food in three forms: (1) carbohydrates, (2) proteins, and (3) lipids. Moreover, each form consists of building blocks: monosaccharides (glucose, fructose, and galactose) for carbohydrates, amino acids for proteins, and fatty acids (FAs) for lipids.

Carbohydrates, which exist in the body mainly in the form of glucose, contain 4.1 kcal/g of energy. The major storage form is **glycogen,** a polymer of glucose (10^6 to 10^8 Da) that consists of glucose molecules linked together by α-1,4 linkages in the straight portions of the polymer (Fig. 58-1) and by α-1,6 linkages at the frequent branch points (see Fig. 45-3). Virtually all cells of the body store glycogen; the highest concentrations occur in liver and muscle. Cells store glycogen in cytoplasmic granules that also contain the enzymes needed for glycogen synthesis and degradation, Glycogen is highly hydrophilic; 1 to 2 g of water is stored with each gram of glycogen, thus providing a handy storage depot for glucose without affecting the osmotic pressure of the intracellular space. However, this packaging of glycogen with water makes glycogen a relatively inefficient means of storing energy because it yields only 1 to 2 kcal for each gram of *hydrated* glycogen instead of the theoretical 4.1 kcal/g of *dry* carbohydrate. In contrast to the other potential stored forms of energy (lipid and protein), the liver can quickly break down glycogen by glycogenolysis to provide glucose for the brain during hypoglycemia. Muscle can quickly break

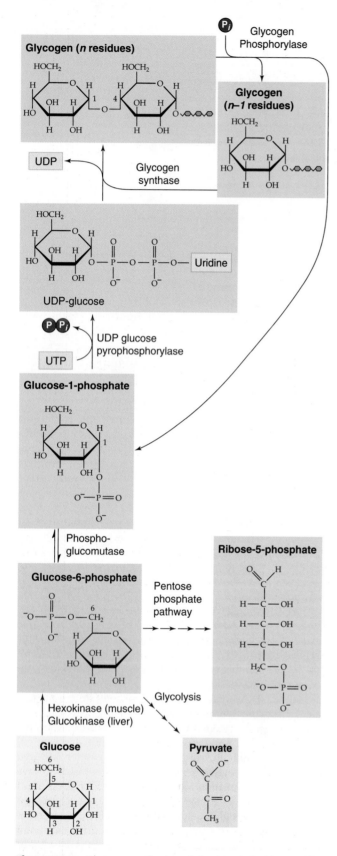

Table 58-1   Energy of Body Stores

Chemical	Weight (kg)	Energy Density (kcal/g)	Energy (kcal)
Glycogen	0.7 kg	4.1	2,870
Protein	9.8/2 = 4.9*	4.3	21,000
Lipid	14 kg	9.4	131,600

*Because only half of this protein can be mobilized as a fuel source, the total yield is only ~21,000 kcal.

down glycogen to glucose-6-phosphate (G6P) to provide the energy necessary to run a high-intensity anaerobic sprint.

The liver normally contains 75 to 100 g of glycogen but can store up to 120 g (8% of its weight) as glycogen. Muscle stores glycogen at much lower concentrations (1% to 2% of its weight). However, because of its larger mass, skeletal muscle has the largest store of glycogen in the body (300 to 400 g). A typical 70-kg human has up to ~700 g of glycogen (~1% of body weight). Thus, the total energy stored in the body in the form of glycogen can be nearly 3000 kcal (Table 58-1), which is still only a tiny fraction of that stored in the form of lipid, enough to supply resting metabolism for less than a day and a half, assuming 100% efficiency. Nonetheless, carbohydrate stores are essential because certain tissues, particularly the brain, rely heavily on carbohydrates for their fuel. Whereas muscle contains the largest store of glycogen in the body, this pool of glycogen cannot contribute directly to blood glucose in response to hypoglycemia because muscles lack G6Pase, which is necessary to convert G6P derived from glycogenolysis to glucose. Instead, the primary role of muscle glycogen is to supply energy locally for muscle contraction during intense exercise.

Proteins are linear polymers of L-amino acids (Fig. 58-2), which have the general molecular structure $^+H_3N—HC(R)—COO^-$. Different functional R groups distinguish the 20 amino acids incorporated into nascent proteins during mRNA translation. In addition, four other amino acids are present in mature proteins: γ-carboxyglutamic acid, hydroxylysine, 4-hydroxyproline, and 3-hydroxyproline. However, these amino acids result from post-translational modification of amino acids that are already in the polypeptide chain. In α-amino acids, the amino group ($—NH_3^+$), the carboxyl group ($—COO^-$), and R all attach to the central or α-carbon atom. In proteins, the amino acids are linked together by peptide bonds that join the α-amino group of one amino acid with the α-carboxyl group of another. Nine of the amino acids are termed **essential amino acids** (Table 58-2) because the body cannot synthesize them at rates sufficient to sustain growth and normal functions. Thus, we must obtain these amino acids in the diet. Proteins contain 4.3 kcal/g, which is approximately the same as carbohydrates. A typical 70-kg human with 14% protein (9.8 kg)— only about half of which is available as a fuel source—can thus store ~21,000 kcal (Table 58-1) in the form of available protein—which could potentially provide ~10 days' worth of energy. Unlike carbohydrate, protein is not a primary

Figure 58-1   Glycogen synthesis and glycogenolysis. After entering a liver or skeletal muscle cell, glucose is immediately phosphorylated to G6P, which can have three fates: glycolysis, breakdown through the pentose phosphate shunt, and glycogen synthesis. Glycogenolysis directly yields G1P and is thus not simply the reverse of glycogen synthesis.

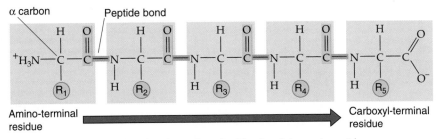

Figure 58-2   Structure of proteins. The chemistry of R determines the identity of the amino acid.

Table 58-2   Essential and Nonessential α-Amino Acids

Essential	Nonessential
Histidine	Alanine
Isoleucine	Arginine
Leucine	Asparagine
Lysine	Aspartate
Methionine	Cysteine
Phenylalanine	Glutamate
Threonine	Glutamine
Tryptophan	Glycine
Valine	Proline
	Serine
	Tyrosine

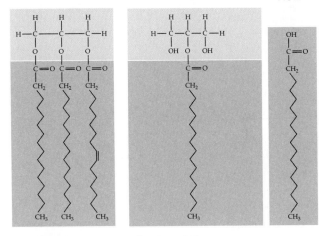

Figure 58-3   Structures of TAGs and FAs.

energy reserve in human. Instead, proteins serve other important structural and functional roles. Structural proteins make up skin, collagen, ligaments, and tendons. Functional proteins include enzymes that catalyze reactions, muscle filaments such as myosin and actin, and various hormones. The body constantly breaks down proteins to amino acids, and vice versa, thereby allowing cells to change their protein make-up as demands change. Thus, it is not surprising that protein catabolism makes only a small contribution—much less than 5%—to normal resting energy requirements. In contrast, during starvation, when carbohydrate reserves are exhausted, protein catabolism can contribute as much as 15% of the energy necessary to sustain the resting metabolic requirements by acting as major substrates for gluconeogenesis (see later).

In the healthy human adult who is eating a weight-maintaining diet, amino acids derived from ingested protein replenish those proteins that have been oxidized in normal daily protein turnover. Once these protein requirements have been met, the body first oxidizes excess protein to CO_2 and then converts the remainder to glycogen or **triacylglycerols (TAGs)**.

Lipids are the most concentrated form of energy storage because they represent, on average, 9.4 kcal/g. **Lipids** are dietary substances that are soluble in organic solvents but not in water and typically occur in the form of TAGs (Fig. 58-3A). The gastrointestinal (GI) tract breaks down ingested TAGs (see Chapter 45) into FAs and 2-monoacylglycerols (Fig. 58-3B). **FAs** are composed of long carbon chains (14 to 24) with a carboxyl terminus, and they can be either *saturated* with hydrogen atoms or *unsaturated* (i.e., double bonds may connect one or more pairs of carbon atoms). When fully saturated, FAs have the general form $CH_3—(CH_2)_n—COOH$ (Fig. 58-3C).

In contrast to glycogen and protein, fat is stored in a nonaqueous environment and therefore yields energy very close to its theoretical 9.4 kcal/g of TAGs. This greater efficiency of energy storage provided by fat is crucial for human existence in that it allows for greater mobility and promotes survival during famine. Therefore, although humans have two large storage depots of potential energy (protein and fat), fat serves as the major expendable fuel source. Most of the body's fat depots exist in the subcutaneous adipose tissue layers, although fat also exists to a small extent in muscle and in visceral (deeper) depots in obese individuals. A typical 70-kg human with 20% fat (14 kg) thus carries 131,600 kcal of energy stored in adipose tissue (Table 58-1). Assuming an RMR of 2100 kcal/day and 100% efficiency of converting the fat to energy, mobilization and subsequent oxidation of this

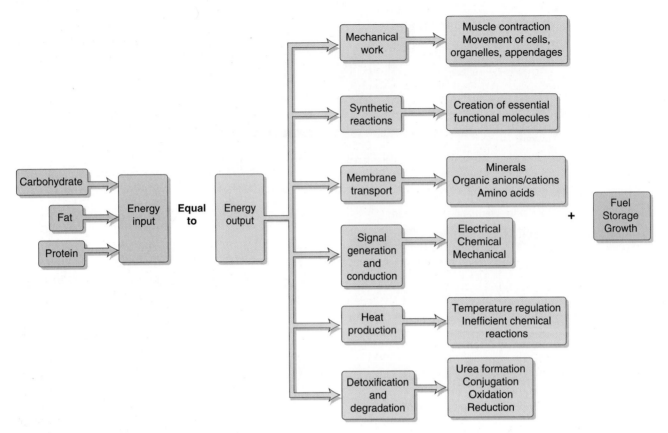

Figure 58-4 Energy balance.

entire depot could theoretically sustain the body's entire resting metabolic requirement for nearly 9 weeks.

ENERGY BALANCE

Energy input to the body is the sum of energy output and storage

The **first law of thermodynamics** states that energy can neither be created nor destroyed; in a closed system, total energy is constant. This concept is illustrated in Figure 58-4. Humans acquire all their energy from ingested food, store it in different forms, and expend it in different ways. In the steady state, energy intake must equal energy output.

The GI tract breaks down ingested carbohydrates, proteins, and fats into smaller components and then absorbs them into the bloodstream for transport to sites of metabolism (see Chapter 45). For example, the GI tract reduces ingested carbohydrates to simple sugars (e.g., glucose), which are then transported to muscle cells and are either oxidized to release energy or are converted to glycogen for storage. Oxidation of fuels generates not only free energy but also waste products and heat (thermal energy).

The body's energy *inputs* must balance the sum of its energy *outputs* and the energy *stored*. When the body takes in more energy than it expends, the person is in **positive energy balance** and gains weight; in the case of adults, this gain is mostly in the form of fat. Healthy children are in positive energy balance during growth periods. Conversely,

when energy intake is less than expenditure, this **negative energy balance** leads to weight loss, mostly from fat and, to a lesser extent, from protein in muscle.

A person can gain or lose weight by manipulating energy intake or output. An optimal strategy to encourage weight loss involves both increasing energy output and reducing energy intake. In most people, a substantial decrease in energy intake alone leads to inadequate nutrient intake, which can compromise bodily function.

Nitrogen balance—the algebraic sum of whole-body protein *degradation* and protein *synthesis*—is an indication of the *change* in whole-body protein stores. It is estimated from dietary protein intake and urinary nitrogen (i.e., urea) excretion. Children eating a balanced diet are in positive nitrogen balance because they store amino acids as protein in the process of growth. Patients who have suffered burns or trauma are usually in negative nitrogen balance because of the loss of lean (mostly muscle) body mass.

The inefficiency of chemical reactions leads to loss of the energy available for metabolic processes

The **second law of thermodynamics** states that chemical transformations always result in a loss of the energy available to drive metabolic processes (**Gibbs free energy, G**). The total internal energy (E) of the human body is the sum of the disposable or free energy (G) plus the unavailable or wasted energy, which ends up as heat (i.e., the product of absolute temperature, T, and entropy, S):

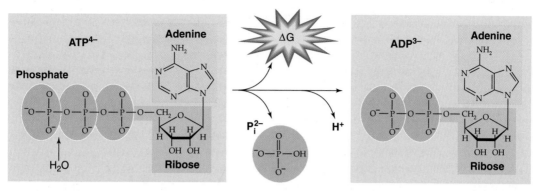

Figure 58-5 Hydrolysis of ATP to ADP, P_i, and H^+.

$$E = G + TS \qquad (58\text{-}1)$$

For example, when you ingest glucose, the total internal energy increases by a small amount (ΔE). Some of this energy will be stored as glycogen (ΔG), and some will be wasted as heat ($T \cdot \Delta S$). According to Equation 58-1, as long as the temperature is constant, the change in total internal energy will have two components:

$$\underset{\substack{\text{Energy of}\\\text{ingested glucose}}}{\underline{\Delta E}} = \underset{\substack{\text{Energy stored}\\\text{as glycogen}}}{\underline{\Delta G}} + \underset{\substack{\text{Energy wasted}\\\text{as heat}}}{\underline{T \cdot \Delta S}} \qquad (58\text{-}2)$$

Thus, some of the increased total energy (ΔE) will be stored as glycogen (ΔG). However, because of the inefficiencies of the chemical reactions that convert glucose to glycogen, some of the ΔE is wasted as heat ($T \cdot \Delta S$). Another way of stating the second law is that $T \cdot \Delta S$ can never be zero or negative, and chemical reactions can never be 100% efficient.

If we add *no energy* to the body (i.e., ΔE is zero), the body's total free energy must decline (i.e., ΔG is negative). This decline in G matches the rise in $T \cdot S$, reflecting inefficiencies inherent in chemical transformations. Consider, for example, what would happen if you took 1 mol of glucose (180 g), put it into a bomb calorimeter with O_2, and completely burned the glucose to CO_2 and H_2O. This combustion would yield 686 kcal in the form of heat but would conserve no usable energy. Now consider what happens if your body burned this same 1 mol of glucose. In contrast to the bomb calorimeter, your mitochondria would not only oxidize glucose to CO_2 and H_2O but also conserve part of the free energy in the form of ATP. Each of the many chemical conversion steps from glucose to CO_2 and H_2O makes available a small amount of the total energy contained in glucose. Converting 1 mol of ADP and P_i to 1 mol of ATP under the conditions prevailing in a cell consumes ~11.5 kcal/mol. Therefore, if a particular step in glucose oxidation releases *at least* 11.5 kcal/mol, it can be coupled to ATP synthesis. The conversion of the lower-energy ADP to the higher-energy ATP traps energy in the system, thus conserving it for later use. The cellular oxidation of 1 mol of glucose conserves ~400 kcal of the potential 686 kcal/mol; the remaining 286 kcal/mol are liberated as heat.

Free energy, conserved as high-energy bonds in ATP, provides the energy for cellular functions

ATP consists of a nitrogenous ring (adenine), a five-carbon sugar (ribose), and three phosphate groups (Fig. 58-5). The last two phosphates are connected to the rest of the molecule by high-energy bonds. The same is true for a related nucleotide, GTP. If we compare the free energies of phosphate bonds of various molecules, we see that the high-energy phosphate bonds of ATP lie toward the middle of the free-energy scale. Thus, in the presence of P_i, ADP can accept energy from compounds that are higher on the free-energy scale (e.g., phosphocreatine), whereas ATP can release energy in the formation of compounds that are lower on the free-energy scale (e.g., G6P). ATP can therefore *store* energy derived from energy-releasing reactions and *release* energy needed to drive other chemical reactions.

Examples of the chemical reactions fueled by converting ATP to ADP and P_i include the bridge formation between actin and myosin during muscle contraction and the pumping of Ca^{2+} against its concentration gradient during muscle relaxation.

ENERGY INTERCONVERSION FROM CYCLING BETWEEN SIX-CARBON AND THREE-CARBON MOLECULES

Some metabolic reactions are neither uniquely anabolic nor catabolic, but they serve to interconvert the carbon skeletons of the building blocks of the three major energy forms—carbohydrates, proteins and lipids. In this major section, we focus on two major pathways of interconversion: glycolysis and gluconeogenesis.

Glycolysis is the conversion of the six-carbon glucose molecule to two three-carbon pyruvate molecules

The breakdown of glucose to pyruvate (Fig. 58-6A) can occur in the presence of O_2 (aerobic glycolysis) or the absence of O_2 (anaerobic glycolysis). This process yields 47 kcal of free energy per mole of glucose. Of this energy, the cell can trap enough to yield directly 2 mol ATP per mole of glucose (Table 58-3), even under the relatively inefficient anaerobic

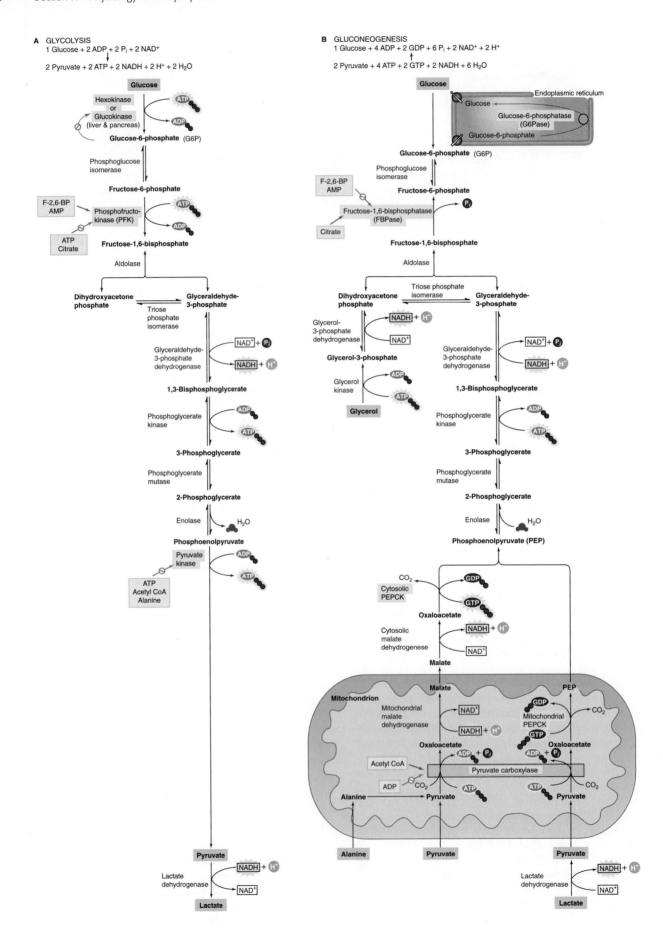

Figure 58-6 Glycolysis and gluconeogenesis. **A**, Highlighted are the three reactions in glycolysis that are essentially irreversible and the corresponding enzymes that are subject to allosteric regulation. **B**, Highlighted are the three gluconeogenic bypasses, which circumvent the three irreversible steps of glycolysis. The precursors for gluconeogenesis include amino acids (illustrated here for alanine), pyruvate, and lactate. The *green arrow* indicates stimulation.

Table 58-3 Generation of ATP from Glycolysis*

Reaction	ATP Change Per Glucose
Glucose → G6P	−1
Fructose-6-phosphate → fructose 1,6-bisphosphate	−1
2× (1,3-Bisphosphoglycerate) → 2× (3-phosphoglycerate)	+2
2× Phosphoenolpyruvate → 2× pyruvate	+2
	Net +2

*Under anaerobic conditions, glycolysis—which takes place in the cytosol—yields two lactate molecules plus two ATP molecules per glucose molecule. Under aerobic conditions, the metabolism of glucose does not proceed to lactate and thus yields a net gain of two NADH molecules per glucose molecule. The oxidative phosphorylation of each NADH molecule will yield 1.5 or 2.5 ATP molecules, depending on which shuttle system the cell uses to transfer the reducing equivalents from the cytosol into the mitochondria. Therefore, under aerobic conditions, glycolysis of one glucose molecule generates two ATP molecules directly plus three or five ATP molecules through the oxidative phosphorylation of the two NADH molecules, for a total of five or seven ATP molecules per glucose molecule. This yield is summarized in the first two rows of Table 58-4.

conditions. Under *aerobic* conditions, the mitochondria can generate an additional three or five ATP molecules per glucose from two reduced nicotinamide adenine dinucleotide (NADH) molecules. Cells that contain few mitochondria (e.g., fast-twitch muscle fibers; see Chapter 9) or no mitochondria (i.e., erythrocytes) rely exclusively on anaerobic glycolysis for energy.

About a century and a half ago, Pasteur recognized that glycolysis by yeast occurs faster in anaerobic conditions than in aerobic conditions. This **Pasteur effect** reflects the cell's attempt to maintain a constant [ATP]$_i$ by controlling the rate at which glycolysis breaks down glucose to generate ATP. The key is the **allosteric regulation** of enzymes that catalyze the three reactions in the glycolytic pathway that are essentially irreversible: **hexokinase** (or glucokinase in liver and pancreas), **phosphofructokinase (PFK)**, and **pyruvate kinase** (highlighted in Fig. 58-6A). In each case, either the direct reaction product (i.e., G6P in the case of hexokinase) or downstream metabolic products (e.g., ATP in the case of the other two) will inhibit the enzyme. If glycolysis should temporarily outstrip the cell's need for ATP, the buildup of products will slow glycolysis. Thus, introducing O_2 activates the citric acid cycle, which, as discussed later, raises [ATP]$_i$, inhibits PFK and pyruvate kinase, and slows glycolysis.

Under anaerobic conditions, cells convert pyruvate to lactate, accompanied by the accumulation of H⁺ (**lactic acidosis**). This acidosis, in turn, can impede muscle contraction by decreasing muscle cell pH, which can result in muscle cramps and inhibition of key glycolytic enzymes needed for ATP synthesis. Thus, sustained skeletal muscle activity depends on the aerobic metabolism of pyruvate as well as FAs.

Gluconeogenesis is the synthesis of the six-carbon glucose molecule from nonhexose precursors

Gluconeogenesis is essential for life because the brain and **anaerobic tissues**—formed elements of blood (erythrocytes, leukocytes), bone marrow, and the renal medulla—normally depend on glucose as the primary fuel source. The daily glucose requirement of the brain in an adult is ~120 g, which accounts for most of the required 180 g of glucose produced by the liver. The major site for gluconeogenesis is the liver; a much smaller amount of glucose is produced in the cortex of the kidney under most conditions. During prolonged fasting (2 to 3 months), the kidney can account for up to 40% of total glucose production.

Although glycolysis converts glucose to pyruvate (Fig. 58-6A) and gluconeogenesis converts pyruvate to glucose (Fig. 58-6B), gluconeogenesis is not simply glycolysis in reverse. The thermodynamic equilibrium of glycolysis lies strongly on the side of pyruvate formation (i.e., the ΔG is very negative). Thus, in contrast to glycolysis, gluconeogenesis requires energy, consuming four ATP, two GTP, and two NADH molecules for every glucose molecule formed. Most of the ΔG decrease in glycolysis occurs in the three essentially irreversible steps indicated by single arrows in Figure 58-6A. Gluconeogenesis bypasses these three irreversible, high-ΔG glycolytic reactions by using four enzymes: **pyruvate carboxylase, phosphoenolpyruvate carboxykinase (PEPCK), fructose-1,6-bisphosphatase (FBPase)** and **G6Pase** (Fig. 58-6B). The enzymes of gluconeogenesis and glycolysis are present in separate cellular compartments to minimize futile cycling of substrates between glycolysis and gluconeogenesis with the glycolytic enzymes residing in the cytosolic compartment, whereas the gluconeogenic enzymes are present in the mitochondria (pyruvate carboxylase) or in the lumen of the endoplasmic reticulum (G6P).

The liver accomplishes gluconeogenesis by taking up, and converting to glucose, several nonhexose precursors (Fig. 58-6B). These include two breakdown products of glycolysis (lactate and pyruvate), all the intermediates of the citric acid cycle, 18 of the 20 amino acids, and glycerol. Regardless of the precursor—except for glycerol—all pathways go through **oxaloacetate (OA)**. Thus, the liver can convert **lactate** to pyruvate and can then use **pyruvate carboxylase** to convert pyruvate to OA, thus consuming one ATP. Similarly, the citric acid cycle can convert all its intermediates to OA. Finally, the liver can deaminate all amino acids—except leucine and lysine—to form pyruvate, OA, or three other intermediates of the citric acid cycle (α-ketoglutarate, succinyl coenzyme A [CoA], or fumarate). The major gluconeogenic amino acids are **alanine** and **glutamine**. Leucine and lysine are not gluconeogenic because their deamination leads to acetyl CoA, which—as shown later—cannot generate net pyruvate or OA. Similarly FAs are not gluconeogenic because their breakdown products are almost exclusively acetyl CoA. In contrast, leucine and lysine are **ketogenic** because cells can convert acetyl CoA to FAs or ketone bodies.

Once the liver has converted the precursor to OA, the next step is the conversion of OA to phosphoenolpyruvate (PEP) by **PEPCK**, thus consuming one GTP molecule (Fig. 58-6B). The liver can convert PEP to FBP by using the glycolytic enzymes in reverse. The gluconeogenic precursor **glycerol** enters the pathway at dihydroxyacetone phosphate. **FBPase** converts FBP to fructose-6-phosphate, and **G6Pase** completes gluconeogenesis by converting G6P to glucose. The major gluconeogenic precursors are as follows: (1) lactate, which is derived from glycolysis in muscle and anaerobic tissues; (2) alanine, which is mostly derived from glycolysis and transamination of pyruvate in skeletal muscle; and (3) glycerol, which is derived from lipolysis in adipocytes.

Reciprocal regulation of glycolysis and gluconeogenesis minimizes futile cycling

We already noted that key glycolytic and gluconeogenic enzymes are located in separate compartments. The liver also reciprocally and coordinately *regulates* these processes so that when one pathway is active, the other pathway is relatively inactive. This regulation is important because both glycolysis and gluconeogenesis are highly exergonic and therefore no thermodynamic barrier prevents futile cycling of substrates between these two pathways. Because glycolysis creates two ATP molecules and gluconeogenesis consumes four ATP and two GTP molecules, a full cycle from one glucose to two pyruvates and back again would have a net cost of two ATP and two GTP molecules. Acutely, the liver regulates flux through these pathways mostly by allosteric regulation of enzyme activity and, chronically, by transcriptional regulation of gene expression.

Allosteric Regulation PFK (glycolysis) is stimulated by AMP, whereas it is inhibited by citrate and ATP (Fig. 58-6A). **FBPase** (gluconeogenesis) is inhibited by AMP and is activated by citrate (Fig. 58-6B). Fructose-2,6-bisphosphate, which is under the reciprocal control of glucagon and insulin, also reciprocally regulates these two enzymes, thus stimulating PFK and inhibiting FBPase. In the fed state, when glucagon is low and insulin is high (see Chapter 51), [fructose-2,6-bisphosphate] is high; this situation promotes consumption of glucose. Conversely, in the fasted state, [fructose-2,6-bisphosphate] is low, a condition promoting gluconeogenesis.

Similarly, the liver reciprocally regulates **pyruvate kinase** (glycolysis) and **pyruvate carboxylase/PEPCK** (gluconeogenesis). High concentrations of ATP and alanine inhibit pyruvate kinase, whereas ADP inhibits pyruvate carboxylase. Furthermore, acetyl CoA inhibits pyruvate kinase but activates pyruvate carboxylase. In this way, high concentrations of biosynthetic precursors and ATP favor gluconeogenesis and suppress glycolysis. Conversely, high concentrations of AMP, reflecting a low energy charge of the liver, suppress gluconeogenesis and favor glycolysis.

Transcriptional Regulation More chronic regulation of gluconeogenesis and glycolysis occurs by hormonal regulation of gene expression. The major hormones involved in this process are insulin, glucagon, epinephrine, and cortisol. In contrast to allosteric regulation, which occurs in seconds to minutes, transcriptional regulation occurs over hours to days. Insulin, which increases following a meal (see Chapter 51), stimulates the expression of the glycolytic enzymes **PFK** and pyruvate kinase, as well as the enzyme that makes fructose-2,6-bisphosphate. In addition, as noted in Figure 51-8, insulin suppresses the expression of the key gluconeogenic enzymes PEPCK, FBPase, and G6Pase. Insulin leads to the phosphorylation of the Foxo1 transcription factor, thus preventing Foxo1 from entering the nucleus and activating transcription of genes that encode these enzymes.

Conversely, glucagon, the levels of which increase during starvation, inhibits the expression of the glycolytic enzymes PFK and pyruvate kinase, as well as the enzyme that makes fructose-2,6-bisphosphate. Epinephrine and norepinephrine, released under conditions of stress, have actions similar to those of glucagon. At the same time, these hormones stimulate the expression of the gluconeogenic enzymes PEPCK and G6Pase through cAMP and protein kinase A (PKA). Phosphorylation of the transcriptional factor CREB then increases the production of the transcriptional cofactor **PGC-1α** (which then binds and activates the transcription factors HNF4 and Foxo1), which promotes the transcription of these key gluconeogenic enzymes.

Cells can convert glucose or amino acids into fatty acids

The body—principally the liver—can convert glucose to FAs. As shown in Figure 58-6A, glycolysis converts glucose to pyruvate, which can enter the mitochondrion through the **mitochondrial pyruvate carrier (MPC)** (Fig. 58-7). When ATP demand is low, high levels of ATP, acetyl CoA, and NADH inside the mitochondria inhibit pyruvate dehydrogenase, which converts pyruvate to acetyl CoA—the normal entry point into the citric acid cycle. Conversely, high levels of ATP and acetyl CoA stimulate pyruvate carboxylase, which instead converts pyruvate to OA, the last element in the citric acid cycle. The mitochondrion then converts the OA and acetyl CoA to citrate, which it exports to the cytosol through the exchanger ClC (SLC25A1). A cytosolic enzyme called **citrate lyase** converts the citrate back to OA and CoA. The hepatocyte converts the cytosolic OA to malate or pyruvate, each of which can re-enter the mitochondrion. Thus, the net effect is to make acetyl CoA disappear from the mitochondrion and appear in the cytosol for FA synthesis.

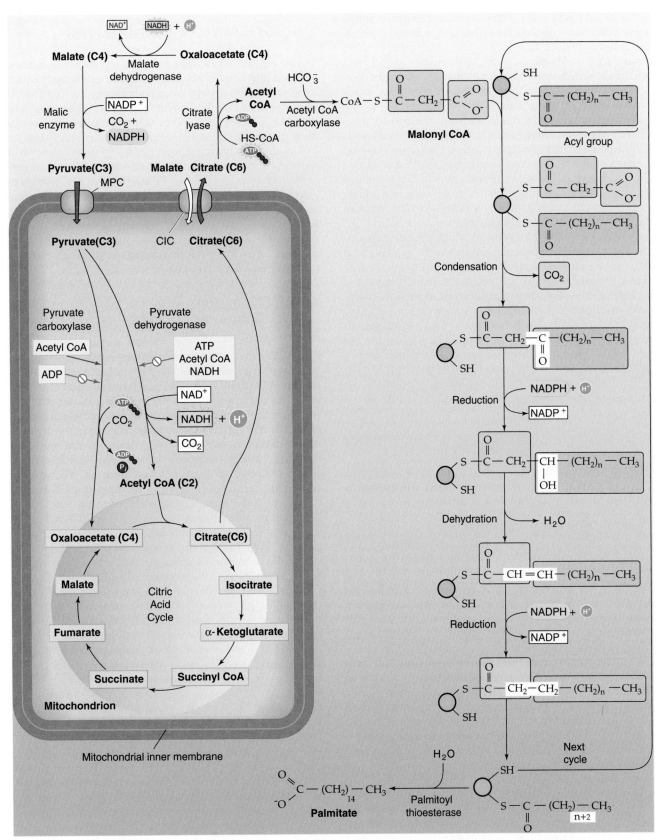

Figure 58-7 FA synthesis. The *left side* of the figure shows how the cell effectively transports acetyl CoA from the inside of the mitochondrion to the cytoplasm—exporting citrate and then taking up pyruvate. The key enzyme is citrate lyase. The *right side* of the figure shows how the cell generates FAs, two carbons at a time. Glucose can feed into the system through pyruvate. Amino acids can feed into the system through acetyl CoA (ketogenic amino acids), pyruvate, or intermediates of the citric acid cycle.

As noted earlier, the breakdown of ketogenic amino acids yields acetyl CoA. This acetyl CoA can also contribute to FA synthesis. In addition, the breakdown of other amino acids yields pyruvate or intermediates of the citric acid cycle, which again can contribute to FA synthesis.

The synthesis of FAs from acetyl CoA takes place in the cytosol, whereas, as discussed later, the oxidation of FAs to acetyl CoA occurs in the mitochondrion. The first committed step—and the rate-limiting step—in FA synthesis is the ATP-dependent carboxylation of acetyl CoA (two carbons) to form **malonyl CoA** (three carbons), catalyzed by **acetyl CoA carboxylase (ACC)**. The next step is the sequential addition of two-carbon units to a growing acyl chain, shown as $-CO-(CH_2)_n-CH_3$ in Figure 58-7, to produce an FA. With each round of elongation, a malonyl CoA molecule reacts with **FA synthase**, which then decarboxylates the malonyl moiety and condenses the growing acyl chain to the remaining two-carbon malonyl fragment. The subsequent reduction, dehydration, and reduction steps—all catalyzed by the same multifunctional peptide—complete one round of elongation. Starting from a priming acetyl group (which comes from acetyl CoA), seven rounds of addition—in addition to a hydrolysis step to remove the acyl chain from the enzyme—are required to produce palmitate:

$$\text{Acetyl CoA} + 7 \text{ malonyl CoA} + 14 \text{ NADPH} + 7H^+ \rightarrow$$
$$\text{Palmitate} + 7\,CO_2 + 14\,NADP^+ + 8\,CoA + 6\,H_2O$$

$$(58\text{-}3)$$

The cell esterifies the FAs to glycerol to make **TAGs**. The liver can package TAGs as **very-low-density lipoproteins (VLDLs)** for export to the blood.

The body permits only certain energy interconversions

The body has a hierarchy for energy interconversion. As discussed earlier, it can convert amino acids to glucose (gluconeogenesis) and fat. It can convert glucose to fat. In addition, the body can convert glucose to certain amino acids. However, the body cannot convert fat to either glucose or amino acids. Fats can only be stored or oxidized. The reason is that cells oxidize FAs two carbons at a time to acetyl CoA (a two-carbon molecule), which they cannot convert into pyruvate (a three-carbon molecule) or OA (a four-carbon molecule). The only exceptions are the uncommon FAs that have an odd number of carbon atoms, and even with these, only the terminal three-carbon unit escapes oxidation to acetyl CoA. Thus, almost all carbon atoms in FAs end up as acetyl CoA, which enters the citric acid cycle. There, isocitrate dehydrogenase and α-ketoglutarate dehydrogenase release the two carbon atoms of acetyl CoA as two CO_2 molecules, thus yielding no net production of OA or pyruvate. In contrast, plants have two additional enzymes (the glyoxylate cycle) that allow them to convert two molecules of acetyl CoA to OA and glucose.

ENERGY CAPTURE (ANABOLISM)

During feeding, when more energy is ingested than is being oxidized, the body stores excess calories as glycogen or fat. However, storing energy has a cost, although it is relatively inexpensive from a total energy standpoint. The process of digesting a mixed meal in the GI tract elevates the whole-body metabolic rate 20% to 25% higher than the RMR for ~90 minutes following a meal. In addition to this cost of digesting and absorbing, the energy cost of *storing* dietary carbohydrate as glycogen or dietary lipid as TAGs is 3% to 7% of the energy taken in. The cost of storing amino acids as protein is nearly 25% of the energy taken in. Moreover, storage after *interconversions* among dietary categories is particularly expensive. The cost of storing dietary carbohydrate as TAGs, or of storing amino acids as glycogen, is nearly 25% of the intake energy.

After a carbohydrate meal, the body burns some ingested glucose and stores the rest as glycogen or TAGs

Three mechanisms maintain normoglycemia following carbohydrate ingestion: (1) suppression of hepatic glucose production; (2) stimulation of hepatic glucose uptake; and (3) stimulation of glucose uptake by peripheral tissues, predominantly muscle. **Insulin** is the primary signal, which orchestrates the storage and metabolism of glucose through the insulin receptor (see Fig. 51-6). Glucose is the dominant signal for insulin secretion. However, with meals, other signals converge on the β cells of the pancreatic islets to coordinate insulin secretion, as becomes apparent when comparing the insulin responses in identical amounts of glucose loads given intravenously versus orally (see Fig. 51-3). Viewed differently, for similar plasma glucose levels, oral glucose raises insulin concentrations several-fold higher than does intravenous glucose. This differential insulin response results from the secretion of multiple incretins (see Chapter 51)—especially glucagon-like peptide (GLP-1) and GI peptide (GIP)—as well as from parasympathetic innervation of the pancreatic β cells. The incretins and neural signals prime the β cells and thus magnify insulin release following meal-induced increases in blood glucose. This priming is absent when blood glucose increases as a result of increased hepatic glycogenolysis in response to stress, thereby avoiding potentially detrimental hyperinsulinemia under these conditions.

Liver Following a carbohydrate meal, levels of insulin and glucose rise in the portal vein (similar to Fig. 51-3A), whereas glucagon levels fall. These changes suppress hepatic glucose production and promote net hepatic glucose uptake. Thus, the liver buffers the entry of glucose from the portal vein into the systemic circulation, thereby minimizing fluctuations in plasma [glucose] while promoting glucose storage. Once plasma [glucose] returns to baseline, the liver resumes net glucose production to maintain normoglycemia. Depending on the size of the carbohydrate load, the liver may take up one fourth to one third of the ingested exogenous glucose load. Because the liver not only decreases its *production* of glucose, but also takes up a significant amount of glucose, the contribution of the liver to postprandial glucose homeostasis is substantial and approaches that of muscle.

Glucose taken up by the liver during the meal is predominantly stored as **glycogen**. The liver synthesizes glycogen by both a **direct pathway** from exogenous glucose and an **indirect pathway** from gluconeogenesis (Fig. 58-8A). When we ingest a meal following an overnight fast, these pathways contribute roughly equally to hepatic glycogen synthesis. However, the relative contribution of these pathways depends on the composition of diet, the level of glycemia achieved during the meal, and the relative concentrations of insulin and glucagon. A high-carbohydrate diet, hyperglycemia, and insulin promote the direct pathway, whereas reduced carbohydrate intake, lower glucose levels, and elevations in circulating glucagon stimulate the indirect pathway.

Hepatic glycogen stores peak 4 to 6 hours following a meal. Thus, when we ingest three meals per day at 4- to 6-hour intervals, hepatic glycogen stores increase throughout the day in a staircase fashion, whereas most of the glucose required for metabolism comes from exogenous glucose (see Fig. 58-8A). Glycogen stores reach their peak around midnight, after which hepatic glycogenolysis contributes ~50% to whole-body glucose production, and the other 50% derives from hepatic gluconeogenesis.

Because the liver has citrate lyase, it can also convert glucose that it takes up following a meal to FAs (Fig. 58-8A). This process is illustrated in Figure 58-7. The hepatocyte esterifies these FAs to glycerol to make TAGs, which it packages as VLDLs for export to the blood.

Muscle Glucose escaping the splanchnic (liver and gut) circulation is cleared predominantly by striated muscle, which stores most of this glucose as glycogen (Fig. 58-8A). Muscle metabolizes the remaining glucose through the glycolytic pathway and then either oxidizes the products or recycles them to the liver, mostly as lactate and alanine.

The uptake of glucose into muscle—as well as adipose tissue—is regulated predominantly by a rise in insulin concentration and, to a lesser extent, by the hyperglycemia per se. Insulin, through the **phosphatidylinositol 3-kinase (PI3K)** pathway (see Chapter 51), promotes translocation of the **GLUT4** transporter to the plasma membrane and consequently stimulates glucose uptake by muscle and fat. In addition, insulin modulates the subsequent metabolism of glucose by increasing the activity of glycogen synthase, thereby promoting glucose storage, and by increasing the activity of pyruvate dehydrogenase, thereby increasing glucose oxidation as well.

Adipose Tissue Whereas adipose tissue typically represents a large component of the peripheral mass (10% to 15% of body weight in men, 25% to 30% in women), adipocytes metabolize only a minor fraction of ingested glucose (Fig. 58-8C). The reason is that, in contrast to the liver, human adipocytes have relatively little **citrate lyase** and can thus synthesize de novo relatively little FA from glucose. However,

adipocytes use glucose as the starting material for generating **glycerol-3-phosphate**, which is required for TAG synthesis, by using FAs that come from the liver (Fig. 58-8A). As we saw earlier, in times of caloric and carbohydrate excess, the liver (which has an abundance of citrate lyase) synthesizes FAs de novo from glucose and esterifies the FAs to generate TAGs, which it then exports in the form of VLDL particles (see Fig. 46-15). Endothelial **lipoprotein lipase (LPL)** hydrolyzes the TAGs in VLDLs to FAs. Subsequently, the FAs enter adipocytes, which re-esterify them to form TAGs for storage. These adipocytes are mostly in the subcutaneous and visceral tissues and, to a much smaller extent, around muscle.

The larger the meal, the greater is the rate of glucose uptake by liver, muscle, and adipose tissue—because of higher levels of circulating insulin and glucose. In contrast, the brain uses glucose, its major oxidative fuel, at a constant rate, despite these fluctuations in plasma glucose during feeding. GLUT1 facilitates glucose uptake across the blood-brain barrier, and GLUT3 mediates glucose uptake into neurons, independent of insulin.

After a protein meal, the body burns some ingested amino acids and incorporates the rest into proteins

Following a protein meal, the amino acids absorbed by the GI tract (see Chapter 45) have two major fates: they can be either oxidized to yield energy or incorporated into protein. The liver removes a large fraction of amino acids that enter portal blood following a meal, particularly the gluconeogenic amino acids (Fig. 58-8B). In contrast, the liver less avidly removes the branched-chain amino acids (leucine, isoleucine, and valine), which muscle predominantly captures. Indeed, branched-chain amino acids are critical for the immediate repletion of muscle protein because they have a unique capacity to promote net protein accumulation, predominantly by inhibiting protein breakdown and to some extent by stimulating protein synthesis.

Insulin plays a major role in orchestrating protein anabolism, mostly by suppressing protein degradation. Therefore, the combination of the hyperinsulinemia and hyperaminoacidemia that follows a protein meal not only blocks proteolysis but also stimulates protein synthesis, thus resulting in net protein accumulation. Because some amino acids (e.g., arginine, leucine) are weak insulin secretagogues (see Chapter 51), a protein meal stimulates insulin release even when the meal lacks carbohydrate. Under such conditions, glucagon plays a critical role to prevent potential hypoglycemia by maintaining hepatic glucose production in the presence of hyperinsulinemia. In a *mixed* meal, the presence of carbohydrates augments insulin secretion beyond the effect of protein alone and further enhances protein anabolism.

After a fatty meal, the body burns some ingested fatty acids and incorporates the rest into TAGs

Following a fat-containing meal (Fig. 58-8C), lipases in the duodenum hydrolyze the TAGs to FAs and glycerol, which enterocytes in the small intestine take up, re-esterified into

A CARBOHYDRATE MEAL

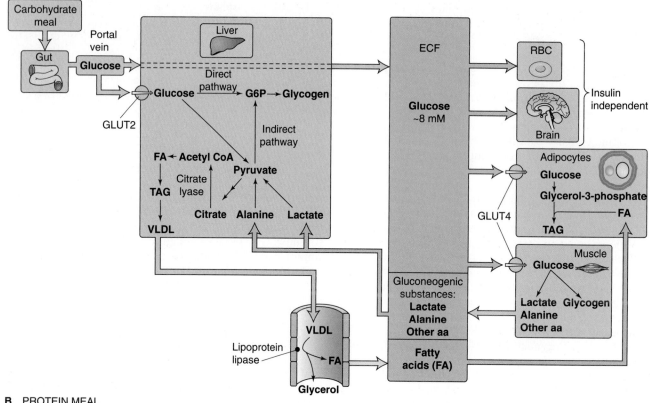

B PROTEIN MEAL

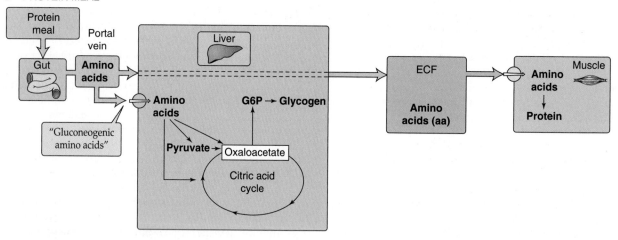

C FATTY MEAL

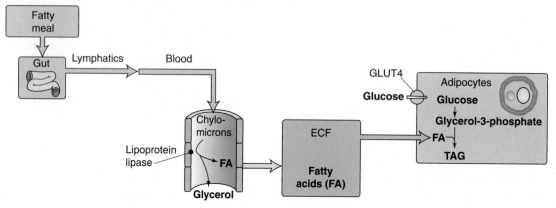

Figure 58-8   Energy storage following meals. In **A**, three major organs handle the glucose assimilated by the small intestine. Liver stores some glucose as glycogen and converts some to FA—packaged as VLDLs—for export to adipocytes. Muscle stores some glucose as glycogen and converts some to lactate and gluconeogenic amino acids for export to the liver. Adipocytes convert glucose to glycerol-3-phosphate, a precursor of TAGs. In **B**, two major organs handle the amino acids assimilated by the small intestine. Liver converts gluconeogenic amino acids to glycogen. Muscle converts amino acids to glycogen. In **C**, chylomicrons from the small intestine undergo hydrolysis in systemic blood vessels. Adipocytes re-esterify the resulting FAs (together with glycerol-3-phosphate generated from glucose) for storage as TAGs. aa, amino acids; ECF, extracellular fluid.

TAGs, and secrete as chylomicrons. The chylomicrons enter the lymphatics and then the systemic circulation.

Insulin, secreted in response to the carbohydrate or protein components of the meal, has three major effects on lipid metabolism (see Chapter 51). First, insulin stimulates **LPL**. LPL promotes hydrolysis of TAGs to FAs and glycerol. The breakdown products enter the adipocytes for re-esterification into TAGs. Insulin promotes storage in muscle and adipose tissue of both *exogenous* TAGs (derived from a meal and carried in chylomicrons) and *endogenous* TAGs (produced by the liver and carried in VLDLs).

Second, insulin stimulates glucose uptake into adipocytes by stimulating **GLUT4**. The adipocytes transform the glucose to glycerol-3-phosphate, which is the backbone required for the re-esterification of FAs into TAGs. Adipocytes lack glycerol kinase and therefore, unlike liver and kidney, are unable to phosphorylate glycerol directly.

Third, insulin inhibits **hormone-sensitive lipase (HSL)** within the fat cell. HSL—not to be confused with LPL—catalyzes the hydrolysis of *stored* TAGs in adipocytes. By suppressing lipolysis, insulin markedly decreases plasma FA concentrations and promotes net storage of absorbed fat into the adipocyte.

In a mixed meal—when glucose, amino acids, and FAs are all available—an increase in plasma [insulin] augments their net storage as glycogen, protein, and fat. This is accomplished by inhibiting glycogenolysis, proteolysis, and lipolysis as well as by promoting the opposite three processes. Because of the dose-response relationships, low levels of insulin preferentially inhibit the breakdown of energy stores, whereas high levels preferentially stimulate energy accumulation. Thus, small meals (associated with smaller insulin responses) mainly conserve depots by reducing breakdown, whereas larger meals (and concomitant greater insulin responses) increase depots by stimulating storage.

ENERGY LIBERATION (CATABOLISM)

The general principle in energy catabolism is that the body first breaks down a complex storage polymer (e.g., glycogen or TAGs) to simpler compounds (e.g., glucose, FAs, lactate) that the cells can then metabolize to provide energy, mostly in the form of ATP, for cellular function.

The first step in energy catabolism is to break down glycogen or TAGs to simpler compounds

Skeletal Muscle   Glycogenolysis in skeletal muscle is catalyzed by glycogen phosphorylase (GP; Fig. 58-9A). **Epinephrine** triggers glycogenolysis by binding to a β-adrenergic receptor, thus promoting the formation of cAMP (see Chapter 3). The cAMP activates PKA, which, in turn, phosphorylates phosphorylase kinase (PK). The now active form of PK then converts the inactive **GPb** to the active **GPa**. In skeletal muscle, a second way of activating GPb is for it to bind AMP allosterically; $[AMP]_i$ increases during muscle activity owing to increased turnover of ATP. Conversely, ATP competes with AMP for this nucleotide-binding site and thus inhibits GPb. Yet a third way of activating GPb is for Ca^{2+} to activate PK allosterically. Thus, during intense activity of skeletal muscle, the accompanying increase in $[Ca^{2+}]_i$ directly promotes muscle glycogenolysis. Skeletal muscle converts the glucose-1-phosphate (G1P) generated from glycogen breakdown to G6P, which, in turn, enters the glycolytic pathway within the muscle cell.

Liver   As is the case in muscle, phosphorylase converts glycogen to G1P in hepatocytes. The mechanism for determining the ratio of GPa to GPb is the same as in muscle, except in the liver, **glucagon** (and, to a lesser extent, epinephrine), which is secreted by the α cells of the pancreas into the portal vein, triggers the increase in $[cAMP]_i$ (Fig. 58-9B). In the presence of glucagon, the liver converts glycogen to G1P and then converts G1P, as in muscle, to G6P. However, unlike muscle, liver contains the enzyme G6Pase, which cleaves the phosphate from G6P, to yield glucose, which is free to enter the bloodstream. Thus, whereas glycogenolysis in skeletal muscle serves to meet *local* energy demands by releasing G6P, glycogenolysis in the liver serves to meet whole-body energy demands—mainly those of the central nervous system (CNS)—by releasing glucose to the *blood*.

Adipocytes   Adipocytes release stored TAGs by using HSL to hydrolyze TAGs to FAs and glycerol. Nearly all (95%) of the available energy of TAGs resides in the FA moieties. Two hormones can stimulate lipolysis: **epinephrine**, which the adrenal medulla secretes under conditions of low blood glucose or stress, and **growth hormone** (see Chapter 48). As in skeletal muscle and hepatocytes, epinephrine acts through

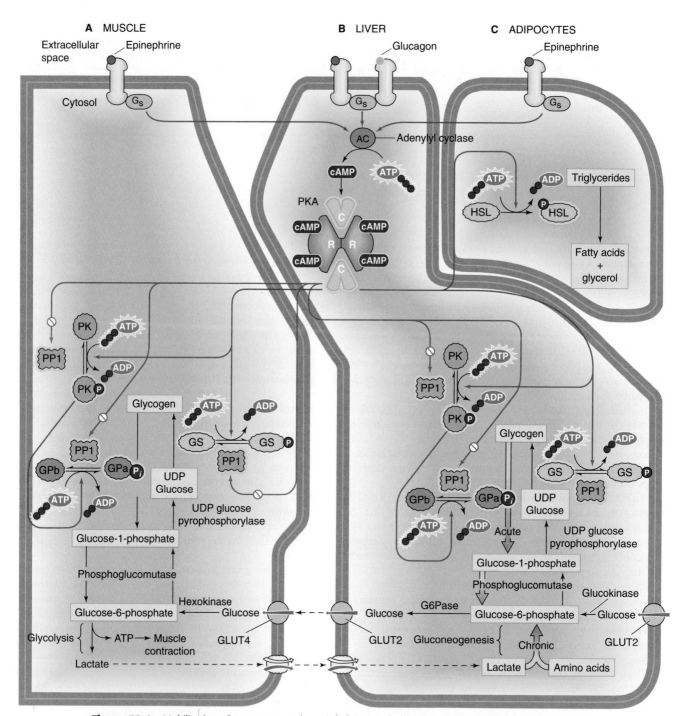

Figure 58-9 Mobilization of energy stores by epinephrine and glucagon. **A**, In muscle, epinephrine promotes glycogenolysis and glycolysis, thereby producing ATP (for muscle contraction) and lactate. See Figure 3-7 for a discussion of how PKA inactivates phosphoprotein phosphatase 1 (PP1). **B**, In liver, primarily glucagon and also epinephrine trigger glucose production acutely through glycogenolysis and chronically through gluconeogenesis. Because they have G6Pase, hepatocytes can generate glucose and can export it to the blood. **C**, In adipocytes, epinephrine triggers production of FAs and glycerol, which leave the adipocytes and enter the blood. GLUT2 and GLUT4, glucose transporters; G6Pase, glucose-6-phosphatase; GPa, active form of glycogen phosphorylase; GPb, inactive form of glycogen phosphorylase; GS, glycogen synthase; HSL, hormone-sensitive lipase; PK, phosphorylase kinase; PKA, protein kinase A; PP1, phosphoprotein phosphatase. Yellow halos indicate the active forms of enzymes.

cAMP (Fig. 58-9C). The result is activation of HSL, which hydrolyzes the ester linkages of TAG molecules, thus releasing FAs, which diffuse out of the adipocytes into the bloodstream. There, the poorly soluble FAs bind to circulating **albumin**, which releases them at the sites of energy demand.

The second step in TAG catabolism is β oxidation of fatty acids

In carbohydrate catabolism, after the breakdown of glycogen, the second step is glycolysis. In TAG metabolism, after the breakdown to FAs, the second step is the β oxidation of FAs in the mitochondrial matrix. (FA synthesis takes place in the cytoplasm). Before β oxidation, however, the hepatocyte uses an **FA transport protein** (**FATP**, member of SLC27 family) to transport the FA into the cytosol (Fig. 58-10), where **acyl CoA synthase** activates the FA to **acyl CoA** (i.e., the FA chain coupled to CoA). To deliver acyl CoA to the mitochondrial matrix, the cell uses **carnitine acyl transferase I** (**CAT I**) on the cytosolic side of the mitochondrial outer membrane to transfer the acyl group to carnitine. The resulting acyl carnitine moves through a **porin** in the mitochondrial outer membrane to enter the intermembrane space. The **carnitine/acyl carnitine transporter** (**CAC**, SLC25A20) on the mitochondrial inner membrane moves acyl carnitine into the mitochondrial matrix. There, CAT II transfers the acyl group back to CoA, to form acyl CoA and carnitine. The carnitine recycles to the cytosol through CAC and the porin, whereas acyl CoA undergoes β oxidation.

β Oxidation is a multistep process that removes a two-carbon fragment from the end of an acyl CoA and releases the fragment as an acetyl CoA (Fig. 58-10). The process also releases one $FADH_2$, one NADH, and the remainder of the acyl chain (beginning with the original β carbon), which serves as the starting point for the next cycle. β Oxidation continues until it consumes the entire FA chain. For an FA chain containing n carbons, the number of cycles is ([n/2]—1). The final cycle generates two acetyl CoA molecules. Unlike the breakdown of glucose, which can yield ATP even in the absence of O_2 (through glycolysis), the catabolism of FAs to yield energy in the form of ATP can occur only in the presence of O_2.

Malonyl CoA plays a central role in regulating the balance between FA synthesis and β oxidation. When energy levels are high, the enzyme ACC generates malonyl CoA from acetyl CoA, as shown in Figure 58-7. In turn, malonyl CoA provides the two-carbon building blocks for FA synthesis. In contrast, malonyl inhibits CAT I and thereby inhibits β oxidation (Fig. 58-10). Mice deficient in ACC2—even those fed a high-fat/high-carbohydrate diet—are thinner than their normal littermates on the same diet.

The final common pathway in the complete oxidation of carbohydrates, TAGs, and proteins to CO_2 comprises the citric acid cycle and oxidative phosphorylation

Under aerobic conditions, cells containing mitochondria typically convert most of the pyruvate they generate from carbohydrate metabolism to acetyl CoA, rather than to lactate. Pyruvate—a three-carbon piece of glucose's carbon skeleton—moves from the cytoplasm into the mitochondrial matrix (Fig. 58-11). There, pyruvate is oxidatively decarboxylated to **acetyl CoA**, thus releasing CO_2 as well as an NADH. Acetyl CoA also forms in the mitochondria as the end product of the β oxidation of FAs, as well as amino acid breakdown. The metabolism of the acetate moiety of acetyl CoA, as well as the oxidation of NADH and $FADH_2$, is the final common pathway of **aerobic catabolism**, which releases CO_2, H_2O, ATP, and heat.

Citric Acid Cycle Acetyl CoA—representing a two-carbon fragment derived from glucose, FA, or amino acid metabolism—enters the citric acid cycle phase of catabolism, also called *internal respiration* (see Chapter 26) or *oxidative decarboxylation* because the two-carbon fragment ends up as two CO_2 molecules (Fig. 58-11). The citric acid cycle conserves the liberated energy as GTP and the reduced electron carriers NADH and $FADH_2$.

Cells tightly control the citric acid cycle by three *mechanisms* that limit substrate flux through the citric acid cycle: substrate availability, product accumulation, and feedback inhibition of key enzymes. Cells regulate the citric acid cycle at four *sites*. The two entry-point enzymes, pyruvate dehydrogenase and citrate synthase, are the most important. **Pyruvate dehydrogenase** is inhibited allosterically by two of its immediate products (NADH and acetyl CoA) and one downstream product (ATP). The second primary site of regulation in the citric acid cycle is **citrate synthase**, which is under feedback inhibition of several immediate and downstream products (citrate, NADH, succinyl CoA, ATP). The citrate produced in this reaction feeds back negatively on PFK, as discussed earlier, thus effectively coupling glycolysis and oxidative metabolism (Fig. 58-6). Two other enzymes, isocitrate dehydrogenase and α-ketoglutarate dehydrogenase, may also be rate limiting for the citric acid cycle under the right conditions.

Oxidative Phosphorylation The process by which mitochondria retrieve energy from $FADH_2$ and NADH is oxidative phosphorylation. These reduced nucleotides are products of glycolysis (Fig. 58-6), β oxidation (Fig. 58-10), conversion of pyruvate to acetyl CoA (Fig. 58-11), and the citric acid cycle. Oxidative phosphorylation involves the transfer of electrons along a chain of molecules, and it ultimately traps the releasing energy in the formation of 1.5 ATP molecules per $FADH_2$ and 2.5 ATP molecules per NADH (see Fig. 5-9).

Ketogenesis Conditions such as prolonged fasting, a low-carbohydrate diet, or untreated diabetes mellitus lead to the production of three water-soluble byproducts of incomplete FA oxidation, substances collectively known as **ketone bodies**: acetoacetate, β-hydroxybutyrate, and acetone. What the conditions have in common is the accelerated β oxidation of FAs that produces acetyl CoA faster than the citric acid cycle can consume them. In addition, accelerated gluconeogenesis steals the OA (Fig. 58-6B) that would be the entry point for acetyl CoA to enter the citric acid cycle (Fig. 58-11). As a result, excess acetyl CoA spills over into the production of the three ketone bodies, primarily by liver

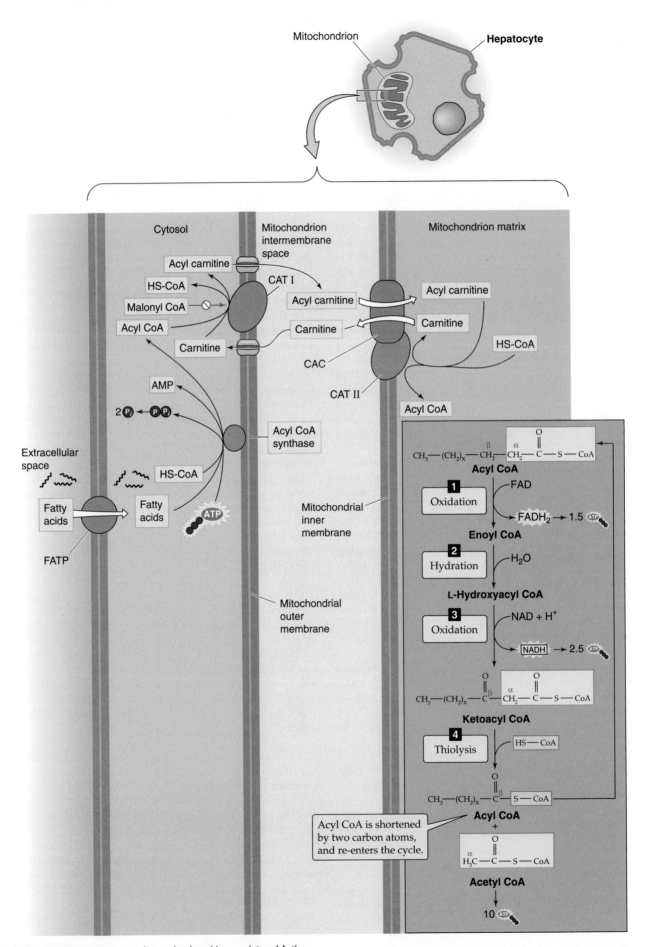

Figure 58-10   FA transport into mitochondrion and β oxidation.

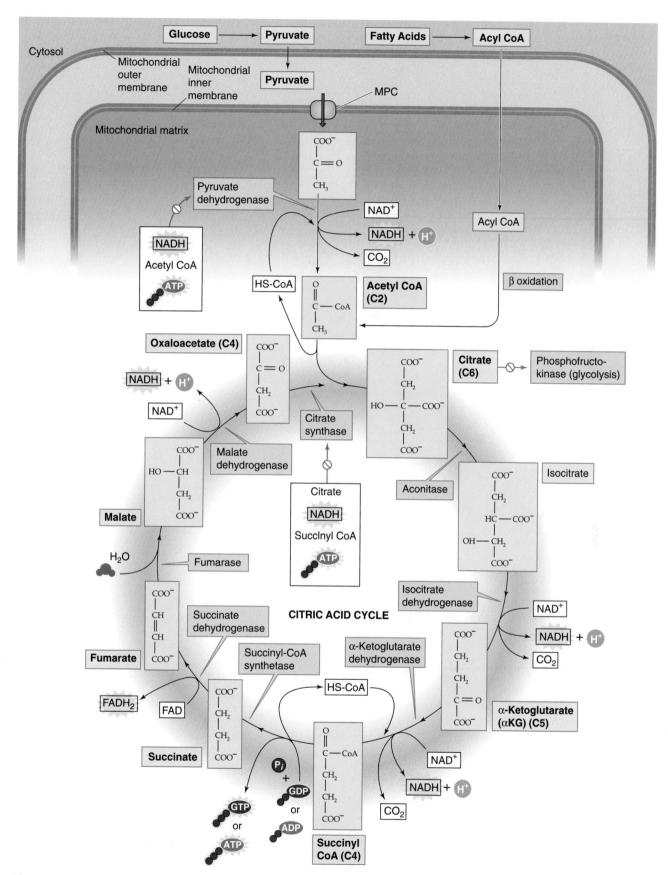

Figure 58-11   Citric acid cycle.

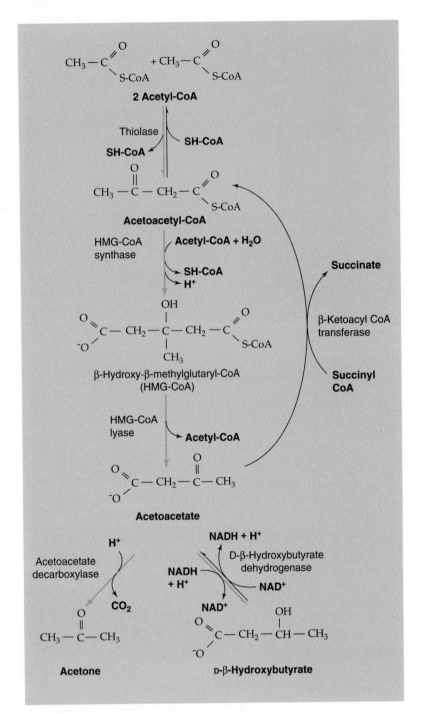

Figure 58-12 Ketogenesis and metabolism of ketone bodies.

mitochondria. As summarized by the downward orange arrows in Figure 58-12, the first three reactions in ketogenesis have the net effect of condensing two molecules of acetyl CoA and one H_2O to one molecule of **acetoacetate,** two molecules of HS-CoA, and one H^+. Thus, ketogenesis causes net metabolic acidosis (see Chapter 28). The second and third reactions are essentially irreversible. Next, the liver can either reduce acetoacetate to D-β-**hydroxybutyrate** or decarboxylate the acetoacetate to **acetone**. The body rids itself of the volatile acetone and CO_2 molecules in the expired air.

The acetone gives the breath a fruity odor that can be useful in the physical diagnosis of diabetic ketoacidosis.

Extrahepatic tissues—especially the CNS and skeletal or cardiac muscle—can consume either one D-β-hydroxybutyrate or one acetoacetate molecule, as shown by the upward purple arrows in Figure 58-12, to produce two acetyl CoA molecules that can then enter the citric acid cycle (Fig. 58-11). The key reaction—catalyzed by β-**ketoacyl CoA transferase**—bypasses the two irreversible ketogenic reactions by transferring a CoA from succinyl CoA to acetoacetate. This reaction is itself essentially irreversible. The reason that ketone bodies flow from the liver to extra-hepatic tissues is that β-ketoacyl CoA transferase is not present in hepatocytes.

Oxidizing different fuels yields similar amounts of energy per unit O₂ consumed

The source with the greatest energy density (kcal/g) is saturated FAs (Table 58-1), which have a high density of carbon and hydrogen that can be oxidized to CO_2 and H_2O. Accordingly, the complete combustion of 1 g of an energy-rich fuel (i.e., lipid) requires more O_2. However, the energy yield per O_2 is similar among fuels, because about the same amount of O_2 is needed to oxidize each carbon and hydrogen. The energy yield per unit of O_2 is only slightly greater for carbohydrate (5.0 kcal/L of O_2) than for lipid (4.7 kcal/L O_2). Carbohydrate, with its greater energy yield per O_2, is the body's preferred fuel for combustion during maximal exercise when O_2 availability is limited. However, fat is the preferred fuel during prolonged activity, when O_2 is available and fuel sources are abundant.

The metabolism of glucose by *aerobic* glycolysis and the citric acid cycle is far more efficient in providing energy in the form of ATP than *anaerobic* glycolysis in that complete oxidation of 1 molecule of glucose to CO_2 and H_2O through oxidative metabolism provides 30 to 32 molecules of ATP, whereas metabolism of 1 molecule of glucose to lactate by anaerobic glycolysis yields only ~2 molecules of ATP (Table 58-4). However, anaerobic glycolysis has the major advantage of being able to supply much more ATP *per unit time* compared with oxidative metabolism of glucose or fat. In this way, energy from glycogen supplies energy for muscle contraction during intense activities, such as sprinting.

Table 58-4 Generation of ATP from the Complete Oxidation of Glucose*

Glycolysis $\xrightarrow{\text{direct}}$	2 ATP
Glycolysis → 2×1 NADH $\xrightarrow{\text{ox. phos.}}$	3 or 5 ATP
2× (Pyruvate → acetyl CoA) → 2 NADH $\xrightarrow{\text{ox. phos.}}$	5 ATP
Citric acid cycle → 2×1 GTP $\xrightarrow{\text{ox. phos.}}$	2 ATP
Citric acid cycle → 2×3 = 6 NADH $\xrightarrow{\text{ox. phos.}}$	15 ATP
Citric acid cycle → 2×1 = 2 FADH₂ $\xrightarrow{\text{ox. phos.}}$	3 ATP
Total (per glucose):	30 or 32 ATP

*The calculation in this table assumes that the oxidative phosphorylation (ox. phos.) of each NADH molecule produced in the cytosol (row 2) will yield 1.5 or 2.5 ATP molecules, depending on which shuttle system that the cell uses transfer the reducing equivalents from the cytosol into the mitochondria. The calculation also assumes that the oxidative phosphorylation of each NADH produced in the mitochondria (rows 3 and 5) yields 2.5 ATPs, and the oxidative phosphorylation of each FADH₂ produced in the mitochondria (row 6) yields 1.5 ATPs.

Responsible for this intense work are fast-twitch type 2 fibers, which have a much lower mitochondrial density than slow-twitch type 1 fibers. Unfortunately, muscle can support this type of activity only for several minutes before lactate accumulates and the muscle cramps, or the muscle exhausts its stored glycogen. In contrast, oxidative metabolism of FAs is the major mechanism for supporting exercising muscle during prolonged activity, such as running a marathon, which is mostly the work of the slow-twitch type 1 muscle fibers (see Chapter 60).

In the case of FA metabolism (Fig. 58-10), each cycle of β oxidation yields a total of 14 ATP molecules (Table 58-5). The total number of ATP molecules generated from an FA depends on the number of carbon atoms in the FA chain. For example, palmitic acid, a 16-carbon FA, needs 7 β-oxidation cycles to form 8 acetyl CoA molecules. The 7 cycles generate $7 \times 14 = 98$ ATPs. The leftover acetyl CoA represents an additional 10 ATPs, for a total of 108 ATPs. Because the initial activation of the palmitate to palmitoyl CoA involves converting an ATP to AMP plus pyrophosphate—and regenerating ATP from AMP requires forming 2 high-energy phosphate bonds—the net ATP production is $108 - 2 = 106$ ATPs per palmitate oxidized.

For each primary fuel source, Table 58-6 provides the **respiratory quotient (RQ)** or ratio of moles of CO_2 produced per mole of O_2 consumed at the tissue level. The RQ reflects the density of oxygen atoms in the fuel source. For example, with carbohydrates, the cell needs to supply only enough external O_2 to oxidize the carbon atoms to CO_2. The H_2O is already built into the carbohydrate molecule, which has a ratio of H to O of 2:1.

Carbohydrate oxidation

$$C_6H_{12}O_6 + 6\,O_2 + 30 \text{ or } 32\,ADP + 30 \text{ or } 32\,P_i \rightarrow$$
$$\textit{Glucose}$$
$$6\,CO_2 + 6\,H_2O + 30 \text{ or } 32\,ATP + \text{heat} \quad (58\text{-}4)$$
$$(RQ = 6\,CO_2/6\,O_2 = 1.00)$$

However, because lipids contain so many fewer oxygen atoms, lipid oxidation requires more external O_2.

Lipid oxidation

$$C_{15}H_{31}COOH + 23\,O_2 + 106\,ADP + 106\,P_i \rightarrow$$
$$\textit{Palmitic acid}$$
$$16\,CO_2 + 16\,H_2O + 106\,ATP + \text{heat} \quad (58\text{-}5)$$
$$(RQ = 16\,CO_2/23\,O_2 = 0.70)$$

The RQ for protein oxidation is 0.80 to 0.85.

Protein oxidation constitutes a very minor fraction of the total fuel oxidation in any tissue. The brain and anaerobic tissues normally use carbohydrate nearly exclusively and have an RQ of 1.0. Most tissues oxidize both carbohydrate and fat, and the RQ reflects this mixture. The whole-body RQ following an overnight fast is ~0.8 for people eating a typical Western diet; individuals with less lipid intake have a higher RQ (i.e., approaching the value of 1 for carbohydrates).

Table 58-5 Generation of ATP in One Cycle of β Oxidation of a Fatty Acid*

(Acyl CoA → enoyl CoA) → 1 FADH₂ $\xrightarrow{\text{ox. phos.}}$	1.5 ATP
(L-Hydroxyacyl CoA → ketoacyl CoA) → 1 NADH $\xrightarrow{\text{ox. phos.}}$	2.5 ATP
1 Acetyl CoA → { Citric acid cycle $\xrightarrow{\text{direct}}$ 1 GTP $\xrightarrow{\text{ox. phos.}}$	1 ATP
citric acid cycle → 3 NADH $\xrightarrow{\text{ox. phos.}}$	7.5 ATP
Citric acid cycle → 1 FADH₂ $\xrightarrow{\text{ox. phos.}}$ }	1.5 ATP
Total (per cycle):	14 ATP

*The foregoing calculation assumes that oxidative phosphorylation (ox. phos.) generates 2.5 ATP/NADH, and 1.5 ATP/FADH2.

Table 58-6 Respiratory Quotients of the Major Foodstuffs

	Energy Density (kcal/g)	Respiratory Quotient
Carbohydrate	4.1	1.00
Protein	4.3	0.80-0.85
Lipid	9.4	0.70

INTEGRATIVE METABOLISM OF FASTING

The human body has two main priorities for energy liberation during fasting. The first priority is to maintain a stable supply of energy for CNS function. The brain has little stored energy in the form of glycogen or TAGs and therefore depends on the liver (and under some circumstances the kidney) for a constant supply of energy in the form of glucose or ketone bodies. In the fed state and early in the fasting state, the brain derives essentially all its energy from oxidation of glucose because ketone bodies are not present and the blood-brain barrier is mostly impermeable to FAs. Most other major organs of the body (liver, skeletal muscle, heart) fill their energy needs at this time by oxidizing FAs. Because a continuous supply of glucose is required to meet the energy demands of the CNS, humans have evolved elaborate, redundant mechanisms to maintain plasma [glucose] within a very narrow range, between 60 and 140 mg/dL (3.3 to 7.8 mM), between fasting and fed states. Lower [glucose] impairs brain function, whereas elevated plasma [glucose] exceeds the renal glucose threshold, results in polyuria, and leads to the multiple complications associated with poorly controlled diabetes mellitus (retinopathy, neuropathy, and nephropathy). In contrast, FAs and ketone bodies can vary in concentration by 10- and 100-fold, respectively, depending on the fed or fasted conditions. During prolonged fasting (>2 days), the liver metabolizes FAs to raise plasma levels of ketone bodies sufficiently to supply much of the brain's oxidative fuel needs. The second priority for the body is to maintain its protein reserves (e.g., contractile proteins, enzymes, nervous tissue) in times of fasting.

The body also has two main priorities for energy repletion after fasting. First, following a meal, liver and muscle replenish their limited glycogen reserves. Once these stores are full, liver and muscle convert any excess energy in the form of carbohydrate and protein to fat. Muscle glycogen is the most readily available form of energy for muscle contraction, especially when intense bursts of physical activity are required. Therefore, maintaining an adequate supply of muscle glycogen at all times also has obvious survival benefits in times of fight or flight. The second priority during feeding is to replenish protein reserves.

During an overnight fast, glycogenolysis and gluconeogenesis maintain plasma glucose levels

The period after an overnight fast serves as a useful reference point because it represents the period before the transition from the fasted to the fed state. At this time, the concentrations of insulin, glucagon, and metabolic substrates that were altered by meal ingestion during the preceding day have returned to some baseline. Moreover, the body is in a relative steady state in which the rate of release of endogenous fuels from storage depots closely matches fuel consumption.

Requirement for Glucose After an overnight fast, the decline in circulating insulin leads to a marked decrease in glucose uptake by insulin-sensitive tissues (e.g., muscle) and a shift toward the use by these tissues of FAs mobilized from fat stores. Nevertheless, the average adult continues to metabolize glucose at a rate of 7 to 10 g/hr. Total body stores of free glucose, which exists mostly in the extracellular space, amount to only 15 to 20 g or ~2 hours' worth of glucose fuel. However, the useful glucose store is even less if we consider that the plasma [glucose]—normally ~90 mg/dL (5.0 mM) after an overnight fast—may not fall to less than ~55 mg/dL (3.0 mM) before brain function becomes abnormal. Thus, maintaining plasma [glucose] in the presence of this ongoing glucose use, particularly by the brain, requires that the body produce glucose at rates sufficient to match its ongoing consumption.

Gluconeogenesis Versus Glycogenolysis Four to 5 hours after a meal (perhaps longer for a very large meal), a fall in plasma [insulin] and a rise in [glucagon] cause the liver to begin breaking down its stores of glycogen and releasing it as glucose (see Chapter 51). Moreover, both the liver and, to a lesser extent, the kidney generate glucose by gluconeogenesis. The release of glucose by these two organs is possible

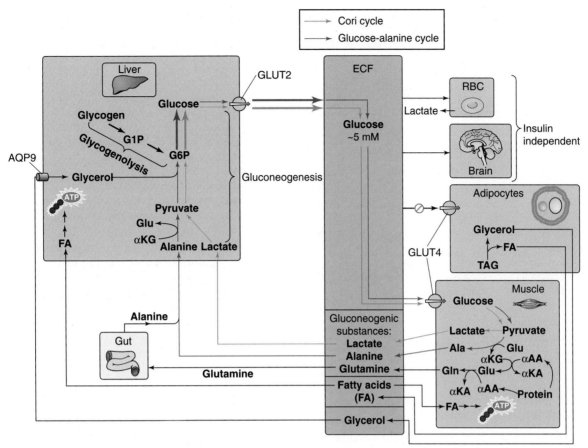

Figure 58-13 Overnight fast. αAA, α-amino acid; AQP9, aquaporin 9; ECF, extracellular fluid; αKA, α-keto acid; αKG, α-ketoglutarate.

because they are the only two with significant amounts of G6Pase, which catalyzes the conversion of G6P to glucose. Net hepatic glycogenolysis and gluconeogenesis each contribute ~50% whole-body glucose production during the first several hours of a fast.

Gluconeogenesis: The Cori Cycle In the first several hours of a fast, the brain consumes glucose at the rate of 4 to 5 g/hr, which is two thirds the rate of hepatic glucose production (~180 g/day). Obligate anaerobic tissues also metabolize glucose but convert it primarily to lactate and pyruvate. The liver takes up these products and uses gluconeogenesis to regenerate glucose at the expense of energy. The liver releases the glucose for uptake by the glucose-requiring tissues, thus completing the **Cori cycle** (Fig. 58-13).

Gluconeogenesis: The Glucose-Alanine Cycle After an overnight fast, the body as a whole is in negative nitrogen balance. Muscle and splanchnic tissues are the principal sites of protein degradation and release of amino acids into the blood. **Alanine** and **glutamine**, which are particularly important, represent ~50% of total amino acid released by muscle, even though these amino acids represent only 10% to 13% of total amino acids in muscle protein. The reason that alanine and glutamine are overrepresented is that muscle synthesizes them (Fig. 58-13). During fasting, breakdown of muscle protein yields amino acids, which subsequently transfer their amino groups to α-ketoglutarate (supplied by

the citric acid cycle) to form glutamate. Glutamine synthase can then add a second amino group to glutamate, thus producing glutamine. Alternatively, alanine aminotransferase can transfer the amino group of glutamate to pyruvate (the product of glucose breakdown), thereby generating alanine and α-ketoglutarate. Both glutamine and alanine enter the blood. The intestine uses some of the glutamine as an oxidative fuel and releases the amino groups into portal blood as either alanine or ammonia.

The amino acids taken up by the liver provide carbon for gluconeogenesis. On a molar basis, alanine is the principal amino acid taken up by the liver. In the first several hours of fasting, the liver principally uses alanine for gluconeogenesis. Because the carbon backbone of alanine came from glucose metabolism in muscle, and the liver regenerates glucose from this alanine, the net effect is a **glucose-alanine cycle** between muscle and liver, analogous to the Cori cycle.

In addition to its role in gluconeogenesis, the glucose-alanine cycle is critical for **nitrogen metabolism**, thus providing a nontoxic alternative to ammonia for transferring amino groups—derived from muscle amino acid catabolism—to the liver (Fig. 58-13). The hepatocytes now detoxify the amino groups on alanine and other amino acids by generating urea, which the kidney then excretes (see Figs. 39-6 and 46-14). Another key amino acid in nitrogen metabolism is glutamine, which muscle releases into the blood for uptake by the gut and liver as well as the kidney. The kidney uses the carbon skeleton of glutamine for renal gluconeogenesis and converts the amino group to ammonia, which it excretes (see Chapter 39). This ammonia excretion is particularly important in maintaining body acid-base balance during fasting. Combined, alanine and glutamine account for more than 40% of the amino acid carbon used by liver and kidneys in gluconeogenesis.

Neither the Cori cycle nor the glucose-alanine cycle in muscle yields new carbon skeletons. Rather, both cycles transfer energy—and the glucose-alanine cycle also transfers nitrogen—between muscle and liver. The energy for hepatic glucose synthesis comes from oxidation of fat in the liver.

Lipolysis Finally, the fall in plasma [insulin] after an overnight fast permits the release of FAs and glycerol from fat stores (see Fig. 51-10). This response appears to be more pronounced in visceral than peripheral fat depots. The decline in [insulin] and the ensuing lipolysis are sufficient to supply FAs to extracerebral tissues (e.g., muscle, heart, liver) for fuel and glycerol to the liver for gluconeogenesis. However, these changes are not sufficient to stimulate the hepatic conversion of FA to ketone bodies.

The body never completely suppresses gluconeogenesis. When an individual ingests a meal, gluconeogenic flux provides glucose for hepatic glycogen stores (*indirect pathway*). During fasting, the liver redirects the gluconeogenic flux to provide glucose for delivery to the circulation.

Starvation beyond an overnight fast enhances gluconeogenesis and lipolysis

We have just seen that, during an overnight fast, glycogenolysis and gluconeogenesis contribute about equally to maintain a fasting plasma glucose concentration of ~90 mg/dL (5.0 mM). What happens if we extend our fast for 1 or 2 days? Because the glucose utilization rate is 7 to 10 g/hr, if half of this were provided by *glycolysis* (as is true for an overnight fast), the hepatic glycogen stores of ~70 g that remain after an overnight fast would be sufficient to last only an additional day. However, in the early stages of starvation, the body compensates by accelerating *gluconeogenesis*.

Orchestrating the metabolic adaptations in the early stages of starvation—increased gluconeogenesis, but also increased proteolysis and lipolysis—are a decline in [insulin] to a level lower than that seen after an overnight fast and a modest increase in portal vein [glucagon]. Insulin deficiency promotes all aspects of the metabolic response, whereas the effect of glucagon is confined to the liver (see Chapter 51).

Enhanced Gluconeogenesis Adaptations in both liver and muscle are responsible for increasing gluconeogenesis (Fig. 58-13). In muscle, acceleration of proteolysis leads to the release of alanine and other glycogenic amino acids, whereas the liver accelerates its conversion of gluconeogenic amino acids into glucose. This enhanced gluconeogenesis, however, is not the result of increased availability of substrates, because plasma levels of alanine and other glycogenic amino acids decline. Instead, fasting upregulates key gluconeogenic enzymes (see Chapter 51) and thus makes gluconeogenesis *more efficient*.

The dependence of gluconeogenesis on proteolysis is reflected by an increase in urinary nitrogen excretion in the early phase of starvation. During the first 24 hours of a fast, the average 70-kg person excretes 7 to 12 g of elemental nitrogen in the urine, equivalent to 50 to 75 g of protein. Because tissue protein content does not exceed 20% by weight for any tissue, 50 to 75 g of protein translates to 250 to 375 g of lean body mass lost on the first day of a fast.

Enhanced Lipolysis The activation of HSL increases release of FAs and glycerol from TAG stores in adipose tissue and muscle (Fig. 58-13). The increased availability of glycerol provides the liver with an additional substrate for gluconeogenesis, as discussed earlier, that contributes to glucose homeostasis. Moreover, the increased availability of FAs to muscle and other peripheral tissues limits their use of glucose, preserves glucose for the CNS and other obligate glucose-using tissues, and thereby diminishes the demands for gluconeogenesis and proteolysis.

Elevated levels of FAs cause **insulin resistance** in skeletal muscle by directly interfering with the activation of GLUT4 (Fig. 58-13) by insulin. FAs activate a serine/threonine kinase cascade, leading to increased *serine* phosphorylation of insulin receptor substrate 1 (IRS-1; see Chapter 51), which, in turn, leads to decreased *tyrosine* phosphorylation of IRS-1 and thus a decrease in the PI3K that is necessary for the insertion of GLUT4 in muscle. This FA-induced decrease in glucose consumption and the parallel increased availability of FAs as a fuel for muscle spare glucose for other tissues under fasting conditions. However, this adaptation may play an important pathologic role in mediating the insulin resistance associated with obesity and type 2 diabetes.

In addition to their effects on muscle, FAs enter the liver, where they undergo β oxidation and generate energy. A fall in the insulin-glucagon ratio inhibits ACC (see Fig. 51-12), reduces levels of malonyl CoA, and promotes mitochondrial FA oxidation. Thus, the hormonal changes both increase the supply of FAs and activate the enzymes necessary for FA oxidation. This β oxidation furnishes the energy and reducing power required for gluconeogenesis. If the availability of FAs outstrips the ability of the citric acid cycle to oxidize the resulting acetyl CoA, the result may be the accumulation of ketone bodies, which can serve as a fuel for the CNS as well as for cardiac and skeletal muscle.

Prolonged starvation moderates proteolysis but accelerates lipolysis, thereby releasing ketone bodies

As the duration of fasting increases, the body shifts from using its limited protein stores for gluconeogenesis to using fat for ketogenesis (Fig. 58-14). Moreover, the brain shifts from oxidizing glucose to oxidizing two ketone bodies, β-hydroxybutyrate and acetoacetate, to meet most of its energy requirements.

Decreased Proteolysis A fasting human could survive for only ~10 days if totally dependent on protein utilization to meet whole-body energy requirements. Thus, prolonged survival during starvation requires a major reduction in proteolysis. Indeed, urea excretion decreases from 10 to 15 g/day during the initial days of a fast to less than 1 g/day after 6 weeks of fasting. Because urea is the major obligatory osmolyte in the urine (see Chapter 38), this reduced urea

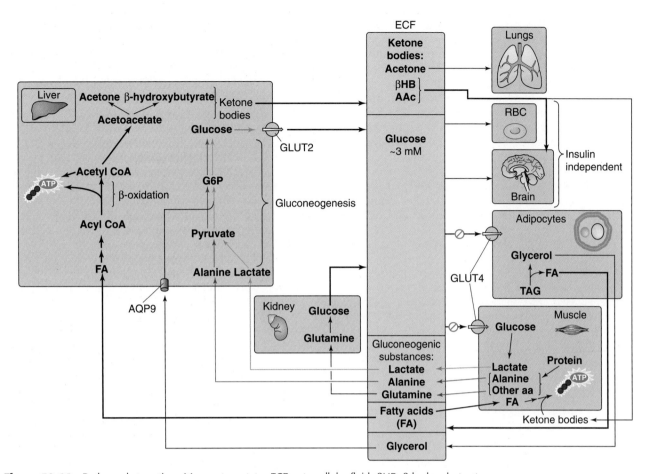

Figure 58-14 Prolonged starvation. AAc, acetoacetate; ECF, extracellular fluid; βHB, β-hydroxybutyrate.

production lessens obligatory water excretion and therefore the daily water requirement. Ammonium excretion also decreases.

Decreased Hepatic Gluconeogenesis The transition from protein to lipid degradation permits humans to extend their survival time during a prolonged fast from weeks to months, as long as fat stores are available and water intake is adequate. During this transition, hepatic gluconeogenesis decreases (Fig. 58-14), mostly because of diminished substrate delivery. During the first few weeks of a fast, muscle releases less alanine, the principal substrate for hepatic gluconeogenesis, thus causing plasma [alanine] to fall markedly, to less than one third of the concentrations seen after the absorption of a meal. Indeed, during a prolonged fast, infusing a small amount of alanine causes plasma [glucose] to rise.

Increased Renal Gluconeogenesis While hepatic gluconeogenesis falls, renal gluconeogenesis rises (Fig. 58-14), to reach as much as 40% of whole-body glucose production. Renal gluconeogenesis, which consumes H^+ (see Fig. 39-5A), most likely is an adaptation to the acidosis that accompanies ketogenesis. Indeed, acidosis stimulates renal ammoniagenesis in parallel with renal gluconeogenesis.

Increased Lipolysis and Ketogenesis During the first 3 to 7 days of fasting, hypoinsulinemia accelerates the mobilization of FAs from adipose tissue and causes plasma levels of FAs to double; FA levels remain stable thereafter. The combination of low insulin and high glucagon levels also increases hepatic oxidation of FAs and leads to a marked increase of hepatic ketogenesis (Fig. 58-14) or *ketogenic capacity*. The liver achieves peak rates of ketone body production (~100 g/day) by the third day and maintains them thereafter. Low insulin levels also progressively reduce the extraction of ketone bodies by peripheral tissues. Thus, despite relatively stable rates of ketone body production, circulating levels of ketone bodies continue to rise throughout the next few weeks. As a result, the CNS receives an increasing supply of these water-soluble substrates, which eventually account for more than one half of the brain's energy requirements. In this way, ketone bodies ultimately supplant the brain's dependency on glucose. Thus, by limiting the brain's gluconeogenic demands, the body preserves protein stores. Besides the CNS, other body tissues, especially the heart and skeletal muscle, can use ketone bodies to cover a significant proportion of their energy demands.

As the fast progresses, and fat stores are depleted, levels of leptin decrease. This decrease in leptin levels is a protective signal that profoundly affects the hypothalamic-pituitary-gonadal axes and reduces the oscillations of luteinizing hormone and follicle-stimulating hormone that cause anovulation. In times of famine, this mechanism protects fertile women from the additional nutritional demands associated with pregnancy.

In summary, the body has evolved powerful adaptive mechanisms that ensure adequate substrate supply in the form of glucose and ketone bodies during a prolonged fast to maintain adequate CNS function. Even during a prolonged fast, humans do not lose consciousness because of decreased substrate supply to the brain. Instead, death under these conditions typically occurs when fat stores are depleted and severe protein wasting causes failure of respiratory muscles, which, in turn, leads to atelectasis and terminal pneumonia.

REFERENCES

Books and Reviews

Hillgartner FB, Salati LM, Goodridge AG: Physiological and molecular mechanisms involved in nutritional regulation of fatty acid synthesis. Physiol Rev 1995; 75:47-76.

Jequier E, Tappy J: Regulation of body weight in humans. Physiol Rev 1999; 79:451-480.

Koretsky AP: Insights into cellular energy metabolism from transgenic mice. Physiol Rev 1995; 75:667-688.

Palmieri F: The mitochondrial transporter family (SLC25): Physiological and pathological implications. Pflugers Arch 2004; 447:689-709.

Shulman GI, Landau BR: Pathways of glycogen repletion. Physiol Rev 1992; 72:1019-1035.

Stahl A: A current review of fatty acid transport proteins (SLC27). Pflugers Arch 2004; 447:722-727.

Wilson JD, Foster DW, Kronenberg HM, Larsen PR (eds): Williams Textbook of Endocrinology, 9th ed. Philadelphia: WB Saunders, 1998.

Journal Article

Abu-Elheiga L, Wonkeun O, Parichher P, Wakil SJ: Acetyl-CoA carboxylase 2 mutant mice are protected against obesity and diabetes induced by high-fat/high-carbohydrate diets. Proc Natl Acad Sci U S A 2003; 100:10207-10212.

CHAPTER 59

REGULATION OF BODY TEMPERATURE

John Stitt

HEAT AND TEMPERATURE: THE ADVANTAGES OF HOMEOTHERMY

Homeothermy enables an organism to maintain its activity over a wide range of environmental temperatures

The ability to regulate internal body temperature has provided higher organisms independence from the environment. Because the rates of most physical and chemical reactions depend on temperature, most physiological functions are sensitive to temperature changes. Thus, the activity levels of **poikilotherms** (species that do not regulate internal body temperature) generally depend on environmental temperature, whereas those of **homeotherms** (species that do regulate internal body temperature) are relatively stable over a broad range of ambient conditions. A lizard, for example, is capable of relatively less movement away from its lair on a cold, overcast day than on a hot, sunny day, whereas a prairie dog may be equally mobile on either day. An arctic fox acclimatizes to the extreme cold of winter by maintaining a thick, insulating coat that enables it to resist body cooling and minimizes the necessity to increase metabolic heat generation, which would require increased food intake.

The thermoregulatory system of homeotherms creates an internal environment in which reaction rates are relatively high and optimal. At the same time, an effective thermoregulatory system avoids the pathologic consequences of wide deviations in body temperature (Table 59-1). The thermoregulatory system incorporates both anticipatory controls and negative feedback controls. The components of this system are as follows: (1) thermal sensors; (2) afferent pathways; (3) an integration system in the central nervous system (CNS); (4) efferent pathways; and (5) target organs that control heat generation and transfer, such as skeletal muscle (e.g., shivering to generate heat), circulation to the skin (to dissipate heat), and the sweat glands (to dissipate heat).

The focus of this chapter is temperature regulation in homeotherms. I examine the physical aspects of heat transfer both within the body and between body and environment, as well as the physiological mechanisms involved in altering these rates of transfer. Finally, I look at the consequences of extreme challenges to the thermoregulatory mechanism, such as hyperthermia, hypothermia, and dehydration.

Body core temperature depends on time of day, physical activity, time in the menstrual cycle, and age

Temperature scales are relative scales of heat content. The centigrade scale is divided into 100 equal increments, referenced to the freezing (0°C) and boiling (100°C) points of water. The "normal" body temperature of an adult human is approximately 37°C (i.e., 98.6°F), but it may be as low as 36°C or as high as 37.5°C in active, healthy people. *Body temperature* usually refers to the temperature of the internal body *core*, measured under the tongue (sublingually), in the ear canal, or in the rectum. For clinical purposes, the most reliable (although the least practical) among these three is the last, because it is least influenced by ambient (air) temperature. Measurement devices range from traditional mercury-in-glass thermometers to electronic, digital readout thermistors. Nearly all such instruments are accurate to 0.1°C. The least invasive approach uses an infrared thermometer to measure the radiant temperature over the temporal artery.

Body core temperature depends on the time of day, the stage of the menstrual cycle in women, the level of the person's activity, and the individual's age. All homeotherms maintain a circadian (24-hour cycle) body temperature rhythm, with variations of ~1°C. In humans, body temperature is usually lowest between 3:00 to 6:00 AM, and it peaks at 3:00 to 6:00 PM. This circadian rhythmicity is inherent in the autonomic nervous system, independent of the sleep-wakefulness cycle, but it is entrained by light-dark cues to a 24-hour cycle.

In many women, body temperature increases approximately 0.5°C during the postovulatory phase of their menstrual cycle (see Chapter 55). An abrupt increase in body temperature of 0.3°C to 0.5°C accompanies ovulation and may be useful as a fertility guide.

Physical activity generates excess heat as a byproduct of elevated metabolic rate. A portion of this excess heat remains

Table 59-1 Consequences of Deviations in Body Temperature

Temperature (°C)	Consequence
40-44	Heat stroke with multiple organ failure and brain lesions
38-40	Hyperthermia (as a result of fever or exercise)
36-38	Normal range
34-36	Mild hypothermia
30-34	Impairment of temperature regulation
27-29	Cardiac fibrillation

in the body, causes the core temperature to rise, and triggers appropriately matching heat loss responses. Core temperature remains elevated during activity and for an extended period after exercise ceases.

Infants and older people are less able to maintain a normal body temperature than are the rest of the population, particularly in the presence of external challenges. Newborns do not readily shiver or sweat and thus behave more like poikilotherms than like homeotherms. These properties, along with a high surface-to-mass ratio, render infants more susceptible to fluctuations in core temperature when exposed to a hot or cold environment. Older people are also subject to greater fluctuations in core temperature. Aging is associated with a progressive deficit in the ability to sense heat and cold, as well as a reduced ability to generate heat (reduced metabolic rate and metabolic potential because of lower muscle mass) and to dissipate heat (reduced cardiovascular reserve and sweat gland atrophy from disuse).

The body's rate of heat production can vary from ~70 kcal/hr at rest to 600 kcal/hr during jogging

The body's rate of heat production is closely linked to the rate of metabolism, the rate of O_2 consumption ($\dot{V}_{O_2}$). Minor variations occur, depending on the mixture of fuels (foods) being oxidized, a process that determines the respiratory quotient (RQ; see Table 58-6). Because of their inherent inefficiency, metabolic transformations generate heat (see Chapter 58). Ultimately, all the energy contained in fuels appears as heat, mass storage or growth, or physical work done on the environment.

The body's metabolic rate, and thus its rate of heat production, is not constant. The **resting metabolic rate** (**RMR**; see Chapter 58) is the rate necessary to maintain the functions of resting cells; these functions include active transport as well as cardiac and respiratory muscle activity. Voluntary or involuntary (e.g., shivering) muscular activity adds to the overall metabolic heat production. Even digesting a meal

increases the metabolic rate (see Chapter 58). An increase in tissue temperature itself raises the metabolic rate, according to the van't Hoff relation (i.e., a 10°C increase in tissue temperature more than doubles the metabolic rate). Furthermore, certain hormones, notably thyroxine and epinephrine, increase the cellular metabolic rate. Because the body's heat production rate is variable, the rate of heat loss must match it closely if the body temperature is to remain constant. At an RQ of 0.8 (see Chapter 58), the average person under sedentary (i.e., RMR) conditions has a resting $\dot{V}_{O_2}$ of 250 mL/min, which corresponds to a heat production of 72 kcal/hr (~85 watts). In other words, an adult of average size generates the heat of an 85-watt light bulb (see Chapter 58).

During physical exercise, the rate of energy production—and hence, heat generation—increases in proportion to the intensity of exercise. An average adult can comfortably sustain an energy production rate of 400 to 600 kcal/hr for extended periods (e.g., a fast walk or a modest jog). Nearly all this increased heat generation occurs in active skeletal muscle, although a portion arises from increased cardiac and respiratory muscle activity. A thermal load of this magnitude would raise core temperature by 1.0°C every 8 to 10 minutes if the extra heat could not escape the body. Physical activity would be limited to 25 to 30 minutes, at which time the effects of excessive hyperthermia (>40°C) would begin to impair body function. This impairment, of course, does not occur, primarily because of the effectiveness of the thermoregulatory system. Within a relatively short period, the increase in body temperature resulting from exercise leads to an increased rate of heat dissipation that matches heat production. Thereafter, the body maintains a new, elevated steady temperature. When exercise ceases, body temperature gradually decreases to its pre-exercise level.

MODES OF HEAT TRANSFER

Maintaining a relatively constant body temperature requires a fine balance between heat production and heat losses

Temperature homeostasis requires that increases or decreases in heat production balance increases or decreases in heat loss. Physiologists usually express this concept in terms of a whole-body **heat balance equation**, which, for an adult of constant mass, is as follows:

$$\underbrace{(M - W)}_{\text{Heat production (H)}} - \underbrace{(R + C + E)}_{\text{Heat losses}} = S$$

where M = Metabolism, W = Work done on environment, R = Radiative heat loss, C = Convective heat loss, E = Evaporative heat loss, S = Storage of heat.

(59-1)

All terms in the foregoing equation have the units kcal/hr.

Several physiological processes contribute to temperature homeostasis, including modulation of metabolic heat production, physical heat transfer, and elimination of heat.

Table 59-2   Contribution of Body Systems to Resting Metabolism

System	RMR
Respiration and circulation	15%
CNS and nerves	20%
Musculature (at rest)	20%
Abdominal viscera	45%
RMR	100% (~70 kcal/hr)

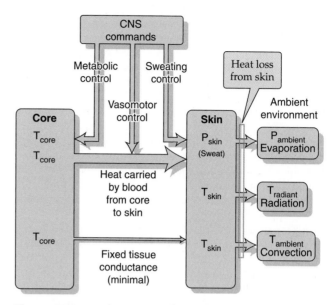

Figure 59-1   Passive or unregulated heat transfer. In the steady state, the rate of heat production by the body core must be matched by the flow of heat from the core to the skin, and from skin to environment. Various homeostatic controls—systems not directly involved in temperature regulation—can affect heat flow. Examples include sweating in response to hypoglycemia, changes in blood flow patterns in response to a fall in blood pressure, and changes in metabolism in response to alterations in thyroid metabolism.

These processes operate at the level of cells, tissues, and organ systems. Let us discuss in order the terms in Equation 59-1.

The **rate of metabolism (M)** arises from the cellular oxidation of carbohydrates, fats, and proteins. Because of their inherent inefficiency, metabolic transformations generate heat (see Chapter 58). Table 59-2 shows the fractional contributions of different body systems to total heat production under sedentary, resting conditions.

Heat production by skeletal muscle can play a vital emergency role in temperature regulation in the cold. **Shivering**—the rhythmic, clonic activation of the major muscle masses surrounding the head, torso, and upper limbs—can increase total body heat production by as much as 400%. The body can grade the intensity of shivering and heat production to match heat loss. **Physical exercise** can generate even more heat than shivering. Under conditions of maximal exercise, $\dot{V}_{O_{2max}}$ may correspond to a total energy expenditure (M in Equation 59-1) of 1300 kcal/hr for an endurance athlete. If 75% to 80% of this energy evolves as heat—so that the athlete does ~300 kcal/hr of **useful work on the environment (W)**—the **rate of heat production (H = M − W)** would be 1000 kcal/hr (~1200 watts) for a brief period of time. This change is equivalent to changing from an 85-watt light bulb to a 1200-watt space heater. Unless the body can dissipate this heat, death from hyperthermia and heat stroke (see box on Heat Stroke) will ensue rapidly.

Virtually all heat leaving the body must exit through the skin surface. In the following three sections, the three major routes of heat elimination are discussed: **radiation (R)**, **convection (C)**, and **evaporation (E)**. As the heat balance equation shows, the difference between (M − W) and (R + C + E) is the **rate of heat storage (S)** within the body. The value of S may be positive or negative, depending on whether (M − W) > (R + C + E) or vice versa. A positive value of S results in a rise of body core temperature, and a negative value results in a fall.

Heat moves from the body core to the skin, primarily by convection

Generally, all heat production occurs within the body's tissues, and all heat elimination occurs at the body surface. Figure 59-1 illustrates a **passive system** in which heat flows

depend on the size, shape, and composition of the body, as well as on the laws of physics. The circulation carries excess heat away from active tissues, such as muscle, to the body core—represented by the heart, lungs, and their central circulating blood volume. How does the body prevents its core from overheating? The answer is that the core transfers this heat to a dissipating heat sink. The organ serving as the body's greatest potential heat sink is the relatively cool **skin**, which is the largest organ in the body. Only a minor amount of the body's generated heat flows *directly* from the underlying body core to the skin by **conduction** across the body tissues. Most of the generated body heat flows to the skin by **convection** in the blood, and blood flow to the skin can increase markedly. There, nearly all the heat transferred to the skin must flow to the environment, facilitated by the skin's large surface area.

The transfer of heat from core to skin occurs by two routes:

$$
\begin{bmatrix} \text{Heat} \\ \text{transfer} \\ \text{from core} \\ \text{to skin} \end{bmatrix} = \begin{bmatrix} \text{Heat} \\ \text{passively } conducted \\ \text{from core to} \\ \text{skin} \end{bmatrix} + \begin{bmatrix} \text{Heat} \\ convected \text{ by blood} \\ \text{from core to} \\ \text{skin} \end{bmatrix}
$$

$$(59\text{-}2)$$

Both the conduction and convection terms in the previous equation are proportional to the temperature gradient from core to skin ($T_{core} - \overline{T}_{skin}$), where $\overline{T}_{skin}$ is the average temperature of at least four representative skin sites. The *proportionality constant* for passive conduction across the subcutaneous fat (the body's insulation) is relatively fixed. However, the proportionality constant for heat convection by blood is a variable term, reflecting the variability of the blood flow to the skin. The ability to alter skin blood flow, under autonomic control, is therefore the primary determinant of heat flow from core to skin. The capacity to *limit* blood flow to the skin is an essential defense against body cooling in the cold (hypothermia). A side effect, however, is that skin temperature falls. Conversely, the capacity to *elevate* skin blood flow is an essential defense against hyperthermia. On very hot days when skin temperature may be very high and close to body core temperature, even high skin blood flow may not be adequate to transfer sufficient heat to allow body core temperature to stabilize because the temperature gradient ($T_{core} - \bar{T}_{skin}$) is too small.

Although most of the heat leaving the core moves to the skin, a small amount also leaves the body core by the evaporation of water from the respiratory tract. The evaporative rate is primarily a function of the rate of ventilation (see Chapter 31), which, in turn, increases linearly with the metabolic rate over a wide range of exercise intensities.

Heat moves from the skin to the environment by radiation, conduction, convection, and evaporation

Figure 59-2 is a graphic summary of the heat balance equation (Equation 59-1) for an athlete exercising in an outdoor environment. This illustration depicts the movement of heat within the body, its delivery to the skin surface, and its subsequent elimination to the environment by radiation, convection, and evaporation.

Radiation Heat transfer by radiation occurs between the skin and solid bodies in the environment. The infrared portion of the electromagnetic energy spectrum carries this energy, which is why infrared cameras can detect warm bodies at night. The body gains or loses heat by radiation at a rate that is proportional to the temperature difference between the skin and the radiating body:

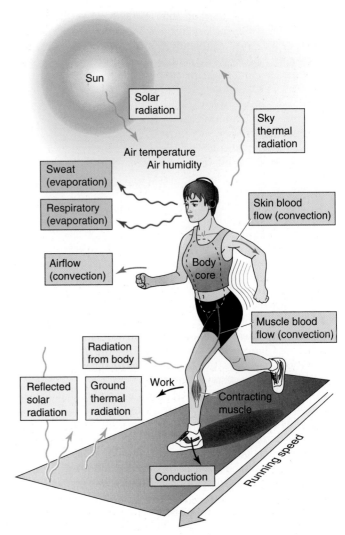

Figure 59-2 Model of energy transfer from the body to the environment.

Rate of radiative heat loss		*Radiative heat-transfer coefficient*		Mean skin temp	Radiant temp of another object	Body surface area available for *radiative* heat exchange	

$$\underbrace{\frac{R}{\frac{kcal}{h}}} = \underbrace{h_{radiative}}_{\frac{kcal}{h \times °C \times m^2}} \cdot \underbrace{(\bar{T}_{skin} - T_{radiant})}_{°C} \cdot \underbrace{A_{radiative}}_{m^2} \qquad \text{(59-3)}$$

R is positive when the body loses heat and negative when it gains heat.

One may not be so aware of radiative heat fluxes to and from the body, particularly when the radiating body temperature ($T_{radiant}$) differs from the ambient environmental temperature ($T_{ambient}$) that tends to dominate our attention. Indoors, $T_{radiant}$ is the same as $T_{ambient}$ because surrounding objects thermally equilibrate with one another. Outdoors, radiating bodies may be at widely different temperatures. The **radiant heat load** from the sun to the body on a cloud-

less summer day may exceed the RMR by a considerable amount. The radiant heat load from a fire or a radiant lamp can provide substantial warming of bodies in the radiant field. Conversely, on a winter evening, the **radiant heat loss** from the body to a cloudless, dark sky—which has a low radiant temperature—may exceed RMR. Thus, one may feel a sudden chill when walking past an uncurtained window. This chill is caused by the sudden fall in skin temperature owing to increased radiant heat loss. Radiation of heat from the body accounts for ~60% of heat lost when the body is at rest in a neutral thermal indoor environment. A **neutral thermal environment** is a set of conditions (air temperature, airflow and humidity, and temperatures of surrounding radiating surfaces) in which the temperature of the body does not change when the subject is at rest (i.e., RMR) and is not shivering.

Conduction Heat transfer by conduction occurs when the body touches a solid material of different temperature. For example, lying on the hot sand causes one to gain heat by conduction. Conversely, placing an ice pack on a sore muscle causes heat loss by conduction. However, under most normal circumstances (e.g., when one is standing and wearing shoes or recumbent and wearing clothes), the heat gain or loss by conduction is minimal.

Convection Heat transfer by convection occurs when a fluid such as air or water carries the heat between the body and the environment. The convective heat loss is proportional to the difference between skin and ambient temperature:

$$\underbrace{C}_{\frac{kcal}{h}} = \underbrace{h_{convective}}_{\frac{kcal}{h \times °C \times m^2}} \cdot \underbrace{(\overline{T}_{skin} - T_{ambient})}_{°C} \cdot \underbrace{A_{convective}}_{m^2}$$

Rate of convective heat loss | Convective heat-transfer coefficient | Mean skin temp | Ambient temp | Body surface area available for convective heat exchange

(59-4)

C is positive when the body loses heat and negative when it gains heat.

Whereas the radiative heat transfer coefficient ($h_{radiative}$) is constant, the convective coefficient ($h_{convective}$) is variable and can increase up to 5-fold when air velocity is high. Thus, even when ($T_{skin} - T_{ambient}$) is fixed, convective heat loss increases markedly as wind speed increases. In the absence of air movement, the air immediately overlying the skin warms as heat leaves the skin. As this warmer and lighter air rises off the skin, cooler ambient air replaces it and, in turn, is warmed by the skin. This is the process of **natural convection**. However, with forced air movement, such as by wind or a fan, the cooler "ambient" air replaces the warmer air overlying the skin more rapidly. This change increases the effective convective heat transfer from the skin, even though the temperature of the ambient air is unchanged. This is a process of **forced convection**, which underlies the **wind chill factor**.

Evaporation Humans can dissipate nearly all the heat produced during exercise by evaporating sweat from the skin surface. The evaporative rate is independent of the temperature gradient between skin and environment. Instead, it is proportional to the water vapor pressure gradient between skin and environment:

$$\underbrace{E}_{\frac{kcal}{h}} = \underbrace{h_{evaporative}}_{\frac{kcal}{h \times mmHg \times m^2}} \cdot \underbrace{(P_{skin} - P_{ambient})}_{mmHg} \cdot \underbrace{A_{evaporative}}_{m^2}$$

Rate of evaporative heat loss | Evaporative heat-transfer coefficient | H_2O vapor pressure of skin | H_2O vapor pressure of environment | Body surface area available for *evaporative* heat exchange

(59-5)

E is positive when the body loses heat by evaporation and negative when it gains heat by condensation.

The evaporation of 1 g of water removes ~0.58 kcal from the body. Because the body's sweat glands can deliver up to 30 g fluid/min or 1.8 L/hr to the skin surface, evaporation can remove 0.58 × 1800 g or ~1000 kcal/hr. Thus, under ideal conditions (i.e., when ambient humidity is sufficiently low to allow efficient evaporation), evaporation could theoretically remove nearly all the heat produced during heavy exercise. As with convection, increased air velocity over the skin increases the effective vapor pressure gradient between skin and the overlying air because of the faster movement of water vapor away from the skin.

The efficiency of heat transfer from the skin to the environment depends on both physiological and environmental factors. If ambient humidity is high, the gradient of water vapor pressure between skin and air will be low, thus slowing evaporation and increasing the body's tendency to accumulate excess heat produced during exercise. This phenomenon underlies the temperature humidity index (**heat index**). Conversely, if ambient humidity is low, as in the desert, net heat loss from the body by evaporation will occur readily, even when ambient temperature exceeds skin temperature and the body is gaining heat by radiation and convection.

When the body is immersed in water, nearly all heat exchange occurs by convection, because essentially no exchanges can occur by radiation or evaporation. Because of the high conductivity and thermal capacity of water, the heat transfer coefficient ($h_{convective}$) is ~100 times greater than that of air. Thus, rate of heat exchange underwater is much greater than it is in air. It is therefore not surprising that nearly all the deaths in the *Titanic* shipwreck disaster resulted from hypothermia in the cold Atlantic waters, rather than from drowning.

When heat gain exceeds heat loss, body core temperature rises

With a knowledge of the transfer coefficients—$h_{radiative}$ (Equation 59-3), $h_{convective}$ (Equation 59-4), and $h_{evaporative}$ (Equation 59-5)—and the gradients of temperature and water vapor pressure between the skin and environment, we can calculate the body heat fluxes (R, C, and E). Knowing M (computed from $\dot{V}_{O_2}$ by indirect calorimetry; see Chapter 49) and W (if any), we can use the heat balance equation (Equation 59-1) to calculate the **heat storage (S)**. From this value, we can predict the rate of change in mean body temperature:

$$\underbrace{\frac{\Delta \overline{T}_{body}}{\Delta t}}_{\substack{\text{Rate of} \\ \text{temperature} \\ \text{increase} \\ \frac{°C}{h}}} = \frac{\overbrace{Rate\ of\ heat\ storage}^{}}{\underbrace{0.83}_{\substack{\text{Specific} \\ \text{heat of} \\ \text{body} \\ \text{tissues}}} \cdot \underbrace{BW}_{\substack{\text{Body} \\ \text{weight}}}}_{\substack{kcal/h \\ [kcal/(kg°C)] \times kg}}$$

(59-6)

We can verify the accuracy of this predicted rate of change in $\overline{T}_{body}$ by comparing it to the $\overline{T}_{body}$ measured by direct thermometry, using a weighted average of the measured T_{core} and average T_{skin}.

The body has to deal with two types of heat loads that tend to make its temperature rise. In the heat balance equation (Equation 59-1), the term (M − W) constitutes an **internal heat load**. In contrast, the term (R + C + E)—normally representing a net heat loss—can represent an **external heat load** if either the radiation or convection terms are heat *gains* rather than heat *losses*. Thus, if we stand in the sun and $T_{radiant}$ exceeds $\overline{T}_{skin}$ (Equation 59-3), we experience a radiant heat load. If we stand in a hot sauna and $T_{ambient}$ exceeds $\overline{T}_{skin}$ (Equation 59-4), we experience a convective heat load. Clearly, both internal and external heat loads can result in net heat storage and thus a rise in body temperature. Changes in environmental temperature ($T_{radiant}$ and $T_{ambient}$) exert their influence from the *outside*, through the body surface. If, starting from relatively low values, $T_{radiant}$ or $T_{ambient}$ rises, at first the rate at which heat leaves the body decreases, so core temperature tends to rise. Further increases in environmental temperature produce a frank heat load rather than a loss.

Conversely, metabolism produces heat *inside* the body. For the athlete, all the terms of the heat balance equation are important because dissipating the thermal load is essential for prolonging exercise. The clinician must understand these principles to treat thermally related illnesses. For example, excessive heat exposure can lead to **heat exhaustion**, in which core temperature rises to as high as 39°C because the body cannot dissipate the heat load. The causes are dehydration (which reduces sweating) and hypovolemia (which reduces blood flow from muscle to core to skin). Heat exhaustion is the most common temperature-related abnormality in athletes. In more severe cases, excessive heat can lead to **heat stroke** (see the box on Heat Stroke), in which core temperature rises to 41°C or more, as a result of impaired thermoregulatory mechanisms.

Clothing insulates the body from the environment and limits heat transfer from the body to the environment

Placing one or more layers of clothing between the skin and the environment insulates the body and retards heat transfer between the core and the environment. In the presence of clothing, heat transfer from a warmer body to a cooler environment occurs by the same means as without clothing (i.e., radiation, conduction, convection, and evaporation), but from the clothing surface rather than from the skin surface. The insulating effect of clothing is described by the **clo unit**. By definition, one clo is the insulation necessary to maintain a resting person at a thermal steady state in comfort at 21°C with minimal air movement. Obviously, clo units increase with a greater area of skin coverage by clothing or with thicker clothing.

ACTIVE REGULATION OF HEAT TRANSFER

The body actively regulates its temperature by a feedback system that includes temperature sensors, afferent nerve fibers that carry sensory information to the brain, a hypothalamic control center, efferent nerve fibers that are prin-

cipally part of the autonomic nervous system, and thermal effectors that either control heat transfer between the body and environment or regulate the body's rate of heat production. This **active system** contrasts with the *passive system*.

Thermal sensors in the skin and in the body core (mainly the hypothalamus) respond to changes in theirlocal temperature

The body has specialized sensory neurons that provide the CNS with information about the body's thermal condition. These thermosensitive elements are free nerve endings that are distributed over the entire skin surface. These elements are also present within the body core, at particularly high densities in the preoptic area and anterior hypothalamus.

Skin receptors, although ideal for sensing changes in environmental temperature, do not serve well during exercise because internal temperatures would rise to intolerably high levels before the skin temperature rose to detect this excess heat. Body core thermoreceptors, in contrast, although ideal for detecting changes in core temperature, are inadequate for sensing changes in the environmental temperature. Because of the thermal inertia of the body's mass, the lag time in using body core sensors to detect externally induced changes in temperature would be too great to achieve effective regulation. Not surprisingly, then, the body is endowed with both peripheral and central thermoreceptors that are integrated within the CNS, to permit a rapid and effective balance of heat loss and heat production while maintaining body core temperature within relatively narrow limits.

Skin Thermoreceptors   The entire surface of the body has a network of sensory nerve endings that serve as thermoreceptors. Peripheral thermoreceptors fall into two categories—**warmth** receptors and **cold** receptors (Fig. 59-3). Each type is anatomically distinct, and each innervates definable warm-sensitive or cold-sensitive spots on the skin surface (see Chapter 15). Thermal discrimination varies over the surface of the body; it is coarsest on the body trunk and

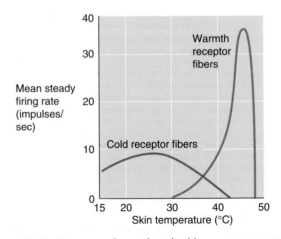

Figure 59-3   Response of warmth and cold receptors to temperature change.

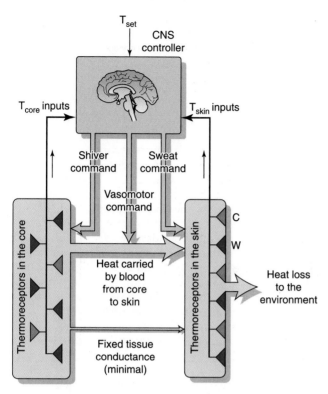

Figure 59-4 Model of negative feedback in temperature regulation.

Body core thermoreceptors are especially important during exercise, which is one of the few conditions in which the body's heat production and dissipation rates can differ dramatically and can lead to rapid changes in core temperature.

The hypothalamic center integrates thermal information and directs changes in efferent activity to modify heat transfer rates

Cooling or warming of the skin alters both the tonic and the phasic components of the activity of cold or warmth receptors (Fig. 59-4). The neural activity of these skin thermoreceptors travels through the spinal cord to the hypothalamus, which integrates thermal information from other parts of the body, including the hypothalamus, compares the prevailing thermal status with an idealized set of thermal conditions, and directs efferent commands to alter the rate of heat generation and to modify heat transfer rates within and from the body.

The skin receptors provide information mainly about environmental temperature, which affects the body's heat loss rate and could ultimately cause core temperature to change, if the body does not initiate the appropriate thermoregulatory responses to skin cooling or warming. Thus, reflex responses to changes in the average skin temperature may be thought of as **anticipatory** rather than negative feedback in nature. Moreover, it is impossible to regulate skin temperature because of the skin's exposure to the ambient environment. However, these anticipatory reflexes are essential elements for an effective thermoregulatory system because the body's thermal inertia is too great to rely on central receptors alone. For example, low skin temperature—enhanced by cutaneous vasoconstriction in the cold—ensures a rapid and continuous cold signal that maintains a drive for shivering and thus thermogenesis. Conversely, thermoregulatory responses to changes in core (i.e., hypothalamic) temperature, such as those that occur during exercise, exhibit **negative feedback**, inasmuch as they modify heat transfer rates that maintain the core temperature at its regulated level.

How do skin and core thermoreceptor inputs interact and how does the CNS integrate these inputs to produce appropriate thermoregulatory responses to both external and internal heat loads? The most plausible explanation is that signals from skin thermoreceptors change the *sensitivity* of the response to signals from core thermoreceptors. For example, in Figure 59-5 a decrease in core temperature produces an effector response (i.e., increased metabolic rate) that depends upon the level of input from skin cold thermoreceptors. Thus, the "gain" of the centrally induced metabolic response increases as skin temperature falls.

Thermal effectors include the cutaneous circulation, sweat glands, and skeletal muscles that are responsible for shivering

Figure 59-4 summarizes the three effectors of the thermoregulatory system. Adjusting the smooth muscle tone of cutaneous arterioles controls **blood flow**, and therefore heat flow, from the core to the skin surface, the primary

limbs and finest on the face, lips, and fingers. Increasing local temperature, up to 44°C to 46°C, causes **warmth receptors** to increase their steady firing rate (Fig. 59-3). **Cold receptors** characteristically increase their steady firing rate as local temperature decreases from ~40°C to 24°C to 28°C. In either case, a sustained temperature change (see Fig. 15-28) may cause a stable change in the sensor's firing rate (i.e., *tonic* or *static* response) or a temporary change (i.e., *phasic* or *dynamic* response).

Because of their location, skin thermoreceptors primarily provide the hypothalamic thermoregulatory center with information about *ambient temperature* (Fig. 59-4). As discussed later, they provide an anticipatory signal in conditions of rapidly changing ambient temperature and allow the autonomic nervous system to exert reflex thermoregulation. Information from skin thermoreceptors also travels through thalamic pathways to the cerebral cortex, thus providing the basis for conscious perception of the thermal environment and appreciation of thermal comfort. We can use this information, for example, to move from the sun to the shade when we sense that we are too hot.

Body Core Thermoreceptors Thermoreceptors are present in the brain, in the spinal cord, and perhaps in the muscles and major blood vessels. However, the hypothalamus clearly plays the major role in detecting changes in deep body temperature (Fig. 59-4). In the preoptic area and anterior hypothalamus (see Chapter 14), ~10% of neurons will show a positive temperature coefficient when local temperature is cycled over a range of 2°C to 4°C about the mean.

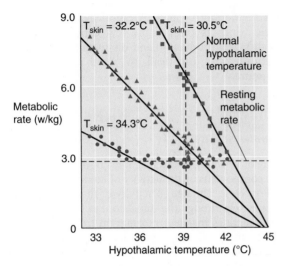

Figure 59-5 Thermoeffector responses. In these experiments on rabbits, the investigators implanted water-perfused thermodes to control the temperature of the preoptic/anterior hypothalamic area (x-axis) at three different skin temperatures (T_{skin}).

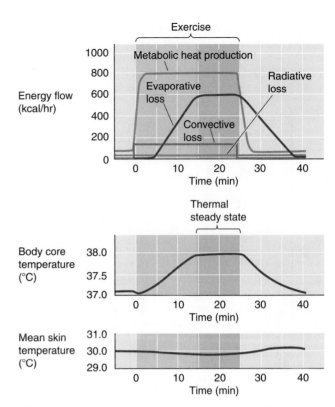

Figure 59-6 Whole-body heat balance during exercise.

site of heat dissipation to the environment. Over most of the skin, the autonomic nervous system controls cutaneous blood flow (see Chapter 24). When it is necessary to increase heat dissipation, active vasodilation can increase cutaneous blood flow up to 10-fold above the resting level. Conversely, when it is necessary to conserve heat in a cold environment, cutaneous vasoconstriction—mediated by sympathetic nerves—can elicit a relatively minor reduction in cutaneous blood flow, to half the resting rate. This vasoconstriction occurs at the expense of allowing skin temperature to drop closer to ambient temperature. Even with maximal vasoconstriction in effect, heat losses to a very cold environment do not fall to zero of the minimum tissue conductance.

With a moderate heat load, the autonomic response primarily increases the heat transfer rate from core to skin by increasing cutaneous blood flow. However, when the heat load is sufficiently great, the autonomic nervous system also activates the **eccrine sweat glands** (see Chapter 60), which secrete sweat onto the skin surface, thus elevating the partial pressure of water vapor there and promoting increased evaporation. The innervation of the secretory segment of the sweat gland is sympathetic, but it is unusual in that acetylcholine is the neurotransmitter (see Chapter 14).

When a cold stress is sufficiently great, the physiological response includes increasing heat production by involuntary, clonic, rhythmic contractions and relaxations of skeletal muscle. This **shivering** can double the metabolic rate for extended periods (hours) before fatigue occurs; for brief intervals, shivering can triple or quadruple the metabolic rate. Nonshivering thermogenesis in newborn infants and hibernating animals can also produce substantial amounts of heat, primarily in brown fat cells (see Chapter 57).

HYPERTHERMIA, HYPOTHERMIA, AND FEVER

Exercise raises heat production, followed by a matching rise in heat loss, but at the cost of a steady-state hyperthermia of exercise

At the onset of muscular exercise, the rate of heat production increases in proportion to the exercise intensity and exceeds the current rate of heat dissipation, thus causing heat storage and a rise in core temperature (Fig. 59-6). Hypothalamic thermoreceptors sense this increase in core temperature. The hypothalamic integrator compares this temperature signal with a reference signal, detects an error between the two, and directs neural output that activates heat dissipation (Fig. 59-4). As a result, skin blood flow and sweating increase as core temperature rises. These processes thus promote an increase in the rate of heat transfer from core to environment and slow the rate of temperature rise. At some point, the rising rate of heat dissipation equals the rate of heat production, and the rate of heat storage falls to zero. However, the now elevated steady-state core temperature persists as long as exercise continues.

The steady-state core temperature during exercise is not "regulated" at the elevated level; rather, the hyperthermia of exercise is the consequence of the initial imbalance between rates of heat production and dissipation. This imbalance is unavoidable because temperature must increase to provide the error signal that culminates in increased heat dissipation and because the response is not instantaneous. In Figure 59-6, metabolic heat production rises rapidly to its maximal level. However, evaporative heat loss increases only after a delay and then rises slowly to its maximal level, driven by increasing body temperature. The result is net storage during the first 15 minutes. The slight initial drop in core temperature at the onset of exercise is caused by flushing out of blood from the cooler peripheral circulation when the muscle and skin beds vasodilate in response to the onset of exercise. In addition, mean skin temperature *decreases* during exercise because of the increased evaporative cooling of the skin caused by sweating.

Hyperthermia or hypothermia occurs when heat transfer from or to the environment overwhelms the body's regulatory capacity

Although the body's temperature regulating machinery is impressive, its capabilities are not limitless. Any factor that causes sufficiently large shifts—either positive or negative—in the rate of heat storage (Equation 59-1) could result in progressive hyperthermia or hypothermia (Equation 59-6). Because humans must operate within a fairly narrow core temperature range, such temperature changes could become life-threatening.

The most common environmental condition that results in excessive **hyperthermia** is prolonged exposure to heat and high ambient humidity, particularly when accompanied by physical activity (i.e., elevated heat production rate). The ability to dissipate heat by *radiation* falls as the radiant temperature of nearby objects increases (Equation 59-3), and the ability to dissipate heat by *convection* falls as ambient temperature increases (Equation 59-4). When ambient temperature reaches the mid-30s (°C), evaporation becomes the only effective avenue for heat dissipation. However, high ambient humidity reduces the skin-to-environment gradient for water vapor pressure and thus reduces *evaporation* (Equation 59-5). The combined reduction of heat loss by these three pathways can markedly increase the rate of heat storage (Equation 59-6) and can cause progressive hyperthermia.

It is uncommon for radiative or convective heat gain to cause hyperthermia under conditions of low ambient humidity, because the body has a high capacity for dissipating the absorbed heat by evaporation. Radiative heat gain can be excessively high during full exposure to the desert sun or during exposure to heat sources such as large furnaces. The most obvious protections against radiative hyperthermia are avoiding radiant sources (e.g., sitting in the shade) and covering the skin with loose clothing. Loose clothing screens the radiation while allowing air circulation and thereby maintaining evaporative and convective losses.

The most common environmental condition causing excessive **hypothermia** is prolonged immersion in cold water. Water has a specific heat per unit volume that is approximately 4000 times that of air and a thermal conductivity that is approximately 25 times that of air. Both properties contribute to a convective heat transfer coefficient ($h_{convective}$ in Equation 59-4) that is approximately 100-fold greater in water than it is in air. The $h_{convective}$ is ~200 kcal/(m²/hr/°C) at rest in still water but ~500 kcal/(m²/hr/°C) while swimming. The body's physiological defenses against hypothermia include peripheral vasoconstriction (increasing

insulation) and shivering (increasing heat production), but even these measures do not prevent hypothermia during prolonged exposure because of water's high thermal conductivity. A thick layer of insulating fat retards heat loss to the water and postpones or even prevents hypothermia during prolonged exposures. Endurance swimmers used this knowledge to protect themselves when they applied a thick layer of grease to the skin surface (now, more commonly, they don a wet suit) before an event. Herman Melville noted this principle in 1851, when he referred to the low thermal conductivity of fat:

> For the whale is indeed wrapt up in his blubber as in a real blanket. . . . It is by reason of this cozy blanketing that the whale is enabled to keep himself comfortable in all seas. . . . this great monster, to whom corporeal warmth is as indispensable as it is to man. . . .
>
> — *Moby Dick*

Like blubber, clothing adds insulation between skin and environment and thus reduces heat loss during exposure to the cold. The more skin one covers, the more one reduces the surface area for direct heat loss from skin to environment by convection and radiation. Adding *layers* of clothing increases the resistance of heat flow by trapping air, which is an excellent insulator. During heat exposure, the major avenue for heat loss is evaporation of sweat. Because evaporation also depends on the surface area available, the amount of clothing should be minimized. Wetting the clothing increases the rate of heat loss from the skin because water is a better conductor than air. Water also can evaporate from the clothing surface, thereby removing heat from the outer layers and increasing the temperature gradient (and rate of heat loss) from skin to clothing.

Heat Stroke

As body core temperature rises, excessive cutaneous vasodilation can lead to a fall in arterial pressure (see Chapter 25) and therefore to a decrease in brain perfusion. As core temperature approaches 41°C, confusion and, ultimately, loss of consciousness occur. Excessive hyperthermia (>41°C) leads to the clinical condition known as **heat stroke**. High temperature can cause fibrinolysis and consumption of clotting factors and thus disseminated intravascular coagulation (DIC), which results in uncontrolled vascular thrombosis and hemorrhage. Heat-induced damage to the cell membranes of skeletal and myocardial muscle leads to rhabdomyolysis (in which disrupted muscle cells release their intracellular contents, including myoglobin, into the circulation) and myocardial necrosis. Cell damage may also cause acute hepatic insufficiency and pancreatitis. Renal function, already compromised by low renal blood flow, may be further disrupted by the high plasma levels of myoglobin. Ultimately, the CNS is affected by the combination of high brain temperature, DIC, and metabolic disturbances.

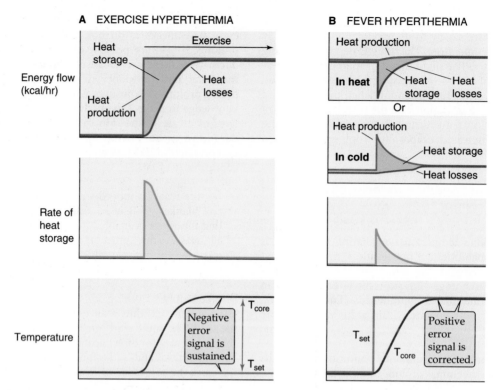

Figure 59-7 Exercise hyperthermia versus fever. **A,** The top panel shows how, during exercise, heat production temporarily exceeds heat loss, thus resulting in net heat storage. The middle panel shows that the rate of heat storage is highest initially and falls to zero in the new steady state. Finally, the bottom panel shows that as body core temperature rises away from the set-point, the error signal gradually increases. In the new steady state, the error signal is maximal and sustained. **B,** The top two panels show how, during fever, net heat storage can occur because of either reduced heat loss or increased heat production. The third panel from the top shows that, as in exercise, the rate of heat storage is highest initially. The bottom panel shows that as body core temperature rises, it approaches the new elevated set-point. Thus, the error signal is initially maximal and gradually decreases to zero in the new steady state.

Fever, unlike other types of hyperthermia, reflects an increase in the set point for temperature regulation

Fever is a *regulated* elevation of core temperature resulting from effects associated with infection or disease. Fever is caused by the action of circulating cytokines called **pyrogens,** which are low-molecular-weight polypeptides produced by cells of the immune system. As for the hyperthermia of exercise, fever begins when heat production temporarily exceeds heat dissipation. However, fever differs from other hyperthermias in that the hypothalamus actively regulates core temperature to an elevated set point.

Figure 59-7 illustrates the basic differences between the events leading to exercise hyperthermia and those leading to fever. During the genesis of exercise hyperthermia (Fig. 59-7A), the rate of heat production increases to more than the rate of heat dissipation for a period and causes net heat storage. Moreover, the temperature set point (T_{set}) is unchanged, and thus the error signal gradually increases to a new, sustained level. During the genesis of a fever (Fig. 59-7B), T_{set} suddenly increases to a value higher than the normal temperature, so the integrator interprets the normal temperature as being lower than the new T_{set}. The fever is an

appropriate response to this condition and develops as the heat loss rate from the body falls or the heat production rate rises until such time as core temperature increases to the new "regulated" level. Thus, the error signal is initially large but becomes smaller as the fever develops. In the new steady state, core temperature remains elevated until the signals responsible for the fever (i.e., pyrogens) subside and T_{set} returns to normal.

The subjective assessments of thermal comfort support this description. During exercise, one perceives the rise in core temperature as body heating and may choose to remove clothing to cool the body. During the onset of a fever, however, the individual feels cold and may choose to put on additional clothing and warm the body. If fever strikes when the patient is in a warm environment in which the cutaneous vessels are dilated (Fig. 59-7B, top panel), the response to the T_{set} increase will be to vasoconstrict, which decreases heat loss. In contrast, if the patient is in a cold environment in which the cutaneous vessels are already constricted (Fig. 59-7B, second panel), the response will be to shiver.

Figure 59-8 summarizes the responses to fever-producing stimuli. Macrophages and, to a lesser extent, lymphocytes release cytokines into the circulation in response to a variety of infectious and inflammatory stimuli. Cytokines, the

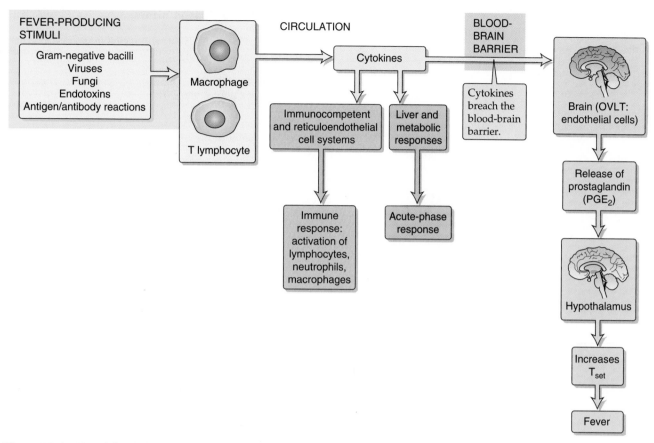

Figure 59-8 Host defense response.

messenger molecules of the immune system, are a diverse group of proteins involved in numerous tasks in the host defense response. The first is the *immune response* to foreign substances including stimulation of T-lymphocyte proliferation, natural killer cells, and antibody production. The second is the *acute-phase response* to foreign substances, a diffuse collection of nonspecific host reactions to infection or trauma. Finally, cytokines may act as endogenous pyrogens (Table 59-3). However, no one cytokine, administered experimentally, can fully mimic the temperature increase that occurs during fever. Fever production may occur through a cascade that is initiated when interleukin (IL-1β), for example, interacts with the endothelial cells in a leaky portion of the blood-brain barrier (see Chapter 11) located in the capillary bed of the *organum vasculosum laminae terminalis* (OVLT). The OVLT is highly vascular tissue that lies in the wall of the third ventricle (above the optic chiasm) in the brain. IL-1β triggers endothelial cells within the OVLT to release prostaglandin E_2 (see Chapter 3), which then diffuses into the adjacent hypothalamus and—in a manner not yet understood—elevates T_{set} and initiates the febrile response.

The value of fever in fighting infection is still debated. A popular hypothesis is that the elevated temperature enhances the host's response to infection. This view is supported

Table 59-3 Endogenous Pyrogens

Pyrogen	Symbol
Interleukin 1α	IL-1α
Interleukin 1β	IL-1β
Interleukin 6	IL-6
Interleukin 8	IL-8
Tumor necrosis factor α	TNF-α
Tumor necrosis factor β	TNF-β
Macrophage inflammatory protein 1α	MIP-1α
Macrophage inflammatory protein 1β	MIP-1β
Interferon α	INF-α
Interferon β	INF-β
Interferon γ	INF-γ

by the in vitro observation that the rate of T-lymphocyte proliferation in response to interleukins is many-fold higher at 39ºC than it is at 37ºC.

REFERENCES

Books and Reviews

Blatteis CM, Sehic E: Fever: How may circulating pyrogens signal the brain? News Physiol Sci 1997; 12:1-9.

Block BA: Thermogenesis in muscle. Annu Rev Physiol 1994; 56:535-577.

Horowitz M: Do cellular heat acclimation responses modulate central thermoregulatory activity? News Physiol Sci 1998; 13:218-225.

Lee-Chiong TL, Stitt JT Jr: Disorders of temperature regulation: Compr Ther 1995; 21:697-704.

Simon HB: Current concepts: Hyperthermia. N Engl J Med 1993; 329:483-487.

CHAPTER 60

EXERCISE PHYSIOLOGY AND SPORTS SCIENCE

Steven S. Segal

Physical exercise is often the greatest stress that the body encounters in the course of daily life. Skeletal muscle typically accounts for 30% to 50% of the total body mass. Thus, with each bout of muscular activity, the body must make rapid, integrated adjustments at the level of cells and organ systems—and must modulate these adjustments over time. The subdiscipline of exercise physiology and sports science focuses on the integrated responses that enable the conversion of chemical energy into mechanical work. To understand these interdependent processes, one must appreciate where regulation occurs, the factors that limit performance, and the adaptations that occur with repetitive use.

The cross-bridge cycle that underlies contraction of skeletal muscle requires energy in the form of ATP (see Chapter 9). To supply this energy, skeletal muscle converts ~25% of the energy stored in foodstuffs into mechanical work. The rest appears as heat as a result of the inefficiencies of the biochemical reactions (see Chapter 58). Thus, the dissipation of this heat is central to cardiovascular function, fluid balance, and the ability to sustain physical effort—an example of an integrated organ system response. Moreover, because muscle stores of ATP, phosphocreatine (PCr), and glycogen are limited, the ability to sustain physical activity requires another set of integrated cellular and organ system responses to supply O_2 and energy sources to active muscles.

MOTOR UNITS AND MUSCLE FUNCTION

In Chapter 9, the cellular and molecular physiology of skeletal muscle contraction is discussed. In this major section, we examine the way in which these smaller elements integrate into a contracting whole muscle.

The motor unit is the functional element of muscle contraction

A typical skeletal muscle receives innervation from ~100 somatic motor neurons. The **motor unit** consists of a single motor neuron and all the muscle fibers that it activates.

When the motor neuron generates an action potential, all the fibers in the motor unit fire simultaneously. Thus, the fineness of control for movement varies with the **innervation ratio**—the number of muscle fibers per motor neuron. As discussed later, the small motor units that are recruited during sustained activity contain a high proportion of type I muscle fibers, which are highly oxidative and resistant to fatigue. In contrast, the large motor units that are recruited for brief periods—for rapid, powerful activity—typically consist of type IIa and IIb (see Chapter 9) muscle fibers, which are glycolytic and are much more susceptible to fatigue.

Within a whole muscle, muscle fibers of each motor unit intermingle with those of other motor units so extensively that—in a volume of muscle that contains 100 muscle fibers—nerve endings from perhaps 50 different motor neurons synapse on the 100 end plates. Within some muscles, the fibers of a motor unit are constrained to discrete compartments. This anatomical organization enables different regions of a muscle to exert force in somewhat different directions, thereby enabling more precise control of movement.

Muscle force rises with the recruitment of motor units and an increase in their firing frequency

During contraction, the force exerted by a muscle depends on (1) how many motor units are recruited and (2) how frequently each of the active motor neurons fire action potentials. Motor units are recruited in a progressive order, from the smallest (i.e., fewest number of muscle fibers) and therefore the weakest motor units to the largest and strongest. This intrinsic behavior of motor unit recruitment is known as the **size principle** and reflects inherent differences in the biophysical properties of respective motor neurons. For a given amount of excitatory input (i.e., depolarizing synaptic current; I_{syn} in Fig. 60-1), a neuronal cell body with smaller volume and surface area has a higher membrane input resistance. Therefore, the depolarizing voltage in a neuron with a smaller neuronal cell body rises to threshold more quickly than in a neuron with a larger cell body (Fig. 60-1). Because the neurons with the small cell bodies tend to innervate a small number of slow-twitch (type I) muscle

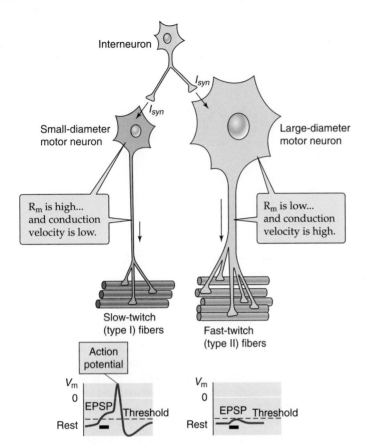

Figure 60-1 The size principle for motor units. Small motor neurons are more excitable, conduct action potentials more slowly, and excite fewer fibers that tend to be slow twitch (type I). Conversely, large motor neurons are less excitable, conduct action potentials more rapidly, and excite many fibers that tend to be fast twitch (type II). EPSP, excitatory postsynaptic potential. I_{syn}, depolarizing synaptic current; V_m, membrane potential. *(Adapted from Kandel ER, Schwartz JH, Jessell TM. Principles of Neural Science, 4th ed. New York: McGraw-Hill, 2000.)*

fibers, the motor units with the greatest resistance to fatigue are the first to be recruited. Conversely, the neurons with the larger cell bodies tend to innervate a larger number of fast-twitch (type II) fibers, so the largest and most fatigable motor units are the last to be recruited. Because the relative timing of action potentials in different motor units is asynchronous, the force developed by individual motor units integrates into a smooth contraction. As a muscle relaxes, the firing of respective motor units diminishes in reverse order.

At levels of force production lower than the upper limit of recruitment, gradations in force are accomplished through concurrent changes in the number of active motor units and the firing rate of those that have been recruited—**rate coding**. Once all the motor units in a muscle have been recruited, any further increase in force results from an increase in firing rate. The relative contribution of motor unit recruitment and rate coding varies among muscles. In some cases, recruitment is maximal by the time muscle force reaches ~50% of maximum, whereas in others, recruitment continues until the muscle reaches nearly 90% of maximal force.

In addition to the intrinsic membrane properties of motor neurons (i.e., the size principle), other neurons that originate in the brainstem project to the motor neurons and

release the neuromodulatory neurotransmitters serotonin and norepinephrine (see Fig. 13-6). For example, this neuromodulatory input, acting on the motor neurons of small, slow-twitch motor units, can promote self-sustained levels of firing of the motor neurons during the maintenance of posture. In contrast, the withdrawal of this excitatory neuromodulatory input during sleep promotes muscle relaxation. Thus, the brain can control the overall gain of a pool of motor neurons.

Compared with type I motor units, type IIb units are faster and stronger but more fatigable

Within a given motor unit, each muscle fiber is of the same **functional** type. As summarized in Tables 9-1 and 9-2, the three muscle fiber types—type I, type IIa, and type IIb—differ in contractile and regulatory proteins, the content of myoglobin (and thus color) and mitochondria and glycogen, and the metabolic pathways used to generate ATP (i.e., oxidative versus glycolytic metabolism). These biochemical properties determine a range of functional parameters, including (1) speeds of contraction and relaxation, (2) maximal force, and (3) susceptibility to fatigue (Fig. 60-2).

In response to an action potential evoked through the motor axon, **slow-twitch** (type I) motor units (top row of Fig. 60-2A) require relatively long times to develop tension and return to rest. In contrast, **fast-twitch** (types IIa and IIb) motor units exhibit relatively short contraction and relaxation times (top row of Fig. 60-2B, C). Accordingly, during repetitive stimulation (middle row of Fig. 60-2), slow-twitch motor units summate to a fused tetanus at lower stimulation frequencies than do fast-twitch motor units. Indeed, the α motor neurons in the spinal cord that drive slow motor units fire at frequencies of 10 to 50 Hz, whereas those that drive fast motor units fire at frequencies ranging from 30 Hz to more than 100 Hz.

The maximal force that can develop per cross-sectional area of muscle tissue is constant across fiber types (~25 N/cm²). Therefore, the ability of different motor units to develop active force is directly proportional to the number and diameter of fibers each motor unit contains. In accord with the innervation ratios of motor units, peak force production (middle row of Fig. 60-2) increases from type I motor units (used for fine control of movement) to type II motor units (recruited during more intense activities).

The susceptibility to fatigue of a motor unit depends on the metabolic profile of its muscle fibers. The red type I muscle fibers have greater mitochondria content and can rely largely on the aerobic metabolism of sugars and lipid for energy because they are well supplied with capillaries for delivery of O_2 and nutrients. Type I motor units, although smaller in size (and innervation ratio), are recruited during sustained activity of moderate intensity and are highly resistant to fatigue (bottom row of Fig. 60-2A). In contrast, the larger type II motor units are recruited less often—during brief periods of intense activity—and rely to a greater extent on short-term energy stores (e.g., glycogen stored within the muscle fiber). Among type II motor units, **type IIa** motor units have a greater mitochondrial content, a larger capacity for aerobic energy metabolism, a greater O_2 supply, and a

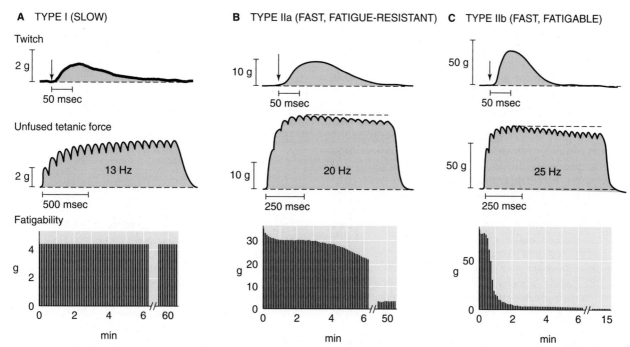

Figure 60-2 **A** to **C,** Properties of fiber types (i.e., motor units in gastrocnemius muscle). The *top row* shows the tension developed during single twitches for each of the muscle types; the *arrows* indicate the time of the electrical stimulus. The *middle row* shows the tension developed during an unfused tetanus at the indicated stimulus frequency (pps, pulses per second). The *bottom row* shows the degree to which each of the fiber types can sustain force during continuous stimulation. The time scales become progressively larger from the top to bottom rows, with a break in the bottom row. In addition, the tension scales become progressively larger from *left* (fewer fibers per motor unit) to *right* (more fibers per motor unit). *(Data from Burke RE, Levine DN, Tsairis P, et al. J Physiol 1977; 234:723–748.)*

higher endurance capacity and hence are classified as **fast fatigue-resistant units** (bottom row of Fig. 60-2B). In contrast, **type IIb** motor units have greater capacity for rapid energy production through nonoxidative (i.e., anaerobic) glycolysis, so they can produce rapid and powerful contractions. However, type IIb units tire more rapidly and are therefore classified as **fast fatigable units** (bottom row of Fig. 60-2C).

As external forces stretch muscle, series elastic elements contribute a larger fraction of total tension

As sarcomeres contract, some of their force acts laterally—through membrane-associated and transmembrane proteins—on the extracellular matrix and connective tissue that surrounds each muscle fiber. Ultimately, the force is transmitted to bone, typically (but not always) through a tendinous insertion. The structural elements that transmit force from the cross-bridges to the skeleton comprise the **series elastic elements** of the muscle and behave as a spring with a characteristic stiffness. Stretching resting muscle causes **passive tension** to increase exponentially with length (see Fig. 9-9C). Thus, muscle stiffness increases with length. During an **isometric contraction** (see Chapter 9), when the external length of a muscle (or muscle fiber) is held constant, the sarcomeres shorten at the expense of stretching the series

elastic elements. An isometric contraction can occur at modest levels of force development, such as holding a cup of coffee, as well as during maximal force development, such as when opposing wrestlers push and pull against each other, with neither gaining ground. Physical activity typically involves contractions in which muscles are shortening and lengthening, as well as periods during which muscle fibers are contracting isometrically.

During cyclic activity such as running, muscles undergo a stretch-shorten cycle that may increase total tension while decreasing active tension. For example, as the calf muscles relax as the foot lands and decelerates, the series elastic elements of the calf muscles (e.g., the Achilles tendon, connective tissue within muscles) are stretched and develop increased passive tension (see Fig. 9-9C). Thus, when the calf muscles contract to begin the next cycle, they start from a higher *passive* tension and thus use a smaller increment in *active* tension to reach a higher *total* tension. This increased force helps to propel the runner forward.

In a **concentric** contraction (e.g., climbing stairs), the force developed by the cross-bridges exceeds the external load, and the sarcomeres shorten. During a concentric contraction, a muscle performs **positive work** (force × distance) and produces power (work/time; see Chapter 9). As shown in Figure 9-9E, the muscle achieves peak power at relatively moderate loads (30% to 40% of isometric tension) and velocities (30% to 40% of maximum shortening velocity).

The capacity of a muscle to perform positive work determines physical performance. For example, a stronger muscle can shorten more rapidly against a given load, and a muscle that is metabolically adapted to a particular activity can sustain performance for a longer period of time before it succumbs to fatigue.

In an **eccentric** contraction (e.g., descending stairs), the force developed by the cross-bridges is less than the imposed load, and the sarcomeres lengthen. During an eccentric contraction, the muscle performs **negative work**, thus providing a brake to decelerate the applied force being applied, and absorbs power. Eccentric contractions can occur with light loads, such as lowering a cup of coffee to the table, as well as with much heavier loads, such as decelerating after jumping off a bench onto the floor. At the same absolute level of *total* force production, eccentric contractions—with increasingly stretched sarcomeres—develop less active tension than do concentric or isometric contractions. Conversely, the passive tension developed by the series elastic elements make a greater contribution to total tension. As a result, the tension generated eccentrically is greater than that generated isometrically. When the external force stretches the muscle sufficiently, all the tension is passive, and the limit is the breaking point (see Fig. 19-9B) of the series elastic elements. Thus, eccentric contractions are much more likely than isometric or isotonic contractions to damage muscle fibers and connective tissue.

The action of a muscle depends on the axis of its fibers and its origin and insertion on the skeleton

In addition to the contractile and metabolic properties of muscle fibers discussed earlier, two anatomical features determine the characteristics of the force produced by a muscle. The first anatomical determinant of muscle function is the arrangement of fibers with respect to the axis of force production (i.e., the angle of pennation). With other determinants of performance (e.g., fiber type and muscle mass) being equal, muscles that have a relatively small number of long fibers oriented parallel to the axis of shortening (e.g. the sartorius muscle of the thigh, Fig. 60-3A, top) shorten more rapidly. Indeed, the more sarcomeres are arranged in *series*, the more rapidly the two ends of the muscle will approach each other. In contrast, muscles that have many short fibers at an angle to the axis (e.g. the soleus muscle of the calf, Fig. 60-3A, bottom) develop more force. Indeed, the greater the number of fibers (and sarcomeres) in *parallel* with each other, the greater is the total cross-sectional area for developing force.

The second anatomical determinant of limb movement consists of the locations of the origin and insertion of the muscle to the skeleton. Consider, for example, the action of the brachialis muscle on the elbow joint. The distance between the insertion of the muscle on the ulna and the joint's center of rotation is D, which may be 5 cm. The **torque** that the muscle produces on the joint is the *component* of total muscle force that is perpendicular to the ulna, multiplied by D (Fig. 60-3B). An equivalent definition is that *torque* is the product of the total muscle force multiplied by the **moment arm**, which is the length of the line segment

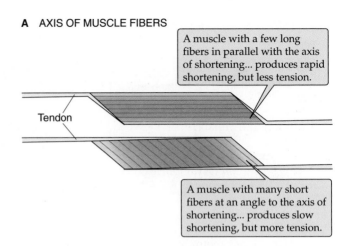

A AXIS OF MUSCLE FIBERS

A muscle with a few long fibers in parallel with the axis of shortening... produces rapid shortening, but less tension.

Tendon

A muscle with many short fibers at an angle to the axis of shortening... produces slow shortening, but more tension.

B ORIGIN AND INSERTION OF A MUSCLE

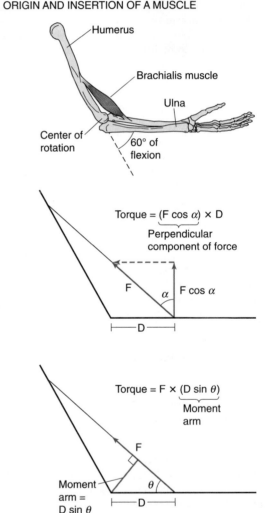

Humerus

Brachialis muscle

Ulna

Center of rotation

60° of flexion

Torque = (F cos α) × D
Perpendicular component of force

F

α

F cos α

D

Torque = F × (D sin θ)
Moment arm

F

Moment arm = D sin θ

θ

D

Figure 60-3 **A** and **B,** Determinants of the mechanical action of a muscle.

that runs perpendicular to the muscle and through the center of rotation (Fig. 60-3B). As we flex our elbow, the moment arm is constantly changing, and muscle force changes as well. For this joint, we achieve maximum torque at 60 degrees of flexion.

Fluid and energetically efficient movements require learning

To perform a desired movement—whether playing the piano or serving a tennis ball—the nervous system must activate a combination of muscles with the appropriate contractile properties, recruit motor units in defined patterns, and thereby create suitable mechanical interactions among body segments. When we perform movements with uncertainty—as in learning a new skill—actions tend to be stiff because of concurrent recruitment of motor units in antagonistic muscles that produce force in opposite directions. Such superfluous muscle fiber activity also increases the energy requirements for the activity. Even in someone who is skilled, the fatigue of small motor units leads to the recruitment of larger motor units in the attempt to maintain activity, but with loss of fine control and greater energy expenditure. With learning, recruitment patterns become refined and coordinated, and muscle fibers adapt to the task. Thus, movements become fluid and more energetically efficient, as exemplified by highly trained musicians and athletes who can make difficult maneuvers appear almost effortless.

Strength versus endurance training differentially alters the properties of motor units

The firing pattern of the α motor neuron—over time—ultimately determines the contractile and metabolic properties of the muscle fibers in the corresponding motor unit. This principle was demonstrated elegantly by classic experiments in which the motor nerve to a muscle consisting primarily of fast motor units was cut and switched with that of a muscle consisting primarily of slow motor units. As the axons regenerated and the muscles recovered contractile function over several weeks, the fast muscle became progressively slower and more fatigue resistant, whereas the slow muscle became faster and more susceptible to fatigue. Varying the pattern of efferent nerve impulses through chronic stimulation of implanted electrodes elicits similar changes in muscle properties. A corollary of this principle is that physical activity leads to adaptation only in those motor units that are actually recruited during the activity.

The effects of physical activity on motor unit physiology depend on the intensity and duration of the exercise. In general, sustained periods of low to moderate intensity performed several times per week—**endurance training**—result in a greater oxidative capacity of muscle fibers and are manifested by increases in O_2 delivery, capillary supply, and mitochondrial content. These adaptations reduce the susceptibility of the affected muscle fibers to fatigue. The lean and slender build of long-distance runners reflects highly oxidative muscle fibers of relatively small diameter that promote O_2 and CO_2 diffusion between capillaries and mitochondria for high levels of aerobic energy production. Further, the high ratio of surface area to volume of the slender body also facilitates cooling of the body during prolonged activity and in hot environments.

In contrast, brief sets of high-intensity contractions performed several times per week—**strength training**—result in motor units that can produce more force and can shorten

against a given load at greater velocity by increasing the amount of contractile protein. The hypertrophied muscles of sprinters and weight lifters exemplify this type of adaptation, which relies more on rapid, anaerobic sources of energy production.

CONVERSION OF CHEMICAL ENERGY TO MECHANICAL WORK

At rest, skeletal muscle has a low metabolic rate. In response to contractile activity, the energy consumption of skeletal muscle can easily rise more than 100-fold. The body meets this increased energy demand by mobilizing energy stores both locally from muscle glycogen and triacylglycerols and systemically from liver glycogen and adipose tissue triacylglycerols. The integrated physiological response to exercise involves the delivery of sufficient O_2 and fuel to ensure that the rate of **ATP** synthesis rises in parallel with the rate of ATP breakdown. Indeed, skeletal muscle precisely regulates the ratio of ATP to ADP even with these large increases in ATP turnover.

Physical performance can be defined in terms of power (work/time), speed, or endurance. Skeletal muscle has three energy systems, each designed to support a particular type of performance (Fig. 60-4). For power events, which typically last a few seconds or less (e.g., hitting a ball with a bat), the immediate energy sources include ATP and **PCr**. For spurts of activity that last several seconds to a minute (e.g., sprinting 100 m), muscles rely primarily on the rapid nonoxidative breakdown of carbohydrate stored as muscle glycogen to form ATP. For activities that last 2 minutes or longer but have low power requirements (e.g., jogging several kilometers), the generation of ATP through the oxidation of fat and glucose derived from the circulation becomes increasingly important. Next I consider the key metabolic pathways for producing the energy that enables skeletal muscle to have such a tremendous dynamic range of activity.

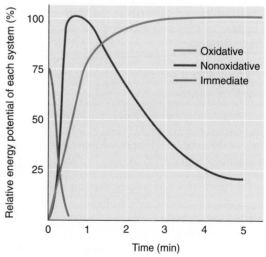

Figure 60-4 Energy sources for muscle contraction. (*Modified from Edington DW, Edgerton VR: The Biology of Physical Activity. Boston: Houghton Mifflin, 1976.*)

ATP and phosphocreatine provide immediate but limited energy

At the onset of exercise, or during the transition to a higher intensity of contractile activity, the immediate energy sources are ATP and PCr. As for any other cell, muscle cells break down ATP to ADP and inorganic phosphate (P_i) and release ~11.5 kcal/mol of free energy (ΔG) under physiological conditions:

$$ATP \rightarrow ADP + P_i + \Delta G \qquad (60\text{-}1)$$

Muscle cells rapidly regenerate ATP from PCr in a reaction that is catalyzed by **creatine kinase**:

$$ADP + PCr \xrightarrow{\text{creatine kinase}} ATP + Creatine \qquad (60\text{-}2)$$

Resting skeletal muscle cells contain 5 to 6 mmol/kg of ATP but 25 to 30 mmol/kg of PCr—representing nearly 5-fold more energy. These two energy stores are sufficient to support intense contractile activity only for a few seconds. When rates of ATP breakdown (Equation 60-1) are high, ADP levels (normally very low) increase and can actually interfere with muscle contraction. Under such conditions, **adenylate kinase** (also known as **myokinase**) transfers the second phosphate group from one ADP to another and thereby regenerates ATP:

$$ADP + ADP \xrightarrow{\text{adenylate kinase}} ATP + AMP \qquad (60\text{-}3)$$

The foregoing reaction is limited by the initial pool of ADP, which is small. In contrast, creatine kinase (Equation 60-2) so effectively buffers ATP that $[ATP]_i$ changes very little. Although changes in $[ATP]_i$ cannot provide an effective signal to stimulate metabolic pathways of energy production, the products of ATP hydrolysis—P_i, ADP, and AMP—are powerful signals.

The high-energy phosphates ATP + PCr are historically referred to as **phosphagens** and are recognized as the immediate energy supply because they are readily available, albeit for only several seconds (Fig. 60-4). This role is of particular importance at the onset of exercise and during transitions to more intense activity, before other metabolic pathways have time to respond.

Anaerobic glycolysis provides a rapid but self-limited source of ATP

When high-intensity exercise continues for more than several seconds, the breakdown of ATP and PCr is followed almost instantly by the accelerated breakdown of intramuscular glycogen to glucose and then to lactate. This anaerobic metabolism of glucose has the major advantage of providing energy quickly to meet the increased metabolic demands of an intense workload, even before O_2, glucose, or fatty acid delivery from blood increases. However, because of the low ATP yield of this pathway, muscle rapidly depletes its glycogen stores and thereby limits intense activity to durations of ~1 minute (Fig. 60-4).

Muscle fibers store 300 to 400 g of carbohydrate in the form of glycogen and, particularly in the case of type II fibers, are rich in the enzymes required for glycogenolysis and glycolysis. In **glycogenolysis**, phosphorylase breaks down glycogen to glucose-1-phosphate. Activation of the sympathetic nervous system during exercise elevates levels of epinephrine and promotes the breakdown of muscle glycogen. Subsequently, phosphoglucomutase converts glucose-1-phosphate to glucose-6-phosphate (G6P). Muscle fibers can also take up blood-borne glucose using the GLUT4 transporter (see Chapter 58) and use hexokinase to phosphorylate it to G6P. Intracellular glycogen is more important than blood-borne glucose in rapidly contributing G6P for entry into **glycolysis**—breakdown of glucose to pyruvate (see Fig. 59-6A).

In the absence of O_2, or when glycolysis generates pyruvate more rapidly than the mitochondria can oxidize it (see later), muscle cells can divert pyruvate to lactic acid, which readily dissociates into H^+ and lactate. The overall process generates two ATP molecules/glucose:

$$\underset{\text{Glucose}}{C_6H_{12}O_6} + 2\,ADP + 2\,P_i \rightarrow \underset{\text{Lactate}}{2\,C_3H_5O_3^-}$$
$$+\ 2\,ATP + 2\,H^+ + heat \qquad (60\text{-}4)$$

This anaerobic regeneration of ATP through breakdown of intramuscular glycogen, although faster than oxidative metabolism, captures only a fraction of the energy stored in glucose. Moreover, the process is self-limiting because the H^+ generated from the dissociation of lactic acid can lower pH_i from 7.1 to nearly 6.2, a process that inhibits glycolysis, impairs the contractile process, and thereby contributes to muscle fatigue.

Oxidation of glucose, lactate, and fatty acids provides a slower but long-term source of ATP

The body stores only a small amount of O_2 in the blood, and the cardiovascular and respiratory systems require 1 to 2 minutes to increase O_2 delivery to muscle to support oxidative metabolism. Endurance training speeds these adjustments. Nevertheless, before the increase in O_2 delivery is complete, muscle must rely on the immediate release of energy from ATP and PCr, as well as anaerobic glycolysis, as just discussed. To sustain light and intermediate physical activity for more than ~1 minute, muscle regenerates ATP through oxidative metabolism in the mitochondria of type I and type IIa muscle fibers (Fig. 60-4). Muscle also uses oxidative metabolism to recover from intense activities of short duration that relied on the immediate and anaerobic systems of energy supply.

The anaerobic metabolism of glucose provides nearly 100-fold more energy than is available through the immediate breakdown of ATP and PCr. Oxidative metabolism of glucose, lactate, and fat provides far more than even the anaerobic metabolism of glucose.

Oxidation of Non-Muscle Glucose The aerobic metabolism of glucose, although slower than anaerobic glycolysis (Equation 60-4), provides nearly 15-fold more ATP molecules per glucose (see Table 58-4):

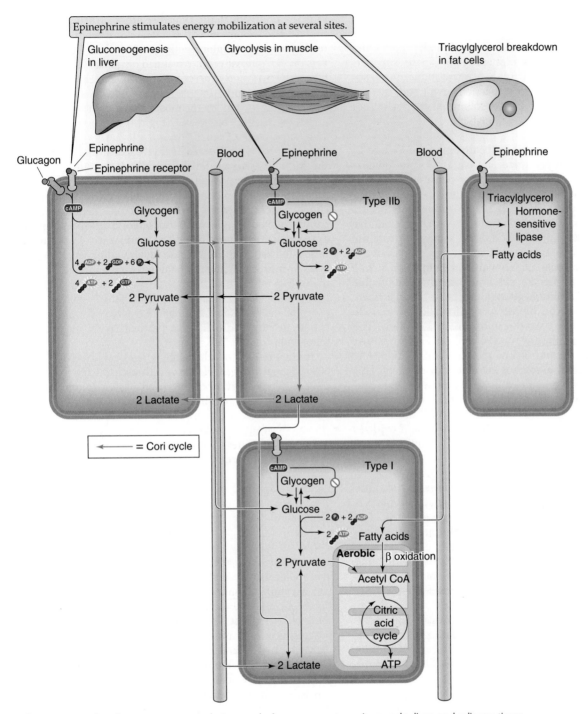

Figure 60-5 Steady-state energy supply to muscle from energy stores in muscle, liver, and adipose tissue.

$$\overset{\text{Glucose}}{C_6H_{12}O_6} + 6\,O_2 + 30\,ADP + 30\,P_i \rightarrow \qquad (60\text{-}5)$$
$$6\,CO_2 + 6\,H_2O + 30\,ATP + heat$$

The glucose that muscle oxidizes comes from the breakdown of hepatic glycogen stores of 75 to 100 g. Glucose uptake by exercising muscle can increase 7- to 40-fold above rest. However, increased glucose release from liver (through glycogenolysis) balances the glucose uptake from the blood by active muscle, thereby stabilizing blood [glucose]. An increase in portal vein levels of **glucagon** in particular (see Fig. 51-12) and a decrease in **insulin**—together with an increase in **epinephrine**—are the main signals for this elevated hepatic glucose output during exercise. However, hepatic denervation in dogs does not prevent accelerated rates of glucose production during exercise, a finding showing that sympathetic innervation of the liver is not essential.

Contracting skeletal muscle is an important sink for blood-borne glucose (Fig. 60-5). Moreover, contractile activity triggers the translocation of additional GLUT4 transporters (see Chapter 51) from the cytosol to the plasma membrane. This process, which is insulin independent and is likely mediated by activation of AMP kinase, supports increased glucose uptake. Because exercise-induced translocation of GLUT4 is insulin independent, endurance exercise is an important adjunct in controlling elevated levels of blood [glucose] in patients with diabetes.

Oxidation of Lactate   During the first minutes of exercise, active muscle fibers use glycogenolysis to liberate glucose and then use glycolysis to form either pyruvate or lactate, depending on the relative activities of glycolysis and mitochondrial respiration. Indeed, lactate production occurs even in fully aerobic contracting muscles with high oxidative capacity. As blood flow and O_2 delivery increase during the initial minutes of the cardiovascular and respiratory adjustments to exercise, muscle fibers convert accumulated lactate back to pyruvate for uptake and subsequent oxidation by the mitochondria. In addition, glycolytic (type IIb) muscle fibers release lactate that can diffuse to nearby oxidative muscle fibers (type I and IIa), which can oxidize it (Fig. 60-5). The lactate that escapes into the bloodstream can enter the heart for oxidation, the distant skeletal muscles for oxidation (Fig. 60-5), or the liver for gluconeogenesis (discussed later). This shuttling of lactate provides a link between anaerobic and oxidative cells. After the initial few minutes of moderate-intensity exercise—and after the cardiovascular and respiratory adjustments—exercising muscle takes up and oxidizes blood-borne glucose and simultaneously diminishes its release of lactic acid.

Gluconeogenesis   Hepatic gluconeogenesis becomes increasingly important as exercise is prolonged beyond an hour and hepatic glycogen stores become depleted. The most important substrates for hepatic gluconeogenesis are lactate and alanine. During prolonged exercise, the key substrate is lactate released into the circulation by contracting skeletal muscle (see later) for uptake by the liver, which resynthesizes glucose for uptake by the muscle—the **Cori cycle** (see Fig. 58-13 and 60-5).

At workloads exceeding 65% of maximal O_2 uptake by the lungs ($\dot{V}_{O_{2max}}$), lactate production rises faster than removal and causes an exponential increase in blood [lactate]. Endurance training increases the rate of lactate clearance from the blood at any given [lactate]. Oxidation is responsible for ~75% of lactate removal, and hepatic gluconeogenesis is responsible for the remainder. Also during prolonged exercise, the oxidation of branched-chain amino acids by skeletal muscle leads to the release of alanine into the circulation for uptake by the liver, followed by hepatic gluconeogenesis and the release of glucose into the blood for uptake by muscle—the **glucose-alanine cycle** (see Fig. 58-13).

The Cori and glucose-alanine cycles play an important role in redistributing glycogen from resting muscle to exercising muscle during prolonged exercise and during recovery from exercise. For example, after prolonged arm exercise, lactate release from leg muscle is 6- to 7-fold greater than in the pre-exercise basal state. Conversely, after leg exercise, lactate release from forearm muscle increases. Thus, the Cori cycle redistributes glycogen from resting muscle to fuel

muscles undergoing prolonged exercise. During recovery, muscle glycogenolysis and lactate release from previously resting muscle continue, and lactate enters the liver for conversion to glucose and release. The subsequent glucose uptake by previously exercising muscles thereby replenishes their glycogen stores. In this way, the body ensures an adequate supply of fuel for the next fight or flight response.

Oxidation of Non-Muscle Lipid   Most stored energy is in the form of triglycerides. In the prototypic 70-kg person, adipocytes store ~132,000 kcal of potential energy. The mobilization of lipid from adipocytes during exercise is largely under the control of the sympathetic nervous system, complemented by the release of growth hormone during exercise lasting longer than 30 to 40 minutes. The result of this mobilization is an increase in circulating levels of fatty acids, which can enter skeletal muscle—especially type I fibers (Fig. 60-5). In addition to fatty acids that enter muscle from adipocytes, skeletal muscle itself stores ~8000 kcal of potential energy as intracellular triacylglycerols, which contribute to fatty acid oxidation, particularly during recovery following prolonged exertion.

In the presence of adequate O_2, fatty acids provide up to 60% of the oxidized fuel supply of muscle during prolonged exercise. The oxidation of fatty acids, using palmitate as an example, has a very high yield of ATP:

$$\overbrace{C_{15}H_{31}COOH}^{\text{Palmitic acid}} + 23\,O_2 + 106\,ADP + 106\,P_i \rightarrow \quad (60\text{-}6)$$
$$16\,CO_2 + 16\,H_2O + 106\,ATP + \text{heat}$$

Lipids are an important source of energy when O_2 is available, that is, during prolonged low- to moderate-intensity activity and during recovery following exercise.

Choice of Fuel Sources   For sustained activity of moderate intensity, fat is the preferred substrate, given ample O_2 availability. For example, at 50% of $\dot{V}_{O_{2max}}$, fatty acid oxidation accounts for more than half of muscle energy production, and glucose accounts for the remainder. As the *duration* of exercise further lengthens, fatty acid oxidation progressively increases, and it becomes the dominant oxidative fuel as glucose utilization by the muscle declines. However, as exercise *intensity* increases, active muscle relies increasingly on glucose derived from intramuscular glycogen as well as on blood-borne glucose. This crossover from lipid to carbohydrate metabolism has the advantage that, per liter of O_2 consumed, carbohydrate provides slightly more energy than lipid. Conversely, as muscle depletes its glycogen stores, it loses its ability to consume O_2 at high rates.

At a given metabolic demand, the increased availability and utilization of fatty acids translate to lower rates of glucose oxidation and muscle glycogenolysis, thereby prolonging the ability to sustain activity. Endurance training promotes these adaptations of skeletal muscle. Under conditions of carbohydrate deprivation (e.g., starvation), extremely prolonged exercise (e.g., ultramarathon), and impaired glucose utilization (e.g., diabetes), muscle can also oxidize ketone bodies as their plasma levels rise.

MUSCLE FATIGUE

Fatigued muscle produces less force and has a reduced velocity of shortening

Muscle fatigue is defined as the inability to maintain a desired power output—resulting from muscle contraction against a load—with a decline in both force and velocity of shortening. A decline in maximal force production with fatigue results from a reduction in the number of active cross-bridges as well as the force produced per cross-bridge. As fatigue develops, the production of force usually declines earlier and to a greater extent than shortening velocity. Other characteristics of fatigued skeletal muscle are lower rates of both force production and relaxation, owing to impaired release and reuptake of Ca^{2+} from the sarcoplasmic reticulum (SR). As a result, fast movements become difficult or impossible, and athletic performance suffers accordingly. Nevertheless, fatigue may serve an important protective role in allowing contractions at reduced rates and lower forces while preventing extreme changes in cell composition that could cause damage. Muscle fatigue is reversible with rest, which contrasts with muscle damage or weakness, in which even muscles that are well rested are compromised in their ability to develop force. For example, muscle damage induced by eccentric contractions can easily be mistaken for fatigue, except the recovery period can last for days.

Factors contributing to fatigue include motivation, physical fitness, nutritional status, and the types of motor units (i.e., fibers) recruited with respect to the intensity and duration of activity. As discussed in this major section, fatigue during *prolonged* activity of *moderate* intensity involving relatively *low* frequencies of motor unit activation is caused by different factors than fatigue during *bursts* of *high* intensity involving *high* frequencies of motor unit activation. Moreover, fatigue can result from events occurring in the central nervous system (CNS; central fatigue) as well as from changes within the muscle (peripheral fatigue).

Changes in the CNS produce central fatigue

Central fatigue reflects changes in the CNS and may involve altered input from muscle sensory nerve fibers, reduced excitatory input to motor control centers of the brain and spinal cord, and altered excitability of α and γ motor neurons (see Fig. 15-30). The contributions of these factors vary with the individual and with the nature of activity. For example, central fatigue is likely to play only a minor role in limiting performance of highly trained athletes who have learned to pace themselves according to the task and are mentally conditioned to discomfort and stress. In contrast, central fatigue is likely of greater importance in novice athletes and during repetitive (i.e., boring) tasks. The identification of specific sites involved in central fatigue is difficult because of the complexity of the CNS. Nevertheless, external sensory input, such as shouting and cheering, can often increase muscle force production and physical performance, a finding indicating that pathways proximal to corticospinal outputs can oppose central fatigue.

Impaired excitability and impaired Ca^{2+} release can produce peripheral fatigue

Transmission block at the neuromuscular junction does not cause muscle fatigue, even though the release of neurotransmitter can decline. **Peripheral fatigue** reflects a spectrum of events at the level of the muscle fiber, including impairments in the initiation and propagation of muscle action potentials, the release and handling of intracellular Ca^{2+} for cross-bridge activation, depletion of substrates for energy metabolism, and the accumulation of metabolic byproducts. The nature of fatigue and the time required for recovery vary with the recruitment pattern of motor units and the metabolic properties of their constitutive muscle fibers (Fig. 60-2).

High-Frequency Fatigue With continuous firing of action potentials during intense exercise, Na^+ entry and K^+ exit exceed the ability of the Na-K pump to restore and maintain normal resting ion concentration gradients. As a result, $[K^+]_o$ and $[Na^+]_i$ increase, thus making the resting membrane potential of muscle fibers more positive by 10 to 20 mV. This depolarization inactivates voltage-gated Na^+ channels and makes it more difficult to initiate and propagate action potentials. Within the T tubule, such depolarization impairs the ability of L-type Ca^{2+} channels to activate Ca^{2+} release channels in the SR (see Fig. 9-3). Fatigue resulting from *impaired membrane excitability* is particularly apparent at high frequencies of stimulation during recruitment of *type II* motor units—**high-frequency fatigue**. On cessation of contractile activity, ionic and ATP homeostasis recovers within 30 minutes; thus, the recovery from high-frequency fatigue occurs relatively quickly.

Low-Frequency Fatigue In prolonged, moderate-intensity exercise, the release of Ca^{2+} from the SR falls—perhaps reflecting change in either the Ca^{2+} release channel or its associated proteins—thus leading to a depression in the amplitude of the $[Ca^{2+}]_i$ transient that accompanies the muscle twitch. A diminution of Ca^{2+} release is apparent at all stimulation frequencies. However, the effect on force development is most apparent at low stimulation frequencies, for the following reason. During unfused tetanus (see Fig. 9-11), $[Ca^{2+}]_i$ does not continuously remain at high enough levels to saturate troponin C (see Chapter 9). As a result, cross-bridge formation is highly sensitive to the amount of Ca^{2+} released from the SR with each stimulus. In contrast, with high frequencies of stimulation that produce fused tetanus, $[Ca^{2+}]_i$ is at such high levels that Ca^{2+} continuously saturates troponin C and thereby maximizes cross-bridge interactions and masks the effects of impaired Ca^{2+} release with each stimulus. Fatigue resulting from *impaired Ca^{2+} release* is thus particularly apparent at low frequencies of stimulation during recruitment of *type I* motor units—**low-frequency fatigue**. Recovery requires several hours.

Fatigue can result from ATP depletion, lactic acid accumulation, and glycogen depletion

ATP Depletion As outlined in Chapter 9, muscle fibers require ATP for contraction, relaxation, and the activity of the membrane pumps that maintain ionic homeostasis. Therefore, the cells must maintain $[ATP]_i$ to avoid fatigue (see Chapter 9).

Intense stimulation of muscle fibers (particularly type IIb) requires high rates of ATP utilization, with PCr initially buffering $[ATP]_i$. As fatigue develops, $[PCr]_i$ diminishes and $[ATP]_i$ can fall from 5 mM to less than 2 mM, particularly at sites of cross-bridge interaction and in the vicinity of membrane pumps, thereby impairing respective ATPase activities. Simultaneously, P_i, ADP, Mg^{2+}, lactate, and H^+ accumulate in the sarcoplasm. Impairment of the Ca^{2+} pump at the SR prolongs the Ca^{2+} transient while reducing the electrochemical driving force for Ca^{2+} release from the SR. Independently, the fall in $[ATP]_i$ and the increase in $[Mg^{2+}]$ can also inhibit Ca^{2+} release through the ryanodine receptor (see Chapter 9).

Lactic Acid Accumulation   Intense activity also activates glycolysis—again, particularly in type IIb fibers—resulting in a high rate of lactic acid production and thus reducing pH_i to as low as 6.2 (Equation 60-4). This fall in pH_i inhibits myosin ATPase activity and thereby reduces the velocity of shortening. The fall in pH_i also inhibits cross-bridge interaction and the binding of Ca^{2+} to troponin, the Na-K pump, as well as to phosphofructokinase (see Chapter 51), the rate-limiting step of muscle glycolysis. The combined effects of low pH_i and high P_i interact to impair the peak force production of muscle fibers more than either agent alone. The mechanisms are reductions in the number of cross-bridges and in the force per cross-bridge by impairing the transition from weak to strong binding states between actin and myosin. In addition, both H^+ and P_i reduce Ca^{2+} sensitivity of contractile proteins, such that higher free $[Ca^{2+}]_i$ is required for a given level of force production.

Glycogen Depletion   During prolonged exercise of moderate intensity (~50% of maximal aerobic power), and with well maintained O_2 delivery, the eventual decrease in glycogen stores in oxidative (type I and IIa) muscle fibers decreases power output. Long-distance runners describe this phenomenon as "hitting the wall." Muscle glycogen stores are critical because the combination of blood-borne delivery of substrates and the availability of intramuscular fatty acids is inadequate to accommodate the energy requirements. In long-distance running, endurance depends on the absolute amount of glycogen stored in the leg muscles before exercise. To postpone hitting the wall, the athlete must either begin the event with an elevated level of muscle glycogen or race more slowly. Because glycogen storage is primarily a function of diet, carbohydrate loading can increase resting muscle glycogen stores and can postpone the onset of fatigue. Low-carbohydrate diets have the opposite effect. Although physical training has little effect on the capacity for glycolysis, it can promote glycogen storage, particularly if it is combined with a carbohydrate-rich diet. Aerobic training can spare muscle glycogen by adaptations such as mitochondrial proliferation that shift the mix of oxidized fuels toward fatty acids. Indeed, well-trained athletes can maintain moderate-intensity exercise for hours.

During exercise at *relatively high* intensities (>65% of maximal aerobic power), fatigue develops on the order of tens of minutes. One explanation for this decrement in performance is that type IIb muscle fibers fatigue when their glycogen supplies become exhausted, and the result is a decline in whole-muscle power output.

DETERMINANTS OF MAXIMAL O₂ UPTAKE AND CONSUMPTION

The O_2 required for oxidative metabolism by exercising muscle travels from the atmosphere to the muscle mitochondria in three discrete steps:

1. The **uptake** of O_2 by the lungs depends on pulmonary ventilation.
2. O_2 **delivery** to muscle depends on blood flow and O_2 content.
3. The **extraction** of O_2 from blood by muscle depends on O_2 delivery and the P_{O_2} gradient between blood and mitochondria.

Maximal O₂ uptake by the lungs can exceed resting O₂ uptake by more than 20-fold

The respiratory and cardiovascular systems can readily deliver O_2 to active skeletal muscle at mild and moderate exercise intensities. As power output increases, the body eventually reaches a point at which the capacity of O_2 transport systems can no longer keep pace with demand, so the rate of O_2 uptake by the lungs ($\dot{V}_{O_2}$) plateaus (Fig. 60-6). At rest, $\dot{V}_{O_2}$ is typically 250 mL/min for a 70-kg person (see Chapter 29), a value that corresponds to 3.6 mL of O_2 consumed per minute for each kg of body mass [mL O_2/(min × kg)]. $\dot{V}_{O_{2max}}$ is an objective index of the functional capacity of the body's ability to generate aerobic power. In people who have a deficiency in any part of the O_2 transport system (e.g., chronic obstructive pulmonary disease or advanced heart disease), $\dot{V}_{O_{2max}}$ can be as low as 10 to 20 mL O_2/(min × kg). The range for mildly active middle-aged adults is 30 to

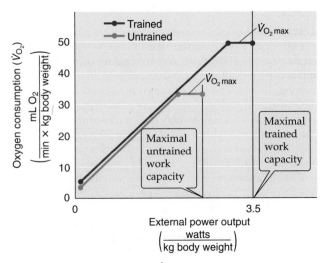

Figure 60-6   Dependence of $\dot{V}_{O_2}$ on mechanical power output. Training increases $V_{O_{2max}}$.

40 mL $O_2/(min \times kg)$; for people in this category, a 3-month program of physical conditioning can increase $\dot{V}_{O_{2max}}$ by 20%. In elite endurance athletes, $\dot{V}_{O_{2max}}$ may be as high as 80 to 90 mL $O_2/(min \times kg)$, more than a 20-fold elevation above the resting $\dot{V}_{O_2}$. Hemorrhage or high altitude decreases $\dot{V}_{O_{2max}}$, whereas blood transfusion or training increases it.

The typical method for determining $\dot{V}_{O_{2max}}$ is an incremental exercise test on a stationary cycle ergometer or treadmill. Such tests assess training status, predict performance in athletes, and provide an index of functional impairment in patients. During the test, the technician monitors the P_{O_2} and P_{CO_2} of the subject's expired air, as well as total ventilation. The criteria for achieving $\dot{V}_{O_{2max}}$ include (1) an inability to continue the pace at the prescribed power requirement, (2) a leveling off of $\dot{V}_{O_2}$ with an increasing power requirement (Fig. 60-6), and (3) a *respiratory exchange ratio* ($\dot{V}_{CO_2}/\dot{V}_{O_2}$) greater than 1.15. This $\dot{V}_{CO_2}/\dot{V}_{O_2}$ is a transient/non–steady-state occurrence (i.e., not a real respiratory quotient, see Chapter 54) and indicates that a significant hyperventilation, triggered by low blood pH (see Chapter 32), is reducing the body's CO_2 stores.

O_2 uptake by muscle is the product of muscle blood flow and O_2 extraction

The body's total store of O_2 is ~1 L (mainly in the form of O_2 bound to hemoglobin), a volume that (if used completely) could support moderate exercise for 30 seconds at best, heavy exercise for not more than 15 seconds, and maximal exercise for less than 10 seconds. If activity is to persist, the body must continually transport O_2 from the ambient air to the muscle mitochondria at a rate that is equivalent to the O_2 utilization by the muscle. This increased O_2 transport is accomplished by increasing alveolar ventilation to maintain alveolar P_{O_2} levels that are sufficient to saturate arterial blood fully (see Chapter 31) and by increasing cardiac output to ensure a sufficiently high flow of oxygenated blood to the muscles (see Chapter 20). The integrated organ system response to the new, elevated metabolic load involves the close coupling of the pulmonary and the cardiovascular O_2 delivery systems to the O_2 acceptor mechanisms in the muscle; the response includes sophisticated reflexes to ensure matching of the two processes.

The convective O_2 delivery rate is the product of cardiac output (i.e., heart rate × stroke volume) and arterial O_2 content:

Arterial O_2 delivery rate to whole body		Heart rate		Cardiac stroke volume		Arterial O_2 content	
$\underbrace{\dot{V}a_{O_2}}_{\dfrac{mL\,O_2}{min}}$	$=$	$\underbrace{HR}_{\dfrac{beats}{min}}$	$\cdot$	$\underbrace{SV}_{\dfrac{mL\,blood}{beat}}$	$\cdot$	$\underbrace{Ca_{O_2}}_{\dfrac{mL\,O_2}{mL\,blood}}$	**(60-7)**

The rate of O_2 uptake by skeletal muscle ($\dot{V}_{O_2}$) depends on both the O_2 delivery to skeletal muscle and the **extraction** of O_2 by the muscle. According to the Fick equation (see Chapter 17), $\dot{V}_{O_2}$ is the product of blood flow to muscle (F) and the arteriovenous (a-v) difference for O_2:

Rate of O_2 uptake by skeletal muscle		Blood flow to skeletal muscle		a – v difference of O_2 content	
$\underbrace{\dot{V}_{O_2}}_{\dfrac{mL\,O_2}{min}}$	$=$	$\underbrace{F}_{\dfrac{mL\,blood}{min}}$	$\cdot$	$\underbrace{(Ca_{O_2} - Cv_{O_2})}_{\dfrac{mL\,O_2}{mL\,blood}}$	**(60-8)**

The $\dot{V}_{O_2}$, established by the rate of oxidative phosphorylation in muscle mitochondria, requires an adequate rate of O_2 delivery to the active muscle. Exercise triggers a complicated series of changes in the cardiovascular system that has the net effect of increasing F and redistributing cardiac output away from the splanchnic and renal vascular beds, as well as from inactive to active muscle (see Chapter 25). Increased O_2 extraction from the blood by active skeletal muscle occurs at the onset of exercise in response to elevated mitochondrial respiration and the attendant fall in intracellular P_{O_2}, which increases the gradient for O_2 diffusion from blood to mitochondria.

At the onset of exercise, the content of O_2 in the arterial blood (Ca_{O_2}) actually increases somewhat (e.g., from 20.0 to 20.4 mL O_2/mL blood; see Table 29-3) secondary to the increase in alveolar ventilation triggered by the CNS (see Chapter 14). Also as a consequence of the anticipatory hyperventilation, P_{CO_2} actually falls with the onset of exercise. Possible mechanisms of this ventilatory increase include a response to mechanoreceptors in joints and muscles, descending cortical input, or resetting of peripheral chemoreceptors by a reduction in their blood supply (see Chapter 32). The increase in ventilation in anticipation of future needs is enhanced in well-trained athletes.

O_2 delivery by the cardiovascular system is the limiting step for maximal O_2 utilization

For years, exercise and sports scientists have debated over the factors that limit $\dot{V}_{O_{2max}}$ and thus contribute to performance limitations. As noted earlier, the transport of O_2 from atmosphere to muscle mitochondria occurs in three steps: uptake, delivery, and extraction. A limitation in any step could be rate limiting for maximal O_2 utilization by muscle.

Limited O_2 Uptake by Lungs One view is that the lungs limit $\dot{V}_{O_{2max}}$. An inability of alveolar O_2 diffusion to saturate arterial blood fully occurs in a subset of elite athletes (including race horses). Thus, a decrease in Ca_{O_2} occurs at maximal effort on an incremental test. The inability to saturate arterial blood in athletes could be the consequence of a ventilation-perfusion mismatch at very high cardiac outputs (see Chapter 31).

Limited O_2 Delivery by Cardiovascular System According to the prevalent view, a limitation in O_2 transport by the cardiovascular system determines $\dot{V}_{O_{2max}}$. That is, according to the **convective flow model**, maximal cardiac output, and hence O_2 delivery, is the limiting step. Support for this view comes from the observation that training can considerably augment maximal cardiac output and muscle blood flow

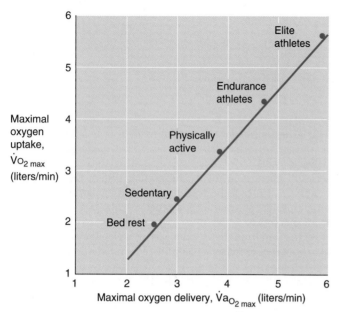

Figure 60-7 Dependence of maximal O_2 utilization on O_2 delivery. The graph illustrates the relationship between maximal O_2 delivery to the peripheral tissues ($\dot{V}a_{O_{2max}}$) and $\dot{V}_{O_{2max}}$ for five individuals with different lifestyles. Training increases both O_2 delivery and O_2 uptake. *(Data from Saltin B, Strange S: Med Sci Sports Exerc 1992; 24:30-37.)*

(see the following section). Moreover, $\dot{V}_{O_{2max}}$ largely increases in parallel with these adaptations (Fig. 60-7).

Limited O_2 Extraction by Muscle A third point of view is that, with increasing demand, extraction by muscle of O_2 from blood becomes inadequate despite adequate O_2 delivery. According to this **diffusive flow model**, a major limitation in O_2 transport is the kinetics of O_2 diffusion from hemoglobin in the red blood cell to the muscle mitochondrial matrix. Thus, anything that lowers either the muscle's diffusing capacity for O_2 or the P_{O_2} gradient between hemoglobin and mitochondria reduces $\dot{V}_{O_{2max}}$.

Effective circulating volume takes priority over cutaneous blood flow for thermoregulation

When we exercise in the heat, our circulatory systems must simultaneously support a large blood flow to both the skin (see Chapter 59) and the contracting muscles, an effort that taxes the cardiac output and effective circulating volume (see Chapter 40). During exercise, the ability to maintain both arterial blood pressure and body core temperature (T_{core}) within acceptable physiological limits depends on maintaining an adequate effective circulating volume. Effective circulating volume depends on total blood volume, which, in turn, relies on extracellular fluid volume and on overall vasomotor (primarily venomotor) tone, which is important for distributing blood between central and peripheral pools. Effective circulating volume tends to fall during prolonged exercise, especially exercise in the heat, for three reasons (Fig. 60-8).

First, exercise causes a **shift in plasma water** from the intravascular to the interstitial space. This transcapillary movement of fluid during exercise primarily reflects increased capillary hydrostatic pressure (see Chapter 20). In addition, increased osmolality within muscle cells removes water from the extracellular space. When exercise intensity exceeds 40% of $\dot{V}_{O_{2max}}$, this loss of plasma water is proportional to the exercise intensity. In extreme conditions, the loss of plasma water can amount to more than 500 mL, or approximately one sixth of the total plasma volume.

Second, exercise causes a loss of total body water through **sweating** (discussed in the next major section). If exercise is prolonged, without concomitant water intake, sweat loss will cost the body an important fraction of its total water. A loss of body water in excess of 3% of body weight is associated with early signs of heat-related illness, including lightheadedness and disorientation, and it constitutes **clinical dehydration**.

Third, exercise causes a **redistribution of blood volume** to the skin because of the increase in cutaneous blood flow in response to body heating (Fig. 60-8). Venous volume *in the skin* increases as a result of the increased pressure in the compliant vessels as blood flow to the skin rises. No compensatory venoconstriction occurs in the skin because of the overriding action of the temperature control system.

In response to this decrease in effective circulating volume that occurs during exercise, the cardiopulmonary, low-pressure baroreceptors (see Chapter 19) initiate compensatory responses to increase total vascular resistance (Fig. 60-8). This increase in resistance is accomplished through the sympathetic nervous system by (1) increasing the splanchnic vascular resistance, (2) offsetting some of the vasodilatory drive to the skin initiated by the temperature control system, and (3) offsetting some of the vasodilatory drive to the active skeletal muscles.

In conditions of heavy thermal demand, the restriction of peripheral blood flow has the benefit of helping to maintain arterial blood pressure and effective circulating volume, but it carries two liabilities. First, it reduces convective heat transfer from the core to the skin because of the reduced skin blood flow and consequently contributes to excessive heat storage and, in the extreme, heat stroke (see Chapter 59 for the box on this topic). Second, the limitation of blood flow to active muscle may compromise O_2 delivery and hence aerobic performance.

In conditions of low thermal and metabolic demand, no serious conflict arises among the systems that regulate effective circulating volume, arterial blood pressure, and body temperature. The cutaneous circulation is capable of handling the heat transfer requirements of the temperature regulatory mechanism without impairing muscle blood flow or cardiac filling pressure.

SWEATING

Eccrine, but not apocrine, sweat glands contribute to temperature regulation

Sweat glands are exocrine glands of the skin, formed by specialized infoldings of the epidermis into the underlying dermis. Sweat glands are of two types: apocrine and eccrine (Fig. 60-9A). The **apocrine** sweat glands, located in the

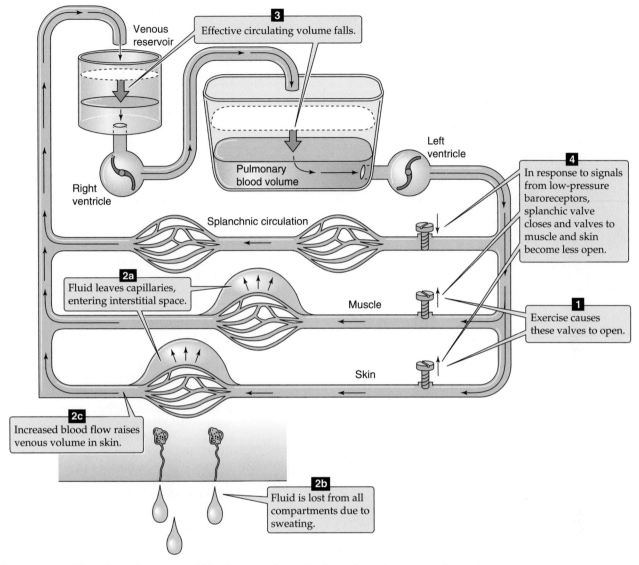

Figure 60-8 Effect of exercise on central blood volume. "Valves" refer to the resistance vasculature of respective organs.

axillary and anogenital regions of the body, are relatively few in number (~100,000) and large in diameter (2 to 3 mm). Their ducts empty into hair follicles. These glands, which often become active during puberty, produce a turbid and viscous secretion that is rich in lipids and carbohydrates and carries a characteristic body odor that has spawned an entire industry to conceal. Apocrine sweat glands have no role in temperature regulation in humans, although they may act as a source of pheromones.

Eccrine sweat glands are distributed over the majority of the body surface, are numerous (several million), and are small in diameter (50 to 100 μm). The palms of the hands and soles of the feet tend to have both larger and more densely distributed eccrine glands than elsewhere. The full complement of eccrine sweat glands is present at birth and becomes functional within a few months, and the density of these glands decreases as the skin enlarges during normal growth. The essential role of eccrine sweating is temperature regulation, although stimuli such as food, emotion, and pain

can evoke secretory activity. Regionally, the trunk, head, and neck show more profuse sweating than the extremities. Sweat production is quantitatively less in women than in men, a finding reflecting less output per gland rather than fewer eccrine sweat glands.

Eccrine sweat glands are tubules comprising a secretory coiled gland and a reabsorptive duct

An eccrine sweat gland is a simple tubular epithelium composed of a coiled gland and a duct (Fig. 60-9B). A rich microvascular network surrounds the entire sweat gland. The **coiled gland**, located deep in the dermis (see Fig. 15-26), begins at a single blind acinus innervated by postganglionic sympathetic fibers that are cholinergic. The release of acetylcholine stimulates muscarinic receptors on the acinar cells and causes them to secrete into the lumen a clear, odorless solution, similar in composition to protein-free plasma. This

A APOCRINE AND ECCRINE SWEAT GLANDS

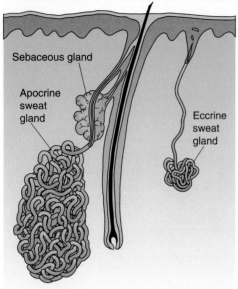

Sebaceous gland

Apocrine sweat gland

Eccrine sweat gland

B COMPONENTS OF AN ECCRINE SWEAT GLAND

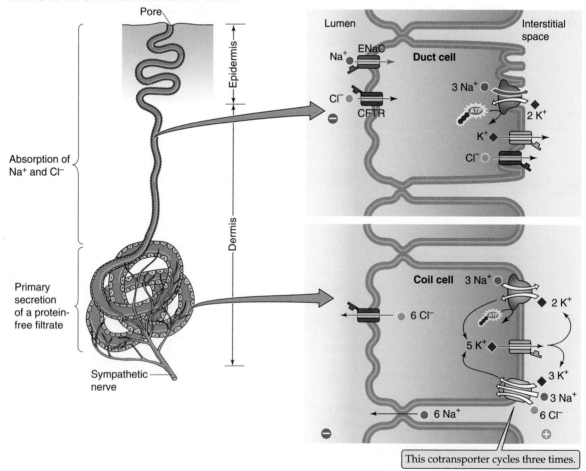

Pore

Epidermis

Dermis

Absorption of Na⁺ and Cl⁻

Primary secretion of a protein-free filtrate

Sympathetic nerve

Lumen

Interstitial space

Na^+ ENaC **Duct cell**

Cl^- CFTR

$3\,Na^+$

ATP

$2\,K^+$

K^+

Cl^-

Coil cell $3\,Na^+$

$2\,K^+$

ATP

$6\,Cl^-$

$5\,K^+$

$3\,K^+$

$3\,Na^+$

$6\,Na^+$

$6\,Cl^-$

This cotransporter cycles three times.

Figure 60-9 A and **B,** Sweat glands. The sebaceous gland—the duct of which empties into the hair follicle independently of the duct apocrine sweat gland—secretes sebum, a mixture of fat and the remnants of the cells that secrete the fat.

primary secretion flows through a long, wavy **duct** that passes outward through the dermis and epidermis. Along the way, duct cells reabsorb salt and water until the fluid reaches the skin surface through an opening, the **sweat pore**. Although these pores are too small to be seen with the naked eye, the location of sweat pores is readily identified as sweat droplets form on the skin surface. Both the secretory cells in the coil and the reabsorptive cells in the duct are rich in mitochondria, which are essential for providing sustained energy for the high rates of ion transport necessary for prolonged periods of intense sweating, for example, during exercise in hot environments.

Surrounding the secretory cells in the coil is a layer of myoepithelial cells that resemble smooth muscle and may contract, thereby expressing sweat to the skin surface in a pulsatile fashion. However, this action is not essential because the hydrostatic pressures generated within the gland can exceed 500 mm Hg.

Secretion by Coil Cells The release of acetylcholine onto the secretory coil cells activates muscarinic G protein–coupled receptors (see Chapter 3) and thus leads to the activation of phospholipase C, which, in turn, stimulates protein kinase C and raises $[Ca^{2+}]_i$. These signals somehow trigger the primary secretion, which follows the general mechanism for Cl^- secretion (see Chapter 5). A Na/K/Cl cotransporter (see Chapter 5) mediates the uptake of Cl^- across the basolateral membrane, and the Cl^- exits across the apical membrane through a Cl^- channel (Fig. 60-9B, lower inset). As Cl^- diffuses into the lumen, the resulting lumen-negative voltage drives Na^+ secretion through the paracellular pathway.

The secretion of NaCl, as well as of urea and lactate, into the lumen sets up an osmotic gradient that drives the secretion of water, so the secreted fluid is nearly isotonic with plasma. This secretion of fluid into the lumen increases hydrostatic pressure at the base of the gland and thereby provides the driving force for moving the fluid along the duct to reach the skin surface.

Reabsorption by Duct Cells As the secreted solution flows along the sweat gland duct, the duct cells reabsorb Na^+ and Cl^- (Fig. 60-9B, upper inset). Na^+ enters the duct cells across the apical membrane through epithelial Na^+ channels (ENaCs), and Cl^- enters through the cystic fibrosis transmembrane regulator (CFTR). The Na-K pump is responsible for the extrusion of Na^+ across the basolateral membrane, and Cl^- exits through a pathway such as a Cl^- channel. Because the water permeability of the epithelium lining the sweat duct is low, water reabsorption is limited, resulting in a final secretory fluid that is always hypotonic to plasma.

Because sweat is hypotonic, sweating leads to the loss of **solute-free water**, that is, the loss of more water than salt. As a result, the extracellular fluid contracts and becomes hyperosmolar, thereby causing water to exit from cells. Thus, intracellular fluid volume decreases, and *intracellular* osmolality increases (see Chapter 5). This water movement helps to correct the fall in extracellular fluid volume. The solute-free water lost in perspiration therefore is ultimately derived from all body fluid compartments.

The NaCl content of sweat increases with the rate of secretion but decreases with acclimatization to heat

Flow Dependence With mild stimulation of acinar cells, the small volume of primary secretion travels slowly along the duct, and the ducts reabsorb nearly all the Na^+ and Cl^-, which can fall to final concentrations as low as ~5 mM (Fig. 60-10). In contrast, with strong cholinergic stimulation, a large volume of primary secretion travels rapidly along the duct, so the load exceeds the capacity of the ductal epithelium to reabsorb Na^+ and Cl^-. Thus, a greater fraction of the secreted Na^+ and Cl^- remains within the lumen, with resulting levels of 50 to 60 mM. In contrast, $[K^+]$ in the sweat remains nearly independent of flow at 5 to 10 mM.

Cystic Fibrosis In patients with cystic fibrosis (see Chapter 43 for the box on this topic), abnormal sweat gland function is attributable to a defect in the CFTR, a cAMP-regulated Cl^- channel that is normally present in the apical membrane of sweat gland duct cells. These individuals secrete normal volumes of sweat into the acinus but have a defect in Cl^- (and, therefore, Na^+) absorption as the fluid travels along the duct. As a result, the sweat is relatively rich in NaCl (Fig. 60-10).

Replenishment During a thermoregulatory response in a healthy individual, the rate of sweat production can commonly reach 1 to 2 L/hour, which, after a sufficient time, can represent a substantial fraction of total body water. Such a loss of water and salt requires adequate repletion to pre-

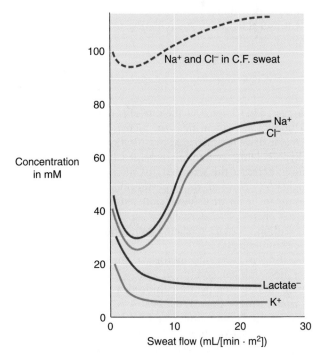

Figure 60-10 Flow dependence of sweat composition. Defective Cl^- (and therefore Na^+) reabsorption in cystic fibrosis (CF) patients leads to greater salt loss in sweat.

serve fluid and electrolyte balance. Restoring body fluid volume following dehydration is often delayed in humans despite the consumption of fluids. The reason for this delay is that dehydrated persons drink *free water*, which reduces the osmolality of the extracellular fluid and thus reduces the osmotic drive for drinking (see Chapter 40). This consumed free water distributes into the cells as well as the extracellular space and dilutes the solutes. In addition, the reduced plasma osmolality leads to decreased secretion of arginine vasopressin (i.e., antidiuretic hormone), thus increasing free water excretion by the kidney (see Fig. 40-7).

A more effective means of restoring body fluid volume is to ingest NaCl with water. When Na^+ is taken with water (as in many exercise drinks), plasma $[Na^+]$ remains elevated throughout a greater duration of the rehydration period and is significantly higher than with the ingestion of water alone. In such conditions, the salt-dependent thirst drive is maintained, and the stimulation of urine production is delayed, thereby leading to more complete restoration of body water content.

Acclimatization With ample, continuing hydration, a heat-acclimatized individual can sweat up to 4 L/hour during maximal sweating. Over several weeks, as the body acclimates to high rates of eccrine sweat production, the ability to reabsorb NaCl increases, and the result is more hypotonic sweat. This adaptation is mediated by **aldosterone** (see Chapter 35) in response to the net loss of Na^+ from the body during the early stages of acclimatization. For example, an individual who is not acclimatized and who sweats profusely can lose more than 30 g of salt per day for the first few days. In contrast, after several weeks of acclimatization, salt loss falls to several grams per day. Thus, an important benefit of physical training and heat acclimatization is the development of more dilute perspiration, which conserves NaCl content and thus effective circulating volume (see Chapter 5) during dehydration.

The hyperthermia of exercise stimulates eccrine sweat glands

As discussed in Chapter 59, the rate of perspiration increases with body T_{core}, which, in turn, increases during exercise. The major drive for increased perspiration is the sensing by the hypothalamic centers of increased body T_{core}. Physical training increases the sensitivity of the hypothalamic drive to higher T_{core}. Indeed, the hyperthermia of exercise causes sweating to begin at a lower skin temperature than does sweating elicited by external heating. The efferent limb of the sweating reflex is mediated by postganglionic sympathetic cholinergic fibers.

Sweating is especially important for thermoregulation under hot ambient conditions and with exercise-induced increases in body temperature. Indeed, as ambient temperature rises to more than 30°C, heat loss through radiation, convection, and conduction (see Chapter 59) becomes progressively ineffective, and evaporative cooling becomes by far the most important mechanism of regulating body temperature. Conversely, evaporative cooling becomes progressively less effective as ambient humidity rises (see Equation 59-5).

AEROBIC TRAINING

Aerobic training requires regular periods of stress and recovery

The body improves its capacity to perform work through physical exertion. However, one must meet four conditions to achieve a **training effect**, or *adaptation* to exercise. First, the intensity of the activity must be higher than a critical threshold. For aerobic training (e.g., running, cycling, and swimming), the level of stress increases with the speed of the activity. Second, each period of activity must be of sufficient duration. Third, one must repeat the activity over time on a regular basis (e.g., several times per week). Finally, sufficient rest must occur between each training session because adaptations occur during the recovery period.

A great deal of research has focused on optimizing the foregoing four factors, as well as task specificity for individual athletes competing in specific events. Increasing levels of exertion progressively recruit and thereby adapt type I muscle fibers, followed by type IIa and then type IIb fibers. However, regardless of how long or intensely an individual trains, inactivity reverses these adaptations with an associated decrement in performance. Aerobic conditioning increases $\dot{V}_{O_{2max}}$ as well as the body's ability to eliminate excess heat that is produced during exercise (see Fig. 59-5).

Aerobic training increases maximal O_2 delivery by increasing plasma volume and maximal cardiac output

$\dot{V}_{O_{2max}}$ could increase as the result of either optimizing O_2 delivery to active muscle or optimizing O_2 extraction by active muscle, as demonstrated in the following modification of Equation 60-7:

$$\underbrace{\dot{V}_{aO_{2max}}}_{\frac{mL\ O_2}{min}} = \underbrace{HR_{opt}}_{\substack{Maximal \\ cardiac\ output}} \cdot \underbrace{SV_{opt}}_{\frac{mL\ blood}{min}} \cdot \underbrace{(Ca_{O_2} - Cv_{O_2})_{max}}_{\frac{mL\ O_2}{mL\ blood}}$$

| Maximal rate of O_2 uptake | Optimal heart rate | Optimal stroke volume | Maximal a−v difference of O_2 content |

$$(60\text{-}9)$$

In fact, aerobic training improves both O_2 delivery and O_2 extraction; the problem for physiologists has been to determine to what extent each system contributes to the whole-body response. For example, an increase in the circulatory system's capacity to deliver O_2 could reflect an increase in either the maximal arterial O_2 content or the maximal cardiac output, or both.

Maximizing Arterial O_2 Content Several factors could theoretically contribute to maximizing Ca_{O_2}:

1. Increasing the maximal alveolar ventilation enhances the driving force for O_2 uptake by the lungs (see Fig. 31-4).
2. Increasing the capacity for gases to diffuse across the alveolar-capillary barrier in the lungs could enhance O_2

uptake at very high cardiac output, particularly at high altitude (see Fig. 27-7).
3. Improving the matching of pulmonary ventilation to perfusion should increase arterial P_{O_2} and the saturation of hemoglobin (see Chapter 31).
4. Increasing the concentration of hemoglobin enables a given volume of arterial blood to carry a greater amount of O_2 (see Chapter 29).

In nearly all conditions of exercise, the pulmonary system maintains alveolar P_{O_2} at levels that are sufficiently high to ensure nearly complete (i.e., ~97%) saturation of hemoglobin with O_2, even at maximal power output. Thus, it is unlikely that an increase in the maximal alveolar ventilation or pulmonary diffusing capacity could explain the large increase in $\dot{V}_{O_{2max}}$ that occurs with training.

Ca_{O_2} would be increased by elevating the blood's hemoglobin concentration. However, no evidence indicates that physical training induces such an increase. On the contrary, [hemoglobin] tends to be slightly lower in endurance athletes, a phenomenon called *sports anemia*, which reflects an expansion of the plasma compartment (discussed later). Whereas increasing [hemoglobin] provides a greater O_2-carrying capacity in blood, maximal O_2 transport does not necessarily increase accordingly because blood viscosity and therefore total vascular resistance also increase. The heart would be required to develop higher arterial pressure to generate an equivalent cardiac output. The resultant increased cardiac work would thus be counterproductive to the overall adaptive response. Blood doping—transfusion of blood before competition—is thus not only illegal, but also hazardous to athletes, particularly when water loss through sweating leads to further hemoconcentration.

Maximizing Cardiac Output Factors that contribute to increasing maximal cardiac output include optimizing the increases in heart rate and cardiac stroke volume so their product (i.e., cardiac output) is maximal (Equation 60-9; see Chapter 25). Because training does not increase maximal heart rate and has a relatively small effect on O_2 extraction, nearly all the increase in $\dot{V}_{O_{2max}}$ that occurs with training must be the result of an increase in maximal cardiac output, the product of optimal heart rate and optimal stroke volume (Equation 60-9). The athlete achieves this increased cardiac output by increasing **maximal cardiac stroke volume.** Maximal cardiac output can increase by ~40% during physical conditioning that also increases maximal aerobic power by 50%. The difference between 40% and 50% is accounted for by increased extraction: $(Ca_{O_2} - Cv_{O_2})_{max}$. This increased extraction is the consequence of capillary proliferation and of increasing the content of mitochondria in muscle fibers that have adapted to endurance training, thereby creating a greater O_2 sink under maximal aerobic conditions.

Maximal cardiac stroke volume increases during aerobic training because expansion of the plasma compartment increases the heart's preload (see Chapter 22), with concomitant hypertrophy of the heart. An increase in preload increases ventricular filling and proportionally increases stroke volume (Starling's law of the heart), thereby elevating maximal cardiac output accordingly. An additional benefit is that a trained athlete achieves a given cardiac output at a

lower heart rate, both at rest and during moderate exercise. Because it is more efficient to increase stroke volume than heart rate, increasing stroke volume reduces the myocardial metabolic load for any particular level of activity.

The expansion of plasma volume probably reflects an increase in albumin content (1 g albumin is dissolved in 18 g of plasma H_2O). This increase appears to be caused both by translocation from the interstitial compartment and by increased synthesis by the liver. The result of more colloid in the capillaries is a shift of fluid from the interstitium to the blood. Although the total volume of red blood cells also increases with aerobic training, the plasma volume expansion is greater than the red blood cell expansion, thus reducing the hemoglobin concentration. This **sports anemia** occurs in highly trained endurance athletes, particularly those acclimatized to hot environments.

The increased blood volume has another beneficial effect. It enhances the ability to maintain high skin blood flow in potentially compromising conditions (e.g., heavy exercise in the heat), thus providing greater heat transport from core to skin and relatively lower storage of heat (see Chapter 59).

Aerobic training enhances O_2 diffusion into muscle

Whereas an increase in maximal cardiac output accounts for most of the increased O_2 delivery to muscle with training, a lesser fraction reflects increased O_2 extraction from blood. Fick's law describes the diffusion of O_2 between the alveolar air and pulmonary capillary blood (see Equation 30-7). A similar relationship describes the diffusion of O_2 from the systemic capillary blood to the mitochondria.

The factors that contribute to O_2 diffusion are analogous to those that affect the diffusing capacity in the lung. Trained muscle can accommodate a greater maximal blood flow because of the growth of new microvessels, particularly capillaries. Indeed, well-conditioned individuals have a 60% greater number of capillaries per cross-sectional area of muscle than do sedentary people. This increased capillary density increases O_2 delivery and thus provides a greater surface area for diffusion. Increase in capillary density also reduces the diffusion distance for O_2 between the capillary and muscle fibers (see Fig. 20-4). In addition, training increases total capillary length and volume, prolongs the transit time of red blood cells along capillaries, and thereby promotes the extraction of O_2 and nutrients from the blood as well as the removal of metabolic byproducts. Finally, training increases cardiac output and muscle blood flow and preserves a relatively high capillary P_{O_2} throughout the muscle that maintains the driving force for O_2 diffusion from capillaries to mitochondria.

Aerobic training increases mitochondrial content

In untrained (but otherwise healthy) individuals, the maximum ability of mitochondria to consume O_2 is considerably greater than that of the cardiovascular system to supply O_2. Thus, mitochondrial content does not limit $\dot{V}_{O_{2max}}$. We have already seen that endurance training markedly increases O_2 delivery. In parallel, endurance training

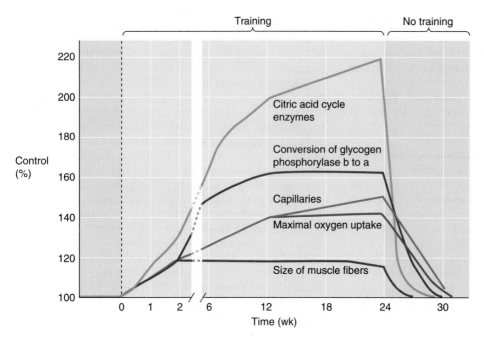

Figure 60-11 Enzyme adaptation during training. Training causes a slow increase in the level of several enzymes, as well as in the number of capillaries, $\dot{V}_{O_{2max}}$, and size of muscle fibers. These changes reverse rapidly on the cessation of training. *(Data from Saltin B, Henriksson J, Nygaard E, Andersen P: Ann N Y Acad Sci 1977; 301:3-29.)*

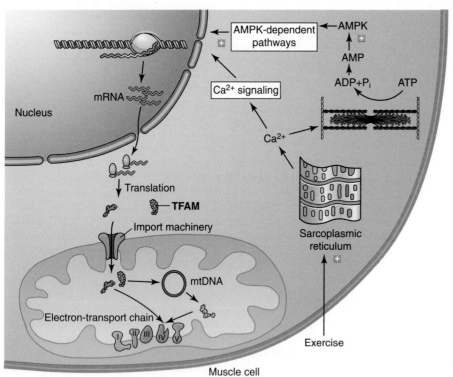

Figure 60-12 Exercise-induced mitochondrial biogenesis. *(Data from Chabi B, Adhihetty PJ, Ljubicic V, Hood DA: Med Sci Sports Exerc 2005; 37:2102-2110.)*

can also increase the mitochondrial content of skeletal muscle fibers nearly 2-fold by stimulating the synthesis of mitochondrial enzymes and other proteins (Fig. 60-11). The stimulus for mitochondrial biogenesis is the repeated activity of the muscle fiber during training, leading to increases in the time-averaged $[Ca^{2+}]_i$, which may act in two ways (Fig. 60-12). One is by directly modulating the transcription of nuclear genes. The other is by increasing cross-bridge cycling and raising $[AMP]_i$, thereby stimulating the fuel sensor AMP

kinase—**AMPK**—which, in turn, can modulate transcription. Some of the newly synthesized proteins are themselves transcription factors that modulate the transcription of nuclear genes. At least one protein (T_{fam}) enters the mitochondrion and stimulates the transcription and translation of mitochondrial genes for key elements of the electron transport chain. Finally, some newly synthesized proteins encoded by genomic DNA, guided by cytoplasmic chaperones, target the mitochondrial import machinery and become part of multiple subunit complexes—together with proteins of mitochondrial origin.

Because mitochondria create the sink for O_2 consumption during the oxidative phosphorylation of ADP to ATP, increased mitochondrial content promotes O_2 extraction from the blood. However, the primary benefit from mitochondrial adaptation in aerobic conditioning is the capacity to oxidize substrates, particularly fat, an ability that enhances endurance of muscle. Recall that mitochondria are responsible not only for the citric acid cycle and oxidative phosphorylation but also for β oxidation of fatty acids. In athletes trained for endurance, the greater reliance on fat at a given level of $\dot{V}_{O_2}$ is the metabolic basis of **glycogen sparing** and thus reduced production of lactate and H^+.

REFERENCES

Books and Reviews

Brooks GA, Fahey TD, Baldwin KM: Exercise Physiology: Human Bioenergetics and Its Applications, 4th ed. Boston: McGraw-Hill, 2004.

Freinkel RK, Woodley DT (eds): The Biology of the Skin. New York: Parthenon, 2001, pp 47-76.

Hurley HJ: The eccrine sweat gland: Structure and function. In Freinkel RK, Woodley DT (eds): The Biology of the Skin. New York: Parthenon, 2001, pp 47-76.

Rowell LR, Shepherd JT (eds): American Physiological Society's Handbook of Physiology, sect 12: Exercise: Regulation and Integration of Multiple Systems. New York: Oxford University Press, 1995.

Tipton CM (ed): American College of Sports Medicine's Advanced Exercise Physiology. Baltimore: Lippincott Williams & Wilkins, 2005.

Journal Articles

Burke RE, Levine DN, Tsairis P, Zajac FE 3rd: Physiological types and histochemical profiles in motor units of the cat gastrocnemius. J Physiol 1973; 234:723-748.

Chabi B, Adhihetty PJ, Ljubicic V, Hood DA: How is mitochondrial biogenesis affected in mitochondrial disease? Med Sci Sports Exerc 2005; 37:2102-2110.

Enoka RM: Morphological features and activation patterns of motor units. J Clin Neurophysiol 1995; 12:538-559.

Holloszy JO: Biochemical adaptations in muscle: Effects of exercise on mitochondrial oxygen uptake and respiratory enzyme activity in skeletal muscle. J Biol Chem 1967; 242:2278-2282.

Salmons S, Sreter FA: Significance of impulse activity in the transformation of skeletal muscle type. Nature 1976; 263:30-34.

Saltin B, Henriksson J, Nygaard E, Andersen P: Fiber types and metabolic potentials of skeletal muscles in sedentary man and endurance runners. Ann N Y Acad Sci 1977; 301:3-29.

Saltin B, Strange S: Maximal oxygen uptake: Old and new arguments for a cardiovascular limitation. Med Sci Sports Exerc 1992; 24:30-37.

Sato K, Kang WH, Saga K, Sato KT: Biology of sweat glands and their disorders. I. Normal sweat gland function. J Am Acad Dermatol 1989; 20:537-563.

Thomas GD, Segal SS: Neural control of muscle blood flow during exercise. J Appl Physiol 2004; 97:731-738.

CHAPTER 61

ENVIRONMENTAL PHYSIOLOGY

Arthur DuBois

The earth and its atmosphere provide environments that are compatible with an extraordinary number of diverse life forms, each adapted to its particular ecologic niche. However, not all the earth's surface is equally friendly for *human* survival, let alone comfort and function. Mountain climbers and deep sea divers know the profound effects of **barometric pressure** (P_B) on human physiology, and astronauts quickly learn how the physically equivalent forces of **gravity** and **acceleration** affect the body. Humans can adapt to changes in P_B and gravity up to a point, but survival under extreme conditions requires special equipment; otherwise, our physiological limitations would restrict our occupancy of this planet to its lowland surfaces.

Much can be learned from exposure to extreme environmental conditions. Although most people do not seek out these extreme environments, the same physiological responses that occur under extreme environmental conditions may also occur, to a lesser extent, in everyday life. In this chapter, I first discuss general principles of environmental physiology and then focus on extreme environments encountered in three activities: deep sea diving, mountain climbing, and space flight.

THE ENVIRONMENT

Voluntary feedback-control mechanisms can modulate the many layers of our external environment

Chapter 1 describes Claude Bernard's concept of the *milieu intérieur* (basically, the extracellular fluid in which cells of the organism live) and his notion that "fixité du milieu intérieur" (the constancy of this extracellular fluid) is the condition of "free, independent life." Chapters 2 through 57 focus mainly on the interaction between cells and their extracellular fluid. In this chapter, I consider how the *milieu extérieur*, which physically surrounds the whole organism, affects our body functions and how we, in turn, modify our surroundings when it is necessary to improve our comfort or to extend the range of habitable environments.

The *milieu extérieur*, in fact, has several layers: the skin surface, the air that surrounds the skin, clothing that may surround that air, additional air that may surround the clothing, a structure (e.g., a house) that may surround that air, and finally a natural environment that surrounds that structure. As we interact with our multilayered environment, sensors monitor multiple aspects of the *milieu intérieur*, and *involuntary* physiological feedback-control mechanisms— operating at a *subconscious* level—make appropriate adjustments to systems that control a panoply of parameters, including blood pressure, ventilation, effective circulating volume, gastric secretions, blood glucose levels, and temperature.

The sensory input can also rise to a *conscious* level and, if perceived as discomfort, can motivate us to take *voluntary* actions that make the surroundings more comfortable. For example, if we sense that we are uncomfortably hot, we may move out of the sun or, if indoors, turn on the air conditioning. If we then sense that we are too cool, we may move into the sun or turn off the air conditioning. Such conscious actions are part of the effector limb in a complex negative feedback system that includes sensors, afferent pathways, integration and conscious decision making in the brain, efferent pathways to our muscles, and perhaps inanimate objects such as air conditioners.

For a voluntary feedback system to operate properly, the person must be aware of a signal from the surroundings and must be able to determine the error by which this signal deviates from a desirable set-point condition. Moreover, the person must respond to this error signal by taking actions that reduce the error signal and thereby restore the *milieu intérieur* to within a normal range. Humans respond to discomfort by a wide variety of activities that may involve any layer of the environment. Thus, we may adjust our clothing, build housing, and eventually even make equipment that allows us to explore the ocean depths, mountain heights, and outer space.

Physiological control mechanisms—involuntary or voluntary—do not always work well. Physicians are acutely aware that factors such as medication, disease, or the extremes of age can interfere with involuntary feedback systems. These same factors can also interfere with voluntary feedback systems. For example, turning on the air conditioning is a difficult or even impossible task for an unconscious person, a bedridden patient, or a perfectly healthy baby. In these situations, a caregiver substitutes for the voluntary physiological control mechanisms. However, to perform this role effectively, the caregiver must understand how the environment would normally affect the care recipient and must anticipate how the involuntary and voluntary physiological control mechanisms would respond.

Environmental temperature provides conscious clues for triggering voluntary feedback mechanisms

Involuntary control mechanisms—discussed in Chapter 60—can only go so far in stabilizing body core temperature in the presence of extreme environmental temperatures. Thus, voluntary control mechanisms can become extremely important.

As summarized in Table 60-1, the usual range of body core temperature is 36°C to 38°C. At an environmental temperature of 26°C to 27°C and a relative humidity of 50%, a naked person is in a **neutral thermal environment** (see Chapter 60), feeling comfortable and being within the zone of vasomotor regulation of body temperature. At 28°C to 29°C, the person feels warm, and ~25% of the skin surface becomes wet with perspiration. At 30°C to 32°C, the person becomes slightly uncomfortable. At 35°C to 37°C, one becomes hot and uncomfortable, ~50% of the skin area is wet, and heat stroke (see the box on heat stroke in Chapter 60) may be possible. The environmental temperature range of 39°C to 43°C is very hot and uncomfortable, and the body may fail to regulate core temperature. At 46°C, the heat is unbearable, and heat stroke is imminent—the body heats rapidly, and the loss of extracellular fluid to sweat may lead to circulatory collapse and death (see Chapter 60).

At the other extreme, we regard environmental temperatures of 24°C to 25°C as cool and 21°C to 22°C as slightly uncomfortable. At temperatures of 19°C to 20°C, we feel cold, vasoconstriction occurs in the hands and feet, and muscles may be painful.

Room ventilation should maintain P$_{O_2}$, P$_{CO_2}$, and toxic substances within acceptable limits

Ventilation of a room ($\dot{V}_{Room}$) must be sufficient to supply enough O_2 and to remove enough CO_2 to keep the partial pressures of these gases within acceptable limits. In addition, it may be necessary to increase $\dot{V}_{Room}$ even more, to lower relative humidity and to reduce odors. As outlined in Table 26-1, dry air in the natural environment at sea level has a P$_{O_2}$ of ~159 mm Hg (20.95%) and a P$_{CO_2}$ of ~0.2 mm Hg (0.03%).

Acceptable limits for P$_{O_2}$ and P$_{CO_2}$

The **acceptable lower limit for** P$_{O_2}$ for work environments is 148 mm Hg in dry air, which is 19.5% of dry air at sea level. The environmental atmosphere of a submarine may be kept at this slightly low P$_{O_2}$ to minimize the chance of fires, yet retain the mental capacity of the occupants.

An **acceptable upper limit for** P$_{CO_2}$ in working environments is 3.8 mm Hg, or 0.5% of dry air at sea level. This level of CO_2 would increase total ventilation by ~7%, a hardly

noticeable rise. Exposures to 3% CO_2 in the ambient air—which initially would cause more substantial respiratory acidosis—could be tolerated for at least 15 minutes, by the end of which it would nearly double total ventilation. With longer exposures to 3% CO_2, the metabolic compensation to respiratory acidosis (see Chapters 28 and 39) would have already begun to increase plasma [HCO$_3^-$] noticeably.

Measuring Room Ventilation Two approaches are available for determining $\dot{V}_{Room}$. The first is a **steady-state method** that requires knowing (1) the rate of CO_2 production ($\dot{V}_{CO_2}$) by the occupants of the room and (2) the fraction of the room air that is CO_2. The equation is analogous to the one introduced for determining *alveolar* ventilation, beginning with Equation 31-9:

$$\dot{V}_{Room} = \frac{\dot{V}_{CO_2}}{\begin{pmatrix} \text{Fraction of} \\ \text{room air} \\ \text{that is } CO_2 \end{pmatrix}} \qquad (61\text{-}1)$$

We could use a similar equation based on P$_{O_2}$ and the rate of O_2 extraction by the occupants.

In the **exponential decay method**, the second approach for determining $\dot{V}_{Room}$, one monitors the washout of a gas from the room. The approach is to add a test gas (e.g., CO_2) to the room and then measure the concentrations of the gas at time zero ($C_{initial}$) and—as $\dot{V}_{Room}$ washes out the gas over some time interval (Δt)—at some later time (C_{final}). The equation for exponential decay is as follows:

$$\dot{V}_{Room} = \frac{V_{Room}}{\Delta t} \ln\left(\frac{C_{initial}}{C_{final}}\right) \qquad (61\text{-}2)$$

For example, imagine that we wish to measure the ventilation of a room that is $3 \times 3 \times 3$ m—a volume of 27 m^3 or 27,000 L. Into this room, we place a tank of 100% CO_2 and a fan to mix the air. We then open the valve on the tank until an infrared CO_2 meter reads 3% CO_2 ($C_{initial}$ = 3%), at which point we shut off the valve on the tank. Ten minutes later (Δt = 10 minutes), the meter reads 1.5% (C_{final} = 1.5%). Substituting these measured values into Equation 61-2 leads to the following:

$$\dot{V}_{Room} = \frac{27,000 \text{ liters}}{10 \text{ min}} \ln\left(\frac{3.0\%}{1.5\%}\right) = 1871 \text{ liters/min} \quad (61\text{-}3)$$

This approach requires that the incoming air contain virtually no CO_2 and that the room contain no CO_2 sources (e.g., people).

Carbon Monoxide More insidious than hypoxia, and less noticeable, is the symptomless encroachment of carbon monoxide (CO) gas on the oxyhemoglobin dissociation curve (see Chapter 29). CO—which can come from incomplete combustion of fuel in furnaces, charcoal burners, or during house fires—suffocates people without their being aware of its presence. Detectors for this gas are thus essential for providing an early warning. CO can be lethal when it occupies approximately half of the binding sites on hemoglobin (Hb), which occurs at a P$_{CO}$ of ~0.13 mm Hg or

$0.13/760 \cong 170$ parts per million (ppm). However, the half-time for washing CO into or out of the body is ~4 hours. Thus, if the ambient CO level were high enough to achieve a 50% saturation of Hb at equilibrium, then after a 2-hour exposure (i.e., one half of the half-time), the CO saturation would be $\frac{1}{2} \times \frac{1}{2} \times 50\%$ or 12.5%. The symptoms at this point would be mild and nonspecific and would include headache, nausea, vomiting, drowsiness, and interference with night vision. Victims with limited coronary blood flow could experience angina. After a 4-hour exposure (i.e., one half-time), the CO saturation would be $\frac{1}{2} \times 50\%$, or 25%. The symptoms would be more severe and would include impaired mental function and perhaps unconsciousness.

Threshold Limit Values and Biological Exposure Indices Threshold limit values (TLVs) are reasonable environmental levels of toxic substances or physical agents (e.g., heat or noise) to which industrial workers can be exposed without causing predictable harm. Rather than depending on concentrations measured in air or food, we can use biological exposure indices (BEIs) to limit exposure to toxic substances by measuring the effects of these substances on animals and humans. The changes detected in the body are called *biomarkers of exposure* and correlate with the intensity and duration of exposure to toxic substances.

Tissues must resist the G force produced by gravity and other mechanisms of acceleration

Standing motionless on the earth's surface at sea level, we experience a gravitational force—our weight—that is the product of our mass and the acceleration resulting from gravity ($g = 9.8 \text{ ms}^{-2}$):

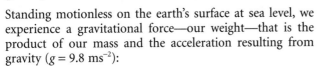

$$\underset{\text{newtons}}{F} = \underset{\text{kg}}{m} \times \underset{\text{ms}^{-2}}{g} \qquad (61\text{-}4)$$

In a particular condition, we may experience a different acceleration (a) from that caused by gravity. The **G force** is a dimensionless number that describes force (m · a) that we experience under a particular condition, relative to the gravitational force (m · g):

$$G = \frac{m \cdot a}{m \cdot g} = \frac{a}{g} \qquad (61\text{-}5)$$

Thus, we normally experience a force of +1G that would cause us to fall with an acceleration of 9.8 ms^{-2} if we were not supported in some way.

Accelerations besides that caused by gravity also affect physiology. An accelerometer, placed on a belt, would show that we can jump upward with an acceleration of ~3G. It would also show that, on landing, we would strike the ground with a force of 3G—a force that our bones and other tissues must be able to tolerate. Later, we discuss G forces from the perspective of air and space flight.

At +1G, each cm^2 of the cross section of a vertebral body, for example, can withstand the compressive force generated by a mass of ~20 kg before the trabeculae begin to be crushed. Thus, at +1G, a vertebral body with a surface area of 10 cm^2 could support the compressive force generated by a mass of

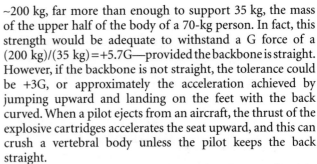

~200 kg, far more than enough to support 35 kg, the mass of the upper half of the body of a 70-kg person. In fact, this strength would be adequate to withstand a G force of a (200 kg)/(35 kg)=+5.7G—provided the backbone is straight. However, if the backbone is not straight, the tolerance could be +3G, or approximately the acceleration achieved by jumping upward and landing on the feet with the back curved. When a pilot ejects from an aircraft, the thrust of the explosive cartridges accelerates the seat upward, and this can crush a vertebral body unless the pilot keeps the back straight.

With increasing age, our bones tend to demineralize (see Chapter 60), a process that weakens them and also causes us to grow shorter because of the demineralization of the vertebrae. Stepping off a curb, an elderly person with demineralized bones may fracture the neck of the femur or crush a vertebra. Demineralization also occurs with immobilization and space flight. In one study, a 6- to 7-week period of immobilization from bed rest led to losses of 14 g of calcium from bones, 1.7 kg of muscle cytoplasm, 21% in the strength of the gastrocnemius muscle, and 6% in average blood volume. The subjects became faint when they were suddenly tilted on a board, head above feet. Although the changes were reversible after these subjects resumed ambulation, it took 4 weeks for muscle strength to return to normal during remobilization.

The partial pressures of gases—other than water—inside the body depend on barometric pressure

As discussed in the next two major sections of this chapter, extremely high or extremely low values of P_B create special challenges for the physiology of the body, particularly the physiology of gases. **Dalton's law** (see Chapter 26 for the box on this topic) states that P_B is the sum of the **partial pressures** of the individual gases in the air mixture. Thus, in the case of ordinary *dry* air (see Table 26-1), most of the sea level P_B of 760 mm Hg is the result of N_2 (~593 mm Hg) and O_2 (~159 mm Hg), with smaller contributions from trace gases such as argon (~7 mm Hg) and CO_2 (~0.2 mm Hg). As P_B increases during diving beneath the water, or as P_B decreases during ascent to high altitude, the partial pressure of each constituent gas in dry ambient air changes in proportion to the change in P_B. At high values of P_B, this relationship is especially important for ambient P_{N_2} and P_{O_2}, which can rise to toxic levels. At low values of P_B, this relationship is important for ambient P_{O_2}, which can fall to levels low enough to compromise the O_2 saturation of Hb (see Chapter 31) and thus the delivery of O_2 to the tissues.

The proportionality between P_B and the partial pressure of constituent gases breaks down in the presence of liquid water. When a gas is in equilibrium with liquid water—as it is for inspired air by the time it reaches the trachea (see Chapter 26)—the partial pressure of water vapor (P_{H_2O}) depends not on P_B but on temperature. Thus, at the very high pressures associated with deep sea diving, P_{H_2O} becomes a negligible fraction of P_B, whereas P_{H_2O} becomes an increasingly dominant factor as we ascend to altitude.

DIVING PHYSIOLOGY

For every 10 m of depth of immersion, barometric pressure increases by 1 atm, thereby compressing gases in the lungs

The average P_B at sea level is 760 mm Hg. In other words, if you stand at sea level, the column of air extending from your feet upward for several tens of kilometers through the atmosphere exerts a pressure of 1 atmosphere (atm). In a deep mine shaft, over which the column of air is even taller, P_B is higher still. However, it is only when diving under water that humans can experience extreme increases in P_B. A column of fresh water extending from the earth's surface upward 10.3 m exerts an additional pressure of 760 mm Hg—as much as a column of air extending from sea level to tens of kilometers skyward. The same is true for a column of water extending from the surface of a lake to a depth of 10.3 m. For seawater, which has a density ~2.5% greater than that of fresh water, the column must be only 10 m to exert 1 atm of pressure. Because liquid water is virtually incompressible, P_B increases linearly with the height (weight) of the column of water (Fig. 61-1). Ten meters below the surface of the sea, P_B is 2 atm, 1 atm for the atmospheric pressure plus 1 atm for the column of water. As the depth increases to 20 m and then to 30 m, P_B increases to 3 atm, then 4 atm, and so on.

Increased external water pressure does not noticeably compress the body's *fluid and solid components* until a depth of ~1.5 km. However, external pressure compresses each of the body's *air* compartments to an extent that depends on the compliance of the compartment. In compliant cavities such as the intestines, external pressure readily compresses internal gases. In relatively stiff cavities, or those that cannot equilibrate readily with external pressure, increases of external pressure can distort the cavity wall, with resulting pain

or damage. For example, when the eustachian tube is blocked, the middle ear pressure cannot equilibrate with external pressure, and blood fills the space in the middle ear or the tympanic membrane ruptures.

According to Boyle's law, pressure and volume vary inversely with each other. Thus, if the chest wall were perfectly compliant, a breath-holding dive to 10 m below the surface would double the pressure and compress the air in the lungs to half its original volume. Aquatic mammals can dive to extreme depths because rib flexibility allows the lungs to empty. Whales, for example, can extend a breath-hold dive for up to 2 hours and can descend to depths as great as 900 m (91 atm) without suffering any ill effects. The human chest wall does not allow complete emptying of the lungs, and, indeed, the human record for a breath-hold dive is 160 m below the surface.

In a **breath-hold dive** that is deep enough to double P_B, alveolar P_{CO_2} could also double to 80 mm Hg. Because this value is substantially higher than the P_{CO_2} of mixed venous blood at sea level (46 mm Hg), the direction of CO_2 diffusion across the blood-gas barrier reverses, and alveolar CO_2 enters pulmonary capillary blood and increases arterial P_{CO_2}. In time, metabolically generated CO_2 accumulates in the blood and eventually raises mixed venous P_{CO_2} to values higher than alveolar P_{CO_2} so CO_2 diffusion again reverses direction, and CO_2 accumulates in the alveoli. The increase in arterial P_{CO_2} can reduce the duration of the dive by increasing ventilatory drive (see Chapter 32). During the ascent phase of the dive, the fall in P_B leads to a fall in alveolar P_{CO_2} and P_{O_2}, promoting the exit of both gases from the blood, and thus a fall in arterial P_{CO_2} and P_{O_2}. The fall in arterial P_{O_2} can lead to **shallow water blackout**.

Divers breathe compressed air to keep their lungs normally expanded

Technical advances have made it possible for divers to remain beneath the water surface for periods longer than permitted by a single breath-hold. One of the earliest devices was a **diving bell** that surrounded the diver on all sides except the bottom. Such a bell was reportedly used by Alexander the Great in 330 BC and then improved by Sir Edmund Halley in 1716 (Fig. 61-2). By the early 19th century, pumping compressed air from above the water surface through a hose to the space underneath the bell kept water out of the bell. In all these cases, the diver breathed air at the same pressure as the surrounding water. Although the pressures both surrounding the diver's chest and inside the airways were far higher than at sea level, the pressure *gradient* across the chest wall was normal. Thus, the lungs were normally expanded.

The conditions are essentially the same in a modern-day **caisson**, a massive, hollow, pressurized structure that functions like a large diving bell. Once again, the pressure inside the caisson (3 to 4 atm) has to be high enough to prevent water at the bottom of the caisson from entering. Several workers ("sand hogs") at the bottom of the caisson may excavate material from the bottom of a river for constructing tunnels or foundations of bridges.

Technical advances also extended to individual divers, who first wore diving suits with spherical helmets over their heads (Fig. 61-3A). The air inside these helmets was pressur-

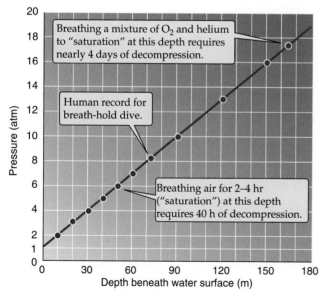

Figure 61-1 Pressures at increasing depth of immersion. The pressure at the surface of the ocean is 1 atm and increases by 1 atm for each 10 m of immersion in sea water.

Breathing a mixture of O_2 and helium to "saturation" at this depth requires nearly 4 days of decompression.

Human record for breath-hold dive.

Breathing air for 2–4 hr ("saturation") at this depth requires 40 h of decompression.

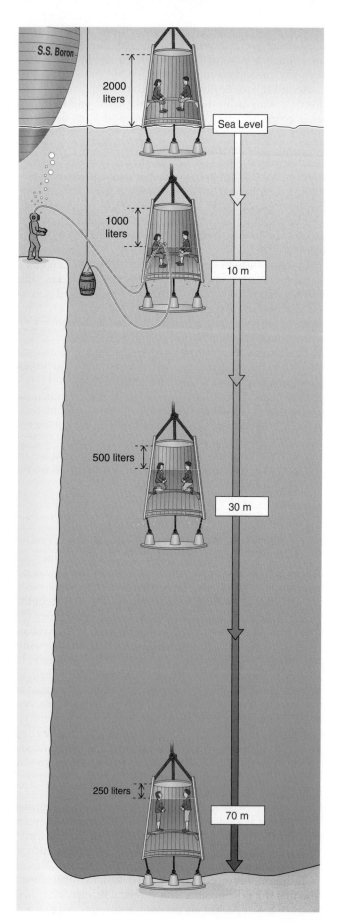

ized to match exactly the pressure of the water in which they were diving. In 1943, Jacques Cousteau perfected the self-contained underwater breathing apparatus, or **SCUBA**, that replaced cumbersome gear and increased the mobility and convenience of an underwater dive (Fig. 61-3B).

Although the foregoing techniques permit deep dives for extended periods of time, they require training and carry the risk of drowning secondary to muscle fatigue and hypothermia. Air floatation and thermal insulation of the diving suit lessen these hazards. For reasons that will become apparent, use of any of these techniques while breathing *room air* carries additional hazards, including nitrogen narcosis, O_2 toxicity, and problems with decompression.

Increasing alveolar P_{N_2} can cause narcosis

Descending beneath the water causes the inspired P_{N_2}—nearly 600 mm Hg at sea level (see Table 26-1)—to increase as P_B increases. According to Henry's law (see Chapter 26 for the box on this topic), the increased P_{N_2} will cause more N_2 to dissolve in pulmonary capillary blood and, eventually, the body's tissues. The dissolved $[N_2]$ in various compartments begins to increase immediately but may take many hours to reach the values predicted by Henry's law, as discussed later. Because of its high lipid solubility, N_2 dissolves readily in adipocytes and in membrane lipids. A high P_{N_2} reduces the ion conductance of membranes, and therefore neuronal excitability, by mechanisms that are similar to those of gas anesthetics. Diving to increased depths (e.g., 4 to 5 atm) while breathing compressed air causes **nitrogen narcosis**. Mild nitrogen narcosis resembles alcohol intoxication (e.g., loss of psychosocial inhibitions). According to "Martini's law," each 15 m of depth has the effects of drinking an additional martini. Progressive narcosis occurs with increasing depth or time of the dive and is accompanied by lethargy and drowsiness, rapid onset of fatigue, and, eventually, loss of consciousness. Because it develops insidiously, nitrogen narcosis poses a potentially fatal threat to divers who are not aware of the risks.

Increasing alveolar P_{O_2} can lead to O_2 toxicity

At sea level, dry inspired air has a P_{O_2} of 159 mm Hg. However, the *alveolar* P_{O_2} of a healthy person at sea level air

---

Figure 61-2 Diving bell. Between 1716 and 1721, Halley, the astronomer who gave his name to the comet, designed and built a wooden diving bell with an open bottom. Because the bell was at a relatively shallow depth (~12 m), the water level rose only partly into the bell. In Halley's system, the air was replenished from a barrel that was open at the bottom and weighted with lead to sink beneath the diving bell. Thus, the air pressure in the barrel was higher than in the bell. The diver used a valve to regulate airflow into the bell. This design was in use for a century, until a practical pump was available for pumping air directly from the surface. The *lower part* of the figure illustrates what would have happened if Halley's bell had been lowered to much greater depths. The greater the depth, the greater the water pressure. Because the air pressure inside the bell must be the same as the water pressure, the air volume progressively decreases at greater depths, and the water level rises inside the bell.

A DIVING HELMET

B SCUBA SYSTEM

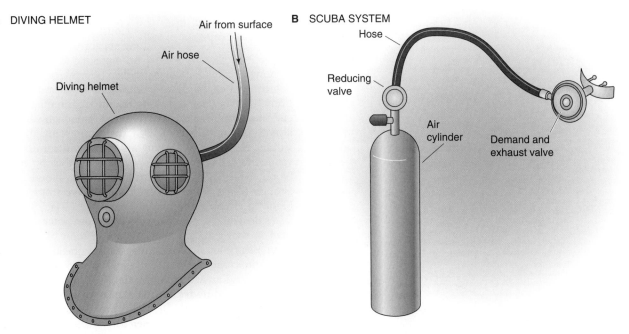

Figure 61-3 Devices for breathing under water. **A,** Compressed air, pumped from the surface to the diver, keeps the pressure inside the helmet slightly higher than that of the surrounding water. **B,** SCUBA is an acronym for self-contained underwater breathing apparatus.

is ~101 mm Hg, reduced from 159 mm Hg by humidification in the airways and removal of O_2 by gas exchange with the blood (see Chapter 31). Arterial P_{O_2} at sea level is very close to alveolar P_{O_2} (within ~10 mm Hg) and nearly saturates Hb, to yield an arterial O_2 content of ~20 mL/dL blood (Fig. 61-4, red curve). As P_B—and therefore arterial P_{O_2}—increases at greater depths, the O_2 bound to Hb increases very little. However, according to Henry's law (see Chapter 26 for the box on this topic), the O_2 that is physically dissolved in the water of blood increases linearly (Fig. 61-4, black line). Thus, the increment of total O_2 content at depth reflects dissolved O_2 (Fig. 61-4, blue curve).

During a breath-hold dive to 5 atm, or in a hyperbaric chamber pressurized to 5 atm, arterial P_{O_2} increases to ~700 mm Hg, slightly higher than breathing 100% O_2 at sea level. Exposure to such a high P_{O_2} has no ill effects for up to several hours. However, prolonged exposure damages the airway epithelium and smooth muscle and causes bronchiolar and alveolar membrane inflammation and, ultimately, pulmonary edema, atelectasis, fibrin formation, and lung consolidation. These effects are the result of inactivating several structural repair enzymes and oxidizing certain cellular constituents.

A prolonged, elevated P_{O_2} also has detrimental effects on nonpulmonary tissues, including the central nervous system (CNS). Exposure to an ambient P_{O_2} of ~1500 mm Hg (e.g., breathing room air at ~10 atm) for as little as 30 to 45 minutes can cause seizures and coma. Preliminary symptoms of **O_2 toxicity** include muscle twitching, nausea, disorientation, and irritability. The toxic effects of O_2 occur because O_2 free radicals (e.g., superoxide and peroxide free radicals) oxidize the polyunsaturated fatty acid component of cell membranes as well as enzymes that are involved in energy metabolism. At the more modest P_{O_2} levels that normally

prevail at sea level, scavenger enzymes (see Chapter 62) eliminate the relatively few radicals formed.

Using helium to replace inspired N_2 and O_2 avoids nitrogen narcosis and O_2 toxicity

Several occupations—including deep mining caisson work and deep diving—require people to spend extended periods at a P_B greater than that at sea level. During an extended dive or other exposure to high pressure (one exceeding several hours), the body's tissues gradually *equilibrate* with the high-pressure gases that one has been breathing. This equilibrated state is referred to by the misnomer **saturation**. At sea level, the human body normally contains ~1 L of dissolved N_2, equally distributed between the body's water and fat compartments. As P_{N_2} rises, the N_2 equilibrates only slowly with the body's lipid stores because adipose tissue is relatively underperfused. Although a deep dive of several minutes does not provide sufficient time to equilibrate the fat with N_2, one of several hours' duration does. At equilibrium—as required by Henry's law—the volume of N_2 dissolved in the tissues is proportional to alveolar P_{N_2}. Thus, if the body normally dissolves 1 L of N_2 at a P_B of 1 atm, it will ultimately dissolve 4 L of N_2 at a P_B of 4 atm. These same principles apply to O_2, although the degree to which O_2 dissolves in various tissues, and the speed at which equilibration takes place, is different.

The adverse effects of N_2 and O_2 depend on the amount of gas that is dissolved in tissues. The amount, in turn, increases with the dive's depth (i.e., partial pressure of the gas) and duration (i.e., how close the gas is to achieving equilibrium with various tissues). Thus, the length of time that a diver can spend safely underwater is inversely proportional to the depth of the dive.

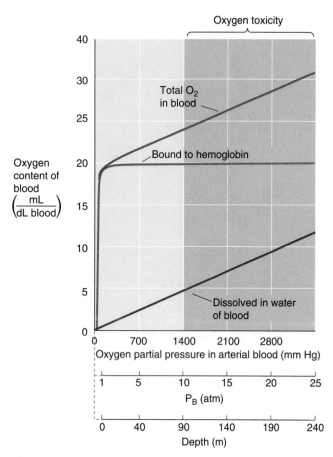

Figure 61-4 O_2 content of blood at high pressures. The *red curve* is the same Hb-O_2 dissociation curve as that in Figure 29-3, except the range is extended to very high values of P_{O_2}.

To prevent **nitrogen narcosis** in saturation diving conditions, divers must partly or completely replace N_2 with another inert gas. Helium is the replacement gas of choice for four reasons:

1. Helium has only a fraction of the narcotizing effect of N_2.
2. Helium dissolves in the tissues to a lesser extent than N_2.
3. Helium has a lower density than N_2, and this lowers effective airway resistance. However, the low density of helium facilitates convective "air" cooling around the body, thereby increasing heat loss. Thus, ambient temperature must be higher in a high-helium compression chamber.
4. During the decompression phase of a dive, helium diffuses out of the tissues more rapidly than does N_2 and thereby alleviates most of the problems associated with decompression.

To prevent **O_2 toxicity** in saturation diving conditions, divers must reduce the fraction of inspired air that is O_2 in the compressed gas mixture. Thus, at a P_B of 10 atm, a mixture of 2% O_2 in helium will provide the same inspired P_{O_2} as room air does at sea level (i.e., ~20% O_2 at a P_B of 1 atm).

Following an extended dive, a diver must decompress slowly to avoid decompression sickness

Although I have focused on problems divers face *while* at great depths, serious difficulties also arise if—*after* a deep saturation dive—the diver *returns* to the surface too quickly. At the end of a saturation dive, P_{N_2} is at the same high value in the alveoli and most tissues. As P_B falls during ascent, alveolar P_{N_2} will fall as well, thus creating a P_{N_2} gradient from the mixed venous blood to the alveolar air. Washout of N_2 from the blood creates a P_{N_2} gradient from tissues to blood. To allow enough time for the dissolved N_2 to move from tissues to blood to alveoli, a diver must rise to the surface slowly (no faster than ~3 m/hr). Because N_2 exits from water much faster than it does from fat, the total elimination of N_2 has two components: some compartments empty quickly (e.g., blood), and some empty slowly (e.g., joints, fat, eyeballs).

Too rapid an ascent causes the N_2 in the tissues—previously dissolved under high pressure—to leave solution and to form bubbles as P_B falls. This process is identical to the formation of gas bubbles when one opens a bottle of a carbonated beverage that had been capped under high pressure. Similar problems can occur in pilots who bail out from a pressurized aircraft at high altitude or in divers who ascend to altitude or become aircraft passengers (i.e., exposed to a lower-than-normal P_B) too soon after completing a dive that, by itself, would not cause difficulties.

During a too-rapid decompression, bubble formation can occur in any tissue in which N_2 has previously dissolved. **Decompression sickness (DCS)** is the general term for the clinical disorder. The pathologic process has three general causes: (1) local formation of bubbles in tissue; (2) bubbles that form emboli in blood; the blood can carry them along until they become wedged in and obstruct a vessel, and a patent foramen ovale can allow bubbles to enter the arterial circulation; and (3) arterial gas embolization; if air is trapped behind an obstructed bronchus, expansion can cause it to tear the lung tissue, enter a pulmonary vein and then a systemic artery, and lodge in the brain or other organ.

Clinicians recognize three categories of DCS. Mild or **type I DCS** can include short-lived mild pains ("niggles"), pruritus, a skin rash, and deep throbbing pain ("bends") resulting from bubbles that form in muscles and joints. Serious or **type II DCS** can include symptoms in the CNS, lungs, and circulatory system. The CNS disorder—most commonly involving the spinal cord—reflects bubble formation in the myelin sheath of axons that compromises nerve conduction. Symptoms may range from dizziness ("staggers") to paralysis. Pulmonary symptoms ("chokes")—resulting from gas emboli in the pulmonary circulation—include burning pain on inspiration, cough, and respiratory distress. In the circulatory system, bubbles can not only obstruct blood flow but also trigger the coagulation cascade and lead to the release of vasoactive substances. Hypovolemic shock is also a part of this syndrome. The third category is **arterial gas embolization**, in which large gas emboli can have catastrophic consequences unless the victim receives immediate recompression treatment.

Figure 61-5 shows how long a diver can spend at various depths—breathing room air—without having to undergo a

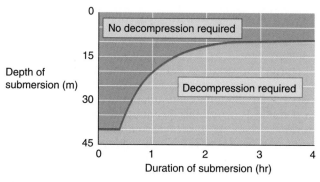

Figure 61-5 The need for decompression as a function of depth and duration of dive. If the dive is sufficiently brief or sufficiently shallow, no decompression is required *(teal area)*. For deeper depths or longer durations, a decompression protocol is required *(salmon area)*. (Data from Duffner GJ: Ciba Clin Symp 1958; 10:99-117.)

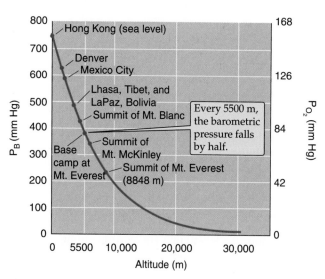

Figure 61-6 Altitude dependence of P_B and P_{O_2} in dry air.

decompression protocol during the ascent. For example, a dive to 8 m can last indefinitely without any ill effects during the ascent. A dive of 25 minutes' duration will not provide sufficient time to saturate the tissues unless the dive exceeds 40 m. However, a longer dive at 40 m will require a decompression program. For instance, a 20-minute dive to a depth of 90 m requires nearly 3 hours of decompression time. Thus, the rate at which a diver should ascend to avoid DCS depends on both the depth and the duration of the dive. Divers use detailed tables to plan their rate of ascent from a deep dive.

The best treatment for DCS is to *recompress* the diver in a hyperbaric chamber. Recompression places the gases back under high pressure and forces them to dissolve again in the tissues, a process that instantly relieves many symptoms. Once the diver is placed under high pressure, decompression can be carried out at a deliberate and supervised pace.

HIGH-ALTITUDE PHYSIOLOGY

Barometric pressure and ambient P_{O_2} on top of Mount Everest are approximately one third of their sea level values

Unlike a column of water, which is relatively noncompressible and has a uniform density, the column of air in the atmosphere is compressible and has a density that decreases exponentially ascending from sea level. Half of the mass of the earth's atmosphere is contained in the lowest 5500 m. Another fourth is contained in the next 5500 m (i.e., 5500 to 11,000 m of altitude). In other words, at higher and higher altitudes, the number of gas molecules pressing down on a mountain climber also falls exponentially; P_B falls by half for each ~5500 m of ascent (Fig. 61-6).

Everest Base Camp   At an altitude of 5500 m—which also happens to be the altitude of the first base camp used in most ascents of Mount Everest—P_B is half the value at sea level ($P_B \cong 380$ mm Hg), as is the ambient P_{O_2} ($P_{O_2} \cong 80$ mm Hg). At this altitude, arterial O_2 delivery (arterial blood O_2 content

× cardiac output) can still meet O_2 demands in most healthy, active persons, even during mild physical activity. However, the body's compensatory responses to reduced ambient P_{O_2} at high altitude vary among different people. Thus, exposure to an altitude of 5500 m is problematic for a significant portion of the population.

Peak of Mount Everest   The peak of Mount Everest—8848 m above sea level—is the highest point on earth. P_B at the peak is ~255 mm Hg, approximately one third that at sea level, and the ambient P_{O_2} is only ~53 mm Hg. For a climber at the peak of Mount Everest, the P_{O_2} of the *humidified* inspired air entering the alveoli is even lower because of the effects of water vapor ($P_{H_2O} = 47$ mm Hg at 37°C). Therefore, the inspired $P_{O_2} = 21\% \times (255 - 47) = 44$ mm Hg, compared with 149 mm Hg at sea level (see Table 26-1). Hypoxia is thus a major problem at the summit of Mount Everest.

Air Travel   Pressurized cabins in passenger planes maintain an ambient pressure equivalent to ~1800 m of altitude (~79% of sea level pressure) in cross-continental flights, or ~2400 m of altitude (~74% of sea level pressure) in transoceanic flights. Considering that most people do not need supplemental O_2 in the inspired air at Denver (~1500 m) or at some ski resorts (~3000 m), most airline passengers are not bothered by the slight reduction in arterial O_2 saturation (89% saturation at 3000 m) associated with these airline cabin pressures. However, passengers with chronic obstructive pulmonary disease may need to carry supplemental O_2 onto the plane even if they do not require it at sea level.

Up to an altitude of ~3000 m, arterial O_2 content falls proportionally less than P_B because of the shape of the hemoglobin-O_2 dissociation curve

Although P_B and ambient P_{O_2} decrease by the same fraction with increasing altitude, the O_2 saturation of Hb in arterial blood decreases relatively little at altitudes up to ~3000 m.

The reason is that, at this altitude, arterial P_{O_2} is 60 to 70 mm Hg, which corresponds to the relatively flat portion of the O_2-Hb dissociation curve (see Fig. 29-3), where almost all the O_2 in blood is bound to Hb. Decreasing arterial P_{O_2} has relatively little effect on arterial O_2 *content* until arterial P_{O_2} falls to less than this flat portion of the curve. Thus, the characteristics of Hb protect the arterial O_2 content, despite modest reductions of P_{O_2}. At higher altitudes, aviators are advised to breathe supplemental O_2.

Although the amount of O_2 in the blood leaving the lung is important, even more important is the amount of O_2 taken up by systemic tissues. This uptake is the product of cardiac output and the arteriovenous (a-v) difference in O_2 content (see Chapter 29). At sea level, arterial P_{O_2} is ~100 mm Hg, corresponding to an Hb saturation of ~97.5%, whereas the mixed venous P_{O_2} is ~40 mm Hg, corresponding to an Hb saturation of ~75%. The difference between the arterial and the venous O_2 contents is ~22.5% of Hb's maximal carrying capacity for O_2. However, at an altitude of 3000 m, arterial P_{O_2} is only ~60 mm Hg, which may correspond to an Hb saturation of only 88%. This reduction in blood O_2 content is called **hypoxemia**. Assuming that everything else remains the same (e.g., O_2 utilization by the tissues, hematocrit, 2,3-diphosphoglycerate levels, pH, cardiac output), then the mixed a-v difference in Hb saturation must still be 22.5%. Thus, the mixed venous blood at 3000 m must have an Hb saturation of 88% − 22.5% = 65.5%, which corresponds to a P_{O_2} of ~33 mm Hg. As a result, the a-v difference of P_{O_2} is much larger at sea level (100 − 40 = 60 mm Hg) than at 3000 m (60 − 33 = 27 mm Hg), even though the a-v difference in O_2 *content* is the same. The reason for the discrepancy is that the O_2-Hb dissociation curve is steeper in the region covered by the P_{O_2} values at high altitude.

At very high altitudes, still another factor comes into play. The uptake of O_2 by pulmonary capillary blood slows at high altitudes and thereby reflects the smaller O_2 gradient from alveolus to blood (see Fig. 30-10D). As a result, at sufficiently high altitudes, particularly during exercise, O_2 may no longer reach diffusion equilibrium between alveolar air and pulmonary capillary blood by the time the blood reaches the end of the capillary. Thus, at increasing altitude, not only does alveolar P_{O_2}—and hence the maximal attainable arterial P_{O_2}—fall in a predictable way, but also the actual arterial P_{O_2} may fall to even a greater extent because of a failure of pulmonary capillary blood to equilibrate with alveolar air.

During the first few days at altitude, compensatory adjustments to hypoxemia include tachycardia and hyperventilation

A reduction in arterial P_{O_2} stimulates the peripheral chemoreceptors and causes an immediate increase in ventilation. Increased ventilation has two effects. First, it brings alveolar P_{O_2} (and thus arterial P_{O_2}) closer to the ambient P_{O_2}. Second, hyperventilation blows off CO_2, the effect of which is respiratory alkalosis that inhibits the peripheral but especially the central chemoreceptors and decreases ventilatory drive (see Chapters 31 and 32). Thus, total ventilation during an acute exposure to 4500 m is only about twice that at sea level, whereas the hypoxia by itself would have produced a much larger stimulation. Accompanying the increased ventilatory

drive during acute altitude exposure is an increase in heart rate, probably owing to the heightened sympathetic drive that accompanies acute hypoxemia (see Chapter 23). The resultant increase in cardiac output enhances O_2 delivery.

During the next few days to weeks at an elevation of 4500 m, **acclimatization** causes ventilation to increase progressively by about the same amount as the acute response. As a result, P_{O_2} continues to improve, and P_{CO_2} falls. Two mechanisms appear to cause this slower phase of increased ventilation. First, the pH of the cerebrospinal fluid (CSF) decreases, an effect that counteracts the respiratory alkalosis induced by the increase in ventilation and thus offsets the inhibition of central chemoreceptors. However, the time course of the pH increase in CSF does not correlate tightly with the time course of the increase in ventilation. The pH at the actual site of the central chemoreceptors may fall with the appropriate time course. Long-term hypoxia appears to increase the sensitivity of the peripheral chemoreceptors to hypoxia, and this effect may better account for acclimatization.

In the second mechanism for acclimatization, the kidneys respond over a period of several days to the respiratory alkalosis by decreasing their rate of acid secretion (see Chapter 39) so blood pH decreases toward normal (i.e., metabolic compensation for respiratory alkalosis). Another result of this compensation is spillage of HCO_3^- into the urine that leads to osmotic diuresis and production of alkaline urine. The consequence of reducing both CSF and plasma pH is to remove part of the inhibition caused by alkaline pH and thus allow hypoxia to drive ventilation to higher values.

An extreme case of adaptation to high altitude occurs in people climbing very high mountains. In 1981, a team of physiologists ascended to the peak of Mount Everest. Although on their way up to the summit the climbers breathed supplemental O_2, at the summit they obtained alveolar gas samples while breathing ambient air—trapping exhaled air in an evacuated metal container. The alveolar P_{CO_2} at the summit was a minuscule 7 to 8 mm Hg, or ~20% of the value of 40 mm Hg at sea level. Thus, assuming a normal rate of CO_2 production, the climber's alveolar ventilation must have been 5-fold higher than normal (see Chapter 31). Because the work of heavy breathing and increased cardiac output at the summit (driven by hypoxia) would increase CO_2 production substantially, the increase in alveolar ventilation must have been much greater than 5-fold.

The climbers' alveolar P_{O_2} at the peak of Mount Everest was ~28 mm Hg, which is marginally adequate to provide a sufficient arterial O_2 content to sustain "resting" metabolic requirement at the summit. However, the term *resting* is somewhat of a misnomer, because the work of breathing and the cardiac output are markedly elevated.

Long-term adaptations to altitude include increases in hematocrit, pulmonary diffusing capacity, capillarity, and oxidative enzymes

Although the increases in ventilation and cardiac output help to maintain O_2 delivery during acute hypoxia, they are costly from an energy standpoint and cannot be sustained for extended periods. During prolonged residence at a high altitude, the reduced arterial P_{O_2} triggers profound adaptations that enhance O_2 delivery to tissues at a cost that is lower than that exacted by short-term compensatory strategies. Many of these adaptations are mediated by an increase in **hypoxia-inducible factor 1 (HIF-1)**, a transcription factor that activates genes involved in erythropoiesis, angiogenesis, and other processes.

Hematocrit   Red blood cell (RBC) mass slowly increases with prolonged hypoxemia. The Hb concentration of blood increases from a sea level value of 14 to 15 g/dL to more than 18 g/dL, and hematocrit increases from 40% to 45% to more than 55%. Normally, the body regulates RBC mass within fairly tight limits. However, renal hypoxia and norepinephrine stimulate the production and release of **erythropoietin (EPO)** from fibroblast-like cells in the kidney (see p. 453 for the box on EPO). EPO is a growth factor that stimulates production of proerythroblasts in bone marrow and also promotes accelerated development of RBCs from their progenitor cells.

Pulmonary Diffusing Capacity   Acclimatization to high altitude also causes a 2- to 3-fold increase in pulmonary diffusing capacity. Much of this increase appears to result from a rise in the blood volume of pulmonary capillaries and from the associated increase in capillary surface area available for diffusion (see Chapter 30). This surface area expands even further because hypoxia stimulates an increase in the depth of inspiration. Finally, right ventricular hypertrophy raises pulmonary arterial pressure and increases perfusion to the upper, well-ventilated regions of the lungs (see Chapter 31).

Capillary Density   Hypoxia causes a dramatic increase in tissue vascularity. Tissue **angiogenesis** (see Chapter 20) occurs within days of exposure to hypoxia, triggered by growth factors released by hypoxic tissues. Among these angiogenic factors are vascular endothelial growth factor (VEGF), fibroblast growth factor (FGF), and angiogenin.

Oxidative Enzymes   Hypoxia promotes expression of oxidative enzymes in the mitochondria and thereby enhances the tissues' ability to extract O_2 from the blood (see Chapter 60). Thus, acclimatization to high altitude increases not only O_2 delivery to the periphery, but also O_2 uptake by the tissues.

Altitude causes mild symptoms in most people and acute or chronic mountain sickness in susceptible individuals

Symptoms of Hypoxia   The first documented evidence of the ill effects of high altitude was in 35 BC, when Chinese travelers called the Himalayas the "Headache Mountains." Recreational mountain climbing became popular in the mid-19th century, and with modern transportation, many people can now travel rapidly to mountain resorts. In fact, it is possible to ascend passively from sea level to high altitude in a matter of minutes (e.g., in a balloon) to hours. A rapid ascent may precipitate a constellation of relatively *mild symptoms*: drowsiness, fatigue, headache, nausea, and a gradual decline in cognition. These uncomfortable effects of

acute hypoxia are progressive with increasing altitude. They occur in some people at altitudes as low as 2100 m and occur in most people at altitudes higher than 3500 m. Initially, these symptoms reflect an inadequate compensatory response to hypoxemia that results in reduced O_2 delivery to the brain. In the longer term, symptoms may stem from mild *cerebral edema*, which probably results from dilation of the cerebral arterioles, thus leading to increased capillary filtration pressure and enhanced transudation (see Chapter 20).

Acute Mountain Sickness   Some people who ascend rapidly to altitudes as seemingly moderate as 3000 to 3500 m develop acute mountain sickness (AMS). The constellation of symptoms is more severe than those described in the previous paragraph and includes headache, fatigue, dizziness, dyspnea, sleep disturbance, peripheral edema, nausea, and vomiting. The symptoms usually develop within the first day and last for 3 to 5 days. The primary problem in AMS is hypoxia, and the symptoms probably have two causes. The first is thought to be a progressive, more severe case of **cerebral edema**. The second cause of the symptoms is **pulmonary edema**, which occurs as hypoxia leads to hypoxic pulmonary vasoconstriction (see Chapter 31), which, in turn, increases total pulmonary vascular resistance, pulmonary capillary pressure, and transudation. Certain people have an exaggerated pulmonary vascular response to hypoxia, and they are especially susceptible to AMS. Cerebral or pulmonary edema can be fatal if the exposure to hypoxia is not rapidly reversed, first by providing supplemental O_2 to breathe and then by removing the individual from the high altitude.

Although being physically fit provides some protection against AMS, the most important factor is an undefined constitutional difference. Persons who are least likely to develop symptoms ventilate more in response to the hypoxia and therefore tend to have a higher P_{O_2} and a lower P_{CO_2}. The higher P_{O_2} and lower P_{CO_2} lead to less cerebral vasodilation, and the higher P_{O_2} minimizes pulmonary vasoconstriction.

Chronic Mountain Sickness   After prolonged residence at high altitude, chronic mountain sickness may develop. The cause of this disorder is an overproduction of RBCs—an exaggerated response to hypoxia. In such conditions, the hematocrit can exceed 60% (**polycythemia**), thereby dramatically increasing blood viscosity and vascular resistance and increasing the risk of intravascular thrombosis. The combination of pulmonary hypoxic vasoconstriction and increased blood viscosity is especially onerous for the right side of the heart, which experiences a greatly increased load. These conditions eventually lead to *congestive heart failure* of the right ventricle.

FLIGHT AND SPACE PHYSIOLOGY

Acceleration in one direction shifts the blood volume in the opposite direction

To accelerate a rocket from rest, we must apply enough force to overcome its inertial force (i.e., its weight, the product of

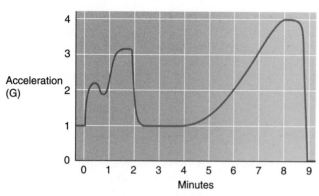

Figure 61-7 G forces during ascent into space on the space shuttle. Before liftoff, astronauts experience +1G, the acceleration that results from the earth's gravity. After liftoff, the solid rockets burn for ~2 minutes, during which time the G force increases to slightly more than +3G. After the solid-rocket burn, the G force falls back to +1G. Thereafter, the main engine gradually builds up the G force to ~+4G before engine cut-off. These G-force data were generated in a human centrifuge to simulate the profile of a shuttle launch. *(Data from Buckey JC, Goble RL, Blomqvist CG: Med Instrum 1987; 87:238-243.)*

 its mass, and the acceleration caused by gravity), as well as the frictional forces of the environment. This requirement is merely a restatement of Newton's *second law* of motion. With the rocket accelerating vertically, astronauts inside experience an inertial *G force*, as required by Newton's *third law*, a force that presses the astronauts into their seats in the direction opposite that of the rocket's acceleration.

Before liftoff, an astronaut experiences only the force of gravity, +1G. As a rocket blasts off from earth, the astronaut experiences higher G forces. In early rockets, astronauts sometimes experienced G forces as high as +10G. Maximal G forces in the space shuttle are only ~+4G (Fig. 61-7). Similarly, pilots of high-performance aircraft experience *positive* G forces as they pull out of a dive, and we all experience *negative* G forces when an aircraft hits turbulence, suddenly loses altitude, and lifts us out of our seats. Although G forces can frequently have potentially large effects on aircraft pilots, they affect astronauts only during the liftoff and re-entry phases of space flight. To ensure that acceleration effects have a minimal influence on body function, astronauts sit with their backs perpendicular to the direction of the accelerating force, so the G force acts across the chest from front to back.

G forces propel the body's tissues in the direction opposite that of acceleration; these forces compress soft tissues against underlying structural elements (e.g., bone) or pull these tissues away from overlying structural elements. In addition, G forces tend to shift the blood volume away from the direction of acceleration, thereby adding to the other component forces that determine blood pressure (see Chapter 17).

In high-performance aircraft, the rapid motions associated with changes in flight direction or altitude produce G forces that can be considerable for several minutes, exceeding 8Gs. Even in relatively primitive aircraft, aerobatic maneuvers can shift blood volume away from the head and can result in transient reductions in cerebral blood flow and O_2

delivery. If these reductions are sufficiently large, they can result in loss of consciousness. The early warnings of such an event are narrowing of the visual field (i.e., loss of peripheral vision) and loss of color perception as the retina is deprived of O_2, a phenomenon called **gray-out**. The term **blackout** describes a total loss of consciousness that occurs during acceleration that lasts for tens of seconds or minutes. Pilots experiencing gray-out or blackout are at extreme risk. As early as World War II, fighter pilots used G-suits that provided counterpressure to the lower extremities during repeated tight maneuvers during dogfights. The counterpressure opposed the pooling of blood in the extremities and maintained sufficient cardiac filling, cardiac output, and blood flow to the brain, thereby eliminating the tendency toward gray-out.

"Weightlessness" causes a cephalad shift of the blood volume

An astronaut in an orbiting spacecraft experiences "weightlessness," a state of near-zero G force, also called a **microgravity** environment. Although an astronaut at an altitude of 200 km still experiences ~94% of the force of the earth's gravity at sea level (i.e., the astronaut truly has weight), the centrifugal force of the spacecraft's orbital trajectory balances the earth's gravitational force, and the astronaut experiences no net acceleration forces and thus has the sensation of weightlessness. This weightlessness, however, differs from the true near-zero-gravity environment in "outer space."

We are adapted to life at +1G, and arteriolar tone in the lower extremities prevents pooling of blood in the capacitance vessels (see Chapter 25), thereby ensuring adequate venous return to the right heart. The acute effects of microgravity on the circulatory system are exactly what you would expect for a system designed to oppose the effect of gravity in a standing person: blood volume redistributes toward the head. This cephalad shift of blood volume—away from the capacitance vessels of the legs—expands the **central blood volume**, increases the cardiac preload, and increases the filtration of plasma water into the interstitium of the facial region. The resulting edema explains the dramatically bloated facial appearance of astronauts in microgravity within 24 hours of the launch. From this discussion, you would think that the **central venous pressure (CVP)** is higher in space. However, such an increase in CVP has been difficult to confirm.

In laboratory studies involving prolonged head-down tilt (i.e., a model intended to simulate microgravity exposure), the cephalad shift of blood volume produces the expected increase in CVP and rapid reflex responses to the apparent volume overload. First, the increased stretch on the right atrium causes release of **atrial natriuretic peptide (ANP)**. Second, stimulation of the low-pressure baroreceptors inhibits secretion of **arginine vasopressin** or antidiuretic hormone from the posterior pituitary (see Chapter 23). These two events increase excretion of salt and water by the kidneys (see Chapter 40). They also correct the perceived volume overload and explain the tendency for astronauts to remain relatively underhydrated during space flight.

In orbiting spacecraft, the cephalad shift of blood volume, even without an increase in CVP, causes a small increase in cerebral arterial pressure and thus in blood flow to the brain. Such regional alterations in blood volume and flow do not substantially affect *total* peripheral resistance in space. Thus, mean arterial pressure and cardiac output are not significantly different from their values on the earth's surface.

Space flight leads to motion sickness and to decreases in muscle and bone mass

Despite training (e.g., in three-dimensional motion simulators), more than half of all astronauts experience motion sickness during the initial days of microgravity. **Motion sickness** (i.e., nausea and vomiting) results from conflicting sensory input to the brain regarding the position of the body. In space flight, motion sickness is the consequence of altered inertial stimulation of the vestibular system in the absence of normal gravitational forces. Nearly all cases of motion sickness resolve within the first 96 hours of microgravity exposure as the vestibular system or the CNS accommodates to the novel input.

The increased cerebral blood flow and blood volume in microgravity, accompanied by increased capillary filtration of fluid from the intravascular space, contribute to the increased incidence of headache, nausea, and motion sickness, at least during the transition period to microgravity. These symptoms reduce performance. Astronauts attempt to minimize these effects by restricting water intake before launch.

Numerous other changes occur during prolonged residence in microgravity, many of which are related to the markedly diminished aerobic power output in space, where the force of gravity does not oppose muscle contraction. The major physiological alterations include reductions in body water content, plasma and RBC volume, total body N_2 stores, muscle mass, and total body Ca^{2+} and phosphate (associated with a loss in bone mass). The bone loss appears to be continuous with time in a weightless environment, whereas the other changes occur only during the first weeks in space. The reductions in plasma and RBC volumes result in a marked decrease in *maximum* cardiac output, a determinant of maximal aerobic power. The reduction of muscle mass decreases the maximal force developed by muscle. The reduction in bone mass similarly decreases bone strength. Although these changes are appropriate adaptations to a microgravity environment, in which great strength and high aerobic capacity have little inherent value, they are decidedly disadvantageous on return to the earth's surface.

Exercise partially overcomes the deconditioning of muscles during space flight

The intermittent loading of muscles, bone, and the cardiovascular system prevents—to some extent—the *deconditioning* effects of space flight on muscle mass and performance. Astronauts have used bungee (i.e., elastic) cords and ergometric (i.e., work-measuring) stationary bicycles to provide resistance against which to exert force. The most effective exercise regimen appears to be walking on a motor-driven treadmill with the lower body encased in a **negative-pressure chamber**. Reducing the chamber pressure to 100 mm Hg lower than ambient pressure creates transmu-

ral pressure differences—across the blood vessels in the feet—that are similar to pressure differences when standing upright on the earth's surface. However, this arrangement greatly exaggerates transmural pressure differences near the waist. For this reason, these astronauts also wear positive-pressure pants that compress the tissues by 70 mm Hg at the level of the waist and—decrementally—by 0 mm Hg at the feet. The net effect of the negative-pressure chamber and the graded positive-pressure pants is to create a physiological toe-to-waist gradient of transmural pressures across the blood vessels of the lower body. The aerobic activity, the impact of the feet on the treadmill, and the generation of physiological transmural pressure gradients appear to be sufficient to simulate exercise at +1G. This regimen can reduce or even eliminate the deconditioning effects of space flight.

Return to earth requires special measures to maintain arterial blood pressure

The problems associated with re-entry reflect a return to full gravity on earth's surface. The most dramatic effects result from reduced blood volume and decreased tone of the leg vessels. Both factors contribute to reductions in cardiac preload, orthostatic tolerance, and exercise capacity. It has been common practice to shield astronauts from public view immediately after return to the earth's surface, until they have regained a good orthostatic response.

In recent years, astronauts have employed various strategies just before re-entry to counter the adaptations to microgravity. The countermeasure to orthostatic intolerance is restoration of blood volume before re-entry. One means of attenuating the reduction of blood volume in space flight is an exercise program. Even a brief period (e.g., 30 minutes) of intense exercise expands plasma albumin content and increases plasma oncotic pressure and plasma volume by 10% within 24 hours. The problems with exercise programs are difficulties in logistics and the astronauts' lack of motivation. A second means of minimizing the reduced blood volume is increasing salt and fluid intake. However, this practice has proven difficult to implement because of the consequent increase in urine flow. Currently, astronauts are educated about the effects of prolonged space flight and are then maintained under continuous scrutiny after re-entry until they have regained a normal orthostatic response. This usually occurs within hours, and certainly within 1 day, of re-entry.

REFERENCES

Books and Reviews

Bunn HF, Poyton RO: Oxygen sensing and molecular adaptation to hypoxia. Physiol Rev 1996; 76:839-885.

Crystal RG, West JB: The Lung. New York: Raven Press, 1991.

Duffner GJ: Medical problems involved in underwater compression and decompression. Ciba Clin Symp 1958; 10:99-117.

Krakauer J: Into Thin Air. New York: Anchor Books–Doubleday, 1997.

Monge C: Chronic mountain sickness. Physiol Rev 1943; 23:166-184.

West JB: Man in space. News Physiol Sci 1986; 1:189-192.

Journal Articles

Buckey JC, Goble RL, Blomqvist CG: A new device for continuous ambulatory central venous pressure measurement. Med Instrum 1987; 87:238-243.

Cain SM, Dunn JE II: Low doses of acetazolamide to aid the accommodation of men to altitude. J Appl Physiol 1966; 21:1195-1200.

Schoene RB, Lahiri S, Hackett PH, et al: Relationship of hypoxic ventilatory response to exercise performance on Mount Everest. J Appl Physiol 1984; 56:1478-1483.

West JB: Human physiology at extreme altitudes on Mount Everest. Science 1984; 223:784-788.

CHAPTER 62

THE PHYSIOLOGY OF AGING

Edward J. Masoro

Biomedical science paid surprisingly little attention to a remarkable change in human biology during the 20th century—the marked increase in human **life expectancy** in developed nations. For example, in the United States, life expectancy for men progressively increased from 47.9 years in 1900 to 74.5 years in 2002, and for women, it increased from 50.7 years in 1900 to 79.9 years in 2002. Not until 1974 did the United States establish the National Institute on Aging (NIA) in the National Institutes of Health. The NIA has had a major impact in the United States and throughout the world in the promotion of research on aging and on the development of geriatric medicine.

CONCEPTS IN AGING

During the 20th century, the age structure of populations in developed nations shifted toward older individuals

The fraction of the U.S. population 65 years of age or older was only 4% in 1900 but 13% in 1990. This trend in age structure is projected to continue (Fig. 62-1). Moreover, because women have a greater life expectancy, they comprised 70.5% of the population that was more than 80 years old in 1990 in developed nations.

The shift in age structure of the U.S. population during the 20th century depended only modestly on an increase in life expectancy from birth. More important was the progressive decrease in birth rates, which led the elderly to become an ever-increasing fraction of the population, particularly in developed nations. Indeed, the effect of the post-World War II "Baby Boom Generation" on population age structure is clearly apparent in Figure 62-1. However, because birth rates are unlikely to fall much further, future changes in the age structure of the U.S. population will depend mainly on further projected increases in life expectancy.

The definition, occurrence, and measurement of aging are fundamental but controversial issues

The **age** of an organism usually refers to the length of time the individual has existed. Biogerontologists and members of the general public alike usually use aging to mean the process of **senescence**. For example, we may say that a person is young for her age, an expression meaning that the processes of senescence appear to be occurring slowly in that person. **Aging**—the synonym for senescence that we use throughout this chapter—*is the progressive deteriorative changes, during the adult period of life, which underlie an increasing vulnerability to challenges and thereby decrease the ability of the organism to survive.*

Biogerontologists distinguish **biological age** from **chronologic age**. Although we easily recognize the biological aging of family members, friends, and pets, it would be helpful to have a quantitative measure of the rate of aging of an *individual*. **Biomarkers of aging**—morphologic and functional changes that occur with time in the adult organism—could in principle serve as a measure of senescent deterioration. Alas, a generally agreed on panel of biomarkers of aging has yet to emerge, so it is currently impossible to quantitate the aging of individuals.

In contrast to the aging of *individuals*, it has long been possible to measure the rate of aging of *populations*. In 1825, Benjamin Gompertz, a British actuary, published a report on human **age-specific death rate**—the fraction of the population entering an age interval (e.g., 60 to 61 years of age) that dies during the age interval. Gompertz found that, after early adulthood, the age-specific death rate increases exponentially with increasing adult age. The same is true for other human populations (Fig. 62-2) and for many animal populations. Based on the assumption that the death rate reflects the vulnerability caused by senescence, it has generally been accepted that the slope in Figure 62-2 reflects the rate of population aging. Although gompertzian and related analyses had long been viewed as the "gold standard" for measuring population aging, some biogerontologists have challenged this approach.

Aging is an evolved trait

Most evolutionary biologists no longer accept the once popular belief that aging is an evolutionary adaptation with a genetic program similar to that for development. The current view is that aging evolved by default and reflected the absence of **forces of natural selection** that would

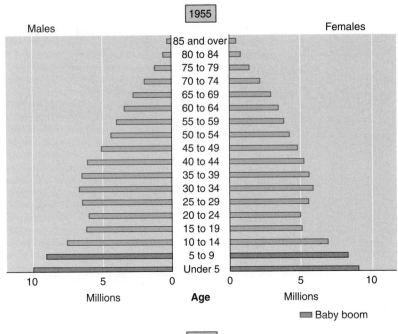

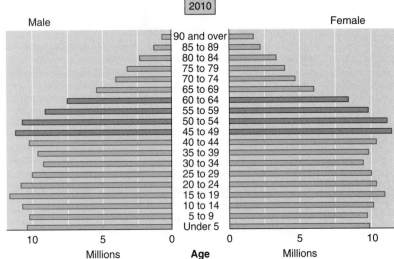

Figure 62-1 The age structure of the 1955 U.S. population and the projected age structure of the 2010 U.S. population. *(From Tauber C: Sixty-Five Plus in America. Washington, DC: U. S. Bureau of the Census, 1992, rev. 1993.)*

otherwise eliminate mutations that promote senescence. For example, consider a cohort of a species that reaches reproductive maturity at age X. At that age, all members of the cohort will be involved in generating progeny. Furthermore, assume that this species is evolving in a hostile environment—the case for most species. As the age of this cohort increases past X, fewer and fewer members survive, so that all members of the cohort die before exhibiting senescence. In this cohort, genes with detrimental actions—expressed only at advanced ages—would not be subjected to natural selection. If we now move the progeny of our cohort to a highly protective environment, many may well live to ages at which the deleterious genes can express their effects, thereby giving rise to the **aging phenotype**. This general concept led to three genetic mechanisms, discussed in the following paragraphs. These mechanisms are not mutually exclusive, and each has experimental support.

In 1952, Peter Medawar proposed a variant of the foregoing model, now referred to as the **mutation-accumulation mechanism**. He proposed that most deleterious mutations in gametes will result in progeny that are defective during most of life, and natural selection removes such genes from the population. However, a very few mutated genes will not have deleterious effects until advanced ages, and natural selection would fail to eliminate such genes.

George Williams proposed another variant in 1957. He postulated that the genes with deleterious actions in late life actually increase evolutionary fitness in early adulthood. Natural selection will strongly favor such alleles because they promote the ability of the young adult to generate progeny and because they have a negative impact only after reproduction—**antagonistic pleiotropy**. In this situation, aging is a byproduct of natural selection.

In 1977, Tom Kirkwood proposed the **Disposable Soma Theory**, according to which the fundamental life role of organisms is to generate progeny. Natural selection would apportion the use of available energy between reproduction and body (i.e., somatic) maintenance, to maximize the individual's lifetime yield of progeny. As a consequence, less energy is available for somatic maintenance than is needed

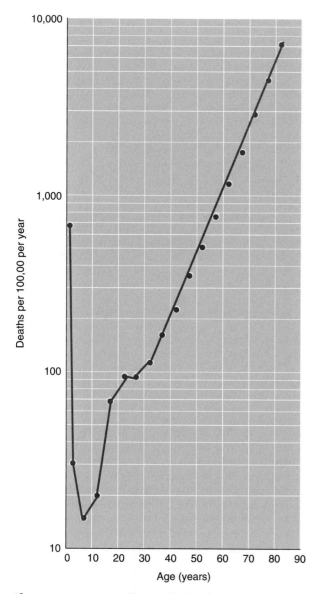

Figure 62-2 Age-specific mortality for the U.S. population (men and women) for 2002. Data are projections from the 2000 U.S. census.

for indefinite survival. This theory further proposes that a hostile environment increases the fraction of energy expended in reproduction and leaves a smaller fraction for somatic maintenance.

Measurements of human aging can be either cross sectional or longitudinal

Measuring the effects of aging on the human physiology presents investigators with a difficulty—the subjects' life span is greater than the investigator's scientific life span.

Cross-Sectional Design The usual approach to the foregoing difficulty is a cross-sectional design in which investigators study cohorts with several different age ranges (e.g., 20 to 29 year olds, 30 to 39 year olds) over a brief period (e.g., a calendar year). However, this design suffers from two serious potential confounders. One is the **cohort effect**; that

is, different cohorts have had different environmental experiences. For example, in studies of the effects of aging on cognition, a confounding factor could be that younger cohorts have had the benefit of a relatively higher level of education. If aware of a potential confounder, the investigator may be able to modify the study's design to avoid the confounder.

The second potential confounder is **selective mortality**—individuals with risk factors for diseases that cause death at a relatively young age are underrepresented in older age groups. For example, in a study on the effect of age on plasma lipoproteins, mortality at a young age from cardiovascular disease would preferentially eliminate individuals with the highest low-density lipoprotein levels.

Longitudinal Design To circumvent the confounders encountered in cross-sectional designs, investigators can repeatedly study a subject over a significant portion of his or her lifetime. However, this longitudinal design has other problems. Long-term longitudinal studies require a special organizational structure that can outlive an individual investigator and complete the study. Even shorter longitudinal studies are very costly. Some problems are inherent in the course of longitudinal studies, including the effect of repeated measurements on the function assessed, changes in subjects' lifestyle (e.g., diet), dropout of subjects from the study, and changes in professional personnel and technology.

Whether age-associated diseases are an integral part of aging remains controversial

Age-associated diseases are those that do not cause morbidity or mortality until advanced ages. Examples are coronary artery disease, stroke, many cancers, type 2 diabetes, osteoarthritis, osteoporosis, cataracts, Alzheimer disease, and Parkinson disease. These are either chronic diseases or acute diseases that result from long-term processes (e.g., atherogenesis).

Most gerontologists have held the view that age-associated diseases are *not* an integral part of aging. These gerontologists developed the concept of primary and secondary aging to explain why age-associated diseases occur in almost all elderly people. **Primary aging** refers to intrinsic changes occurring with age, unrelated to disease or environmental influences. **Secondary aging** refers to changes caused by the interaction of primary aging with environmental influences or disease processes.

In contrast, some gerontologists adhere to the following view, expressed by Robin Holliday: "The distinction between age-related changes that are not pathological and those that are pathological is not at all fundamental." Moreover, the genetic mechanisms proposed for the evolution of aging may apply equally to the processes underlying both primary and secondary aging.

CELLULAR AND MOLECULAR MECHANISMS OF AGING

In this major section, I consider three major classes of cellular and molecular processes that may be proximate causes of organismic aging: (1) damage caused by oxidative stress and other factors, (2) inadequate repair of damage, and (3) dysregulation of cell number. No single one of these processes is *the* underlying mechanism of aging. The basic mechanism of aging is likely to be the long-term imbalance between damage and repair. During growth and development, the genetic program not only creates a complex structure, but also repairs damaged molecules that arise in the process. Following development is a brief adult period when damage and repair are in balance, and then begins long-term imbalance in favor of damage.

The factors underlying the imbalance vary among species and among individuals within species, as a result of both genetic and environmental variability. For example, oxidative stress is one of many damaging processes that underlie aging, and the genome of the animal as well as the environment will determine the extent to which it is an important causal factor.

Oxidative stress and related processes that damage macromolecules may have a causal role in aging

One gram of tissue from a small mammal has a higher resting metabolic rate (RMR; see Chapter 58) than the same mass of tissue from a larger mammal (e.g., a human). Because smaller mammals have a shorter life span than humans, Max Rubner reported in 1908 that a gram of tissue from diverse domestic animals and humans has similar lifetime energy expenditure. Based on these findings, Raymond Pearl in 1928 proposed that organisms have a finite amount of a "vital principle" that they deplete at a rate proportional to the rate of energy expenditure. However, later experimental evidence did not support this *Rate of Living Theory of Aging.*

Reactive O₂ Species As illustrated in Figure 62-3A, reactive oxygen species (ROS) include molecules such as **hydrogen peroxide (H_2O_2)**, neutral free radicals such as the **hydroxyl radical ($^\bullet OH$)**, and anionic radicals such as the **superoxide anion radical (O_2^-)**. **Free radicals** have an unpaired electron in the outer orbital, shown in red in Figure 62-3A. These free radicals are extremely unstable because they react with a target molecule to capture an electron and thus become a stable molecule with only paired electrons in the outer shell. However, the target molecule left behind becomes a free radical, initiating a chain reaction that continues until two free radicals meet to create a product with a covalent bond. ROS—particularly $^\bullet OH$, which is the most reactive of them all—have the potential to damage important biological molecules, such as proteins, lipids and DNA. However, ROS also play important physiological roles in the oxidation of iodide anions by thyroid peroxidase in the formation of thyroid hormone (see Chapter 49), as well as in the destruction of certain bacteria by NADPH oxidase and myeloperoxidase in phagocytic cells. Finally, the highly reactive signaling molecule nitric oxide (see Chapter 3) is a free radical (Fig. 62-3A).

ROS can also form as the result of ionizing radiation. Quantitatively, the most important source of ROS is the mitochondrial electron transport chain (see Chapter 5).

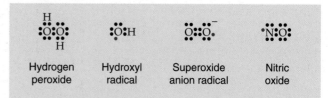

Hydrogen peroxide   Hydroxyl radical   Superoxide anion radical   Nitric oxide

B MITOCHONDRIAL GENERATION OF ROS

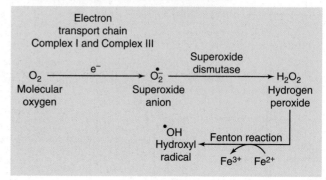

Figure 62-3 ROS. **A**, Structures. **B**, Mitochondrial generation.

Complex I and complex III of the electron transport chain generate O_2^- as byproducts (Fig. 62-3B). The enzyme **superoxide dismutase (SOD)** converts O_2^- to H_2O_2, which, in turn, can yield the highly reactive $^\bullet OH$.

Only a small fraction of the oxygen (<1%) used in aerobic metabolism generates ROS. However, even that amount would be lethal in the absence of protective mechanisms. Fortunately, organisms have two potent antioxidant defenses. The major defense is enzymatic, specifically SODs, catalase, and glutathione peroxidase (Fig. 62-4). In addition, low-molecular-weight antioxidants, such as vitamins C and E, play a minor role in the defense against the metabolically produced radicals.

Because these defense mechanisms are not fully protective, some investigators have suggested that ROS may cause the molecular damage observed in aging. According to the **oxidative stress theory**, an imbalance between the production and removal of ROS is the major cause of aging.

Glycation and Glycoxidation **Glycation** refers to nonenzymatic reactions between the carbonyl groups of reducing sugars (e.g., glucose) and the amino groups of macromolecules (e.g., proteins, DNA) to form **advanced glycation end products (AGEs)**. Figure 62-5 shows an interaction of open-chain D-glucose with a lysine residue on a protein, yielding a Schiff base, and water. The Schiff base undergoes an intramolecular rearrangement to form an open-chain Amadori compound that undergoes the Amadori rearrangement to form a ring structure called an **Amadori product**. In cooking, Amadori products undergo a series of further reactions to produce polymers and copolymers called melanoidins, which give a brown color to cooked food. In humans, the Amadori product can undergo a series of intramolecular and intermolecular rearrangements that include oxidation (**glycoxidation**) to form AGE molecules. For example, the Amadori product in Figure 62-5 can either form **carboxymethyllysine** or react with an arginine residue on the same or a different protein to form a cross-link called **pentosidine**.

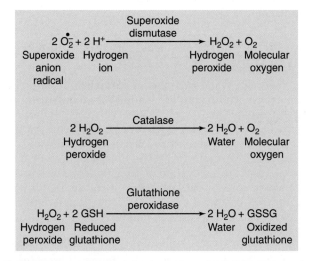

Figure 62-4 Enzymatic defenses against ROS. SODs eliminate the O_2^- but generate H_2O_2, which, as shown in Figure 62-3B, can yield the highly reactive ·OH through the Fenton reaction. The H_2O_2 is eliminated by catalase or glutathione peroxidase, which yield relatively nonreactive products: water, molecular O_2, and oxidized glutathione.

The formation of AGEs is especially important for long-lived proteins, and it appears to play a role in the long-term complications of diabetes. The similarity between the aging phenotype and that of the diabetic patient led Anthony Cerami to propose the **Glycation Hypothesis of Aging**. Although glucose is not the only reducing sugar involved in glycation, it is an important one. Thus, the level of **glycemia** is a major factor in glycation, and periods of hyperglycemia are probably the reason glycation—including the glycation of hemoglobin—is enhanced in patients with diabetes. Proteins containing AGEs exhibit altered structural and functional properties. For example, AGE formation in lens proteins of the eye probably contribute to age-associated opacification. Moreover, with advancing age, the increased stiffness of collagen in connective tissues (e.g., blood vessels; see Chapter 19) may also, in part, contribute to AGE-mediated collagen cross-links. AGE-induced DNA damage may lead to alterations in genomic function.

Mitochondrial Damage Because mitochondria are the major *source* of ROS, they are also likely to be a major *target* of oxidative damage. Damage to mitochondrial DNA (mtDNA) increases greatly with age because, unlike genomic DNA, mtDNA is not protected by histones (see Chapter 4). According to the **Mitochondrial Theory of Aging**, the damage to mtDNA reduces ability of the mitochondria to generate ATP, and this decreased production of ATP results in the loss of cell function and hence aging.

Somatic Mutations Damage to genomic DNA and mtDNA can occur as the result of radiation and other

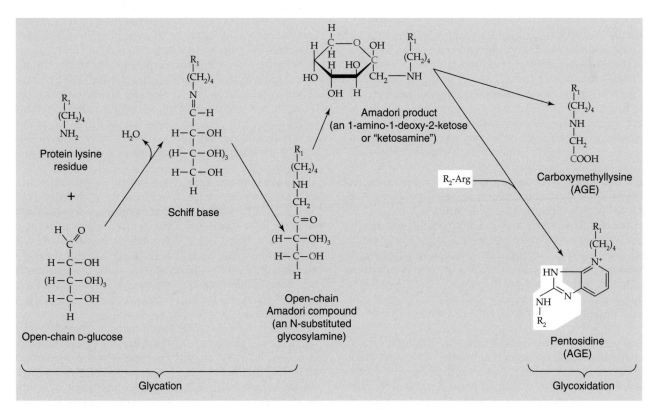

Figure 62-5 Examples of glycation, glycoxidation, and the formation of AGEs. R_1 and R_2, two different proteins or two different domains of the same protein.

environmental agents, such as toxic chemicals. In recent years, oxidative stress has been recognized as a major source of DNA damage. Cells can repair much of the damage to DNA, and the level of damage is in a steady state between damaging and repair processes. According to the **DNA Damage Theory of Aging**, accumulated DNA damage interferes with DNA replication and transcription, thereby impairing the ability of cells to function and causing aging. Moreover, this loss of function increases as the steady-state level of DNA damage increases. Although oxidative stress results in DNA damage, it is not clear that DNA damage and mutations in somatic cells are sufficient to cause the organismic functional deterioration that characterizes the aging phenotype.

Age-associated inadequacy of repair processes may contribute to the aging phenotype

Many biogerontologists believe that agents that cause damage throughout life are not really the cause of aging. Rather, they believe that aging occurs because of the progressive age-associated loss in the ability to repair such damage.

DNA Repair   As noted earlier, the steady-state level of damaged DNA depends on the balance between damaging and repair processes. The **DNA Repair Theory of Aging** proposes that DNA repair declines with advancing age and eventually falls, the steady-state level of DNA damage consequently rises, and the integrity of the genome is thereby compromised. Investigators have tested the effects of aging on only some of the cell's multiple repair pathways in some species. For example, evidence suggests that the repair of nucleotide excision decreases with advancing age in laboratory rodents.

Protein Turnover   In addition to oxidative stress and non-enzymatic glycation, many other processes occur, including deamidation, racemization, and isomerization. These many different alterations result in changes in the secondary and tertiary structures as well as aggregation and fragmentation of protein molecules, all of which can interfere with protein function. Protecting the organism from an excessive accumulation of altered proteins are proteolytic degradation and subsequent biosynthetic replacement—**protein turnover**.

The rate of total body protein turnover in humans decreases with age. Thus, the average lifetime of most, but not all protein, species increases with age. Especially susceptible to damage are the long-lived proteins in the extracellular matrix, particularly collagen and elastin, which with increasing age undergo changes such as oxidation, glycation, and cross-linking. For the cells embedded in the matrix, these changes probably alter properties such as proliferation, migration, and the response to cytokines. It is possible that an increased level of altered proteins results in loss of functional proteins and may contribute to aging.

Membrane Deterioration   Because of the high level of polyunsaturated fatty acids (i.e., those with many double bonds) in the phospholipid bilayer of many membranes, oxidative processes generate **lipid peroxides** that accumulate with age in the membranes. Moreover, lipid peroxides can undergo cleavage to yield reactive lipid aldehydes that further damage the membrane, including its proteins. Although the

cell rapidly replaces membrane lipids with new molecules, these replacements alter the membranes. Thus, the number of double bonds in the fatty acids gradually falls, and the ratio of cholesterol to phospholipid in the membrane lipids gradually rises. Therefore, with increasing age, membrane fluidity (see Chapter 2) gradually decreases. It is possible that these age-associated changes may interfere with important membrane functions, such as the barrier function, transport, and signaling processes.

Dysfunction of the homeostasis of cell number may be a major factor in aging

For most cell types, the number of cells remains nearly constant over much of adult life. An imbalance in favor of *cell division* results in hyperplasia (see Chapter 48), such as occurs in the prostate of elderly men, or in neoplasia (i.e., formation of new, abnormal cells), a disease process that increases in frequency with age. An imbalance in favor of *cell removal* results in a reduction of cell number, such as occurs with age in some skeletal muscles. Of course, in cell types that are truly postmitotic in adult life, any age-associated loss of cells results in a decrease in number.

Limitations in Cell Division   In 1961, Leonard Hayflick and Paul Moorhead reported that human fibroblasts in culture could divide only a limited number of times, a phenomenon known as the *Hayflick limit*. This concept also applies to many other somatic cell types in culture. Although Hayflick hypothesized that this limited cell proliferation in culture was a "test tube" model of aging, more recent findings indicated that the in vitro cell culture system falls short as a valid model of organismic aging. Nevertheless, intensive study of the Hayflick limit led to consideration of the role of telomeres in aging.

Telomeres are elements at the ends of linear chromosomes and are composed of repeated specific DNA sequences and associated proteins. In the late 1980s, Calvin Harley found that the telomeres of human cells in culture shortened with each mitotic division. When the telomeres shorten to a critical length, the cell can no longer divide—a probable basis of the Hayflick limit. Such cells also exhibit other functional changes.

Are the telomere findings in culture systems relevant to organismic senescence? A reduction in telomere length could play a role for cell types that exhibit an age-associated decrease in cell number. Clearly, a reduction in telomere length cannot be a factor in the aging of cells that are truly postmitotic during adult life. Telomeres do not shorten in the germline, which, unlike somatic cells, contains significant levels of **telomerase**, an enzyme that catalyzes the extension of telomere length. Cancer cells are also rich in telomerase.

Although not associated with a major dysregulation of cell number, aging may impair the burst in proliferation that is needed to meet certain challenges. For example, with increasing age, the immune system is less effective in protecting the organism from infection. An important factor may be that an antigenic challenge may trigger a proliferation of T lymphocytes, perhaps because of an age-associated decrease in the length of T-lymphocyte telomeres.

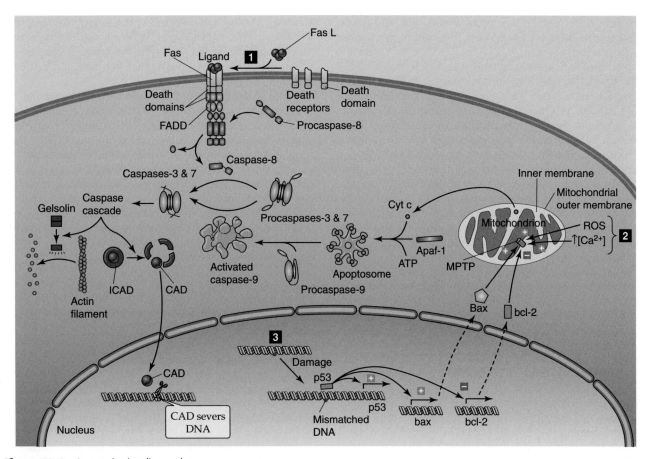

Figure 62-6 Apoptotic signaling pathways.

Cell Removal   Necrosis and apoptosis are two major processes by which the body loses cells. **Necrosis,** a cellular response to severe trauma, is manifested by uncontrolled breakdown of cellular structure, cell lysis, and an inflammatory response. The morphologic characteristics of necrosis are cell swelling and loss of membrane integrity.

Apoptosis is programmed cell death (see Chapter 2). It plays a key role in organogenesis and tissue renewal, and it also occurs in response to relatively mild damage. Apoptosis requires ATP, is gene driven, and is characterized by preservation of organelles, maintenance of membrane integrity, absence of inflammation, cell shrinkage, and fragmentation of the cell into multiple membrane-enclosed apoptotic bodies. Macrophages or neighboring cells remove the apoptotic bodies by phagocytosis.

Three interacting pathways (see Fig. 25-1C) lead to apoptosis (Fig. 62-6). First, in the **extrinsic pathway,** extracellular signals bind to cell surface receptors—**death receptors (DRs)**—of the tumor necrosis factor receptor (TNFR) family, which are examples of receptors that act at least in part through regulated proteolysis (see Table 3-1). The DRs include Fas, TNFR1, DR3, DR4, and DR5, all of which have a cytosolic **death domain.** In the case of the receptor **Fas,** the homotrimeric ligand called **FasL** binds to three Fas molecules and results in the formation of a trimer of ligand-receptor complexes. This clustering allows the death domains on Fas to bind to death domains of an intracellular adapter protein called FADD (Fas-associated death domain). Death-

effector domains of FADD recruit several copies of **procaspase 8,** the aggregation of which leads to the autoproteolytic cleavage of procaspase 8, thereby releasing active **caspase 8.** This *initiator* caspase is a member of the **caspase** family of proteolytic enzymes. Relatively small numbers of caspase 8 molecules, by proteolytic cleavage, activate much larger numbers of *effector* caspases, including caspases 3 and 7, as well as another initiator caspase called caspase 9. This amplified cascade results in the proteolysis of numerous cytosolic and nuclear proteins and leads to apoptosis. One of the cytosolic caspase targets is a **gelsolin,** which, when cleaved, severs actin filaments and leads to a loss of normal cell shape. One of the nuclear caspase targets is **inhibitor of caspase-activated DNase (ICAD),** which normally binds to and thereby inactivates **caspase-activated DNase (CAD).** Cleavage of ICAD releases active CAD, which then severs chromosomal DNA.

The second pathway involves damage to the mitochondria (Fig. 62-6), triggered by such agents as ROS, increases in $[Ca^{2+}]$ in the mitochondrial matrix, and caspases. The result is the opening of a large pore in the mitochondrial inner membrane—the **mitochondrial permeability transition pore (MPTP)**—followed by mitochondrial swelling, rupture of the outer mitochondrial membrane, and release of cytochrome c into the cytosol. There, the **apoptotic protease-activating factor (Apaf-1)** complexes with the cytochrome c and ATP, to form a wheel-like structure that contains seven of each molecule—an **apoptosome.** This structure recruits seven procaspase 9 molecules and results in the formation of active caspase 9, thus committing the cell to apoptosis.

The third pathway is triggered by damage to nuclear DNA (Fig. 62-6). The tumor suppressor p53, a nuclear protein, recognizes certain base-pair mismatches. In cases of modest DNA damage, p53 increases the transcription of p21, which, in turn, halts the cell cycle. In cases of more severe DNA damage, p53 upregulates its own transcription. In addition, p53 increases the transcription of the proapoptotic protein **bax** (Bcl–2-associated X protein) and decreases the transcription of the antiapoptotic protein **bcl-2** (B-cell chronic lymphocytic lymphoma/lymphoma 2). The increase in the ratio of bax to bcl-2 appears to activate MPTP, thereby precipitating the events leading to apoptosis described in the second pathway. Finally, p53 also upregulates Fas and thus reinforces the first pathway.

Dysregulation of apoptosis promotes aging. Failure of apoptosis to remove damaged cells could result in abnormal function or increase the risk of cancer. Excess apoptosis would unnecessarily decrease cell number.

AGING OF THE HUMAN PHYSIOLOGICAL SYSTEMS

The age-related changes just described at cellular and molecular levels can also manifest as deterioration of entire physiological systems. Although I discuss *typical* age-related changes in physiological systems, the extent of change among individuals may range from barely perceptible to very marked. Indeed, a subset of individuals shows minimal physiological deterioration—these people have undergone "successful" aging. Many individuals show marked deterioration with age in all physiological systems, whereas other individuals exhibit little or no deterioration in one or more systems. Although the nature of the aging process is similar in the two sexes—except, of course, for the reproductive system—important quantitative differences exist. For example, women lose bone mass much faster with increasing age than do men. Because of the great reserve capacity or redundancy of some physiological systems, the effect of aging on a physiological process is often not apparent until either the individual faces an unusual challenge or function has fallen to less than some critical level.

Aging people lose height and lean body mass but gain and redistribute fat

Women reach peak height by age 16 to 17 years and men by 18 to 19 years. After these peaks, height starts to decline, primarily because of compression of the cartilaginous disks between the vertebrae and loss of vertebral bone. This decline begins at ~20 years of age in women and at 25 years of age in men. By the age of 70 years, height has fallen 2.5% to 5% lower than peak level.

In most Americans, **body mass** increases until middle age in both sexes and begins to decrease after age 70 years. **Fat-free mass** is defined as body mass minus **adipose tissue fat mass**, and **lean body mass** is defined as fat-free mass minus both bone mass and non–adipose tissue fat mass. Both fat-free mass and lean body mass progressively decrease over most of adult life in both sexes. Although a sedentary lifestyle may contribute to this loss, lifelong athletes also show a progressive age-associated loss in fat-free mass and lean body mass.

Adipose tissue fat mass increases with adult age, but the extent differs markedly among individuals. Although a sedentary lifestyle may be a factor, even physically fit individuals who do not exhibit an age-associated increase in body mass show a small but progressive increase in adipose tissue fat mass (in parallel with the aforementioned decrease in fat-free body mass). In addition, the distribution of body fat changes with increasing age, with an accumulation of fat around abdominal viscera and in abdominal subcutaneous tissue. At the same time, a decrease occurs in the extremities and the face; facial fat loss can give rise to the gaunt look that characterizes many elderly persons.

Aging thins the skin and causes the musculoskeletal system to become weak, brittle, and stiff

Skin   As is clearly evident from cosmetic advertisements, most of us use the skin as an indicator of aging. Intrinsic aging is manifest in skin areas protected from the sun, such as the buttocks. The additional damage caused by long-term exposure to the sun's ultraviolet radiation is called *photoaging*.

In intrinsic aging, the thickness of the **epidermis** (see Chapter 15) decreases slightly, with no change in the outermost epidermal layer, the stratum corneum. The rate of generation of keratinocytes, which end their lives as the stratum corneum, slows with age, thereby increasing the dwell time of stratum corneum components. The decreasing number of melanocytes reduces photoprotection, and the decreasing number of Langerhans' cells reduces immune surveillance.

Intrinsic aging of the **dermis** affects mainly the extracellular matrix. The amount of elastin and collagen decreases, and their structure changes. Glycosaminoglycan composition also changes. As a result, the dermis thins by ~20% and becomes stiffer, less malleable, and thus more vulnerable to injury.

Photoaging increases the extent of most intrinsic age changes in both the epidermis and dermis, and it has additional effects. For example, photoaging causes coarse wrinkles, which occur minimally or not at all because of intrinsic aging.

Aging also reduces the number and function of sweat glands as well as the production of sebum by sebaceous glands. The number of active melanocytes in hair follicles decreases, resulting in graying of hair. Nail growth also slows with increasing age.

Skeletal Muscle   A steady loss in skeletal muscle mass—**sarcopenia**—occurs with aging, particularly beyond 50 years, and it primarily reflects a loss of number and, to a lesser extent, size of muscle fibers. The sarcopenia partly results from inactivity, but it is also caused by a progressive loss of the motor neurons innervating type II motor units, which are recruited less frequently. With loss of their motor nerve, affected muscle fibers either atrophy and die or become innervated by a sprout that emerges from a healthy axon nearby. This process of reinnervation ultimately results in larger motor units and thus a decrement in fine motor control (see Chapter 9). The reduction in muscle strength and power is often a major cause of disability in elderly persons. However, strength training in elderly persons can increase the *size* of the fibers and can thereby increase muscle mass.

Bone   Remodeling of bone occurs throughout adult life; it involves the coordinated activity of **osteoclasts**, which resorb bone, and **osteoblasts**, which form bone. Until middle age, bone resorption and formation are in balance. However, starting in middle age, resorption exceeds formation, thus leading to a progressive loss in bone mass. In women, bone loss accelerates during the first few years following menopause. Bone loss can progress to **osteoporosis**, defined by the World Health Organization as a bone mineral density 2.5 standard deviations or more lower than mean values for young adults (see Chapter 52). Osteoporosis, a major problem in geriatric medicine, carries a heightened risk of bone fractures.

Synovial Joints   Synovial joints permit free movement of the bones linked to them. With increasing adult age, joint flexibility declines, mainly because of the aging of **articular cartilage**. This cartilage thins and exhibits altered mechanical features, including decreases in tensile stiffness, fatigue resistance, and strength. These changes are partly the result of decreased water content. Aging impairs the function of **chondrocytes**, increases the cross-linking of collagen, and causes a loss of proteoglycans. The age-related changes in joint cartilage undoubtedly play a major role in the development of **osteoarthritis**.

Healthy elderly persons experience deficits in sensory transduction and speed of central processing

It is a common misconception that advancing age causes marked deterioration in the nervous system. However, in the absence of neurodegenerative disorders such as Alzheimer disease and Parkinson disease, impairment of the nervous system with age is much less severe.

Sensory Functions   Most sensory systems exhibit some deterioration with age. Sensitivity to **touch** decreases, as do the abilities to sense vibration and to distinguish two spatially distinct points of contact. Proprioception, including the vestibular system of the inner ear, also deteriorates somewhat. As discussed in Chapter 59, the loss of thermoregulatory ability, a serious problem for many elderly people, occurs in part because of an impaired ability to sense heat and cold.

Hearing loss, particularly of high-frequency sound, is almost an invariable consequence of advancing age. This impairment is usually caused by loss of hair cells of the organ of Corti (see Chapter 15), but it can also stem from loss of nerve cells of the auditory nerve or from reduced blood supply to the cochlea. A deficit in central processing can make it difficult for some elderly people to distinguish spoken words from background noise.

Vision also deteriorates with increasing age. A progressive loss in the power of accommodation (**presbyopia**) occurs during adult life. Almost all elderly persons have a reduced number of retinal cones, lessened ability to alter pupil size in response to light intensity, and decreased ability of retinal rods to adapt to low-intensity light (see Chapter 15). In addition, age-associated diseases—cataracts, glaucoma, and macular degeneration—can markedly decrease vision in many elderly persons.

The ability to detect and discriminate among sweet, sour, salty, and bitter **taste** qualities deteriorates somewhat at advanced ages, along with a marked reduction in **olfaction** (see Chapter 15). Because taste involves both gustation and olfaction, many elderly persons live in a world of "pastel" food flavors.

Motor Functions   A major effect of aging is the slowing of **reaction time**: the time elapsed between the stimulus and the motor response. This delay is observable in simple responses and becomes more pronounced as the complexity of the response increases (e.g., the need to make a choice among responses). Thus, a hallmark of nervous system aging is the slowing of **central processing**. One result is that elderly people tend to execute movements more slowly than do young people.

The ability to maintain posture and balance deteriorates with increasing age. Slowing of central processing is a factor, but decreased muscle strength and deterioration of vision and proprioception also play important roles. Not surprisingly, elderly persons have a high incidence of falls. Even when *capable* of walking at normal speeds, healthy elderly people *tend* to walk more slowly than the young and take shorter and more frequent steps. This walking pattern is less taxing for a person with knee and ankle joints that are less flexible, aids in maintaining balance, and enables a deteriorating sensory system to monitor hazards more effectively.

Cognitive Functions   Although most people generally believe that cognitive functions (e.g., intelligence, memory, learning) decline with advancing age, the cognitive decline is not marked in the absence of dementia. The decline that does occur in healthy elderly persons may reflect the slowing of central processing. The capacity to use knowledge is not decreased in the healthy aged, but the ability to solve novel problems does decline. Certain types of memory deteriorate with advancing age, such as remembering where the car keys were left, but other types are not lost, such as retrieving conceptual information. Older people are capable of learning, but they do so less quickly than younger people.

Aging causes decreased arterial compliance and increased ventilation-perfusion mismatching

Atherosclerosis can cause marked deterioration of cardiovascular function in elderly persons, and chronic obstructive pulmonary disease (see Chapter 27) can do the same for pulmonary function. However, in the absence of such diseases, age-associated changes in these physiological systems are modest.

Cardiovascular Function As discussed in Chapter 19, aging decreases the distensibility of arteries. The decreased compliance elevates systolic pressure, slightly decreases diastolic pressure, and thus widens pulse pressure. Afterload (see Chapter 22), the resistance to ejection of blood from the left ventricle, increases with advancing age, primarily because of reduced arterial compliance. The increased afterload causes thickening of the left ventricular wall, which involves an increase in size but not number of myocytes.

Preload, the end-diastolic volume of blood in the left ventricle (see Chapter 22), does not change with age in subjects at rest. Although early diastolic filling falls, a compensatory increase in left atrial contraction enhances late-diastolic filling. Many elderly persons suffer from postural hypotension (see Chapter 25) because of age-associated blunting of the arterial baroreceptor reflex.

Pulmonary Function The strength and endurance of the respiratory muscles decrease with age, primarily because of atrophy of type IIa muscle fibers. Lung volumes—both static volume and forced expiratory volume (see Chapter 27) gradually decrease with age. With age, small airways have an increased tendency to collapse (atelectasis) because of degeneration of the collagen and elastin support structure. This situation results in impaired ventilation of dependent lung regions, ventilation-perfusion mismatch (see Chapter 31), and reduced resting arterial P_{O_2}.

Exercise Maximal O_2 uptake ($\dot{V}_{O_{2max}}$) declines progressively with aging in physically trained individuals and even more so in untrained individuals of the same chronologic age. Decreasing muscle mass and reduced cardiovascular and pulmonary function probably contribute to the decline in $\dot{V}_{O_{2max}}$, and the relative importance of each factor varies among individuals.

The cardiovascular system of elderly persons responds to exercise differently than in the young. For a given increase in cardiac output, heart rate rises less and stroke volume rises more in elderly people. Because the heart is less responsive to adrenergic stimulation, the increase in stroke volume is primarily the result of the Frank-Starling mechanism. Thus, during exercise, the left ventricular end-diastolic and end-systolic volumes increase, and maximal left ventricular ejection fraction falls.

Elderly persons exhibit a decrease in the pulmonary diffusing capacity and alveolar capillary volume, and ventilation-perfusion mismatch increases. These alterations in pulmonary function have been implicated in the decrease in $\dot{V}_{O_{2max}}$.

The ability of the body to respond to physical conditioning decreases with aging. Nevertheless, skeletal muscle and the cardiovascular system remain responsive to exercise into the 10th decade of life.

Glomerular filtration rate falls with age in many but not all people

Cross-sectional studies show that glomerular filtration rate (GFR) starts to decline at 30 years of age and thereafter falls linearly with age. However, longitudinal analysis revealed that one third of the participants of the Baltimore Longitudinal Study of Aging exhibited the GFR decline predicted from cross-sectional analysis, one third had a steeper decline, and one third had no decline at all. Thus, an age-associated decline in GFR is not inevitable.

Cross-sectional studies indicate that renal tubule transport functions decrease with age. The kidneys do not respond as effectively to changes in sodium load, do not dilute or concentrate urine as effectively, and also have a somewhat impaired ability to excrete potassium, phosphate, and acid.

The capacity and compliance of the urinary bladder decrease with advancing age, and the number of uninhibited contractions increases, thus making it more difficult to postpone voiding. The rate of bladder emptying decreases, and the residual bladder volume after voiding increases.

Aging has only minor effects on gastrointestinal function

Although gastrointestinal problems are the second most common reason for hospital admission of elderly patients, the gastrointestinal system functions in healthy elderly persons about as well as in the young. Although a loss of ability to secrete gastric acid was previously thought to be part of aging, it is now clear that this loss is limited to persons infected with *Helicobacter pylori* (see the box in Chapter 42 for more on that topic). The loss of skeletal muscle at both ends of the gastrointestinal tract can lead to minor age-related decreases in function (i.e., chewing, swallowing, fecal continence). Minor decreases occur in secretion by exocrine glands. Liver mass and hepatic blood flow, as well as the clearance of certain drugs, decrease significantly. Moreover, elderly people experience a delay in hepatic regeneration following damage.

Aging causes modest declines in most endocrine functions

Total energy expenditure decreases with age, primarily because of decreases in physical activity. An age-associated decrease in the **RMR** (see Chapter 58) reflects a decrease in fat-free mass; that is, the RMR per kilogram of fat-free mass does not decrease.

Endocrine Pancreas The impaired **glucose tolerance** (see Chapter 51) that usually occurs with aging is caused by increased **insulin resistance**, which, in turn, results mainly from increased adiposity. However, aging per se does play a small role. An increase in serum **low-density lipoproteins** (see Chapter 46) occurs in both genders with advancing age.

Pituitary Aging diminishes peak concentrations of hormone generated by the pulsatile action of somatotrophs. Greatly reduced plasma insulin-like growth factor 1 (IGF-1) concentrations result (see Chapter 48).

Adrenal Cortex The basal, circadian, and stimulated secretion of **cortisol** exhibits little age-related change. **Aldosterone** secretion is also well preserved. In contrast, the plasma concentration of the adrenal cortical hormone

dehydroepiandrosterone (see Chapter 54) decreases markedly with increasing age.

Thyroid Gland   Thyroid function appears to be unaffected by age into the ninth decade of life. However, in centenarians, plasma thyroid-stimulating hormone (TSH) levels may decline because of decreased secretion, and free triiodothyronine levels may fall because of impaired 5'/3'-deiodinase (see Chapter 49). Plasma **parathyroid** hormone levels increase with advancing age.

Gonads   Reproductive ability in women abruptly ceases at ~50 years of age with the occurrence of the **menopause** (see Chapter 55). Men do not undergo an abrupt change in reproductive function during middle age. However, a progressive decrease in male reproductive and related functions does occur, often referred to as the **andropause** (see the box on testosterone and aging in Chapter 54).

AGING SLOWLY

Slowing the aging process and thereby extending life have been human goals throughout recorded history and probably in preliterate times as well. The marked increase in human life expectancy in the 20th century could be viewed as achieving this goal. However, much of that increase results from prevention of premature deaths related to infections and other environmental hazards. It remains to be established how much, if any, of the increase relates to slowing the aging process. Indeed, over the centuries, the life span of the oldest of the old in human populations has changed little, although the fraction of the population reaching these advanced ages has increased significantly. In contrast, both environmental and genetic manipulations can markedly extend the maximal life span of a population in several other species.

Caloric restriction slows aging and extends life of several species, including some mammals

Restricting the food intake of rats, starting soon after weaning, increases both mean and maximum life span of several strains of rats and of both genders, as first reported by Clive McCay in 1935. The marked increase in rat longevity is graphically illustrated by the survival curves in Figure 62-7. Manipulation of the components (protein, fat, carbohydrate, minerals, and vitamins) of a purified rat diet revealed that the life-extending action of food restriction resulted from caloric restriction, rather than from a specific dietary component.

Reducing food intake also extends the life of mice, hamsters, dogs, fish, several invertebrate animal species, and yeast. Studies of rhesus monkeys, still in progress, indicate that food restriction may also extend the life of nonhuman primates.

Does food restriction extend life by slowing aging processes? This is a difficult question to answer because of the lack of consensus on how to measure the aging of individuals or populations. However, for two reasons, most biogerontologists believe that food restriction does retard the aging

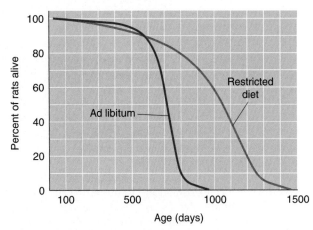

Figure 62-7   Survival curves for a population of 115 male F344 rats fed ad libitum and 115 male F344 rats with restricted food intake (i.e., 60% of the ad libitum intake) starting at 6 weeks of age. Both the median length of life and the maximum length of life are markedly greater in the restricted population. *(Data from Yu BP, Masoro EJ, Murata I, et al: J Gerontol 1982; 37:130-141.)*

processes. First, compared with rodents of the same age who were fed ad libitum, rodents on food-restriction regimens maintained physiological processes more like those of young animals. Second, food restriction delayed the onset or the progression of most age-associated diseases, including neoplastic, degenerative, and immune diseases.

During the past 70 years, many hypotheses have been proposed for the biological mechanisms underlying the life-prolonging action of food restriction, but none is firmly established. McCay proposed that caloric restriction extended life by retarding growth. However, later observations showed that food restriction, even when initiated in young adult rats or middle-aged mice, significantly extended life. Another early hypothesis was that food restriction extends life by markedly reducing adipose fat mass. However, it is possible to dissociate the effects of food restriction on longevity from the effects on fat mass in rats and mice.

Currently, the most popular view is that food restriction extends life by decreasing oxidative stress. Indeed, food restriction does decrease the accumulation of age-associated oxidative damage. Food restriction also causes a sustained reduction in plasma glucose levels, which could reduce glycation and glycoxidation. Food restriction also causes marked and sustained reductions in plasma levels of insulin and IGF-1. Genetic studies strongly indicate that decreasing insulin-like signaling (see Chapters 48 and 51) extends life. Thus, decreasing the levels of insulin and IGF-1 may well play an important role in life extension.

Another theory of the antiaging action of caloric restriction is **hormesis**, defined as the beneficial effects resulting from cellular responses to mild repeated stress, which would stimulate maintenance and repair processes and thereby retard aging. Food restriction, at the level that extends life, is a mild stress repeated daily. Moreover, food-restricted rodents have an increased ability to cope with acute, intense damaging agents, such as surgery, toxic chemicals, and high environmental temperatures.

Genetic alterations can extend life in several species

Caloric restriction is an example of environmental factors that determine longevity. It is also clear that genetics has a major role. For example, the large difference in life span among species (from <100 days in *Drosophila melanogaster* to <5 years in mice to >100 years in humans) is primarily, if not exclusively, the result of genetic differences. Moreover, selective breeding within a species can produce populations that differ significantly in longevity.

Longevity probably depends on multiple genes. Thus, it was a surprise when Friedman and Johnson reported in 1988 that mutation of the *age-1* gene of the nematode worm, *Caenorhabditis elegans*, resulted in a marked increase in longevity. The *age-1* gene encodes a phosphatidylinositol-3-kinase, which is a component of the insulin-like signaling pathway. *C. elegans*, like other invertebrates, does not have separate signaling pathways for insulin and IGF-1, as do mammals (see Chapters 48 and 51). The mutation of *age-1* in the Friedman and Johnson study caused some loss of function—that is, it was a weak mutation. Among other single-gene manipulations found to extend the life of *C. elegans*, *D. melanogaster*, *Saccharomyces cerevisiae*, and mice, many but not all involve a partial loss of function of the insulin-like signaling pathway.

Ames dwarf mice have a recessive point mutation in the *Prop-1* gene, which results in the inability of the pituitary to produce growth hormone (GH), TSH, and prolactin. These mice have low levels of thyroid hormone, IGF-1, and insulin. Significantly, these dwarf mice have an increased life span compared with littermates not homozygous for this mutation.

Further support for a role of reduced insulin-like signaling in life extension comes from studies of mice with a knockout of the *GHR/BP* gene, which encodes the GH receptor and its proteolytic cleavage product, GH-binding protein. This knockout mouse exhibits growth retardation, high plasma GH levels, low plasma IGF-1 levels, and significant life extension. Reducing the expression of the insulin receptor by 85% to 90% in the adipose tissue of mice resulted in significant life extension. Finally, overexpression of the **Klotho** gene in mice increased the plasma level of Klotho protein, which suppressed insulin and IGF-1 signaling and extended the life of the mice.

In yeast, overexpression of the *sir2* gene increases the level of a sirtuin protein called Sir2 and extends the replicative life of *S. cerevisiae*. Sir2 is a deacetylase that stabilizes ribosomal DNA. Sir2 may play a role in other species. Indeed, stimulating Sir2 orthologues extends the life span of *C. elegans*, *D. melanogaster*, and human cell lines. However, it is not yet clear whether sirtuin proteins play an important role in the life-prolonging action of caloric restriction.

Proposed interventions to slow aging and extend human life are controversial

The practice of **antiaging medicine** is becoming popular and plays an important role in preventing the occurrence and progression of certain age-associated diseases. For example, exercise and diet can reduce the incidence of coronary heart disease, stroke, and type 2 diabetes. However, some practitioners of antiaging medicine, as well as suppliers of pharmaceuticals and nutriceuticals, claim to have "magic bullets" that slow or even reverse aging. The magic bullets include antioxidants (e.g., vitamins E and C), amino acids (e.g., methionine), drugs (e.g., deprenyl), and hormones (e.g., melatonin, dehydroepiandrosterone, GH, estrogen and testosterone). No credible evidence indicates that any of these agents will reverse or even slow human aging. Aside from the question of efficacy is the possibility of long-term adverse effects of these magic bullets. Combined estrogen and progestin therapy is a case in point. Although hailed for relieving the symptoms of menopause, this hormone replacement therapy was long in use before a well-designed study uncovered its harmful effects on the cardiovascular system. In light of the animal studies that strongly indicate that insulin-like signaling promotes aging, the current use of recombinant GH is of concern. Although GH increases lean body mass in elderly persons, well-designed studies will be needed before GH is used as an antiaging agent.

REFERENCES

Books and Reviews
Finkel T, Holbrook NJ: Oxidants, oxidative stress, and the biology of aging. Nature 2000; 408:239-247.

Kim S-H, Komiker P, Campisi J: Telomeres, aging, and cancer: In search of a happy ending. Oncogene 2002; 21:503-511.

Liang H, Masoro EJ, Nelson JF, et al: Genetic mouse models of extended lifespan. Exp Gerontol 2003, 38:1353-1364.

Masoro EJ: Caloric Restriction: A Key to Understanding and Modulating Aging. Amsterdam: Elsevier, 2002.

Tauber C: Sixty-Five Plus in America. Washington, DC: U. S. Bureau of the Census, 1992, rev. 1993.

Zhang Y, Herman B: Ageing and apoptosis. Mech Ageing Dev 2002; 123:245-260.

Journal Articles
Cristofalo VJ, Allen RG, Pignolo RJ, et al: Relationship between donor age and the replicative lifespan of human cells in culture: A reevaluation. Proc Natl Acad Sci U S A 1998; 95:10620-10625.

Hughes KA, Alipaz JA, Drnevich JM, Reynolds RM: A test of evolutionary theories of aging. Proc Natl Acad Sci U S A 2002; 99:14286-14291.

Kurosu H, Yamamoto M, Clark JD, et al: Suppression of aging in mice by the hormone Klotho. Science 2005; 309:1829-1833.

Lindeman RD, Tobin J, Shock NW: Longitudinal studies on the rate of decline in renal function with age. J Am Geriatr Soc 1985; 33:278-285.

Pongor S, Ulrich PC, Bencsath FA, Cerami A: Aging of proteins: Isolation and identification of a fluorescent chromophore from the reaction of polypeptides with glucose. Proc Natl Acad Sci U S A 1984; 81:2684-2688.

Yu BP, Masoro EJ, Murata I, et al: Life span of SPF Fischer 344 male rats fed ad libitum or restricted diets: Longevity, growth, lean body mass, and disease. J Gerontol 1982; 37:130-141.

INDEX

Note: Page numbers followed by f indicate figures; those followed by t indicate tables; and those followed by b indicate boxed material.